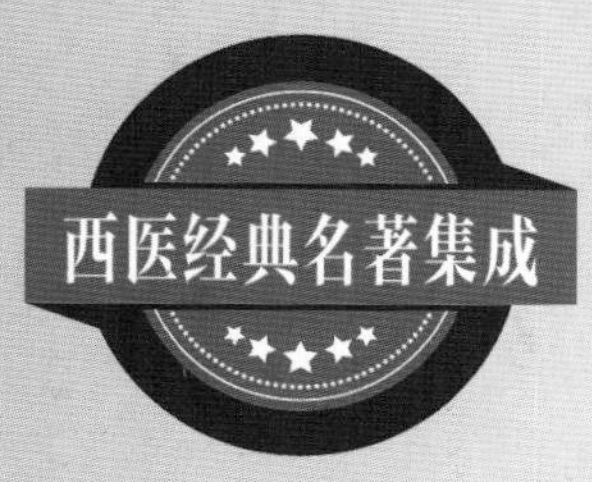

古德曼·吉尔曼治疗学的药理学基础

Goodman & Gilman's THE PHARMACOLOGICAL BASIS OF THERAPEUTICS

13TH EDITION

LAURENCE L. BRUNTON

RANDA HILAL-DANDAN

BJÖRN C. KNOLLMANN

第13版（双语版）

编译委员会主任委员　周宏灏

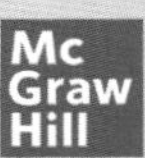

CS | K 湖南科学技术出版社

西医经典名著集成

古德曼·吉尔曼治疗学的药理学基础

第13版（双语版）

编译委员会

主任委员	周宏灏	中南大学
副主任委员	舒　焱	马里兰大学
	郭　莹	中南大学
	彭名菁	中南大学
	曹　杉	中南大学
委　　员	何　楠	堪萨斯大学
	肖洲生	田纳西大学
	伍忠銮	香港大学
	戴菱菱	哈佛大学
	李　清	中南大学
	周　淦	中南大学
	贺毅憬	中南大学
	成　瑜	中南大学
	范　岚	中南大学

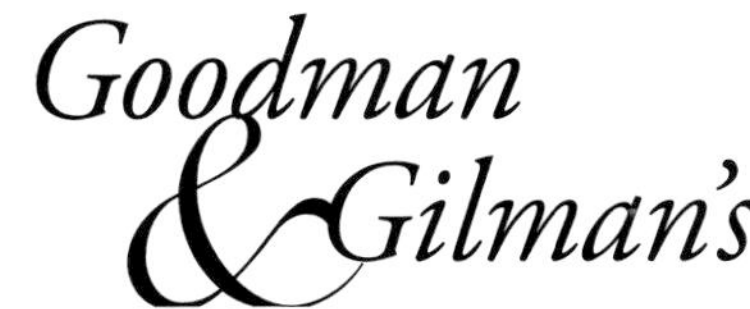

THE PHARMACOLOGICAL BASIS OF THERAPEUTICS

THIRTEENTH EDITION

Editor-in-chief

Laurence L. Brunton, PhD
Professor of Pharmacology and Medicine
School of Medicine, University of California, San Diego
La Jolla, California

Editors

Randa Hilal-Dandan, PhD
Lecturer in Pharmacology
School of Medicine, University of California, San Diego
La Jolla, California

Björn C. Knollmann, MD, PhD
William Stokes Professor of Medicine and Pharmacology
Director, Vanderbilt Center for Arrhythmia Research and Therapeutics
Division of Clinical Pharmacology
Vanderbilt University School of Medicine
Nashville, Tennessee

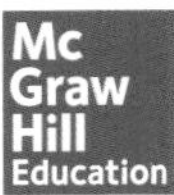

New York Chicago San Francisco Athens London Madrid Mexico City
Milan New Delhi Singapore Sydney Toronto

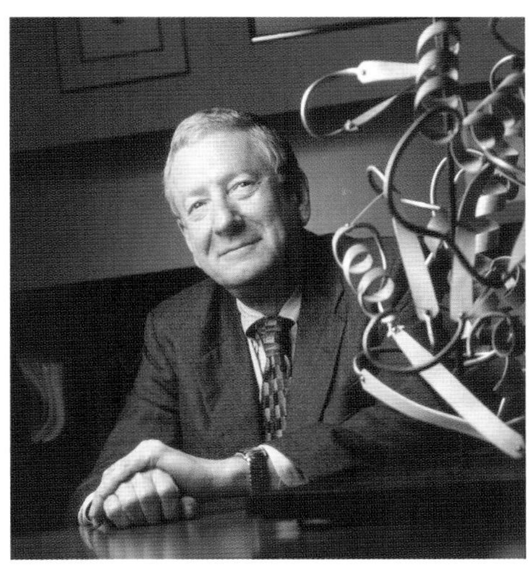

In Memoriam

Alfred Goodman Gilman

(1941-2015)

Mentor, teacher, researcher, Nobel laureate, raconteur, mensch,
and longtime editor of this book

Contributors

Edward P. Acosta, PharmD
Professor and Director, Division of Clinical Pharmacology
University of Alabama at Birmingham School of Medicine
Birmingham, Alabama

Susan G. Amara, PhD
Scientific Director
National Institute of Mental Health
National Institutes of Health
Bethesda, Maryland

Michael B. Atkins, MD
Professor of Oncology and Medicine
Georgetown University, School of Medicine
Washington DC

Jamil Azzi, MD, FAST
Assistant Professor of Medicine
Transplantation Research Center
Harvard Medical School
Boston, Massachusetts

Peter J. Barnes, DM, DSc, FRCP, FMedSci, FRS
Professor and Head of Respiratory Medicine
National Heart & Lung Institute
Imperial College, London

Robert R. Bies, PharmD, PhD
Associate Professor
School of Pharmacy and Pharmaceutical Sciences
University at Buffalo
The State University of New York
Buffalo, New York

Donald K. Blumenthal, PhD
Associate Professor of Pharmacology & Toxicology
College of Pharmacy
University of Utah
Salt Lake City, Utah

Katharina Brandl, PhD
Assistant Professor of Pharmacy
University of California San Diego
Skaggs School of Pharmacy and Pharmaceutical Sciences
La Jolla, California

Gregory A. Brent, MD
Professor of Medicine and Physiology
Geffen School of Medicine
University of California
Los Angeles, California

Joan Heller Brown, PhD
Professor and Chair of Pharmacology
University of California
San Diego, California

Craig N. Burkhart, MD
Associate Professor of Dermatology, School of Medicine
University of North Carolina
Chapel Hill, North Carolina

Iain L. O. Buxton, PharmD
Foundation Professor and Chair
Department of Pharmacology
University of Nevada, Reno School of Medicine
Reno, Nevada

Michael C. Byrns, PhD
Associate Professor of Environmental Health
Illinois State University
Normal, Illinois

William A. Catterall, PhD
Professor and Chair of Pharmacology
University of Washington School of Medicine
Seattle, Washington

Janet A. Clark, PhD
Director, Office of Fellowship Training
Intramural Research Program
National Institute of Mental Health
National Institutes of Health
Bethesda, Maryland

Michael W. H. Coughtrie, PhD
Professor and Dean
Faculty of Pharmaceutical Sciences
University of British Columbia
Vancouver, Canada

James E. Crowe, Jr.
Professor of Pediatrics, Pathology, Microbiology and Immunology
Director, Vanderbilt Vaccine Center
Vanderbilt University Medical Center
Nashville, Tennessee

David D'Alessio, MD
Professor, Department of Medicine
Director, Division of Endocrinology
Duke University Medical Center
Durham, North Carolina

Michael David, PharmD, PhD
Professor of Biology and Moores Cancer Center
University of California, San Diego
La Jolla, California

Ankit A. Desai, MD
Assistant Professor of Medicine
University of Arizona
Tucson, Arizona

Michelle Erickson, PhD
Research Assistant Professor of Gerontology and Geriatric Medicine, School of Medicine
University of Washington
Seattle, Washington

Thomas Eschenhagen, MD
Professor of Pharmacology and Toxicology
Chair of Pharmacology
University Medical Center Hamburg Eppendorf
Hamburg, Germany

Nancy Fares-Frederickson, PhD
Division of Biology and Moores Cancer Center
University of California, San Diego
La Jolla, California

Garret A. FitzGerald, MD
Professor of Medicine, Pharmacology and Translational Medicine and Therapeutics;
Chair of Pharmacology
University of Pennsylvania School of Medicine
Philadelphia, Pennsylvania

Charles W. Flexner, MD
Professor of Medicine, Pharmacology and Molecular Sciences, and International Health
The Johns Hopkins University School of Medicine and Bloomberg School of Public Health
Baltimore, Maryland

Dustin R. Fraidenburg, MD
Assistant Professor of Medicine
University of Illinois at Chicago
Chicago, Illinois

R. Benjamin Free, PhD
Staff Scientist, Molecular Neuropharmacology Section
National Institute of Neurological Disorders and Stroke
National Institutes of Health
Bethesda, Maryland

Peter A. Friedman, PhD
Professor of Pharmacology and Chemical Biology, and of Structural Biology
University of Pittsburgh School of Medicine
Pittsburgh, Pennsylvania

John W. Funder, AC, MD, BS, PhD, FRACP
Professor of Medicine, Prince Henry's Institute
Monash Medical Centre
Clayton, Victoria, Australia

Giuseppe Giaccone, MD, PhD
Professor of Medical Oncology and Pharmacology
Georgetown University
Washington DC

Kathleen M. Giacomini, PhD
Professor of Bioengineering and Therapeutic Sciences, School of Pharmacy
University of California
San Francisco, California

Alfred G. Gilman, MD, PhD (deceased)
Professor (Emeritus) of Pharmacology
University of Texas Southwestern Medical School
Dallas, Texas

Frank J. Gonzalez, PhD
Chief, Laboratory of Metabolism
Center for Cancer Research, National Cancer Institute
Bethesda, Maryland

Tilo Grosser, MD
Research Associate Professor of Pharmacology
Institute for Translational Medicine and Therapeutics
University of Pennsylvania
Philadelphia, Pennsylvania

Tawanda Gumbo, MD
Director, Center for Infectious Diseases Research and Experimental Therapeutics
Baylor Research Institute
Baylor University Medical Center
Dallas, Texas

Holly Gurgle, PharmD, BCACP, CDE
Assistant Professor (Clinical) of Pharmacotherapy
College of Pharmacy
University of Utah
Salt Lake City, Utah

David A. Hafler, MD
William S. and Lois Stiles Edgerly Professor of Neurology and Immunobiology
Chairman, Department of Neurology
Yale School of Medicine
New Haven, Connecticut

Stephen R. Hammes, MD, PhD
Professor of Medicine, Chief of Endocrinology and Metabolism
School of Medicine and Dentistry
University of Rochester
Rochester, New York

R. Adron Harris, PhD
Professor of Neuroscience and Pharmacology
Waggoner Center for Alcohol and Addiction Research
University of Texas
Austin, Texas

Lisa A. Hazelwood, PhD
Principal Research Scientist, Liver Disease and Fibrosis, AbbVie
North Chicago, Illinois

Jeffrey D. Henderer, MD
Professor of Ophthalmology
Dr. Edward Hagop Bedrossian Chair of Ophthalmology
Lewis Katz School of Medicine at Temple University
Philadelphia, Pennsylvania

Ryan E. Hibbs, PhD
Assistant Professor of Neuroscience
University of Texas Southwestern Medical School
Dallas, Texas

Randa Hilal-Dandan, PhD
Lecturer in Pharmacology
University of California
San Diego, California

Peter J. Hotez, MD, PhD
Professor of Pediatrics and Molecular Virology & Microbiology
Texas Children's Hospital Endowed Chair in Tropical Pediatrics
Dean, National School of Tropical Medicine
Baylor College of Medicine
Houston, Texas

Claudine Isaacs, MD, FRCPC
Professor of Medicine and Oncology
Georgetown University, School of Medicine
Washington DC

Nina Isoherranen, PhD
Professor of Pharmaceutics, School of Pharmacy
University of Washington
Seattle, Washington

Edwin K. Jackson, PhD
Professor of Pharmacology and Chemical Biology
University of Pittsburgh School of Medicine
Pittsburgh, Pennsylvania

Kenneth Kaushansky, MD
Dean, School of Medicine and Senior Vice President of Health Sciences
SUNY Stony Brook
New York, New York

Jennifer Keiser, PhD
Professor of Neglected Tropical Diseases
Swiss Tropical and Public Health Institute
Basel, Switzerland

Thomas J. Kipps, MD, PhD
Professor of Medicine, Moores Cancer Center
University of California
San Diego, California

Jennifer J. Kiser, PharmD
Associate Professor, Pharmaceutical Sciences
University of Colorado
Denver, Colorado

Ronald J. Koenig, MD, PhD
Professor of Metabolism, Endocrinology and Diabetes
Department of Internal Medicine
University of Michigan Health System
Ann Arbor, Michigan

George F. Koob, PhD
Director, National Institute on Alcohol Abuse and Alcoholism
National Institutes of Health
Rockville, Maryland

Alan M. Krensky, MD
Vice Dean
Professor of Pediatrics and Microbiology & Immunology
Feinberg School of Medicine
Northwestern University
Chicago, Illinois

Ellis R. Levin, MD
Professor of Medicine; Chief of Endocrinology
Diabetes and Metabolism
University of California, Irvine, and Long Beach
VA Medical Center
Long Beach, California

Heather Macarthur, PhD
Associate Professor of Pharmacology and Physiology
Saint Louis University School of Medicine
St. Louis, Missouri

Conan MacDougall, PharmD, MAS
Professor of Clinical Pharmacy
School of Pharmacy
University of California
San Francisco, California

Wallace K. MacNaughton, PhD
Professor and Head of Physiology and Pharmacology
Cumming School of Medicine,
University of Calgary
Calgary, Alberta, Canada

Kenneth P. Mackie, MD
Professor of Psychological and Brain Sciences
Indiana University
Bloomington, Indiana

Jody Mayfield, PhD
Science Writer and Editor
Waggoner Center for Alcohol and Addiction Research
University of Texas
Austin, Texas

James McCarthy, MD
Senior Scientist QIMR Berghofer Intitute of Medical Research
Department of Infectious Diseases, Royal Brisbane
and Womens Hospital
Brisbane, Queensland, Australia

James O. McNamara, MD
Professor and Chair of Neurobiology
Director of Center for Translational Neuroscience
Duke University Medical Center
Durham, North Carolina

Cameron S. Metcalf, PhD
Research Assistant Professor
Associate Director, Anticonvulsant Drug Development Program
Department of Pharmacology & Toxicology
College of Pharmacy
University of Utah
Salt Lake City, Utah

Jonathan M. Meyer, MD
Psychopharmacology Consultant
California Department of State Hospitals
Assistant Clinical Professor of Psychiatry
University of California
San Diego, California

S. John Mihic, PhD
Professor of Neuroscience
Waggoner Center for Alcohol & Addiction Research
University of Texas
Austin, Texas

Mark E. Molitch, MD
Martha Leland Sherwin Professor of Endocrinology
Northwestern University
Chicago, Illinois

Dean S. Morrell, MD
Professor of Dermatology
University of North Carolina
Chapel Hill, North Carolina

Thomas D. Nolin, PharmD, PhD
Associate Professor of Pharmacy and Therapeutics, and of Medicine
University of Pittsburgh School of Pharmacy and School of Medicine
Pittsburgh, Pennsylvania

Charles P. O'Brien, MD, PhD
Professor of Psychiatry, School of Medicine
University of Pennsylvania
Philadelphia, Pennsylvania

James O'Donnell, PhD
Dean and Professor
School of Pharmacy & Pharmaceutical Sciences
University at Buffalo
The State University of New York
Buffalo, New York

Hemal H. Patel, PhD
Professor of Anesthesiology
University of California, San Diego
VA-San Diego Healthcare System
San Diego, California

Piyush M. Patel, MD, FRCPC
Professor of Anesthesiology
University of California, San Diego
VA-San Diego Healthcare System
San Diego, California

Matthew L. Pearn, MD
Associate Professor of Anesthesiology
University of California, San Diego
VA-San Diego Healthcare System
San Diego, California

Trevor M. Penning, PhD
Professor of Systems Pharmacology & Translational Therapeutics
Director, Center of Excellence in Environmental Toxicology
School of Medicine
University of Pennsylvania
Philadelphia, Pennsylvania

Margaret A. Phillips, PhD
Professor of Pharmacology
University of Texas Southwestern Medical School
Dallas, Texas

Alvin C. Powers, MD
Professor of Medicine, Molecular Physiology and Biophysics
Director, Vanderbilt Diabetes Center
Chief, Division of Diabetes, Endocrinology, and Metabolism
Vanderbilt University School of Medicine
Nashville, Tennessee

Christopher J. Rapuano, MD
Director, Cornea Service and Refractive Surgery
Wills Eye Hospital
Philadelphia, Pennsylvania

Anna T. Riegel, PhD
Professor of Oncology and Pharmacology
Georgetown University, School of Medicine
Washington DC

Suzanne M. Rivera, PhD, MSW
Assistant Professor of Bioethics
Case Western Reserve University
Cleveland, Ohio

Erik D. Roberson, MD, PhD
Associate Professor of Neurology and Neurobiology
Co-Director, Center for Neurodegeneration and
Experimental Therapeutics
University of Alabama at Birmingham
Birmingham, Alabama

Dan M. Roden, MD
Professor of Medicine, Pharmacology, and Biomedical Informatics
Senior Vice President for Personalized Medicine
Vanderbilt University Medical Center
Nashville, Tennessee

P. David Rogers, PharmD, PhD, FCCP
First Tennessee Endowed Chair of Excellence in Clinical Pharmacy
Vice-Chair for Research
Director, Clinical and Experimental Therapeutics
Co-Director, Center for Pediatric Pharmacokinetics and Therapeutics
Professor of Clinical Pharmacy and Pediatrics
University of Tennessee College of Pharmacy
Memphis, Tennessee

David M. Roth, MD, PhD
Professor of Anesthesiology
University of California, San Diego
VA-San Diego Healthcare System
San Diego, California

Edward A. Sausville, MD, PhD
Professor of Medicine; Adjunct Professor, Pharmacology &
Experimental Therapeutics
University of Maryland School of Medicine
Baltimore, Maryland

Matthew J. Sewell, MD
Pediatric Dermatology Fellow
Department of Dermatology
University of North Carolina
Chapel Hill, North Carolina

Bernard P. Schimmer, PhD
Professor (Emeritus) of Pharmacology and Toxicology
University of Toronto
Ontario, Canada

Keith A. Sharkey, PhD, CAGF, FCAHS
Professor of Physiology and Pharmacology
Cumming School of Medicine
University of Calgary
Calgary, Alberta, Canada

Richard C. Shelton, MD
Professor, Department of Psychiatry and Behavioral Neurobiology
The University of Alabama at Birmingham
Birmingham, Alabama

Danny Shen, PhD
Professor of Pharmaceutics, School of Pharmacy
University of Washington
Seattle, Washington

David R. Sibley, PhD
Senior Investigator, Molecular Neuropharmacology Section
National Institute of Neurological Disorders & Stroke
National Institutes of Health
Bethesda, Maryland

Randal A. Skidgel, PhD
Professor of Pharmacology
College of Medicine, University of Illinois-Chicago
Chicago, Illinois

Misty D. Smith, PhD
Research Assistant Professor, Department of Pharmacology & Toxicology;
Research Assistant Professor, School of Dentistry
Co-Investigator, Anticonvulsant Drug Development Program
University of Utah
Salt Lake City, Utah

Emer M. Smyth, PhD
Director, Cancer Research Alliances
Assistant Dean for Cancer Research
Assistant Professor, Pathology and Cell Biology
Herbert Irving Comprehensive Cancer Center
Columbia University Medical Center
New York, New York

Peter J. Snyder, MD
Professor of Medicine
University of Pennsylvania
Philadelphia, Pennsylvania

Yuichi Sugiyama, PhD
Head of Sugiyama Laboratory
RIKEN Innovation Center
RIKEN Yokohama
Yokohama, Japan

Palmer Taylor, PhD
Sandra & Monroe Trout Professor of Pharmacology, School of Medicine
Dean Emeritus, Skaggs School of Pharmacy and Pharmaceutical Sciences
University of California
San Diego, California

Kenneth E. Thummel, PhD
Professor and Chair, Department of Pharmaceutics
University of Washington
Seattle, Washington

Roberto Tinoco, PhD
Research Assistant Professor
Infectious and Inflammatory Diseases Center
Sanford Burnham Prebys Medical Discovery Institute
La Jolla, California

Robert H. Tukey, PhD
Professor of Pharmacology and Chemistry/Biochemistry
University of California
San Diego, California

Joseph M. Vinetz, MD
Professor of Medicine, Division of Infectious Diseases
University of California
San Diego, California

Wendy Vitek, MD
Assistant Professor of Obstetrics and Gynecology
University of Rochester School of Medicine and Dentistry
Rochester, New York

Mark S. Wallace, MD
Professor of Clinical Anesthesiology
University of California
San Diego, California

Jeffrey I. Weitz, MD, FRCP(C), FACP
Professor of Medicine
Biochemistry and Biomedical Sciences McMaster University
Executive Director, Thrombosis & Atherosclerosis Research Institute
Hamilton, Ontario, Canada

Anton Wellstein, MD, PhD
Professor of Oncology and Pharmacology
Georgetown University, School of Medicine
Washington DC

Jürgen Wess, PhD
Chief, Molecular Signaling Section
Lab. of Bioorganic Chemistry
National Institute of Diabetes and Digestive and Kidney Diseases
Bethesda, Maryland

David P. Westfall, PhD
Professor (Emeritus) of Pharmacology
University of Nevada School of Medicine
Reno, Nevada

Thomas C. Westfall, PhD
Professor and Chair Emeritus, Department of Pharmacology and Physiology
Saint Louis University School of Medicine
St. Louis, Missouri

Dawn M. Wetzel, MD, PhD
Assistant Professor of Pediatrics (Division of Infectious Diseases) and Pharmacology
University of Texas Southwestern Medical Center
Dallas, Texas

Karen S. Wilcox, PhD
Professor and Chair, Department of Pharmacology
Director, Anticonvulsant Drug Development Program
University of Utah
Salt Lake City, Utah

Kerstin de Wit, MD
Department of Medicine
Divisions of Emergency and Haematology
McMaster University, Canada;
Thrombosis and Emergency Physician
Hamilton Health Sciences
Hamilton, Ontario, Canada

Tony L. Yaksh, PhD
Professor of Anesthesiology and Pharmacology
University of California, San Diego
La Jolla, California

Jason X.-J. Yuan, MD, PhD
Professor of Medicine and Physiology;
Chief, Division of Translational and Regenerative Medicine
University of Arizona
Tucson, Arizona

Alexander C. Zambon, PhD
Assistant Professor of Biopharmaceutical Sciences
Keck Graduate Institute
Claremont, California

Preface

The first edition of this book appeared in 1941, the product of a collaboration between two friends and professors at Yale, Louis Goodman and Alfred Gilman. Their purpose, stated in the preface to that edition, was to correlate pharmacology with related medical sciences, to reinterpret the actions and uses of drugs in light of advances in medicine and the basic biomedical sciences, to emphasize the applications of pharmacodynamics to therapeutics, and to create a book that would be useful to students of pharmacology and to physicians. We continue to follow these principles in the 13th edition.

The 1st edition was quite successful despite its high price, $12.50, and soon became known as the "blue bible of pharmacology." The book was evidence of the deep friendship between its authors, and when the Gilmans' son was born in 1941, he was named Alfred Goodman Gilman. World War II and the relocation of both authors—Goodman to Utah, Gilman to Columbia—postponed a second edition until 1955. The experience of writing the second edition during a period of accelerating basic research and drug development persuaded the authors to become editors, relying on experts whose scholarship they trusted to contribute individual chapters, a pattern that has been followed ever since.

Alfred G. Gilman, the son, served as an associate editor for the 5th edition (1975), became the principal editor for the 6th (1980), 7th (1985), and 8th (1990) editions, and consulting editor for the 9th and 10th editions that were edited by Lee Limbird and Joel Hardman. After an absence in the 11th edition, Al Gilman agreed to co-author the introductory chapter in the 12th edition. His final contribution to G&G, a revision of that chapter, is the first chapter in this edition, which we dedicate to his memory.

A multi-authored text of this sort grows by accretion, posing challenges to editors but also offering 75 years of wisdom, memorable pearls, and flashes of wit. Portions of prior editions persist in the current edition, and we have given credit to recent former contributors at the end of each chapter. Such a text also tends to grow in length with each edition, as contributors add to existing text and as pharmacotherapy advances. To keep the length manageable and in a single volume, Dr. Randa Hilal-Dandan and I prepared a shortened version of each chapter and then invited contributors to add back old material that was essential and to add new material. We also elected to discard the use of extract (very small) type and to use more figures to explain signaling pathways and mechanisms of drug action. Not wanting to favor one company's preparation of an agent over that of another, we have ceased to use trade names except as needed to refer to drug combinations or to distinguish multiple formulations of the same agent with distinctive pharmacokinetic or pharmacodynamic properties. Counter-balancing this shortening are five new chapters that reflect advances in the therapeutic manipulation of the immune system, the treatment of viral hepatitis, and the pharmacotherapy of cardiovascular disease and pulmonary artery hypertension.

Editing such a book brings into view a number of overarching issues: Over-prescribing of antibiotics and their excessive use in agricultural animal husbandry continues to promote the development of antimicrobial resistance; the application of CRISPR/cas9 will likely provide new therapeutic avenues; global warming and the sheer size of the human population require medical scientists and practitioners to promote remedial and preventive action based on data, not ideology.

A number of people have made invaluable contributions to the preparation of this edition. My thanks to Randa Hilal-Dandan and Bjorn Knollmann for their editorial work; to Harriet Lebowitz of McGraw-Hill, who guided our work, prescribed the updated style, and kept the project moving to completion; to Vastavikta Sharma of Cenveo Publishers Services, who oversaw the copy editing, typesetting, and preparation of the artwork; to Nelda Murri, our consulting pharmacist, whose familiarity with clinical pharmacy is evident throughout the book; to James Shanahan, publisher at McGraw-Hill, for supporting the project; and to the many readers who have written to critique the book and offer suggestions.

Laurence L. Brunton
San Diego, CA
1 September 2017

Acknowledgments

The editors appreciate the assistance of:

Harriet Lebowitz
Senior Project Development Editor
McGraw-Hill Education

Laura Libretti
Administrative Assistant
McGraw-Hill Education

Bryan Mott, PhD
Consulting Medicinal Chemist

Nelda Murri, PharmD, MBA
Consulting Pharmacist

Christie Naglieri
Senior Project Development Editor
McGraw-Hill Education

Joseph K. Prinsen, DO, PhD
Jason D. Morrow Chief Fellow in Clinical Pharmacology
Vanderbilt University School of Medicine

David Aaron Rice
Administrative Assistant
University of California, San Diego

James F. Shanahan
Publisher, Medical Textbooks
McGraw-Hill Education

Vastavikta Sharma
Lead Project Manager
Cenveo Publisher Services

Roberto Tinoco, PhD
Research Assistant Professor
Sanford-Burnham-Prebys Medical Discovery Institute

Contents 目 录

Section III
Modulation of Pulmonary, Renal, and Cardiovascular Function 463
第三篇　肺、肾和心血管功能的调节

Section IV
Inflammation, Immunomodulation, and Hematopoiesis 645
第四篇　炎症、免疫调节和造血

Section V
Hormones and Hormone Antagonists 797
第五篇　激素和激素拮抗药

Section VI
Gastrointestinal Pharmacology 935
第六篇　胃肠药理学

Section VII
Chemotherapy of Infectious Diseases 985
第七篇 传染病的化学治疗

Section VIII
Pharmacotherapy of Neoplastic Disease 1191
第八篇 肿瘤的药物治疗

Section IX
Special Systems Pharmacology 1283
第九篇 特殊系统药理学

Appendices
附录

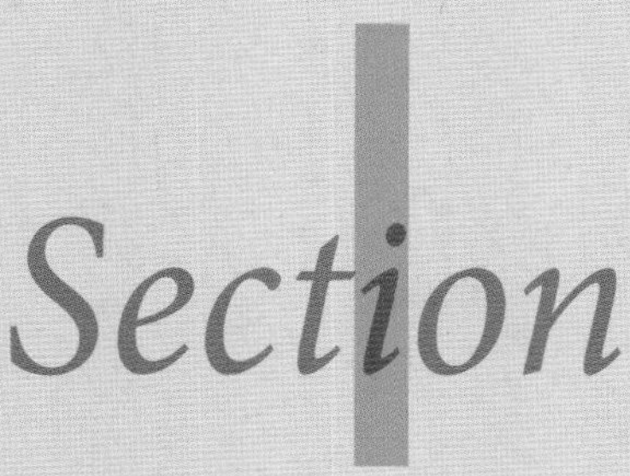

General Principles

第一篇　总　则

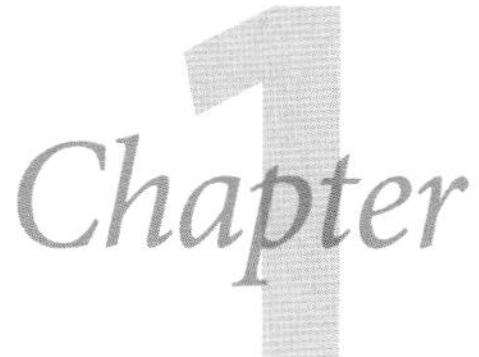

Drug Invention and the Pharmaceutical Industry

Suzanne M. Rivera and Alfred Goodman Gilman*

第一章　药物研发和制药业

中文导读

本章主要介绍：人类早期植物药的应用经验到现代化学的发展历程；药物来源，包括传统小分子化合物、活性分子来源的先导化合物和重要性日益突显的大分子药物；药物作用靶点，提出了“靶点是否可‘成药’？”“靶点是否已经过验证？”“药物研发投入是否有经济效益？”3个关键问题；临床前辅助研究；临床试验，包括美国食品药品监督管理局（FDA）的职能、临床试验的实施、“安全性”和“有效性”的确定；个体化医疗；对药品行业公共政策的思考与批判，包括“谁买单？”、知识产权和专利、药品营销、对国际不公正的担忧、产品责任、仿制与真正的发明——新药研发之路。

*Deceased, December 23, 2015. AGG served on the Board of Directors of Regeneron Pharmaceuticals, Inc., a potential conflict of interest.

Abbreviations

ADME: absorption, distribution, metabolism, excretion
AHFS-DI: American Hospital Formulary Service-Drug Information
BLA: Biologics License Application
CDC: Centers for Disease Control and Prevention
CDER: Center for Drug Evaluation and Research
DHHS: U.S. Department of Health and Human Services
FDA: U.S. Food and Drug Administration
HCV: hepatitis C virus
HMG CoA: 3-hydroxy-3-methylglutaryl coenzyme A
IND: Investigational New Drug
LDL: low-density lipoprotein
NDA: New Drug Application
NIH: National Institutes of Health
NMEs: New Molecular Entities
NMR: nuclear magnetic resonance
PCSK9: proprotein convertase subtilisin/kexin type 9
PDUFA: Prescription Drug User Fee Act
PhRMA: Pharmaceutical Research and Manufacturers of America
R&D: research and development
SCHIP: State Children's Health Insurance Program
siRNAs: small interfering RNAs

The first edition of *Goodman & Gilman*, published in 1941, helped to organize the field of pharmacology, giving it intellectual validity and an academic identity. That edition began: "The subject of pharmacology is a broad one and embraces the knowledge of the source, physical and chemical properties, compounding, physiological actions, absorption, fate, and excretion, and therapeutic uses of drugs. A *drug* may be broadly defined as any chemical agent that affects living protoplasm, and few substances would escape inclusion by this definition." This General Principles section provides the underpinnings for these definitions by exploring the processes of drug invention, development, and regulation, followed by the basic properties of the interactions between the drug and biological systems: *pharmacodynamics*, *pharmacokinetics* (including drug transport and metabolism), and *pharmacogenomics*, with a brief foray into *drug toxicity and poisoning*. Subsequent sections deal with the use of drugs as therapeutic agents in human subjects.

Use of the term *invention* to describe the process by which a new drug is identified and brought to medical practice, rather than the more conventional term *discovery,* is intentional. Today, useful drugs are rarely discovered hiding somewhere waiting to be found. The term *invention* emphasizes the process by which drugs are sculpted and brought into being based on experimentation and optimization of many independent properties; there is little serendipity.

From Early Experiences With Plants to Modern Chemistry

The human fascination—and sometimes infatuation—with chemicals that alter biological function is ancient and results from long experience with and dependence on plants. Because most plants are root bound, many of them produce harmful compounds for defense that animals have learned to avoid and humans to exploit (or abuse).

Earlier editions of this text described examples: the appreciation of coffee (caffeine) by the prior of an Arabian convent, who noted the behavior of goats that gamboled and frisked through the night after eating the berries of the coffee plant; the use of mushrooms and the deadly nightshade plant by professional poisoners; of belladonna ("beautiful lady") to dilate pupils; of the Chinese herb ma huang (containing ephedrine) as a circulatory stimulant; of curare by South American Indians to paralyze and kill animals hunted for food; and of poppy juice (opium) containing morphine (from the Greek *Morpheus*, the God of dreams) for pain relief and control of dysentery. Morphine, of course, has well-known addicting properties, mimicked in some ways by other problematic ("recreational") natural products—nicotine, cocaine, and ethanol.

Although terrestrial and marine organisms remain valuable sources of compounds with pharmacological activities, drug invention became more allied with synthetic organic chemistry as that discipline flourished over the past 150 years, beginning in the dye industry. Dyes are colored compounds with selective affinity for biological tissues. Study of these interactions stimulated Paul Ehrlich to postulate the existence of chemical receptors in tissues that interacted with and "fixed" the dyes. Similarly, Ehrlich thought that unique receptors on microorganisms or parasites might react specifically with certain dyes and that such selectivity could spare normal tissue. Ehrlich's work culminated in the invention of arsphenamine in 1907, which was patented as "salvarsan," suggestive of the hope that the chemical would be the salvation of humankind. This and other organic arsenicals were used for the chemotherapy of syphilis until the discovery of penicillin. The work of Gerhard Domagk demonstrated that another dye, prontosil (the first clinically useful sulfonamide), was dramatically effective in treating streptococcal infections, launching the era of antimicrobial chemotherapy.

The collaboration of pharmacology with chemistry on the one hand and with clinical medicine on the other has been a major contributor to the effective treatment of disease, especially since the middle of the 20th century.

Sources of Drugs

Small Molecules Are the Tradition

With the exception of a few naturally occurring hormones (e.g., insulin), most drugs were small organic molecules (typically <500 Da) until recombinant DNA technology permitted synthesis of proteins by various organisms (bacteria, yeast) and mammalian cells. The usual approach to invention of a small-molecule drug is to screen a collection of chemicals ("library") for compounds with the desired features. An alternative is to synthesize and focus on close chemical relatives of a substance known to participate in a biological reaction of interest (e.g., congeners of a specific enzyme substrate chosen to be possible inhibitors of the enzymatic reaction), a particularly important strategy in the discovery of anticancer drugs.

Drug discovery in the past often resulted from serendipitous observations of the effects of plant extracts or individual chemicals on animals or humans; today's approach relies more on high-throughput screening of libraries containing hundreds of thousands or even millions of compounds for their capacity to interact with a specific molecular target or elicit a specific biological response. Ideally, the target molecules are of human origin, obtained by transcription and translation of the cloned human gene. The potential drugs that are identified in the screen ("hits") are thus known to react with the human protein and not just with its relative (ortholog) obtained from the mouse or another species.

Among the variables considered in screening are the "drugability" of the target and the stringency of the screen in terms of the concentrations of compounds that are tested. *Drugability* refers to the ease with which the function of a target can be altered in the desired fashion by a small organic molecule. If the protein target has a well-defined binding site for a small molecule (e.g., a catalytic or allosteric site), chances are excellent that hits will be obtained. If the goal is to employ a small molecule to mimic or disrupt the interaction between two proteins, the challenge is much greater.

From Hits to Leads

Initial hits in a screen are rarely marketable drugs, often having modest affinity for the target and lacking the desired specificity and pharmacological properties. Medicinal chemists synthesize derivatives of the hits, thereby defining the structure-activity relationship and optimizing parameters such as affinity for the target, agonist/antagonist activity, permeability across cell membranes, absorption and distribution in the body, metabolism, and unwanted effects.

This approach was driven largely by instinct and trial and error in the past; modern drug development frequently takes advantage of determination of a high-resolution structure of the putative drug bound to its target. X-ray crystallography offers the most detailed structural information if the target protein can be crystallized with the lead drug bound to it. Using techniques of molecular modeling and computational chemistry, the structure provides the chemist with information about substitutions likely to improve the "fit" of the drug with the target and thus enhance the affinity of the drug for its target. Nuclear magnetic resonance (NMR) studies of the drug-receptor complex also can provide useful information (albeit usually at lower resolution), with the advantage that the complex need not be crystallized.

The holy grail of this approach to drug invention is to achieve success entirely through computation. Imagine a database containing detailed chemical information about millions of chemicals and a second database containing detailed structural information about all human proteins. The computational approach is to "roll" all the chemicals over the protein of interest to find those with high-affinity interactions. The dream becomes bolder if we acquire the ability to roll the chemicals that bind to the target of interest over all other human proteins to discard compounds that have unwanted interactions. Finally, we also will want to predict the structural and functional consequences of a drug binding to its target (a huge challenge), as well as all relevant pharmacokinetic properties of the molecules of interest. Indeed, computational approaches have suggested new uses for old drugs and offered explanations for recent failures of drugs in the later stages of clinical development (e.g., torcetrapib; see Box 1-2) (Xie et al., 2007, 2009).

Large Molecules Are Increasingly Important

Protein therapeutics were uncommon before the advent of recombinant DNA technology. Insulin was introduced into clinical medicine for the treatment of diabetes following the experiments of Banting and Best in 1921. Insulins purified from porcine or bovine pancreas are active in humans, although antibodies to the foreign proteins are occasionally problematic. Growth hormone, used to treat pituitary dwarfism, exhibits more stringent species specificity. Only the human hormone could be used after purification from pituitary glands harvested during autopsy, and such use had its dangers—some patients who received the human hormone developed Creutzfeldt-Jakob disease (the human equivalent of mad cow disease), a fatal degenerative neurological disease caused by prion proteins that contaminated the drug preparation. Thanks to gene cloning and the production of large quantities of proteins by expressing the cloned gene in bacteria or eukaryotic cells, protein therapeutics now use highly purified preparations of human (or humanized) proteins. Rare proteins can be produced in quantity, and immunological reactions are minimized. Proteins can be designed, customized, and optimized using genetic engineering techniques. Other types of macromolecules may also be used therapeutically. For example, antisense oligonucleotides are used to block gene transcription or translation, as are siRNAs.

Proteins used therapeutically include hormones; growth factors (e.g., erythropoietin, granulocyte colony-stimulating factor); cytokines; and a number of monoclonal antibodies used in the treatment of cancer and autoimmune diseases (Chapters 34–36 and 67). Murine monoclonal antibodies can be "humanized" (by substituting human for mouse amino acid sequences). Alternatively, mice have been engineered by replacement of critical mouse genes with their human equivalents, such that they make completely human antibodies. Protein therapeutics are administered parenterally, and their receptors or targets must be accessible extracellularly.

Targets of Drug Action

Early drugs came from observation of the effects of plants after their ingestion by animals, with no knowledge of the drug's mechanism or site of action. Although this approach is still useful (e.g., in screening for the capacity of natural products to kill microorganisms or malignant cells), modern drug invention usually takes the opposite approach, starting with a statement (or hypothesis) that a certain protein or pathway plays a critical role in the pathogenesis of a certain disease, and that altering the protein's activity would be effective against that disease. Crucial questions arise:

- Can one find a drug that will have the desired effect against its target?
- Does modulation of the target protein affect the course of disease?
- Does this project make sense economically?

The effort expended to find the desired drug will be determined by the degree of confidence in the answers to the last two questions.

Is the Target Drugable?

The drugability of a target with a low-molecular-weight organic molecule relies on the presence of a binding site for the drug that exhibits considerable affinity and selectivity.

If the target is an enzyme or a receptor for a small ligand, one is encouraged. If the target is related to another protein that is known to have, for example, a binding site for a regulatory ligand, one is hopeful. However, if the known ligands are large peptides or proteins with an extensive set of contacts with their receptor, the challenge is much greater. If the goal is to disrupt interactions between two proteins, it may be necessary to find a "hot spot" that is crucial for the protein-protein interaction, and such a region may not be detected. Accessibility of the drug to its target also is critical. Extracellular targets are intrinsically easier to approach, and, in general, only extracellular targets are accessible to macromolecular drugs.

Has the Target Been Validated?

The question of whether the target has been validated is obviously a critical one. A negative answer, frequently obtained only retrospectively, is a common cause of failure in drug invention (Box 1–1). Modern techniques of molecular biology offer powerful tools for validation of potential drug targets, to the extent that the biology of model systems resembles human biology. Genes can be inserted, disrupted, and altered in mice. One can thereby create models of disease in animals or mimic the effects of long-term disruption or activation of a given biological process. If, for example, disruption of the gene encoding a specific enzyme or receptor has a beneficial effect in a valid murine model of a human disease, one may believe that the potential drug target has been validated. Mutations in humans also can provide extraordinarily valuable information.

For example, loss-of-function mutations in the *PCSK9* gene (encoding proprotein convertase subtilisin/kexin type 9) greatly lower concentrations of LDL cholesterol in blood and reduce the risk of myocardial infarction (Horton et al., 2009; Poirier and Mayer, 2013). Based on these

BOX 1-1 ■ Target Validation: The Lesson of Leptin

Biological systems frequently contain redundant elements or can alter expression of drug-regulated elements to compensate for the effect of the drug. *In general, the more important the function, the greater the complexity of the system.* For example, many mechanisms control feeding and appetite, and drugs to control obesity have been notoriously difficult to find. The discovery of the hormone leptin, which suppresses appetite, was based on mutations in mice that cause loss of either leptin or its receptor; either kind of mutation results in enormous obesity in both mice and people. Leptin thus appeared to be a marvelous opportunity to treat obesity. However, on investigation, it was discovered that obese individuals have high circulating concentrations of leptin and appear insensitive to its action.

findings, two companies now market antibodies that inhibit the action of *PCSK9*. These antibodies lower the concentration of LDL cholesterol in blood substantially and are essentially additive to the effects of statins; long-term outcome studies are in progress to determine whether the risk of significant cardiovascular events also is reduced. Additional molecules are in the queue.

Is This Drug Invention Effort Economically Viable?

Drug invention and development is expensive (see Table 1-1), and economic realities influence the direction of pharmaceutical research. For example, investor-owned companies generally cannot afford to develop products for rare diseases or for diseases that are common only in economically underdeveloped parts of the world. Funds to invent drugs targeting rare diseases or diseases primarily affecting developing countries (especially parasitic diseases) often come from taxpayers or wealthy philanthropists.

Additional Preclinical Research

Following the path just described can yield a potential drug molecule that interacts with a validated target and alters its function in the desired fashion. Now, one must consider all aspects of the molecule in question—its affinity and selectivity for interaction with the target; its pharmacokinetic properties (ADME); issues of its large-scale synthesis or purification; its pharmaceutical properties (stability, solubility, questions of formulation); and its safety. One hopes to correct, to the extent possible, any obvious deficiencies by modification of the molecule itself or by changes in the way the molecule is presented for use.

Before being administered to people, potential drugs are tested for general toxicity by long-term monitoring of the activity of various systems in two species of animals, generally one rodent (usually the mouse) and one nonrodent (often the rabbit). Compounds also are evaluated for carcinogenicity, genotoxicity, and reproductive toxicity (see Chapter 4). In vitro and ex vivo assays are used when possible, both to spare animals and to minimize cost. If an unwanted effect is observed, an obvious question is whether it is mechanism based (i.e., caused by interaction of the drug with its intended target) or caused by an off-target effect of the drug, which might be minimized by further optimization of the molecule.

Before the drug candidate can be administered to human subjects in a clinical trial, the sponsor must file an IND application, a request to the U.S. FDA (see "Clinical Trials") for permission to use the drug for human research. The IND describes the rationale and preliminary evidence for efficacy in experimental systems, as well as pharmacology, toxicology, chemistry, manufacturing, and so forth. It also describes the plan (protocol) for investigating the drug in human subjects. The FDA has 30 days to review the IND application, by which time the agency may disapprove it, ask for more data, or allow initial clinical testing to proceed.

Clinical Trials

Role of the FDA

The FDA is a federal regulatory agency within the U.S. DHHS. It is responsible for protecting the public health by ensuring the safety, efficacy, and security of human and veterinary drugs, biological products, medical devices, our nation's food supply, cosmetics, and products that emit radiation (FDA, 2014). The FDA also is responsible for advancing public health by helping to speed innovations that make medicines and foods more effective, safer, and more affordable and by helping people obtain the accurate, science-based information they need to use medicines and foods to improve their health.

New governmental regulations often result from tragedies. The first drug-related legislation in the U.S., the Federal Food and Drug Act of 1906, was concerned only with the interstate transport of adulterated or misbranded foods and drugs. There were no obligations to establish drug efficacy or safety. This act was amended in 1938 after the deaths of over 100 children from "elixir sulfanilamide," a solution of sulfanilamide in diethylene glycol, an excellent but highly toxic solvent and an ingredient in antifreeze. The enforcement of the amended act was entrusted to the FDA, which began requiring toxicity studies as well as approval of an NDA (see "The Conduct of Clinical Trials") before a drug could be promoted and distributed. Although a new drug's safety had to be demonstrated, no proof of efficacy was required.

In the 1960s, thalidomide, a hypnotic drug with no obvious advantages over others, was introduced in Europe. Epidemiological research eventually established that this drug, taken early in pregnancy, was responsible for an epidemic of what otherwise is a relatively rare and severe birth defect, phocomelia, in which limbs are malformed. In reaction to this catastrophe, the U.S. Congress passed the Harris-Kefauver amendments to the Food, Drug, and Cosmetic Act in 1962. These amendments established the requirement for proof of efficacy as well as documentation of relative safety in terms of the risk-to-benefit ratio for the disease entity to be treated (the more serious the disease, the greater the acceptable risk).

Today, the FDA faces an enormous challenge, especially in view of the widely held belief that its mission cannot possibly be accomplished with the resources allocated by Congress. Moreover, harm from drugs that cause unanticipated adverse effects is not the only risk of an imperfect system; harm also occurs when the approval process delays the approval of a new drug with important beneficial effects.

The Conduct of Clinical Trials

Clinical trials of drugs are designed to acquire information about the pharmacokinetic and pharmacodynamic properties of a candidate drug in humans. Efficacy must be proven and an adequate margin of safety established for a drug to be approved for sale in the U.S.

The U.S. NIH identifies seven ethical principles that must be satisfied before a clinical trial can begin:

1. Social and clinical value
2. Scientific validity
3. Fair selection of subjects
4. Informed consent
5. Favorable risk-benefit ratio
6. Independent review
7. Respect for potential and enrolled subjects (NIH, 2011).

The FDA-regulated clinical trials typically are conducted in four phases. Phases I-III are designed to establish safety and efficacy, while phase IV postmarketing trials delineate additional information regarding new indications, risks, and optimal doses and schedules. Table 1–1 and Figure 1–1 summarize the important features of each phase of clinical trials; note the attrition at each successive stage over a relatively long and costly process. When initial phase III trials are complete, the sponsor (usually a pharmaceutical company) applies to the FDA for approval to market the drug; this application is called either an NDA or a BLA. These applications contain comprehensive information, including individual case report forms from the hundreds or thousands of individuals who have received the drug during its phase III testing. Applications are reviewed by teams of specialists, and the FDA may call on the help of panels of external experts in complex cases.

Under the provisions of the PDUFA (enacted in 1992 and renewed every 5 years, most recently in 2012), pharmaceutical companies now provide a significant portion of the FDA budget via user fees, a legislative effort to expedite the drug approval review process by providing increased resources. The PDUFA also broadened the FDA's drug safety program and increased resources for review of television drug advertising. Under the PDUFA, once an NDA is submitted to the FDA, review typically takes 6–10 months. During this time, numerous review functions are usually performed, including advisory committee meetings, amendments, manufacturing facility inspections, and proprietary name reviews (FDA, 2013a). Before a drug is approved for marketing, the company and the FDA must agree on the content of the "label" (package insert)—the official prescribing information. This label describes the approved indications for

TABLE 1–1 ■ TYPICAL CHARACTERISTICS OF THE VARIOUS PHASES OF THE CLINICAL TRIALS REQUIRED FOR MARKETING OF NEW DRUGS

PHASE I FIRST IN HUMAN	PHASE II FIRST IN PATIENT	PHASE III MULTISITE TRIAL	PHASE IV POSTMARKETING SURVEILLANCE
10–100 participants	50–500 participants	A few hundred to a few thousand participants	Many thousands of participants
Usually healthy volunteers; occasionally patients with advanced or rare disease	Patient-subjects receiving experimental drug	Patient-subjects receiving experimental drug	Patients in treatment with approved drug
Open label	Randomized and controlled (can be placebo controlled); may be blinded	Randomized and controlled (can be placebo controlled) or uncontrolled; may be blinded	Open label
Safety and tolerability	Efficacy and dose ranging	Confirm efficacy in larger population	Adverse events, compliance, drug-drug interactions
1–2 years	2–3 years	3–5 years	No fixed duration
U.S. $10 million	U.S. $20 million	U.S. $50–100 million	—
Success rate: 50%	Success rate: 30%	Success rate: 25%–50%	—

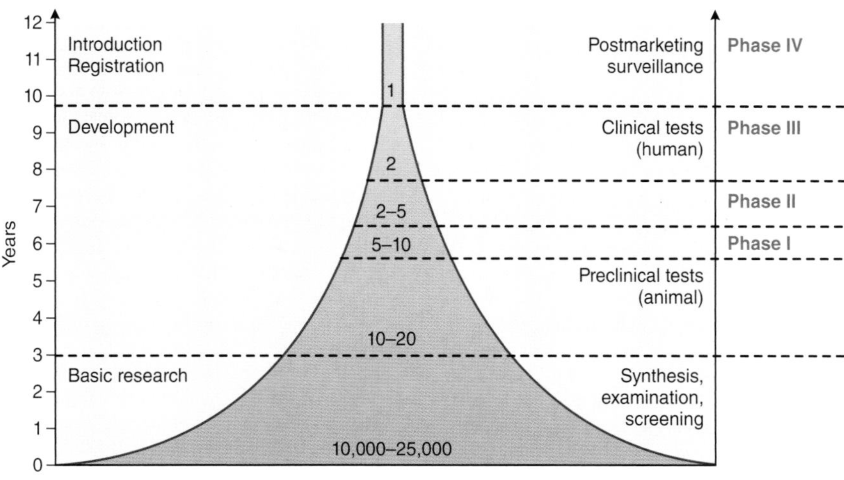

Figure 1–1 *The phases, time lines, and attrition that characterize the invention of new drugs.* See also Table 1–1.

use of the drug and clinical pharmacological information, including dosage, adverse reactions, and special warnings and precautions (sometimes posted in a "black box").

Promotional materials used by pharmaceutical companies cannot deviate from information contained in the package insert. Importantly, the physician is not bound by the package insert; a physician in the U.S. *may* legally prescribe a drug for any purpose that he or she deems reasonable. However, third-party payers (insurance companies, Medicare, and so on) generally will not reimburse a patient for the cost of a drug used for an "off-label" indication unless the new use is supported by a statutorily named compendium (e.g., the AHFS-DI). Furthermore, a physician may be vulnerable to litigation if untoward effects result from an unapproved use of a drug.

Determining "Safe" and "Effective"

Demonstrating efficacy to the FDA requires performing "adequate and well-controlled investigations," generally interpreted to mean two replicate clinical trials that are usually, but not always, randomized, double blind, and placebo (or otherwise) controlled.

Is a placebo the proper control? The World Medical Association's *Declaration of Helsinki* (World Medical Association 2013) discourages use of placebo controls when an alternative treatment is available for comparison because of the concern that study participants randomized to placebo in such a circumstance would, in effect, be denied treatment during the conduct of the trial.

What must be measured in the trials? In a straightforward trial, a readily quantifiable parameter (a secondary or surrogate end point), thought to be predictive of relevant clinical outcomes, is measured in matched drug- and placebo-treated groups. Examples of surrogate end points include LDL cholesterol as a predictor of myocardial infarction, bone mineral density as a predictor of fractures, or hemoglobin A_{1c} as a predictor of the complications of diabetes mellitus. More stringent trials would require demonstration of reduction of the incidence of myocardial infarction in patients taking a candidate drug in comparison with those taking an HMG CoA reductase inhibitor (statin) or other LDL cholesterol-lowering agent or reduction in the incidence of fractures in comparison with those taking a bisphosphonate. Use of surrogate end points significantly reduces cost and time required to complete trials, but there are many mitigating factors, including the significance of the surrogate end point to the disease that the candidate drug is intended to treat.

Some of the difficulties are well illustrated by experiences with ezetimibe, a drug that inhibits absorption of cholesterol from the gastrointestinal tract and lowers LDL cholesterol concentrations in blood, especially when used in combination with a statin. Lowering of LDL cholesterol was assumed to be an appropriate surrogate end point for the effectiveness of ezetimibe to reduce myocardial infarction and stroke, and the drug was approved based on such data. Surprisingly, a subsequent clinical trial (ENHANCE) demonstrated that the combination of ezetimibe and a statin did not reduce intima media thickness of carotid arteries (a more direct measure of subendothelial cholesterol accumulation) compared with the statin alone, despite the fact that the drug combination lowered LDL cholesterol concentrations substantially more than did either drug alone (Kastelein et al., 2008).

Critics of ENHANCE argued that the patients in the study had familial hypercholesterolemia, had been treated with statins for years, and did not have carotid artery thickening at the initiation of the study. Should ezetimibe have been approved? Must we return to measurement of true clinical end points (e.g., myocardial infarction) before approval of drugs that lower cholesterol by novel mechanisms? The costs involved in such extensive and expensive trials must be borne somehow (see below). A follow-up 7-year study involving over 18,000 patients (IMPROVE-IT) vindicated the decision to approve ezetimibe (Jarcho and Keaney, 2015). Taken in conjunction with a statin, the drug significantly reduced the incidence of myocardial infarction and stroke in high-risk patients (Box 1–2).

No drug is totally safe; all drugs produce unwanted effects in at least some people at some dose. Many unwanted and serious effects of drugs occur so infrequently, perhaps only once in several thousand patients, that they go undetected in the relatively small populations (a few thousand) in the standard phase III clinical trial (see Table 1–1). To detect and verify that such events are, in fact, drug-related would require administration of the drug to tens or hundreds of thousands of people during clinical trials, adding enormous expense and time to drug development and delaying access to potentially beneficial therapies. In general, the true spectrum and incidence of untoward effects become known only after a drug is released to the broader market and used by a large number of people (phase IV, postmarketing surveillance). Drug development costs and drug prices could be reduced substantially if the public were willing to accept more risk. This would require changing the way we think about a pharmaceutical company's liability for damages from an unwanted effect of a drug that was not detected in clinical trials deemed adequate by the FDA. While the concept is obvious, many lose sight of the fact that extremely severe unwanted effects of a drug, including death, may be deemed acceptable if its therapeutic effect is sufficiently unique and valuable. Such dilemmas are not simple and can become issues for great debate.

Several strategies exist to detect adverse reactions after marketing of a drug. Formal approaches for estimation of the magnitude of an adverse drug response include the follow-up or "cohort" study of patients who are receiving a particular drug; the "case-control" study, in which the frequency of drug use in cases of adverse responses is compared to controls; and meta-analysis of pre- and postmarketing studies. Voluntary reporting of adverse events has proven to be an effective way to generate an early signal that a drug may be causing an adverse reaction (Aagard and Hansen, 2009). The primary sources for the reports are responsible, alert physicians; third-party payers (pharmacy benefit managers, insurance companies) and consumers also play important roles. Other useful sources are nurses, pharmacists, and students in these disciplines. In addition, hospital-based pharmacy and therapeutics committees and quality assurance committees frequently are charged with monitoring adverse drug reactions in hospitalized patients. In 2013, the reporting system in the U.S., called *MedWatch,* celebrated its 20th anniversary and announced improvements designed to encourage reporting by consumers (FDA, 2013b). The simple forms for reporting may be obtained 24 hours a day, 7 days a week, by calling 800-FDA-1088; alternatively, adverse reactions can be reported directly using the Internet (http://www.fda.gov/Safety/MedWatch/default.htm). Health professionals also may contact the pharmaceutical manufacturer, who is legally obligated to file reports with the FDA.

BOX 1–2 ■ A Late Surprise in the Development of a Blockbuster

Torcetrapib elevates high-density lipoprotein (HDL) cholesterol (the "good cholesterol"), and higher levels of HDL cholesterol are statistically associated with (are a surrogate end point for) a lower incidence of myocardial infarction. Surprisingly, clinical administration of torcetrapib caused a significant *increase* in mortality from cardiovascular events, ending a development path of 15 years and $800 million. In this case, approval of the drug based on this secondary end point would have been a mistake (Cutler, 2007). A computational systems analysis suggested a mechanistic explanation of this failure (Xie et al., 2009).

Personalized (Individualized, Precision) Medicine

Drug inventors strive to "fit" the drug to the individual patient. To realize the full potential of this approach, however, requires intimate knowledge of the considerable heterogeneity of both the patient population and the targeted disease process. Why does one antidepressant appear to ameliorate depression in a given patient, while another with the same or very similar presumed mechanism of action does not? Is this a difference in the patient's response to the drug; in patient susceptibility to the drug's unwanted effects; in the drug's ADME; or in the etiology of the depression? By contrast, how much of this variability is attributable to environmental factors and possibly their interactions with patient-specific genetic variability? Recent advances, especially in genetics and genomics, provide powerful tools for understanding this heterogeneity. The single most powerful tool for unraveling these myriad mysteries is the ability to sequence DNA rapidly and economically. The cost of sequencing a human genome has fallen by six orders of magnitude since the turn of the 21st century, and the speed of the process has increased correspondingly. The current focus is on the extraordinarily complex analysis of the enormous amounts of data now being obtained from many thousands of individuals, ideally in conjunction with deep knowledge of their phenotypic characteristics, especially including their medical history.

Readily measured biomarkers of disease are powerful adjuncts to DNA sequence information. Simple blood or other tests can be developed to monitor real-time progress or failure of treatment, and many such examples already exist. Similarly, chemical, radiological, or genetic tests may be useful not only to monitor therapy but also to predict success or failure, anticipate unwanted effects of treatment, or appreciate pharmacokinetic variables that may require adjustments of dosage or choice of drugs. Such tests already play a significant role in the choice of drugs for cancer chemotherapy, and the list of drugs specifically designed to "hit" a mutated target in a specific cancer is growing. Such information is also becoming increasing useful in the choice of patients for clinical trials of specific agents—thereby reducing the time required for such trials and their cost, to say nothing of better defining the patient population who may benefit from the drug. These important subjects are discussed in detail in Chapter 7, Pharmacogenetics.

Public Policy Considerations and Criticisms of the Pharmaceutical Industry

Drugs can save lives, prolong lives, and improve the quality of people's lives. However, in a free-market economy, access to drugs is not equitable. Not surprisingly, there is tension between those who treat drugs as entitlements and those who view drugs as high-tech products of a capitalistic society. Supporters of the entitlement position argue that a constitutional right to life should guarantee access to drugs and other healthcare, and they are critical of pharmaceutical companies and others who profit from the business of making and selling drugs. Free-marketers point out that, without a profit motive, it would be difficult to generate the resources and innovation required for new drug development. Given the public interest in the pharmaceutical industry, drug development is both a scientific process and a political one in which attitudes can change quickly. Two decades ago, Merck was named as America's most admired company by *Fortune* magazine 7 years in a row—a record that still stands. In the 2015 survey of the most admired companies in the U.S., no pharmaceutical company ranked in the top 10.

Critics of the pharmaceutical industry frequently begin from the position that people (and animals) need to be protected from greedy and unscrupulous companies and scientists (Kassirer, 2005). In the absence of a government-controlled drug development enterprise, our current system relies predominantly on investor-owned pharmaceutical companies that, like other companies, have a profit motive and an obligation to shareholders. The price of prescription drugs causes great consternation among consumers, especially as many health insurers seek to control costs by choosing not to cover certain "brand-name" products (discussed later). Further, a few drugs (especially for treatment of cancer) have been introduced to the market in recent years at prices that greatly exceeded the costs of development, manufacture, and marketing of the product. Many of these products were discovered in government laboratories or in university laboratories supported by federal grants.

The U.S. is the only large country that places no controls on drug prices and where price plays no role in the drug approval process. Many U.S. drugs cost much more in the U.S. than overseas; thus, U.S. consumers subsidize drug costs for the rest of the world, and they are irritated by that fact. The example of new agents for the treatment of hepatitis C infection brings many conflicting priorities into perspective (Box 1–3).

The drug development process is long, expensive, and risky (see Figure 1–1 and Table 1–1). Consequently, drugs must be priced to recover the substantial costs of invention and development and to fund the marketing efforts needed to introduce new products to physicians and patients.

BOX 1–3 ■ The Cost of Treating Hepatitis C

Infection with hepatitis C virus (HCV) is a chronic disease afflicting millions of people. Some suffer little from this condition; many others eventually develop cirrhosis or hepatocellular carcinoma. Who should be treated? The answer is unknown. Until recently, the treatment of choice for people with genotype 1 HCV involved year-long administration of an interferon (by injection) in combination with ribavirin and a protease inhibitor. Unwanted effects of this regimen are frequent and severe (some say worse than the disease); cure rates range from 50% to 75%. A newer treatment involves an oral tablet containing a combination of sofosbuvir and ledipasvir (see Chapter 63). Treatment usually requires daily ingestion of one tablet, for 8–12 weeks; cure rates exceed 95%, and side effects are minimal.

Controversy surrounds the price of the treatment, about $1000/d. Some insurers refused to reimburse this high cost, relegating many patients to less-effective, more toxic, but less-expensive treatment. However, these third-party payers have negotiated substantial discounts of the price, based on the availability of a competing product. Is the cost exorbitant? Should insurers, rather than patients and their physicians, be making such important decisions?

Continued and excessive escalation of drug and other healthcare costs will bankrupt the healthcare system. The question of appropriate cost involves complex pharmacoeconomic considerations. What are the relative costs of the two treatment regimens? What are the savings from elimination of the serious sequelae of chronic HCV infection? How does one place value to the patient on the less-toxic and more effective and convenient regimen? What are the profit margins of the company involved? Who should make decisions about costs and choices of patients to receive various treatments? How should we consider cases (unlike that for HCV) for which the benefits are quite modest, such as when a very expensive cancer drug extends life only briefly? One astute observer (and an industry critic of many drug prices) summarized the situation as follows: "great, important problem; wrong example."

Nevertheless, as U.S. healthcare spending continues to rise at an alarming pace, prescription drugs account for only about 10% of total U.S. healthcare expenditures (CDC, 2013), and a significant fraction of this drug cost is for low-priced, nonproprietary medicines. Although the increase in prices is significant in certain classes of drugs (e.g., anticancer agents), the total price of prescription drugs is growing at a slower rate than other healthcare costs. Even drastic reductions in drug prices that would severely limit new drug invention would not lower the overall healthcare budget by more than a few percent.

Are profit margins excessive among the major pharmaceutical companies? There is no objective answer to this question. Pragmatic answers come from the markets and from company survival statistics. The U.S. free-market system provides greater rewards for particularly risky and important fields of endeavor, and many people agree that the rewards should be greater for those willing to take the risk. The pharmaceutical industry is clearly one of the more risky:

- The costs to bring products to market are enormous.
- The success rate is low (accounting for much of the cost).
- Accounting for the long development time, effective patent protection for marketing a new drug is only about a decade (see Intellectual Property and Patents), requiring every company to completely reinvent itself on roughly a 10-year cycle.
- Regulation is stringent.
- Product liability is great.
- Competition is fierce.
- With mergers and acquisitions, the number of companies in the pharmaceutical world is shrinking.

Many feel that drug prices should be driven more by their therapeutic impact and their medical need, rather than by simpler free-market considerations; there is movement in this direction. Difficulties involve estimation or measurement of value, and there are many elements in this equation (Schnipper et al., 2015). There is no well-accepted approach to answer the question of value.

Who Pays?

The cost of prescription drugs is borne by consumers ("out of pocket"), private insurers, and public insurance programs such as Medicare, Medicaid, and the SCHIP. Recent initiatives by major retailers and mail-order pharmacies run by private insurers to offer consumer incentives for purchase of generic drugs have helped to contain the portion of household expenses spent on pharmaceuticals; however, more than one-third of total retail drug costs in the U.S. are paid with public funds—tax dollars.

Healthcare in the U.S. is more expensive than everywhere else, but it is not, on average, demonstrably better than everywhere else. One way in which the U.S. system falls short is with regard to healthcare access. Although the Patient Protection and Affordable Care Act of 2010 has reduced the percentage of Americans without health insurance to a historic low, practical solutions to the challenge of providing healthcare for all who need it must recognize the importance of incentivizing innovation.

Intellectual Property and Patents

Drug invention produces intellectual property eligible for patent protection, protection that is enormously important for innovation. As noted in 1859 by Abraham Lincoln, the only U.S. president to ever hold a patent (for a device to lift boats over shoals), by giving the inventor exclusive use of his or her invention for a limited time, the patent system "added the fuel of interest to the fire of genius in the discovery and production of useful things (Lincoln, 1859)." The U.S. patent protection system provides protection for 20 years from the time the patent is filed. During this period, the patent owner has exclusive rights to market and sell the drug. When the patent expires, equivalent nonproprietary products can come on the market; a generic product must be therapeutically equivalent to the original, contain equal amounts of the same active chemical ingredient, and achieve equal concentrations in blood when administered by the same routes. These generic preparations are sold much more cheaply than the original drug and without the huge development costs borne by the original patent holder.

The long time course of drug development, usually more than 10 years (see Figure 1–1), reduces the time during which patent protection functions as intended. The Drug Price Competition and Patent Term Restoration Act of 1984 (Public Law 98-417, informally called the Hatch-Waxman Act) permits a patent holder to apply for extension of a patent term to compensate for delays in marketing caused by FDA approval processes; nonetheless, the average new drug brought to market now enjoys only about 10–12 years of patent protection. Some argue that patent protection for drugs should be shortened, so that earlier generic competition will lower healthcare costs. The counterargument is that new drugs would have to bear even higher prices to provide adequate compensation to companies during a shorter period of protected time. If that is true, lengthening patent protection would actually permit lower prices. Recall that patent protection is worth little if a superior competitive product is invented and brought to market.

Bayh-Dole Act

The Bayh-Dole Act (35 U.S.C. § 200) of 1980 created strong incentives for federally funded scientists at academic medical centers to approach drug invention with an entrepreneurial spirit. The act transferred intellectual property rights to the researchers and their respective institutions (rather than to the government) to encourage partnerships with industry that would bring new products to market for the public's benefit. While the need to protect intellectual property is generally accepted, this encouragement of public-private research collaborations has given rise to concerns about conflicts of interest by scientists and universities (Kaiser, 2009).

Biosimilars

As noted previously, the path to approval of a chemically synthesized small molecule that is identical to an approved compound whose patent protection has expired is relatively straightforward. The same is not true for large molecules (usually proteins), which are generally derived from a living organism (e.g., eukaryotic cell or bacterial culture). Covalent modification of proteins (e.g., glycosylation) or conformational differences may influence pharmacokinetics, pharmacodynamics, immunogenicity, or other properties, and demonstration of therapeutic equivalence may be a complex process.

The Biologics Price Competition and Innovation Act was enacted as part of the Patient Protection and Affordable Care Act in 2010. The intent was to implement an abbreviated licensure pathway for certain "similar" biological products. *Biosimilarity* is defined to mean "that the biological product is highly similar to a reference product notwithstanding minor differences in clinically inactive components" and that "there are no clinically meaningful differences between the biological product and the reference product in terms of the safety, purity, and potency of the product." In general, an application for licensure of a biosimilar must provide satisfactory data from analytical studies, animal studies, and a clinical study or studies. The interpretation of this language has involved seemingly endless discussion, and hard-and-fast rules seem unlikely.

Drug Promotion

In an ideal world, physicians would learn all they need to know about drugs from the medical literature, and good drugs would thereby sell themselves. Instead, we have print advertising and visits from salespeople directed at physicians and extensive direct-to-consumer advertising aimed at the public (in print, on the radio, and especially on television). There are roughly 80,000 pharmaceutical sales representatives in the U.S. who target about 10 times that number of physicians. This figure is down from about 100,000 in 2010, and the decline is likely related to increased attention to real and actual conflicting interests caused by their practices. It has been noted that college cheerleading squads are attractive sources for recruitment of this sales force. The amount spent on promotion of drugs approximates or perhaps even exceeds that spent on research and development. Pharmaceutical companies have been especially vulnerable to criticism for some of their marketing practices.

Promotional materials used by pharmaceutical companies cannot deviate from information contained in the package insert. In addition, there must be an acceptable balance between presentation of therapeutic claims for a product and discussion of unwanted effects. Nevertheless, direct-to-consumer advertising of prescription drugs remains controversial and is permitted only in the U.S. and New Zealand. Canada allows a modified form of advertising in which either the product or the indication can be mentioned, but not both. Physicians frequently succumb with misgivings to patients' advertising-driven requests for specific medications. The counterargument is that patients are educated by such marketing efforts and in many cases will then seek medical care, especially for conditions (e.g., depression) that they may have been denying (Avery et al., 2012).

The major criticism of drug marketing involves some of the unsavory approaches used to influence physician behavior. Gifts of value (e.g., sports tickets) are now forbidden, but dinners where drug-prescribing information is presented by non-sales representatives are widespread. Large numbers of physicians are paid as "consultants" to make presentations in such settings. The acceptance of any gift, no matter how small, from a drug company by a physician is now forbidden at many academic medical centers and by law in several states. In 2009, the board of directors of PhRMA adopted an enhanced Code on Interactions With Healthcare Professionals that prohibits the distribution of noneducational items, prohibits company sales representatives from providing restaurant meals to healthcare professionals (although exceptions are granted when a third-party speaker makes the presentation), and requires companies to ensure that their representatives are trained about laws and regulations that govern interactions with healthcare professionals.

Concerns About Global Injustice

Because development of new drugs is so expensive, private-sector investment in pharmaceutical innovation has focused on products that will have lucrative markets in wealthy countries such as the U.S., which combines patent protection with a free-market economy. Accordingly, there is concern about the degree to which U.S. and European patent protection laws have restricted access to potentially lifesaving drugs in developing countries.

To lower costs, pharmaceutical companies increasingly test their experimental drugs outside the U.S. and the E.U., in developing countries where there is less regulation and easier access to large numbers of patients. According to the U.S. DHHS, there has been a 2000% increase in foreign trials of U.S. drugs over the past 25 years. When these drugs are successful in obtaining marketing approval, consumers in the countries where the trials were conducted often cannot afford them. Some ethicists have argued that this practice violates the justice principle articulated in the Belmont Report (DHHS, 1979, p10), which states that "research should not unduly involve persons from groups unlikely to be among the beneficiaries of subsequent applications of the research." A counterargument is that the conduct of trials in developing nations also frequently brings needed medical attention to underserved populations. This is another controversial issue.

Product Liability

Product liability laws are intended to protect consumers from defective products. Pharmaceutical companies can be sued for faulty design or manufacturing, deceptive promotional practices, violation of regulatory requirements, or failure to warn consumers of known risks. So-called failure-to-warn claims can be made against drug makers even when the product is approved by the FDA. With greater frequency, courts are finding companies that market prescription drugs directly to consumers responsible when these advertisements fail to provide an adequate warning of potential adverse effects.

Although injured patients are entitled to pursue legal remedies, the negative effects of product liability lawsuits against pharmaceutical companies may be considerable. First, fear of liability may cause pharmaceutical companies to be overly cautious about testing, thereby delaying access to the drug. Second, the cost of drugs increases for consumers when pharmaceutical companies increase the length and number of trials they perform to identify even the smallest risks and when regulatory agencies increase the number or intensity of regulatory reviews. Third, excessive liability costs create disincentives for development of so-called orphan drugs, pharmaceuticals that benefit a small number of patients. Should pharmaceutical companies be liable for failure to warn when all of the rules were followed and the product was approved by the FDA but the unwanted effect was not detected because of its rarity or another confounding factor? The only way to find "all" of the unwanted effects that a drug may have is to market it—to conduct a phase IV "clinical trial" or observational study. This basic friction between risk to patients and the financial risk of drug development does not seem likely to be resolved except on a case-by-case basis, in the courts.

The U.S. Supreme Court added further fuel to these fiery issues in 2009 in the case *Wyeth v. Levine*. A patient (Levine) suffered gangrene of an arm following inadvertent arterial administration of the antinausea drug promethazine. She subsequently lost her hand. The healthcare provider had intended to administer the drug by so-called intravenous push. The FDA-approved label for the drug *warned against*, but did not prohibit, administration by intravenous push. The state court and then the U.S. Supreme Court held both the healthcare provider *and the company* liable for damages. Specifically, the Vermont court found that Wyeth had inadequately labeled the drug. This means that FDA approval of the label does not protect a company from liability or prevent individual states from imposing regulations more stringent than those required by the federal government.

"Me Too" Versus True Innovation: The Pace of New Drug Development

Me-too drug is a term used to describe a pharmaceutical that is usually structurally similar to a drug already on the market. Other names used are *derivative medications, molecular modifications*, and *follow-up drugs*. In some cases, a me-too drug is a different molecule developed deliberately by a competitor company to take market share from the company with existing drugs on the market. When the market for a class of drugs is especially large, several companies can share the market and make a profit. Other me-too drugs result coincidentally from numerous companies developing products simultaneously without knowing which drugs will be approved for sale (Box 1–4).

BOX 1–4 ■ A Not-So-New Drug

Some me-too drugs are only slightly altered formulations of a company's own drug, packaged and promoted as if really offering something new. An example is the heartburn medication esomeprazole, marketed by the same company that makes omeprazole. Omeprazole is a mixture of two stereoisomers; esomeprazole contains only one of the isomers and is eliminated less rapidly. Development of esomeprazole created a new period of market exclusivity, although generic versions of omeprazole are marketed, as are branded congeners of omeprazole/esomeprazole. Both omeprazole and esomeprazole are now available over the counter—narrowing the previous price difference.

There are valid criticisms of me-too drugs. First, an excessive emphasis on profit may stifle true innovation. Of the 487 drugs approved by the FDA between 1998 and 2003, only 67 (14%) were considered by the FDA to be NMEs. Between 1998 and 2011, on average only 24 NMEs were approved by the FDA's CDER. Second, some me-too drugs are more expensive than the older versions they seek to replace, increasing the costs of healthcare without corresponding benefit to patients. Nevertheless, for some patients, me-too drugs may have better efficacy or fewer side effects or promote compliance with the treatment regimen. For example, the me-too that can be taken once a day rather than more frequently is convenient and promotes compliance. Some me-too drugs add great value from a business and medical point of view. Atorvastatin was the seventh statin to be introduced to market; it subsequently became the best-selling drug in the world.

Critics argue that pharmaceutical companies are not innovative and do not take risks, and, further, that medical progress is actually slowed by their excessive concentration on me-too products. Figure 1–2 summarizes a few of the facts behind this and other arguments. Clearly, only a modest

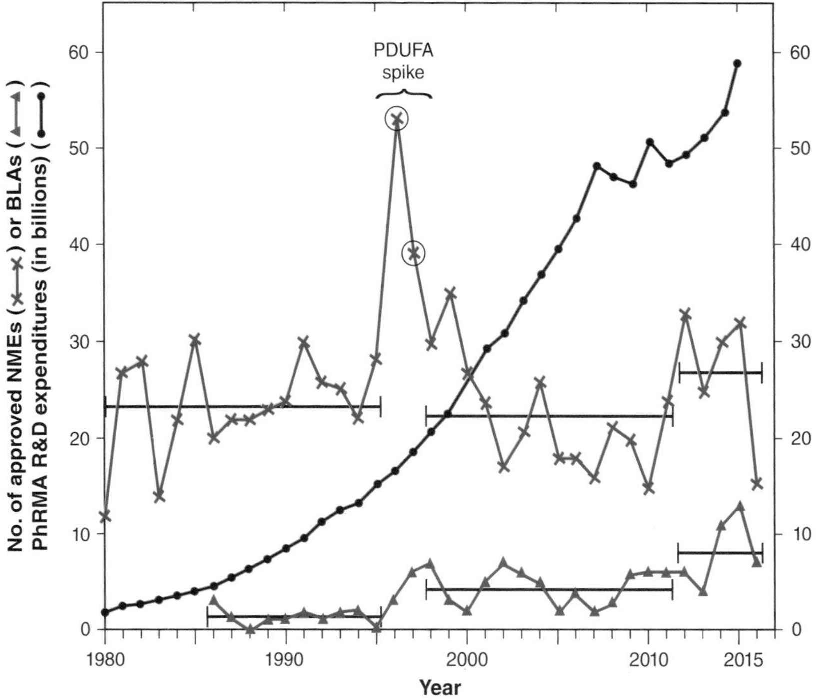

Figure 1–2 *The cost of drug invention is rising. Is productivity?* Each horizontal black line shows the average annual number of NMEs or BLAs for the time period bracketed by the line's length.

number of NMEs, about two dozen a year, achieved FDA approval in the years 1980 to 2011, with the exception of the several-year spike in approvals following the introduction of PDUFA. Yet, from 1980 to 2010, the industry's annual investment in research and development grew from \$2 billion to \$50 billion. This disconnect between research and development investment and new drugs approved occurred at a time when combinatorial chemistry was blooming, the human genome was being sequenced, highly automated techniques of screening were being developed, and new techniques of molecular biology and genetics were offering novel insights into the pathophysiology of human disease.

In recent years, there has been a modest increase in approval of NMEs (inhibitors of a number of protein kinases) and new biologics (numerous therapeutic antibodies) (see Figure 1–2). A continued increase in productivity will be needed to sustain today's pharmaceutical companies as they face waves of patent expirations. There are strong arguments that development of much more targeted, individualized drugs, based on a new generation of molecular diagnostic techniques and improved understanding of disease in individual patients, will improve both medical care and the survival of pharmaceutical companies.

Finally, many of the advances in genetics and molecular biology are still new, particularly when measured in the time frame required for drug development. One can hope that modern molecular medicine will sustain the development of more efficacious and more specific pharmacological treatments for an ever-wider spectrum of human diseases.

Bibliography

Aagard L, Hansen EH. Information about ADRs explored by pharmacovigilance approaches: a qualitative review of studies on antibiotics, SSRIs and NSAIDs. *BMC Clin Pharmacol*, **2009**, *9*:4.

Avery RJ, et al. The impact of direct-to-consumer television and magazine advertising on antidepressant use. *J Health Econ*, **2012**, *31*:705–718.

CDC. Health expenditures. **2013**. Available at: http://www.cdc.gov/nchs/fastats/health-expenditures.htm. Accessed July 8, 2015.

Cutler DM. The demise of a blockbuster? *N Engl J Med*, **2007**, *356*:1292–1293.

DHHS. The Belmont Report. Ethical Principles and Guidelines for the Protection of Human Subjects of Research. The National Commission for the Protection of Human Subjects of Biomedical and Behavioral Research, **1979**.

FDA. An evaluation of the PDUFA Workload Adjuster: Fiscal Years 2009–2013. **2013a**. Available at: http://www.fda.gov/downloads/ForIndustry/UserFees/PrescriptionDrugUserFee/UCM350567.pdf. Accessed June 19, 2015.

FDA. MedWatch: Improving on 20 Years of Excellence. *FDA Voice*. **2013b**. Available at: http://blogs.fda.gov/fdavoice/index.php/2013/06/medwatch-improving-on-20-years-of-excellence/. Accessed May 11, 2017.

FDA. What we do. **2014**. Available at: http://www.fda.gov/AboutFDA/WhatWeDo/. Accessed June 19, 2015.

Horton JD, et al. PCSK9: a convertase that coordinates LDL catabolism. *Lipid Res*, **2009**, *50*:S172–S177.

Jarcho JA, Keaney JF Jr. Proof that lower is better—LDL cholesterol and IMPROVE-IT. *N Engl J Med*, **2015**, *372*:2448–2450.

Kaiser J. Private money, public disclosure. *Science*, **2009**, *325*:28–30.

Kassirer JP. *On the Take. How Medicine's Complicity With Big Business Can Endanger Your Health.* Oxford University Press, New York, **2005**.

Kastelein JJ, et al. Simvastatin with or without ezetimibe in familial hypercholesterolemia. *N Engl J Med*, **2008**, *358*:1421–1443.

Lincoln A. Second speech on discoveries and inventions. **1859**. Available at: http://quod.lib.umich.edu/l/lincoln/lincoln3/1:87?rgn=div1;view=fulltext. Accessed May 8, 2017.

NIH. Ethics in clinical research. **2011**. Available at: http://clinicalcenter.nih.gov/recruit/ethics.html. Accessed July 8, 2015.

Poirier S, Mayer G. The biology of PCSK9 from the endoplasmic reticulum to lysosomes: new and emerging therapeutics to control low-density lipoprotein cholesterol. *Drug Design Dev Ther*, **2013**, *7*:1135.

Schnipper LE, et al. American Society of Clinical Oncology Statement: a conceptual framework to assess the value of cancer treatment options. *J Clin Oncol*, **2015**, *33*:2563–2577.

World Medical Association. World Medical Association Declaration of Helsinki: ethical principles for medical research involving human subjects. *JAMA*, **2013**, *310*:2191–2194.

Xie L, et al. Drug discovery using chemical systems biology: identification of the protein-ligand binding network to explain the side effects of CETP inhibitors. *PLoS Comput Biol*, **2009**, *5*:e1000387.

Xie L, et al. In silico elucidation of the molecular mechanism defining the adverse effect of selective estrogen receptor modulators. *PLoS Comput Biol*, **2007**, *3*:e217.

Pharmacokinetics: The Dynamics of Drug Absorption, Distribution, Metabolism, and Elimination

Iain L. O. Buxton

第二章　药物代谢动力学：药物吸收、分布、代谢和排泄动力学

PASSAGE OF DRUGS ACROSS MEMBRANE BARRIERS
- The Plasma Membrane Is Selectively Permeable
- Modes of Permeation and Transport

DRUG ABSORPTION, BIOAVAILABILITY, AND ROUTES OF ADMINISTRATION
- Absorption and Bioavailability
- Routes of Administration
- Novel Methods of Drug Delivery

BIOEQUIVALENCE

DISTRIBUTION OF DRUGS
- Not All Tissues Are Equal
- Binding to Plasma Proteins
- Tissue Binding

METABOLISM OF DRUGS
- A Few Principles of Metabolism and Elimination
- Prodrugs; Pharmacogenomics

EXCRETION OF DRUGS
- Renal Excretion
- Biliary and Fecal Excretion
- Excretion by Other Routes

CLINICAL PHARMACOKINETICS
- Clearance
- Distribution
- Steady-State Concentration
- Half-Life
- Extent and Rate of Absorption
- Nonlinear Pharmacokinetics
- Design and Optimization of Dosage Regimens

THERAPEUTIC DRUG MONITORING

中文导读

本章主要介绍：药物跨膜转运，包括质膜选择透过性、渗透和转运模式；药物的吸收、生物利用度、给药途径和新的给药方法；生物等效性；药物的分布，包括药物分布的组织差异、药物与血浆蛋白和组织的结合；药物的新陈代谢，包括药物代谢和消除的原理、前药和药物基因组学；药物的排泄，包括肾脏、胆道和粪便及其他途径的排泄；临床药物动力学，包括药物的清除、分配、稳态浓度、半衰期、吸收程度和速率、非线性药代动力学、剂量方案的设计和优化；治疗药物监测。

Abbreviations

ABC: ATP-binding cassette
ACE: angiotensin-converting enzyme
AUC: area under the concentration-time curve of drug absorption and elimination
BBB: blood-brain barrier
CL: clearance
CNS: central nervous system
CNT1: concentrative nucleoside transporter 1
C_p: plasma concentration
CSF: cerebrospinal fluid
C_{ss}: steady-state concentration
CYP: cytochrome P450
F: bioavailability
GI: gastrointestinal
h: hours
k: a rate constant
MDR1: multidrug resistance protein
MEC: minimum effective concentration
min: minutes
SLC: solute carrier
T, t: time
$t_{1/2}$: half-life
V: volume of distribution
V_{ss}: volume of distribution at steady state

The human body restricts access to foreign molecules; therefore, to reach its target within the body and have a therapeutic effect, a drug molecule must cross a number of restrictive barriers en route to its target site. Following administration, the drug must be absorbed and then distributed, usually via vessels of the circulatory and lymphatic systems; in addition to crossing membrane barriers, the drug must survive metabolism (primarily hepatic) and elimination (by the kidney and liver and in the feces). ADME, the absorption, distribution, metabolism, and elimination of drugs, are the processes of *pharmacokinetics* (Figure 2–1). Understanding these processes and their interplay and employing pharmacokinetic principles increase the probability of therapeutic success and reduce the occurrence of adverse drug events.

The absorption, distribution, metabolism, and excretion of a drug involve its passage across numerous cell membranes. Mechanisms by which drugs cross membranes and the physicochemical properties of molecules and membranes that influence this transfer are critical to understanding the disposition of drugs in the human body. The characteristics of a drug that predict its movement and availability at sites of action are its molecular size and structural features, degree of ionization, relative lipid solubility of its ionized and nonionized forms, and its binding to serum and tissue proteins. Although physical barriers to drug movement may be a single layer of cells (e.g., intestinal epithelium) or several layers of cells and associated extracellular protein (e.g., skin), the plasma membrane is the basic barrier.

Passage of Drugs Across Membrane Barriers

The Plasma Membrane Is Selectively Permeable

The plasma membrane consists of a bilayer of amphipathic lipids with their hydrocarbon chains oriented inward to the center of the bilayer to form a continuous hydrophobic phase, with their hydrophilic heads oriented outward. Individual lipid molecules in the bilayer vary according to the particular membrane and can move laterally and organize themselves into microdomains (e.g., regions with sphingolipids and cholesterol, forming lipid rafts), endowing the membrane with fluidity, flexibility, organization, high electrical resistance, and relative impermeability to highly polar molecules. Membrane proteins embedded in the bilayer serve as structural anchors, receptors, ion channels, or transporters to transduce electrical or chemical signaling pathways and provide selective targets for drug actions. Far from being a sea of lipids with proteins floating randomly about, membranes are ordered and compartmented (Suetsugu et al., 2014), with structural scaffolding elements linking to the cell interior. Membrane proteins may be associated with caveolin and sequestered within caveolae, be excluded from caveolae, or be organized in signaling domains rich in cholesterol and sphingolipid not containing caveolin or other scaffolding proteins.

Modes of Permeation and Transport

Passive diffusion dominates transmembrane movement of most drugs. However, carrier-mediated mechanisms (*active transport* and *facilitated diffusion*) play important roles (Figure 2–2; Figure 5–4).

Passive Diffusion

In passive transport, the drug molecule usually penetrates by diffusion along a concentration gradient by virtue of its solubility in the lipid bilayer. Such transfer is directly proportional to the magnitude of the concentration gradient across the membrane, to the lipid:water partition coefficient of the drug, and to the membrane surface area exposed to the drug. At steady state, the concentration of the unbound drug is the same on both sides of the membrane if the drug is a nonelectrolyte. For ionic compounds, the steady-state concentrations depend on the electrochemical gradient for the ion and on differences in pH across the membrane, which will influence the state of ionization of the molecule disparately on either side of the membrane and can effectively trap ionized drug on one side of the membrane.

Influence of pH on Ionizable Drugs

Many drugs are weak acids or bases that are present in solution as both the lipid-soluble, diffusible nonionized form and the ionized species that is relatively lipid insoluble and poorly diffusible across a membrane. Among the common ionizable groups are carboxylic acids and amino groups (primary, secondary, and tertiary; quaternary amines hold a permanent positive charge). The transmembrane distribution of a weak electrolyte is influenced by its pK_a and the pH gradient across the membrane. The pK_a is the pH at which half the drug (weak acid or base electrolyte) is in its ionized form. The ratio of nonionized to ionized drug at any pH may be calculated from the Henderson-Hasselbalch equation:

$$\log \frac{[\text{protonated form}]}{[\text{unprotonated form}]} = pK_a - pH \qquad \text{(Equation 2–1)}$$

Equation 2–1 relates the pH of the medium around the drug and the drug's acid dissociation constant (pK_a) to the ratio of the protonated (HA or BH^+) and unprotonated (A^- or B) forms, where

$$HA \leftrightarrow A^- + H^+, \text{ where } K_a = \frac{[A^-][H^+]}{[HA]}$$

describes the dissociation of an acid, and

$$BH^+ \leftrightarrow B + H^+, \text{ where } K_a = \frac{[B][H^+]}{[BH^+]}$$

describes the dissociation of the protonated form of a base.

At steady state, an acidic drug will accumulate on the more basic side of the membrane and a basic drug on the more acidic side. This phenomenon, known as *ion trapping*, is an important process in drug distribution with potential therapeutic benefit (Perletti et al., 2009). Figure 2–3 illustrates this effect and shows the calculated values for the distribution of a weak acid between the plasma and gastric compartments.

One can take advantage of the effect of pH on transmembrane partitioning to alter drug excretion. In the kidney tubules, urine pH can vary over a wide range, from 4.5 to 8. As urine pH drops (as $[H^+]$ increases), weak acids (A^-) and weak bases (B) will exist to a greater extent in their

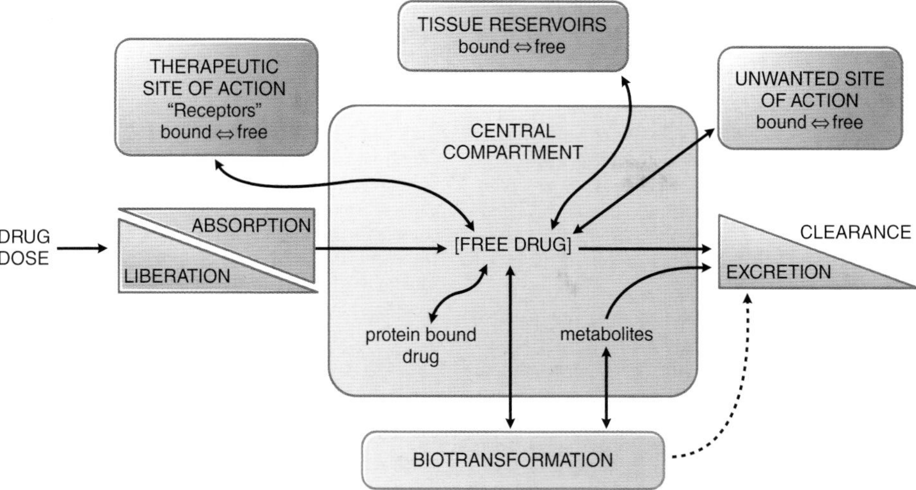

Figure 2–1 *The interrelationship of the absorption, distribution, binding, metabolism, and excretion of a drug and its concentration at its sites of action.* Possible distribution and binding of metabolites in relation to their potential actions at receptors are not depicted.

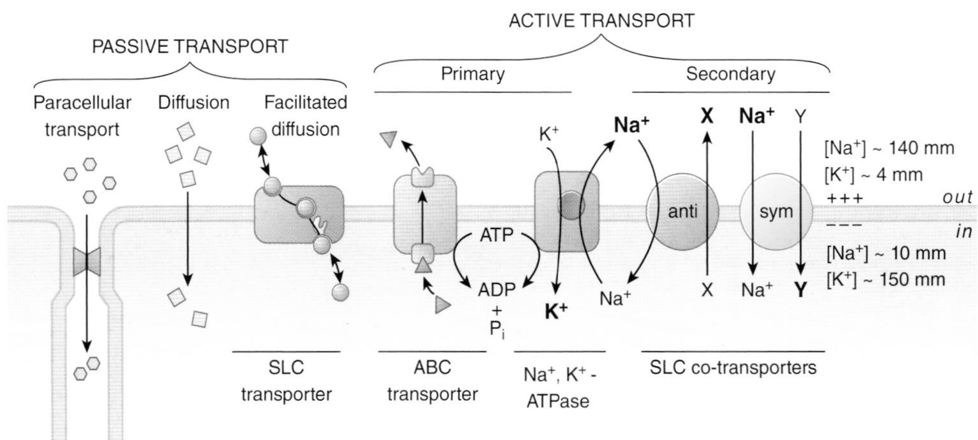

Figure 2–2 *Drugs move across membrane and cellular barriers in a variety of ways.* See details in Figures 5–1 through 5–5.

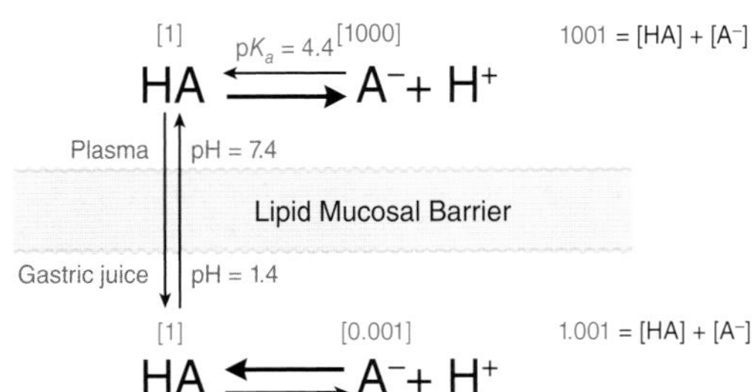

Figure 2–3 *Influence of pH on the distribution of a weak acid* (pK_a = 4.4) *between plasma and gastric juice separated by a lipid barrier.* **A weak acid dissociates to different extents** in plasma (pH 7.4) and gastric acid (pH 1.4): The higher pH facilitates dissociation; the lower pH reduces dissociation. The uncharged form, HA, equilibrates across the membrane. Blue numbers in brackets show relative equilibrium concentrations of HA and A^-, as calculated from Equation 2–1.

protonated forms (HA and BH^+); the reverse is true as pH rises, where A^- and B will be favored. Thus, alkaline urine favors excretion of weak acids; acid urine favors excretion of weak bases. Elevation of urine pH (by giving sodium bicarbonate) will promote urinary excretion of weak acids such as aspirin ($pK_a \sim 3.5$) and urate ($pK_a \sim 5.8$). Another useful consequence of a drug's being ionized at physiological pH is illustrated by the relative lack of sedative effects of second-generation histamine H_1 antagonists (e.g., loratadine): Second-generation antihistamines are ionized molecules (less lipophilic, more hydrophilic) that cross the BBB poorly compared to first-generation agents such as diphenhydramine, which are now used as sleep aids.

Carrier-Mediated Membrane Transport

Proteins in the plasma membrane mediate transmembrane movements of many physiological solutes; these proteins also mediate transmembrane movements of drugs and can be targets of drug action. Mediated transport is broadly characterized as *facilitated diffusion* or *active transport* (see Figure 2–2; Figure 5–4). Membrane transporters and their roles in drug response are presented in detail in Chapter 5.

Facilitated Diffusion. *Facilitated diffusion* is a carrier-mediated transport process in which the driving force is simply the electrochemical gradient of the transported solute; thus, these carriers can facilitate solute movement either in or out of cells, depending on the direction of the electrochemical gradient. The carrier protein may be highly selective for a specific conformational structure of an endogenous solute or a drug whose rate of transport by passive diffusion through the membrane would otherwise be quite slow. For instance, the organic cation transporter OCT1 (SLC22A1) facilitates the movement of a physiologic solute, thiamine, and also of drugs, including metformin, which is used in treating type 2 diabetes. Chapter 5 describes OCT1 and other members of the human SLC superfamily of transporters.

Active Transport. *Active transport* is characterized by a direct requirement for energy, capacity to move solute against an electrochemical gradient, saturability, selectivity, and competitive inhibition by cotransported compounds. Na^+,K^+-ATPase is an important example of an active transport mechanism that is also a therapeutic target of digoxin in the treatment of heart failure (Chapter 29). A group of primary active transporters, the ABC family, hydrolyze ATP to export substrates across membranes. For example, the P-glycoprotein, also called ABCB1 and MDR1, exports bulky neutral or cationic compounds from cells; its physiologic substrates include steroid hormones such as testosterone and progesterone. MDR1 exports many drugs as well, including digoxin, and a great variety of other agents (see Table 5–4). P-glycoprotein in the enterocyte limits the absorption of some orally administered drugs by exporting compounds into the lumen of the GI tract subsequent to their absorption. ABC transporters perform a similar function in the cells of the BBB, effectively reducing net accumulation of some compounds in the brain. By the same mechanism, P-glycoprotein also can confer resistance to some cancer chemotherapeutic agents (see Chapters 65–68).

Members of the SLC superfamily can mediate secondary active transport using the electrochemical energy stored in a gradient (usually Na^+) to translocate both biological solutes and drugs across membranes. For instance, the Na^+–Ca^{2+} exchange protein (SLC8) uses the energy stored in the Na^+ gradient established by Na^+,K^+-ATPase to export cytosolic Ca^{2+} and maintain it at a low basal level, about 100 nM in most cells. SLC8 is thus an *antiporter*, using the inward flow of Na^+ to drive an outward flow of Ca^{++}; SLC8 also helps to mediate the positive inotropic effects of digoxin and other cardiac glycosides that inhibit the activity of Na^+,K^+-ATPase and thereby reduce the driving force for the extrusion of Ca^{++} from the ventricular cardiac myocyte. Other SLC cotransporters are *symporters*, in which driving force ion and solute move in the same direction. The CNT1 (SLC28A1), driven by the Na^+ gradient, moves pyrimidine nucleosides and the cancer chemotherapeutic agents gemcitabine and cytarabine into cells. DAT, NET, and SERT, transporters for the neurotransmitters dopamine, norepinephrine, and serotonin, respectively, are secondary active transporters that also rely on the energy stored in the transmembrane Na^+ gradient, symporters that coordinate movement of Na^+ and neurotransmitter in the same direction (into the neuron); they are also the targets of CNS-active agents used in therapy of depression. Members of the SLC superfamily are active in drug transport in the GI tract, liver, and kidney, among other sites.

Paracellular Transport

In the vascular compartment, paracellular passage of solutes and fluid through intercellular gaps is sufficiently large that passive transfer across the endothelium of capillaries and postcapillary venules is generally limited by blood flow. Capillaries of the CNS and a variety of epithelial tissues have tight junctions that limit paracellular movement of drugs (Spector et al., 2015).

Drug Absorption, Bioavailability, and Routes of Administration

Absorption and Bioavailability

Absorption is the movement of a drug from its site of administration into the central compartment (see Figure 2–1). For solid dosage forms, absorption first requires dissolution of the tablet or capsule, thus liberating the drug. Except in cases of malabsorption syndromes, the clinician is concerned primarily with bioavailability rather than absorption (Tran et al., 2013).

Bioavailability describes the fractional extent to which an administered dose of drug reaches its site of action or a biological fluid (usually the systemic circulation) from which the drug has access to its site of action. A drug given orally must be absorbed first from the GI tract, but net absorption may be limited by the characteristics of the dosage form, by the drug's physicochemical properties, by metabolic attack in the intestine, and by transport across the intestinal epithelium and into the portal circulation. The absorbed drug then passes through the liver, where metabolism and biliary excretion may occur before the drug enters the systemic circulation. Accordingly, less than all of the administered dose may reach the systemic circulation and be distributed to the drug's sites of action. If the metabolic or excretory capacity of the liver and the intestine for the drug is large, bioavailability will be reduced substantially (*first-pass effect*). This decrease in availability is a function of the anatomical site from which absorption takes place; for instance, intravenous administration generally permits all of the drug to enter the systemic circulation. Other anatomical, physiological, and pathological factors can influence bioavailability (described further in this chapter), and the choice of the route of drug administration must be based on an understanding of these conditions. We can define bioavailability F as:

$$F = \frac{\text{Quantity of drug reaching systemic circulation}}{\text{Quantity of drug administered}} \quad \text{(Equation 2–2)}$$

where $0 < F \leq 1$.

Factors modifying bioavailability apply as well to prodrugs that are activated by the liver, in which case availability results from metabolism that produces the form of the active drug.

Routes of Administration

Some characteristics of the major routes employed for systemic drug effect are compared in Table 2–1.

Oral Administration

Oral ingestion is the most common method of drug administration. It also is the safest, most convenient, and most economical. Its disadvantages include limited absorption of some drugs because of their physical characteristics (e.g., low water solubility or poor membrane permeability), emesis as a result of irritation to the GI mucosa, destruction of some drugs by digestive enzymes or low gastric pH, irregularities in absorption or propulsion in the presence of food or other drugs, and the need for cooperation on the part of the patient. In addition, drugs in the GI tract may be metabolized by the enzymes of the intestinal microbiome, mucosa, or liver before they gain access to the general circulation.

Absorption from the GI tract is governed by factors such as surface area for absorption; blood flow to the site of absorption; the physical state of the drug (solution, suspension, or solid dosage form); its aqueous solubility; and the drug's concentration at the site of absorption. For drugs given in solid form, the rate of dissolution may limit their absorption. Because most drug absorption from the GI tract occurs by passive diffusion, absorption is favored when the drug is in the nonionized, more lipophilic form. Based on the pH-partition concept (see Figure 2–3), one would predict that drugs that are weak acids would be better absorbed from the stomach (pH 1–2) than from the upper intestine (pH 3–6), and vice versa for weak bases. However, the surface area of the stomach is relatively small, and a mucus layer covers the gastric epithelium. By contrast, the villi of the upper intestine provide an extremely large surface area (~200 m^2). Accordingly, the rate of absorption of a drug from the intestine will be greater than that from the stomach even if the drug is predominantly ionized in the intestine and largely nonionized in the stomach. Thus, any factor that accelerates gastric emptying (recumbent position right side) will generally increase the rate of drug absorption, whereas any factor that delays gastric emptying will have the opposite effect. The gastric emptying rate is influenced by numerous factors, including the caloric

TABLE 2–1 ■ SOME CHARACTERISTICS OF COMMON ROUTES OF DRUG ADMINISTRATION[a]

ROUTE AND BIOAVAILABILTY (*F*)	ABSORPTION PATTERN	SPECIAL UTILITY	LIMITATIONS AND PRECAUTIONS
Intravenous	Absorption circumvented	Valuable for emergency use	Increased risk of adverse effects
$F = 1$ by definition	Potentially immediate effects	Permits titration of dosage	Must inject solutions *slowly* as a rule
	Suitable for large volumes and for irritating substances, or complex mixtures, when diluted	Usually required for high-molecular-weight protein and peptide drugs	Not suitable for oily solutions or poorly soluble substances
Subcutaneous $0.75 < F < 1$	Prompt from aqueous solution	Suitable for some poorly soluble suspensions and for instillation of slow-release implants	Not suitable for large volumes
	Slow and sustained from repository preparations		Possible pain or necrosis from irritating substances
Intramuscular $0.75 < F < 1$	Prompt from aqueous solution	Suitable for moderate volumes, oily vehicles, and some irritating substances	Precluded during anticoagulant therapy
	Slow and sustained from repository preparations	Appropriate for self-administration (e.g., insulin)	May interfere with interpretation of certain diagnostic tests (e.g., creatine kinase)
Oral ingestion $.05 < F < 1$	Variable, depends on many factors (see text)	Most convenient and economical; usually safer	Requires patient compliance
			Bioavailability potentially erratic and incomplete

[a]See text for more complete discussion and for other routes.

content of food; volume, osmolality, temperature, and pH of ingested fluid; diurnal and interindividual variation; metabolic state (rest or exercise); and the ambient temperature. Gastric emptying is influenced in women by the effects of estrogen (i.e., compared to men, emptying is slower for premenopausal women and those taking estrogen replacement therapy).

Drugs that are destroyed by gastric secretions and low pH or that cause gastric irritation sometimes are administered in dosage forms with an enteric coating that prevents dissolution in the acidic gastric contents. Enteric coatings are useful for drugs that can cause gastric irritation and for presenting a drug such as mesalamine to sites of action in the ileum and colon (see Figure 51–4).

Controlled-Release Preparations. The rate of absorption of a drug administered as a tablet or other solid oral dosage form is partly dependent on its rate of dissolution in GI fluids. This is the basis for *controlled-release, extended-release, sustained-release,* and *prolonged-action* pharmaceutical preparations that are designed to produce slow, uniform absorption of the drug for 8 h or longer. Potential advantages of such preparations are reduction in the frequency of administration compared with conventional dosage forms (often with improved compliance by the patient), maintenance of a therapeutic effect overnight, and decreased incidence and intensity of undesired effects (by dampening of the peaks in drug concentration) and nontherapeutic blood levels of the drug (by elimination of troughs in concentration) that often occur after administration of immediate-release dosage forms. Controlled-release dosage forms are most appropriate for drugs with short half-lives ($t_{1/2} < 4$ h) or in select patient groups, such as those receiving antiepileptic or antipsychotic agents (Bera, 2014).

Sublingual Administration. Absorption from the oral mucosa has special significance for certain drugs despite the fact that the surface area available is small. Venous drainage from the mouth is to the superior vena cava, thus bypassing the portal circulation. As a consequence, a drug held sublingually and absorbed from that site is protected from rapid intestinal and hepatic first-pass metabolism. For example, sublingual nitroglycerin (see Chapter 27) is rapidly effective because it is nonionic, has high lipid solubility, and is not subject to the first-pass effect prior to reaching the heart and arterial system.

Parenteral Injection

Parenteral (i.e., not via the GI tract) injection of drugs has distinct advantages over oral administration. In some instances, parenteral administration is essential for delivery of a drug in its active form, as in the case of monoclonal antibodies. Availability usually is more rapid, extensive, and predictable when a drug is given by injection; the effective dose can be delivered more accurately to a precise dose; this route is suitable for the loading dose of medications prior to initiation of oral maintenance dosing (e.g., digoxin). In emergency therapy and when a patient is unconscious, uncooperative, or unable to retain anything given by mouth, parenteral therapy may be necessary. Parenteral administration also has disadvantages: Asepsis must be maintained, especially when drugs are given over time (e.g., intravenous or intrathecal administration); pain may accompany the injection; and it is sometimes difficult for patients to perform the injections themselves if self-medication is necessary.

The major routes of parenteral administration are intravenous, subcutaneous, and intramuscular. Absorption from subcutaneous and intramuscular sites occurs by simple diffusion along the gradient from drug depot to plasma. The rate is limited by the area of the absorbing capillary membranes and by the solubility of the substance in the interstitial fluid. Relatively large aqueous channels in the endothelial layer account for the indiscriminate diffusion of molecules regardless of their lipid solubility. Larger molecules, such as proteins, slowly gain access to the circulation by way of lymphatic channels. Drugs administered into the systemic circulation by any route, excluding the intra-arterial route, are subject to possible first-pass elimination in the lung prior to distribution to the rest of the body. The lungs also serve as a filter for particulate matter that may be given intravenously and provide a route of elimination for volatile substances.

Intravenous. Factors limiting absorption are circumvented by intravenous injection of drugs in aqueous solution because bioavailability is complete ($F = 1.0$) and distribution is rapid. Also, drug delivery is controlled and achieved with an accuracy and immediacy not possible by any other procedures. Certain irritating solutions can be given only in this manner because the drug, when injected slowly, is greatly diluted by the blood.

There are advantages and disadvantages to intravenous administration. Unfavorable reactions can occur because high concentrations of drug may be attained rapidly in plasma and tissues. There are therapeutic circumstances for which it is advisable to administer a drug by bolus injection (e.g., tissue plasminogen activator) and other circumstances where slower or prolonged administration of drug is advisable (e.g., antibiotics). Intravenous administration of drugs warrants careful determination of dose and close monitoring of the patient's response; once the drug is injected, there is often no retreat. Repeated intravenous injections depend on the ability to maintain a patent vein. Drugs in an oily vehicle, those that precipitate blood constituents or hemolyze erythrocytes, and drug combinations that cause precipitates to form *must not* be given intravenously.

Subcutaneous. Injection into a subcutaneous site can be done only with drugs that are not irritating to tissue; otherwise, severe pain, necrosis, and tissue sloughing may occur. The rate of absorption following subcutaneous injection of a drug often is sufficiently constant and slow to provide a sustained effect. Moreover, altering the period over which a drug is absorbed may be varied intentionally, as is accomplished with insulin for injection using particle size, protein complexation, and pH. The incorporation of a vasoconstrictor agent in a solution of a drug to be injected subcutaneously also retards absorption. Absorption of drugs implanted under the skin in a solid pellet form occurs slowly over a period of weeks or months; some hormones (e.g., contraceptives) are administered effectively in this manner.

Intramuscular. Absorption of drugs in aqueous solution after intramuscular injection depends on the rate of blood flow to the injection site and can be relatively rapid. Absorption may be modulated to some extent by local heating, massage, or exercise. Generally, the rate of absorption following injection of an aqueous preparation into the deltoid or vastus lateralis is faster than when the injection is made into the gluteus maximus. The rate is particularly slower for females after injection into the gluteus maximus, a feature attributed to the different distribution of subcutaneous fat in males and females and because fat is relatively poorly perfused. Slow, constant absorption from the intramuscular site results if the drug is injected in solution in oil or suspended in various other repository (depot) vehicles.

Intra-arterial. Occasionally, a drug is injected directly into an artery to localize its effect in a particular tissue or organ, such as in the treatment of liver tumors and head and neck cancers. Diagnostic agents sometimes are administered by this route (e.g., technetium-labeled human serum albumin). Inadvertent intra-arterial administration can cause serious complications and requires careful management (Sen et al., 2005).

Intrathecal. The BBB and the blood-CSF barrier often preclude or slow the entrance of drugs into the CNS, reflecting the activity of P-glycoprotein (MDR1) and other transporters to export xenobiotics from the CNS. Therefore, when local and rapid effects of drugs on the meninges or cerebrospinal axis are desired, as in spinal anesthesia, drugs sometimes are injected directly into the spinal subarachnoid space. Brain tumors (Calias et al., 2014) or serious CNS infections (Imberti et al., 2014) also may be treated by direct intraventricular drug administration, increasingly through the use of specialized long-term indwelling reservoir devices. Injections into the CSF and epidural space are covered in chapters on analgesia and local anesthesia (Chapters 20 and 22, respectively).

Pulmonary Absorption

Gaseous and volatile drugs may be inhaled and absorbed through the pulmonary epithelium and mucous membranes of the respiratory tract. Access to the circulation is rapid by this route because the lung's surface area is large. In addition, solutions of drugs can be atomized and the fine droplets in air (aerosol) inhaled. Advantages are the almost instantaneous absorption of a drug into the blood, avoidance of hepatic first-pass loss, and in the case of pulmonary disease, local application of the drug at the desired site of action (see Chapters 21 and 40), as in the use of inhaled nitric oxide for pulmonary hypertension in term and near-term infants and adults (see Chapter 31).

Topical Application

Mucous Membranes. Drugs are applied to the mucous membranes of the conjunctiva, nasopharynx, oropharynx, vagina, colon, urethra, and urinary bladder primarily for their local effects. Absorption from these sites is generally excellent and may provide advantages for immunotherapy because vaccination of mucosal surfaces using mucosal vaccines provides the basis for generating protective immunity in both the mucosal and systemic immune compartments.

Eye. Topically applied ophthalmic drugs are used primarily for their local effects (see Chapter 69). The use of drug-loaded contact lenses and ocular inserts allows drugs to be better placed where they are needed for direct delivery.

Skin: Transdermal Absorption. Absorption of drugs able to penetrate the intact skin is dependent on the surface area over which they are applied and their lipid solubility (see Chapter 70). Systemic absorption of drugs occurs much more readily through abraded, burned, or denuded skin. Toxic effects result from absorption through the skin of highly lipid-soluble substances (e.g., a lipid-soluble insecticide in an organic solvent). Absorption through the skin can be enhanced by suspending the drug in an oily vehicle and rubbing the resulting preparation into the skin. Hydration of the skin with an occlusive dressing may be used to facilitate absorption. Controlled-release topical patches are increasingly available, with nicotine for tobacco-smoking withdrawal, scopolamine for motion sickness, nitroglycerin for angina pectoris, testosterone and estrogen for replacement therapy, various estrogens and progestins for birth control, and fentanyl for pain relief.

Rectal Administration

Approximately 50% of the drug that is absorbed from the rectum will bypass the liver, thereby reducing hepatic first-pass metabolism. However, rectal absorption can be irregular and incomplete, and certain drugs can cause irritation of the rectal mucosa. Rectal administration may be desirable, as in the use of opioids in hospice care.

Novel Methods of Drug Delivery

Drug-eluting stents and other devices are being used to target drugs locally to maximize efficacy and minimize systemic exposure. Recent advances in drug delivery include the use of biocompatible polymers and nanoparticles for drug delivery (Yohan and Chithrani, 2014).

Bioequivalence

Drug products are considered to be pharmaceutical equivalents if they contain the same active ingredients and are identical in strength or concentration, dosage form, and route of administration. Two pharmaceutically equivalent drug products are considered to be *bioequivalent* when the rates and extents of bioavailability of the active ingredient in the two products are not significantly different under suitable and identical test conditions. Generic versus brand name prescribing is further discussed in connection with drug nomenclature and the choice of drug name in writing prescription orders (see Appendix I). Courts have not always found generic and brand name drugs to be legally equivalent (see Chapter 1).

Distribution of Drugs

Not All Tissues Are Equal

Following absorption or systemic administration into the bloodstream, a drug distributes into interstitial and intracellular fluids as functions of the physicochemical properties of the drug, the rate of drug delivery to individual organs and compartments, and the differing capacities of those regions to interact with the drug. Cardiac output, regional blood flow, capillary permeability, and tissue volume affect the rate of delivery and amount of drug distributed into tissues (Table 2–2 and Figure 2–4). Initially, liver, kidney, brain, and other well-perfused organs receive most of the drug; delivery to muscle, most viscera, skin, and fat is slower. This second distribution phase may require minutes to several hours before the concentration of drug in tissue is in equilibrium with that in blood. The second phase also involves a far larger fraction of body mass (e.g., muscle) than does the initial phase and generally accounts for most of the extravascular distribution. With exceptions such as the brain, diffusion of

TABLE 2–2 ■ DISTRIBUTION OF BLOOD FLOW IN 70-KG MALE AT REST

	KIDNEYS	HEART	LIVER	BRAIN	SKELETAL MUSCLE	FAT	REMAINDER	Σ
Blood Flow (mL/min)	1100	250	1700	800	900	250	500	5500
Mass (kg)	0.3	0.3	2.6	1.3	34	10	21.5	70
Flow/Mass (mL/min/kg)	3667	833	654	615	26	25	23	
% Cardiac Output	20	4.5	31	14.5	16.4	4.5	9.1	100

drug into the interstitial fluid occurs rapidly because of the highly permeable nature of the capillary endothelium. Thus, tissue distribution is determined by the partitioning of drug between blood and the particular tissue.

Binding to Plasma Proteins

Many drugs circulate in the bloodstream bound to plasma proteins. Albumin is a major carrier for acidic drugs; α_1-acid glycoprotein binds basic drugs. Nonspecific binding to other plasma proteins generally occurs to a much smaller extent. The binding is usually reversible. In addition, certain drugs may bind to proteins that function as specific hormone carrier proteins, such as the binding of estrogen or testosterone to sex hormone–binding globulin or the binding of thyroid hormone to thyroxin-binding globulin.

The fraction of total drug in plasma that is bound is determined by the drug concentration, the affinity of binding sites for the drug, and the concentration of available binding sites. For most drugs, the therapeutic range of plasma concentrations is limited; thus, the extent of binding and the unbound fraction are relatively constant. The extent of plasma protein binding also may be affected by disease-related factors (e.g., hypoalbuminemia). Conditions resulting in the acute-phase reaction response (e.g., cancer, arthritis, myocardial infarction, Crohn's disease) lead to elevated levels of α_1-acid glycoprotein and enhanced binding of basic drugs. Changes in protein binding caused by disease states and drug-drug interactions are clinically relevant mainly for a small subset of so-called high-clearance drugs of narrow therapeutic index that are administered intravenously, such as lidocaine. When changes in plasma protein binding occur in patients, unbound drug rapidly equilibrates throughout the body and only a transient significant change in unbound plasma concentration will occur. Only drugs that show an almost-instantaneous relationship between free plasma concentration and effect (e.g., antiarrhythmics) will show a measurable effect. Thus, unbound plasma drug concentrations will exhibit significant changes only when either drug input or clearance of unbound drug occurs as a consequence of metabolism or active transport. A more common problem resulting from competition of drugs for plasma

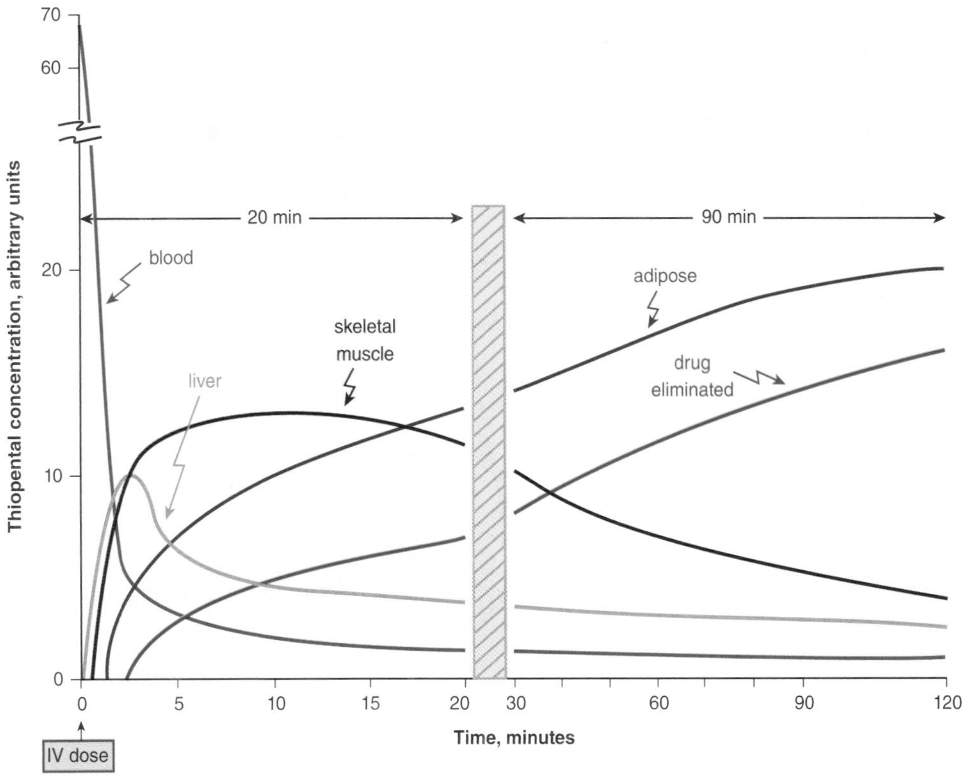

Figure 2–4 *Redistribution.* Curves depict the distribution of the barbiturate anesthetic thiopental into different body compartments following a single rapid intravenous dose. Note breaks and changes of scale on both axes. The drug level at thiopental's site of action in the brain closely mirrors the plasma level of the drug. The rate of accumulation in the various body compartments depends on regional blood flow; the extent of accumulation reflects the differing capacities of the compartments and the steady but slow effect of elimination to reduce the amount of drug available. Emergence from the anesthetic influence of this single dose of thiopental relies on redistribution, not on metabolism. The drug will partition out of tissue depots as metabolism and elimination take their course. Depletion of compartments will follow the same order as accumulation, as a function of their perfusion.

protein-binding sites is misinterpretation of measured concentrations of drugs in plasma because most assays do not distinguish free drug from bound drug. Competition for plasma protein-binding sites may cause one drug to elevate the concentration of one bound less avidly.

Binding of a drug to plasma proteins limits its concentration in tissues and at its site of action because only unbound drug is in equilibrium across membranes. Accordingly, after distribution equilibrium is achieved, the concentration of unbound drug in intracellular water is the same as that in plasma except when carrier-mediated active transport is involved. Binding of a drug to plasma protein limits the drug's glomerular filtration and may also limit drug transport and metabolism.

Tissue Binding

Many drugs accumulate in tissues at higher concentrations than those in the extracellular fluids and blood. Tissue binding of drugs usually occurs with cellular constituents such as proteins, phospholipids, or nuclear proteins and generally is reversible. A large fraction of drug in the body may be bound in this fashion and serve as a reservoir that prolongs drug action in that same tissue or at a distant site reached through the circulation. Such tissue binding and accumulation also can produce local toxicity (e.g., renal and ototoxicity associated with aminoglycoside antibiotics).

CNS, the BBB, and CSF

The brain capillary endothelial cells have continuous tight junctions; therefore, drug penetration into the brain depends on transcellular rather than paracellular transport. The unique characteristics of brain capillary endothelial cells and pericapillary glial cells constitute the BBB. At the choroid plexus, a similar blood-CSF barrier is present, formed by epithelial cells that are joined by tight junctions. The lipid solubility of the nonionized and unbound species of a drug is therefore an important determinant of its uptake by the brain; the more lipophilic a drug, the more likely it is to cross the BBB. In general, the BBB's function is well maintained; however, meningeal and encephalic inflammation increase local permeability. Drugs may also be imported to and exported from the CNS by specific transporters (see Chapter 5).

Bone

The tetracycline antibiotics (and other divalent metal-ion chelating agents) and heavy metals may accumulate in bone by adsorption onto the bone crystal surface and eventual incorporation into the crystal lattice. Bone can become a reservoir for the slow release of toxic agents such as lead or radium; their effects thus can persist long after exposure has ceased. Local destruction of the bone medulla also may result in reduced blood flow and prolongation of the reservoir effect as the toxic agent becomes sealed off from the circulation; this may further enhance the direct local damage to the bone. A vicious cycle results, whereby the greater the exposure to the toxic agent, the slower is its rate of elimination. The adsorption of drug onto the bone crystal surface and incorporation into the crystal lattice have therapeutic advantages for the treatment of osteoporosis.

Fat as a Reservoir

Many lipid-soluble drugs are stored by physical solution in the neutral fat. In obese persons, the fat content of the body may be as high as 50%, and even in lean individuals, fat constitutes 10% of body weight; hence, fat may serve as a reservoir for lipid-soluble drugs. Fat is a rather stable reservoir because it has a relatively low blood flow.

Redistribution

Termination of drug effect after withdrawal of a drug usually is by metabolism and excretion but also may result from redistribution of the drug from its site of action into other tissues or sites. Redistribution is a factor in terminating drug effect primarily when a highly lipid-soluble drug that acts on the brain or cardiovascular system is administered rapidly by intravenous injection or inhalation. Such is the case of the intravenous anesthetic thiopental, a lipid-soluble drug. Because blood flow to the brain is high and thiopental readily crosses the BBB, thiopental reaches its maximal concentration in brain rapidly after its intravenous injection. Subsequently, the plasma and brain concentrations decrease as thiopental redistributes to other tissues, such as muscle and, finally, adipose tissue. This redistribution is the mechanism by which thiopental anesthesia is terminated (see Figure 2–4) because its clearance is rather slow (elimination $t_{1/2}$ after a single dose is 3–8 h). The concentration of the drug in brain follows that of the plasma because there is little binding of the drug to brain constituents. Thus, both the onset and the termination of thiopental anesthesia are relatively rapid, and both are related directly to the concentration of drug in the brain.

Placental Transfer of Drugs

The transfer of drugs across the placenta is of critical importance because drugs may cause anomalies in the developing fetus; thus, the burden for evidenced-based drug use in pregnancy is paramount (see Appendix I). Lipid solubility, extent of plasma binding, and degree of ionization of weak acids and bases are important general determinants in drug transfer across the placenta. The placenta functions as a selective barrier to protect the fetus against the harmful effects of drugs. Members of the ABC family of transporters limit the entry of drugs and other xenobiotics into the fetal circulation via vectorial efflux from the placenta to the maternal circulation (see Figure 2–2 and Chapter 5). The fetal plasma is slightly more acidic than that of the mother (pH 7.0–7.2 vs. 7.4), so that ion trapping of basic drugs occurs. The view that the placenta is an absolute barrier to drugs is inaccurate, in part because a number of influx transporters are also present. The fetus is to some extent exposed to all drugs taken by the mother. The Food and Drug Administration categorizes the relative safety of drugs that may be used in pregnant women (see Appendix I).

Metabolism of Drugs

A Few Principles of Metabolism and Elimination

The many therapeutic agents that are lipophilic do not pass readily into the aqueous environment of the urine. The metabolism of drugs and other xenobiotics into more hydrophilic metabolites is essential for their renal elimination from the body, as well as for termination of their biological and pharmacological activity.

From the point of view of pharmacokinetics, the following are the three essential aspects of drug metabolism:

- **First-order kinetics.** For most drugs in their therapeutic concentration ranges, the amount of drug metabolized per unit time is proportional to the plasma concentration of the drug (C_p) and *the fraction of drug removed by metabolism is constant (i.e., first-order kinetics).*
- **Zero-order kinetics.** For some drugs, such as ethanol and phenytoin, metabolic capacity is saturated at the concentrations usually employed, and drug metabolism becomes *zero order; that is, a constant amount of drug is metabolized per unit time.* Zero-order kinetics can also occur at high (toxic) concentrations as drug-metabolizing capacity becomes saturated.
- **Inducible biotransforming enzymes.** The major drug-metabolizing systems are inducible, broad-spectrum enzymes with some predictable genetic variations. Drugs that are substrates in common for a metabolizing enzyme may interfere with each other's metabolism, or a drug may induce or enhance metabolism of itself or other drugs.

In general, drug-metabolizing reactions generate more polar, inactive metabolites that are readily excreted from the body. However, in some cases, metabolites with potent biological activity or toxic properties are generated. Many of the enzyme systems that transform drugs to inactive metabolites also generate biologically active metabolites of endogenous compounds, as in steroid biosynthesis. The biotransformation of drugs occurs primarily in the liver and involves *phase 1 reactions* (oxidation, reduction, or hydrolytic reactions and the activities of CYPs) and *phase 2 reactions* (conjugations of the phase 1 product with a second molecule) and a few other reactions. Other organs with significant drug-metabolizing capacity include the GI tract, kidneys, and lungs. Drug-metabolizing enzymes, especially CYPs, are inducible by some drugs and inhibited by drugs and competing substrates. Chapter 6 covers drug metabolism at length. Knowing which CYP metabolizes a given drug and which other drugs may affect that metabolism is crucial to good drug therapy.

Prodrugs; Pharmacogenomics

Prodrugs are pharmacologically inactive compounds that are converted to their active forms by metabolism. This approach can maximize the amount of the active species that reaches its site of action. Inactive prodrugs are converted rapidly to biologically active metabolites, often by the hydrolysis of an ester or amide linkage. Such is the case with a number of ACE inhibitors employed in the management of high blood pressure. Enalapril, for instance, is relatively inactive until converted by esterase activity to the diacid enalaprilat (see Chapters 6 and 26).

For a number of therapeutic areas, clinical pharmacogenomics, the study of the impact of genetic variations or genotypes of individuals on their drug response or drug metabolism, allows for improved treatment of individuals or groups (Ramamoorthy et al., 2015; Zhang et al., 2015; see Chapter 7).

Excretion of Drugs

Drugs are eliminated from the body either unchanged or as metabolites. Excretory organs, the lung excluded, eliminate polar compounds more efficiently than substances with high lipid solubility. Thus, lipid-soluble drugs are not readily eliminated until they are metabolized to more polar compounds. The kidney is the most important organ for excreting drugs and their metabolites. Renal excretion of unchanged drug is a major route of elimination for 25%–30% of drugs administered to humans. Substances excreted in the feces are principally unabsorbed orally ingested drugs or drug metabolites either excreted in the bile or secreted directly into the intestinal tract and not reabsorbed. Excretion of drugs in breast milk is important not because of the amounts eliminated (which are small) but because the excreted drugs may affect the nursing infant (also small, and with poorly developed capacity to metabolize xenobiotics). Excretion from the lung is important mainly for the elimination of anesthetic gases (see Chapter 21).

Renal Excretion

Excretion of drugs and metabolites in the urine involves three distinct processes: glomerular filtration, active tubular secretion, and passive tubular reabsorption (Figure 2–5). The amount of drug entering the tubular lumen by filtration depends on the glomerular filtration rate and the extent of plasma binding of the drug; only unbound drug is filtered. In the proximal renal tubule, active, carrier-mediated tubular secretion also may add drug to the tubular fluid (see Chapters 5 and 25). Drug from the tubular lumen may be reabsorbed back into the systemic circulation. In the renal tubules, especially on the distal side, the nonionized forms of weak acids and bases undergo net passive reabsorption. Because the tubular cells are less permeable to the ionized forms of weak electrolytes, passive reabsorption of these substances depends on the pH. When the tubular urine is made more alkaline, weak acids are largely ionized and are excreted more rapidly and to a greater extent; conversely, acidification of the urine will reduce fractional ionization and excretion of weak acids. Effects of changing urine pH are opposite for weak bases. In the treatment of drug poisoning, the excretion of some drugs can be hastened by appropriate alkalinization or acidification of the urine (see Figure 2–3 and Chapter 4).

In neonates, renal function is low compared with body mass but matures rapidly within the first few months after birth. During adulthood, there is a slow decline in renal function, about 1% per year, so that in elderly patients a substantial degree of functional impairment may be present, and medication adjustments are often needed.

Biliary and Fecal Excretion

Transporters present in the canalicular membrane of the hepatocyte (see Figure 5–6) actively secrete drugs and metabolites into bile. Ultimately, drugs and metabolites present in bile are released into the GI tract during

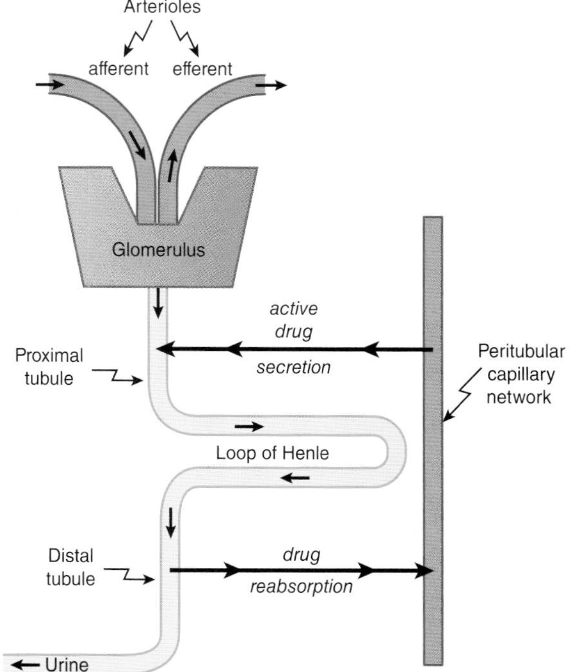

Figure 2–5 *Renal drug handling.* Drugs may be filtered from the blood in the renal glomerulus, secreted into the proximal tubule, reabsorbed from the distal tubular fluid back into the systemic circulation, and collected in the urine. Membrane transporters (OAT, OCT, MDR1, and MRP2, among others) mediate secretion into the proximal tubule (see Figures 5–12 and 5–13 for details). Reabsorption of compounds from the distal tubular fluid (generally acidic) is pH sensitive: Ionizable drugs are subject to ion trapping, and altering urinary pH to favor ionization can enhance excretion of charged species (see Figure 2–2).

the digestive process. Subsequently, the drugs and metabolites can be reabsorbed into the body from the intestine, which, in the case of conjugated metabolites such as glucuronides, may require enzymatic hydrolysis by the intestinal microflora. Such *enterohepatic recycling*, if extensive, may prolong significantly the presence of a drug (or toxin) and its effects within the body prior to elimination by other pathways. To interrupt enterohepatic cycling, substances may be given orally to bind metabolites excreted in the bile (for instance, see bile acid sequestrants and ezetimibe, Chapter 33). Biliary excretions and unabsorbed drug are excreted in the feces.

Excretion by Other Routes

Excretion of drugs into sweat, saliva, and tears is quantitatively unimportant. Because milk is more acidic than plasma, basic compounds may be slightly concentrated in this fluid; conversely, the concentration of acidic compounds in the milk is lower than in plasma. Nonelectrolytes (e.g., ethanol and urea) readily enter breast milk and reach the same concentration as in plasma, independent of the pH of the milk (Rowe et al., 2015). Breast milk can also contain heavy metals from environmental exposures. The administration of drugs to breastfeeding women carries the general caution that the suckling infant will be exposed to some extent to the medication or its metabolites. Although excretion into hair and skin is quantitatively unimportant, sensitive methods of detection of drugs in these tissues have forensic significance.

Clinical Pharmacokinetics

Clinical pharmacokinetics relate the pharmacological effects of a drug and concentration of the drug in an accessible body compartment (e.g., in blood or plasma) as these change in time. In most cases, the concentration of drug at its sites of action will be related to the concentration of drug in the systemic circulation (see Figure 2–1). The pharmacological effect that results may be the clinical effect desired or an adverse or toxic effect. Clinical pharmacokinetics attempts to provide

- a quantitative relationship between dose and effect, and
- a framework within which to interpret measurements of drug concentration in biological fluids and their adjustment through changes in dosing for the benefit of the patient.

The importance of pharmacokinetics in patient care is based on the improvement in therapeutic efficacy and the avoidance of unwanted effects that can be attained by application of its principles when dosage regimens are chosen and modified.

The following are the four most important parameters governing drug disposition:

1. *Bioavailability,* the fraction of drug absorbed as such into the systemic circulation.
2. *Volume of distribution,* a measure of the apparent space in the body available to contain the drug based on how much is given versus what is found in the systemic circulation.
3. *Clearance,* a measure of the body's efficiency in eliminating drug from the systemic circulation.
4. *Elimination* $t_{1/2}$, a measure of the rate of removal of drug from the systemic circulation.

Clearance

Clearance is the most important concept to consider when designing a rational regimen for long-term drug administration. The clinician usually wants to maintain steady-state concentrations of a drug within a *therapeutic window* or range associated with therapeutic efficacy and a minimum of toxicity for a given agent. Assuming complete bioavailability, the steady-state concentration of drug in the body will be achieved when the rate of drug elimination equals the rate of drug administration. Thus,

$$\text{Dosing rate} = CL \cdot C_{ss} \quad \text{(Equation 2–3)}$$

where CL is clearance of drug from the systemic circulation, and C_{ss} is the steady-state concentration of drug. When the desired steady-state concentration of drug in plasma or blood is known, the rate of clearance of drug will dictate the rate at which the drug should be administered.

Knowing the clearance of a drug is useful because its value for a particular drug usually is constant over the range of concentrations encountered clinically. This is true because metabolizing enzymes and transporters usually are not saturated; thus, the absolute rate of elimination of the drug is essentially a linear function of its concentration in plasma (first-order kinetics), where a *constant fraction* of drug in the body is eliminated per unit of time. If mechanisms for elimination of a given drug become saturated, the kinetics approach zero order (the case for ethanol and high doses of phenytoin), in which case a *constant amount* of drug is eliminated per unit of time.

With first-order kinetics, clearance CL will vary with the concentration of drug (C), often according to Equation 2–4:

$$CL = \frac{v_m}{(K_m + C)} \quad \text{(Equation 2–4)}$$

where K_m represents the concentration at which half the maximal rate of elimination is reached (in units of mass/volume), and v_m is equal to the maximal rate of elimination (in units of mass/time). Thus, clearance is derived in units of volume cleared of drug/time. This equation is analogous to the Michaelis-Menten equation for enzyme kinetics.

Clearance of a drug is its rate of elimination by all routes normalized to the concentration of drug C in some biological fluid where measurement can be made:

$$CL = \text{Rate of elimination}/C \quad \text{(Equation 2–5)}$$

Thus, when clearance is constant, the rate of drug elimination is directly proportional to drug concentration. Clearance indicates the volume of biological fluid such as blood or plasma from which drug would have to be completely removed to account for the clearance per unit of body weight (e.g., mL/min per kg). Clearance can be defined further as blood clearance CL_b, plasma clearance CL_p, or clearance based on the concentration of unbound drug CL_u, depending on the measurement made (C_b, C_p, or C_u). Clearance of drug by several organs is additive. Elimination of drug from the systemic circulation may occur as a result of processes that occur in the kidney, liver, and other organs. Division of the rate of elimination by each organ by a concentration of drug (e.g., plasma concentration) will yield the respective clearance by that organ. Added together, these separate clearances will equal systemic clearance:

$$CL_{renal} + CL_{hepatic} + CL_{other} = CL \quad \text{(Equation 2–6)}$$

Any significant alteration in renal or hepatic function can result in decreased clearance for those drugs with high renal or hepatic clearance. Systemic clearance may be determined at steady state by using Equation 2–3. For a single dose of a drug with complete bioavailability and first-order kinetics of elimination, systemic clearance may be determined from mass balance and the integration of Equation 2–5 over time:

$$CL = \text{Dose}/AUC \quad \text{(Equation 2–7)}$$

AUC is the total area under the curve that describes the measured concentration of drug in the systemic circulation as a function of time (from zero to infinity), as in Figure 2–9.

Examples of Clearance

The plasma clearance for the antibiotic cephalexin is 4.3 mL/min/kg, with 90% of the drug excreted unchanged in the urine. For a 70-kg man, the clearance from plasma would be 301 mL/min, with renal clearance accounting for 90% of this elimination. In other words, the kidney is able to excrete cephalexin at a rate such that the drug is completely removed (cleared) from about 270 mL of plasma every minute (renal clearance = 90% of total clearance). Because clearance usually is assumed to remain constant in a medically stable patient (e.g., no acute decline in kidney function), the rate of elimination of cephalexin will depend on the concentration of drug in the plasma (see Equation 2–5).

The β adrenergic receptor antagonist propranolol is cleared from the blood at a rate of 16 mL/min/kg (or 1600 mL/min in a 100-kg man), almost exclusively by the liver. Thus, the liver is able to remove the amount of propranolol contained in 1600 mL of blood in 1 min, roughly equal to total hepatic blood (see Table 2–2). In fact, the plasma clearance of some drugs exceeds the rate of blood flow to this organ. Often, this is so because the drug partitions readily into and out of red blood cells (rbc), and the rate of drug delivered to the eliminating organ is considerably higher than expected from measurement of its concentration in plasma. The relationship between plasma clearance (subscript p) and blood clearance (subscript b; all components of blood) at steady state is given by

$$\frac{CL_p}{CL_b} = \frac{C_b}{C_p} = 1 + H\left[\frac{C_{rbc}}{C_p} - 1\right] \quad \text{(Equation 2–8)}$$

Clearance from the blood therefore may be estimated by dividing the plasma clearance by the drug's blood-to-plasma concentration ratio, obtained from knowledge of the hematocrit (H = 0.45) and concentration ratio of red cells to plasma. In most instances, the blood clearance will be less than liver blood flow (1.5–1.7 L/min) or, if renal excretion also is involved, the sum of the blood flows to each eliminating organ. For example, the plasma clearance of the immunomodulator tacrolimus, about 2 L/min, is more than twice the hepatic plasma flow rate and even exceeds the organ's blood flow despite the fact that the liver is the predominant site of this drug's extensive metabolism. However, after taking into account the extensive distribution of tacrolimus into red cells, its clearance from the blood is only about 63 mL/min, and it is actually a drug with a rather low clearance, not a high-clearance agent as might be expected from the plasma clearance value alone. Clearance from the blood by metabolism can exceed liver blood flow, and this indicates extrahepatic metabolism. In the case of the β_1 receptor antagonist esmolol, the blood clearance value (11.9 L/min) is greater than cardiac output (~5.5 L/min) because the drug is metabolized efficiently by esterases present in red blood cells.

A further definition of clearance is useful for understanding the effects of pathological and physiological variables on drug elimination, particularly with respect to an individual organ. The rate of presentation of drug to the organ is the product of blood flow Q and the arterial drug concentration C_A, and the rate of exit of drug from the organ is the product of blood flow and the venous drug concentration C_V. The difference between these rates at steady state is the rate of drug elimination by that organ:

$$\text{Rate of elimination} = Q\cdot C_A - Q\cdot C_V = Q(C_A - C_V) \qquad \text{(Equation 2–9)}$$

Dividing Equation 2–8 by the concentration of drug entering the organ of elimination, C_A, yields an expression for clearance of the drug by the organ in question:

$$CL_{organ} = Q\left[\frac{C_A - C_V}{C_A}\right] = Q\cdot E \qquad \text{(Equation 2–10)}$$

The expression $(C_A - C_V)/C_A$ in Equation 2–10 can be referred to as the extraction ratio E of the drug. While not employed in general medical practice, calculations of a drug's extraction ratio(s) are useful for modeling the effects of disease of a given metabolizing organ on clearance and in the design of ideal therapeutic properties of drugs in development.

Hepatic Clearance

For a drug that is removed efficiently from the blood by hepatic processes (metabolism or excretion of drug into the bile), the concentration of drug in the blood leaving the liver will be low, the extraction ratio will approach unity, and the clearance of the drug from blood will become limited by hepatic blood flow. Drugs that are cleared efficiently by the liver (e.g., drugs with systemic clearances > 6 mL/min/kg, such as diltiazem, imipramine, lidocaine, morphine, and propranolol) are restricted in their rate of elimination not by intrahepatic processes but by the rate at which they can be transported in the blood to the liver.

Pharmacokinetic models indicate that when the capacity of the eliminating organ to metabolize the drug is large in comparison with the rate of presentation of drug to the organ, clearance will approximate the organ's blood flow. By contrast, when the drug-metabolizing capacity is small in comparison with the rate of drug presentation, clearance will be proportional to the unbound fraction of drug in blood and the drug's intrinsic clearance, where intrinsic clearance represents drug binding to components of blood and tissues or the intrinsic capacity of the liver to eliminate a drug in the absence of limitations imposed by blood flow (Guner and Bowen, 2013).

Renal Clearance

Renal clearance of a drug results in its appearance in the urine. In considering the clearance of a drug from the body by the kidney, glomerular filtration, secretion, reabsorption, and glomerular blood flow must be considered (see Figure 2–5). The rate of filtration of a drug depends on the volume of fluid that is filtered in the glomerulus and the concentration of unbound drug in plasma (because drug bound to protein is not filtered). The rate of secretion of drug into the tubular fluid will depend on the drug's intrinsic clearance by the transporters involved in active secretion as affected by the drug's binding to plasma proteins, the degree of saturation of these transporters, the rate of delivery of the drug to the secretory site, and the presence of drugs that can compete for these transporters. In addition, one must consider processes of drug reabsorption from the tubular fluid back into the bloodstream. The influences of changes in protein binding, blood flow, and the functional state of nephrons will affect renal clearance.

Aspirin demonstrates the interplay among these processes. Aspirin has a bimodal effect on the renal handling of uric acid: High doses of aspirin (>3 g/d) are uricosuric (probably by blocking urate reabsorption), while low dosages (1–2 g/d) cause uric acid retention (probably via inhibiting urate secretion). Low-dose aspirin, indicated for the prophylaxis of cardiovascular events, can cause changes in renal function and uric acid handling in elderly patients.

Distribution

Volume of Distribution

The volume of distribution V relates the amount of drug in the body to the concentration of drug C in the blood or plasma, depending on the fluid measured. This volume does not necessarily refer to an identifiable physiological volume but rather to the fluid volume that would be required to contain all of the drug in the body at the same concentration measured in the blood or plasma:

$$\text{Amount of drug in body}/V = C$$

or

$$V = \text{Amount of drug in body}/C \qquad \text{(Equation 2–11)}$$

View V as an imaginary volume because for many drugs V exceeds the known volume of any and all body compartments (Box 2–1). For example, the value of V for the highly lipophilic antimalarial chloroquine is some 15,000 L, whereas the volume of total-body water is about 42 L in a 70-kg male.

For drugs that are bound extensively to plasma proteins but are not bound to tissue components, the volume of distribution will approach that of the plasma volume because drug bound to plasma protein is measurable in the assay of most drugs. In contrast, certain drugs have high volumes of distribution even though most of the drug in the circulation is bound to albumin because these drugs are also sequestered elsewhere.

The volume of distribution defined in Equation 2–11 considers the body as a single homogeneous compartment. In this one-compartment model, all drug administration occurs directly into the central compartment, and distribution of drug is instantaneous throughout the volume V. Clearance of drug from this compartment occurs in a first-order fashion, as defined in Equation 2–5; that is, the amount of drug eliminated per unit of time depends on the amount (concentration) of drug in the body

BOX 2–1 ■ *V* Values May Exceed Any Physiological Volume

For many drugs, Equation 2–11 will give V values that exceed any physiological volume. For example, if 500 μg of the cardiac glycoside digoxin were added into the body of a 70-kg subject, a plasma concentration of about 0.75 ng/mL would be observed. Dividing the amount of drug in the body by the plasma concentration yields a volume of distribution for digoxin of about 667 L, or a value about 15 times greater than the total-body volume of a 70-kg man. In fact, digoxin distributes preferentially to muscle and adipose tissue and binds to its specific receptors, the Na^+,K^+-ATPase, leaving a very small amount of drug in the plasma to be measured. A drug's volume of distribution therefore can reflect the extent to which it is present in extravascular tissues and not in the plasma.

Thus, V may vary widely depending on the relative degrees of binding to high-affinity receptor sites, plasma and tissue proteins, the partition coefficient of the drug in fat, and accumulation in poorly perfused tissues. The volume of distribution for a given drug can differ according to a patient's age, gender, body composition, and presence of disease. Total-body water of infants younger than 1 year of age, for example, is 75%–80% of body weight, whereas that of adult males is 60% and that of females is 55%.

compartment at that time. Figure 2–6A and Equation 2–9 describe the decline of plasma concentration with time for a drug introduced into this central compartment:

$$C = \left[\frac{\text{Dose}}{V}\right][e^{-kt}] \qquad \text{(Equation 2–12)}$$

where k is the rate constant for elimination that reflects the fraction of drug removed from the compartment per unit of time. This rate constant is inversely related to the $t_{1/2}$ of the drug [$kt_{1/2} = \ln 2 = 0.693$]. The idealized one-compartment model does not describe the entire time course of the plasma concentration. Certain tissue reservoirs can be distinguished from the central compartment, and the drug concentration appears to decay in a manner that can be described by multiple exponential terms (Figure 2–6B).

Rates of Distribution

In many cases, groups of tissues with similar perfusion-to-partition ratios all equilibrate at essentially the same rate such that only one apparent phase of distribution is seen (rapid initial decrease in concentration of intravenously injected drug, as in Figure 2–6B). It is as though the drug starts in a "central" volume (see Figure 2–1), which consists of plasma and tissue reservoirs that are in rapid equilibrium, and distributes to a "final" volume, at which point concentrations in plasma decrease in a log-linear fashion with a rate constant of k (see Figure 2–6B). The multicompartment model of drug disposition can be viewed as though the blood and highly perfused lean organs such as heart, brain, liver, lung, and kidneys cluster as a single central compartment, whereas more slowly perfused tissues such as muscle, skin, fat, and bone behave as the final compartment (the tissue compartment).

If blood flow to certain tissues changes within an individual, rates of drug distribution to these tissues also will change. Changes in blood flow may cause some tissues that were originally in the "central" volume to equilibrate sufficiently more slowly so they appear only in the "final" volume. This means that central volumes will appear to vary with disease states that cause altered regional blood flow (such as would be seen in cirrhosis of the liver). After an intravenous bolus dose, drug concentrations in plasma may be higher in individuals with poor perfusion (e.g., shock) than they would be if perfusion were better. These higher systemic concentrations may in turn cause higher concentrations (and greater effects) in tissues such as brain and heart, whose usually high perfusion has not been reduced. Thus, the effect of a drug at various sites of action can vary depending on perfusion of these sites.

Multicompartment Volumes

In multicompartment kinetics, a volume of distribution term is useful especially when the effect of disease states on pharmacokinetics is to be determined. The volume of distribution at steady state V_{ss} represents the volume in which a drug would appear to be distributed during steady state if the drug existed throughout that volume at the same concentration as that in the measured fluid (plasma or blood). V_{ss} also may be appreciated as shown in Equation 2–13, where V_C is the volume of distribution of drug in the central compartment and V_T is the volume term for drug in the tissue compartment:

$$V_{ss} = V_C + V_T \qquad \text{(Equation 2–13)}$$

Steady-State Concentration

Equation 2–3 (Dosing rate = $CL \cdot C_{ss}$) indicates that a steady-state concentration eventually will be achieved when a drug is administered at a constant rate. At this point, drug elimination (the product of clearance and concentration; Equation 2–5) will equal the rate of drug availability. This concept also extends to regular intermittent dosage (e.g., 250 mg of drug every 8 h). During each interdose interval, the concentration of drug rises with absorption and falls by elimination. At steady state, the entire cycle is repeated identically in each interval (Figure 2–7). Equation 2–3 still applies for intermittent dosing, but it now describes the average steady-state drug concentration during an interdose interval. Note the extension of this idea to derive $\bar{C}_{ss}$ during continuous intravenous drug infusion, as explained in the legend to Figure 2–7.

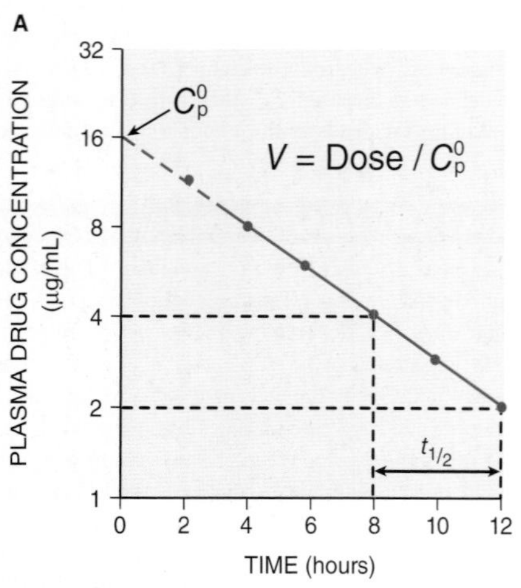

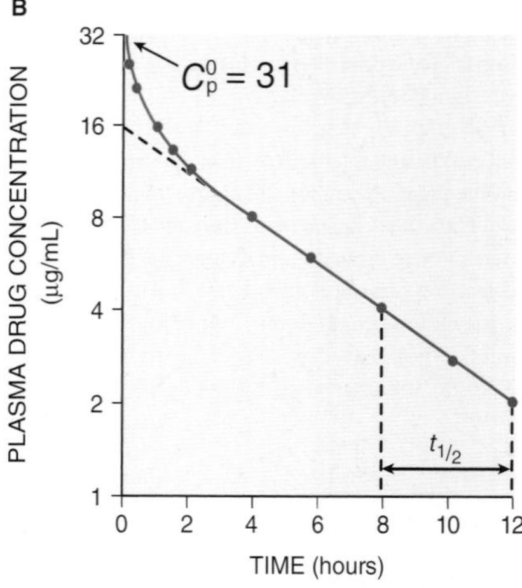

Figure 2–6 *Plasma concentration-time curves following intravenous administration of a drug (500 mg) to a 70-kg patient.* **A.** Drug concentrations are measured in plasma at 2-hour intervals following drug administration. The semilogarithmic plot of plasma concentration C_p versus time suggests that the drug is eliminated from a single compartment by a first-order process (see Equation 2–12) with a $t_{1/2}$ of 4 h ($k = 0.693/t_{1/2} = 0.173\ \text{h}^{1}$). The volume of distribution V may be determined from the value of C_p obtained by extrapolation to zero-time. Volume of distribution (see Equation 2–11) for the one-compartment model is 31.3 L, or 0.45 L/kg ($V = \text{dose}/C_p^0$). The clearance for this drug is 90 mL/min; for a one-compartment model, $CL = kV$.
B. Sampling before 2 h indicates that the drug follows multiexponential kinetics. The terminal disposition $t_{1/2}$ is 4 h, clearance is 84 mL/min (see Equation 2–7), and V_{ss} is 26.8 L (see Equation 2–13). The initial or "central" distribution volume for the drug (V = dose/C0p) is 16.1 L. The example indicates that multicompartment kinetics may be overlooked when sampling at early times is neglected. In this particular case, there is only a 10% error in the estimate of clearance when the multicompartment characteristics are ignored. For many drugs, multicompartment kinetics may be observed for significant periods of time, and failure to consider the distribution phase can lead to significant errors in estimates of clearance and in predictions of appropriate dosage.

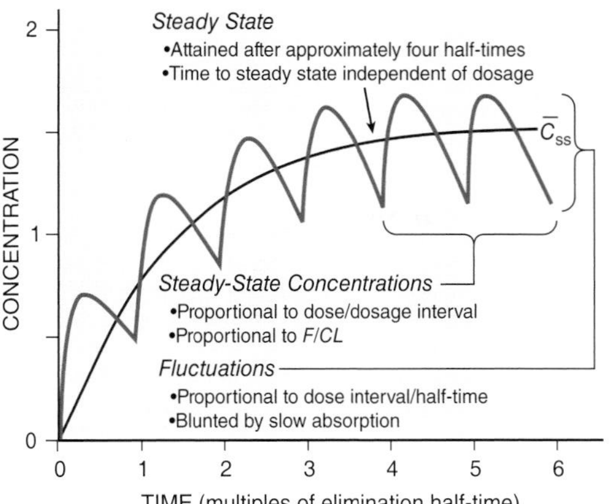

Figure 2–7 *Fundamental pharmacokinetic relationships for repeated administration of drugs.* The red line is the pattern of drug accumulation during repeated administration of a drug at intervals equal to its elimination half-time. With instantaneous absorption, each dose would add 1 concentration unit to C_p at the time of administration, and then half of that would be eliminated prior to administration of the next dose, resulting in the oscillation of C_p between 1 and 2 after four or five elimination half-times. However, this more realistic simulation uses a rate of drug absorption that is not instantaneous but is 10 times as rapid as elimination; drug is eliminated throughout the absorption process, blunting the maximal blood level achieved after each dose. With repeated administration, C_p achieves steady state, oscillating around the blue line at 1.5 units. The blue line depicts the pattern during administration of equivalent dosage by continuous intravenous infusion. Curves are based on the one-compartment model. Average drug concentration at steady state $\bar{C}_{ss}$ is:

$$C_{ss} = \frac{F \cdot \text{dose}}{CL \cdot T} = \frac{F \cdot \text{dosing rate}}{CL}$$

where the dosing rate is the dose per time interval and is dose/T, F is the fractional bioavailability, and CL is clearance. Note that substitution of infusion rate for [F · dose/T] provides the concentration maintained at steady state during continuous intravenous infusion (F = 1 with intravenous administration).

Half-Life

The $t_{1/2}$ is the time it takes for the plasma concentration to be reduced by 50%. For the one-compartment model of Figure 2–6A, $t_{1/2}$ may be determined readily by inspection of the data and used to make decisions about drug dosage. However, as indicated in Figure 2–6B, drug concentrations in plasma often follow a multicomponent pattern of decline.

Half-Life, Volume of Distribution, and Clearance

When using pharmacokinetics to calculate drug dosing in disease, note that $t_{1/2}$ changes as a function of both clearance and volume of distribution:

$$t_{1/2} \cong 0.693 \cdot V_{ss}/CL \qquad \text{(Equation 2–14)}$$

This $t_{1/2}$ reflects the decline of systemic drug concentrations during a dosing interval at steady state as depicted in Figure 2–7.

Terminal Half-Life

With prolonged dosing (or with high drug concentrations), a drug may penetrate beyond the central compartment into "deep" or secondary body compartments that equilibrate only slowly with the plasma. When the infusion or dosing stops, the drug will be initially cleared from plasma as expected but will eventually drop to a point at which net diffusion from the secondary compartments begins, and this slow equilibration will produce a prolongation of the half-life of the drug, referred to as the terminal half-life.

Steady-State $t_{1/2}$ and Terminal $t_{1/2}$ Compared

Examples of drugs with marked differences in terminal $t_{1/2}$ versus steady-state $t_{1/2}$ are gentamicin and indomethacin. Gentamicin has a $t_{1/2}$ of 2–3 h following a single administration, but a terminal $t_{1/2}$ of 53 h because drug accumulates in spaces such as kidney parenchyma (where this accumulation can result in toxicity). Biliary cycling probably is responsible for the 120-h terminal value for indomethacin (compared to the steady-state value of 2.4 h). Intravenous anesthetics provide a good example; many have *context-sensitive* half-times; these agents, with short half-times after single intravenous doses, exhibit longer half-times in proportion to the duration of exposure when used in maintenance anesthesia (see Figure 21–2).

Clearance is the measure of the body's capacity to eliminate a drug; thus, as clearance decreases, owing to a disease process, for example, $t_{1/2}$ will increase as long as the volume of distribution remains unchanged; alternately, the volume of distribution may change but CL remains constant or a combination of the two changes. For example, the $t_{1/2}$ of diazepam increases with increasing age; however, this does not reflect a change in clearance but rather a change in the volume of distribution. Similarly, changes in protein binding of a drug (e.g., hypoalbuminemia) may affect its clearance as well as its volume of distribution, leading to unpredictable changes in $t_{1/2}$ as a function of disease. The $t_{1/2}$ defined in Equation 2–14 provides an approximation of the time required to reach steady state after a dosage regimen is initiated or changed (e.g., four half-lives to reach ~ 94% of a new steady state).

Extent and Rate of Absorption

Bioavailability

It is important to distinguish between the amount of drug that is administered and the quantity of drug that ultimately reaches the systemic circulation. Dissolution and absorption of drug may be incomplete; some drug may be destroyed prior to entering the systemic circulation, especially by hepatic first-pass metabolism. The first-pass effect is extensive for many oral medications that enter the portal vein and pass directly to the liver. The fraction of a dose F that is absorbed and escapes first-pass elimination measures the drug's *bioavailability*; thus, $0 < F \leq 1$ (see Equation 2–2).

For some drugs, extensive first-pass metabolism greatly reduces their effectiveness or precludes their use as oral agents (e.g., lidocaine, propranolol, naloxone, and glyceryl trinitrate). For other agents, the extent of absorption may be very low, thereby reducing bioavailability. When drugs are administered by a route that is subject to significant first-pass loss or incomplete absorption, the equations presented previously that contain the terms *dose* or *dosing rate* (see Equations 2–3, 2–7, and 2–12) also must include the bioavailability term F such that the available dose or dosing rate is used (Box 2–2). For example, Equation 2–2 is modified to

$$F \cdot \text{Dosing rate} = CL \cdot C_{ss} \qquad \text{(Equation 2–15)}$$

where the value of F is between 0 and 1.

Rate of Absorption

The rate of absorption can be important with a drug given as a single dose, such as a sleep-inducing medication that must act in a reasonable time frame and achieve an effective blood level that is maintained for an appropriate duration. However, with periodic and repeated dosing, the rate of drug absorption does not, in general, influence the average steady-state concentration of the drug in plasma, provided the drug is stable before it is absorbed; the rate of absorption may, however, still influence drug therapy. If a drug is absorbed rapidly (e.g., a dose given as an intravenous bolus) and has a small "central" volume, the concentration of drug initially will be high. It will then fall as the drug is distributed to its "final" (larger) volume (see Figure 2–6B). If the same drug is absorbed more slowly (e.g., by slow infusion), a significant amount of the drug will be distributed while it is being administered, and peak concentrations will be lower and will occur later. Controlled-release oral preparations are designed to provide a slow and sustained rate of absorption to produce smaller fluctuations in the plasma concentration-time profile during the dosage interval compared with more immediate-release formulations. Because the beneficial, nontoxic effects of drugs are based on knowledge of an ideal or desired plasma concentration range, maintaining that range while avoiding large swings between peak and trough concentrations can improve therapeutic outcome.

Nonlinear Pharmacokinetics

Nonlinearity in pharmacokinetics (i.e., changes in such parameters as clearance, volume of distribution, and $t_{1/2}$ as a function of dose or concentration of drug) is usually caused by saturation of protein binding, hepatic metabolism, or active renal transport of the drug.

Saturable Protein Binding

As the molar concentration of small drug molecules increases, the unbound fraction eventually also must increase (as all binding sites become saturated when drug concentrations in plasma are in the range of tens to hundreds of micrograms per milliliter). For a drug that is metabolized by the liver with a low intrinsic clearance-extraction ratio, saturation of plasma-protein binding will cause both V and CL to increase as drug concentrations increase; $t_{1/2}$ thus may remain constant (see Equation 2–14). For such a drug, C_{ss} will not increase linearly as the rate of drug administration is increased. For drugs that are cleared with high intrinsic clearance-extraction ratios, C_{ss} can remain linearly proportional to the rate of drug administration. In this case, hepatic clearance will not change, and the increase in V will increase the half-time of disappearance by reducing the fraction of the total drug in the body that is delivered to the liver per unit of time. Most drugs fall between these two extremes.

Saturable Elimination

In the case of saturable elimination, the Michaelis-Menten equation (see Equation 2–4) usually describes the nonlinearity. All active processes are undoubtedly saturable, but they will appear to be linear if values of drug concentrations encountered in practice are much less than K_m for that process (Box 2–3). When drug concentrations exceeds K_m, nonlinear kinetics are observed. Saturable metabolism causes oral first-pass metabolism to be less than expected (higher *fractional bioavailability*), resulting in a greater fractional increase in C_{ss} than the corresponding fractional increase in the rate of drug administration; basically, the rate of drug entry into the systemic circulation exceeds the maximum possible rate of drug metabolism, and elimination becomes zero order. The major consequences of saturation of metabolism or transport are the opposite of those for saturation of protein binding. Saturation of protein binding will lead to increased CL because CL increases as drug concentration increases, whereas saturation of metabolism or transport may decrease CL.

C_{ss} can be computed by substituting Equation 2–4 (with $C = C_{ss}$) into Equation 2–3 and solving for the steady-state concentration:

$$C_{ss} = \frac{\text{Dosing rate} \cdot K_m}{v_m - \text{dosing rate}} \quad \text{(Equation 2–16)}$$

BOX 2–2 ■ Poor Absorption Notwithstanding, Some Agents With Low Bioavailability Are Effective Orally

The value of F varies widely for drugs administered by mouth, and successful therapy can still be achieved for some drugs with F values as low as 0.03 (e.g., etidronate and aliskiren). Aliskiren is the first orally applicable direct renin inhibitor approved for treatment of hypertension; its bioavailability is 2.6%. Etidronate, a bisphosphonate used to stabilize bone matrix in the treatment of Paget's disease and osteoporosis, has a similarly low bioavailability of 0.03, meaning that only 3% of the drug appears in the bloodstream following oral dosing. In these cases, therapy using oral administration is still useful, although the administered dose of the drug per kilogram is larger than would be given by injection.

As the dosing rate approaches the maximal elimination rate v_m, the denominator of Equation 2–16 approaches zero, and C_{ss} increases disproportionately. Because saturation of metabolism should have no effect on the volume of distribution, clearance and the relative rate of drug elimination decrease as the concentration increases; therefore, the log C_p time curve is concave-downward until metabolism becomes sufficiently desaturated such that first-order elimination is observed (Figure 2–8).

Thus, in the region of saturation of metabolism, the concept of a constant $t_{1/2}$ is not applicable. Consequently, changing the dosing rate for a drug with nonlinear metabolism is difficult and unpredictable because the resulting steady state is reached more slowly, and importantly, the effect is disproportionate to the alteration in the dosing rate.

Figure 2–8 compares the effects of first-order and zero-order elimination kinetics on important pharmacokinetic parameters.

Design and Optimization of Dosage Regimens

The Therapeutic Window

The intensity of a drug's effect is related to its concentration (usually C_p) above a minimum effective concentration, whereas the duration of the drug's effect reflects the length of time the drug level is above this value (Figure 2–9). These considerations, in general, apply to both desired and undesired (adverse) drug effects; as a result, a *therapeutic window*

BOX 2–3 ■ Saturable Metabolism: Phenytoin

The antiseizure medication phenytoin is a drug for which metabolism can become saturated by levels of the drug in the therapeutic range. Factors contributing to this are phenytoin's variable half-life and clearance and an effective concentration that varies and can saturate clearance mechanisms, such that the C_{ss} may be saturating clearance mechanisms or be well above or below that value. The $t_{1/2}$ of phenytoin is 6–24 h. For clearance, K_m (5–10 mg/L) is typically near the lower end of the therapeutic range (10–20 mg/L). For some individuals, especially young children and newborns being treated for emergent seizures, K_m may be as low as 1 mg/L. Consider an extreme case of a 70kg adult in whom the target concentration (C_{ss}) is 15 mg/L, K_m = 1 mg/L, and the maximal elimination rate, v_m, (from Appendix II) is 5.9 mg/kg/day, or 413 mg/day/70kg. Substituting into Equation 2–16:

$$15\text{mg/L} = (\text{dosing rate})(1\text{mg/L})/(413\text{mg/day} - \text{dosing rate})$$
$$\text{dosing rate} = 387 \text{ mg/day}$$

In this case, the dosing rate is just below the elimination capacity. If the dosing rate were to vary upward by 10% (to 387 + 38.7 or ~426 mg/day), the dosing rate would exceed the elimination capacity by 13 mg/day and the C_p of phenytoin would begin a slow climb to toxic levels. Conversely, if the dosing rate were to vary downward by 10% (to 387-38.7 or ~348 mg/day), the C_{ss} achieved would be 5.4 mg/L, a drastic reduction to a level below the therapeutic range.

Consider a more common K_m, 8 mg/L, such that the desired C_{ss} of 15mg/L is farther from saturating the elimination capacity. In a 70 kg subject (v_m = 413 mg/day), these data require a dosing rate of only 269 mg/day. An increase in this rate by 10% (to 296 mg/day) would not saturate the elimination capacity but would lead to a C_{ss} = 20.2 mg/L. A 10% downward variance in the dosing rate (to 242 mg/day) will produce a C_{ss} = 11.3 mg/L, a much less drastic decrease than above and still in the therapeutic range.

Factoring in all the variables, predicting and controlling dosage so precisely (<10% error) can be difficult. Therefore, for patients in whom the target concentration for phenytoin is ≥10 times the K_m, alternating between inefficacious therapy and toxicity is common, careful monitoring is essential, and a pharmacokinetic consult to establish or revise dosing may be appropriate.

Other agents exhibiting saturated metabolism at or near the commonly employed concentrations include aspirin, fluoxetine, verapamil, and ethanol.

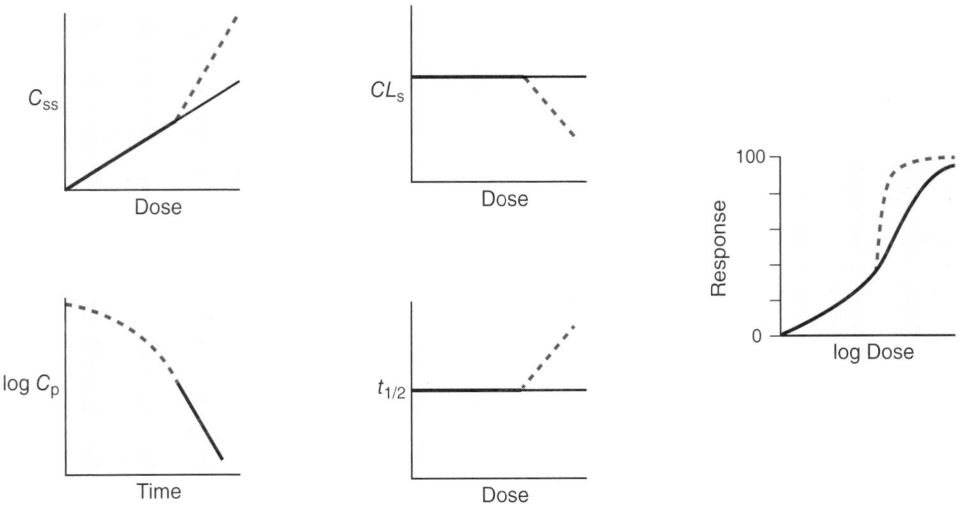

Figure 2–8 *Comparative pharmacokinetic parameters with first-order and zero-order elimination.* Black lines represent the relationships under first-order kinetics of elimination. Dashed red lines indicate the effects of transitioning to a region of saturated elimination (zero-order kinetics).

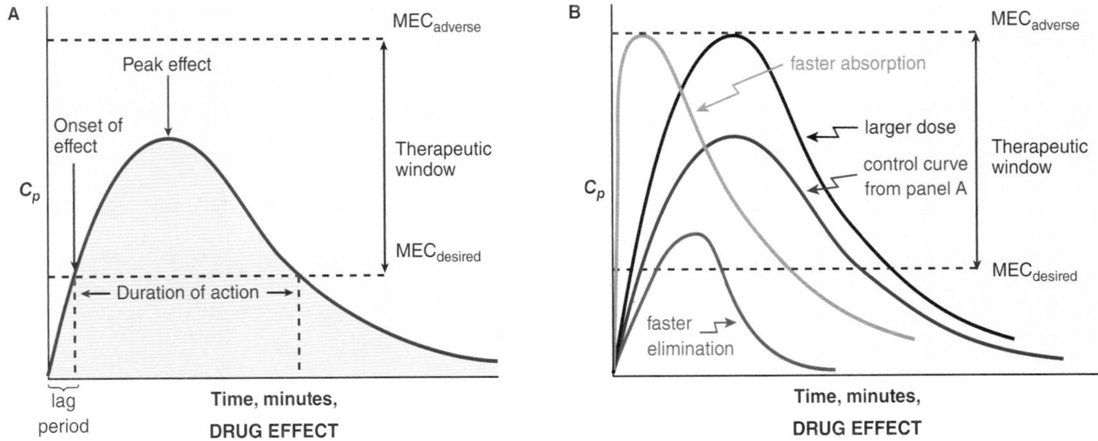

Figure 2–9 **A.** *Temporal characteristics of drug effect and relationship to the therapeutic window (e.g., single dose, oral administration).* A lag period is present before the plasma drug concentration C_p exceeds the MEC for the desired effect $MEC_{desired}$. Following onset of the response, the intensity of the effect increases as the drug continues to be absorbed and distributed. This reaches a peak, after which drug elimination results in a decline in C_p and in the effect's intensity. Effect disappears when the drug concentration falls below the $MEC_{desired}$. The duration of a drug's action is determined by the time period over which concentrations exceed the $MEC_{desired}$. An MEC also exists for each adverse response ($MEC_{adverse}$), and if the drug concentration exceeds this, toxicity will result. The therapeutic goal is to obtain and maintain concentrations within the therapeutic window for the desired response with a minimum of toxicity. Drug response *below* the $MEC_{desired}$ will be subtherapeutic; *above* the $MEC_{adverse}$, the probability of toxicity will increase. The AUC (pale red) can be used to calculate the clearance (see Equation 2–7) for first-order elimination. The AUC is also used as a measure of bioavailability (defined as 100% for an intravenously administered drug). Bioavailability is less than 100% for orally administered drugs, due mainly to incomplete absorption and first-pass metabolism and elimination. Changing drug dosage shifts the curve up or down the C_p scale and is used to modulate the drug's effect, as shown in panel B.
B. *Effects of altered absorption, elimination, and dosage and the temporal profile of a single dose administered orally.* The bold green curve is the same as that shown in panel A. Increasing the dose (blue line) decreases the lag period and prolongs the drug's duration of effectivess but at the risk of increasing the likelihood of adverse effects. Unless the drug is nontoxic (e.g., penicillins), increasing the dose is not a useful strategy for extending the duration of action if the increase puts the drug level near $MEC_{adverse}$. Instead, another dose of drug should be given, timed to maintain concentrations within the therapeutic window (see Figure 2–7). An increased rate of absorption of the dose (orange line) reduces the lag period, leads to a higher maximum C_p at an earlier time, but results in a shorter duration of action (time above $MEC_{desired}$). Increasing the rate of elimination of the dose decreases the maximum C_p and reduces the time of $C_p > MEC_{desired}$.

exists that reflects a concentration range that provides efficacy without unacceptable toxicity. Following administration of a single dose, a lag period precedes the onset of the drug effect, after which the magnitude of the effect increases to a maximum and then declines; if a subsequent dose is not administered, the effect eventually disappears as the drug is eliminated. This time course reflects changes in the drug's concentration as determined by the pharmacokinetics of its absorption, distribution, and elimination.

Similar considerations apply after multiple dosing associated with long-term therapy, and they determine the amount and frequency of drug administration to achieve an optimal therapeutic effect. *In general, the lower limit of a drug's therapeutic range is approximately equal to the drug concentration that produces about half the greatest possible therapeutic effect, and the upper limit of the therapeutic range is such that no more than 5%–10% of patients will experience a toxic effect.* For some drugs, this may mean that the upper limit of the range is no more than twice the lower limit. Of course, these figures can be highly variable, and some patients may benefit greatly from drug concentrations that exceed the therapeutic range, whereas others may suffer significant toxicity at much lower values (e.g., with digoxin).

For a limited number of drugs, some effect of the drug is easily measured (e.g., blood pressure, blood glucose) and can be used to optimize dosage using a trial-and-error approach. Even in an ideal case, certain quantitative issues arise, such as how often to change dosage and by how much. These usually can be settled with simple rules of thumb based on the principles presented (e.g., change dosage by no more than 50% and no more often than every three or four half-lives). Alternatively, some drugs have little dose-related toxicity, and maximum efficacy usually is desired. In such cases, doses well in excess of the average required will ensure efficacy (if this is possible) and prolong drug action. Such a "maximal dose" strategy typically is used for penicillins. For many drugs, however, the effects are difficult to measure (or the drug is given for prophylaxis), toxicity and lack of efficacy are both potential dangers, or the therapeutic index is narrow. In these circumstances, doses must be titrated carefully, and drug dosage is limited by toxicity rather than efficacy.

Thus, the therapeutic goal is to maintain steady-state drug levels within the therapeutic window. When the concentrations associated with this desired range are not known, it is sufficient to understand that efficacy and toxicity depend on concentration and how drug dosage and frequency of administration affect the drug level. However, for a small number of drugs for which there is a small (2- to 3-fold) difference between concentrations resulting in efficacy and toxicity (e.g., digoxin, theophylline, lidocaine, aminoglycosides, cyclosporine, tacrolimus, sirolimus, warfarin, and some anticonvulsants), a plasma concentration range associated with effective therapy has been defined. In these cases, a desired (target) steady-state concentration of the drug (usually in plasma) associated with efficacy and minimal toxicity is chosen, and a dosage is computed that is expected to achieve this value. Drug concentrations are subsequently measured, and dosage is adjusted if necessary (described further in the chapter).

Maintenance Dose

In most clinical situations, drugs are administered in a series of repetitive doses or as a continuous infusion to maintain a steady-state concentration of drug associated with the therapeutic window. Calculation of the appropriate maintenance dosage is a primary goal. To maintain the chosen steady-state or target concentration, the rate of drug administration is adjusted such that the rate of input equals the rate of loss. This relationship is expressed here in terms of the desired target concentration:

$$\text{Dosing rate} = \text{Target } C_p \cdot CL/F \qquad \text{(Equation 2–17)}$$

If the clinician chooses the desired concentration of drug in plasma and knows the clearance and bioavailability for that drug in a particular patient, the appropriate dose and dosing interval can be calculated (Box 2–4).

Dosing Interval for Intermittent Dosage

In general, marked fluctuations in drug concentrations between doses are not desirable. If absorption and distribution were instantaneous, fluctuations in drug concentrations between doses would be governed entirely by the drug's elimination $t_{1/2}$. If the dosing interval t were chosen to be equal to the $t_{1/2}$, then the total fluctuation would be 2-fold; this is often a tolerable variation. Pharmacodynamic considerations modify this. If a drug is relatively nontoxic such that a concentration many times that necessary for therapy can be tolerated easily, the maximal dose strategy can be used, and the dosing interval can be much longer than the elimination $t_{1/2}$ (for convenience). The $t_{1/2}$ of amoxicillin is about 2 h, but dosing every 2 h would be impractical. Instead, amoxicillin often is given in large doses every 8 or 12 h.

For some drugs with a narrow therapeutic range, it may be important to estimate the maximal and minimal concentrations that will occur for a particular dosing interval. The minimal steady-state concentration $C_{ss,\,min}$ may be reasonably determined by:

$$C_{ss,\,min} = \frac{F \cdot dose/V_{ss}}{1-e^{-kT}} \cdot e^{-kT} \qquad \text{(Equation 2–18)}$$

where k equals 0.693 divided by the clinically relevant plasma $t_{1/2}$, and T is the dosing interval. The term e^{-kT} is the fraction of the last dose (corrected for bioavailability) that remains in the body at the end of a dosing interval.

For drugs that follow multiexponential kinetics (administered orally), estimation of the maximal steady-state concentration $C_{ss,max}$ involves a set of parameters for distribution and absorption (Box 2–5). If these terms are ignored for multiple oral dosing, one easily may estimate a maximal steady-state concentration by omitting the e^{-kT} term in the numerator of Equation 2–18 (see Equation 2–19 in Box 2–5). Because of the approximation, the predicted maximal concentration from Equation 2–19 will be greater than that actually observed.

BOX 2–4 ■ Calculating Dosage of Digoxin in Heart Failure

Oral digoxin is to be used as a maintenance dose to gradually "digitalize" a 63-year-old, 84-kg patient with congestive heart failure. A steady-state plasma concentration of 0.7–0.9 ng/mL is selected as a conservative target based on prior knowledge of the action of the drug in patients with heart failure to maintain levels at or below the 0.5- to 1.0-ng/mL range (Bauman et al., 2006). This patient's creatinine clearance CL_{Cr} is given as 56 mL/min/84 kg; knowing that digoxin's clearance may be estimated by consulting the entry for digoxin in Appendix II: $CL = 0.88\ CL_{Cr} + 0.33$ mL/min/kg. Thus,

$$\begin{aligned} CL &= 0.88\ CL_{Cr} + 0.33 \text{ mL/min/kg} \\ &= 0.88 \times 56/84 + 0.33 \text{ mL/min/kg} \\ &= 0.92 \text{ mL/min/kg} \end{aligned}$$

For this 84-kg patient:

$$CL = (84 \text{ kg})(0.92 \text{ mL/min/kg}) = 77 \text{ mL/min} = 4.6 \text{ L/h}$$

Knowing that the oral bioavailability of digoxin is 70% ($F = 0.7$) and with a target C_p of 0.75 ng/mL, one can use Equation 2–17 to calculate an appropriate dose rate for this 84-kg patient:

$$\begin{aligned} &\text{Dosing rate} = \text{Target } C_p \cdot CL/F \\ &= [0.75 \text{ ng/mL} \times 77 \text{ mL/min}] \div [0.7] = 82.5 \text{ ng/min} \\ &\text{or } 82.5 \text{ ng/min} \times 60 \text{ min/h} \times 24 \text{ h/d} = 119\ \mu\text{g/d} \end{aligned}$$

In practice, the dosing rate is rounded to the closest oral dosage size, 0.125 mg/d, which would result in a C_{ss} of 0.79 ng/mL (0.75 × 125/119, or using Equation 2–15). Digoxin is a well-characterized example of a drug that is difficult to dose, has a low therapeutic index (~2–3), and has a large coefficient of variation for the clearance equation in patients with heart failure (52%); the effective blood level in one patient may be toxic or ineffective in another. Thus, monitoring the clinical status of patients (new or increased ankle edema, inability to sleep in a recumbent position, decreased exercise tolerance), whether accomplished by home health follow-up or regular visits to the clinician, is essential to avoid untoward results (see Chapter 29).

Loading Dose

As noted, repeated administration of a drug more frequently than its complete elimination will result in accumulation of the drug to or around a steady-state level (see Figure 2–7). When a constant dosage is given, reaching a steady-state drug level (the desired therapeutic concentration) will take four to five elimination half-times. This period can be too long when treatment demands a more immediate therapeutic response. In such

BOX 2–5 ■ Estimating Maximal and Minimal Blood Levels of Digoxin

In the 84-kg patient with congestive heart failure discussed in Box 2–4, an oral maintenance dose of 0.125 mg digoxin per 24 h was calculated to achieve an average plasma concentration of 0.79 ng/mL during the dosage interval. Digoxin has a narrow therapeutic index, and plasma levels ≤ 1.0 ng/mL usually are associated with efficacy and minimal toxicity. What are the maximum and minimum plasma concentrations associated with this regimen? This first requires estimation of digoxin's volume of distribution based on pharmacokinetic data (Appendix II).

$$V_{ss} = 3.12\ CL_{Cr} + 3.84\ \text{L} \cdot \text{kg}^{-1}$$
$$= 3.12 \times (56/84) + 3.84\ \text{L} \cdot \text{kg}^{-1}$$
$$= 5.92\ \text{L/kg}$$

or 497 L in this 84-kg patient.

Combining this value with that of digoxin's clearance provides an estimate of digoxin's elimination $t_{1/2}$ in the patient (Equation 2–14).

$$t_{1/2} = 0.693\ V_{ss}/CL$$
$$= \frac{0.693 \times 497\ \text{L}}{4.6\ \text{L/h}} = 75\ \text{h} = 3.1\ \text{days}$$

Accordingly, the fractional rate constant of elimination k is equal to 0.22 day^{-1} (0.693/3.1 days). Maximum and minimum digoxin plasma concentrations then may be predicted depending on the dosage interval. With T = 1 day (i.e., 0.125 mg given every day),

$$C_{ss,max} = \frac{F \cdot \text{dose}/V_{ss}}{1 - e^{-kT}} \quad \text{(Equation 2–19)}$$
$$= \frac{0.7 \times 0.125\ \text{mg}/497\ \text{L}}{0.2}$$
$$= 0.88\ \text{ng/mL}\ (\sim 0.9\ \text{ng/mL})$$

$$C_{ss,\,min} = C_{ss,\,max} \cdot e^{-kt} \quad \text{(Equation 2–20)}$$
$$= (0.88\ \text{ng/mL})(0.8) = 0.7\ \text{ng/mL}$$

Thus, the plasma concentrations would fluctuate minimally about the steady-state concentration of 0.79 ng/mL, well within the recommended therapeutic range of 0.5–1.0 ng/mL.

a case, one can employ a *loading dose*, one or a series of doses given at the onset of therapy with the aim of achieving the target concentration rapidly. The loading dose is calculated as

$$\text{Loading dose} = \text{Target}\ C_p \cdot V_{ss}/F \quad \text{(Equation 2–21)}$$

Consider the case for treatment of arrhythmias with lidocaine, for example. The $t_{1/2}$ of lidocaine is usually 1–2 h. Arrhythmias encountered after myocardial infarction may be life threatening, and one cannot wait four half-times (4–8 h) to achieve a therapeutic concentration of lidocaine by infusion of the drug at the rate required to attain this concentration. Hence, use of a loading dose of lidocaine in the coronary care unit is standard.

The use of a loading dose also has significant disadvantages. First, the particularly sensitive individual may be exposed abruptly to a toxic concentration of a drug that may take a long time to decrease (i.e., long $t_{1/2}$). Loading doses tend to be large, and they are often given parenterally and rapidly; this can be particularly dangerous if toxic effects occur as a result of actions of the drug at sites that are in rapid equilibrium with plasma. This occurs because the loading dose calculated on the basis of V_{ss} subsequent to drug distribution is at first constrained within the initial and smaller "central" volume of distribution. It is therefore usually advisable to divide the loading dose into a number of smaller fractional doses that are administered over a period of time (Box 2–6). Alternatively, the loading dose should be administered as a continuous intravenous infusion over a period of time using computerized infusion pumps.

Therapeutic Drug Monitoring

The major use of measured concentrations of drugs (at steady state) is to refine the estimate of *CL*/*F* for the patient being treated, using Equation 2–15 as rearranged:

$$CL/F_{patient} = \text{Dosing rate}/C_{ss}(\text{measured}) \quad \text{(Equation 2–22)}$$

The new estimate of *CL*/*F* can be used in Equation 2–17 to adjust the maintenance dose to achieve the desired target concentration (Box 2–7).

Practical details associated with therapeutic drug monitoring should be kept in mind. The first of these relates to the time of sampling for measurement of the drug concentration.

The purpose of sampling during supposed steady state is to modify the estimate of *CL*/*F* and thus the choice of dosage. Early postabsorptive concentrations do not reflect clearance; they are determined primarily by the rate of absorption, the "central" (rather than the steady-state) volume of distribution, and the rate of distribution, all of which are pharmacokinetic features of virtually no relevance in choosing the long-term maintenance dosage. When the goal of measurement is adjustment of dosage,

BOX 2–6 ■ A Loading Dose of Digoxin

In the 84-kg patient described previously, accumulation of digoxin to an effective steady-state level was gradual when a daily maintenance dose of 0.125 mg was administered (for at least 12.4 days, based on $t_{1/2}$ = 3.1 days). A more rapid response could be obtained (if deemed necessary) by using a loading dose strategy and Equation 2–21. Choosing a target C_p of 0.9 ng/mL (the $C_{ss,\,max}$ calculated in Box 2–5 and below the recommended maximum of 1.0 ng/mL):

$$\text{Loading dose} = 0.9\ \text{ng} \cdot \text{mL}^{-1} \times 497\ \text{L}/0.7 = 639\ \mu\text{g}$$

Using standard dosage sizes, one would use a loading dose of 0.625 mg given in divided doses. To avoid toxicity, this oral loading dose would be given as an initial 0.25-mg dose followed by a 0.25-mg dose 6–8 h later, with careful monitoring of the patient, and the final 0.125-mg dose given another 6–8 h later.

BOX 2–7 ■ Adjusting the Dose at Steady State

If a drug follows first-order kinetics, the average, minimum, and maximum concentrations at steady state are linearly related to dose and dosing rate (see Equations 2–15, 2–18, and 2–19). Therefore, the ratio between the measured and desired concentrations can be used to adjust the dose, consistent with available dosage sizes:

$$\frac{C_{ss}(\text{measured})}{C_{ss}(\text{predicted})} = \frac{\text{Dose (previous)}}{\text{Dose (new)}} \quad \text{(Equation 2–23)}$$

Consider the previously described patient given 0.125 mg digoxin every 24 h, for example. If the measured minimum (trough) steady-state concentration were found to be 0.35 ng/mL rather than the predicted level of 0.7 ng/mL, an appropriate, practical change in the dosage regimen would be to increase the daily dose by 0.125 mg to 0.25 mg digoxin daily.

the sample should be taken just before the next planned dose, when the concentration is at its minimum.

If it is unclear whether efficacious concentrations of drug are being achieved, a sample taken shortly after a dose may be helpful. On the other hand, if a concern is whether low clearance (as in renal failure) may cause accumulation of drug, concentrations measured just before the next dose will reveal such accumulation and are considerably more useful for this purpose than is knowledge of the maximal concentration.

Determination of both maximal and minimal concentrations is recommended. These two values can offer a more complete picture of the behavior of the drug in a specific patient (particularly if obtained over more than one dosing period) and can better support pharmacokinetic modeling to adjust treatment.

When constant dosage is given, steady state is reached after four to five elimination half-times. If a sample is obtained too soon after dosage is begun, it will not reflect this state and the drug's clearance accurately. Yet, for toxic drugs, if sampling is delayed until steady state, the damage may have been done. In such cases, the first sample should be taken after two $t_{1/2}$ assuming that no loading dose has been given. If the concentration already exceeds 90% of the eventual expected mean steady-state concentration, the dosage rate should be halved, another sample obtained in another two (supposed) $t_{1/2}$, and the dosage halved again if this sample exceeds the target. If the first concentration is not too high, the initial rate of dosage is continued; even if the concentration is lower than expected, it is usually reasonable to await the attainment of steady state in another two estimated $t_{1/2}$ and then to proceed to adjust dosage as described in Box 2-7.

Acknowledgment: *Grant R. Wilkinson, Leslie Z. Benet, Deanna L. Kroetz, and Lewis B. Sheiner contributed to this chapter in recent editions of this book. We have retained some of their text in the current edition.*

Bibliography

Bauman JL, et al. A method of determining the dose of digoxin for heart failure in the modern era. *Arch Intern Med,* **2006**, *166*:2539–2545.

Bera RB. Patient outcomes within schizophrenia treatment: a look at the role of long-acting injectable antipsychotics. *J Clin Psychiatry,* **2014**, *75*(suppl 2):30–33.

Calias P, et al. Intrathecal delivery of protein therapeutics to the brain: a critical reassessment. *Pharmacol Ther,* **2014**, *144*:114–122.

Guner OF, Bowen JP. Pharmacophore modeling for ADME. *Curr Top Med Chem,* **2013**, *13*:1327–1342.

Imberti R, et al. Intraventricular or intrathecal colistin for the treatment of central nervous system infections caused by multidrug-resistant gram-negative bacteria. *Expert Rev Anti Infect Ther,* **2014**, *12*:471–478.

Perletti G, et al. Enhanced distribution of fourth-generation fluoroquinolones in prostatic tissue. *Int J Antimicrob Agents,* **2009**, *33*:206–210.

Ramamoorthy A, et al. Racial/ethnic differences in drug disposition and response: review of recently approved drugs. *Clin Pharmacol Ther,* **2015**, *97*:263–273.

Rowe H, et al. Maternal medication, drug use, and breastfeeding. *Child Adolesc Psychiatr Clin N Am,* **2015**, *24*:1–20.

Sen S, et al. Complications after unintentional intra-arterial injection of drugs: risks, outcomes, and management strategies. *Mayo Clin Proc,* **2005**, *80*:783–795.

Spector R, et al. A balanced view of choroid plexus structure and function: focus on adult humans. *Exp Neurol,* **2015**, *267*:78–86.

Suetsugu S, et al. Dynamic shaping of cellular membranes by phospholipids and membrane-deforming proteins. *Physiol Rev,* **2014**, *94*:1219–1248.

Tran TH, et al. Drug absorption in celiac disease. *Am J Health Syst Pharm,* **2013**, *70*:2199–2206.

Yohan D, Chithrani BD. Applications of nanoparticles in nanomedicine. *J Biomed Nanotechnol,* **2014**, *10*:2371–2392.

Zhang G, et al. Web resources for pharmacogenomics. *Genomics Proteomics Bioinformatics,* **2015**, *13*:51–54.

Pharmacodynamics: Molecular Mechanisms of Drug Action

Donald K. Blumenthal

第三章　药物效应动力学：药物作用的分子机制

中文导读

本章主要介绍：药物效应动力学的相关概念，包括生理性受体、药物反应的特异性、构效关系与药物设计、药物与受体相互作用的定量、药物效应动力学的变异——个体和群体药物效应动力学；药物作用机制，包括影响内源性配体浓度的受体、与细胞外过程相关的药物受体、抗感染药利用的受体、调节离子环境的受体、生理性受体激活的细胞内途径、生理性受体的结构和功能家族、凋亡和自噬途径、受体脱敏和受体调节、受体和通路功能障碍导致的疾病、生理系统对多种信号的整合；信号通路和药物作用。

Pharmacodynamic Concepts

Pharmacodynamics is the study of the biochemical, cellular, and physiological effects of drugs and their mechanisms of action. The effects of most drugs result from their interaction with macromolecular components of the organism. The term drug *receptor* or drug *target* denotes the cellular macromolecule or macromolecular complex with which the drug interacts to elicit a cellular or systemic response. Drugs commonly alter the rate or magnitude of an intrinsic cellular or physiological response rather than create new responses. Drug receptors are often located on the surface of cells but may also be located in specific intracellular compartments, such as the nucleus, or in the extracellular compartment, as in the case of drugs that target coagulation factors and inflammatory mediators. Many drugs also interact with *acceptors* (e.g., serum albumin), which are entities that do not directly cause any change in biochemical or physiological response but can alter the pharmacokinetics of a drug's actions.

A large percentage of the new drugs approved in recent years are *therapeutic biologics*, including genetically engineered enzymes and monoclonal antibodies. Going far beyond the traditional concept of a drug are genetically modified viruses and microbes. One recently approved agent for treating melanoma is a genetically modified live oncolytic herpes virus that is injected into tumors that cannot be removed completely by surgery. *Gene therapy products* using viruses as vectors to replace genetic mutations that give rise to lethal and debilitating diseases have already been approved in China and Europe. The next generation of gene therapy products will be those capable of targeted genome editing using antisense oligonucleotides and RNAi and by delivering the CRISPR/Cas9 genome-editing system using viruses or genetically modified microorganisms. These new agents will have pharmacological properties that are distinctly different from traditional small-molecule drugs.

Physiological Receptors

Many drug receptors are proteins that normally serve as receptors for endogenous regulatory ligands. These drug targets are termed *physiological receptors*. Drugs that bind to physiological receptors and mimic the regulatory effects of the endogenous signaling compounds are termed *agonists*. If the drug binds to the same *recognition site* as the endogenous agonist, the drug is said to be a *primary agonist*. *Allosteric* (or *allotopic*) *agonists* bind to a different region on the receptor, referred to as an allosteric or allotopic site. Drugs that block or reduce the action of an agonist are termed *antagonists*. Antagonism generally results from competition with an agonist for the same or overlapping site on the receptor (a *syntopic interaction*), but can also occur by interacting with other sites on the receptor (*allosteric antagonism*), by combining with the agonist (*chemical antagonism*), or by *functional antagonism* by indirectly inhibiting the cellular or physiological effects of the agonist. Agents that are only partially as effective as agonists are termed *partial agonists*. Many receptors exhibit some constitutive activity in the absence of a regulatory ligand; drugs that stabilize such receptors in an inactive conformation are termed *inverse agonists* (Figure 3–1) (Kenakin, 2004; Milligan, 2003). In the presence of a full agonist, partial and inverse agonists will behave as competitive antagonists.

Specificity of Drug Responses

The strength of the reversible interaction between a drug and its receptor, as measured by the **dissociation constant**, is defined as the *affinity* of one for the other. (By tradition, only rarely will the inverse of the dissociation constant, the association constant, be used, even though both carry the same information.) Both the *affinity* of a drug for its receptor and its *intrinsic activity* are determined by its *chemical structure*. The chemical structure of a drug also contributes to the drug's *specificity*. A drug that interacts with a single type of receptor that is expressed on only a limited number of differentiated cells will exhibit high specificity. Conversely, a drug acting on a receptor expressed ubiquitously throughout the body will exhibit widespread effects.

Many clinically important drugs exhibit a broad (low) specificity because they interact with multiple receptors in different tissues. Such broad specificity might not only enhance the clinical utility of a drug but also contribute to a spectrum of adverse side effects because of off-target interactions. One example of a drug that interacts with multiple receptors is *amiodarone*, an agent used to treat cardiac arrhythmias. Amiodarone also has a number of serious toxicities, some of which are caused by the drug's structural similarity to thyroid hormone and, as a result, its capacity to interact with nuclear thyroid receptors. Amiodarone's salutary effects and toxicities may also be mediated through interactions with receptors that are poorly characterized or unknown.

Some drugs are administered as racemic mixtures of stereoisomers. The stereoisomers can exhibit different pharmacodynamic as well as pharmacokinetic properties. For example, the antiarrhythmic drug *sotalol* is prescribed as a racemic mixture; the D- and L-enantiomers are equipotent as K^+ channel blockers, but the L-enantiomer is a much more potent β adrenergic antagonist (see Chapter 30). A drug may have multiple mechanisms of action that depend on receptor specificity, the tissue-specific expression of the receptor(s), drug access to target tissues, different drug concentrations in different tissues, pharmacogenetics, and interactions with other drugs.

Chronic administration of a drug may cause a *downregulation* of receptors or *desensitization* of response that can require dose adjustments to maintain adequate therapy. Chronic administration of nitrovasodilators to treat angina results in the rapid development of *complete tolerance*, a process known as *tachyphylaxis*. *Drug resistance* may also develop because of pharmacokinetic mechanisms (i.e., the drug is metabolized more rapidly with chronic exposure), the development of mechanisms that prevent the drug from reaching its receptor (i.e., increased expression of the multidrug resistance transporter in drug-resistant cancer cells; see Chapter 5), or the clonal expansion of cancer cells containing drug-resistant mutations in the drug receptor.

Some drug effects do not occur by means of macromolecular receptors. For instance, aluminum and magnesium hydroxides [$Al(OH)_3$ and $Mg(OH)_2$] reduce gastric acid chemically, neutralizing H^+ with OH^+ and raising gastric pH. Mannitol acts osmotically to cause changes in the distribution of water to promote diuresis, catharsis, expansion of circulating volume in the vascular compartment, or reduction of cerebral edema (see Chapter 25). Anti-infective drugs such as antibiotics, antivirals, and antiparasitics achieve specificity by targeting receptors or cell processes that are critical for the growth or survival of the infective agent but are nonessential or lacking in the host organism. Resistance to antibiotics, antivirals, and other drugs can occur through a variety of mechanisms, including mutation of the target receptor, increased expression of enzymes that degrade or increase efflux of the drug from the infective agent, and development of alternative biochemical pathways that circumvent the drug's effects on the infective agent.

Structure-Activity Relationships and Drug Design

The receptors responsible for the clinical effects of many drugs have yet to be identified. Conversely, sequencing of the entire human genome has identified novel genes related by sequence to known receptors, for which endogenous and exogenous ligands are unknown; these are called *orphan receptors*.

Both the affinity of a drug for its receptor and its intrinsic activity are determined by its chemical structure. This relationship frequently is stringent. Relatively minor modifications in the drug molecule may result in major changes in its pharmacological properties based on altered affinity for one or more receptors. Exploitation of structure-activity relationships has frequently led to the synthesis of valuable therapeutic agents. Because changes in molecular configuration need not alter all actions and effects of a drug equally, it is sometimes possible to develop a congener with a more favorable ratio of therapeutic to adverse effects, enhanced selectivity amongst different cells or tissues, or more acceptable secondary characteristics than those of the parent drug. Therapeutically useful antagonists of hormones or neurotransmitters have been developed by chemical modification of the structure of the physiological agonist.

Abbreviations

AAV: adeno-associated virus
AC: adenylyl cyclase
ACE: angiotensin-converting enzyme
ACh: acetylcholine
AChE: acetylcholinesterase
AKAP: A-kinase anchoring protein
AMPA: α-amino-3-hydroxy-5-methyl-4-isoxazole propionic acid
AngII: angiotensin II
ANP: atrial natriuretic peptide
Apaf-1: apoptotic activating protease factor 1
ASO: antisense oligonucleotide
***ATG*:** autophagy gene
AT_1R: AT_1 receptor
BNP: brain natriuretic peptide
cAMP: cyclic adenosine monophosphate
cAMP-GEF: cAMP-guanine exchange factor
cGMP: cyclic guanosine monophosphate
CNG: cyclic nucleotide–gated channel
CNP: C-type natriuretic peptide
CREB: cAMP response element–binding protein
CRISPR/Cas9: clustered regularly interspersed short palindromic repeats/CRISPR-associated protein 9
DA: dopamine
DAG: diacylglycerol
DMD: Duchenne muscular dystrophy
DRAM: damage-regulated autophagy modulator
4EBP: eukaryotic initiation factor 4e (eif-4E)–binding protein
EC_{50}: half-maximally effective concentration
EGF: epidermal growth factor
eNOS: endothelial NOS (NOS3)
EPAC: exchange protein activated by cAMP
FADD: Fas-associated death domain
FGF: fibroblast growth factor
FKBP12: immunophilin target (binding protein) for tacrolimus (FK506)
FXR: farnesoid X receptor
GABA: γ-aminobutyric acid
GAP: GTPase-activating protein
GC: guanylyl cyclase
GEF: guanine nucleotide exchange factor
GI: gastrointestinal
GPCR: G protein–coupled receptor
GRK: GPCR kinase
HCN: hyperpolarization-activated, cyclic nucleotide–gated channel
HRE: hormone response element
5HT: serotonin
IGF1R: insulinlike growth factor 1 receptor
IKK: IκB kinase
iNOS: inducible NOS (NOS2)
IP_3: inositol 1,4,5-trisphosphate
IRAK: interleukin-1 receptor-associated kinase
Jak: Janus kinase
JNK: c-Jun N-terminal kinase
K_{ATP}: ATP-dependent K^+ channel
K_i: affinity of a competitive antagonist
LBD: ligand-binding domain
LDLR: low-density lipoprotein receptor
LXR: liver X receptor
MAO: monoamine oxidase
MAPK: mitogen-activated protein kinase
MHC: major histocompatibility complex
MLCK: myosin light chain kinase
mTOR: mammalian target of rapamycin
MyD88: myeloid differentiation protein 88
NE: norepinephrine
NF-κB: nuclear factor kappa B
NGF: nerve growth factor
NGG: 5′-(any Nucleotide)-Guanosine-Guanosine-3′
NMDA: *N*-methyl-D-aspartate
nmDMD: nonsense mutation Duchenne muscular dystrophy
nNOS: neuronal NOS (NOS1)
NO: nitric oxide
NOS: NO synthase
NPR-A: ANP receptor
NPR-B: natriuretic peptide B receptor
NPR-C: natriuretic peptide C receptor
NSAID: nonsteroidal anti-inflammatory drug
PDE: cyclic nucleotide phosphodiesterase
PAM: protospacer-adjacent motif
PDGF: platelet-derived growth factor
PDGF-R: PDGR receptor
PI3K: phosphatidylinositol 3-kinase
PIP_3: phosphatidylinositol 3,4,5-trisphosphate
PK_: protein kinase _ (e.g., PKA)
PKB: protein kinase B (also known as Akt)
PLC: phospholipase C
PPAR: peroxisome proliferator-activated receptor
RGS: regulator of G protein signaling
RIP1: receptor interacting protein 1
RISC: RNA-induced silencing complex
RNAi: RNA interference
RXR: retinoic acid receptor
SERCA: SR Ca^{2+}-ATPase
sGC: soluble guanylyl cyclase
sgRNA: single "guide" RNA
siRNA: small interfering RNA
S6K: S6 kinase
SMAC: second mitochondria-derived activator of caspase
SMC: smooth muscle cell
SR: sarcoplasmic reticulum
STAT: signal transducer and activator of transcription
TAK1: transforming growth factor β–activated kinase 1
TCR: T cell receptor
TGF-β: transforming growth factor β
TLR: Toll-like receptor
TNF-α: tumor necrosis factor α
TRADD: TNF receptor–associated death domain
TRAF: TNF receptor–associated factor
TRAIL: TNF-related apoptosis-inducing ligand
TRP: transient receptor potential
VEGF: vascular endothelial growth factor

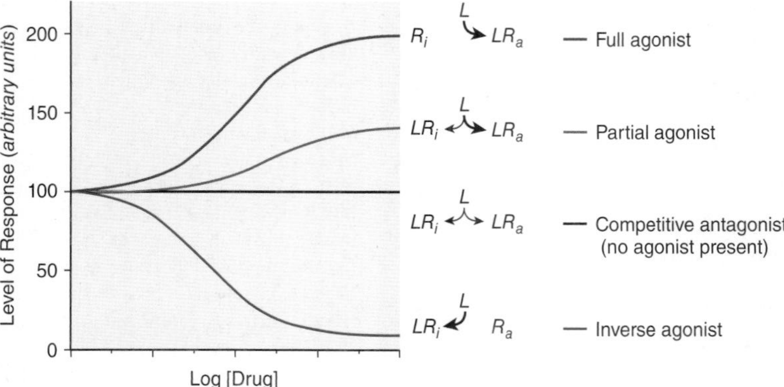

Figure 3–1 *Regulation of the activity of a receptor with conformation-selective drugs.* In this model, receptor R can exist in active (R_a) and inactive (R_i) conformations, and drugs binding to one, the other, or both states of R can influence the balance of the two forms of R and the net effect of receptor-controlled events. The ordinate is the activity of the receptor produced by R_a, the active receptor conformation (e.g., stimulation of AC by an activated β adrenergic receptor). If a drug L selectively binds to R_a, it will produce a maximal response. If L has equal affinity for R_i and R_a, it will not perturb the equilibrium between them and will have no effect on net activity; L would appear as a competitive antagonist if it blocks an agonist binding site (see Figure 3–4). If the drug selectively binds to R_i, then the net influence and amount of R_a will be diminished. If L can bind to receptor in an active conformation R_a but also bind to inactive receptor R_i with lower affinity, the drug will produce a partial response; L will be a partial agonist. If there is sufficient R_a to produce an elevated basal response in the absence of ligand (agonist-independent constitutive activity), and L binds to R_i, then that basal activity will be inhibited; L will then be an inverse agonist. Inverse agonists selectively bind to the inactive form of the receptor and shift the conformational equilibrium toward the inactive state. In systems that are not constitutively active, inverse agonists will behave like competitive antagonists, which helps explain that the properties of inverse agonists and the number of such agents previously described as competitive antagonists were only recently appreciated. Receptors that have constitutive activity and are sensitive to inverse agonists include benzodiazepine, histamine, opioid, cannabinoid, dopamine, bradykinin, and adenosine receptors.

With information about the molecular structures and pharmacological activities of a relatively large group of congeners, it is possible to use computer analysis to identify the chemical properties (i.e., the *pharmacophore*) required for optimal action at the receptor: size, shape, position, and orientation of charged groups or hydrogen bond donors, and so on. Advances in molecular modeling of organic compounds and the methods for drug target (receptor) discovery and biochemical measurement of the primary actions of drugs at their receptors have enriched the quantitation of structure-activity relationships and its use in drug design (Carlson and McCammon, 2000). Such information increasingly is allowing the optimization or design of chemicals that can bind to a receptor with improved affinity, selectivity, or regulatory effect. Similar structure-based approaches also are used to improve pharmacokinetic properties of drugs, particularly if knowledge of their metabolism is known. Knowledge of the structures of receptors and of drug-receptor complexes, determined at atomic resolution by X-ray crystallography, is even more helpful in the design of ligands and in understanding the molecular basis of drug resistance and circumventing it. Emerging technology in the field of pharmacogenetics (see Chapter 7) is improving our understanding of the nature of and variation in receptors and their impact on pharmacotherapy (Jain, 2004).

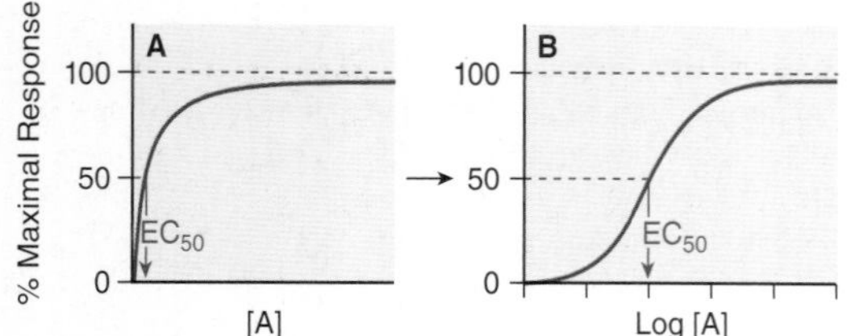

Figure 3–2 *Graded responses. On the y axis, the response is expressed as a percentage of maximal response plotted as a function of the concentration of drug A present at the receptor (x axis).* The hyperbolic shape of the curve in panel **A** becomes sigmoid when plotted semilogarithmically, as in panel **B**. The concentration of drug that produces 50% of the maximal response quantifies drug activity and is referred to as the EC_{50} (effective concentration of agonist for 50% response). The range of concentrations needed to fully depict the dose-response relationship (~3 $\log_{10}$ [10] units) is too wide to be useful in the linear format of Figure 3–2A; thus, most dose-response curves use *log [Drug]* on the *x* axis, as in Figure 3–2B. Dose-response curves presented in this way are sigmoidal in shape and have three noteworthy properties: threshold, slope, and maximal asymptote. These three parameters quantitate the activity of the drug.

Quantitative Aspects of Drug Interactions With Receptors

Receptor occupancy theory assumes that a drug's response emanates from a receptor occupied by the drug, a concept that has its basis in the law of mass action. The *dose-response curve* depicts the observed effect of a drug as a function of its concentration in the receptor compartment. Figure 3–2 shows a typical dose-response curve, usually plotted as in Figure 3-2B.

Some drugs cause low-dose stimulation and high-dose inhibition. Such U-shaped relationships are said to display *hormesis*. Several drug-receptor systems can display this property (e.g., prostaglandins, endothelin, and purinergic and serotonergic agonists), which may be at the root of some drug toxicities (Calabrese and Baldwin, 2003).

Affinity, Efficacy, and Potency

In general, the drug-receptor interaction is characterized by (1) binding of drug to receptor and (2) generation of a response in a biological system, as illustrated in Equation 3–1, where the drug or ligand is denoted as L and the inactive receptor as R. The first reaction, the reversible formation of the ligand-receptor complex LR, is governed by the chemical property of *affinity*.

$$L+R \underset{k_{-1}}{\overset{k_{+1}}{\rightleftharpoons}} LR \underset{k_{-2}}{\overset{k_{+2}}{\rightleftharpoons}} LR^* \qquad \text{(Equation 3–1)}$$

LR^* is produced in proportion to $[LR]$ and leads to a *response*. This simple relationship illustrates the reliance of the affinity of the ligand (L) with receptor (R) on both the forward or *association rate* k_{+1} and the reverse or *dissociation rate* k_{-1}. At any given time, the concentration of ligand-receptor complex $[LR]$ is equal to the product of $k_{+1}[L][R]$, the rate of formation of the bimolecular complex LR, minus the product $k_{-1}[LR]$, the rate of dissociation of LR into L and R. At equilibrium (i.e., when $\delta[LR]/\delta t = 0$),

$k_{+1}[L][R] = k_{-1}[LR]$. The *equilibrium dissociation constant* K_D is then described by ratio of the off and on rate constants, k_{-1}/k_{+1}.

Thus, at equilibrium,

$$K_D = \frac{[L][R]}{[LR]} = \frac{k_{-1}}{k_{+1}} \qquad \text{(Equation 3–2)}$$

The *affinity constant* or *equilibrium association constant* K_A is the reciprocal of the equilibrium dissociation constant (i.e., $K_A = 1/K_D$); thus, *a high-affinity drug has a low* K_D *and will bind a greater number of a particular receptor at a low concentration than a low-affinity drug.* As a practical matter, the affinity of a drug is influenced most often by changes in its off rate (k_{-1}) rather than its on rate (k_{+1}).

Equation 3–2 permits us to describe the *fractional occupancy f* of receptors by agonist *L* as a function of $[R]$ and $[LR]$:

$$f = \frac{[\text{ligand-receptor complexes}]}{[\text{total receptors}]} = \frac{[LR]}{[R]+[LR]} \qquad \text{(Equation 3–3)}$$

f can also be expressed in terms of K_A (or K_D) and $[L]$:

$$f = \frac{K_A[L]}{1+K_A[L]} = \frac{[L]}{1/K_A+[L]} = \frac{[L]}{K_D+[L]} \qquad \text{(Equation 3–4)}$$

From Equation 3–4, it follows that *when the concentration of drug equals the* K_D *(or* $1/K_A$*),* $f = 0.5$*, that is, the drug will occupy 50% of the receptors.* When $[L] = K_D$:

$$f = \frac{K_D}{K_D+K_D} = \frac{1}{2} \qquad \text{(Equation 3–4A)}$$

Equation 3–4 describes only receptor occupancy, not the eventual response that may be amplified by the cell. Because of downstream amplification, many signaling systems can reach a full biological response with only a fraction of receptors occupied.

Potency is defined by example in Figure 3–3. Basically, when two drugs produce equivalent responses, the drug whose dose-response curve (plotted as in Figure 3–3A) lies to the left of the other (i.e., the concentration producing a half-maximal effect [EC50] is smaller) is said to be the more potent.

Efficacy reflects the capacity of a drug to activate a receptor and generate a cellular response. Thus, a drug with high efficacy may be a full agonist, eliciting, at some concentration, a full response. A drug with a lower efficacy at the same receptor may not elicit a full response at any dose (see Figure 3–1). A drug with a low intrinsic efficacy will be a partial agonist. A drug that binds to a receptor and exhibits zero efficacy is an antagonist.

Quantifying Agonism

When the relative potency of two agonists of equal efficacy is measured in the same biological system and downstream signaling events are the same for both drugs, the comparison yields a relative measure of the affinity and efficacy of the two agonists (see Figure 3–3). We often describe agonist response by determining the *half-maximally effective concentration* (EC_{50}) for producing a given effect. We can also compare maximal asymptotes in systems where the agonists do not produce maximal response (Figure 3–3B). The advantage of using maxima is that this property depends solely on efficacy, whereas drug *potency* is a mixed function of both affinity and efficacy.

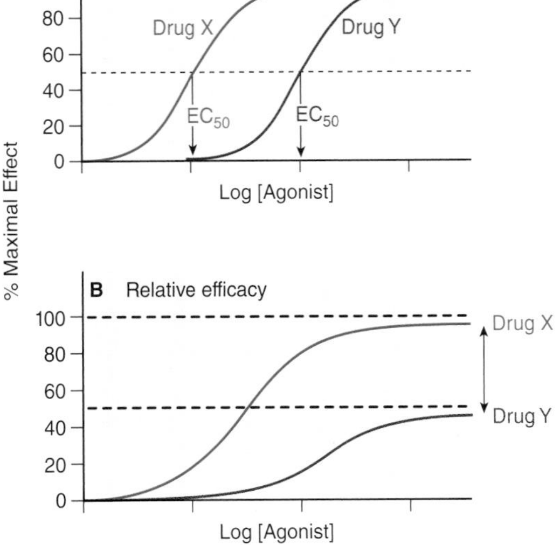

Figure 3–3 *Two ways of quantifying agonism.* **A.** The relative potency of two agonists (drug X, ——; *drug Y*, ——) obtained in the same tissue is a function of their relative affinities and intrinsic efficacies. The EC_{50} of drug X occurs at a concentration that is one-tenth the EC_{50} of drug Y. Thus, drug X is more potent than drug Y. **B.** In systems where the two drugs do not both produce the maximal response characteristic of the tissue, the observed maximal response is a nonlinear function of their relative intrinsic efficacies. Drug X is more efficacious than drug Y; their asymptotic fractional responses are 100% for drug X and 50% for drug Y.

Quantifying Antagonism

Characteristic patterns of antagonism are associated with certain mechanisms of receptor blockade. One is straightforward *competitive antagonism*, whereby a drug with affinity for a receptor but lacking intrinsic efficacy (i.e., an antagonist) competes with the agonist for the primary binding site on the receptor (Ariens, 1954; Gaddum, 1957). *The characteristic pattern of such antagonism is the concentration-dependent production of a parallel shift to the right of the agonist dose-response curve with no change in the maximal response* (Figure 3–4A). The magnitude of the rightward shift of the curve depends on the concentration of the antagonist and its affinity for the receptor (Schild, 1957). *A competitive antagonist will reduce the response to zero.*

A *partial agonist* similarly can compete with a "full" agonist for binding to the receptor. *However, increasing concentrations of a partial agonist will inhibit response to a finite level characteristic of the intrinsic efficacy of the partial agonist.* Partial agonists may be used therapeutically to buffer a response by inhibiting excessive receptor stimulation without totally abolishing receptor stimulation. For example, varenicline is a nicotinic receptor partial agonist used in smoking cessation therapy. Its utility derives from the fact that it activates brain nicotinic receptors sufficiently to prevent craving, but blocks the effects of high-dose nicotine delivered by smoking a cigarette.

An antagonist may dissociate so slowly from the receptor that its action is exceedingly prolonged. In the presence of a slowly dissociating antagonist, the maximal response to the agonist will be depressed at some antagonist concentrations (Figure 3–4B). Operationally, this is referred to as *noncompetitive antagonism*, although the molecular mechanism of action cannot be inferred unequivocally from the effect on the dose-response curve. An *irreversible antagonist* competing for the same binding site as the agonist can produce the same pattern of antagonism shown in Figure 3–4B. Noncompetitive antagonism can be produced by an *allosteric* or *allotopic antagonist*, which binds to a site on the receptor distinct from that of the primary agonist, thereby changing the affinity of the receptor for the agonist. *In the case of an allosteric antagonist, the affinity of the receptor for the agonist is decreased by the antagonist* (Figure 3–4C). In contrast, a drug binding at an allosteric site could potentiate the effects of primary agonists (Figure 3–4D); such a drug would be referred to as an *allosteric agonist* or *coagonist* (May et al., 2007).

The affinity of a competitive antagonist (K_i) for its receptor can be determined in radioligand binding assays or by measuring the functional response of a system to a drug in the presence of the antagonist (Cheng, 2004; Cheng and Prusoff, 1973; Limbird, 2005). Measuring a functional

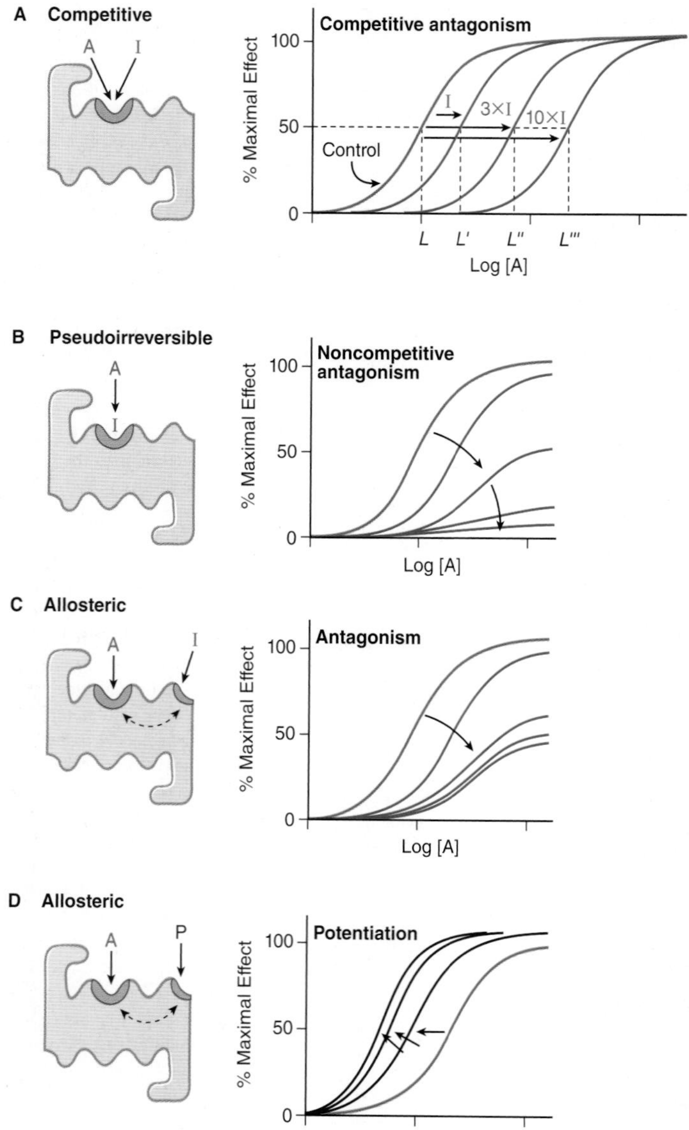

Figure 3–4 *Mechanisms of receptor antagonism.* In each set of curves, the green curve represents the effect of orthosteric agonist, unmodulated by any antagonist or potentiator. **A.** Competitive antagonism occurs when the agonist **A** and antagonist **I** compete for the same binding site on the receptor. Response curves for the agonist are shifted to the right in a concentration-related manner by the antagonist such that the EC_{50} for the agonist increases (e.g., *L* versus *L′*, *L″*, and *L‴*) with the concentration of the antagonist. **B.** If the antagonist binds to the same site as the agonist but does so irreversibly or pseudoirreversibly (slow dissociation but no covalent bond), it causes a shift of the dose-response curve to the right, with progressive depression of the maximal response as [**I**] increases. Allosteric effects occur when an allosteric ligand **I** or **P** binds to a different site on the receptor to either inhibit (I) the response (panel **C.** Increasing concentrations of I shift the curves progressively to right and downward.) or potentiate (**P**) the response (panel **D.** Increasing concentrations of P shift the curves progressively to left.). This allosteric effect is saturable; inhibition or potentiation reaches a limiting value when the allosteric site is fully occupied.

response, concentration curves are run with the agonist alone and with the agonist plus an effective concentration of the antagonist (see Figure 3–4A). As more antagonist (I) is added, a higher concentration of the agonist is needed to produce an equivalent response (the half-maximal, or 50%, response is a convenient and accurately determined level of response). *The extent of the rightward shift of the concentration-dependence curve is a measure of the affinity of the inhibitor, and a high-affinity inhibitor will cause a greater rightward shift than a low-affinity inhibitor at the same inhibitor concentration.*

Using Equations 3–3 and 3–4, one may write mathematical expressions of *fractional occupancy* ***f*** of the receptor R by an agonist ligand (L) for the agonist alone [$f_{control}$] and agonist in the presence of inhibitor [f_{+I}].

For the agonist drug alone, the fractional occupancy is given by Equations 3–3 and 3–4:

$$f_{control} = \frac{[L]}{[L]+K_D} \qquad \text{(Equation 3–5)}$$

For the case of agonist plus antagonist, the problem involves two equilibria:

$R + L \rightleftharpoons RL$ (fractional occupancy is expressed by Eq 3–5)

$$R + I \rightleftharpoons RI;\ K_i = \frac{[R][I]}{[RI]} \text{ or } [RI] = \frac{[R][I]}{K_i} \quad \text{(Equation 3–6)}$$

Fractional occupancy by the agonist L in the presence of I is:

$$f_{+I} = \frac{[RL]}{[RL]+[RI]+[R]} \quad \text{(Equation 3–7)}$$

Equal fractional occupancies can occur in the absence and presence of a competitive inhibitor, but at different concentrations of agonist. The concentration of agonist needed to achieve a designated fractional occupancy in the presence of antagonist (**[L′]**) will be greater than the concentration of agonist needed in the inhibitor's absence (**[L]**). Using the expressions for dissociation constants for the agonist and antagonist ligands (Equations 3-2 and 3-6) and applying a little algebraic tinkering to the righthand side of Equation 3-7, the fractional occupancy in the presence of the competitive inhibitor [f_{+I}] can be expressed in terms of L′, K_D, K_i, and I:

$$f_{+I} = \frac{[L']}{[L']+K_D\left(1+\frac{[I]}{K_i}\right)} \quad \text{(Equation 3–8)}$$

Assuming that equal responses result from equal fractional receptor occupancies in both the absence and presence of antagonist, one can set the fractional occupancies equal at experimentally determined agonist concentrations (**[L]** and **[L′]**) that generate equivalent responses, as depicted in Figure 3–4A. Thus,

$$f_{control} = f_{+I} \quad \text{(Equation 3–9)}$$

$$\frac{[L]}{[L]+K_D} = \frac{[L']}{[L']+K_D\left(1+\frac{[I]}{K_i}\right)} \quad \text{(Equation 3–10)}$$

Simplifying, one obtains

$$\frac{[L']}{[L]} - 1 = \frac{[I]}{K_i} \quad \text{(Equation 3–11)}$$

where all values are known except K_i. *Thus, one can determine the K_i for a reversible, competitive antagonist without knowing the K_D for the agonist and without needing to define the precise relationship between receptor and response.*

Additivity and Synergism: Isobolograms

Drugs with different mechanisms of action are often used in combination to achieve *additive* and *positive synergistic* effects (Figure 3–5). Such positive interactions of two agents may permit use of reduced concentrations of each drug, thereby reducing concentration-dependent adverse effects. *Positive synergism* refers to the *superadditive* effects of drugs used in combination. Drugs used in combination can also demonstrate *negative synergism* or *subadditive effects*, where the efficacy of the drug combination is less than would be expected if the effects were additive. Figure 3–5 is a plot known as an *isobologram*, which shows that a line connecting the EC_{50} values of two drugs, A and B, describes the relative concentrations of each drug that will achieve a half-maximal response *when A and B are used in combination, if the effects of A and B are additive*. Similar lines drawn parallel to the 50% additive line can be used to determine the relative

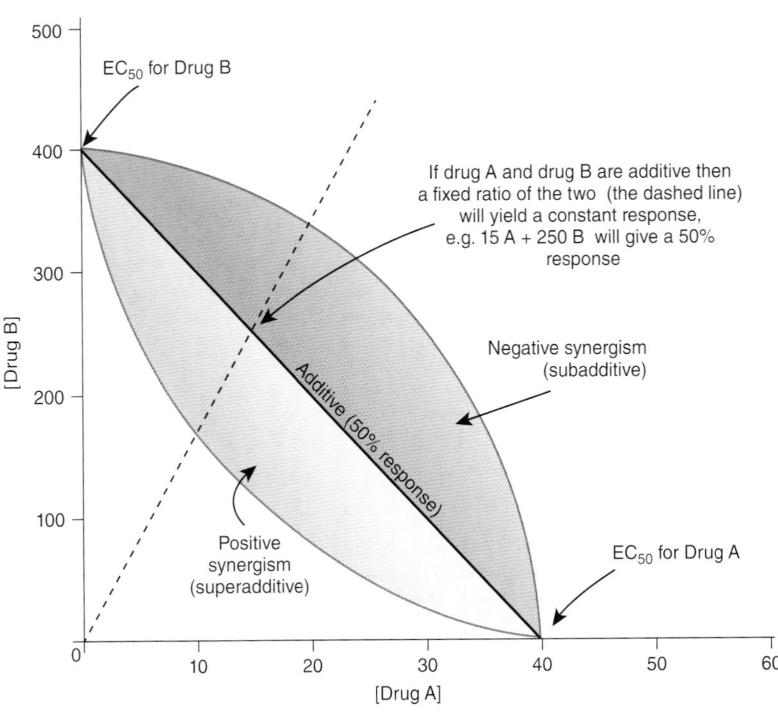

Figure 3–5 *Isobologram showing additivity and synergism of a drug combination.* The isobologram shows the line of additivity for a 50% effect obtained with a combination of two drugs (concentrations of drug A are on the *x* axis, concentrations of drug B are on the *y* axis) that have similar effects but different mechanisms of action. The intercept of the line of additivity (50% effect) with the *x* axis is the EC_{50} for A, while the intercept on the *y* axis is the EC_{50} for B. If the combination of A and B exhibits positive synergism (superadditivity), then the 50% effect with a combination of the two drugs will fall somewhere below the line of additivity, whereas negative synergism (subadditivity) will fall above the line of additivity. Lines of additivity for different percentage effects (e.g., 90% effect) are parallel to the 50% line of additivity. The isobologram can be used to estimate the concentrations of two drugs needed to obtain a given effect when used in combination. For a full explanation of the concept and utility of isoboles, consult Tallarida (2006, 2012).

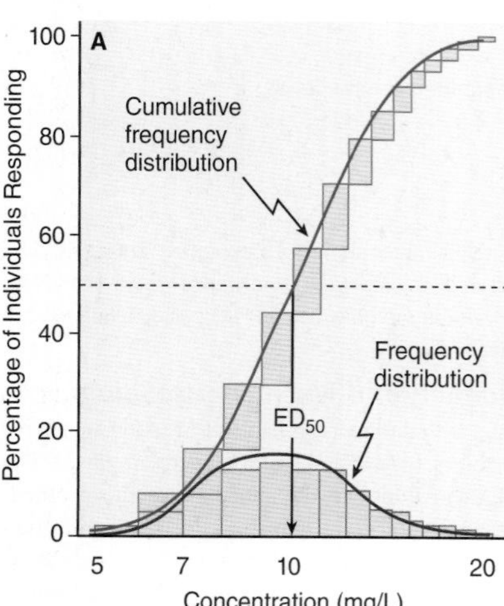

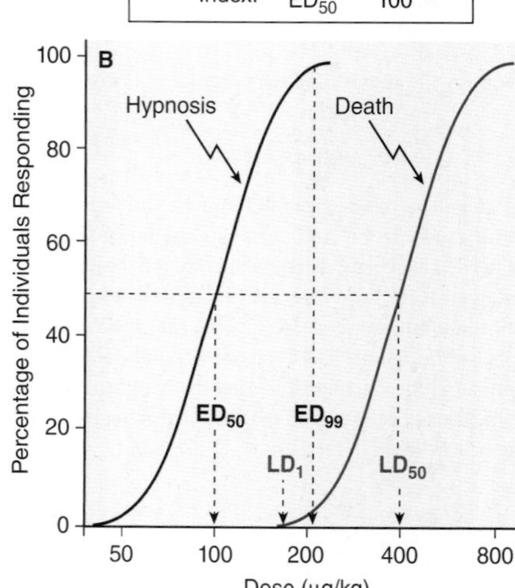

Figure 3–6 *Frequency distribution curves and quantal concentration-effect and dose-effect curves.* **A.** *Frequency distribution curves.* An experiment was performed on 100 subjects, and the effective plasma concentration that produced a quantal response was determined for each individual. The number of subjects who required each dose was plotted, giving a log-normal frequency distribution (**purple bars**). The normal frequency distribution, when summated, yields the cumulative frequency distribution—a sigmoidal curve that is a quantal concentration-effect curve (red bars, red line). **B.** *Quantal dose-effect curves.* Animals were injected with varying doses of a drug, and the responses were determined and plotted. The therapeutic index, the ratio of the LD_{50} to the ED_{50}, is an indication of how selective a drug is in producing its desired effects relative to its toxicity. See text for additional explanation.

concentrations of A and B required to achieve other responses (e.g., 10%, 20%, 80%, 90%, etc.). If A and B are superadditive (positive synergism), the relative concentrations of A and B needed to achieve a given response will fall below the additive response line. Conversely, if A and B are subadditive (negative synergism), their relative concentrations will lie above the additive response line. The basis for the use of isobolograms in characterizing the effects of drug combinations has been developed and reviewed by Tallarida (2006, 2012).

Pharmacodynamic Variability: Individual and Population Pharmacodynamics

Individuals vary in the magnitude of their response to the same concentration of a single drug, and a given individual may not always respond in the same way to the same drug concentration. Drug responsiveness may change because of disease, age, or previous drug administration. Receptors are dynamic, and their concentrations and functions may be up- or downregulated by endogenous and exogenous factors.

Data on the correlation of drug levels with efficacy and toxicity must be interpreted in the context of the pharmacodynamic variability in the population (e.g., genetics, age, disease, and the presence of coadministered drugs). The variability in pharmacodynamic response in the population may be analyzed by constructing a *quantal concentration-effect curve* (Figure 3–6A). The dose of a drug required to produce a specified effect in 50% of the population is the *median effective dose* (*ED_{50}*; see Figure 3–6A). In preclinical studies of drugs, the *median lethal dose* (*LD_{50}*) is determined in experimental animals (Figure 3–6B). The LD_{50}/ED_{50} ratio is an indication of the *therapeutic index*, a term that reflects how selective the drug is in producing its desired effects versus its adverse effects. A similar term, the *therapeutic window*, is the range of steady-state concentrations of drug that provides therapeutic efficacy with minimal toxicity (Figures 2–9 and 3–7). In clinical studies, the dose, or preferably the concentration, of a drug required to produce toxic effects can be compared with the concentration required for therapeutic effects in the population to evaluate the *clinical therapeutic index*. The concentration or dose of drug required to produce a therapeutic effect in most of the population usually will overlap the concentration required to produce toxicity in some of the population, even though the drug's therapeutic index in an individual patient may be large. Thus, a *population therapeutic window* expresses a range of concentrations at which the likelihood of efficacy is high and the probability of adverse effects is low (see Figure 3–7); it does not guarantee efficacy or safety. *Therefore, use of the population therapeutic window to optimize the dosage of a drug should be complemented by monitoring appropriate clinical and surrogate markers for drug effect(s) in a given patient.*

Factors Modifying Drug Action

Numerous factors contribute to the wide patient-to-patient variability in the dose required for optimal therapy observed with many drugs (Figure 3–8). The effects of these factors on variability of drug pharmacokinetics are described more thoroughly in Chapters 2, 5, 6, and 7.

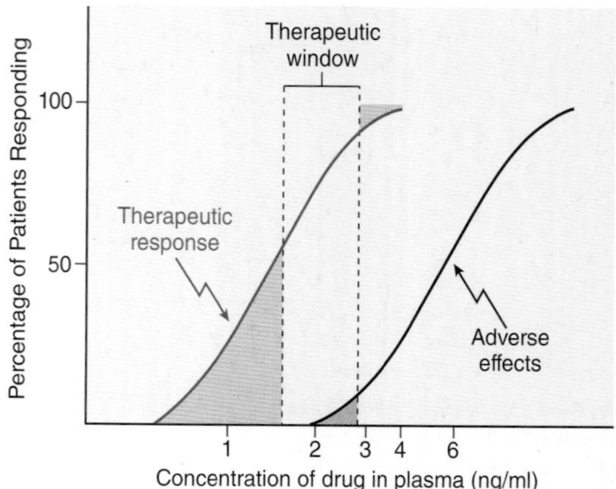

Figure 3–7 *Relation of the therapeutic window of drug concentrations to therapeutic and adverse effects in the population.* The ordinate is linear; the abscissa is logarithmic.

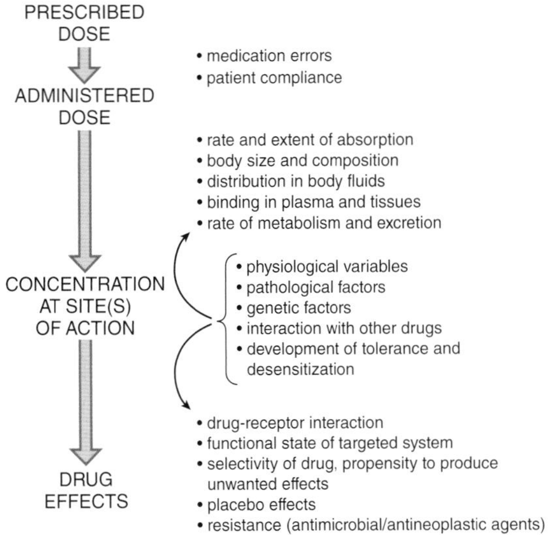

Figure 3–8 *Factors influencing the response to a prescribed drug dose.*

Drug Interactions and Combination Therapy

Drugs are commonly used in combination with other drugs, sometimes to achieve an additive or synergistic effect, but more often because two or more drugs are needed to treat multiple conditions. When drugs are used in combination, one cannot assume that their effects are the same as when each agent is administered by itself. Marked alterations in the effects of some drugs can result from coadministration with other agents, including prescription and nonprescription drugs, supplements, and nutraceuticals. Such interactions can cause toxicity or inhibit the drug effect and the therapeutic benefit. Drug interactions always should be considered when unexpected responses to drugs occur. Understanding the mechanisms of drug interactions provides a framework for preventing them.

Drug interactions may be pharmacokinetic (the delivery of a drug to its site of action is altered by a second drug) or pharmacodynamic (the response of the drug target is modified by a second drug). Examples of pharmacokinetic interactions that can enhance or diminish the delivery of drug to its site of action are provided in Chapter 2. In a patient with multiple comorbidities requiring a variety of medications, it may be difficult to identify adverse effects due to medication interactions and to determine whether these are pharmacokinetic, pharmacodynamic, or some combination of interactions.

Combination therapy constitutes optimal treatment of many conditions, including heart failure (see Chapter 29), hypertension (see Chapter 28), and cancer (see Chapters 65–68). However, some drug combinations produce pharmacodynamic interactions that result in adverse effects. For example, nitrovasodilators produce vasodilation via NO-dependent elevation of cGMP in vascular smooth muscle. The pharmacologic effects of sildenafil, tadalafil, and vardenafil result from inhibition of the PDE5 that hydrolyzes cGMP to 5′GMP in the vasculature. Thus, coadministration of an NO donor (e.g., nitroglycerin) with a PDE5 inhibitor can cause potentially catastrophic vasodilation and severe hypotension.

The oral anticoagulant warfarin has a narrow margin between therapeutic inhibition of clot formation and bleeding complications and is subject to numerous important pharmacokinetic and pharmacodynamic drug interactions. Alterations in dietary vitamin K intake may significantly affect the pharmacodynamics of warfarin and mandate altered dosing; antibiotics that alter the intestinal flora reduce the bacterial synthesis of vitamin K, thereby enhancing the effect of warfarin; concurrent administration of NSAIDs with warfarin increases the risk of GI bleeding almost 4-fold compared with warfarin alone. By inhibiting platelet aggregation, aspirin increases the incidence of bleeding in warfarin-treated patients.

Most drugs are evaluated in young and middle-aged adults, and data on their use in children and the elderly are sparse. At the extremes of age, drug pharmacokinetics and pharmacodynamics can be altered, possibly requiring avoidance of selected drugs or substantial alteration in the dose or dosing regimen to safely produce the desired clinical effect. The American Geriatrics Society publishes the Beers Criteria for Potentially Inappropriate Medication Use in Older Adults, an explicit list of drugs that should be avoided in older adults, drugs that should be avoided or be used at lower doses in patients with reduced kidney function, and specific drug-disease and drug-drug interactions that are known to be harmful in older adults (Beers Update Panel, 2015).

Mechanisms of Drug Action

Receptors That Affect Concentrations of Endogenous Ligands

A large number of drugs act by altering the synthesis, storage, release, transport, or metabolism of endogenous ligands such as neurotransmitters, hormones, and other intercellular mediators. For example, some of the drugs acting on adrenergic neurotransmission include *α-methyltyrosine* (inhibits synthesis of NE), *cocaine* (blocks NE reuptake), *amphetamine* (promotes NE release), and *selegiline* (inhibits NE breakdown by MAO) (see Chapters 8 and 12). There are similar examples for other neurotransmitter systems, including ACh (see Chapters 8 and 10), DA, and 5HT (see Chapters 13–16). Drugs that affect the synthesis and degradation of circulating mediators such as vasoactive peptides (e.g., ACE inhibitors; see Chapter 26) and lipid-derived autocoids (e.g., cyclooxygenase inhibitors; see Chapter 37) are also widely used in the treatment of hypertension, inflammation, myocardial ischemia, and heart failure.

Drug Receptors Associated With Extracellular Processes

Many widely used drugs target enzymes and molecules that control extracellular processes such as thrombosis, inflammation, and immune responses. For instance, the coagulation system is highly regulated and has a number of drug targets that control the formation and degradation of clots, including several coagulation factors (thrombin and factor Xa), antithrombin, and glycoproteins on the surface of platelets that control platelet activation and aggregation (see Chapter 32).

Receptors Utilized by Anti-infective Agents

Anti-infective agents such as antibacterials, antivirals, antifungals, and antiparasitic agents target receptors that are microbial proteins. These proteins are key enzymes in biochemical pathways that are required by the infectious agent but are not critical for the host. Examples of the various mechanisms of action of antibiotics are described in Chapters 52 through 64. A novel approach to preventing infections such as that of the mosquito-borne malaria parasite is to genetically engineer the vector organism to be resistant to infection by the parasite using techniques such as the CRISPR-Cas9 system. Although this approach is just being tested outside the laboratory and must undergo numerous regulatory hurdles before being used on a wide scale, it provides proof of principle that interrupting the life cycle of a parasite in the vector could be as effective as treating the infected host (see Chapter 53).

Receptors That Regulate the Ionic Milieu

A relatively small number of drugs act by affecting the ionic milieu of blood, urine, and the GI tract. The receptors for these drugs are ion pumps and transporters, many of which are expressed only in specialized cells of the kidney and GI tract. Most of the diuretics (e.g., furosemide, chlorothiazide, amiloride) act by directly affecting ion pumps and transporters in epithelial cells of the nephron that increase the movement of Na^+ into the urine or by altering the expression of ion pumps in these cells (e.g., aldosterone). Another therapeutically important target is the H^+,K^+-ATPase (proton pump) of gastric parietal cells. Irreversible inhibition of this proton pump by drugs such as esomeprazole reduces gastric acid secretion by 80%–95% (see Chapter 49).

Intracellular Pathways Activated by Physiological Receptors

Signal Transduction Pathways

The largest number of drug receptors are physiological receptors expressed on the surface of cells that transduce extracellular signals to signals within cells that alter cellular processes. Physiological receptors on the surface of cells have two major functions, ligand binding and message propagation (i.e., transmembrane and intracellular signaling). These functions imply the existence of at least two functional domains within the receptor: a *LBD* and an *effector domain*.

The regulatory actions of a receptor may be exerted directly on its cellular target(s), on *effector protein(s)*, or on intermediary cellular signaling molecules called *transducers*. The receptor, its cellular target, and any intermediary molecules are referred to as a *receptor-effector system* or *signal transduction pathway*. Frequently, the proximal cellular effector protein is not the ultimate physiological target but rather is an enzyme, ion channel, or transport protein that creates, moves, or degrades a small molecule (e.g., a cyclic nucleotide, IP_3, or NO) or ion (e.g., Ca^{2+}) termed a *second messenger*. Second messengers can diffuse in the proximity of their synthesis or release and convey information to a variety of targets that may integrate multiple signals. Even though these second messengers originally were thought of as freely diffusible molecules within the cell, biochemical and imaging studies show that their diffusion and intracellular actions are constrained by *compartmentation*—selective localization of receptor/transducer/effector/signal/signal termination complexes—established by protein-lipid and protein-protein interactions (Baillie, 2009). All cells express multiple forms of proteins designed to localize signaling pathways by protein-protein interactions; these proteins are termed *scaffolds* or *anchoring proteins* (Carnegie et al., 2009).

Receptors and their associated effector and transducer proteins also act as integrators of information as they coordinate signals from multiple ligands with each other and with the differentiated activity of the target cell. For example, signal transduction systems regulated by changes in cAMP and intracellular Ca^{2+} are integrated in many excitable tissues. In cardiac myocytes, an increase in cellular cAMP caused by activation of β adrenergic receptors enhances cardiac contractility by augmenting the rate and amount of Ca^{2+} delivered to the contractile apparatus; thus, cAMP and Ca^{2+} are positive contractile signals in cardiac myocytes. By contrast, cAMP and Ca^{2+} produce opposing effects on the contraction of SMCs: As usual, Ca^{2+} is a contractile signal; however, activation of β receptor-cAMP-PKA pathway in these cells leads to relaxation through the phosphorylation of proteins that mediate Ca^{2+} signaling, such as MLCK and ion channels that hyperpolarize the cell membrane.

Another important property of physiological receptors is their capacity to significantly amplify a physiological signal. Neurotransmitters, hormones, and other extracellular ligands are often present at the LBD of a receptor in very low concentrations (nanomolar to micromolar levels). However, the effector domain or the signal transduction pathway often contains enzymes and enzyme cascades that catalytically amplify the intended signal. These signaling systems are excellent targets for drugs.

Structural and Functional Families of Physiological Receptors

Receptors for physiological regulatory molecules can be assigned to functional families that share common molecular structures and biochemical mechanisms. Table 3–1 outlines six major families of receptors with examples of their physiological ligands, signal transduction systems, and drugs that affect these systems.

G Protein–Coupled Receptors

The GPCRs comprise a large family of transmembrane receptors (Figure 3–9) that span the plasma membrane as a bundle of seven α helices (Palczewski et al., 2000) (Figure 3–10). Amongst the ligands for GPCRs are neurotransmitters such as ACh, biogenic amines such as NE, all eicosanoids and other lipid-signaling molecules, peptide hormones, opioids, amino acids such as GABA, and many other peptide and protein ligands. GPCRs are important regulators of nerve activity in the CNS and are the receptors for the neurotransmitters of the peripheral autonomic nervous system (GPCR Network; Stevens et al., 2013). Because of their number and physiological importance, GPCRs are the targets for many drugs.

GPCR Subtypes. There are multiple receptor subtypes within families of receptors. Ligand-binding studies initially identified receptor subtypes; molecular cloning has greatly accelerated the discovery and definition of additional receptor subtypes; their expression as recombinant proteins has facilitated the discovery of subtype-selective drugs. The distinction between classes and subtypes of receptors, however, is often arbitrary or historical. The α_1, α_2, and β adrenergic receptors differ from each other both in ligand selectivity and in coupling to G proteins (G_q, G_i, and G_s, respectively), yet α and β are considered receptor classes and α_1 and α_2 are considered subtypes. Pharmacological differences amongst receptor subtypes are exploited therapeutically through the development and use of receptor-selective drugs. For example, β_2 adrenergic agonists such as terbutaline are used for bronchodilation in the treatment of asthma in the hope of minimizing cardiac side effects caused by stimulation of the β_1 adrenergic receptor (see Chapter 12). Conversely, the use of β_1-selective antagonists minimizes the likelihood of bronchoconstriction in patients being treated for hypertension or angina (see Chapters 12, 27, and 28).

Receptor Dimerization. GPCRs undergo both homo- and heterodimerization and possibly oligomerization. Dimerization of receptors may regulate the affinity and specificity of the complex for G proteins and the sensitivity of the receptor to phosphorylation by receptor kinases and the binding of arrestin, events important in termination of the action of agonists and removal of receptors from the cell surface. Dimerization also may permit binding of receptors to other regulatory proteins, such as transcription factors.

G Proteins. GPCRs couple to a family of heterotrimeric GTP-binding regulatory proteins termed *G proteins*. G proteins are signal transducers that convey the information from the agonist-bound receptor to one or more effector proteins. G protein–regulated effectors include enzymes such as AC, PLC, cGMP PDE6, and membrane ion channels selective for Ca^{2+} and K^+ (see Table 3–1 and Figure 3–10).

The G protein heterotrimer consists of a guanine nucleotide-binding α subunit, which confers specific recognition to both receptors and effectors, and an associated dimer of β and γ subunits that helps confer membrane localization of the G protein heterotrimer by prenylation of the γ subunit. In the basal state of the receptor-heterotrimer complex, the α subunit contains bound GDP, and the α-GDP:βγ complex is bound to the unliganded receptor (Gilman, 1987) (see Figure 3–9). The α subunits fall into four families (G_s, G_i, G_q, and $G_{12/13}$), which are responsible for coupling GPCRs to relatively distinct effectors. The $G_s\alpha$ subunit uniformly activates AC; the $G_i\alpha$ subunit inhibits certain isoforms of AC; the $G_q\alpha$ subunit activates all forms of PLCβ; and the $G_{12/13}\alpha$ subunits couple to GEFs, such as p115RhoGEF for the small GTP-binding proteins Rho and Rac (Etienne-Manneville and Hall, 2002). The signaling specificity of the large number of possible βγ combinations is not yet clear; nonetheless, it is known that K^+ channels, Ca^{2+} channels, and PI3K are some of the effectors of free βγ dimer. In the instance of cAMP signaling, endocytosis of GPCRs can prolong aspects of signaling and lend "spatial coding" to distal signaling and regulation of transcription (Irannejad et al., 2015). Figure 3–10 and its legend summarize the basic activation/inactivation scheme for GPCR-linked systems.

Second-Messenger Systems. ***Cyclic AMP.*** cAMP is synthesized by the enzyme AC; stimulation is mediated by the $G_s\alpha$ subunit, inhibition by the $G_i\alpha$ subunit. There are nine membrane-bound isoforms of AC and one soluble isoform found in mammals (Dessauer et al., 2017; Hanoune and Defer, 2001). cAMP generated by ACs has three major targets in most cells: the cAMP-dependent PKA; cAMP-regulated GEFs termed EPACs (Cheng et al., 2008; Roscioni et al., 2008); and, via PKA phosphorylation, a transcription factor termed CREB (Mayr and Montminy, 2001; Sands and Palmer, 2008). In cells with specialized functions, cAMP can have additional targets, such as CNG and HCN (Wahl-Schott and Biel, 2009), and cyclic nucleotide-regulated PDEs. For an overview

TABLE 3-1 ■ PHYSIOLOGICAL RECEPTORS

STRUCTURAL FAMILY	FUNCTIONAL FAMILY	PHYSIOLOGICAL LIGANDS	EFFECTORS AND TRANSDUCERS	EXAMPLE DRUGS
GPCR	β Adrenergic receptors	NE, EPI, DA	G_s; AC	Dobutamine, propranolol
	Muscarinic cholinergic receptors	ACh	G_i and G_q; AC, ion channels, PLC	Atropine
	Eicosanoid receptors	Prostaglandins, leukotrienes, thromboxanes	G_s, G_i, and G_q proteins	Misoprostol, montelukast
	Thrombin receptors (PAR)	Receptor peptide	$G_{12/13}$, GEFs	(In development)
Ion channels	Ligand gated	ACh (M_2), GABA, 5HT	Na^+, Ca^{2+}, K^+, Cl^-	Nicotine, gabapentin
	Voltage gated	None (activated by membrane depolarization)	Na^+, Ca^{2+}, K^+, other ions	Lidocaine, verapamil
Transmembrane enzymes	Receptor tyrosine kinases	Insulin, PDGF, EGF, VEGF, growth factors	SH2 domain and PTB-containing proteins	Herceptin, imatinib
	Membrane bound GC	Natriuretic peptides	cGMP	Nesiritide
	Tyrosine phosphatases	Pleiotrophin, contactins	Tyr-phosphorylated proteins	
Transmembrane, nonenzymes	Cytokine receptors	Interleukins and other cytokines	Jak/STAT, soluble tyrosine kinases	Interferons, anakinra
	Toll-like receptors	Lipopolysaccharide, bacterial products	MyD88, IRAKs, NF-kB	(In development)
Nuclear receptors	Steroid receptors	Estrogen, testosterone	Coactivators	Estrogens, androgens, cortisol
	Thyroid hormone receptors	Thyroid hormone		Thyroid hormone
	PPARγ	PPARγ		Thiazolidinediones
Intracellular enzymes	Soluble GC	NO, Ca^{2+}	cGMP	Nitrovasodilators

of cyclic nucleotide action and a historical perspective, see Beavo and Brunton (2002).

- **PKA.** The PKA holoenzyme consists of two catalytic (C) subunits reversibly bound to a regulatory (R) subunit dimer to form a heterotetrameric complex (R_2C_2). When AC is activated and cAMP concentrations increase, four cAMP molecules bind to the R_2C_2 complex, two to each R subunit, causing a conformational change in the R subunits that lowers their affinity for the C subunits, resulting in their activation. The active C subunits phosphorylate serine and threonine residues on specific protein substrates. There are multiple isoforms of PKA; molecular cloning has revealed α and β isoforms of both the regulatory subunits (RI and RII), as well as three C subunit isoforms Cα, Cβ, and Cγ. The R subunits exhibit different subcellular localization and binding affinities for cAMP, giving rise to PKA holoenzymes with different thresholds for activation (Taylor et al., 2008). PKA function also is modulated by subcellular localization mediated by AKAPs (Carnegie et al., 2009).
- **PKG.** Stimulation of receptors that raise intracellular cGMP concentrations (see Figure 3–13) leads to the activation of the cGMP-dependent PKG that phosphorylates some of the same substrates as PKA and some that are PKG-specific. Unlike the heterotetramer (R_2C_2) structure of the PKA holoenzyme, the catalytic domain and cyclic nucleotide-binding domains of PKG are expressed as a single polypeptide, which dimerizes to form the PKG holoenzyme.

  Protein kinase G exists in two homologous forms, PKG-I and PKG-II. PKG-I has an acetylated N terminus, is associated with the cytoplasm, and has two isoforms (Iα and Iβ) that arise from alternate splicing. PKG-II has a myristylated N-terminus, is membrane-associated, and can be localized by PKG-anchoring proteins in a manner analogous to that for PKA, although the docking domains of PKA and PKG differ structurally. Pharmacologically important effects of elevated cGMP include modulation of platelet activation and relaxation of smooth muscle (Rybalkin et al., 2003). Receptors linked to cGMP synthesis are covered in a separate section that follows.
- **PDEs.** Cyclic nucleotide PDEs form another family of important signaling proteins whose activities are regulated via the rate of gene transcription as well as by second messengers (cyclic nucleotides or Ca^{2+}) and interactions with other signaling proteins such as β arrestin and PKs. PDEs hydrolyze the cyclic 3′,5′-phosphodiester bond in cAMP and cGMP, thereby terminating their action. The PDEs comprise a superfamily with more than 50 different proteins (Conti and Beavo, 2007). The substrate specificities of the different PDEs include those specific for cAMP hydrolysis and for cGMP hydrolysis and some that hydrolyze both cyclic nucleotides. PDEs (mainly PDE3 forms) are drug targets for treatment of diseases such as asthma, cardiovascular diseases such as heart failure, atherosclerotic coronary and peripheral arterial disease, and neurological disorders. PDE5 inhibitors (e.g., sildenafil) are used in treating chronic obstructive pulmonary disease and erectile dysfunction (Mehats et al., 2002).
- **EPACs.** EPAC, also known as cAMP-GEF, is a novel cAMP-dependent signaling protein that plays unique roles in cAMP signaling. cAMP signaling through EPAC can occur in isolation or in concert with PKA signaling (Schmidt et al., 2013). EPAC serves as a cAMP-regulated GEF for the family of small Ras GTPases (especially the Rap small GTPases), catalyzing the exchange of GTP for GDP, thus activating the small GTPase by promoting formation of the GTP-bound form. Two isoforms of EPAC are known, EPAC1 and EPAC2; they differ in their architecture and tissue expression. Both EPAC isoforms are multidomain proteins that contain a regulatory cAMP-binding domain, a catalytic domain, and domains that determine the intracellular localization of EPAC. Compared to EPAC2, EPAC1 contains an additional N-terminal low-affinity cAMP-binding domain. The expression of EPAC1 and EPAC2 are differentially regulated during development

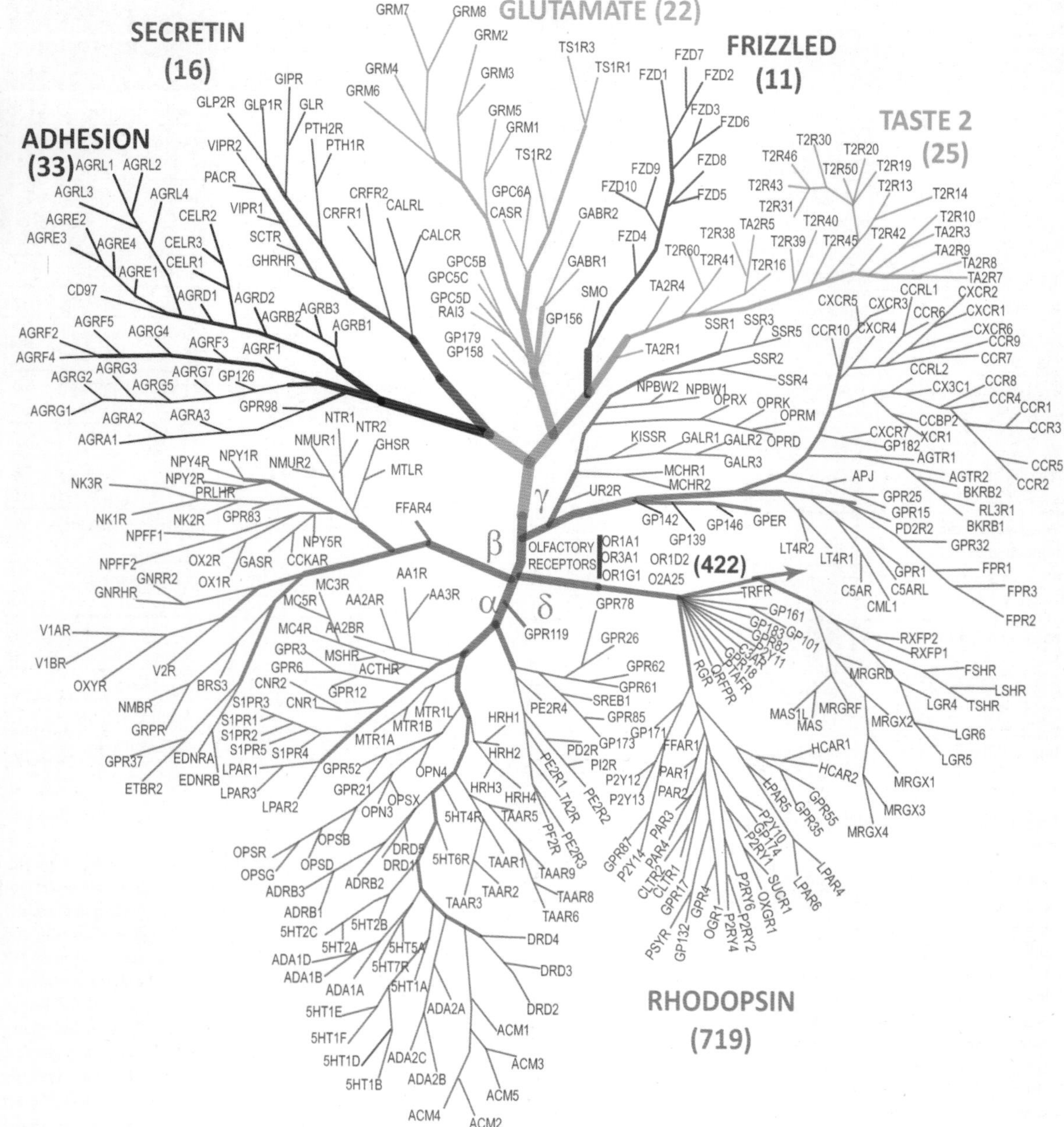

Figure 3–9 *The human GPCR superfamily.* Human GPCRs are targeted by about 30% of marketed drugs. This dendrogram, constructed using sequence similarities within the seven-transmembrane region, identifies GPCRs by their names in the UniProt database. There are over 825 human GPCRs, which can be subdivided into the color-coded groups named by the capitalized words on the outer edge of the dendrogram (number of group members in parentheses). These groups can be further subdivided on the basis of sequence similarity. The large Rhodopsin class is subdivided into four broad groups: α, β, δ, and γ. Olfactory receptors constitute the largest fraction of the Rhodopsin class of GPCRs, with 422 members. Receptors on the dendrogram that readers will frequently encounter include AA2AR, A_{2A} adenosine receptor; ACM3, M_3 muscarinic acetylcholine receptor; ADRB1, β_1 adrenergic receptor; AGTR1, AT_1 angiotensin receptor; CNR1, CB_1 cannabinoid receptor; CXCR4, CXC_4 chemokine receptor; DRD2, D_2 dopamine receptor; EDNRA, ET_A endothelin receptor; FPR1, f-Met-Leu-Phe receptor; GCGR, glucagon receptor; GRM1, $mGluR_1$ metabotropic glutamate receptor; HRH1, H_1 histamine receptor; 5HT2B, the $5HT_{2B}$ serotonin receptor; OPRM, μ opioid receptor; RHO, rhodopsin; SMO, smoothened homolog; S1PR1, $S1P_1$ sphingosine-1-phosphate receptor, also known as EDG_1; TSHR, thyrotropin (TSH) receptor; and VIPR1, V_1 vasoactive intestinal peptide receptor. Details of entries on the dendrogram are available from the GPCR Network (http://gpcr.usc.edu). Additional information on GPCRs is available from the IUPHAR/BPS Guide to Pharmacology (http://www.guidetopharmacology.org). (Reproduced with permission from Angela Walker, Vsevolod Katrich, and Raymond Stevens of the GPCR Network at the University of Southern California, as created in the Stevens lab by Yekaterina Kadyshevskaya.)

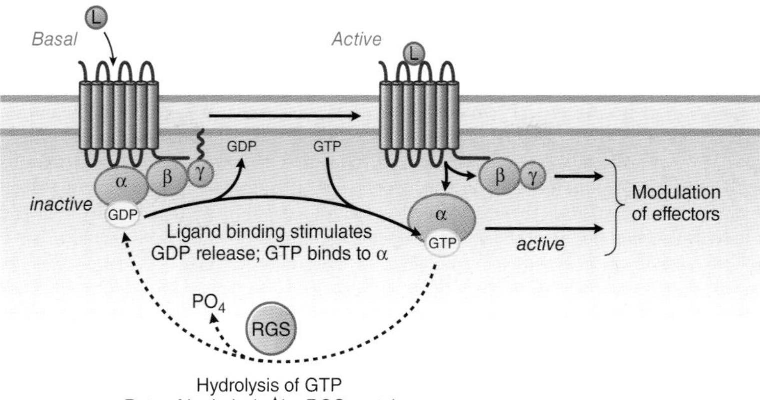

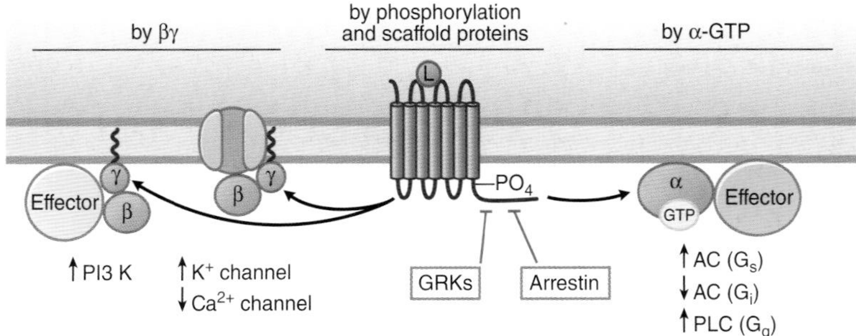

Figure 3–10 *The basic GPCR-G_s protein-effector pathway.* In the absence of ligand, the GPCR and G protein heterotrimer form a complex in the membrane with the Gα subunit bound to GDP. Following binding of ligand, the receptor and G protein α subunit undergo a conformational change leading to release of GDP, binding of GTP, and dissociation of the complex. The activated GTP-bound Gα subunit and the freed βγ dimer bind to and regulate effectors. The system is returned to the basal state by hydrolysis of the GTP on the α subunit, a reaction that is markedly enhanced by the RGS proteins. Prolonged stimulation of the receptor can lead to downregulation of the receptor. This event is initiated by GRKs that phosphorylate the C-terminal tail of the receptor, leading to recruitment of proteins termed arrestins; arrestins bind to the receptor on the internal surface, displacing G proteins and inhibiting signaling. Detailed descriptions of these signaling pathways are given throughout the text in relation to the therapeutic actions of drugs affecting these pathways.

and in a variety of disease states. EPAC2 can promote incretin-stimulated insulin secretion from pancreatic β cells through activation of Rap1 (Figure 47–3). Sulfonylureas, important oral drugs used to treat type II diabetes mellitus, may act in part by activating EPAC2 in β cells and increasing insulin release.

G_q-PLC-DAG/IP_3-Ca^{2+} Pathway. Calcium is an important messenger in all cells and can regulate diverse responses, including gene expression, contraction, secretion, metabolism, and electrical activity. Ca^{2+} can enter the cell through Ca^{2+} channels in the plasma membrane (see the Ion Channels section) or be released by hormones or growth factors from intracellular stores. In keeping with its role as a signal, the basal Ca^{2+} level in cells is maintained in the 100-nM range by membrane Ca^{2+} pumps that extrude Ca^{2+} to the extracellular space and a SERCA in the membrane of the ER that accumulates Ca^{2+} into its storage site in the ER/SR.

Hormones and growth factors release Ca^{2+} from its intracellular storage site, the ER, via a signaling pathway that begins with activation of PLC, of which there are two primary forms, PLCβ and PLCγ. GPCRs that couple to G_q or G_i activate PLCβ by activating the Gα subunit (see Figure 3–10) and releasing the βγ dimer. Both the active, G_q-GTP–bound α subunit and the βγ dimer can activate certain isoforms of PLCβ. PLCγ isoforms are activated by tyrosine phosphorylation, including phosphorylation by receptor and nonreceptor tyrosine kinases.

The PLCs are cytosolic enzymes that translocate to the plasma membrane on receptor stimulation. When activated, they hydrolyze a minor membrane phospholipid, phosphatidylinositol-4,5-bisphosphate, to generate two intracellular signals, IP_3 and the lipid DAG. DAG directly activates some members of the PKC family. IP_3 diffuses to the ER, where it activates the IP_3 receptor in the ER membrane, causing release of stored Ca^{2+} from the ER (Patterson et al., 2004). Release of Ca^{2+} from these intracellular stores raises Ca^{2+} levels in the cytoplasm many-fold within seconds and activates Ca^{2+}-dependent enzymes such as some of the PKCs and Ca^{2+}/calmodulin-sensitive enzymes such as one of the cAMP-hydrolyzing PDEs and a family of Ca^{2+}/calmodulin-sensitive PKs (e.g., phosphorylase kinase, MLCK, and CaM kinases II and IV) (Hudmon and Schulman, 2002). Depending on the cell's differentiated function, the Ca^{2+}/calmodulin kinases and PKC may regulate the bulk of the downstream events in the activated cells.

Ion Channels

Changes in the flux of ions across the plasma membrane are critical regulatory events in both excitable and nonexcitable cells. To establish the electrochemical gradients required to maintain a membrane potential, all cells express ion transporters for Na^+, K^+, Ca^{2+}, and Cl^-. For example, the Na^+,K^+-ATPase expends cellular ATP to pump Na^+ out of the cell and K^+ into the cell. The electrochemical gradients thus established are used by excitable tissues such as nerve and muscle to generate and transmit electrical impulses, by nonexcitable cells to trigger biochemical and secretory events, and by all cells to support a variety of secondary symport and antiport processes (see Figures 2–2 and 5–4).

Passive ion fluxes down cellular electrochemical gradients are regulated by a large family of ion channels located in the membrane. Humans express about 232 distinct ion channels to precisely regulate the flow of Na^+, K^+, Ca^{2+}, and Cl^- across the cell membrane (Jegla et al., 2009). Because of their roles as regulators of cell function, these proteins are important drug targets. The diverse ion channel family can be divided into subfamilies based on the mechanisms that open the channels, their architecture, and the ions they conduct. They can also be classified as *voltage-activated, ligand-activated, store-activated, stretch-activated,* and *temperature-activated channels.*

Voltage-Gated Channels. Humans express multiple isoforms of voltage-gated channels for Na^+, K^+, Ca^{2+}, and Cl^- ions. In nerve and muscle cells, voltage-gated Na^+ channels are responsible for the generation of robust action potentials that depolarize the membrane from its resting potential of −70 mV up to a potential of +20 mV within a few milliseconds. These Na^+ channels are composed of three subunits, a pore-forming α subunit and two regulatory β subunits (Purves et al., 2011). The α subunit is a 260-kDa protein containing four domains that form a Na^+ ion–selective pore by arranging into a pseudotetramer shape. The β subunits are 36-kDa proteins that span the membrane once (Figure 3–11A). Each domain of the α subunit contains six membrane-spanning helices (S1–S6) with an extracellular loop between S5 and S6, termed the pore-forming or P loop; the P loop dips back into the pore and, combined with residues from the corresponding P loops from the other domains, provides a selectivity filter for the Na^+ ion (see Figure 14–2). Four other helices surrounding the pore (one S4 helix from each of the domains) contain a set of charged amino acids that form the voltage sensor and cause a conformational change in the pore at more positive voltages, leading to opening of the pore and depolarization of the membrane (Figure 11–2). The voltage-activated Na^+ channels in pain neurons are targets for local anesthetics, such as lidocaine and tetracaine, which block the pore, inhibit depolarization, and thus block the sensation of pain (see Chapter 22). They are also the targets of the naturally occurring marine toxins *tetrodotoxin* and *saxitoxin*. Voltage-activated Na^+ channels are also important targets of many drugs used to treat cardiac arrhythmias (see Chapter 30).

Voltage-gated Ca^{2+} channels have a similar architecture to voltage-gated Na^+ channels with a large α subunit (four domains of five membrane-spanning helices) and three regulatory subunits (the β, δ, and γ subunits).

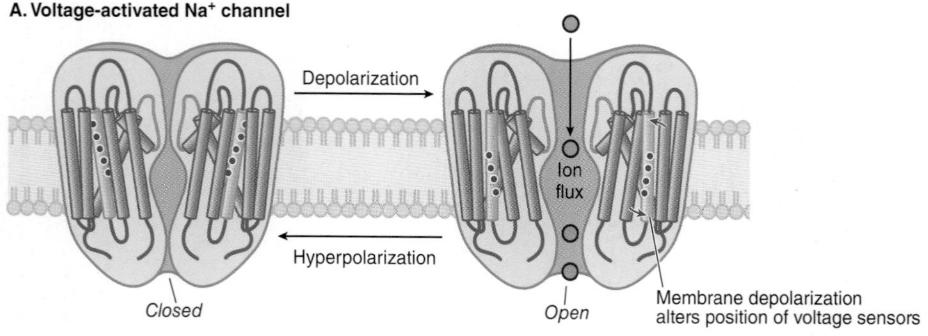

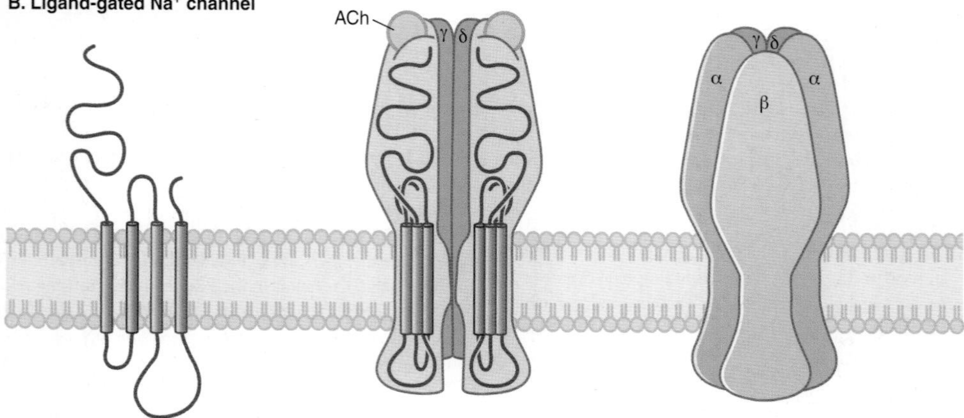

Figure 3–11 *Two types of ion channels regulated by receptors and drugs.* **A.** A voltage-activated Na^+ channel with the pore in the closed and open states. The pore-forming P loops are shown in blue, angled into the pore to form the selectivity filter. The S4 helices forming the voltage sensor are shown in orange, with the positively charged amino acids displayed as red dots. **B.** Ligand-gated nicotinic ACh receptor expressed in the skeletal muscle neuromuscular junction. The pore is made up of five subunits, each with a large extracellular domain and four transmembrane helices (one of these subunits is shown at the left of panel **B**). The helix that lines the pore is shown in blue. The receptor is composed of two α subunits and β, γ, and δ subunits. See text for discussion of other ligand-gated ion channels. Detailed descriptions of specific channels are given throughout the text in relation to the therapeutic actions of drugs affecting these channels (see especially Chapters 11, 14, and 22). (Adapted with permission from Purves D et al., eds. *Neuroscience*. 5th ed. Sinauer Associates, Inc., Sunderland, MA, **2011**. By permission of Oxford University Press, USA.)

Ca^{2+} channels can be responsible for initiating an action potential (as in the pacemaker cells of the heart) but are more commonly responsible for modifying the shape and duration of an action potential initiated by fast voltage-gated Na^+ channels. These channels initiate the influx of Ca^{2+} that stimulates the release of neurotransmitters in the central, enteric, and autonomic nervous systems and that control heart rate and impulse conduction in cardiac tissue (see Chapters 8, 14, and 30). The L-type voltage-gated Ca^{2+} channels are subject to additional regulation via phosphorylation by PKA. Voltage-gated Ca^{2+} channels expressed in smooth muscle regulate vascular tone; the intracellular concentration of Ca^{2+} is critical to regulating the phosphorylation state of the contractile apparatus via the activity of the Ca^{2+}/calmodulin-sensitive MLCK. Ca^{2+} channel antagonists such as nifedipine, diltiazem, and verapamil are effective vasodilators and are widely used to treat hypertension, angina, and certain cardiac arrhythmias (see Chapters 27, 28, and 30).

Voltage-gated K^+ channels are the most numerous and structurally diverse members of the voltage-gated channel family and include the voltage-gated K_v channels, the inwardly rectifying K^+ channel, and the tandem or two-pore domain "leak" K^+ channels (Jegla et al., 2009). The inwardly rectifying channels and the two-pore channels are voltage insensitive, regulated by G proteins and H^+ ions, and greatly stimulated by general anesthetics. Increasing K^+ conductance through these channels drives the membrane potential more negative (closer to the equilibrium potential for K^+); thus, these channels are important in regulating resting membrane potential and restoring the resting membrane at -70 to -90 mV following depolarization.

Ligand-Gated Channels. Channels activated by the binding of a ligand to a specific site in the channel protein have a diverse architecture and set of ligands. Major ligand-gated channels in the nervous system are those that respond to excitatory neurotransmitters such as ACh (Figures 3–11B and 11–1) or glutamate (or agonists such as AMPA and NMDA) and inhibitory neurotransmitters such as glycine or GABA (Purves et al., 2011). Activation of these channels is responsible for the majority of synaptic transmission by neurons both in the CNS and in the periphery (see Chapters 8, 11, and 14). In addition, there are a variety of more specialized ion channels that are activated by intracellular small molecules and are structurally distinct from conventional ligand-gated ion channels. These include ion channels that are formally members of the K_v family, such as the HCN channel expressed in the heart that is responsible for the slow depolarization seen in phase 4 of atrioventricular and sinoatrial nodal cell action potentials (Wahl-Schott and Biel, 2009) (see Chapter 30) and the CNG channel that is important for vision (see Chapter 69). The intracellular small-molecule category of ion channels also includes the IP_3-sensitive Ca^{2+} channel responsible for release of Ca^{2+} from the ER and the sulfonylurea "receptor" (SUR1) that associates with the $K_{ir}6.2$ channel to regulate the K_{ATP} in pancreatic β cells. The K_{ATP} channel is the target of oral hypoglycemic drugs such as sulfonylureas and meglitinides that stimulate insulin release from pancreatic β cells and are used to treat type 2 diabetes (see Chapter 47).

The nicotinic ACh receptor is an instructive example of a ligand-gated ion channel. Isoforms of this channel are expressed in the CNS, in autonomic ganglia, and at the neuromuscular junction (Figures 3–11B and 11–2). The pentameric channel consists of four different subunits (2α, β, δ, γ) in the neuromuscular junction or two different subunits (2α, 3β) in autonomic ganglia (Purves et al., 2011). Each α subunit has an identical ACh binding site; the different compositions of the other three subunits between the neuronal and neuromuscular junction receptors account for the ability of competitive antagonists such as rocuronium to inhibit the receptor in the neuromuscular junction without effect on the ganglionic receptor. This property is exploited to provide muscle relaxation during surgery with minimal autonomic side effects (Chapter 11). Each subunit of the receptor contains a large, extracellular N-terminal domain, four membrane-spanning helices (one of which lines the pore in the assembled complex), and an internal loop between helices 3 and 4 that forms the intracellular domain of the channel. The pore opening in the channel measures about 3 nm, whereas the diameter of a Na^+ or K^+ ion is only 0.3 nm or less. Accordingly, ligand-gated ion channels do not possess the exquisite ion selectivity found in most voltage-activated channels, and activation of the nicotinic ACh receptor allows passage of both Na^+ and K^+ ions.

Transient Receptor Potential Channels. The TRP cation channels are involved in a variety of physiological and pathophysiological sensory processes, including nociception, heat and cold sensation, mechanosensation, and sensation of chemicals such as capsaicin and menthol. The TRP channel superfamily is diverse and consists of 28 channels in six families (Cao et al., 2013; Ramsey et al., 2006; Venkatachalam and Montell, 2007). The typical TRP channel structure consists of monomers predicted to have six transmembrane helices (S1–S6) with a pore-forming loop between S5 and S6 and large intracellular regions at the amino and carboxyl termini. Most of the functional TRP channels are homotetramers, but heteromultimers are also formed. Genetic mutations in TRP channels are related to channelopathies that are associated with inherited pain syndrome, several different kidney and bladder diseases, and skeletal dysplasias. Agonists and antagonists are being developed and are in clinical trials for a wide variety of indications, including pain, gastroesophageal reflux disorder, respiratory disorders, osteoarthritis, skin disorders, and overactive bladder.

Transmembrane Receptors Linked to Intracellular Enzymes

Receptor Tyrosine Kinases. The receptor tyrosine kinases include receptors for hormones such as insulin; growth factors such EGF, PDGF, NGF, FGF, VEGF; and ephrins. With the exception of the insulin receptor, which has α and β chains (see Chapter 47), these macromolecules consist of single polypeptide chains with large, cysteine-rich extracellular domains, short transmembrane domains, and an intracellular region containing one or two protein tyrosine kinase domains. Activation of growth factor receptors leads to cell survival, cell proliferation, and differentiation. Activation of the ephrin receptors leads to neuronal angiogenesis, axonal migration, and guidance (Ferguson, 2008).

The inactive state of growth factor receptors is monomeric; binding of ligand induces dimerization of the receptor and cross-phosphorylation of the kinase domains on multiple tyrosine residues (Figure 3–12A). The phosphorylation of other tyrosine residues forms docking sites for the SH2 domains contained in a large number of signaling proteins. There are over 100 proteins encoded in the human genome containing SH2 domains, and following receptor activation, large signaling complexes are formed on the receptor that eventually lead to cell proliferation.

Molecules recruited to phosphotyrosine-containing proteins by their SH2 domains include PLCγ, the activity of which raises intracellular levels of Ca^{2+} and activates PKC. The α and β isoforms of PI3K contain SH2 domains, dock at the phosphorylated receptor, are activated, and increase the level of PIP_3 and PKB (also known as Akt). PKB can regulate mTOR, which is upstream of various signaling pathways, and the *Bad* protein that is important in apoptosis.

In addition to recruiting enzymes, phosphotyrosine-presenting proteins can interact with SH2 domain-containing adaptor molecules without activity (e.g., Grb2), which in turn attract GEFs such as Sos that can activate the small GTP-binding protein Ras. The small GTP-binding proteins Ras and Rho belong to a large family of small monomeric GTPases. All of the small GTPases are activated by GEFs regulated by a variety of mechanisms and inhibited by GAPs (Etienne-Manneville and Hall, 2002). Activation of members of the Ras family leads in turn to activation of a PK cascade termed the Ras-MAPK pathway. Activation of the MAPK pathway is one of the major routes used by growth factor receptors to signal to the nucleus and stimulate cell growth (Figure 3–12A). Oncogenic mutations that result in constitutively activated growth factor receptors and Ras can also activate the MAPK pathway and drive tumor proliferation. Anticancer agents that target the MAPK pathway and the protein tyrosine kinase activity of oncogenic growth factors are now important agents in treating several forms of cancer (see Chapter 65 and 67).

Jak-STAT Receptor Pathway. Cells express a family of receptors for cytokines such as γ-interferon and hormones such as growth hormone and prolactin, which signal to the nucleus by a more direct manner than the receptor tyrosine kinases. These receptors have no intrinsic enzymatic activity; rather, the intracellular domain binds a separate, intracellular tyrosine kinase termed a Jak. On dimerization induced by ligand binding, Jaks phosphorylate other proteins termed STATs, which translocate to the nucleus and regulate transcription (Figure 3–12B). The entire pathway is termed the Jak-STAT pathway (Gough et al., 2008; Wang et al., 2009). There are four Jaks and six STATs in mammals that, depending on the cell type and signal, combine differentially to activate gene transcription.

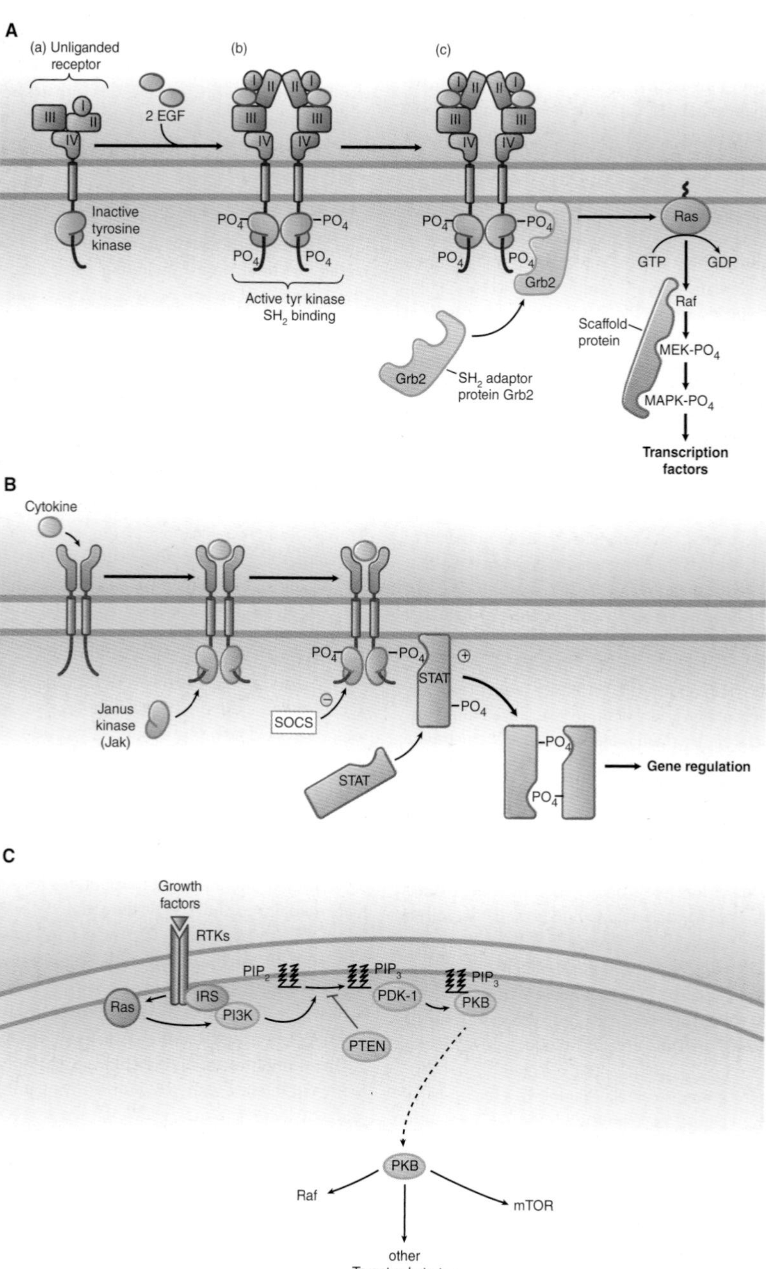

Figure 3–12 *Mechanism of activation of a receptor tyrosine kinase and a cytokine receptor.* **A.** *Activation of the EGF receptor.* The extracellular structure of the unliganded receptor (a) contains four domains (I–IV), which rearrange significantly on binding two EGF molecules. In (b), the conformational changes lead to activation of the cytoplasmic tyrosine kinase domains and tyrosine phosphorylation of intracellular regions to form SH2 binding sites. (c). The adapter molecule Grb2 binds to the phosphorylated tyrosine residues and activates the Ras-MAPK cascade. **B.** *Activation of a cytokine receptor.* Binding of the cytokine causes dimerization of the receptor and recruits the Jaks to the cytoplasmic tails of the receptor. Jaks transphosphorylate and lead to the phosphorylation of the STATs. The phosphorylated STATs translocate to the nucleus and regulate transcription. There are proteins termed SOCS (suppressors of cytokine signaling) that inhibit the Jak-STAT pathway. **C.** *Activation of the mTOR pathway.* Signaling via this pathway promotes growth, proliferation, and survival of cells via a complex web of signaling pathways (see Figures 35–2 and 67–4 and Guri and Hall, 2016). mTOR signaling is emerging as a major consideration in immunosuppression and cancer pharmacotherapy, and inhibitors of mTOR signaling are sometimes included as adjunct therapy.

Receptor Serine-Threonine Kinases. Protein ligands such as TGF-β activate a family of receptors that are analogous to the receptor tyrosine kinases except that they have a serine-threonine kinase domain in the cytoplasmic region of the protein. There are two isoforms of the monomeric receptor protein, type I (seven forms) and type II (five forms). In the basal state, these proteins exist as monomers; upon binding an agonist ligand, they dimerize, leading to phosphorylation of the kinase domain of the type I monomer, which activates the receptor. The activated receptor then phosphorylates a gene regulatory protein termed a *Smad*. Once phosphorylated by the activated receptor on a serine residue, Smad dissociates from the receptor, migrates to the nucleus, associates with transcription factors, and regulates genes leading to morphogenesis and transformation. There are also inhibitory Smads (the Smad6 and Smad7 isoforms) that compete with the phosphorylated Smads to terminate signaling.

Toll-like Receptors. Signaling related to the innate immune system is carried out by a family of more than 10 single membrane-spanning receptors termed TLRs, which are highly expressed in hematopoietic cells. In a single polypeptide chain, these receptors contain a large extracellular LBD, a short membrane-spanning domain, and a cytoplasmic region termed the TIR domain that lacks intrinsic enzymatic activity. *Ligands for TLRs comprise a multitude of pathogen products, including lipids, peptidoglycans, lipopeptides, and viruses.* Activation of TLRs produces an inflammatory response to the pathogenic microorganisms.

The first step in activation of TLRs by ligands is dimerization, which in turn causes signaling proteins to bind to the receptor to form a signaling complex. Ligand-induced dimerization recruits a series of adaptor proteins, including Mal and MyD88 to the intracellular TIR domain; these proteins in turn recruit the IRAKs. The IRAKs autophosphorylate in the complex and subsequently form a more stable complex with MyD88. The phosphorylation event also recruits TRAF6 to the complex, which facilitates interaction with a ubiquitin ligase that attaches a polyubiquitin molecule to TRAF6. This complex can now interact with TAK1 and the adaptor protein TAB1. TAK1 is a member of the MAPK family, which activates the NF-κB kinases; phosphorylation of the NF-κB transcription factors causes their translocation to the nucleus and transcriptional activation of a variety of inflammatory genes (Gay and Gangloff, 2007).

TNF-α Receptors. The mechanism of action of TNF-α signaling to the NF-κB transcription factors is similar to that used by TLRs in that the intracellular domain of the receptor has no enzymatic activity. The TNF-α receptor is another membrane monospan protein with an extracellular LBD, a transmembrane domain, and a cytoplasmic domain termed the *death domain*. TNF-α binds a complex composed of TNF receptor 1 and TNF receptor 2. Upon trimerization, the death domains bind the adaptor protein TRADD, which recruits the RIP1 to form a receptor-adaptor complex at the membrane. RIP1 is polyubiquinated, resulting in recruitment of the TAK1 kinase and the IKK complex to the ubiquinated molecules (Skaug et al., 2009). The activation loop of IKK is phosphorylated in the complex, eventually resulting in the release of IκBα from the complex, allowing the p50/p65 heterodimer of the complex to translocate to the nucleus and activate the transcription of inflammatory genes (Ghosh and Hayden, 2008; Hayden and Ghosh, 2008; Kataoka, 2009). While there currently are no drugs that interdict the cytoplasmic portions of the TNF-α signaling pathway, humanized monoclonal antibodies to TNF-α itself, such as *infliximab* and *adalimumab*, are important for the treatment of rheumatoid arthritis and Crohn disease (see Chapters 34, 35, 37, and 51).

Receptors That Stimulate Synthesis of cGMP

The signaling pathways that regulate the synthesis of cGMP in cells include hormonal regulation of transmembrane guanylyl cyclases such as the ANP receptor and the activation of sGC by NO (Figure 3–13). The downstream effects of cGMP are carried out by multiple isoforms of PKG, cGMP-gated ion channels, and cGMP-modulated PDEs that degrade cAMP.

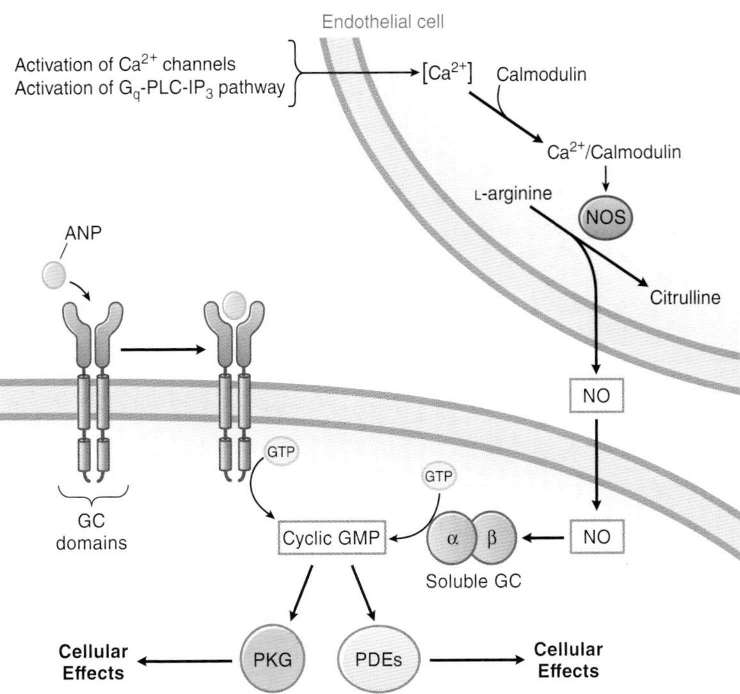

Figure 3–13 *Cyclic GMP signaling pathways.* Formation of cGMP is regulated by cell surface receptors with intrinsic GC activity and by soluble forms of GC. The cell surface receptors respond to natriuretic peptides such as ANP with an increase in cGMP. sGC responds to NO generated from L-arginine by NOS. Cellular effects of cGMP are carried out by PKG and cGMP-regulated PDEs. In this diagram, NO is produced by a Ca^{2+}/calmodulin–dependent NOS in an adjacent endothelial cell. Detailed descriptions of these signaling pathways are given throughout the text in relation to the therapeutic actions of drugs affecting these pathways.

Natriuretic Peptide Receptors: Ligand-Activated Guanylyl Cyclases. The class of membrane receptors with intrinsic enzymatic activity includes the receptors for three small peptide ligands released from cells in cardiac tissues and the vascular system, the natriuretic peptides: ANP, released from atrial storage granules following expansion of intravascular volume or stimulation with pressor hormones; BNP, synthesized and released in large amounts from ventricular tissue in response to volume overload; and CNP, synthesized in the brain and endothelial cells. Like BNP, CNP is not stored in granules; rather, its synthesis and release are increased by growth factors and sheer stress on vascular ECs. The major physiological effects of these hormones are to decrease blood pressure (ANP, BNP), to reduce cardiac hypertrophy and fibrosis (BNP), and to stimulate long-bone growth (CNP). The transmembrane receptors for ANP, BNP, and CNP are ligand-activated guanylyl cyclases. The NPR-A is the molecule that responds to ANP and BNP. The protein is widely expressed and prominent in kidney, lung, adipose, and cardiac and vascular SMCs. ANP and BNP play a role in maintaining the normal state of the cardiovascular system; NPR-A knockout mice develop hypertension and hypertrophic hearts. The synthetic BNP agonist *nesiritide* and the neprilysin inhibitor *sacubitril* (blocks ANP and BNP breakdown) are used in the treatment of acute decompensated heart failure (Chapter 29).

The NPR-B receptor responds to CNP, is widely expressed, and has a physical structure similar to the NPR-A receptor. A role for CNP in bone is suggested by the observation that NPR-B knockout mice exhibit dwarfism. The NPR-C has an extracellular domain similar to those of NPR-A and NPR-B but does not contain the guanylyl cyclase domain. NPR-C has no enzymatic activity and is thought to function as a clearance receptor, removing excess natriuretic peptide from the circulation (Potter et al., 2009).

NO Synthase and Soluble Guanylyl Cyclase. NO is produced locally in cells by forms of the enzyme NOS. NO stimulates sGC to produce cGMP. There are three forms of NOS: nNOS (or NOS1), eNOS (or NOS3), and iNOS (or NOS2). All three forms are widely expressed but are especially important in the cardiovascular system, where they are found in myocytes, vascular smooth muscle cells, endothelial cells, hematopoietic cells, and platelets. Elevated cell Ca^{2+}, acting via calmodulin, markedly activates nNOS and eNOS; the inducible form is less sensitive to Ca^{2+}, but synthesis of iNOS protein in cells can be induced more than 1000-fold by inflammatory stimuli such as endotoxin, TNF-α, interleukin 1β, and interferon γ.

Nitric oxide synthase produces NO by catalyzing the oxidation of the guanido nitrogen of L-arginine, producing L-citrulline and NO. NO activates sGC, a heterodimer that contains a protoporphyrin-IX heme domain. NO binds to this domain at low nanomolar concentrations and produces a 200- to 400-fold increase in the V_{max} of guanylyl cyclase, leading to an elevation of cellular cGMP (Tsai and Kass, 2009). The cellular effects of cGMP on the vascular system are mediated by a number of mechanisms, but especially by PKG. In vascular smooth muscle, activation of PKG leads to vasodilation by

- Inhibiting IP_3-mediated Ca^{2+} release from intracellular stores
- Phosphorylating voltage-gated Ca^{2+} channels to inhibit Ca^{2+} influx
- Phosphorylating phospholamban, a modulator of the sarcoplasmic Ca^{2+} pump, leading to a more rapid reuptake of Ca^{2+} into intracellular stores
- Phosphorylating and opening the Ca^{2+}-activated K^+ channel, leading to hyperpolarization of the cell membrane, which closes L-type Ca^{2+} channels and reduces the flux of Ca^{2+} into the cell

Nuclear Hormone Receptors and Transcription Factors

Nuclear hormone receptors comprise a superfamily of 48 receptors that respond to a diverse set of ligands. The nuclear receptor proteins are transcription factors able to regulate the expression of genes controlling numerous physiological processes, such as reproduction, development, and metabolism. Members of the family include receptors for circulating steroid hormones such as androgens, estrogens, glucocorticoids, thyroid hormone, and vitamin D. Other members of the family are receptors for a diverse group of fatty acids, bile acids, lipids, and lipid metabolites (McEwan, 2009).

Examples include the RXR; the LXR (the ligand is 22-OH cholesterol); the FXR (the ligand is chenodeoxycholic acid); and the PPARs α, β, and γ; 15-deoxy prostaglandin J2 is a possible ligand for PPARγ; the cholesterol-lowering fibrates bind to and regulate PPARγ. In the inactive state, receptors for steroids such as glucocorticoids reside in the cytoplasm and translocate to the nucleus on binding ligand. Other members of the family, such as the LXRs and FXRs reside in the nucleus and are activated by changes in the concentration of hydrophobic lipid molecules.

Nuclear hormone receptors contain four major domains in a single polypeptide chain. The N-terminal domain can contain an *activation region* (AF-1) essential for transcriptional regulation, followed by a very conserved region with two zinc fingers that bind to DNA (the *DNA-binding domain*). The N-terminal activation region (AF-1) is subject to regulation by phosphorylation and other mechanisms that stimulate or inhibit transcription. The C-terminal half of the molecule contains a *hinge region* (which can be involved in binding DNA), the domain responsible for binding the hormone or ligand (the LBD), and specific sets of amino acid residues for binding *coactivators* and *corepressors* in a second activation region (AF-2). The LBD is formed from a bundle of 12 helices; ligand binding induces a major conformational change in helix 12 that affects the binding of the coregulatory proteins essential for activation of the receptor-DNA complex (Figure 3–14) (Privalsky, 2004; Tontonoz and Spiegelman, 2008).

When binding to DNA, most of the nuclear hormone receptors act as dimers—some as homodimers, others as heterodimers. Steroid hormone receptors such as the glucocorticoid receptor are commonly homodimers, whereas those for lipids are heterodimers with the RXR receptor. The receptor dimers bind to repetitive DNA sequences, either direct repeat sequences or inverted repeats termed *HREs* that are specific for each type of receptor. The HREs in DNA are found upstream of the regulated genes or in some cases within the regulated genes. An agonist-bound nuclear

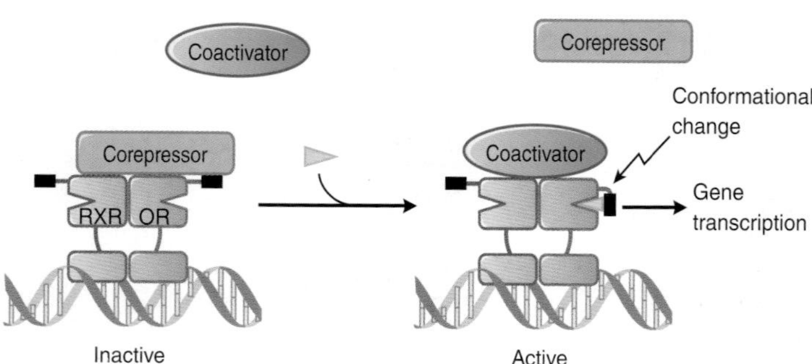

Figure 3–14 *Activation of nuclear hormone receptors.* A nuclear hormone receptor (OR) is shown in complex with the RXR. When an agonist (yellow triangle) and coactivator bind, a conformational change occurs in helix 12 (black bar), and gene transcription is stimulated. If corepressors are bound, activation does not occur. See text for details; see also Figure 6–12.

hormone receptor often activates a large number of genes to carry out a program of cellular differentiation or metabolic regulation. *An important property of these receptors is that they must bind their ligand, the appropriate HRE, and a coregulator, to regulate their target genes.* The activity of the nuclear hormone receptors in a given cell depends not only on the ligand but also on the ratio of coactivators and corepressors recruited to the complex. Coactivators recruit enzymes to the transcription complex that modify chromatin, such as histone acetylase that serves to unravel DNA for transcription. Corepressors recruit proteins such as histone deacetylase, which keeps DNA tightly packed and inhibits transcription.

Apoptosis and Autophagy Pathways

Organ development and renewal requires a balance between cell population survival and expansion versus cell death and removal. One process by which cells are genetically programmed for death is termed *apoptosis*. Defective apoptosis is an important characteristic of many cancers that contributes to both tumorigenesis and resistance to anticancer therapies. *Autophagy* an intracellular degradation pathway that may have evolved before apoptosis, can also lead to programmed cell death. The pharmacological perturbation of these processes could be of importance in many diseases.

Apoptosis

Apoptosis is a highly regulated program of biochemical reactions that leads to cell rounding, shrinking of the cytoplasm, condensation of the nucleus and nuclear material, and changes in the cell membrane that eventually lead to presentation of phosphatidylserine on the outer surface of the cell. Phosphatidylserine is recognized as a sign of apoptosis by macrophages, which engulf and phagocytize the dying cell. During this process, the membrane of the apoptotic cell remains intact, and the cell does not release its cytoplasm or nuclear material. Thus, unlike necrotic cell death, the apoptotic process does not initiate an inflammatory response. Alterations in apoptotic pathways are implicated in cancer, neurodegenerative diseases, autoimmune diseases. Thus, maintaining or restoring normal apoptotic pathways is the goal of major drug development efforts to treat diseases that involve dysregulated apoptotic pathways. Resistance to many cancer chemotherapies is associated with reduced function of apoptotic pathways.

Two major signaling pathways induce apoptosis. Apoptosis can be initiated by external signals that have features in common with those used by ligands such as TNF-α or by an internal pathway activated by DNA damage, improperly folded proteins, or withdrawal of cell survival factors (Figure 3–15). The apoptotic program is carried out by a large family of cysteine proteases termed *caspases*. The caspases are highly specific cytoplasmic proteases that are inactive in normal cells but become activated by apoptotic signals (Bremer et al., 2006; Ghavami et al., 2009).

The external apoptosis signaling pathway can be activated by ligands such as TNF, Fas (also called Apo-1), or TRAIL. The receptors for Fas and TRAIL are transmembrane receptors with no enzymatic activity, similar to the organization of the TNF receptor described previously. On binding TNF, Fas ligand, or TRAIL, these receptors form a receptor dimer, undergo a conformational change, and recruit adapter proteins to the death domain. The adaptor proteins then recruit RIP1 and caspase 8 to form a complex that results in the activation of caspase 8. Activation of caspase 8 leads to the activation of caspase 3, which initiates the apoptotic program. The final steps of apoptosis are carried out by caspases 6 and 7, leading to degradation of enzymes, structural proteins, and DNA fragmentation characteristic of cell death (Danial and Korsmeyer, 2004; Wilson et al., 2009) (see Figure 3–15).

The internal apoptosis pathway can be activated by signals such as DNA damage, leading to increased transcription of the p53 gene, and involves damage to the mitochondria by proapoptotic members of the

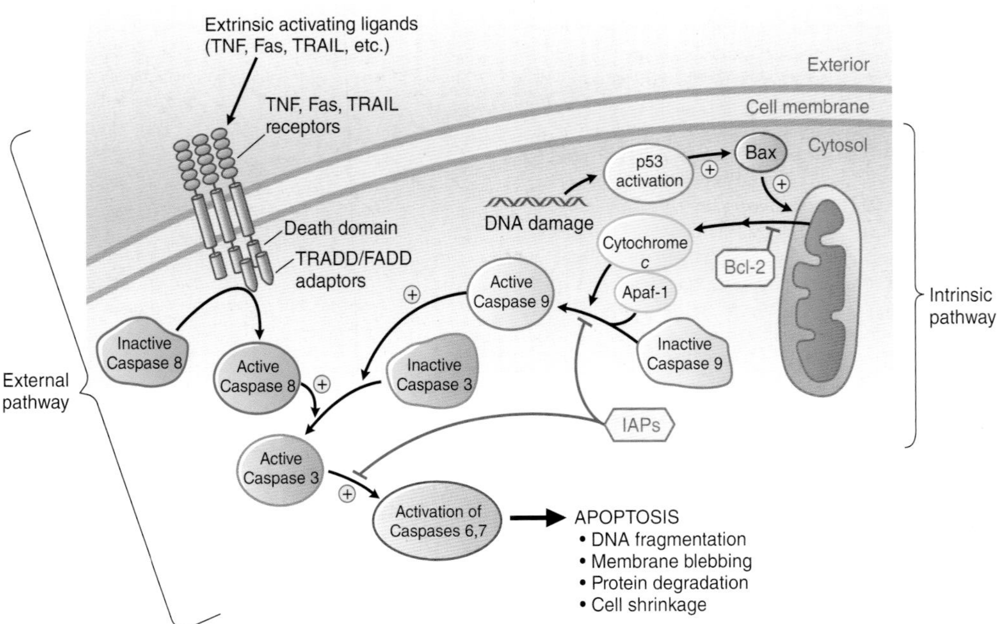

Figure 3–15 *Two pathways leading to apoptosis.* Apoptosis can be initiated by external ligands such as TNF, Fas, or TRAIL at specific transmembrane receptors (left half of figure). Activation leads to trimerization of the receptor, and binding of adaptor molecules such as TRADD, to the intracellular death domain. The adaptors recruit caspase 8 and activate it, leading to cleavage and activation of the effector caspase, caspase 3, which activates the caspase pathway, leading to apoptosis. Apoptosis can also be initiated by an *intrinsic pathway* regulated by Bcl-2 family members such as Bax and Bcl-2. Bax is activated by DNA damage or malformed proteins via p53 (right half of figure). Activation of this pathway leads to release of cytochrome *c* from the mitochondria, formation of a complex with Apaf-1 and caspase 9. Caspase 9 is activated in the complex and initiates apoptosis through activation of caspase 3. Either the extrinsic or the intrinsic pathway can overwhelm the inhibitor of apoptosis proteins (IAPs), which otherwise keep apoptosis in check.

Bcl-2 family of proteins. This family includes proapoptotic members such as Bax, Bak, and Bad, which induce damage at the mitochondrial membrane. There are also antiapoptotic Bcl-2 members, such as Bcl-2, Bcl-X, and Bcl-W, which serve to inhibit mitochondrial damage and are negative regulators of the system (Rong and Distelhorst, 2008). When DNA damage occurs, p53 transcription is activated and holds the cell at a cell cycle checkpoint until the damage is repaired. If the damage cannot be repaired, apoptosis is initiated through the proapoptotic Bcl-2 members, such as Bax. Bax is activated, translocates to the mitochondria, overcomes the antiapoptotic proteins, and induces the release of cytochrome *c* and a protein termed the SMAC. SMAC binds to and inactivates the inhibitor of apoptosis proteins (IAPs) that normally prevent caspase activation. Cytochrome *c* combines in the cytosol with another protein, Apaf-1, and with caspase 9. This complex leads to activation of caspase 9 and ultimately to the activation of caspase 3 (Ghobrial et al., 2005; Wilson et al., 2009). Once activated, caspase 3 activates the same downstream pathways as the external pathway described previously, leading to the cleavage of proteins, cytoskeletal elements, and DNA repair proteins, with subsequent DNA condensation and membrane blebbing that eventually lead to cell death and engulfment by macrophages.

Autophagy

Autophagy is a highly regulated, multistep, catabolic pathway in which cellular contents (including aggregate-prone proteins, organelles such as mitochondria and peroxisomes, and infectious agents) are sequestered within double-membrane vesicles known as autophagosomes, then delivered to lysosomes, where fusion occurs and autophagosome contents are degraded by lysosomal proteases (Bento et al., 2016; Hurley and Young, 2017). The functions of autophagy are to remove cell contents that are damaged and provide cells with substrates for energy and biosynthesis under conditions of stress and starvation. Autophagy plays an important protective role in a number of diseases, including neurodegenerative diseases (e.g., Alzheimer, Parkinson, and Huntington diseases) caused by aggregate-prone proteins and certain infectious diseases (*Salmonella typhi* and *Mycobacterium tuberculosis*). Autophagy-related genes may also play a role in tumor suppression, and decreased autophagic capacity is correlated with poor prognosis in brain tumors. However, in breast, ovarian, and prostate cancers, autophagy can function as a tumor promoter and may enhance the survival of metastatic cells at sites where nutrients are limited.

Autophagy is a highly conserved process controlled by autophagy-related genes (known as *ATGs*, AuTophaGy genes). More than 30 *ATGs* have been identified in eukaryotes, and the ATG proteins function at various steps in autophagy, including induction of cargo packaging, vesicle formation, vesicle fusion with lysosomes, and degradation of vesicular contents. Autophagy is primarily regulated by various cellular stress-mediated and growth factor signaling pathways that integrate signaling output via the PI3K-PKB-mTOR pathway (Figure 3–16). Activated mTORC1 inhibits autophagy. Another important regulator of autophagy is the antiapoptotic protein Bcl-2 through its interaction with Beclin-1, an ATG protein. The binding of Bcl-2 to Beclin-1 inhibits autophagy. Phosphorylation of Beclin-1 by JNK1 promotes the dissociation of Beclin-1 from Bcl-2, which promotes autophagy. The ubiquitin-proteasome system is a major protein degradation system that functionally complements autophagy and also regulates autophagy. Ubiquitination of Beclin-1 disrupts its interaction with Bcl-2 and initiates autophagy, but Beclin-1 degradation by the proteasome downregulates autophagy. The tumor suppressor p53 is also a regulator of autophagy through its inhibitory interactions with an ATG on the lysosomal membrane, DRAM.

Receptor Desensitization and Regulation of Receptors

Receptors are almost always subject to feedback regulation by their own signaling outputs. Continued stimulation of cells with agonists generally results in a state of *desensitization* (also referred to as *adaptation, refractoriness,* or *downregulation*) such that the effect of continued or repeated exposure to the same concentration of drug is diminished. This phenomenon, called *tachyphylaxis*, occurs rapidly and is important therapeutically; an example is attenuated response to the repeated use of β adrenergic receptor agonists as bronchodilators for the treatment of asthma (see Chapters 12 and 40).

Desensitization can result from temporary inaccessibility of the receptor to agonist or from fewer receptors being synthesized (e.g., downregulation of receptor number). Phosphorylation of GPCRs by specific GRKs plays a key role in triggering rapid desensitization. Phosphorylation of agonist-occupied GPCRs by GRKs facilitates the binding of cytosolic proteins termed *arrestins* to the receptor, resulting in the uncoupling of G

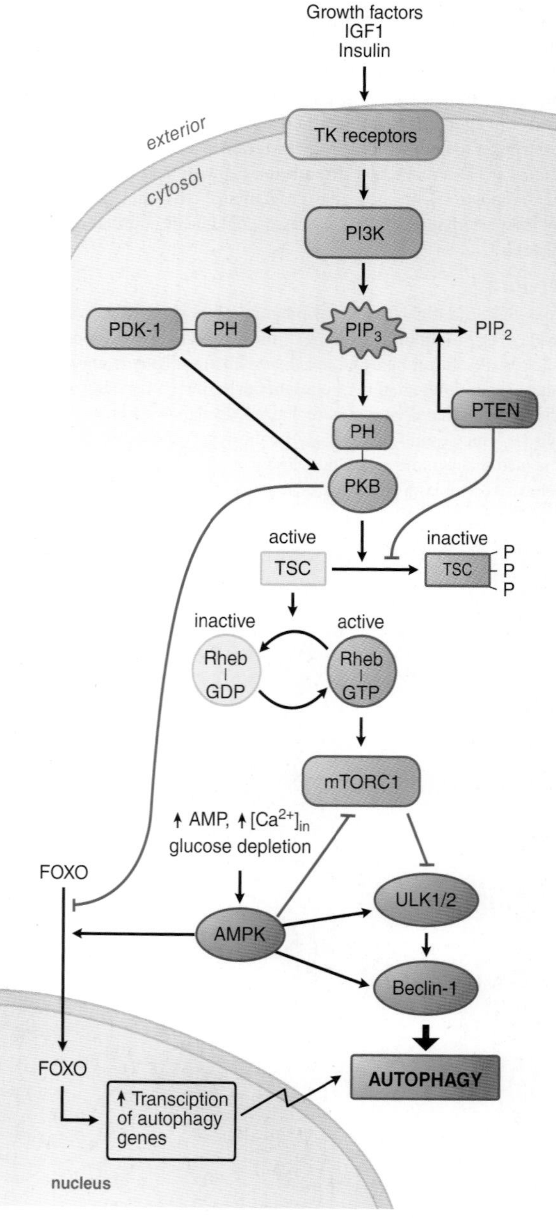

Figure 3–16 *Pathways regulating autophagy.* Two of the primary regulators of autophagy are growth factor signaling and cellular stress. Growth factor signaling pathways that lead to activation of mTORC1 (green boxes) inhibit autophagy, whereas cellular stress caused by nutrient starvation enhance autophagy through activation of AMPK (red boxes). These pathways not only interact with one another, but also with other pathways including apoptosis pathways as described in the text. See Figure 35–5 for the effect of mTOR inhibitors as immunosuppressants.

protein from the receptor. The β arrestins recruit proteins, such as PDE4, which limit cAMP signaling, and clathrin and β_2 adaptin, which promote sequestration of receptor from the membrane (*internalization*), thereby providing a scaffold that permits additional signaling steps.

Conversely, *supersensitivity* to agonists also frequently follows chronic reduction of receptor stimulation. As an example, supersensitivity can be noticeable following withdrawal from prolonged receptor blockade (e.g., the long-term administration of β adrenergic receptor antagonists such as metoprolol) or in the case where chronic denervation of a preganglionic fiber induces an increase in neurotransmitter release per pulse and to greater postsynaptic effect, indicating postganglionic neuronal supersensitivity.

Diseases Resulting From Receptor and Pathway Dysfunction

Alteration in receptors and their downstream signaling pathways can be the cause of disease. The loss of a receptor in a highly specialized signaling system may cause a phenotypic disorder (e.g., deficiency of the androgen receptor and testicular feminization syndrome; see Chapter 45). Deficiencies in widely employed signaling pathways have broad effects, as are seen in myasthenia gravis (due to autoimmune disruption of nicotinic cholinergic receptor function; Chapter 11) and in some forms of insulin-resistant diabetes mellitus (as a result of autoimmune depletion of insulin and interference with insulin receptor function; Chapter 47). The expression of constitutively active, aberrant, or ectopic receptors, effectors, and coupling proteins potentially can lead to *supersensitivity, subsensitivity*, or *other untoward responses* (Smit et al., 2007). For example, many forms of cancer are now known to arise from mutations that result in constitutive activity of growth factor receptors and downstream signaling enzymes in the Ras-MAPK pathway, or loss of tumor suppressors and other proteins that regulate cell proliferation (see Chapter 67).

Common polymorphisms in receptors and proteins downstream of the receptor can also lead to variability in therapeutic responses in patient populations from different geographic and ethnic origins. An example is the variability in therapeutic response to β blockers in patients with heart failure. African American patients with heart failure do not respond as well to β blockade therapy as do patients of European and Asian descent, and at least part of the lower efficacy in African Americans is attributable to polymorphisms in several components of the myocardial β adrenergic receptor signaling pathway, including β_1 adrenergic receptor polymorphisms that increase its constitutive activity and sensitivity to activation by NE. Interestingly, a GRK5 gain-of-function polymorphism that is more common in African Americans increases the ability of GRK5 to desensitize β_1 receptors and provides a β_1 antiadrenergic effect that increases survival in patients with heart failure not receiving blocker therapy.

Pharmacotherapies That Modify Specific Genes and Their Transcription and Translation

Many hereditary diseases result from mutations in physiologically important proteins that are not receptors or proteins associated with downstream signaling. Until recently, it was difficult or impossible to treat many of these diseases except to provide supportive therapy. However, various gene therapies currently being tested in animal models and humans hold promise of curing or significantly ameliorating the effects of a mutation in a protein that is key to an important physiological process. Examples of diseases that might be treated or cured by gene therapies include DMD, cystic fibrosis, metabolic disorders, and various disorders of the eye.

Approximately 11% of genetic mutations in inherited disease are nonsense mutations that introduce a premature stop codon in the mRNA gene transcript. The first drug approved (in the E.U., but not yet in the U.S.) for the treatment of nmDMD is *ataluren*. This small-molecule drug is thought to act on the ribosome to override the premature stop (nonsense) codon in nonsense mutations, allowing the ribosome to "read through" the transcript and produce normal full-length protein. In the case of nmDMD, ataluren improves synthesis of functional dystrophin, a cytosolic socket protein that is a component of the complex that connects intracellular fibers of a muscle cell with the extracellular matrix. This effect of ataluren modestly improves the symptoms of patients. Ataluren is currently in clinical trials for treatment of other inherited diseases caused by nonsense mutations, including cystic fibrosis (nonsense mutation in the *CFTR* gene) and anaridia (nonsense mutation in the *PAX6* gene).

A different approach to treating diseases resulting from gene mutations is through the use of nucleic acids, including ASOs and RNAi. ASOs are synthetic nucleic acids that are complementary to the mRNA "sense" strand of the disease-causing gene and act by binding to the mRNA, preventing its translation. Examples of ASOs that have been approved include *fomivirsen* for treatment of cytomegalovirus retinitis viral infections of the eye (this agent has been discontinued in the U.S.) and *mipomersen* for treatment of homozygous familial hypercholesterolemia. The target gene for mipomersen is apolipoprotein B100.

Another way to selectively silence gene expression is using siRNA. RNAi is a ubiquitous cellular mechanism for small RNA-guided suppression of gene expression that uses the RISC. The antisense strand of the siRNA guides the RISC to destroy the target mRNA and is protected from degradation by the RISC, resulting in elimination of many copies of the target mRNA and gene knockdown effects that can persist for days to weeks. A number of clinical trials are in progress to treat cancer using naked siRNAs as well as siRNA delivery systems using adenovirus, liposomes, polymers, and various kinds of nanoparticles.

Perhaps the therapeutic approach with the greatest potential to treat patients with a hereditary disease is the CRISPR/Cas9 genome-editing system using viruses or genetically modified microorganisms. The CRISPR/Cas9 system allows precise and imprecise editing of the genome using sgRNAs that target the Cas9 double-stranded DNA nuclease to specific sites in the genome that contain an adjacent NGG PAM sequence. The CRISPR/Cas9 system allows targeted replacement and modification of disease-causing genes. Recent proof-of-principle experiments in mouse models of DMD demonstrated that CRISPR/Cas9 delivered systemically using AAV vectors can correct disease-causing mutations in the dystrophin gene in young and adult mice. Although there are many technical, regulatory, and ethical hurdles to overcome before genome editing is approved for use in patients, the results of preclinical studies demonstrated the potential impact on treating and curing diseases that previously had no pharmacotherapeutic options.

Physiological Systems Integrate Multiple Signals

Consider the vascular wall of an arteriole (Figure 3–17). Several cell types interact at this site, including vascular smooth muscle cells, endothelial cells, platelets, and postganglionic sympathetic neurons. A variety of physiological receptors and ligands are present, including ligands that cause SMCs to contract (AngII, NE) and relax (NO, BNP, and epinephrine), as well as ligands that alter SMC gene expression (PDGF, AngII, NE, and eicosanoids).

Angiotensin II has both acute and chronic effects on SMCs. Interaction of AngII with AT_1Rs mobilizes stored Ca^{2+} via the G_q-PLC-IP_3-Ca^{2+} pathway. The Ca^{2+} binds and activates calmodulin and its target protein, MLCK. The activation of MLCK results in the phosphorylation of myosin, leading to SMC contraction. Activation of the sympathetic nervous system also regulates SMC tone through release of NE from postganglionic sympathetic neurons. NE binds α_1 adrenergic receptors, which also activate the G_q-PLC-IP_3-Ca^{2+} pathway, resulting in SMC contraction, an effect that is additive to that of AngII.

The contraction of SMCs is opposed by mediators that promote relaxation, including NO, BNP, and catecholamines acting at β_2 adrenergic receptors. NO is formed in endothelial cells by eNOS when the G_q-PLC-IP_3-Ca^{2+} pathway is activated and by iNOS when that isoform is induced. The NO formed in the endothelium diffuses into SMCs and activates the sGC, which catalyzes the formation of cGMP, which leads to activation of PKG and phosphorylation of proteins in SMCs that reduce intracellular concentrations of Ca^{2+} and thereby promote relaxation. Intracellular

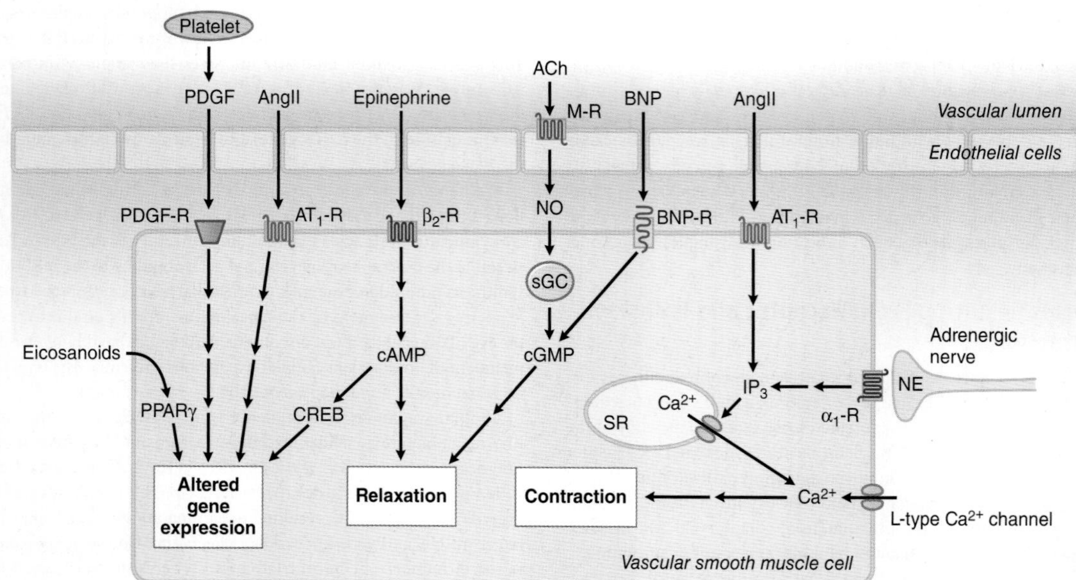

Figure 3–17 *Interaction of multiple signaling systems regulating vascular SMCs.* See text for explanation of signaling and contractile pathways and abbreviations.

concentrations of cGMP are also increased by activation of transmembrane BNP receptors (NPR-A, and to a lesser extent to NPR-B), whose guanylyl cyclase activity is increased when BNP binds.

As a consequence of the variety of pathways that affect arteriolar tone, a patient with hypertension may be treated with one or several drugs that alter signaling through these pathways. Drugs commonly used to treat hypertension include β_1 adrenergic receptor antagonists to reduce secretion of renin (the rate-limiting first step in AngII synthesis); a direct renin inhibitor (aliskiren) to block the rate-limiting step in AngII production; ACE inhibitors (e.g., enalapril) to reduce the concentrations of circulating AngII; AT_1R blockers (e.g., losartan) to block AngII binding to AT_1Rs on SMCs; α_1 adrenergic blockers to block NE binding to SMCs; sodium nitroprusside to increase the quantities of NO produced; or a Ca^{2+} channel blocker (e.g., nifedipine) to block Ca^{2+} entry into SMCs. The β_1 adrenergic receptor antagonists would also block the baroreceptor reflex increase in heart rate and blood pressure elicited by a drop in blood pressure induced by the therapy. ACE inhibitors also inhibit the degradation of a vasodilating peptide, bradykinin (see Chapter 26). Thus, the choices and mechanisms are complex, and the appropriate therapy in a given patient depends on many considerations, including the diagnosed causes of hypertension in the patient, possible side effects of the drug, efficacy in a given patient, and cost.

Signaling Pathways and Drug Action

Throughout this text, cellular signaling pathways figure prominently in explaining the actions of therapeutic agents. Not all pathways have been mentioned or fully explored in this chapter. To aid readers in finding more information on signaling and drug action, Table 3–2 lists relevant figures that appear in other chapters.

Acknowledgment: *Elliot M. Ross, Terry P. Kenakin, Iain L. O. Buxton, and James C. Garrison contributed to this chapter in recent editions of this book. We have retained some of their text in the current edition.*

Bibliography

Ariens EJ. Affinity and intrinsic activity in the theory of competitive inhibition. I. Problems and theory. *Arch Int Pharmacodyn Ther*, **1954**, *99*:32–49.

Baillie GS. Compartmentalized signalling: spatial regulation of cAMP by the action of compartmentalized phosphodiesterases. *FEBS J*, **2009**, *276*:1790–1799.

Beavo JA, Brunton LL. Cyclic nucleotide research—still expanding after half a century. *Nat Rev Mol Cell Biol*, **2002**, *3*:710–718.

Beers Update Panel. American Geriatrics Society 2015 updated Beers Criteria for Potentially Inappropriate Medication Use in Older Adults. *J Am Geriatr Soc*, **2015**, *63*:2227–2246.

Bento CF, et al. Mammalian autophagy: how does it work? *Annu Rev Biochem*, **2016**, *85*:685–713.

Bremer E, et al. Targeted induction of apoptosis for cancer therapy: current progress and prospects. *Trends Mol Med*, **2006**, *12*: 382–393.

Calabrese EJ, Baldwin LA. Hormesis: the dose-response revolution. *Annu Rev Pharmacol Toxicol*, **2003**, *43*:175–197.

Cao E, et al. TRPV1 structures in distinct conformations reveal activation mechanisms. *Nature*, **2013**, *504*:113–118.

Carlson HA, McCammon JA. Accommodating protein flexibility in computational drug design. *Mol Pharmacol*, **2000**, *57*:213–218.

Carnegie GK, et al. A-kinase anchoring proteins: from protein complexes to physiology and disease. *IUBMB Life*, **2009**, *61*:394–406.

Cheng HC. The influence of cooperativity on the determination of dissociation constants: examination of the Cheng-Prusoff equation, the Scatchard analysis, the Schild analysis and related power equations. *Pharmacol Res*, **2004**, *50*:21–40.

Cheng X, et al. Epac and PKA: a tale of two intracellular cAMP receptors. *Acta Biochim Biophys Sin (Shanghai)*, **2008**, *40*:651–662.

Cheng Y, Prusoff WH. Relationship between the inhibition constant (K_I) and the concentration of inhibitor which causes 50 per cent inhibition (I_{50}) of an enzymatic reaction. *Biochem Pharmacol*, **1973**, *22*: 3099–3108.

TABLE 3–2 ■ SUMMARY: RECEPTOR-SIGNALING PATHWAYS AS SITES OF DRUG ACTION

RECEPTOR/PATHWAY	FIGURE TITLE	FIGURE NUMBER
Drug transport proteins	Major mechanisms by which transporters mediate adverse drug responses	**Figure 5–3**
CYPs, drug metabolism	Location of CYPs in the cell	**Figure 6–2**
Nuclear receptors	Induction of drug metabolism by nuclear receptor–mediated signal transduction	**Figure 6–13**
General neurotransmission	Steps involved in excitatory and inhibitory neurotransmission	**Figure 8–3**
Exocytosis	Molecular basis of exocytosis: docking and fusion of synaptic vesicles with neuronal membranes	**Figure 8–4**
Cholinergic neurotransmission	A typical cholinergic neuroeffector junction	**Figure 8–6**
Adrenergic neurotransmission	A typical adrenergic neuroeffector junction	**Figure 8–8**
AChE and its inhibition	Steps involved in the hydrolysis of ACh by AChE and in the inhibition and reactivation of the enzyme	**Figure 10–2**
Transmission at the NMJ	A pharmacologist's view of the motor end plate	**Figure 11–4**
β Blockers and vasodilation	Mechanisms underlying actions of vasodilating β blockers in blood vessels	**Figure 12–4**
Serotonergic neurotransmission	A serotonergic synapse	**Figure 13–4**
Dopaminergic neurotransmission	A dopaminergic synapse	**Figure 13–9**
Voltage-sensitive cation channels	Voltage-sensitive Na^+, Ca^{2+}, and K^+ channels	**Figure 14–2**
Neurotransmission	Transmitter release, action, and inactivation	**Figure 14–4**
Ligand-gated ion channels	Pentameric ligand-gated ion channels	**Figure 14–5**
$GABA_A$ receptor	Pharmacologic binding sites on the $GABA_A$ receptor	**Figure 14–11**
NMDA receptor	Pharmacologic binding sites on the NMDA receptor	**Figure 14–12**
Glutamate toxicity	Mechanisms contributing to glutamate-induced cytotoxicity/neuronal injury during ischemia-reperfusion–induced glutamate release	**Figure 14–13**
Histamine signaling	Signal transduction pathways for histamine receptors	**Figure 14–14**
Cannabinoids in CNS	Anandamide synthesis and signaling	**Figure 14–17**
Neurotrophin signaling	Neurotrophic factor signaling in the CNS	**Figure 14–18**
Actions of antidepressants	Sites of action of antidepressants at noradrenergic and serotonergic nerve terminals	**Figure 15–1**
Na^+ channel	Antiseizure drug–enhanced Na^+ channel inactivation	**Figure 17–2**
$GABA_A$ receptor/channel	Some antiseizure drugs enhance GABA synaptic transmission	**Figure 17–3**
T-type Ca^{2+} channel	Antiseizure drug–induced reduction of current through T-type Ca^{2+} channels	**Figure 17–4**
Dopaminergic signaling	Dopaminergic nerve terminal	**Figure 18–1**
Endogenous opioid signaling	Receptor specificity of endogenous opioids; effects of receptor activation on neurons.	**Figure 20–3**
Biased opioid signaling	Biased signaling via opioid receptors	**Figure 20–4**
Cation signaling	Structure and function of voltage-gated Na^+ channels	**Figure 22–2**
Local anesthetic action on Na^+ channels	A pharmacologist's view of the interaction of a local anesthetic with a voltage-gated Na^+ channel	**Figure 22–3**
Aldosterone signaling	Effects of aldosterone on late distal tubule and collecting duct and diuretic mechanism of aldosterone antagonists	**Figure 25–6**
ANP signaling	Inter medullary collecting duct Na^+ transport and its regulation	**Figure 25–7**
V_1 receptor signaling	Mechanism of V_1 receptor-effector coupling	**Figure 25–11**
V_2 receptor signaling	Mechanism of V_2 receptor-effector coupling	**Figure 25–12**
Signals regulating renin release	Mechanisms by which the macula densa regulates renin release	**Figure 26–4**
Signals regulating blood pressure	Principles of blood pressure regulation and its modification by drugs	**Figure 28–2**
E-C coupling	Cardiac excitation-contraction coupling and its regulation by positive inotropic drugs	**Figure 29–6**
NO/cGMP signaling in pulmonary hypertension	Stimulators of NO/cGMP signaling	**Figure 31–3**
cAMP signaling in pulmonary hypertension	Membrane receptor agonists that increase cAMP	**Figure 31–4**
PLC signaling in pulmonary hypertension	Membrane receptor antagonists that inhibit activation of phospholipase C	**Figure 31–5**

(Continued)

TABLE 3–2 ■ SUMMARY: RECEPTOR-SIGNALING PATHWAYS AS SITES OF DRUG ACTION (*CONTINUED*)

RECEPTOR/PATHWAY	FIGURE TITLE	FIGURE NUMBER
Endothelium–smooth muscle signaling	Interactions between endothelium and vascular smooth muscle in pulmonary artery hypertension	**Figure 31–7**
Aggregatory signaling	Platelet adhesion and aggregation	**Figure 32–1**
Coagulatory signaling	Major reactions of blood coagulation	**Figure 32–2**
Fibrinolytic signaling	Fibrinolysis	**Figure 32–3**
Blood clotting and its prevention	Sites of action of antiplatelet drugs	**Figure 32–7**
LDLR and endocytosis	LDL catabolism: effects of PCSK9, antibody to PCSK9, and statins	**Figure 33–4**
T cell receptor (TCR) ligands	TCR signaling and its modulation by co-receptors and antibodies	**Figure 34–4**
MHC/antigen complexes leading to TCR signaling	Professional antigen-presenting cells (APCs)	**Figure 34–5**
T cell receptor signaling, immunophilins	T cell activation and sites of action of immunosuppressive agents	**Figure 35–2**
T cell activation	T cell activation: costimulation and coinhibitory checkpoints	**Figure 35–4**
Prostanoid receptors	Prostanoid receptors and their primary signaling pathways	**Figure 37–4**
Eicosanoid signaling	Human Eicosanoid Receptors	**Table 37–2**
Bradykinin/kallikrein signaling	Synthesis and receptor interactions of active peptides generated by the kallikrein-kinin and renin-angiotensin systems	**Figure 39–4**
Inflammatory signaling and glucocorticoid receptors	Mechanism of anti-inflammatory action of corticosteroids in asthma	**Figure 40–7**
Growth hormone receptor (GHR)	Mechanisms of GH and PRL action and of GHR antagonism	**Figure 42–5**
Oxytocin receptor signaling	Sites of action of oxytocin and tocolytic drugs in the uterine myometrium	**Figure 42–8**
Estrogen receptor (ER), nuclear signaling	Molecular mechanism of action of nuclear ER	**Figure 44–4**
Soluble guanylyl cyclase and PDE5	Mechanism of action of PDE5 inhibitors in the corpus cavernosum	**Figure 45–6**
Glucocorticoid receptor (GR)	Intracellular mechanism of action of the GR	**Figure 46–5**
Insulin secretion	Regulation of insulin secretion from a pancreatic β cell	**Figure 47–3**
Insulin receptor	Pathways of insulin signaling	**Figure 47–4**
FGF receptor	FGF23-FGFR-Klotho complex	**Figure 48–4**
H_2 and gastrin receptors; gastric secretion	Pharmacologist's view of gastric secretion and its regulation: the basis for therapy of acid-peptic disorders	**Figure 49–1**
EP_2 and EP_4 receptors; GI ion transporters; cAMP, cGMP	Mechanism of action of drugs that alter intestinal epithelial secretion and absorption	**Figure 50–4**
Emetic signaling	Pharmacologist's view of emetic stimuli	**Figure 50–5**
EGF receptor	Targeting the EGFR in cancer	**Figure 67–1**
Growth factor receptors	Cancer cell signaling pathway and drug targets	**Figure 67–2**
IGFIR	Caveat mTOR: effect of rapamycin on growth factor signaling	**Figure 67–4**
T cell/APC signaling	Targeting of immune checkpoints	**Figure 67–5**
IL-2 receptor	A pharmacologist's view of IL-2 receptors, their cellular signaling pathways, and their inhibition	**Figure 67–6**
Apoptotic signaling	BH3 mimetics enhance apoptosis	**Figure 67–7**
Rhodopsin	Pharmacologist's view of photoreceptor signaling	**Figure 69–9**

Conti M, Beavo J. Biochemistry and physiology of cyclic nucleotide phosphodiesterases: essential components in cyclic nucleotide signaling. *Annu Rev Biochem*, **2007**, *76*:481–511.

Danial NN, Korsmeyer SJ. Cell death: critical control points. *Cell*, **2004**, *116*:205–219.

Dessauer CW, et al. International Union of Basic and Clinical Pharmacology. CI. Structures and small molecule modulators of mammalian adenylyl cyclases. *Pharmacol Rev*, **2017**, *69*:93–139.

Etienne-Manneville S, Hall A. Rho GTPases in cell biology. *Nature*, **2002**, *420*:629–635.

Ferguson KM. Structure-based view of epidermal growth factor receptor regulation. *Annu Rev Biophys*, **2008**, *37*:353–373.

Gaddum JH. Theories of drug antagonism. *Pharmacol Rev*, **1957**, *9*:211–218.

Gay NJ, Gangloff M. Structure and function of toll receptors and their ligands. *Annu Rev Biochem*, **2007**, *76*:141–165.

Ghavami S, et al. Apoptosis and cancer: mutations within caspase genes. *J Med Genet*, **2009**, *46*:497–510.

Ghobrial IM, et al. Targeting apoptosis pathways in cancer therapy. *CA Cancer J Clin*, **2005**, *55*:178–194.

Ghosh S, Hayden MS. New regulators of NFκB in inflammation. *Nat Rev Immunol*, **2008**, *8*:837–848.

Gilman AG. G proteins: transducers of receptor-generated signals. *Annu Rev Biochem*, **1987**, *56*:615–649.

Gough DJ, et al. IFN-γ signaling—does it mean JAK-STAT? *Cytokine Growth Factor Rev*, **2008**, *19*:383–394.

GPCR Network. Understanding human GPCR biology. Home page. Available at: http://gpcr.usc.edu. Accessed March 15, 2017.

Hanoune J, Defer N. Regulation and role of adenylyl cyclase isoforms. *Annu Rev Pharmacol Toxicol*, **2001**, *41*:145–174.

Hayden MS, Ghosh S. Shared principles in NFκB signaling. *Cell*, **2008**, *132*:344–362.

Hudmon A, Schulman H. Structure-function of the multifunctional Ca^{2+}/calmodulin-dependent protein kinase II. *Biochem J*, **2002**, *364*:593–611.

Hurley JH, Young LN. Mechanisms of autophagy initiation. *Annu Rev Biochem*, **2017**, March 2017. doi:10.1146/annurev-biochem-061516-044820.

Irannejad R, et al. Effects of endocytosis on receptor-mediated signaling. *Curr Opin Cell Biol*, **2015**, *35*:137–114.

Jain KK. Role of pharmacoproteomics in the development of personalized medicine. *Pharmacogenomics*, **2004**, *5*:331–336.

Jegla TJ, et al. Evolution of the human ion channel set. *Comb Chem High Throughput Screen*, **2009**, *12*:2–23.

Kataoka T. Chemical biology of inflammatory cytokine signaling. *J Antibiot (Tokyo)*, **2009**, *62*:655–667.

Kenakin T. Efficacy as a vector: the relative prevalence and paucity of inverse agonism. *Mol Pharmacol*, **2004**, *65*:2–11.

Limbird LE. *Cell Surface Receptors: A Short Course on Theory and Methods*. Springer-Verlag, New York, **2005**.

May LT, et al. Allosteric modulation of G protein–coupled receptors. *Annu Rev Pharmacol Toxicol*, **2007**, *47*:1–51.

Mayr B, Montminy M. Transcriptional regulation by the phosphorylation-dependent factor creb. *Nat Rev Mol Cell Biol*, **2001**, *2*: 599–609.

McEwan IJ. Nuclear receptors: one big family. *Methods Mol Biol*, **2009**, *505*:3–18.

Mehats C, et al. Cyclic nucleotide phosphodiesterases and their role in endocrine cell signaling. *Trends Endocrinol Metab*, **2002**, *13*: 29–35.

Milligan G. Constitutive activity and inverse agonists of G protein-coupled receptors: a current perspective. *Mol Pharmacol*, **2003**, *64*: 1271–1276.

Palczewski K, et al. Crystal structure of rhodopsin: a G protein-coupled receptor. *Science*, **2000**, *289*:739–745.

Patterson RL, et al. Inositol 1,4,5-trisphosphate receptors as signal integrators. *Annu Rev Biochem*, **2004**, *73*:437–465.

Potter LR, et al. Natriuretic peptides: their structures, receptors, physiologic functions and therapeutic applications. *Handb Exp Pharmacol*, **2009**, 341–366.

Privalsky ML. The role of corepressors in transcriptional regulation by nuclear hormone receptors. *Annu Rev Physiol*, **2004**, *66*: 315–360.

Purves D, et al. Channels and transporters. In: Purves D, et al., eds. *Neuroscience*. 5th ed. Sinauer, Sunderland, MA, **2011**, 61–84.

Ramsey IS, et al. An introduction to TRP channels. *Annu Rev Physiol*, **2006**, 68:619–647.

Rong Y, Distelhorst CW. Bcl-2 protein family members: versatile regulators of calcium signaling in cell survival and apoptosis. *Annu Rev Physiol*, **2008**, *70*:73–91.

Roscioni SS, et al. Epac: effectors and biological functions. *Naunyn Schmiedebergs Arch Pharmacol*, **2008**, *377*:345–357.

Rybalkin SD, et al. Cyclic GMP phosphodiesterases and regulation of smooth muscle function. *Circ Res*, **2003**, *93*:280–291.

Sands WA, Palmer TM. Regulating gene transcription in response to cyclic AMP elevation. *Cell Signal*, **2008**, *20*:460–466.

Schild HO. Drug antagonism and pA_2. *Pharmacol Rev*, **1957**, *9*: 242–246.

Schmidt M, et al. Exchange protein directly activated by cAMP (Epac): a multidomain cAMP mediator in the regulation of diverse biological functions. *Pharmacol Rev*, **2013**, *65*:670–709.

Skaug B, et al. The role of ubiquitin in NFκB regulatory pathways. *Annu Rev Biochem*, **2009**, *78*:769–796.

Smit MJ, et al. Pharmacogenomic and structural analysis of constitutive G protein-coupled receptor activity. *Annu Rev Pharmacol Toxicol*, **2007**, *47*:53–87.

Stevens RC, et al. The GPCR Network: a large-scale collaboration to determine human GPCR structure and function. *Nat Rev Drug Discov*, **2013**, *12*:25–34.

Tallarida RJ. An overview of drug combination analysis with isobolograms. *J Pharmacol Exp Ther*, **2006**, *319*:1–7.

Tallarida RJ. Revisiting the isobole and related quantitative methods for assessing drug synergism. *J Pharmacol Exp Ther*, **2012**, *342*:2–8.

Taylor SS, et al. Signaling through cAMP and cAMP-dependent protein kinase: diverse strategies for drug design. *Biochim Biophys Acta*, **2008**, *1784*:16–26.

Tontonoz P, Spiegelman BM. Fat and beyond: the diverse biology of PPARγ. *Annu Rev Biochem*, **2008**, *77*:289–312.

Tsai EJ, Kass DA. Cyclic GMP signaling in cardiovascular pathophysiology and therapeutics. *Pharmacol Ther*, **2009**, *122*:216–238.

Venkatachalam K, Montell C. TRP channels. *Annu Rev Biochem*, **2007**, *76*:387–417.

Wahl-Schott C, Biel M. HCN channels: Structure, cellular regulation and physiological function. *Cell Mol Life Sci*, **2009**, *66*:470–494.

Wang X, et al. Structural biology of shared cytokine receptors. *Annu Rev Immunol*, **2009**, *27*:29–60.

Wilson NS, et al. Death receptor signal transducers: nodes of coordination in immune signaling networks. *Nat Immunol*, **2009**, *10*:348–355.

Drug Toxicity and Poisoning

Michelle A. Erickson and Trevor M. Penning

第四章　药物毒性和中毒

中文导读

本章主要介绍：药物的剂量-效应关系，包括常规剂量-效应曲线、非单调剂量-效应曲线；药物代谢动力学与毒物代谢动力学，包括药物体内过程（ADME）的变化、治疗药物毒性的类型；描述性动物毒理试验；安全药理学和临床试验；药物不良反应和药物中毒的流行病学；中毒的预防，包括减少用药错误、家庭中毒预防；中毒治疗原则，包括临床中毒类型的鉴别、中毒患者的解毒、加强毒物的消除；药物毒性和中毒相关的信息资源。

Abbreviations

ADEs: adverse drug events
ADME: absorption, distribution, metabolism, and elimination
CYP: cytochrome P450
ECG: electrocardiogram
ED_{50}: median effective dose
FDA: U.S. Food and Drug Administration
GI: gastrointestinal
Ig: immunoglobulin
IND: investigational new drug
IRB: institutional review board
LD_{50}: median lethal dose
SSRI: selective serotonin reuptake inhibitor
TI: therapeutic index
WBI: whole-bowel irrigation

Pharmacology intersects with *toxicology* when the physiological response to a drug is an *adverse effect*. A *poison* is any substance, including any drug, that has the capacity to harm a living organism. *Poisoning* generally implies that damaging physiological effects result from exposure to pharmaceuticals, illicit drugs, or chemicals.

Dose-Response

Conventional Dose-Response Curves

There is a graded dose-response relationship in an *individual* and a quantal dose-response relationship in the *population* (see Figures 3–2, 3–3, and 3–6). Graded doses of a drug given to an individual usually result in a greater magnitude of response as the dose increases. In a quantal dose-response relationship, the percentage of the population affected increases as the dose is increased; the relationship is quantal in that the effect is judged to be either present or absent in a given individual. This quantal dose-response phenomenon is used to determine the LD_{50} of drugs, as defined in Figure 4–1A.

One can also determine a quantal dose-response curve for the therapeutic effect of a drug to generate ED_{50}, the concentration of drug at which 50% of the population will have the desired response, and a quantal dose-response curve for lethality by the same agent (Figure 4–1B). These two curves can be used to generate a TI, which quantifies the relative safety of a drug:

$$TI = \frac{LD_{50}}{ED_{50}} \quad \text{(Equation 4–1)}$$

Clearly, the higher the ratio, the safer the drug.

Values of TI vary widely, from 1–2 to more than 100. Drugs with a low TI must be administered with caution (e.g., the cardiac glycoside digoxin and cancer chemotherapeutic agents). Agents with very high TI (e.g., penicillin) are extremely safe in the absence of a known allergic response in a given patient. Note that use of median doses fails to consider that the slopes of the dose-response curves for therapeutic and lethal (toxic) effects may differ (Figure 4–1). As an alternative the ED_{99} for the therapeutic effect can be compared to the LD_1 for lethality (toxic effect), to yield a *margin of safety*.

$$\text{Margin of safety} = \frac{LD_1}{ED_{99}} \quad \text{(Equation 4–2)}$$

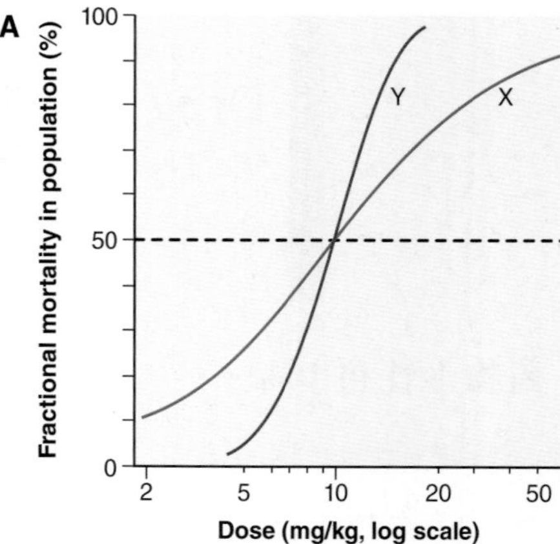

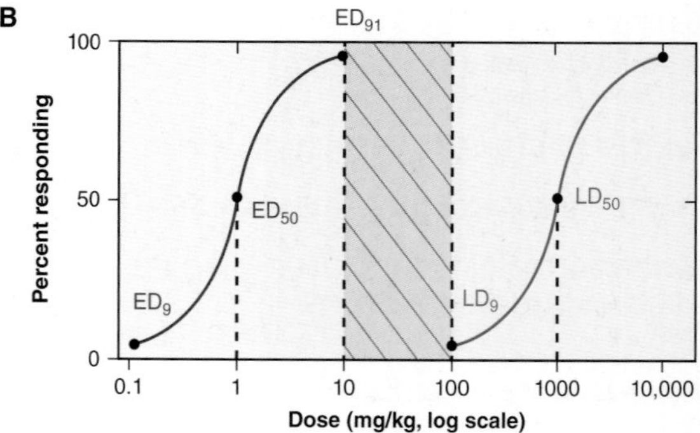

Figure 4–1 *Dose-response relationships.* **A.** The LD_{50} of a compound is determined experimentally, usually by administration of the chemical to mice or rats (orally or intraperitoneally). The midpoint of the curve representing percentage of population responding (response here is death) versus dose (log scale) represents the LD_{50}, or the dose of drug that is lethal in 50% of the population. The LD_{50} values for both compounds are the same (~10 mg/kg); however, the slopes of the dose-response curves are quite different. Thus, at a dose equal to one-half the LD_{50} (5 mg/kg), fewer than 5% of the animals exposed to compound Y would die, but about 25% of the animals given compound X would die. **B.** Depiction of ED and LD. The crosshatched area between the ED_{91} (10 mg/kg) and the LD_9 (100 mg/kg) gives an estimate of the margin of safety.

Nonmonotonic Dose-Response Curves

Not all dose-response curves follow a typical sigmoidal shape. Three examples of these are shown in Figure 4–2. *U-shaped dose-response curves* can be observed for essential metals and vitamins (Figure 4–2A). At low dose, adverse effects are observed because there is a deficiency of these nutrients to maintain homeostasis. As dose increases, homeostasis is achieved, and the bottom of the U-shaped dose-response curve is reached. As dose increases to surpass the amount required to maintain homeostasis, overdose toxicity can ensue. Thus, adverse effects are seen at both low and high doses.

Some toxicants, such as formaldehyde, are also metabolic by-products for which cells have detoxifying mechanisms. Thus, very low doses of exogenous formaldehyde do not sufficiently exceed levels produced physiologically to elicit a significant adverse response, and do not saturate the detoxifying mechanisms, in this instance, alcohol dehydrogenase (ADH5/GSNOR; Pontel et al., 2015). When these endogenous protective mechanisms are overwhelmed, one will observe a toxic response. Toxicologists represent this type of response as a "hockey stick" (Figure 4–2B), a region of no response followed by an adverse response as the toxicant exceeds

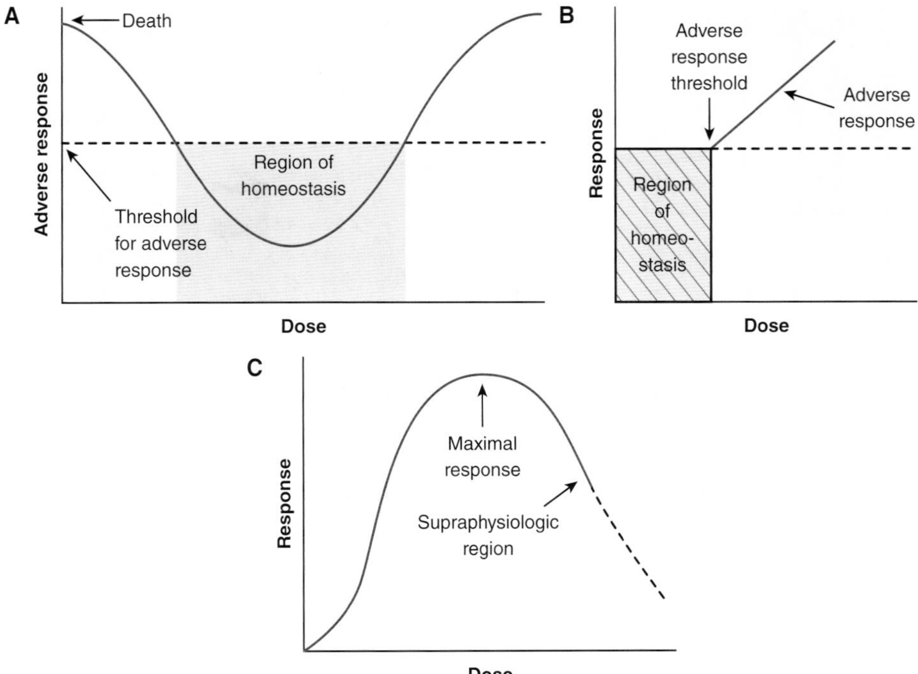

Figure 4–2 *Nonmonotonic dose-response relationships.* **A.** U-shaped dose-response curve for essential metals and vitamins. **B.** Hockey stick-shaped dose-response curve for toxicants that are also metabolic by-products. **C.** Inverted U-shaped dose-response curve for ligands that downregulate their receptors.

the endogenous protective mechanisms and rises sufficiently to cause an adverse response.

Inverted U-shaped dose response curves are observed when receptor downregulation/desensitization occurs following exposure to a ligand or when an additional and distinct negative effect occurs at a concentration beyond that which produces the primary positive effect.

For example, estrogen at high levels can have maximal effects. However, at supraphysiologic levels, the effects of estrogen are reduced, presumably due to downregulation of estrogen receptors. Many endocrine-disrupting chemicals are thought to have inverted U-shaped dose-response curves similar to that of estrogen. Indeed, multiphasic and U-shaped curves are common in complex systems in which an administered compound elicits multiple effects, first one effect and then another, possibly opposing, effect as the concentration increases. This phenomenon highlights a necessity for using an extensive dose range and a sufficient response time to ensure detection of the full spectrum of responsiveness and toxicity for a given substance.

Pharmacokinetics Versus Toxicokinetics

Alterations in ADME

Poisoning may significantly alter the functions of ADME (see Chapters 2, 5, and 6), and these alterations can profoundly alter treatment decisions and prognosis. The pharmacokinetics of a drug under circumstances that produce toxicity or excessive exposure are referred to as *toxicokinetics*. Ingesting larger-than-therapeutic doses of a pharmaceutical may prolong its absorption, alter its protein binding and apparent volume of distribution, and change its metabolic fate. When confronted with potential poisoning, two questions should be foremost in the clinician's mind:

- How long will an asymptomatic patient need to be monitored (drug absorption and dynamics)?
- How long will it take an intoxicated patient to get better (drug elimination and dynamics)?

Drug Absorption

Aspirin poisoning is a leading cause of overdose morbidity and mortality as reported to U.S. poison control centers (Bronstein et al., 2008). In therapeutic dosing, aspirin reaches peak plasma concentrations in about 1 h. However, aspirin overdose may cause spasm of the pyloric valve, delaying entry of the drug into the small intestine. Aspirin, especially enteric-coated forms, may coalesce into bezoars, reducing the effective surface area for absorption. Peak plasma salicylate concentrations from aspirin overdose may not be reached for 4–35 h after ingestion (Rivera et al., 2004).

Drug Elimination

Table 4–1 lists some pharmaceuticals notorious for their predilection to have initial symptoms develop *after* a typical 4- to 6-hour emergency medical observation period (Box 4–1).

TABLE 4–1 ■ DRUGS THAT COMMONLY MANIFEST INITIAL SYMPTOMS MORE THAN 4–6 HOURS AFTER ORAL OVERDOSE[a]
Acetaminophen
Aspirin
Illicit drugs in rubber or plastic packages
Monoamine oxidase inhibitors
Sulfonylureas
Sustained-release formulation drugs
Thyroid hormones
Valproic acid
Warfarin-like anticoagulants

[a]Drugs coingested with agents having anticholinergic activity, as manifest by diminished GI motility, may also exhibit delayed onset of action.

BOX 4–1 ■ Valproic Acid

After therapeutic dosing, valproic acid has an elimination $t_{1/2}$ of about 14 h. Valproic acid poisoning may lead to coma. In predicting the duration of the coma, it is important to consider that, after overdose, first-order metabolic processes for valproate appear to become saturated, and the apparent elimination $t_{1/2}$ may exceed 30–45 h (Sztajnkrycer, 2002), putting the patient at risk for a much longer time.

Types of Therapeutic Drug Toxicity

In therapeutics, a drug typically produces numerous effects, but usually only one is sought as the primary goal of treatment; most of the other effects are undesirable effects for that therapeutic indication. *Side effects* of drugs usually are bothersome but not deleterious. Other undesirable effects may be characterized as toxic effects (Figure 4–3).

Dose-Dependent Reactions

Toxic effects of drugs may be classified as *pharmacological*, *pathological*, or *genotoxic*. Typically, the incidence and seriousness of the toxicity is proportionately related to the concentration of the drug in the body and to the duration of the exposure.

Pharmacological Toxicity. The CNS depression produced by barbiturates is largely predictable in a dose-dependent fashion. The progression of clinical effects goes from anxiolysis to sedation to somnolence to coma. Similarly, the degree of hypotension produced by nifedipine is related to the dose of the drug administered. Tardive dyskinesia (see Chapter 16), an extrapyramidal motor disorder associated with use of antipsychotic medications, seems to be dependent on duration of exposure. Pharmacological toxicity can also occur when the correct dose is given; for example, there is phototoxicity associated with exposure to sunlight in patients treated with tetracyclines, sulfonamides, chlorpromazine, and nalidixic acid.

Pathological Toxicity. Acetaminophen is metabolized to nontoxic glucuronide and sulfate conjugates and to a highly reactive metabolite NAPQI via CYP isoforms. At a therapeutic dose of acetaminophen, NAPQI binds to nucleophilic glutathione, but in acetaminophen overdose, glutathione depletion may lead to the pathological finding of hepatic necrosis due to shunting of NAPQI toward interactions with nucleophilic cellular macromolecules (Figure 4–4).

Genotoxic Effects. Ionizing radiation and many environmental chemicals are known to injure DNA and may lead to mutagenic or carcinogenic toxicities. Many of the cancer chemotherapeutic agents (see Chapters 65–68) may be genotoxic (see Chapters 6 and 7).

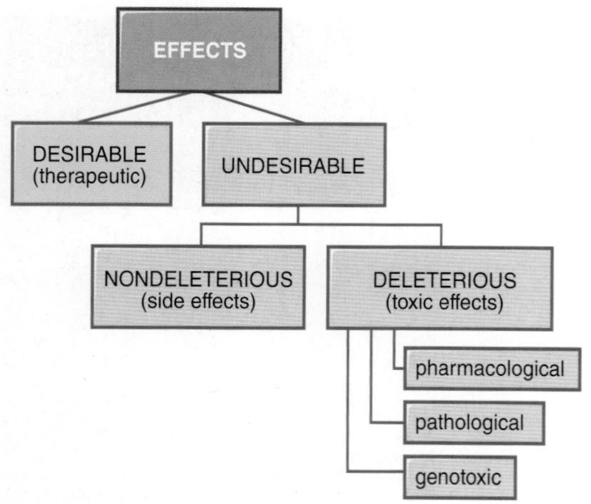

Figure 4–3 *Spectrum of the effects of pharmaceuticals.*

Allergic Reactions

An *allergy* is an adverse reaction, mediated by the immune system, that results from previous sensitization to a particular chemical or to one that is structurally similar (see Chapter 34). Allergic responses have been divided into four general categories based on the mechanism of immunological involvement.

Type I: Anaphylactic Reactions. Anaphylaxis is mediated by IgE antibodies. The Fc portion of IgE can bind to receptors on mast cells and basophils. If the Fab portion of the antibody molecule then binds an antigen, various mediators (e.g., histamine, leukotrienes, and prostaglandins) are released and cause vasodilation, edema, and an inflammatory response. The main targets of this type of reaction are the GI tract (food allergies), the skin (urticaria and atopic dermatitis), the respiratory system (rhinitis and asthma), and the vasculature (anaphylactic shock). These responses tend to occur quickly after challenge with an antigen to which the individual has been sensitized and are termed *immediate hypersensitivity reactions.*

Type II: Cytolytic Reactions. Type II allergies are mediated by both IgG and IgM antibodies and usually are attributed to their capacity to activate the complement system. The major target tissues for cytolytic reactions are the cells in the circulatory system. Examples of type II allergic responses include penicillin-induced hemolytic anemia, quinidine-induced thrombocytopenic purpura, and sulfonamide-induced granulocytopenia. These autoimmune reactions to drugs usually subside within several months after removal of the offending agent.

Type III: Arthus Reactions. Type III allergic reactions are mediated predominantly by IgG; the mechanism involves the generation of antigen-antibody complexes that subsequently fix complement. The complexes are deposited in the vascular endothelium, where a destructive inflammatory response called *serum sickness* occurs. The clinical symptoms of serum sickness include urticarial skin eruptions, arthralgia or arthritis, lymphadenopathy, and fever. Several drugs, including commonly used antibiotics, can induce serum sickness-like reactions. These

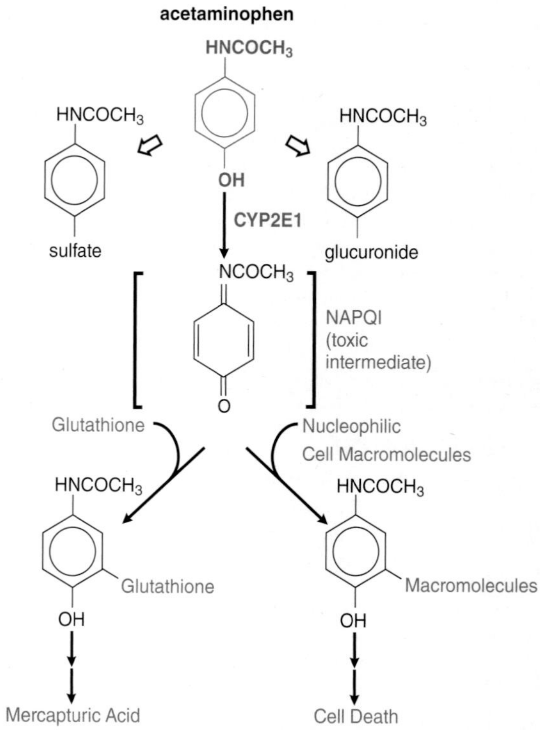

acetaminophen
$HNCOCH_3$
OH
CYP2E1
$HNCOCH_3$ sulfate
$HNCOCH_3$ glucuronide
$NCOCH_3$
O
NAPQI (toxic intermediate)
Glutathione
Nucleophilic Cell Macromolecules
$HNCOCH_3$ Glutathione OH
$HNCOCH_3$ Macromolecules OH
Mercapturic Acid
Cell Death

Figure 4–4 *Pathways of acetaminophen metabolism and toxicity.* The toxic intermediate NAPQI is *N*-acetyl-*p*-benzoquinoneimine.

reactions usually last 6–12 days and then subside after the offending agent is eliminated.

Type IV: Delayed Hypersensitivity Reactions. These reactions are mediated by sensitized T lymphocytes and macrophages. When sensitized cells come in contact with antigen, an inflammatory reaction is generated by the production of lymphokines and the subsequent influx of neutrophils and macrophages. An example of type IV or delayed hypersensitivity is the contact dermatitis caused by poison ivy.

Idiosyncratic Reactions and Pharmacogenetic Contributions

Idiosyncrasy is an abnormal reactivity to a chemical that is peculiar to a given individual; the idiosyncratic response may be extreme sensitivity to low doses or extreme insensitivity to high doses of drugs. A common mechanism is covalent drug binding to serum proteins that leads to the presentation of a foreign hapten, resulting in an immunotoxicological response.

Many interindividual differences in drug responses have a *pharmacogenetic basis* (see Chapter 7). A fraction of black males (~10%) develop a serious hemolytic anemia when they receive primaquine as an antimalarial therapy; this development is due to a genetic deficiency of erythrocyte glucose-6-phosphate dehydrogenase. Polymorphisms in NAT2 lead to a multimodal distribution of isoniazid acetylation and clearance (Figures 60–3 and 60–4). Variability in the anticoagulant response to warfarin is due to polymorphisms in CYP2C9 and VKORC1 (see Figure 7–7, Figure 32–6, and Table 32–2). In addition, CYP3A4 and CYP2D6 metabolize a large number of drugs in the liver (see Figure 6–3). Single nucleotide polymorphic variants in CYP3A4 and CYP2D6 can affect enzyme activity and thus alter drug $t_{1/2}$. Administration of a drug that is a CYP substrate in combination with a drug that is an inhibitor of the same CYP can lead to drug overdose toxicity. Many package inserts for drugs provide prescribing information warning of these drug-drug interactions.

Drug-Drug Interactions

Patients are commonly treated with more than one drug may also be using over-the-counter medications, vitamins, and other "natural" supplements; and may have unusual diets. All of these factors can contribute to drug interactions, a failure of therapy, and toxicity. Figure 4–5 summarizes the mechanisms and types of interactions.

Interaction of Absorption. A drug may cause either an increase or a decrease in the absorption of another drug from the intestinal lumen. Ranitidine, an antagonist of histamine H_2 receptors, raises gastrointestinal pH and may increase the absorption of basic drugs such as triazolam (O'Connor-Semmes et al., 2001). Conversely, the bile acid sequestrant cholestyramine leads to significantly reduced serum concentrations of propranolol (Hibbard et al., 1984).

Interaction of Protein Binding. Many drugs, such as aspirin, barbiturates, phenytoin, sulfonamides, valproic acid, and warfarin, are highly protein bound in the plasma, and it is the free (unbound) drug that produces the clinical effects. These drugs may have enhanced toxicity in overdose if protein-binding sites become saturated in physiological states that lead to hypoalbuminemia, or when displaced from plasma proteins by other drugs (Guthrie et al., 1995).

Interaction of Metabolism. A drug can frequently influence the metabolism of one or several other drugs (see Chapter 6), especially when hepatic CYPs are involved. Acetaminophen is partially transformed by CYP2E1 to the toxic metabolite NAPQI (see Figure 4–4). Intake of ethanol, a potent inducer of CYP2E1, may lead to increased susceptibility to acetaminophen poisoning after overdose (Dart et al., 2006).

Interaction of Receptor Binding. Buprenorphine is an opioid with partial agonist and antagonist receptor activities, commonly used to treat opioid addiction. The drug binds to opiate receptors with high affinity and can prevent euphoria from concomitant use of narcotic drugs of abuse.

Interaction of Therapeutic Action. Aspirin is an inhibitor of platelet aggregation, heparin is an anticoagulant; given together, they may increase risk for bleeding. Sulfonylureas cause hypoglycemia by stimulating pancreatic insulin release, whereas biguanide drugs (e.g., metformin) lead to decreased hepatic glucose production, and these drugs can be used together to control diabetic hyperglycemia.

Such drug interactions are *additive* when the combined effect of two drugs equals the sum of the effect of each agent given alone and *synergistic* when the combined effect exceeds the sum of the effects of each drug given alone. *Potentiation of toxicity* describes the creation of a toxic effect from one drug due to the presence of another drug. *Antagonism* is the interference of one drug with the action of another. *Functional* or *physiological antagonism* occurs when two chemicals produce opposite effects on the same physiological function. *Chemical antagonism*, or *inactivation*, is a reaction between two chemicals to neutralize their effects, such as is seen with chelation therapy. *Dispositional antagonism* is the alteration of the disposition of a substance (its absorption, biotransformation, distribution, or excretion) so that less of the agent reaches the target organ or its persistence in the target organ is reduced. *Receptor* (meaning receptor, enzyme, drug transporter, ion channel, etc.) *antagonism* is the blockade of the effect of one drug by another drug that competes at the receptor site.

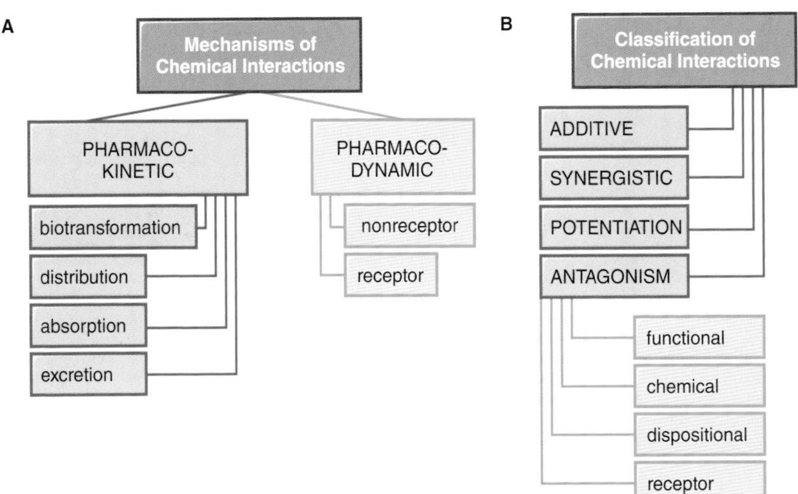

Figure 4–5 *Mechanisms and classification of drug interactions.*

SECTION I GENERAL PRINCIPLES

Descriptive Toxicity Testing in Animals

Two main principles or assumptions underlie all descriptive toxicity tests performed in animals.

First, those effects of chemicals produced in laboratory animals, when properly qualified, apply to human toxicity. When calculated on the basis of dose per unit of body surface, toxic effects in human beings usually are encountered in the same range of concentrations as those in experimental animals. On the basis of body weight, human beings generally are more vulnerable than experimental animals.

Second, exposure of experimental animals to toxic agents in high doses is a necessary and valid method to discover possible hazards to human beings who are exposed to much lower doses. This principle is based on the quantal dose-response concept. As a matter of practicality, the number of animals used in experiments on toxic materials usually will be small compared with the size of human populations potentially at risk. For example, 0.01% incidence of a serious toxic effect (such as cancer) represents 25,000 people in a population of 250 million. Such an incidence is unacceptably high. Yet, detecting an incidence of 0.01% experimentally probably would require a minimum of 30,000 animals. To estimate risk at low dosage, large doses must be given to relatively small groups instead. *The validity of the necessary extrapolation is clearly a crucial question.*

Chemicals are first tested for toxicity by estimation of the LD_{50} in two animal species by two routes of administration; one of these is the expected route of exposure of human beings to the chemical being tested. The number of animals that die in a 14-day period after a single dose is recorded. The animals also are examined for signs of intoxication, lethargy, behavioral modification, and morbidity. The chemical is next tested for toxicity by repeat exposure, usually for 90 days. This study is performed most often in two species by the route of intended use or exposure with at least three doses. A number of parameters are monitored during this period, and at the end of the study, organs and tissues are examined by a pathologist.

Long-term or chronic studies are carried out in animals at the same time that clinical trials are undertaken. For drugs, the length of exposure depends somewhat on the intended clinical use. If the drug normally would be used for short periods under medical supervision, as would an antimicrobial agent, a chronic exposure of animals for 6 months might suffice. If the drug would be used in human beings for longer periods, a study of chronic use for 2 years may be required.

Studies of chronic exposure often are used to determine the carcinogenic potential of chemicals. These studies usually are performed in rats and mice for the average lifetime of the species. Other tests are designed to evaluate teratogenicity (congenital malformations), perinatal and postnatal toxicity, and effects on fertility. Teratogenicity studies usually are performed by administering drugs to pregnant rats and rabbits during the period of organogenesis. *In silico* computational methods of systems chemical biology may soon contribute to such studies.

Safety Pharmacology and Clinical Trials

Fewer than one-third of the drugs tested in clinical trials reach the marketplace. U.S. federal law and ethical considerations require that the study of new drugs in humans be conducted in accordance with stringent guidelines.

Once a drug is judged ready to be studied in humans, an IND application must be filed with the FDA. The IND includes (1) information on the composition and source of the drug; (2) chemical and manufacturing information; (3) all data from animal studies; (4) proposed clinical plans and protocols; (5) the names and credentials of physicians who will conduct the clinical trials; and (6) a compilation of the key data relevant to study the drug in humans made available to investigators and their IRBs.

Testing in humans begins only after sufficient acute and subacute animal toxicity studies have been completed. Chronic safety testing in animals, including carcinogenicity studies, is usually done concurrently with clinical trials. Accumulating and analyzing all necessary data often requires 4–6 years of clinical testing. In each of the three formal phases of clinical trials, volunteers or patients must be informed of the investigational status of the drug as well as the possible risks and must be allowed to decline or to consent to participate and receive the drug. These regulations are based on the ethical principles set forth in the Declaration of Helsinki. In addition, an interdisciplinary IRB at the facility where the clinical drug trial will be conducted must review and approve the scientific and ethical plans for testing in humans. The prescribed phases, time lines, and costs for developing a new drug are presented in Table 1–1 and Figure 1–1.

Epidemiology of Adverse Drug Responses and Pharmaceutical Poisoning

Poisoning can occur in many ways following therapeutic and nontherapeutic exposures to drugs or chemicals (Table 4–2). In the U.S., an estimated 2 million hospitalized patients have serious adverse drug reactions each year, and about 100,000 suffer fatal adverse drug reactions (Lazarou et al., 1998). Use of good principles of prescribing, as described in Appendix I and Table 4–5, can aid in avoiding such adverse outcomes.

Some toxicities of pharmaceuticals can be predicted based on their known pharmacological mechanism; often, however, the therapeutic toxicity profile of a drug becomes apparent only during the postmarketing period. The Adverse Event Reporting System of the FDA relies on two signals to detect rarer ADEs. First, the FDA requires drug manufacturers to perform postmarketing surveillance of prescription drugs and nonprescription products. Second, the FDA operates a voluntary reporting system (MedWatch, at http://www.fda.gov/Safety/MedWatch) available to both health professionals and consumers. Hospitals may also support committees to investigate potential ADEs. Unfortunately, any national data set will likely underestimate the morbidity and mortality attributable to ADEs due to underreporting and the difficulty of estimating the denominator of total patient exposures.

Therapeutic drug toxicity is only a subset of poisoning, as noted in Table 4–2. Misuse and abuse of both prescription and illicit drugs are major public health problems. The incidence of unintentional, noniatrogenic poisoning is bimodal, primarily affecting exploratory young children, ages 1–5 years, and the elderly. *Intentional* overdose with pharmaceuticals is most common in adolescence and through adulthood. The substances most frequently involved in human exposures and fatalities are presented in Tables 4–3 and 4–4, respectively.

Prevention of Poisoning

Reduction of Medication Errors

Over the past decade, considerable attention has been given to the reduction of medication errors and ADEs. Medication errors can occur in any part of the medication prescribing or use process, whereas ADEs are injuries related to the use or nonuse of medications. It is believed that medication errors are 50–100 times more common than ADEs (Bates et al., 1995). The "five rights" noted in Box 4–2 can serve as a corrective.

TABLE 4–2 ■ POTENTIAL SCENARIOS FOR THE OCCURRENCE OF POISONING
Therapeutic drug toxicity
Exploratory exposure by young children
Environmental exposure
Occupational exposure
Recreational abuse
Errors of prescribing, dispensing, or administering
Purposeful administration for self-harm
Purposeful administration to harm another

TABLE 4–3 ■ SUBSTANCES MOST FREQUENTLY INVOLVED IN HUMAN POISONING EXPOSURES

SUBSTANCE	%
Analgesics	11.3
Personal care products	7.7
Cleaning substances	7.7
Sedatives/hypnotics/antipsychotics	5.9
Antidepressants	4.4
Antihistamines	4.0
Cardiovascular drugs	4.0
Foreign bodies/toys/miscellaneous	3.9
Pesticides	3.2

In the subset of pediatric exposures (age < 5 years), cosmetic/personal care products and household cleaning products accounted for 25% of cases, followed by analgesics (9.3%), foreign bodies/toys (6.7%), topical preparations (5.8%), vitamins (4.5%), and antihistamines (4.3%).
Source: Data from Mowry et al., 2015.

TABLE 4–4 ■ POISONS ASSOCIATED WITH THE LARGEST NUMBER OF HUMAN FATALITIES

Sedatives/hypnotics/antipsychotics	Stimulants and street drugs
Cardiovascular drugs	Alcohols
Acetaminophen (alone and in combinations)	SSRIs
Opioids	

As reported in Mowry et al., 2015.

BOX 4–2 ■ Five Principles of Safe Medication

Following the "five rights" of safe medication administration can help practitioners avoid medication errors:

Right drug, right patient, right dose, right route, right time

In practice, accomplishing a reduction in medication errors involves scrutiny of the systems involved in prescribing, documenting, transcribing, dispensing, administering, and monitoring a therapy, as presented in Appendix I. Good medication use practices have mandatory and redundant checkpoints (Figure 4–6), such as having a pharmacist, a doctor, and a nurse, all review and confirm, prior to the drug's administration, that an ordered dose of a medication is appropriate for the patient. Several practical strategies can help to reduce medication errors within health care settings (Table 4–5).

Poisoning Prevention in the Home

There are several contexts into which poisoning prevention can be directed (Table 4-2). Depression and suicidal ideation need to be identified and treated. Exposure to hazards in the home, outdoor, and work environments need to be reduced to reasonably achievable levels. Poisoning prevention strategies may be categorized as *passive*, requiring no behavior change on the part of the individual, or *active*, requiring sustained adaptation to be successful. Passive prevention strategies are the most effective (Table 4-6). The incidence of poisoning in children has decreased dramatically over the past four decades, largely due to improved safety packaging of drugs, drain cleaners, turpentine, and other household chemicals; improved medical training and care; and increased public awareness of potential poisons.

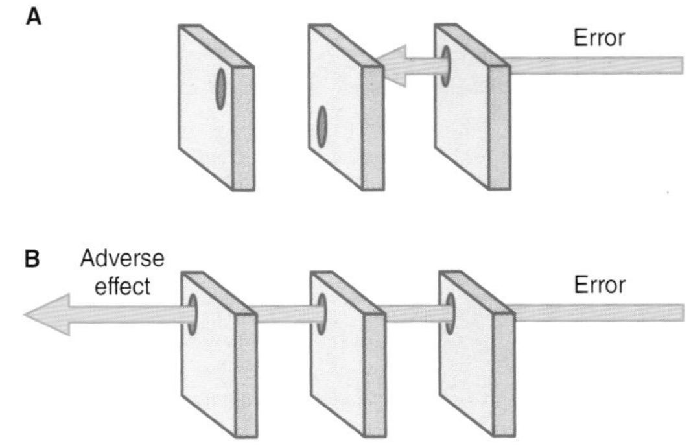

Figure 4–6 *The "Swiss cheese" model of medication error.* Several checkpoints typically exist to identify and prevent an adverse drug event, and that adverse event can only occur if holes in several systems align. **A.** One systematic error does not lead to an adverse event because it is prevented by another check in the system. **B.** Several systematic errors can align to allow an adverse event to occur. (Data from Reason J, *Br Med J*, 2000;320:768–770.)

Principles of Treatment of Poisoning

When toxicity is expected or occurs, the priorities of poisoning treatment are to

- *Maintain vital physiological functions*
- *Reduce or prevent absorption and enhance elimination to minimize the tissue concentration of the poison*
- *Combat the toxicological effects of the poison at the effector sites (Box 4–3)*

Identification of Clinical Patterns of Toxicity

A medical history may allow for the creation of a list of available medications or chemicals implicated in a poisoning event. Often, an observation of physical symptoms and signs may be the only additional clues to a poisoning diagnosis. Groups of physical signs and symptoms associated with specific poisoning syndromes are known as *toxidromes* (Erickson et al., 2007; Osterhoudt, 2004) (Table 4–7).

TABLE 4–5 ■ BEST PRACTICE RECOMMENDATIONS TO REDUCE MEDICATION ADMINISTRATION ERRORS[a]

SHORT TERM

- Maintain unit-dose distribution systems for nonemergency medications
- Have pharmacies prepare intravenous solutions
- Remove inherently dangerous medications (e.g., concentrated KCl) from patient care areas
- Develop special procedures for high-risk drugs
- Improve drug-related clinical information resources
- Improve medication administration education for clinicians
- Educate patients about the safe and accurate use of medications
- Improve access of bedside clinicians to pharmacists

LONG TERM

Implement technology-based safeguards:

- Computerized order entry
- Computerized dose and allergy checking
- Computerized medication tracking
- Use of bar codes or electronic readers for medication preparation and administration

[a]See Massachusetts Coalition for the Prevention of Medical Errors, 2017.

TABLE 4–6 ■ PASSIVE POISONING PREVENTION STRATEGIES AND EXAMPLES

Reduce manufacture/sale of poisons *Withdrawal of phenformin from U.S. pharmaceutical market*
Decrease amount of poison in a consumer product *Limiting number of pills in a single bottle of baby aspirin*
Prevent access to poison *Using child-resistant packaging*
Change product formulation *Removing ethanol from mouthwash*

The urine drug toxicology test is an immunoassay designed to detect common drugs of abuse, such as amphetamines, barbiturates, benzodiazepines, cannabis, cocaine, and opiates. Acute poisoning with these substances can usually be determined on clinical grounds, and the results of these assays are infrequently available fast enough to guide stabilization. In addition, detection of drugs or their metabolites on a urine immunoassay does not mean that the detected drug is responsible for the currently observed poisoning illness. When ingestion of acetaminophen or aspirin cannot clearly be excluded via the exposure history, serum quantification of these drugs is recommended. An ECG may be useful at detecting heart blocks, Na^+ channel blockade, or K^+ channel blockade associated with specific medication classes (Table 4–8). Further laboratory analysis should be tailored to the individual poisoning circumstance.

Decontamination of the Poisoned Patient

Poisoning exposures may be by inhalation, by dermal or mucosal absorption, by injection, or by ingestion. The first step in preventing absorption of poison is to stop any ongoing exposure. If necessary, eyes and skin should be washed copiously. GI decontamination prevents or reduces absorption of a substance after it has been ingested. The strategies for GI decontamination are *gastric emptying, adsorption of poison, WBI,* and *catharsis*. Minimal indications for considering GI decontamination include

- The poison must be potentially dangerous.
- The poison must still be unabsorbed in the stomach or intestine, so it must be soon after ingestion.
- The procedure must be able to be performed safely and with proper technique.

Gastric emptying is rarely recommended anymore (Manoguerra and Cobaugh, 2005), but the administration of activated charcoal and the performance of WBI remain therapeutic options. Gastric emptying reduces drug absorption by about one-third under optimal conditions (American Academy of Clinical Toxicology, 2004; Tenenbein et al., 1987) (see Syrup of Ipecac section that follows).

BOX 4–3 ■ Initial Stabilization of the Poisoned Patient

The "ABCDE" mnemonic of emergency care applies to the treatment of acute poisoning:

Airway	Maintain patency
Breathing	Maintain adequate oxygenation and ventilation
Circulation	Maintain perfusion of vital organs
Disability	Assess for CNS dysfunction *If neurological disability is noted, consider* • *O_2 administration (check pulse oximetry)* • *Dextrose administration (check [glucose] in blood)* • *Naloxone administration (consider empiric trial)* • *Thiamine (for adult patients receiving dextrose)*
Exposure	Assess "toxidrome" (see Table 4–7)

In severe cases, endotracheal intubation, mechanical ventilation, pharmacological blood pressure support, or extracorporeal circulatory support may be necessary and appropriate.

Adsorption

Adsorption of a poison refers to the binding of a poison to the surface of another substance so that the poison is less available for absorption into the body. Fuller's earth has been suggested as an adsorbent for paraquat, Prussian blue binds thallium and cesium, and sodium polystyrene can adsorb lithium. The most common adsorbent used in the treatment of acute drug overdose is activated charcoal.

Activated Charcoal. Charcoal is created through controlled pyrolysis of organic matter and is *activated* through steam or chemical treatment, which increases its internal pore structure and adsorptive surface capacity. The surface of activated charcoal contains carbon moieties that are capable of binding poisons. The recommended dose is typically 0.5–2 g/kg of body weight, up to a maximum tolerated dose of about 75–100 g. As a rough estimate, 10 g of activated charcoal is expected to bind about 1 g of drug. Alcohols, corrosives, hydrocarbons, and metals are not well adsorbed by charcoal. Complications of activated charcoal therapy include vomiting, constipation, pulmonary aspiration, and death. Nasogastric administration of charcoal increases the incidence of vomiting (Osterhoudt et al., 2004) and may increase the risk for pulmonary aspiration. Charcoal should not be given to patients with suspected GI perforation or to patients who may be candidates for endoscopy. Use of activated charcoal in the treatment of poisoning has declined over the last 20 years to 2.1% of cases in 2014 (Mowry et al., 2015).

Whole-Bowel Irrigation

Whole-bowel irrigation involves the enteral administration of large amounts of a high-molecular-weight, iso-osmotic polyethylene glycol electrolyte solution with the goal of passing poison by the rectum before it can be absorbed. Potential candidates for WBI include:

- "body packers" with intestinal packets of illicit drugs
- patients with iron overdose
- patients who have ingested patch pharmaceuticals
- patients with overdoses of sustained-release or bezoar-forming drugs

Polyethylene glycol electrolyte solution is typically administered at a rate of 25–40 mL/kg/h until the rectal effluent is clear and no more drug is being passed. To achieve these high administration rates, a nasogastric tube may be used. WBI is contraindicated in the presence of bowel obstruction or perforation and may be complicated by abdominal distention or pulmonary aspiration.

Cathartics. The two most common categories of simple cathartics are the Mg^{2+} salts, such as magnesium citrate and magnesium sulfate, and the nondigestible carbohydrates, such as sorbitol. The use of simple cathartics has been abandoned as a GI decontamination strategy.

Gastric Lavage. The procedure for gastric lavage involves passing an orogastric tube into the stomach with the patient in the left lateral decubitus position with head lower than feet. After withdrawing stomach contents, 10–15 mL/kg (up to 250 mL) of saline lavage fluid is administered and withdrawn. This process continues until the lavage fluid returns clear. Complications of the procedure include mechanical trauma to the stomach or esophagus, pulmonary aspiration of stomach contents, and vagus nerve stimulation.

Syrup of Ipecac. The alkaloids cephaeline and emetine within syrup of ipecac act as emetics because of both a local irritant effect on the enteric tract and a central effect on the chemoreceptor trigger zone in the area postrema of the medulla. *Based on review of existing evidence, the American Academy of Pediatrics no longer recommends syrup of ipecac as part of its childhood injury prevention program, and the American Academy of Clinical Toxicology dissuades routine use of gastric emptying in the poisoned patient.* As a result, ipecac was administered in only 0.006% of all human poisonings in the U.S. in 2014 (Mowry et al., 2015).

TABLE 4–7 ■ COMMON TOXIDROMES

DRUG CLASS	EXAMPLE(S)	MENTAL STATUS	HR	BP	RR	T	PUPIL SIZE	OTHER
Sympathomimetic	Cocaine Amphetamine	Agitation	↑	↑		↑	↑	Tremor, diaphoresis
Anticholinergic	Diphenhydramine Atropine	Delirium	↑	↑		↑	↑	Ileus, flushing
Cholinergic	Organophosphates	Somnolence Coma			↑		↓	SLUDGE,[a] fasciculation
Opioid	Heroin Oxycodone	Somnolence Coma	↓		↓		↓	
Sedative-hypnotic	Benzodiazepines Barbiturates	Somnolence Coma		↓	↓			
Salicylate	Aspirin	Confusion	↑		↑	↑		Diaphoresis, vomiting
Ca^{2+} channel blocker	Verapamil		↓	↓				

BP, blood pressure; HR, heart rate; RR, respiratory rate; T, temperature.
[a]SLUDGE, muscarinic effects of salivation, lacrimation, urination, defecation, gastric cramping, and emesis.

Enhancing the Elimination of Poisons

Once absorbed, the deleterious toxicodynamic effects of some drugs may be reduced by methods that hasten their elimination from the body, as described next.

Manipulating Urinary pH: Urinary Alkalinization

Drugs subject to renal clearance are excreted into the urine by glomerular filtration and active tubular secretion; nonionized compounds may be reabsorbed far more rapidly than ionized polar molecules (see Chapter 2). Weakly acidic drugs are susceptible to "ion trapping" in the urine. Aspirin is a weak acid with a $pK_a = 3.0$. As the pH of the urine increases, more salicylate is in its ionized form at equilibrium, and more salicylic acid diffuses into the tubular lumen of the kidney. Urinary alkalinization is also believed to speed clearance of phenobarbital, chlorpropamide, methotrexate, and chlorophenoxy herbicides. The American Academy of Clinical Toxicologists recommends urine alkalinization as first-line treatment only for moderately severe salicylate poisoning that does not meet criteria for hemodialysis (Proudfoot et al., 2004).

To achieve alkalinization of the urine, 100–150 mEq of sodium bicarbonate in 1 L of 5% dextrose in water (D5W) is infused intravenously at twice the maintenance fluid requirements and then titrated to effect. Hypokalemia should be treated because it will hamper efforts to alkalinize the urine due to H^+-K^+ exchange in the kidney. Urine alkalinization is contraindicated in renal failure or if fluid administration may worsen pulmonary edema or congestive heart failure. Acetazolamide is not used to alkalinize urine as it promotes acidemia.

TABLE 4–8 ■ DIFFERENTIAL POISONING DIAGNOSIS (PARTIAL LISTING) FOR ELECTROCARDIOGRAPHIC MANIFESTATIONS OF TOXICITY

BRADYCARDIA/HEART BLOCK	QRS INTERVAL PROLONGATION	QTc INTERVAL PROLONGATION
Cholinergic agents Physostigmine Neostigmine Organophosphates, Carbamates *Sympatholytic agents* β Receptor antagonists Clonidine Opioids *Other* Digoxin Ca^{2+} channel blockers Lithium	Antiarrhythmia drugs Bupropion Chloroquine Diphenhydramine Lamotrigine Phenothiazines Propranolol Tricyclic antidepressants	See CredibleMeds® QTDrugs List: https://www.crediblemeds.org/new-drug-list/

Multiple-Dose Activated Charcoal

Activated charcoal adsorbs drug to its surface and promotes enteral elimination. Multiple doses of activated charcoal can speed elimination of absorbed drug by two mechanisms: Charcoal may interrupt enterohepatic circulation of hepatically metabolized drug excreted in the bile, and charcoal may create a diffusion gradient across the GI mucosa and promote movement of drug from the bloodstream onto the charcoal in the intestinal lumen. Activated charcoal may be administered in multiple doses, 12.5 g/h every 1, 2, or 4 h (smaller doses may be used for children). Charcoal enhances the clearance of many drugs of low molecular weight, small volume of distribution, and long elimination $t_{1/2}$. Multiple-dose activated charcoal is believed to have the highest potential utility in overdoses of carbamazepine, dapsone, phenobarbital, quinine, theophylline, and yellow oleander (American Academy of Clinical Toxicology, 1999; de Silva et al., 2003).

Extracorporeal Drug Removal

The ideal drug amenable to removal by hemodialysis has a low molecular weight, a low volume of distribution, high solubility in water, and minimal protein binding. Hemoperfusion involves passing blood through a cartridge containing adsorbent particles. The most common poisonings for which hemodialysis is sometimes used include salicylate, methanol, ethylene glycol, lithium, carbamazepine, and valproate.

Antidotal Therapies

Antidotal therapy involves antagonism or chemical inactivation of an absorbed poison. Among the most common specific antidotes used are *N*-acetyl-*L*-cysteine for acetaminophen poisoning, opioid antagonists for opioid overdose, and chelating agents for poisoning from certain metal ions. A list of antidotes used is presented in Table 4–9.

The pharmacodynamics of a poison can be altered by competition at a receptor, as in the antagonism provided by naloxone therapy in the setting of heroin overdose. A physiological antidote may use a different cellular mechanism to overcome the effects of a poison, as in the use of glucagon to circumvent a blocked β adrenergic receptor and increase cellular cyclic AMP in the setting of an overdose of a β adrenergic antagonist. Antivenoms and chelating agents bind and directly inactivate poisons.

TABLE 4–9 ■ COMMON ANTIDOTES AND THEIR INDICATIONS

ANTIDOTE	POISONING INDICATION(S)
Acetylcysteine	Acetaminophen
Atropine sulfate	Organophosphorus and carbamate pesticides
Benztropine	Drug-induced dystonia
Bicarbonate, sodium	Na^+ channel blocking drugs
Bromocriptine	Neuroleptic malignant syndrome
Calcium gluconate or chloride	Ca^{2+} channel blocking drugs, fluoride
Carnitine	Valproate hyperammonemia
Crotalidae polyvalent immune Fab	North American crotaline snake envenomation
Dantrolene	Malignant hyperthermia
Deferoxamine	Iron
Digoxin immune Fab	Cardiac glycosides
Diphenhydramine	Drug-induced dystonia
Dimercaprol (BAL)	Lead, mercury, arsenic
EDTA, $CaNa_2$	Lead
Ethanol	Methanol, ethylene glycol
Fomepizole	Methanol, ethylene glycol
Flumazenil	Benzodiazepines
Glucagon hydrochloride	β adrenergic antagonists
Hydroxocobalamin hydrochloride	Cyanide
Insulin (high dose)	Ca^{2+} channel blockers
Leucovorin calcium	Methotrexate
Methylene blue	Methemoglobinemia
Naloxone hydrochloride	Opioids
Octreotide acetate	Sulfonylurea-induced hypoglycemia
Oxygen, hyperbaric	Carbon monoxide
Penicillamine	Lead, mercury, copper
Physostigmine salicylate	Anticholinergic syndrome
Pralidoxime chloride (2-PAM)	Organophosphorus pesticides
Pyridoxine hydrochloride	Isoniazid seizures
Succimer (DMSA)	Lead, mercury, arsenic
Thiosulfate, sodium	Cyanide
Vitamin K_1 (phytonadione)	Coumarin, indanedione

The biotransformation of a drug can also be altered by an antidote; for example, fomepizole will inhibit alcohol dehydrogenase and stop the formation of toxic acid metabolites from ethylene glycol and methanol. Many drugs used in the supportive care of a poisoned patient (anticonvulsants, vasoconstricting agents, etc.) may be considered nonspecific functional antidotes.

The mainstay of therapy for poisoning is good support of the airway, breathing, circulation, and vital metabolic processes of the poisoned patient until the poison is eliminated from the body.

Resources for Information on Drug Toxicity and Poisoning

Additional information on poisoning from drugs and chemicals can be found in many dedicated books of toxicology (Flomenbaum et al., 2006; Klaassen, 2013; Olson, 2011; Shannon et al., 2007). A popular computer database for information on toxic substances is POISINDEX® (Micromedex, Inc., Denver, CO). The National Library of Medicine offers information on toxicology and environmental health (http://sis.nlm.nih.gov/enviro.html), including a link to TOXNET® (http://toxnet.nlm.nih.gov/). Regional poison control centers are a resource for valuable poisoning information and may be contacted within the U.S. through the national Poison Help hotline: 1-800-222-1222.

Acknowledgment: *Curtis D. Klaassen and Kevin Osterhoudt contributed to this chapter in recent editions of this book. We have retained some of their text in the current edition.*

Bibliography

American Academy of Clinical Toxicology and the European Association of Poisons Centres and Clinical Toxicologists. Position paper: gastric lavage. *J Toxicol Clin Toxicol*, **2004**, *42*:933–943.

American Academy of Clinical Toxicology and the European Association of Poisons Centres and Clinical Toxicologists. Position statement and practice guidelines on the use of multi-dose activated charcoal in the treatment of acute poisoning. *Clin Toxicol*, **1999**, *37*:731–751.

Bates DW, et al. Relationship between medication errors and adverse drug events. *J Gen Intern Med*, **1995**, *10*:199–205.

Bronstein AC, et al. 2007 Annual report of the American Association of Poison Control Centers' National Poison Data System (NPDS): 25th annual report. *Clin Toxicol*, **2008**, *46*:927–1057.

CredibleMeds®. QTDrugs List. Available at: https://crediblemeds.org. Accessed May 24, 2017.

Dart RC, et al. Acetaminophen poisoning: an evidence-based consensus guideline for out-of-hospital management. *Clin Toxicol*, **2006**, *44*:1–18.

de Silva HA, et al. Multiple-dose activated charcoal for treatment of yellow oleander poisoning: a single-blind, randomized, placebo-controlled trial. *Lancet*, **2003**, *361*:1935–1938.

Erickson TE, et al. The approach to the patient with an unknown overdose. *Emerg Med Clin North Am*, **2007**, *25*:249–281.

Flomenbaum NE, et al., eds. *Goldfrank's Toxicologic Emergencies*, 8th ed. McGraw-Hill, New York, **2006**.

Guthrie SK, et al. Hypothesized interaction between valproic acid and warfarin. *J Clin Psychopharmacol*, **1995**, *15*:138–139.

Hibbard DM, et al. Effects of cholestyramine and colestipol on the plasma concentrations of propralolol. *Br J Clin Pharmacol*, **1984**, *18*:337–342.

Klaassen CD, ed. *Casarett and Doull's Toxicology: The Basic Science of Poisons*, 8th ed. McGraw-Hill, New York, **2013**.

Lazarou J, et al. Incidence of adverse drug reactions in hospitalized patients: a meta-analysis of prospective studies. *JAMA*, **1998**, *279*:1200–1205.

Manoguerra AS, Cobaugh DJ. Guidelines for the Management of Poisonings Consensus Panel. *Clin Toxicol*, **2005**, *43*:1–10.

Massachusetts Coalition for the Prevention of Medical Errors. **2017**. Available at: macoalition.org. Accessed May 24, 2017.

Mowry JB, et al. 2014 Annual report of the American Association of Poison Control Centers' National Poison Data System (NPDS): 32nd annual report. *Clin Toxicol*, **2015**, *53*:962–1147.

O'Connor-Semmes RL, et al. Effect of ranitidine on the pharmacokinetics of triazolam and alpha-hydroxytriazolam in both young and older people. *Clin Pharmacol Ther*, **2001**, *70*:126–131.

Olson KR, ed. *Poisoning & Drug Overdose*, 6th ed. McGraw-Hill, New York, **2011**.

Osterhoudt KC. No sympathy for a boy with obtundation. *Pediatr Emerg Care*, **2004**, *20*:403–406.

Osterhoudt KC, et al. Risk factors for emesis after therapeutic use of activated charcoal in acutely poisoned children. *Pediatrics*, **2004**, *113*:806–810.

Proudfoot AT, et al. Position paper on urine alkalinization. *J Toxicol Clin Toxicol*, **2004**, *42*:1–26.

Pontel LA, et al. Endogenous formaldehyde is a hematopoietic stem cell genotoxin and metabolic carcinogen. *Mol Cell*, **2015**, *60*:177–188.

Reason J. Human error: models and management. *Br Med J*, **2000**, *320*:768–770.

Rivera W, et al. Delayed salicylate toxicity at 35 hours without early manifestations following a single salicylate ingestion. *Ann Pharmacother*, **2004**, *38*:1186–1188.

Shannon MW, et al., eds. *Haddad and Winchester's Clinical Management of Poisoning and Drug Overdose*, 4th ed. Saunders/Elsevier, Philadelphia, **2007**.

Sztajnkrycer MD. Valproic acid toxicity: overview and management. *Clin Toxicol*, **2002**, *40*:789–801.

Tenenbein M, et al. Efficacy of ipecac-induced emesis, orogastric lavage, and activated charcoal for acute drug overdose. *Ann Emerg Med*, **1987**, *16*:838–841.

Membrane Transporters and Drug Response

Kathleen M. Giacomini and Yuichi Sugiyama

第五章 膜转运体和药物效应

中文导读

本章主要介绍：膜转运体在治疗药物效应中的作用，包括对药物代谢动力学、药物效应动力学和耐药性的影响；膜转运体与药物不良反应；膜转运的基本机制，包括转运体与通道、被动扩散、易化扩散和主动转运；转运动力学；ABC转运体和SLC转运体的结构与机制；向量转运体；人类基因组中的转运体超家族，包括SLC超家族、ABC超家族、ABC转运体的生理作用及其在药物吸收和消除中的作用；肝脏和肾脏中与药物代谢动力学相关的转运体；脑部药物转运体和药物效应动力学，包括GABA摄取与GAT_1、GAT_3和GAT_2，儿茶酚胺摄取与NET，多巴胺摄取与DAT，以及血清素摄取与SERT；血脑屏障——药理学观点；扩展的清除概念和基于生理的药物代谢动力学模型；膜转运体的遗传变异对临床药物效应的影响；转运体对监管科学的影响。

Abbreviations

ABC: ATP *b*inding *c*assette
ABCC: ATP binding cassette family C
ACE inhibitor: angiotensin-converting enzyme inhibitor
AUC: area under the concentration-time curve
BBB: blood-brain barrier
BCRP: breast cancer resistance protein
BSEP: *b*ile *s*alt *e*xport *p*ump
CFTR: cystic fibrosis transmembrane regulator
$CL_{int,all}$: overall hepatic intrinsic clearance
CL_{met}: metabolic clearance
CPT-11: irinotecan hydrochloride
CSF: cerebrospinal fluid
DA: dopamine
DAT: dopamine transporter
FDA: U.S. Food and Drug Administration
GABA: γ-aminobutyric acid
GAT: GABA reuptake transporter
GSH, GSSG: reduced and oxidized glutathione
HIV: human immunodeficiency virus
HMG-CoA: 3-hydroxy-3-methylglutaryl coenzyme A
5HT: serotonin
α-KG: α-ketoglutarate
LAT: large amino acid transporter
MAO: monoamine oxidase
MATE1: multidrug and toxin extrusion protein 1
MDMA: 3,4-methylenedioxymethamphetamine
MRP: multidrug resistance protein
NBDs: nucleotide-binding domains
NE: norepinephrine
NET: NE transporter
NME: new molecular entity
NTCP: Na^+-*t*aurocholate *c*otransporting *p*olypeptide
OAT1: organic anion transporter 1
OCT1: organic cation transporter 1
OCTN: novel organic cation transporter
PAH: *p*-aminohippurate
PGE_2: prostaglandin E_2
Pgp: P-glycoprotein
PPARα: peroxisome proliferator-activated receptor α
RAR: retinoic acid receptor
RXR: retinoid X receptor
SERT: serotonin transporter
SLC: *so*lute *c*arrier
SNP: single-nucleotide polymorphism
SXR: steroid X receptor
URAT1: uric acid transporter 1
XOI: xanthine oxidase inhibitor

Membrane transport proteins are present in all organisms. These proteins control the influx of essential nutrients and ions and the efflux of cellular waste, environmental toxins, drugs, and other xenobiotics (Figure 5–1). Consistent with their critical roles in cellular homeostasis, about 2000 genes in the human genome, ~7% of the total number of genes, code for transporters or transporter-related proteins. The functions of membrane transporters may be facilitated (equilibrative, not requiring energy) or active (requiring energy). In considering the transport of drugs, pharmacologists generally focus on transporters from two major superfamilies, ABC and SLC transporters (Nigam, 2015).

Most ABC proteins are primary active transporters, which rely on ATP hydrolysis to actively pump their substrates across membranes. Among the best-recognized transporters in the ABC superfamily are Pgp (encoded by *ABCB1*, also termed *MDR1*) and CFTR (encoded by *ABCC7*).

The SLC superfamily includes genes that encode facilitated transporters and ion-coupled secondary active transporters. Fifty-two SLC families with about 395 transporters have been identified in the human genome (Hediger et al., 2013; Nigam et al., 2015). Many SLC transporters serve as drug targets or in drug absorption and disposition. Widely recognized SLC transporters include SERT and DAT, both targets for antidepressant medications.

Membrane Transporters in Therapeutic Drug Responses

Pharmacokinetics

Transporters important in pharmacokinetics generally are located in intestinal, renal, and hepatic epithelia, where they function in the selective absorption and elimination of endogenous substances and xenobiotics, including drugs. Transporters work in concert with drug-metabolizing enzymes to eliminate drugs and their metabolites (Figure 5–2). In addition, transporters in various cell types mediate tissue-specific drug distribution (drug targeting). Conversely, transporters also may serve as protective barriers to particular organs and cell types. For example, Pgp in the BBB protects the CNS from a variety of structurally diverse drugs through its efflux mechanisms.

Pharmacodynamics: Transporters as Drug Targets

Membrane transporters are the targets of many clinically used drugs. SERT (*SLC6A4*) is a target for a major class of antidepressant drugs, the SSRIs. Other neurotransmitter reuptake transporters serve as drug targets for the tricyclic antidepressants, various amphetamines (including amphetamine-like drugs used in the treatment of attention-deficit disorder in children), and anticonvulsants.

These transporters also may be involved in the pathogenesis of neuropsychiatric disorders, including Alzheimer and Parkinson diseases. An inhibitor of the vesicular monoamine transporter VMAT2 (SLC18A2), tetrabenazine, is approved for the symptomatic treatment of Huntington disease; the antichorea effect of tetrabenazine appears to relate to its capacity to deplete stores of biogenic amines by inhibiting their uptake into storage vesicles by VMAT2. Transporters that are nonneuronal also may be potential drug targets (e.g., cholesterol transporters in cardiovascular disease, nucleoside transporters in cancers, glucose transporters in metabolic syndromes, and Na^+-Cl^- cotransporters in the SLC12 family in hypertension).

Recently, first-in-class drugs that inhibit Na^+-glucose transporters in the SLC5 family (SGLT1 and SGLT2) have been approved for the treatment of type 2 diabetes. These drugs, which include canagliflozin, dapagliflozin, and empagliflozin, reduce renal reabsorption of glucose, thereby facilitating glucose elimination in the kidney. All three are prescribed as second-line therapy for treatment of inadequately controlled diabetes. In addition, lesinurad, a first-in-class drug that targets URAT1 (SLC22A12), was recently approved by the FDA for the treatment of gout when used with an XOI; other URAT1 inhibitors are in clinical trial. These drugs are uricosurics and act by selectively inhibiting uric acid reabsorption in the kidney.

Finally, a first-in-class drug, ivacaftor, was recently approved for the treatment of patients with cystic fibrosis who harbor a coding mutation in CFTR (ABCC7), CFTR-G551D. Ivacaftor, termed a potentiator, increases the probability that the mutant chloride channel, CFTR-G551D, remains in the open state. Other drugs in clinical trials for CFTR include both potentiators and correctors, compounds that enhance trafficking of mutant proteins to the plasma membrane.

Drug Resistance

Membrane transporters play critical roles in the development of resistance to anticancer drugs, antiviral agents, and anticonvulsants. *Decreased uptake of drugs*, such as folate antagonists, nucleoside analogues, and platinum complexes, is mediated by reduced expression of influx transporters required for these drugs to access the tumor. *Enhanced efflux of*

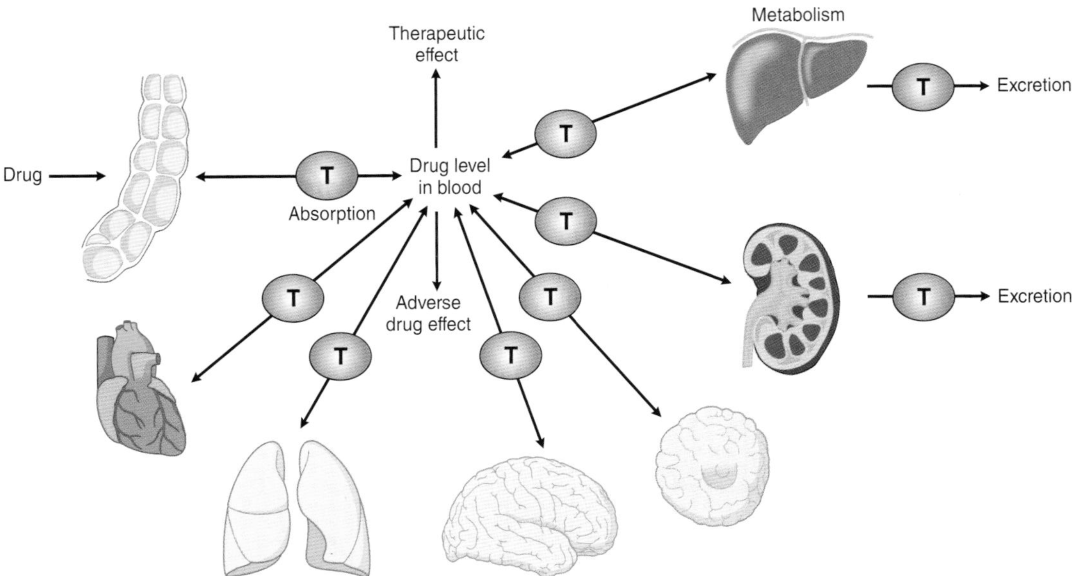

Figure 5–1 *Membrane transporters in pharmacokinetic pathways.* Membrane transporters (T) play roles in pharmacokinetic pathways (drug absorption, distribution, metabolism, and excretion), thereby setting systemic drug levels. Drug levels often drive therapeutic and adverse drug effects.

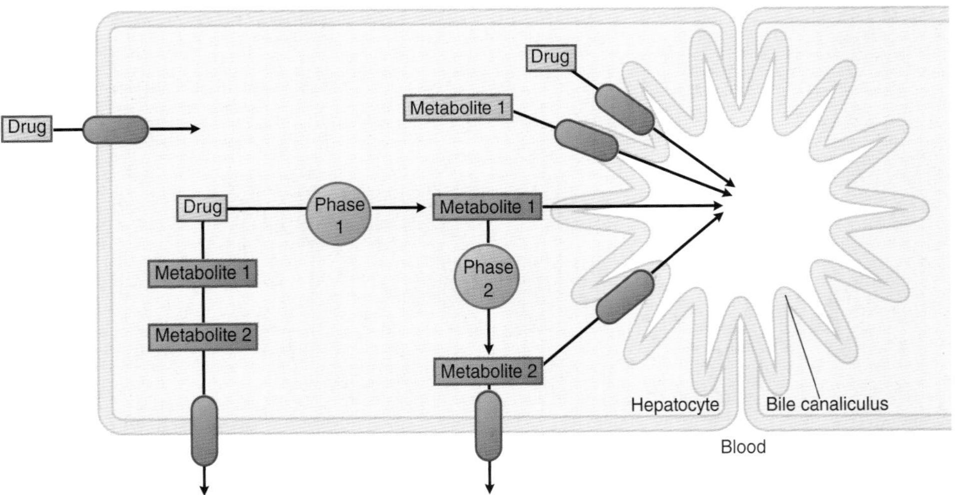

Figure 5–2 *Hepatic drug transporters.* Membrane transporters (red ovals with arrows) work in concert with phase 1 and phase 2 drug-metabolizing enzymes in the hepatocyte to mediate the uptake and efflux of drugs and their metabolites.

hydrophobic drugs is one mechanism of antitumor resistance in cellular assays of resistance. The overexpression of MRP4 is associated with resistance to antiviral nucleoside analogues (Aceti et al., 2015). Pgp (MDR1, ABCB1) and BCRP (ABCG2) can be overexpressed in tumor cells after exposure to cytotoxic anticancer agents and are implicated in resistance to these agents, exporting anticancer drugs, reducing their intracellular concentration, and rendering cells resistant to the drugs' cytotoxic effects. Modulation of MDR1 expression and activity to regulate drug resistance could be a useful adjunct in pharmacotherapy (Gu and Manautou, 2010; He et al., 2011; Toyoda et al., 2008).

Membrane Transporters and Adverse Drug Responses

As controllers of import and export, transporters ultimately control the exposure of cells to chemical carcinogens, environmental toxins, and drugs. Thus, transporters play crucial roles in the cellular activities and toxicities of these agents. Transporter-mediated adverse drug responses generally can be classified into three categories (Figure 5–3):

- Decreased uptake or excretion at clearance organs
- Increased uptake or decreased efflux at target organs

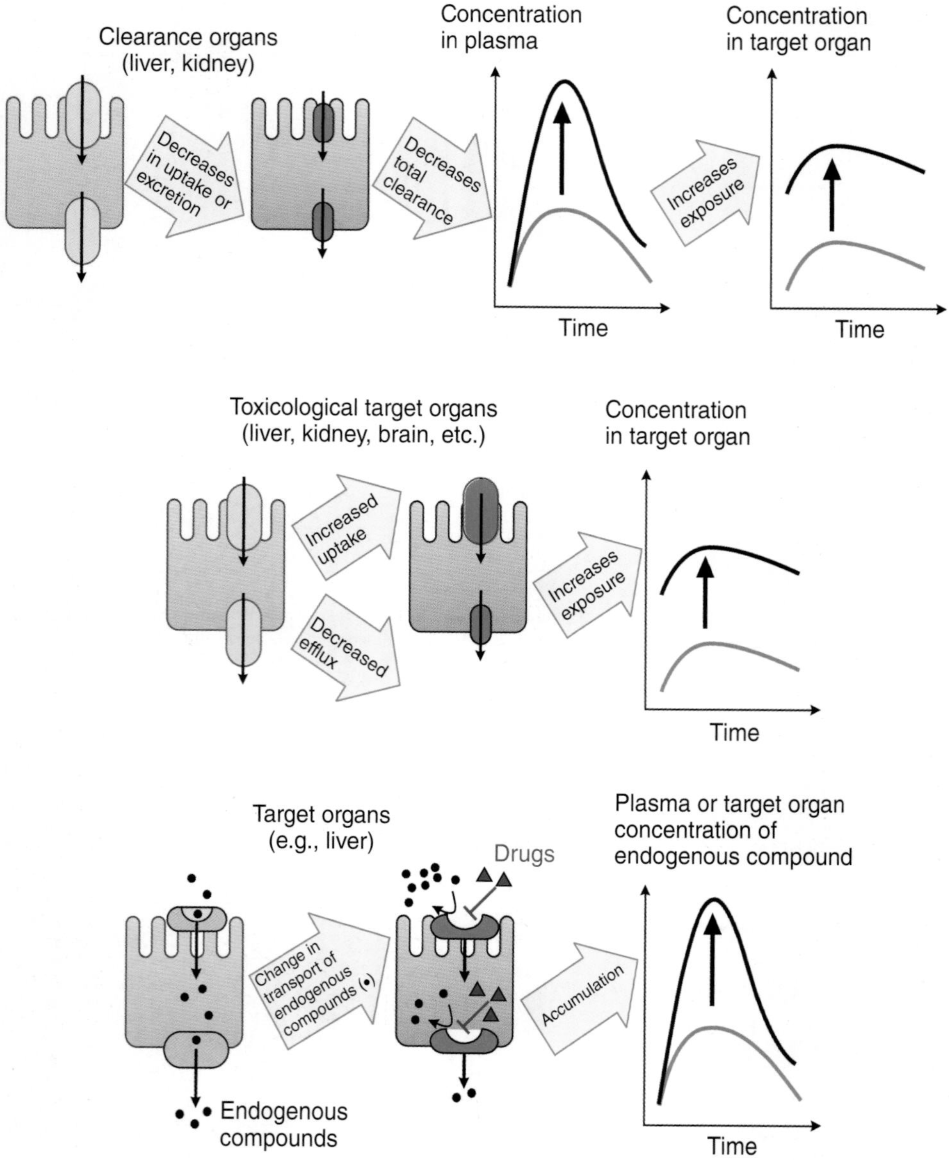

Figure 5–3 *Major mechanisms by which transporters mediate adverse drug responses.* Three cases are given. The left panel of each case provides a representation of the mechanism; the right panel shows the resulting effect on drug levels. (*Top panel*) Increase in the plasma concentrations of drug due to a decrease in the uptake or secretion in clearance organs (e.g., liver and kidney). (*Middle panel*) Increase in the concentration of drug in toxicological target organs due to enhanced uptake or reduced efflux. (*Bottom panel*) Increase in the plasma concentration of an endogenous compound (e.g., a bile acid) due to a drug inhibiting the influx of the endogenous compound in its eliminating or target organ. The diagram also may represent an increase in the concentration of the endogenous compound in the target organ owing to drug-inhibited efflux of the endogenous compound.

- Altered transport of endogenous compounds at target organs

Transporters expressed in the liver and kidney, as well as metabolic enzymes, are key determinants of drug exposure in the systemic circulation, thereby affecting exposure, and hence toxicity, in all organs (Figure 5–3, top panel). For example, after oral administration of an HMG-CoA reductase inhibitor (e.g., pravastatin), the efficient first-pass hepatic uptake of the drug by the SLC OATP1B1 maximizes the effects of such drugs on hepatic HMG-CoA reductase. Uptake by OATP1B1 also minimizes the escape of these drugs into the systemic circulation, where they can cause adverse responses, such as skeletal muscle myopathy.

Transporters expressed in tissues that may be targets for drug toxicity (e.g., brain) or in barriers to such tissues (e.g., the BBB) can tightly control local drug concentrations and thus control the exposure of these tissues to the drug (Figure 5–3, middle panel). For example, endothelial cells in the BBB are linked by tight junctions, and some efflux transporters are expressed on the blood-facing (luminal) side, thereby restricting the penetration of compounds into the brain. The interactions of loperamide and quinidine are good examples of transporter control of drug exposure at this site. Loperamide is a peripheral opioid used in the treatment of diarrhea and is a substrate of Pgp, which prevents accumulation of loperamide in the CNS. Inhibition of Pgp-mediated efflux in the BBB would cause an increase in the concentration of loperamide in the CNS and potentiate adverse effects. Indeed, coadministration of loperamide and the potent Pgp inhibitor quinidine results in significant respiratory depression, an adverse response to loperamide. Pgp is also expressed in the intestine, where inhibition of Pgp will reduce intestinal efflux of loperamide, increase its systemic concentrations, and contribute to increased concentrations in the CNS.

Drug-induced toxicity sometimes is caused by the concentrative tissue distribution mediated by influx transporters. For example, biguanides (e.g., metformin), used for the treatment of type 2 diabetes mellitus, can produce lactic acidosis, a lethal side effect. Biguanides are substrates of the OCT1 (SLC22A1), which is highly expressed in the liver; of OCT2 (SLC22A2), expressed in the kidney; and of OCT3 (SLC22A3) in adipocytes and skeletal muscle. In experimental animals lacking OCT1, hepatic uptake of biguanides and development of lactic acidosis are greatly reduced. These results indicate that OCT1-mediated hepatic uptake of biguanides and uptake into tissues such as kidney and skeletal muscle mediated by other OCTs play an important role in facilitating tissue concentrations of biguanides and thus the development of lactic acidosis (Wang et al., 2003), which may result from biguanide-induced impairment of mitochondrial function and consequent increased glycolytic flux (Dykens et al., 2008). Biguanides are exported by the MATE1 transporter, and inhibition of this efflux by a variety of drugs, including tyrosine kinase inhibitors, enhances biguanide toxicity (DeCorter et al., 2012).

OAT1 (SLC22A1), OCT1, and OCT2 provide other examples of transporter-related toxicity. OAT1 is expressed mainly in the kidney and is responsible for the renal tubular secretion of anionic compounds. Substrates of OAT1, such as cephaloridine (a β-lactam antibiotic) and adefovir and cidofovir (antiviral drugs), reportedly cause nephrotoxicity. Exogenous expression of OCT1 and OCT2 enhances the sensitivities of tumor cells to the cytotoxic effect of oxaliplatin for OCT1 and cisplatin and oxaliplatin for OCT2 (Zhang et al., 2006a). Renal toxicity of cisplatin is modulated by OCT2 present on the basolateral membrane of the proximal tubule as well as by transporters in the SLC47 family, MATE1 (SLC47A1) and MATE2 (SLC47A2), on the apical membrane (Harrach and Ciarimboli, 2015).

Drugs may modulate transporters for endogenous ligands and thereby exert adverse effects (Figure 5–3, bottom panel). For example, bile acids are taken up mainly by NTCP and excreted into the bile by BSEP (*ABCB11*). Bilirubin is taken up by OATP1B1 and conjugated with glucuronic acid; bilirubin glucuronide is excreted into the bile by the MRP2 (*ABCC2*) and transported into the blood by MRP3. Bilirubin glucuronide in the blood undergoes reuptake into the liver by OATP1B1. Inhibition of these transporters by drugs may cause cholestasis or hyperbilirubinemia.

Uptake and efflux transporters determine the plasma and tissue concentrations of endogenous compounds and xenobiotics, thereby influencing the systemic or site-specific toxicity of drugs.

Basic Mechanisms of Membrane Transport

Transporters Versus Channels

Both channels and transporters facilitate the membrane permeation of inorganic ions and organic compounds. In general, channels have two primary states, open and closed, that are stochastic phenomena. Only in the open state do channels appear to act as pores for the selected ions flowing down an electrochemical gradient. After opening, channels return to the closed state as a function of time. As noted, drugs termed *potentiators* (e.g., ivacaftor) may increase the probability that a channel is in the open state. By contrast, a transporter forms an intermediate complex with the substrate (solute), and a subsequent conformational change in the transporter induces translocation of the substrate to the other side of the membrane. As a consequence, the kinetics of solute movement differ between transporters and channels. Typical turnover rate constants of channels are 10^6 to 10^8 s^{-1}; those of transporters are, at most, 10^1 to 10^3 s^{-1}. Because a particular transporter forms intermediate complexes with specific compounds (referred to as *substrates*), transporter-mediated membrane transport is characterized by saturability and inhibition by substrate analogues, as described in the section Kinetics of Transport.

The basic mechanisms involved in solute transport across biological membranes include passive diffusion, facilitated diffusion, and active transport. Active transport can be further subdivided into primary and secondary active transport. These mechanisms are depicted in Figure 5–4.

Passive Diffusion

Simple diffusion of a solute across the plasma membrane consists of three processes: partition from the aqueous to the lipid phase, diffusion across the lipid bilayer, and repartition into the aqueous phase on the opposite side. Passive diffusion of any solute (including drugs) occurs down an electrochemical potential gradient of the solute.

Facilitated Diffusion

Diffusion of ions and organic compounds across the plasma membrane may be facilitated by a membrane transporter. Facilitated diffusion is a form of transporter-mediated membrane transport that does not require energy input. Just as in passive diffusion, the transport of ionized and nonionized compounds across the plasma membrane occurs down their electrochemical potential gradients. Therefore, steady state will be achieved when the electrochemical potentials of a compound on both sides of the membrane become equal.

Active Transport

Active transport is the form of membrane transport that requires the input of energy. It is the transport of solutes against their electrochemical gradients, leading to the concentration of solutes on one side of the plasma membrane and the creation of potential energy in the electrochemical gradient formed. Active transport plays an important role in the uptake and efflux of drugs and other solutes. Depending on the driving force, active transport can be subdivided into primary active transport in which ATP hydrolysis is coupled directly to solute transport, and secondary active transport, in which transport uses the energy in an existing electrochemical gradient established by an ATP-using process to move a solute uphill against its electrochemical gradient. Secondary active transport is further subdivided into symport and antiport. Symport describes movement of driving ion and transported solute in the same direction. Antiport occurs when the driving ion and the transported solute move in opposite directions, as when the sodium/calcium exchanger (SLC8A1) transports $3Na^+$ *into* and $1Ca^{2+}$ *out of* a cardiac ventricular myocyte (see Figure 5–4).

Primary Active Transport

Membrane transport that directly couples with ATP hydrolysis is called *primary active transport*. ABC transporters are examples of primary active transporters. In mammalian cells, ABC transporters mediate the unidirectional efflux of solutes across biological membranes. Another example of primary active transport that establishes the inward Na^+ gradient and outward K^+ gradient across the plasma membrane, found in all mammalian cells, is the Na^+,K^+-ATPase.

Secondary Active Transport

In secondary active transport, the transport across a biological membrane of a solute S_1 against its concentration gradient is energetically driven by the transport of another solute S_2 in accordance with its electrochemical gradient. Depending on the transport direction of the solute, secondary active transporters are classified as either symporters or antiporters. For example, using the inwardly directed Na^+ concentration gradient across the plasma membrane that the Na^+,K^+-ATPase maintains, the inward movement of 3 Na^+ can drive the outward movement of 1 Ca^{++} via the Na^+/Ca^{++} exchanger, NCX. This is an example of antiport, or exchange transport, in which the transporter moves S_2 and S_1 in opposite directions. *Symporters*, also termed *cotransporters*, transport S_2 and S_1 in the same direction, as for glucose transport into the body from the lumen of the small intestine by the Na^+-glucose transporter SGLT1 (see Figure 5–4).

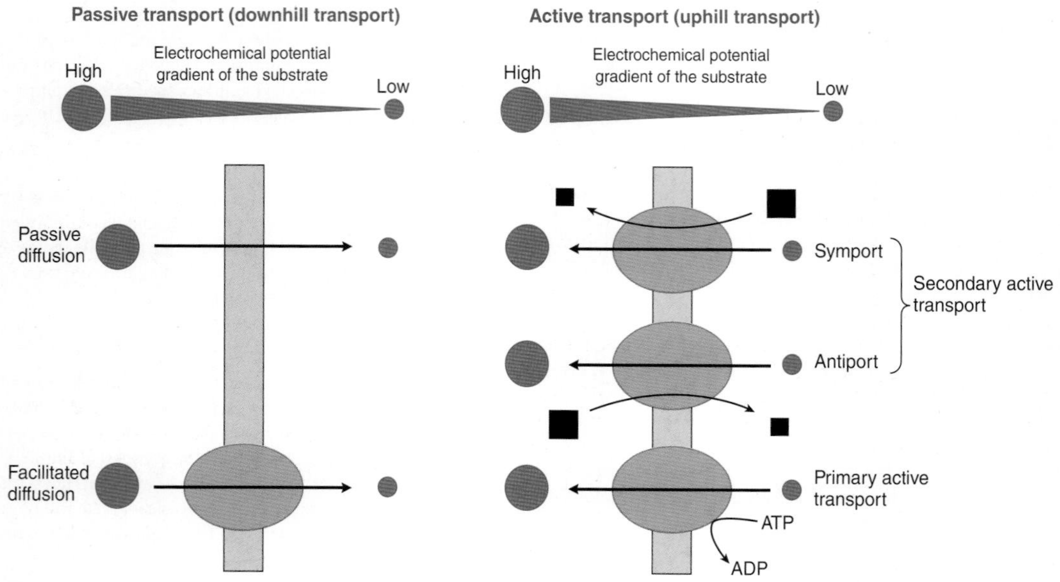

Figure 5–4 *Classification of membrane transport mechanisms.* Red circles depict the substrate. Size of the circles is proportional to the concentration of the substrate. Arrows show the direction of flux. Black squares represent the ion that supplies the driving force for transport (size is proportional to the concentration of the ion). Blue ovals depict transport proteins.

Kinetics of Transport

The flux of a substrate (rate of transport) across a biological membrane via a transporter-mediated process is characterized by saturability. The relationship between the flux v and substrate concentration C in a transporter-mediated process is given by the Michaelis-Menten equation:

$$v = \frac{V_{max}C}{K_m + C} \qquad \text{(Equation 5–1)}$$

where V_{max} is the maximum transport rate and is proportional to the density of transporters on the plasma membrane, and K_m is the Michaelis constant, which represents the substrate concentration at which the flux is half the V_{max} value. K_m is an approximation of the dissociation constant of the substrate from the intermediate complex. The K_m and V_{max} values can be determined by examining the flux at different substrate concentrations. Rearranging Equation 5–1 gives

$$v = -K_m \frac{v}{C} + V_{max} \qquad \text{(Equation 5–2)}$$

Plotting v versus v/C provides a convenient graphical method for determining the V_{max} and K_m values, the Eadie-Hofstee plot (Figure 5–5): The slope is $-K_m$ and the y intercept is V_{max}.

Transporter-mediated membrane transport of a substrate is also characterized by inhibition by other compounds. The manner of inhibition can be categorized as one of three types: *competitive*, *noncompetitive*, and *uncompetitive*. Competitive inhibition occurs when substrates and inhibitors share a common binding site on the transporter, resulting in an increase in the apparent K_m value in the presence of inhibitor. The flux of a substrate in the presence of a competitive inhibitor is

$$v = \frac{V_{max}C}{K_m(1 + I/K_i) + C} \qquad \text{(Equation 5–3)}$$

where I is the concentration of inhibitor, and K_i is the inhibition constant. Noncompetitive inhibition assumes that the inhibitor has an allosteric effect on the transporter, does not inhibit the formation of an intermediate complex of substrate and transporter, but does inhibit the subsequent translocation process.

$$v = \frac{V_{max}C}{K_m(1 + I/K_i) + C(1 + I/K_i)} \qquad \text{(Equation 5–4)}$$

Uncompetitive inhibition assumes that inhibitors can form a complex only with an intermediate complex of the substrate and transporter and inhibit subsequent translocation.

$$v = \frac{V_{max}C}{K_m + C(1 + I/K_i)} \qquad \text{(Equation 5–5)}$$

Transporter Structure and Mechanism

Predictions of secondary structure of membrane transport proteins based on hydropathy analysis indicate that membrane transporters in the SLC and ABC superfamilies are multimembrane-spanning proteins. Emerging crystals structures are adding to our ideas of the mechanisms of transport via these proteins.

ABC Transporters

The ABC superfamily includes 49 genes, each containing one or two conserved ABC regions. The core catalytic ABC regions of these proteins bind and hydrolyze ATP, using the energy for uphill transport of their substrates across the membrane. Most ABC transporters in eukaryotes move compounds from the cytoplasm to the cell exterior or into an intracellular compartment (endoplasmic reticulum, mitochondria, peroxisomes). ABC transporters also are found in prokaryotes, where they are involved predominantly in the import of essential compounds that cannot be obtained by passive diffusion (sugars, vitamins, metals, etc.).

ABC transporters have NBDs on the cytoplasmic side. The NBDs are considered the motor domains of ABC transporters and contain conserved motifs (e.g., Walker-A motif, ABC signature motif) that participate in binding and hydrolysis of ATP. Crystal structures of all four full

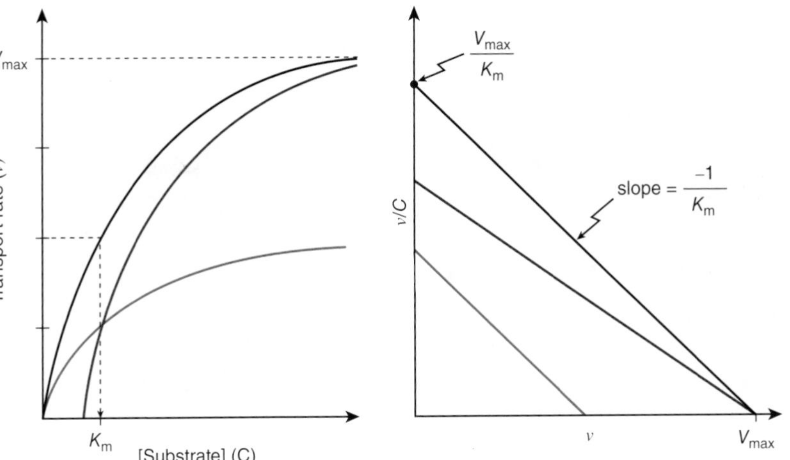

Figure 5–5 *Eadie-Hofstee plot of transport data.* The black lines show the hyperbolic concentration-dependence curve (v vs. C, left panel) and the Eadie-Hofstee transformation of the transport data (v/C vs. v, right panel) for a simple transport system. The blue lines depict transport in the presence of a competitive inhibitor (surmountable inhibition; achieves same V_{max}). The red lines depict the system in the presence of a noncompetitive inhibitor that effectively reduces the number of transporting sites but leaves the K_m of the functional sites unchanged. Involvement of multiple transporters with different K_m values gives an Eadie-Hofstee plot that is curved and can be resolved into multiple components. Algebraically, the Eadie-Hofstee plot of kinetic data is equivalent to the Scatchard plot of equilibrium binding data (see Chapter 3).

ABC transporters show two NBDs, which are in contact with each other, and a conserved fold. The mechanism, shared by these ABC transporters, appears to involve binding of ATP to the NBDs, which subsequently triggers an outward-facing conformation of the transporters. Dissociation of the hydrolysis products of ATP appears to result in an inward-facing conformation. In the case of drug extrusion, when ATP binds, the transporters open to the outside, releasing their substrates to the extracellular media. On dissociation of the hydrolysis products, the transporters return to the inward-facing conformation, permitting the binding of ATP and substrate (Figure 5–6). Although some ABC superfamily transporters contain only a single ABC motif, they form homodimers (BCRP/ABCG2) or heterodimers (ABCG5 and ABCG8) that exhibit a transport function.

SLC Transporters

The SLC superfamily of transporters comprises a structurally diverse group that includes channels, facilitators, and secondary active transporters (Hediger et al., 2013). SLC substrates include ionic and nonionic species and a variety of xenobiotics and drugs. Nonetheless, for a number of SLC transporters that are important to pharmacokinetics and pharmacodynamics, there are a few common structural and mechanistic aspects. Human SLC transporters may use an alternating access, the gated pore mechanism, whereby the transporter exposes a single solute binding site interchangeably at either side of the membrane barrier (Figure 5–7).

In general terms, the transporter undergoes a reversible conformational change between the two sides of the membrane during the translocation process. The transport cycle would be as follows: The substrate accesses the substrate binding site on one side of the membrane; substrate binding induces structural changes in the carrier protein, reorienting the opening of the binding site to the opposite side. The substrate dissociates from the transport site, allowing another substrate to be bound and transported in the opposite direction. Such a mechanism requires that binding of different substrates (the "outbound" and "inbound" substrates) that is mutually exclusive; that is, there is a single reorienting binding site. Variations of the model are possible, and some are based on crystal structures of bacterial homologs of human transporters, where two distinctive protomers are joined in the cytoplasmic side by a connecting loop, supporting a rocker switch mechanism (Figure 5–7).

Vectorial Transport

Asymmetrical transport across a monolayer of polarized cells, such as the epithelial and endothelial cells of brain capillaries, is called *vectorial transport* (Figure 5–8). Vectorial transport is important for the absorption of nutrients and bile acids in the intestine in the intestinal absorption of drugs (from lumen to blood). Vectorial transport also plays a major role in hepatobiliary and urinary excretion of drugs from the blood to the lumen. In addition, efflux of drugs from the brain via brain endothelial cells and brain choroid plexus epithelial cells involves vectorial transport. The ABC transporters mediate only unidirectional efflux, whereas SLC transporters mediate either drug uptake or drug efflux. For lipophilic compounds that have sufficient membrane permeability, ABC transporters alone are able to achieve vectorial transport without the help of influx transporters. For relatively hydrophilic organic anions and cations, coordinated uptake and efflux transporters in the polarized plasma membranes are necessary to achieve the vectorial movement of solutes across an epithelium. A typical configuration involves a primary or secondary active transporter at one membrane and a passive transporter at the other. In this way, common substrates of coordinated transporters are transferred efficiently across the epithelial barrier.

In the liver, a number of transporters with different substrate specificities are localized on the sinusoidal membrane (facing blood). These transporters are involved in the uptake of bile acids, amphipathic organic anions, and hydrophilic organic cations into the hepatocytes. Similarly, ABC transporters on the canalicular membrane (facing bile) export such compounds into the bile. Multiple combinations of uptake (OATP1B1, OATP1B3, OATP2B1) and efflux transporters (MDR1, MRP2, and BCRP) are involved in the efficient transcellular transport of a wide variety of compounds in the liver by using a system called "doubly transfected cells"; these cells express both uptake and efflux transporters on each side. In many cases, overlapping substrate specificities between the uptake transporters (OATP family) and efflux transporters (MRP family) make the vectorial transport of organic anions highly efficient. Similar transport systems also are present in the intestine, renal tubules, and endothelial cells of the brain capillaries (see Figure 5–8).

Transporter expression can be regulated transcriptionally in response to drug treatment and pathophysiological conditions, resulting in induction or downregulation of transporter mRNAs. Type II nuclear receptors,

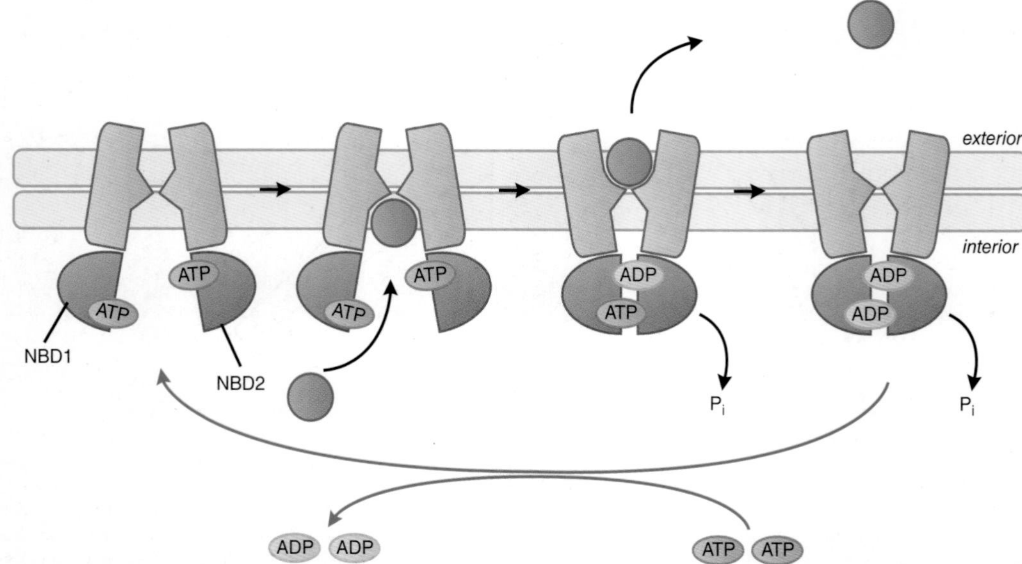

Figure 5–6 *Model of ABC transporter function.* The transporter accepts a solute molecule at the cytoplasmic membrane surface when its nucleotide NBDs are fully charged with ATP. Sequential hydrolysis of the ATP molecules produces steric change and leads to the translocation and release of the solute at the exterior membrane surface. Exchange of ADP for ATP on both NBDs completes the cycle and restores the system for readiness to transport another solute molecule.

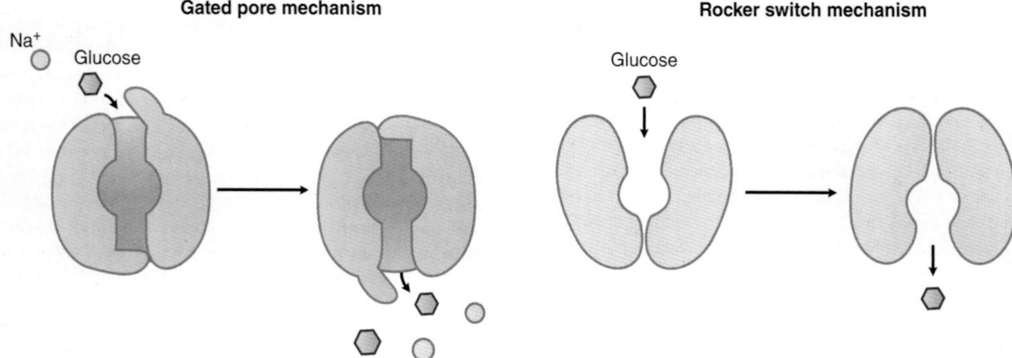

Figure 5–7 *Alternating access models of the transport of two transporters.* The gated pore represents the model for SGLT in which the rotation of two broken helices facilitates alternating access of substrates to the intracellular and extracellular sides of the plasma membrane. The rocker switch represents the model by which major facilitator superfamily (MFS) proteins, such as Lac Y, work. This example models a facilitated glucose transporter, GLUT2.

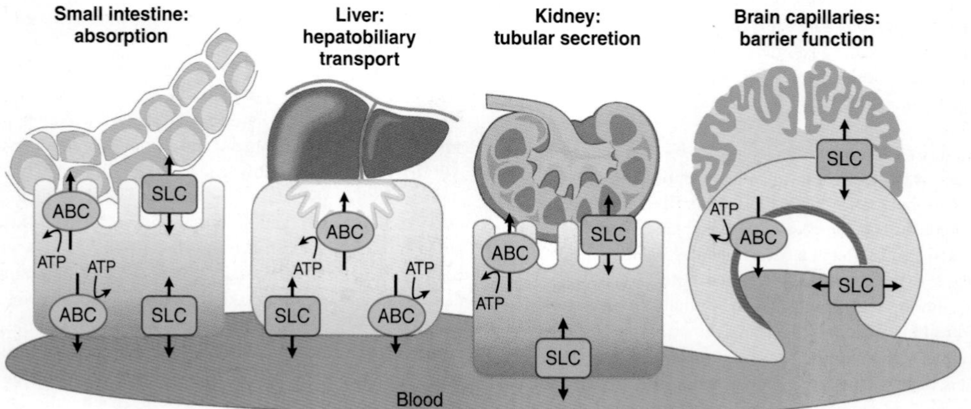

Figure 5–8 *Transepithelial and transendothelial flux.* Transepithelial or transendothelial flux of drugs requires distinct transporters at the two surfaces of the epithelial or endothelial barrier. These are depicted diagrammatically for transport across the small intestine (absorption), the kidney, liver (elimination), and brain capillary endothelial cells that comprise the BBB.

which form heterodimers with the 9-*cis*-retinoic acid receptor (RXR), can regulate transcription of genes for drug-metabolizing enzymes and transporters (see Table 6–4, Figure 6–8, and Urquhart et al., 2007). Such receptors include PXR (NR1I2), CAR (NR1I3), FXR (NR1H4), PPARα, and RAR. Except for CAR, these are ligand-activated nuclear receptors that, as heterodimers with RXR, bind specific elements in the enhancer regions of target genes. CAR has constitutive transcriptional activity that is antagonized by inverse agonists, such as androstenol and androstanol, and induced by barbiturates. PXR, also referred to as SXR in humans, is activated by synthetic and endogenous steroids, bile acids, and drugs such as clotrimazole, phenobarbital, rifampicin, sulfinpyrazone, ritonavir, carbamazepine, phenytoin, sulfadimidine, paclitaxel, and hyperforin (a constituent of St. John's wort) (Guo and Zhou, 2015). The potency of activators of PXR varies among species, such that rodents are not necessarily a model for effects in humans. There is an overlap of substrates between CYP3A4 and Pgp, and PXR mediates coinduction of CYP3A4 and Pgp, supporting their synergy in efficient detoxification. Recent studies in human hepatocytes treated with an activator of PXR suggested that the expression levels of enzymes in the CYP family are much more highly increased than the levels of transporters in the SLC or ABC families (Smith et al., 2014). Table 5–1 summarizes the effects of drug activation of type II nuclear receptors on expression of transporters.

DNA methylation is one mechanism underlying the epigenetic control of gene expression. Reportedly, the tissue-selective expression of transporters is achieved by DNA methylation (silencing in the transporter-negative tissues) as well as by transactivation in the transporter-positive tissues. Transporters subjected to epigenetic control include OAT3, URAT1, OCT2, OATP1B2, NTCP, and PEPT2 in the SLC families and MDR1, BCRP, BSEP, and ABCG5/ABCG8 (Imai et al., 2009).

Transporter Superfamilies in the Human Genome

The SLC Superfamily

The SLC superfamily includes 52 families and represents about 395 genes in the human genome, the products of which are membrane-spanning proteins, some of which are associated with genetic diseases (Table 5–2). Myriad substrates, including inorganic and organic ions, interact with SLC transporters. There are highly selective transporters that interact with structurally similar molecules, such as transporters in the SLC18 family that interact with monoamines. On the other hand, there are transporters that accept a broad range of chemically diverse substrates, such as organic ion transporters in the SLC22 family. Unlike ABC transporters that rely on ATP hydrolysis to actively translocate their substrates, SLC transporters are mostly facilitative transporters, although some are secondary active transporters (see Figure 5–4). Knowledge of the superfamily continues to grow; in the past decade, about 100 new human SLC transporters have been identified (Lin et al., 2015).

The physiologic roles of SLC transporters are important and diverse. For example, transporters in the SLC1, SLC3, SLC6, SLC7, SLC25, and SLC36 families, which are expressed in the intestine and kidney, among other organs, transport an array of amino acids critical in protein synthesis and energy homeostasis. Glucose and other sugars interact with transporters in the SLC2, SLC5, and SLC50 families for absorption, elimination, and cellular distribution. Proteins in the SLC11, SLC30, SLC39, and SLC40 families transport zinc, iron, and other metals. Members of the SLC19, SLC46, and SLC52 families transport water-soluble vitamins. Transporters in the SLC6 family move neurotransmitters across the plasma membrane;

TABLE 5–1 ■ REGULATION OF TRANSPORTER EXPRESSION BY NUCLEAR RECEPTORS IN HUMANS

TRANSPORTER	TRANSCRIPTION FACTOR	LIGAND	EFFECT
MDR1 (Pgp)	PXR	Rifampin	↑ Transcription activity
			↑ Expression in duodenum
			↓ Oral bioavailability of digoxin
			↓ AUC of talinolol
			↑ Expression in primary hepatocyte
		St John's wort	↑ Expression in duodenum
			↓ Oral bioavailability of digoxin
	CAR	Phenobarbital	↑ Expression in primary hepatocyte
MRP2	PXR	Rifampin	↑ Expression in duodenum
		Rifampin/hyperforin	↑ Expression in primary hepatocyte
	FXR	GW4064/chenodeoxycholate	↑ Expression in HepG2-FXR
	CAR	Phenobarbital	↑ Expression in hepatocyte
BCR	PXR	Rifampin }	↑ Expression in primary hepatocyte
	CAR	Phenobarbital }	
MRP3	PXR	Rifampin	↑ Expression in hepatocyte
OATP1B1	SHP1	Cholic acid	Indirect effect on HNF1α expression
	PXR	Rifampin	↑ Expression in hepatocyte
OATP1B3	FXR	Chenodeoxycholate	↑ Expression in hepatoma cells
BSEP	FXR	Chenodeoxycholate	↑ Transcription activity
OSTα/β	FXR	Chenodeoxycholate/GW4064	↑ Transcription activity
		Chenodeoxycholate	↑ Expression in ileal biopsies

CAR, constitutive androstane receptor; FXR, farnesoid X receptor; HNF1a, hepatocyte nuclear factor 1a; PXR, pregnane X receptor; SHP1, small heterodimer partner 1.

TABLE 5–2 ■ THE HUMAN SOLUTE CARRIER SUPERFAMILY

GENE	FAMILY	SELECTED DRUG SUBSTRATES	EXAMPLES OF LINKED HUMAN DISEASES
SLC1	Low-K_m glu/neutral aa T		Dicarboxylic aminoaciduria
SLC2	Facilitative GLUT		Fanconi-Bickel syndrome
SLC3	Heavy subunits, heteromeric aa Ts	Melphalan	Classic cystinuria type I
SLC4	Bicarbonate T		Distal renal tubule acidosis
SLC5	Na^+ glucose co-T	Dapagliflozin	Glucose-galactose malabsorption
SLC6	Na^+/Cl^--dependent neurotransmitter T	Paroxetine, fluoxetine	Cerebral creatine deficiency syndrome
SLC7	Cationic aa T	Melphalan	Lysinuric protein intolerance
SLC8	Na^+/Ca^{2+} Exch	Di-CH_3-arg	
SLC9	Na^+/H^+ Exch	Thiazide diuretics	Hypophosphatemic nephrolithiasis
SLC10	Na^+ bile salt co-T	Benzothiazepines (diltiazem)	Primary bile acid malabsorption
SLC11	H^+-coupled metal ion T		Hereditary hemochromatosis
SLC12	Electroneutral cation–Cl^- co-T		Gitelman syndrome
SLC13	Na^+–SO_4^-/COO^- co-T	SO_4^-/cys conjugates	
SLC14	Urea T		Kidd antigen blood group
SLC15	H^+–oligopeptide co-T	Valacyclovir	
SLC16	Monocarboxylate T	Salicylate, T_3/T_4, atorvastatin	Familial hyperinsulinemic hypoglycemia 7
SLC17	Vesicular glu T		Sialic acid storage disease
SLC18	Vesicular amine T	Reserpine	Myasthenic syndromes
SLC19	Folate/thiamine T	Methotrexate	Thiamine-responsive megaloblastic anemia
SLC20	Type III Na^+–PO_4^- co-T		
SLC21 (SLCO)	Organic anion T	Pravastatin	Rotor syndrome, hyperbilirubinemia
SLC22	Organic ion T	Pravastatin, metformin	Primary systemic carnitine deficiency
SLC23	Na^+-dependent ascorbate T	Vitamin C	
SLC24	$Na^+/(Ca^{2+}$-$K^+)$ Exch		Congenital stationary night blindness type 1D
SLC25	Mitochondrial carrier		Familial hypertrophic cardiomyopathy
SLC26	Multifunctional anion Exch	Salicylate, ciprofloxacin	Multiple epiphyseal dysplasia 4
SLC27	Fatty acid T		Ichthyosis prematurity syndrome
SLC28	Na^+-coupled nucleoside T	Gemcitabine, cladribine	
SLC29	Facilitative nucleoside T	Dipyridamole, gemcitabine	
SLC30	Zn efflux		Hypermanganesemia with dystonia
SLC31	Cu T	Cisplatin	
SLC32	Vesicular inhibitory aa T	Vigabatrin	
SLC33	Acetyl-CoA T		Congenital cataracts
SLC34	Type II Na^+–PO_4^-/ co-T		Hypercalciuric rickets
SLC35	Nucleoside-sugar T		Leukocyte adhesion deficiency II
SLC36	H^+-coupled aa T	D-Serine, cycloserine	Iminoglycinuria
SLC37	Sugar-phosphate/PO_4^- Exch		Glycogen storage disease
SLC38	Na^+-coupled neutral aa T		
SLC39	Metal ion T		Acrodermatitis enteropathica
SLC40	Basolateral Fe T		Hemochromatosis type IV
SLC41	MgtE-like Mg^{2+} T		
SLC42	Rh ammonium T		Rh-null regulator type disease
SLC43 *SLC45* *SLC52*	Na^+-independent L-like aa T Unknown substrate Riboflavin transporter family	Riboflavin	Oculocutaneous albinism type 4 Riboflavin deficiency

aa, amino acid; Exch, exchanger; T, transporter T_3/T_4, thyroid hormone.

SLC18 family members transport neurotransmitters into storage vesicles.

Pharmacologically, SLC transporters have been characterized for their role in drug absorption, elimination, and tissue distribution and importantly as mediators of drug-drug interactions. Notably, transporters in the solute carrier organic anion family, SLCO, interact with diverse substrates, including statins and antidiabetic drugs. Transporters in the SLC22 family interact with anionic and cationic drugs, including many antibiotics and antiviral agents, to mediate active renal secretion. SLC transporters are increasingly being targeted for treatment of human disease. Over 100 SLC transporters are associated with monogenic disorders and therefore may be usefully targeted in the treatment of rare diseases. Many SNPs in SLC transporters have reached a genome-wide level of significance in association studies of human disease. Notably, polymorphisms in *SLC30A8* are associated with type 1 diabetes mellitus, and polymorphisms in *SLC22A4* and *SLC22A5* are associated with inflammatory bowel disease.

The ABC Superfamily

The seven groups of ABC transporters are essential for many cellular processes, and mutations in at least 13 of the genes for ABC transporters cause or contribute to human genetic disorders (Table 5–3). In addition to conferring multidrug resistance, an important pharmacological aspect of these transporters is xenobiotic export from healthy tissues. In particular, MDR1/*ABCB1*, MRP2/*ABCC2*, and BCRP/*ABCG2* are involved in overall drug disposition.

Tissue Distribution of Drug-Related ABC Transporters

Table 5–4 summarizes the tissue distribution of drug-related ABC transporters in humans along with information about typical substrates. MDR1 (*ABCB1*), MRP2 (*ABCC2*), and BCRP (*ABCG2*) are all expressed in the apical side of the intestinal epithelia, where they serve to pump out xenobiotics, including many orally administered drugs. MRP3 (*ABCC3*) is expressed in the basal side of the epithelial cells.

Key to the vectorial excretion of drugs into urine or bile, ABC transporters are expressed in the polarized tissues of kidney and liver: MDR1, MRP2, BCRP, and MRP4 (*ABCC4*) on the brush border membrane of renal epithelia; MDR1, MRP2, and BCRP on the bile canalicular membrane of hepatocytes; and MRP3 and MRP4 on the sinusoidal membrane of hepatocytes. Some ABC transporters are expressed specifically on the blood side of the endothelial or epithelial cells that form barriers to the free entrance of toxic compounds into tissues: the BBB (MDR1 and MRP4 on the luminal side of brain capillary endothelial cells), the blood-CSF barrier (MRP1 and MRP4 on the basolateral blood side of choroid plexus epithelia), the blood-testis barrier (MRP1 on the basolateral membrane of mouse Sertoli cells and MDR1 in several types of human testicular cells), and the blood-placenta barrier (MDR1, MRP2, and BCRP on the luminal maternal side and MRP1 on the antiluminal fetal side of placental trophoblasts).

MRP/ABCC Family

The substrates of transporters in the MRP/ABCC family are mostly organic anions. Both MRP1 and MRP2 accept glutathione and glucuronide conjugates, sulfated conjugates of bile salts, and nonconjugated organic anions of an amphipathic nature (at least one negative charge and some degree of hydrophobicity). They also transport neutral or cationic anticancer drugs, such as vinca alkaloids and anthracyclines, possibly by means of a cotransport or symport mechanism with GSH. MRP3 also has a substrate specificity that is similar to that of MRP2 but with a lower transport affinity for glutathione conjugates compared with MRP1 and MRP2. MRP3 is expressed on the sinusoidal side of hepatocytes and is induced under cholestatic conditions. MRP3 functions to return toxic bile salts and bilirubin glucuronides into the blood circulation. MRP4 accepts negatively charged molecules, including cytotoxic compounds (e.g., 6-mercaptopurine and methotrexate), cyclic nucleotides, antiviral drugs (e.g., adefovir and tenofovir), diuretics (e.g., furosemide and trichlormethiazide), and cephalosporins (e.g., ceftizoxime and cefazolin). Glutathione enables MRP4 to accept taurocholate and leukotriene B_4. MRP5 has a narrower substrate specificity and accepts nucleotide analogue and clinically important anti-HIV drugs. No substrates have been identified that explain the mechanism of the MRP6-associated disease pseudoxanthoma.

BCRP/ABCG2

BCRP accepts both neutral and negatively charged molecules, including cytotoxic compounds (e.g., topotecan, flavopiridol, and methotrexate); sulfated conjugates of therapeutic drugs and hormones (e.g., estrogen sulfate); antibiotics (e.g., nitrofurantoin and fluoroquinolones); statins (e.g., pitavastatin and rosuvastatin); and toxic compounds found in normal food [phytoestrogens, (2-amino-1-methyl-6-phenylimidazo[4,5-*b*] pyridine), and pheophorbide A, a chlorophyll catabolite]. In addition, genetic variants in the transporter have been implicated in hyperuricemia and gout and in the disposition of uric acid and the XOIs allopurinol and oxypurinol.

TABLE 5–3 ■ THE HUMAN ATP BINDING CASSETTE (ABC) SUPERFAMILY

GENE	FAMILY	NUMBER OF MEMBERS	EXAMPLES OF LINKED HUMAN DISEASES
ABCA	ABC A	12	Tangier disease (defect in cholesterol transport; ABCA1), Stargardt syndrome (defect in retinal metabolism; ABCA4)
ABCB	ABC B	11	Bare lymphocyte syndrome type 1 (defect in antigen presenting; ABCB3 and ABCB4), progressive familial intrahepatic cholestasis type 3 (defect in biliary lipid secretion; MDR3/ABCB4), X-linked sideroblastic anemia with ataxia (a possible defect in iron homeostasis in mitochondria; ABCB7), progressive familial intrahepatic cholestasis type 2 (defect in biliary bile acid excretion; BSEP/*ABCB11*)
ABCC	ABC C	13	Dubin-Johnson syndrome (defect in biliary bilirubin glucuronide excretion; MRP2/*ABCC2*), pseudoxanthoma (unknown mechanism; *ABCC6*), cystic fibrosis (defect in Cl^- channel regulation; *ABCC7*), persistent hyperinsulinemic hypoglycemia of infancy (defect in inwardly rectifying K^+ conductance regulation in pancreatic B cells; SUR1/*ABCC8*)
ABCD	ABC D	4	Adrenoleukodystrophy (a possible defect in peroxisomal transport or catabolism of very long-chain fatty acids; ABCD1)
ABCE	ABC E	1	
ABCF	ABC F	3	
ABCG	ABC G	5	Sitosterolemia (defect in biliary and intestinal excretion of plant sterols; ABCG5 and ABCG8)

TABLE 5–4 ■ ABC TRANSPORTERS INVOLVED IN DRUG ABSORPTION, DISTRIBUTION, AND EXCRETION PROCESSES

NAME TISSUE DISTRIBUTION	SUBSTRATES
MDR1 (ABCB1) Liver, kidney, intestine, BBB, BTB, BPB	**Characteristics:** Bulky neutral or cationic compounds (many xenobiotics)—etoposide, doxorubicin, vincristine; diltiazem, verapamil; indinavir, ritonavir; erythromycin, ketoconazole; testosterone, progesterone; cyclosporine, tacrolimus; digoxin, quinidine, fexofenadine, loperamide
MRP1 (ABCC1) Ubiquitous	**Characteristics:** Negatively charged amphiphiles—vincristine (with GSH), methotrexate; GSH conjugate of LTC_4, ethacrynic acid; glucuronide of estradiol, bilirubin; estrone-3-sulfate; saquinavir; grepafloxacin; folate, GSH, GSSG
MRP2 (ABCC2) Liver, kidney, intestine, BPB	**Characteristics:** Negatively charged amphiphiles—methotrexate, vincristine; GSH conjugates of LTC_4, ethacrynic acid; glucuronides of estradiol, bilirubin; taurolithocholate sulfate; statins, AngII receptor antagonists, temocaprilat; indinavir, ritonavir; GSH, GSSG
MRP3 (ABCC3) Liver, kidney, intestine	**Characteristics:** Negatively charged amphiphiles—etoposide, methotrexate; GSH conjugates of LTC_4, PGJ_2; glucuronides of estradiol, etoposide, morphine, acetaminophen, hymecromone, harmol; sulfate conjugates of bile salts; glycocholate, taurocholate; folate, leucovorin
MRP4 (ABCC4) Ubiquitous, including BBB and BCSFB	**Characteristics:** Nucleotide analogues, 6-mercaptopurine, methotrexate; estradiol glucuronide; dehydroepiandrosterone sulfate; cyclic AMP/GMP; furosemide, trichlormethiazide; adefovir, tenofovir; cefazolin, ceftizoxime; folate, leucovorin, taurocholate (with GSH)
MRP5 (ABCC5) Ubiquitous	**Characteristics:** Nucleotide analogues 6-mercaptopurine; cyclic AMP/GMP; adefovir
MRP6 (ABCC6) Liver, kidney	**Characteristics:** Doxorubicin,[a] etoposide,[a] GSH conjugate of LTC_4; BQ-123 (cyclic penta peptide antagonist at the ETA endothelin receptor)
BCRP(MXR) (ABCG2) Liver, intestine, BBB	**Characteristics:** Neutral and anionic compounds—methotrexate, mitoxantrone, camptothecins, SN-38, topotecan, imatinib; glucuronides of 4-methylumbelliferone, estradiol; sulfate conjugates of dehydroepiandrosterone, estrone; nitrofurantoin, fluoroquinolones; pitavastatin, rosuvastatin; cholesterol, estradiol, dantrolene, prazosin, sulfasalazine, uric acid, allopurinol, oxypurinol
MDR3 (ABCB4) Liver	**Characteristics:** Phospholipids
BSEP (ABCB11) Liver	**Characteristics:** Bile salts
ABCG5, ABCG8 Liver, intestine	**Characteristics:** Plant sterols

BBB, blood-brain barrier; BTB, blood-testis barrier; BPB, blood-placenta barrier; BCSFB, blood-cerebrospinal fluid barrier; LTC, Leukotriene C; PGJ, prostaglandin J.

[a]Substrates and cytotoxic drugs with increased resistance (cytotoxicity with increased resistance is usually caused by the decreased accumulation of the drugs). Although MDR3 (ABCB4), BSEP (ABCB11), ABCG5, and ABCG8 are not directly involved in drug disposition, their inhibition will lead to unfavorable side effects.

Physiological Roles of ABC Transporters

The physiological significance of the ABC transporters has been amply illustrated by studies involving knockout animals or patients with genetic defects in these transporters. For instance, mice deficient in MDR1 function are viable and fertile and do not display obvious phenotypic abnormalities other than hypersensitivity to the toxicity of drugs. There are equally remarkable data for MRP1, MRP4, BCRP, and BSEP. The lesson is this: Complete absence of these drug-related ABC transporters is not lethal and can remain unrecognized in the absence of exogenous perturbations due to food, drugs, or toxins. However, inhibition of physiologically important ABC transporters (especially those related directly to the genetic diseases described in Table 5–3) by drugs should be avoided to reduce the incidence of drug-induced side effects.

ABC Transporters in Drug Absorption and Elimination

With respect to clinical medicine, MDR1 is the most renowned ABC transporter yet identified. The systemic exposure to orally administered digoxin is decreased by coadministration of rifampin (an MDR1 inducer) and is negatively correlated with the MDR1 protein expression in the human intestine. MDR1 is also expressed on the brush border membrane of renal epithelia, and its function can be monitored using digoxin (> 70% excreted in the urine). MDR1 inhibitors (e.g., quinidine, verapamil, valspodar, spironolactone, clarithromycin, and ritonavir) all markedly reduce renal excretion of digoxin. Drugs with narrow therapeutic windows (e.g., digoxin, cyclosporine, tacrolimus) should be used with great care if MDR1-based drug-drug interactions are likely.

In the intestine, MRP3 can mediate intestinal absorption in conjunction with uptake transporters. MRP3 mediates sinusoidal efflux in the liver, decreasing the efficacy of the biliary excretion from the blood and excretion of intracellularly formed metabolites, particularly glucuronide conjugates. Thus, dysfunction of MRP3 results in shortening of the elimination $t_{1/2}$. MRP4 substrates also can be transported by OAT1 and OAT3 on the basolateral membrane of the epithelial cells in the kidney. The rate-limiting process in renal tubular secretion is likely the uptake process at the basolateral surface. Dysfunction of MRP4 enhances the renal concentration but has limited effect on the blood concentration.

Transporters Involved in Pharmacokinetics

Drug transporters play a prominent role in pharmacokinetics (see Figure 5–1 and Table 5–4). Transporters in the liver and kidney have important roles in removal of drugs from the blood and hence in metabolism and excretion.

Hepatic Transporters

Hepatic uptake of organic anions (e.g., drugs, leukotrienes, and bilirubin), cations, and bile salts is mediated by SLC-type transporters in the basolateral (sinusoidal) membrane of hepatocytes: OATPs (SLCO), OCTs (SLC22), and NTCP (SLC10A1), respectively. These transporters mediate uptake by either facilitated or secondary active mechanisms.

ABC transporters such as MRP2, MDR1, BCRP, BSEP, and MDR2 in the bile canalicular membrane of hepatocytes mediate the efflux (excretion) of drugs and their metabolites, bile salts, and phospholipids against a steep concentration gradient from liver to bile. This primary active transport is driven by ATP hydrolysis.

Vectorial transport of drugs from the circulating blood to the bile using an uptake transporter (OATP family) and an efflux transporter (MRP2, BCRP) is important for determining drug exposure in the circulating blood and liver. Moreover, there are many other uptake and efflux transporters in the liver (Figure 5–9).

The following examples illustrate the importance of vectorial transport in determining drug exposure in the circulating blood and liver and the role of transporters in drug-drug interactions.

HMG-CoA Reductase Inhibitors

Statins are cholesterol-lowering agents that reversibly inhibit HMG-CoA reductase, which catalyzes a rate-limiting step in cholesterol biosynthesis (see Chapter 33). Most of the statins in their acid form are substrates of hepatic uptake transporters and undergo enterohepatic recirculation (see Figure 5–6). In this process, hepatic uptake transporters such as OATP1B1 and efflux transporters such as MRP2 act cooperatively to produce *bisubstrate vectorial transcellular transport*. The efficient first-pass hepatic uptake of these statins by OATP1B1 helps concentrate them in the liver where they produce their pharmacological effects, thus minimizing their systemic levels and adverse effects in smooth muscle. Genetic polymorphisms of OATP1B1 also affect the function of this transporter (Meyer zu Schwabedissen et al., 2015).

Gemfibrozil

The cholesterol-lowering agent gemfibrozil, a PPARα activator, can enhance toxicity (myopathy) to several statins by a mechanism that involves transport. Gemfibrozil and its glucuronide inhibit the uptake of the active hydroxy forms of statins into hepatocytes by OATP1B1, resulting in an increase in the plasma concentration of the statin and a concomitant increase in toxicity.

Irinotecan

CPT-11 is a potent anticancer drug, but late-onset GI toxicities, such as severe diarrhea, make this a difficult agent to use safely. After intravenous administration of CPT-11, a carboxylesterase converts the drug to SN-38, an active metabolite. SN-38 is subsequently conjugated with glucuronic acid in the liver. SN-38 and SN-38 glucuronide are then excreted into the bile by MRP2, entering the GI tract and causing adverse effects. The inhibition of MRP2-mediated biliary excretion of SN-38 and its glucuronide by coadministration of probenecid reduces the drug-induced diarrhea in experimental systems and may prove useful in humans (Horikawa et al., 2002). For additional details, see Figures 6–6, 6–8, 6–9.

Bosentan

Bosentan is an endothelin antagonist used to treat pulmonary arterial hypertension. It is taken up in the liver by OATP1B1 and OATP1B3 and subsequently metabolized by CYP2C9 and CYP3A4. Transporter-mediated hepatic uptake can be a determinant of elimination of bosentan, and inhibition of its hepatic uptake by cyclosporine, rifampicin, and sildenafil can affect its pharmacokinetics.

Temocapril and other ACE inhibitors

Temocapril is an ACE inhibitor (see Chapter 26). Its active metabolite, temocaprilat, is excreted both in the bile and in the urine by the liver and kidney, respectively, whereas other ACE inhibitors are excreted mainly by the kidney. A special feature of temocapril among ACE inhibitors is that the plasma concentration of temocaprilat remains relatively unchanged even in patients with renal failure. However, the plasma AUC of enalaprilat and other ACE inhibitors is markedly increased in patients with renal disorders. Temocaprilat is a bisubstrate of the OATP family and MRP2, whereas other ACE inhibitors are not good substrates of MRP2 (although they are taken up into the liver by the OATP family). Taking these findings into consideration, the affinity for MRP2 may dominate in determining the biliary excretion of any series of ACE inhibitors. Drugs that are

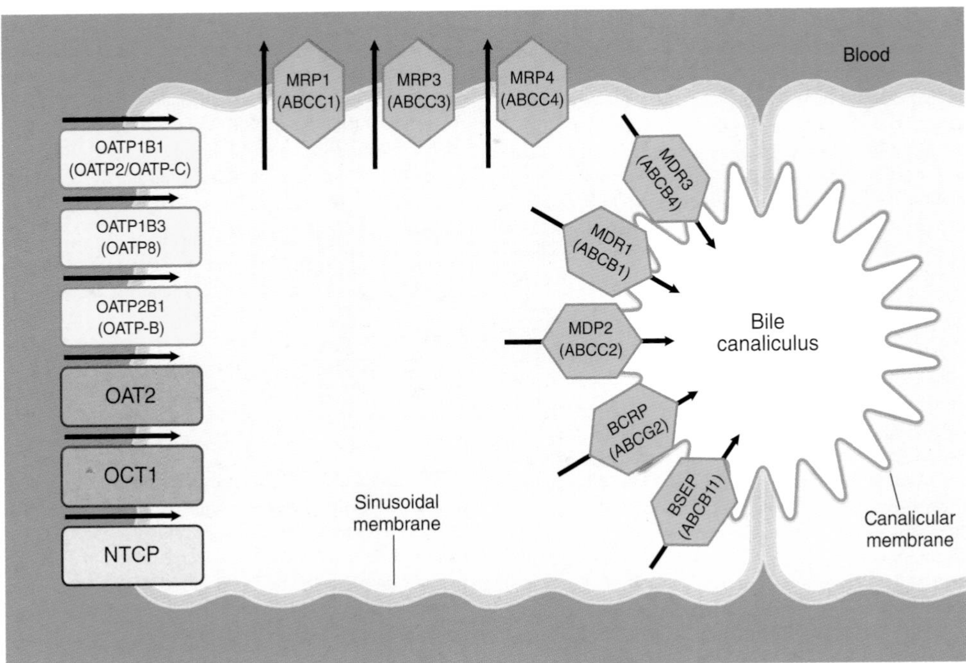

Figure 5–9 *Transporters in the hepatocyte that function in the uptake and efflux of drugs across the sinusoidal membrane and efflux of drugs into the bile across the canalicular membrane.* Arrows show the primary direction of transport. See text for details of the transporters pictured.

excreted into both the bile and urine to the same degree thus are expected to exhibit minimum interindividual differences in their pharmacokinetics.

Angiotensin II Receptor Antagonists

Angiotensin II receptor antagonists are used for the treatment of hypertension, acting on AT_1 receptors expressed in vascular smooth muscle, proximal tubule, adrenal medullary cells, and elsewhere. For most of these drugs, hepatic uptake and biliary excretion are important factors for their pharmacokinetics and pharmacological effects. Telmisartan is taken up into human hepatocytes in a saturable manner, predominantly via OATP1B3 (Ishiguro et al., 2006). On the other hand, both OATPs 1B1 and 1B3 are responsible for the hepatic uptake of valsartan and olmesartan, although the relative contributions of these transporters are unclear. Studies using doubly transfected cells with hepatic uptake transporters and biliary excretion transporters have clarified that MRP2 plays the most important role in the biliary excretion of valsartan and olmesartan.

Repaglinide and Nateglinide

Repaglinide is a meglitinide analogue antidiabetic drug. Although it is eliminated almost completely by the metabolism mediated by CYPs 2C8 and 3A4, transporter-mediated hepatic uptake is one of the determinants of its elimination rate. In subjects with the OATP1B1 (*SLCO1B1*) 521CC genotype, a significant change in the pharmacokinetics of repaglinide was observed (Niemi et al., 2005). Genetic polymorphism in *SLCO1B1* 521T>C results in altered pharmacokinetics of nateglinide, suggesting OATP1B1 is a determinant of its elimination, although it is subsequently metabolized by CYPs 2C9, 3A4, and 2D6 (Zhang et al., 2006b).

Renal Transporters

Organic Cation Transport

Structurally diverse organic cations are secreted in the proximal tubule. Many secreted organic cations are endogenous compounds (e.g., choline, *N*-methylnicotinamide, and DA), and renal secretion helps to eliminate excess concentrations of these substances. Another function of organic cation secretion is ridding the body of xenobiotics, including many positively charged drugs and their metabolites (e.g., cimetidine, ranitidine, metformin, varenicline, and trospium) and toxins from the environment (e.g., nicotine and paraquat). Organic cations that are secreted by the kidney may be either hydrophobic or hydrophilic. Hydrophilic organic drug cations generally have molecular weights less than 400 Da; a current model for their secretion in the proximal tubule of the nephron is shown in Figure 5–10 involving the transporters described next.

For the transepithelial flux of a compound (e.g., secretion), the compound must traverse two membranes sequentially, the basolateral membrane facing the blood side and the apical membrane facing the tubular lumen. Organic cations appear to cross the basolateral membrane in the human proximal tubule by two distinct transporters in the SLC family 22 (SCL22): OCT2 (*SLC22A2*) and OCT3 (*SLC22A3*). Organic cations are transported across this membrane down an electrochemical gradient.

Transport of organic cations from cell to tubular lumen across the apical membrane occurs through an electroneutral proton–organic cation exchange, which is mediated by transporters in the SLC47 family, which comprises members of the MATE family. Transporters in the MATE family, assigned to the apical membrane of the proximal tubule, appear to play a key role in moving hydrophilic organic cations from tubule cell to lumen. In addition, OCTNs, located on the apical membrane, appear to contribute to organic cation flux across the proximal tubule. In humans, these include *OCTN1* (SLC22A4) and *OCTN2* (SLC22A5). These bifunctional transporters are involved not only in organic cation secretion but also in carnitine reabsorption. In the reuptake mode, the transporters function as Na^+ cotransporters, relying on the inwardly driven Na^+ gradient created by Na^+,K^+-ATPase to move carnitine from tubular lumen to cell. In the secretory mode, the transporters appear to function as proton–organic cation exchangers. That is, protons move from tubular lumen to cell interior in exchange for organic cations, which move from cytosol to tubular lumen. The inwardly directed proton gradient (tubular lumen → cytosol) is maintained by transporters in the SLC9 family, which are Na^+/K^+ exchangers (NHEs, antiporters). Of the two steps involved in secretory transport, transport across the luminal membrane appears to be rate limiting.

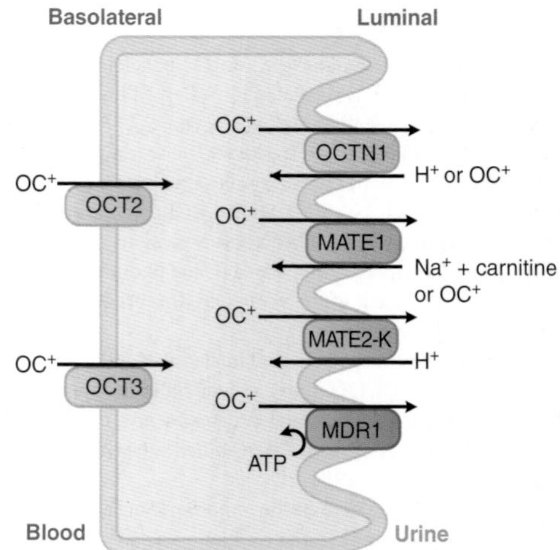

Figure 5–10 *Organic cation secretory transporters in the proximal tubule.* OC^+, organic cation. See text for details of the transporters pictured.

***OCT2* (SLC22A2).** Human, mouse, and rat orthologs of OCT2 are expressed in abundance in human kidney and to some extent in neuronal tissue such as choroid plexus. In the kidney, OCT2 is localized in the proximal and distal tubules and collecting ducts. In the proximal tubule, OCT2 is restricted to the basolateral membrane. OCT2-mediated transport of model organic cations MPP^+ (1-methyl-4-phenylpyridinium) and TEA (tetraethylammonium) is electrogenic, and both OCT2 and OCT1 can support organic cation–organic cation exchange. OCT2 generally accepts a wide array of monovalent organic cations with molecular weights below 400 Da. OCT2 is also present in neuronal tissues; however, monoamine neurotransmitters have low affinities for OCT2.

***OCT3* (SLC22A3).** The OCT3 gene is located in tandem with genes for OCT1 and OCT2 on chromosome 6. Tissue distribution studies suggest that human OCT3 is expressed in liver, kidney, intestine, placenta, skeletal muscle, and adipose tissue, although in the kidney it appears to be expressed in considerably less abundance than OCT2, and in the liver it is less abundant than OCT1. Like OCT1 and OCT2, OCT3 appears to support electrogenic potential-sensitive organic cation transport. OCT3 plays a role in both the renal elimination and the intestinal absorption of metformin.

***OCTN1* (SLC22A4).** OCTN1 seems to operate as an organic cation–proton exchanger. OCTN1-mediated influx of model organic cations is enhanced at alkaline pH, whereas efflux is increased by an inwardly directed proton gradient. OCTN1 contains a nucleotide-binding sequence motif, and transport of its substrates appears to be stimulated by cellular ATP. OCTN1 also can function as an organic cation–organic cation exchanger. OCTN1 functions as a bidirectional pH- and ATP-dependent transporter at the apical membrane in renal tubular epithelial cells and appears to be important in renal transport of gabapentin.

***OCTN2* (SLC22A5).** OCTN2 is a bifunctional transporter; it functions as both an Na^+-dependent carnitine transporter and an Na^+-independent OCT. OCTN2 transport of organic cations is sensitive to pH, suggesting that OCTN2 may function as an organic cation exchanger. The transport of *L*-carnitine by OCTN2 is an Na^+-dependent electrogenic process. Mutations in OCTN2 can result in insufficient renal reabsorption of carnitine and appear to be the cause of primary systemic carnitine deficiency (Tamai, 2013)

***MATE1* and *MATE2-K* (SLC47A1, SLC47A2).** Multidrug and toxin extrusion family members MATE1 and MATE2-K interact with structurally diverse hydrophilic organic cations, including the antidiabetic drug metformin, the H_2 antagonist cimetidine, and the anticancer drug topotecan. In addition to cationic compounds, the transporters recognize some anions, including the antiviral agents acyclovir and ganciclovir. The zwitterions cephalexin and cephradine are specific substrates of MATE1. The herbicide paraquat, a bis-quaternary ammonium compound that is nephrotoxic in humans, is a high-affinity substrate of MATE1. Both MATE1 and MATE2-K have been localized to the apical membrane of the proximal tubule. MATE1, but not MATE2-K, is also expressed on the canalicular membrane of the hepatocyte. These transporters appear to be the long-searched-for organic cation–proton antiporters on the apical membrane of the proximal tubule; that is, an oppositely directed proton gradient can drive the movement of organic cations via MATE1 or MATE2-K. The antibiotics levofloxacin and ciprofloxacin, though potent inhibitors, are not translocated by either MATE1 or MATE2-K.

Polymorphisms of OCTs and MATEs. OCT1 exhibits the greatest number of amino acid polymorphisms, followed by OCT2 and then OCT3. Recent studies suggest that genetic variants of OCT1 and OCT2 are associated with alterations in the renal elimination and response to the antidiabetic drug metformin. MATEs have fewer amino acid polymorphisms; however, recent studies suggested that noncoding region variants of SLC47A1 and SLC47A2 are associated with variation in response to metformin.

Organic Anion Transport

As with organic cation transport, a primary function of organic anion secretion appears to be the removal of xenobiotics from the body. The candidate substrates are structurally diverse and include many weakly acidic drugs (e.g., pravastatin, captopril, PAH, and penicillins) and toxins (e.g., ochratoxin). OATs not only move both hydrophobic and hydrophilic anions but also may interact with cations and neutral compounds.

Figure 5–11 shows a current model for the transepithelial flux of organic anions in the proximal tubule. Two primary transporters on the basolateral membrane mediate the flux of organic anions from interstitial fluid to tubule cell: OAT1 (*SLC22A6*) and OAT3 (*SLC22A8*). Energetically, hydrophilic organic anions are transported across the basolateral membrane against an electrochemical gradient, exchanging with intracellular α-ketoglutarate, which moves down its concentration gradient from cytosol to blood. The outwardly directed gradient of α-ketoglutarate is maintained at least in part by a basolateral Na^+-dicarboxylate transporter (NaDC3), using the Na^+ gradient established by Na^+,K^+-ATPase. Transport of low-molecular-weight organic anions by the cloned transporters OAT1 and OAT3 can be driven by α-ketoglutarate; coupled transport of α-ketoglutarate and low-molecular-weight organic anions (e.g., PAH) occurs in isolated basolateral membrane vesicles. The molecular pharmacology and molecular biology of OATs have recently been reviewed (Srimaroeng et al., 2008).

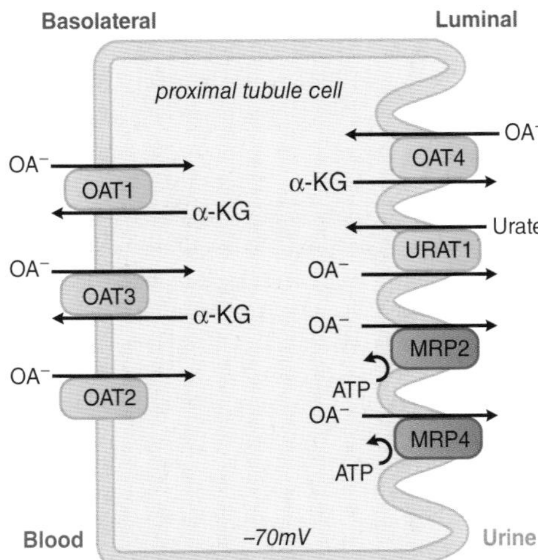

Figure 5–11 *Organic anion secretory transporters in the proximal tubule.* Two primary transporters on the basolateral membrane mediate the flux of OAs from interstitial fluid to tubule cell: OAT1 (*SLC22A6*) and OAT3 (*SLC22A8*). Hydrophilic OAs are transported across the basolateral membrane against an electrochemical gradient in exchange with intracellular α-ketoglutarate (α-KG), which moves down its concentration gradient from cytosol to blood. The outwardly directed gradient of α-KG is maintained at least in part by a basolateral Na^+-dicarboxylate uptake transporter (NaDC3). The Na^+ gradient that drives NaDC3 is maintained by Na^+,K^+-ATPase.

The mechanism responsible for the apical membrane transport of organic anions from tubule cell cytosol to tubular lumen remains controversial. OAT4 may serve as the luminal membrane transporter for organic anions, but the movement of substrates via this transporter can be driven by exchange with a α-ketoglutarate, suggesting that OAT4 may function in the reabsorptive, rather than secretory, flux of organic anions. NaPT1, originally cloned as a phosphate transporter, can support the low-affinity transport of hydrophilic organic anions such as PAH. MRP2 and MRP4, multidrug resistance transporters in the ABCC, can interact with some organic anions and may actively pump them from tubule cell cytosol to tubular lumen.

***OAT1* (SLC22A6).** Mammalian isoforms of OAT1 are expressed primarily in the kidney, with some expression in brain and skeletal muscle. Immunohistochemical studies suggest that OAT1 is expressed on the basolateral membrane of the proximal tubule in humans, with highest expression in the middle segment, S2 (see Figure 25-1). Based on quantitative PCR, OAT1 is expressed at a third of the level of OAT3. OAT1 exhibits saturable transport of organic anions such as PAH. This transport is trans-stimulated by other organic anions, including α-ketoglutarate. Thus, the inside negative-potential difference drives the efflux of the dicarboxylate α-ketoglutarate, which in turn supports the influx of monocarboxylates such as PAH. Sex steroids regulate expression of OAT1 in the kidney. OAT1 generally transports low-molecular-weight organic anions, either endogenous (e.g., PGE_2 and urate) or exogenous (ingested drugs and toxins). Some neutral compounds are also transported by OAT1 at a lower affinity (e.g., cimetidine).

***OAT2* (SLC22A7).** OAT2 is present in both kidney and liver; renal OAT2 is localized to the basolateral membrane of the proximal tubule. OAT2 functions as a transporter for nucleotides, particularly guanine nucleotides such as cyclic GMP, for which it is a bidirectional facilitative transporter (Cropp et al., 2008). Cellular studies indicate that OAT2 functions in both the influx and the efflux of guanine nucleotides. OAT2 transports organic anions such as PAH and methotrexate with low affinity, PGE_2 with high affinity, and some neutral compounds but with lower affinity (e.g., cimetidine).

***OAT3* (SLC22A8).** Human OAT3 is confined to the basolateral membrane of the proximal tubule. This protein consists of two variants, one of which transports a wide variety of organic anions, including PAH, estrone sulfate, and many drugs (e.g., pravastatin, cimetidine, 6-mercaptopurine, and methotrexate) (Srimaroeng et al., 2008). The longer variant does not support transport. The specificities of OAT3 and OAT1 overlap, although kinetic parameters differ: Estrone sulfate is transported by both but by OAT3 with a much higher affinity; OAT1 transports the H_2 receptor antagonist cimetidine with high affinity.

***OAT4* (SLC22A11).** Human OAT4 is expressed in placenta and kidney (on the luminal membrane of the proximal tubule). Organic anion transport by OAT4 can be stimulated by transgradients of α-ketoglutarate, suggesting that OAT4 may be involved in the reabsorption of organic anions from tubular lumen into cell (see Figure 5–11). The specificity of OAT4 includes the model compounds estrone sulfate and PAH, as well as zidovudine, tetracycline, and methotrexate. Collectively, emerging studies suggest that OAT4 may be involved not in secretory flux of organic anions but in reabsorption instead.

Other Anion Transporters. URAT1 (*SLC22A12*) is a kidney-specific transporter confined to the apical membrane of the proximal tubule.

URAT1 is primarily responsible for urate reabsorption, mediating electroneutral urate transport that can be transstimulated by Cl^- gradients. NPT1, Na^+-dependent phosphate transport protein 1 (SLC17A1), is expressed on the luminal membrane of the proximal tubule as well as in the brain. NPT1 transports PAH, probenecid, and penicillin G. It appears to be involved in organic anion efflux from tubule cell to lumen and interacts with uric acid.

MRP2 (*ABCC2*) is considered to be the primary transporter involved in efflux of many drug conjugates (such as GSH conjugates) across the canalicular membrane of the hepatocyte. MRP2 is also found on the apical membrane of the proximal tubule, where it is thought to play a role in the efflux of organic anions into the tubular lumen. In general, MRP2 transports larger, bulkier compounds than do most of the OATs in the SLC22 family. MRP4 (*ABCC4*), localized on the apical membrane of the proximal tubule, transports a wide array of conjugated anions, including glucuronides and GSH conjugates. MRP4 appears to interact with methotrexate, cyclic nucleotide analogues, and antiviral nucleoside analogues. BCRP (ABCG2) is localized to the apical membrane of the proximal tubule and duodenum and is involved in uric acid secretion and secretion of the XOIs allopurinol and oxypurinol.

Polymorphisms in OAT1 and OAT3 have been identified in ethnic human subpopulations (see https://www.pharmgkb.org). Notably, polymorphisms in ABCG2 have been associated with reduced response to allopurinol and oxypurinol.

Transporters and Pharmacodynamics: Drug Action in the Brain

Biogenic amine neurotransmitters are packaged in vesicles in presynaptic neurons, released in the synapse by fusion of the vesicles with the plasma membrane, and then taken back into the presynaptic neurons or postsynaptic cells (see Chapters 8 and 14). Transporters involved in the neuronal reuptake of the neurotransmitters and the regulation of their levels in the synaptic cleft belong to two major superfamilies, SLC1 and SLC6. Transporters in both families play roles in reuptake of GABA, glutamate, and the monoamine neurotransmitters NE, 5HT, and DA. These transporters may serve as pharmacologic targets for neuropsychiatric drugs. SLC6 family members localized in the brain and involved in the reuptake of neurotransmitters into presynaptic neurons include NET (*SLC6A2*), DAT (*SLC6A3*), SERT (*SLC6A4*), and several GATs (GAT1, GAT2, and GAT3). Each of these transporters appears to have 12 transmembrane (TM) regions and a large extracellular loop with glycosylation sites between TM3 and TM4.

SLC6 family members are secondary active transporters, depending on the Na^+ gradient to transport their substrates into cells. Cl^- is also required, although to a variable extent depending on the family member. Through their reuptake mechanisms, the neurotransmitter transporters in the SLC6A family regulate the concentrations and dwell times of neurotransmitters in the synaptic cleft; the extent of transmitter uptake also influences subsequent vesicular storage of transmitters. Many of these transporters are present in other tissues (e.g., intestine, kidney, and platelets) and may serve other roles. Further, the transporters can function in the reverse direction; that is, the transporters can export neurotransmitters in a Na^{2+}-independent fashion.

GABA Uptake: GAT1 (*SLC6A1*), GAT3 (*SLC6A11*), GAT2 (*SLC6A13*), and BGT1 (*SLC6A12*)

GAT1 is the most important GABA transporter in the brain, expressed in GABAergic neurons and found largely on presynaptic neurons. GAT1 is abundant in the neocortex, cerebellum, basal ganglia, brainstem, spinal cord, retina, and olfactory bulb. GAT3 is found only in the brain, largely in glial cells. GAT2 is found in peripheral tissues, including the kidney and liver, and within the CNS in the choroid plexus and meninges. Physiologically, GAT1 appears to be responsible for regulating the interaction of GABA at receptors. The presence of GAT2 in the choroid plexus and its absence in presynaptic neurons suggest that this transporter may play a primary role in maintaining the homeostasis of GABA in the CSF. GAT1 is the target of the antiepileptic drug tiagabine (a nipecotic acid derivative), which presumably acts to prolong the dwell time of GABA in the synaptic cleft of GABAergic neurons by inhibiting the reuptake of GABA. A fourth GAT, BGT1, occurs in extrasynaptic regions of the hippocampus and cortex (Madsen et al., 2011).

Catecholamine Uptake: NET (*SLC6A2*)

NET is found in central and peripheral nervous tissues as well as in adrenal chromaffin tissue. NET colocalizes with neuronal markers, consistent with a role in reuptake of monoamine neurotransmitters. NET provides reuptake of NE (and DA) into neurons, thereby limiting the synaptic dwell time of NE and terminating its actions, salvaging NE for subsequent repackaging. NET serves as a drug target for the antidepressant desipramine, other tricyclic antidepressants, and cocaine. Orthostatic intolerance, a rare familial disorder characterized by an abnormal blood pressure and heart rate response to changes in posture, has been associated with a mutation in NET.

Dopamine Uptake: DAT (*SLC6A3*)

DAT is located primarily in the brain in dopaminergic neurons. The primary function of DAT is the reuptake of DA, terminating its actions. Although present on presynaptic neurons at the neurosynaptic junction, DAT is also present in abundance along the neurons, away from the synaptic cleft. Physiologically, DAT is involved in functions attributed to the dopaminergic system, including mood, behavior, reward, and cognition. Drugs that interact with DAT include cocaine and its analogues, amphetamines, and the neurotoxin MPTP (methylphenyltetrahydropyridine).

Serotonin Uptake: SERT (*SLC6A4*)

SERT is responsible for the reuptake and clearance of 5HT in the brain. Like the other SLC6A family members, SERT transports its substrates in a Na^+-dependent fashion and is dependent on Cl^- and possibly on the countertransport of K^+. Substrates of SERT include 5HT, various tryptamine derivatives, and neurotoxins such as MDMA (ecstasy) and fenfluramine. SERT is the specific target of the SSRI antidepressants (e.g., fluoxetine and paroxetine) and one of several targets of tricyclic antidepressants (e.g., amitriptyline). Genetic variants of SERT have been associated with an array of behavioral and neurological disorders. The precise mechanism by which reduced activity of SERT, caused by either a genetic variant or an antidepressant, ultimately affects behavior, including depression, is not known.

The Blood-Brain Barrier: A Pharmacological View

The CNS is well protected from circulating neurotransmitters, well supplied with necessary nutrients and ions, and able to exclude many toxins, bacteria, and xenobiotics. This careful set of conditions is achieved by a barrier called the BBB. This barrier results from the specialized properties of the microvasculature of the CNS. Functionally, the BBB is partly physical, partly a consequence of selective permeability (export of undesirable molecules and import of necessary molecules), and partly a consequence of the enzymatic destruction of certain permeants by enzymes in the barrier. There are some neurosensory and neurosecretory regions of the brain that lack the barrier: posterior pituitary, median eminence, area postrema, subfornical organ, subcommissural organ, and laminar terminalis.

The *physical part* of the BBB derives from the distinctive structure of the capillary endothelium in the brain and choroid plexus. Unlike the endothelial cells of peripheral microvasculature that have gaps between them that permit flow of water and small molecules to the interstitial space, endothelial cells in the CNS have tight junctions that limit paracellular flow and generally have very low rates of vesicular transport (transcytosis) compared to peripheral endothelium. Moreover, CNS endothelium is wrapped by basement membrane, pericytes, and the pseudopodial processes of astroglia. Lipophilic molecules and gases such as O_2 and CO_2 can readily diffuse across these layers from blood to brain. Hydrophilic molecules (nutrients, ions, charged molecules, many drugs) cannot cross these multiple membrane barriers by diffusion at sufficient rates.

Thus, the system relies on *selective permeability*. For instance, there are transport systems: for ions; for nutrients, many in the SLC family of transport proteins, such as SLC2A1/GLUT1 (glucose), SLC7A1 and SLC7A5/LAT1 (amino acids); for nucleosides; and for metabolic by-products such as lactate and pyruvate (SLC16A1). Members of the SLC22 family (OAT1 and OAT3) play a role in the efflux of xenobiotics from CSF to plasma. There are receptor-mediated transport systems for ferritin and insulin, and there is a low level of transcytosis (caveolin-dependent vesicle trafficking). The endothelial membranes also express exporters that basically prevent molecules such as drugs from crossing the endothelium. There are transporters such as Pgp (ABCB1/MDR1), the well-characterized efflux transporter that extrudes its substrates across the luminal membrane of the brain capillary endothelial cells into the blood, thereby limiting penetration into the brain. There is accumulating evidence for similar roles of BCRP and MRP4. The physiological compounds that need to cross the BBB are able to cross.

There is a *metabolic barrier* for some compounds. For instance, circulating catecholamines are inactivated by MAO in the endothelial cells and endothelial MAO and dopa decarboxylase (aromatic amino acid decarboxylase; see Chapter 8) metabolizes L-dopa to 3,4-dihydroxyphenylacetate (hence the necessity of including a dopa decarboxylase inhibitor when giving L-dopa to treat Parkinson disease). The metabolic barrier enzyme γ-glutamyl transpeptidase cleaves the leukotriene mediator produced by the 5-lipoxygenase pathway, LTC_4, and other glutathione adducts.

What about drug molecules? Once they reach the systemic circulation, delivery to the general region of the brain is not a problem: The brain receives about 15% of cardiac output (see Table 2–2). What about crossing the BBB? Small drugs can diffuse across the BBB as a function of their lipid solubility (oil/water partition coefficient). Thus, anesthetics such as nitrous oxide and thiopental move readily across the BBB. Some drugs may resemble substrates that are transported into the brain (e.g., amino acids, nucleosides) and thereby gain entry. LAT1 (SLC7A5) is involved in the influx of several drugs, such as L-dopa and gabapentin across the BBB. OAT1 and OAT3, which generally play a role in the efflux of drugs from the CSF, mediate the uptake of organic compounds such as β-lactam antibiotics, statins, and H_2 receptor antagonists. Charged and large drugs, on the other hand, generally do not penetrate so easily into the brain. The transport proteins, especially MDR1, BCRP, and MRP4, actively extrude many drugs; clearly, recognition by these transporters is a major disadvantage for a drug used to treat CNS disease.

There are methods of permeation under development: nanoparticles and liposomes containing drugs, drugs adducted to ferritin, and development of drug forms with suitable lipophilicity. Basic biomedical research is advancing our understanding of the role of nuclear receptors in the regulation of drug transporters in the BBB (Chan et al., 2013) and of the development of the BBB and the interaction of its cellular and subcellular components to maintain barrier function (Daneman and Prat, 2015). Kim and Bynoe (2015) reported that activation of the adenosine A_{2A} receptor in an in vitro human brain endothelial barrier model permeabilized the barrier sufficiently to permit passage of T cells and the chemotherapeutic agent gemcitabine. Such studies and techniques may provide progress in putting the control of BBB permeability into the hands of physicians.

The Extended Clearance Concept and Physiologically Based Pharmacokinetic (PBPK) Modeling

Based on the "extended clearance concept," hepatic clearance consists of some intrinsic processes, such as hepatic uptake PS_1, backflux from hepatocytes to blood PS_2, hepatic metabolism CL_{met}, and biliary sequestration PS_3 (Figure 5–12) (Shitara et al., 2006, 2013).

The overall hepatic intrinsic clearance $CL_{int,all}$ is expressed as

$$CL_{int,all} = PS_1 \cdot \frac{CL_{met} + PS_3}{PS_2 + CL_{met} + PS_3} \quad \text{(Equation 5–6)}$$

If the sum of the intrinsic clearance of metabolism and biliary sequestration is much larger than the backflux clearance ($PS_2 << (CL_{met} + PS_3)$), $CL_{int,all}$ approximates PS_1, and uptake is a rate-determining process of the overall hepatic intrinsic clearance. In general, many transporter substrates are efficiently excreted into bile or extensively metabolized rather than fluxed back into blood, so their uptake clearances often determine their overall intrinsic hepatic clearance. Assuming that an orally administered drug is completely absorbed from the small intestine and predominantly cleared by the liver, its blood AUC based on the "well-stirred model" can be described as

$$AUC_{blood} = \frac{Dose}{f_B \cdot CL_{int,all}} = \frac{Dose}{f_B \cdot PS_1 \cdot \frac{CL_{met} + PS_3}{PS_2 + CL_{met} + PS_3}} \quad \text{(Equation 5–7)}$$

where f_B represents the unbound fraction in blood.

The AUC_{liver} is described as (Shitara et al., 2013)

$$\begin{aligned} AUC_{liver} &= \frac{PS_1}{PS_2 + CL_{met} + PS_3} \cdot AUC_{blood} \\ &= \frac{PS_1}{PS_2 + CL_{met} + PS_3} \cdot \frac{Dose}{f_B \cdot PS_1 \cdot \frac{CL_{met} + PS_3}{PS_2 + CL_{met} + PS_3}} \\ &= \frac{Dose}{f_B \cdot (CL_{met} + PS_3)} \end{aligned} \quad \text{(Equation 5–8)}$$

Equations 5–6 through 5–8 suggest that if the uptake clearance PS_1 is decreased, AUC_{blood} is increased in inverse proportion to PS_1, while AUC_{liver} is not affected. On the other hand, if drug uptake is a rate-determining process of the overall hepatic intrinsic clearance, the decrease in the function of metabolism or biliary sequestration causes the increase in AUC_{liver}, but not AUC_{blood}. Therefore, if the molecular targets of pharmacological effect and adverse effect induced by drugs are located inside and outside hepatocytes, respectively, as in the case of statins, decrease in the hepatic uptake clearance of drugs caused by drug-drug interaction or genetic polymorphism of transporters affect mainly adverse effect and not so much pharmacological effect.

To simulate the impact of variations in the transporter activities on the systemic and liver exposure of a statin, which is eliminated mainly via OATP1B1 and MRP2, a PBPK model has been used (Jamei et al., 2014; Watanabe et al., 2009).

In a PBPK model, compartments representing actual tissues are connected by blood flow to predict the time course of drug disposition in

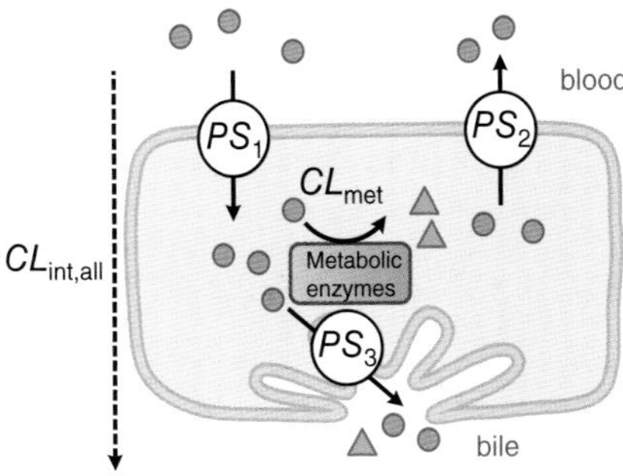

Figure 5–12 *Extended clearance concept: hepatic uptake, backflux into blood, metabolism, and efflux into bile.* The red circles represent parent drugs; the green triangles represent drug metabolites.

the body. A PBPK model allows deep insight into the factors governing the systemic exposure and tissue distribution of drugs and simulates the impact of variations in physiological or drug-dependent parameters on drug disposition. Sensitivity analyses based on the PBPK model indicate that the variation in OATP1B1 activities will have a minimal impact on the therapeutic efficacy but a large impact on the side effect (myopathy) of pravastatin; the opposite will be true for variations in MRP2 activities: a large impact on efficacy, a small impact on the side effect (Watanabe et al., 2009) (Figure 5–13). Such characteristics have been demonstrated for some statins (e.g., simvastatin and rosuvastatin): Pharmacogenomic variation of OATP1B1 activity is associated with the risk of adverse reactions, whereas variation of biliary excretion and intestinal absorption mechanisms result in variation in therapeutic response (Chasman et al., 2012; SEARCH Collaborative Group, 2008).

Genetic Variation in Membrane Transporters: Implications for Clinical Drug Response

There are inherited defects in SLC transporters (see Table 5–2) and ABC transporters (see Table 5–3). Polymorphisms in membrane transporters play roles in drug response and are yielding new insights in pharmacogenetics and pharmacology (see Chapter 7).

Clinical studies have focused on a limited number of transporters, relating genetic variation in membrane transporters to drug disposition and response. For example, two common SNPs in *SLCO1B1* (OATP1B1) are associated with elevated plasma levels of pravastatin (Niemi et al., 2011), a widely used drug for the treatment of hypercholesterolemia (see Chapter 33). Recent studies using genome-wide association methods

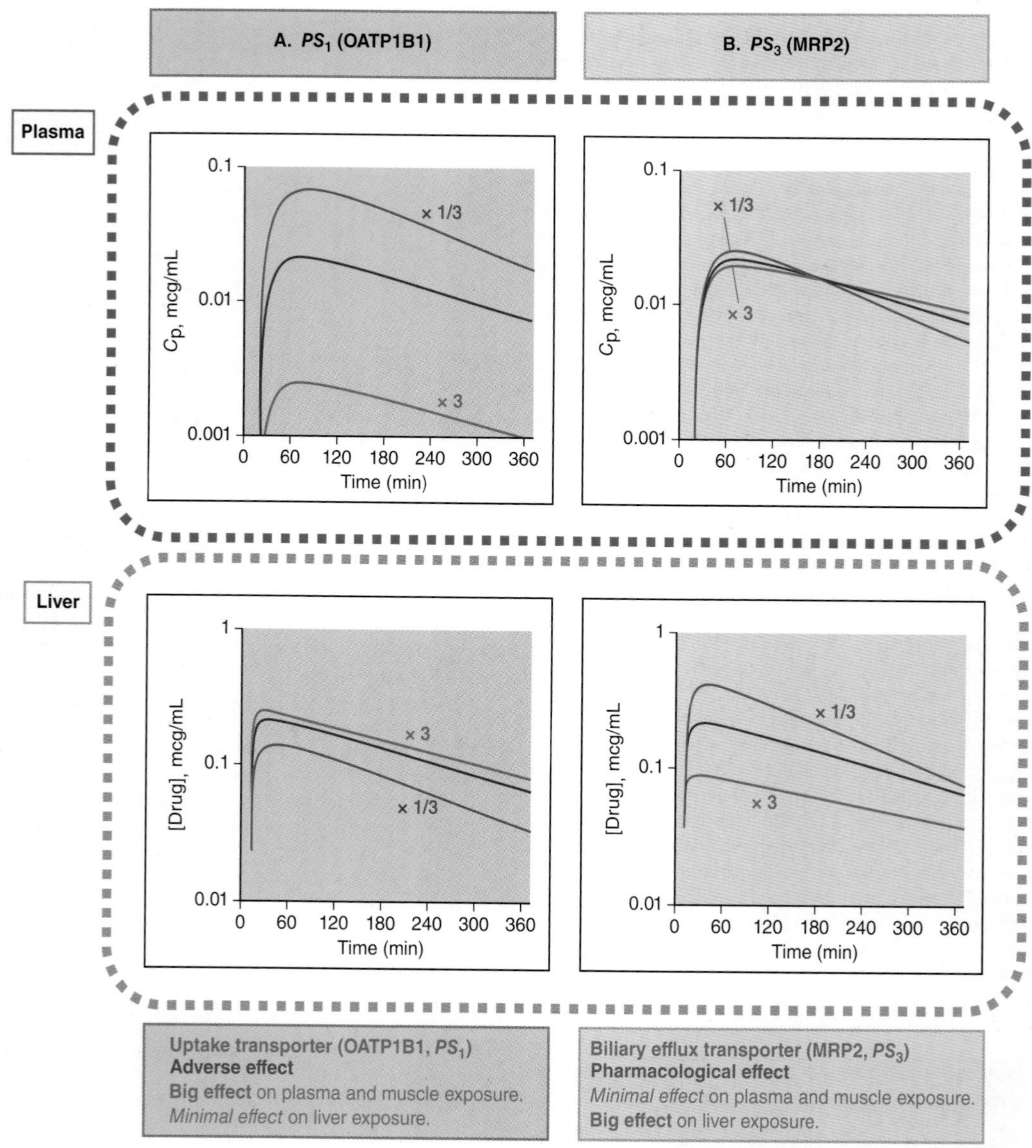

Figure 5–13 *Sensitivity analysis of the effect of functional changes of hepatic uptake clearance* PS_1*(A) and biliary excretion clearance* PS_3*(B) on the plasma and liver concentrations of pravastatin* (Watanabe et al., 2009). These sensitivity analyses were made based on the PBPK model, which connected five sequential liver compartments by blood flow so that this model can be used for drugs exhibiting transporter-mediated high clearance. Plasma and liver concentrations after oral administration (40 mg) were simulated with varying hepatic transport activities over a 1/3- to 3-fold range of the initial values.

show that genetic variants in *SLCO1B1* (OATP1B1) predispose patients to risk for muscle toxicity associated with use of simvastatin as well as altered response to selected statins. Other studies indicate that genetic variants in transporters in the SLC22A family are associated with variation in renal clearance and response to various drugs, including the antidiabetic drug metformin (Chen et al. 2013). Responses to the XOI allopurinol and to rosuvastatin have recently been associated with genetic variants in ABCG2 (BCRP) (Chasman et al., 2012; Wen et al., 2015). For both drugs, a pharmacokinetic mechanism is responsible for the altered pharmacodynamics. Likewise, genetic variants of MRP2 and MRP4 are associated with drug-related phenotypes (Rungtivasuwan et al., 2015). For example, the disposition of tenofovir, an antiviral agent, has been associated with polymorphisms in both ABCC2 and ABCC4 (MRP2 and MRP4, respectively).

Transporters in Regulatory Sciences

Because of their importance in drug disposition and action, transporters are major determinants of variation in therapeutic and adverse drug reactions. As a result, transporters may mediate drug-drug interactions that result in drug safety issues. A notable example is the interaction between gemfibrozil and cerivastatin. Gemfibrozil glucuronide formed in hepatocytes reduces the hepatic uptake and metabolism of cerivastatin; the result is a high C_p for cerivastatin. Elevated statin levels result in statin-induced myopathies, including rhabdomyolysis, a life-threatening adverse effect. This interaction resulted in the removal of cerivastatin from the market because of deaths due to rhabdomyolysis. The U.S. FDA has issued a draft clinical pharmacology guidance on performing drug-drug interaction studies during clinical drug development (FDA, 2012). The guidance presents information on how to use in vitro data for transporter studies to make decisions about whether to conduct a clinical drug-drug interaction study. For example, if a new molecular entity (NME) inhibits the in vitro uptake of a canonical substrate of OCT2 at clinically relevant (unbound) concentrations, the guidance recommends that the sponsor consider performing a clinical drug-drug interaction study to determine whether the NME inhibits the renal clearance of an OCT2 substrate (e.g., metformin) in vivo. On the other hand, if the NME does not inhibit OCT2-mediated uptake in in vitro assays at therapeutic concentrations, the guidance does not recommend a clinical study. Although only a handful of transporters (OATP1B1, OATP1B3, Pgp, BCRP, OCT2, MATE1, OAT1, and OAT3) are included in the FDA guidance, an increasing number of studies are being performed to identify and characterize transporters that mediate clinical drug-drug interactions.

Bibliography

Aceti A, et al. Pharmacogenetics as a tool to tailor antiretroviral therapy: a review. *World J Virol*, **2015**, *4*:198–208.

Chan GN, et al. Role of nuclear receptors in the regulation of drug transporters in the brain. *Trends Pharmacol Sci*, **2013**, *34*:361–372.

Chasman DI, et al. Genetic determinants of statin-induced low-density lipoprotein cholesterol reduction: the Justification for the Use of Statins in Prevention: an Intervention Trial Evaluating Rosuvastatin (JUPITER) trial. *Circ Cardiovasc Genet*, **2012**, *5*:257–264.

Chen S, et al. Pharmacogenetic variation and metformin response. *Curr Drug Metab*, **2013**, *14*:1070–1082.

Cropp CD, et al. Organic anion transporter 2 (SLC22A7) is a facilitative transporter of cGMP. *Mol Pharmacol*, **2008**, *73*:1151–1158.

Daneman R, Prat A. The blood-brain barrier. *Cold Spring Harb Perspect Biol*, **2015**, *7*:1–23.

DeCorter MK, et al. Drug transporters in drug efficacy and toxicity. *Ann Rev Pharmacol Toxicol*, **2012**, *52*:249–273.

Dykens JA, et al. Biguanide-induced mitochondrial dysfunction yields increased lactate production and cytotoxicity of aerobically-poised HepG2 cells and human hepatocytes in vitro. *Toxicol Appl Pharmacol*, **2008**, *233*:203–210.

FDA. Draft guidance for industry: drug interaction studies—study design, data analysis, implications for dosing, and labeling recommendations, 2012. Available at: http://www.fda.gov/downloads/Drugs/Guidances/ucm292362.pdf. Accessed May 29, **2017**.

Gu X, Manautou JE. Regulation of hepatic ABC transporters by xenobiotics and in disease states. *Drug Metab Rev*, **2010**, *42*:482–538.

Guo GL, Zhou H-P. Bile acids and nuclear receptors in the digestive system and therapy. *Acta Pharm Sin B*, **2015**, *5*:89–168.

Harrach S, Ciarimboli G. Role of transporters in the distribution of platinum-based drugs. *Front Pharmacol*, **2015**, 6:85. doi:10.3389/fphar.2015.00085

He S-M, et al. Structural and functional properties of human multidrug resistance protein 1 (MRP1/ABCC1). *Curr Med Chem*, **2011**, *18*:439–481.

Hediger MA, et al. The ABCs of membrane transporters in health and disease (SLC series): introduction. *Mol Aspects Med*, **2013**, *34*:95–107.

Horikawa M, et al. The potential for an interaction between MRP2 (ABCC2) and various therapeutic agents: probenecid as a candidate inhibitor of the biliary excretion of irinotecan metabolites. *Drug Metab Pharmacokinet*, **2002**, *17*:23–33.

Imai S, et al. Analysis of DNA methylation and histone modification profiles of liver-specific transporters. *Mol Pharmacol*, **2009**, *75*:568–576.

Ishiguro N, et al. Predominant contribution of OATP1B3 to the hepatic uptake of telmisartan, an angiotensin II receptor antagonist, in humans. *Drug Metab Dispos*, **2006**, *34*:1109–1115.

Jamei M, et al. A mechanistic framework for in vitro–in vivo extrapolation of liver membrane transporters: prediction of drug–drug interaction between rosuvastatin and cyclosporine. *Clin Pharmacokinet*, **2014**, *53*:73–87.

Kim DG, Bynoe MS. A2A adenosine receptor regulates the human blood-brain barrier permeability. *Mol Neurobiol*, **2015**, *52*:664–678.

Lin L, et al. SLC transporters as therapeutic targets: emerging opportunities. *Nat Rev Drug Discov*, **2015**, *14*:543–560.

Madsen KK et al. Selective GABA transporter inhibitors Tiagabine and EF1502 exhibit mechanistic differences in their ability to modulate the ataxia and anticonvulsant action of the extrasynaptic GABAA receptor agonist Gaboxadol. *J Pharmacol Exp Therap*, **2011**, *338*:214–219.

Meyer zu Schwabedissen HE, et al. Function-impairing polymorphisms of the hepatic uptake transporter SLCO1B1 modify the therapeutic efficacy of statins in a population-based cohort. *Pharmacogenet Genomics*, **2015**, *25*:8–18.

Niemi M, et al. Organic anion transporting polypeptide 1B1: a genetically polymorphic transporter of major importance for hepatic drug uptake. *Pharmacol Rev*, **2011**, *63*:157–181.

Niemi M, et al. Polymorphic organic anion transporting polypeptide 1B1 is a major determinant of repaglinide pharmacokinetics. *Clin Pharmacol Ther*, **2005**, *77*:468–478.

Nigam S. What do drug transporters really do? *Nat Drug Discov*, **2015**, *14*:29–44.

Nigam S, et al. The organic anion transporter (OAT) family: a systems biology perspective. *Physiol Rev*, **2015**, *95*:83–123.

Rungtivasuwan K, et al. Influence of ABCC2 and ABCC4 polymorphisms on tenofovir plasma concentrations in Thai HIV-infected patients. *Antimicrob Agents Chemother*, **2015**, *59*:3240–3245.

SEARCH Collaborative Group. SLCO1B1 variants and statin-induced myopathy—a genomewide study. *N Engl J Med*, **2008**, *359*:789–799.

Shitara Y, et al. Transporters as a determinant of drug clearance and tissue distribution. *Eur J Pharm Sci*, **2006**, *27*:425–446.

Shitara Y, et al. Clinical significance of organic anion transporting polypeptides (OATPs) in drug disposition: their roles in hepatic clearance and intestinal absorption. *Biopharm Drug Dispos*, **2013**, *34*:45–78.

Srimaroeng C, et al. Physiology, structure, and regulation of the cloned organic anion transporters. *Xenobiotica*, **2008**, *38*:889–935.

Smith RP, et al. Genome-wide discovery of drug-dependent human liver regulatory elements. *PLoS Genet*, **2014**, *10*:e1004648.

Tamai I. Pharmacological and pathophysiological roles of carnitine/organic cation transporters (OCTNs: SLC22A4, SLC22A5 and Slc22a21). *Biopharm Drug Dispos*, **2013**, *34*:29–44.

Toyoda Y, et al. MRP class of human ATP binding cassette (ABC) transporters: historical background and new research directions. *Xenobiotica*, **2008**, *38*:833–862.

Urquhart BL, et al. Nuclear receptors and the regulation of drug-metabolizing enzymes and drug transporters: implications for interindividual variability in response to drugs. *J Clin Pharmacol*, **2007**, *47*:566–578.

Wang DS, et al. Involvement of organic cation transporter 1 in the lactic acidosis caused by metformin. *Mol Pharmacol*, **2003**, *63*:844–848.

Watanabe T, et al. Physiologically based pharmacokinetic modeling to predict transporter-mediated clearance and distribution of pravastatin in humans. *J Pharmacol Exp Ther*, **2009**, *328*:652–662.

Wen CC, et al. Genome-wide association study identifies ABCG2 (BCRP) as an allopurinol transporter and a determinant of drug response. *Clin Pharmacol Ther*, **2015**, *97*:518–525.

Zhang S, et al. Organic cation transporters are determinants of oxaliplatin cytotoxicity. *Cancer Res*, **2006a**, *66*:8847–8857.

Zhang W, et al. Effect of SLCO1B1 genetic polymorphism on the pharmacokinetics of nateglinide. *Br J Clin Pharmacol*, **2006b**, *62*:567–572.

Drug Metabolism

Frank J. Gonzalez, Michael Coughtrie, and Robert H. Tukey

第六章　药物代谢

中文导读

本章主要介绍：机体对外源性物质的应对；药物代谢相；药物代谢的部位；Ⅰ相反应，包括细胞色素P450家族、黄素单加氧酶、水解酶；Ⅱ相反应，包括连接酶催化的葡萄糖醛酸化、硫酸化、谷胱甘肽结合、N-乙酰化和甲基化反应；外源性物质代谢在药物安全和有效应用中的作用；药物代谢的诱导；药物代谢在药品研发中的作用。

Abbreviations

ADR: adverse drug reaction
AUC: area under the plasma concentration–time curve
AZA: azathioprine
CAR: constitutive androstane receptor
CES2: carboxylesterase 2
COMT: catechol-*O*-methyltransferase
CPT-11: irinotecan
CYP: cytochrome P450
DPYD: dihydropyrimidine dehydrogenase
EH: epoxide hydrolase
FMO: flavin-containing monooxygenase
GI: gastrointestinal
GSH and GSSG: reduced and oxidized glutathione
GST: glutathione-*S*-transferase
HGPRT: hypoxanthine guanine phosphoribosyl transferase
HIF: hypoxia-inducible factor
HIV: human immunodeficiency virus
HNMT: histamine *N*-methyltransferase
HPPH: 5-(-4-hydroxyphenyl)-5-phenylhydantoin
INH: isonicotinic acid hydrazide (isoniazid)
MAO: monoamine oxidase
MAPK: mitogen-activated protein kinase
mEH: microsomal epoxide hydrolase
6-MP: 6-mercaptopurine
MRP: multidrug resistance protein
MT: methyltransferase
NADPH: nicotinamide adenine dinucleotide phosphate
NAPQI: *N*-acetyl-*p*-benzoquinone imine
NAT: *N*-acetyltransferase
NNMT: nicotinamide *N*-methyltransferase
PAPS: 3′-phosphoadenosine-5′-phosphosulfate
Per: Period
Pgp: P-glycoprotein
PNMT: phenylethanolamine *N*-methyltransferase
POMT: phenol-*O*-methyltransferase
PPAR: peroxisome proliferator–activated receptor
PXR: pregnane X receptor
RXR: retinoid X receptor
SAM: *S*-adenosyl-methionine
sEH: soluble epoxide hydrolase
SULT: sulfotransferase
TBP: TATA box–binding protein
6-TGN: 6-thioguanine nucleotide
TMA: trimethylamine
TPMT: thiopurine methyltransferase
TPT: thiol methyltransferase
UDP-GA: uridine diphosphate-glucuronic acid
UGT: uridine diphosphate–glucuronosyltransferase

Coping With Xenobiotics

Humans come into contact with thousands of foreign chemicals or xenobiotics (substances foreign to the body) through diet and exposure to environmental contaminants. Fortunately, humans have developed a means to rapidly eliminate xenobiotics so that they do not accumulate in the tissues and cause harm. Plants are a common source of dietary xenobiotics, providing many structurally diverse chemicals, some of which are associated with pigment production and others that are actually toxins (called *phytoalexins*) that protect plants against predators. Poisonous mushrooms are a common example: They have many toxins that are lethal to mammals, including amanitin, gyromitrin, orellanine, muscarine, ibotenic acid, muscimol, psilocybin, and coprine. Animals must be able to metabolize and eliminate such chemicals to consume vegetation. While humans can now choose their dietary sources, a typical animal does not have this luxury and as a result is subject to its environment and the vegetation that exists in that environment. Thus, the ability to metabolize unusual chemicals in plants and other food sources is critical for adaptation to a changing environment and ultimately the survival of animals.

Enzymes that metabolize xenobiotics have historically been called drug-metabolizing enzymes; however, these enzymes are involved in the metabolism of many foreign chemicals to which humans are exposed and are more appropriately called *xenobiotic-metabolizing enzymes.* Myriad diverse enzymes have evolved in animals to metabolize foreign chemicals. Dietary differences among species during the course of evolution could account for the marked species variation in the complexity of the xenobiotic-metabolizing enzymes. Additional diversity within these enzyme systems has also derived from the necessity to "detoxify" a host of endogenous chemicals that would otherwise prove harmful to the organism, such as bilirubin, steroid hormones, and catecholamines. Many of these endogenous biochemicals are detoxified by the same or closely related xenobiotic-metabolizing enzymes.

Drugs are xenobiotics, and the capacity to metabolize and clear drugs involves the same enzymatic pathways and transport systems that are used for normal metabolism of dietary constituents. Indeed, many drugs are derived from chemicals found in plants, some of which have been used in Chinese herbal medicines for thousands of years. Of the prescription drugs in use today for cancer treatment, some are also derived from plants (see Chapter 68); investigating folkloric claims led to the discovery of most of these drugs. The capacity to metabolize xenobiotics, although largely beneficial, has made development of drugs more time consuming and costly due in part to:

- species differences in expression of enzymes that metabolize drugs and thereby limit the utility of animal models to predict drug effects in humans
- interindividual variations in the capacity of humans to metabolize drugs
- drug-drug interactions involving xenobiotic metabolizing enzymes
- metabolic activation of chemicals to toxic and carcinogenic derivatives

Today, most xenobiotics to which humans are exposed come from sources that include environmental pollution, food additives, cosmetic products, agrochemicals, processed foods, and drugs.

In general, most xenobiotics are lipophilic chemicals; in the absence of metabolism, these would not be efficiently eliminated and thus would accumulate in the body, potentially resulting in toxicity. With few exceptions, all xenobiotics are subjected to one or multiple enzymatic pathways that constitute *phase 1 oxidation* and *phase 2 conjugation.* As a general paradigm, metabolism serves to convert these hydrophobic chemicals into more hydrophilic derivatives that can easily be eliminated from the body through the urine or the bile.

To enter cells and reach their sites of action, drugs generally must possess physical properties that allow them to move down a concentration gradient and across cell membranes. Many drugs are hydrophobic, a property that allows entry via diffusion across lipid bilayers into the systemic circulation and then into cells. With some compounds, transporters on the plasma membrane facilitate entry (see Chapter 5). This property of hydrophobicity renders drugs difficult to eliminate because, in the absence of metabolism, they accumulate in fat and cellular phospholipid bilayers. The xenobiotic-metabolizing enzymes convert drugs and other xenobiotics into derivatives that are more hydrophilic and thus easily eliminated via excretion into the aqueous compartments of the tissues and ultimately into the urine.

Metabolism of a drug can begin even before a drug is absorbed: Gut bacteria represent the first metabolic interface between orally administered drugs and the body. The microbiome of the GI tract can metabolize xenobiotics; interindividual differences in composition of the gut flora could influence drug action and contribute to differences in drug response. Indeed, diurnal oscillations in GI bacteria and their metabolic capacity, superposed on host clock gene oscillations, appear to affect drug disposition and effect (FitzGerald et al., 2015).

The process of drug metabolism that leads to elimination also plays a major role in diminishing the biological activity of a drug. For example, *(S)-phenytoin*, an anticonvulsant used in the treatment of epilepsy, is virtually insoluble in water. Metabolism by the phase 1 CYPs followed by phase 2 UGT enzymes produces a metabolite that is highly water soluble and readily eliminated from the body (Figure 6–1). Metabolism also terminates the biological activity of the drug. Because conjugates are generally hydrophilic, elimination via the bile or urine is dependent on the actions of many efflux transporters to facilitate transmembrane passage (see Chapter 5).

While xenobiotic-metabolizing enzymes facilitate the elimination of chemicals from the body, paradoxically these same enzymes can also convert certain chemicals to highly reactive, toxic, and carcinogenic metabolites. This occurs when an unstable intermediate is formed that has reactivity toward other compounds found in the cell. Chemicals that can be converted by xenobiotic metabolism to cancer-causing derivatives are called carcinogens. Depending on the structure of the chemical substrate, xenobiotic-metabolizing enzymes can produce electrophilic metabolites that react with nucleophilic cellular macromolecules such as DNA, RNA, and protein. This can cause cell death and organ toxicity. Most drugs and other xenobiotics that cause hepatotoxicity damage mitochondria and lead to hepatocyte death. Reaction of these electrophiles with DNA can sometimes result in cancer through the mutation of genes, such as oncogenes or tumor suppressor genes. It is generally believed that most human cancers are due to exposure to chemical carcinogens.

This potential for carcinogenic activity makes testing the safety of drug candidates of vital importance. Testing for cancer-causing potential is particularly critical for drugs that will be used for the treatment of chronic diseases. Because each species has evolved a unique combination of xenobiotic-metabolizing enzymes, nonprimate models (mostly rodents) cannot be solely used for testing the safety of new drug candidates targeted for human diseases. Nevertheless, testing in rodent models (e.g., mice and rats) can usually identify potential carcinogens. Fortunately, there are no instances of drugs that test negative in rodents but cause cancer in humans, albeit some rodent carcinogens are not associated with human cancer. However, many cytotoxic cancer drugs have the potential to cause cancer; this risk is minimized by their acute, rather than chronic, use in cancer therapy.

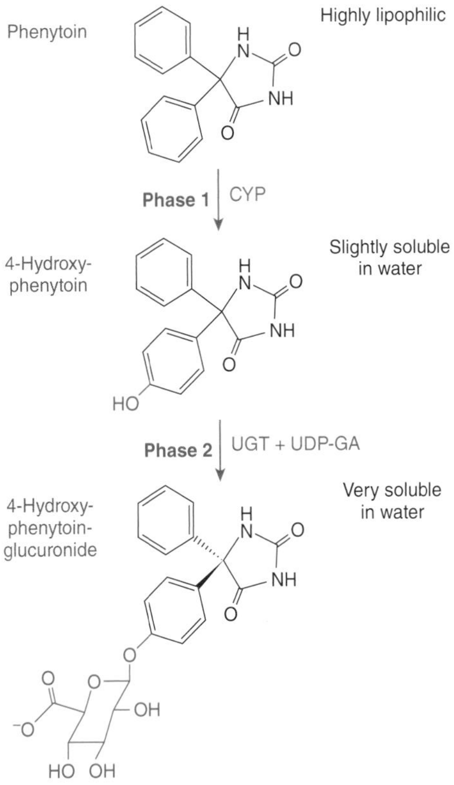

Figure 6–1 *Metabolism of phenytoin.* In phase 1, CYP facilitates 4-hydroxylation of phenytoin to yield HPPH. In phase 2, the hydroxy group serves as a substrate for UGT, which conjugates a molecule of glucuronic acid using UDP-GA as a cofactor. Together, phase 1 and phase 2 reactions convert a very hydrophobic molecule to a larger hydrophilic derivative that is eliminated via the bile.

The Phases of Drug Metabolism

Xenobiotic-metabolizing enzymes have historically been categorized as

- *phase 1 reactions*, which include oxidation, reduction, or hydrolytic reactions; or
- *phase 2 reactions*, in which enzymes catalyze the conjugation of the substrate (the phase 1 product) with a second molecule.

The *phase 1 enzymes* lead to the introduction of what are called functional groups, such as –OH, –COOH, –SH, –O–, or NH_2 (Table 6–1). The addition of functional groups does little to increase the water solubility of the drug but can dramatically alter the biological properties of the drug. Reactions carried out by phase 1 enzymes usually lead to the inactivation of a drug. However, in certain instances, metabolism, usually the hydrolysis of an ester or amide linkage, results in bioactivation of a drug. Inactive drugs that undergo metabolism to an active drug are called prodrugs (Huttenen et al., 2011). Examples of prodrugs bioactivated by CYPs are the antitumor drug *cyclophosphamide*, which is bioactivated to a cell-killing electrophilic derivative (see Chapter 66), and the anti-thrombotic agent clopidogrel, which activated to 2-oxo-clopidogrel, which is further metabolized to an irreversible inhibitor of platelet ADP P2Y12 receptors. *Phase 2 enzymes* produce a metabolite with improved water solubility and thereby facilitate the elimination of the drug from the tissue, normally via efflux transporters described in Chapter 5. Thus, in general, phase 1 reactions result in biological inactivation of a drug, and phase 2 reactions

TABLE 6–1 ■ XENOBIOTIC-METABOLIZING ENZYMES

ENZYMES	REACTIONS
Phase 1 enzymes (CYPs, FMOs, EHs)	
Cytochrome P450s (P450 or CYP)	C and O oxidation, dealkylation, others
Flavin-containing monooxygenases (FMOs)	N, S, and P oxidation
Epoxide hydrolases (EHs)	Hydrolysis of epoxides
Phase 2 "transferases"	
Sulfotransferases (SULT)	Addition of sulfate
UDP-glucuronosyltransferases (UGTs)	Addition of glucuronic acid
Glutathione-*S*-transferases (GSTs)	Addition of glutathione
N-Acetyltransferases (NATs)	Addition of acetyl group
Methyltransferases (MTs)	Addition of methyl group
Other enzymes	
Alcohol dehydrogenases	Reduction of alcohols
Aldehyde dehydrogenases	Reduction of aldehydes
NADPH-quinone oxidoreductase (NQO)	Reduction of quinones

mEH and sEH, microsomal and soluble epoxide hydrolase, respectively; NADPH, reduced nicotinamide adenine dinucleotide phosphate; UDP, uridine diphosphate.

facilitate the drug elimination and the inactivation of electrophilic and potentially toxic metabolites produced by oxidation.

Superfamilies of evolutionarily related enzymes and receptors are common in the mammalian genome; the enzyme systems responsible for drug metabolism are good examples. The phase 1 oxidation reactions are carried out by CYPs, FMOs, and EHs. The CYPs and FMOs are composed of superfamilies of enzymes. Each superfamily contains multiple genes. The phase 2 enzymes include several superfamilies of conjugating enzymes. Among the more important are the GSTs, UGTs, SULTs, NATs, and MTs (Table 6-1).

These conjugation reactions usually require the substrate to have oxygen (hydroxyl or epoxide groups), nitrogen, and sulfur atoms that serve as acceptor sites for a hydrophilic moiety, such as glutathione, glucuronic acid, sulfate, or an acetyl group, that is covalently conjugated to an acceptor site on the molecule. Examine the phase 1 and phase 2 metabolism of phenytoin (Figure 6–1). The oxidation by phase 1 enzymes either adds or exposes a functional group, permitting the products of phase 1 metabolism to serve as substrates for the phase 2 conjugating or synthetic enzymes. In the case of the UGTs, glucuronic acid is delivered to the functional group, forming a glucuronide metabolite that is more water soluble and is targeted for excretion in the urine or bile. When the substrate is a drug, these reactions usually convert the original drug to a form that is not able to bind to its target receptor, thus attenuating the biological response to the drug.

Sites of Drug Metabolism

Xenobiotic-metabolizing enzymes are found in most tissues in the body, with the highest levels located in the GI tract (liver, small and large intestines). The small intestine plays a crucial role in drug metabolism. Orally administered drugs first are exposed to the GI flora, which can metabolize some drugs. During absorption, drugs are exposed to xenobiotic-metabolizing enzymes in the epithelial cells of the GI tract; this is the initial site of drug metabolism. Once absorbed, drugs enter the portal circulation and are taken to the liver, where they can be extensively metabolized (the "first-pass effect"). The liver is the major "metabolic clearinghouse" for both endogenous chemicals (e.g., cholesterol, steroid hormones, fatty acids, and proteins) and xenobiotics. While a portion of active drug escapes metabolism in the GI tract and liver, subsequent passes through the liver result in more metabolism of the parent drug until the agent is eliminated. Thus, drugs that are poorly metabolized remain in the body for longer periods of time, and their pharmacokinetic profiles show much longer elimination half-lives than drugs that are rapidly metabolized.

During drug development, compounds are sought that have a favorable pharmacokinetic profile in which they are eliminated over the course of 24 h after administration. This allows the use of daily single dosing. If a compound with a favorable efficacy cannot be modified to improve its pharmacokinetic profile, twice-a-day or even three times-a-day dosing needs to be used. Other organs that contain significant xenobiotic-metabolizing enzymes include tissues of the nasal mucosa and lung, which play important roles in the metabolism of drugs that are administered through aerosol sprays. These tissues are also the first line of contact with hazardous chemicals that are airborne.

Within the cell, xenobiotic-metabolizing enzymes are found in the intracellular membranes and in the cytosol. The phase 1 CYPs, FMOs, and EHs and some phase 2 conjugating enzymes, notably the UGTs, are all located in the endoplasmic reticulum (ER) of the cell (Figure 6–2). The endoplasmic reticulum consists of phospholipid bilayers organized as tubes and sheets throughout the cytoplasm. This network has an inner lumen that is physically distinct from the rest of the cytosolic components of the cell and has connections to the plasma membrane and nuclear envelope. This membrane localization is ideally suited for the metabolic function of these enzymes: Hydrophobic molecules enter the cell and become embedded in the lipid bilayer, where they come into direct contact with the phase 1 enzymes. Once subjected to oxidation, drugs can be directly conjugated by the UGTs (in the lumen of the endoplasmic reticulum) or by the cytosolic transferases, such as GST and SULT. Glucuronide conjugates must be transported out

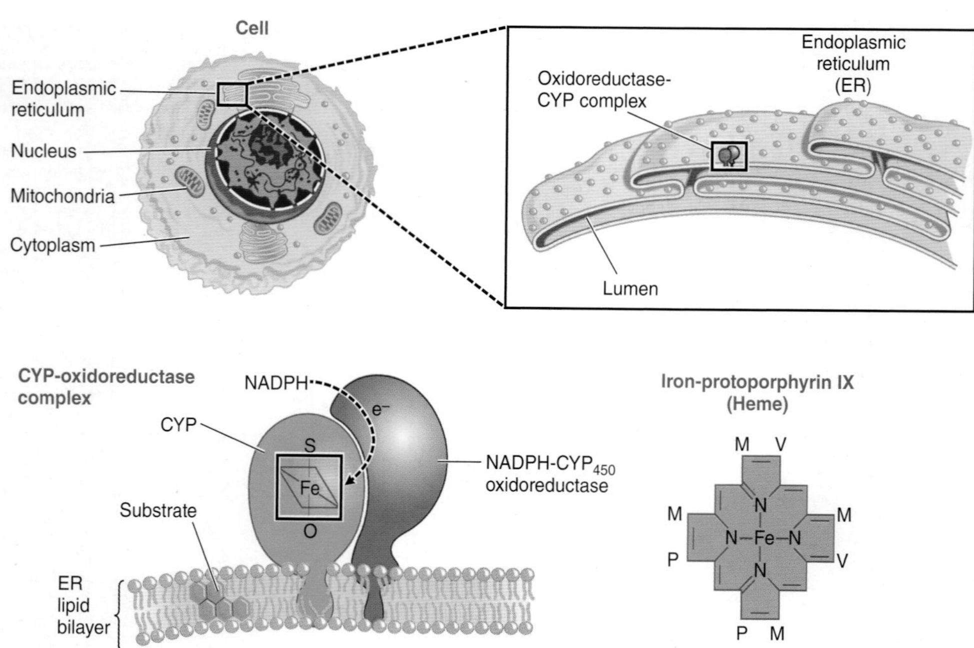

Figure 6–2 *Location of CYPs in the cell.* Increasingly microscopic levels of detail are shown, sequentially expanding the areas within the black boxes. CYPs are embedded in the phospholipid bilayer of the ER. Most of the enzyme is located on the cytosolic surface of the ER. A second enzyme, NADPH-CYP oxidoreductase, transfers electrons to the CYP where it can, in the presence of O_2, oxidize xenobiotic substrates, many of which are hydrophobic and dissolved in the ER. A single NADPH-CYP oxidoreductase species transfers electrons to all CYP isoforms in the ER. Each CYP contains a molecule of iron-protoporphyrin IX that functions to bind and activate O_2. Substituents on the porphyrin ring are methyl (M), propionyl (P), and vinyl (V) groups.

of the endoplasmic reticulum. The metabolites are transported across the plasma membrane and into the bloodstream, then conveyed to the liver and into the bile through the bile canaliculus, from which they are deposited in the gut (see Figure 5–9).

Phase 1 Reactions

CYPs: The Cytochrome P450 Superfamily

The CYPs are a superfamily of enzymes, each of which contains a molecule of heme bound noncovalently to the polypeptide chain (Figure 6–2). Many enzymes that use O_2 as a substrate for their reactions contain heme, and heme is the oxygen-binding moiety in hemoglobin. Heme contains one atom of iron in a hydrocarbon cage that functions to bind O_2 in the active site of the CYP as part of the catalytic cycle of these enzymes. CYPs use O_2, plus H^+ derived from the cofactor-reduced NADPH, to carry out the oxidation of substrates. The H^+ is supplied through the enzyme NADPH-CYP oxidoreductase. Metabolism of a substrate by a CYP consumes one molecule of O_2 and produces an oxidized substrate and a molecule of H_2O as a by-product. However, for most CYPs, depending on the nature of the substrate, the reaction is "uncoupled," consuming more O_2 than substrate metabolized and producing what is called activated oxygen or O_2^-. The O_2^- is usually converted to water by the enzyme superoxide dismutase. When elevated, O_2^-, also called a reactive oxygen species (ROS), can cause oxidative stress that is detrimental to cellular physiology and is associated with diseases such as hepatic cirrhosis.

Among the diverse reactions carried out by mammalian CYPs are *N*-dealkylation, *O*-dealkylation, aromatic hydroxylation, *N*-oxidation, *S*-oxidation, deamination, and dehalogenation (Table 6–2). More than 50 individual CYPs have been identified in humans. As a family of enzymes, CYPs are involved in the metabolism of dietary and xenobiotic chemicals, as well as the synthesis of endogenous compounds such as steroids and fatty acid signaling molecules such as epoxyeicosatrienoic acids. CYPs also participate in the production of bile acids from cholesterol.

In contrast to the drug-metabolizing CYPs, the CYPs that catalyze steroid and bile acid synthesis have specific substrate preferences. For example, the CYP that produces estrogen from testosterone, CYP19 or aromatase, can metabolize only testosterone or androstenedione and does not metabolize xenobiotics. Specific inhibitors for aromatase, such as *anastrozole*, have been developed for use in the treatment of estrogen-dependent tumors (see Chapters 44 and 66).

The synthesis of bile acids from cholesterol occurs in the liver, where, subsequent to CYP-catalyzed oxidation, the bile acids are conjugated with amino acids and transported through the bile duct and gallbladder into the small intestine. Bile acids are emulsifiers that facilitate the elimination of conjugated drugs from the liver and the absorption of fatty acids and vitamins from the diet. In this capacity, more than 90% of bile acids are reabsorbed by the gut and transported back to the hepatocytes. Similar to the steroid biosynthetic CYPs, CYPs involved in bile acid production have strict substrate requirements and do not participate in xenobiotic or drug metabolism.

The CYPs that carry out xenobiotic metabolism have a tremendous capacity to metabolize a large number of structurally diverse chemicals. This is due to multiple forms of CYPs and to the capacity of a single CYP to metabolize many structurally distinct chemicals. There is also significant overlapping substrate specificity among CYPs; a single compound may be metabolized, albeit at different rates, by different CYPs. In addition, CYPs can metabolize a single compound at different positions on the molecule. In contrast to enzymes in the body that carry out highly specific reactions in which there is a single substrate and one or more products or two simultaneous substrates, the CYPs are considered promiscuous in their capacity to bind and metabolize multiple substrates (Table 6–2).

This accommodating property, due to large and fluid substrate-binding sites in the CYP, sacrifices metabolic turnover rates: CYPs metabolize substrates at a fraction of the rate of more typical enzymes involved in intermediary metabolism and mitochondrial electron transfer. As a result, drugs generally have half-lives on the order of 3–30 h, while endogenous compounds have half-lives on the order of seconds or minutes (e.g., dopamine and insulin). Even though CYPs have slow catalytic rates, their activities are sufficient to metabolize drugs that are administered at high concentrations in the body.

This unusual feature of extensive overlapping substrate specificities by the CYPs is one of the underlying reasons for the predominance of drug-drug interactions. When two coadministered drugs are both metabolized by a single CYP, they compete for binding to the enzyme's active site. This can result in the inhibition of metabolism of one or both of the drugs, leading to elevated plasma levels. If there is a narrow therapeutic index for the drugs, the elevated serum levels may elicit unwanted toxicities. Drug-drug interactions are among the leading causes of ADRs.

The Naming of CYPs

The CYPs, responsible for metabolizing the vast majority of therapeutic drugs, are the most actively studied of the xenobiotic-metabolizing enzymes. CYPs are complex and diverse in their regulation and catalytic activities. Genome sequencing has revealed the existence of 102 putatively functional CYP genes and 88 pseudogenes in the mouse and 57 putatively functional genes and 58 pseudogenes in humans. These genes are grouped, based on amino acid sequence similarity, into a superfamily composed of families and subfamilies with increasing sequence similarity. CYPs are named with the root CYP followed by a number designating the family, a letter denoting the subfamily, and another number designating the CYP form. Thus, CYP3A4 is family 3, subfamily A, and gene number 4.

A Small Number of CYPs Metabolize the Majority of Drugs

A limited number of CYPs (15 in humans) that fall into families 1, 2, and 3 are primarily involved in xenobiotic metabolism. Because a single CYP can metabolize a large number of structurally diverse compounds, these enzymes can collectively metabolize scores of chemicals found in the diet, environment, and pharmaceuticals. In humans, 12 CYPs (CYP1A1, 1A2, 1B1, 2A6, 2B6, 2C8, 2C9, 2C19, 2D6, 2E1, 3A4, and 3A5) are important for metabolism of xenobiotics. The liver contains the greatest abundance of xenobiotic-metabolizing CYPs, thus ensuring efficient first-pass metabolism of drugs. CYPs are also expressed throughout the GI tract and in lower amounts in lung, kidney, and even in the CNS.

The expression of the different CYPs can differ markedly as a result of dietary and environmental exposure to inducers or through interindividual changes resulting from heritable polymorphic differences in gene structure, and tissue-specific expression patterns can affect overall drug metabolism and clearance. The most active CYPs for drug metabolism are those in the CYP2C, CYP2D, and CYP3A subfamilies. CYP3A4, the most abundantly expressed in liver, is involved in the metabolism of over 50% of clinically used drugs (Figure 6–3A). The CYP1A, CYP1B, CYP2A, CYP2B, and CYP2E subfamilies are not significantly involved in the metabolism of therapeutic drugs, but they do catalyze the metabolic activation of many protoxins and procarcinogens to their ultimate reactive metabolites.

There are large differences in levels of expression of each CYP between individuals as assessed by both clinical pharmacologic studies and analysis of expression in human liver samples. This large interindividual variability in CYP expression is due to the presence of genetic polymorphisms and differences in gene regulation (see discussion that follows). Several human CYP genes exhibit polymorphisms, including *CYP2A6*, *CYP2C9*, *CYP2C19*, and *CYP2D6*. Allelic variants have been found in the *CYP1B1* and *CYP3A4* genes, but they are present at low frequencies in humans and appear not to have a major role in interindividual levels of expression of these enzymes. However, homozygous mutations in the *CYP1B1* gene are associated with primary congenital glaucoma.

Drug-Drug Interactions

Differences in the rate of metabolism of a drug can be due to drug interactions. Most commonly, this occurs when two drugs (e.g., a statin and a macrolide antibiotic or antifungal agent) are coadministered and subjected to metabolism by the same enzyme. Because most of these drug-drug interactions are due to CYPs, it thus becomes important to determine the identity of the CYP that metabolizes a particular drug and to avoid

TABLE 6–2 ■ MAJOR REACTIONS INVOLVED IN DRUG METABOLISM

	REACTION	EXAMPLES
I. Oxidative reactions		
N-Dealkylation	$R{-}NH{-}CH_3 \rightarrow R{-}NH_2 + CH_2O$	Imipramine, diazepam, codeine, erythromycin, morphine, tamoxifen, theophylline, caffeine
O-Dealkylation	$R{-}O{-}CH_3 \rightarrow R{-}OH + CH_2O$	Codeine, indomethacin, dextromethorphan
Aliphatic hydroxylation	$R{-}CH_2{-}CH_3 \rightarrow R{-}CH(OH){-}CH_3$	Tolbutamide, ibuprofen, phenobarbital, meprobamate, cyclosporine, midazolam
Aromatic hydroxylation	$R{-}C_6H_4{-}H \rightarrow$ arene epoxide (H, O, H) $\rightarrow R{-}C_6H_4{-}OH$	Phenytoin, phenobarbital, propanolol, ethinyl estradiol, amphetamine, warfarin
N-Oxidation	$R{-}NH_2 \rightarrow R{-}NH{-}OH$ $R_1{-}NH{-}R_2 \rightarrow R_1{-}N(OH){-}R_2$	Chlorpheniramine, dapsone, meperidine
S-Oxidation	$R_1{-}S{-}R_2 \rightarrow R_1{-}S(=O){-}R_2$	Cimetidine, chlorpromazine, thioridazine omeprazole
Deamination	$C(CH_3)(H)(NH_2) \rightarrow C(CH_3)(OH)(NH_2) \rightarrow C(CH_3){=}O + NH_3$	Diazepam, amphetamine
II. Hydrolysis reactions		
	Epoxide (R, R, H, O, H) $\rightarrow$ trans-dihydrodiol (R, R, H, OH, H, OH)	Carbamazepine (see Figure 6-4)
	$R_1{-}C(=O){-}O{-}R_2 \rightarrow R_1{-}C(=O){-}O{-}H + HO{-}R_2$	Procaine, aspirin, clofibrate, meperidine, enalapril, cocaine
	$R_1{-}C(=O){-}NH{-}R_2 \rightarrow R_1{-}C(=O){-}O{-}H + H_2N{-}R_2$	Lidocaine, procainamide, indomethacin
III. Conjugation reactions		
Glucuronidation	UDP-glucuronic acid (^{-}OOC, HO, HO, HO, O–UDP) $+ HO{-}R \rightarrow$ glucuronide (^{-}OOC, HO, HO, HO, O–R)	Acetaminophen, morphine, oxazepam, lorazepam
Sulfation	$PAPS + HO{-}R \rightarrow HO_3S{-}O{-}R + PAP$	Acetaminophen, steroids, methyldopa
Acetylation	$CoA{-}S{-}C(=O){-}CH_3 + R{-}NH_2 \rightarrow R{-}NH{-}C(=O){-}CH_3$	Sulfonamides, isoniazid, dapsone, clonazepam
Methylation*	$R{-}OH + AdoMet \rightarrow R{-}O{-}CH_3 + AdoHomCys$	L-dopa, methyldopa, mercaptopurine, captopril
Glutathionylation	$GSH + R \rightarrow R{-}GSH$	Adriamycin, fosfomycin, busulfan

PAPS, 3′-phosphoadenosine-5′ phosphosulfate; PAP, 3′-phosphoadenosine-5′-phosphate; AdoMet, S-adenosylmethionine; AdoHomCys, S-adenosylhomocysteine.
*also for RS-, RN-.

A. Phase 1 Enzymes

CYP1A1/2
Esterases
CYP1B1
Epoxide hydrolase
Others
CYP2A6
CYP2B6
DPYD
CYP2C8/9
CYP2C10
CYP2D6
CYP3A4/5
CYP2E1

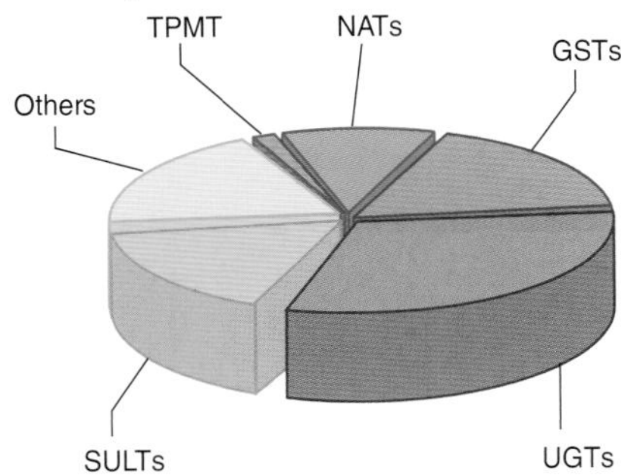

Figure 6–3 *The fraction of clinically used drugs metabolized by the major phase 1 and phase 2 enzymes.* The relative size of each pie section represents the estimated percentage of drugs metabolized by the major phase 1 (**A**) and phase 2 (**B**) enzymes, based on studies in the literature. In some cases, more than a single enzyme is responsible for metabolism of a single drug.

coadministering drugs that are metabolized by the same enzyme. Some drugs can also inhibit CYPs independently of being substrates for a CYP. For example, the common antifungal agent *ketoconazole* is a potent inhibitor of CYP3A4 and other CYPs, and coadministration of ketoconazole with the anti-HIV viral protease inhibitors reduces the clearance of the protease inhibitor and increases its plasma concentration and the risk of toxicity.

Some drugs are CYP inducers that not only can increase their own rates of metabolism but also can induce metabolism of other coadministered drugs (see the following discussion and Figure 6–12). Steroid hormones and herbal products such as St. John's wort can increase hepatic levels of CYP3A4, thereby increasing the metabolism of many orally administered drugs. Drug metabolism can also be influenced by diet. CYP inhibitors and inducers are commonly found in foods, and in some cases these can influence the toxicity and efficacy of a drug. For most drugs, descriptive information found on the package insert lists the CYP that carries out its metabolism and the potential for drug interactions. Components found in grapefruit juice (e.g., naringin, furanocoumarins) are potent inhibitors of CYP3A4, and thus some drug inserts recommend not taking medication with grapefruit juice because it could increase the bioavailability of a drug.

Terfenadine, a once-popular antihistamine, was removed from the market because its metabolism was inhibited by CYP3A4 substrates such as *erythromycin* and grapefruit juice. Terfenadine is actually a prodrug that requires oxidation by CYP3A4 to its active metabolite, and at high doses the parent compound caused arrhythmias. Elevated plasma levels of the parent drug resulting from CYP3A4 inhibition caused ventricular tachycardia in some individuals, which ultimately led to the withdrawal of terfenadine from the market.

Interindividual differences in drug metabolism are significantly influenced by polymorphisms in CYPs. The CYP2D6 polymorphism has led to the withdrawal of several clinically used drugs (e.g., *debrisoquine* and *perhexiline*) and the cautious use of others that are known CYP2D6 substrates (e.g., *encainide* and *flecainide* [antiarrhythmics], *desipramine* and *nortriptyline* [antidepressants], and *codeine*).

Flavin-Containing Monooxygenases

The FMOs are another superfamily of phase 1 enzymes involved in drug metabolism. Similar to CYPs, the FMOs are expressed at high levels in the liver and are bound to the endoplasmic reticulum, a site that favors interaction with and metabolism of hydrophobic drug substrates. There are six families of FMOs, with FMO3 the most abundant in liver. FMO3 is able to metabolize nicotine, as well as H_2-receptor antagonists (*cimetidine* and *ranitidine*), antipsychotics (*clozapine*), and antiemetics (*itopride*). Trimethylamine *N*-oxide (TMAO) occurs in high concentrations, up to 15% by weight, in marine animals, where it acts as an osmotic regulator. In humans, FMO3 normally metabolizes TMAO to TMA, but a genetic deficiency of FMO3 causes the fish-odor syndrome, in which unmetabolized TMAO accumulates in the body and causes a socially offensive fish odor.

FMOs are considered minor contributors to drug metabolism, and they almost always produce benign metabolites. In addition, FMOs are not readily inhibited and are not induced by any of the xenobiotic receptors (see discussion that follows); thus, in contrast to CYPs, FMOs would not be expected to be involved in drug-drug interactions. In fact, this has been demonstrated by comparing the pathways of metabolism of two drugs used in the control of gastric motility: itopride and cisapride. Itopride is metabolized by FMO3; cisapride is metabolized by CYP3A4. As predicted, itopride is less likely to be involved in drug-drug interactions than is cisapride. CYP3A4 participates in drug-drug interactions through induction and inhibition of metabolism, whereas FMO3 is not induced or inhibited by any clinically used drugs. It is possible that FMOs may be important in the development of new drugs. A candidate drug could be designed by introducing a site for FMO oxidation with the knowledge that selected metabolism and pharmacokinetic properties could be accurately calculated for efficient drug-based biological efficacy.

Hydrolytic Enzymes

Two forms of EH carry out hydrolysis of epoxides, most of which are produced by CYPs. The sEH is expressed in the cytosol; mEH is localized to the membrane of the endoplasmic reticulum. Epoxides are highly reactive electrophiles that can bind to cellular nucleophiles found in protein, RNA, and DNA, resulting in cell toxicity and transformation. Thus, EHs participate in the deactivation of potentially toxic metabolites generated by CYPs.

There are a few examples of the influence of mEH on drug metabolism. The antiepileptic drug *carbamazepine* is a prodrug that is converted to its pharmacologically active derivative carbamazepine-10,11-epoxide, by CYP. This metabolite is efficiently hydrolyzed to a dihydrodiol by mEH, resulting in inactivation of the drug (Figure 6–4). Inhibition of mEH can cause an elevation in plasma concentrations of the active metabolite and consequent side effects. The tranquilizer *valnoctamide* and anticonvulsant *valproate* inhibit mEH, resulting in clinically significant drug interactions with carbamazepine. This has led to efforts to develop new antiepileptic drugs, such as *gabapentin* and *levetiracetam*, that are metabolized by CYPs and not by EHs.

In general, the sEH complements the mEH in terms of substrate selectivity, with mEH degrading epoxides on cyclic systems and sEH having a high V_m and low K_m for fatty acid epoxides. Fatty acid epoxides are chemical mediators in the CYP branch of the arachidonic acid cascade. Simplistically, they can be thought of as balancing the generally pro-inflammatory and hypertensive prostaglandins, thromboxanes, and leukotrienes. The epoxides of arachidonic acid and docosahexaenoic acid

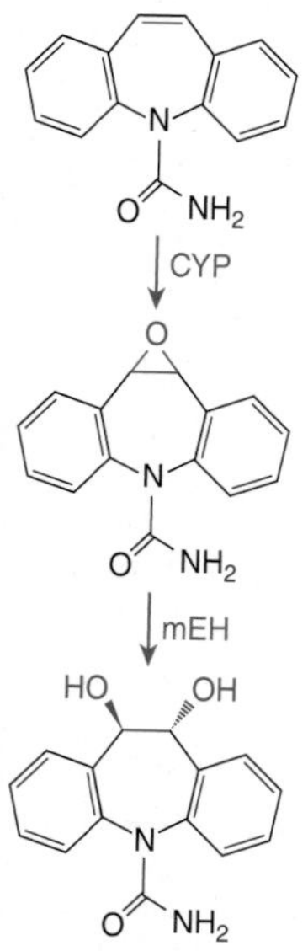

Figure 6–4 *Metabolism of carbamazepine by CYP and mEH.* Carbamazepine is oxidized to the pharmacologically active metabolite carbamazepine-10,11-epoxide by CYP. The epoxide is converted to a trans-dihydrodiol by mEH. This metabolite is biologically inactive and can be conjugated by phase 2 enzymes.

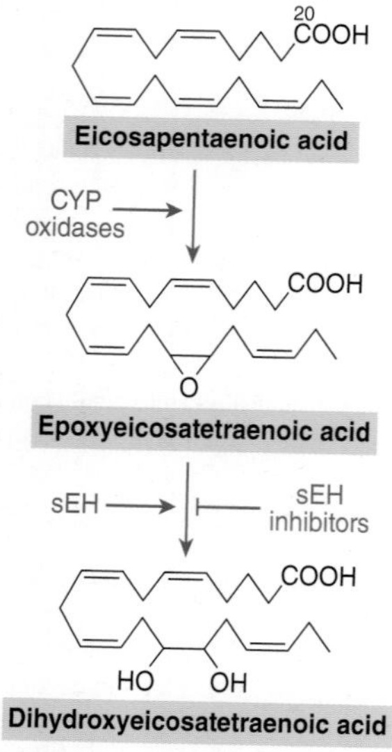

Figure 6–5 *Production and metabolism of an omega-3 fatty acid epoxide.* Fatty acid epoxides, such as the epoxide of the omega-3 fatty acid shown here, have a variety of anti-inflammatory and antinociceptive properties in test systems but are usually evanescent, metabolized to biologically less-active dihydroxy forms by sEH. Inhibition of sEH may promote the salutary effects of these epoxides.

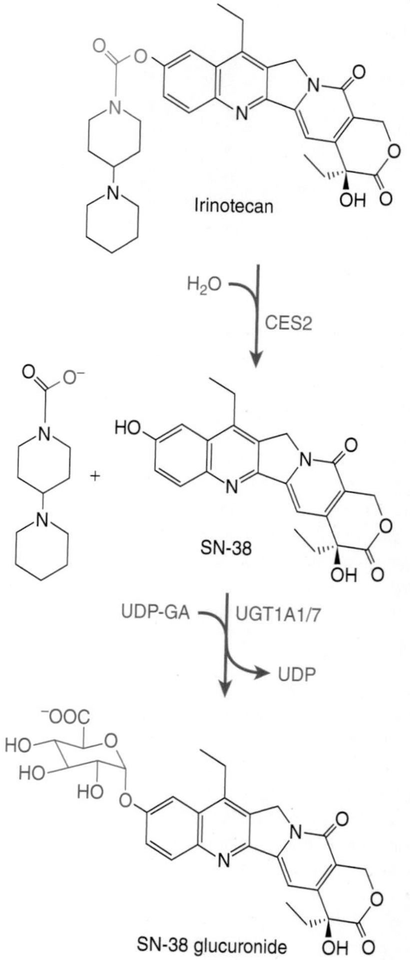

reduce inflammation, hypertension, and pain but are normally degraded quickly by sEH to vicinal diols that are generally less biologically active (Figure 6–5). Thus, by inhibiting sEH, one can obtain dramatic biological effects. Recent work has focused on pain, where sEH inhibitors reduce both inflammatory and neuropathic pain and synergize with nonsteroidal anti-inflammatory drugs (Kodani and Hammock, 2015). In experimental systems, epoxides of dietary omega-3 and omega-6 fatty acids have anti-inflammatory properties, moderating inflammation and autophagy in insulin-sensitive tissues, effects that inhibitors of sEH promote (Lopez-Vicario et al., 2015).

The *carboxylesterases* comprise a superfamily of enzymes that catalyze the hydrolysis of ester- and amide-containing chemicals. These enzymes are found in both the endoplasmic reticulum and the cytosol of many cell types and are involved in detoxification or metabolic activation of various drugs, environmental toxicants, and carcinogens. Carboxylesterases also catalyze the activation of prodrugs to their respective free acids. For example, the prodrug and cancer chemotherapeutic agent *irinotecan* is a camptothecin analogue that is bioactivated by intracellular carboxylesterases to the potent topoisomerase inhibitor SN-38 (Figure 6–6).

Figure 6–6 *Metabolism of irinotecan (CPT-11).* The prodrug CPT-11 is initially metabolized by a serum esterase (CES2) to the topoisomerase inhibitor SN-38, which is the active camptothecin analogue that slows tumor growth. SN-38 is then subject to glucuronidation, which results in loss of biological activity and facilitates elimination of SN-38 in the bile.

Phase 2 Reactions: Conjugating Enzymes

There are a large number of phase 2 conjugating enzymes, all of which are considered to be synthetic in nature because they result in the formation of metabolites with increased molecular mass. Phase 2 reactions also normally terminate the biological activity of the drug, although there are exceptions: For *morphine* and *minoxidil*, glucuronide and sulfate conjugates, respectively, are more pharmacologically active than the parent. The contributions of different phase 2 reactions to drug metabolism are shown in Figure 6–3B.

Two of the phase 2 reactions, glucuronidation and sulfation, result in the formation of metabolites with a significantly increased water-to-lipid partition coefficients. Sulfation and acetylation generally terminate the biological activity of drugs, and the minor change in overall charge increases the aqueous solubility of the metabolite. The enhanced hydrophilicity facilitates metabolite transport into the aqueous compartments of the cell and the body. Characteristic of the phase 2 reactions is the dependency on the catalytic reactions for cofactors (or, more correctly, cosubstrate): UDP-GA for UGT and PAPS for SULTs, which react with available functional groups on the substrates. The reactive functional groups are often generated by the phase 1 CYPs, although there are many drugs (e.g., *acetaminophen*) for which glucuronidation and sulfation occur directly without prior oxidative metabolism. All of the phase 2 reactions are carried out in the cytosol of the cell, with the exception of glucuronidation, which is localized to the luminal side of the endoplasmic reticulum.

The catalytic rates of phase 2 reactions are significantly faster than the rates of the CYPs. Thus, if a drug is targeted for phase 1 oxidation through the CYPs, followed by a phase 2 conjugation reaction, usually the rate of elimination will depend on the initial (phase 1) oxidation reaction. Because the rate of conjugation is faster and the process leads to an increase in hydrophilicity of the drug, phase 2 reactions are generally considered to ensure efficient elimination and detoxification of most drugs.

Glucuronidation

Among the more important of the phase 2 reactions in drug metabolism is those catalyzed by UGTs (Figure 6–3B). These enzymes catalyze the transfer of glucuronic acid from the cofactor UDP-GA to a substrate to form β-d-glucopyranosiduronic acids (glucuronides), metabolites that are sensitive to cleavage by β-glucuronidase. Glucuronides can be formed via alcoholic and phenolic hydroxyl groups; carboxyl, sulfuryl, and carbonyl moieties; and primary, secondary, and tertiary amines. UGT substrates include many hundreds of chemically unique pharmaceuticals; dietary substances; environmental agents; humoral agents such as circulating hormones (androgens, estrogens, mineralocorticoids, glucocorticoids, thyroxine); bile acids; retinoids; and bilirubin, the end product of heme catabolism.

Examples of glucuronidation reactions are shown in Table 6–2 and Figures 6–1 and 6–6. The structural diversity of the drugs and other xenobiotics that are processed through glucuronidation ensures that most clinically efficacious therapeutic agents will be excreted as glucuronides.

The UGTs are expressed in a highly coordinated tissue-specific and often inducible fashion, with the highest concentration found in the GI tract and liver. Per tissue weight, there are a greater number and higher concentration of the UGTs in the small intestine compared to the liver, so efficient first-pass metabolism plays a role in predicting bioavailability of many orally administered medications. Formation of glucuronides and their increased polarity can result in their passage into the circulation, from which they are excreted into the urine. Alternatively, as xenobiotics enter the liver and are absorbed into hepatocytes, glucuronide formation provides substrates for active transport into the bile canaliculi and ultimate excretion with components of the bile (see Figure 5–9). Many of the glucuronides that are excreted into the bile eventually become substrates for soluble microbial β-glucuronidase in the large intestine, resulting in the formation of free glucuronic acid and the initial substrate. The colon actively absorbs water and a variety of other compounds (see Figure 50–3); depending on its solubility, the glucuronide or the original substrate may be reabsorbed via passive diffusion or by apical transporters in the colon and reenter the systemic circulation. This process, called *enterohepatic recirculation*, can extend the half-life of a xenobiotic that is conjugated in the liver because the compound's ultimate excretion is delayed (see Figures 6–8 and 6–9).

There are 19 human genes that encode the UGT proteins. Nine are encoded by the *UGT1A* locus on chromosome 2q37 (1A1, 1A3, 1A4, 1A5, 1A6, 1A7, 1A8, 1A9, and 1A10), while 10 genes are encoded by the *UGT2* family of genes on chromosome 4q13.2 (2B17, 2B15, 2B10, 2A3, 2B7, 2B11, 2B2, 2B4, 2A1, 2A2, and 2A3). Of these proteins, the major UGTs involved in drug metabolism are UGT1A1, 1A3, 1A4, 1A6, 1A9, and 2B7 (for a list of common UGT drug substrates, see Rowland et al., 2013). Although both families of proteins are associated with metabolism of drugs and xenobiotics, the UGT2 family of proteins appears to have greater specificity for the glucuronidation of endogenous substances.

The *UGT1* locus on chromosome 2 (Figure 6–7) spans nearly 200 kb, with over 150 kb of a tandem array of cassette exonic regions that encode approximately 280 amino acids of the amino terminal portion of the UGT1A proteins. Four exons are located at the 3′ end of the locus; these encode the carboxyl 245 amino acids that combine with one of the consecutively numbered array of first exons to form the individual *UGT1A* gene products. Because exons 2 to 5 encode the same sequence for each UGT1A protein, the variability in substrate specificity for each of the UGT1A proteins results from the significant divergence in sequence encoded by the exon 1 regions. Reduced UGT activity resulting from allelic mutations in exons 2 to 5 affect all of the UGT1A proteins, whereas inactivating mutations in the exon 1 region lead to reduced glucuronidation by only the affected UGT1A protein. Over 100 allelic variants targeting the divergent exon 1 regions have been identified, many of which result in lowered UGT activity.

From a clinical perspective, the expression of UGT1A1 assumes an important role in drug metabolism because the glucuronidation of bilirubin by UGT1A1 is the rate-limiting step in ensuring efficient bilirubin clearance, and this rate can be affected by both genetic variation and competing substrates (drugs). Bilirubin is the breakdown product of heme, 80% of which originates from circulating hemoglobin and 20% from other heme-containing proteins, such as the CYPs. Bilirubin is hydrophobic, associates with serum albumin, and must be metabolized further by glucuronidation to ensure its elimination. The failure to efficiently metabolize bilirubin by glucuronidation leads to elevated serum levels and a clinical symptom called hyperbilirubinemia or jaundice. Delayed expression of the *UGT1A1* gene in newborns is the primary reason for neonatal hyperbilirubinemia.

There are more than 40 genetic lesions in the *UGT1A1* gene that can lead to inheritable unconjugated hyperbilirubinemia. Crigler-Najjar

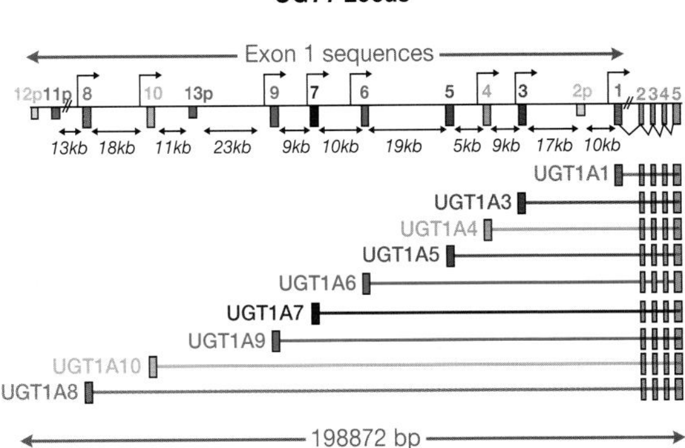

Figure 6–7 *Organization of the UGT1A locus.* Transcription of the *UGT1A* genes commences with the activation of PolII, which is controlled through tissue-specific events. Conserved exons 2 to 5 are spliced to each respective exon 1 sequence, resulting in the production of unique *UGT1A* sequences. The *UGT1A* locus encodes nine functional proteins.

syndrome-type 1 (CN-1) is diagnosed as a complete lack of bilirubin glucuronidation and results from inactivating mutations in exon 1 or in the common exons of the *UGT1A1* gene. CN-2 is differentiated by the detection of low amounts of bilirubin glucuronides in duodenal secretions and is linked to promoter mutations or reading frame mutations in the *UGT1A1* gene that lead to greatly reduced glucuronide formation. The danger associated with CN-1 and CN-2 is the accumulation of toxic levels of unconjugated bilirubin, which can lead to CNS toxicity. Children diagnosed with CN-1 require immediate and extensive blue light therapy to break down circulating bilirubin; these patients eventually require liver transplantation. Agents that induce *UGT1A1* gene expression, such as phenobarbital, can improve bilirubin glucuronidation and its elimination in patients with CN-2. The *UGT1A1* gene is the only gene associated with xenobiotic metabolism that is essential for life because there is an absolute requirement for the daily elimination of serum bilirubin. Allelic variants associated with other xenobiotic-metabolizing genes (phase 1 and phase 2) can enhance disease and toxicity associated with drug use but show few or no phenotypic effects.

Gilbert syndrome is a generally benign condition that is present in 8%–23% of the population, based on ethnic diversity. It is diagnosed clinically by circulating bilirubin levels that are 100%–300% higher than normal. There is increasing epidemiological evidence to suggest that Gilbert syndrome may be protective against cardiovascular disease, potentially as a result of the antioxidant properties of bilirubin. The most common genetic polymorphism associated with Gilbert syndrome is a mutation in the *UGT1A1* gene promoter, identified as the *UGT1A1*28* allele, that leads to an $A(TA)_7TAA$ promoter sequence that differs from the more common $A(TA)_6TAA$ sequence. The elevated total serum bilirubin levels are associated with significantly reduced expression levels of hepatic UGT1A1.

Subjects diagnosed with Gilbert syndrome may be predisposed to ADRs (Table 6–3) resulting from a reduced capacity to metabolize drugs by UGT1A1. If a drug undergoes selective metabolism by UGT1A1, competition for drug metabolism with bilirubin glucuronidation will exist, resulting in pronounced hyperbilirubinemia as well as reduced clearance of the metabolized drug. *Tranilast* [*N*-(3′4′-demethoxycinnamoyl)-anthranilic acid] is an investigational drug used for the prevention of restenosis in patients who have undergone transluminal coronary revascularization (intracoronary stents). Tranilast therapy in patients with Gilbert syndrome can lead to hyperbilirubinemia, as well as potential hepatic complications resulting from elevated levels of tranilast.

Gilbert syndrome also alters patient responses to irinotecan. Irinotecan, a prodrug used in chemotherapy of solid tumors (see Chapter 66) is metabolized to its active form, SN-38, by tissue carboxylesterases (Figure 6–6). SN-38, a potent topoisomerase inhibitor, is inactivated by UGT1A1 and excreted in the bile (Figures 6–8 and 6–9). Once in the lumen of the intestine, the SN-38 glucuronide undergoes cleavage by bacterial β-glucuronidase and reenters the circulation through intestinal absorption. Elevated levels of SN-38 in the blood lead to hematological toxicities characterized by leukopenia and neutropenia, as well as damage to the intestinal epithelial cells, resulting in acute and life-threatening ileocolitis. Patients with Gilbert syndrome who are receiving irinotecan therapy are predisposed to the hematological and GI toxicities resulting from elevated serum levels of SN-38, the net result of insufficient UGT1A activity and the consequent accumulation of a toxic drug in the GI epithelium.

While most of the drugs that are metabolized by UGT1A1 compete for glucuronidation with bilirubin, patients with Gilbert syndrome who are HIV positive and on protease inhibitor therapy with atazanavir develop hyperbilirubinemia because atazanavir inhibits UGT1A1 function even though atazanavir is not a substrate for glucuronidation. Severe hyperbilirubinemia can develop in patients with Gilbert syndrome who have also been genotyped to contain inactivating mutations in the *UGT1A3* and *UGT1A7* genes. Clearly, drug-induced side effects attributed to the inhibition of the UGT enzymes can be a significant concern and can be complicated in the presence of gene-inactivating polymorphisms.

TABLE 6–3 ■ DRUG TOXICITY AND GILBERT SYNDROME

PROBLEM	FEATURE
Gilbert syndrome	UGT1A1*28 (main variant in Caucasians)
Established toxicity reactions	Irinotecan, atazanavir
UGT1A1 substrates (potential risk?)	Gemfibrozil,[a] ezetimibe Simvastatin, atorvastatin, cerivastatin[a] Ethinylestradiol, buprenorphine, fulvestrant Ibuprofen, ketoprofen

[a]A severe drug reaction owing to the inhibition of glucuronidation (UGT1A1) and CYP2C8 and CYP2C9 when both drugs were combined led to the withdrawal of cerivastatin.

Source: Reproduced with permission from Strassburg CP. Pharmacogenetics of Gilbert's syndrome. *Pharmacogenomics*, **2008**, 9:703–715.

Sulfation

The SULTs, located in the cytosol, conjugate sulfate derived from PAPS to hydroxyl and, less frequently, amine groups of aromatic and aliphatic compounds. Like all of the xenobiotic-metabolizing enzymes, the SULTs metabolize a wide variety of endogenous and exogenous substrates. In humans, 13 SULT isoforms have been identified; based on sequence comparisons, they are classified into the SULT1 (SULT1A1, SULT1A2, SULT1A3/4, SULT1B1, SULT1C2, SULT1C3, SULT1C4, SULT1E1); SULT2 (SULT2A1, SULT2B1a, SULT2B1b); SULT4 (SULT4A1); and SULT6 (SULT6A1) families. There are major interspecies differences in the expressed complement of SULTs, which makes extrapolation of data on xenobiotic sulfation in animals to humans particularly unreliable.

SULTs play an important role in normal human homeostasis. For example, SULT2B1b is a predominant form expressed in skin, carrying out the catalysis of cholesterol. Cholesterol sulfate is an essential metabolite in regulating keratinocyte differentiation and skin development. SULT2A1 is highly expressed in the fetal adrenal gland, where it produces the large quantities of dehydroepiandrosterone sulfate that are required for placental estrogen biosynthesis during the second half of pregnancy. SULTs 1A3 and 1A4 are highly selective for catecholamines, while estrogens (in particular 17β-estradiol) are sulfated by SULT1E1. In humans, significant fractions of circulating catecholamines, estrogens, iodothyronines, and DHEA exist in the sulfated form.

Some human SULTs display unique substrate specificities, whereas others are promiscuous. Members of the SULT1 family are the major isoforms involved in xenobiotic metabolism, with SULT1A1 quantitatively and qualitatively the most important in the liver. SULT1A1 displays extensive diversity in its capacity to catalyze the sulfation of a broad variety of structurally heterogeneous xenobiotics with high affinity. The isoforms in the SULT1 family are recognized as phenol SULTs; they catalyze the sulfation of phenolic molecules such as *acetaminophen*, *minoxidil*, and *17α-ethinyl estradiol*. SULT1B1 is similar to SULT1A1 in its wide range of substrates, although it is much more abundant in the intestine than the liver. Three SULT1C isoforms exist in humans, but little is known of their substrate specificity. In rodents, SULT1C enzymes are capable of sulfating the hepatic carcinogen *N*-OH-2-acetylaminofluorene and are responsible for the bioactivation of this and related carcinogens. Their role in this pathway in humans is not clear. SULT1C enzymes are expressed abundantly in human fetal tissues, yet decline in abundance in adults. SULT1E catalyzes the sulfation of endogenous and exogenous steroids and is localized in liver and in hormone-responsive tissues such as the testis, breast, adrenal gland, and placenta. In the upper GI tract, SULT1A3/4 and SULT1B1 are particularly abundant.

The conjugation of drugs and xenobiotics is considered primarily a detoxification step, ensuring that the metabolites enter the aqueous compartments of the body and are targeted for elimination. However, drug metabolism through sulfation often leads to the generation of chemically reactive metabolites, wherein the sulfate is electron withdrawing and may be heterolytically cleaved, leading to the formation of an electrophilic

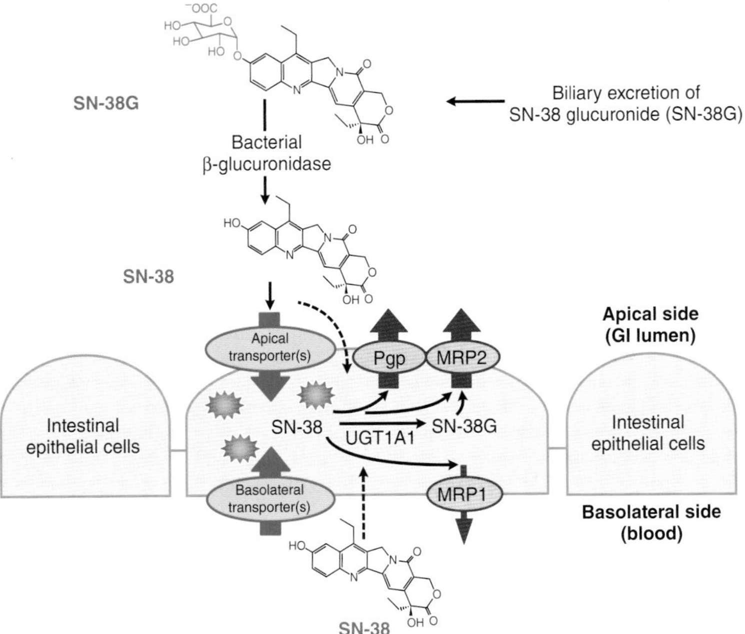

Figure 6–8 *Routes of SN-38 transport and exposure to intestinal epithelial cells.* SN-38 is transported into the bile following glucuronidation by liver UGT1A1 and extrahepatic UGT1A7. Following cleavage of luminal SN-38 glucuronide (SN-38G) by bacterial β-glucuronidase, reabsorption into epithelial cells can occur by passive diffusion (indicated by the dashed arrows entering the cell) as well as by apical transporters. Movement into epithelial cells may also occur from the blood by basolateral transporters. Intestinal SN-38 can efflux into the lumen through Pgp and MRP2 and into the blood via MRP1. Excessive accumulation of the SN-38 in intestinal epithelial cells, resulting from reduced glucuronidation, can lead to cellular damage and toxicity. (Modified and reproduced with permission from Tukey RH et al. Pharmacogenomics of human UDP-glucuronosyltransferases and irinotecan toxicity. *Mol Pharmacol,* **2002**, *62*:446–450. Copyright © 2002 The American Society for Pharmacology and Experimental Therapeutics.)

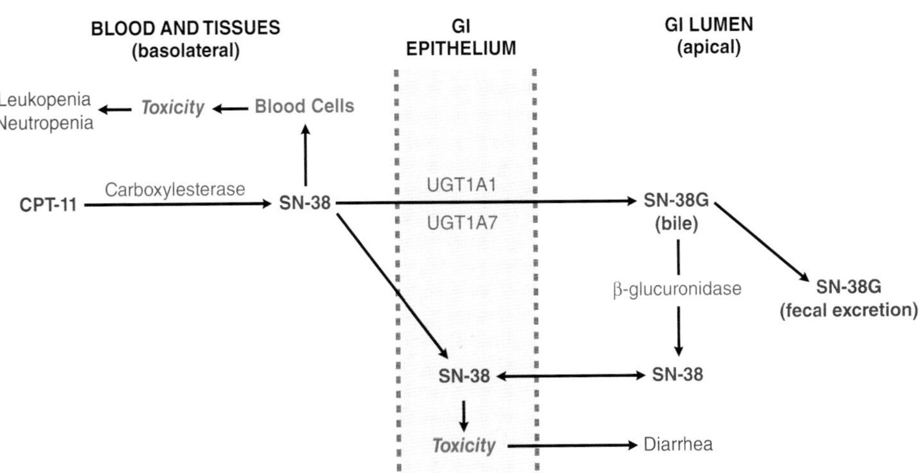

Figure 6–9 *Cellular targets of SN-38 in the blood and intestinal tissues.* Excessive accumulation of SN-38 can lead to blood toxicities, such as leukopenia and neutropenia, as well as damage to the intestinal epithelium. These toxicities are pronounced in individuals who have reduced capacity to form the SN-38 glucuronide, such as patients with Gilbert syndrome. Note the different body compartments and cell types involved. (Modified and reproduced with permission from Tukey RH et al. Pharmacogenomics of human UDP-glucuronosyltransferases and irinotecan toxicity. *Mol Pharmacol*, **2002**, 62:446–450. Copyright © 2002 The American Society for Pharmacology and Experimental Therapeutics.)

cation. Most examples of the generation by sulfation of a carcinogenic or toxic response in animal or mutagenicity assays have been documented with chemicals derived from the environment or from heterocyclic arylamine food mutagens generated from well-cooked meat. Thus, it is important to understand whether genetic linkages can be made by associating known human SULT polymorphisms to cancers that are believed to originate from environmental sources. Because SULT1A1 is the most abundant SULT form in human tissues and displays broad substrate specificity, the polymorphic profiles associated with this gene and their associations with various human cancers are of considerable interest.

Gene copy number polymorphisms within the SULT1A1, SULT1A3, and SULT1A4 genes have been identified, which may help explain much of the interindividual variation in the expression and activity of these enzymes. Knowledge of the structure, activities, regulation, and polymorphisms of the SULT superfamily will aid in understanding the linkages between sulfation and cancer susceptibility, reproduction, and development. Structural data, the results of kinetic studies, and molecular dynamics simulations are beginning to provide a picture of the mechanisms by which the SULTs express their unique patterns of substrate specificity (Tibbs et al., 2015).

Glutathione Conjugation

The GSTs catalyze the transfer of glutathione to reactive electrophiles, a function that serves to protect cellular macromolecules from interacting with electrophiles that contain electrophilic heteroatoms (–O, –N, and –S) and in turn protects the cellular environment from damage (Hayes et al., 2005). The cosubstrate in the reaction is glutathione, a tripeptide consisting of γ-glutamic acid, cysteine, and glycine (Figure 6–10). Glutathione exists in the cell in oxidized (GSSG) and reduced (GSH) forms, and the GSH:GSSG ratio is critical in maintaining a cellular environment in the reduced state. In addition to affecting xenobiotic conjugation with GSH, a severe reduction in GSH content can predispose cells to oxidative damage, a state that has been linked to a number of human health issues.

In the formation of glutathione conjugates, the GST reaction generates a thioether linkage with drug or xenobiotic to the cysteine moiety of the tripeptide. Characteristically, all GST substrates contain an electrophilic atom and are hydrophobic; by nature, they will associate with cellular proteins. Because the concentration of glutathione in cells is usually high, typically 7 μmol/g of liver or in the 10-mM range, many drugs and xenobiotics can react nonenzymatically with glutathione. However, the GSTs have been found to occupy up to 10% of the total hepatocellular protein concentration, a property that ensures efficient conjugation of glutathione to reactive electrophiles. The high concentration of GSTs also provides the cells with a sink of cytosolic protein, a property that facilitates noncovalent and sometimes covalent interactions with compounds that are not substrates for glutathione conjugation. The cytosolic pool of GSTs, once identified as *ligandin*, binds steroids, bile acids, bilirubin, cellular hormones, and environmental toxicants, in addition to complexing with other cellular proteins.

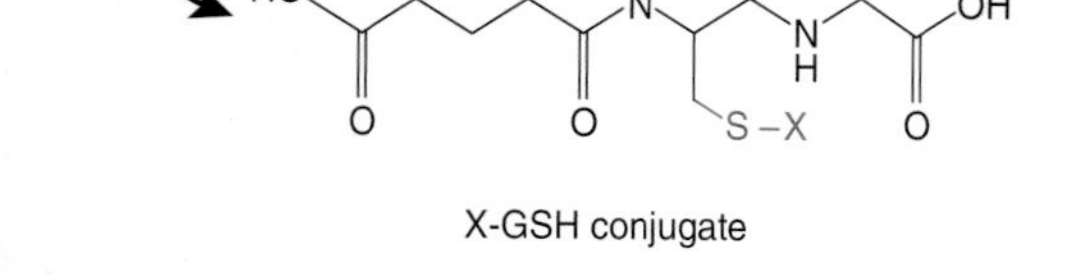

Figure 6–10 *Glutathione is a cosubstrate in the conjugation of a xenobiotic (X) by GST.*

There are in excess of 20 human GSTs, divided into two subfamilies: the *cytosolic* and the *microsomal* forms. The major differences in function between the microsomal and cytosolic GSTs reside in the selection of substrates for conjugation; the cytosolic forms have more importance in the metabolism of drugs and xenobiotics, whereas the microsomal GSTs are important in the endogenous metabolism of leukotrienes and prostaglandins. The cytosolic GSTs are divided into seven classes termed alpha (GSTA1 and 2), mu (GSTM1 through 5), omega (GSTO1), pi (GSTP1), sigma (GSTS1), theta (GSTT1 and GSTT2), and zeta (GSTZ1). Those in the alpha and mu classes can form heterodimers, allowing for a large number of active transferases to form. The cytosolic forms of GST catalyze conjugation, reduction, and isomerization reactions.

The high concentrations of GSH in the cell, as well as the overabundance of GSTs, means that few reactive molecules escape detoxification. Despite the appearance of overcapacity of enzyme and reducing equivalents, there is always concern that some reactive intermediates will escape detoxification and, by nature of their electrophilicity, will bind to cellular components and cause havoc. The potential for such an occurrence is heightened if GSH is depleted or if a specific form of GST is polymorphic and dysfunctional. While it is difficult to deplete cellular GSH levels, therapeutic agents that require large doses to be clinically efficacious have the greatest potential to lower cellular GSH levels.

Acetaminophen, normally metabolized by glucuronidation and sulfation, is also a substrate for oxidative metabolism by CYP2E1 and CYP3A4, which generate the toxic metabolite NAPQI, which, under normal dosing, is readily neutralized through conjugation with GSH. However, an overdose of acetaminophen can deplete cellular GSH levels and thereby increase the potential for NAPQI to interact with other cellular components, resulting in toxicity and cell death. Acetaminophen toxicity is associated with increased levels of NAPQI and hepatic necrosis, although it may be treated in a time- and drug concentration–dependent manner by administration of *N*-acetylcysteine (see Figure 4–4).

All of the GSTs are polymorphic. The mu (GSTM1*0) and theta (GSTT1*0) genotypes express a null phenotype; thus, individuals who are polymorphic at these loci are predisposed to toxicities by agents that are selective substrates for these GSTs. For example, the mutant GSTM1*0 allele is observed in 50% of the Caucasian population and links genetically to human malignancies of the lung, colon, and bladder. Null activity in the *GSTT1* gene associates with adverse side effects and toxicity in cancer chemotherapy with cytostatic drugs; the toxicities result from insufficient clearance of the drugs via GSH conjugation. Expression of the null genotype can be as high as 60% in Chinese and Korean populations. GST polymorphisms may influence efficacies and severity of adverse side effects of drugs.

While the GSTs play an important role in cellular detoxification, their activities in cancerous tissues have been linked to the development of drug resistance toward chemotherapeutic agents that are both substrates and nonsubstrates for the GSTs. Many anticancer drugs are effective because they initiate cell death or apoptosis, which is linked to the activation of MAPKs such as JNK and p38. Investigational studies demonstrated that overexpression of GSTs is associated with resistance to apoptosis and the inhibition of MAPK activity. In a variety of tumors, GSTs are overexpressed, leading to a reduction in MAPK activity and reduced efficacy of chemotherapy. Taking advantage of the relatively high levels of GST in tumor cells, inhibition of GST activity has been exploited as a therapeutic strategy to modulate drug resistance by sensitizing tumors to anticancer drugs. TLK199, a glutathione analogue, is a prodrug that plasma esterases convert to a GST inhibitor, TLK117, which potentiates the toxicity of different anticancer agents (Figure 6–11).

Alternatively, the elevated GST activity in cancer cells has been utilized to develop prodrugs that can be activated by the GSTs to form electrophilic intermediates. For example, TLK286 is a substrate for GST that undergoes a β-elimination reaction, forming a glutathione conjugate and a nitrogen mustard (Figure 6–12) that is capable of alkylating cellular nucleophiles and resulting in antitumor activity (Townsend and Tew, 2003).

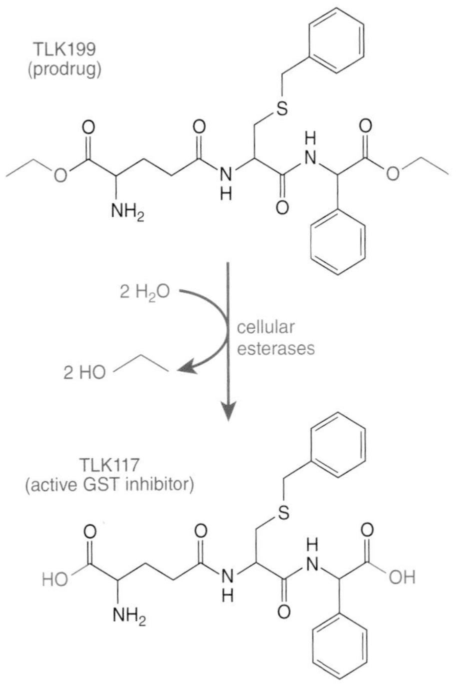

Figure 6–11 *Activation of TLK199 to TLK117, a GST inhibitor.*

N-Acetylation

The cytosolic NATs are responsible for the metabolism of drugs and environmental agents that contain an aromatic amine or hydrazine group. The addition of the acetyl group from the cofactor acetyl-coenzyme A often leads to a metabolite that is *less* water soluble because the potential ionizable amine is neutralized by the covalent addition of the acetyl group. NATs are among the most polymorphic of all the human xenobiotic drug-metabolizing enzymes.

The characterization of an acetylator phenotype in humans was one of the first hereditary traits identified and was responsible for the development of the field of pharmacogenetics (see Chapter 7). Following the discovery that isoniazid (isonicotinic acid hydrazide) could be used to treat tuberculosis, a significant proportion of the patients (5%–15%) experienced toxicities that ranged from numbness and tingling in their fingers to CNS damage. After finding that isoniazid was metabolized by acetylation and excreted in the urine, researchers noted that individuals who had the toxic effects of the drug excreted the largest amount of unchanged drug and the least amount of acetylated isoniazid. Pharmacogenetic studies led to the classification of "rapid" and "slow" acetylators, with the slow phenotype predisposed to toxicity (see Figure 60–4). Purification and characterization of NAT and the eventual cloning of its RNA provided sequence characterization of the gene for slow and fast acetylators, revealing polymorphisms that correspond to the slow acetylator phenotype.

There are two functional NAT genes in humans, *NAT1* and *NAT2*. Over 25 allelic variants of *NAT1* and *NAT2* have been characterized. In individuals in whom acetylation of drugs is compromised, homozygous genotypes for at least two variant alleles are required to predispose a patient to slower drug metabolism. Polymorphism in the *NAT2* gene and its association with the slow acetylation of isoniazid were one of the first completely characterized genotypes shown to affect drug metabolism, thereby linking pharmacogenetic phenotype to a genetic polymorphism. Although nearly as many mutations have been identified in the *NAT1* gene as the *NAT2* gene, the frequency of the slow acetylation patterns is attributed mostly to the polymorphism in the *NAT2* gene.

Some common drug substrates of NAT and their known toxicities are listed in Table 6–4 (see Meisel, 2002, for details). The therapeutic relevance of NAT polymorphisms is in avoiding drug-induced toxicities. The adverse drug response in a slow acetylator resembles a drug overdose; thus, reducing the dose or increasing the dosing interval is recommended. Aromatic amine or hydrazine groups exist in many classes of clinically used drugs, and if a drug is known to be subjected to metabolism through acetylation, determining an individual's phenotype can be important in maximizing a positive therapeutic outcome. For example, *hydralazine*, a once-popular orally active antihypertensive (vasodilator)

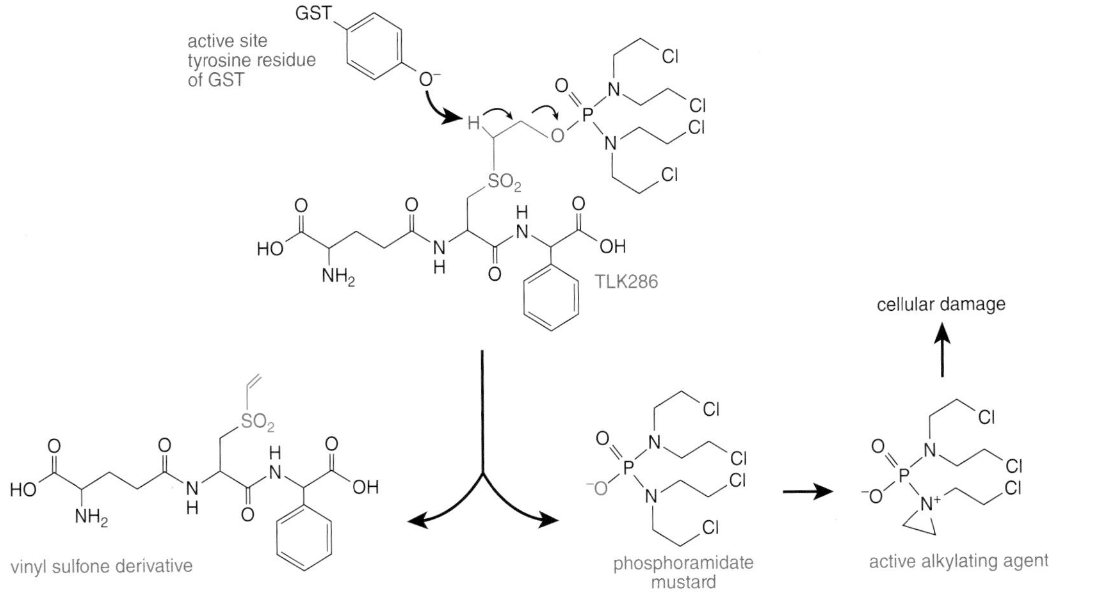

Figure 6–12 *Generation of the reactive alkylating agent following the conjugation of glutathione to TLK286.* GST interacts with the prodrug and GSH analogue TLK286 via a tyrosine in the active site of GST. The GSH portion is shown in blue. The interaction promotes β-elimination and cleavage of the prodrug to a vinyl sulfone and an active alkylating fragment.

TABLE 6–4 ■ THERAPEUTIC USES AND ADVERSE EFFECTS OF COMMON *N*-ACETYLTRANSFERASE SUBSTRATES

NAT SUBSTRATE	THERAPEUTIC USES	ADVERSE EFFECTS
Acebutolol	Adrenal cortex carcinoma, breast cancer	Drowsiness, weakness, insomnia
Aminoglutethimide	β Blockade, arrhythmias, hypertension	Clumsiness, nausea, dizziness, agranulocytosis
Aminosalicylic acid	Ulcerative colitis	Allergic fever, itching, leukopenia
Amrinone	Positive inotrope in heart failure	Thrombocytopenia, arrhythmias
Benzocaine	Local anesthesia	Dermatitis, itching, rash, methemoglobinemia
Caffeine	Neonatal respiratory distress syndrome	Dizziness, insomnia, tachycardia
Clonazepam	Seizures, anxiety	Drowsiness, ataxia, dizziness, slurred speech
Dapsone	Leprosy, dermatitis	Hemolysis, methemoglobinemia, nausea, dermatitis
Hydralazine	Hypertension (acts via vasodilation)	Hypotension, sympathetic baroreceptor reflex effects
Isoniazid	Tuberculosis	Peripheral neuritis, hepatotoxicity
Nitrazepam	Insomnia	Dizziness, somnolence
Phenelzine	Depression (acts via MAO inhibition)	Dizziness, CNS excitation, insomnia, orthostatic hypotension, hepatotoxicity
Procainamide	Ventricular tachyarrhythmia	Hypotension, bradycardia, lupus erythematosus
Sulfonamides	As bacteriostatic agents	Hypersensitivity, acute hemolytic anemia, reversible bone marrow suppression (with AIDS or myelosuppressive chemotherapy)

drug, is metabolized by NAT2. The administration of therapeutic doses of hydralazine to a slow acetylator can result in extreme hypotension and tachycardia.

Several known targets for acetylation, such as the sulfonamides, have been implicated in idiosyncratic hypersensitivity reactions; in such instances, an appreciation of a patient's acetylation phenotype is particularly important. Sulfonamides are transformed into hydroxylamines that interact with cellular proteins, generating haptens that can elicit autoimmune responses, to which slow acetylators are predisposed.

Tissue-specific expression patterns of NAT1 and NAT2 have a significant impact on the fate of drug metabolism and the potential for eliciting a toxic episode. NAT1 is ubiquitously expressed among most human tissues, whereas NAT2 is found predominantly in liver and the GI tract. Characteristic of both NAT1 and NAT2 is the ability to form *N*-hydroxy–acetylated metabolites from bicyclic aromatic hydrocarbons, a reaction that leads to the nonenzymatic release of acetyl groups and the generation of highly reactive nitrenium ions. Thus, *N*-hydroxy acetylation is thought to activate certain environmental toxicants. In contrast, direct *N*-acetylation of bicyclic aromatic amines is stable and leads to detoxification. Individuals who are NAT2 fast acetylators are able to efficiently metabolize and detoxify bicyclic aromatic amines through liver-dependent acetylation. However, slow acetylators (NAT2 deficient) accumulate bicyclic aromatic amines that become substrates for CYP-dependent *N*-oxidation. These N-OH metabolites are eliminated in the urine. In tissues such as bladder epithelium, NAT1 is highly expressed and can efficiently catalyze the *N*-hydroxy acetylation of bicyclic aromatic amines, a process that leads to deacetylation and the formation of the mutagenic nitrenium ion, especially in NAT2-deficient subjects. Epidemiological studies have shown that slow acetylators are predisposed to bladder cancer if exposed environmentally to bicyclic aromatic amines.

Methylation

In humans, drugs and xenobiotics can undergo *O*-, *N*-, and *S*-methylation. Humans express two COMTs, three *N*-methyl transferases, a POMT, a TPMT, and a TMT. All of the MTs exist as monomers and use S-adenosylmethionine (AdoMet) as the methyl donor. With the exception of a signature sequence that is conserved among the MTs, there is limited conservation in sequence, indicating that each MT has evolved to display a unique catalytic function. Although the common theme among the MTs is the generation of a methylated product, substrate specificity is high and distinguishes the individual enzymes.

Among the *N*-methyl transferases, NNMT methylates serotonin and tryptophan as well as pyridine-containing compounds such as nicotinamide and nicotine. PNMT is responsible for the methylation of the neurotransmitter norepinephrine to form epinephrine; the HNMT metabolizes drugs containing an imidazole ring. COMT, which exists as two protein isoforms generated by alternate exon usage, methylates neurotransmitters containing a catechol moiety, such as dopamine and norepinephrine, as well as methyldopa and *ecstasy* (3,4-methylenedioxy-methamphetamine, MDMA).

From a clinical perspective, the most important MT may be TPMT, which catalyzes the *S*-methylation of aromatic and heterocyclic sulfhydryl compounds, including the thiopurine drugs *AZA*, *6-MP*, and *thioguanine*. AZA and 6-MP are used for the management of inflammatory bowel disease (see Chapter 51), as well as autoimmune disorders such as systemic lupus erythematosus and rheumatoid arthritis. Thioguanine is used in the treatment of acute myeloid leukemia, and 6-MP is used worldwide for the treatment of childhood acute lymphoblastic leukemia (see Chapter 66). Because TPMT is responsible for the detoxification of 6-MP, a genetic deficiency in TPMT can result in severe toxicities in patients taking the drug (see metabolic scheme in Figure 51-5). When given orally at clinically established doses, 6-MP serves as a prodrug that is metabolized by HGPRT to 6-TGNs, which become incorporated into DNA and RNA, resulting in arrest of DNA replication and cytotoxicity.

Toxic side effects arise when a lack of 6-MP methylation by TPMT causes a buildup of 6-MP and the consequent generation of toxic levels of 6-TGNs. The identification of the inactive TPMT alleles and the development of a genotyping test to identify homozygous carriers of the defective allele permit identification of individuals who may be predisposed to the toxic side effects of 6-MP therapy. Simple adjustments in the patient's dosage regimen are a lifesaving intervention for those with TPMT deficiencies.

Role of Xenobiotic Metabolism in Safe and Effective Use of Drugs

Any xenobiotics entering the body must be eliminated through metabolism and excretion via the urine or bile/feces. Mechanisms of metabolism and excretion prevent foreign compounds from accumulating in the body and possibly causing toxicity. In the case of drugs, metabolism normally results in the inactivation of their therapeutic effectiveness and facilitates their elimination. The extent of metabolism can determine the efficacy and toxicity of a drug by controlling its biological half-life. Among the most serious considerations in the clinical use of drugs are ADRs. If a drug is metabolized too quickly, it rapidly loses its therapeutic efficacy. This can occur if specific enzymes involved in metabolism are overly active or are induced by dietary or environmental factors. If a drug is metabolized too slowly, the drug can accumulate in the bloodstream; as a consequence, the plasma clearance of the drug is decreased, the AUC (see Figure 5–3) is elevated, and exposure to the drug may exceed clinically appropriate levels. An increase in AUC often results when specific xenobiotic-metabolizing enzymes are inhibited, which can occur when an individual is taking a combination of different therapeutic agents and one of those drugs targets the enzyme involved in drug metabolism. For example, the consumption of grapefruit juice with drugs taken orally can inhibit intestinal CYP3A4, blocking the metabolism of many of these drugs. The inhibition of specific CYPs in the gut by dietary consumption of grapefruit juice alters the oral bioavailability of many classes of drugs, including certain antihypertensives, immunosuppressants, antidepressants, antihistamines, and the statins, to name a few. Among the components of grapefruit juice that inhibit CYP3A4 are *naringin* and *furanocoumarins*.

While environmental factors can alter the steady-state levels of specific enzymes or inhibit their catalytic potential, these phenotypic changes in drug metabolism are also observed clinically in groups of individuals who are genetically predisposed to ADRs because of pharmacogenetic differences in the expression of xenobiotic-metabolizing enzymes (see Chapter 7). Most of the xenobiotic-metabolizing enzymes display polymorphic differences in their expression, resulting from heritable changes in the structure of the genes. For example, hyperbilirubinemia can result from a reduction in the ability to glucuronidate circulating bilirubin due to a lowered expression of the *UGT1A1* gene (Gilbert syndrome). Drugs that are subject to glucuronidation by UGT1A1, such as the topoisomerase inhibitor SN-38 (Figures 6–6, 6–8, and 6–9), will display an increased AUC in individuals with Gilbert syndrome because such patients cannot detoxify these drugs. Most cancer chemotherapeutic agents have a narrow therapeutic index, and increases in the circulating levels of the active form due to a deficiency in drug clearance can result in significant toxicities.

Nearly every class of therapeutic agent has been reported to initiate an ADR. In the United States, ADRs annually cost an estimated at $100 billion and cause over 100,000 deaths. An estimated 56% of drugs associated with ADRs are substrates for xenobiotic-metabolizing enzymes, notably CYPs and UGTs. Because many of the CYPs and UGTs are subject to induction as well as inhibition by drugs, dietary factors, and other environmental agents, these enzymes play an important role in most ADRs. Thus, prior to filing a New Drug Application (NDA), a new drug's route of metabolism must be known. Thus, it is routine practice in the pharmaceutical industry to establish which enzymes are involved in metabolism of a drug candidate and to identify the metabolites and determine their potential toxicity. In consideration of the major role of CYPs in the generation of ADRs, there is likely to be a move to avoid the major oxidative routes of metabolism when developing new small-molecule drugs.

Induction of Drug Metabolism

Xenobiotics can influence drug metabolism by activating transcription and inducing the expression of genes encoding drug-metabolizing enzymes. Thus, a foreign compound may induce its own metabolism, as may certain drugs. One potential consequence of this is a decrease in plasma drug concentration over the course of treatment, resulting in loss of efficacy, as the autoinduced metabolism of the drug exceeds the rate at which new drug enters the body. A list of ligands and the receptors through which they induce drug metabolism is shown in Table 6–5. A particular receptor, when activated by a ligand, can induce the transcription of a battery of target genes. Among these target genes are certain CYPs and drug transporters. Thus, any drug that is a ligand for a receptor that induces CYPs and transporters could lead to drug interactions. Figure 6–13 shows the scheme by which a drug may interact with nuclear receptors to induce its own metabolism.

The aryl hydrocarbon receptor (AHR) is a member of a superfamily of transcription factors with diverse roles in mammals, such as serving a regulatory role in the development of the mammalian CNS and modulating the response to chemical and oxidative stress. This superfamily of transcription factors includes (Period) and Sim (Simpleminded), two transcription factors involved in development of the CNS, and HIF1α, HIF2α, and their dimerization partner HIF1β, which activate genes in response to low cellular O_2 levels.

The AHR induces expression of genes encoding CYP1A1, CYP1A2, and CYP1B1, which are able to metabolically activate chemical carcinogens, including environmental contaminants and carcinogens derived from food. Many of these substances are inert unless metabolized by CYPs. Thus, induction of these CYPs by a drug could potentially result in an increase in the toxicity and carcinogenicity of procarcinogens. For example, *omeprazole*, a proton pump inhibitor used to treat gastric and duodenal ulcers (see Chapter 49), is a ligand for the AHR and can induce CYP1A1 and CYP1A2, with the possible consequences of toxin/carcinogen activation as well as drug-drug interactions in patients receiving agents that are substrates for either of these CYPs.

Another important induction mechanism is due to type 2 nuclear receptors that are in the same superfamily as the steroid hormone receptors. Many of these receptors, identified on the basis of their structural similarity to steroid hormone receptors, were originally termed *orphan receptors* because no endogenous ligands were known to interact with them. Subsequent studies revealed that some of these receptors are activated by xenobiotics, including drugs. The type 2 nuclear receptors of most importance to drug metabolism and drug therapy include PXR, CAR, and PPARs. PXR, discovered because it is activated by the synthetic steroid pregnenolone-16α-carbonitrile, is also activated by a number of other drugs, including antibiotics (*rifampicin* and *troleandomycin*), Ca^{2+} channel blockers (*nifedipine*), statins (*mevastatin*), antidiabetic drugs (*troglitazone*), HIV protease inhibitors (*ritonavir*), and anticancer drugs (*paclitaxel*).

Hyperforin, a component of St. John's wort, an over-the-counter herbal remedy used for depression, also activates PXR. This activation is thought to be the basis for the increase in failure of oral contraceptives in individuals taking St. John's wort: Activated PXR is an inducer of CYP3A4, which can metabolize steroids found in oral contraceptives. PXR also induces the expression of genes encoding certain drug transporters and phase 2 enzymes, including SULTs and UGTs. Thus, PXR facilitates the

TABLE 6–5 ■ NUCLEAR RECEPTORS THAT INDUCE DRUG METABOLISM

RECEPTOR	LIGANDS
Aryl hydrocarbon receptor (AHR)	Omeprazole
Constitutive androstane receptor (CAR)	Phenobarbital
Pregnane X receptor (PXR)	Rifampin
Farnesoid X receptor (FXR)	Bile acids
Vitamin D receptor (VDR)	Vitamin D
Peroxisome proliferator–activated receptor (PPARs)	Fibrates
Retinoic acid receptor (RAR)	*all-trans*-Retinoic acid
Retinoid X receptor (RXR)	9-*cis*-Retinoic acid

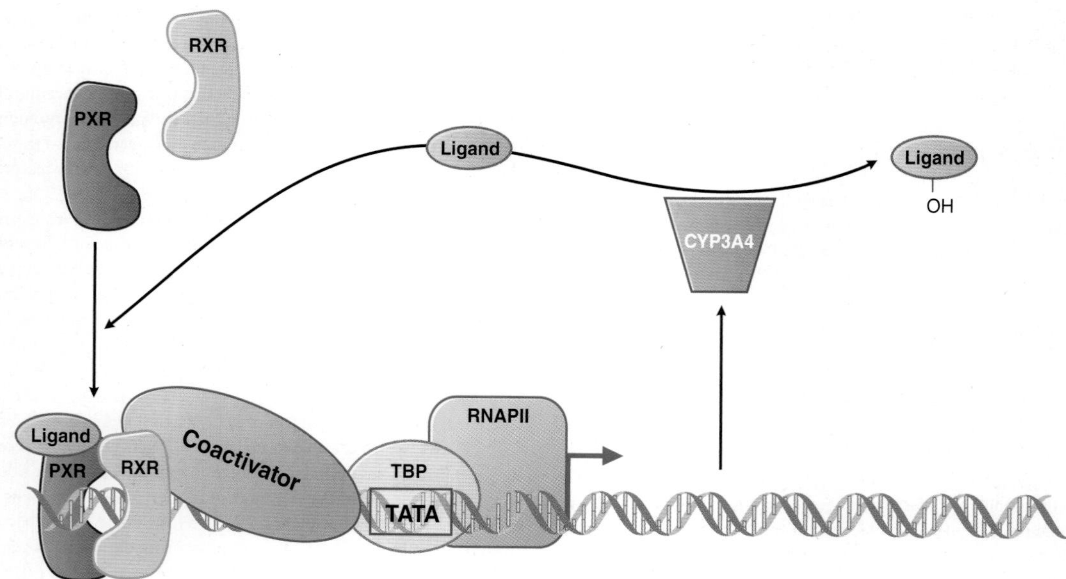

Figure 6–13 *Induction of drug metabolism by nuclear receptor–mediated signal transduction.* When a drug such as atorvastatin (Ligand) enters the cell, it can bind to a nuclear receptor such as the PXR. The PXR then forms a complex with the RXR, binds to DNA upstream of target genes, recruits coactivator (which binds to the TBP), and activates transcription. Among PXR target genes are *CYP3A4*, which can metabolize the atorvastatin and decrease its cellular concentration. Thus, atorvastatin induces its own metabolism. Atorvastatin undergoes both ortho- and parahydroxylation.

metabolism and elimination of xenobiotics, including drugs, with notable consequences.

The nuclear receptor CAR was discovered based on its ability to activate genes in the absence of ligand. Steroids such as *androstanol*, the antifungal agent *clotrimazole*, and the antiemetic *meclizine* are inverse agonists that inhibit gene activation by CAR, while the pesticide 1,4-bis[2-(3,5-dichloropyridyloxy)]benzene, the steroid 5-β-pregnane-3,20-dione, and probably other endogenous compounds are agonists that activate gene expression when bound to CAR. Genes induced by CAR include those encoding several CYPs (CYP2B6, CYP2C9, and CYP3A4); various phase 2 enzymes (including GSTs, UGTs, and SULTs); and drug and endobiotic transporters. CYP3A4 is induced by both PXR and CAR; thus, its level is highly influenced by a number of drugs and other xenobiotics. In addition to a potential role in inducing the degradation of drugs, including the over-the-counter analgesic acetaminophen, this receptor may function in the control of bilirubin degradation, the process by which the liver decomposes heme.

Clearly, PXR and CAR can bind a great variety of ligands. As with the xenobiotic-metabolizing enzymes, species differences also exist in the ligand specificities of these receptors. For example, rifampicin activates human PXR, but not mouse or rat PXR, while pregnenolone-16α-carbonitrile preferentially activates the mouse and rat PXR. Paradoxically, meclizine activates mouse CAR but inhibits gene induction by human CAR. These findings further underscore that in some cases studies with rodent model systems do not reflect the response of humans to drugs.

The PPAR family is composed of three members: α, β, and γ. PPARα is the target for the fibrate class of hyperlipidemic drugs, including the widely prescribed *gemfibrozil* and *fenofibrate*. Activation of PPARα results in induction of target genes encoding fatty acid–metabolizing enzymes, resulting in lowering of serum triglycerides; in addition, activation of PPARα induces CYP4 enzymes that carry out the oxidation of fatty acids and drugs with fatty acid–containing side chains, such as *leukotriene* and arachidonate analogues. PPARγ is the target for the thiazolidinedione class of anti–type 2 diabetic drugs, including rosiglitazone and pioglitazone. PPARγ does not induce xenobiotic metabolism.

The UGT genes, in particular UGT1A1, are a target for AHR, PXR, CAR, PPARα, and Nrf2 (nuclear factor 2 (erythroid-derived 2-like factor), a major transcriptional regulator of cytoprotective genes induced by an antioxidant response). Because the UGTs are abundant in the GI tract and liver, regulation of the UGTs by drug-induced activation of these receptors would be expected to play a role concerning the pharmacokinetic parameters of many orally administered therapeutics.

Role of Drug Metabolism in Drug Development

There are two key elements associated with successful drug development: *efficacy* and *safety*. Both depend on drug metabolism. It is necessary to determine which enzymes metabolize a new drug candidate to predict whether the compound may cause drug-drug interactions or be susceptible to marked interindividual variation in metabolism due to genetic polymorphisms.

For determination of metabolism, the compound is subjected to analysis by human liver cells or extracts from these cells that contain the drug-metabolizing enzymes. Such studies determine how humans will metabolize a particular drug and, to a limited extent, predict the rate of metabolism. If a CYP is involved, a panel of recombinant CYPs can be used to determine which CYP predominates in the metabolism of the drug. If a single CYP, such as CYP3A4, is found to be the sole CYP that metabolizes a drug candidate, then a decision can be made about the likelihood of drug interactions.

Interactions become a problem when multiple drugs are simultaneously administered, for example, in elderly patients, who on a daily basis may take prescribed anti-inflammatory drugs, cholesterol-lowering drugs, blood pressure medications, a gastric acid suppressant, an anticoagulant, and a number of over-the-counter medications. Ideally, the best drug candidate would be metabolized by several CYPs so that variability in expression levels of one CYP or drug-drug interactions would not significantly affect its metabolism and pharmacokinetics.

Similar studies can be carried out with phase 2 enzymes and drug transporters to predict the metabolic fate of a drug. In addition to the use of recombinant human xenobiotic-metabolizing enzymes in predicting drug metabolism, human receptor-based (PXR and CAR) systems or cell lines expressing these receptors are used to determine whether a particular drug candidate could be a ligand or activator of PXR, CAR, or PPARα. For example, a drug that activates PXR may result in rapid clearance of other drugs that are CYP3A4 substrates, thus decreasing their bioavailability and efficacy.

Computer-based computational (in silico) prediction of drug metabolism is a prospect for the near future. The structures of several CYPs have been determined, including those of CYPs 2A6, 2C9, and 3A4. These structures may be used to predict metabolism of a drug candidate by fitting the compound to the enzyme's active site and determining oxidation potentials of sites on the molecule. However, the structures, determined by X-ray analysis of crystals of enzyme-substrate complexes, are static, whereas enzymes are flexible; this vital distinction may be limiting. The large size of the CYP active sites, which permits them to metabolize many different compounds, also renders them difficult to model. The potential for modeling ligand or activator interactions with nuclear receptors also exists with limitations similar to those discussed for the CYPs.

Determining the potential for a drug candidate to produce acute toxicity in preclinical studies is vital and routine in drug development. This is typically done by administering the drug candidate to rodents at escalating doses, usually above the predicted human therapeutic dose. For drug candidates proposed for chronic use in humans, such as for lowering serum triglycerides and cholesterol or for treatment of type 2 diabetes, long-term carcinogenicity studies are carried out in rodent models. Signs of toxicity are monitored and organ damage assessed by postmortem pathologies. This process is not high throughput and can be a bottleneck in development of lead compounds.

A new technology of high-throughput screening for biomarkers of toxicity is being adopted for drug development using *metabolomics*. Metabolomics is the systematic identification and quantification of all metabolites in a given organism or biological sample. Analytical platforms such as ^{1}H nuclear magnetic resonance and liquid chromatography or gas chromatography coupled to mass spectrometry, in conjunction with chemometric and multivariate data analysis, allow the simultaneous determination and comparison of thousands of chemicals in biological fluids such as serum and urine, as well as the chemical constituents of cells and tissues. This technology can be a screen for drug toxicity in whole-animal systems during preclinical drug development and can obviate the need for time-consuming and expensive necropsies and pathologies on thousands of animals.

Using metabolomics, animals, either treated or not treated with a drug candidate, can be analyzed for the presence of one or more metabolites in urine that correlate with drug efficacy or toxicity. Urine metabolites that are fingerprints for liver, kidney, and CNS toxicity have been identified using known chemical toxicants. Metabolic fingerprints of specific compounds that are elevated in urine can be used to determine, in dose escalation studies, whether a particular drug causes toxicity and can also be employed in early clinical trials to monitor for potential toxicities. Metabolomics can be used to find biomarkers for drug efficacy and toxicity that can be of value in clinical trials to identify responders and nonresponders. Drug metabolism can be studied in whole-animal model systems and in humans to determine the metabolites of a drug or indicate the presence of a polymorphism in drug metabolism that might signal an adverse clinical outcome. Finally, biomarkers developed from experimental metabolomics could eventually be developed for routine monitoring for signs of toxicity in patients receiving pharmacotherapy.

Bibliography

FitzGerald GA, et al. Molecular clocks and the human condition: approaching their characterization in human physiology and disease. *Diabetes Obes Metab*, **2015**, *17*:139–142.

Hayes JD, et al. Glutathione transferases. *Annu Rev Pharmacol Toxicol*, **2005**, *45*:51–88.

Huttenen KM, et al. Prodrugs-from serendipity to rational design. *Pharmacol Rev*, **2011**, *63*:750–71.

Kodani S, Hammock BD. Epoxide hydrolases: drug metabolism to therapeutics for chronic pain. *Drug Metab Dispos*, **2015**, *43*:788–802.

Lopez-Vicario C, et al. Inhibition of soluble epoxide hydrolase modulates inflammation and autophagy in obese adipose tissue and liver. Role for omega-3 epoxides. *Proc Natl Acad Sci USA*, **2015**, *112*:536–541.

Meisel P. Arylamine *N*-acetyltransferases and drug response. *Pharmacogenomics*, **2002**, *3*:349–366.

Rowland A, et al. The UDP-glucuronosyltransferases: their role in drug metabolism and detoxification. *Int J Biochem Cell Biol*, **2013**, *45*:1121–1132.

Strassburg CP. Pharmacogenetics of Gilbert's syndrome. *Pharmacogenomics*, **2008**, *9*:703–715.

Tibbs ZE, et al. Structural plasticity in the human cytosolic sulfotransferase dimer and its role in substrate selectivity and catalysis. *Drug Metab Pharmacokinet*, **2015**, *30*:3–20.

Townsend DM, Tew KD. The role of glutathione-*S*-transferase in anticancer drug resistance. *Oncogene*, **2003**, *22*:7369–7375.

Tukey RH, et al. Pharmacogenomics of human UDP-glucuronosyltransferases and irinotecan toxicity. *Mol Pharmacol*, **2002**, *62*:446–450.

Pharmacogenetics

Dan M. Roden

第七章　遗传药理学

中文导读

本章主要介绍：遗传药理学在药物反应差异中的重要作用；遗传药理学的基本概念，包括表型驱动术语、遗传变异的类型、共祖多样性；遗传药理学研究设计基本原则，包括遗传药理学特征、基因分型、候选基因与全基因组关联方法、大规模“跨平台”方法、多态性的功能研究、遗传药理学表型、基因组学作为发现新药物靶点的途径；遗传药理学在临床实践中的运用。

Abbreviations

ABCB1: multidrug resistance transporter (P-glycoprotein)
ACE: angiotensin-converting enzyme
ADR: adverse drug reaction
AUC: area under the curve
CBS: cystathionine β-synthase
CF: cystic fibrosis
CNV: copy number variation
cSNP: coding SNP
CYP: cytochrome P450
EGFR: epidermal growth factor receptor
EMR: electronic medical record
FDA: U.S. Food and Drug Administration
FH: familial hypercholesterolemia
GI: gastrointestinal
G6PD: glucose-6-phosphate dehydrogenase
GST: glutathione-S-transferase
GSTM1: glutathione-*S*-transferase M1
GWAS: genome-wide association study
HIV: human immunodeficiency virus
HMG-CoA: 3-hydroxy-3-methylglutaryl coenzyme A
5HT: 5-hydroxytryptamine, serotonin
indels: insertions or deletions
INR: international normalized ratio
iPSC: induced pluripotent stem cell
LDL: low-density lipoprotein
MAF: minor allele frequency
MDR1: multidrug resistance protein 1
mRNA: messenger RNA
MTHFR: methylenetetrahydrofolate reductase
nsSNP: nonsynonymous SNP
PharmGKB: Pharmacogenomics Knowledgebase
PheWAS: phenome-wide association study
PM: poor metabolizer
RCT: randomized clinical trial
SNP: single-nucleotide polymorphism
SNV: single-nucleotide variant
sSNP: synonymous or sense SNP
TPMT: thiopurine methyltransferase
TYMS: thymidylate synthase
UDP: uridine diphosphate
UGT: UDP-glucuronosyltransferase
UTR: untranslated region
VKORC1: vitamin K epoxide reductase

It is a given that patients vary in their responses to drug therapy. Some patients derive striking and sustained benefits from drug administration; others may display no benefit, and still others display mild, severe, or even fatal adverse drug reactions (ADRs). Common sources of such variability include noncompliance, medication errors, drug interactions (see Chapter 4 and Appendix I), and genetic factors. *Pharmacogenetics* is the study of the genetic basis for variation in drug response and often implies large effects of a small number of DNA variants. *Pharmacogenomics*, on the other hand, studies larger numbers of variants, in an individual or across a population, to explain the genetic component of variable drug responses. Discovering which variants or combinations of variants have functional consequences for drug effects, validating those discoveries, and ultimately applying them to patient care and to drug discovery are the tasks of modern pharmacogenetics and pharmacogenomics.

Importance of Pharmacogenetics to Variability in Drug Response

An individual's response to a drug depends on the complex interplay among environmental factors (e.g., diet, age, infections, other drugs, exercise level, occupation, exposure to toxins, and tobacco and alcohol use) and genetic factors. Genetic variation may result in altered protein sequence and function or in altered protein levels through regulatory variation. Key genes involved in driving variable drug actions include those encoding drug-metabolizing enzymes, drug transport molecules, the molecular targets with which drugs interact, and a host of other genes that modulate the molecular context within which drugs act, notably genes dysregulated in the disease for which the drug is administered. In some situations, variation in nongermline genomes (e.g., in cancers or in infectious agents) can be critical determinants of variable drug responses.

Drug metabolism is highly heritable, as assessed using drug exposures in monozygotic versus fraternal twins, drug exposures in cell lines from related subjects, or analysis of very large data sets using technologies such as genome-wide genotyping, discussed further in this chapter. Twin studies suggested that up to 75% of the variability in elimination half-lives for metabolized drugs can be heritable. Some drug metabolism traits behave in a conventional "monogenic" fashion with three clearly definable (and separable) groups of drug response phenotypes: heterozygotes as well as major and minor allele homozygotes. The study of these types of responses has helped define key genetic variants that contribute to the striking variability in responses described in this chapter. However, large effect size single variants are the exception, and for many (most) drug responses, the genetic component of variable responses—although substantial—likely reflects interacting influences of many genetic variants. A major challenge to the field is to accrue large numbers of subjects with well-phenotyped drug responses to enable discovery, and subsequent replication and validation, of multigene effects or of interactions of gene(s) with environmental factors.

Principles of Pharmacogenetics

Phenotype-Driven Terminology

A trait (e.g., the CYP2D6 "poor metabolizer" [PM], as opposed to "extensive metabolizer" [EM]) may be apparent only with nonfunctional alleles on both the maternal and the paternal chromosomes. If the gene is on a nonsex chromosome, the trait is autosomal. The nonfunctional alleles may be the same; the trait is then termed *autosomal recessive*, or different, in which case the subject is a *compound heterozygote*. A trait is deemed *codominant* if heterozygotes exhibit a phenotype that is intermediate to that of homozygotes for the common allele and homozygotes for the variant allele. Many polymorphic traits (e.g., CYP2C19 metabolism of drugs such as clopidogrel and omeprazole) are now recognized to exhibit some degree of codominance; as a result, heterozygotes exhibit metabolizing activity that is intermediate between that of EM and PM subjects.

In some instances, such as clopidogrel, codeine, and irinotecan (described further in this chapter), variants in a single gene produce clearly defined and clinically important differences in drug response. However, these high effect size examples are the exception for two reasons. First, even within a single gene, a vast array of polymorphisms (promoter, coding, noncoding, completely inactivating, or modestly modifying) is possible. Each polymorphism may produce a different effect on gene function and therefore differentially affect a measured trait. Second, even if the designations of recessive, codominant, and dominant are informative for a given gene, their utility in describing the genetic variability that underlies variability in drug response phenotype is diminished because variability is often multigenic.

Types of Genetic Variants

The major types of sequence variation are *single-nucleotide polymorphisms* (SNPs, sometimes termed *single-nucleotide variants*, SNVs), and *insertions*

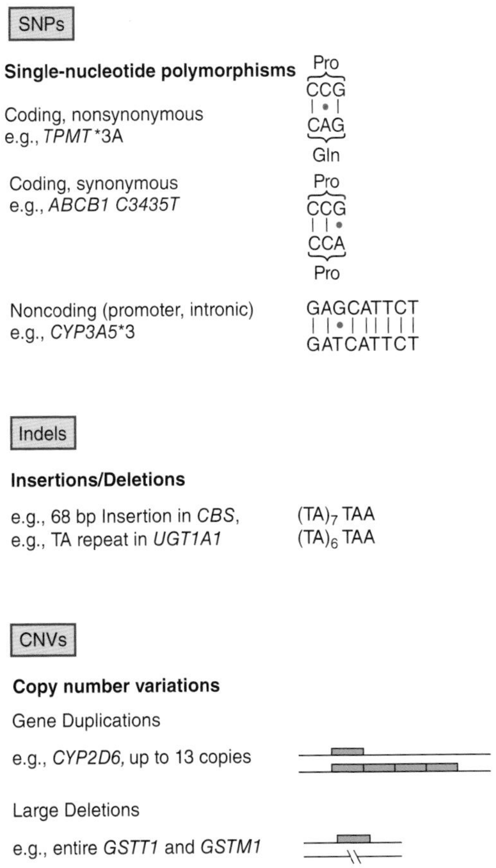

SNPs

Single-nucleotide polymorphisms

Coding, nonsynonymous e.g., *TPMT**3A — Pro CCG / CAG Gln

Coding, synonymous e.g., *ABCB1 C3435T* — Pro CCG / CCA Pro

Noncoding (promoter, intronic) e.g., *CYP3A5**3 — GAGCATTCT / GATCATTCT

Indels

Insertions/Deletions

e.g., 68 bp Insertion in *CBS*, e.g., TA repeat in *UGT1A1* — $(TA)_7$ TAA / $(TA)_6$ TAA

CNVs

Copy number variations

Gene Duplications

e.g., *CYP2D6*, up to 13 copies

Large Deletions

e.g., entire *GSTT1* and *GSTM1*

Figure 7–1 *Molecular mechanisms of genetic polymorphisms.* The most common genetic variants are SNP substitutions. Coding nonsynonymous SNPs result in a nucleotide substitution that changes the amino acid codon (here proline to glutamine), which could change protein structure, stability, or substrate affinities or introduce a stop codon. Coding synonymous SNPs do not change the amino acid codon but may have functional consequences (transcript stability, splicing). Noncoding SNPs may be in promoters, introns, or other regulatory regions that may affect transcription factor binding, enhancers, transcript stability, or splicing. The second major type of polymorphism is indels. SNP indels can have any of the same effects as SNP substitutions: short repeats in the promoter (which can affect transcript amount) or indels that add or subtract amino acids. CNVs involve large segments of genomic DNA that may involve gene duplications (stably transmitted inherited germline gene replication that causes increased protein expression and activity), gene deletions that result in the complete lack of protein production, or inversions of genes that may disrupt gene function. All of these mechanisms have been implicated in common germline pharmacogenetic polymorphisms.

or deletions, which can range in size from a single nucleotide to an entire chromosome; smaller ones are generally termed *indels*, and larger ones are designated CNVs. SNPs are much more common than indels or CNVs (Figure 7–1). The term *polymorphism* was formerly applied to variants occurring at a frequency greater than 1%. However, the application of genome sequencing to large numbers of subjects has made it clear that each individual has more than 10 million sites across their genome at which they differ from some reference sequence (i.e., ~ 1 variant per 1000 base pairs). While some of these are "common" (>1% frequency), the vast majority are much rarer. For rare variants clearly associated with a genetic disease, the term *mutation* may also be used, but distinguishing between a very rare variant and a mutation may be difficult. Publically available web-based databases (e.g., http://gnomad.broadinstitute.org) aggregate sequence data in tens of thousands of subjects and highlight that MAFs may vary strikingly across ancestries (discussed later), and that for the vast majority of variants is much less than 1%.

The SNPs in the coding region are termed *cSNPs* and are further classified as *nonsynonymous* (changing the encoded amino acid sequence) or *synonymous* (or *sense*, with no amino acid change). A nucleotide substitution in an nsSNP that changes the amino acid codon (e.g., proline [CCG] to glutamine [CAG]) can as a result change protein structure, stability, or substrate affinities. There are 64 trinucleotide codons and only 20 amino acids, so multiple codons encode the same amino acid. Often, substitutions of the third base pair, termed the *wobble position*, in a codon with 3 base pairs, such as the G-to-A substitution in proline (CCG → CCA), do not alter the encoded amino acid. Up to about 10% of SNPs display more than two possible alleles (e.g., a C can be replaced by either an A or a G), so that the same polymorphic site can be associated with amino acid substitutions in some alleles but not others. As discussed in the material that follows, assessing the functional consequences of nsSNPs can be challenging. SNPs that introduce a premature stop codon, and small indels in a coding region that disrupt the open reading frame and thereby introduce abnormal 3′ protein sequences often with early stop codons, are termed *nonsense* variants, and these are thought to be most likely to display abnormal protein function.

Synonymous polymorphisms have been reported to contribute to a phenotypic trait. One example is a polymorphism in *ABCB1*, which encodes MDR1 (also termed P-glycoprotein), an efflux pump that interacts with many clinically used drugs. In *MDR1*, a synonymous polymorphism, C3435T, is associated with various phenotypes, and some evidence indicates that the one of the resulting mRNAs is translated at a slower rate, thereby altering folding of the protein, its insertion into the membrane, and thus its interaction with drugs (Kimchi-Sarfaty et al., 2007).

The vast majority (>97%–99%) of human DNA is noncoding, and the regulatory functions of noncoding sequences are only now being defined. Polymorphisms in noncoding regions may occur in the 3′ and 5′ untranslated regions, in promoter or enhancer regions, in intronic regions, or in large regions between genes, intergenic regions (for nomenclature guide, see Figure 7–2). Noncoding SNPs in promoter or enhancer sequences are thought to alter DNA binding by regulatory proteins to affect transcription. 3′ SNPs may alter binding of microRNAs that affect transcript

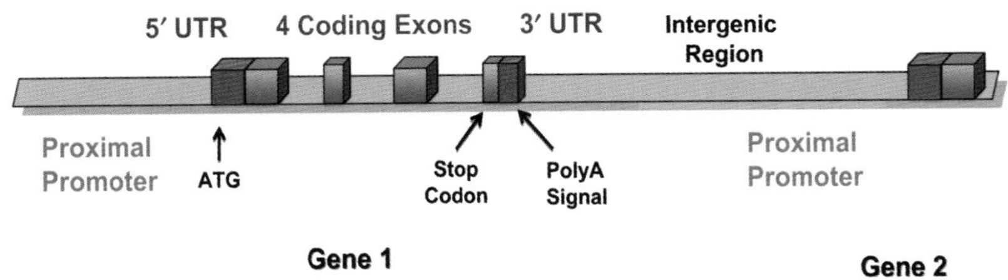

Figure 7–2 *Nomenclature of genomic regions.*

stability. Noncoding SNPs may also create alternative intron-exon splicing sites, and the altered transcript may have fewer or more exons, or shorter or longer exons, than the wild-type transcript. Large consortia are defining the functions of noncoding DNA: The ENCODE project identifies functional elements (enhancers, promoters, etc.) in genome sequences; and GTEx relates genome sequence variation to tissue-specific variability in gene expression (ENCODE Project Consortium, 2012; GTEx Consortium, 2015).

Like SNPs, indels can be short repeats in the promoter (which can affect transcript amount) or insertions/deletions that add or subtract amino acids in the coding region. The number of TA repeats in the *UGT1A1* promoter affects the quantitative expression of this important glucuronosyltransferase in liver; the most common allele has six repeats and the seven-repeat variant (*UGT1A1**28*) decreases *UGT1A1* expression. The frequency of the *28 allele is up to 30%, with up to 10% of subjects (depending on ancestry) being homozygous. Decreased *UGT1A1* transcription can modulate drug actions as described further in the chapter and also accounts for a common form of mild hyperbilirubinemia (Gilbert syndrome; see Table 6–3 and Figure 6–7).

The CNVs appear to occur in about 10% of the human genome and in one study accounted for about 18% of the detected genetic variation in expression of about 15,000 genes in lymphoblastoid cell lines (Stranger et al., 2007). The ultrarapid CYP2D6 metabolizer phenotype arises as a result of *CYP2D6* duplication(s), and individuals with more than 10 functional copies of the gene have been described. A common *GSTM1* polymorphism is caused by a large (50-kb) deletion, and the null allele has a population frequency of 30%–50%. Biochemical studies indicated that livers from homozygous null individuals have only about 50% of the glutathione-conjugating capacity of those with at least one copy of the *GSTM1* gene.

A *haplotype*—a series of alleles found at a linked locus on a chromosome—specifies the DNA sequence variation in a gene or a gene region on one chromosome. For example, consider two SNPs in *ABCB1*. One SNP is a T-to-A base-pair substitution at position 3421, and the other is a C-to-T change at position 3435. Possible haplotypes would be $T_{3421}C_{3435}$, $T_{3421}T_{3435}$, $A_{3421}C_{3435}$, and $A_{3421}T_{3435}$. For any gene, individuals will have two haplotypes, one maternal and one paternal in origin. A haplotype represents the constellation of variants that occur together for the gene on each chromosome. In some cases, this constellation of variants, rather than the individual variant or allele, may be functionally important. In others, however, a single variant may be functionally important regardless of other linked variants within the haplotype(s).

Linkage disequilibrium is the term used to describe the situation in which genotypes at the two loci are not independent of one another. With complete linkage disequilibrium, genotype at one site is a perfect predictor of genotype at the linked site. Patterns of linkage disequilibrium are population specific, and as recombination occurs, linkage disequilibrium between two alleles will decay and linkage equilibrium will result. Linkage disequilibrium has been enabling for genome-wide association studies because genotyping at a small number of SNPs ("tag SNPs") in linkage disequilibrium with many others can capture common variation across regions.

Ancestral Diversity

Polymorphisms differ in their frequencies within human populations and have been classified as either cosmopolitan or population (or race and ethnic) specific. *Cosmopolitan polymorphisms* are those polymorphisms present in all ethnic groups and are likely to be ancient, having arisen before migrations of humans from Africa, although present-day frequencies may differ among ancestral groups. The presence of *ancestry-specific polymorphisms* is consistent with geographical isolation of human populations. These polymorphisms probably arose in isolated populations and then reached a certain frequency because they are either advantageous in some way (positive selection) or neutral to a population. Individuals descended from multiple ancestries may display haplotype structures and allele frequencies intermediate between their parents. In the U.S., African Americans have the highest number of population-specific polymorphisms (and the smallest haplotype blocks) in comparison to European Americans, Mexican Americans, and Asian Americans.

Pharmacogenetic Study Design Considerations

There are many important considerations for the conduct of an experiment designed to identify sources of genetic variation contributing to variable drug responses. These include material to be studied (e.g., cells, organs, human subjects); the subjects' genetic backgrounds; the presence of confounders such as diet or variable experimental conditions; the selection of variants to be studied (ranging from a single high-likelihood candidate SNP to "agnostic" approaches that interrogate the whole genome); the methods used for genotyping and quality control; statistical analysis considerations, including effect size estimates and consideration of ancestry; and replication of findings.

Pharmacogenetic Traits

A *pharmacogenetic trait* is any measurable or discernible trait associated with a drug. Some traits reflect the beneficial or adverse effect of a drug in a patient; lowering of blood pressure or reduction in tumor size are examples. These have the disadvantage that they reflect many genetic and nongenetic influences, but the advantage that they indicate a drug's clinical effects. Other traits represent drug response "endophenotypes," measures that may more directly reflect the action of a drug in a biologic system and thus be more amenable to genetic study but may be removed from the whole patient or a whole population. Examples of the latter include enzyme activity, drug or metabolite levels in plasma or urine, or drug-induced changes in gene expression patterns.

A variant drug metabolizer phenotype can be inferred from genotype data or in some cases directly measured by administering a "probe drug" (one thought to be metabolized by a single pathway) and measuring drug and metabolite concentrations. For example, one method to determine *CYP2D6* metabolizer status is to measure the urinary ratio of parent drug to metabolite after a single oral dose of the *CYP2D6* substrate dextromethorphan. Similarly, mephenytoin can be used as a probe drug for *CYP2C19* metabolizer phenotype. An important caveat is that other drugs can interfere with this assessment: If dextromethorphan is given with a potent inhibitor of CYP2D6, such as quinidine or fluoxetine, the phenotype may be consistent with or a "phenocopy of" the poor metabolizer genotype, even though the subject carries wild-type *CYP2D6* alleles. In this case, the assignment of a *CYP2D6* poor metabolizer phenotype would not be accurate. Another pharmacogenetic endophenotype, the erythromycin breath test (for CYP3A activity), can sometimes be unstable within a subject, indicating that the phenotype is highly influenced by nongenetic or multigenic factors. *Most pharmacogenetic traits are multigenic rather than monogenic* (Figure 7–3), and considerable effort is being made to identify the important polymorphisms that influence variability in drug response.

Genotyping

Most genotyping methods use DNA extracted from somatic, diploid cells, usually white blood cells or buccal cells. This "germline" DNA is extremely stable if appropriately extracted and stored, and the DNA sequence is generally (but likely not totally) invariant throughout an individual's lifetime. Any genotyping result should be subject to standard and rigorous quality control, which may include inspection of source genotyping experimental data, exclusion of SNPs with a high genotyping failure rate, exclusion of subjects in which many SNP analyses failed, assessment of Hardy-Weinberg equilibrium, and ensuring the absence of important substructure (e.g., many related individuals) in a general population study. *Hardy-Weinberg* equilibrium is maintained when mating within a population is random and there is no natural selection effect on the variant. Such assumptions are described mathematically when the proportions of the population that are observed to be homozygous for the variant genotype (q^2), homozygous for the wild-type genotype (p^2), and heterozygous (2^*p^*q) are not significantly different from that predicted from the overall allele frequencies

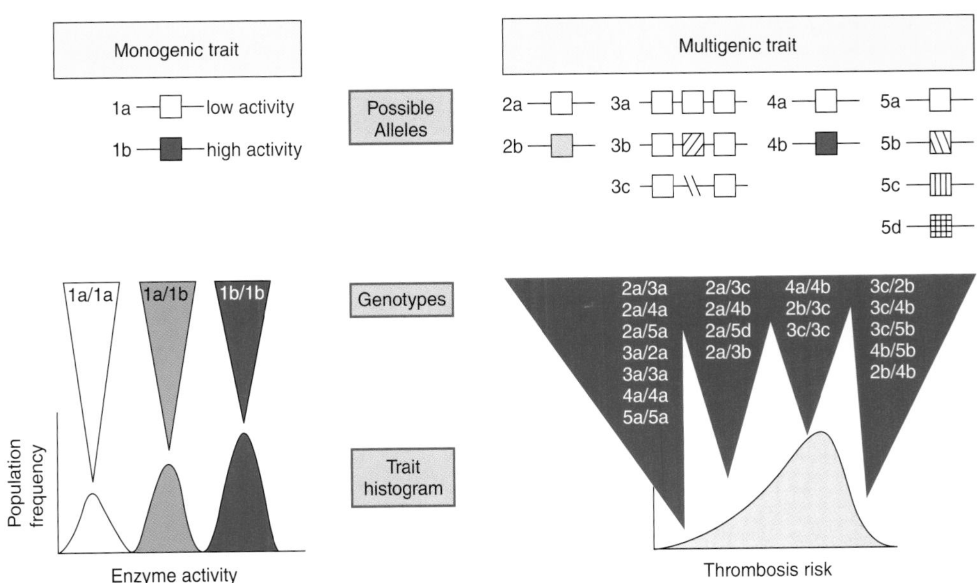

Figure 7–3 *Monogenic versus multigenic pharmacogenetic traits.* Possible alleles for a monogenic trait (*upper left*), in which a single gene has a low-activity (*1a*) and a high-activity (*1b*) allele. The population frequency distribution of a monogenic trait (*bottom left*), here depicted as enzyme activity, may exhibit a trimodal frequency distribution among low activity (homozygosity for *1a*), intermediate activity (heterozygote for *1a* and *1b*), and high activity (homozygosity for *1b*). This is contrasted with multigenic traits (e.g., an activity influenced by up to four different genes, genes 2 through 5), each of which has two, three, or four alleles (*a* through *d*). The population histogram for activity is unimodal skewed, with no distinct differences among the genotypic groups. Multiple combinations of alleles coding for low activity and high activity at several of the genes can translate into low-, medium-, and high-activity phenotypes.

(p = frequency of wild-type allele; q = frequency of variant allele) in the population. A deviation from Hardy-Weinberg equilibrium (i.e., from the rule that $p^2 + 2pq + q^2 = 1$) suggests a specific survival disadvantage for a particular genotype or a genotyping or other experimental error.

Candidate Gene Versus Genome-Wide Approaches

A candidate gene study uses what is known about a drug (e.g., its metabolism, transport, or mechanism of action) to test the hypothesis that variants in the underlying genes account for variable drug response phenotypes. Variants may be chosen because they are common, known (or thought) to be functional, or tag haplotype blocks. After assays are developed for a set of such variants, statistical methods are used to relate genotype to phenotype. There are several databases that contain information on polymorphisms in human genes (Table 7–1); these databases allow the investigator to search by gene for reported polymorphisms. Some of the databases, such as PharmGKB, include phenotypic as well as genotypic data.

Large-Scale "Agnostic" Approaches

While the candidate gene approach has the intuitive appeal that known drug response pathways are studied, it has the drawback of looking only in regions of known biologic activity. Indeed, candidate genetic studies for susceptibility to common diseases have a remarkably high rate of failure to replicate, and this has been attributed to naïveté about the polygenic nature of most traits, small sizes with underpowering, and a "winner's curse" in which only positive results are published (Ioannidis et al., 2001). It has been argued that, unlike common disease studies, precedent has shown that drug responses may indeed reflect large effect sizes of a small number of genes, but these limitations should nevertheless be borne in mind in the conduct of these studies.

An alternate approach to the candidate gene approach is a GWAS, in

TABLE 7–1 ■ DATABASES CONTAINING INFORMATION ON HUMAN GENETIC VARIATION

DATABASE NAME	URL (AGENCY)	DESCRIPTION OF CONTENTS
Pharmacogenomics Knowledgebase (PharmGKB)	www.pharmgkb.org (National Institutes of Health–sponsored research network and knowledge database)	Genotype and phenotype data related to drug response
dbSNP	www.ncbi.nlm.nih.gov/projects/SNP (National Center for Biotechnology Information [NCBI])	SNPs and frequencies
GWAS Central	www.gwascentral.org	Genotype/phenotype associations
Genome Aggregation Database	www.gnomad.broadinstitute.org	Variants identified by sequencing >120,000 exomes and >15,000 whole genomes
Online Mendelian Inheritance in Man (OMIM)	www.ncbi.nlm.nih.gov/omim	Human genes and genetic disorders
University of California Santa Cruz (UCSC) Genome Browser	http://genome.ucsc.edu	Sequence of the human genome; variant alleles
GTEx	www.gtexportal.org/home/	Genetics of gene expression
Broad Institute Software	www.broadinstitute.org/data-software-and-tools	Software tools for the analysis of genetic studies

which genotypes at more than 500,000 SNP sites (generally tagging haplotype blocks across the genome) are compared across a continuous trait or between cases and controls (e.g., those with or without a therapeutic response or an ADR). A GWAS requires large numbers of subjects, must consider the appropriate statistical approaches to minimize type I (false-positive) errors, and, if successful, identifies loci of interest that require further investigation to identify causative variants and the underlying biology. While associations identified by GWASs generally have modest effect sizes (odds ratios < 2), even with very low *P* values, pharmacogenetic GWASs provide some exceptions; for example, a GWAS in 51 cases of flucloxacillin-induced hepatotoxicity and 282 controls identified risk SNPs in the HLA-B locus with an odds ratio greater than 80 (Daly et al., 2009). Not all pharmacogenetic GWASs have successfully identified signals with this strength, but the approach has some promise and is increasingly used (Karnes et al., 2015; Mosley et al., 2015; Motsinger-Reif et al., 2013; Van Driest et al., 2015).

The GWAS analyses have also provided strong support for candidate gene studies that implicate variants in *CYP2C9* and *VKORC1* in warfarin dose requirement (Cooper et al., 2008; Takeuchi et al., 2009; see Figure 32–6 and Table 32–2) and variants in CYP2C19 in clopidogrel clinical response (Shuldiner et al., 2009). Newer genotyping platforms can capture both rare coding region variants and tags for common haplotype blocks, and the availability of increasing amounts of sequence data allows reasonable inferences (by a statistical method called imputation) of up to 10 million genotypes from a GWAS genotyping experiment.

While single experimental approaches can suggest a relationship between variable drug responses and a variant in a specific locus or gene, the use of multiple complementary approaches provides the strongest evidence supporting such relationships. One method is to establish that putative variants do in fact display altered function in an in vitro system, as discussed in the material that follows. Another approach is to integrate genotype data (by GWAS) with other large-scale measures of gene function, such as the abundance of mRNAs (transcriptomics) or proteins (proteomics). This has the advantage that the abundance of signal may itself directly reflect some of the relevant genetic variation. One such study identified six loci at which exposure to simvastatin in cell lines changed gene expression, and variants in one of these genes, glycine amidinotransferase, was associated with simvastatin myotoxicity in a clinical trial (Mangravite et al., 2013). However, both mRNA and protein expression are highly influenced by choice of tissue type, which may not be available; for example, it may not be feasible to obtain biopsies of brain tissue for studies of CNS toxicity. The GTEx project described previously couples whole-genome sequence to mRNA transcript levels across multiple tissues and should enable further such studies.

Large-scale coupling of genotypes to phenotypes in EMR systems with associated DNA biobanks represents another potential resource for pharmacogenomic studies. One interesting approach using such biobanks is to turn the GWAS paradigm "on its head" and to ask with what human phenotype is a particular genetic variant associated. This PheWAS can be used to replicate a GWAS result or to identify entirely new associations (Denny et al., 2013) and has been used to "repurpose" (suggest new indications for) marketed drugs (Rastegar-Mojarad et al., 2015).

Functional Studies of Polymorphisms

Once a gene or a locus modulating a drug response phenotype is identified, a major challenge is to establish which coding or regulatory variants contribute. Comparative genomics and functional studies of individual polymorphisms in vitro and in animal models are commonly used approaches. Precedents from Mendelian diseases suggest that the variants with the greatest potential effect sizes are rare nonsense variants or missense variants that drastically alter evolutionarily conserved residues. For example, studies of variants in membrane transporters and ion channels suggested that those conferring with the greatest change in function are at low allele frequencies and change an evolutionarily conserved amino acid residue. These data indicate that SNPs that alter evolutionarily conserved residues are most deleterious. For example, substitution of a charged amino acid (Arg) for a nonpolar, uncharged amino acid (Cys) is more likely to affect function than substitution of residues that are more chemically similar (e.g., Arg to Lys). The data also suggest that rare nsSNPs are more likely to alter function than common ones.

The link between Mendelian disease and variant drug responses is highlighted by the fact that one of the first pharmacogenetic examples to be discovered was G6PD deficiency, an X-linked monogenic trait that results in severe hemolytic anemia in individuals after ingestion of fava beans or various drugs, including many antimalarial agents. G6PD is normally present in red blood cells and regulates levels of the antioxidant glutathione. Antimalarials such as primaquine increase red blood cell fragility in individuals with G6PD deficiency, leading to profound hemolytic anemia; the trait is more common in African Americans. The severity of the deficiency syndrome varies among individuals and is related to the amino acid variant in G6PD. The severe form of G6PD deficiency is associated with changes at residues that are highly conserved across evolutionary history. *The information in* Table 7–2 *on genetic polymorphisms influencing drug response at the end of the chapter can be used as a guide for prioritizing polymorphisms in candidate gene association studies.*

With increasing application of exome or whole-genome sequencing in populations, millions of DNA variants are being identified, and methods to establish their function are evolving. One approach uses computational algorithms to identify potentially deleterious amino acid substitutions. Earlier methods (e.g., BLOSUM62, SIFT, and PolyPhen) use sequence comparisons across multiple species to identify and score substitutions, especially at highly conserved residues. More recent approaches use structural predictions (Kircher et al., 2014) or integrate multiple predictors (e.g., CADD). While these programs are becoming increasingly sophisticated, they have not yet reached the point that they can substitute for experimental verification.

The functional activity of amino acid variants for many proteins can be studied in isolation, in cellular assays, or in animal models. A traditional step in a cellular study of a nonsynonymous variant is to isolate the variant gene or to construct the variant by site-directed mutagenesis, express it in cells, and compare its functional activity (enzymatic activity, transport kinetics, ion channel gating, etc.) to that of the reference or most common form of the protein (Figure 7–4). Figure 7–5 shows an example of how the combination of population studies, in vitro functional assays, and in silico simulations can be integrated to identify a variant that modulates the risk of drug-induced arrhythmias.

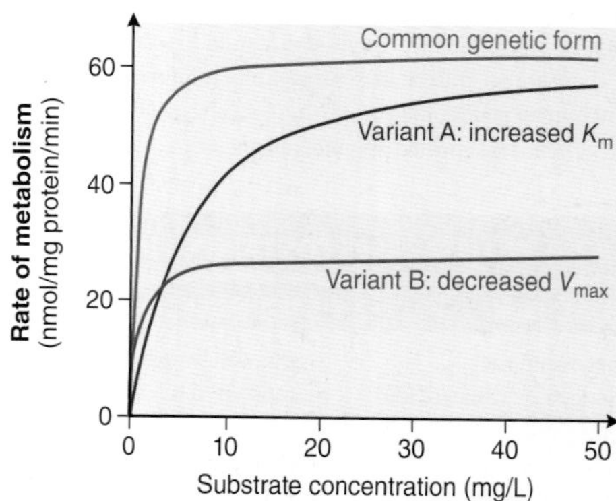

Figure 7–4 *Simulated concentration-dependence curves for the common genetic form of an enzyme and two nonsynonymous variants.* Compared to the common form of the enzyme, variant A exhibits an increased K_m, likely reflecting an altered substrate-binding site of the protein by the substituted amino acid. Variant B exhibits the same K_m as the common form but a reduced maximum rate of metabolism of the substrate (V_{max}). Because these measurements were made on cell extracts, the reduced V_{max} may be due to a reduced expression level of the enzyme. If similar data were obtained with purified protein, then the reduced activity of variant B could be ascribed to a structural alteration in the enzyme that affects its maximal catalytic rate but not its affinity for the substrate under these assay conditions.

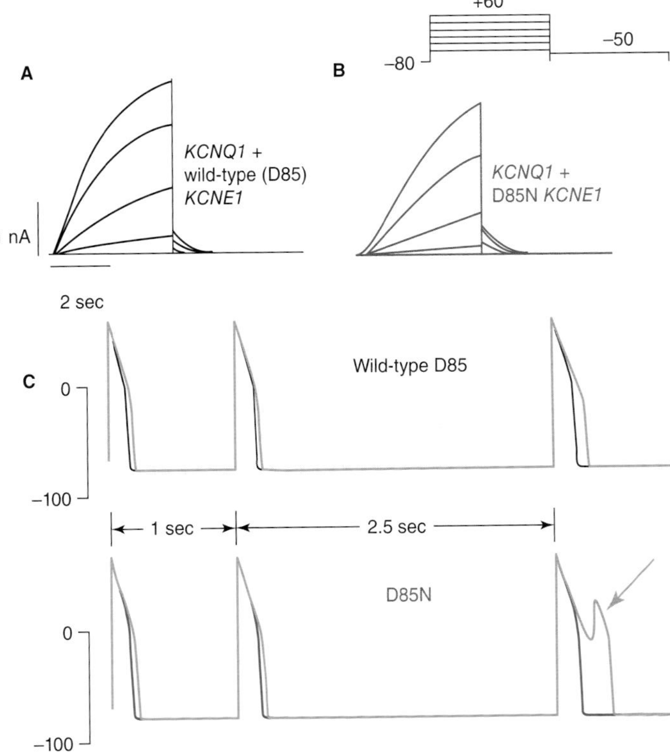

Figure 7–5 *Functional evaluation of an ion channel variant.* A population study implicated an nsSNP resulting in D85N in *KCNE1* as a modulator of the risk for arrhythmias when blockers of the KCNH2 K^+ channel are administered to patients (Kääb et al., 2012). *KCNE1* encodes a function-modifying subunit for a different cardiac K^+ channel (encoded by *KCNQ1*), and the ion currents generated at a range of voltages by heterologous coexpression of *KCNQ1* plus the wild-type or mutant *KCNE1* are shown in **A** and **B**, respectively. While there are subtle differences in activation kinetics and overall current amplitude, it is not clear whether these are functionally important. **C.** Results of numerical action potential simulations incorporating either the experimentally determined wild-type or variant K^+ current. At baseline (black and green tracings), there is no difference in computed action potential duration. However, when drug block of the KCNH2 K^+ channel is superimposed and the stimulation rate is slowed (orange tracings), an arrhythmogenic afterpotential (*arrow*) is seen with the mutant but not the wild-type *KCNE1*. Taken together, these functional data therefore provide support for the population study. (Data from Drs. Al George and Yoram Rudy.)

The SNPs identified in GWASs as associated with clinical phenotypes, including drug response phenotypes, have largely been in noncoding regions. An example of profound functional effect of a noncoding SNP is provided by *CYP3A5*; a common noncoding intronic SNP in *CYP3A5* accounts for its polymorphic expression in humans. The SNP accounting for variation in CYP3A5 protein creates an alternative splice site, resulting in not only a transcript with a larger exon 3 but also the introduction of an early stop codon (Figure 7–6). The nonfunctional allele is more common in subjects of European ancestry compared to those of African ancestry; as a result, CYP3A5 activity is lower in individuals expressing the noncoding intronic SNP (i.e., for a given dose of a drug that is a substrate of CYP3A5, concentrations of the drug will be higher in Europeans). Increased rates of transplant rejection in subjects of African descent may reflect decreased plasma concentrations of the antirejection drug tacrolimus, a substrate for CYP3A5 (the higher activity form lacking the noncoding intronic SNP) (Birdwell et al., 2012).

Two new technologies appear poised to revolutionize functional studies. The first is the ability to generate iPSCs from any individual and then use the cells to generate specific cell types (hepatocytes, cardiomyocytes, neurons, etc.), thereby enabling studies of that individual's cellular physiology. The second is rapid and efficient genome editing using CRISPR/cas9 in iPSCs or any other cell system (see Chapter 3). Multiple exciting applications of genome-editing technology, from rapid generation of genetically modified animals to curing genetic disease in humans, are being explored. Genome editing holds the promise that the function of individual coding or noncoding variants, alone or in combination, can be rapidly assessed in cellular systems.

Pharmacogenetic Phenotypes

Candidate genes for therapeutic and adverse response can be divided into three categories:

- those modifying drug disposition (*pharmacokinetic*)
- those altering the function of the molecules with which drugs interact to produce their beneficial or adverse effects (*receptor/target*)
- those altering the broad *biologic milieu* in which the drugs interact with target molecules, including the changes associated with the diseases for which the drug is being prescribed

This section summarizes important examples of each type but cannot be all inclusive. Web-based resources such as PharmGKB (Table 7–1) can be consulted for specific genes, variants, drugs, and diseases.

Pharmacokinetic Alterations

Germline variability in genes that encode determinants of the pharmacokinetics of a drug, in particular metabolizing enzymes and transporters, affect drug concentrations and are therefore major determinants of therapeutic and adverse drug response (at the end of the chapter, see Table 7–2 on genetic polymorphisms influencing drug response). A particularly high-risk situation is a drug with a narrow therapeutic margin eliminated by a single pathway: Loss of function in that pathway can lead to drastic increases in drug concentrations (and decreases in metabolite concentrations) with attendant loss of efficacy and an increased likelihood of ADRs (Roden and Stein, 2009). The loss of function can be genetic or can arise as a result of drug interactions or dysfunction of excretory organs

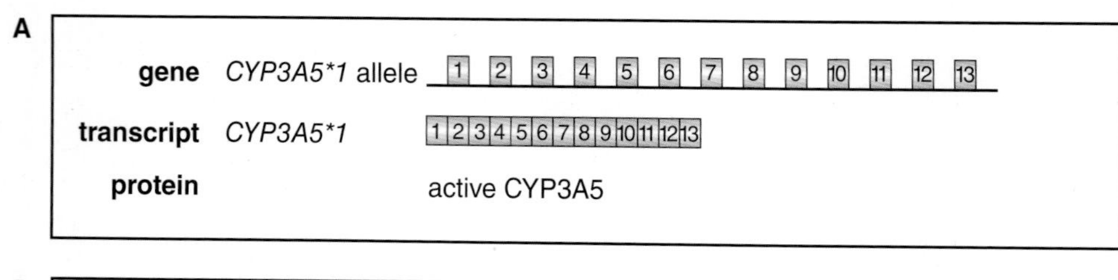

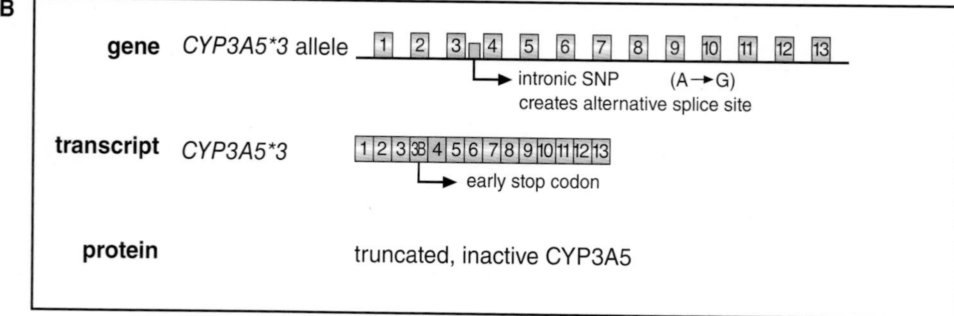

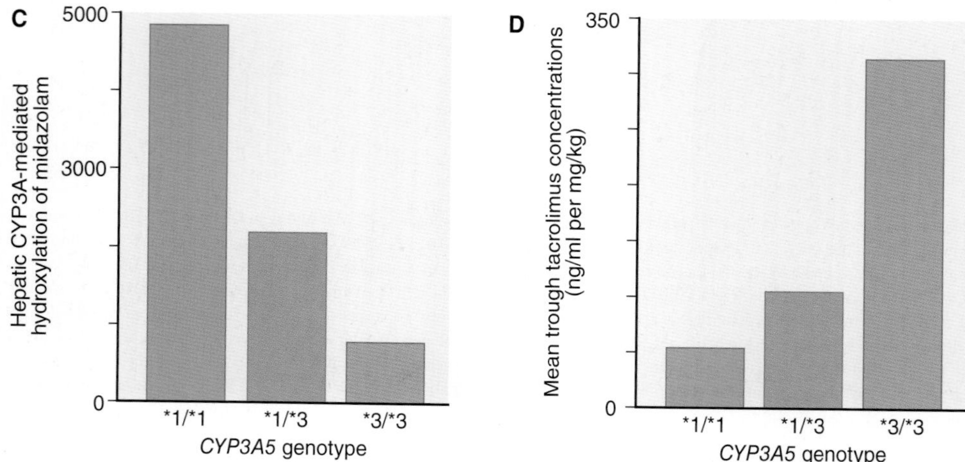

Figure 7–6 *An intronic SNP can affect splicing and account for polymorphic expression of CYP3A5.* A common polymorphism (A > G) in intron 3 of CYP3A5 defines the genotypes associated with the wild-type CYP3A5*1 allele or the variant nonfunctional CYP3A5*3 allele. This intronic SNP creates an alternative splice site that results in the production of an alternative CYP3A5 transcript carrying an additional intron 3B (**B**), with an early stop codon and truncated CYP3A5 protein. The wild-type gene (more common in African than Caucasian or Asian populations) results in production of active CYP3A5 protein (**A**); the *3 variant results in a truncated and inactive protein. Thus, metabolism of CYP3A5 substrates is diminished in vitro (**C**), and blood concentrations of such substrates (medications) are higher in vivo (**D**) for those with the *3 than the *1 allele. (Data from Haufroid et al., 2004; Kuehl et al., 2001; Lin et al., 2002.)

(e.g., renal failure will elevate plasma concentrations of renally excreted drugs unless dosages are reduced).

CYP2C9-mediated metabolism of the more active *S*-enantiomer of warfarin is an example. Individuals with the loss of function *3 allele require lower steady-state warfarin dosages and are at increased risk of bleeding (Aithal et al., 1999; Kawai et al., 2014; see also Table 32–2). When multiple enzymes and transporters are involved in the pharmacokinetics of a drug, single variants are unlikely to produce large clinical effects.

Another high-risk situation is a drug that requires bioactivation to achieve pharmacological effect. Individuals with increased or decreased bioactivation, because of genetic variants or drug interactions, are at risk for variant drug responses. Clopidogrel, bioactivated by CYP2C19, and tamoxifen, bioactivated by CYP2D6, are examples (see Table 7–2 and Figure 6–3A). PM subjects homozygous for a common loss function variant in *CYP2C19* display decreased antiplatelet effects and increased stent thrombosis during clopidogrel treatment (Mega et al., 2010; Shuldiner et al., 2009). In heterozygotes (~20%) receiving clopidogrel, adequate antiplatelet effects can be achieved by increasing the dose, whereas in homozygotes (2%–3%) an alternate antiplatelet drug should be used because even large dose increases do not affect platelet function. Other loss-of-function variants (notably *3) are common in Chinese and Japanese populations. Several proton pump inhibitors, including omeprazole and lansoprazole, are inactivated by CYP2C19. Thus, PM patients have higher exposure to active parent drug, a greater pharmacodynamic effect (higher gastric pH), and a higher probability of ulcer cure than heterozygotes or homozygous wild-type individuals.

A variation on this theme is the use of codeine (a prodrug bioactivated to morphine by CYP2D6). In PMs, analgesia is absent. Perhaps more important, excess morphine is generated in ultrarapid metabolizers, and death due to respiratory arrest has been reported (Ciszkowski et al., 2009). A large number of medications (estimated at 15%–25% of all medicines in use) are substrates for CYP2D6.

The *UGT1A1*28* variant, encoding the 7-TA reduced function *UGT1A1* promoter mentioned previously, has been associated with higher levels of the active metabolite SN-38 of the cancer chemotherapeutic agent *irinotecan* (see Chapter 66), and this increased concentration has been associated with an increased risk of serious toxicities (see Figures 6–6, 6–8, and 6–9).

Drug Receptor/Target Alterations

Warfarin exerts its anticoagulant effect by interfering with the synthesis of vitamin K–dependent clotting factors, and the target molecule with which warfarin interacts to exert this effect is encoded by *VKORC1*, an enzyme in the vitamin K cycle (Figure 7–7). Rare coding region variants in the gene lead to partial or complete warfarin resistance; interestingly, these variants are common (5% allele frequency) in Ashkenazi patients and may account for high dosage requirements in carrier subjects. The *VKORC1* promoter includes common variants that strongly modulate its expression; in subjects with reduced expression, lower steady-state warfarin doses are required. These variants are more common in Asian subjects than in Caucasians or Africans. Inherited variation in *CYP2C9* and *VKORC1* account for more than 50% of the variability in warfarin doses needed to achieve the desired coagulation level. *VKORC1* is one example of how both rare and common variants in genes encoding drug targets can exert important effects on drug actions.

In some instances, highly penetrant variants with profound functional consequences may cause disease phenotypes that confer negative selective pressure; more subtle variations in the same genes can be maintained in the population without causing disease but nonetheless causing variation in drug response. For example, rare loss-of-function mutations in MTHFR cause severe mental retardation, cardiovascular disease, and a shortened life span. Conversely, the 677C→T SNP causes an amino acid substitution that is maintained in the population at a high frequency (40% allele frequency in most white populations) and is associated with modestly lower MTHFR activity (~30% less than the 677C allele) and modest but significantly elevated plasma homocysteine concentrations (~25% higher). This polymorphism does not alter drug pharmacokinetics but does appear to modulate pharmacodynamics by predisposing to GI toxicity to the antifolate drug methotrexate in stem cell transplant recipients.

Like warfarin, methotrexate's clinical effects are dependent on a number of polymorphisms affecting metabolism, transport, drug modifiers, and drug targets. Several of the direct targets (dihydrofolate reductase, purine transformylases, and TYMS) are also subject to common polymorphisms. A polymorphic indel in *TYMS* (two vs. three repeats of a 28–base pair sequence in the enhancer) affects the amount of enzyme expression in both normal and tumor cells. The *TYMS* polymorphism can affect both toxicity and efficacy of anticancer agents (e.g., fluorouracil and methotrexate) that target TYMS. Thus, the genetic contribution to variability in the pharmacokinetics and pharmacodynamics of methotrexate cannot be understood without assessing genotypes at a number of different loci.

Other examples of drug target variants affecting drug response are presented in Table 7–2 at the end of the chapter. Serotonin receptor polymorphisms have been implicated as predictors of responsiveness to antidepressants and of the overall risk of depression. β adrenergic receptor polymorphisms have been linked to asthma responsiveness, changes in renal function following ACE inhibitors, sinus heart rate following β blockers, and the incidence of atrial fibrillation during β blocker therapy. The degree of lowering of LDL by statins has been linked to polymorphisms in HMG-CoA reductase, the statin target (see Chapter 31). Ion channel polymorphisms have been linked by both candidate gene and exome sequencing approaches to a risk of cardiac arrhythmias in the presence and absence of drug triggers (Kääb et al., 2012; Weeke et al., 2014).

Modifiers of the Biologic Milieu

The *MTHFR* polymorphism is linked to homocysteinemia, which in turn affects thrombosis risk. The risk of drug-induced thrombosis is dependent not only on the use of prothrombotic drugs but also on environmental and genetic predisposition to thrombosis, which may be affected by germline polymorphisms in *MTHFR*, factor V, and prothrombin. These polymorphisms do not directly act on the pharmacokinetics or pharmacodynamics of prothrombotic drugs such as glucocorticoids, estrogens, and asparaginase but may modify the risk of the phenotypic event (thrombosis) in the presence of the drug. Likewise, polymorphisms in ion channels (e.g., *KCNQ1, KCNE1, KCNE2*) that are not themselves the targets of drugs that prolong QT intervals may affect the duration of the baseline QT interval and the overall risk of cardiac arrhythmias; this may in turn increase risk of long QT arrhythmias seen with antiarrhythmics and a number of other "noncardiovascular" drugs (e.g., macrolide antibiotics, antihistamines).

Cancer as a Special Case

Cancer appears to be a disease of genomic instability. In addition to the underlying variation in the germline of the host, tumor cells exhibit

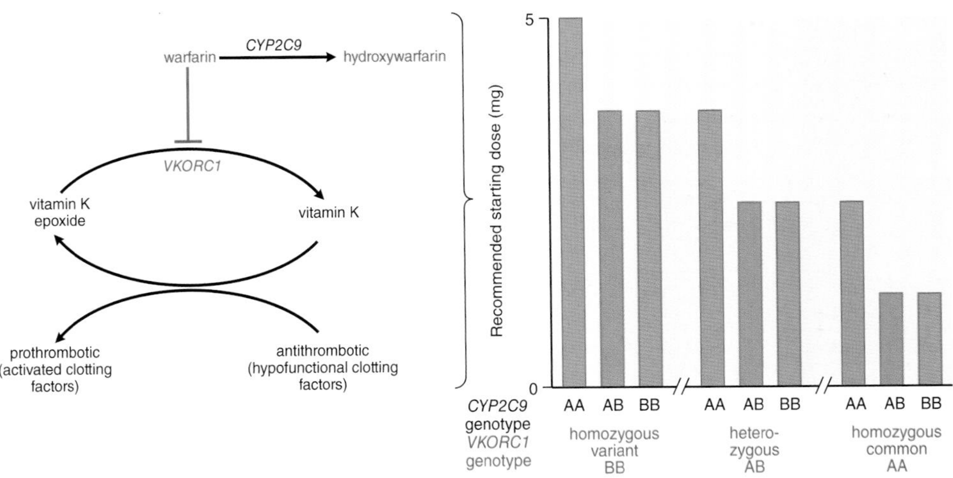

Figure 7–7 *Pharmacogenetics of warfarin dosing.* Warfarin is metabolized by *CYP2C9* to inactive metabolites and exerts its anticoagulant effect partly via inhibition of *VKORC1*, an enzyme necessary for reduction of inactive to active vitamin K. Common polymorphisms in both genes, *CYP2C9* and *VKORC1*, have an effect on warfarin pharmacokinetics and pharmacodynamics, respectively, to affect the population mean therapeutic doses of warfarin necessary to maintain the desired degree of anticoagulation (often measured by the INR blood test) and minimize the risk of too little anticoagulation (thrombosis) or too much anticoagulation (bleeding). See also Figure 32–6 and Table 32–2. (Data from Caraco et al., 2008; Schwarz et al., 2008; Wen et al., 2008.)

somatically acquired mutations, some of which generate mutant protein kinases that are drivers for the development of cancer. Thus, tumor sequencing is becoming standard of care for choosing among anticancer drugs in certain settings (see Chapters 65–68).

For example, patients with lung cancer with activating mutations in *EGFR*, encoding the epidermal growth factor receptor, display increased responses to the EGFR inhibitor gefitinib (Maemondo et al., 2010). Thus, the EGFR is altered, and patients with the activating mutation have, in treatment terms, a distinct pharmacogenetic category of lung cancer. The Her2 antibody trastuzumab can produce cardiomyopathy in all exposed patients. Patients with breast cancer whose tumors express the Her2 antigen may benefit from trastuzumab, whereas those whose tumors do not express Her2 do not benefit but are nevertheless susceptible to cardiomyopathy. Similarly, only patients with melanoma whose tumors express the mutant BRAF V600E respond to vemurafinib; interestingly, vemurafinib may also be effective in other tumors (thyroid cancer, hairy cell leukemia) that express BRAF V600E. Some genetic alterations affect both tumor and host: The presence of two instead of three copies of a *TYMS* enhancer repeat polymorphism not only increases the risk of host toxicity but also increases the chance of tumor susceptibility to TYMS inhibitors (Evans and McLeod, 2003).

Genomics as a Pathway to Identification of New Drug Targets

The identification of genetic pathways in normal physiology and in disease can provide important clues to new drug targets. Seminal studies of patients with the rare disease FH identified HMG-CoA reductase as the key rate-limiting enzyme in LDL cholesterol biosynthesis; now, inhibitors of that enzyme (the statins) are among the most effective and widely used medications in cardiovascular therapy (see Chapter 33). PCSK9 contributes to the degradation of LDL receptors, which are responsible

TABLE 7–2 ■ EXAMPLES OF GENETIC POLYMORPHISMS INFLUENCING DRUG RESPONSE

GENE PRODUCT (*GENE*)	DRUGS[a]	RESPONSES AFFECTED
Drug metabolism and transport		
CYP2C9	Tolbutamide, warfarin,[a] phenytoin, nonsteroidal anti-inflammatory	Anticoagulant effect of warfarin
CYP2C19	Mephenytoin, omeprazole, voriconazole,[a] hexobarbital, mephobarbital, propranolol, proguanil, phenytoin, clopidogrel	Peptic ulcer response to omeprazole; cardiovascular events after clopidogrel
CYP2D6	β blockers, antidepressants, antipsychotics, codeine, debrisoquine, atomoxetine,[a] dextromethorphan, encainide, flecainide, fluoxetine, guanoxan, *N*-propylajmaline, perhexiline, phenacetin, phenformin, propafenone, sparteine, tamoxifen	Tardive dyskinesia from antipsychotics, narcotic side effects, codeine efficacy, imipramine dose requirement, β-blocker effect; breast cancer recurrence after tamoxifen
CYP3A4/3A5/3A7	Macrolides, cyclosporine, tacrolimus, Ca^{2+} channel blockers, midazolam, terfenadine, lidocaine, dapsone, quinidine, triazolam, etoposide, teniposide, lovastatin, alfentanil, tamoxifen, steroids	Efficacy of immunosuppressive effects of tacrolimus
Dihydropyrimidine dehydrogenase	Fluorouracil, capecitabine[a]	5-Fluorouracil toxicity
N-acetyltransferase (*NAT2*)	Isoniazid, hydralazine, sulfonamides, amonafide, procainamide, dapsone, caffeine	Hypersensitivity to sulfonamides, amonafide toxicity, hydralazine-induced lupus, isoniazid neurotoxicity
Glutathione transferases (*GSTM1, GSTT1, GSTP1*)	Several anticancer agents	Decreased response in breast cancer, more toxicity and worse response in acute myelogenous leukemia
Thiopurine methyltransferase (*TPMT*)	Mercaptopurine,[a] thioguanine,[a] azathioprine[a]	Thiopurine toxicity and efficacy, risk of second cancers
UDP-glucuronosyl-transferase (*UGT1A1*)	Irinotecan,[a] bilirubin	Irinotecan toxicity
P-glycoprotein (*ABCB1*)	Natural product anticancer drugs, HIV protease inhibitors, digoxin	Decreased CD4 response in HIV-infected patients, decreased digoxin AUC, drug resistance in epilepsy
UGT2B7	Morphine	Morphine plasma levels
Organic anion transporter (*SLC01B1*)	Statins, methotrexate, ACE inhibitors	Statin plasma levels, myopathy; methotrexate plasma levels, mucositis
Catechol-*O*-methyltransferase	Levodopa	Enhanced drug effect
Organic cation transporter (*SLC22A1, OCT1*)	Metformin	Pharmacologic effect and pharmacokinetics
Organic cation transporter (*SLC22A2, OCT2*)	Metformin	Renal clearance
Novel organic cation transporter (*SLC22A4, OCTN1*)	Gabapentin	Renal clearance
CYP2B6	Cyclophosphamide	Ovarian failure

(*Continued*)

TABLE 7–2 ■ EXAMPLES OF GENETIC POLYMORPHISMS INFLUENCING DRUG RESPONSE (*CONTINUED*)

GENE PRODUCT (*GENE*)	DRUGS[a]	RESPONSES AFFECTED
Targets and receptors		
Angiotensin-converting enzyme (ACE)	ACE inhibitors (e.g., enalapril)	Renoprotective effects, hypotension, left ventricular mass reduction, cough
Thymidylate synthase	5-Fluorouracil	Colorectal cancer response
Chemokine receptor 5 (CCR5)	Antiretrovirals, interferon	Antiviral response
β_2 adrenergic receptor (*ADBR2*)	β_2-Antagonists (e.g., albuterol, terbutaline)	Bronchodilation, susceptibility to agonist-induced desensitization, cardiovascular effects (e.g., increased heart rate, cardiac index, peripheral vasodilation)
β_1 adrenergic receptor (*ADBR1*)	β_1-Antagonists	Blood pressure and heart rate after β_1 antagonists
5-Lipoxygenase (ALOX5)	Leukotriene receptor antagonists	Asthma response
Dopamine receptors (D_2, D_3, D_4)	Antipsychotics (e.g., haloperidol, clozapine, thioridazine, nemonapride)	Antipsychotic response (D_2, D_3 D_4), antipsychotic-induced tardive dyskinesia (D_3) and acute akathisia (D_3), hyperprolactinemia in females (D_2)
Estrogen receptor α	Estrogen hormone replacement therapy	High-density lipoprotein cholesterol
Serotonin transporter (5HTT)	Antidepressants (e.g., clomipramine, fluoxetine, paroxetine, fluvoxamine)	Clozapine effects, 5HT neurotransmission, antidepressant response
Serotonin receptor ($5HT_{2A}$)	Antipsychotics	Clozapine antipsychotic response, tardive dyskinesia, paroxetine antidepression response, drug discrimination
HMG-CoA reductase	Pravastatin	Reduction in serum cholesterol
Vitamin K oxidoreductase (VKORC1)	Warfarin[a]	Anticoagulant effect, bleeding risk
Corticotropin-releasing hormone receptor (CRHR1)	Glucocorticoids	Bronchodilation, osteopenia
Ryanodine receptor (RYR1)	General anesthetics	Malignant hyperthermia
Modifiers		
Adducin	Diuretics	Myocardial infarction or strokes, blood pressure
Apolipoprotein E	Statins (e.g., simvastatin), tacrine	Lipid lowering; clinical improvement in Alzheimer disease
Human leukocyte antigen	Abacavir, carbamazepine, phenytoin	Hypersensitivity reactions
G6PD deficiency	Rasburicase,[a] dapsone[a]	Methemoglobinemia
Cholesteryl ester transfer protein	Statins (e.g., pravastatin)	Slowing atherosclerosis progression
Ion channels (*HERG, KvLQT1, Mink, MiRP1*)	Erythromycin, cisapride, clarithromycin, quinidine	Increased risk of drug-induced torsades de pointes, increased QT interval (Roden, 2003, 2004)
Methylguanine-methyltransferase	DNA methylating agents	Response of glioma to chemotherapy
Parkin	Levodopa	Parkinson disease response
MTHFR	Methotrexate	GI toxicity (Ulrich et al., 2001)
Prothrombin, factor V	Oral contraceptives	Venous thrombosis risk
Stromelysin-1	Statins (e.g., pravastatin)	Reduction in cardiovascular events and in repeat angioplasty
Inosine triphosphatase	Azathioprine, mercaptopurine	Myelosuppression
Vitamin D receptor	Estrogen	Bone mineral density

[a]Information on genetics-based dosing, adverse events, or testing added to FDA-approved drug label (Grossman, 2007).

for removing LDL cholesterol from the circulation; an increase in PCSK9 activity results in reduction of LDL receptor function and an increase in LDL cholesterol. One rare cause of FH is gain-of-function mutations in *PCSK9*. Conversely, work in the Dallas Heart Study showed that individuals carrying nonsense mutations in *PCSK9* had lower LDL cholesterol values and decreased risk for coronary artery disease compared to noncarriers (Cohen et al., 2006). This result, in turn, identified PCSK9 as a potential drug target. In 2015, two antibodies that target PCSK9, alirocumab and evolocumab, were approved by the FDA for clinical use in FH and other lipid disorders. These PCSK9 inhibitors prevent degradation of LDL receptors and enhance their recycling to the hepatocyte membrane, thereby facilitating removal of LDL cholesterol and lowering blood LDL cholesterol levels (see Figure 33–4).

In a similar fashion, new drug targets have been identified by work showing that rare loss-of-function variants in *APOC3* lower triglycerides and reduce the risk of coronary artery disease (Stitziel et al., 2014), and loss-of-function variants in *SLC30A8* reduce risk for type 2 diabetes (Flannick et al., 2014). Patients homozygous for *SCN9A* loss-of-function variants are pain insensitive (Cox et al., 2006); inhibitors of SCN9A might be useful analgesics. Hundreds of mutations in the chloride transporter encoded by CFTR cause CF, but through diverse mechanisms. Ivacaftor partially corrects abnormal gating of certain rare variants of CFTR (G551D and others), while lumacaftor improves cell surface expression of the most common variant, ΔF508. Ivacaftor (Ramsey et al., 2011) and the ivacaftor/lumacaftor combination (Wainwright et al., 2015) improve symptoms and outcomes in patients with CF; both agents have now been approved in genotyped patients.

Pharmacogenetics in Clinical Practice

The increasing understanding of genetic contributors to variable drug actions raises questions of how these data might be used by healthcare providers to choose among drugs, doses, and dosing regimens. One approach is point-of-care testing, in which genotyping is ordered at the time of drug prescription; platforms that reliably deliver relevant genotypes rapidly (often in less than an hour) now make such approaches feasible. However, one difficulty in this approach is that each drug requires a separate assay. An alternate approach envisions genotyping at multiple loci relevant for responses to large numbers of drugs, embedding this information in each patient's EMR, and using clinical decision support to advise on drug selection and dosing when a relevant drug is prescribed to a patient with a variant genotype. This approach is being tested in a number of "early adopter" sites (Pulley et al., 2012; Rasmussen-Torvik et al., 2014).

There are several barriers that must be addressed if such an approach is to become widely adopted. First, the evidence linking a variant to a variable drug response must be solid, the variable outcome must be clinically important, and some form of genetically guided advice should be provided (choose another drug, choose another dose, etc.). Drug gene pairs such as *CYP2C19*2*/clopidogrel or *CYP2C9*3*/warfarin may fall into this category; the Clinical Pharmacogenomics Implementation Consortium provides guidelines on such advice by genotype across multiple drugs (Relling and Klein, 2011). Second, the strength of the evidence supporting a genotype-specific prescribing strategy varies. The strongest level of evidence comes from RCTs, in which a clinically important, genotype-guided treatment strategy is compared to a standard of care. Using this approach, genotyping for HLA-B5701 has been shown to eliminate the risk for severe skin reactions (such as the Stevens-Johnson syndrome) during treatment with the antiretroviral agent abacavir (Mallal et al., 2008). A number of trials have studied the utility of genotyping for *CYP2C9* and *VKORC1* variants during warfarin therapy. The main outcome metric has been duration of drug exposure in therapeutic range during the first 30–90 days of therapy; the results have been inconsistent, with none showing a huge effect (Kimmel et al., 2013; Pirmohamed et al., 2013). These studies have few bleeding events, but EMR-based case-control studies looking at this problem have implicated variants in CYP2C9 or CYP4F2 as risk alleles (Kawai et al., 2014; Roth et al., 2014). Nonrandomized study designs are weaker than RCTs, but performing RCTs to target small subsets of patients carrying uncommon variants may not be feasible.

Acknowledgment: *Mary V. Relling and Kathleen M. Giacomini contributed to this chapter in recent editions of this book. We have retained some of their text in the current edition.*

Bibliography

Aithal GP, et al. Association of polymorphisms in the cytochrome P450 CYP2C9 with warfarin dose requirement and risk of bleeding complications. *Lancet*, **1999**, *353*:717–719.

Birdwell KA, et al. The use of a DNA biobank linked to electronic medical records to characterize pharmacogenomic predictors of tacrolimus dose requirement in kidney transplant recipients. *Pharmacogenet Genomics*, **2012**, *22*:32–42.

Caraco Y, et al. CYP2C9 genotype-guided warfarin prescribing enhances the efficacy and safety of anticoagulation: a prospective randomized controlled study. *Clin Pharmacol Ther*, **2008**, *83*:460–470.

Ciszkowski C, et al. Codeine, ultrarapid-metabolism genotype, and postoperative death. *N Engl J Med*, **2009**, *361*:827–828.

Cohen JC, et al. Sequence variations in PCSK9, low LDL, and protection against coronary heart disease. *N Engl J Med*, **2006**, *354*:1264–1272.

Cooper GM, et al. A genome-wide scan for common genetic variants with a large influence on warfarin maintenance dose. *Blood*, **2008**, *112*:1022–1027.

Cox JJ, et al. An SCN9A channelopathy causes congenital inability to experience pain. *Nature*, **2006**, *444*:894–898.

Daly AK, et al. HLA-B*5701 genotype is a major determinant of drug-induced liver injury due to flucloxacillin. *Nat Genet*, **2009**, *41*:816–819.

Denny JC, et al. Systematic comparison of phenome-wide association study of electronic medical record data and genome-wide association study data. *Nat Biotechnol*, **2013**, *31*:1102–1111.

ENCODE Project Consortium. An integrated encyclopedia of DNA elements in the human genome. *Nature*, **2012**, *489*:57–74.

Evans WE, McLeod HL. Pharmacogenomics—drug disposition, drug targets, and side effects. *N Engl J Med*, **2003**, *348*:538–49.

Flannick J, et al. Loss-of-function mutations in SLC30A8 protect against type 2 diabetes. *Nat Genet*, **2014**, *46*:357–363.

GTEx Consortium. The Genotype-Tissue Expression (GTEx) pilot analysis: multitissue gene regulation in humans. *Science*, **2015**, *348*: 648–660.

Grossman I. Routine pharmacogenetic testing in clinical practice: Dream or reality? *Pharmacogenomics*, **2007**, *8*:1449–1459.

Haufroid V, et al. The effect of CYP3A5 and MDR1 (ABCB1) polymorphisms on cyclosporine and tacrolimus dose requirements and trough blood levels in stable renal transplant patients. *Pharmacogenetics*, **2004**, *14*:147–154.

Ioannidis JP, et al. Replication validity of genetic association studies. *Nat Genet*, **2001**, *29*:306–309.

Kääb S, et al. A large candidate gene survey identifies the KCNE1 D85N polymorphism as a possible modulator of drug-induced torsades de pointes. *Circ Cardiovasc Genet*, **2012**, *5*:91–99.

Karnes JH, et al. A genome-wide association study of heparin-induced thrombocytopenia using an electronic medical record. *Thromb Haemost*, **2015**, *113*:772–781.

Kawai VK, et al. Genotype and risk of major bleeding during warfarin treatment. *Pharmacogenomics*, **2014**, *15*:1973–1983.

Kimchi-Sarfaty C, et al. A "silent" polymorphism in the MDR1 gene changes substrate specificity. *Science*, **2007**, *315*:525–528.

Kimmel SE, et al. A pharmacogenetic versus a clinical algorithm for warfarin dosing. *N Engl J Med*, **2013**, *369*:2283–2293.

Kircher M, et al. A general framework for estimating the relative pathogenicity of human genetic variants. *Nat Genet*, **2014**, *46*:310–315.

Kuehl P, et al. Sequence diversity in CYP3A promoters and characterization of the genetic basis of polymorphic CYP3A5 expression. *Nat Genet*, **2001**, *27*:383–391.

Lin YS, et al. Co-regulation of CYP3A4 and CYP3A5 and contribution to hepatic and intestinal midazolam metabolism. *Mol Pharmacol*, **2002**, *62*:162–172.

Maemondo M, et al. Gefitinib or chemotherapy for non–small-cell lung cancer with mutated EGFR. *N Engl J Med*, **2010**, *362*:2380–2388.

Mallal S, et al. HLA-B*5701 screening for hypersensitivity to abacavir. *N Engl J Med*, **2008**, *358*:568–579.

Mangravite LM, et al. A statin-dependent QTL for GATM expression is associated with statin-induced myopathy. *Nature*, **2013**, *502*:377–380.

Mega JL, et al. Reduced-function CYP2C19 genotype and risk of adverse clinical outcomes among patients treated with clopidogrel predominantly for PCI: a meta-analysis. *JAMA*, **2010**, *304*:1821–1830.

Mosley JD, et al. A genome-wide association study identifies variants in KCNIP4 associated with ACE inhibitor-induced cough. *Pharmacogenomics J*, **2015**,

Motsinger-Reif AA, et al. Genome-wide association studies in pharmacogenomics: successes and lessons. *Pharmacogenet Genomics*, **2013**, *23*:383–394.

Pirmohamed M, et al. A randomized trial of genotype-guided dosing of warfarin. *N Engl J Med*, **2013**, *369*:2294–2303.

Pulley JM, et al. Operational implementation of prospective genotyping for personalized medicine: the design of the Vanderbilt PREDICT project. *Clin Pharmacol Ther*, **2012**, *92*:87–95.

Ramsey BW, et al. A CFTR potentiator in patients with cystic fibrosis and the G551D mutation. *N Engl J Med*, **2011**, *365*:1663–1672.

Rasmussen-Torvik LJ, et al. Design and anticipated outcomes of the eMERGE-PGx project: a multi-center pilot for pre-emptive pharmacogenomics in electronic health record systems. *Clin Pharmacol Ther*, **2014**, *96*:482–489.

Rastegar-Mojarad M, et al. Opportunities for drug repositioning from phenome-wide association studies. *Nat Biotechnol*, **2015**, *33*:342–345.

Relling MV, Klein TE. CPIC: Clinical Pharmacogenetics Implementation Consortium of the Pharmacogenomics Research Network. *Clin Pharmacol Ther*, **2011**, *89*:464–467.

Roden DM. Cardiovascular pharmacogenomics. *Circulation*, **2003**, *108*: 3071–3074.

Roden DM. Drug-induced prolongation of the QT interval. *N Engl J Med*, **2004**, *350*:1013–1022.

Roden DM, Stein CM. Clopidogrel and the concept of high-risk pharmacokinetics. *Circulation*, **2009**, *119*:2127–2130.

Roth JA, et al. Genetic risk factors for major bleeding in warfarin patients in a community setting. *Clin Pharmacol Ther*, **2014**, *95*:636–643.

Schwarz UI, et al. Genetic determinants of response to warfarin during initial anticoagulation. *N Engl J Med*, **2008**, *358*:999–1008.

Shuldiner AR, et al. Association of cytochrome P450 2C19 genotype with the antiplatelet effect and clinical efficacy of clopidogrel therapy. *JAMA*, **2009**, *302*:849–857.

Stitziel NO, et al. Inactivating mutations in NPC1L1 and protection from coronary heart disease. *N Engl J Med*, **2014**, *371*:2072–2082.

Stranger BE, et al. Relative impact of nucleotide and copy number variation on gene expression phenotypes. *Science*, **2007**, *315*:848–853.

Takeuchi F, et al. A genome-wide association study confirms *VKORC1*, *CYP2C9*, and *CYP4F2* as principal genetic determinants of warfarin dose. *PLoS Genet*, **2009**, *5*:e1000433.

Ulrich CN, et al. Pharmacogenetics of methotrexate: toxicity among marrow transplantation patients varies with the methylenetetrahydrofolate reductase C677T polymorphism. *Blood*, **2001**, *9*:231–234.

Van Driest SL, et al. Genome-wide association study of serum creatinine levels during vancomycin therapy. *PLoS One*, **2015**, *10*:e0127791.

Wainwright CE, et al. Lumacaftor–ivacaftor in patients with cystic fibrosis homozygous for Phe508del CFTR. *N Engl J Med*, **2015**, *373*:220–231.

Weeke P, et al. Exome sequencing implicates an increased burden of rare potassium channel variants in the risk of drug-induced long QT interval syndrome. *J Am Coll Cardiol*, **2014**, *63*:1430–1437.

Wen MS, et al. Prospective study of warfarin dosage requirements based on CYP2C9 and VKORC1 genotypes. *Clin Pharmacol Ther*, **2008**, *84*:83–89.

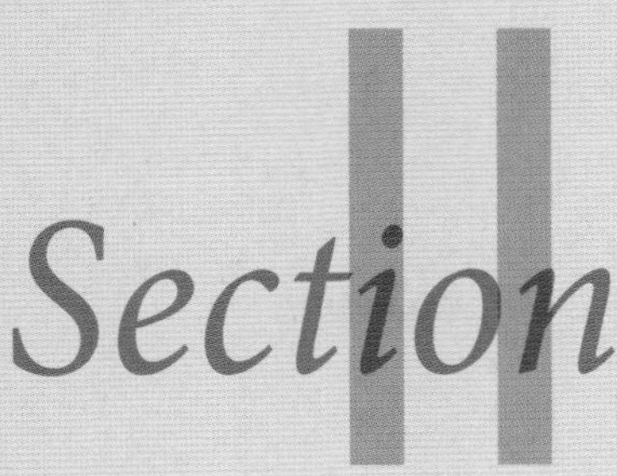

Section II

Neuropharmacology

第二篇　神经药理学

Neurotransmission: The Autonomic and Somatic Motor Nervous Systems

Thomas C. Westfall, Heather Macarthur, and David P. Westfall

第八章　神经传递：自主和躯体运动神经系统

中文导读

本章主要介绍：神经系统的解剖学和一般功能，包括自主神经与躯体神经之间的差异，外周自主神经系统的分类，交感神经、副交感神经和运动神经的区别；神经递质传递，包括神经递质传递的证据、神经传递的步骤、胆碱能神经传递、肾上腺素能神经传递；药理学方面的思考，包括干扰递质的合成或释放、促进递质释放、对受体的激动和拮抗作用、干扰递质的降解；自主神经系统其他递质，包括自主神经系统的协同递质，非肾上腺素能非胆碱能的嘌呤能传递，介导信号整合与血管反应调节的内皮源性因子NO和内皮素。

Abbreviations

AA: arachidonic acid
AAADC: aromatic L-amino acid decarboxylase
α-BTX: α-bungarotoxin
AC: adenylyl cyclase
ACh: acetylcholine
AChE: acetylcholinesterase
AD: aldehyde dehydrogenase
ADH: alcohol dehydrogenase
anti-ChE: anti-cholinesterase
AP: action potential
AR: aldehyde reductase
AV: atrioventricular
CaM: calmodulin
CCK: cholecystokinin
CGRP: calcitonin gene–related peptide
ChAT: choline acetyl transferase
CHT1: Choline transporter
CNS: central nervous system
COMT: catechol-*O*-methyltransferase
CSF: cerebrospinal fluid
DA: dopamine
DAG: diacylglycerol
DAT: DA transporter
DβH: dopamine β-hydroxylase
DOMA: 3,4-dihydroxymandelic acid
DOPEG: 3,4-dihydroxyphenyl glycol
DOPGAL: dihydroxyphenylglycolaldehyde
ENS: enteric nervous system
ENT: extraneuronal transporter
EPI: epinephrine
EPP: end-plate potential
EPSP: excitatory postsynaptic potential
ET: endothelin
GABA: γ-aminobutyric acid
GI: gastrointestinal
GRK: G protein-coupled receptor kinase
GPCR: G protein–coupled receptor
HR: heart rate
5HT: serotonin (5-hydroxytryptamine)
HVA: homovanillic acid
IP_3: inositol 1,4,5-trisphosphate
IPSP: inhibitory postsynaptic potential
KO: knockout
mAChR: muscarinic acetylcholine receptor
MAO: monoamine oxidase
MAPK: mitogen-activated protein kinase
mepps: miniature end-plate potentials
MOPEG: 3-methyl,4-hydroxyphenylglycol
MOPGAL: monohydroxyphenylglycolaldehyde
nAChR: nicotinic ACh receptor
NANC: nonadrenergic, noncholinergic
NE: norepinephrine (noradrenaline)
NET: norepinephrine transporter
NMJ: neuromuscular junction (of skeletal muscle)
NO: nitric oxide
NOS: nitric oxide synthase
NPY: neuropeptide Y
NSF: *N*-ethylmaleamide sensitive factor
PACAP: pituitary adenylyl cyclase–activating peptide
PG_: prostaglandin _, as in PGE_2
PK_: protein kinase _, as in PKA
PL_: phospholipase _, as in PLA_2, PLC, etc.
PNMT: phenylethanolamine-*N*-methyltransferase
PTX: pertussis toxin
rNTPase: releasable nucleotidase
SA: sinoatrial
SERT: serotonin transporter
SLC: solute carrier
SNAP: soluble NSF attachment protein, synaptosome-associated protein
SNARE: SNAP receptor
SST: somatostatin
STN: solitary tract nucleus
TH: tyrosine hydroxylase
VAChT: vesicular ACh transporter
VAT: vesicle-associated transporter
VIP: vasoactive intestinal polypeptide
VMA: vanillyl mandelic acid
VMAT2: vesicular uptake transporter

Anatomy and General Functions

The autonomic nervous system, also called the *visceral, vegetative,* or *involuntary nervous system,* is distributed widely throughout the body and regulates autonomic functions that occur without conscious control. In the periphery, it consists of nerves, ganglia, and plexuses that innervate the heart, blood vessels, glands, other visceral organs, and smooth muscle in various tissues.

Differences Between Autonomic and Somatic Nerves

- The *efferent nerves* of the autonomic nervous system supply all innervated structures of the body except skeletal muscle, which is served by *somatic nerves.*
- The most distal synaptic junctions in the autonomic reflex arc occur in *ganglia* that are entirely *outside the cerebrospinal axis.* Somatic nerves contain no peripheral *ganglia,* and the synapses are located entirely *within the cerebrospinal axis.*
- Many autonomic nerves form extensive peripheral plexuses; such networks are absent from the somatic system.
- Postganglionic autonomic nerves generally are *nonmyelinated;* motor nerves to skeletal muscles are *myelinated.*
- When the spinal efferent nerves are interrupted, smooth muscles and glands generally retain some level of spontaneous activity, whereas the *denervated* skeletal muscles are paralyzed.

Sensory Information: Afferent Fibers and Reflex Arcs

Afferent fibers from visceral structures are the first link in the reflex arcs of the autonomic system. With certain exceptions, such as local axon reflexes, most visceral reflexes are mediated through the CNS.

Visceral Afferent Fibers. Information on the status of the visceral organs is transmitted to the CNS through two main sensory systems: the *cranial nerve (parasympathetic) visceral sensory system* and the *spinal (sympathetic) visceral afferent system.* The cranial visceral sensory system carries mainly mechanoreceptor and chemosensory information, whereas the afferents of the spinal visceral system principally convey sensations related to temperature and tissue injury of mechanical, chemical, or thermal origin.

Cranial visceral sensory information enters the CNS by four cranial nerves: the trigeminal (V), facial (VII), glossopharyngeal (IX), and vagus (X) nerves. These four cranial nerves transmit visceral sensory information from the internal face and head (V); tongue (taste, VII); hard palate and upper part of the oropharynx (IX); and carotid body, lower part of the oropharynx, larynx, trachea, esophagus, and thoracic and abdominal organs (X), with the exception of the pelvic viscera. The pelvic viscera are innervated by nerves from the second through fourth sacral spinal segments. The visceral afferents from these four cranial nerves terminate topographically in the STN (Altschuler et al., 1989).

Sensory afferents from visceral organs also enter the CNS from the spinal nerves. Those concerned with muscle chemosensation may arise at all spinal levels, whereas sympathetic visceral sensory afferents generally arise at the thoracic levels where sympathetic preganglionic neurons are found. Pelvic sensory afferents from spinal segments S2–S4 enter at that level and are important for the regulation of sacral parasympathetic outflow. In general, visceral afferents that enter the spinal nerves convey information concerned with temperature as well as nociceptive visceral inputs related to mechanical, chemical, and thermal stimulation. The primary pathways taken by ascending spinal visceral afferents are complex (Saper, 2002). An important feature of the ascending pathways is that they provide collaterals that converge with the cranial visceral sensory pathway at virtually every level (Saper, 2000).

The neurotransmitters that mediate transmission from sensory fibers have not been characterized unequivocally. Substance P and CGRP, present in afferent sensory fibers, dorsal root ganglia, and the dorsal horn of the spinal cord, likely communicate nociceptive stimuli from the periphery to the spinal cord and higher structures. SST, VIP, and CCK also occur in sensory neurons (Hökfelt et al., 2000). ATP appears to be a neurotransmitter in certain sensory neurons (e.g., the urinary bladder). Enkephalins, present in interneurons in the dorsal spinal cord (within the *substantia gelatinosa*), have antinociceptive effects both pre- and postsynaptically to inhibit the release of substance P and diminish the activity of cells that project from the spinal cord to higher centers in the CNS. The excitatory amino acids glutamate and aspartate also play major roles in transmission of sensory responses to the spinal cord. These transmitters and their signaling pathways are reviewed in Chapter 14.

Central Autonomic Connections

There probably are no purely autonomic or somatic centers of integration, and extensive overlap occurs. Somatic responses always are accompanied by visceral responses and vice versa. Autonomic reflexes can be elicited at the level of the spinal cord. They clearly are demonstrable in experimental animals or humans with spinal cord transection and are manifested by sweating, blood pressure alterations, vasomotor responses to temperature changes, and reflex emptying of the urinary bladder, rectum, and seminal vesicles. Extensive central ramifications of the autonomic nervous system exist above the level of the spinal cord. For example, integration of the control of respiration in the medulla oblongata is well known. The hypothalamus and the STN generally are regarded as principal loci of integration of autonomic nervous system functions, which include regulation of body temperature, water balance, carbohydrate and fat metabolism, blood pressure, emotions, sleep, respiration, and reproduction. Signals are received through ascending spinobulbar pathways, the limbic system, neostriatum, cortex, and to a lesser extent other higher brain centers. Stimulation of the STN and the hypothalamus activates bulbospinal pathways and hormonal output to mediate autonomic and motor responses (Andresen and Kunze, 1994) (see Chapter 14). The hypothalamic nuclei that lie posteriorly and laterally are sympathetic in their main connections, whereas parasympathetic functions evidently are integrated by the midline nuclei in the region of the tuber cinereum and by nuclei lying anteriorly.

Highly integrated patterns of response generally are organized at a hypothalamic level and involve autonomic, endocrine, and behavioral components. More limited patterned responses are organized at other levels of basal forebrain, brainstem, and spinal cord.

Divisions of the Peripheral Autonomic System

On the efferent side, the autonomic nervous system consists of two large divisions: (1) the *sympathetic* or *thoracolumbar outflow* and (2) the *parasympathetic* or *craniosacral outflow*. Figure 8–1 schematically summarizes the arrangement of the principal parts of the peripheral autonomic nervous system.

The neurotransmitter of all preganglionic autonomic fibers, most postganglionic parasympathetic fibers, and a few postganglionic sympathetic fibers is ACh. Some postganglionic parasympathetic nerves use NO as a neurotransmitter and are termed *nitrergic* (Toda and Okamura, 2003). The majority of the postganglionic sympathetic fibers are *adrenergic,* in which the transmitter is NE (also called noradrenaline). The terms *cholinergic* and *adrenergic* describe neurons that liberate ACh or NE, respectively. Not all the transmitters of the primary afferent fibers, such as those from the mechano- and chemoreceptors of the carotid body and aortic arch, have been identified conclusively. Substance P and glutamate may mediate many afferent impulses; both are present in high concentrations in the dorsal spinal cord.

Sympathetic Nervous System

The cells that give rise to the preganglionic fibers of the sympathetic nervous system division lie mainly in the intermediolateral columns of the spinal cord and extend from the first thoracic to the second or third lumbar segment. The axons from these cells are carried in the anterior (ventral) nerve roots and synapse, with neurons lying in sympathetic ganglia outside the cerebrospinal axis. Sympathetic ganglia are found in three locations: paravertebral, prevertebral, and terminal.

The 22 pairs of paravertebral sympathetic ganglia form the lateral chains on either side of the vertebral column. The ganglia are connected to each other by nerve trunks and to the spinal nerves by *rami communicantes.* The white rami are restricted to the segments of the thoracolumbar outflow; they carry the preganglionic myelinated fibers that exit the spinal cord by the anterior spinal roots. The gray rami arise from the ganglia and carry postganglionic fibers back to the spinal nerves for distribution to sweat glands and pilomotor muscles and to blood vessels of skeletal muscle and skin. The prevertebral ganglia lie in the abdomen and the pelvis near the ventral surface of the bony vertebral column and consist mainly of the celiac (solar), superior mesenteric, aorticorenal, and inferior mesenteric ganglia. The terminal ganglia are few in number, lie near the organs they innervate, and include ganglia connected with the urinary bladder and rectum and the cervical ganglia in the region of the neck. In addition, small intermediate ganglia lie outside the conventional vertebral chain, especially in the thoracolumbar region. They are variable in number and location but usually are in proximity to the communicating rami and the anterior spinal nerve roots.

Preganglionic fibers issuing from the spinal cord may synapse with the neurons of more than one sympathetic ganglion. Their principal ganglia of termination need not correspond to the original level from which the preganglionic fiber exits the spinal cord. Many of the preganglionic fibers from the fifth to the last thoracic segment pass through the paravertebral ganglia to form the splanchnic nerves. Most of the splanchnic nerve fibers do not synapse until they reach the celiac ganglion; others directly innervate the adrenal medulla.

Postganglionic fibers arising from sympathetic ganglia innervate visceral structures of the thorax, abdomen, head, and neck. The trunk and the limbs are supplied by the sympathetic fibers in spinal nerves. The prevertebral ganglia contain cell bodies whose axons innervate the glands and smooth muscles of the abdominal and the pelvic viscera. Many of the upper thoracic sympathetic fibers from the vertebral ganglia form terminal plexuses, such as the cardiac, esophageal, and pulmonary plexuses. The sympathetic distribution to the head and the neck (vasomotor, pupillodilator, secretory, and pilomotor) is by means of the cervical sympathetic chain and its three ganglia. All postganglionic fibers in this chain arise from cell bodies located in these three ganglia. All preganglionic fibers arise from the upper thoracic segments of the spinal cord, there being no sympathetic fibers that leave the CNS above the first thoracic level.

Pharmacologically, anatomically, and embryologically, the chromaffin cells of the adrenal medulla resemble a collection of postganglionic sympathetic nerve cells. Typical preganglionic fibers that release ACh innervate these chromaffin cells, stimulating the release of EPI (also called adrenaline), in distinction to the NE released by postganglionic sympathetic fibers.

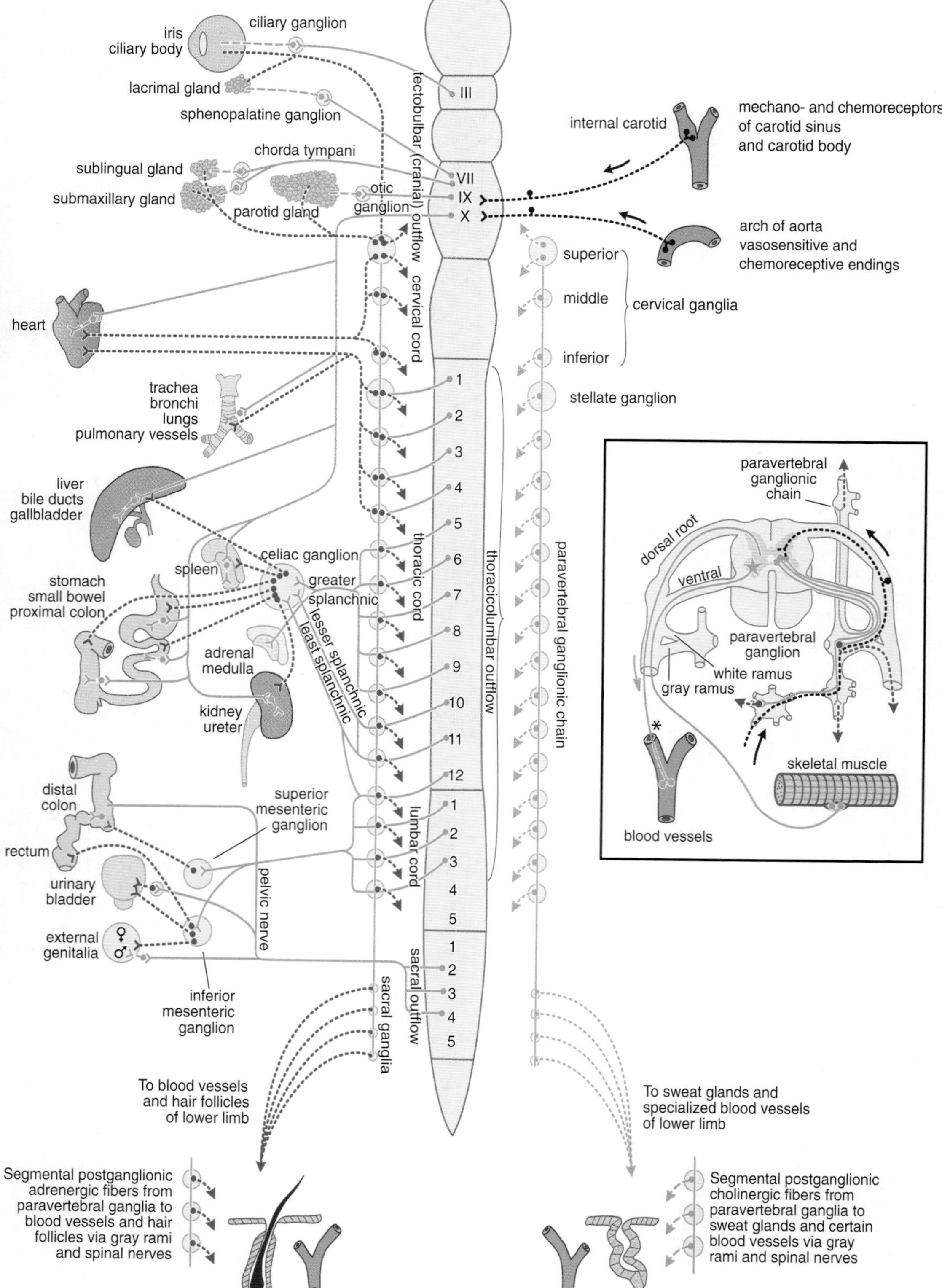

Figure 8–1 *The autonomic nervous system.* Schematic representation of the autonomic nerves and effector organs based on chemical mediation of nerve impulses. Yellow (————), cholinergic; red (————), adrenergic; dotted blue (- - - - - - - -), visceral afferent; solid lines, preganglionic; broken lines, postganglionic. The rectangle at right shows the finer details of the ramifications of adrenergic fibers at any one segment of the spinal cord, the path of the visceral afferent nerves, the cholinergic nature of somatic motor nerves to skeletal muscle, and the presumed cholinergic nature of the vasodilator fibers in the dorsal roots of the spinal nerves. The asterisk (*) indicates that it is not known whether these vasodilator fibers are motor or sensory or where their cell bodies are situated.

Parasympathetic Nervous System

The parasympathetic nervous system consists of preganglionic fibers that originate in the CNS and their postganglionic connections. The regions of central origin are the midbrain, the medulla oblongata, and the sacral part of the spinal cord. The midbrain, or tectal, outflow consists of fibers arising from the Edinger-Westphal nucleus of the third cranial nerve and going to the ciliary ganglion in the orbit. The medullary outflow consists of the parasympathetic components of the VII, IX, and X cranial nerves.

The fibers in the VII (facial) cranial nerve form the chorda tympani, which innervates the ganglia lying on the submaxillary and sublingual glands. They also form the greater superficial petrosal nerve, which innervates the sphenopalatine ganglion. The autonomic components of the IX (glossopharyngeal) cranial nerve innervate the otic ganglia. Postganglionic parasympathetic fibers from these ganglia supply the sphincter of the iris (pupillary constrictor muscle), the ciliary muscle, the salivary and lacrimal glands, and the mucous glands of the nose, mouth, and pharynx. These fibers also include vasodilator nerves to these same organs. Cranial nerve X (vagus) arises in the medulla and contains preganglionic fibers, most of which do not synapse until they reach the many small ganglia lying directly on or in the viscera of the thorax and abdomen. In the intestinal wall, the vagal fibers terminate around ganglion cells in the myenteric and submucosal plexuses. *Thus, in the parasympathetic branch of the autonomic nervous system, preganglionic fibers are very long, whereas postganglionic fibers are very short.* The vagus nerve also carries a far greater number of afferent fibers (but apparently no pain fibers) from the viscera into the medulla. The parasympathetic sacral outflow consists of axons that arise from cells in the second, third, and fourth segments of the sacral cord and proceed as preganglionic fibers to form the pelvic nerves (*nervi erigentes*). They synapse in terminal ganglia lying near or within the bladder, rectum, and sexual organs. The vagal and sacral outflows provide motor and secretory fibers to thoracic, abdominal, and pelvic organs (see Figure 8–1).

Enteric Nervous System

The processes of mixing, propulsion, and absorption of nutrients in the GI tract are controlled locally through a restricted part of the peripheral nervous system called the *ENS*. The ENS comprises components of the sympathetic and parasympathetic nervous systems and has sensory nerve connections through the spinal and nodose ganglia (see Chapter 46 and Furness et al., 2014). The ENS is involved in sensorimotor control and thus consists of both afferent sensory neurons and a number of motor nerves and interneurons that are organized principally into two nerve plexuses: the myenteric (Auerbach) plexus and the submucosal (Meissner) plexus. The myenteric plexus, located between the longitudinal and circular muscle layers, plays an important role in the contraction and relaxation of GI smooth muscle. The submucosal plexus is involved with secretory and absorptive functions of the GI epithelium, local blood flow, and neuroimmune activities.

Parasympathetic preganglionic inputs are provided to the GI tract via the vagus and pelvic nerves. ACh released from *preganglionic neurons* activates nAChRs on postganglionic neurons within the enteric ganglia. Excitatory preganglionic input activates both excitatory and inhibitory motor neurons that control processes such as muscle contraction and secretion/absorption. *Postganglionic sympathetic nerves* also synapse with intrinsic neurons and generally induce relaxation. Sympathetic input is excitatory (contractile) at some sphincters. Information from afferent and preganglionic neural inputs to the enteric ganglia is integrated and distributed by a network of interneurons. ACh is the primary neurotransmitter providing excitatory inputs between interneurons, but other substances, such as ATP (via postjunctional P2X receptors), substance P (by NK_3 receptors), and 5HT (via 5HT3 receptors) are also important in mediating integrative processing via interneurons.

The muscle layers of the GI tract are dually innervated by excitatory and inhibitory motor neurons, with cell bodies primarily in the myenteric ganglia. ACh is a primary excitatory motor neurotransmitter released from postganglionic neurons. ACh activates M_2 and M_3 receptors in postjunctional cells to elicit motor responses. Pharmacological blockade of mAChRs does not block all excitatory neurotransmission, however, because neurokinins (neurokinin A and substance P) are also coreleased by excitatory motor neurons and contribute to postjunctional excitation. Inhibitory motor neurons in the GI tract regulate motility events such as accommodation, sphincter relaxation, and descending receptive relaxation. Inhibitory responses are elicited by a purine derivative (either ATP or β-nicotinamide adenine dinucleotide) acting at postjunctional $P2Y_1$ receptors) and NO. Inhibitory neuropeptides, such as VIP and PACAP, may also be released from inhibitory motor neurons under conditions of strong stimulation.

In general, motor neurons do not directly innervate smooth muscle cells in the GI tract. Nerve terminals make synaptic connections with the interstitial cells of Cajal (ICCs), and these cells make electrical connections (gap junctions) with smooth muscle cells (Ward et al., 2000). Thus, the ICCs are the receptive, postjunctional transducers of inputs from enteric motor neurons, and loss of these cells has been associated with conditions that appear to be neuropathies. ICCs have all of the major receptors and effectors necessary to transduce both excitatory and inhibitory neurotransmitters into postjunctional responses (Chen et al., 2007).

Comparison of Sympathetic, Parasympathetic, and Motor Nerves

Differences among somatic motor, sympathetic, and parasympathetic nerves are shown schematically in Figure 8–2. To summarize:

- The *sympathetic* system is distributed to effectors throughout the body, whereas *parasympathetic* distribution is much more limited.
- A *preganglionic sympathetic fiber* may traverse a considerable distance of the sympathetic chain and pass through several ganglia before it finally synapses with a postganglionic neuron; also, its terminals make contact with a large number of postganglionic neurons. The *parasympathetic system* has terminal ganglia very near or within the organs innervated and is generally more circumscribed in its influences.
- The cell bodies of *somatic motor neurons* reside in the ventral horn of the spinal cord; the axon divides into many branches, each of which innervates a single muscle fiber; more than 100 muscle fibers may be supplied by one motor neuron to form a motor unit. At each NMJ, the axonal terminal loses its myelin sheath and forms a terminal arborization that lies in apposition to a specialized surface of the muscle membrane, termed the *motor end plate* (see Figure 11–3). Reciprocal trophic signals between muscle and nerve regulate the development of the NMJ (Witzemann, 2006).
- Ganglionic organization can differ among the different types of nerves and locales. In some organs innervated by the parasympathetic branch, a 1:1 relationship between the number of preganglionic and postganglionic fibers has been suggested. In sympathetic ganglia, one ganglion cell may be supplied by several preganglionic fibers, and the ratio of preganglionic axons to ganglion cells may be 1:20 or more; this organization permits diffuse discharge of the sympathetic system. The ratio of preganglionic vagal fibers to ganglion cells in the myenteric plexus has been estimated as 1:8000.

A Few Details About Innervation

The terminations of the postganglionic autonomic fibers in smooth muscle and glands form a rich plexus, or terminal reticulum. The terminal reticulum (sometimes called the *autonomic ground plexus*) consists of the final ramifications of the postganglionic sympathetic, parasympathetic, and visceral afferent fibers, all of which are enclosed within a frequently interrupted sheath of satellite or Schwann cells. At these interruptions, varicosities packed with vesicles are seen in the efferent fibers. Such varicosities occur repeatedly but at variable distances along the course of the ramifications of the axon.

"Protoplasmic bridges" occur between the smooth muscle fibers themselves at points of contact between their plasma membranes. They are believed to permit the direct conduction of impulses from cell to cell

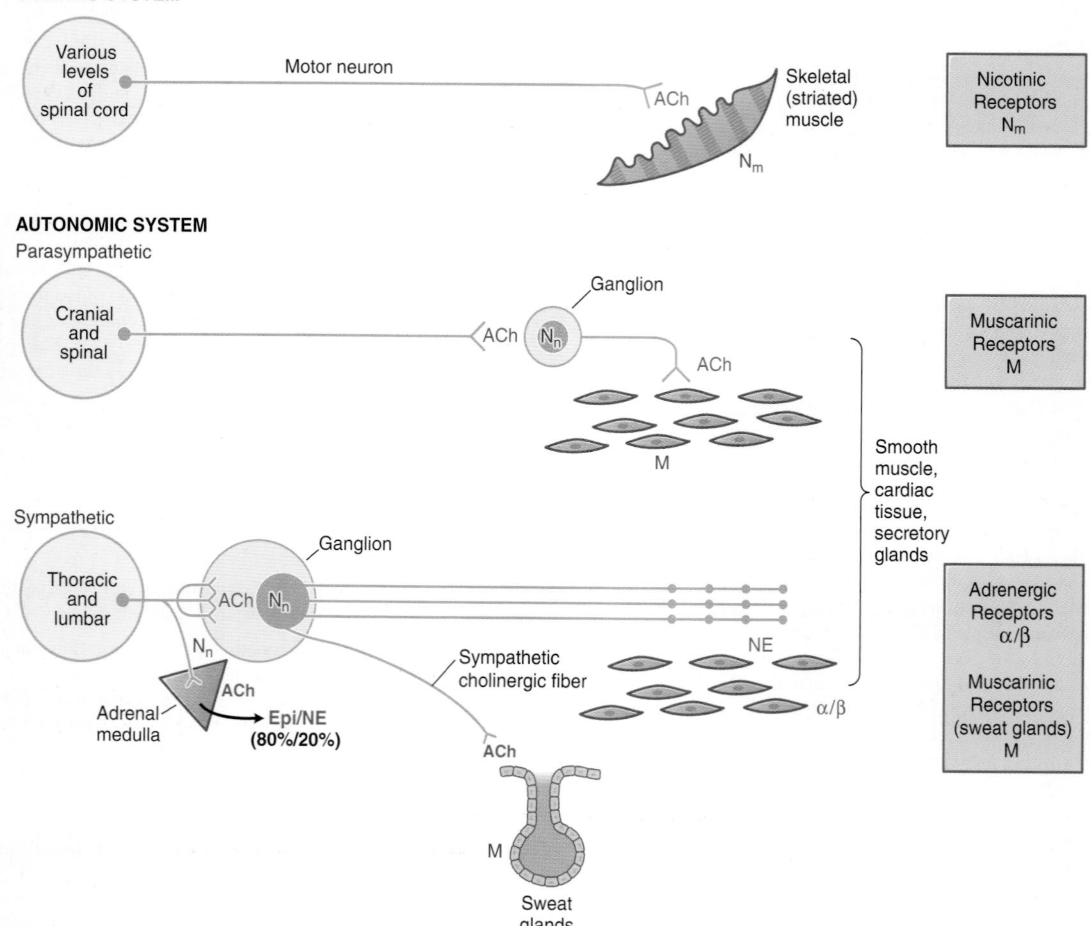

Figure 8–2 *Comparative features of somatic motor nerves and efferent nerves of the autonomic nervous system.* The principal neurotransmitters, ACh and NE, are shown in *red*. The receptors for these transmitters, nicotinic (N) and muscarinic (M) cholinergic receptors, α and β adrenergic receptors, are shown in *green*. Somatic nerves innervate skeletal muscle directly at a specialized synaptic junction, the motor end plate, where ACh activates N_m receptors. Autonomic nerves innervate smooth muscles, cardiac tissue, and glands. Both parasympathetic and sympathetic systems have ganglia, where ACh is released by the preganglionic fibers; ACh acts on N_n receptors on the postganglionic nerves. ACh is also the neurotransmitter at cells of the adrenal medulla, where it acts on N_n receptors to cause release of EPI and NE into the circulation. ACh is the dominant neurotransmitter released by postganglionic parasympathetic nerves and acts on muscarinic receptors. The ganglia in the parasympathetic system are near or within the organ being innervated, with generally a one-to-one relationship between pre- and postganglionic fibers. NE is the principal neurotransmitter of postganglionic sympathetic nerves, acting on α or β adrenergic receptors. Autonomic nerves form a diffuse pattern with multiple synaptic sites. In the sympathetic system, the ganglia are generally far from the effector cells (e.g., within the sympathetic chain ganglia). Preganglionic sympathetic fibers may make contact with a large number of postganglionic fibers.

without the need for chemical transmission. These structures have been termed *nexuses,* or *tight junctions,* and they enable the smooth muscle fibers to function as a syncytial unit.

Sympathetic ganglia are extremely complex anatomically and pharmacologically (see Chapter 11). The preganglionic fibers lose their myelin sheaths and divide repeatedly into a vast number of end fibers with diameters ranging from 0.1 to 0.3 μm; except at points of synaptic contact, they retain their satellite cell sheaths. The vast majority of synapses are axodendritic. Apparently, a given axonal terminal may synapse with multiple dendritic processes.

Responses of Effector Organs to Autonomic Nerve Impulses. *In many instances, the sympathetic and parasympathetic neurotransmitters can be viewed as physiological or functional antagonists* (Table 8–1). Most viscera are innervated by both divisions of the autonomic nervous system, and their activities on specific structures may be either discrete and independent or integrated and interdependent. The effects of sympathetic and parasympathetic stimulation of the heart and the iris show a pattern of functional antagonism in controlling heart rate and pupillary aperture, respectively, whereas their actions on male sexual organs are complementary and are integrated to promote sexual function.

From the responses of the various effector organs to autonomic nerve impulses and the knowledge of the intrinsic autonomic tone, one can predict the actions of drugs that mimic or inhibit the actions of these nerves.

General Functions of the Autonomic Nervous System. *The autonomic nervous system is the primary regulator of the constancy of the internal environment of the organism.*

The *sympathetic system* and its associated adrenal medulla are not essential to life in a controlled environment, but the lack of sympathoadrenal functions becomes evident under circumstances of stress. In the absence of the sympathetic system, body temperature cannot be regulated

HISTORICAL PERSPECTIVE

The earliest concrete proposal of a neurohumoral mechanism was made shortly after the turn of the 20th century. Lewandowsky and Langley independently noted the similarity between the effects of injection of extracts of the adrenal gland and stimulation of sympathetic nerves. In 1905, T. R. Elliott, while a student with Langley at Cambridge, postulated that sympathetic nerve impulses release minute amounts of an EPI-like substance in immediate contact with effector cells. He considered this substance to be the chemical step in the process of transmission. He also noted that long after sympathetic nerves had degenerated, the effector organs still responded characteristically to the hormone of the adrenal medulla. Langley suggested that effector cells have excitatory and inhibitory "receptive substances," and that the response to EPI depended on which type of substance was present. In 1907, Dixon, impressed by the correspondence between the effects of the alkaloid muscarine and the responses to vagal stimulation, advanced the concept that the vagus nerve liberated a muscarine-like substance that acted as a chemical transmitter of its impulses. In the same year, Reid Hunt described the actions of ACh and other choline esters. In 1914, Dale investigated the pharmacological properties of ACh and other choline esters and distinguished its nicotine-like and muscarine-like actions. Intrigued with the remarkable fidelity with which this drug reproduced the responses to stimulation of parasympathetic nerves, he introduced the term *parasympathomimetic* to characterize its effects. Dale also noted the brief duration of action of this chemical and proposed that an esterase in the tissues rapidly splits ACh to acetic acid and choline, thereby terminating its action.

The studies of Loewi, begun in 1921, provided the first direct evidence for the chemical mediation of nerve impulses by the release of specific chemical agents. Loewi stimulated the vagus nerve of a perfused (donor) frog heart and allowed the perfusion fluid to come in contact with a second (recipient) frog heart used as a test object. The recipient frog heart was found to respond, after a short lag, in the same way as the donor heart. It thus was evident that a substance was liberated from the first organ that slowed the rate of the second. Loewi referred to this chemical substance as *Vagusstoff* ("vagus substance," "parasympathin"); subsequently, Loewi and Navratil presented evidence to identify it as ACh. Loewi also discovered that an accelerator substance similar to EPI and called *Acceleranstoff* was liberated into the perfusion fluid in summer, when the action of the sympathetic fibers in the frog's vagus, a mixed nerve, predominated over that of the inhibitory fibers. Feldberg and Krayer demonstrated in 1933 that the cardiac "vagus substance" also is ACh in mammals.

In the same year as Loewi's discovery, Cannon and Uridil reported that stimulation of the sympathetic hepatic nerves resulted in the release of an EPI-like substance that increased blood pressure and heart rate. Subsequent experiments firmly established that this substance is the chemical mediator liberated by sympathetic nerve impulses at neuroeffector junctions. Cannon called this substance "sympathin." In many of its pharmacological and chemical properties, sympathin closely resembled EPI, but also differed in certain important respects. As early as 1910, Barger and Dale noted that the effects of sympathetic nerve stimulation were reproduced more closely by the injection of sympathomimetic primary amines than by that of EPI or other secondary amines. The possibility that demethylated EPI (NE) might be sympathin had been advanced repeatedly, but definitive evidence for its being the sympathetic nerve mediator was not obtained until specific assays were developed for the determination of sympathomimetic amines in extracts of tissues and body fluids. In 1946, von Euler found that the sympathomimetic substance in highly purified extracts of bovine splenic nerve resembled NE by all criteria used (von Euler, 1946).

We now know that NE is the predominant sympathomimetic substance in the postganglionic sympathetic nerves of mammals and is the adrenergic mediator liberated by their stimulation. NE, its immediate precursor DA, and its *N*-methylated derivative EPI also are neurotransmitters in the CNS (see Chapter 14). As for ACh, in addition to its role as the transmitter of most postganglionic parasympathetic fibers and of a few postganglionic sympathetic fibers, ACh functions as a neurotransmitter in three additional classes of nerves: preganglionic fibers of both the sympathetic and the parasympathetic systems, motor nerves to skeletal muscle, and certain neurons within the CNS.

when environmental temperature varies; the concentration of glucose in blood does not rise in response to urgent need; compensatory vascular responses to hemorrhage, oxygen deprivation, excitement, and exercise are lacking; and resistance to fatigue is lessened. Sympathetic components of instinctive reactions to the external environment are lost, and other serious deficiencies in the protective forces of the body are discernible. The sympathetic system normally is continuously active, the degree of activity varying from moment to moment and from organ to organ, adjusting to a constantly changing environment. The sympathoadrenal system can discharge as a unit. Heart rate is accelerated; blood pressure rises; blood flow is shifted from the skin and splanchnic region to the skeletal muscles; blood glucose rises; the bronchioles and pupils dilate; and the organism is better prepared for "fight or flight." Many of these effects result primarily from or are reinforced by the actions of EPI secreted by the adrenal medulla.

The *parasympathetic system* is organized mainly for discrete and localized discharge. Although it is concerned primarily with conservation of energy and maintenance of organ function during periods of minimal activity, its elimination is not compatible with life. The parasympathetic system slows the heart rate, lowers the blood pressure, stimulates GI movements and secretions, aids absorption of nutrients, protects the retina from excessive light, and empties the urinary bladder and rectum.

Neurochemical Transmission

Nerve impulses elicit responses in smooth, cardiac, and skeletal muscles; exocrine glands; and postsynaptic neurons by liberating specific chemical neurotransmitters.

Evidence for Neurohumoral Transmission

The concept of neurohumoral transmission or chemical neurotransmission was developed primarily to explain observations relating to the transmission of impulses from postganglionic autonomic fibers to effector cells. Evidence supporting this concept includes the following:

- demonstration of the presence of a physiologically active compound and its biosynthetic enzymes at appropriate sites;
- recovery of the compound from the perfusate of an innervated structure during periods of nerve stimulation but not (or in greatly reduced amounts) in the absence of stimulation;
- demonstration that the compound is capable of producing responses identical to responses to nerve stimulation; and
- demonstration that the responses to nerve stimulation and to the administered compound are modified in the same manner by various drugs, usually competitive antagonists

While these criteria are applicable for most neurotransmitters, includ-

TABLE 8–1 ■ RESPONSES OF EFFECTOR ORGANS TO AUTONOMIC NERVE IMPULSES

ORGAN SYSTEM	SYMPATHETIC EFFECT[a]	ADRENERGIC RECEPTOR SUBTYPE[b]	PARASYMPATHETIC EFFECT[a]	CHOLINERGIC RECEPTOR SUBTYPE[b]
Eye				
Radial muscle, iris	Contraction (mydriasis)++	α_1		
Sphincter muscle, iris			Contraction (miosis)+++	M_3, M_2
Ciliary muscle	Relaxation for far vision+	β_2	Contraction for near vision+++	M_3, M_2
Lacrimal glands	Secretion+	α	Secretion+++	M_3, M_2
Heart[c]				
Sinoatrial node	↑ heart rate++	$\beta_1 > \beta_2$	↓ heart rate+++	$M_2 >> M_3$
Atria	↑ contractility and conduction velocity++	$\beta_1 > \beta_2$	↓ contractility++ and shortened AP duration	$M_2 >> M_3$
Atrioventricular node	↑ automaticity and conduction velocity++	$\beta_1 > \beta_2$	↓ conduction velocity; AV block+++	$M_2 >> M_3$
His-Purkinje system	↑ automaticity and conduction velocity	$\beta_1 > \beta_2$	Little effect	$M_2 >> M_3$
Ventricle	↑ contractility, conduction velocity, automaticity, and rate of idioventricular pacemakers+++	$\beta_1 > \beta_2$	Slight ↓ in contractility	$M_2 >> M_3$
Blood vessels				
Arteries and arterioles[d]				
Coronary	Constriction+; dilation[e]++	α_1, α_2; β_2	No innervation[h]	—
Skin and mucosa	Constriction+++	α_1, α_2	No innervation[h]	—
Skeletal muscle	Constriction; dilation[e,f]++	α_1; β_2	Dilation[h] (?)	—
Cerebral	Constriction (slight)	α_1	No innervation[h]	—
Pulmonary	Constriction+; dilation	α_1; β_2	No innervation[h]	—
Abdominal viscera	Constriction+++; dilation+	α_1; β_2	No innervation[h]	—
Salivary glands	Constriction+++	α_1, α_2	Dilation[h]++	M_3
Renal	Constriction++; dilation++	α_1, α_2; β_1, β_2	No innervation[h]	
(Veins)[d]	Constriction; dilation	α_1, α_2; β_2		
Endothelium	—	—	↑ NO synthase[h]	M_3
Lung				
Tracheal and bronchial smooth muscle	Relaxation	β_2	Contraction	$M_2 = M_3$
Bronchial glands	↓ secretion, ↑ secretion	α_1	Stimulation	M_2, M_3
		β_2		
Stomach				
Motility and tone	↓ (usually)[i]+	α_1, α_2, β_1, β_2	↑[i]+++	$M_2 = M_3$
Sphincters	Contraction (usually)+	α_1	Relaxation (usually)+	M_3, M_2
Secretion	Inhibition	α_2	Stimulation++	M_3, M_2
Intestine				
Motility and tone	Decrease[h]+	α_1, α_2, β_1, β_2	↑[i]+++	M_3, M_2
Sphincters	Contraction+	α_1	Relaxation (usually)+	M_3, M_2
Secretion	↓	α_2	↑++	M_3, M_2
Gallbladder and ducts kidney	Relaxation+	β_2	Contraction+	M
Renin secretion	↓+; ↑++	α_1; β_1	No innervation	—
Urinary bladder				
Detrusor	Relaxation+	β_2	Contraction+++	$M_3 > M_2$
Trigone and sphincter	Contraction++	α_1	Relaxation++	$M_3 > M_2$

(Continued)

TABLE 8–1 ■ RESPONSES OF EFFECTOR ORGANS TO AUTONOMIC NERVE IMPULSES(*CONTINUED*)

ORGAN SYSTEM	SYMPATHETIC EFFECT[a]	ADRENERGIC RECEPTOR SUBTYPE[b]	PARASYMPATHETIC EFFECT[a]	CHOLINERGIC RECEPTOR SUBTYPE[b]
Ureter				
Motility and tone	↑	α_1	↑ (?)	M
Uterus	Pregnant contraction	α_1		
	Relaxation	β_2	Variable[j]	M
	Nonpregnant relaxation	β_2		
Sex organs, male skin	Ejaculation+++	α_1	Erection+++	M_3
Pilomotor muscles	Contraction++	α_1	—	
Sweat glands	Localized secretion[k]++	α_1	—	
	—		Generalized secretion+++	M_3, M_2
Spleen capsule	Contraction+++	α_1	—	—
	Relaxation+	β_2	—	
Adrenal medulla	—		Secretion of EPI and NE	N $(\alpha_3)_2(\beta_4)_3$; M (secondarily)
Skeletal muscle	Increased contractility; glycogenolysis; K^+ uptake	β_2	—	—
Liver	Glycogenolysis and gluconeogenesis+++	α_1	—	—
		β_2		
Pancreas				
Acini	↓ secretion+	α	Secretion++	M_3, M_2
Islets (β cells)	↓ secretion+++	α_2	—	
	↑ secretion+	β_2		
Fat cells[l]	Lipolysis+++; thermogenesis	α_1, β_1, β_2, β_3	—	—
	Inhibition of lipolysis	α_2		
Salivary glands	K^+ and water secretion+	α_1	K^+ and water secretion+++	M_3, M_2
Nasopharyngeal glands	—		Secretion++	M_3, M_2
Pineal glands	Melatonin synthesis	β	—	
Posterior pituitary	ADH secretion	β_1	—	
Autonomic nerve endings				
Sympathetic terminal				
Autoreceptor	Inhibition of NE release	$\alpha_{2A} > \alpha_{2C}(\alpha_{2B})$		
Heteroreceptor	—		Inhibition of NE release	M_2, M_4
Parasympathetic terminal				
Autoreceptor	—	—	Inhibition of ACh release	M_2, M_4
Heteroreceptor	Inhibition ACh release	$\alpha_{2A} > \alpha_{2C}$	—	—

[a]Responses are designated + to +++ to provide an approximate indication of the importance of sympathetic and parasympathetic nerve activity in the control of the various organs and functions listed.

[b]Adrenergic receptors: α_1, α_2 and subtypes thereof; β_1, β_2, β_3. Cholinergic receptors: nicotinic (N); muscarinic (M), with subtypes 1–4. The receptor subtypes are described more fully in Chapters 9 and 12 and in Tables 8–2, 8–3, 8–6, and 8–7. When a designation of subtype is not provided, the nature of the subtype has not been determined unequivocally. Only the principal receptor subtypes are shown. Transmitters other than ACh and NE contribute to many of the responses.

[c]In the human heart, the ratio of β_1 to β_2 is about 3:2 in atria and 4:1 in ventricles. While M_2 receptors predominate, M_3 receptors are also present (Wang et al., 2004).

[d]The predominant α_1 receptor subtype in most blood vessels (both arteries and veins) is α_{1A}, although other α_1 subtypes are present in specific blood vessels. The α_{1D} is the predominant subtype in the aorta (Michelotti et al., 2000).

[e]Dilation predominates in situ owing to metabolic autoregulatory mechanisms.

[f]Over the usual concentration range of physiologically released circulating EPI, the β receptor response (vasodilation) predominates in blood vessels of skeletal muscle and liver; β receptor response (vasoconstriction) predominates in blood vessels of other abdominal viscera. The renal and mesenteric vessels also contain specific dopaminergic receptors whose activation causes dilation.

[g]Sympathetic cholinergic neurons cause vasodilation in skeletal muscle beds, but this is not involved in most physiological responses.

[h]The endothelium of most blood vessels releases NO, which causes vasodilation in response to muscarinic stimuli. However, unlike the receptors innervated by sympathetic cholinergic fibers in skeletal muscle blood vessels, these muscarinic receptors are not innervated and respond only to exogenously added muscarinic agonists in the circulation.

[i]While adrenergic fibers terminate at inhibitory β receptors on smooth muscle fibers and at inhibitory β receptors on parasympathetic (cholinergic) excitatory ganglion cells of the myenteric plexus, the primary inhibitory response is mediated via enteric neurons through NO, P2Y receptors, and peptide receptors.

[j]Uterine responses depend on stages of menstrual cycle, amount of circulating estrogen and progesterone, and other factors.

[k]Palms of hands and some other sites ("adrenergic sweating").

[l]There is significant variation among species in the receptor types that mediate certain metabolic responses. All three β adrenergic receptors have been found in human fat cells. Activation of β_3 receptors produces a vigorous thermogenic response as well as lipolysis. The significance is unclear. Activation of β receptors also inhibits leptin release from adipose tissue.

ing NE and ACh, there are now exceptions to these general rules. For instance, NO has been found to be a neurotransmitter, in a few postganglionic parasympathetic nerves; in NANC neurons in the periphery; in the ENS; and in the CNS. However, NO is not stored in neurons and released by exocytosis. Rather, it is synthesized when needed and readily diffuses across membranes.

Neurotransmission in the peripheral nervous system and CNS once was believed to conform to the hypothesis that each neuron contains only one transmitter substance. However, we now find that synaptic transmission may be mediated by the release of more than one neurotransmitter. Additional peptides, such as enkephalin, substance P, NPY, VIP, and SST; purines such as ATP and adenosine; and small molecules such as NO have been found in nerve endings along with the "classical" biogenic amine neurotransmitters. These additional substances can depolarize or hyperpolarize nerve terminals or postsynaptic cells. For example, enkephalins are found in postganglionic sympathetic neurons and adrenal medullary chromaffin cells. VIP is localized selectively in peripheral cholinergic neurons that innervate exocrine glands, and NPY is found in sympathetic nerve endings. These observations suggest that synaptic transmission in many instances may be mediated by the release of more than one neurotransmitter (see the next section).

Steps Involved in Neurotransmission

The sequence of events involved in neurotransmission is of particular importance because pharmacologically active agents modulate the individual steps.

Axonal Conduction

Conduction refers to the passage of an electrical impulse along an axon or muscle fiber. At rest, the interior of the typical mammalian axon is about 70 mV negative to the exterior. In response to depolarization to a threshold level, an action potential is initiated at a local region of the membrane. The action potential consists of two phases. Following depolarization that induces an open conformation of the channel, the *initial phase* is caused by a rapid increase in the permeability and inward movement of Na^+ through voltage-sensitive Na^+ channels, and a rapid depolarization from the resting potential continues to a positive overshoot. The *second phase* results from the rapid inactivation of the Na^+ channel and the delayed opening of a K^+ channel, which permits outward movement of K^+ to terminate the depolarization. Although not important in axonal conduction, Ca^{2+} channels in other tissues (e.g., L-type Ca^{2+} channels in heart) contribute to the action potential by prolonging depolarization by an inward movement of Ca^{2+}. This influx of Ca^{2+} also serves as a stimulus to initiate intracellular events (Catterall, 2000), and Ca^{2+} influx is important in excitation-exocytosis coupling (transmitter release).

The transmembrane ionic currents produce local circuit currents such that adjacent resting channels in the axon are activated, and excitation of an adjacent portion of the axonal membrane occurs, leading to propagation of the action potential without decrement along the axon. The region that has undergone depolarization remains momentarily in a refractory state.

With the exception of the local anesthetics, few drugs modify axonal conduction in the doses employed therapeutically. The puffer fish poison,

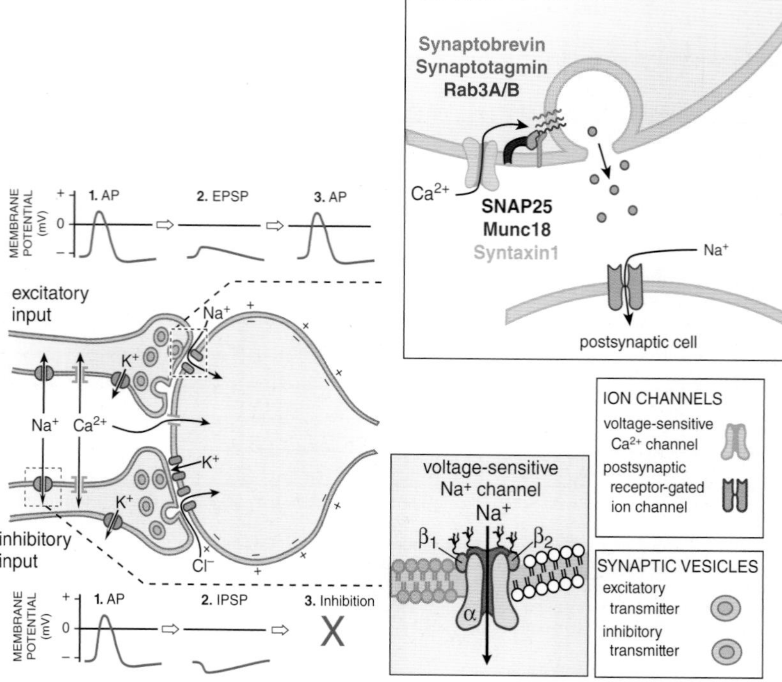

Figure 8–3 *Steps involved in excitatory and inhibitory neurotransmission.* ***1.*** The nerve AP consists of a transient self-propagated reversal of charge on the axonal membrane. (The internal potential E_i goes from a negative value, through zero potential, to a slightly positive value, primarily through increases in Na^+ permeability, and then returns to resting values by an increase in K^+ permeability.) When the AP arrives at the presynaptic terminal, it initiates release of the excitatory or inhibitory transmitter. Depolarization at the nerve ending and entry of Ca^{2+} initiate docking and then fusion of the synaptic vesicle with the membrane of the nerve ending. Some of the SNARE proteins involved in docking and fusion are shown. Figures 8–4 and 8–5 show some additional details of the life cycle of neurotransmitter storage vesicle and exocytosis. ***2.*** Interaction of the excitatory transmitter with postsynaptic receptors produces a localized depolarization, the EPSP, through an increase in permeability to cations, most notably Na^+. The inhibitory transmitter causes a selective increase in permeability to K^+ or Cl^-, resulting in a localized hyperpolarization, the IPSP. ***3.*** The EPSP initiates a conducted AP in the postsynaptic neuron; this can be prevented, however, by the hyperpolarization induced by a concurrent IPSP. The transmitter is dissipated by enzymatic destruction, by reuptake into the presynaptic terminal or adjacent glial cells, or by diffusion. Depolarization of the postsynaptic membrane can permit Ca^{2+} entry if voltage-gated Ca^{2+} channels are present.

tetrodotoxin, and a close congener found in some shellfish, *saxitoxin*, selectively block axonal conduction by blocking the voltage-sensitive Na^+ channel and preventing the increase in Na^+ permeability associated with the rising phase of the action potential. In contrast, *batrachotoxin*, an extremely potent steroidal alkaloid secreted by a South American frog, produces paralysis through a selective increase in permeability of the Na^+ channel, which induces a persistent depolarization. Scorpion toxins are peptides that also cause persistent depolarization by inhibiting the inactivation process (Catterall, 2000). Na^+ and Ca^{2+} channels are discussed in more detail in Chapters 11, 14, and 22.

Junctional Transmission

The term *transmission* refers to the passage of an impulse across a synaptic or neuroeffector junction. The arrival of the action potential at the axonal terminals initiates a series of events that trigger transmission of an excitatory or inhibitory biochemical message across the synapse or neuroeffector junction. These events, diagrammed in Figures 8–3, 8–4, and 8–5, are the following:

5. *Storage and release of transmitter.* The nonpeptide (small-molecule) neurotransmitters, such as biogenic amines, are largely synthesized in the region of the axonal terminals and stored there in synaptic vesicles. Neurotransmitter transport into storage vesicles is driven by an electrochemical gradient generated by the vesicular proton pump (vesicular ATPase) (Figures 8–5 and 8–6). Synaptic vesicles cluster in discrete areas underlying the presynaptic plasma membrane, termed *active zones*, often aligning with the tips of postsynaptic folds. Proteins in the vesicular membrane (e.g., synapsin, synaptophysin, synaptogyrin) are involved in development and trafficking of the storage vesicle to the active zone. The processes of priming, docking, fusion, and exocytosis involve the interactions of proteins in the vesicular and plasma membranes and the rapid entry of extracellular Ca^{2+} and its binding to synaptotagmins (Figure 8–4).

Life Cycle of a Storage Vesicle; Molecular Mechanism of Exocytosis. Fusion of the storage vesicle and plasma membrane involves formation of a multiprotein complex that includes proteins in the membrane of the synaptic vesicle, proteins embedded in the inner surface of the plasma membrane, and several cytosolic components. These proteins are referred to as SNARE proteins. Through the assembly of these proteins, vesicles draw near the membrane (priming, docking), spatially prepared for the next step, which the entry of Ca^{2+} initiates. When Ca^{2+} enters with the action potential, fusion and exocytosis occur rapidly. After fusion, the chaperone ATPase NSF and its SNAP adapters catalyze dissociation of the SNARE complex. Figures 8–4 and 8–5 depict this life cycle. Figure 8–4 shows some details of the assembly of the SNARE protein complex leading to fusion and exocytosis of neurotransmitter. The isoforms of the participating proteins may differ in different neurotransmitter systems, but the general mechanism seems to be conserved.

During the resting state, there is continual slow release of isolated quanta of the transmitter; this produces electrical responses (*miniature*

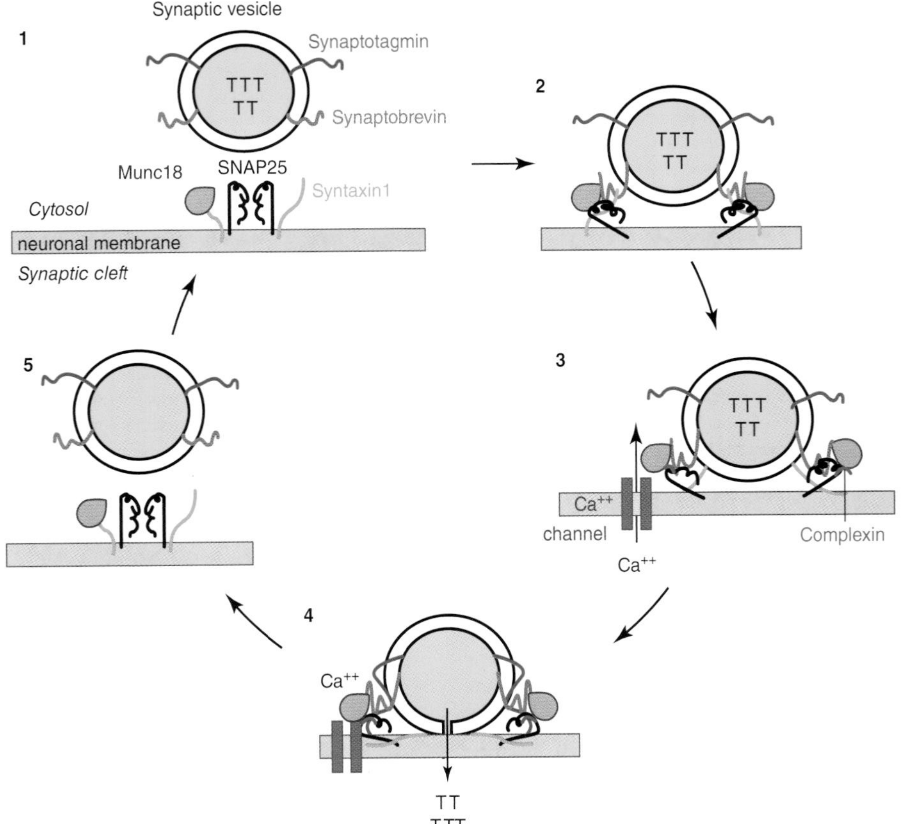

Figure 8–4 *Molecular basis of exocytosis: docking and fusion of synaptic vesicles with neuronal membranes.* **1.** *Vesicular docking in the active zone*: Munc18 binds to syntaxin 1, stabilizing the neuronal membrane SNARE proteins. **2.** *Priming I*: Syntaxin assembles with SNAP25, allowing for the vesicle SNARE protein synaptobrevin to bind to the complex. **3.** *Priming II*: Complexin binds to the SNARE complex and allows for the vesicular synaptotagmin to bind Ca^{2+} that drives the full fusion process. **4.** *Fusion pore opening*: Synaptotagmin interacts with the SNARE complex and binds Ca^{2+}, permitting pore fusion and exocytosis of neurotransmitter. Other components, not shown, are the vesicular GTP-binding Rab3/27; the linking proteins Munc13, RIM, and RIM-BP; and tethering to the Ca^{2+} channel. **5.** *Return to ground state*: After fusion, the chaperone ATPase NSF and its SNAP adapters catalyze dissociation of the SNARE-complex. For a more detailed view of this process, see Südhof (2014).

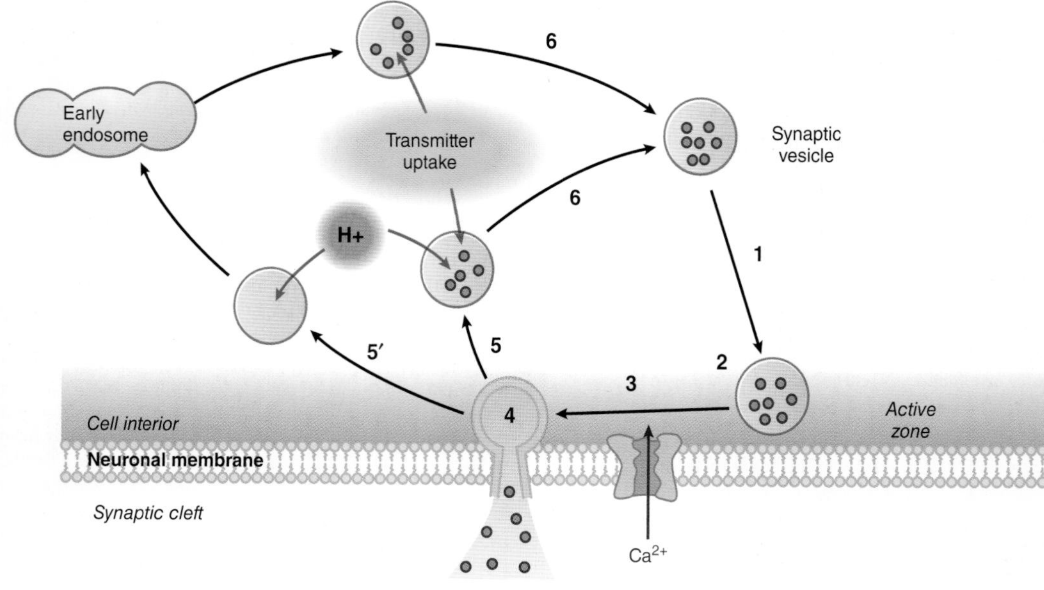

Figure 8–5 *Life cycle of a synaptic vesicle.* A mature storage vesicle, replete with transmitter, is translocated to the perimembrane space (*active zone*) (**1**). Once in the active zone (**2**), the vesicle undergoes docking and priming (see Figure 8–4), as proteins from the cytosol and the vesicular and plasma membranes (SNARE proteins) interact to tether the vesicle in a prefusion stage. The rapid entry of Ca^{2+} via voltage-sensitive channels located in the active zone (**3**) activates the calcium sensor synaptotagmin and initiates the process of fusion and exocytosis of the vesicular contents into the synaptic space (**4**). After transmitter release, the vesicle is endocytosed, the SNARE protein complex is disassembled by the action of the chaperone ATPase NSF and its SNAP adapters, and the empty vesicle is recycled, either trafficked directly back into use (**5**) or routed through an early endosomal pathway (**5′**). In either event, the vesicular ATPase is at work, promoting H^+ uptake to establish the gradient that drives transmitter uptake and repletion of the vesicle (**6**). For a more detailed view of the exocytotic process, see Südhof (2014). Secreted neuropeptides are stored in larger, dense core vesicles (see text). Their secretory process is similar; however, there are no uptake transporters for peptide neurotransmitters; rather, vesicles containing releasable peptides are formed in the trans-Golgi network of the nerve cell body and transported to the release site by molecular motors (kinesins, F-actin, etc.); nonsecreted vesicle components are recycled. Park and Loh (2008), Heaslip et al. (2014), and Salogiannis and Reck-Peterson (2016) have reviewed aspects of the transport of such vesicles.

end-plate potentials or *mepps*) at the postjunctional membrane that are associated with the maintenance of the physiological responsiveness of the effector organ. A low level of spontaneous activity within the motor units of skeletal muscle is particularly important because skeletal muscle lacks inherent tone.

The action potential causes the synchronous release of several hundred quanta of neurotransmitter. In the fusion/exocytosis process, the contents of the vesicles, including enzymes and other proteins, are discharged to the synaptic space. Synaptic vesicles may either fully exocytose with complete fusion or form a transient, nanometer-size pore that closes after transmitter has escaped, "kiss-and-run" exocytosis. In full-fusion exocytosis, the pit formed by the vesicle's fusing with the plasma membrane is clathrin-coated and retrieved from the membrane via endocytosis and transported to an endosome for full recycling. During kiss-and-run exocytosis, the pore closes, and the vesicle is immediately and locally recycled for reuse in neurotransmitter repackaging (Alabi and Tsien, 2013; Südhof, 2014).

Modulation of Transmitter Release. A number of autocrine and paracrine factors may influence the exocytotic process, including the released neurotransmitter itself. Adenosine, DA, glutamate, GABA, prostaglandins, and enkephalins influence neurally mediated release of neurotransmitters. Receptors for these factors exist in the membranes of the soma, dendrites, and axons of neurons (Miller, 1998; Westfall, 2004): *Soma-dendritic receptors*, when activated, primarily modify functions of the soma-dendritic region, such as protein synthesis and generation of action potentials. *Presynaptic receptors*, when activated, modify functions of the terminal region, such as synthesis and release of transmitters.

Two main classes of presynaptic receptors have been identified on most neurons: *Heteroreceptors* are presynaptic receptors that respond to neurotransmitters, neuromodulators, or neurohormones released from adjacent neurons or cells. For example, NE can influence the release of ACh from parasympathetic neurons by acting on α_{2A}, α_{2B}, and α_{2C} receptors, whereas ACh can influence the release of NE from sympathetic neurons by acting on M_2 and M_4 receptors. *Autoreceptors* are receptors located on or close to axon terminals of a neuron through which the neuron's own transmitter can modify transmitter synthesis and release (see Figures 8–6 and 8–8). For example, NE released from sympathetic neurons may interact with α_{2A} and α_{2C} receptors to inhibit neurally released NE. Similarly, ACh released from parasympathetic neurons may interact with M_2 and M_4 receptors to inhibit neurally released ACh.

6. *Interaction of the transmitter with postjunctional receptors and production of the postjunctional potential.* The transmitter diffuses across the synaptic or junctional cleft and combines with specialized receptors on the postjunctional membrane; this often results in a localized increase in the ionic permeability, or conductance, of the membrane. With certain exceptions (noted in the following discussion), one of three types of permeability change can occur:

- Generalized increase in the permeability to cations (notably Na^+ but occasionally Ca^{2+}), resulting in a localized depolarization of the membrane, that is, an EPSP.

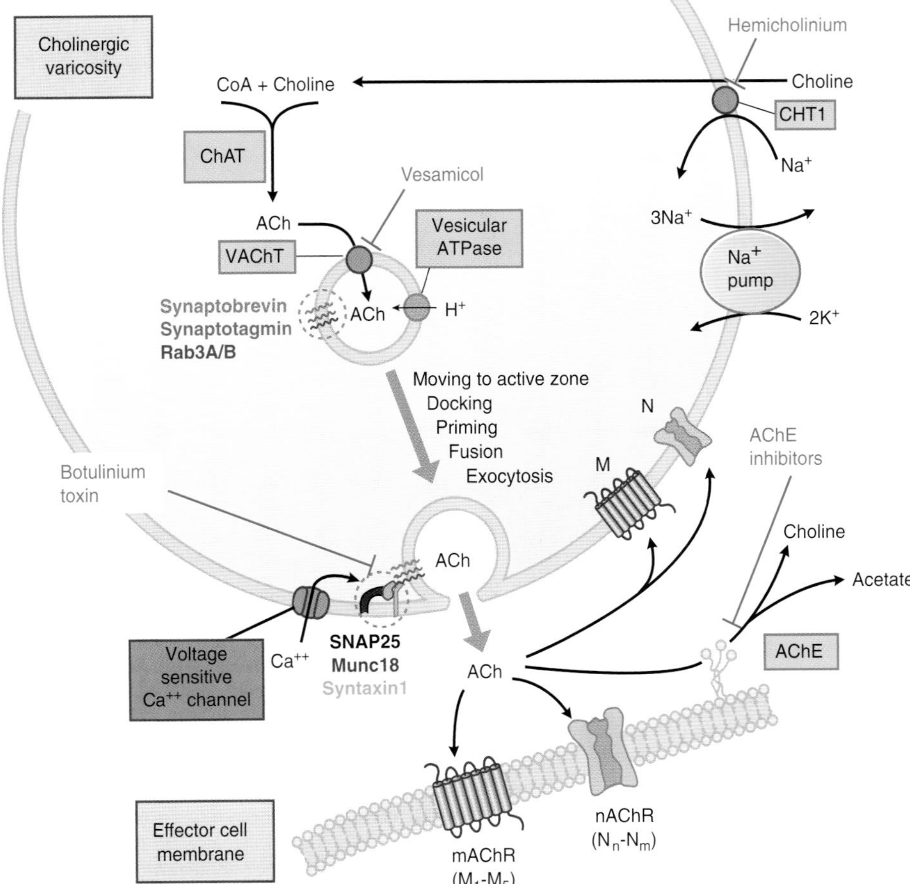

Figure 8–6 *A typical cholinergic neuroeffector junction.* The synthesis of ACh in the varicosity depends on the uptake of choline via a Na^+-dependent carrier, CHT1, that hemicholinium can block. The enzyme ChAT catalyzes the synthesis of ACh from choline and the acetyl moiety of acetyl CoA. ACh is transported into the storage vesicle by VAChT, which can be inhibited by vesamicol. ACh is stored in vesicles (along with other potential cotransmitters, such as ATP and VIP, at certain neuroeffector junctions). Release of ACh and any cotransmitters occurs via exocytosis (the stages are itemized along the gray arrow), triggered by Ca^{2+} entry via a voltage-sensitive Ca^{2+} channel in response to membrane depolarization, as described in Figures 8–3, 8–4, and 8–5. Exocytotic release of ACh at the NMJ can be blocked by botulinum toxins, the active fragments of which are endopeptidases that cleave synaptobrevin, an essential member of the SNARE proteins that mediate docking/priming/exocytosis. Once released, ACh can interact with the muscarinic receptors (M), which are GPCRs, or nicotinic receptors (N), which are ligand-gated ion channels, to produce the characteristic response of the postsynaptic cell. ACh also can act on presynaptic mAChRs or nAChRs to modify its own release. The action of ACh is terminated by extracellular metabolism to choline and acetate by AChE, which is associated with synaptic membranes.

- Selective increase in permeability to anions, usually Cl^-, resulting in stabilization or actual hyperpolarization of the membrane, which constitutes an IPSP.
- Increased permeability to K^+. Because the K^+ gradient is directed out of the cell, hyperpolarization and stabilization of the membrane potential occur (an IPSP).

Electric potential changes associated with the EPSP and IPSP at most sites are the results of passive fluxes of ions down their concentration gradients. The changes in channel permeability that cause these potential changes are specifically regulated by the specialized postjunctional receptors for the neurotransmitter that initiates the response (see Figures 8–6, 8–8, and 11–4 and Chapter 14). These receptors may be clustered on the effector cell surface, as seen at the NMJs of skeletal muscle and other discrete synapses, or distributed more uniformly, as observed in smooth muscle. These *high-conductance, ligand-gated ion channels* usually permit passage of Na^+ or Cl^-; K^+ and Ca^{2+} are involved less frequently. In the presence of an appropriate neurotransmitter, the channel opens rapidly to a high-conductance state, remains open for about a millisecond, and then closes. A short square-wave pulse of current is observed as a result of the channel's opening and closing. The summation of these microscopic events gives rise to the EPSP.

The ligand-gated channels belong to a superfamily of ionotropic receptor proteins that includes the nicotinic, glutamate, and certain 5HT3 and purine receptors, which conduct primarily Na^+, cause depolarization, and are excitatory; and GABA acid and glycine receptors, which conduct Cl^-, cause hyperpolarization, and are inhibitory. Neurotransmitters also can modulate the permeability of K^+ and Ca^{2+} channels indirectly. In these cases, the receptor and channel are separate proteins, and information is conveyed between them by G proteins (see Chapter 3).

The nicotinic, GABA, glycine, and 5HT3 receptors are closely related, whereas the glutamate and purinergic ionotropic receptors have distinct structures (see Figure 11–1 and Chapter 14). Neurotransmitters also can modulate the permeability of K^+ and Ca^{2+} channels indirectly. In these cases, the receptor and channel are separate proteins, and information is conveyed between them by G proteins. Other receptors for neurotransmitters act by influencing the synthesis of intracellular second messengers and do not necessarily cause a change in membrane potential. The most widely documented examples of receptor regulation of second-messenger systems are the activation or inhibition of adenylyl cyclase to modulate cellular cAMP concentrations and the increase in cytosolic concentrations of Ca^{2+} that results from release of the ion from internal stores by inositol trisphosphate (see Chapter 3).

7. *Initiation of postjunctional activity*. If an EPSP exceeds a certain threshold value, it initiates a propagated action potential in a postsynaptic neuron or a muscle action potential in skeletal or cardiac muscle by activating voltage-sensitive channels in the immediate vicinity. In certain smooth muscle types in which propagated impulses are minimal, an EPSP may increase the rate of spontaneous depolarization, cause Ca^{2+} release, and enhance muscle tone; in gland cells, the EPSP initiates secretion through Ca^{2+} mobilization. An IPSP, which is found in neurons and smooth muscle but not in skeletal muscle, will tend to oppose excitatory potentials simultaneously initiated by other neuronal sources. Whether a propagated impulse or other response ensues depends on the summation of all the potentials.
8. *Destruction or dissipation of the transmitter*. When impulses can be transmitted across junctions at frequencies up to several hundred per second, there must be an efficient means of disposing of the transmitter following each impulse. At cholinergic synapses involved in rapid neurotransmission, high and localized concentrations of AChE are available for this purpose. When AChE activity is inhibited, removal of the transmitter is accomplished principally by diffusion. Under these circumstances, the effects of released ACh are potentiated and prolonged (see Chapter 10).

   Rapid termination of NE occurs by a combination of simple diffusion and reuptake by the axonal terminals of most of the released NE. Termination of the action of amino acid transmitters results from their active transport into neurons and surrounding glia. Peptide neurotransmitters are hydrolyzed by various peptidases and dissipated by diffusion.
9. *Nonelectrogenic functions*. The activity and turnover of enzymes involved in the synthesis and inactivation of neurotransmitters, the density of presynaptic and postsynaptic receptors, and other characteristics of synapses are controlled by trophic actions of neurotransmitters or other trophic factors released by the neuron or target cells.

Cholinergic Transmission

The neurochemical events that underlie cholinergic neurotransmission are summarized in Figure 8–6.

Synthesis and Storage of ACh

Two enzymes, choline acetyltransferase and AChE, are involved in ACh synthesis and degradation, respectively.

Choline Acetyltransferase. *Choline acetyltransferase* catalyzes the synthesis of ACh—the acetylation of choline with acetyl CoA. Choline acetyltransferase is synthesized within the perikaryon and then is transported along the length of the axon to its terminal. Axonal terminals contain a large number of mitochondria, where acetyl CoA is synthesized. Choline is taken up from the extracellular fluid into the axoplasm by active transport. The final step in the synthesis occurs within the cytoplasm, following which most of the ACh is sequestered within synaptic vesicles. Although moderately potent inhibitors of choline acetyltransferase exist, they have no therapeutic utility, in part because the rate-limiting step in ACh biosynthesis is the uptake of choline.

Choline and Choline Transport. The availability of choline is critical to the synthesis of ACh. Choline must be derived primarily from the diet (there is little de novo synthesis of choline in cholinergic neurons) or, secondarily, from recycling of choline. Once ACh is released from cholinergic neurons in response to an action potential, ACh is hydrolyzed by AChE to acetate and choline. Much of the choline is taken up at cholinergic nerve terminals and reused for ACh synthesis. Under many circumstances, this reuptake and availability of choline appear to be rate limiting in ACh synthesis. There are three mammalian transport systems for choline; all three are transmembrane proteins with multiple TM segments; all are inhibited by hemicholinium but at distinct concentrations in the same order as their affinities for choline (Haga, 2014):

- The high-affinity (4-μM) choline transporter CHT1 (SLC5A7) present on presynaptic membranes of cholinergic neurons. This transporter is a member of the SLC5 family of solute carrier proteins that includes Na^+-glucose cotransporters and shares about 25% homology with those transporters (Haga, 2014). Choline transport by CHT1 is Na^+ and Cl^- dependent. This system provides choline for ACh synthesis and is the high-affinity hemicholinium-binding protein (K_i = 0.05 μM).
- A low-affinity (40-μM), Na^+-independent transporter, CTL1 (SLC44A), which is widely distributed and appears to supply choline for phospholipid synthesis (e.g., phosphatidyl choline, sphigomyelin).
- A lower-affinity (100-μM) Na^+-independent transporter, OCT2 (SLC22A2), a nonspecific organic cation secretory transporter found in renal proximal tubules (see Figures 5–8 and 5–9), hepatocytes, the choroid plexus, the lumenal membrane of brain endothelium, and synaptic vesicles from cholinergic neurons. Its role in neurons remains to be clarified.

In model systems, CHT1 localizes mainly to intracellular organelles, including transmitter storage vesicles; neural activity increases the fraction of CHT1 in the plasma membrane, and phosphorylation by PKC enhances internalization (Haga, 2014).

Storage of ACh. ACh is transported into synaptic vesicles by the VAChT (a solute carrier protein, SLC18A3) using the potential energy of a proton electrochemical gradient that a vacuolar ATPase establishes, such that the transport of protons out of the vesicle is coupled to uptake of ACh into the vesicle and against a concentration gradient. The process is inhibited by the noncompetitive and reversible inhibitor *vesamicol*, which does not affect the vesicular ATPase (Figure 8–6). The gene for choline acetyltransferase and the vesicular transporter are found at the same locus, with the transporter gene positioned in the first intron of the transferase gene. Hence, a common promoter regulates the expression of both genes (Eiden, 1998).

There appear to be two types of vesicles in cholinergic terminals: electron-lucent vesicles (40–50 nm in diameter) and dense-cored vesicles (80–150 nm). The core of the vesicles contains both ACh and ATP, at a ratio of about 11:1, which are dissolved in the fluid phase with metal ions (Ca^{2+} and Mg^{2+}) and a proteoglycan called vesiculin. Vesiculin, negatively charged and thought to sequester the Ca^{2+} or ACh, is bound within the vesicle, with the protein moiety anchoring it to the vesicular membrane. In some cholinergic terminals, there are peptides, such as VIP, that act as *cotransmitters*. The peptides usually are located in the dense-cored vesicles.

Estimates of the ACh content of synaptic vesicles range from 1000 to over 50,000 molecules per vesicle, with a single motor nerve terminal containing 300,000 or more vesicles. In addition, an uncertain but possibly significant amount of ACh is present in the extravesicular cytoplasm. Recording the electrical events associated with the opening of single channels at the motor end plate during continuous application of ACh has permitted estimation of the potential change induced by a single molecule of ACh (3×10^{-7} V); from such calculations, it is evident that even the lower estimate of the ACh content per vesicle (1000 molecules) is sufficient to account for the magnitude of the miniature end-plate potentials.

Release of ACh. Exocytotic release of ACh and cotransmitters (e.g., ATP, VIP) occurs on depolarization of the nerve terminals. Depolarization of the terminals allows the entry of Ca^{2+} through voltage-gated Ca^{2+} channels and promotes fusion of the vesicular membrane with the plasma membrane, allowing exocytosis to occur, as described previously and in Figure 8–6.

Two pools of ACh appear to exist. One pool, the "depot" or "readily releasable" pool, consists of vesicles located near the plasma membrane of the nerve terminals; these vesicles contain newly synthesized transmitter. Depolarization of the terminals causes these vesicles to release ACh rapidly or readily. The other pool, the "reserve pool," seems to replenish the readily releasable pool and may be required to sustain ACh release during periods of prolonged or intense nerve stimulation.

Botulinum toxin blocks ACh release by interfering with the machinery of transmitter release. The active fragments of botulinum toxins are endopeptidases; the SNARE proteins are their substrates. There are eight isotypes of botulinum toxin, each cleaving a specific site on SNARE proteins. Tetanus toxins act similarly, but in the CNS. The active fragments of these toxins cleave synaptobrevin and block exocytosis in specific sets of neurons (inhibitory neurons in the CNS for tetanus, the NMJ for botulinum).

Acetylcholinesterase. At the NMJ, immediate hydrolysis of ACh by AChE reduces lateral diffusion of the transmitter and activation of adjacent receptors. Rapid release of ACh onto the nAChRs of the motor end plate, followed by rapid hydrolysis of the neurotransmitter, spatially limits receptor activation and facilitates rapid control of responses. The time required for hydrolysis of ACh at the NMJ is less than a millisecond. Chapter 10 presents details of the structure, mechanism, and inhibition of AChE.

AChE is found in cholinergic neurons and is highly concentrated at the postsynaptic end plate of the NMJ. BuChE (butyrylcholinesterase, also called pseudocholinesterase) is virtually absent in neuronal elements of the central and peripheral nervous systems. BuChE is synthesized primarily in the liver and is found in liver and plasma; its likely physiological function is the hydrolysis of ingested esters from plant sources. AChE and BuChE typically are distinguished by the relative rates of ACh and butyrylcholine hydrolysis and by effects of selective inhibitors (see Chapter 10).

Almost all pharmacological effects of the anti-ChE agents are due to the inhibition of AChE, with the consequent accumulation of endogenous ACh in the vicinity of the nerve terminal. Distinct but single genes encode AChE and BuChE in mammals; the diversity of molecular structure of AChE arises from alternative mRNA processing (Taylor et al., 2000).

Numerous reports suggest that AChE plays roles in addition to its classical function in terminating impulse transmission at cholinergic synapses. Nonclassical functions of AChE might include hydrolysis of ACh in a nonsynaptic context, action as an adhesion protein involved in synaptic development and maintenance or as a bone matrix protein, involvement in neurite outgrowth, and acceleration of the assembly of Aβ peptide into amyloid fibrils (Silman and Sussman, 2005).

Characteristics of Cholinergic Transmission at Various Sites

There are marked differences amongst various sites of cholinergic transmission with respect to architecture and fine structure, the distributions of AChE and receptors, and the temporal factors involved in normal function. In skeletal muscle, for example, the junctional sites occupy a small, discrete portion of the surface of the individual fibers and are relatively isolated from those of adjacent fibers; in the superior cervical ganglion, about 100,000 ganglion cells are packed within a volume of a few cubic millimeters, and both the presynaptic and the postsynaptic neuronal processes form complex networks.

Skeletal Muscle. At the NMJ, ACh stimulates the nicotinic receptor's intrinsic channel, which opens for about 1 ms, admitting about 50,000 Na^+ ions. The channel-opening process is the basis for the localized depolarizing EPP within the end plate, which triggers the muscle action potential and leads to contraction. The amount of ACh (10^{-17} mol) required to elicit an EPP following its microiontophoretic application to the motor end plate of a rat diaphragm muscle fiber is equivalent to that recovered from each fiber following stimulation of the phrenic nerve.

Following sectioning and degeneration of the motor nerve to skeletal muscle or of the postganglionic fibers to autonomic effectors, there is a marked reduction in the threshold doses of the transmitters and of certain other drugs required to elicit a response; that is, denervation supersensitivity occurs. In skeletal muscle, this change is accompanied by a spread of the receptor molecules from the end-plate region to the adjacent portions of the sarcoplasmic membrane, which eventually involves the entire muscle surface. Embryonic muscle also exhibits this uniform sensitivity to ACh prior to innervation. Hence, innervation represses the expression of the receptor gene by the nuclei that lie in extrajunctional regions of the muscle fiber and directs the subsynaptic nuclei to express the structural and functional proteins of the synapse.

Autonomic Effector Cells. Stimulation or inhibition of autonomic effector cells occurs on activation of muscarinic ACh receptors (discussed below). In this case, the effector is coupled to the receptor by a G protein (Chapter 3). In contrast to skeletal muscle and neurons, smooth muscle and the cardiac conduction system sinoatrial (SA node, atrium, AV node, and the His-Purkinje system) normally exhibit intrinsic activity, both electrical and mechanical, that is modulated but not initiated by nerve impulses.

In the basal condition, unitary smooth muscle exhibits waves of depolarization or spikes that are propagated from cell to cell at rates considerably slower than the action potential of axons or skeletal muscle. The spikes apparently are initiated by rhythmic fluctuations in the membrane resting potential. Application of ACh (0.1 to 1 μM) to isolated intestinal muscle causes the membrane potential to become less negative and increases the frequency of spike production, accompanied by a rise in tension. A primary action of ACh in initiating these effects through muscarinic receptors is probably partial depolarization of the cell membrane brought about by an increase in Na^+ and, in some instances, Ca^{2+} conductance. ACh also can produce contraction of some smooth muscles when the membrane has been depolarized completely by high concentrations of K^+, provided that Ca^{2+} is present. Hence, ACh stimulates ion fluxes across membranes or mobilizes intracellular Ca^{2+} to cause contraction.

In the heart, spontaneous depolarizations normally arise from the SA node. In the cardiac conduction system, particularly in the SA and AV nodes, stimulation of the cholinergic innervation or the direct application of ACh causes inhibition, associated with hyperpolarization of the membrane and a marked decrease in the rate of depolarization. These effects are due, at least in part, to a selective increase in permeability to K^+.

Autonomic Ganglia. The primary pathway of cholinergic transmission in autonomic ganglia is similar to that at the NMJ of skeletal muscle. The initial depolarization is the result of activation of nAChRs, which are ligand-gated cation channels with properties similar to those found at the NMJ. Several secondary transmitters or modulators either enhance or diminish the sensitivity of the postganglionic cell to ACh (see Figure 11–5).

Prejunctional Sites. ACh release is subject to complex regulation by mediators, including ACh itself acting on M_2 and M_4 *autoreceptors*, and activation of *heteroreceptors* (e.g., NE acting on α_{2A} and α_{2C} adrenergic receptors) or substances produced locally in tissues (e.g., NO) (Philipp and Hein, 2004; Wess et al., 2007). ACh-mediated inhibition of ACh release following activation of M_2 and M_4 autoreceptors is a physiological negative-feedback control mechanism. At some neuroeffector junctions (e.g., the myenteric plexus in the GI tract or the cardiac SA node), sympathetic and parasympathetic nerve terminals often lie juxtaposed to each other. There, opposing effects of NE and ACh result not only from the opposite effects of the two neurotransmitters on the smooth muscle or cardiac cells but also from the inhibition of ACh release by NE or inhibition of NE release by ACh acting on heteroreceptors on parasympathetic or sympathetic terminals.

Inhibitory heteroreceptors on parasympathetic terminals include adenosine A_1 receptors, histamine H_3 receptors, opioid receptors, and α_{2A} and α_{2C} adrenergic receptors. The parasympathetic nerve terminal varicosities also may contain additional heteroreceptors that could respond by inhibition or enhancement of ACh release by locally formed autacoids, hormones, or administered drugs.

Extraneuronal Sites. All elements of the cholinergic system are functionally expressed independently of cholinergic innervation in numerous nonneuronal cells. These *nonneuronal cholinergic* systems can both modify and control phenotypic cell functions such as proliferation, differentiation, formation of physical barriers, migration, and ion and water movements.

The widespread synthesis of ACh in nonneuronal cells has changed the thinking that ACh acts only as a neurotransmitter. Each component of the cholinergic system in nonneuronal cells can be affected by pathophysiological conditions. Dysfunctions of nonneuronal cholinergic systems may be involved in the pathogenesis of diseases (e.g., inflammatory processes) (Wessler and Kirkpatrick, 2008).

HISTORICAL PERSPECTIVE

Sir Henry Dale noted that the various esters of choline elicited responses that were similar to those of either nicotine or muscarine depending on the pharmacological preparation. A similarity in response also was noted between muscarine and nerve stimulation in those organs innervated by the craniosacral divisions of the autonomic nervous system. Thus, Dale suggested that ACh or another ester of choline was a neurotransmitter in the autonomic nervous system; he also stated that the compound had dual actions, which he termed a "nicotine action" (*nicotinic*) and a "muscarine action" (*muscarinic*).

The capacities of tubocurarine and atropine to block nicotinic and muscarinic effects of ACh, respectively, provided further support for the proposal of two distinct types of cholinergic receptors. Although Dale had access only to crude plant alkaloids of then-unknown structure from *Amanita muscaria* and *Nicotiana tabacum*, this classification remains the primary subdivision of cholinergic receptors. Its utility has survived the discovery of several distinct subtypes of nicotinic and muscarinic receptors.

Cholinergic Receptors and Signal Transduction

Nicotinic receptors are ligand-gated ion channels whose activation always causes a rapid (millisecond) increase in cellular permeability to Na^+ and Ca^{2+}, depolarization, and excitation. *Muscarinic receptors* are GPCRs. Responses to muscarinic agonists are slower; they may be either excitatory or inhibitory, and they are not necessarily linked to changes in ion permeability. The muscarinic and nicotinic receptors for ACh belong to two different families whose features are described in Chapters 9 and 11, respectively.

Subtypes of nAChRs. The *nAChRs* exist at the skeletal NMJ, autonomic ganglia, adrenal medulla, and CNS and in nonneuronal tissues. The nAChRs are composed of five homologous subunits organized around a central pore (see Table 8–2 and Figure 11–2). In general, the nAChRs are further divided into two groups:

- *Muscle type* (N_m), found in the vertebrate skeletal muscle, where they mediate transmission at the NMJ
- *Neuronal type* (N_n), found mainly throughout the peripheral nervous system, CNS, and nonneuronal tissues

Neuronal nAChRs are widely distributed in the CNS and are found at presynaptic, perisynaptic, and postsynaptic sites. At pre- and perisynaptic sites, nAChRs appear to act as autoreceptors or heteroreceptors to regulate the release of several neurotransmitters (ACh, DA, NE, glutamate, and 5HT) at diverse sites in the brain (Albuquerque et al., 2009).

Muscle-Type nAChRs. In fetal muscle prior to innervation, in adult muscle after denervation, and in fish electric organs, the nAChR subunit stoichiometry is $(\alpha1)_2\beta1\gamma\delta$, whereas in adult muscle the γ subunit is replaced by ε to give the $(\alpha1)_2\beta1\varepsilon\delta$ stoichiometry (Table 8–2). The γ/ε and δ subunits are involved together with the α1 subunits in forming the ligand-binding sites and in the maintenance of cooperative interactions between the α1 subunit. Different affinities to the two binding sites are conferred by the presence of different non-α subunits. Binding of ACh to the αγ and αδ sites is thought to induce a conformational change predominantly in the α1 subunits that interacts with the transmembrane region to cause channel opening.

Neuronal-Type nAChRs. Neuronal nAChRs are widely expressed in peripheral ganglia, the adrenal medulla, numerous areas of the brain, and nonneuronal cells, such as epithelial cells and cells of the immune system. To date, nine α (α2–α10) and three β (β2–β4) subunit genes have been cloned. The α7–α10 subunits are found either as homopentamers (of five α7, α8, and α9 subunits) or as heteropentamers of α7, α8, and α9/α10. By contrast, the α2–α6 and β2–β4 subunits form heteropentamers usually with $(\alpha x)_2(\beta y)_3$ stoichiometry. The α5 and β3 subunits do not appear to be able to form functional receptors when expressed alone or in paired combinations with α or β subunits, respectively (Kalamida et al., 2007).

TABLE 8–2 ■ CHARACTERISTICS OF SUBTYPES OF NICOTINIC ACETYLCHOLINE RECEPTORS (NACHRS)

RECEPTOR (Primary Receptor Subtype)[a]	MAIN SYNAPTIC LOCATION	MEMBRANE RESPONSE	MOLECULAR MECHANISM	AGONISTS	ANTAGONISTS
Skeletal Muscle (N_m) $(\alpha1)_2\beta1\varepsilon\delta$ adult $(\alpha1)_2\beta1\gamma\delta$ fetal	Skeletal neuromuscular junction (postjunctional)	Excitatory; end-plate depolarization; skeletal muscle contraction	Increased cation permeability (Na^+; K^+)	ACh Nicotine Succinylcholine	Atracurium Vecuronium *d*-Tubocurarine Pancuronium α-Conotoxin α-Bungarotoxin
Peripheral neuronal (N_n) $(\alpha3)_2(\beta4)_3$	Autonomic ganglia; adrenal medulla	Excitatory; depolarization; firing of postganglion neuron; depolarization and secretion of catecholamines	Increased cation permeability (Na^+; K^+)	ACh Nicotine Epibatidine Dimethylphenyl-piperazinium	Trimethaphan Mecamylamine
CNS neuronal $(\alpha4)_2(\beta4)_3$ (*α-BTX-insensitive*)	CNS; pre- and postjunctional	Pre- and postsynaptic excitation; prejunctional control of transmitter release	Increased cation permeability (Na^+; K^+)	Cytosine, epibatidine Anatoxin A	Mecamylamine DHbE Erysodine Lophotoxin
$(\alpha7)_5$ (*α-BTX-sensitive*)	CNS; pre- and postsynaptic	Pre- and postsynaptic excitation; prejunctional control of transmitter release	Increased permeability (Ca^{2+})	Anatoxin A	Methyllycaconitine α-Bungarotoxin α-Conotoxin ImI

[a]Nine α (α2–α10) and three β (β2–β4) subunits have been identified and cloned in human brain, which combine in various conformations to form individual receptor subtypes. The structure of individual receptors and the subtype composition are incompletely understood. Only a finite number of naturally occurring functional nAChR constructs have been identified. DHbE, dihydro-β-erythroidine.

TABLE 8–3 ■ CHARACTERISTICS OF MUSCARINIC ACETYLCHOLINE RECEPTOR (mAChRs) SUBTYPES

RECEPTOR	CELLULAR AND TISSUE LOCATION[a]	CELLULAR RESPONSE[b]	FUNCTIONAL RESPONSE[c]	DISEASE RELEVANCE
M_1	CNS; most abundant in cerebral cortex, hippocampus, striatum, and thalamus Autonomic ganglia Glands (gastric and salivary) Enteric nerves	Couples by $G_{q/11}$ to activate PLC-IP_3-Ca^{2+}-PKC pathway Depolarization and excitation (↑ sEPSP) Activation of PLD_2, PLA_2; ↑AA	Increased cognitive function (learning and memory) Increased seizure activity Decrease in dopamine release and locomotion Increase in depolarization of autonomic ganglia Increase in secretions	Alzheimer disease Cognitive dysfunction Schizophrenia
M_2	Widely expressed in CNS, hindbrain, thalamus, cerebral cortex, hippocampus, striatum, heart, smooth muscle, autonomic nerve terminals	Couples by G_i/G_o (PTX sensitive) Inhibition of AC, ↓ cAMP Activation of inwardly rectifying K^+ channels Inhibition of voltage-gated Ca^{2+} channels Hyperpolarization and inhibition	***Heart:*** SA node: slowed spontaneous depolarization; hyperpolarization, ↓ HR AV node: decrease in conduction velocity Atrium: ↓ refractory period, ↓ contraction Ventricle: slight ↓ contraction ***Smooth muscle:*** ↑ Contraction ***Peripheral nerves:*** Neural inhibition via autoreceptors and heteroreceptor ↓ Ganglionic transmission. ***CNS:*** Neural inhibition ↑ Tremors; hypothermia; analgesia	Alzheimer disease Cognitive dysfunction Pain
M_3	Widely expressed in CNS (<other mAChRs), cerebral cortex, hippocampus Abundant in smooth muscle and glands Heart	Couples by $G_{q/11}$ to activate PLC-IP_3/DAG-Ca^{2+}-PKC pathway Depolarization and excitation (↑ sEPSP) Activation of PLD_2, PLA_2; ↑AA	***Smooth muscle:*** ↑ Contraction (predominant in some, e.g., bladder) ***Glands:*** ↑ Secretion (predominant in salivary gland) Increases food intake, body weight, fat deposits Inhibition of DA release Synthesis of NO	Chronic obstructive pulmonary disease (COPD) Urinary incontinence Irritable bowel disease
M_4	Preferentially expressed in CNS, particularly forebrain, also striatum, cerebral cortex, hippocampus	Couples by G_i/G_0 (PTX sensitive) Inhibition of AC, ↓ cAMP Activation of inwardly rectifying K^+ channels Inhibition of voltage-gated Ca^{2+} channels Hyperpolarization and inhibition	Autoreceptor- and heteroreceptor-mediated inhibition of transmitter release in CNS and periphery Analgesia; cataleptic activity Facilitation of DA release	Parkinson disease Schizophrenia Neuropathic pain
M_5	Substantia nigra Expressed in low levels in CNS and periphery Predominant mAchR in neurons in VTA and substantia nigra	Couples by $G_{q/11}$ to activate PLC-IP_3-Ca^{2+}-PKC pathway Depolarization and excitation (↑ sEPSP) Activation of PLD_2, PLA_2; ↑AA	Mediator of dilation in cerebral arteries and arterioles (?) Facilitates DA release Augmentation of drug-seeking behavior and reward (e.g., opiates, cocaine)	Drug dependence Parkinson disease Schizophrenia

[a]Most organs, tissues, and cells express multiple mAChRs.

[b]M_1, M_3, and M_5 mAChRs appear to couple to the same G proteins and signal through similar pathways. Likewise, M_2 and M_4 mAChRs couple through similar G proteins and signal through similar pathways.

[c]Despite the fact that in many tissues, organs, and cells multiple subtypes of mAChRs coexist, one subtype may predominate in producing a particular function; in others, there may be equal predominance.

VTA, ventral tegmentum area.

The precise function of many of the neuronal nAChRs in the brain is not known; they appear to act more as synaptic modulators, the molecular diversity of the subunits putatively resulting in numerous nAChR subtypes with different physiological properties. Neuronal nAChRs are widely distributed in the CNS and are found at presynaptic, perisynaptic, and postsynaptic sites. At pre- and perisynaptic sites, nAChRs appear to act as autoreceptors or heteroreceptors to regulate the release of several neurotransmitters (ACh, DA, NE, glutamate, and 5HT) at sites throughout the brain (Exley and Cragg, 2008). The synaptic release of a particular neurotransmitter can be regulated by different neuronal-type nAChR subtypes in different CNS regions. For instance, DA release from striatal and thalamic DA neurons can be controlled by the α4β2 subtype or both α4β2 and α6β2β3 subtypes, respectively. In contrast, glutametergic neurotransmission is regulated everywhere by α7 nAChRs (Kalamida et al., 2007).

Subtypes of Muscarinic Receptors. In mammals, there are five distinct subtypes of mAChRs, each produced by a different gene. These variants have distinct anatomic locations in the periphery and CNS and differing chemical specificities. The mAChRs are GPCRs (see Table 8–3 and Chapter 9), present in virtually all organs, tissues, and cell types (Table 8–3 and Chapter 9). Most cell types have multiple mAChR subtypes, but certain subtypes often predominate in specific sites (Wess et al., 2007). For example, the M_2 receptor is the predominant subtype in the heart and in CNS neurons is mostly located presynaptically, whereas the M_3 receptor is the predominant subtype in the detrusor muscle of the bladder (Dhein et al., 2001; Fetscher et al., 2002).

In the periphery, mAChRs mediate the classical muscarinic actions of ACh in organs and tissues innervated by parasympathetic nerves, although receptors may be present at sites that lack parasympathetic innervation (e.g., most blood vessels). In the CNS, mAChRs are involved in regulating a large number of cognitive, behavioral, sensory, motor, and autonomic functions. Owing to the lack of specific muscarinic agonists and antagonists that demonstrate selectivity for individual mAChRs and the fact that most organs and tissues express multiple mAChRs, it has been a challenge to assign specific pharmacological functions to distinct mAChRs. The development of gene-targeting techniques in mice has been helpful in defining specific functions (Table 8–3) (Wess et al., 2007).

The functions of mAChRs are mediated by interactions with G proteins. The M_1, M_3, and M_5 subtypes couple through $G_{q/11}$ to stimulate the PLC-IP_3/DAG-Ca^{2+} pathway, leading to activation of PKC and Ca^{2+}-sensitive enzymes. Activation of M_1, M_3, and M_5 receptors can also cause the activation of PLA_2, leading to the release of arachidonic acid and consequent eicosanoid synthesis; these effects of M_1, M_3, and M_5 mAChRs are generally secondary to elevation of intracellular Ca^{2+}. Stimulated M_2 and M_4 cholinergic receptors couple to G_i and G_o, with resulting inhibition of adenylyl cyclase, leading to a decrease in cellular cAMP, activation of inwardly rectifying K^+ channels, and inhibition of voltage-gated Ca^{2+} channels (van Koppen and Kaiser, 2003). The functional consequences of these effects are hyperpolarization and inhibition of excitable membranes. In the myocardium, inhibition of adenylyl cyclase and activation of K^+ conductances account for the negative inotropic and chronotropic effects of ACh. In addition, heterologous systems may produce different receptor-transducer-effector interactions (Nathanson, 2008).

Following activation by classical or allosteric agonists, mAChRs can be phosphorylated by a variety of receptor kinases and second-messenger regulated kinases; the phosphorylated mAChR subtypes then can interact with β-arrestin and possibly other adapter proteins. As a result, mAChR signaling pathways may be differentially altered. Agonist activation of mAChRs also may induce receptor internalization and downregulation (van Koppen and Kaiser, 2003). Muscarinic AChRs can also regulate other signal transduction pathways that have diverse effects on cell growth, survival, and physiology, such as MAPK, phosphoinositide-3-kinase, RhoA, and Rac1 (Nathanson, 2008).

Changes in mAChR levels and activity have been implicated in the pathophysiology of numerous major diseases in the CNS and in the autonomic nervous system (Table 8–3). Phenotypic analysis of mAChR-mutant mice as well as the development of selective agonists and antagonists has led to a wealth of new information regarding the physiological and potential pathophysiological roles of the individual mAChR subtype (Langmead et al., 2008; Wess et al., 2007).

Adrenergic Transmission

Norepinephrine (NE) is the principal transmitter of most sympathetic postganglionic fibers and of certain tracts in the CNS; DA is the predominant transmitter of the mammalian extrapyramidal system and of several mesocortical and mesolimbic neuronal pathways; and EPI is the major hormone of the adrenal medulla. Collectively, these three amines are called *catecholamines*. Drugs affecting these endogenous amines and their actions are used in the treatment of hypertension, mental disorders, and a variety of other conditions. The details of these interactions and of the pharmacology of the sympathomimetic amines themselves can be found in subsequent chapters. The basic physiological, biochemical, and pharmacological features are presented here.

Synthesis of Catecholamines

The steps in the synthesis of catecholamines and the characteristics of the enzymes involved are shown in Figure 8–7 and Table 8–4. Tyrosine is sequentially 3-hydroxylated and decarboxylated to form DA. DA is β-hydroxylated to yield NE, which is *N*-methylated in chromaffin tissue to give EPI. The enzymes involved have been identified, cloned, and characterized (Nagatsu, 2006). Table 8–4 summarizes some of the important characteristics of the four enzymes. These enzymes are not completely specific; consequently, other endogenous substances, as well as certain drugs, are also substrates. For example, 5HT can be produced from 5-hydroxy-*L*-tryptophan by aromatic *L*-amino acid decarboxylase (or dopa decarboxylase). Dopa decarboxylase also converts dopa into DA (Chapter 13) and methyldopa to α-methyldopamine, which in turn is converted by DβH to methylnorepinephrine.

The hydroxylation of tyrosine by TH is the rate-limiting step in the biosynthesis of catecholamines (Zigmond et al., 1989). This enzyme is activated following stimulation of sympathetic nerves or the adrenal medulla. The enzyme is a substrate for PKA, PKC, and CaM kinase; phosphorylation is associated with increased hydroxylase activity. In addition, there is a delayed increase in TH gene expression after nerve stimulation. These mechanisms serve to maintain the content of catecholamines in response to increased transmitter release. TH also is subject to feedback inhibition by catechol compounds.

Deficiency of TH has been reported in humans and is characterized by generalized rigidity, hypokinesia, and low CSF levels of NE and DA metabolites HVA and 3-methoxy-4-hydroxyphenylethylene glycol (Wevers et al., 1999). TH knockout is embryonically lethal in mice, presumably because the loss of catecholamines results in altered cardiac function. Interestingly, residual levels of DA are present in these mice. Tyrosinase may be an alternate source for catecholamines, although tyrosinase-derived catecholamines are clearly not sufficient for survival (Carson and Robertson, 2002).

Deficiency of DβH in humans is characterized by orthostatic hypotension, ptosis of the eyelids, retrograde ejaculation, and elevated plasma levels of DA. In the case of DβH-deficient mice, there is about 90% embryonic mortality (Carson and Robertson, 2002).

Our understanding of the cellular sites and mechanisms of synthesis, storage, and release of catecholamines derives from studies of sympathetically innervated organs and the adrenal medulla. Nearly all the NE content of innervated organs is confined to the postganglionic sympathetic fibers; it disappears within a few days after section of the nerves. In the adrenal medulla, catecholamines are stored in chromaffin granules (Aunis, 1998). These vesicles contain extremely high concentrations of catecholamines (~21% dry weight), ascorbic acid, and ATP, as well as specific proteins, such as chromogranins, DβH, and peptides, including enkephalin and neuropeptide Y. Vasostatin 1, the *N*-terminal fragment of chromogranin A, has been found to have antibacterial and antifungal activity (Lugardon et al., 2000), as have other chromogranin A fragments, such as chromofungin, vasostatin II, prochromacin, and chromacins I and II (Taupenot et al., 2003). Two types of storage vesicles are found in sympathetic nerve

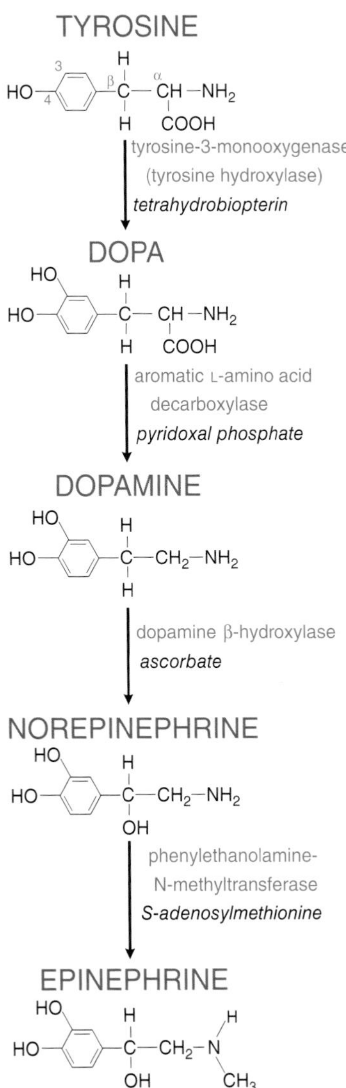

Figure 8–7 *Steps in the enzymatic synthesis of dopamine, norepinephrine and epinephrine.* The enzymes involved are shown in red; essential cofactors in italics. The final step occurs only in the adrenal medulla and in a few epinephrine-containing neuronal pathways in the brainstem.

terminals: large dense-core vesicles corresponding to chromaffin granules and small dense-core vesicles containing NE, ATP, and membrane-bound DβH.

The main features of the mechanisms of synthesis, storage, and release of catecholamines at an adrenergic neuroeffector junction and their modifications by drugs are summarized in Figure 8–8 and its legend. The *adrenal medulla* has two distinct catecholamine-containing cell types: those with NE and those with primarily EPI. The latter cell population contains the enzyme PNMT. In these cells, the NE formed in the granules leaves these structures and is methylated in the cytoplasm to EPI. EPI then reenters the chromaffin granules, where it is stored until released. EPI accounts for about 80% of the catecholamines of the adrenal medulla and NE about 20%.

A major factor that controls the rate of synthesis of EPI, and hence the size of the store available for release from the adrenal medulla, is the level of glucocorticoids secreted by the adrenal cortex. The intra-adrenal portal vascular system carries the corticosteroids directly to the adrenal medullary chromaffin cells, where they induce the synthesis of PNMT (Figure 8–7). The activities of both TH and DβH also are increased in the adrenal medulla when the secretion of glucocorticoids is stimulated (Viskupic et al., 1994). Thus, any stress that persists sufficiently to evoke an enhanced secretion of corticotropin mobilizes the appropriate hormones of both the adrenal cortex (predominantly cortisol in humans) and medulla (EPI). This remarkable relationship is present only in certain mammals, including humans, in which the adrenal chromaffin cells are enveloped entirely by steroid-secreting cortical cells. PMNT is expressed in mammalian tissues such as brain, heart, and lung, leading to extra-adrenal EPI synthesis (Ziegler et al., 2002).

In addition to de novo synthesis, NE stores in the terminal portions of the adrenergic fibers are replenished by reuptake and restorage of NE following its release (see discussion in the following material).

Storage, Release, and Reuptake of Catecholamines; Termination of Action

Storage. NE, ATP, and NPY are stored frequently in the same nerve endings.

Catecholamines. Catecholamines are stored in vesicles, thereby ensuring their regulated release, protecting them from metabolism by cellular enzymes, and preventing their leakage out of the neuron. The vesicular monoamine transporter VMAT2, a vesicular membrane protein, moves NE and other catecholamines from the cytosol into neuronal storage vesicles (Chaudhry et al., 2008). VMAT2 is driven by a pH gradient established by an ATP-dependent proton translocase in the vesicular membrane; for each molecule of amine taken up, two H^+ ions are extruded. VMAT2 is a member of the SLC protein superfamily and is designated SLC18A. Monoamine transporters in the SLC18 family are relatively promiscuous and transport DA, NE, EPI, and 5HT, as well as metaiodobenzylguanidine, which can be used to image chromaffin cell tumors (Schuldiner, 1994). *Reserpine* inhibits monoamine transport into storage vesicles and ultimately leads to depletion of catecholamine from sympathetic nerve endings and in the brain.

ATP. ATP is an essential component of catecholamine storage; the capacity of ATP and catecholamines to form relatively stable complexes apparently facilitates accumulation of high concentrations of neurotransmitter within the adrenergic storage granule. The granule accumulates ATP via another vesicular nucleotide carrier, VNUT, a member of the SLC superfamily. VNUT is a Na^+/anion cotransporter, designated as SLC17A9 (see Chapter 5). The frequency and quantal size of exocytotic release mirror VNUT activity (Estévez-Herrera et al., 2016). Thus, vesicular ATP has multiple actions beyond its role as a cellular energy source and energy storage molecule: Vesicular ATP facilitates vesicular storage of high concentrations of catecholamines and, when released with the vesicular contents, acts as a transmitter at purinergic receptors (Burnstock et al., 2015).

Neuropeptide Y. NPY, a peptide with 36 amino acids, is synthesized in the endoplasmic reticulum, first as a 97-amino-acid precursor, prepro-NPY, that is processed by three steps of proteolysis and a final C-terminal amidation; the resultant NPY_{1-36} is stored in large, dense-core vesicles that may also contain NE. NE and ATP are more generally stored in smaller dense-core vesicles, but NPY, ATP, and NE are often coreleased following nerve stimulation, albeit in proportions that change with the pattern and intensity of stimulation (Westfall, 2004). NPY is abundant in the brain and is a powerful orexigenic. In the peripheral nervous system, NPY occurs in sympathetic nerves and adrenal chromaffin cells; it can also be found in platelets, endothelium, and the GI tract and is inducible in the immune system (Hirsch et al., 2012).

Release. Details of excitation-secretion coupling in sympathetic neurons and adrenal medulla are becoming known and are summarized in Figures 8–3 and 8–8. The triggering event is the entry of Ca^{2+}, which results in the exocytosis of the granular contents, including the catecholamine, ATP, some neuroactive peptides (e.g., NPY) or their precursors, chromogranins, and DβH. The various SNARE proteins (e.g., SNAP-25, syntaxin, and synaptobrevin) described for exocytosis of ACh are also involved here (Figures 8–3 through 8–6).

TABLE 8–4 ■ ENZYMES FOR SYNTHESIS OF CATECHOLAMINES

ENZYME	OCCURRENCE	SUBCELLULAR DISTRIBUTION	COFACTORS	SUBSTRATE SPECIFICITY	COMMENTS
TH	Widespread	Cytoplasm	tetradrobiopterin (BH_4), O_2, Fe^{2+}	Specific for L-tyrosine	Rate-limiting step. Inhibition can deplete NE.
AAADC	Widespread	Cytoplasm	Pyridoxal PO_4	Nonspecific	Inhibition does not alter tissue NE and EPI appreciably.
DβH	Widespread	Synaptic vesicles	Ascorbate, O_2 (DβH contains Cu)	Nonspecific	Inhibition can ↓ NE and EPI levels.
PNMT	Largely in adrenal gland	Cytoplasm	S-adenosyl methionine (SAM) as (CH_3 donor)	Nonspecific	Inhibition can ↓ adrenal EPI/NE; regulated by glucocorticoids.

Reuptake and Termination of Action. Following its release from a sympathetic nerve varicosity, NE interacts with presynaptic and postsynaptic membrane receptors. Adrenergic fibers can sustain the output of NE during prolonged periods of stimulation without exhausting their supply, provided that synthesis and reuptake of the transmitter are unimpaired. Acute regulation of transmitter synthesis involving activation of TH and DβH has been described previously in this chapter. Recycling of transmitter is also essential, and this is provided by reuptake, restorage, and reuse of transmitter. *The actions of catecholamines are terminated by reuptake into the nerve and postjunctional cells and to a smaller extent by diffusion out of the synaptic cleft.* Two distinct carrier-mediated transport systems are involved in reuptake (see Figure 8–8; Table 8–5):

- NET: This transporter, previously called *uptake 1*, moves NE across the neuronal membrane from the extracellular fluid to the cytoplasm. NET has a higher affinity for NE than for EPI (see Table 8–5). NET is a member of an SLC family of similar transporters and is designated as SLC6A2. This family of proteins transports amino acids and their derivatives into cells using cotransport of extracellular Na^+ as a driving force for substrate translocation against chemical gradients (see Chapter 5). The SLC6A monoamine transporters include NET, DAT (SLC6A3), and SERT (SLC6A4).
- ENT: This transporter, previously called *uptake 2,* is an organic cation transporter, OCT3, designated as SLC22A3. OCT3 facilitates passive transmembrane movement of organic anions down their electrochemical gradients, including the movement of catecholamines into nonneuronal cells. Compared to NET, it has a lower affinity for catecholamines, favors EPI over NE and DA, has a higher maximum uptake rate for catecholamines, is not Na^+ dependent, and has a different profile for pharmacological inhibition. The synthetic β adrenergic receptor agonist isoproterenol is not a substrate for this system. OCT3 activity is altered by MAPK and Ca^{2+}-CaM signaling (Roth et al., 2012). In addition to catecholamines, OCT3 can transport a wide variety of other organic cations, including 5HT, histamine, choline, spermine, guanidine, and creatinine, as can the closely related OCT1 and OCT2. The characteristics and locations of the nonneuronal transporters are summarized in Table 8–5.

For NE released by neurons, uptake by NET is more important than uptake by ENT. Sympathetic nerves as a whole remove about 87% of released NE by NET, compared with 5% by extraneuronal uptake (ENT) and 8% by diffusion to the circulation. In contrast, clearance of circulating catecholamines, such as those released from the adrenal medulla, is primarily by nonneuronal mechanisms, with liver and kidney accounting for over 60% of the clearance of circulating catecholamines. Because VMAT2 has a much higher affinity for NE than does MAO, over 70% of recaptured NE is resequestered into storage vesicles (Eisenhofer, 2001).

The NET is also present in the adrenal medulla, the liver, and the placenta, whereas DAT is present in the stomach, pancreas, and kidney (Eisenhofer, 2001). These plasma membrane transporters appear to have greater substrate specificity than does VMAT2. NET and DAT are targets for drugs such as cocaine and tricyclic antidepressants (e.g., imipramine); selective 5HT reuptake inhibitors such as fluoxetine inhibit SERT. Inhibitors of OCT3 include normetanephrine (an O-methylated metabolite of NE; see Figure 8–9), Pharmacological probes of OCT3 include corticosterone (an inhibitor), and the substrates metformin and cimetidine; the interaction of substrates and inhibitors at renal OCT3 can lead to adverse drug effects (see Chapter 5).

The use of selective inhibitors of NET in animal and human studies and data from analysis of mice with targeted deletions (KO) of the NET and DAT genes reveal the impact of these uptake systems. The NET-KO and DAT-KO animals exhibit increased extracellular levels and decreased intracellular levels of NE despite increased or unaltered neurotransmitter synthesis (Xu et al., 2000; Gainetdinov and Caron, 2003). NET-KO mice also display marked behavioral alterations (Xu et al., 2000) and show characteristic hemodynamic changes (e.g., excessive tachycardia and increased blood pressure during sympathetic activation with wakefulness and activity), whereas resting mean arterial pressure and heart rate are maintained at nearly normal levels, most likely because of increased central sympathoinhibition (Keller et al., 2004). A coding mutation in humans (A457P in TM9) reduces NET activity and yields marked hemodynamic changes and orthostatic intolerance. When expressed in a heterologous cell line, the mutation resulted in a 98% loss of NET function compared with the wild-type transporter (Shannon et al., 2000). Furthermore, when coexpressed with wild-type NET, the A457P mutant exerts a dominant negative effect on wild-type NET, likely reflecting transporter oligomerization (Hahn et al., 2003), providing an explanation for the phenotype observed in heterozygous carriers. Another human variant of NET with an F528C mutation displays increased membrane expression of NET associated with increased NE uptake compared with wild-type NET (Hahn et al., 2005); this variant may be associated with an increased incidence of depression (Haenisch et al., 2009).

Certain sympathomimetic drugs (e.g., ephedrine and tyramine) produce some of their effects indirectly by displacing NE from the nerve terminals to the extracellular fluid, where it then acts at receptor sites of the effector cells. The mechanisms by which these drugs release NE from nerve endings are complex. All such agents are substrates for NET. As a result of their uptake by NET, they make carrier available at the inner surface of the membrane for the outward transport of NE ("facilitated exchange diffusion"). In addition, these amines are able to mobilize NE stored in the vesicles by competing for the vesicular uptake process (VMAT2).

The actions of indirect-acting sympathomimetic amines are subject to *tachyphylaxis.* For example, repeated administration of tyramine results in rapidly decreasing effectiveness, whereas repeated administration of NE does not reduce effectiveness and, in fact, reverses the tachyphylaxis to tyramine. These phenomena have not been explained fully. One hypothesis is that the pool of neurotransmitter available for displacement by these drugs is small relative to the total amount stored in the sympathetic nerve ending. This pool is presumed to reside close to the plasma membrane, and the NE of such vesicles may be replaced by the less-potent amine following repeated

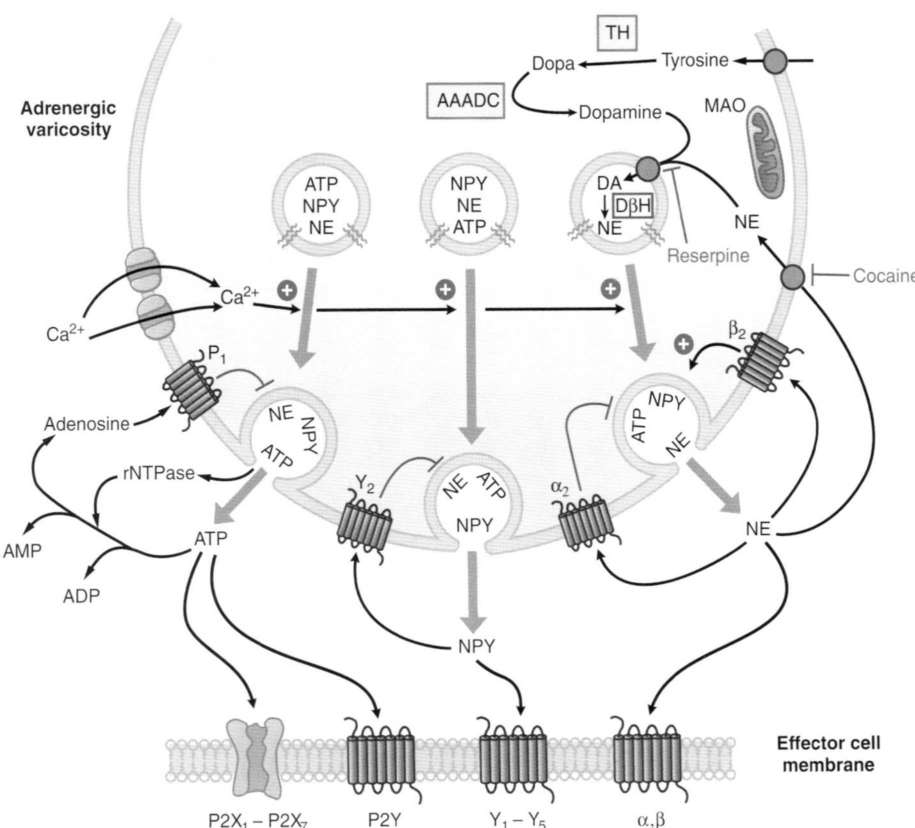

Figure 8–8 *A typical adrenergic neuroeffector junction.* Tyrosine is transported into the varicosity and is converted to DOPA by TH and DOPA to DA by the action of AAADC. DA is taken up into the vesicles of the varicosity by a transporter, VMAT2, that can be blocked by reserpine. Cytoplasmic NE also can be taken up by this transporter. DA is converted to NE within the vesicle via the action of DβH. NE is stored in vesicles along with other cotransmitters, NPY and ATP, depending on the particular neuroeffector junction. Release of the transmitters occurs via exocytosis, a process activated by depolarization of the varicosity, which allows entry of Ca^{2+} through voltage-dependent Ca^{2+} channels and the interaction of numerous docking and fusion proteins located in the vesicle and the neuronal cell membrane, as described in Figures 8–3, 8–4, and 8–5. In this schematic representation, NE, NPY, and ATP are stored in the same vesicles. Different populations of vesicles, however, may preferentially store different proportions of the cotransmitters. Once in the synapse, NE can interact with α and β adrenergic receptors (GPCRs) to produce the responses characteristic of the particular postsynaptic cell. The α and β receptors also can be located presynaptically, via which NE can either diminish ($α_2$) or facilitate (β) its own release and that of the cotransmitters. The principal mechanism by which NE is cleared from the synapse is via a cocaine-sensitive neuronal uptake transporter, NET. Once transported into the cytosol, NE can be re-stored in the vesicle or metabolized by MAO. NPY produces its effects by activating NPY receptors (also GCPRs), of which there are at least five types (Y_1 through Y_5). NPY can modify its own release and that of the other transmitters via presynaptic Y_2 receptors. NPY action is terminated by the actions of peptidases. ATP produces its effects by activating P2X receptors (ligand-gated ion channels) or P2Y receptors (GPCRs). There are multiple subtypes of both P2X and P2Y receptors. As with other cotransmitters, ATP can act prejunctionally to modify its own release via receptors for ATP or via its metabolic breakdown to adenosine that acts on P1 (adenosine) receptors. ATP is cleared from the synapse primarily by rNTPases and by cell-fixed ectonucleotidases.

administration of the latter substance. In any case, neurotransmitter release by displacement is not associated with the release of DβH and does not require extracellular Ca^{2+}; thus, it is presumed not to involve exocytosis.

Prejunctional Regulation of NE Release. The release of the three sympathetic cotransmitters can be modulated by prejunctional autoreceptors and heteroreceptors. Following their release from sympathetic terminals, all three cotransmitters—NE, NPY, and ATP—can feed back on prejunctional receptors to inhibit the release of each other (Westfall, 2004; Westfall et al., 2002). The most thoroughly studied have been prejunctional $α_2$ adrenergic receptors. The $α_{2A}$ and $α_{2C}$ adrenergic receptors are the principal prejunctional receptors that inhibit sympathetic neurotransmitter release, whereas the $α_{2B}$ adrenergic receptors also may inhibit transmitter release at selected sites. Antagonists of this receptor, in turn, can enhance the electrically evoked release of sympathetic neurotransmitter. NPY, acting on Y_2 receptors, and ATP-derived adenosine, acting on P1 receptors, also can inhibit sympathetic neurotransmitter release. Activation of numerous heteroreceptors on sympathetic nerve varicosities can inhibit the release of sympathetic neurotransmitters; these include M_2 and M_4 muscarinic, 5HT, PGE_2, histamine, enkephalin, and DA receptors. Enhancement of sympathetic neurotransmitter release can be produced by activation of $β_2$ adrenergic receptors, angiotensin AT_2 receptors, and nAChRs. All of these receptors can be targets for agonists and antagonists (Kubista and Boehm, 2006).

Metabolism of Catecholamines. Uptake of released catecholamine terminates the neurotransmitter's effects at the synaptic junction. Following uptake, catecholamines can be metabolized (in neuronal and nonneuronal cells) or re-stored in vesicles (in neurons). Two enzymes are important in the initial steps of metabolic transformation of catecholamines—MAO and COMT.

TABLE 8–5 ■ CHARACTERISTICS OF PLASMA MEMBRANE TRANSPORTERS FOR ENDOGENOUS CATECHOLAMINES

TYPE OF TRANSPORTER	SUBSTRATE SPECIFICITY	TISSUE	REGION/CELL TYPE	INHIBITORS
Neuronal				
NET	DA > NE > EPI	All sympathetically innervated tissue	Sympathetic nerves	Desipramine Cocaine Nisoxetine
		Adrenal medulla	Chromaffin cells	
		Liver	Capillary endothelial cells	
		Placenta	Syncytiotrophoblast	
DAT	DA > NE > EPI	Kidney	Endothelium	Cocaine Imazindol
		Stomach	Parietal and endothelial cells	
		Pancreas	Pancreatic duct	
Nonneuronal				
OCT1	DA > EPI >> NE	Liver	Hepatocytes	Isocyanines Corticosterone
		Intestine	Epithelial cells	
		Kidney (not human)	Distal tubule	
OCT2	DA >> NE > EPI	Kidney	Medullary proximal and distal tubules	Isocyanines Corticosterone
		Brain	Glial cells of DA-rich regions, some nonadrenergic neurons	
ENT (OCT3)	EPI >> NE > DA	Liver	Hepatocytes	Isocyanines Corticosterone *O*-methyl-isoproterenol
		Brain	Glial cells, others	
		Heart	Myocytes	
		Blood vessels	Endothelial cells	
		Kidney	Cortex, proximal and distal tubules	
		Placenta	Syncytiotrophoblasts (basal membrane)	
		Retina	Photoreceptors, ganglion amacrine cells	

MAO and COMT. MAO metabolizes transmitter that is released within the nerve terminal or that is in the cytosol as a result of reuptake and has not yet reached the safety of the storage vesicle. COMT, particularly in the liver, plays a major role in the metabolism of endogenous circulating and administered catecholamines. The importance of neuronal reuptake of catecholamines is shown by observations that inhibitors of uptake (e.g., cocaine and imipramine) potentiate the effects of the neurotransmitter; inhibitors of MAO and COMT have less effect.

Both MAO and COMT are distributed widely throughout the body, including the brain; their highest concentrations are in the liver and the kidney. However, little or no COMT is found in sympathetic neurons. In the brain, there is no significant COMT in presynaptic terminals, but it is found in some postsynaptic neurons and glial cells. In the kidney, COMT is localized in proximal tubular epithelial cells, where DA is synthesized and is thought to exert local diuretic and natriuretic effects.

There are distinct differences in the localizations of the two enzymes; MAO is associated chiefly with the outer surface of mitochondria, including those within the terminals of sympathetic or central noradrenergic neuronal fibers, whereas COMT is largely cytosolic, except in the chromaffin cells of the adrenal medulla, where COMT is membrane bound. These factors are of importance both in determining the primary metabolic pathways followed by catecholamines in various circumstances and in explaining the effects of certain drugs. The physiological substrates for COMT include L-dopa, all three endogenous catecholamines (DA, NE, and EPI), their hydroxylated metabolites, catecholestrogens, ascorbic acid, and dihydroxyindolic intermediates of melanin (Männistö and Kaakkola, 1999).

Two different isozymes of MAO (MAO-A and MAO-B) are found in widely varying proportions in different cells in the CNS and in peripheral tissues. In the periphery, MAO-A is located in the syncytiotrophoblast layer of term placenta and liver, whereas MAO-B is located in platelets, lymphocytes, and liver. In the brain, MAO-A is located in all regions containing catecholamines, with the highest abundance in the locus ceruleus. MAO-B, on the other hand, is found primarily in regions that are known to synthesize and store 5HT. MAO-B is most prominent not only in the nucleus raphe dorsalis but also in the posterior hypothalamus and in glial cells in regions known to contain nerve terminals. MAO-B is also present in osteocytes around blood vessels (Abell and Kwan, 2001).

Many MAO inhibitors are not selective for MAO-A or MAO-B, and these nonselective agents (e.g., phenelzine, tranylcypromine, and isocarboxazid) enhance the bioavailability of tyramine contained in many foods; tyramine-induced NE release from sympathetic neurons may lead to markedly increased blood pressure (hypertensive crisis). Drugs with selectivity for MAO-B (e.g., selegiline, rasagiline, pargyline) or reversible inhibitors of MAO-A (e.g., moclobemide) are less likely to cause this potential interaction (Volz and Gleiter, 1998; Wouters, 1998).

Inhibitors of MAO activity can cause an increase in the concentration of NE, DA, and 5HT in the brain and other tissues accompanied by a variety of pharmacological effects. No striking pharmacological action in the periphery can be attributed to the inhibition of COMT. However, the COMT inhibitors entacapone and tocapone are efficacious in the therapy of Parkinson disease (Chong and Mersfelder, 2000, and Chapter 18).

The Metabolic Pathway (Figure 8–9). There is ongoing passive leakage of catecholamines from vesicular storage granules of sympathetic neurons and adrenal medullary chromaffin cells. As a consequence, most metabolism of catecholamines takes place in the same cells where the amines are synthesized and stored. VMAT2 effectively sequesters about 90% of the

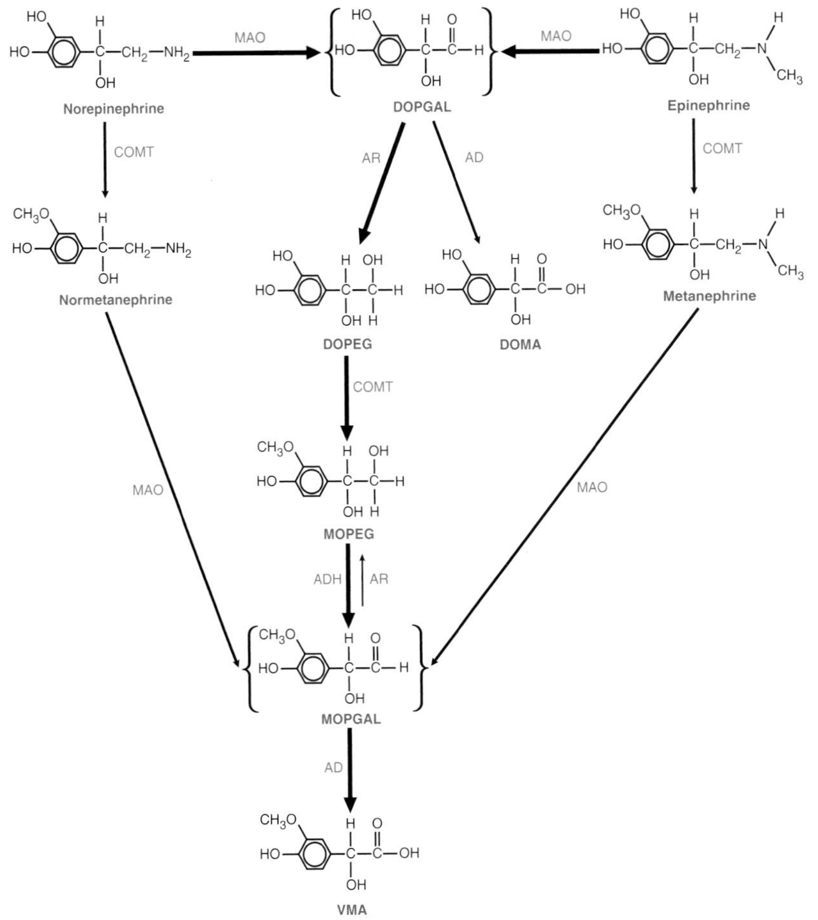

Figure 8–9 *Metabolism of catecholamines.* NE and EPI are first oxidatively deaminated to a short-lived intermediate (DOPGAL) by MAO. DOPGAL then undergoes further metabolism to more stable alcohol- or acid-deaminated metabolites. AD metabolizes DOPGAL to DOMA, while AR metabolizes DOPGAL to DOPEG. Under normal circumstances, DOMA is a minor metabolite, with DOPEG being the major metabolite produced from NE and EPI. Once DOPEG leaves the major sites of its formation (sympathetic nerves; adrenal medulla), it is converted to MOPEG by COMT. MOPEG is then converted to the unstable aldehyde (MOPGAL) by ADH and finally to VMA by AD. VMA is the major end product. Another route for the formation of VMA is conversion of NE or EPI into normetanephrine or metanephrine by COMT in either the adrenal medulla or extraneuronal sites, with subsequent metabolism to MOPGAL and thence to VMA. Catecholamines are also metabolized by *sulfotransferases.* AD, aldehyde dehydrogenase; ADH, alcohol dehydrogenase; AR, aldehyde reductase; COMT, catechol-*O*-methyltransferease; DOMA, 3,4-dihydroxymandelic acid; DOPEG, 3,4-dihydroxyphenyl glycol; DOPGAL, dihydroxyphenylglycolaldehyde; MAO, monoamine oxidase; MOPEG, 3-methyl,4-hydroxyphenylglycol; MOPGAL, monohydroxyphenylglycol aldehyde; VMA, vanillyl mandelic acid.

amines leaking into the cytoplasm back into storage vesicles; about 10% escapes sequestration and is metabolized (Eisenhofer et al., 2004).

Sympathetic nerves contain MAO but not COMT, and this MAO catalyzes only the first step of a two-step reaction. MAO converts NE or EPI into a short-lived intermediate, DOPGAL, which undergoes further metabolism in a second step catalyzed by another group of enzymes forming more stable alcohol- or acid-deaminated metabolites. Aldehyde dehydrogenase metabolizes DOPGAL to DOMA, while aldehyde reductase metabolizes DOPGAL to DOPEG. In addition to aldehyde reductase, a related enzyme, aldose reductase, can reduce a catecholamine to its corresponding alcohol. This latter enzyme is present in sympathetic neurons and adrenal chromaffin cells. Under normal circumstances, DOMA is an insignificant metabolite of NE and EPI, with DOPEG being the main metabolite produced by deamination in sympathetic neurons and adrenal medullary chromaffin cells.

Once it leaves the sites of formation (sympathetic neurons, adrenal medulla), DOPEG is converted to MOPEG by COMT. Thus, most MOPEG comes from extraneuronal *O*-methylation of DOPEG produced in and diffusing rapidly from sympathetic neurons into the extracellular fluid. MOPEG is then converted to VMA by the sequential actions of alcohol and aldehyde dehydrogenases. MOPEG is first converted to the unstable aldehyde metabolite MOPGAL and then to VMA, with VMA being the major end product of NE and EPI metabolism. Another route for the formation of VMA is conversion by COMT of NE and EPI into normetanephrine and metaneprhine, respectively, followed by deamination to MOPGAL and thence to VMA. This is now thought to be only a minor pathway, as indicated by the size of the arrows on Figure 8–9.

In contrast to sympathetic neurons, adrenal medullary chromaffin cells contain both MAO and COMT, the COMT mainly as the membrane-bound form. This isoform of COMT has a higher affinity for catecholamines than does the soluble form found in most other tissues (e.g., liver and kidney). In adrenal medullary chromaffin cells, leakage of NE and EPI from storage vesicles leads to substantial intracellular production of the *O*-methylated metabolites normetanephrine and metanephrine. In humans, over 90% of circulating metanephrine and 25%–40% of circulating normetanephrine are derived from catecholamines metabolized within adrenal chromaffin cells.

The sequence of cellular uptake and metabolism of catecholamines

TABLE 8–6 ■ CHARACTERISTICS FOR ADRENERGIC RECEPTOR SUBTYPES[a]

	G PROTEIN COUPLING	PRINCIPLE EFFECTORS	TISSUE LOCALIZATION	DOMINANT EFFECTS[b]
α_{1A}	$G\alpha_q$ ($\alpha_{11}/\alpha_{14}/\alpha_{16}$)	↑ PLC, ↑ PLA_2 ↑ Ca^{2+} channels ↑ Na^+/H^+ exchanger Modulation of K^+ channels ↑ MAPK Signaling	Heart, lung Liver Smooth muscle Blood vessels Vas deferens, prostate Cerebellum, cortex Hippocampus	• Dominant receptor for contraction of vascular smooth muscle • Promotes cardiac growth and structure • Vasoconstriction of large resistant arterioles in skeletal muscle
α_{1B}	$G\alpha_q$ ($\alpha_{11}/\alpha_{14}/\alpha_{16}$)	↑ PLC, ↑ PLA_2 ↑ Ca^{2+} channels ↑ Na^+/H^+ exchanger Modulation of K^+ channels ↑ MAPK signaling	Kidney, lung Spleen Blood vessels Cortex Brainstem	• Most abundant subtype in heart • Promotes cardiac growth and structure
α_{1D}	$G\alpha_q$ ($\alpha_{11}/\alpha_{14}/\alpha_{16}$)	↑ PLC, ↑ PLA_2 ↑ Ca^{2+} channels ↑ Na^+/H^+ exchanger Modulation of K^+ channels ↑ MAPK signaling	Platelets, aorta Coronary artery Prostate Cortex Hippocampus	• Dominant receptor for vasoconstriction in aorta and coronaries
α_{2A}	$G\alpha_i$ $G\alpha_o$ (α_{o1}/α_{o2})	↓ AC-cAMP-PKA pathway	Platelets Sympathetic neurons Autonomic ganglia Pancreas Coronary/CNS vessels Locus ceruleus Brainstem, spinal cord	• Dominant inhibitory receptor on sympathetic neurons • Vasoconstriction of precapillary vessels in skeletal muscle
α_{2B}	$G\alpha_i$ $G\alpha_o$ (α_{o1}/α_{o2})	↓ AC-cAMP-PKA pathway	Liver, kidney Blood vessels Coronary/CNS vessels Diencephalon Pancreas, platelets	• Dominant mediator of α_2 vasoconstriction
α_{2C}	$G\alpha_i$ ($\alpha_{11}/\alpha_{12}/\alpha_{13}$) $G\alpha_o$ (α_{o1}/α_{o2})	↓ AC-cAMP-PKA pathway	Basal ganglia Cortex, cerebellum Hippocampus	• Dominant receptor modulating DA neurotransmission • Dominant receptor inhibiting hormone release from adrenal medulla
β_1	$G\alpha_s$	↑ AC-cAMP-PKA pathway ↑ L-type Ca^{2+} channels	Heart, kidney Adipocytes Skeletal muscle Olfactory nucleus Cortex, brainstem Cerebellar nuclei Spinal cord	• Dominant mediator of positive inotropic and chronotropic effects in heart
β_2[c]	$G\alpha_s$	↑ AC-cAMP-PKA pathway ↑ Ca^{2+} channels	Heart, lung, kidney Blood vessels Bronchial smooth muscle GI smooth muscle Skeletal muscle Olfactory bulb Cortex, hippocampus	• Smooth muscle relaxation • Skeletal muscle hypertrophy
β_3[c,d]	$G\alpha_s$	↑ AC-cAMP-PKA pathway ↑ Ca^{2+} channels	Adipose tissue GI tract, heart	• Metabolic effects

[a]At least three subtypes each of α_1 and α_2 adrenergic receptors are known, but distinctions in their mechanisms of action have not been clearly defined.

[b]In some species (e.g., rat), metabolic responses in the liver are mediated by α_1 adrenergic receptors, whereas in others (e.g., dog) β_2 adrenergic receptors are predominantly involved. Both types of receptors appear to contribute to responses in human beings.

[c]β Receptor coupling to cell signaling can be more complex. In addition to coupling to G_s to stimulate AC, β_2 receptors can activate signaling via a GRK/β-arrestin pathway. β_2 and β_3 receptors can couple to both G_s and G_i in a manner that may reflect agonist stereochemistry. See also Chapter 12.

[d]Metabolic responses in tissues with atypical pharmacological characteristics (e.g., adipocytes) may be mediated by β_3 receptors. Most β receptor antagonists (including propranolol) do not block these responses.

in extraneuronal tissues contributes only modestly (~25%) to the total metabolism of endogenously produced NE in sympathetic neurons or the adrenal medulla. However, extraneuronal metabolism is an important mechanism for the clearance of circulating and exogenously administered catecholamines.

Classification of Adrenergic Receptors

Adrenergic receptors are broadly classified as either α or β, with subtypes within each group (Table 8–6). The original subclassification was based on the rank order of agonist potency:

- EPI ≥ NE >> isoproterenol for α adrenergic receptors.
- Isoproterenol > EPI ≥ NE for β adrenergic receptors.

Elucidation of the characteristics of these receptors and the biochemical and physiological pathways they regulate has increased our understanding of the seemingly contradictory and variable effects of catecholamines on various organ systems. Although structurally related (discussed further in the chapter), different receptors regulate distinct physiological processes by controlling the synthesis or mobilization of a variety of second messengers.

Raymond Ahlquist and the Functional Definition of α and β Receptors. Based on studies of the capacities of EPI, NE, and related agonists to regulate various physiological processes, Ahlquist (1948) proposed the existence of more than one adrenergic receptor. It was known that adrenergic agents could cause either contraction or relaxation of smooth muscle depending on the site, the dose, and the agent chosen. For example, NE was known to have potent excitatory effects on smooth muscle and correspondingly low activity as an inhibitor; isoproterenol displayed the opposite pattern of activity. EPI could both excite and inhibit smooth muscle. Thus, Ahlquist proposed the designations α and β for receptors on smooth muscle where catecholamines produce excitatory and inhibitory responses, respectively (an exception was the gut, which generally is relaxed by activation of either α or β receptors). He developed the rank orders of potency that define α and β receptor–mediated responses, as noted above. This initial classification was corroborated by the finding that certain antagonists produced selective blockade of the effects of adrenergic nerve impulses and sympathomimetic agents at α receptors (e.g., phenoxybenzamine), whereas others produced selective β receptor blockade (e.g., propranolol).

α and β Receptor Subtypes. Subsequent to Ahlquist's functional description of α and β receptors, adrenergic pharmacologists used increasingly sophisticated probes, tools, and methods to elucidate subtypes of α and β receptors. The β receptors were subclassified as β_1 (e.g., those in the myocardium) and β_2 (smooth muscle and most other sites), reflecting the finding that EPI and NE essentially are equipotent at β_1 sites, whereas EPI is 10–50 times more potent than NE at β_2 sites. Antagonists that discriminate between β_1 and β_2 receptors were subsequently developed (Chapter 12). Cloning confirmed that these β subtypes are products of different genes, and a human gene that encodes a third β receptor (designated β_3) was isolated (Emorine et al., 1989). Because the β_3 receptor is about 10-fold more sensitive to NE than to EPI and is relatively resistant to blockade by antagonists such as propranolol, the β_3 receptor may mediate responses to catecholamine at sites with "atypical" pharmacological characteristics (e.g., adipose tissue, which expresses all three β receptor subtypes). Animals treated with β_3 receptor agonists exhibit a vigorous thermogenic response as well as lipolysis (Robidoux et al., 2004). Polymorphisms in the β_3 receptor gene may be related to risk of obesity or type 2 diabetes in some populations (Arner and Hoffstedt, 1999), and Weyer and colleagues (1999) suggested that β_3 receptor–selective agonists may be beneficial in treating these disorders. The existence of a fourth β adrenergic receptor, β_4 was proposed but no such receptor has been cloned; rather, the "β_4 receptor" seems to be an affinity state of the β_1 adrenergic receptor rather than a distinct new protein (Gherbi et al., 2015; Hieble, 2007).

There is also heterogeneity among α adrenergic receptors. The initial distinction was based on functional and anatomic considerations: NE and other α adrenergic agonists profoundly inhibit the release of NE from neurons (Westfall, 1977) (Figure 8–8); conversely, certain α receptor antagonists markedly increase NE release when sympathetic nerves are stimulated. This feedback-inhibitory effect of NE on its release from nerve terminals is mediated by α receptors that are pharmacologically distinct from the classical postsynaptic α receptors. Accordingly, these presynaptic α adrenergic receptors were designated α_2, whereas the postsynaptic "excitatory" α receptors were designated α_1 (Langer, 1997). Compounds such as clonidine are more potent agonists at α_2 than at α_1 receptors; by contrast, phenylephrine and methoxamine selectively activate postsynaptic α_1 receptors.

Although there is little evidence to suggest that α_1 adrenergic receptors function presynaptically in the autonomic nervous system, α_2 receptors are present at postjunctional or nonjunctional sites in several tissues. For example, stimulation of postjunctional α_2 receptors in the brain is associated with reduced sympathetic outflow from the CNS and appears to be responsible for a significant component of the antihypertensive effect of drugs such as clonidine (Chapter 12). Thus, the anatomic concept of prejunctional α_2 and postjunctional α_1 adrenergic receptors has been abandoned in favor of a pharmacological and functional classification (Tables 8–6 and 8–7).

Cloning revealed additional heterogeneity of both α_1 and α_2 adrenergic receptors (Bylund, 1992). There are three pharmacologically defined α_1 receptors (α_{1A}, α_{1B}, and α_{1D}) with distinct sequences and tissue distributions and three cloned subtypes of α_2 receptors (α_{2A}, α_{2B}, and α_{2C}) (Table 8–6). A fourth type of α_1 receptor, α_{1L}, has been defined on the basis of a low affinity for the selective antagonists prazosin and 5-methyl urapidil but a high affinity for tamsulosin and silodosin. This phenotype could be of physiological significance; the α_{1L} profile has been identified in myriad tissues across a number of species, where it appears to regulate smooth muscle contractility in the vasculature and lower urinary tract. Despite intense efforts, the α_{1L} adrenergic receptor has not been cloned; currently, it is viewed as a second phenotype originating from the α_{1A} receptor gene (Hieble, 2007; Yoshiki et al., 2013). Distinct pharmacological phenotypes of the α_{1B} receptor have also been described (Yoshiki et al., 2014).

Owing to the lack of sufficiently subtype-selective ligands, the precise physiological function and therapeutic potential of the subtypes of adrenergic receptors have not been elucidated fully. Genetic approaches using transgenic and receptor knockout experiments in mice (discussed further in the chapter) have advanced our understanding. These mouse models have been used to identify and localize particular receptor subtypes and to describe the pathophysiological relevance of individual adrenergic receptor subtypes (Philipp and Hein, 2004; Tanoue et al., 2002a, 2002b; Xiao et al., 2006).

Molecular Basis of Adrenergic Receptor Function

Structural Features. All adrenergic receptors are GPCRs that link to heterotrimeric G proteins. Structurally, there are similarities in the regions for ligand binding and modulation by intracellular protein kinases (Figure 8–10). The coding region of each of the three β adrenergic receptor genes and the three α_2 adrenergic receptor genes is contained in a single exon, whereas each of the three α_1 adrenergic receptor genes has a single large intron separating regions that encode the body of the receptor from those that encode the seventh transmembrane domain and carboxy terminus (Dorn, 2010). Each major receptor type shows preference for a particular class of G proteins, that is, α_1 to G_q, α_2 to G_i, and β to G_s (see Table 8–6). The responses that follow receptor activation result from G protein–mediated effects on the generation of second messengers and on the activity of ion channels (see Chapter 3). The signaling pathways overlap broadly with those discussed for muscarinic ACh receptors.

α Adrenergic Receptors. The α_1 receptors (α_{1A}, α_{1B}, and α_{1D}) and the α_2 receptors (α_{2A}, α_{2B}, and α_{2C}) are heptahelical proteins that couple differentially to a variety of G proteins to regulate smooth muscle contraction, secretory pathways, and cell growth (see Table 8–6). Within the membrane-spanning domains, the three α_1 adrenergic receptors share about 75% identity in amino acid residues, as do the three α_2 receptors, but the α_1 and α_2 subtypes are no more similar than are the α and β subtypes (~30%–40%).

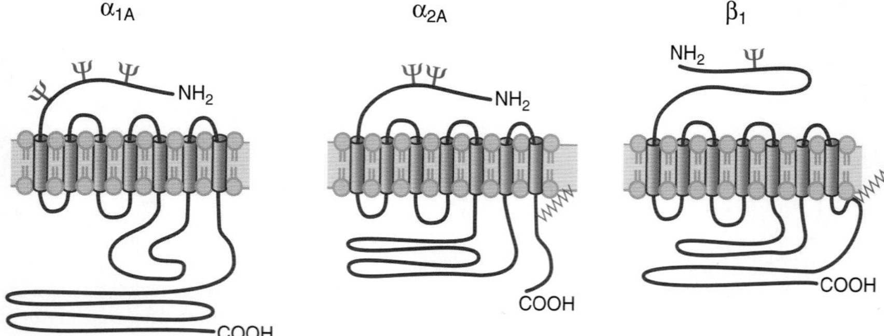

Figure 8–10 *Structural features of adrenergic receptor subtypes.* All of the adrenergic receptors are hepta-spanning GPCRs. A representative of each type is shown; each type has three subtypes: α_{1A}, α_{1B}, and α_{1D}; α_{2A}, α_{2B}, and α_{2C}; and β_1, β_2, and β_3. The principle effector systems affected by α_1, α_2 and β receptors are depicted in Table 8–6. ψ indicates a site for *N*-glycosylation.

***α_1* Adrenergic Receptors.** Stimulation of α_1 receptors activates the G_q-PLC_β-IP_3/DAG-Ca^{2+} pathway and results in the activation of PKC and other Ca^{2+} and CaM-sensitive pathways, such as CaM kinases, with sequelae depending on cell differentiation (e.g., contraction of vascular smooth muscle, stimulation of growth in smooth muscles and hypertrophy in cardiac myocytes, and activation of endothelial NOS in vascular endothelium) (see Chapter 3). PKC phosphorylates many substrates, including membrane proteins such as channels, pumps, and ion exchange proteins (e.g., Ca^{2+}-transport ATPase). α_1 Receptor stimulation of PLA_2 leads to the release of free arachidonate, which is then metabolized by cyclooxygenase (yielding prostaglandins) and lipoxygenase (yielding leukotrienes) (see Chapter 37); PLD hydrolyzes phosphatidylcholine to yield phosphatidic acid, which can yield diacylglycerol, a cofactor for PKC activation. PLD is an effector for ADP-ribosylating factor, suggesting that PLD may play a role in membrane trafficking. In most smooth muscles, the increased concentration of intracellular Ca^{2+} causes contraction (see Figure 3–17). In contrast, the increased concentration of intracellular Ca^{2+} following α_1 stimulation of GI smooth muscle causes hyperpolarization and relaxation by activation of Ca^{2+}-dependent K^+ channels. Stimulation of α_1 receptors can activate p38/p42/p44, PI3K, JNK, and others to affect cell growth and proliferation, albeit in receptor subtype-specific and tissue-specific manners.

The α_{1A} receptor is the predominant receptor causing vasoconstriction in many vascular beds, including the following arteries: mammary, mesenteric, splenic, hepatic, omental, renal, pulmonary, and epicardial coronary. It is also the predominant subtype in the vena cava and the saphenous and pulmonary veins (Michelotti et al., 2000). Together with the α_{1B} receptor subtype, it promotes cardiac growth and structure. The α_{1B} receptor subtype is the most abundant subtype in the heart, whereas the α_{1D} receptor subtype is the predominant receptor causing vasoconstriction in the aorta. There is evidence to support the idea that α_{1B} receptors mediate behaviors such as reaction to novelty and exploration and are involved in behavioral sensitizations and in the vulnerability to addiction (see Chapter 24).

In addition to their traditional localization in the plasma membrane, α_1 receptors have nuclear localization signals (as do β receptors and receptors for endothelin and angiotensin) and have been found on the nuclear membrane of adult mouse cardiac myocytes, where they activate intranuclear signaling and appear to play a cardioprotective role (Wu and O'Connell, 2015).

***α_2* Adrenergic Receptors.** The α_2 receptors couple to a variety of effectors (Tan and Limbird, 2005). Inhibition of adenylyl cyclase activity was the first effect observed, but in some systems the enzyme actually is stimulated by α_2 adrenergic receptors, either by G_i βγ subunits or by weak direct stimulation of G_s. The physiological significance of these last processes is not currently clear. The α_2 receptors activate G protein–gated K^+ channels, resulting in membrane hyperpolarization. In some cases (e.g., cholinergic neurons in the myenteric plexus), this may be Ca^{2+} dependent, whereas in others (e.g., muscarinic ACh receptors in atrial myocytes) it results from direct interaction of βγ subunits with K^+ channels. The α_2 receptors also can inhibit voltage-gated Ca^{2+} channels; this is mediated by G_o. Other second-messenger systems linked to α_2 receptor activation include acceleration of Na^+/H^+ exchange, stimulation of $PLC\beta_2$ activity and arachidonic acid mobilization, increased phosphoinositide hydrolysis, and increased intracellular availability of Ca^{2+}. The last is involved in the smooth muscle–contracting effect of α_2 adrenergic receptor agonists. In addition, the α_2 receptors activate MAPKs via mechanisms dependent on both the α and βγ components of G_i, with involvement of protein tyrosine kinases and small GTPases (Goldsmith and Dhanasekaran, 2007). These pathways are reminiscent of pathways activated by tyrosine kinase activities of growth factor receptors. The α_{2A} and α_{2C} receptors play a major role in inhibiting NE release from sympathetic nerve endings and suppressing sympathetic outflow from the brain, leading to hypotension (Kable et al., 2000).

Thus, depending on subtype, the major biological effects of α_2 adrenergic receptors can be on platelet aggregation, regulation of sympathetic outflow from the CNS, reuptake of NE from within peripheral sympathetic nerve synapses, insulin secretion and lipolysis, or, to a limited extent, vasoconstriction (Gavras and Gavras, 2001). Similar studies with knockout mice have been carried out as was done with α_1 adrenergic receptors.

In the CNS, α_{2A} receptors, which appear to be the dominant adrenergic receptor, probably mediate the antinociceptive effects, sedation, hypothermia, hypotension, and behavioral actions of α_2 agonists (Lakhlani et al., 1997). The α_{2C} receptor occurs in the ventral and dorsal striatum and hippocampus. It appears to modulate DA neurotransmission and various behavioral responses. The α_{2B} receptor is the main receptor mediating α_2-induced vasoconstriction, whereas the α_{2C} receptor is the predominant receptor inhibiting the release of catecholamines from the adrenal medulla and modulating DA neurotransmission in the brain.

β Adrenergic Receptors

Subtypes. The three β receptor subtypes share about 60% amino acid sequence identity within the putative membrane-spanning domains where the ligand-binding pockets for EPI and NE are found. Based on results of site-directed mutagenesis, individual amino acids in the β_2 receptor that interact with each of the functional groups on the catecholamine agonist molecule have been identified. Figure 8–10 depicts the general hepta-spanning structure of adrenergic receptors and notes some differences in the sizes of the third and fourth intracellular loops.

The β receptors regulate numerous functional responses, including heart rate and contractility, smooth muscle relaxation, and myriad metabolic events in numerous tissues, including skeletal muscle, liver, and adipose tissue (Lynch and Ryall, 2008) (Table 8–1).

β Receptor Signaling. All three of the β receptor subtypes (β_1, β_2, and β_3) couple to G_s and activate adenylyl cyclase (Table 8–7). Stimulation of β adrenergic receptors leads to the accumulation of cAMP, activation of the PKA, and altered function of numerous cellular proteins as a result of their phosphorylation (Chapter 3). In addition, G_s subunits can enhance directly the activation of voltage-sensitive Ca^{2+} channels in the plasma membrane of skeletal and cardiac muscle cells.

The β_1, β_2, and β_3 receptors can differ in their intracellular signaling pathways and subcellular location (Brodde et al., 2006; Violin and Lefkowitz, 2007; Woo et al., 2009). While the positive chronotropic effects of β_1 receptor activation are clearly mediated by G_s in myocytes, dual coupling of β_2 receptors to G_s and G_i occurs in myocytes from newborn mice. Stimulation of β_2 receptors causes a transient increase in heart rate that is followed by a prolonged decrease. Following pretreatment with pertussis toxin, which prevents activation of G_i, the negative chronotropic effect of β_2 activation is abolished. These specific signaling properties of β receptor subtypes likely result from subtype-selective association with intracellular scaffolding and signaling proteins (Baillie and Houslay, 2005). The β_2 receptors normally are confined to caveolae in cardiac myocyte membranes. The activation of PKA by cAMP and the importance of compartmentation of components of the cAMP pathway are discussed in Chapter 3.

Refractoriness to Catecholamines. Exposure of catecholamine-sensitive cells and tissues to adrenergic agonists causes a progressive diminution in their capacity to respond to such agents. This phenomenon, variously termed *refractoriness, desensitization,* or *tachyphylaxis,* can limit the therapeutic efficacy and duration of action of catecholamines and other agents (Chapter 3). An understanding of the mechanisms involved in regulation of GPCR desensitization and the roles of GRKs and β-arrestins has developed over the last two decades due to the efforts of Lefkowitz and colleagues (Violin and Lefkowitz, 2007) and Houslay and colleagues (Baillie and Houslay, 2005), among others. For a perspective on refractoriness and on the roles of GRKs and β-arrestins in biased agonism, see the discussion that follows.

Desensitization has functional correlates in human health. Long-term exposure to catecholamines can cause cardiac dysfunction and contribute to the course of deterioration in heart failure. Data support the idea that the β_1 receptor is the primary mediator of catecholamine cardiotoxicity (Communal et al., 1999). Studies in genetically manipulated mice indicate that β_1 receptor signaling has greater potential than β_2 receptor signaling to contribute to heart failure.

Desensitization, Downregulation, Sustained Signaling. Catecholamines promote β receptor feedback regulation, that is, desensitization, receptor downregulation, and internalization into endosomes. The β receptors differ in the extent to which they undergo such regulation, with the β_2 receptor being the most susceptible, as described in Chapter 3. Post-stimulatory interactions of the agonist-liganded β_2 receptor with a GRK produces a phosphorylated receptor that readily interacts with β-arrestin, which blocks receptor access to the G protein and directs the receptor toward an endocytotic pathway, thereby reducing the number of receptors available at the cell surface. As a scaffolding protein, β-arrestin can also anchor proteins such as phosphodiesterase 4, which can modulate cAMP accumulation. The β receptor–β-arrestin complexes localize to coated pits and are subsequently internalized reversibly into endosomes (where the receptors may be dephosphorylated; such receptors can reenter the plasma membrane to aid resensitization), some complexes reaching lysosomes, where they are degraded (see Chapter 3). β-Arrestin also serves as an organizing center for the formation of a complex of a phospho-GPCR, a G protein, and β-arrestin, and this complex may provide sustained intracellular signaling from the internalized GPCR (Thomsen et al., 2016).

Biased Agonism and Selective Responsiveness. The original idea that a β adrenergic agonist activates just the G_s-AC-cAMP-PKA pathway is incomplete. Recent data demonstrate differences in downstream signals and events activated by the three β receptors and differences when various ligands activate a single receptor subtype. This concept, termed *biased agonism*, follows from four findings:

- signaling resulting from GPCR activation can be complex and involve a host of pathways
- ligand-activated GPCRs can adopt a multiplicity of conformations
- GRKs and β-arrestins are signal transducers, independently of G proteins
- distinct GRKs are recruited to and phosphorylate receptors based on specific ligand-induced receptor conformations, leading to specific signaling mediated by β-arrestin

A biased agonist stabilizes one or a subset of possible GPCR conformations and thereby activates a subset of all possible responses; these responses may involve signaling mechanisms mediated by β-arrestins through its myriad scaffolding partners. In work leading to the Nobel Prize in 2012, Lefkowitz and colleagues described this "pluridimensionality of β-arrestin–dependent signaling" at GPCRs (Reiter et al., 2012). This idea raises the possibility that one may design biased agonists that have unusually precise specificity. Biased agonism is discussed at greater length in Chapter 20 with regard to mu opioid agonists.

Adrenergic Receptor Polymorphism

Numerous polymorphisms and splice variants of adrenergic receptors continue to be identified. Such polymorphisms in adrenergic receptors could result in altered physiological responses to activation of the sympathetic nervous system, contribute to disease states, and alter the responses to adrenergic agonists or antagonists (Brodde, 2008). Knowledge of the functional consequences of specific polymorphisms could theoretically result in the individualization of drug therapy based on a patient's genetic makeup and could explain marked interindividual variability within the human population.

α_1 Adrenergic Receptor Polymorphisms. The α_1 adrenergic receptor is abundant in vascular smooth muscle and is implicated in regulating arterial resistance and blood pressure (Rokosh and Simpson, 2002). The α_1 adrenergic receptor polymorphism most often studied in human hypertension is α_{1A} Arg347Cys; the accumulated data so far suggest only a marginal effect of this polymorphism in cardiovascular responses to sympathetic stimulation or human hypertension. There are no functional phenotypes or cardiovascular disease associations reported for the α_{1B} and α_{1D} adrenergic receptors.

α_{2A} Adrenergic Receptor Polymorphisms. As with the α_{1A} adrenergic receptor, there is insufficient evidence supporting a major effect of α_2 receptor polymorphisms in hypertension. Likewise, although there are interesting and provocative studies suggesting an association between α_{2A}, α_{2BA}, and α_{2C} polymorphisms and coronary heart disease, heart failure, and sudden death, these linkages are not yet definitive. In contrast, a convincing role for α_{2A} adrenergic receptor polymorphisms in human type 2 diabetes has been elucidated. Moreover, in mice, deletion of the α_{2A} adrenergic receptor results in enhanced insulin secretion (Fagerholm et al., 2004) and β-cell–specific overexpression of α_{2A}R mimics diabetes (Devedjian et al., 2000).

β_1 Adrenergic Receptor Polymorphisms. Evidence does support the notion that increased cardiomyocyte β_1 receptor signaling by any means, including chronic agonist stimulation (Mobine et al., 2009), increased receptor expression (Dorn et al., 1999; Liggett et al., 2000), or enhanced receptor signaling (Mialet et al., 2003), can ultimately result in cardiac toxicity and contribute to heart failure. On the other hand, β_1 adrenergic receptor polymorphisms do not seem to be major risk factors in human hypertension.

Biochemical, functional, and structural studies in cultured cell expression systems and genetic mouse models indicate that the Gly389Arg β_1 adrenergic receptor exhibits a gain-of-signaling function that can initially improve cardiac contractility but ultimately predisposes to cardiomyopathic decompensation. This abnormally active Arg389 receptor is more sensitive to pharmacological blockade and exhibits distinctive pharmacological properties of different β blockers. This polymorphism may affect heart failure risk or progression, but the β blockers currently in use are sufficient to overcome the subtle differences that polymorphic receptor function may have on heart failure survival (Dorn, 2010).

β_2 Adrenergic Receptor Polymorphisms. Data supporting an interaction between β_2 adrenergic receptor polymorphisms and hypertension are inconclusive and suggest that effects of β_2 adrenergic receptor polymorphisms on blood pressure are modest. Similarly, there is no consensus about β_2 adrenergic receptor polymorphisms and heart disease (Dorn, 2010).

β_3 Adrenergic Receptor Polymorphisms. Polymorphisms of the β_3 adrenergic receptor appear to be associated with diabetes phenotypes, but there have been few clinical cardiac studies (Dorn, 2010).

Localization of Adrenergic Receptors

Presynaptic α_2 and β_2 receptors regulate neurotransmitter release from sympathetic nerve endings. Presynaptic α_2 receptors also may mediate inhibition of release of neurotransmitters other than NE in the central and peripheral nervous systems. Both α_2 and β_2 receptors are located at postsynaptic sites (Table 8–6), such as on many types of neurons in the brain. In peripheral tissues, postsynaptic α_2 receptors are found in vascular and other smooth muscle cells (where they mediate contraction), adipocytes, and various secretory epithelial cells (intestinal, renal, endocrine). Postsynaptic β_2 receptors can be found in the myocardium (where they mediate contraction) as well as on vascular and other smooth muscle cells (where they mediate relaxation), and skeletal muscle (where they can mediate hypertrophy). Indeed, most normal human cell types express β_2 receptors. Both α_2 and β_2 receptors may be situated at sites that are relatively remote from nerve terminals that release NE. Such extrajunctional receptors typically are found on vascular smooth muscle cells and blood elements (platelets and leukocytes) and may be activated preferentially by circulating catecholamines, particularly EPI.

In contrast, α_1 and β_1 receptors appear to be located mainly in the immediate vicinity of sympathetic adrenergic nerve terminals in peripheral target organs, strategically placed to be activated during stimulation of these nerves. These receptors also are distributed widely in the mammalian brain (Table 8–6).

The cellular distributions of the three α_1 and three α_2 receptor subtypes still are incompletely understood. Studies using in situ hybridization with receptor mRNA and receptor subtype-specific antibodies indicate that α_{2A} receptors in the brain may be both pre- and postsynaptic, suggesting that this receptor subtype may also function as a presynaptic autoreceptor in central noradrenergic neurons (Aantaa et al., 1995; Lakhlani et al., 1997). Using similar approaches, α_{1A} mRNA was found to be the dominant subtype message expressed in prostatic smooth muscle (Walden et al., 1997).

Pharmacological Considerations

Each step involved in neurotransmission is a potential point of pharmacological intervention. The diagrams of the cholinergic and adrenergic terminals and their postjunctional sites (Figure 8–6 and 8–8) show these points of intervention. Drugs that affect processes involved in the steps of transmission at both cholinergic and adrenergic junctions are summarized in Table 8–7, which lists representative agents that act through the mechanisms below.

Interference With the Synthesis or Release of the Transmitter

Cholinergic

Hemicholinium, a synthetic compound, blocks the transport system by which choline accumulates in the terminals of cholinergic fibers, thus limiting the synthesis of ACh. Vesamicol blocks the transport of ACh into its storage vesicles, thereby preventing repletion of ACh stores following transmitter release and thus reducing ACh available for subsequent release. The site on the presynaptic nerve terminal for block of ACh release by botulinum toxin was discussed previously; death usually results from respiratory paralysis unless patients with respiratory failure receive artificial ventilation. Injected locally, botulinum toxin type A is used in the treatment of certain ophthalmic conditions associated with spasms of ocular muscles (e.g., strabismus and blepharospasm) (Chapter 69) and for a wide variety of unlabeled uses, ranging from treatment of muscle dystonias and palsy (Chapter 11) to cosmetic erasure of facial lines and wrinkles (a modern medical testament to the vanity of human wishes; Chapter 70).

Adrenergic

α-Methyltyrosine (metyrosine) blocks the synthesis of NE by inhibiting TH, the enzyme that catalyzes the rate-limiting step in catecholamine synthesis. This drug occasionally may be useful in treating selected patients with pheochromocytoma. On the other hand, methyldopa, an inhibitor of aromatic *L*-amino acid decarboxylase, is—like dopa itself—successively decarboxylated and hydroxylated in its side chain to form the putative "false neurotransmitter" α-methylnorepinephrine. The use of methyldopa in the treatment of hypertension is discussed in Chapter 28. Bretylium, guanadrel, and guanethidine act by preventing the release of NE by the nerve impulse. However, such agents can transiently stimulate the release of NE because of their capacity to displace the amine from storage sites.

Promotion of Release of the Transmitter

Cholinergic

The ability of pharmacological agents to promote the release of ACh is limited. The latrotoxins from black widow spider venom and stonefish are known to promote neuroexocytosis by binding to receptors on the neuronal membrane.

Adrenergic

Several drugs that promote the release of NE already have been discussed. On the basis of the rate and duration of the drug-induced release of NE from adrenergic terminals, one of two opposing effects can predominate. Tyramine, ephedrine, amphetamine, and related drugs cause a relatively rapid, brief liberation of the transmitter and produce a sympathomimetic effect. On the other hand, reserpine, by blocking the uptake of amines by VMAT2, produces a slow, prolonged depletion of the adrenergic transmitter from adrenergic storage vesicles, where it is largely metabolized by intraneuronal MAO. The resulting depletion of transmitter produces the equivalent of adrenergic blockade. Reserpine also causes the depletion of 5HT, DA, and possibly other, unidentified, amines from central and peripheral sites, and many of its major effects may be a consequence of the depletion of transmitters other than NE.

As discussed previously, deficiencies of TH in humans cause a neurologic disorder (Carson and Robertson, 2002) that can be treated by supplementation with the DA precursor levodopa.

A syndrome caused by congenital DβH deficiency is characterized by the absence of NE and EPI, elevated concentrations of DA, intact baroreceptor reflex afferent fibers and cholinergic innervation, and undetectable concentrations of plasma DβH activity (Carson and Robertson, 2002). Patients with this syndrome have severe orthostatic hypotension, ptosis of the eyelids, and retrograde ejaculations. Dihydroxyphenylserine (L-DOPS) improves postural hypotension in this rare disorder. This therapeutic approach takes advantage of the nonspecificity of aromatic *L*-amino acid decarboxylase, which synthesizes NE directly from this drug in the absence of DβH (Man in't Veld et al., 1988; Robertson et al., 1991). Despite the restoration of plasma NE in humans with L-DOPS, EPI levels are not restored, leading to speculation that PNMT may require DβH for appropriate functioning (Carson and Robertson, 2002).

Agonist and Antagonist Actions at Receptors

Cholinergic

The nicotinic receptors of autonomic ganglia and skeletal muscle are not identical; they respond differently to certain stimulating and blocking agents, and their pentameric structures contain different combinations of homologous subunits (Table 8–2). *Dimethylphenylpiperazinium*

TABLE 8–7 ■ REPRESENTATIVE AGENTS ACTING AT PERIPHERAL CHOLINERGIC AND ADRENERGIC NEUROEFFECTOR JUNCTIONS

MECHANISM OF ACTION	SYSTEM	AGENTS	EFFECT
1. Interference with synthesis of transmitter	Cholinergic	Choline acetyl transferase inhibitors	Minimal depletion of ACh
	Adrenergic	α-Methyltyrosine (inhibition of tyrosine hydroxylase)	Depletion of NE
2. Metabolic transformation by same pathway as precursor of transmitter	Adrenergic	Methyldopa	Displacement of NE by α-methyl-NE, which is an α_2 agonist, similar to clonidine, that reduces sympathetic outflow from CNS
3. Blockade of transport system at nerve terminal membrane	Cholinergic	Hemicholinium	Block of choline uptake with consequent depletion of ACh
	Adrenergic	Cocaine, imipramine	Accumulation of NE at receptors
4. Blockade of transport system of storage vesicle	Cholinergic	Vesamicol	Block of ACh storage
	Adrenergic	Reserpine	Destruction of NE by mitochondrial MAO and depletion from adrenergic terminals
5. Promotion of exocytosis or displacement of transmitter from storage sites	Cholinergic	Latrotoxins	Cholinomimetic followed by anticholinergic
	Adrenergic	Amphetamine, tyramine	Sympathomimetic
6. Prevention of release of transmitter	Cholinergic	Botulinum toxin (BTX, endopeptidase, acts on synaptobrevin)	Anticholinergic (prevents skeletal muscle contraction)
	Adrenergic	Bretylium, guanadrel	Antiadrenergic
7. Mimicry of transmitter at postjunctional sites	Cholinergic		
	Muscarinic[a]	Methacholine, bethanachol	Cholinomimetic
	Nicotinic[b]	Nicotine, epibatidine, cytisine	Cholinomimetic
	Adrenergic		
	α_1	Phenylephrine	Selective α_1 agonist
	α_2	Clonidine	Sympathomimetic (periphery); reduced sympathetic outflow (CNS)
	α_1, α_2	Oxymetazoline	Nonselective α adrenomimetic
	β_1	Dobutamine	Selective cardiac stimulation (also activates α_1 receptors)
	β_2	Terbutaline, albuterol metaproterenol	Selective β_2 receptor agonist (selective inhibition of smooth muscle contraction)
	β_1, β_2	Isoproterenol	Nonselective β agonist
8. Blockade of postsynaptic receptor	Cholinergic		
	Muscarinic[a]	Atropine	Muscarinic blockade
	Nicotinic (N_m)[b]	*d*-Tubucurarine, atracurium	Neuromuscular blockade
	Nicotinic (N_n)[b]	Trimethaphan	Ganglionic blockade
	Adrenergic		
	α_1, α_2	Phenoxybenzamine	Nonselective α receptor blockade (irreversible)
	α_1, α_2	Phentolamine	Nonselective α receptor blockade (reversible)
	α_1	Prazosin, terazosin, doxasozin	Selective α_1 receptor blockade (reversible)
	α_2	Yohimbine	Selective α_2 receptor blockade
	β_1, β_2	Propranolol	Nonselective β receptor blockade
	β_1	Metoprolol, atenolol	Selective β_1 receptor blockade (cardiomyocytes; renal j-g cells)
	β_2	—	Selective β_2 receptor blockade (smooth muscle)

(Continued)

TABLE 8–7 ■ REPRESENTATIVE AGENTS ACTING AT PERIPHERAL CHOLINERGIC AND ADRENERGIC NEUROEFFECTOR JUNCTIONS (*CONTINUED*)

MECHANISM OF ACTION	SYSTEM	AGENTS	EFFECT
9. Inhibition of enzymatic breakdown of transmitter	Cholinergic	AChE inhibitors edrophonium, neostigmine, pyridostigmine	Cholinomimetic (muscarinic sites) Depolarization blockade (nicotinic sites)
	Adrenergic	Nonselective MAO inhibitors: pargyline, nialamide	Little direct effect on NE or sympathetic response; potentiation of tyramine
		Selective MAO-B inhibitor: selegeline	Adjunct in Parkinson disease
		Peripheral COMT inhibitor: Entacapone	Adjunct in Parkinson disease
		COMT inhibitor: Tolcapone	

The j-g cells are renin-secreting cells in the juxtaglomerular complex of the kidney.
[a]At least five subtypes of muscarinic receptors exist (see Table 8–3). Agonists show little subtype selectivity; several antagonists show partial subtype selectivity (see Chapter 9).
[b]Two subtypes of muscle acetylcholine nicotinic receptors and several subtypes of neuronal receptors have been identified (see Table 8–2).

(DMPP) and phenyltrimethylammonium (PTMA) show some selectivity for stimulation of autonomic ganglion cells and muscle motor end plates. Trimethaphan and hexamethonium are relatively selective competitive and noncompetitive ganglionic blocking agents, respectively. Although tubocurarine effectively blocks transmission at both motor end plates and autonomic ganglia, its action at the former site predominates. Succinylcholine, a depolarizing agent, produces selective neuromuscular blockade. Transmission at autonomic ganglia and the adrenal medulla is complicated further by the presence of muscarinic receptors in addition to the principal nicotinic receptors (see Chapter 11).

Various toxins in snake venoms exhibit a high degree of specificity toward cholinergic receptors. The α-neurotoxins from the Elapidae family interact with the agonist-binding site on the nicotinic receptor. α-Bungarotoxin is selective for the muscle receptor and interacts with only certain neuronal receptors, such as those containing α7 through α9 subunits. Neuronal bungarotoxin shows a wider range of inhibition of neuronal receptors. A second group of toxins, called the *fasciculins,* inhibits AChE. A third group of toxins, termed the *muscarinic toxins* (MT_1 through MT_4), includes partial agonists and antagonists for muscarinic receptors. Venoms from the Viperidae family of snakes and the fish-hunting cone snails also have relatively selective toxins for nicotinic receptors.

Muscarinic ACh receptors, which mediate the effects of ACh at autonomic effector cells, now can be divided into five subclasses. Atropine blocks all the muscarinic responses to injected ACh and related cholinomimetic drugs whether they are excitatory, as in the intestine, or inhibitory, as in the heart. Newer muscarinic agonists, pirenzepine for M_1, tripitramine for M_2, and darifenacin for M_3, show selectivity as muscarinic-blocking agents. Several muscarinic antagonists show sufficient selectivity in the clinical setting to minimize the bothersome side effects seen with the nonselective agents at therapeutic doses (see Chapter 9).

Adrenergic

A vast number of synthetic compounds that bear structural resemblance to the naturally occurring catecholamines can interact with α and β adrenergic receptors to produce sympathomimetic effects (see Chapter 12). Phenylephrine acts selectively at α_1 receptors, whereas clonidine is a selective α_2 adrenergic agonist. Isoproterenol exhibits agonist activity at both β_1 and β_2 receptors. Preferential stimulation of cardiac β_1 receptors follows the administration of dobutamine. Terbutaline exerts relatively selective action on β_2 receptors; it produces effective bronchodilation with minimal effects on the heart. The main features of adrenergic blockade, including the selectivity of various blocking agents for α and β adrenergic receptors, are considered in detail in Chapter 12. Partial dissociation of effects at β_1 and β_2 receptors has been achieved by subtype-selective antagonists, as exemplified by the β_1 receptor antagonists metoprolol and atenolol, which antagonize the cardiac actions of catecholamines while causing somewhat less antagonism at bronchioles. Prazosin and yohimbine are representative of α_1 and α_2 receptor antagonists, respectively; prazosin has a relatively high affinity at α_{2B} and α_{2C} subtypes compared with α_{2A} receptors. Several important drugs that promote the release of NE (e.g., tyramine) or deplete the transmitter (e.g., reserpine) resemble, in their effects, activators or blockers of postjunctional receptors.

Interference With the Destruction of the Transmitter

Cholinergic

The anti-ChE agents (see Chapter 10) constitute a chemically diverse group of compounds, the primary action of which is inhibition of AChE, with the consequent accumulation of endogenous ACh. At the NMJ, accumulation of ACh produces depolarization of end plates and flaccid paralysis. At postganglionic muscarinic effector sites, the response is either excessive stimulation resulting in contraction and secretion or an inhibitory response mediated by hyperpolarization. At ganglia, depolarization and enhanced transmission are observed.

Adrenergic

The reuptake of NE by the adrenergic nerve terminals by means of NET is the major mechanism for terminating NE's transmitter action. Interference with this process is the basis of the potentiating effect of cocaine on responses to adrenergic impulses and injected catecholamines. The antidepressant actions and some of the adverse effects of imipramine and related drugs may be due to a similar action at adrenergic synapses in the CNS (Chapter 15).

Entacapone and tolcapone are nitro catechol-type COMT inhibitors. Entacapone is a peripherally acting COMT inhibitor, whereas tolcapone also inhibits COMT activity in the brain. COMT inhibition has been shown to attenuate levodopa toxicity on dopaminergic neurons and enhance DA's action in the brain of patients with Parkinson disease (Chapter 18). On the other hand, nonselective MAO inhibitors, such as tranylcypromine, potentiate the effects of tyramine and may potentiate effects of neurotransmitters. While most MAO inhibitors used as antidepressants inhibit both MAO-A and MAO-B, selective MAO-A and MAO-B inhibitors are available. Selegiline is a selective and irreversible MAO-B inhibitor that also has been used as an adjunct in the treatment of Parkinson disease.

Other Autonomic Neurotransmitters

ATP and ACh coexist in cholinergic vesicles (Dowdall et al., 1974), and ATP, NPY, and catecholamines are found within storage granules in nerves and the adrenal medulla (see previous discussion). ATP is released along with the transmitters, and it and its metabolites can play significant roles in synaptic transmission in some circumstances (see further discussion). Recently, attention has focused on the growing list of peptides that are found in the adrenal medulla, nerve fibers, or ganglia of the autonomic nervous system or in the structures that are innervated by the autonomic nervous system. This list includes enkephalins, substance P and other tachykinins, SST, gonadotropin-releasing hormone, CCK, CGRP, galanin, PACAP, VIP, chromogranins, and NPY (Hökfelt et al., 2000). Some of the orphan GPCRs discovered in the course of genome-sequencing projects may represent receptors for undiscovered peptides or other cotransmitters.

Cotransmission in the Autonomic Nervous System

There is a large body of literature on cotransmission in the autonomic nervous system. Much of the research in this area has focused on co-release of ATP by adrenergic and cholinergic nerves. Co-release of NPY, VIP, CGRP, substance P, and NO has also been studied. Whether these co-released factors act as neurotransmitters, neuromodulators, or trophic factors remains a topic of debate (Burnstock, 2013, 2015; Mutafova-Yambolieva et al, 2014).

The evidence is substantial that ATP plays a role in sympathetic nerves as a cotransmitter with NE (Silinsky et al., 1998; Westfall et al., 1991, 2002). For example, the rodent vas deferens is supplied with dense sympathetic innervation, and stimulation of the nerves results in a biphasic mechanical response that consists of an initial rapid twitch followed by a sustained contraction. The first phase of the response is mediated by ATP acting on postjunctional P2X receptors, whereas the second phase is mediated mainly by NE acting on α_1 receptors (Sneddon and Westfall, 1984). The cotransmitters apparently are released from the same types of nerves because pretreatment with 6-hydroxydopamine, an agent that specifically destroys adrenergic nerves, abolishes both phases of the neurogenically induced biphasic contraction. Whether ATP and NE originate from the same populations of vesicles within a nerve ending is still open to debate and experimentation (Todorov et al., 1996; Mutafova-Yambolieva et al, 2014; Burnstock, 2015).

Once ATP is released into the neuroeffector junction, some of it is metabolized by extracellularly directed membrane-bound nucleotidases to ADP, AMP, and adenosine (Gordon, 1986). However, the majority of its metabolism occurs by the actions of releasable nucleotidases. There is also evidence that ATP and its metabolites exert presynaptic modulatory effects on transmitter release by P2 receptors and receptors for adenosine. In addition to evidence showing that ATP is a cotransmitter with NE, there is evidence that ATP may be a cotransmitter with ACh in certain postganglionic parasympathetic nerves, such as those in the urinary bladder.

The NPY family of peptides is distributed widely in the central and peripheral nervous systems and consists of three members: NPY, pancreatic polypeptide, and peptide YY. NPY is colocalized and coreleased with NE and ATP in most sympathetic nerves in the peripheral nervous system, especially those innervating blood vessels (Westfall, 2004). There is also convincing evidence that NPY exerts prejunctional modulatory effects on transmitter release and synthesis. Moreover, there are numerous examples of postjunctional interactions that are consistent with a cotransmitter role for NPY at various sympathetic neuroeffector junctions. Thus, NPY, together with NE and ATP, qualifies as the third sympathetic cotransmitter of the sympathetic branch of the autonomic nervous system. Functions of NPY include

- direct postjunctional contractile effects
- potentiation of the contractile effects of the other sympathetic cotransmitters
- inhibitory modulation of the nerve stimulation–induced release of all three sympathetic cotransmitters, including actions on autoreceptors to inhibit its own release

Studies with selective NPY-Y_1 antagonists provided evidence that the principal postjunctional receptor is of the Y_1 subtype, although other receptors are also present at some sites and may exert physiological actions. Studies with selective NPY-Y_2 antagonists suggested that the principal prejunctional receptor is of the Y_2 subtype both in the periphery and in the CNS. There is evidence for a role for other NPY receptors, and clarification awaits the further development of selective antagonists. NPY also can act prejunctionally to inhibit the release of ACh, CGRP, and substance P. In the CNS, NPY exists as a cotransmitter with catecholamine in some neurons and with peptides and mediators in others. A prominent action of NPY is the presynaptic inhibition of the release of various neurotransmitters, including NE, DA, GABA, glutamate, and 5HT, as well as inhibition or stimulation of the release of neurohormones such as gonadotropin-releasing hormone, vasopressin, and oxytocin. Evidence also exists for stimulation of NE and DA release by NPY.

The NPY may use several mechanisms to produce its presynaptic effects, including inhibition of Ca^{2+} channels, activation of K^+ channels, and regulation of the vesicle release complex at some point distal to Ca^{2+} entry. NPY also may play a role in several pathophysiological conditions. The further development of selective NPY agonists and antagonists should enhance understanding about the physiological and pathophysiological roles of NPY.

The pioneering studies of Hökfelt and coworkers, which demonstrated the existence of VIP and ACh in peripheral autonomic neurons, initiated interest in the possibility of peptidergic cotransmission in the autonomic nervous system. Subsequent work has confirmed the frequent association of these two substances in autonomic fibers, including parasympathetic fibers that innervate smooth muscle and exocrine glands and cholinergic sympathetic neurons that innervate sweat glands (Hökfelt et al., 2000).

The role of VIP in parasympathetic transmission has been studied most extensively in the regulation of salivary secretion. The evidence for cotransmission includes the release of VIP following stimulation of the chorda lingual nerve and the incomplete blockade by atropine of vasodilation when the frequency of stimulation is raised; the last observation may indicate independent release of the two substances, which is consistent with histochemical evidence for storage of ACh and VIP in separate populations of vesicles. Synergism between ACh and VIP in stimulating vasodilation and secretion also has been described. VIP may be involved in parasympathetic responses in the trachea and in the GI tract, where it may facilitate sphincter relaxation.

Nonadrenergic, Noncholinergic (NANC) Transmission by Purines

The smooth muscle of many tissues that are innervated by the autonomic nervous system shows inhibitory junction potentials following stimulation by field electrodes. Because such responses frequently are undiminished in the presence of adrenergic and muscarinic cholinergic antagonists, these observations have been taken as evidence for the existence of NANC transmission in the autonomic nervous system.

Burnstock and colleagues have compiled compelling evidence for the existence of purinergic neurotransmission in the GI tract, genitourinary tract, and certain blood vessels; ATP fulfills all the criteria for a neurotransmitter. In at least some circumstances, primary sensory axons may be an important source of ATP (Burnstock et al., 2015). Although adenosine is generated from the released ATP by ectoenzymes and releasable nucleotidases, its primary function appears to be modulatory by causing feedback inhibition of transmitter release.

Adenosine can be transported from the cell cytoplasm to activate extracellular receptors on adjacent cells. The efficient uptake of adenosine by cellular transporters and its rapid metabolism to inosine or to adenine nucleotides contribute to its rapid turnover. Several inhibitors of adenosine transport and metabolism can influence concentrations of extracellular adenosine and ATP (Sneddon et al., 1999).

The purinergic receptors found on the cell surface may be divided into the adenosine (P1) receptors and the receptors for ATP (P2X and P2Y receptors) (Fredholm et al., 2000). Both P1 and P2 receptors have various subtypes. There are four adenosine receptors (A_1, A_{2A}, A_{2B}, and A_3) and multiple subtypes of P2X and P2Y receptors throughout the body. The adenosine receptors and the P2Y receptors mediate their responses via G proteins, whereas the P2X receptors are a subfamily of ligand-gated ion channels (Burnstock et al., 2015). Methylxanthines such as caffeine and theophylline preferentially block P1 adenosine receptors (Chapter 40).

Signal Integration and Modulation of Vascular Responses by Endothelium-Derived Factors: NO and Endothelin

The contents of adrenergic storage vesicles are not alone in regulating vascular tone. Many other factors modulate vascular contractility, including kinins, angiotensin, natriuretic peptides, substance P, VIP, CGRP, and eicosanoids, all described elsewhere in this volume. There are additional factors generated by the vascular endothelium that influence vascular reactivity: NO and endothelin.

Furchgott and colleagues demonstrated that an intact endothelium is necessary to achieve vascular relaxation in response to ACh (Furchgott, 1999). This inner cellular layer of the blood vessel now is known to modulate autonomic and hormonal effects on the contractility of blood vessels. In response to a variety of vasoactive agents and physical stimuli, endothelial cells release a short-lived vasodilator termed endothelium-derived relaxing factor, now identified as NO. Less commonly, an endothelium-derived hyperpolarizing factor and endothelium-derived contracting factor are released (Vanhoutte, 1996). Formation of endothelium-derived contracting factor depends on cyclooxygenase activity.

Products of inflammation and platelet aggregation (e.g., 5HT, histamine, bradykinin, purines, and thrombin) exert all or part of their action by stimulating the production of NO. Endothelium-dependent mechanisms of relaxation are important in a variety of vascular beds, including the coronary circulation (Hobbs et al., 1999). Activation of specific GPCRs linking to G_q and the mobilization of Ca^{2+} within endothelial cells promotes NO production. NO diffuses readily to the underlying smooth muscle and induces relaxation of vascular smooth muscle by activating the soluble form of guanylyl cyclase, which increases cyclic GMP concentrations (Figures 3–13 and 3–17). Nitrovasodilating drugs used to lower blood pressure or to treat ischemic heart disease probably act through conversion to or release of NO (Chapter 27). Certain nerves (termed *nitrergic*) innervating blood vessels and smooth muscles of the GI tract also release NO. NO has a negative inotropic action on the heart.

Alterations in the release or action of NO may affect a number of major clinical situations, such as atherosclerosis (Hobbs et al., 1999; Ignarro et al., 1999). Furthermore, there is evidence suggesting that the hypotension of endotoxemia or that induced by cytokines is mediated by induction of NOS2 (the inducible form of NOS) and the enhanced production NO; consequently, increased NO production may have pathological significance in septic shock.

Full contractile responses of cerebral arteries also require an intact endothelium. A family of peptides, termed *endothelins,* is stored in vascular endothelial cells. Endothelin contributes to the maintenance of vascular homeostasis by acting via multiple endothelin receptors that are GPCRs (Sokolovsky, 1995; Hilal-Dandan et al., 1997). The release of endothelin-1 (21 amino acids) onto smooth muscle promotes contraction by stimulation of the ET_A receptor. Endothelin antagonists are now employed in treating pulmonary artery hypertension (Chapter 31).

Bibliography

Aantaa R, et al. Molecular pharmacology of α_2-adrenoceptor subtypes. *Ann Med*, **1995**, *27*:439–449.

Abell CW, Kwan SW. Molecular characterization of monoamine oxidases A and B. *Prog Nucleic Acid Res Mol Biol*, **2001**, *65*:129–156.

Ahlquist RP. A study of the adrenotropic receptors. *Am J Physiol*, **1948**, *153*:586–600.

Alabi AA, Tsien RW. Perspectives on kiss-and-run: role in exocytosis, endocytosis, and neurotransmission. *Annu Rev Physiol*, **2013**, *75*:393–422.

Albuquerque EX, et al. Mammalian nicotinic acetylcholine receptors: from structure to function. *Physiol Rev*, **2009**, *89*:73–120.

Altschuler SM, et al. Viscerotopic representation of the upper alimentary tract in the rat: sensory ganglia and nuclei of the solitary and spinal trigeminal tracts. *J Comp Neurol*, **1989**, *283*:248–268.

Andresen MC, Kunze DL. Nucleus tractus solitarius: gateway to neural circulatory control. *Annu Rev Physiol*, **1994**, *56*:93–116.

Arner P, Hoffstedt J. Adrenoceptor genes in human obesity. *J Intern Med*, **1999**, *245*:667–672.

Aunis D. Exocytosis in chromaffin cells of the adrenal medulla. *Int Rev Cytol*, **1998**, *181*:213–320.

Baillie G, Houslay M. Arrestin times for compartmentalized cAMP signalling and phosphodiesterase-4 enzymes. *Curr Opin Cell Biol*, **2005**, *17*:129–134.

Brodde OE. β_1 and β_2 adrenoceptor polymorphisms: functional importance, impact on cardiovascular disease and drug responses. *Pharmacol Ther*, **2008**, *117*:1–29.

Brodde OE, et al. Cardiac adrenoceptors: physiological and pathophysiological relevance. *J Pharmacol Sci*, **2006**, *100*:323–337.

Burnstock G. Cotransmission in the autonomic nervous system. *Handb Clin Neurol*, **2013**, *117*:23–35.

Burnstock G, et al. Purinergic signalling and the autonomic nervous system. *Autonomic Neurosci*, **2015**, *191*:1–147.

Carson RP, Robertson D. Genetic manipulation of noradrenergic neurons. *J Pharmacol Exp Ther*, **2002**, *301*:407–410.

Catterall WA. From ionic currents to molecular mechanisms: the structure and function of voltage-gated sodium channels. *Neuron*, **2000**, *26*:13–25.

Chaudhry FA, et al. Vesicular neurotransmitter transporters as targets for endogenous and exogenous toxic substances. *Annu Rev Pharmacol Toxicol*, **2008**, *48*:277–301.

Chen H, et al. Differential gene expression in functional classes of interstitial cells of Cajal in murine small intestine. *Physiol Genomics*, **2007**, *31*:492–509.

Chong BS, Mersfelder TL. Entacapone. *Ann Pharmacother*, **2000**, *34*:1056–1065.

Communal C, et al. Opposing effects of beta(1)- and beta(2)-adrenergic receptors on cardiac myocyte apoptosis: role of a pertussis toxin-sensitive G protein. *Circulation*, **1999**, *100*:2210–2212.

Devedjian JC, et al. Transgenic mice overexpressing alpha2a-adrenoceptors in pancreatic beta-cells show altered regulation of glucose homeostasis. *Diabetologia*, **2000**, *43*:899–906.

Dhein S, et al. Muscarinic receptors in the mammalian heart. *Pharmacol Res*, **2001**, *44*:161–182.

Dorn GW. Adrenergic signaling polymorphisms and their impact on cardiovascular disease. *Phys Rev*, **2010**, *90*:1013–1062.

Dorn GW, et al. Low- and high-level transgenic expression of beta2-adrenergic receptors differentially affect cardiac hypertrophy and function in galphaq-overexpressing mice. *Proc Natl Acad Sci U S A*, **1999**, *96*:6400–6405.

Dowdall MJ, et al. Adenosine triphosphate, a constituent of cholinergic synaptic vesicles. *Biochem J*, **1974**, *140*:1–12.

Eiden LE. The cholinergic gene locus. *J Neurochem*, **1998**, *70*:2227–2240.

Eisenhofer G. The role of neuronal and extraneuronal plasma membrane transporters in the inactivation of peripheral catecholamine. *Pharmacol Ther*, **2001**, *91*:35–62.

Eisenhofer G, et al. Catecholamine metabolism: a contemporary view with implications for physiology and medicine. *Pharmacol Rev*, **2004**, *56*:331–349.

Emorine LJ, et al. Molecular characterization of the human β_3-adrenergic receptor. *Science*, **1989**, *245*:1118–1121.

Estévez-Herrera J, et al. ATP: the crucial component of secretory vesicles. *Proc Natl Acad Sci U S A*, **2016**, *113*:E4098–E4106.

Exley R, Cragg SJ. Presynaptic nicotinic receptors: a dynamic and diverse cholinergic filter of striatal dopamine neurotransmission. *Br J Pharmacol*, **2008**, *153*:S283–S297.

Fagerholm V, et al. Altered glucose homeostasis in alpha2a-adrenoceptor knockout mice. *Eur J Pharmacol*, **2004**, *505*:243–252.

Fetscher C, et al. M_3 muscarinic receptors mediate contraction of human urinary bladder. *Br J Pharmacol*, **2002**, *136*:641–643.

Fredholm BB, et al. Adenosine receptors. In Girdleston D, ed. *The IUPHAR Compendium of Receptor Characterization and Classification.* IUPHAR Media, London; **2000**, 78–87.

Furchgott RF. Endothelium-derived relaxing factor: discovery, early studies, and identification as nitric oxide. *Biosci Rep*, **1999**, *19*: 235–251.

Furness JB, et al. The enteric nervous system and gastrointestinal innervation: integrated local and central control. *Adv Exp Med Biol*, **2014**, *817*:39–71.

Gainetdinov RR, Caron MG. Monoamine transporters: from genes to behavior. *Ann Rev Pharmacol Toxicol*, **2003**, *43*:261–284.

Gavras I, Gavras H. Role of alpha2-adrenergic receptors in hypertension. *Am J Hyper*, **2001**, *14*:171S-177S.

Gherbi K, et al. Negative cooperativity across β_1-adrenoceptor homodimers provides insights into the nature of the secondary low-affinity CGP 12177 β_1-adrenoceptor binding conformation. *FASEB J*, **2015**, *29*:2859–2871.

Goldsmith ZG, Dhanasekaran DN. G protein regulation of MAPK networks. *Oncogene*, **2007**, *26*:3122–3142.

Gordon JL. Extracellular ATP: effects, sources and fate. *Biochem J*, **1986**, *233*:309–319.

Haenisch B, et al. Association of major depression with rare functional variants in norepinephrine transporter and serotonin1a receptor genes. *Am J Med Gen Pt B Neuropsych Gen*, **2009**, *150B*:1013–1016.

Haga T. Molecular properties of the high-affinity choline transporter CHT1. *J Biochem*, **2014**, *156*:181–194.

Hahn MK, et al. Single nucleotide polymorphisms in the human norepinephrine transporter gene affect expression, trafficking, antidepressant interaction, and protein kinase c regulation. *Mol Pharmacol*, **2005**, *68*:457–466.

Hahn MK, et al. A mutation in the human norepinephrine transporter gene (slc6a2) associated with orthostatic intolerance disrupts surface expression of mutant and wild-type transporters. *J Neurosci*, **2003**, *23*:4470–4478.

Heaslip AT, et al. Cytoskeletal dependence of insulin granule movement dynamics in INS-1 beta-cells in response to glucose. *PLoS One*, **2014**, 9:e109082.

Hieble JP. Subclassification and nomenclature of α- and β-adrenoceptors. *Curr Top Med Chem*, **2007**, *7*:129–134.

Hilal-Dandan R, et al. The quasi-irreversible nature of endothelin binding and G protein-linked signaling in cardiac myocytes. *J Pharmacol Exp Ther*, **1997**, *281*:267–273.

Hirsch D, et al. NPY and stress 30 years later: the peripheral view. *Cell Mol Neurobiol*, **2012**, *32*:645–659.

Hobbs AJ, et al. Inhibition of nitric oxide synthase as a potential therapeutic target. *Annu Rev Pharmacol Toxicol*, **1999**, *39*:191–220.

Hökfelt T, et al. Neuropeptides: an overview. *Neuropharmacology*, **2000**, *39*:1337–1356.

Ignarro LJ, et al. Nitric oxide as a signaling molecule in the vascular system: an overview. *J Cardiovasc Pharmacol*, **1999**, *34*:879–886.

Kable JW, et al. In vivo gene modification elucidates subtype-specific functions of α_2-adrenergic receptors. *J Pharmacol Exp Ther*, **2000**, *293*:1–7.

Kalamida D, et al. Muscle and neuronal nicotinic acetylcholine receptors structure function and pathogenicity. *FEBS J*, **2007**, *274*:3799–3845.

Keller NR, et al. Norepinephrine transporter-deficient mice exhibit excessive tachycardia and elevated blood pressure with wakefulness and activity. *Circulation*, **2004**, *110*:1191–1196.

Kubista H, Boehm S. Molecular mechanisms underlying the modulation of exocytoxic noradrenaline release via presynaptic receptors. *Pharmacol Ther*, **2006**, *112*:213–242.

Lakhlani PP, et al. Substitution of a mutant α_{2A}-adrenergic receptor via "hit and run" gene targeting reveals the role of this subtype in sedative, analgesic, and anesthetic-sparing responses in vivo. *Proc Natl Acad Sci U S A*, **1997**, *94*:9950–9955.

Langer SZ. 25 years since the discovery of presynaptic receptors: present knowledge and future perspectives. *Trends Pharmacol Sci*, **1997**, *18*:95–99.

Langmead CJ, et al. Muscarinic acetylcholine receptors as CNS drug targets. *Pharmacol Ther*, **2008**, *117*:232–243.

Liggett SB, et al. Early and delayed consequences of beta(2)-adrenergic receptor overexpression in mouse hearts: critical role for expression level. *Circulation*, **2000**, *101*:1707–1714.

Lugardon K, et al. Antibacterial and anti-fungal activities of vasostatin-1, the N-terminal fragment of chromogranin A. *J Biol Chem*, **2000**, *275*:10745–10753.

Lynch GS, Ryall JG. Role of β-adrenoceptor signaling in skeletal muscle: implications for muscle wasting and disease. *Physiol Rev*, **2008**, *88*:729–767.

Man in't Veld A, et al. Patients with congenital dopamine β-hydroxylase deficiency: a lesson in catecholamine physiology. *Am J Hypertens*, **1988**, *1*:231–238.

Männistö PT, Kaakkola S. Catechol-O-methyltransferase (COMT): biochemistry, molecular biology, pharmacology, and clinical efficacy of the new selective COMT inhibitors. *Pharmacol Rev*, **1999**, *51*: 593–628.

Mialet Perez J, et al. Beta 1-adrenergic receptor polymorphisms confer differential function and predisposition to heart failure. *Nat Med*, **2003**, *9*:1300–1305.

Michelotti GA, et al. α_1-Adrenergic receptor regulation: basic science and clinical implications. *Pharmacol Ther*, **2000**, *88*:281–309.

Miller RJ. Presynaptic receptors. *Annu Rev Pharmacol Toxicol*, **1998**, *38*:201–227.

Mobine HR, et al. Pheochromocytoma-induced cardiomyopathy is modulated by the synergistic effects of cell-secreted factors. *Circ Heart Fail*, **2009**, *2*:121–128.

Mutafova-Yambolieva VN, Durnin L. The purinergic neurotransmitter revisited: A single substance or multiple players? *Pharmacol Ther*, **2014**, 144:162–191.

Nagatsu T. The catecholamine system in health and disease—relation to tyrosine 3-monooxygenase and other catecholamine-synthesizing enzymes. *Proc Jpn Acad Ser B Phys Biol Sci*, **2006**, *82*:388–415.

Nathanson NM. Synthesis, trafficking and localization of muscarinic acetylcholine receptors. *Pharmacol Ther*, **2008**, *119*:33–43.

Philipp M, Hein L. Adrenergic receptor knockout mice: distinct functions of 9 receptor subtypes. *Pharmacol Ther*, **2004**, *101*:65–74.

Reiter E, et al. Molecular mechanism of β-arrestin-biased agonism at seven-transmembrane receptors. *Annu Rev Pharmacol Toxicol*, **2012**, *52*:179–197.

Robertson D, et al. Dopamine β-hydroxylase deficiency: a genetic disorder of cardiovascular regulation. *Hypertension*, **1991**, *18*:1–8.

Robidoux J, et al. β-Adrenergic receptors and regulation of energy expenditure: a family affair. *Annu Rev Pharmacol Toxicol*, **2004**, *44*:297–323.

Rokosh DG, Simpson PC. Knockout of the alpha $1_{a/c}$-adrenergic receptor subtype: the alpha 1a/c is expressed in resistance arteries and is required to maintain arterial blood pressure. *Proc Natl Acad Sci U S A*, **2002**, *99*:9474–9479.

Roth M, et al. OATPs, OATs and OCTs: the organic anion and cation transporters of the *SLCO* and *SLC22A* gene superfamilies. *Br J Pharmacol*, **2012**, *165*:1260–1287.

Salogiannis J, Reck-Peterson SL. Hitchhiking: a non-canonical mode of microtubule-based transport. *Trends Cell Biol*, **2016**. http://dx.doi.org/10.1016/j.tcb.2016.09.005.

Saper CB. Pain as a visceral sensation. *Prog Brain Res*, **2000**, *122*:237–243.

Saper CB. The central autonomic nervous system: conscious visceral perception and autonomic pattern generation. *Annu Rev Neurosci*, **2002**, *25*:433–469.

Schuldiner S. A molecular glimpse of vesicular monoamine transporters. *J Neurochem*, **1994**, *62*:2067–2078.

Shannon JR, et al. Orthostatic intolerance and tachycardia associated with norepinephrine-transporter deficiency. *N Engl J Med*, **2000**, *342*:541–549.

Silinsky EM, et al. Functions of extracellular nucleotides in peripheral and central neuronal tissues. In Turner JT, Weisman GA, Fedan JS, eds. *The P_2 Nucleotide Receptors*. Humana Press, Totowa, NJ, **1998**, 259–290.

Silman I, Sussman JL. Acetylcholinesterase: "classical and non-classical" functions and pharmacology. *Curr Opin Pharmacol*, **2005**, *5*:293–302.

Sneddon P, Westfall DP. Pharmacological evidence that adenosine trisphosphate and noradrenaline are co-transmitters in the guinea-pig vas deferens. *J Physiol*, **1984**, *347*:561–580.

Sneddon P, et al. Modulation of purinergic neurotransmission. *Prog Brain Res*, **1999**, *120*:11–20.

Sokolovsky M. Endothelin receptor subtypes and their role in transmembrane signaling mechanisms. *Pharmacol Ther*, **1995**, *68*:435–471.

Südhof TC. The molecular machine of neurotransmitter release. In Grandin K, ed. *The Nobel Prizes, 2013*. Nobel Foundation, Stockholm, **2014**.

Tan CM, Limbird LE. *The α_2-Adrenergic Receptors: Lessons From Knockouts*. Humana, Clifton, NJ, **2005**, 241–266.

Tanoue A, et al. Transgenic studies of α_1-adrenergic receptor subtype function. *Life Sci*, **2002a**, *71*:2207–2215.

Tanoue A, et al. The α_{1D}-adrenergic receptor directly regulates arterial blood pressure via vasoconstriction. *J Clin Invest*, **2002b**, *109*:765–775.

Taupenot L, et al. The chromogranin–secretogranin family. *N Engl J Med*, **2003**, *348*:1134–1149.

Taylor P, et al. The genes encoding the cholinesterases: structure, evolutionary relationships and regulation of their expression. In Giacobini E, ed. *Cholinesterase and Cholinesterase Inhibitors*. Martin Dunitz, London, **2000**, 63–80.

Thomsen AR, et al. GPCR-G protein-β-arrestin super-complex mediates sustained G protein signaling. *Cell*, **2016**, *166*:907–919.

Toda N, Okamura J. The pharmacology of nitric oxide in the peripheral nervous system of blood vessels. *Pharmacol Rev*, **2003**, *55*:271–324.

Todorov LD, et al. Evidence for the differential release of the cotransmitters ATP and noradrenaline from sympathetic nerves of the guinea-pig vas deferens. *J Physiol*, **1996**, *496*:731–748.

Vanhoutte PM. Endothelium-dependent responses in congestive heart failure. *J Mol Cell Cardiol*, **1996**, *28*:2233–2240.

van Koppen CJ, Kaiser B. Regulation of muscarinic acetylcholine signaling. *Pharmacol Ther*, **2003**, *98*:197–220.

Violin JD, Lefkowitz RJ. β-Arrestin-biased ligands at seven-transmembrane receptors. *Trends Pharmacol Sci*, **2007**, *28*:416–422.

Viskupic E, et al. Increase in rat adrenal phenylethanolamine *N*-methyltransferase mRNA level caused by immobilization stress depends on intact pituitary-adrenocortical axis. *J Neurochem*, **1994**, *63*:808–814.

Volz HP, Gleiter CH. Monoamine oxidase inhibitors: a perspective on their use in the elderly. *Drugs Aging*, **1998**, *13*:341–355.

Von Euler US. A substance with sympathin E properties in spleen extracts. *Nature*, **1946**, *157*:369.

Walden PD, et al. Localization of mRNA and receptor binding sites for the α_{1A}-adrenoceptor subtype in the rat, monkey and human urinary bladder and prostate. *J Urol*, **1997**, *157*:1032–1038.

Wang Z, et al. Functional M_3 muscarinic acetylcholine receptors in mammalian hearts. *Br J Pharmacol*, **2004**, *142*:395–408.

Ward SE, et al. Interstitial cells of cajal mediate cholinergic neurotransmission from enteric motor neurons *J Neurosci*, **2000**, *20*:1393–1403.

Wess J, et al. Muscarinic acetylcholine receptors: mutant mice provide new insights for drug development. *Nat Rev/Drug Discov*, **2007**, *6*:721–733.

Wessler I, Kirkpatrick CJ. Acetylcholine beyond neurons: the non-neuronal cholinergic system in humans. *Br J Pharmacol*, **2008**, *154*:1558–1571.

Westfall DP, et al. ATP as neurotransmitter, cotransmitter and neuromodulator. In Phillis T, ed. *Adenosine and Adenine Nucleotides as Regulators of Cellular Function*. CRC Press, Boca Raton, FL, **1991**, 295–305.

Westfall DP, et al. ATP as a cotransmitter in sympathetic nerves and its inactivation by releasable enzymes. *J Pharmacol Exp Ther*, **2002**, *303*:439–444.

Westfall TC. Local regulation of adrenergic neurotransmission. *Physiol Rev*, **1977**, *57*:659–728.

Westfall TC. Prejunctional effects of neuropeptide Y and its role as a cotransmitter. In Michel MC, ed. *Neuropeptide Y and Related Peptides, Handbook of Experimental Pharmacology*, vol. 162. Springer, Berlin, **2004**, 137–183.

Wevers RA, et al. A review of biochemical and molecular genetic aspects of tyrosine hydroxylase deficiency including a novel mutation (291delC). *J Inherit Metab Dis*, **1999**, *22*:364–373.

Weyer C, et al. Development of β_3-adrenoceptor agonists for the treatment of obesity and diabetes: an update. *Diabetes Metab*, **1999**, *25*:11–21.

Witzemann V. Development of the neuromuscular junction. *Cell Tissue Res*, **2006**, *326*:263–71.

Woo AY-H, et al. Stereochemistry of an agonist determines coupling preference of β_2-adrenoceptor to different G proteins in cardiomyocytes. *Mol Pharmacol*, **2009**, *75*:158–165.

Wouters J. Structural aspects of monoamine oxidase and its reversible inhibition. *Curr Med Chem*, **1998**, *5*:137–162.

Wu SC, O'Connell TD. Nuclear compartmentalization of α1-adrenergic receptor signaling in adult cardiac myocytes. *Cardiovasc Pharmacol*, **2015**, *65*:91–100.

Yoshiki H, et al. Agonist pharmacology at recombinant α1A- and α1L-adrenoceptors and in lower urinary tract α1-adrenoceptors. *Br J Pharmacol*, **2013**, *170*:1242–1252.

Yoshiki H, et al. Pharmacologically distinct phenotypes of α1B-adrenoceptors: variation in binding and functional affinities for antagonists. *Br J Pharmacol*, **2014**, *171*:4890–4901.

Xiao RP, et al. Sutype-specific α_1- and β-adrenoceptor signaling in the heart. *Trends Pharm Sci*, **2006**, *27*:330–337.

Xu F, et al. Mice lacking the norepinephrine transporter are supersensitive to psychostimulants. *Nat Neurosci*, **2000**, *3*:465–471.

Ziegler MG, et al. Location, development, control, and function of extraadrenal phenylethanolamine *N*-methyltransferase. *Ann N Y Acad Sci*, **2002**, *971*:76–82.

Zigmond RE, et al. Acute regulation of tyrosine hydroxylase by nerve activity and by neurotransmitters via phosphorylation. *Annu Rev Neurosci*, **1989**, *12*:415–461.

Muscarinic Receptor Agonists and Antagonists

Joan Heller Brown, Katharina Brandl, and Jürgen Wess

第九章　毒蕈碱受体激动药和拮抗药

中文导读

本章主要介绍：乙酰胆碱及其毒蕈碱受体靶点，包括毒蕈碱受体的性质和亚型、乙酰胆碱的药理作用；毒蕈碱受体激动药的ADME、治疗用途、禁忌证、预防措施、不良反应和毒理学；毒蕈碱受体拮抗药的构-效关系、作用机制、药理作用、治疗用途、禁忌证和不良反应以及具有抗毒蕈碱特性药物的毒理学。

Abbreviations

ACh: acetylcholine
AChE: acetylcholinesterase
AV: atrioventricular
COPD: chronic obstructive pulmonary disease
eNOS: endothelial NO synthase
HCN: hyperpolarization-activated, cyclic nucleotide–gated (channels)
5HT: serotonin
$I_{Ca\text{-}L}$: L-type Ca^{2+} current
I_f: cardiac pacemaker current
$I_{K\text{-}ACh}$: ACh-activated K^+ current
M_1, M_2, M_3: muscarinic receptor subclasses
NO: nitric oxide

Acetylcholine and Its Muscarinic Receptor Target

Muscarinic acetylcholine receptors in the peripheral nervous system are found primarily on autonomic effector cells innervated by postganglionic parasympathetic nerves. Muscarinic receptors are also present in autonomic ganglia and on some cells (e.g., vascular endothelial cells) that, paradoxically, receive little or no cholinergic innervation. Within the CNS, the hippocampus, cortex, and thalamus have high densities of muscarinic receptors.

Acetylcholine, the naturally occurring neurotransmitter for these receptors, has virtually no systemic therapeutic applications because its actions are diffuse, and its hydrolysis, catalyzed by both AChE and plasma butyrylcholinesterase, is rapid. Muscarinic agonists mimic the effects of ACh at these sites. These agonists typically are longer-acting congeners of ACh or natural alkaloids, some of which stimulate nicotinic as well as muscarinic receptors.

The mechanisms of action of endogenous ACh at the postjunctional membranes of the effector cells and neurons that represent different types of cholinergic synapses are discussed in Chapter 8. Cholinergic synapses occur at:

- autonomic effector sites innervated by postganglionic parasympathetic nerves (or, in the sweat glands, by postganglionic sympathetic nerves)
- sympathetic and parasympathetic ganglia and the adrenal medulla, innervated by preganglionic autonomic nerves
- motor end plates on skeletal muscle, innervated by somatic motor nerves
- certain synapses in the CNS (Krnjevíc, 2004) where ACh can have either pre- or postsynaptic actions

When ACh is administered systemically, it can potentially act at all of these sites; however, as a quaternary ammonium compound, its penetration to the CNS is limited, and the amount of ACh that reaches peripheral areas with low blood flow is limited due to hydrolysis by plasma butyrylcholinesterase.

The actions of ACh and related drugs at autonomic effector sites are referred to as *muscarinic*, based on the observation that the alkaloid muscarine acts selectively at those sites and produces the same qualitative effects as ACh. The muscarinic, or parasympathomimetic, actions of the drugs considered in this chapter are practically equivalent to the parasympathetic effects of ACh listed in Table 8–1. Muscarinic receptors are present in autonomic ganglia and the adrenal medulla but primarily function to modulate the nicotinic actions of ACh at these sites (Chapter 11). In the CNS, muscarinic receptors are widely distributed and have a role in mediating many important responses. The differences between the actions of ACh and other muscarinic agonists are largely quantitative, with limited selectivity for one organ system or another. All of the actions of ACh and its congeners at muscarinic receptors can be competitively inhibited by atropine.

Properties and Subtypes of Muscarinic Receptors

Muscarinic receptors were characterized initially by analysis of the responses of cells and organ systems in the periphery and the CNS. For example, differential effects of two muscarinic agonists, bethanechol and McN-A-343, on the tone of the lower esophageal sphincter led to the initial designation of muscarinic receptors as M_1 (ganglionic) and M_2 (effector cell) (Goyal and Rattan, 1978). Molecular cloning of muscarinic receptors has identified five distinct gene products (Bonner et al., 1987), now designated as M_1 through M_5 muscarinic receptors (Chapter 8). All of the known muscarinic receptors are G protein–coupled receptors that in turn couple to various cellular effectors (Chapter 3). Although selectivity is not absolute, stimulation of M_1, M_3, and M_5 receptors causes hydrolysis of polyphosphoinositides and mobilization of intracellular Ca^{2+} as a consequence of activation of the G_q-PLC pathway, resulting in a variety of Ca^{2+}-mediated responses. In contrast, M_2 and M_4 muscarinic receptors inhibit adenylyl cyclase and regulate specific ion channels via their coupling to the pertussis toxin–sensitive G proteins, G_i and G_o (Chapter 3).

Recent X-ray crystallographic studies convincingly demonstrated that the classical (*orthosteric*) binding site for muscarinic agonists and antagonists is highly conserved among muscarinic receptor subtypes (Haga et al., 2012; Kruse et al., 2012, 2013). The orthosteric binding site consists of a cleft deeply buried within the membrane, formed by conserved amino acid chains located on several of the receptors' seven TM helices (TM1–TM7). A key feature shared by other receptors for biogenic amine ligands is the presence of a charge-charge interaction between the tertiary or quaternary nitrogen of the orthosteric ligands and a conserved TM3 aspartic acid side chain. A feature unique to muscarinic receptors is hydrogen bond interactions between the orthosteric ligand and a TM6 asparagine residue. Agonist binding to the receptor leads to considerable contraction of the ligand-binding pocket, reflecting the relatively small size of muscarinic agonists, as compared to muscarinic antagonists. Because the residues that line the orthosteric binding site are highly conserved among all muscarinic receptors, developing orthosteric muscarinic ligands endowed with a high degree of receptor subtype selectivity has proven difficult.

The five muscarinic receptor subtypes are widely distributed in both the CNS and peripheral tissues; most cells express at least two subtypes (Abrams et al., 2006; Wess, 1996; Wess et al., 2007). Identifying the role of a specific subtype in mediating a particular muscarinic response to ACh has been difficult due to the lack of subtype-specific agonists and antagonists. More recently, studies with M_1–M_5 receptor knockout mice have yielded novel information about the physiological roles of the individual muscarinic receptor subtypes (Kruse et al., 2014; Wess et al., 2007; Table 8–3); these studies demonstrated that multiple receptor subtypes are involved in mediating a specific muscarinic response in most cases. For example, abolition of cholinergic bronchoconstriction, salivation, pupillary constriction, and bladder contraction generally requires deletion of more than one receptor subtype.

Various lines of evidence suggest that muscarinic receptors possess one or more topographically distinct allosteric binding sites formed by amino acid side chains located within the extracellular loops or the outer segments of different transmembrane (TM) helices (Birdsall and Lazareno, 2005; May et al., 2007). Because these regions show a considerable degree of sequence variation among the M_1–M_5 receptors, considerable progress has been made in developing so-called allosteric modulators that show high selectivity for distinct muscarinic receptor subtypes (Conn et al., 2009, 2014; Gentry et al., 2015). These agents exert their pharmacological actions by altering the affinity or efficacy of orthosteric muscarinic ligands. Positive allosteric modulators (PAMs) enhance orthosteric activity, while negative allosteric modulators (NAMs) inhibit it. Allosteric agents that can directly activate muscarinic receptors are termed *allosteric agonists*. However, these designations are not absolute; they depend on the nature of the orthosteric ligand, receptor subtype under investigation, and assay system used. The remarkable progress that has been made recently in identifying subtype-selective muscarinic allosteric agents may lead to the development of new therapeutic agents with increased efficacy and reduced side effects. Currently, much research is focused on the potential of such agents for the treatment of several severe disorders of the CNS, including Alzheimer disease and schizophrenia.

A recent X-ray structure revealed the molecular details of a PAM–muscarinic receptor complex; the binding pocket for muscarinic PAMs is located just above the orthosteric binding crevice (Kruse et al., 2013). This new structure also illustrates that the bound PAM interferes with the dissociation of the bound orthosteric agonist from the receptor. Another potential strategy for achieving receptor subtype selectivity is the development of hybrid, bitopic orthosteric/allosteric ligands that interact with both the orthosteric binding cavity and an allosteric site (Lane et al., 2013; Mohr et al., 2010). By targeting orthosteric and allosteric sites simultaneously, bitopic ligands achieve both high affinity and receptor subtype selectivity.

Pharmacological Effects of Acetylcholine

The influence of ACh and parasympathetic innervation on various organs and tissues was introduced in Chapter 8; a more detailed description of the effects of ACh is presented here as background for understanding the physiological basis for the therapeutic uses of the muscarinic receptor agonists and antagonists.

Cardiovascular System

Acetylcholine has four primary effects on the cardiovascular system:

- vasodilation
- decrease in heart rate (negative chronotropic effect)
- decrease in the conduction velocity in the AV node (negative dromotropic effect)
- decrease in the force of cardiac contraction (negative inotropic effect)

The negative inotropic effect is of less significance in the ventricles than in the atria. In addition, some of these effects can be obscured by baroreceptor and other reflexes that dampen the direct responses to ACh.

Although ACh rarely is given systemically, its cardiac actions are important because the effects of cardiac glycosides, antiarrhythmic agents, and many other drugs are at least partly due to changes in parasympathetic (vagal) stimulation of the heart; in addition, afferent stimulation of the viscera during surgical interventions can reflexly increase the vagal stimulation of the heart.

The intravenous injection of a small dose of ACh produces a transient fall in blood pressure owing to generalized vasodilation (mediated by vascular endothelial NO), which is usually accompanied by reflex tachycardia. The generalized vasodilation produced by exogenously administered ACh is due to the stimulation of muscarinic receptors, primarily of the M_3 subtype located on vascular endothelial cells. Occupation of these receptors activates the G_q-PLC-IP_3 pathway, leading to Ca^{2+}-calmodulin–dependent activation of endothelial eNOS (NOS3) and production of NO (endothelium-derived relaxing factor) (Moncada and Higgs, 1995), which diffuses to adjacent vascular smooth muscle cells, where it stimulates guanylyl cyclase, thereby promoting relaxation via a cyclic GMP–dependent mechanism (see Figure 3-11; Furchgott, 1999; Ignarro et al., 1999). Baroreceptor or chemoreceptor reflexes or direct stimulation of the vagus can also elicit parasympathetic coronary vasodilation mediated by ACh and the consequent production of NO by the endothelium (Feigl, 1998). If the endothelium is damaged, however, as occurs under various pathophysiological conditions, ACh acts predominantly on M_3 receptors located on the underlying vascular smooth muscle cells, causing vasoconstriction.This capacity to both relax and constrict vessels is shared by many hormones that act via the G_q-PLC-IP_3-Ca^{2+} pathway and for which both endothelial cells and vascular smooth muscle cells express receptors. If the agonist can reach both cell types, each cell type will respond in its differentiated way to an elevation of intracellular Ca^{2+}, endothelium with a stimulation of NO synthase, smooth muscle with contraction.

Acetylcholine has direct effects on cardiac function at doses higher than those required for vasodilation. The cardiac effects of ACh are mediated primarily by M_2 muscarinic receptors (Stengel et al., 2000), which couple to G_i/G_o. Direct effects of ACh include an increase in the $I_{K\text{-}ACh}$ due to activation of K-ACh channels, a decrease in the $I_{Ca\text{-}L}$ due to inhibition of L-type Ca^{2+} channels, and a decrease in the I_f due to inhibition of HCN (pacemaker) channels (DiFrancesco and Tromba, 1987). ACh acting on M_2 receptors also leads to a G_i-mediated decrease in cyclic AMP, which opposes and counteracts the β_1 adrenergic/G_s–mediated increase in cyclic AMP, and an inhibition of the release of norepinephrine from sympathetic nerve terminals. The inhibition of norepinephrine release is mediated by presynaptic M_2 and M_3 receptors, which are activated by ACh released from adjacent parasympathetic postganglionic nerve terminals (Trendelenburg et al., 2005). There are also presynaptic M_2 receptors that inhibit ACh release from parasympathetic postganglionic nerve terminals in the human heart (Oberhauser et al., 2001).

In the SA node, each normal cardiac impulse is initiated by the spontaneous depolarization of the pacemaker cells (Chapter 30). At a critical level (the threshold potential), this depolarization initiates an action potential. ACh slows the heart rate primarily by decreasing the rate of spontaneous depolarization; attainment of the threshold potential and the succeeding events in the cardiac cycle are therefore delayed. Until recently, it was widely accepted that β_1 adrenergic and muscarinic cholinergic effects on heart rate resulted from regulation of the cardiac pacemaker current mentioned previously (I_f). Unexpected findings made through genetic deletion of HCN4 and pharmacological inhibition of I_f have generated an alternative theory involving a pace-making function for an intracellular Ca^{2+} "clock" (Lakatta and DiFrancesco, 2009) that might mediate effects of ACh on heart rate (Lyashkov et al., 2009).

In the atria, ACh causes hyperpolarization and decreased action potential duration by increasing $I_{K\text{-}ACh}$. ACh also inhibits cyclic AMP formation and norepinephrine release, decreasing atrial contractility. In the AV node, ACh slows conduction and increases the refractory period by inhibiting $I_{Ca\text{-}L}$; the decrement in AV conduction is responsible for the complete heart block that may be observed when large quantities of cholinergic agonists are administered systemically. When parasympathetic (vagal) tone to the resting heart is increased (e.g., by digoxin), the prolonged refractory period of the AV node can reduce the frequency with which aberrant atrial impulses are transmitted to the ventricles and thereby decrease the ventricular rate during atrial flutter or fibrillation.

The ventricular myocardium and His-Purkinje system receive only sparse cholinergic (vagal) innervation (Levy and Schwartz, 1994), and the effects of ACh are smaller than those observed in the atria and nodal tissues. The modest negative inotropic effect of ACh in the ventricle is most apparent when there is concomitant adrenergic stimulation or underlying sympathetic tone (Brodde and Michel, 1999; Levy and Schwartz, 1994; Lewis et al., 2001). Automaticity of Purkinje fibers is suppressed, and the threshold for ventricular fibrillation is increased.

Respiratory Tract

The parasympathetic nervous system plays a major role in regulating bronchomotor tone. A diverse set of stimuli cause reflex increases in parasympathetic activity that contributes to bronchoconstriction. The effects of ACh on the respiratory system include bronchoconstriction, increased tracheobronchial secretion, and stimulation of the chemoreceptors of the carotid and aortic bodies. These effects are mediated primarily by M_3 muscarinic receptors located on bronchial and tracheal smooth muscle (Eglen et al., 1996; Fisher et al., 2004).

Urinary Tract

Parasympathetic sacral innervation causes detrusor muscle contraction, increased voiding pressure, and ureteral peristalsis. These responses are difficult to observe with administered ACh because poor perfusion of visceral organs and rapid hydrolysis by plasma butyrylcholinesterase limit access of systemically administered ACh to visceral muscarinic receptors. Control of bladder contraction apparently is mediated by multiple muscarinic receptor subtypes. Muscarinic stimulation of bladder contraction is mediated primarily by M_3 receptors expressed by detrusor smooth muscle cells. Smooth muscle M_2 receptors also seem to make a small contribution to this response. M_2 receptors may also cause bladder contractions indirectly by reversing β receptor–cyclic AMP–mediated relaxation of the detrusor muscle (Hegde, 2006; Matsui et al, 2002).

GI Tract

Although stimulation of vagal input to the GI tract increases tone, amplitude of contractions, and secretory activity of the stomach and intestine, such responses are inconsistently seen with administered ACh for the same reasons that urinary tract responses are difficult to observe. As in the urinary tract, M_3 receptors appear to be primarily responsible for mediating cholinergic control of GI motility, but M_2 receptors also contribute to this activity (Matsui et al., 2002).

Secretory Effects

In addition to its stimulatory effects on the tracheobronchial and GI secretions, ACh stimulates secretion from other glands that receive parasympathetic or sympathetic cholinergic innervation, including the lacrimal, nasopharyngeal, salivary, and sweat glands. All of these effects are mediated primarily by M_3 muscarinic receptors (Caulfield and Birdsall, 1998); M_1 receptors also contribute significantly to the cholinergic stimulation of salivary secretion (Gautam et al., 2004).

Eye

When instilled into the eye, ACh produces miosis by contracting the pupillary sphincter muscle and accommodation for near vision by contracting the ciliary muscle; both of these effects are mediated primarily by M_3 muscarinic receptors, but other subtypes may contribute to the ocular effects of cholinergic stimulation.

CNS Effects

While systemically administered ACh has limited CNS penetration, muscarinic agonists that can cross the blood-brain barrier evoke a characteristic cortical arousal or activation response similar to that produced by injection of cholinesterase inhibitors or by electrical stimulation of the brainstem reticular formation. All five muscarinic receptor subtypes are expressed in the brain (Volpicelli and Levey, 2004), and recent studies suggest that muscarinic receptor–regulated pathways may have an important role in cognitive function, motor control, appetite regulation, nociception, and other processes (Wess et al., 2007).

Muscarinic Receptor Agonists

Muscarinic cholinergic receptor agonists can be divided into two groups:

- choline esters, including ACh and several synthetic esters
- the naturally occurring cholinomimetic alkaloids (particularly pilocarpine, muscarine, and arecoline) and their synthetic congeners

Of several hundred synthetic choline derivatives investigated, only methacholine, carbachol, and bethanechol (Figure 9–1) have had clinical applications.

Methacholine (acetyl-β-methylcholine), the β-methyl analogue of ACh, is a synthetic choline ester that differs from ACh chiefly in its greater duration and selectivity of action. Its action is more prolonged because the added methyl group increases its resistance to hydrolysis by cholinesterases. Its selectivity is reflected in a predominance of muscarinic with only minor nicotinic actions, the former manifest most clearly in the cardiovascular system (Table 9–1).

Carbachol, and its β-methyl analogue, bethanechol, are unsubstituted carbamoyl esters that are almost completely resistant to hydrolysis by cholinesterases; their $t_{1/2}$ values are thus sufficiently long that they become distributed to areas of low blood flow. Carbachol retains substantial nicotinic activity, particularly on autonomic ganglia. Bethanechol has mainly muscarinic actions, with prominent effects on motility of the GI tract and urinary bladder.

The major natural alkaloid muscarinic agonists—muscarine, pilocarpine, and arecoline—have the same principal sites of action as the choline esters. Muscarine acts almost exclusively at muscarinic receptor sites, and the classification of these receptors derives from the actions of this alkaloid. Pilocarpine has a dominant muscarinic action but is a partial rather than full agonist; the sweat glands are particularly sensitive to pilocarpine. Arecoline also acts at nicotinic receptors. Although these naturally occurring alkaloids are of great value as pharmacological tools and muscarine has toxicological significance (discussed further in the chapter), present clinical use is restricted largely to the employment of pilocarpine as a sialagogue and miotic agent (Chapter 69).

HISTORY AND SOURCES

The alkaloid muscarine was isolated from the mushroom *Amanita muscaria* by Schmiedeberg in 1869. Pilocarpine is the chief alkaloid obtained from the leaflets of South American shrubs of the genus *Pilocarpus*. Although the natives had long known that the chewing of leaves of *Pilocarpus* plants caused salivation, the active compound, pilocarpine, was isolated only in 1875 and shown to affect the pupil and sweat and salivary glands. Arecoline is the main alkaloid of areca or betel nuts, which are consumed as a euphoretic masticatory mixture by the natives of the Indian subcontinent and East Indies. Hunt and Taveau synthesized and studied methacholine as early as 1911. Carbachol and bethanechol were synthesized and investigated in the 1930s.

ADME

The absorption and distribution of these compounds may be predicted from their structures. Muscarine and the choline esters are quaternary amines; pilocarpine and arecoline are tertiary amines (see examples in Figure 9–1). The choline esters, as quaternary amines, are poorly absorbed following oral administration and have limited ability to cross the blood-brain barrier. Even though these drugs resist hydrolysis, the choline

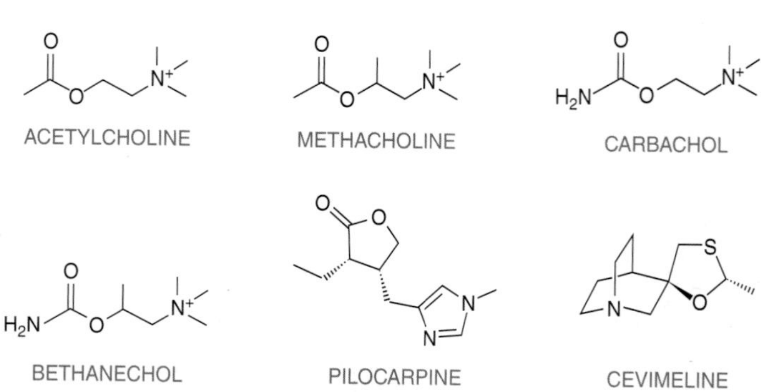

ACETYLCHOLINE METHACHOLINE CARBACHOL BETHANECHOL PILOCARPINE CEVIMELINE

Figure 9–1 *Structural formulas of ACh, choline esters, and natural alkaloids that stimulate muscarinic receptors.*

TABLE 9–1 ■ PHARMACOLOGICAL PROPERTIES OF CHOLINE ESTERS AND NATURAL ALKALOIDS

	HYDROLYSIS BY AChE	NICOTINIC ACTIVITY
Acetylcholine	+++	++
Methacholine	+	+
Carbachol	–	+++
Bethanechol	–	–
Muscarine	–	–
Pilocarpine	–	–

esters are short-acting agents due to rapid renal elimination. Pilocarpine and arecoline, as tertiary amines, are readily absorbed and can cross the blood-brain barrier. While muscarine is a quaternary amine and is poorly absorbed, it can still be toxic when ingested and can even have CNS effects. The natural alkaloids are primarily eliminated by the kidneys; excretion of the tertiary amines can be accelerated by acidification of the urine to trap the cationic form in the urine.

Therapeutic Uses of Muscarinic Receptor Agonists

Muscarinic agonists are currently used in the treatment of urinary bladder disorders and xerostomia and in the diagnosis of bronchial hyperreactivity. They are also used in ophthalmology as miotic agents and for the treatment of glaucoma. There is growing interest in the use of M_1 agonists in treating the cognitive impairment associated with Alzheimer disease. Other receptor subtypes, including M_2 and M_5, also appear to be involved in the regulation of cognitive function, at least in animal models (Wess et al., 2007).

Acetylcholine

Although rarely given systemically, ACh is used topically for the induction of miosis during ophthalmologic surgery, instilled into the eye as a 1% solution (Chapter 69).

Methacholine

Methacholine is administered by inhalation for the diagnosis of bronchial airway hyperreactivity in patients who do not have clinically apparent asthma (Crapo et al., 2000). It is available as a powder that is diluted with 0.9% NaCl and administered via a nebulizer. While muscarinic agonists can cause bronchoconstriction and increased tracheobronchial secretions in all individuals, asthmatic patients respond with intense bronchoconstriction and a reduction in vital capacity. The response to methacholine may be exaggerated or prolonged in patients taking β adrenergic receptor antagonists. Contraindications to methacholine testing include severe airflow limitation, recent myocardial infarction or stroke, uncontrolled hypertension, or pregnancy. Emergency resuscitation equipment, oxygen, and medications to treat severe bronchospasm (e.g., β_2 adrenergic receptor agonists for inhalation) should be available during testing.

Bethanechol

Bethanechol primarily affects the urinary and GI tracts. In the urinary tract, bethanechol has utility in treating urinary retention and inadequate emptying of the bladder when organic obstruction is absent, as in postoperative urinary retention, diabetic autonomic neuropathy, and certain cases of chronic hypotonic, myogenic, or neurogenic bladder; catheterization can thus be avoided. When used chronically, 10–50 mg of the drug is given orally three to four times daily; the drug should be administered on an empty stomach (i.e., 1 h before or 2 h after a meal) to minimize nausea and vomiting.

In the GI tract, bethanechol stimulates peristalsis, increases motility, and increases resting lower esophageal sphincter pressure. Bethanechol formerly was used to treat postoperative abdominal distention, gastric atony, gastroparesis, adynamic ileus, and gastroesophageal reflux; more efficacious therapies for these disorders are now available (Chapters 49 and 50).

Carbachol

Carbachol is used topically in ophthalmology for the treatment of glaucoma and the induction of miosis during surgery; it is instilled into the eye as a 0.01%–3% solution (Chapter 69).

Pilocarpine

Pilocarpine hydrochloride is used for the treatment of xerostomia that follows head and neck radiation treatments or that is associated with Sjögren syndrome (Porter et al., 2004; Wiseman and Faulds, 1995), an autoimmune disorder occurring primarily in women in whom secretions, particularly salivary and lacrimal, are compromised. Treatment can enhance salivary secretion, ease of swallowing, and subjective improvement in hydration of the oral cavity provided salivary parenchyma maintains residual function. Side effects typify cholinergic stimulation, with sweating the most common complaint. The usual dose is 5–10 mg three times daily; the dose should be lowered in patients with hepatic impairment.

Pilocarpine is used topically in ophthalmology for the treatment of glaucoma and as a miotic agent; it is instilled in the eye as a 0.5%–6% solution and also can be delivered via an ocular insert (Chapter 69).

Cevimeline

Cevimeline is a muscarinic agonist that seems to preferentially activate M_1 and M_3 receptors on lacrimal and salivary gland epithelia. The drug has a long-lasting sialogogic action and may have fewer side effects and better patient compliance than pilocarpine (Noaiseh et al., 2014). The usual dose is 30 mg three times daily.

Contraindications, Precautions, and Adverse Effects

Most contraindications, precautions, and adverse effects are predictable consequences of muscarinic receptor stimulation. Thus, important contraindications to the use of muscarinic agonists include asthma, chronic obstructive pulmonary disease, urinary or GI tract obstruction, acid-peptic disease, cardiovascular disease accompanied by bradycardia, hypotension, and hyperthyroidism (muscarinic agonists may precipitate atrial fibrillation in hyperthyroid patients). Common adverse effects include diaphoresis; diarrhea, abdominal cramps, nausea/vomiting, and other GI side effects; a sensation of tightness in the urinary bladder; difficulty in visual accommodation; and hypotension, which can severely reduce coronary blood flow, especially if it is already compromised. These contraindications and adverse effects are generally of limited concern with topical administration for ophthalmic use.

Toxicology

Poisoning from the ingestion of plants containing pilocarpine, muscarine, or arecoline is characterized chiefly by exaggeration of their various parasympathomimetic effects. Treatment consists of the parenteral administration of atropine in doses sufficient to cross the blood-brain barrier and measures to support the respiratory and cardiovascular systems and to counteract pulmonary edema.

Muscarinic Receptor Antagonists

The muscarinic receptor antagonists include

- the naturally occurring alkaloids atropine and scopolamine
- semisynthetic derivatives of these alkaloids, which primarily differ from the parent compounds in their disposition in the body or their duration of action

- synthetic derivatives, some of which show a limited degree of selectivity for certain muscarinic receptor subtypes

Noteworthy agents among the last two categories are homatropine and tropicamide, which have a shorter duration of action than atropine, and methscopolamine, ipratropium, tiotropium, aclidinium, and umeclidinium, which are quaternary amines that do not cross the blood-brain barrier or readily cross membranes. The synthetic derivatives possessing some degree of receptor subtype selectivity include pirenzepine, an M_1 receptor–preferring antagonist, and darifenacin and solifenacin, two M_3 receptor–preferring agents.

Muscarinic antagonists prevent the effects of ACh by blocking its binding to muscarinic receptors on effector cells at parasympathetic (and sympathetic cholinergic) neuroeffector junctions in peripheral ganglia and the CNS. In general, muscarinic antagonists cause little blockade of nicotinic receptors. However, the quaternary ammonium antagonists generally exhibit a greater degree of nicotinic-blocking activity and therefore are more likely to interfere with ganglionic or neuromuscular transmission.

While many effects of muscarinic antagonists can be predicted from an understanding of the physiological responses mediated by muscarinic receptors at parasympathetic and sympathetic cholinergic neuroeffector junctions, paradoxical responses can occur. For example, presynaptic muscarinic receptors of variable subtype are present on postganglionic parasympathetic nerve terminals. Because blockade of presynaptic receptors generally augments neurotransmitter release, the presynaptic effects of muscarinic antagonists may counteract their postsynaptic receptor blockade. Blockade of the modulatory muscarinic receptors in peripheral ganglia represents an additional mechanism for paradoxical responses.

An important consideration in the therapeutic use of muscarinic antagonists is the fact that physiological functions in different organs vary in their sensitivity to muscarinic receptor blockade (Table 9–2). Small doses of atropine depress salivary and bronchial secretion and sweating. With larger doses, the pupil dilates, accommodation of the lens to near vision is inhibited, and vagal effects on the heart are blocked so that the heart rate increases. Larger doses antagonize parasympathetic control of the urinary bladder and GI tract, thereby inhibiting micturition and decreasing intestinal tone and motility. Still larger doses are required to inhibit gastric motility and particularly secretion. Thus, doses of atropine and most related muscarinic antagonists that depress gastric secretion also almost invariably affect salivary secretion, ocular accommodation, micturition, and GI motility. This hierarchy of relative sensitivities is not a consequence of differences in the affinity of atropine for the muscarinic receptors at these sites because atropine lacks selectivity toward different muscarinic receptor subtypes. More likely determinants include the degree to which the functions of various end organs are regulated by parasympathetic tone, the "spareness" of receptors and signaling mechanisms, the involvement of intramural neurons and reflexes, and the presence of other regulatory mechanisms.

Most clinically available muscarinic antagonists lack receptor subtype selectivity and their actions differ little from those of atropine, the prototype of the group. Notably, the clinical efficacy of some agents may actually depend on antagonistic actions on two or more receptor subtypes.

TABLE 9–2 ■ EFFECTS OF ATROPINE IN RELATION TO DOSE

DOSE (mg)	EFFECTS
0.5	Slight cardiac slowing; some dryness of mouth; inhibition of sweating
1	Definite dryness of mouth; thirst; acceleration of heart, sometimes preceded by slowing; mild dilation of pupils
2	Rapid heart rate; palpitation; marked dryness of mouth; dilated pupils; some blurring of near vision
5	Previous symptoms marked; difficulty in speaking and swallowing; restlessness and fatigue; headache; dry, hot skin; difficulty in micturition; reduced intestinal peristalsis
≥10	Previous symptoms more marked; pulse rapid and weak; iris practically obliterated; vision very blurred; skin flushed, hot, dry, and scarlet; ataxia, restlessness, and excitement; hallucinations and delirium; coma

The clinical picture of a high (toxic) dose of atropine may be remembered by an old mnemonic device that summarizes the symptoms: *Red as a beet, Dry as a bone, Blind as a bat, Hot as firestone, and Mad as a hatter.*

Structure-Activity Relationships

An intact ester of tropine and tropic acid (Figure 9–2) is essential for antimuscarinic action because neither the free acid nor the basic alcohol exhibits significant antimuscarinic activity. The presence of a free OH group in the acyl portion of the ester also is important for activity. Quaternary ammonium derivatives of atropine and scopolamine are generally more potent than their parent compounds in both muscarinic- and ganglionic- (nicotinic-) blocking activities when given parenterally. These derivatives are poorly and unreliably absorbed when given orally.

Mechanism of Action

Atropine and related compounds compete with ACh and other muscarinic agonists for the orthosteric ACh site on the muscarinic receptor. The antagonism by atropine is competitive; thus, it is surmountable by ACh if the concentration of ACh at muscarinic receptors is increased sufficiently. Muscarinic receptor antagonists inhibit responses to postganglionic cholinergic nerve stimulation less effectively than they inhibit responses to injected choline esters. The difference may be explained by the fact that release of ACh by cholinergic nerve terminals occurs in close proximity to the receptors, resulting in very high concentrations of the transmitter at the receptors.

Pharmacological Effects of Muscarinic Antagonists

The pharmacological effects of atropine, the prototypical muscarinic antagonist, provide a good background for understanding the therapeutic uses of the various muscarinic antagonists. The effects of other muscarinic antagonists will be mentioned only when they differ significantly from those of atropine. The major pharmacological effects of increasing doses of atropine, summarized in Table 9–2, offer a general guide to the problems associated with administration of this class of agents.

HISTORY

The naturally occurring muscarinic receptor antagonists atropine and scopolamine are alkaloids of the belladonna (Solanaceae) plants. Preparations of belladonna were known to the ancient Hindus and have long been used by physicians. During the time of the Roman Empire and in the Middle Ages, the deadly nightshade shrub was frequently used to produce an obscure and often-prolonged poisoning, prompting Linnaeus to name the shrub *Atropa belladonna*, after Atropos, the oldest of the three Fates, who cuts the thread of life. The name *belladonna* derives from the alleged use of this preparation by Italian women to dilate their pupils; modern-day fashion models are known to use this same device for visual appeal. Atropine (D,L-hyoscyamine) also is found in *Datura stramonium* (Jamestown or jimson weed). Scopolamine (L-hyoscine) is found chiefly in *Hyoscyamus niger* (henbane). In India, the root and leaves of jimson weed were burned and the smoke inhaled to treat asthma. British colonists observed this ritual and introduced the belladonna alkaloids into Western medicine in the early 1800s. Atropine was isolated in pure form in 1831.

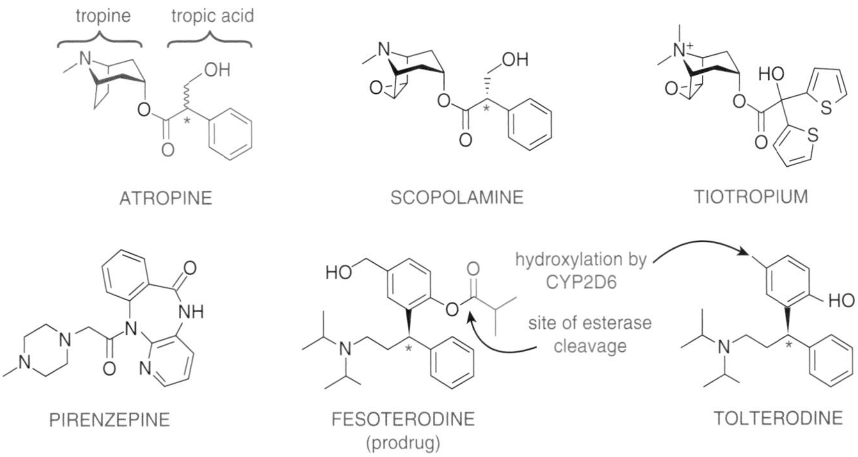

Figure 9–2 *Structural formulas of the belladonna alkaloids and semisynthetic and synthetic analogues.* Fesoterodine is converted to an active 5-hydroxymeythyl metabolite by esterase activity. CYP2D6 converts tolterodine to the same metabolite. Note that atropine, scopolamine, tolterodine, and fesoterodine each contain an asymmetric carbon atom (indicated by red asterisk); these compounds therefore exist as racemic mixtures. Clinically, only the (R)-enantiomers of tolterodine and fesoterodine are used.

Cardiovascular System

Heart. The main effect of atropine on the heart is to alter the rate. Although the dominant response is tachycardia, there is often a transient bradycardia with average clinical doses (0.4–0.6 mg; Table 9–2). The slowing is modest (4–8 beats per min), occurs with no accompanying changes in blood pressure or cardiac output, and is usually absent after rapid intravenous injection. This unexpected effect has been attributed to the block of presynaptic M_1 muscarinic receptors on parasympathetic postganglionic nerve terminals in the SA node, which normally inhibit ACh release (Wellstein and Pitschner, 1988).

Larger doses of atropine cause progressive tachycardia by blocking M_2 receptors on the SA nodal pacemaker cells, thereby antagonizing parasympathetic (vagal) tone to the heart. The resting heart rate is increased by about 35–40 beats per min in young men given 2 mg of atropine intramuscularly. The maximal heart rate (e.g., in response to exercise) is not altered by atropine. The influence of atropine is most noticeable in healthy young adults, in whom vagal tone is considerable. In infants, the elderly, and patients with heart failure, even large doses of atropine may fail to accelerate the heart.

Atropine can abolish many types of reflex vagal cardiac slowing or asystole, such as that occurring from inhalation of irritant vapors, stimulation of the carotid sinus, pressure on the eyeballs, peritoneal stimulation, or injection of contrast dye during cardiac catheterization. Atropine also prevents or abruptly abolishes bradycardia or asystole caused by choline esters, acetylcholinesterase inhibitors, or other parasympathomimetic drugs, as well as cardiac arrest from electrical stimulation of the vagus.

The removal of vagal tone to the heart by atropine may facilitate AV conduction. Atropine shortens the functional refractory period of the AV node and can increase the ventricular rate in patients who have atrial fibrillation or flutter. In certain cases of second-degree AV block (e.g., Wenckebach AV block) in which vagal activity is an etiological factor (as with digoxin toxicity), atropine may lessen the degree of block. In some patients with complete AV block, the idioventricular rate may be accelerated by atropine; in others, it is stabilized. Atropine may improve the clinical condition of patients with inferior or posterior wall myocardial infarction by relieving severe sinus or nodal bradycardia or AV block.

Circulation. Atropine alone has little effect on blood pressure because most vessels lack significant cholinergic innervation. However, in clinical doses, atropine completely counteracts the peripheral vasodilation and sharp fall in blood pressure caused by choline esters. In toxic and occasionally in therapeutic doses, atropine can dilate cutaneous blood vessels, especially those in the blush area (atropine flush). This may be a compensatory reaction permitting the radiation of heat to offset the atropine-induced rise in temperature that can accompany inhibition of sweating.

Respiratory System

Although atropine can cause some bronchodilation and decrease in tracheobronchial secretion in normal individuals by blocking parasympathetic (vagal) tone to the lungs, its effects on the respiratory system are most significant in patients with respiratory disease. Atropine can inhibit the bronchoconstriction caused by histamine, bradykinin, and the eicosanoids, which presumably reflects the participation of reflex parasympathetic (vagal) activity in the bronchoconstriction elicited by these agents. The ability to block the indirect bronchoconstrictive effects of these mediators forms the basis for the use of muscarinic receptor antagonists, along with β adrenergic receptor agonists, in the treatment of asthma. Muscarinic antagonists also have an important role in the treatment of chronic obstructive pulmonary disease (Chapter 40).

Atropine inhibits the secretions of the nose, mouth, pharynx, and bronchi and thus dries the mucous membranes of the respiratory tract. This action is especially marked if secretion is excessive and formed the basis for the use of atropine and other muscarinic antagonists to prevent irritating inhalational anesthetics such as diethyl ether from increasing bronchial secretion; newer inhalational anesthetics are less irritating. Muscarinic antagonists are used to decrease the rhinorrhea ("runny nose") associated with the common cold or with allergic and nonallergic rhinitis. Reduction of mucous secretion and mucociliary clearance can, however, result in mucus plugs, a potentially undesirable side effect of muscarinic antagonists in patients with airway disease.

The quaternary ammonium compounds ipratropium, tiotropium, aclidinium, and umeclidinium are used exclusively for their effects on the respiratory tract. Dry mouth is the only frequently reported side effect, as the absorption of these drugs from the lungs or the GI tract is inefficient. In addition, aclidinium has been shown to undergo rapid hydrolysis in plasma to inactive metabolites, thus reducing systemic exposure to the drug (Gavalda et al., 2009). The degree of bronchodilation achieved by these agents is thought to reflect the level of basal parasympathetic tone, supplemented by reflex activation of cholinergic pathways brought about by various stimuli. A therapeutically important property of ipratropium and tiotropium is their minimal inhibitory effect on mucociliary clearance relative to atropine. Hence, the choice of these agents for use in patients with airway disease minimizes the increased accumulation of lower airway secretions encountered with atropine.

Eye

Muscarinic receptor antagonists block the cholinergic responses of the pupillary sphincter muscle of the iris and the ciliary muscle controlling lens curvature (Chapter 69). Thus, these agents dilate the pupil (mydriasis) and paralyze accommodation (cycloplegia). The wide pupillary dilation results in photophobia; the lens is fixed for far vision, near objects are blurred, and objects may appear smaller than they are. The normal pupillary reflex constriction to light or on convergence of the eyes is abolished. These effects are most evident when the agent is instilled into the eye but can also occur after systemic administration of the alkaloids.

Conventional systemic doses of atropine (0.6 mg) have little ocular effect, in contrast to equal doses of scopolamine, which cause evident mydriasis and loss of accommodation. Locally applied atropine produces ocular effects of considerable duration; accommodation and pupillary reflexes may not fully recover for 7–12 days. Other muscarinic receptor antagonists with shorter durations of action are therefore preferred as mydriatics in ophthalmologic practice. Pilocarpine and choline esters (e.g., carbachol) in sufficient concentrations can reverse the ocular effects of atropine.

Muscarinic receptor antagonists administered systemically have little effect on intraocular pressure except in patients predisposed to angle-closure glaucoma, in whom the pressure may occasionally rise dangerously. The rise in pressure occurs when the anterior chamber is narrow and the iris obstructs outflow of aqueous humor into the trabeculae. Muscarinic antagonists may precipitate a first attack in unrecognized cases of this relatively rare condition. In patients with open-angle glaucoma, an acute rise in pressure is unusual. Atropine-like drugs generally can be used safely in the latter condition, particularly if the glaucoma is being treated appropriately.

GI Tract

Knowledge of the actions of muscarinic receptor agonists on the stomach and intestine led to the use of muscarinic receptor antagonists as antispasmodic agents for GI disorders and to reduce gastric acid secretion in the treatment of peptic ulcer disease.

Motility. Parasympathetic nerves enhance GI tone and motility and relax sphincters, thereby favoring the passage of gastrointestinal contents. In normal subjects and in patients with GI disease, muscarinic antagonists produce prolonged inhibitory effects on the motor activity of the stomach, duodenum, jejunum, ileum, and colon, characterized by a reduction in tone and in amplitude and frequency of peristaltic contractions. Relatively large doses are needed to produce such inhibition, probably because the enteric nervous system can regulate motility independently of parasympathetic control; parasympathetic nerves serve only to modulate the effects of the enteric nervous system. Although atropine can completely abolish the effects of exogenous muscarinic agonists on GI motility and secretion, it does not completely inhibit the GI responses to vagal stimulation. This difference, particularly striking in the effects of atropine on gut motility, can be attributed to the fact that preganglionic vagal fibers innervating the GI tract synapse not only with postganglionic cholinergic fibers, but also with a network of noncholinergic intramural neurons that form the plexuses of the enteric nervous system and utilize neurotransmitters whose effects atropine does not block (e.g., 5HT, dopamine, and various peptides).

Gastric Acid Secretion. Similarly, atropine only partially inhibits the gastric acid secretory responses to vagal activity because vagal stimulation of gastrin secretion is mediated not by ACh but by peptidergic neurons in the vagal trunk that release gastrin-releasing peptide (GRP). GRP stimulates gastrin release from G cells; gastrin can act directly to promote acid secretion by parietal cells and to stimulate histamine release from enterochromaffin-like (ECL) cells (see Figure 49–1). Parietal cells (acid secretors) respond to at least three agonists: gastrin, histamine, and ACh. Atropine will inhibit only the components of acid secretion that result from muscarinic stimulation of parietal cells and from muscarinic stimulation of ECL cells that secrete histamine.

Secretions. Salivary secretion is particularly sensitive to inhibition by muscarinic receptor antagonists, which can completely abolish the copious, watery secretion induced by parasympathetic stimulation. The mouth becomes dry, and swallowing and talking may become difficult. The gastric cells that secrete mucin and proteolytic enzymes are more directly under vagal influence than are the acid-secreting cells, and atropine selectively decreases their secretory function. Although atropine can reduce gastric secretion, the doses required also affect salivary secretion, ocular accommodation, micturition, and GI motility (Table 9–2).

In contrast to most muscarinic receptor antagonists, pirenzepine, which shows some degree of selectivity for M_1 receptors, inhibits gastric acid secretion at doses that have little effect on salivation or heart rate. Because parietal cells primarily express M_3 receptors, perhaps M_1 receptors in intramural ganglia are the primary target of pirenzepine (Eglen et al., 1996). However, this concept has been questioned by the observation that pirenzepine is still able to inhibit carbachol-stimulated gastric acid secretion in M_1 receptor–deficient mice (Aihara et al., 2005). In general, histamine H_2 receptor antagonists and proton pump inhibitors have replaced muscarinic antagonists as inhibitors of acid secretion (Chapter 49).

Other Smooth Muscle

Urinary Tract. Muscarinic antagonists decrease the normal tone and amplitude of contractions of the ureter and bladder and often eliminate drug-induced enhancement of ureteral tone. However, this effect is usually accompanied by reduced salivation and lacrimation and blurred vision (Table 9–2).

Biliary Tract. Atropine exerts mild antispasmodic action on the gallbladder and bile ducts in humans. However, this effect usually is not sufficient to overcome or prevent the marked spasm and increase in biliary duct pressure induced by opioids. The nitrates are more effective than atropine in this respect.

Sweat Glands and Temperature

Small doses of atropine inhibit the activity of sweat glands innervated by sympathetic cholinergic fibers, and the skin becomes hot and dry. Sweating may be depressed enough to raise the body temperature, but only notably so after large doses or at high environmental temperatures.

CNS

Atropine has minimal effects on the CNS at therapeutic doses, although mild stimulation of the parasympathetic medullary centers may occur. With toxic doses of atropine, central excitation becomes more prominent, leading to restlessness, irritability, disorientation, hallucinations, or delirium (see the discussion of atropine poisoning further in the chapter). With still larger doses, stimulation is followed by depression, leading to circulatory collapse and respiratory failure after a period of paralysis and coma.

In contrast to atropine, scopolamine has prominent central effects at low therapeutic doses; atropine therefore is preferred over scopolamine for most purposes. The basis for this difference is probably the greater permeation of scopolamine across the blood-brain barrier. Scopolamine in therapeutic doses normally causes CNS depression, manifest as drowsiness, amnesia, fatigue, and dreamless sleep, with a reduction in REM sleep. It also causes euphoria and can therefore be subject to abuse. The depressant and amnesic effects formerly were sought when scopolamine was used as an adjunct to anesthetic agents or for preanesthetic medication. However, in the presence of severe pain, the same doses of scopolamine can occasionally cause excitement, restlessness, hallucinations, or delirium. These excitatory effects resemble those of toxic doses of atropine. Scopolamine also is effective in preventing motion sickness, probably by blocking neural pathways from the vestibular apparatus in the inner ear to the emetic center in the brainstem.

ADME

The belladonna alkaloids and the *tertiary* synthetic and semisynthetic derivatives are absorbed rapidly from the GI tract. They also enter the circulation when applied locally to the mucosal surfaces of the body.

Absorption from intact skin is limited, although efficient absorption does occur in the postauricular region for some agents (e.g., scopolamine, allowing delivery by transdermal patch). Systemic absorption of inhaled or orally ingested *quaternary* muscarinic receptor antagonists is limited. The quaternary ammonium derivatives of the belladonna alkaloids also penetrate the conjunctiva of the eye less readily, and central effects are lacking because the quaternary agents do not cross the blood-brain barrier. Atropine has a $t_{1/2}$ of about 4 h; hepatic metabolism accounts for the elimination of about half of a dose, and the remainder is excreted unchanged in the urine.

Ipratropium is administered as an aerosol or solution for inhalation, whereas tiotropium is administered as a dry powder. As with most drugs administered by inhalation, about 90% of the dose is swallowed. When inhaled, their action is confined almost completely to the mouth and airways. Most of the swallowed drug appears in the feces. After inhalation, maximal responses usually develop over 30–90 min, with tiotropium having the slower onset. The effects of ipratropium last for 4–6 h; tiotropium's effects persist for 24 h, and the drug is amenable to once-daily dosing.

Therapeutic Uses of Muscarinic Receptor Antagonists

Muscarinic receptor antagonists have been used predominantly to inhibit effects of parasympathetic activity in the respiratory tract, urinary tract, GI tract, eye, and heart. Their CNS effects have resulted in their use in the treatment of Parkinson disease, the management of extrapyramidal side effects of antipsychotic drugs, and the prevention of motion sickness. The major limitation in the use of the nonselective drugs is often failure to obtain desired therapeutic responses without concomitant side effects. While these usually are not serious, they can be sufficiently disturbing to decrease patient compliance, particularly during long-term administration. To date, selectivity is mainly achieved by local administration (e.g., by pulmonary inhalation or instillation in the eye). The development of allosteric modulators that recognize sites unique to particular receptor subtypes is currently considered an important approach to obtain receptor subtype-selective drugs for the treatment of specific clinical conditions (Conn et al., 2009).

Respiratory Tract

Ipratropium, tiotropium, aclidinium, and umeclidinium are important agents in the treatment of chronic obstructive pulmonary disease; they are less effective in most patients with asthma (see Chapter 40). These agents often are used with inhaled long-acting β_2 adrenergic receptor agonists, although there is little evidence of true synergism.

Ipratropium appears to block all subtypes of muscarinic receptors and accordingly also antagonizes the inhibition of ACh release by presynaptic M_2 receptors on parasympathetic postganglionic nerve terminals in the lung; the resulting increase in ACh release may counteract the drug's blockade of M_3 receptor-mediated bronchoconstriction. In contrast, tiotropium shows some selectivity for M_1 and M_3 receptors. In addition, tiotropium and aclidinium have lower affinities for M_2 receptors and dissociate more slowly from M_3 than from M_2 receptors. This minimizes its presynaptic effect to enhance ACh release (Alagha et al., 2014).

Ipratropium is administered four times daily via a metered-dose inhaler or nebulizer; aclidinium is used twice daily via a dry powder inhaler. Tiotropium and umeclidinium are once-daily medications that can be used for maintenance therapy via a dry powder inhaler in patients with moderate-to-severe disease.

In normal individuals, inhalation of antimuscarinic drugs can provide virtually complete protection against the bronchoconstriction produced by the subsequent inhalation of such irritants as sulfur dioxide, ozone, or cigarette smoke. However, patients with atopic asthma or demonstrable bronchial hyperresponsiveness are less well protected. Although these drugs cause a marked reduction in sensitivity to methacholine in asthmatic subjects, more modest inhibition of responses to challenge with histamine, bradykinin, or $PGF_{2\alpha}$ is achieved, and little protection is afforded against the bronchoconstriction induced by 5HT or leukotrienes.

The therapeutic uses of ipratropium and tiotropium are discussed further in Chapter 40.

Ipratropium also is approved by the FDA for use in nasal inhalers for the treatment of the rhinorrhea associated with the common cold or with allergic or nonallergic perennial rhinitis. Although the ability of muscarinic antagonists to reduce nasopharyngeal secretions may provide some symptomatic relief, such therapy does not affect the natural course of the condition. It is probable that the contribution of first-generation antihistamines employed in nonprescription cold medications is due primarily to their antimuscarinic properties, except in conditions with an allergic basis (see Chapters 34 and 39).

Genitourinary Tract

Overactive urinary bladder can be successfully treated with muscarinic receptor antagonists. These agents can lower intravesicular pressure, increase capacity, and reduce the frequency of contractions by antagonizing parasympathetic control of the bladder; they also may alter bladder sensation during filling (Chapple et al., 2005). Muscarinic antagonists can be used to treat enuresis in children, particularly when a progressive increase in bladder capacity is the objective, and to reduce urinary frequency and increase bladder capacity in spastic paraplegia.

The muscarinic receptor antagonists indicated for overactive bladder are oxybutynin, tolterodine, trospium chloride, darifenacin, solifenacin, and fesoterodine. Although some comparison trials have demonstrated small but statistically significant differences in efficacy between these agents (Chapple et al., 2008), the clinical relevance of these differences remains uncertain. The most important adverse reactions are consequences of muscarinic receptor blockade and include xerostomia, blurred vision, and GI side effects such as constipation and dyspepsia. CNS-related antimuscarinic effects, including drowsiness, dizziness, and confusion, can occur and are particularly problematic in elderly patients. CNS effects appear to be less likely with trospium, a quaternary amine, and with darifenacin and solifenacin; the last two agents show some preference for M_3 receptors and therefore seem to have minimal effects on M_1 receptors in the CNS, which appear to play an important role in memory and cognition (Kay et al., 2006). Adverse effects can limit the tolerability of these drugs with continued use, and patient acceptance declines. Xerostomia is the most common reason for discontinuation.

Oxybutynin, the oldest of the antimuscarinics currently used to treat overactive bladder disorders, is associated with a high incidence of antimuscarinic side effects, particularly xerostomia. In an attempt to increase patient acceptance, oxybutynin is marketed as a transdermal system that is associated with a lower incidence of side effects than the oral immediate- and extended-release formulations; a topical gel formulation of oxybutynin also appears to offer a more favorable side-effect profile. Because of the extensive metabolism of oral oxybutynin by enteric and hepatic CYP3A4, higher doses are used in oral than transdermal administration; the dose may need to be reduced in patients taking drugs that inhibit CYP3A4.

Tolterodine shows selectivity for the urinary bladder in animal models and in clinical studies, resulting in greater patient acceptance; however, the drug binds to all muscarinic receptors with similar affinity. Tolterodine is metabolized by CYP2D6 to 5-hydroxymethyltolterodine, a metabolite that possesses similar activity as the parent drug but differs pharmacokinetically. CYP2D6 is a polymorphic enzyme, with significant variability of expression; thus, the production of the 5-hydroxymethyl metabolite can vary, as can the half-life of the parent drug. In patients who poorly metabolize tolterodine via CYP2D6, the CYP3A4 pathway becomes important in tolterodine elimination. Because it is often difficult to assess which patients will be poor metabolizers, tolterodine doses may need to be reduced in patients taking drugs that inhibit CYP3A4 (dosage adjustments generally are not necessary in patients taking drugs that inhibit CYP2D6). Patients with significant renal or hepatic impairment also should receive lower doses of the drug. Fesoterodine is a prodrug that is rapidly hydrolyzed to the active metabolite of tolterodine by esterases (Figure 9-2) rather than CYP2D6, thereby providing a less variable source of the 5-hydroxymethyl metabolite of tolterodine regardless of CYP2D6 status.

Trospium, a quaternary amine, is as effective as oxybutynin and with better tolerability. It is the only antimuscarinic agent used for overactive bladder that is eliminated primarily by the kidneys; 60% of the absorbed trospium dose is excreted unchanged in the urine, and dosage adjustment is necessary for patients with impaired renal function.

Solifenacin shows some preference for M_3 receptors, giving it a favorable ratio of efficacy to side effect (Chapple et al., 2004). Solifenacin is significantly metabolized by CYP3A4; thus, patients taking drugs that inhibit CYP3A4 should receive lower doses.

Like solifenacin, darifenacin shows some degree of selectivity for M_3 receptors (Caulfield and Birdsall, 1998). It is metabolized by CYP2D6 and CYP3A4; as with tolterodine, the latter pathway becomes more important in patients who poorly metabolize the drug by CYP2D6. Darifenacin doses may need to be reduced in patients taking drugs that inhibit either of these CYPs.

GI Tract

Muscarinic receptor antagonists were once widely used for the management of peptic ulcer. Although they can reduce gastric motility and the secretion of gastric acid, antisecretory doses produce pronounced side effects, such as xerostomia, loss of visual accommodation, photophobia, and difficulty in urination (Table 9–2). As a consequence, patient compliance in the long-term management of symptoms of acid-peptic disease with these drugs is poor. H_2 receptor antagonists and proton pump inhibitors generally are considered to be the current drugs of choice to reduce gastric acid secretion (Chapter 49).

Pirenzepine, a tricyclic drug similar in structure to imipramine, displays a limited degree of selectivity for M_1 receptors (Caulfield and Birdsall, 1998). Telenzepine, an analogue of pirenzepine, has higher potency and similar selectivity for M_1 receptors. Both drugs are used in the treatment of acid-peptic disease in Europe, Japan, and Canada, but not currently in the U.S. At therapeutic doses of pirenzepine, the incidence of xerostomia, blurred vision, and central muscarinic disturbances is relatively low. Central effects are not seen because of the drug's limited penetration into the CNS.

Most studies indicate that pirenzepine (100–150 mg per day) produces about the same rate of healing of duodenal and gastric ulcers as the H_2 receptor antagonists cimetidine or ranitidine; pirenzepine also may be effective in preventing the recurrence of ulcers (Tryba and Cook, 1997). Side effects necessitate drug withdrawal in less than 1% of patients.

Myriad conditions known or supposed to involve increased tone (spasticity) or motility of the GI tract are treated with belladonna alkaloids (e.g., atropine, hyoscyamine sulfate, and scopolamine) alone or in combination with sedatives (e.g., phenobarbital) or antianxiety agents (e.g., chlordiazepoxide). The belladonna alkaloids and their synthetic substitutes can reduce tone and motility when administered in maximally tolerated doses. M_3-selective antagonists might achieve more selectivity but are unlikely to be better tolerated, as M_3 receptors also have an important role in the control of salivation, bronchial secretion and contraction, and bladder motility. Glycopyrrolate, a muscarinic antagonist that is structurally unrelated to the belladonna alkaloids, is used to reduce GI tone and motility; as a quaternary amine, it is less likely to cause adverse CNS effects than atropine, scopolamine, and other tertiary amines. Alternative agents for treatment of increased GI motility and its associated symptoms are discussed in Chapter 50.

Diarrhea associated with irritation of the lower bowel, such as mild dysenteries and diverticulitis, may respond to atropine-like drugs, an effect that likely involves actions on ion transport as well as motility. However, more severe conditions such as *Salmonella* dysentery, ulcerative colitis, and Crohn disease respond little, if at all, to muscarinic antagonists.

Dicyclomine hydrochloride is a weak muscarinic receptor antagonist that also has nonspecific direct spasmolytic effects on smooth muscle of the GI tract. It is occasionally used in the treatment of diarrhea-predominant irritable bowel syndrome.

Salivary Secretions

The belladonna alkaloids and synthetic substitutes are effective in reducing excessive salivation, such as drug-induced salivation and that associated with heavy-metal poisoning and Parkinson disease. Glycopyrrolate is a quaternary amine and as mentioned is less likely to penetrate the CNS. Glycopyrrolate (as oral solution) is indicated to reduce drooling (e.g., in patients with Parkinson disease).

Eye

Effects limited to the eye are obtained by topical administration of muscarinic receptor antagonists to produce mydriasis and cycloplegia. Cycloplegia is not attainable without mydriasis and requires higher concentrations or more prolonged application of a given agent. Mydriasis often is necessary for thorough examination of the retina and optic disc and in the therapy of iridocyclitis and keratitis. Homatropine hydrobromide, a semisynthetic derivative of atropine (Figure 9–2), cyclopentolate hydrochloride, and tropicamide are agents used in ophthalmological practice. These agents are preferred to topical atropine or scopolamine because of their shorter duration of action. Additional information on the ophthalmological properties and preparations of these and other drugs is provided in Chapter 69.

Cardiovascular System

The cardiovascular effects of muscarinic receptor antagonists are of limited clinical utility. Generally, these agents are used only in coronary care units for short-term interventions or in surgical settings. They are also sometimes used as an adjunct to stress testing to increase heart rate in the setting of chronotropic incompetence.

Atropine may be considered in the initial treatment of patients with acute myocardial infarction in whom excessive vagal tone causes sinus bradycardia or AV nodal block. Sinus bradycardia is the most common arrhythmia seen during acute myocardial infarction of the inferior or posterior wall. Atropine may prevent further clinical deterioration in cases of high vagal tone or AV block by restoring heart rate to a level sufficient to maintain adequate hemodynamic status and to eliminate AV nodal block. Dosing must be judicious; doses that are too low can cause a paradoxical bradycardia (described previously), while excessive doses will cause tachycardia that may extend the infarct by increasing the demand for O_2.

Atropine occasionally is useful in reducing the severe bradycardia and syncope associated with a hyperactive carotid sinus reflex. It has little effect on most ventricular rhythms. In some patients, atropine may eliminate premature ventricular contractions associated with a very slow atrial rate. It also may reduce the degree of AV block when increased vagal tone is a major factor in the conduction defect, such as the second-degree AV block that can be produced by digoxin. Selective M_2 receptor antagonists would be of potential utility in blocking ACh-mediated bradycardia or AV block; however, no such agents are currently available for clinical use.

Autonomic control of the heart is known to be abnormal in patients with cardiovascular disease, especially in heart failure. Patients with heart failure typically exhibit increased sympathetic tone accompanied by vagal withdrawal, both of which may contribute to the progression of disease. While β-blockers have now emerged as standard of care in heart failure, less is known about whether augmentation of vagal tone may be beneficial. Studies in animals suggest that augmenting vagal tone chronically decreases the inflammatory response and prevents adverse cardiac remodeling in heart failure, and early studies in humans support their use. However, the pivotal clinical trials of such therapy remain ongoing as of this writing (Dunlap et al., 2015; Schwartz and De Ferrari, 2011).

CNS

The belladonna alkaloids were among the first drugs to be used in the prevention of motion sickness. Scopolamine is the most effective of these agents for short (4- to 6-h) exposures to severe motion and probably for exposures of up to several days. All agents used to combat motion sickness should be given prophylactically; they are much less effective after severe nausea or vomiting has developed. A transdermal preparation of scopolamine has been shown to be highly effective when used prophylactically for the prevention of motion sickness. The drug, incorporated into a multilayer adhesive unit, is applied to the postauricular mastoid region, an area where transdermal absorption of the drug is especially efficient, resulting in the delivery of about 0.5 mg of scopolamine over 72 h.

Xerostomia is common, drowsiness is not infrequent, and blurred vision occurs in some individuals using the scopolamine patch. Mydriasis and cycloplegia can occur by inadvertent transfer of the drug to the eye from the fingers after handling the patch. Rare but severe psychotic episodes have been reported.

Muscarinic receptor antagonists have long been used in the treatment of Parkinson disease, which is characterized by reduced dopaminergic input into the striatum, resulting in an imbalance between striatal muscarinic cholinergic and dopaminergic neurotransmission (see Chapter 18). The striatum, the major input area of the basal ganglia, contains multiple cell types, including cholinergic interneurons, all of which express one or more muscarinic receptor subtypes (Goldberg et al., 2012). Studies with muscarinic receptor mutant mice suggested that the beneficial effects of muscarinic antagonists in the treatment of Parkinson disease are primarily due to the blockade of M_1 and M_4 receptors, resulting in the activation or inhibition, respectively, of specific striatal neuronal subpopulations (Wess et al., 2007).

Muscarinic antagonists can be effective in the early stages of Parkinson disease if tremor is predominant, particularly in young patients. Muscarinic receptor antagonists also are used to treat the extrapyramidal symptoms that commonly occur as side effects of conventional antipsychotic drug therapy (Chapter 16). Certain antipsychotic drugs are relatively potent muscarinic receptor antagonists (Roth et al., 2004) and, perhaps for this reason, cause fewer extrapyramidal side effects.

The muscarinic antagonists used for Parkinson disease and drug-induced extrapyramidal symptoms include benztropine mesylate, trihexyphenidyl hydrochloride, and biperiden; all are tertiary amines that readily gain access to the CNS.

Anesthesia

Atropine is commonly given to block responses to vagal reflexes induced by surgical manipulation of visceral organs. Atropine or glycopyrrolate are also used to block the parasympathomimetic effects of neostigmine when it is administered to reverse skeletal muscle relaxation after surgery. Serious cardiac arrhythmias have occasionally occurred, perhaps because of the initial bradycardia produced by atropine combined with the cholinomimetic effects of neostigmine.

Anticholinesterase Poisoning

The use of atropine in large doses for the treatment of poisoning by anticholinesterase organophosphorus insecticides is discussed in Chapter 10. Atropine also may be used to antagonize the parasympathomimetic effects of pyridostigmine or other anticholinesterases administered in the treatment of myasthenia gravis. It does not interfere with the salutary effects at the skeletal neuromuscular junction. It is most useful early in therapy, before tolerance to muscarinic side effects of anticholinesterases has developed.

Other Therapeutic Uses

Methscopolamine bromide is a quaternary ammonium derivative of scopolamine and therefore lacks the central actions of scopolamine. Although formerly used to treat peptic ulcer disease, at present it is primarily used in certain combination products for the temporary relief of symptoms of allergic rhinitis, sinusitis, and the common cold.

Homatropine methylbromide, the methyl derivative of homatropine, is less potent than atropine in antimuscarinic activity but four times more potent as a ganglionic blocking agent. Formerly used for the treatment of irritable bowel syndrome and peptic ulcer disease, at present it is primarily used with hydrocodone as an antitussive combination.

Contraindications and Adverse Effects

Most contraindications, precautions, and adverse effects are predictable consequences of muscarinic receptor blockade: xerostomia, constipation, blurred vision, dyspepsia, and cognitive impairment. Important contraindications to the use of muscarinic antagonists include urinary tract obstruction, GI obstruction, and uncontrolled (or susceptibility to attacks of) angle-closure glaucoma. Muscarinic receptor antagonists also are contraindicated (or should be used with extreme caution) in patients with benign prostatic hyperplasia. These adverse effects and contraindications generally are of more limited concern with muscarinic antagonists that are administered by inhalation or used topically in ophthalmology.

Toxicology of Drugs With Antimuscarinic Properties

The deliberate or accidental ingestion of natural belladonna alkaloids is a major cause of poisonings. Many histamine H_1 receptor antagonists, phenothiazines, and tricyclic antidepressants also block muscarinic receptors and, in sufficient dosage, produce syndromes that include features of atropine intoxication. Among the tricyclic antidepressants, protriptyline and amitriptyline are the most potent muscarinic receptor antagonists, with affinities for muscarinic receptors only an order of magnitude less than that of atropine. Because these drugs are administered in therapeutic doses considerably higher than the effective dose of atropine, antimuscarinic effects are often observed clinically (Chapter 15). In addition, overdose with suicidal intent is a danger in the population using antidepressants. Fortunately, most of the newer antidepressants and selective serotonin reuptake inhibitors have more limited anticholinergic properties.

Like the tricyclic antidepressants, many of the older antipsychotic drugs have antimuscarinic effects. These effects are most likely to be observed with the less-potent drugs (e.g., chlorpromazine and thioridazine), which must be given in higher doses. The newer antipsychotic drugs, classified as "atypical" and characterized by their low propensity for inducing extrapyramidal side effects, also include agents that are potent muscarinic receptor antagonists. In particular, clozapine binds to human brain muscarinic receptors with high affinity (10 nM, compared to 1–2 nM for atropine); olanzapine also is a potent muscarinic receptor antagonist (Roth et al., 2004). Accordingly, xerostomia is a prominent side effect of these drugs. A paradoxical side effect of clozapine is increased salivation and drooling, possibly the result of partial agonist properties of this drug.

Infants and young children are especially susceptible to the toxic effects of muscarinic antagonists. Indeed, cases of intoxication in children have resulted from conjunctival instillation for ophthalmic refraction and other ocular effects. Systemic absorption occurs either from the nasal mucosa after the drug has traversed the nasolacrimal duct or from the GI tract if the drug is swallowed. Poisoning with diphenoxylate-atropine, used to treat diarrhea, has been extensively reported in the pediatric literature. Transdermal preparations of scopolamine used for motion sickness have been noted to cause toxic psychoses, especially in children and in the elderly. Serious intoxication may occur in children who ingest berries or seeds containing belladonna alkaloids. Poisoning from ingestion and smoking of jimson weed is seen with some frequency today.

Table 9–2 shows the oral doses of atropine causing undesirable responses or symptoms of overdosage. These symptoms are predictable results of blockade of parasympathetic innervation. In cases of full-blown atropine poisoning, the syndrome may last 48 h or longer. Intravenous injection of the anticholinesterase agent physostigmine may be used for confirmation. If physostigmine does not elicit the expected salivation, sweating, bradycardia, and intestinal hyperactivity, intoxication with atropine or a related agent is almost certain. Depression and circulatory collapse are evident only in cases of severe intoxication; the blood pressure declines, convulsions may ensue, respiration becomes inadequate, and death due to respiratory failure may follow after a period of paralysis and coma.

If the poison has been taken orally, begin measures to limit intestinal absorption without delay. For symptomatic treatment, slow intravenous injection of physostigmine rapidly abolishes the delirium and coma caused by large doses of atropine, but carries some risk of overdose in mild atropine intoxication. Because physostigmine is metabolized rapidly, the patient may again lapse into coma within 1–2 h, and repeated doses may be needed (Chapter 10). If marked excitement is present and more specific treatment is not available, a benzodiazepine is the most suitable agent for sedation and for control of convulsions. Phenothiazines or agents with

Drug Facts for Your Personal Formulary: *Muscarinic Receptor Agonists and Antagonists*

Drugs	Therapeutic Uses	Clinical Pharmacology and Tips
Muscarinic Receptor Agonists		
Methacholine	• Diagnosis of bronchial airway hyperreactivity	• Muscarinic effects: GI cramps, diarrhea, nausea, vomiting; lacrimation, salivation, sweating; urinary urgency; vision problems; bronchospasm • Do not use in patients with GI obstruction, urinary retention, asthma/COPD
Carbachol	• Glaucoma (topical administration)	• Systemic muscarinic effects minimal with proper topical application, otherwise similar to methacholine
Bethanechol	• Ileus (postoperative, neurogenic) • Urinary retention	• Similar to methacholine • Take on empty stomach to minimize nausea/vomiting

Pilocarpine	• Glaucoma (topical administration)
	• Xerostomia due to
	  • Sjögren syndrome
	  • Head and neck irradiation
		• Systemic muscarinic effects minimal with proper topical application, otherwise similar to methacholine

Cevimeline	• Xerostomia due to • Sjögren syndrome	• Similar to methacholine
Muscarinic Receptor Antagonists		
Atropine	• Acute symptomatic bradycardia (e.g., AV block) • Cholinesterase inhibitor intoxication • Aspiration prophylaxis	• Antimuscarinic adverse effects: xerostomia, constipation, blurred vision, dyspepsia, and cognitive impairment • Contraindicated in patients with urinary tract obstruction (especially in benign prostatic hyperplasia), GI obstruction, and angle-closure glaucoma
Scopolamine	• Motion sickness	• CNS effects (drowsiness, amnesia, fatigue)
Homatropine, cyclopentolate, tropicamide	• Ophthalmological examination (cycloplegia and mydriasis induction)	• Antimuscarinic adverse effects are minimal with proper topical application
Ipratropium, tiotropium, aclidinium, umeclidinium	• COPD • Rhinorrhea (ipratropium)	• Minimal absorption as quaternary amine ⇒ fewer antimuscarinic adverse effects, otherwise similar to atropine
Pirenzepine, telenzepine	• Peptic ulcer disease (not in U.S.)	• Antimuscarinic adverse effects and contraindications similar to atropine
Oxybutynin, trospium, darifenacin, solifenacin, tolterodine, fesoterodine	• Overactive bladder, enuresis, neurogenic bladder	• Antimuscarinic adverse effects and contraindications similar to atropine • CNS-related antimuscarinic effects less likely with trospium (quaternary amine), darifenacin and solifenacin (some selectivity for M_3 receptors), fesoterodine (prodrug of tolterodine), and tolterodine (preference for muscarinic receptors in the bladder)
Glycopyrrolate	• Duodenal ulcer • Sialorrhea	• Antimuscarinic adverse effects and contraindications similar to atropine • Fewer CNS effects as glycopyrrolate is a quaternary amine and therefore unable to cross the blood-brain barrier
Dicyclomine, hyoscyamine	Diarrhea-predominant irritable bowel syndrome (IBS)	• Antimuscarinic adverse effects and contraindications similar to atropine (including constipation-dominant IBS) • Evidence for efficacy is limited
Trihexyphenidyl, benztropine	• Parkinson disease	• Antimuscarinic adverse effects and contraindications similar to atropine • Mainly used to treat the tremor in Parkinson disease • Not recommended for elderly or demented patients

antimuscarinic activity should not be used because their antimuscarinic action is likely to intensify toxicity. Support of respiration and control of hyperthermia may be necessary. Ice bags and alcohol sponges help to reduce fever, especially in children.

Acknowledgment: *Nora Laiken and Palmer W. Taylor contributed to this chapter in recent editions of this book. We have retained some of their text in the current edition.*

Bibliography

Abrams P, et al. Muscarinic receptors: their distribution and function in body systems, and the implications for treating overactive bladder. *Br J Pharmacol*, **2006**, *148*:565–578.

Aihara T, et al. Cholinergically stimulated gastric acid secretion is mediated by M_3 and M_5 but not M_1 muscarinic acetylcholine receptors in mice. *Am J Physiol*, **2005**, *288*:G1199–G1207.

Alagha, et al. Long-acting muscarinic receptor antagonists for the treatment of chronic airways diseases. *Ther Adv Chronic Dis*, **2014**, *2*:85–98.

Birdsall NJM, Lazareno S. Allosterism at muscarinic receptors: ligands and mechanisms. *Mini Rev Med Chem*, **2005**, *5*:523–543.

Bonner TI, et al. Identification of a family of muscarinic acetylcholine receptor genes. *Science*, **1987**, *237*:527–532.

Brodde OE, Michel MC. Adrenergic and muscarinic receptors in the human heart. *Pharmacol Rev*, **1999**, *51*:651–690.

Caulfield MP, Birdsall NJ. International Union of Pharmacology, XVII. Classification of muscarinic acetylcholine receptors. *Pharmacol Rev*, **1998**, *50*:279–290.

Chapple CR, et al. Randomized, double-blind placebo- and tolterodine-controlled trial of the once-daily antimuscarinic agent solifenacin in patients with symptomatic overactive bladder. *BJU Int*, **2004**, 93:303–310.

Chapple CR, et al. The effects of antimuscarinic treatments in overactive bladder: a systematic review and meta-analysis. *Eur Urol*, **2005**, *48*:5–26.

Chapple CR, et al. The effects of antimuscarinic treatments in overactive bladder: an update of a systematic review and meta-analysis. *Eur Urol*, **2008**, *54*(3):543–562.

Conn PJ, et al. Subtype-selective allosteric modulators of muscarinic receptors for the treatment of CNS disorders. *Trends Pharmacol Sci*, **2009**, *30*:148–155.

Conn PJ, et al. Opportunities and challenges in the discovery of allosteric modulators of GPCRs for treating CNS disorders. *Nat Rev Drug Discov*, **2014**, *13*:692–708.

Crapo RO, et al. Guidelines for methacholine and exercise challenge testing—1999. *Am J Respir Crit Care Med*, **2000**, *161*:309–329.

DiFrancesco D, Tromba C. Acetylcholine inhibits activation of the cardiac hyperpolarizing-activated current, i_f. *Pflugers Arch*, **1987**, *410*:139–142.

Dunlap ME, et al. Autonomic modulation in heart failure: ready for prime time? *Curr Cardiol Rep*, **2015**, *17*:103.

Eglen RM, et al. Muscarinic receptor subtypes and smooth muscle function. *Pharmacol Rev*, **1996**, *48*:531–565.

Feigl EO. Neural control of coronary blood flow. *J Vasc Res*, **1998**, *35*:85–92.

Fisher JT, et al. Loss of vagally mediated bradycardia and bronchoconstriction in mice lacking M_2 or M_3 muscarinic acetylcholine receptors. *FASEB J*, **2004**, *18*:711–713.

Furchgott RF. Endothelium-derived relaxing factor: discovery, early studies, and identification as nitric oxide. *Biosci Rep*, **1999**, *19*:235–251.

Gautam D, et al. Cholinergic stimulation of salivary secretion studied with M_1 and M_3 muscarinic receptor single- and double-knockout mice. *Mol Pharmacol*, **2004**, 66:260–267.

Gavalda A, et al. Characterization of aclidinium bromide, a novel inhaled muscarinic antagonist, with long duration of action and a favorable pharmacological profile. *J Pharmacol Exp Ther*, **2009**, *331*(2):740–751.

Gentry PR, et al. Novel allosteric modulators of G protein-coupled receptors. *J Biol Chem*, **2015**, *290*:19478–19488.

Goldberg JA, et al. Muscarinic modulation of striatal function and circuitry. *Handb Exp Pharmacol*, **2012**, *208*:223–241.

Goyal RK, Rattan S. Neurohumoral, hormonal, and drug receptors for the lower esophageal sphincter. *Gastroenterology*, **1978**, *74*:598–619.

Haga K, et al. Structure of the human M_2 muscarinic acetylcholine receptor bound to an antagonist. *Nature*, **2012**, *482*:547–551.

Hegde SS. Muscarinic receptors in the bladder: from basic research to therapeutics. *Br J Pharmacol*, **2006**, *147*(suppl 2):S80–S87.

Ignarro LJ, et al. Nitric oxide as a signaling molecule in the vascular system: an overview. *J Cardiovasc Pharmacol*, **1999**, *34*:879–886.

Kay G, et al. Differential effects of the antimuscarinic agents darifenacin and oxybutynin ER on memory in older subjects. *Eur Urol*, **2006**, *50*:317–326.

Krnjević K. Synaptic mechanisms modulated by acetylcholine in cerebral cortex. *Prog Brain Res*, **2004**, *145*:81–93.

Kruse AC, et al. Structure and dynamics of the M_3 muscarinic acetylcholine receptor. *Nature*, **2012**, *482*:552–556.

Kruse AC, et al. Activation and allosteric modulation of a muscarinic acetylcholine receptor. *Nature*, **2013**, *504*:101–106.

Kruse AC, et al. Muscarinic acetylcholine receptors: novel opportunities for drug development. *Nat Rev Drug Discov*, **2014**, *13*:549–560.

Lakatta EG, DiFrancesco D. What keeps us ticking: a funny current, a calcium clock, or both? *J Mol Cell Cardiol*, **2009**, *47*:157–170.

Lane JR, et al. Bridging the gap: bitopic ligands of G-protein-coupled receptors. *Trends Pharmacol Sci*, **2013**, *34*:59–66.

Levy MN, Schwartz PJ, eds. *Vagal Control of the Heart: Experimental Basis and Clinical Implications*. Futura, Armonk, NY, **1994**.

Lewis ME, et al. Vagus nerve stimulation decreases left ventricular contractility in vivo in the human and pig heart. *J Physiol*, **2001**, *534*:547–552.

Lyashkov AE, et al. Cholinergic receptor signaling modulates spotaneous firing of sinoatrial nodal cells via integrated effects on PKAH-dependent Ca^{2+} cycling and I_{KACh}. *Am J Physiol*, **2009**, *297*:949–959.

Matsui M, et al. Mice lacking M_2 and M_3 muscarinic acetylcholine receptors are devoid of cholinergic smooth muscle contractions but still viable. *J Neurosci*, **2002**, *22*:10627–10632.

May LT, et al. Allosteric modulation of G protein-coupled receptors. *Annu Rev Pharmacol Toxicol*, **2007**, *47*:1–51.

Mohr K, et al. Rational design of dualsteric GPCR ligands: quests and promise. *Br J Pharmacol*, **2010**, *159*:997–1008.

Moncada S, Higgs EA. Molecular mechanisms and therapeutic strategies related to nitric oxide. *FASEB J*, **1995**, *9*:1319–1330.

Noiaseh G, et al. Comparison of the discontinuation rates and side-effect profiles of pilocarpine and cevimeline for xerostomia in primary Sjögren's syndrome. *Clin Exp Rheumatol*, **2014**, *32*:575–577.

Oberhauser V, et al. Acetylcholine release in human heart atrium: influence of muscarinic autoreceptors, diabetes, and age. *Circulation*, **2001**, *103*:1638–1643.

Porter SR, et al. An update of the etiology and management of xerostomia. *Oral Surg Oral Med Oral Pathol Oral Radiol Endod*, **2004**, *97*:28–46.

Roth B, et al. Magic shotguns versus magic bullets: selectively non-selective drugs for mood disorders and schizophrenia. *Nat Rev Drug Discov*, **2004**, *3*:353–359.

Schwartz PJ, De Ferrari GM. Sympathetic—parasympathetic interaction in health and disease: abnormalities and relevance in heart failure. *Heart Fail Rev*, **2011**, *16*:101–107.

Stengel PW, et al. M_2 and M_4 receptor knockout mice: muscarinic receptor function in cardiac and smooth muscle in vitro. *J Pharmacol Exp Ther*, **2000**, *292*:877–885.

Trendelenburg AU, et al. Distinct mixtures of muscarinic receptor subtypes mediate inhibition of noradrenaline release in different mouse peripheral tissues, as studied with receptor knockout mice. *Br J Pharmacol*, **2005**, *145*:1153–1159.

Tryba M, Cook D. Current guidelines on stress ulcer prophylaxis. *Drugs*, **1997**, *54*:581–596.

Volpicelli LA, Levey AI. Muscarinic acetylcholine receptor sub-types in cerebral cortex and hippocampus. *Progr Brain Res*, **2004**, *145*:59–66.

Wellstein A, Pitschner HF. Complex dose-response curves of atropine in man explained by different functions of M_1- and M_2-cholinoceptors. *Naunyn Schmiedebergs Arch Pharmacol*, **1988**, *338*:19–27.

Wess J. Molecular biology of muscarinic acetylcholine receptors. *Crit Rev Neurobiol*, **1996**, *10*:69–99.

Wess J, et al. Muscarinic acetylcholine receptors: mutant mice provide new insights for drug development. *Nature Rev Drug Discov*, **2007**, 6:721–733.

Wiseman LR, Faulds D. Oral pilocarpine: a review of its pharmacological properties and clinical potential in xerostomia. *Drugs*, **1995**, *49*:143–155.

Anticholinesterase Agents

Palmer Taylor

第十章　抗胆碱酯酶药

中文导读

本章主要介绍：乙酰胆碱酯酶，包括乙酰胆碱酯酶的结构及其是否为机体必需；乙酰胆碱酯酶抑制药作用的分子机制、化学和构-效关系、药理作用基础、对生理系统的影响、ADME和毒理学；乙酰胆碱酯酶抑制药的治疗用途，包括可用的治疗制剂，在麻痹性肠梗阻和膀胱松弛、青光眼和其他眼科适应证、重症肌无力、阿尔茨海默病中的应用、胆碱酯酶抑制药中毒的预防、抗胆碱能药物中毒。

Abbreviations

ACh: acetylcholine
AChE: acetylcholinesterase
anti-ChE: anticholinesterase
BChE: butyrylcholinesterase
ChE: cholinesterase
CNS: central nervous system
CYP: cytochrome P450
DFP: diisopropyl fluorophosphate (diisopropyl phosphorofluoridate)
EPA: Environmental Protection Agency
FDA: Food and Drug Administration
2-PAM: pralidoxime
PON1: paraoxonase isoform 1
TOCP: triorthocresyl phosphate

Acetylcholinesterase

The hydrolytic activity of AChE terminates the action of ACh at the junctions of the various cholinergic nerve endings with their effector organs or postsynaptic sites (Chapter 8). Drugs that inhibit AChE are called anti-ChEs, since they inhibit both AChE and BChE. BChE is not found in nerve ending synapses but in liver and plasma, where it metabolizes circulating esters. AChE inhibitors cause ACh to accumulate in the vicinity of cholinergic nerve terminals and thus are potentially capable of producing effects equivalent to excessive stimulation of cholinergic receptors throughout the central and peripheral nervous systems. In view of the widespread distribution of cholinergic neurons across animal species, it is not surprising that the anti-ChE agents have received extensive application as toxic agents, in the form of agricultural insecticides, pesticides, and potential chemical warfare "nerve gases." Moreover, several compounds of this class are used therapeutically; others that cross the blood-brain barrier have been approved or are in clinical trials for the treatment of Alzheimer disease.

Prior to World War II, only the "reversible" anti-ChE agents were generally known, of which physostigmine is the prototype (Box 10-1). Shortly before and during World War II, a new class of highly toxic chemicals, the organophosphates, was developed, first as agricultural insecticides and later as potential chemical warfare agents. The extreme toxicity of these compounds was found to be due to their "irreversible" inactivation of AChE, which resulted in prolonged enzyme inhibition. Because the pharmacological actions of both the reversible and irreversible anti-ChE agents are qualitatively similar, they are discussed here as a group. Interactions of anti-ChE agents with other drugs acting at peripheral autonomic synapses and the neuromuscular junction are described in Chapters 9 and 11.

Structure of Acetylcholinesterase

Acetylcholinesterase exists in two general classes of molecular forms: simple homomeric oligomers of catalytic subunits (monomers, dimers, and tetramers) and heteromeric associations of catalytic subunits with structural subunits (Massoulié, 2000; Taylor et al., 2000). The homomeric forms are found as soluble species in the cell, presumably destined for export or for association with the outer membrane of the cell, typically through an attached glycophospholipid. One heteromeric form, largely found in neuronal synapses, is a tetramer of catalytic subunits disulfide-linked to a 20-kDa lipid-linked subunit and localized to the outer surface of the cell membrane. The other heteromeric form consists of tetramers of catalytic subunits, linked by disulfide bonds to each of three strands of a collagen-like structural subunit. This molecular species, whose molecular mass approaches 10^6 Da, is associated with the basal lamina of neuromuscular junctional areas of skeletal muscle.

Molecular cloning revealed that a single gene encodes vertebrate AChEs (Schumacher et al., 1986; Taylor et al., 2000). However, multiple gene products arise from alternative processing of the mRNA that differ only in their carboxyl termini; the portion of the gene encoding the catalytic core of the enzyme is invariant. Hence, the individual AChE species can be expected to show identical substrate and inhibitor specificities.

A separate, structurally related, gene encodes butyrylcholinesterase, which is synthesized in the liver and is found primarily in plasma (Lockridge, 2015; Lockridge et al., 1987). The cholinesterases define a superfamily of proteins that share a common structural motif, the α,β-hydrolase fold (Cygler et al., 1993). The family includes several esterases, other hydrolases not found in the nervous system, and surprisingly, proteins without hydrolase activity, such as thyroglobulin and members of the tactin and neuroligin families (Taylor et al., 2000).

The three-dimensional structures of AChEs show the active center to be nearly centrosymmetric to each subunit, residing at the base of a narrow gorge about 20 Å in depth (Bourne et al., 1995; Sussman et al., 1991). At the base of the gorge lie the residues of the catalytic triad: Ser203, His447, and Glu334 in mammals (Figure 10–1). The catalytic mechanism resembles that of other hydrolases; the serine hydroxyl group is rendered highly nucleophilic through a charge-relay system involving the carboxylate anion from glutamate, the imidazole of histidine, and the hydroxyl of serine (Figure 10–2A).

During enzymatic attack of ACh, an ester with trigonal geometry, a tetrahedral intermediate between enzyme and substrate is formed (Figure 10–2A) that collapses to an acetyl enzyme conjugate with the concomitant release of choline. The acetyl enzyme is very labile to hydrolysis, which results in the formation of acetate and active enzyme (Froede and Wilson, 1971; Rosenberry, 1975). AChE is one of the most

BOX 10–1 ■ History

Physostigmine, also called *eserine,* is an alkaloid obtained from the Calabar or ordeal bean, the dried, ripe seed of *Physostigma venenosum,* a perennial plant found in tropical West Africa. This Calabar bean once was used by native tribes of West Africa as an "ordeal poison" in trials for witchcraft, in which guilt was judged by death from the poison, innocence by survival after ingestion of a bean. A pure alkaloid was isolated by Jobst and Hesse in 1864 and named physostigmine. The first therapeutic use of the drug was in 1877 by Laqueur in the treatment of glaucoma, one of its clinical uses today. Karczmar (1970) and Holmstedt (2000) have presented accounts of the history of physostigmine.

After basic research elucidated the chemical basis of the activity of physostigmine, scientists began systematic investigations of a series of substituted aromatic esters of alkyl carbamic acids. Neostigmine was introduced in 1931 for its stimulant action on the GI tract and subsequently was reported to be effective in the symptomatic treatment of myasthenia gravis.

Following the synthesis of about 2000 compounds, Schrader defined the structural requirements for insecticidal activity (and, as learned subsequently, for anti-ChE activity). One compound in this early series, parathion (a phosphorothioate), later became the most widely used insecticide of this class. Malathion, which currently is used extensively, also contains the thionophosphorus bond found in parathion. Prior to and during World War II, the efforts of Schrader's group were directed toward the development of chemical warfare agents. The synthesis of several compounds of much greater toxicity than parathion, such as sarin, soman, and tabun, was kept secret by the German government. Investigators in the Allied countries also followed Lange and Krueger's lead in 1932 in the search for potentially toxic compounds; DFP, synthesized by McCombie and Saunders, was studied most extensively by British and American scientists (Giacobini, 2000).

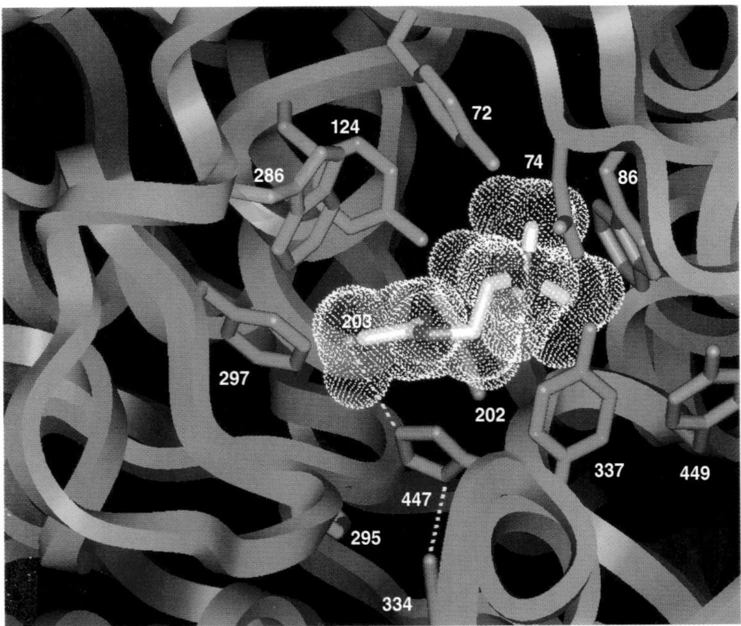

Figure 10–1 *The active center gorge of mammalian AChE, looking from the portal of substrate entry.* Bound ACh is shown by the dotted structure depicting its van der Waals radii. The crystal structure of mouse cholinesterase active center, which is virtually identical to human AChE, is shown (Bourne et al., 1995). Included are the side chains of (a) the catalytic triad: Glu334, His447, Ser203 (hydrogen bonds are denoted by the dotted lines); (b) acyl pocket: Phe295 and Phe297; (c) choline subsite: Trp86, Glu202, and Tyr337; and (d) the peripheral site: Trp286, Tyr72, Tyr124, and Asp74. Tyrosines 337 and 449 are further removed from the active center but likely contribute to stabilization of certain ligands. The catalytic triad, choline subsite, and acyl pocket are located at the base of the gorge, while the peripheral site is at the lip of the gorge. The gorge is 18- to 20-Å deep, with its base centrosymmetric to the subunit.

efficient enzymes known: One molecule of AChE can hydrolyze 6×10^5 ACh molecules per minute; this yields a turnover time of 100 μsec.

Is AChE Essential?

Knockout mice lacking the gene encoding AChE can survive under highly supportive conditions and with a special diet, but they exhibit continuous tremors and are stunted in growth (Xie et al., 2000). Mice that selectively lack AChE expression in skeletal muscle but have normal or near-normal expression in brain and organs innervated by the autonomic nervous system can reproduce but have tremors and severe compromise of skeletal muscle strength. By contrast, mice with selective reductions of CNS AChE by elimination of the exons encoding alternative spliced regions or expression of the structural subunits influencing expression in brain yield no obvious phenotype. This arises from large adaptive responses and compensatory reductions of ACh synthesis and storage and receptor responses (Camp et al., 2008; Dobbertin et al., 2009).

Acetylcholinesterase Inhibitors

Molecular Mechanism of Action of AChE Inhibitors

The mechanisms of action of compounds that typify the three classes of anti-ChE agents are also shown in Figure 10–2.

Three distinct domains on AChE constitute binding sites for inhibitory ligands and form the basis for specificity differences between AChE and butyrylcholinesterase:

- the acyl pocket of the active center;
- the choline subsite of the active center; and
- the peripheral anionic site (Reiner and Radić, 2000; Taylor and Radić, 1994).

Reversible inhibitors, such as edrophonium and tacrine, bind to the choline subsite in the vicinity of Trp86 and Glu202 (Silman and Sussman, 2000) (Figure 10–2B). Edrophonium has a brief duration of action because its quaternary structure facilitates renal elimination, and it binds reversibly to the AChE active center. Additional reversible inhibitors, such as donepezil, bind with higher affinity to the active center gorge. Other reversible inhibitors, such as propidium and the snake peptidic toxin fasciculin, bind to the peripheral anionic site on AChE. This site resides at the rim of the gorge and is defined by Try286 and Tyr72 and Tyr124 (Figure 10–1).

Drugs that have a carbamoyl ester linkage, such as physostigmine and neostigmine, are hydrolyzed by AChE, but much more slowly than is ACh. The quaternary amine neostigmine and the tertiary amine physostigmine exist as cations at physiological pH. By serving as alternate substrates to ACh (Figure 10–2C), their reaction with the active center serine progressively generates the carbamoylated enzyme. The conjugated carbamoyl moiety resides in the acyl pocket outlined by Phe295 and Phe297. In contrast to the acetyl enzyme, methylcarbamoyl AChE and dimethylcarbamoyl AChE are far more stable (the $t_{1/2}$ for hydrolysis of the dimethylcarbamoyl enzyme is 15–30 min). Sequestration of the enzyme in its carbamoylated form thus precludes the enzyme-catalyzed hydrolysis of ACh for extended periods of time. When administered systemically, the duration of inhibition by the carbamoylating agents is 3–4 h.

The organophosphate inhibitors, such as DFP, serve as true hemisubstrates; the resultant conjugate with the active center serine phosphorylated or phosphonylated is extremely stable (Figure 10–2D). The organophosphorus inhibitors are tetrahedral in configuration, a configuration that resembles the transition state formed in carboxyl ester hydrolysis. Similar to the carboxyl esters, the phosphoryl oxygen binds within the oxyanion hole of the active center. If the alkyl groups in the phosphorylated enzyme are ethyl or methyl, spontaneous regeneration of active enzyme requires several hours. Secondary (as in DFP) or tertiary alkyl groups

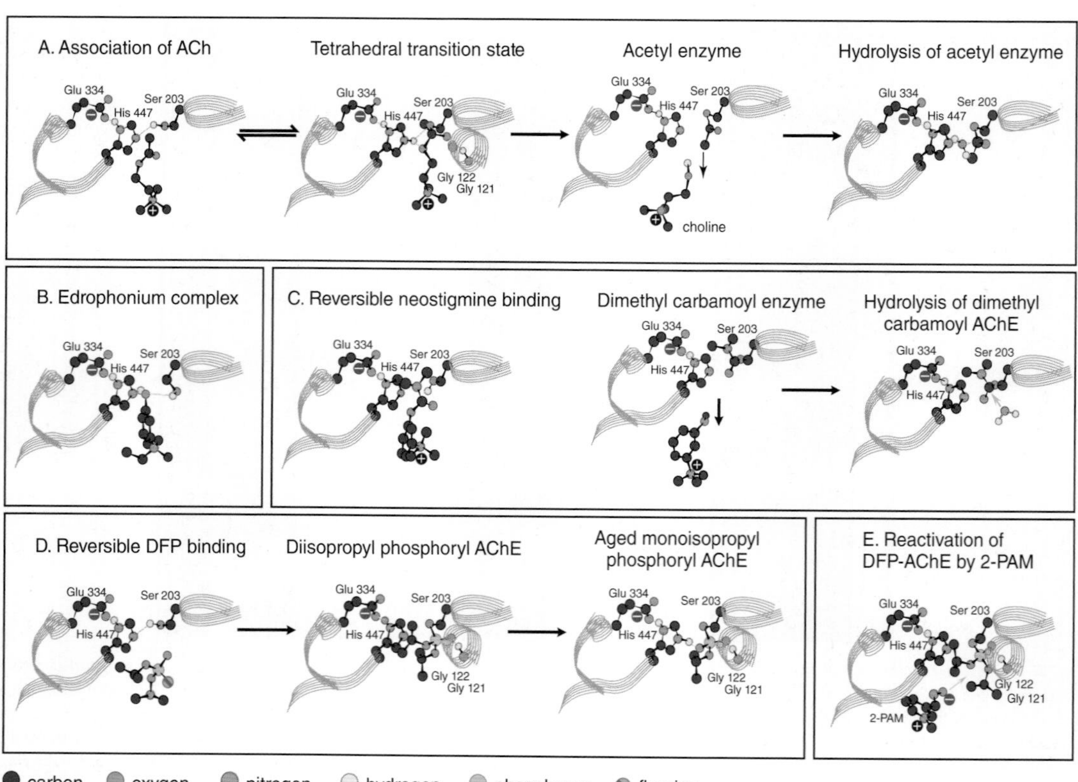

Figure 10–2 *Steps involved in the hydrolysis of ACh by AChE and in the inhibition and reactivation of the enzyme.* Only the three residues of the catalytic triad shown in Figure 10–1 are depicted. Net charge in a region is represented by red and blue circles containing – or + signs, respectively. The associations and reactions shown are as follows: **A.** ACh catalysis: binding of ACh, formation of a tetrahedral transition state, formation of the acetyl enzyme with liberation of choline, rapid hydrolysis of the acetyl enzyme with return to the original state. **B.** Reversible binding and inhibition by edrophonium. **C.** Neostigmine reaction with and inhibition of AChE: reversible binding of neostigmine, formation of the dimethyl carbamoyl enzyme, slow hydrolysis of the dimethyl carbamoyl enzyme. **D.** DFP reaction and inhibition of AChE: reversible binding of DFP, formation of the diisopropyl phosphoryl enzyme, formation of the aged monoisopropyl phosphoryl enzyme. Hydrolysis of the diisopropyl enzyme is very slow and is not shown. The aged monoisopropyl phosphoryl enzyme is virtually resistant to hydrolysis and reactivation. The tetrahedral transition state of ACh hydrolysis resembles the conjugates formed by the tetrahedral phosphate inhibitors and accounts for their potency. Amide bond hydrogens from Gly121 and Gly122 stabilize the carbonyl and phosphoryl oxygens. **E.** Reactivation of the diisopropyl phosphoryl enzyme by 2-PAM. 2-PAM attack of the phosphorus on the phosphorylated enzyme will form a phospho-oxime with regeneration of active enzyme. The individual steps of phosphorylation reaction and oxime reaction have been characterized by mass spectrometry. (Data from Jennings et al, 2003).

further enhance the stability of the phosphorylated enzyme, and significant regeneration of active enzyme usually is not observed. The stability of the phosphorylated enzyme is enhanced through "aging," which results from the loss of one of the alkyl groups. Hence, the return of AChE activity depends on biosynthesis of new AChE protein.

Thus, the terms *reversible* and *irreversible* as applied to the carbamoyl ester and organophosphate anti-ChE agents are relative terms, reflecting only quantitative differences in rates of decarbamoylation or dephosphorylation of the conjugated enzyme. Both chemical classes react covalently with the active center serine in essentially the same manner as does ACh in forming the transient acetyl enzyme.

Chemistry and Structure-Activity Relationships

Structure-activity relationships of anti-ChE agents have been extensively reviewed in the scientific literature. Only agents of general therapeutic or toxicological interest are considered here.

Noncovalent Inhibitors

While these agents interact by reversible and noncovalent association with the active site in AChE, they differ in their disposition in the body and their affinity for the enzyme. Edrophonium, a quaternary drug whose activity is limited to peripheral nervous system synapses, has a moderate affinity for AChE. Its volume of distribution is limited and renal elimination is rapid, accounting for its short duration of action. By contrast, tacrine and donepezil (Figure 10–3) have higher affinities for AChE, are more hydrophobic, and readily cross the blood-brain barrier to inhibit AChE in the CNS. Partitioning into lipid and higher affinities for AChE account for their longer durations of action.

"Reversible" Carbamate Inhibitors

Drugs of this class that are of therapeutic interest are shown in Figure 10–3. Early studies showed that the essential moiety of the physostigmine molecule was the methylcarbmate of an amine-substituted phenol. The quaternary ammonium derivative neostigmine is a compound of equal or greater potency. Pyridostigmine is a close congener also used in myasthenia gravis patients.

Carbamoylating inhibitors with high lipid solubility (rivastigmine) have longer duration of action, cross the blood-brain barrier, and are used as an alternative in the treatment of Alzheimer disease (Cummings, 2004) (Chapter 18). The carbamate insecticides carbaryl, propoxur, and aldicarb, used extensively as garden insecticides, inhibit AChE with a mechanism identical to other carbamoylating agents. While more reversible and less toxic, symptoms parallel those of organophosphates (Eddleston and Clark,

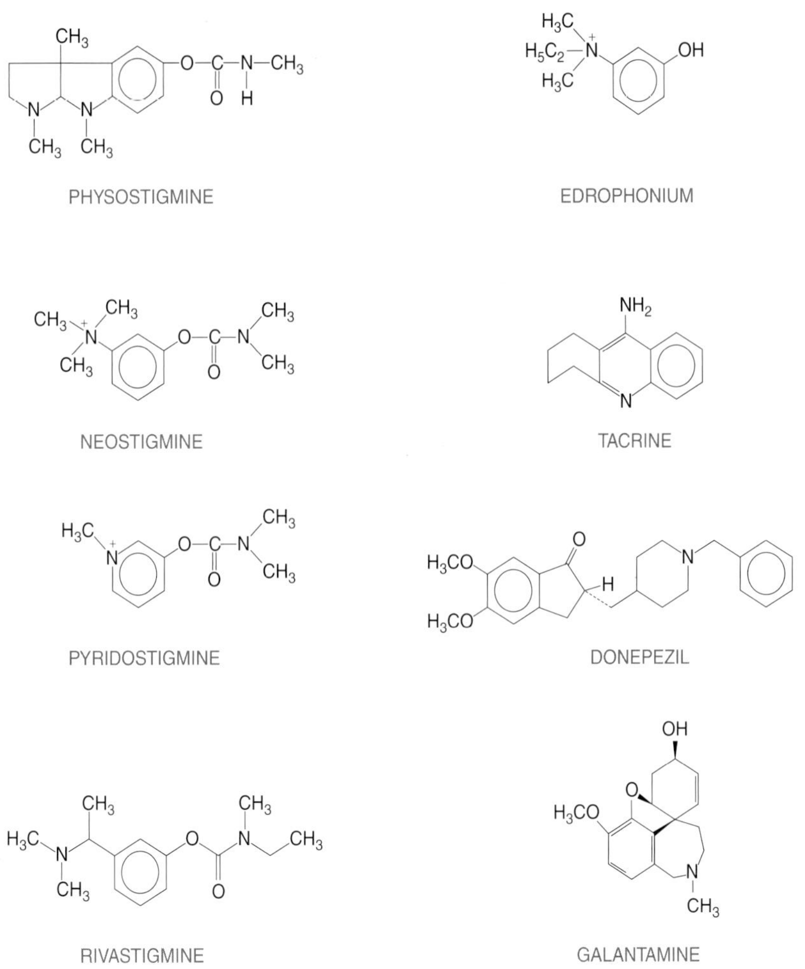

PHYSOSTIGMINE

EDROPHONIUM

NEOSTIGMINE

TACRINE

PYRIDOSTIGMINE

DONEPEZIL

RIVASTIGMINE

GALANTAMINE

Figure 10–3 *"Reversible" carbamate and noncovalent AChE inhibitors used clinically.*

2011; King and Aaron, 2015).

Organophosphorus Compound

The general formula for the organophosphorus compound class of ChE inhibitors is presented in Table 10–1. A great variety of substituents is possible: R_1 and R_2 may be alkyl, alkoxy, aryloxy, amido, mercaptan, or other groups; and X, the leaving group, typically a conjugate base of a weak acid, is a halide, cyanide, thiocyanate, phenoxy, thiophenoxy, phosphate, thiocholine, or carboxylate group. For a compilation of the organophosphorus compounds and their toxicity, see Gallo and Lawryk (1991).

Diisopropyl fluorophosphate produces virtually irreversible inactivation of AChE and other esterases by alkylphosphorylation. Its high lipid solubility, low molecular weight, and volatility facilitate inhalation, transdermal absorption, and penetration into the CNS. After desulfuration, the insecticides in current use form the dimethoxy or diethoxyphosphoryl conjugate of AChE.

The "nerve gases"—tabun, sarin, soman, and VX—are among the most potent synthetic toxins known; they are lethal to laboratory animals in nanogram doses. Insidious employment of these agents occurred in the Matsumoto incident and Tokyo subway terrorism attacks in Japan and against civilians by despotic regimes in the Middle East (Council on Foreign Relations, 2013; Dolgin, 2013; King and Aaron, 2015; Nozaki and Aikawa, 1995). While estimates of lethality in Japan amounted to 8 and 10 people killed, in Syria estimates vary, ranging up to 1000 individuals, with over 3000 showing symptoms of organophosphate toxicity. Attacks continued into 2017 with release of sarin vapor from explosive devices. Toxicity results from inhalation and rapid distribution of sarin to the central and peripheral nervous systems. A assignation homicide also occurred in Malaysia in 2017 via slower dermal absorption of VX.

Parathion and methylparathion were widely used as insecticides because of their favorable properties of low volatility and stability in aqueous solution. Acute and chronic toxicity has limited their use, and potentially less-hazardous compounds have replaced them for home and garden use now largely throughout the world. These compounds are inactive in inhibiting AChE in vitro; paraoxon is the active metabolite. The phosphoryl oxygen for sulfur substitution is carried out predominantly by hepatic CYPs. This reaction also occurs in the insect, typically with more efficiency. Other insecticides possessing the phosphorothioate structure have been widely employed for agricultural use. These include *diazinon* and *chlorpyrifos*. Use of these agents is restricted because of evidence of chronic toxicity in the newborn animal. They have been banned from indoor and outdoor residential use since 2005.

Malathion also requires replacement of a sulfur atom with oxygen in vivo, conferring resistance to mammalian species. Also, this insecticide can be detoxified by hydrolysis of the carboxyl ester linkage by plasma carboxylesterases. Plasma carboxylesterase activity dictates species resistance to malathion: The detoxification reaction is much more rapid in mammals and birds than in insects (Costa et al., 2013). In recent years, malathion has been employed in aerial spraying of relatively populous areas for control of citrus orchard–destructive Mediterranean fruit flies and mosquitoes that harbor and transmit viruses harmful to human beings, such as the West Nile encephalitis virus.

TABLE 10–1 ■ CHEMICAL CLASSIFICATION OF REPRESENTATIVE ORGANOPHOSPHORUS AChE INHIBITORS

General formula R_1 O P R_2 X

Group **A**, X = halogen, cyanide, or thiocyanate leaving group; group **B**, X = alkylthio, arylthio, alkoxy, or aryloxy leaving group; group **C**, thionophosphorus or thio-thionophosphorus compounds; group **D**, quaternary ammonium leaving group. R_1 can be an alkyl (phosphonates), alkoxy (phosphorates) or an alkylamino (phosphoramidates) group.

GROUP	STRUCTURAL FORMULA	COMMON, CHEMICAL, AND OTHER NAMES	COMMENTS
A	i-C_3H_7O O P i-C_3H_7O F	DFP; Isoflurophate; diisopropyl fluorophosphate	Potent, irreversible inactivator
	$(CH_3)_2N$ O P C_2H_5O CN	Tabun Ethyl N-dimethylphosphoramidocyanidate	Extremely toxic "nerve gas"
	i-C_3H_7O O P CH_3 F	Sarin (GB) Isopropyl methylphosphonofluoridate	Extremely toxic "nerve gas"
	CH_3 CH_3 CH_3–C—C CH_3 H O O P CH_3 F	Soman (GD) Pinacolyl methylphosphonofluoridate	Extremely toxic "nerve gas"; greatest potential for irreversible action/rapid aging
B	C_2H_5O O P H_3C S–C_2H_4N i-C_3H_7 i-C_3H_7	VX *O*-ethyl S [2-(diisopropylamino)ethyl] methyl phosponothioate	Potent, slower onset, skin-penetrating nerve agent
	CH_3O O P CH_3O S–$CHCOOC_2H_5$ $CH_2COOC_2H_5$	Malaoxon *O,O*-Dimethyl S-(1,2-dicarboxyethyl)-phosphorothioate	Active metabolite of malathion
C	C_2H_5O S P C_2H_5O O–(phenyl)–NO_2	Parathion *O,O*-Diethyl *O*-(4-nitrophenyl)-phosphorothioate	Agricultural insecticide, resulting in numerous cases of accidental poisoning; phased out in 2003.
	C_2H_5O S P C_2H_5O O–(pyrimidine: CH_3, N, N, CH(CH_3)(CH_3))	Diazinon, Dimpylate *O,O*-Diethyl *O*-(2-isopropyl-6-methyl-4-pyrimidinyl) phosphorothioate	Insecticide; use limited to non-residential agricultural settings
	S ‖ H_5C_2O–P H_5C_2O O–(pyridine: N, Cl, Cl, Cl)	Chlorpyrifos *O,O*-Diethyl *O*-(3,5,6-trichloro-2-pyridyl) phosphorothioate	Insecticide; use limited to non-residential agricultural settings
	CH_3O S P CH_3O S–$CHCOOC_2H_5$ $CH_2COOC_2H_5$	Malathion *O,O*-Dimethyl S-(1,2-dicarbethoxyethyl) phosphorodithioate	Widely employed insecticide of greater safety than parathion or other agents because of rapid detoxification by higher organisms
D	C_2H_5O O I^- P C_2H_5O $SCH_2CH_2\overset{+}{N}(CH_3)_3$	Echothiophate (PHOSPHOLINE IODIDE), MI-217 Diethoxyphosphinylthiocholine iodide	Extremely potent choline derivative; administered locally in treatment of glaucoma; relatively stable in aqueous solution

Evidence of acute toxicity from malathion arises primarily with suicide attempts or deliberate poisoning. The lethal dose in mammals is about 1 g/kg. Exposure to the skin results in a small fraction (<10%) systemically absorbed. Malathion is used topically in the treatment of pediculosis (lice) infestations in cases of permethrin resistance (Centers for Disease Control and Prevention, 2015).

Among the quaternary ammonium organophosphorus compounds (group D in Table 10–1), only echothiophate is useful clinically, and its use is limited to ophthalmic administration. Being positively charged, it is not volatile and does not readily penetrate the skin.

Basis for the Pharmacological Effects of ChE Inhibitors

The characteristic pharmacological effects of the anti-ChE agents are due primarily to the prevention of hydrolysis of ACh by AChE at sites of cholinergic transmission. Transmitter thus accumulates, enhancing the response to ACh that is liberated by cholinergic impulses or that is spontaneously released from the nerve ending. Virtually all acute effects of moderate doses of organophosphates are attributable to this action. For example, the characteristic miosis that follows local application of DFP to the eye is not observed after chronic postganglionic denervation of the eye because there is no source from which to release endogenous ACh. The consequences of enhanced concentrations of ACh at motor end plates are unique to these sites and are discussed below.

Generally, the pharmacological properties of anti-ChE agents can be predicted by knowing those loci where ACh is released physiologically by nerve impulses, the degree of nerve impulse activity, and the responses of the corresponding effector organs to ACh (see Chapter 8). The anti-ChE agents potentially can produce all the following effects:

- stimulation of muscarinic receptor responses at autonomic effector organs;
- stimulation, followed by depression or paralysis, of all autonomic ganglia and skeletal muscle (nicotinic actions); and
- stimulation, with occasional subsequent depression, of pre- and postsynaptic cholinergic receptor sites in the CNS.

At therapeutic doses, several modifying factors are significant. Compounds containing a quaternary ammonium group do not penetrate cell membranes readily; hence, anti-ChE agents in this category are absorbed poorly from the GI tract or across the skin and are excluded from the CNS by the blood-brain barrier after moderate doses. On the other hand, such compounds act preferentially at the neuromuscular junctions of skeletal muscle, exerting their action both as anti-ChE agents and as direct agonists. They have comparatively less effect at autonomic effector sites and ganglia. In contrast, the more lipid-soluble agents are well absorbed after oral administration, have ubiquitous effects at both peripheral and central cholinergic sites, and may be sequestered in lipids for long periods of time. Lipid-soluble organophosphorus agents, such as the chemical warfare agent VX, are well absorbed through the skin, whereas the volatile agents are transferred readily across the alveolar membranes in the lung (King and Aaron, 2015; Storm et al., 2000).

The actions of anti-ChE agents on autonomic effector cells and on cortical and subcortical sites in the CNS, where ACh receptors are largely of the muscarinic type, are blocked by atropine. Likewise, atropine blocks some of the excitatory actions of anti-ChE agents on autonomic ganglia because both nicotinic and muscarinic receptors are involved in ganglionic neurotransmission (Chapter 11).

Effects on Physiological Systems

The sites of action of anti-ChE agents of therapeutic importance are the CNS, eye, intestine, and neuromuscular junction of skeletal muscle; other actions are of toxicological consequence.

Eye

When applied locally to the conjunctiva, anti-ChE agents cause conjunctival hyperemia and constriction of the pupillary sphincter muscle around the pupillary margin of the iris (miosis) and the ciliary muscle (block of accommodation reflex with resultant focusing to near vision). Miosis is apparent in a few minutes and can last several hours to days. Although the pupil may be "pinpoint" in size, it generally contracts further when exposed to light. The block of accommodation is more transient and generally disappears before termination of miosis. Intraocular pressure, when elevated, usually falls as the result of facilitation of outflow of the aqueous humor (Chapter 69).

GI Tract

In humans, neostigmine enhances gastric contractions and increases the secretion of gastric acid. After bilateral vagotomy, the effects of neostigmine on gastric motility are greatly reduced. The lower portion of the esophagus is stimulated by neostigmine; in patients with marked achalasia and dilation of the esophagus, the drug can cause a salutary increase in tone and peristalsis.

Neostigmine also augments motor activity of the small and large bowel; the colon is particularly stimulated. Atony produced by muscarinic receptor antagonists or prior surgical intervention may be overcome, propulsive waves are increased in amplitude and frequency, and movement of intestinal contents is thus promoted. The total effect of anti-ChE agents on intestinal motility probably represents a combination of actions at the ganglion cells of the Auerbach plexus and at the smooth muscle fibers as a result of the preservation of ACh released by the cholinergic preganglionic and postganglionic fibers, respectively (Chapter 50).

Neuromuscular Junction

Most of the effects of potent anti-ChE drugs on skeletal muscle can be explained adequately on the basis of their inhibition of AChE at neuromuscular junctions. However, there is good evidence for an accessory direct action of neostigmine and other quaternary ammonium anti-ChE agents on skeletal muscle. For example, the intra-arterial injection of neostigmine into chronically denervated muscle, or muscle in which AChE has been inactivated by prior administration of DFP, evokes an immediate contraction, whereas physostigmine does not.

Normally, a single nerve impulse in a terminal motor-axon branch liberates enough ACh to produce a localized depolarization (end-plate potential) of sufficient magnitude to initiate a propagated muscle action potential. The ACh released is rapidly hydrolyzed by AChE, such that the lifetime of free ACh within the nerve-muscle synapse (~200 μsec) is shorter than the decay of the end-plate potential or the refractory period of the muscle. Therefore, each nerve impulse gives rise to a single wave of depolarization. After inhibition of AChE, the residence time of ACh in the synapse increases, allowing for lateral diffusion and rebinding of the transmitter to multiple receptors. Successive stimulation of neighboring receptors to the release site in the end plate results in a prolongation of the decay time of the end-plate potential. Quanta released by individual nerve impulses are no longer isolated. This action destroys the synchrony between end-plate depolarizations and the development of the muscle action potentials. Consequently, asynchronous excitation and fasciculations of muscle fibers occur. With sufficient inhibition of AChE, depolarization of the end-plate predominates, and blockade due to depolarization ensues (Chapter 11). When ACh persists in the synapse, it also may depolarize the axon terminal, resulting in antidromic firing of the motoneuron; this stimulation contributes to fasciculations that involve the entire motor unit.

Anti-ChE agents will reverse the antagonism caused by competitive neuromuscular blocking agents. By contrast, neostigmine is not effective against the skeletal muscle paralysis caused by succinylcholine, which produces neuromuscular blockade by depolarization; neostigmine will enhance depolarization and the resultant blockade.

Cardiopulmonary System

The cardiovascular actions of anti-ChE agents are complex because they reflect both ganglionic and postganglionic effects of accumulated ACh on the heart and blood vessels and actions in the CNS. The predominant effect on the heart from the peripheral action of accumulated ACh is bradycardia, resulting in a fall in cardiac output. Higher doses usually enhance the fall in blood pressure, as a consequence of effects of anti-ChE agents on the medullary vasomotor centers of the CNS.

Anti-ChE agents augment vagal influences on the heart. This shortens the effective refractory period of atrial muscle fibers and increases the refractory period and conduction time at the sinoatrial and atrioventricular nodes. At the ganglionic level, accumulating ACh initially is excitatory on nicotinic receptors, but at higher concentrations, ganglionic blockade ensues as a result of persistent depolarization of the postsynaptic nerve. The excitatory action on the parasympathetic ganglion cells would tend to reinforce the diminished cardiac output, whereas the opposite sequence results from the action of ACh on sympathetic ganglion cells. Excitation followed by inhibition also is elicited by ACh at the central medullary vasomotor and cardiac centers. All of these effects are complicated further by the hypoxemia resulting from the bronchoconstrictor and secretory actions of increased ACh on the respiratory system; hypoxemia, in turn, can reinforce both sympathetic tone and ACh-induced discharge of epinephrine from the adrenal medulla. Hence, it is not surprising that an increase in heart rate is seen with severe ChE inhibitor poisoning. Hypoxemia probably is a major factor in the CNS depression that appears after large doses of anti-ChE agents.

Actions at Other Sites

Secretory glands that are innervated by postganglionic cholinergic fibers include the bronchial, lacrimal, sweat, salivary, gastric (antral G cells and parietal cells), intestinal, and pancreatic acinar glands. Low doses of anti-ChE agents augment secretory responses to nerve stimulation, and higher doses actually produce an increase in the resting rate of secretion.

Anti-ChE agents increase contraction of smooth muscle fibers of the bronchioles and ureters, and the ureters may show increased peristaltic activity.

ADME

Physostigmine is absorbed readily from the GI tract, subcutaneous tissues, and mucous membranes. The conjunctival instillation of solutions of the drug may result in systemic effects if measures (e.g., pressure on the inner canthus) are not taken to prevent absorption from the nasal mucosa. Parenterally administered physostigmine is largely destroyed within 2–3 h, mainly by hydrolytic cleavage by plasma esterases.

Neostigmine and pyridostigmine are absorbed poorly after oral administration, such that much larger doses are needed than by the parenteral route. Whereas the effective parenteral dose of neostigmine is 0.5–2 mg, the equivalent oral dose may be 15–30 mg or more. Neostigmine and pyridostigmine are also destroyed by plasma esterases; the half-lives of these drugs are about 1–2 h (Cohan et al., 1976).

Organophosphate anti-ChE agents with the highest risk of toxicity are highly lipid-soluble liquids; others, such as sarin, have high vapor pressures, augmenting their dispersal. The less-volatile agents that are commonly used as agricultural insecticides (e.g., diazinon, malathion) generally are dispersed as aerosols or as dusts adsorbed to an inert, finely particulate material. Consequently, the compounds are absorbed rapidly through the skin and mucous membranes following contact with moisture, by the lungs after inhalation, and by the GI tract after ingestion (Storm et al., 2000).

Following their absorption, most organophosphates are excreted almost entirely as hydrolysis products in the urine. Plasma and liver esterases are responsible for hydrolysis to the corresponding phosphoric and phosphonic acids. However, CYPs are responsible for converting the inactive phosphorothioates containing a phosphorus-sulfur (thiono) bond to phosphorates with a phosphorus-oxygen bond, resulting in their activation. These enzymes also play a role in the inactivation of certain organophosphorus agents, and allelic differences are known to affect rates of metabolism (Furlong, 2007).

The organophosphate anti-ChE agents are hydrolyzed by two families of hepatic enzymes: the carboxylesterases and the paraoxonases (A-esterases). These enzymes are secreted into plasma and scavenge or hydrolyze a large number of organophosphates by cleaving the phosphoester, anhydride, phosphofluoridate, or phosphoryl cyanide bonds. Natural substrates of the paraoxonases appear to be lactones. In addition to catalyzing hydrolysis of organophosphates, the paraoxonase isozyme PON1 associates with high-density lipoproteins and appears to play a role in removing oxidized lipids, thereby exerting a protective effect in atherosclerosis and inflammation (Costa et al., 2013; Harel et al., 2004; Mackness and Mackness, 2015). Wide variations in paraoxonase activity exist among animal species. Young animals are deficient in carboxylesterases and paraoxonases, which may account for age-related toxicities seen in newborn animals and suspected to be a basis for organophosphate toxicity in humans (Padilla et al., 2004).

Plasma and hepatic carboxylesterases (aliesterases) and plasma butyrylcholinesterase are inhibited irreversibly by organophosphates (Costa et al., 2013; Lockridge 2015); their scavenging capacity for organophosphates can afford partial protection against inhibition of AChE in the nervous system. The carboxylesterases also catalyze hydrolysis of malathion and other organophosphates that contain carboxyl-ester linkages, rendering them less active or inactive. Because carboxylesterases are inhibited by organophosphates, toxicity from simultaneous exposure to two organophosphorus insecticides can prove synergistic.

Toxicology

Scope of the Problem

The toxicological aspects of the anti-ChE agents are of practical importance to clinicians. In addition to cases of accidental intoxication from the use and manufacture of organophosphorus compounds as agricultural insecticides, these agents have been used frequently for homicidal and suicidal purposes. Organophosphates account for as many as 80% of pesticide-related hospital admissions. The World Health Organization documents pesticide toxicity as a widespread global problem associated with over 300,000 deaths a year; most poisonings occur in Southeast Asia (Eddleston and Chowdhury, 2015; Eddleston and Clark, 2011). Occupational exposure occurs most commonly by the dermal and pulmonary routes, while oral ingestion is most common in cases of nonoccupational poisoning.

Sources of Information

In the U.S., the EPA, by virtue of revised risk assessments and the Food Quality Protection Act of 1996, has placed several organophosphate insecticides, including diazinon and chlorpyrifos, on restricted use and phased-out status in consumer products for home and garden use. A primary concern relates to exposure in pregnancy and to infants and children because the developing nervous system may be particularly susceptible to certain of these agents (Eaton et al., 2008). The National Pesticide Information Center (http://npic.orst.edu/) and the Office of Pesticide Programs of the EPA (https://www.epa.gov/pesticides) provide continuous reviews of the status of organophosphate pesticides, their tolerance reassessments, and revisions of risk assessments through their websites.

Acute Intoxication

Acute intoxication by anti-ChE agents is manifested by muscarinic and nicotinic signs and symptoms and, except for quaternary compounds of low lipid solubility, by signs referable to the CNS. Systemic effects appear within minutes after inhalation of vapors or aerosols, while onset of symptoms is delayed after GI and percutaneous absorption. The duration of toxic symptoms is determined largely by the properties of the compound: its lipid solubility, whether it must be activated to form the oxon, the stability of the organophosphate-AChE bond, and whether "aging" of the phosphorylated enzyme has occurred.

After local exposure to vapors or aerosols or after their inhalation, ocular and respiratory effects generally appear first. Ocular manifestations include marked miosis, ocular pain, conjunctival congestion, diminished vision, ciliary spasm, and brow ache. With acute systemic absorption, miosis may not be evident due to sympathetic discharge in response to hypotension. In addition to rhinorrhea and hyperemia of the upper respiratory tract, respiratory responses consist of tightness in the chest and wheezing caused by the combination of bronchoconstriction and increased bronchial secretion. GI symptoms occur earliest after ingestion and include anorexia, nausea and vomiting, abdominal cramps, and diarrhea. With percutaneous absorption of liquid, localized sweating and muscle fasciculations in the immediate vicinity are generally the earliest symptoms. Severe intoxication is manifested by extreme salivation, involuntary defecation and urination, sweating, lacrimation, penile erection, bradycardia, and hypotension.

Nicotinic actions at the neuromuscular junctions of skeletal muscle usually consist of fatigability and generalized weakness, involuntary twitchings, scattered fasciculations, and eventually severe weakness and paralysis. The most serious consequence is paralysis of the respiratory muscles.

A broad spectrum of effects of acute AChE inhibition on the CNS includes confusion, ataxia, slurred speech, loss of reflexes, Cheyne-Stokes respiration, generalized convulsions, coma, and central respiratory paralysis. Actions on the vasomotor and other cardiovascular centers in the medulla oblongata lead to hypotension.

The time of death after a single acute exposure may range from less than 5 min to nearly 24 h, depending on the dose, route, and agent. The cause of death primarily is respiratory failure, usually accompanied by a secondary cardiovascular component. Peripheral muscarinic and nicotinic as well as central actions all contribute to respiratory compromise; effects include laryngospasm, bronchoconstriction, increased tracheobronchial and salivary secretions, and compromised voluntary control of the diaphragm and intercostal muscles. Blood pressure may fall to alarmingly low levels, and cardiac arrhythmias may result from hypoxemia.

Delayed symptoms appearing after 1–4 days and marked by persistent low blood ChE and severe muscle weakness are termed the *intermediate syndrome* (Lotti, 2002). Delayed neurotoxicity and recurrent seizures also may be evident after severe intoxication (discussed below in "*Reactivation and Disposition*").

Diagnosis and Treatment

The diagnosis of severe, acute anti-ChE intoxication is made readily from the history of exposure and the characteristic signs and symptoms. In suspected cases of milder acute or chronic intoxication, determination of the ChE activities in erythrocytes and plasma generally will establish the diagnosis (Storm et al., 2000). Although these values vary considerably in the normal population, they usually are depressed well below the normal range before symptoms are evident.

Atropine in sufficient dosage (described further in the chapter) effectively antagonizes the actions at muscarinic receptor sites, including increased tracheobronchial and salivary secretion, bronchoconstriction, and bradycardia. Larger doses are required to get appreciable concentrations of atropine into the CNS. Atropine is virtually without effect against the peripheral neuromuscular compromise, which can be reversed by 2-PAM, a cholinesterase reactivator.

In moderate or severe intoxication with an organophosphorus anti-ChE agent, the recommended adult dose of 2-PAM is 1–2 g, slowly infused intravenously. If weakness is not relieved or if it recurs after 20–60 min, the dose should be repeated. Early treatment is important to ensure that the oxime reaches the phosphorylated AChE while the latter still can be reactivated. Many of the alkylphosphates are extremely lipid soluble, and if extensive partitioning into body fat has occurred and desulfuration is required for inhibition of AChE, toxicity will persist.

General supportive measures also are important, including

- termination of exposure, by removal of the patient or application of a gas mask if the atmosphere remains contaminated, removal and destruction of contaminated clothing, copious washing of contaminated skin or mucous membranes with water, or gastric lavage;
- maintenance of a patent airway, including endobronchial aspiration;
- artificial respiration; administration of O_2, if required;
- alleviation of persistent convulsions with diazepam (5–10 mg IV); and
- treatment of shock.

Atropine should be given in doses sufficient to cross the blood-brain barrier. Following an initial injection of 2–4 mg, given intravenously if possible, otherwise intramuscularly, 2 mg should be given every 5–10 min until muscarinic symptoms disappear, if they reappear, or until signs of atropine toxicity appear. More than 200 mg may be required on the first day. AChE reactivating agents and mild degree of atropine block then should be maintained for as long as symptoms are evident.

Although the phosphorylated esteratic site of AChE undergoes hydrolytic regeneration at a slow or negligible rate, nucleophilic agents, such as hydroxylamine (NH_2OH), hydroxamic acids (RCONH–OH), and oximes (RCH=NOH), reactivate the enzyme more rapidly than does spontaneous hydrolysis. Froede and Wilson (1971) reasoned that selective reactivation could be achieved by a site-directed nucleophile, wherein interaction of a quaternary nitrogen with the negative subsite of the active center would place the nucleophile in close apposition to the phosphorus. The oxime is oriented proximally to exert a nucleophilic attack on the phosphorus; a phosphoryloxime is formed, leaving the regenerated enzyme (Figure 10–2E).

Several *bis*-quaternary aldoximes are even more potent as reactivators for insecticide and nerve gas poisoning; examples are obidoxime and HI-6, which are used in Europe as antidotes (Worek and Thiermann, 2013; Steinritz et al., 2016). However, these compounds do not cross the blood-brain barrier, limiting their effectiveness to peripheral nervous system sites only.

Certain phosphorylated AChEs can undergo a fairly rapid process of "aging," so that within the course of minutes or hours they become completely resistant to the reactivators. Aging is due to the loss of one alkoxy group, leaving a much more stable monoalkyl- or monoalkoxy-phosphoryl-AChE (Figure 10–2D and 10–2E). Organophosphorus compounds containing tertiary alkoxy groups, such as soman, are more prone to aging than are congeners containing the secondary or primary alkoxy groups. The oximes are not effective in antagonizing the toxicity of the more rapidly hydrolyzing carbamoyl ester inhibitors; since 2-PAM itself has weak anti-ChE activity, it is not recommended for the treatment of overdosage with neostigmine or physostigmine or poisoning with carbamoylating insecticides such as carbaryl.

Reactivation and Disposition

The reactivating action of oximes in vivo is most marked at the skeletal neuromuscular junction. Antidotal effects are less striking at autonomic effector sites, and the quaternary ammonium group restricts entry into the CNS (Eddleston et al., 2008; Eddleston and Clark, 2011).

Although high doses or accumulation of oximes can inhibit AChE and cause neuromuscular blockade, they should be given until one can be assured of clearance of the offending organophosphate. Current antidotal therapy for organophosphate exposure resulting from warfare or terrorism includes parenteral atropine, an oxime (2-PAM, HI-6 or obidoxime), and diazepam or midazolam as anticonvulsants (King and Aaron, 2015; Worek and Thiermann, 2013). The oximes and their metabolites are readily eliminated by the kidney.

Parenterally administered human butyrylcholinesterase and recombinant DNA-expressed paraoxonases and phosphotriesterases with selected mutations are under development to scavenge the organophosphate at its portal of entry or plasma before it reaches peripheral and central tissue sites (Cerasoli et al., 2005; Mata et al., 2014; Worek et al., 2014). Because scavenging by butyrylcholinesterase is stoichiometric rather than catalytic, large quantities are required, so a broad spectrum of catalytic activities from other phosphoesterases is sought. Catalytic enzyme scavengers are limited by their slow distribution from intramuscular sites; rapid scavenging by enzymes requires intravenous administration.

Certain fluorine-containing organophosphorus anti-ChE agents (e.g., DFP, mipafox) have the property of inducing delayed neurotoxicity, a property they share with the triarylphosphates, of which TOCP is the classical example. This syndrome first received widespread attention following the demonstration that TOCP, an adulterant of Jamaica ginger, was responsible for an outbreak of thousands of cases of paralysis that occurred in the U.S. during Prohibition.

The clinical picture is that of severe polyneuropathy manifested initially by mild sensory disturbances, ataxia, weakness, muscle fatigue and twitching, reduced tendon reflexes, and tenderness to palpation. In severe cases, the weakness may progress to flaccid paralysis and muscle wasting. Recovery may require several years and may be incomplete.

Toxicity from this organophosphate-induced delayed polyneuropathy is not dependent on inhibition of cholinesterases; instead, a distinct esterase, termed *neurotoxic esterase,* is linked to the lesions (Johnson, 1993). This enzyme has a specificity for hydrophobic esters, but its natural substrate and function remain unknown (Glynn, 2006; Read et al., 2009). Myopathies that result in generalized necrotic lesions and changes in end-plate cytostructure also are found in experimental animals after long-term exposure to organophosphates (De Bleecker et al., 1991).

Therapeutic Uses of AChE Inhibitors

Current use of anti-AChE agents is limited to four conditions in the periphery:

- atony of the smooth muscle of the intestinal tract and urinary bladder
- glaucoma
- myasthenia gravis
- reversal of the paralysis of competitive neuromuscular blocking drugs

Long-acting and hydrophobic ChE inhibitors are the only inhibitors with well-documented efficacy, albeit limited, in the treatment of dementia symptoms of Alzheimer disease. Physostigmine, with its shorter duration of action, is used to treat intoxication by atropine and several drugs with anticholinergic side effects (discussed further in the chapter); it also is indicated for the treatment of Friedreich or other inherited ataxias. Edrophonium has been used for terminating attacks of paroxysmal supraventricular tachycardia.

Available Therapeutic Agents

The compounds described here are those commonly used as anti-ChE drugs and ChE reactivators in the U.S. Preparations used solely for ophthalmic purposes are described in Chapter 69. Conventional dosages and routes of administration are given in the further discussion of therapeutic applications.

Physostigmine salicylate is available for injection. Physostigmine sulfate ophthalmic ointment and physostigmine salicylate ophthalmic solution also are available. Pyridostigmine bromide is available for oral or parenteral use. Neostigmine bromide is available for oral use. Neostigmine methylsulfate is marketed for parenteral injection. Ambenonium chloride is available for oral use. Tacrine, donepezil, rivastigmine, and galantamine have been approved for the treatment of Alzheimer disease.

Pralidoxime chloride is the only AChE reactivator currently available in the U.S. and can be obtained in a parenteral formulation. HI-6 is available in several European and Near Eastern countries.

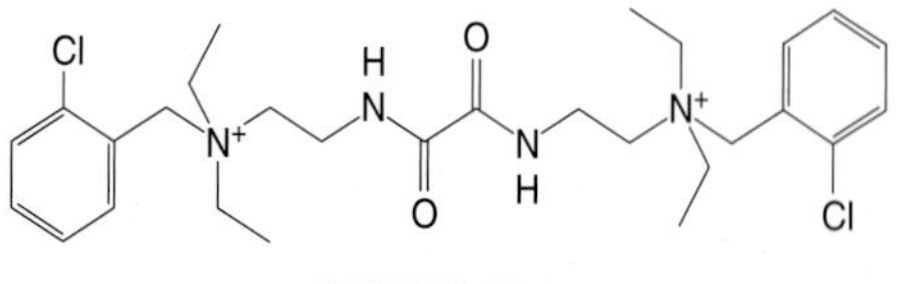

AMBENONIUM

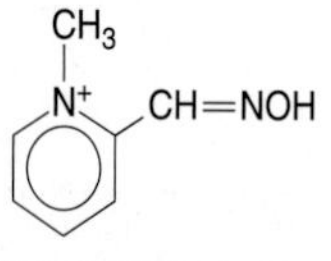

PRALIDOXIME (2-PAM)

Paralytic Ileus and Atony of the Urinary Bladder

In the treatment of both paralytic ileus and urinary bladder atony, neostigmine generally is preferred among the anti-ChE agents. Directly acting muscarinic agonists (Chapter 9) are employed for the same purposes.

Neostigmine is used for the relief of abdominal distension and acute colonic pseudo-obstruction from a variety of medical and surgical causes (Ponec et al., 1999). The usual subcutaneous dose of neostigmine methylsulfate for postoperative paralytic ileus is 0.5 mg, given as needed. Peristaltic activity commences 10–30 min after parenteral administration, whereas 2–4 h are required after oral administration of neostigmine bromide (15–30 mg). It may be necessary to assist evacuation with a small low enema or gas with a rectal tube.

When neostigmine is used for the treatment of atony of the detrusor muscle of the urinary bladder, postoperative dysuria is relieved. The drug is used in a similar dose and manner as in the management of paralytic ileus. Neostigmine should not be used when the intestine or urinary bladder is obstructed, when peritonitis is present, when the viability of the bowel is doubtful, or when bowel dysfunction results from inflammatory bowel disease.

Glaucoma and Other Ophthalmologic Indications

Glaucoma is a complex disease characterized by an increase in intraocular pressure that, if sufficiently high and persistent, will damage the optic disc at the juncture of the optic nerve and the retina; irreversible blindness can result. Of the three types of glaucoma—primary, secondary, and congenital—anti-AChE agents are of value in the management of the primary as well as of certain categories of the secondary type (e.g., aphakic glaucoma, following cataract extraction); congenital glaucoma rarely responds to any therapy other than surgery. Primary glaucoma is subdivided into narrow-angle (acute congestive) and wide-angle (chronic simple) types, based on the configuration of the angle of the anterior chamber where the aqueous humor is reabsorbed.

Narrow-angle glaucoma is nearly always a medical emergency in which drugs are essential in controlling the acute attack, but the long-range management is often surgical (e.g., peripheral or complete iridectomy). Wide-angle glaucoma, on the other hand, has a gradual, insidious onset and is not generally amenable to surgical improvement; in this type, control of intraocular pressure usually is dependent on continuous drug therapy.

Because the cholinergic agonists and ChE inhibitors also block accommodation and induce myopia, these agents produce transient blurring of far vision, limited visual acuity in low light, and loss of vision at the margin when instilled in the eye. With long-term administration of the cholinergic agonists and anti-ChE agents, the compromise of vision diminishes. Nevertheless, other agents without these side effects, such as prostaglandin analogues, β adrenergic receptor antagonists, and carbonic anhydrase inhibitors, have become the primary topical therapies for open-angle glaucoma. AChE inhibitors are held in reserve for the chronic conditions when patients become refractory to the agents mentioned. Topical treatment with long-acting ChE inhibitors such as echothiophate give rise to symptoms characteristic of systemic ChE inhibition. (For a complete account of the use of anti-ChE agents in ocular therapy, see Chapter 69).

Myasthenia Gravis

Myasthenia gravis is a neuromuscular disease of complex genetic etiology characterized by exacerbations and remissions of weakness and marked fatigability of skeletal muscle (Drachman, 1994; Renton et al., 2015).

The relative importance of prejunctional and postjunctional defects in myasthenia gravis was unknown until Patrick and Lindstrom (1973) found that rabbits immunized with nicotinic receptor slowly developed muscular weakness and respiratory difficulties that resembled the symptoms of myasthenia gravis. This animal model prompted intense investigation into whether the natural disease represented an autoimmune response directed toward the ACh receptor. Antireceptor antibodies are detectable in sera of 90% of patients with the disease, although the clinical status of the patient does not correlate precisely with antibody titers (Drachman, 1994). Sequences and the structural location in the α_1 subunit constituting the main immunogenic region are well defined (Lindstrom, 2008).

The picture that emerges is that myasthenia gravis is caused by an autoimmune response primarily to the ACh receptor at the postjunctional end plate. These antibodies reduce the number of receptors detectable either by snake α-neurotoxin–binding assays (Fambrough et al., 1973) or by electrophysiological measurements of ACh sensitivity (Drachman, 1994). Immune complexes along with marked ultrastructural abnormalities appear in the synaptic cleft and enhance receptor degradation through complement-mediated lysis in the end plate.

In a subset of about 10% of patients presenting with a myasthenic syndrome, muscle weakness has a congenital rather than an autoimmune basis. Characterization of biochemical and genetic bases of the congenital condition has demonstrated mutations in the ACh receptor that affect ligand-binding, channel-opening kinetics and durations; receptor biosynthesis; and synaptic location of receptors (Engel et al., 2012; Sine and Engel, 2006). Other mutations occur as a deficiency in the form of AChE that contains the collagen-like tail unit, in presynaptic transporters involved in the uptake of choline, and in vesicular storage of ACh. In this group of patients, identification of the mutation is essential for ascertaining whether a specific pharmacologic treatment is warranted.

Diagnosis

Although the diagnosis of autoimmune myasthenia gravis usually can be made from the history, signs, and symptoms, its differentiation from certain neurasthenic, infectious, endocrine, congenital, neoplastic, and degenerative neuromuscular diseases can be challenging. However, in autoimmune myasthenia gravis, the aforementioned deficiencies and enhancement of muscle strength can be improved dramatically by anti-ChE medication. The edrophonium test for initial diagnosis relies on these responses. The edrophonium test is performed by rapid intravenous injection of 2 mg of edrophonium chloride, followed 45 sec later by an additional 8 mg if the first dose is without effect. A positive response consists of brief improvement in strength, unaccompanied by lingual fasciculation (which generally occurs in nonmyasthenic patients).

An excessive dose of an anti-ChE drug results in a *cholinergic crisis*. The condition is characterized by weakness resulting from generalized depolarization of the motor end plate; other features result from overstimulation of muscarinic receptors. The weakness resulting from depolarization blockade may resemble myasthenic weakness, which is manifest when anti-ChE medication is insufficient. The distinction is of obvious practical importance because the former is treated by withholding, and the latter by administering, the anti-ChE agent. Detection of antireceptor antibodies in muscle biopsies or plasma is now widely employed to establish the diagnosis.

Treatment of Myasthenia Gravis

Pyridostigmine, neostigmine, and ambenonium are the standard anti-ChE drugs used in the symptomatic treatment of myasthenia gravis. All can increase the response of myasthenic muscle to repetitive nerve impulses, primarily by the preservation of endogenous ACh. Following AChE inhibition, receptors over a greater cross-sectional area of the end plate presumably are exposed to concentrations of ACh that are sufficient for channel opening and production of a postsynaptic end-plate potential.

Unpredictable exacerbations and remissions of the myasthenic state may require adjustment of dosage. Pyridostigmine is available in sustained-release tablets containing a total of 180 mg, of which 60 mg are released immediately and 120 mg are released over several hours; this preparation is of value in maintaining patients for 6- to 8-h periods but should be limited to use at bedtime. Muscarinic cardiovascular and GI side effects of anti-ChE agents generally can be controlled by atropine or other anticholinergic drugs (Chapter 9). However, these anticholinergic drugs mask many side effects of an excessive dose of an anti-ChE agent. In most patients, tolerance develops eventually to the muscarinic effects. Several drugs, including curariform agents and certain antibiotics and general anesthetics, interfere with neuromuscular transmission (Chapter 11); their administration to patients with myasthenia gravis requires proper adjustment of anti-ChE dosage and other precautions.

Other therapeutic measures are essential elements in the management of this disease. Glucocorticoids promote clinical improvement in a high percentage of patients. However, when treatment with steroids is continued over prolonged periods, a high incidence of side effects may result (Chapter 46). Initiation of steroid treatment augments muscle weakness; however, as the patient improves with continued administration of steroids, doses of anti-ChE drugs can be reduced (Drachman, 1994). Other immunosuppressive agents, such as azathioprine and cyclosporine and high-dose cyclophosphamide (Drachman et al., 2008), have also been beneficial in more refractory cases (Chapter 35). Thymectomy should be considered in myasthenia associated with a thymoma or when the disease is not controlled adequately by anti-ChE agents and steroids. Because the thymus contains myoid cells with nicotinic receptors (Schluep et al., 1987), and a predominance of patients have thymic abnormalities, the thymus may be responsible for the initial pathogenesis. It also is the source of autoreactive T-helper cells.

Alzheimer Disease

A deficiency of intact cholinergic neurons, particularly those extending from subcortical areas such as the nucleus basalis, has been observed in patients with progressive dementia of the Alzheimer type (Chapter 18). Using a rationale similar to that in other CNS degenerative diseases, therapy for enhancing concentrations of cholinergic and other neurotransmitters in the CNS has been investigated.

In 1993, the FDA approved tacrine (tetrahydroaminoacridine) for use in mild-to-moderate Alzheimer disease, but a high incidence of enhanced alanine aminotransferase and hepatotoxicity limited the utility of this drug.

Subsequently, donepezil was approved for clinical use and has emerged as the primary agent for treatment in multiple countries (Lee et al., 2015). Initially, 5-mg doses are administered daily, and if tolerated, doses are increased to 10 mg for mild-to-moderate conditions. Recent clinical trials in moderate-to-severe Alzheimer disease have confirmed benefits for a 23-mg/d sustained release form. Most studies are carried out for periods of 24 weeks, although treatment periods have been extended, usually extending the treatment baseline, but without further improvement or some decline after 6 months. Adverse side effects have been attributed to excessive peripheral cholinergic stimulation and include nasopharyngitis, diarrhea, nausea, and vomiting. Rhabdomyolysis reportedly occurs, requiring discontinuation of the drug. Cotreatment with memantine did not result in significant improvement over the higher-dose donepezil treatment (Howard et al., 2012).

Rivastigmine, a more lipid soluble, longer-acting carbamylating inhibitor, is approved for use in the U.S. and Europe in both oral and skin patch forms. While having similar side effects to other cholinesterase inhibitors, rivastigmine is reported to have shown a higher incidence of fatalities than other cholinesterase inhibitors used in Alzheimer dementias (Ali et al., 2015). It has not been determined whether the increase relates to misuse of the transdermal form of administration. Galantamine is another FDA-approved agent for Alzheimer dementias, acting as a reversible AChE inhibitor with a side-effect profile similar to that of donepezil.

These three cholinesterase inhibitors, which have the requisite affinity and hydrophobicity to cross the blood-brain barrier and exhibit a prolonged duration of action, along with an excitatory amino acid transmitter mimic, memantine, constitute current modes of therapy. These agents are not disease modifying and lack well-documented actions on the pathology of Alzheimer disease. However, the bulk of the evidence indicates that they slow the decline in cognitive function and behavioral manifestation for limited intervals of time (Chapter 18). Associated symptoms, such as depression, may be preferentially delayed (Lu et al., 2009). Current clinical research efforts are directed to synergistic actions of arresting inflammatory processes or neurodegeneration and combining cholinesterase inhibition with selective cholinergic receptor modulation.

Prophylaxis in Cholinesterase Inhibitor Poisoning

Studies in experimental animals have shown that pretreatment with pyridostigmine reduces the incapacitation and mortality associated with nerve agent poisoning, particularly for agents such as soman that show rapid aging. The first large-scale administration of pyridostigmine to humans occurred in 1990 in anticipation of nerve agent attack in the first Gulf War. At an oral dose of 30 mg every 8 h, the incidence of side effects was around 1%; fewer than 0.1% of the subjects had responses sufficient to warrant discontinuing the drug in the setting of military action (Keeler et al., 1991). Long-term follow-up indicates that veterans of the Gulf War who received pyridostigmine showed a low incidence of a neurologic syndrome, now termed the *Persian Gulf War syndrome.* It is characterized by impaired cognition, ataxia, confusion, myoneuropathy, adenopathy, weakness, and incontinence (Haley et al., 1997).

Controversy still surrounds the basis of Gulf War syndrome or illness, despite multiple reports and reviews by the U.S. Department of Veterans Affairs in 2008 and 2010 and the Institute of Medicine (Committee on Gulf War and Health, 2013; Institute of Medicine, 2013). Although several origins of the syndrome, such as pyridostigmine administration, have been ruled out as unlikely, the constellation of symptoms reflect an interplay of chemical toxicants and psychological factors, encompassing widespread pesticide use, and exposure from postwar demolition bombing of munitions facilities likely containing chemical warfare agents (sarin and mustards). Psychological factors, emerging as post-traumatic stress disorders, have been documented in prolonged wars since the early 20th century.

Intoxication by Anticholinergic Drugs

In addition to atropine and other muscarinic agents, many other drugs, such as the phenothiazines, antihistamines, and tricyclic antidepressants, have central and peripheral anticholinergic activity. Physostigmine is potentially useful in reversing the central anticholinergic syndrome produced by overdosage or an unusual reaction to these drugs (Nilsson, 1982). While the effectiveness of physostigmine in reversing anticholinergic side effects has been documented, other toxic effects of the tricyclic antidepressants and phenothiazines (Chapters 15 and 16), such as intraventricular conduction deficits and ventricular arrhythmias, are not reversed by physostigmine. In addition, physostigmine may precipitate seizures; hence, its usually small potential benefit must be weighed against this risk. The use of anti-ChE agents to reverse the effects of competitive neuromuscular blocking agents is discussed in Chapter 11.

Drug Facts for Your Personal Formulary: *Anticholinesterase Agents*

Drugs	Therapeutic Uses	Major Toxicity and Clinical Pearls
Noncovalent Reversible Inhibitors		
Edrophonium Tacrine Donepezil Propidium Fasciculin Galantamine	• Edrophonium can be used to diagnose myasthenia gravis • Tacrine, donepezil and galantamine used for Alzheimer disease	• Edrophonium and tacrine: bind reversibly to choline subsite near Trp86 and Glu202 • Edrophonium has a short duration of action because of rapid renal elimination; effects are limited to the peripheral nervous system. • Donepezil and tacrine: higher affinity for AChE, more hydrophobic, can cross BBB. • Tacrine: high incidence of hepatotoxicity • Donepezil binds with higher affinity to the active center gorge of AChE. • Propidium & fasciculin: bind peripheral anionic site on AChE
Carbamate Inhibitors		
"Reversible" Carbamate Inhibitors Physostigmine Neostigmine Pyridostigmine Ambenonium Rivastigmine	• Pyridostigmine, neostigmine and ambenonium are used for treatment of myasthenia gravis • Neostigmine is used for paralytic ileus and atony of the urinary bladder • Rivastigmine, a very lipid soluble alternative for treating Alzheimer disease • Pyridostigmine used prophylactically in nerve gas attacks	• Drugs with carbamoyl ester linkage: AChE substrates that block by carbamylation of AChE active center serine, are hydrolyzed slowly; regarded as hemi-substrate blockers • Neostigmine and pyridostigmine are poorly absorbed after oral administration • Pyridostigmine: available in sustained release tablets; oral dose much higher than parenteral dose • Rivastigmine can cross the BBB, has longer duration of action, and is available in oral and epidermal patch formulations
Carbamate insecticides Carbaryl Propoxur Aldicarb	• Garden insecticides	• Symptoms of poisoning resemble those of organophosphates but are more readily reversed and less toxic
Organophosphates		
Echothiophate	• Treatment of glaucoma	• Instilled locally in the eye • Stable in aqueous solution
Nerve Agents DFP Tabun Sarin Soman Cyclosarin VX	• Alkylphosphates are the most potent synthetic toxins • React covalently with the active site serine • Potent and irreversible inactivators of ChE • Recent documented use in terrorism	• Form a stable conjugate with the active site serine by phosphorylátion/phosphonylation • Hydrolyzed by hepatic carboxyesterases and paraoxonases • Low MW, hydrophobic, rapidly penetrates into CNS from pulmonary inhalation • Tabun, sarin, and cyclosarin are volatile and extremely toxic "nerve gases" • VX is absorbed through the skin, has slower onset, but high toxicity • 2-PAM and related aldoximes are used to reactivate organophosphate-ChE conjugates • Resistance to organophosphate-AChE reactivation is enhanced through "aging" that results from loss of one alkyl group

Drug Facts for Your Personal Formulary: *Anticholinesterase Agents (continued)*

Drugs	Therapeutic Uses	Major Toxicity and Clinical Pearls
Organophosphates		
Pesticides Parathion Methylparathion Malathion Diazonin Chlorpyrifos	• Insecticides largely agricultural • Malathion is used topically in the treatment of pediculosis in cases of permethrin resistance • Lethal dose of malathion in mammals is 1g/kg • Diazinon and chlorpyrifos are used widely in agriculture	• Metabolism of these *thion* pesticides to the corresponding *oxon* confers pesticide activity and toxicity, more rapid rate in insects • Malathion: detoxified by plasma carboxylesterases, a detoxification reaction that is more rapid in mammals and birds than insects, yielding a further margin of safety
Antidotal therapy for Organophosphate Exposure		
Cholinesterase reactivators 2-PAM HI-6 Obidoxime	• Quaternary pyridinium aldoxime reactivators indicated for insecticide and nerve gas poisoning • Improved agents in development	• Reactivates organophosphate-AChE conjugate by attacking the conjugated phosphorus to form phospho-oxime and regenerate the active enzyme • Dose is infused IV or IM with autoinjector; dosing should be repeated frequently • Early treatment helps insure that the oxime reaches the phosphorylated enzyme prior to complete "aging" • Reactivators do not cross the blood-brain barrier and do not reactivate CNS AChE
Anticholinergic agents Atropine	• Blocks symptoms mediated through muscarinic receptors	• Given by parenterally in 2-4mg doses every few min until muscarinic symptoms disappear
Benzodiazepines Diazepam Midazolam	• Minimize seizures and associated neuronal toxicity	• Administered parenterally post-exposure

Bibliography

Ali TB, et al. Adverse effects of cholinesterase inhibitors in dementia, according to pharmacovigilance data of the United States and Canada. *PLoS One*, **2015**, *10*:e0144337.

Bourne Y, et al. Acetylcholinesterase inhibition by fasciculin: crystal structure of the complex. *Cell*, **1995**, *83*:493–506.

Burkhart CG. Relationship of treatment resistant head lice to the safety and efficacy of pediculicides. *Mayo Clin Proc*, **2004**, *79*:661–666.

Camp S, et al. Acetylcholinesterase expression in muscle is specifically controlled by a promoter selective enhancesome in the first intron. *J Neurosci*, **2008**, *28*:2459–2470.

Centers for Disease Control and Prevention. Head lice: treatment. **2015**. http://www.cdc.gov/parasites/lice/head/treatment.html. Accessed March 12, 2016.

Cerasoli DM, et al. In vitro and in vivo characterization of recombinant human butyrylcholinesterase (Protexia) as a potential nerve agent scavenger. *Chem Biol Interactions*, **2005**, *157–158*:363–365.

Cohan SL, et al. The pharmacokinetics of pyridostigmine. *Neurology*, **1976**, *26*:536–539.

Committee on Gulf War and Health Reports, *Update of Health Effects of Serving in the Gulf War and Treatment of Chronic Multi-symptom Illness*. National Academies Press, Washington, DC, **2013**.

Costa LG, et al. Paraoxonase 1 (PON1) as a genetic determinant of susceptibility to organophosphate toxicity. *Toxicology*, **2013**, *307*:115–122.

Council on Foreign Relations. UN report on chemical weapons use in Syria. **2013**. http://www.cfr.org/syria/un-report-chemical-weapons-use-syria/p31404. Accessed March 12, 2016.

Cummings JL. Alzheimer's disease. *N Engl J Med*, **2004**, *351*:56–67.

Cygler M, et al. Relationship between sequence conservation and three dimensional structure in a large family of esterases, lipases and related proteins. *Protein Sci*, **1993**, *2*:366–382.

De Bleecker J, et al. Histological and histochemical study of paraoxon myopathy in the rat. *Acta Neurol Belg*, **1991**, *91*:255–270.

Dobbertin A, et al. Targeting acetylcholinesterase in neurons: a dual processing function for the proline-rich membrane anchor and the attachment domain of the catalytic subunit. *J Neurosci*, **2009**, *29*:4519–4530.

Dolgin E. Syrian gas attack reinforces need for better antisarin drugs. *Nat Med*, **2013**, *19*:1194–1195.

Drachman DB. Myasthenia gravis. *N Engl J Med*, **1994**, *330*:1797–1810.

Drachman DB, et al. Robooting the immune system with high-dose cyclophosphamide for treatment of refractory myasthenia gravis. *Ann N Y Acad Sci*, **2008**, *1132*:305–314.

Eaton DL, et al. Review of the toxicology of chlorpyrifos with an emphasis on human exposure and neurodevelopment. *Clin Rev Toxicol*, **2008**, *38*:1–125.

Eddleston M, Chowdhury FR. Pharmacological treatment of organophosphorus insecticide poisoning: the old and the (possible) new. *Brit J Clin Pharm*, **2015**, *81*:462–470.

Eddleston M, Clark R. Insecticides: organophosphorus compounds and carbamates. In Nelson LS, ed. *Goldfrank's Toxicologic Emergencies*. McGraw-Hill Medical, New York, **2011**, 150–166.

Engel AG, et al. New horizons for congenital myasthenic syndromes. *Ann N Y Acad Sci*, **2012**, *1275*:54–62.

Fambrough DM, et al. Neuromuscular junction in myasthenia gravis: decreased acetylcholine receptors. *Science*, **1973**, *182*:293–295.

Froede HC, Wilson IB. Acetylcholinesterase. In Boyer PD, ed. *The Enzymes*, vol. 5. Academic Press, New York, **1971**, 87–114.

Furlong CE. Genetic variability in the cytochrome P450–paraoxonase 1 pathway for detoxication of organophosphorus compounds. *J Biochem Molec Toxicol*, **2007**, *21*:197–205.

Gallo MA, Lawryk NJ. Organic phosphorus pesticides. In Hayes WJ Jr, Laws ER Jr, eds. *Handbook of Pesticide Toxicology*, vol. 2. Academic Press, San Diego, CA, **1991**, 917–1123.

Giacobini E. Cholinesterase inhibitors: from the Calabar bean to Alzheimer's therapy. In Giacobini E, ed. *Cholinesterases and Cholinesterase Inhibitors*. Martin Dunitz, London, **2000**, 181–227.

Glynn P. A mechanism for organophosphate-induced delayed neuropathy. *Toxicol Lett*, **2006**, *162*:94–97.

Haley RW, et al. Is there a Gulf War syndrome? *JAMA*, **1997**, *277*:215–222.

Harel M, et al. Structure and evolution of the serum paraoxonase family of detoxifying and anti-atherosclerotic enzymes. *Nat Struct Mol Biol*, **2004**, *11*:412–419.

Holmstedt B. Cholinesterase inhibitors: an introduction. In Giacobini E, ed. *Cholinesterases and Cholinesterase Inhibitors*. Martin Dunitz, London, **2000**, 1–8.

Institute of Medicine (National Academy of Science–USA). *Gulf War and Health*, vol. 2. National Academies Press, Washington, DC, **2013**.

Howard R, et al. Donepezil and memantine for moderate to severe Alzheimer's disease. *N Eng J Med*, **2012**, *366*:893–903.

Jennings LL, et al. Direct analysis of the kinetic profiles of organophosphate-acetylcholinesterase adducts by MALDI-TOF mass spectrometry. *Biochemistry*, **2003**, *42*:11083–11091.

Johnson MK. Symposium introduction: retrospect and prospects for neuropathy target esterase (NTE) and the delayed polyneuropathy (OPIDP) induced by some organophosphorus esters. *Chem Biol Interact*, **1993**, *87*:339–346.

Karczmar AG. History of the research with anticholinesterase agents. In Karczmar AG, ed. *Anticholinesterase Agents*, vol. 1, *International Encyclopedia of Pharmacology and Therapeutics*, section 13. Pergamon Press, Oxford, UK, **1970**, 1–44.

Keeler JR, et al. Pyridostigmine used as a nerve agent pretreatment under wartime conditions. *JAMA*, **1991**, *266*:693–695.

King AM, Aaron CK. Organophosphate and carbamate poisoning. *Emerg Med Clin N Am*, **2015**, *33*:133–151.

Lee J-H, et al. Donepezil across the spectrum of Alzheimer's disease: dose optimization and clinical relevance. *Acta Neurol Scand*, **2015**, *131*:259–267.

Lindstrom JM. Myasthenia gravis and the tops and bottoms of AChRs-antigenic structure of the MIR and specific immuno-suppression of EAMG using AChR cytoplasmic domains. *Ann N Y Acad Sci*, **2008**, *1132*:29–41.

Lockridge O. Review of human butyrylcholinesterase structure, function genetic variants history of use in the clinic and potential therapeutic uses. *Pharmacol Ther*, **2015**, *148*:34–46.

Lockridge O, et al. Complete amino acid sequence of human serum cholinesterase. *J Biol Chem*, **1987**, *262*:549–557.

Lotti M. Low-level exposures to organophosphorus esters and peripheral nerve function. *Muscle Nerve*, **2002**, *25*:492–504.

Lu PH, et al. Donepezil delays progression of A.D. in MCI subjects with depressive symptoms. *Neurology*, **2009**, *72*:2115–2212.

Mackness M, Mackness B. Human paraoxonase 1 (PON 1): gene structure and expression, promiscuous acitivties and multiple physiological roles. *Gene*, **2015**, *567*:12–21.

Massoulié J. Molecular forms and anchoring of acetylcholinesterase. In Giacobini E, ed. *Cholinesterases and Cholinesterase Inhibitors*. Martin Dunitz, London, **2000**, 81–103.

Mata DG, et al. Investigation of evolved paraoxonase-1 variants for prevention of organophosphate pesticide compound introxication. *J Pharmacol Exp Ther*, **2014**, *349*:549–558.

Nilsson E. Physostigmine treatment in various drug-induced intoxications. *Ann Clin Res*, **1982**, *14*:165–172.

Nozaki H, Aikawa N. Sarin poisoning in Tokyo subway. *Lancet*, **1995**, *346*:1446–1447.

Padilla S, et al. Further assessment of an in vitro screen that may help identify organophosphate insecticides that are more acutely toxic to the young. *J Toxicol Environ Health*, **2004**, *67*:1477–1489.

Patrick J, Lindstrom J. Autoimmune response to acetylcholine receptor. *Science*, **1973**, *180*:871–872.

Ponec RJ, et al. Neostigmine for the treatment of acute colonic pseudo-obstruction. *N Engl J Med*, **1999**, *341*:137–141.

Read DJ, et al. Neuropathy target esterase is required for adult vertebrate axon maintenance. *J Neurosci*, **2009**, *29*:11594–11600.

Reiner E, Radić Z. Mechanism of action of cholinesterase inhibitors. In Giacobini E, ed. *Cholinesterases and Cholinesterase Inhibitors*. Martin Dunitz, London, **2000**, 103–120.

Renton AE, et al. A genome-wide association study of myasthenia gravis. *JAMA Neurol*. **2015**, *72*:394–404.

Rosenberry TL. Acetylcholinesterase. *Adv Enzymol Relat Areas Mol Biol*, **1975**, *43*:103–218.

Schluep M, et al. Acetylcholine receptors in human thymic myoid cells in situ: an immunohistological study. *Ann Neurol*, **1987**, *22*: 212–222.

Schumacher M, et al. Primary structure of *Torpedo californica* acetylcholinesterase deduced from its cDNA sequence. *Nature*, **1986**, *319*: 407–409.

Silman I, Sussman JL. Structural studies on acetylcholinesterase. In Giacobini E, ed. *Cholinesterases and Cholinesterase Inhibitors*. Martin Dunitz, London, **2000**, 9–26.

Sine SM, Engel AG. Recent advances in Cys-loop receptor structure and function. *Nature (London)*, **2006**, *440*:448–455.

Steinritz D et al. Repetitive obidoxime treatment induced increase of red blood cell acetylcholinesterase activity even in a late phase of a severe methamidophos poisoning: A case report. *Toxicol Lett*, **2016**, *244*:121–123.

Storm JE, et al. Occupational exposure limits for 30 organophosphate pesticides based on inhibition of red blood cell acetylcholinesterase. *Toxicology*, **2000**, *150*:1–29.

Sussman JL, et al. Atomic structure of acetylcholinesterase from *Torpedo californica*: a prototypic acetylcholine-binding protein. *Science*, **1991**, *253*:872–879.

Taylor P, et al. The genes encoding the cholinesterases: structure, evolutionary relationships and regulation of their expression. In Giacobini E, ed. *Cholinesterases and Cholinesterase Inhibitors*. Martin Dunitz, London, **2000**, 63–80.

Taylor P, Radic Z. The cholinesterases: from genes to proteins. *Ann Rev Pharmacol*, **1994**, *34*:281–320.

Worek F, et al., Post-exposure treatment of VX poisoned guinea pigs with engineered phosphotriesterase mutant: a proof-of-concept study. *Toxicology Lett*, **2014**, *231*:45–54.

Worek F, Wille T, et al. Toxicology of organophosphorus compounds in view of an increasing terrorist threat. *Arch Toxicol*, **2016**, *90*:2131–2145.

Xie W, et al. Postnatal development delay and supersensitivity to organophosphate in gene-targeted mice lacking acetylcholinesterase. *J Pharmacol Exp Ther*, **2000**, *293*:892–902.

Nicotine and Agents Acting at the Neuromuscular Junction and Autonomic Ganglia

Ryan E. Hibbs and Alexander C. Zambon

第十一章 尼古丁与作用于神经肌肉接头和自主神经节的药物

中文导读

本章主要介绍：烟碱型乙酰胆碱受体，包括作者观点、烟碱型受体的结构；神经肌肉接头处的信号传递，包括神经肌肉阻滞药及其临床药理学；神经节的神经传递，包括神经元烟碱型受体和突触后电位、神经节激动药及神经节阻滞药；尼古丁成瘾和戒除，包括尼古丁替代疗法、瓦伦尼克林和胱氨酸治疗法。

Abbreviations

ACh: acetylcholine
AChE: acetylcholinesterase
anti-ChE: anticholinesterase
CNS: central nervous system
EPP: end-plate potential
EPSP: excitatory postsynaptic potential
FDA: Food and Drug Administration
GABA: γ-aminobutyric acid
GI: gastrointestinal
5HT: 5-hydroxytryptamine (serotonin)
IPSP: inhibitory postsynaptic potential
M_x: muscarinic receptor subtype x (x = 1, 2, 3, 4, or 5)
N_m: nicotinic ACh receptor in skeletal muscle
N_n: nicotinic ACh receptor in neurons
NRT: nicotine replacement therapy
TM: transmembrane
VMAT2: vesicular monoamine transporter 2

The Nicotinic Acetylcholine Receptor

The nicotinic ACh receptor mediates neurotransmission postsynaptically at the neuromuscular junction and peripheral autonomic ganglia; in the CNS, it largely modulates release of neurotransmitters from presynaptic sites. The receptor is called the *nicotinic ACh receptor* because both the alkaloid nicotine and the neurotransmitter ACh can stimulate the receptor. Distinct subtypes of nicotinic receptors exist at the neuromuscular junction (N_m), in autonomic ganglia, and in the CNS (the neuronal form, N_n). The binding of ACh to the nicotinic ACh receptor initiates an EPP in muscle or an EPSP in peripheral ganglia by directly mediating cation influx into the postsynaptic cell (see Chapter 8).

Perspective

Classical studies of the actions of curare and nicotine defined the concept of the nicotinic ACh receptor over a century ago and made this the prototypical pharmacological receptor. By taking advantage of specialized structures that have evolved to mediate cholinergic neurotransmission and of natural toxins that block motor activity, nicotinic receptors were isolated and characterized. These accomplishments represent landmarks in the development of molecular pharmacology.

Cholinergic neurotransmission mediates motor activity in marine vertebrates and mammals, and a large number of peptide, terpinoid, and alkaloid toxins that block the nicotinic receptors have evolved to enhance predation or protect plant and animal species from predation (Taylor et al., 2007). Among these toxins are the α-toxins: peptides of about 7 kDa from venoms of the krait, *Bungarus multicinctus*, and varieties of the cobra, *Naja naja*. These toxins potently inhibit neuromuscular transmission, are readily radiolabeled, and provide excellent probes for the nicotinic receptor.

The electrical organs from the aquatic species of *Electrophorus* and *Torpedo* provide rich sources of nicotinic receptor; up to 40% of the surface of the electric organ's membrane is excitable and contains cholinergic receptors, in contrast to vertebrate skeletal muscle, in which motor end plates occupy 0.1% or less of the cell surface. Using the α-toxin probes, the receptor from *Torpedo* was purified, the cDNAs of the subunits were isolated, and the genes were cloned for the multiple receptor subunits from mammalian neurons and muscle (Numa et al., 1983). By simultaneously expressing various permutations of the genes that encode the individual subunits in cellular systems and then measuring binding and the electrophysiological events that result from activation by agonists, researchers have been able to correlate functional properties with details of primary structures of the receptor subtypes (Changeux and Edelstein, 2005; Karlin, 2002; Sine et al., 2008).

Structure of Nicotinic Receptors

In vertebrates, the nicotinic receptors of skeletal muscle N_m are pentamers composed of four distinct subunits (α, β, γ, and δ) in a stoichiometric ratio of 2:1:1:1 (Changeux and Edelstein, 2005; Karlin, 2002; Unwin, 2005). In mature, innervated muscle end plates, the γ subunit is replaced by ε, a closely related subunit. The individual subunits are about 40% identical in their amino acid sequences. The nicotinic receptor is the prototype for other pentameric ligand-gated ion channels, which include the receptors for the inhibitory amino acids (GABA and glycine; Chapter 14) and $5HT_3$ receptors (Chapter 13). Each of the subunits in the pentameric receptor has a molecular mass of 40–60 kDa. In each subunit, the amino-terminal approximately 210 residues constitute a large extracellular domain. This is followed by four domains that span the membrane; the region between TM3 and TM4 forms most of the cytoplasmic component (Figure 11–1).

The five subunits of the nicotinic ACh receptor are arranged around a pseudoaxis of symmetry to circumscribe a channel. The resulting receptor is an asymmetrical molecule (16 × 8 nm) of 290 kDa, with the bulk of the non-membrane—spanning domain on the extracellular surface. The receptor is present at high densities (10,000/μm^2) in junctional areas (i.e., the motor end plate in skeletal muscle and the ventral surface of the *Torpedo* electrical organ). Agonist-binding sites occur at the subunit interfaces; in muscle, only two of the five subunit interfaces, αγ and αδ, bind ligands (Figure 11–2). Both of the subunits forming the subunit interface contribute to ligand specificity. Neuronal nicotinic N_n receptors found in ganglia and the CNS also exist as pentamers of one or more types of subunits. Subunit types $α_2$ through $α_{10}$ and $β_2$ through $β_4$ are found in neuronal tissues. Although not all pentameric combinations of α and β subunits lead to functional receptors, the diversity in subunit composition is large and exceeds the capacity of ligands to distinguish subtypes on the basis of their selectivity.

Agonist-mediated changes in ion permeability occur through a cation channel intrinsic to the receptor structure. Measurements of membrane conductance demonstrate rates of ion translocation of 5×10^7 ions/s. The channel is generally nonselective among cations; while highly permeable to Na^+, K^+, and in some cases Ca^{2+}, the majority of the current is carried by Na^+ ions. The second of four TM α-helices in each subunit line the ion channel. The agonist-binding site is intimately coupled with the ion channel; in the N_m, simultaneous binding of two agonist molecules results in a rapid conformational change that opens the channel.

Transmission at the Neuromuscular Junction

Neuromuscular Blocking Agents

Modern-day neuromuscular blocking agents fall generally into two classes, depolarizing and competitive/nondepolarizing. At present, only a single depolarizing agent, succinylcholine, is in general clinical use; multiple competitive or nondepolarizing agents are available (see Figure 11–3). Neuromuscular blocking agents are most commonly used for facilitating endotracheal intubation and to relax skeletal muscle during surgery.

Chemistry

Early structure-activity studies led to the development of the polymethylene bis-trimethyl-ammonium series (referred to as the methonium compounds, or depolarizing blockers). The most potent of these agents at the neuromuscular junction was the compound with 10 carbon atoms between the quaternary nitrogens: decamethonium (Figure 11–3). The compound with 6 carbon atoms in the chain, hexamethonium, was found to be essentially devoid of neuromuscular blocking activity but particularly effective as a ganglionic blocking agent (see following discussion).

Several structural features distinguish competitive and depolarizing neuromuscular blocking agents. The competitive agents (e.g., tubocurarine, the benzylisoquinolines, the amino steroids, and the asymmetric mixed-onium chlorofumarates) are relatively bulky, rigid molecules,

HISTORY Curare

In the mid-19th century, Claude Bernard demonstrated that the locus of action of curare was at or near the neuromuscular junction. Curare is a generic term for various South American arrow poisons. The drug has been used for centuries by Indians along the Amazon and Orinoco Rivers for immobilizing and paralyzing wild animals used for food; death results from paralysis of skeletal muscles. The preparation of curare was long shrouded in mystery and was entrusted only to tribal witch doctors. Soon after the discovery of the American continent, European explorers and botanists became interested in curare, and late in the 16th century, samples of the native preparations were brought to Europe. Following the pioneering work of scientist/explorer von Humboldt in 1805, the botanical sources of curare became the object of much field research. The curares from eastern Amazonia come from *Strychnos* species; these and other South American species of *Strychnos* contain chiefly quaternary neuromuscular blocking alkaloids. The Asiatic, African, and Australian species nearly all contain tertiary strychnine-like alkaloids.

Research on curare was accelerated by the work of Gill, who, after prolonged and intimate study of the native methods of preparing curare, brought to the U.S. a sufficient amount of the authentic drug to permit chemical and pharmacological investigations. The modern clinical use of curare apparently dates from 1932, when West employed highly purified fractions in patients with tetanus and spastic disorders. King established the essential structure of tubocurarine in 1935 (Figure 11–3). Griffith and Johnson reported the first trial of curare for promoting muscular relaxation in general anesthesia in 1942.

whereas the depolarizing agents (e.g., decamethonium [no longer marketed in the U.S.] and succinylcholine) generally have more flexible structures that enable free bond rotations. While the distance between quaternary groups in the flexible depolarizing agents can vary up to the limit of the maximal bond distance (1.45 nm for decamethonium), the distance for the rigid competitive blockers is typically 1.0 ± 0.1 nm.

Mechanism of Action

Competitive antagonists bind the N_m and thereby competitively block the binding of ACh. The depolarizing agents, such as succinylcholine, depolarize the membrane by opening channels in the same manner as ACh. However, they persist longer at the neuromuscular junction primarily because of their resistance to AChE. The depolarization is thus longer lasting, resulting in a brief period of repetitive excitation that may elicit transient and repetitive muscle excitation (fasciculations), followed by blocking of neuromuscular transmission and flaccid paralysis (called *phase I block*). The block arises because, after an initial opening, perijunctional Na^+ channels close and will not reopen until the end plate is repolarized. At this point, neural release of ACh results in the binding of ACh to receptors on an already-depolarized end plate. These closed perijunctional channels keep the depolarization signal from affecting downstream channels and effectively shield the rest of the muscle from activity at the motor end plate. This sequence is influenced by such factors as the anesthetic agent used concurrently, the type of muscle, and the rate of drug administration. The characteristics of depolarization and competitive blockade are contrasted in Table 11–1.

Under clinical conditions, with increasing concentrations of succinylcholine and over time, the block may convert slowly from a depolarizing phase I block to a nondepolarizing *phase II block* (Durant and Katz, 1982). While the response to peripheral stimulation during phase II block resembles that of the competitive agents, reversal of phase II block by administration of anti-AChE agents (e.g., with neostigmine) is difficult to predict and should be undertaken cautiously. The characteristics of phase I and phase II blocks are shown in Table 11–2.

Many drugs and toxins block neuromuscular transmission by other mechanisms, such as interference with the synthesis or release of ACh (Figure 8-6), but most of these agents are not employed clinically for neuromuscular blockade. One exception is the group of botulinum toxins, which are administered locally into muscles of the orbit in the management of ocular blepharospasm and strabismus and have been used to control other muscle spasms and to facilitate facial muscle relaxation (Table 8–7 and Chapter 70). This toxin also has been injected into the lower esophageal sphincter to treat achalasia (Chapter 50). The sites of action and interrelationship of several agents that serve as pharmacological tools are shown in Figure 11–4.

Sequence and Characteristics of Paralysis

Following intravenous injection of an appropriate dose of a *competitive blocking agent*, motor weakness progresses to total flaccid paralysis. Small, rapidly moving muscles such as those of the eyes, jaw, and larynx relax before those of the limbs and trunk. Ultimately, the intercostal muscles

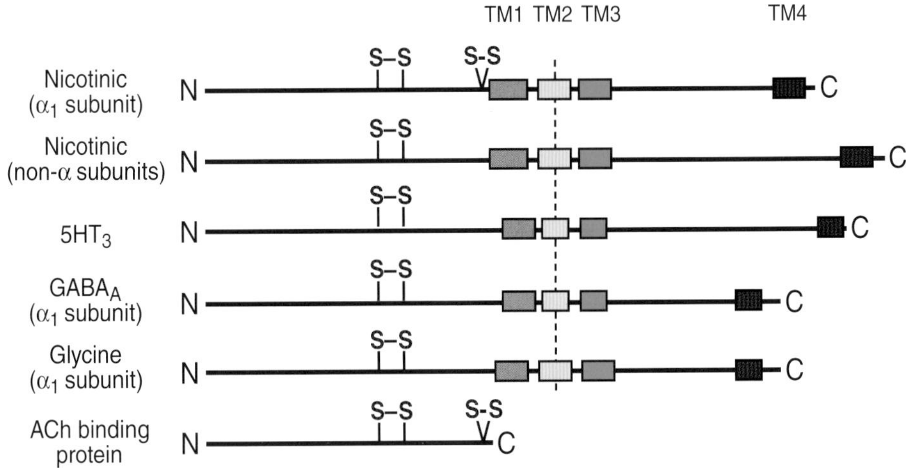

Figure 11–1 *Subunit organization of pentameric ligand-gated ion channels and the ACh-binding protein.* For each subunit of these pentameric receptors, the amino-terminal region of about 210 amino acids is found at the extracellular surface. It is then followed by four hydrophobic regions that span the membrane (TM1–TM4), leaving the small carboxyl terminus on the extracellular surface. The TM2 region is α-helical, and TM2 regions from each subunit of the pentameric receptor line the internal pore of the receptor. Two disulfide loops at positions 128–142 and 192–193 are found in the α subunit of the nicotinic receptor. The 128–142 motif is conserved in the family of receptors, whereas the vicinal cysteines at 192 and 193 distinguish α subunits and the ACh-binding protein from β, γ, δ, and ε in the nicotinic receptor.

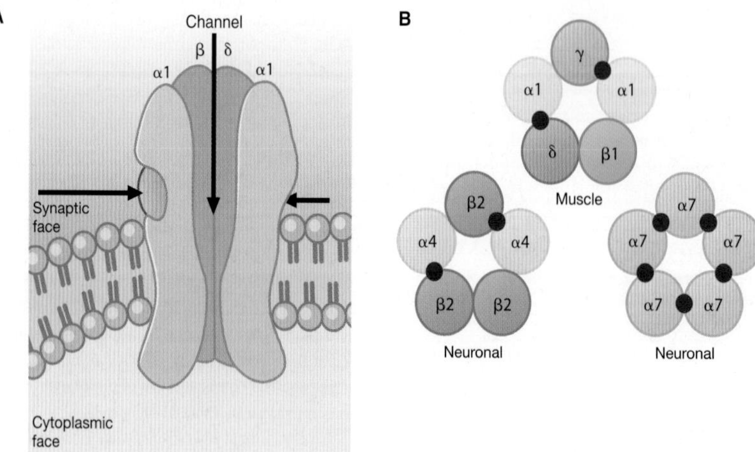

Figure 11–2 *Subunit arrangement and molecular structure of the nicotinic ACh receptor.* **A.** Longitudinal view of receptor schematic with the γ subunit removed. The remaining subunits, two copies of α, one of β, and one of δ, are shown to surround an internal channel with an outer vestibule and its constriction located deep in the membrane bilayer region. Spans of α-helices with slightly bowed structures form the perimeter of the channel and come from the TM2 region of the linear sequence (Figure 11–1). ACh-binding sites, indicated by red arrows, occur at the αγ and αδ (not visible) interfaces. **B.** Nicotinic receptor subunit arrangement, with examples of subunit assembly. Agonist binding sites (*red circles*) occur at α subunit–containing interfaces. A total of 17 functional receptor isoforms have been observed in vivo, with different ligand specificity, relative Ca^{2+}/Na^{+} permeability, and physiological function as determined by their subunit composition. The only isoform found at the neuromuscular junction is that shown here. There are 16 neuronal receptor isoforms found at autonomic ganglia and in the CNS, homo- and heteropentamers of α (α2–α10) and β (β2–β4) subunits.

and finally the diaphragm are paralyzed, and respiration then ceases. Recovery of muscles usually occurs in the reverse order to that of their paralysis, and thus the diaphragm ordinarily is the first muscle to regain function (Naguib et al., 2015).

After a single intravenous dose (10–30 mg) of the *depolarizing blocking agent* succinylcholine, muscle fasciculations, particularly over the chest and abdomen, occur briefly; then, relaxation occurs within 1 min, becomes maximal within 2 min, and generally disappears within 5 min. Transient apnea usually occurs at the time of maximal effect. Muscle relaxation of longer duration is achieved by continuous intravenous infusion. After infusion is discontinued, the effects of the drug usually disappear rapidly because of its efficient hydrolysis by plasma and hepatic butyrylcholinesterase. Muscle soreness may follow the administration of succinylcholine.

During prolonged depolarization, muscle cells may lose significant quantities of K^+ and gain Na^+, Cl^-, and Ca^{2+}. In patients with extensive injury to soft tissues, the efflux of K^+ following continued administration of succinylcholine can be life threatening. There are many conditions for which succinylcholine administration is contraindicated or should be undertaken with great caution. The change in the nature of the blockade produced by succinylcholine (from phase I to phase II) presents an additional complication with long-term infusions.

Effects in CNS and at Ganglia

Tubocurarine and other quaternary neuromuscular blocking agents are virtually devoid of central effects following ordinary clinical doses because of their inability to penetrate the blood-brain barrier.

Neuromuscular blocking agents show variable potencies in producing ganglionic blockade. Ganglionic blockade by tubocurarine and other stabilizing drugs is reversed or antagonized by anti-ChE agents (e.g., edrophonium, neostigmine, pyridostigmine, etc).

Clinical doses of tubocurarine produce partial blockade both at autonomic ganglia and at the adrenal medulla, resulting in a fall in blood pressure and tachycardia. Pancuronium shows less ganglionic blockade at common clinical doses. Atracurium, vecuronium, doxacurium, pipecuronium, mivacurium, and rocuronium are even more selective, showing less ganglionic blockade (Naguib et al., 2015). The maintenance of cardiovascular reflex responses usually is desired during anesthesia. Pancuronium has a vagolytic action, presumably from blockade of muscarinic receptors, which leads to tachycardia.

Of the depolarizing agents, succinylcholine at doses producing neuromuscular relaxation rarely causes effects attributable to ganglionic blockade. However, cardiovascular effects are sometimes observed, probably owing to the successive stimulation of vagal ganglia (manifested by bradycardia) and sympathetic ganglia (resulting in hypertension and tachycardia).

ADME

Quaternary ammonium neuromuscular blocking agents are poorly absorbed from the GI tract. Absorption is adequate from intramuscular sites. Rapid onset is achieved with intravenous administration. The more potent agents must be given in lower concentrations, and diffusional requirements slow their rate of onset.

When long-acting competitive blocking agents such as D-tubocurarine and pancuronium are administered, blockade may diminish after 30 min owing to redistribution of the drug, yet residual blockade and plasma levels of the drug persist. Subsequent doses show diminished redistribution *as tissues become saturated.* Long-acting agents may accumulate with multiple doses.

The amino steroids contain ester groups that are hydrolyzed in the liver. Typically, the metabolites have about one-half the activity of the parent compound and contribute to the total relaxation profile. Amino steroids of intermediate duration of action, such as vecuronium and rocuronium (Table 11–3), are cleared more rapidly by the liver than is pancuronium. The more rapid decay of neuromuscular blockade with compounds of intermediate duration argues for sequential dosing of these agents rather than administering a single dose of a long-duration neuromuscular blocking agent.

Atracurium is converted to less-active metabolites by plasma esterases and by spontaneous degradation in plasma and tissue (Hofmann elimination). Cisatracurium is also subject to this spontaneous degradation. Because of these alternative routes of metabolism, atracurium and cisatracurium do not exhibit an increased $t_{1/2}$ of elimination in patients with impaired renal function and therefore are good choices in this setting (Fisher et al., 1986; Naguib et al., 2015).

The extremely brief duration of action of succinylcholine is due largely to its rapid hydrolysis by the butyrylcholinesterase synthesized by the liver and found in the plasma. Among the occasional patients who exhibit prolonged apnea following the administration of succinylcholine or mivacurium, most have an atypical plasma cholinesterase or a deficiency of the enzyme owing to allelic variations, hepatic or renal disease, or a nutritional

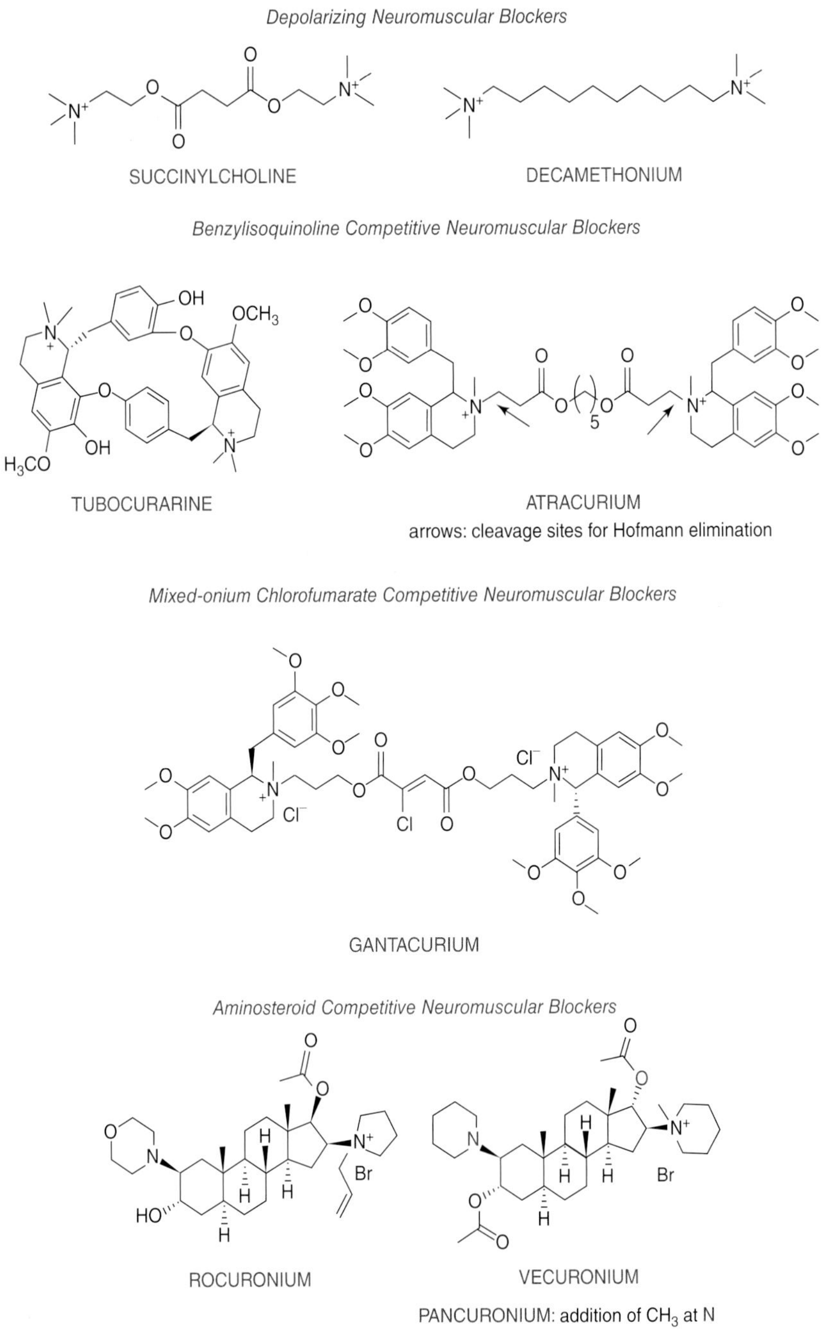

Depolarizing Neuromuscular Blockers

SUCCINYLCHOLINE

DECAMETHONIUM

Benzylisoquinoline Competitive Neuromuscular Blockers

TUBOCURARINE

ATRACURIUM
arrows: cleavage sites for Hofmann elimination

Mixed-onium Chlorofumarate Competitive Neuromuscular Blockers

GANTACURIUM

Aminosteroid Competitive Neuromuscular Blockers

ROCURONIUM

VECURONIUM
PANCURONIUM: addition of CH_3 at N

Figure 11–3 *Structural formulas of major neuromuscular blocking agents.*

disturbance; however, in some, the enzymatic activity in plasma is normal (Naguib et al., 2015).

Gantacurium is degraded by two chemical mechanisms, a rapid cysteine adduction and a slower hydrolysis of the ester bond adjacent to the chlorine. Both processes are purely chemical and hence not dependent on enzymatic activities. The adduction process has a $t_{1/2}$ of 1–2 min and is likely the basis for the ultrashort duration of action of gantacurium. Administration of exogenous cysteine, which may have excitotoxic side effects, can accelerate the antagonism of gantacurium-induced neuromuscular blockade (Naguib and Brull, 2009).

Clinical Pharmacology

Choice of Agent

Therapeutic selection of a neuromuscular blocking agent should be based on achieving a pharmacokinetic profile consistent with the duration of the interventional procedure and minimizing cardiovascular compromise or other side effects, with attention to drug-specific modes of elimination in patients with renal or hepatic failure (see Drug Facts Table).

Two characteristics are useful in distinguishing side effects and pharmacokinetic behavior of neuromuscular blocking agents:

TABLE 11–1 ■ COMPARISON OF COMPETITIVE (D-TUBOCURARINE) AND DEPOLARIZING (DECAMETHONIUM) BLOCKING AGENTS

	D-TUBOCURARINE	DECAMETHONIUM
Effect of D-tubocurarine administered previously	Additive	Antagonistic
Effect of decamethonium administered previously	No effect or antagonistic	Some tachyphylaxis, but may be additive
Effect of anticholinesterase agents on block	Reversal of block	No reversal
Effect on motor end plate	Elevated threshold to acetylcholine; no depolarization	Partial, persisting depolarization
Initial excitatory effect on striated muscle	None	Transient fasciculations
Character of muscle response to indirect tetanic stimulation during *partial* block	Poorly sustained contraction	Well-sustained contraction

TABLE 11–2 ■ CLINICAL RESPONSES AND MONITORING OF PHASE I AND PHASE II NEUROMUSCULAR BLOCKADE BY SUCCINYLCHOLINE INFUSION

RESPONSE	PHASE I	PHASE II
End-plate membrane potential	Depolarized to –55 mV	Repolarization toward –80 mV
Onset	Immediate	Slow transition
Dose dependence	Lower	Usually higher or follows prolonged infusion
Recovery	Rapid	More prolonged
Train of four and tetanic stimulation	No fade	Fade[a]
Acetylcholinesterase inhibition	Augments	Reverses or antagonizes
Muscle response	Fasciculations → flaccid paralysis	Flaccid paralysis

[a]Posttetanic potentiation follows fade.

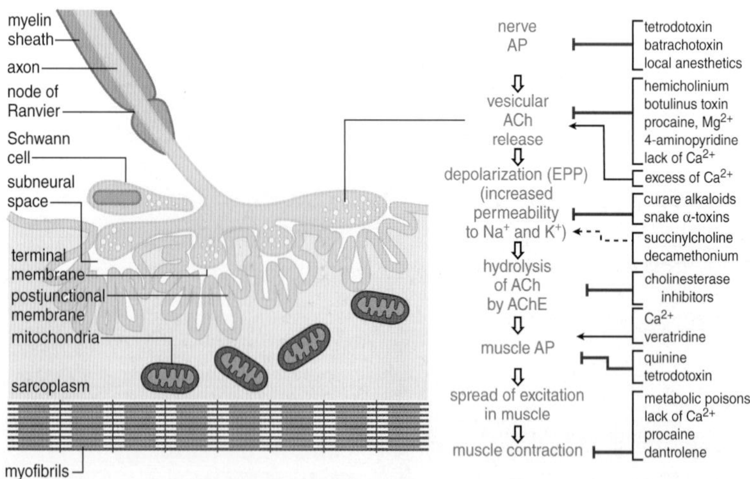

Figure 11–4 *A pharmacologist's view of the motor end plate.* The structures of the motor end plate (left side of figure) facilitate the series of physiological events leading from nerve action potential (AP) to skeletal muscle contraction (center column). Pharmacological agents can modify neurotransmission and excitation-contraction coupling at myriad sites (righthand column). ←——, enhancement; ⊢——, blockade; ←- - - -, depolarization and phase II block.

TABLE 11–3 ■ NEUROMUSCULAR BLOCKING AGENTS

AGENT Chemical Class *Type of action*	ONSET (min)[a]	DURATION (min)[a]	MODE OF ELIMINATION
Ultrashort and short duration			
Succinylcholine DCE, *depolarizing*	0.8–1.4	6–11	Hydrolysis by plasma cholinesterases
Gantacurium[c] MOCF, *competitive*	1–2	5–10	Cysteine adduction, ester hydrolysis
Mivacurium BIQ, *competitive*	2–3	15–21	Hydrolysis by plasma cholinesterases
Intermediate duration			
Vecuronium AS, *competitive*	2–3	25–40	Hepatic and renal elimination
Atracurium BIQ, *competitive*	3	45	Hofmann elimination; ester hydrolysis
Rocuronium AS, *competitive*	0.5–2	36–73	Hepatic elimination
Cisatracurium BIQ, *competitive*	2–8	45–90	Hofmann elimination; renal elimination
Long duration			
Pipecuronium[b] AS, *competitive*	3–6	30–90	Renal elimination; hepatic metabolism/clearance
D-Tubocurarine[b] CBI, *competitive*	6	80	Renal and hepatic elimination
Pancuronium AS, *competitive*	3–4	85–100	Renal and hepatic elimination
Metocurine[b] BIQ, *competitive*	4	110	Renal elimination
Doxacurium[b] BIQ, *competitive*	4–8	120	Renal elimination

[a]As achieved from dose ranges in Table 11–4.

[b]Not commercially available in the U.S.

[c]Gantacurium is in investigational status.

Abbreviations: AS, aminosteroid; BIQ, benzylisoquinoline; CBI (natural alkaloid), cyclic benzylisoquinoline; DCE, dicholine ester;

MOCF, assymetric mixed-onium chlorofumarate.

TABLE 11–4 ■ DOSING RANGES FOR NEUROMUSCULAR BLOCKING AGENTS

AGENT	INITIATION DOSE (mg/kg)	INTERMITTENT INJECTION (mg/kg)	CONTINUOUS INFUSION (μg/kg/min)
Succinylcholine	0.3–1	0.04–0.07	N/A
D-Tubocurarine[a]	0.6	0.25–0.5	2–3
Metocurine[a]	0.4	0.5–1	N/A
Atracurium	0.3–0.5	0.08–0.2	2–15
Cisatracurium	0.15–0.2	0.03	1–3
Mivacurium	0.15–0.25	0.1	9–10
Doxacurium[a]	0.03–0.06	0.005–0.01	N/A
Pancuronium	0.04–0.1	0.01	1[b]
Rocuronium	0.45–1.2	0.1–0.2	10–12
Vecuronium	0.04–0.28	0.01–0.015	0.8–1.2
Gantacurium[a]	0.2–0.5	N/A	N/A

[a]Not commercially available in the U.S.

[b]Off-label use.

- ***The chemical nature of the agents (Figure 11–3 and Table 11–3).*** Apart from a shorter duration of action, newer agents exhibit greatly diminished frequency of side effects, chiefly ganglionic blockade, block of vagal responses, and histamine release.
- ***Duration of drug action.*** These agents are categorized as long-, intermediate-, short-, or ultrashort-acting agents. Often, the long-acting agents are the more potent, requiring the use of low doses (Table 11–4). The necessity of administering potent agents at low concentrations delays their onset.

The prototypical amino steroid pancuronium induces virtually no histamine release; however, it blocks muscarinic receptors, an antagonism manifested primarily by vagal blockade and tachycardia. Tachycardia is eliminated in the newer amino steroids vecuronium and rocuronium. The benzylisoquinolines appear to be devoid of vagolytic and ganglionic blocking actions but show a slight propensity to cause histamine release. The unusual metabolism of the prototype compound atracurium and its congener mivacurium confers special indications for use of these compounds. For example, atracurium's disappearance from the body depends on hydrolysis of the ester moiety by plasma esterases and by a spontaneous or Hofmann degradation (cleavage of the *N*-alkyl portion in the benzylisoquinoline). Hence, two routes for termination of effect are available, both of which remain functional in renal failure. Mivacurium is extremely sensitive to catalysis by cholinesterase or other plasma hydrolases, accounting for its short duration of action. Side effects are not yet fully characterized for gantacurium, but transient adverse cardiovascular effects suggestive of histamine release have been observed at doses over three times the ED_{95} (Belmont et al., 2004).

Muscle Relaxation

The main clinical use of the neuromuscular blocking agents is as an adjuvant in surgical anesthesia to obtain relaxation of skeletal muscle, particularly of the abdominal wall, to facilitate operative manipulations. With muscle relaxation no longer dependent on the depth of general anesthesia, a much lighter level of anesthesia suffices. Thus, the risk of respiratory and cardiovascular depression is minimized, and postanesthetic recovery is shortened. Neuromuscular blocking agents of short duration often are used to facilitate endotracheal intubation and have been used to facilitate laryngoscopy, bronchoscopy, and esophagoscopy in combination with a general anesthetic agent. Neuromuscular blocking agents are administered parenterally, nearly always intravenously. These agents may be administered by continuous infusion in the intensive care setting for improving chest wall compliance and eliminating ventilator dyssynchrony.

Measurement of Neuromuscular Blockade in Humans

Assessment of neuromuscular block usually is performed by stimulation of the ulnar nerve (Naguib et al., 2015). Responses are monitored from compound action potentials or muscle tension developed in the adductor pollicis (thumb) muscle. Responses to repetitive or tetanic stimuli are most useful for evaluation of blockade of transmission. Rates of onset of blockade and recovery are more rapid in the airway musculature (jaw, larynx, and diaphragm) than in the thumb. Hence, tracheal intubation can be performed before onset of complete block at the adductor pollicis, whereas partial recovery of function of this muscle allows sufficient recovery of respiration for extubation.

Preventing Trauma During Electroshock Therapy

Electroconvulsive therapy of psychiatric disorders occasionally is complicated by trauma to the patient; the seizures induced may cause dislocations or fractures. Inasmuch as the muscular component of the convulsion is not essential for benefit from the procedure, neuromuscular blocking agents, usually succinylcholine, and a short-acting barbiturate, usually methohexital, are employed.

Control of Muscle Spasms and Rigidity

Botulinum toxins and dantrolene act peripherally to reduce muscle contraction; a variety of other agents act centrally to reduce skeletal muscle tone and spasm. IncobotulinumtoxinA, onabotulinumtoxinA, abobotulinumtoxinA, and rimabotulinumtoxinB, by blocking ACh release, produce flaccid paralysis of skeletal muscle and diminished activity of parasympathetic and sympathetic cholinergic synapses. Inhibition lasts from several weeks to 3–4 months, and restoration of function requires nerve sprouting.

Originally approved for the treatment of the ocular conditions of strabismus and blepharospasm and for hemifacial spasms, botulinum toxins have been used to treat spasms and dystonias and spasms associated with the lower esophageal sphincter and anal fissures. Botulinum toxin treatments also have become a popular cosmetic procedure for those seeking a wrinkle-free face. Like the bloom of youth, the reduction of wrinkles is temporary; unlike the bloom of youth, the effect of botulinum toxin can be renewed by readministration. The FDA has issued a safety alert, warning of respiratory paralysis from unexpected spread of the toxin from the site of injection (uses are described in Chapter 70).

Dantrolene inhibits Ca^{2+} release from the sarcoplasmic reticulum of skeletal muscle by limiting the capacity of Ca^{2+} and calmodulin to activate the ryanodine receptor, RYR1. Because of its efficacy in managing an acute attack of malignant hyperthermia (described separately in the section Adverse Effects), dantrolene has been used experimentally in the treatment of muscle rigidity and hyperthermia in neuroleptic malignant syndrome. Dantrolene is also used in treatment of spasticity and hyperreflexia. With its peripheral action, it causes generalized weakness. Thus, its use should be reserved to nonambulatory patients with severe spasticity. Hepatotoxicity has been reported with chronic use, requiring frequent liver function tests and use of the lowest possible oral dose.

Several agents, many of limited efficacy, have been used to treat spasticity involving the α-motor neurons originating in the brainstem and spinal cord. Agents that act in the CNS at either higher centers or the spinal cord to block spasms, with the objective of increasing functional capacity and relieving discomfort, include baclofen, the benzodiazepines, tizanidine, and cyclobenzaprine. A number of other agents used as muscle relaxants seem to rely on sedative properties and blockade of nociceptive pathways; this group includes carisoprodol (which is metabolized to meprobamate; see Chapter 19); metaxalone; methocarbamol; and orphenadrine. Tetrabenazine is available for treatment of the chorea associated with Huntington disease; the drug is a VMAT2 inhibitor that depletes vesicular stores of dopamine in the CNS (Chapters 8 and 18).

Synergisms and Antagonisms

The comparison of interactions between competitive and depolarizing neuromuscular blocking agents is instructive (Table 11–1) and a good test of one's understanding of the drugs' actions. In addition, many other drugs affect transmission at the neuromuscular junction and thus can affect the choice and dosage of neuromuscular blocking agent used.

Because the anti-ChE agents neostigmine, pyridostigmine, and edrophonium preserve endogenous ACh and also act at the neuromuscular junction, they have been used in the treatment of overdosage with competitive blocking agents. Similarly, on completion of the surgical procedure, many anesthesiologists employ neostigmine or edrophonium to reverse and decrease the duration of competitive neuromuscular blockade. A muscarinic antagonist (atropine or glycopyrrolate) is used concomitantly to prevent stimulation of muscarinic receptors and thereby to avoid slowing of the heart rate. Anti-ChE agents will not reverse depolarizing neuromuscular blockade and, in fact, can enhance it.

Many inhalational anesthetics exert a stabilizing effect on the postjunctional membrane and therefore potentiate the activity of competitive blocking agents. Consequently, when such blocking drugs are used for muscle relaxation as adjuncts to these anesthetics, their doses should be reduced. The rank order of potentiation is desflurane > sevoflurane > isoflurane > halothane > nitrous oxide-barbiturate-opioid or propofol anesthesia (Naguib et al., 2015).

Aminoglycoside antibiotics produce neuromuscular blockade by inhibiting ACh release from the preganglionic terminal (through competition with Ca^{2+}) and to a lesser extent by noncompetitively blocking the receptor. The blockade is antagonized by Ca^{2+} salts but only inconsistently by anti-ChE agents (see Chapter 58). The tetracyclines also can produce neuromuscular blockade, possibly by chelation of Ca^{2+}. Additional antibiotics that have neuromuscular blocking action, through both presynaptic and postsynaptic actions, include polymyxin B, colistin, clindamycin, and lincomycin. Ca^{2+} channel blockers enhance neuromuscular blockade produced by both competitive and depolarizing antagonists. When neuromuscular blocking agents are administered to patients receiving these agents, dose adjustments should be considered.

Miscellaneous drugs that may have significant interactions with either competitive or depolarizing neuromuscular blocking agents include trimethaphan, lithium, opioid analgesics, procaine, lidocaine, quinidine, phenelzine, carbamazepine, phenytoin, propranolol, dantrolene, azathioprine, tamoxifen, magnesium salts, corticosteroids, digitalis glycosides, chloroquine, catecholamines, and diuretics.

Adverse Effects

The important untoward responses of the neuromuscular blocking agents include prolonged apnea, cardiovascular collapse, those resulting from histamine release, and, rarely, anaphylaxis. Related factors may include alterations in body temperature; electrolyte imbalance, particularly of K^+; low plasma butyrylcholinesterase levels, resulting in a reduction in the rate of destruction of succinylcholine; the presence of latent myasthenia gravis or of malignant disease such as small cell carcinoma of the lung with Eaton-Lambert myasthenic syndrome; reduced blood flow to skeletal muscles, causing delayed removal of the blocking drugs; and decreased elimination of the muscle relaxants secondary to hepatic dysfunction (cisatracurium, rocuronium, vecuronium) or reduced renal function (pancuronium). Great care should be taken when administering neuromuscular blockers to dehydrated or severely ill patients. Depolarizing agents can cause rapid release of K^+ from intracellular sites; this may be a factor in production of the prolonged apnea in patients who receive these drugs while in electrolyte imbalance. Succinylcholine-induced hyperkalemia is a life-threatening complication of that drug.

Malignant Hyperthermia. Malignant hyperthermia is a potentially life-threatening event triggered by the administration of certain anesthetics and neuromuscular blocking agents. The clinical features include contracture, rigidity, and heat production from skeletal muscle, resulting in severe hyperthermia (increases of up to 1°C/5 min), accelerated muscle metabolism, metabolic acidosis, and tachycardia. Uncontrolled release of Ca^{2+} from the sarcoplasmic reticulum of skeletal muscle is the initiating event. Although the halogenated hydrocarbon anesthetics (e.g., halothane, isoflurane, and sevoflurane) and succinylcholine alone have been reported to precipitate the response, most of the incidents arise from the combination of depolarizing blocking agent and anesthetic. Susceptibility to malignant hyperthermia, an autosomal dominant trait, is associated with certain congenital myopathies, such as *central core disease*. In the majority of cases, however, no clinical signs are visible in the absence of anesthetic intervention.

Treatment entails intravenous administration of dantrolene, which blocks Ca^{2+} release from the sarcoplasmic reticulum of skeletal muscle (see previous discussion, Control of Muscle Spasms and Rigidity). Rapid cooling, inhalation of 100% O_2, and control of acidosis should be considered adjunct therapy in malignant hyperthermia.

Respiratory Paralysis. Treatment of respiratory paralysis arising from an adverse reaction or overdose of a neuromuscular blocking agent should be by positive-pressure artificial respiration with O_2 and maintenance of a patent airway until recovery of normal respiration is ensured. With the competitive blocking agents, this may be hastened by the administration of neostigmine methylsulfate (0.5–2 mg IV) or edrophonium (10 mg IV, repeated as required up to a total of 40 mg) (Watkins, 1994). In the case of overdose, a muscarinic cholinergic antagonist (atropine or glycopyrrolate) may be added to prevent undue slowing of the heart (see Synergisms and Antagonisms).

Histamine Release From Mast Cells. Some clinical responses to neuromuscular blocking agents (e.g., bronchospasm, hypotension, excessive bronchial and salivary secretion) appear to be caused by the release of histamine. Succinylcholine, mivacurium, and atracurium cause histamine release, but to a lesser extent than tubocurarine unless administered rapidly. The amino steroids pancuronium, vecuronium, pipecuronium, and rocuronium have even less tendency to release histamine after intradermal or systemic injection (Basta, 1992; Watkins, 1994). Histamine release typically is a direct action of the muscle relaxant on the mast cell rather than anaphylaxis mediated by immunoglobulin E.

Interventional Strategies for Toxic Effects

Neostigmine effectively antagonizes only the skeletal muscular blocking action of the competitive blocking agents and may aggravate such side effects as hypotension or induce bronchospasm. In such circumstances, sympathomimetic amines may be given to support the blood pressure. Atropine or glycopyrrolate is administered to counteract muscarinic stimulation. Antihistamines are definitely beneficial to counteract the responses that follow the release of histamine, particularly when administered before the neuromuscular blocking agent.

Reversal of Effects by Chelation Therapy. Sugammadex, a modified γ-cyclodextrin, is a chelating agent specific for rocuronium and vecuronium. Sugammadex at doses greater than 2 mg/kg is able to reverse neuromuscular blockade from rocuronium within 3 min. Sugammadex clearance is markedly reduced in patients with impaired renal function, and use of this agent should be avoided. Sugammadex is approved for clinical use in Europe but not yet in the U.S. Side effects include dysgeusia and rare hypersensitivity.

Pediatric and Geriatric Indications and Problems

Because the neuromuscular junction is not fully developed at birth, additional care must be taken in administration of neuromuscular blocking agents to infants and children. Succinylcholine is not safe for routine use in pediatric patients, and its use must be reserved for extreme emergency situations where immediate securing of the airway is necessary and other options for neuromuscular blockade are not available. Competitive blocking agents, however, are commonly used in pediatric patients; generally, dosage is similar to adults but both rate of block onset and clearance are faster. Atracurium is an exception: The dosage and duration of action are not significantly different between children older than 2 years and adults, and the same dose (0.25 to 0.5 mg/kg) can be used among these populations for tracheal intubation. Vecuronium, cisatracurium, rocuronium, and mivacurium are also commonly administered to children for short procedures where only a single intubating dose is required.

There are normal changes at the neuromuscular junction in elderly patients that may affect pharmacodynamics of neuromuscular blocking agents. With aging, the distance between the terminus of the motor neuron and the end plate increases, the end-plate invaginations become flatter, the amount of transmitter per synaptic vesicle decreases, the vesicle release probability is lower, and the density of receptors at the end plate decreases. The end result of these changes is decreased efficiency of neuromuscular transmission. General physiological changes in aging patients, including decreases in body water and muscle, increases in total body fat, and decreases in renal and hepatic function, also contribute to the action of neuromuscular blockers. The dosing of succinylcholine is not significantly altered in the geriatric population. Among the competitive blocking agents, initial dose requirements are unchanged, however, the onset of blockade is delayed in an age-related manner, and block is prolonged. For compounds dependent on the kidney, liver, or both for clearance, such as pancuronium, vecuronium, and rocuronium, plasma clearance times are prolonged by 30%–50% (Naguib et al., 2015). For compounds such as atracurium that are not dependent on hepatic or renal blood flow for their elimination, pharmacodynamics and kinetics are largely unaltered.

Ganglionic Neurotransmission

The Neural Nicotinic Receptor and Postsynaptic Potentials

Neurotransmission in autonomic ganglia involves release of ACh by preganglionic fibers and the rapid depolarization of postsynaptic membranes via the activation of neuronal nicotinic (N_n) receptors by ACh. Unlike the neuromuscular junction, ganglia do not have discrete end plates with focal localization of receptors; rather, the dendrites and nerve cell bodies contain the receptors. The characteristics of nicotinic-receptor channels of the ganglia and the neuromuscular junction are similar. There are multiple nicotinic receptor subunits (e.g., α3, α5, α7, β2, and β4) in ganglia, with α3 and β4 most abundant and important. The ganglionic nicotinic ACh receptors are sensitive to classical blocking agents such as hexamethonium and trimethaphan (see discussion that follows). Measurements of single-channel conductances indicate that the characteristics of nicotinic receptor channels of the ganglia and the neuromuscular junction are similar.

Intracellular recordings from postganglionic neurons indicate that at least four different changes in postsynaptic membrane potential can be elicited by stimulation of the preganglionic nerve (Figure 11–5):

- An initial EPSP (via nicotinic receptors) that may result in an action potential
- An IPSP mediated by M_2 (G_i/G_o-coupled) muscarinic receptors

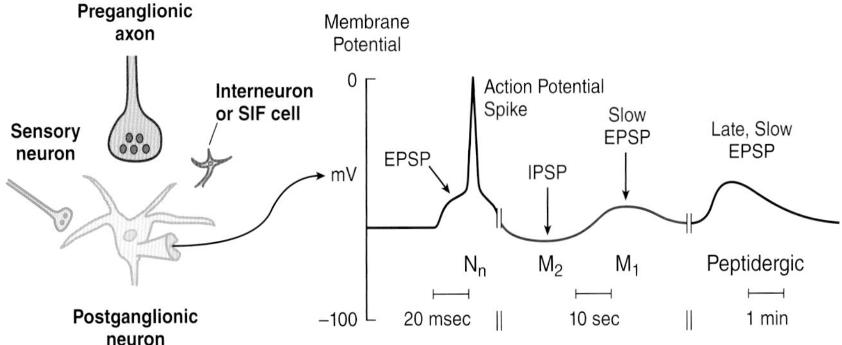

Figure 11–5 *Postsynaptic potentials recorded from an autonomic postganglionic nerve cell body after stimulation of the preganglionic nerve fiber.* The preganglionic nerve releases ACh onto postganglionic cells. The initial EPSP results from the inward Na^+ current (and perhaps Ca^{2+} current) through the nicotinic receptor channel. If the EPSP is of sufficient magnitude, it triggers an action potential spike, which is followed by a slow IPSP, a slow EPSP, and a late, slow EPSP. The slow IPSP and slow EPSP are not seen in all ganglia. The electrical events subsequent to the initial EPSP are thought to modulate the probability that a subsequent EPSP will reach the threshold for triggering a spike. Other interneurons, such as catecholamine-containing SIF cells, and axon terminals from sensory, afferent neurons also release transmitters, which may influence the slow potentials of the postganglionic neuron. A number of cholinergic, peptidergic, adrenergic, and amino acid receptors are found on the dendrites and soma of the postganglionic neuron and the interneurons. The preganglionic fiber releases ACh and peptides; the interneurons store and release catecholamines, amino acids, and peptides; the sensory afferent nerve terminals release peptides. The initial EPSP is mediated through nicotinic (N_n) receptors, the slow IPSP and EPSP through M_2 and M_1 muscarinic receptors, and the late, slow EPSP through several types of peptidergic receptors.

- A secondary slow EPSP mediated by M_1 (G_q/G_{11}-coupled) muscarinic receptors
- A late, slow EPSP mediated by myriad peptides

An action potential is generated in the postganglionic neuron when the initial EPSP achieves a threshold potential. The events that follow the initial depolarization (IPSP; slow EPSP; late, slow EPSP) are insensitive to hexamethonium or other N_n antagonists. Electrophysiological and neurochemical evidence suggests that catecholamines participate in the generation of the IPSP. Dopamine and norepinephrine cause hyperpolarization of ganglia; however, in some ganglia IPSPs are mediated by M_2 muscarinic receptors.

The slow EPSP is generated by ACh activation of M_1 muscarinic receptors and is blocked by atropine and M_1-selective antagonists (see Chapter 9). The slow EPSP has a longer latency and greater duration (10–30 sec) than the initial EPSP. Slow EPSPs result from decreased K^+ conductance, the *M current* that regulates the sensitivity of the cell to repetitive fast-depolarizing events. By contrast, the late, slow EPSP lasts for several minutes and is mediated by peptides released from presynaptic nerve endings or interneurons in specific ganglia (see next section). The peptides and ACh may be coreleased at the presynaptic nerve terminals; the relative stability of the peptides in the ganglion extends its sphere of influence to postsynaptic sites beyond those in the immediate proximity of the nerve ending.

Secondary synaptic events modulate the initial EPSP. A variety of peptides, including gonadotropin-releasing hormone, substance P, angiotensin, calcitonin gene–related peptide, vasoactive intestinal polypeptide, neuropeptide Y, and enkephalins, have been identified in ganglia by immunofluorescence. They appear localized to particular cell bodies, nerve fibers, or small, intensely fluorescent (SIF) cells; are released on nerve stimulation; and are presumed to mediate the late, slow EPSP. Other neurotransmitter substances (e.g., 5HT and GABA) can modify ganglionic transmission.

Ganglionic Stimulating Agents

Drugs that stimulate N_n cholinergic receptors on autonomic ganglia have been essential for analyzing the mechanism of ganglionic function; however, these ganglionic agonists have limited therapeutic use. They can be grouped into two categories. The first group consists of drugs with specificities similar to nicotine: lobeline, tetramethylammonium, and dimethylphenylpiperazinium. Nicotine's excitatory effects on ganglia are rapid in onset, are blocked by ganglionic nicotinic-receptor antagonists, and mimic the initial EPSP. The second group consists of muscarinic receptor agonists such as muscarine, McN-A-343, and methacholine (see Chapter 9); their excitatory effects on ganglia are delayed in onset, blocked by atropine-like drugs, and mimic the slow EPSP.

Nicotine

Nicotine is of considerable medical significance because of its toxicity, presence in tobacco, and propensity for conferring dependence on its users. The chronic effects of nicotine and the untoward effects of the chronic use of tobacco are considered in Chapter 24. Nicotine is one of the few natural liquid alkaloids. It is a colorless, volatile base (pK_a = 8.5) that turns brown and acquires the odor of tobacco on exposure to air.

H N+ N

NICOTINE

Mechanism of Action. In addition to the actions of nicotine on a variety of neuroeffector and chemosensitive sites, the alkaloid can both stimulate and desensitize receptors, making nicotine's effects complex and unpredictable. The ultimate response of any one system represents the summation of stimulatory and inhibitory effects of nicotine. Nicotine can increase heart rate by excitation of sympathetic ganglia or by paralysis of parasympathetic cardiac ganglia, and it can slow heart rate by paralysis of sympathetic or stimulation of parasympathetic cardiac ganglia. The effects of the drug on the chemoreceptors of the carotid and aortic bodies and on regions of the CNS also can influence heart rate, as can the compensatory baroreceptor reflexes resulting from changes in blood pressure caused by nicotine. Finally, nicotine can stimulate secretion of epinephrine from the adrenal medulla, which accelerates heart rate and raises blood pressure.

Effects on Physiological Systems

Peripheral Nervous System. The major action of nicotine consists initially of transient stimulation and then a more persistent depression of all autonomic ganglia. Small doses of nicotine stimulate the ganglion cells directly and may facilitate impulse transmission. Following larger doses, the initial stimulation is followed by a blockade of transmission. Whereas stimulation of the ganglion cells coincides with their depolarization, depression of transmission by adequate doses of nicotine occurs both during the depolarization and after it has subsided. Nicotine also possesses a biphasic action on the adrenal medulla: Small doses evoke the discharge of catecholamines; larger doses prevent their release in response to splanchnic nerve stimulation.

The effects of high doses of nicotine on the neuromuscular junction are similar to those on ganglia. However, the stimulant phase is obscured largely by the rapidly developing paralysis. In the latter stage, nicotine also produces neuromuscular blockade by receptor desensitization. At lower concentrations, such as those typically achieved by recreational tobacco use (~200 nM), nicotine's effects reflect its higher affinity for a neuronal nicotinic receptor ($\alpha4\beta2$) than for the neuromuscular junction receptor ($\alpha_1\beta_1\gamma\delta$) (Xiu et al., 2009).

Nicotine, like ACh, stimulates a number of sensory receptors. These include mechanoreceptors that respond to stretch or pressure of the skin, mesentery, tongue, lung, and stomach; chemoreceptors of the carotid body; thermal receptors of the skin and tongue; and pain receptors. Prior administration of hexamethonium prevents stimulation of the sensory receptors by nicotine but has little, if any, effect on the activation of sensory receptors by physiological stimuli.

Central Nervous System. Nicotine markedly stimulates the CNS. Low doses produce weak analgesia; higher doses cause tremors, leading to convulsions at toxic doses. The excitation of respiration is a prominent action of nicotine: Large doses act directly on the medulla oblongata, whereas smaller doses augment respiration reflexly by excitation of the chemoreceptors of the carotid and aortic bodies. Stimulation of the CNS with large doses is followed by depression, and death results from failure of respiration owing to both central paralysis and peripheral blockade of the diaphragm and intercostal muscles that facilitate respiration.

Nicotine induces vomiting by both central and peripheral actions. The central component of the vomiting response is due to stimulation of the emetic chemoreceptor trigger zone in the area postrema of the medulla oblongata. In addition, nicotine activates vagal and spinal afferent nerves that form the sensory input of the reflex pathways involved in the act of vomiting. The primary sites of action of nicotine in the CNS are prejunctional, causing the release of other transmitters. The stimulatory and pleasure-reward actions of nicotine appear to result from release of excitatory amino acids, dopamine, and other biogenic amines from various CNS centers (Dorostkar and Boehm, 2008).

Chronic exposure to nicotine in several systems causes a marked increase in the density or number of nicotinic receptors, possibly contributing to tolerance and dependence. Nicotine is thought to act as an intracellular pharmacological chaperone; it is uncharged at physiological pH and readily permeates the plasma membrane. Inside the cell, it upregulates receptor expression by stabilizing nascent subunits in pentamers in the endoplasmic reticulum. Chronic low-dose exposure to nicotine also significantly increases the $t_{1/2}$ of nicotinic receptors on the cell surface (Kuryatov et al., 2005; Srinivasan et al., 2014).

Cardiovascular System. In general, the cardiovascular responses to nicotine are due to stimulation of sympathetic ganglia and the adrenal medulla, together with the discharge of catecholamines from sympathetic nerve endings. Contributing to the sympathomimetic response to nicotine is the activation of chemoreceptors of the aortic and carotid bodies, which reflexly results in vasoconstriction, tachycardia, and elevated blood pressure.

GI Tract. The combined activation of parasympathetic ganglia and cholinergic nerve endings by nicotine results in increased tone and motor activity of the bowel. Nausea, vomiting, and occasionally diarrhea are observed following systemic absorption of nicotine in an individual who has not been exposed to nicotine previously.

Exocrine Glands. Nicotine causes an initial stimulation of salivary and bronchial secretions that is followed by inhibition.

ADME. Nicotine is readily absorbed from the respiratory tract, buccal membranes, and skin. Severe poisoning has resulted from percutaneous absorption. As a relatively strong base, nicotine has limited absorption from the stomach. Intestinal absorption is far more efficient. Nicotine in chewing tobacco, because it is absorbed more slowly than inhaled nicotine, has a longer duration of effect. The average cigarette contains 6–11 mg nicotine and delivers about 1–3 mg nicotine systemically to the smoker; bioavailability can increase as much as 3-fold with the intensity of puffing and technique of the smoker (Benowitz, 1998).

Approximately 80%–90% of nicotine is altered in the body, mainly in the liver but also in the kidney and lung. Cotinine is the major metabolite. The $t_{1/2}$ of nicotine following inhalation is about 2 h. Nicotine and its metabolites are eliminated rapidly by the kidney. The rate of urinary excretion of nicotine diminishes when the urine is alkaline. Nicotine also is excreted in the milk of lactating women who smoke; the milk of heavy smokers may contain 0.5 mg/L.

Acute Adverse Effects. Poisoning from nicotine may occur from accidental ingestion of nicotine-containing insecticide sprays or in children from ingestion of tobacco products. The acutely fatal dose of nicotine for an adult is probably about 60 mg. Smoking tobacco usually contains 1%–2% nicotine. The gastric absorption of nicotine from tobacco taken by mouth is delayed because of slowed gastric emptying, so vomiting caused by the central effect of the initially absorbed fraction may remove much of the tobacco remaining in the GI tract.

The onset of symptoms of acute, severe nicotine poisoning is rapid; they include nausea, salivation, abdominal pain, vomiting, diarrhea, cold sweat, headache, dizziness, disturbed hearing and vision, mental confusion, and marked weakness. Faintness and prostration ensue; the blood pressure falls; breathing is difficult; the pulse is weak, rapid, and irregular; and collapse may be followed by terminal convulsions. Death may result within a few minutes from respiratory failure.

For treating nicotine poisoning, vomiting may be induced, or gastric lavage should be performed. Alkaline solutions should be avoided. A slurry of activated charcoal is then passed through the tube and left in the stomach. Respiratory assistance and treatment of shock may be necessary.

Ganglionic Blocking Agents

There are two categories of agents that block ganglionic nicotinic receptors. The prototype of the first group, nicotine, initially stimulates the ganglia by an ACh-like action and then blocks them by causing persistent depolarization (Volle, 1980). Compounds in the second category (e.g., *trimethaphan* and *hexamethonium*) impair transmission. Trimethaphan acts by competition with ACh, analogous to the mechanism of action of curare at the neuromuscular junction. Hexamethonium appears to block the channel after it opens; this action shortens the duration of current flow because the open channel either becomes occluded or closes. Thus, the initial EPSP is blocked, and ganglionic transmission is inhibited. Representative diverse chemicals that block autonomic ganglia without first causing stimulation are shown in Figure 11–6.

Ganglionic blocking agents were the first effective therapy for the treatment of hypertension. However, due to the role of ganglionic transmission in both sympathetic and parasympathetic neurotransmission, the antihypertensive action of ganglionic blocking agents was accompanied by numerous undesirable side effects. Mecamylamine, a secondary amine with a channel block mechanism similar to hexamethonium, is available as an antihypertensive agent with good oral bioavailability.

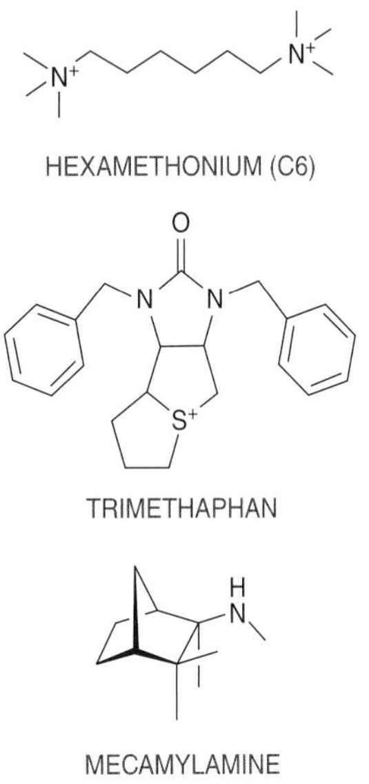

HEXAMETHONIUM (C6)

TRIMETHAPHAN

MECAMYLAMINE

Figure 11–6 *Ganglionic blocking agents.*

Mechanism of Action

Nearly all the physiological alterations observed after the administration of ganglionic blocking agents can be anticipated with reasonable accuracy by a careful inspection of Figure 8–1 and Table 8–1, and by knowing which division of the autonomic nervous system exercises dominant control of various organs (Table 11–5). For example, blockade of sympathetic ganglia interrupts adrenergic control of arterioles and results in vasodilation, improved peripheral blood flow in some vascular beds, and a fall in blood pressure.

Generalized ganglionic blockade also may result in atony of the bladder and GI tract, cycloplegia, xerostomia, diminished perspiration, and, by abolishing circulatory reflex pathways, postural hypotension. These changes represent the generally undesirable features of ganglionic blockade that severely limit the therapeutic efficacy of ganglionic blocking agents.

Cardiovascular Effects

Existing sympathetic tone is a critical determinant of the degree ganglionic blockade will lower blood pressure. Thus, blood pressure may decrease only minimally in recumbent normotensive subjects but may fall markedly in sitting or standing subjects. Postural hypotension limits the use of ganglionic blockers in ambulatory patients. Changes in heart rate following ganglionic blockade depend largely on existing vagal tone. In humans, only mild tachycardia usually accompanies the hypotension, a sign that indicates fairly complete ganglionic blockade. However, a decrease may occur if the heart rate is high initially. Cardiac output often is reduced by ganglionic blocking drugs in patients with normal cardiac function, as a consequence of venodilation, peripheral pooling of blood, and the resulting decrease in venous return. In patients with cardiac failure, ganglionic blockade frequently results in increased cardiac output owing to a reduction in peripheral resistance. In hypertensive subjects, cardiac output, stroke volume, and left ventricular work are diminished. Although total systemic vascular resistance is decreased in patients who receive ganglionic blocking agents, changes in blood flow and vascular resistance of individual vascular beds are variable. Reduction of cerebral blood flow is small unless mean systemic blood pressure falls below 50–60 mm Hg. Skeletal muscle blood flow is unaltered, but splanchnic and renal blood flow decrease.

ADME

The absorption of quaternary ammonium and sulfonium compounds from the enteric tract is incomplete and unpredictable. This is due both

TABLE 11–5 ■ USUAL PREDOMINANCE OF SYMPATHETIC OR PARASYMPATHETIC TONE AT VARIOUS EFFECTOR SITES AND CONSEQUENCES OF AUTONOMIC GANGLIONIC BLOCKADE

SITE	PREDOMINANT TONE	EFFECT OF GANGLIONIC BLOCKADE
Arterioles	Sympathetic (adrenergic)	Vasodilation; increased peripheral blood flow; hypotension
Veins	Sympathetic (adrenergic)	Dilation: peripheral pooling of blood; decreased venous return; decreased cardiac output
Heart	Parasympathetic (cholinergic)	Tachycardia
Iris	Parasympathetic (cholinergic)	Mydriasis
Ciliary muscle	Parasympathetic (cholinergic)	Cycloplegia—focus to far vision
Gastrointestinal tract	Parasympathetic (cholinergic)	Reduced tone and motility; constipation; decreased gastric and pancreatic secretions
Urinary bladder	Parasympathetic (cholinergic)	Urinary retention
Salivary glands	Parasympathetic (cholinergic)	Xerostomia
Sweat glands	Sympathetic (cholinergic)	Anhidrosis
Genital tract	Sympathetic and parasympathetic	Decreased stimulation

to the limited ability of these ionized substances to penetrate cell membranes and to the depression of propulsive movements of the small intestine and gastric emptying. Although the absorption of mecamylamine is less erratic, reduced bowel activity and paralytic ileus are a danger. After absorption, the quaternary ammonium- and sulfonium-blocking agents are confined primarily to the extracellular space and are excreted mostly unchanged by the kidney. Mecamylamine concentrates in the liver and kidney and is excreted slowly in an unchanged form.

Therapeutic Uses; Adverse Effects

Trimethaphan was once used for the induction of controlled hypotension during surgery to reduce bleeding and for the rapid reduction of blood pressure in the treatment of hypertensive emergencies; however, the agent is no longer marketed in the U.S.

Among the milder untoward responses observed are visual disturbances, dry mouth, conjunctival suffusion, urinary hesitancy, decreased potency, subjective chilliness, moderate constipation, occasional diarrhea, abdominal discomfort, anorexia, heartburn, nausea, eructation, and bitter taste and the signs and symptoms of syncope caused by postural hypotension. More severe reactions include marked hypotension, constipation, syncope, paralytic ileus, urinary retention, and cycloplegia.

Nicotine Addiction and Smoking Cessation

As a therapeutic, nicotine is primarily used to aid in smoking cessation. Two goals of the pharmacotherapy of smoking cessation are the reduction of the craving for nicotine and inhibition of the reinforcing effects of smoking. Myriad approaches and drug regimens are used, including NRT, bupropion (a CNS-active nicotinic antagonist; see Chapter 15), and partial agonists of the nicotinic ACh receptor (e.g., varenicline).

Current consensus is that NRT, bupropion, and varenicline all help smokers to quit their smoking habit. Cytisine (not approved for use in Europe or the U.S.) also appears effective. The safety and efficacy of NRT are clear. The highest rates of smoking cessation (~30% success at maintaining abstinence from smoking for 6 months) result from the combination of NRT (e.g., patch plus inhaler) and varenicline (Cahill et al., 2013, 2014).

Nicotine Replacement Therapy

Nicotine replacement therapy is available in several dosage forms to help achieve abstinence from tobacco use. Nicotine is marketed for over-the-counter use as a gum or lozenge or transdermal patch and by prescription as a nasal spray or vapor inhaler. Different nicotine delivery systems produce different patterns of exposure (see Figure 24–2; St. Helen et al., 2016). The efficacy of these dosage forms in producing abstinence from smoking is enhanced when linked to counseling and motivational therapy (Frishman, 2009; Prochaska and Benowitz 2016).

Varenicline

Varenicline has been recently introduced as an aid to smoking cessation. The drug interacts with nicotinic ACh receptors. In model systems, varenicline is a partial agonist at $\alpha4\beta2$ receptors, which is thought to be the principal nicotinic receptor subtype involved in nicotine addiction. Varenicline is a full agonist at the $\alpha7$ subtype and exhibits weak activity toward $\alpha3\beta2$- and $\alpha6$-containing receptors. The drug is effective clinically; however, it is not benign: The FDA has issued a warning about mood and behavioral changes associated with its use, and there is some evidence of increased cardiovascular risk (Chelladurai and Singh, 2014; Singh et al., 2011).

Cytisine

Cytisine is a plant alkaloid and a partial agonist at nicotinic ACh receptors, with an affinity for the $\alpha4\beta2$ subtype. Cytisine is taken orally, has a half-life of about 5 h, and can produce mild GI side effects. In a recent small trial, cytisine was effective in producing effects similar to those of NRT and varenicline (Walker et al., 2014).

Drug Facts for Your Personal Formulary: *Agents Acting at the NMJ and Autonomic Ganglia; Antispasmodics; Nicotine*

Drug	Therapeutic Uses	Clinical Pharmacology and Tips
Nicotinic ACh Receptor Agonists		
Succinylcholine[US] (N_m agonist)	Induction of neuromuscular blockade in surgery and during intubation	• Induces rapid depolarization of motor end plate, inducing phase I block • Resistant to and augments AChE inhibition; induces fasciculations, then flaccid paralysis • Influenced by anesthetic agent, type of muscle, and rate of administration • Leads to phase II block after prolonged use • Metabolized by butyrylcholinestarase; not safe for infants and children • Contraindications: history of malignant hyperthermia, muscular dystrophy
Dexamethonium (depolarizer)	• Not used clinically in the U.S.	
Nicotine (N_n agonist)	• Smoking cessation	• Low dose induces postganglionic depolarization • High doses induce ganglionic transmission blockade
Varenicline (N_n [α4β2 subtype])	• Smoking cessation • FDA warning about mood and behavioral changes	• Partial nicotinic receptor agonist preventing nicotine stimulation and decreasing craving • Potential for neuropsychiatric events, may cause seizures with alcohol use; excreted largely unchanged in urine
Competitive Nicotinic ACh Receptor Antagonists (Nondepolarizing Neuromuscular Blocking Agents)		
D-Tubocurarine[a,L]	• Induction of neuromuscular blockade in surgery and during intubation • All neuromuscular blocking agents are administered parenterally	• No longer used clinically in the U.S. or Canada • Produces partial blockade of ganglionic ACh transmission that can produce hypertension and reflex tachycardia • Can induce histamine release
Mivacurium[S]		• Short acting due to rapid hydrolysis by plasma cholinesterase • Use with caution in patients with renal or hepatic insufficiency
Pancuronium[L]		• Shows antimuscarinic receptor activity • Renal and hepatic elimination • Vagolytic activity may cause tachycardia, hypertension, and increased cardiac output
Rocuronium[I]		• Amino steroid • Stable in solution • More rapid onset than vecuronium and cisatracurium • Hepatic elimination
Vecuronium[I]		• Amino steroid • Not stable in solution • Hepatic and renal elimination
Metocurine[a,L]		• Three times more potent than tubocurarine • Less histamine release
Atracurium[I]	• Preferred agent for patients with renal failure	• Susceptible to Hofmann elimination and ester hydrolysis • Same dosage for infants > 1 month, children, and adults
Cisatracurium[I]		• More potent than atracurium, Hofmann elimination, no histamine release (unlike atracurium)
Doxacurium[a,L]		• Renal elimination
Pipecuronium[a,L]		• Hepatic metabolism; renal elimination
Competitive Nicotinic ACh Receptor Antagonists (Nondepolarizing Neuromuscular Blocking Agents) (continued)		
Gantacurium[b,US]		• New compound class; in clinical trial stage • Fastest onset and shortest acting • Metabolism: rapid cysteine adduction, slow ester hydrolysis
Hexamethonium	• Not used therapeutically	• N_n receptor antagonist; blocks ganglionic transmission
Trimethaphan	• Hypertensive crisis • No longer used	• N_n receptor antagonist; blocks ganglionic transmission
CNS-Active Agents		
Baclofen **Benzodiazepines** **Tizanidine** **Cyclobenzaprine**	• Control of muscle spasms	• See Chapter 22

Drug Facts for Your Personal Formulary: *Agents Acting at the NMJ and Autonomic Ganglia; Antispasmodics; Nicotine (continued)*

Drug	Therapeutic Uses	Clinical Pharmacology and Tips
CNS-Active Agents		
Carisoprodol **Metaxalone** **Methocarbamol** **Orphenadrine** **Tetrabenazine**	• Muscle relaxants acting in CNS, having, in general, a depressant effect	• CYP2C19 metabolizes carisoprodol to largely to meprobamate • Tetrabenazine is a VCAT2 inhibitor and depletes neuronal monoamine stores
Agents That Block ACh Release		
AbobotulinumtoxinA	• Cervical dystonia • Glabellar lines (moderate to severe)	• Spread of toxin effect may induce paralysis of nontargeted muscle, rarely if administered carefully • Paralysis of swallowing and respiration can be life threatening
IncobotulinumtoxinA	• Blepharospasm, cervical dystonia • Glabellar lines (moderate to severe)	
OnabotulinumtoxinA	• Botox: axillary hyperhidrosis (severe) • Blepharospasm associated with dystonia; cervical dystonia; migraine (chronic) prophylaxis • Overactive bladder; strabismus; upper limb spasticity (severe); urinary incontinence (due to detrusor overactivity associated with a neurologic condition)	
RimabotulinumtoxinB	• Cervical dystonia	
Inhibitor of Release of Ca^{2+} From the SR		
Dantrolene	• Management and prevention of malignant hyperthermia • Treatment of spasticity associated with upper motor neuron disorders (e.g., spinal cord injury, stroke, cerebral palsy, or multiple sclerosis)	• Hepatic metabolism • Can cause significant hepatotoxicity

Duration of action: [L]long (> ~ 80 min), [I]intermediate (~20–80 min), [S]short (~15–20 min), [US]ultrashort (< ~ 15 min).
[a]Not available in the U.S.
[b]Gantacurium is in investigational status.

Bibliography

Basta SJ. Modulation of histamine release by neuromuscular blocking drugs. *Curr Opin Anaesthesiol*, **1992**, *5*:512–566.

Belmont MR, et al. Clinical pharmacology of GW280430A in humans. *Anesthesiology*, **2004**, *100*:768–773.

Benowitz NL. Nicotine and cardiovascular disease. In Benowitz NL, ed. *Nicotine Safety and Toxicity*. Oxford University Press, New York, **1998**, 3–28.

Cahill K, et al. Pharmacological interventions for smoking cessation: an overview and network meta-analysis. *Cochrane Database Syst Rev*, **2013**, *5*:CD009329. doi:10.1002/14651858.CD009329.pub2. Accessed February 29, 2016.

Changeux JP, Edelstein SJ. *Nicotinic Acetylcholine Receptors*. Odile Jacob, New York, **2005**.

Chelladurai Y, Singh S. Varenicline and cardiovascular adverse events: a perspective review. *Ther Adv Drug Saf*, **2014**, *5*:167–172.

Dorostkar MM, Boehm S. Presynaptic lonotropic receptors. *Handb Exp Pharmacol*, **2008**, *184*:479–527.

Durant NN, Katz RL. Suxamethonium. *Br J Anaesth*, **1982**, *54*: 195–208.

Fisher DM, et al. Elimination of atracurium in humans: contribution of Hofmann elimination and ester hydrolysis versus organ-based elimination. *Anesthesiology*, **1986**, *65*:6–12.

Frishman WH. Smoking cessation pharmacotherapy. *Ther Adv Cardiovasc Dis*, **2009**, *3*:287–308.

Karlin A. Emerging structures of nicotinic acetylcholine receptors. *Nat Rev Neurosci*, **2002**, *3*:102–114.

Kuryatov A, et al. Nicotine acts as a pharmacological chaperone to up-regulate human a4b2 acetylcholine receptors. *Mol Pharm*, **2005**, *68*:1839–1851.

Naguib M, Brull SJ. Update on neuromuscular pharmacology. *Curr Opin Anaesthesiol*, **2009**, *22*:483–490.

Naguib M, et al. Pharmacology of neuromuscular blocking drugs. In Miller RD, ed. *Miller's Anesthesia*. 8th ed. Saunders, an imprint of Elsevier, Philadelphia, **2015**, 958–994.

Prochaska JJ, Benowitz NL. The past, present, and future of nicotine addiction therapy. *Ann Rev Med*, **2016**, *67*:467–486.

St. Helen G, et al. Nicotine delivery, retention and pharmacokinetics from various electronic cigarettes. *Addiction*, **2016**, *111*:534–544.

Singh S, et al. Risk of serious adverse cardiovascular events associated with varenicline: a systematic review and meta-analysis. *CMAJ*, **2011**, *183*:1359–1366.

Srinivasan R, et al. Pharmacological chaperoning of nAChRs: a therapeutic target for Parkinson's disease. *Pharmacol Res*, **2014**, *83*:20–29.

Unwin N. Refined structure of the nicotinic acetylcholine receptor at 4 Å resolution. *J Mol Biol*, **2005**, *346*:967–989.

Volle RL. Nicotinic ganglion-stimulating agents. In Kharkevich DA, ed. *Pharmacology of Ganglionic Transmission*. Springer-Verlag, Berlin, **1980**, 281–312.

Walker N, et al. Cytisine versus nicotine for smoking cessation. *N Engl J Med*, **2014**, *371*:2353–2362.

Watkins J. Adverse reaction to neuromuscular blockers: frequency, investigation, and epidemiology. *Acta Anaesthesiol Scand Suppl*, **1994**, *102*:6–10.

Xiu X, et al. Nicotine binding to brain receptors requires a strong cation-π interaction. *Nature*, **2009**, *458*:534–537.

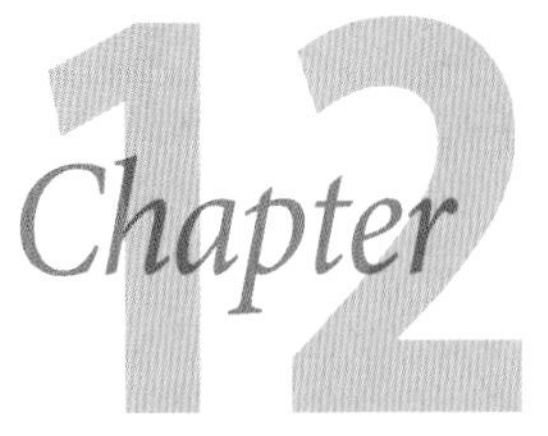

Adrenergic Agonists and Antagonists

Thomas C. Westfall, Heather Macarthur, and David P. Westfall

第十二章　肾上腺素激动药和拮抗药

中文导读

本章主要介绍：儿茶酚胺类和拟交感神经类药的作用概述；拟交感神经类药的分类，包括拟交感神经胺的构-效关系、肾上腺素能反应的生理基础、伪递质概念；内源性儿茶酚胺，包括肾上腺素、去甲肾上腺素和多巴胺；β肾上腺素能受体激动药，包括异丙肾上腺素、多巴酚丁胺、β_2-选择性肾上腺素能受体激动药和β_3-肾上腺素能受体激动药；α肾上腺素能受体激动药，包括α_1-选择性肾上腺素能受体激动药和α_2-选择性肾上腺素能受体激动药；其他交感神经激动药；拟交感神经药的治疗用途；肾上腺素能受体拮抗药；α肾上腺素能受体拮抗药，包括α_1-肾上腺素能受体拮抗药、α_2-肾上腺素能受体拮抗药、非选择性α肾上腺素拮抗药及其他α肾上腺素能受体拮抗药；β肾上腺素能受体拮抗药，包括概述、非选择性β肾上腺素能受体拮抗药、β_1-选择性肾上腺素能受体拮抗药、具有额外心血管效应的β肾上腺素能受体拮抗药（第三代β受体阻滞药）。

Abbreviations

AAAD: L-aromatic amino acid decarboxylase
ACEI: angiotensin-converting enzyme inhibitor
ADHD: attention-deficit/hyperactivity disorder
AV: atrioventricular
BPH: benign prostatic hyperplasia
CNS: central nervous system
COMT: catechol-*O*-methyltransferase
COPD: chronic obstructive pulmonary disease
DA: dopamine
ECG: electrocardiogram
EPI: epinephrine
FDA: Food and Drug Administration
GI: gastrointestinal
HDL: high-density lipoprotein
HMG CoA: 3-hydroxy-3-methylglutaryl coenzyme A
5HT: 5-hydroxytryptamine (serotonin)
INE: isoproterenol (Isopropyl NE)
LABA: long-acting β_2 adrenergic agonist
LDL: low-density lipoprotein
MAO: monoamine oxidase
NE: norepinephrine
NET: NE transporter
NPY: neuropeptide Y
PBZ: phenoxybenzamine
PDE: phosphodiesterase
PVR: peripheral vascular resistance
ROS: reactive oxygen species
SA: sinoatrial
VLABA: very long-acting β_2 adrenergic agonist

Overview: Actions of Catecholamines and Sympathomimetic Drugs

Most of the actions of catecholamines and sympathomimetic agents can be classified into seven broad types:

1. *A peripheral excitatory action* on certain types of smooth muscle, such as those in blood vessels supplying skin, kidney, and mucous membranes; and on gland cells, such as those in salivary and sweat glands.
2. *A peripheral inhibitory action* on certain other types of smooth muscle, such as those in the wall of the gut, in the bronchial tree, and in blood vessels supplying skeletal muscle.
3. *A cardiac excitatory action* that increases heart rate and force of contraction.
4. *Metabolic actions*, such as an increase in the rate of glycogenolysis in liver and muscle and liberation of free fatty acids from adipose tissue.
5. *Endocrine actions*, such as modulation (increasing or decreasing) of the secretion of insulin, renin, and pituitary hormones.
6. *Actions in the CNS*, such as respiratory stimulation, an increase in wakefulness and psychomotor activity, and a reduction in appetite.
7. *Prejunctional actions* that either inhibit or facilitate the release of neurotransmitters, the inhibitory action being physiologically more important.

Many of these actions and the receptors that mediate them are summarized in Tables 8–1 and 8–6. Not all sympathomimetic drugs show each of the types of action to the same degree; however, many of the differences in their effects are only quantitative. The pharmacological properties of these drugs as a class are described in detail for the prototypical agent, epinephrine (EPI). Appreciation of the pharmacological properties of the drugs described in this chapter depends on an understanding of the classification, distribution, and mechanism of action of α and β adrenergic receptors (Chapter 8).

Classification of Sympathomimetic Drugs

Catecholamines and sympathomimetic drugs are classified as *direct-acting, indirect-acting, or mixed-acting sympathomimetics* (Figure 12–1). Direct-acting sympathomimetic drugs act directly on one or more of the adrenergic receptors. These agents may exhibit considerable selectivity for a specific receptor subtype (e.g., phenylephrine for α_1, terbutaline for β_2) or may have no or minimal selectivity and act on several receptor types (e.g., EPI for α_1, α_2, β_1, β_2, and β_3 receptors; NE for α_1, α_2, and β_1 receptors).

Indirect-acting drugs increase the availability of NE or EPI to stimulate adrenergic receptors by several mechanisms:

- By releasing or displacing NE from sympathetic nerve varicosities
- By inhibiting the transport of NE into sympathetic neurons (e.g., cocaine), thereby increasing the dwell time of the transmitter at the receptor
- By blocking the metabolizing enzymes, MAO (e.g., pargyline) or COMT (e.g., entacapone), effectively increasing transmitter supply

Drugs that indirectly release NE and also directly activate receptors are referred to as *mixed-acting sympathomimetic drugs* (e.g., ephedrine). A feature of *direct-acting sympathomimetic drugs* is that their responses are not reduced by prior treatment with reserpine or guanethidine, which deplete NE from sympathetic neurons. After transmitter depletion, the actions of direct-acting sympathomimetic drugs actually may increase because the loss of the neurotransmitter induces compensatory changes that upregulate receptors or enhance the signaling pathway. In contrast, the responses of indirect-acting sympathomimetic drugs (e.g., *amphetamine, tyramine*) are abolished by prior treatment with reserpine or guanethidine. The cardinal feature of mixed-acting sympathomimetic drugs is that their effects are blunted, but not abolished, by prior treatment with reserpine or guanethidine.

Because *the actions of NE are more pronounced on α and β_1 receptors than on β_2 receptors*, many noncatecholamines that release NE have predominantly α receptor–mediated and cardiac effects. However, certain noncatecholamines with both direct and indirect effects on adrenergic receptors show significant β_2 activity and are used clinically for these effects. Thus, ephedrine, although dependent on release of NE for some of its effects, relieves bronchospasm by its action on β_2 receptors in bronchial smooth muscle, an effect not seen with NE. Moreover, some noncatecholamines (e.g., phenylephrine) act primarily and directly on target cells. It therefore is impossible to predict precisely the effects of noncatecholamines solely on their ability to provoke NE release.

Structure-Activity Relationship of Sympathomimetic Amines

β-Phenylethylamine can be viewed as the parent compound of the sympathomimetic amines, *consisting of a benzene ring and an ethylamine side chain* (parent structure in Table 12–1). The structure permits substitutions to be made on the aromatic ring, the α- and β-carbon atoms, and the terminal amino group to yield a variety of compounds with sympathomimetic activity. *NE, EPI, DA, INE*, and a few other agents have hydroxyl groups substituted at positions 3 and 4 of the benzene ring. Because *o-dihydroxybenzene* is also known as *catechol*, sympathomimetic amines with these hydroxyl substitutions in the aromatic ring are termed *catecholamines*.

Many directly acting sympathomimetic drugs influence both α and β receptors, but the ratio of activities varies among drugs in a continuous spectrum from predominantly α activity (phenylephrine) to predominantly β activity (INE). Despite the multiplicity of the sites of action of sympathomimetic amines, several generalizations can be made (Table 12–1).

Separation of Aromatic Ring and Amino Group

By far the greatest sympathomimetic activity occurs when two carbon atoms separate the ring from the amino group. This rule applies with few exceptions to all types of action.

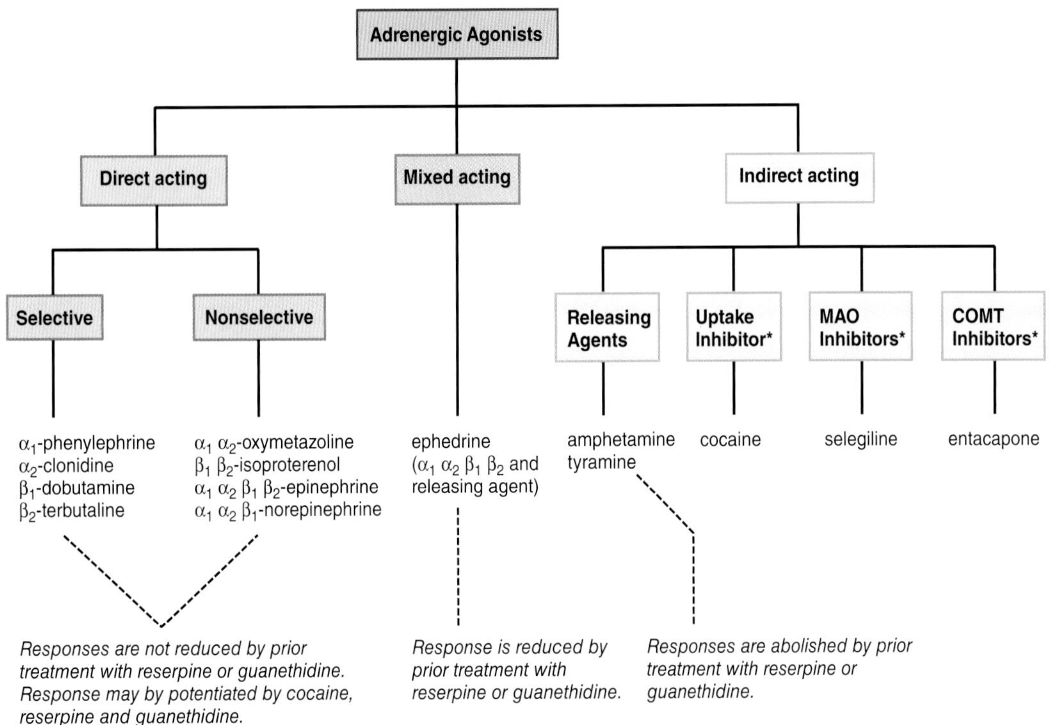

Figure 12–1 *Classification of adrenergic receptor agonists (sympathomimetic amines) or drugs that produce sympathomimetic-like effects.* For each category, a prototypical drug is shown. (*Not actually sympathetic drugs but produce sympathomimetic-like effects.)

TABLE 12–1 ■ STRUCTURES AND MAIN CLINICAL USES OF IMPORTANT SYMPATHOMIMETIC DRUGS

	Ring (positions 2–6)	β CH	α CH	NH	A	N	P	V	B	C	U	CNS
					MAIN CLINICAL USES: α RECEPTOR				β RECEPTOR			
Phenylethylamine		H	H	H								
Epinephrine	3-OH, 4-OH	OH	H	CH_3	A		P	V	B	C		
Norepinephrine	3-OH, 4-OH	OH	H	H			P			C[a]		
Dopamine	3-OH, 4-OH	H	H	H			P					
Droxidopa	3-OH, 4-OH	OH	COOH	H			P			C[a]		
Dobutamine	3-OH, 4-OH	H	H	X						C		
Isoproterenol	3-OH, 4-OH	OH	H	$CH(CH_3)_2$					B	C		
Terbutaline	3-OH, 5-OH	OH	H	$C(CH_3)_3$					B		U	
Metaraminol	3-OH	OH	CH_3	H			P					
Phenylephrine	3-OH	OH	H	CH_3		N	P					
Methoxamine	2-OCH_3, 5-OCH_3	OH	CH_3	H			P					
Albuterol	3-CH_2OH, 4-OH	OH	H	$C(CH_3)_3$					B		U	
Amphetamine		H	CH_3	H								++
Methamphetamine		H	CH_3	CH_3								++
Ephedrine		OH	CH_3	CH_3		N	P		B	C		

X: $-CH(CH_3)-(CH_2)_2-C_6H_4-OH$

α Activity: A, Allergic reactions (includes β action); N, Nasal decongestion; P, Pressor (may include β action); V, Other local vasoconstriction

β Activity: B, Bronchodilator; C, Cardiac; U, Uterus

[a]Direct effects reduced by compensatory baroreceptor reflex.

Substitution on the Amino Group

The effects of amino substitution are most readily seen in the actions of catecholamines on α and β receptors. *Increase in the size of the alkyl substituent increases β receptor activity (e.g., INE).* NE has, in general, rather feeble β_2 activity; this activity is greatly increased in EPI by the addition of a methyl group. A notable exception is phenylephrine, which has an *N*-methyl substituent but is an α-selective agonist. β_2-Selective compounds require a large amino substituent, but depend on other substitutions to define selectivity for β_2 rather than for β_1 receptors. *In general, the smaller the substitution on the amino group, the greater the selectivity for α activity, although N-methylation increases the potency of primary amines. Thus, α activity is maximal in EPI, less in NE, and almost absent in INE.*

Substitution on the Aromatic Nucleus

Maximal α and β activity depends on the presence of hydroxyl groups on positions 3 and 4. When one or both of these groups are absent, with no other aromatic substitution, the overall potency is reduced. Phenylephrine is thus less potent than EPI at both α and β receptors, with β_2 activity almost completely absent. Studies of the β adrenergic receptor suggest that the hydroxyl groups on serine residues 204 and 207 probably form hydrogen bonds with the catechol hydroxyl groups at positions 3 and 4, respectively. It also appears that aspartate 113 is a point of electrostatic interaction with the amine group on the ligand. Because the serines are in the fifth membrane-spanning region and the aspartate is in the third (Chapter 8), it is likely that catecholamines bind parallel to the plane of the membrane, forming a bridge between the two membrane spans. However, models involving DA receptors suggest alternative possibilities.

Hydroxyl groups in positions 3 and 5 confer β_2 receptor selectivity on compounds with large amino substituents. Thus, *terbutaline* and similar compounds relax the bronchial musculature in patients with asthma but cause less-direct cardiac stimulation than do the nonselective drugs. The response to noncatecholamines is partly determined by their capacity to release NE from storage sites. These agents thus cause effects that are mostly mediated by α and β_1 receptors because NE is a weak β_2 agonist. *Phenylethylamines that lack hydroxyl groups on the ring and the β-hydroxyl group on the side chain act almost exclusively by causing the release of NE from sympathetic nerve terminals.*

Because substitution of polar groups on the phenylethylamine structure makes the resultant compounds less lipophilic, *unsubstituted or alkyl-substituted compounds cross the blood-brain barrier more readily and have more central activity.* Thus, ephedrine, amphetamine, and methamphetamine exhibit considerable CNS activity. As noted, the absence of polar hydroxyl groups results in a loss of direct sympathomimetic activity.

Catecholamines have only a brief duration of action and are ineffective when administered orally because they are rapidly inactivated in the intestinal mucosa and in the liver before reaching the systemic circulation (Chapter 8). Compounds without one or both hydroxyl substituents are not acted on by COMT, and their oral effectiveness and duration of action are enhanced.

Groups other than hydroxyls have been substituted on the aromatic ring. In general, potency at α receptors is reduced, and β receptor activity is minimal; the compounds may even block β receptors. For example, methoxamine, with methoxy substituents at positions 2 and 5, has highly selective α stimulating activity and in large doses blocks β receptors. Albuterol, a β_2-selective agonist, has a substituent at position 3 and is an important exception to the general rule of low β receptor activity.

Substitution on the α-Carbon Atom

The substitution on the α-carbon atom blocks oxidation by MAO, greatly prolonging the duration of action of noncatecholamines because their degradation depends largely on the action of this enzyme. The duration of action of drugs such as ephedrine or amphetamine is thus measured in hours rather than in minutes. Similarly, compounds with an α-methyl substituent persist in the nerve terminals and are more likely to release NE from storage sites. Agents such as metaraminol exhibit a greater degree of indirect sympathomimetic activity.

Substitution on the β-Carbon Atom

Substitution of a hydroxyl group on the β-carbon generally decreases actions within the CNS, largely because it lowers lipid solubility. However, such substitution greatly enhances agonist activity at both α and β adrenergic receptors. Although ephedrine is less potent than methamphetamine as a central stimulant, it is more powerful in dilating bronchioles and increasing blood pressure and heart rate.

Optical Isomerism

Substitution on either α- or β-carbon yields optical isomers. Levorotatory substitution on the β-carbon confers the greater peripheral activity, so that the naturally occurring *l*-EPI and *l*-NE are at least 10 times more potent than their unnatural *d*-isomers. Dextrorotatory substitution on the α-carbon generally results in a more potent compound. *d*-Amphetamine is more potent than *l*-amphetamine in central but not peripheral activity.

Physiological Basis of Adrenergic Responsiveness

Important factors in the response of any cell or organ to sympathomimetic amines are the density and relative proportion of α and β adrenergic receptors. For example, NE has relatively little capacity to increase bronchial airflow because the receptors in bronchial smooth muscle are largely of the β_2 subtype. In contrast, INE and EPI are potent bronchodilators. Cutaneous blood vessels physiologically express almost exclusively α receptors; thus, NE and EPI cause constriction of such vessels, whereas INE has little effect. The smooth muscle of blood vessels that supply skeletal muscles has both β_2 and α receptors; activation of β_2 receptors causes vasodilation, and stimulation of α receptors constricts these vessels. In such vessels, the threshold concentration for activation of β_2 receptors by EPI is lower than that for α receptors, but when both types of receptors are activated at high concentrations of EPI, the response to α receptors predominates. Physiological concentrations of EPI primarily cause vasodilation.

The ultimate response of a target organ to sympathomimetic amines is dictated not only by the direct effects of the agents but also by the reflex homeostatic adjustments of the organism. One of the most striking effects of many sympathomimetic amines is a rise in arterial blood pressure caused by stimulation of vascular α adrenergic receptors. This stimulation elicits compensatory reflexes that are mediated by the carotid-aortic baroreceptor system. As a result, sympathetic tone is diminished and vagal tone is enhanced; each of these responses leads to slowing of the heart rate. Conversely, when a drug (e.g., a β_2 agonist) lowers mean blood pressure at the mechanoreceptors of the carotid sinus and aortic arch, the baroreceptor reflex works to restore pressure by reducing parasympathetic (vagal) outflow from the CNS to the heart and increasing sympathetic outflow to the heart and vessels. The baroreceptor reflex effect is of special importance for drugs that have little capacity to activate β receptors directly. With diseases such as atherosclerosis, which may impair baroreceptor mechanisms, the effects of sympathomimetic drugs may be magnified.

False-Transmitter Concept

Indirectly acting amines are taken up into sympathetic nerve terminals and storage vesicles, where they replace NE in the storage complex. Phenylethylamines that lack a β-hydroxyl group are retained there poorly, but β-hydroxylated phenylethylamines and compounds that subsequently become hydroxylated in the synaptic vesicle by DA β-hydroxylase are retained in the synaptic vesicle for relatively long periods of time. Such substances can produce a persistent diminution in the content of NE at functionally critical sites. When the nerve is stimulated, the contents of a relatively constant number of synaptic vesicles are released by exocytosis. If these vesicles contain phenylethylamines that are much less potent than NE, activation of postsynaptic α and β receptors will be diminished.

This hypothesis, known as the *false-transmitter concept*, is a possible explanation for some of the effects of MAO inhibitors. Phenylethylamines normally are synthesized in the GI tract as a result of the action of bacterial tyrosine decarboxylase. The *tyramine* formed in this fashion usually is oxidatively deaminated in the GI tract and the liver, and the amine does not reach the systemic circulation in significant concentrations. However, when a MAO inhibitor is administered, tyramine may be absorbed systemically and transported into sympathetic nerve terminals, where its catabolism again is prevented because of the inhibition of MAO at this site; the tyramine then is β-hydroxylated to octopamine and stored in the vesicles in this form. As a consequence, NE gradually is displaced, and stimulation of the nerve terminal results in the release of a relatively small amount of NE along with a fraction of octopamine. The latter amine has relatively little ability to activate either α or β receptors. Thus, a functional impairment of sympathetic transmission parallels long-term administration of MAO inhibitors.

Despite such functional impairment, patients who have received MAO inhibitors may experience severe hypertensive crises if they ingest cheese, beer, or red wine. These and related foods, which are produced by fermentation, contain a large quantity of tyramine and, to a lesser degree, other phenylethylamines. When GI and hepatic MAO are inhibited, the large quantity of tyramine that is ingested is absorbed rapidly and reaches the systemic circulation in high concentration. A massive and precipitous release of NE can result, causing hypertension severe enough to precipitate a myocardial infarction or a stroke. The properties of various MAO inhibitors (reversible or irreversible; selective or nonselective at MAO-A and MAO-B) are discussed in Chapters 8 and 15.

Endogenous Catecholamines

Epinephrine

Epinephrine (adrenaline) is a potent stimulant of both α and β adrenergic receptors, and its effects on target organs are thus complex. Most of the responses listed in Table 8–1 are seen after injection of EPI, although the occurrence of sweating, piloerection, and mydriasis depends on the physiological state of the subject. Particularly prominent are the actions on the heart and on vascular and other smooth muscle.

Actions on Organ Systems

Effects on Blood Pressure. Epinephrine is one of the most potent vasopressor drugs known. If a pharmacological dose is given rapidly by an intravenous route, it evokes a characteristic effect on blood pressure, which rises rapidly to a peak that is proportional to the dose. The increase in systolic pressure is greater than the increase in diastolic pressure, so that the pulse pressure increases. As the response wanes, the mean pressure may fall below normal before returning to control levels.

The mechanism of the rise in blood pressure due to EPI is a triad of effects:

- a direct myocardial stimulation that increases the strength of ventricular contraction (*positive inotropic action*);
- an increased heart rate (*positive chronotropic action*); and
- vasoconstriction in many vascular beds—especially in the *precapillary resistance vessels* of skin, mucosa, and kidney—along with marked constriction of the veins.

The pulse rate, at first accelerated, may be slowed markedly at the height of the rise of blood pressure by compensatory vagal discharge (baroreceptor reflex). Small doses of EPI (0.1 μg/kg) may cause the blood pressure to fall. The depressor effect of small doses and the biphasic response to larger doses are due to greater sensitivity to EPI of vasodilator β_2 receptors than of constrictor α receptors.

Absorption of EPI after subcutaneous injection is slow due to local vasoconstrictor action; the effects of doses as large as 0.5–1.5 mg can be duplicated by intravenous infusion at a rate of 10–30 μg/min. There is a moderate increase in systolic pressure due to increased cardiac contractile force and a rise in cardiac output (Figure 12–2). Peripheral resistance decreases, owing to a dominant action on β_2 receptors of vessels in skeletal muscle, where blood flow is enhanced; as a consequence, diastolic pressure usually falls. Because the mean blood pressure is not, as a rule, greatly elevated, compensatory baroreceptor reflexes do not appreciably antagonize the direct cardiac actions. Heart rate, cardiac output, stroke volume, and left ventricular work per beat are increased as a result of direct cardiac stimulation and increased venous return to the heart, which is reflected by an increase in right atrial pressure. At slightly higher rates of infusion, there may be no change or a slight rise in peripheral resistance and diastolic pressure, depending on the dose and the resultant ratio of α to β responses in the various vascular beds; compensatory reflexes also may come into play. The details of the effects of intravenous infusion of EPI, NE, and INE in humans are compared in Figure 12–2 and of EPI and NE in Table 12–2.

Vascular Effects. In the vasculature, *EPI acts chiefly on the smaller arterioles and precapillary sphincters*, although veins and large arteries also respond to the drug. Various vascular beds react differently, which results in a substantial redistribution of blood flow. *Injected EPI markedly decreases cutaneous blood flow, constricting precapillary vessels and small venules.* Cutaneous vasoconstriction accounts for a marked decrease in blood flow in the hands and feet. *Blood flow to skeletal muscles is increased by therapeutic doses in humans.* This is due in part to a powerful β_2-mediated vasodilator action that is only partially counterbalanced by a vasoconstrictor action on the α receptors that also are present in the vascular bed.

The effect of EPI on cerebral circulation is related to systemic blood pressure. In usual therapeutic doses, the drug has relatively little constrictor action on cerebral arterioles. Indeed, autoregulatory mechanisms tend to limit the increase in cerebral blood flow caused by increased blood pressure.

Doses of EPI that have little effect on mean arterial pressure consistently increase renal vascular resistance and reduce renal blood flow by as much as 40%. All segments of the renal vascular bed contribute to the increased resistance. Because the glomerular filtration rate is only slightly and variably altered, the filtration fraction is consistently increased. Excretion of Na^+, K^+, and Cl^- is decreased; urine volume may be increased, decreased, or unchanged. Maximal tubular reabsorptive and excretory capacities are unchanged. *The secretion of renin is increased as a consequence of a direct action of EPI on β_1 receptors in the juxtaglomerular apparatus.*

Arterial and venous pulmonary pressures are raised. Although direct pulmonary vasoconstriction occurs, redistribution of blood from the systemic to the pulmonary circulation, due to constriction of the more powerful musculature in the systemic great veins, doubtless plays an important part in the increase in pulmonary pressure. Very high concentrations of EPI may cause pulmonary edema precipitated by elevated pulmonary capillary filtration pressure and possibly by "leaky" capillaries.

Coronary blood flow is enhanced by EPI or by cardiac sympathetic stimulation under physiological conditions. The increased flow, which occurs even with doses that do not increase the aortic blood pressure, is the result of two factors. The first is the increased relative duration of diastole at higher heart rates (described further in the chapter); this is partially

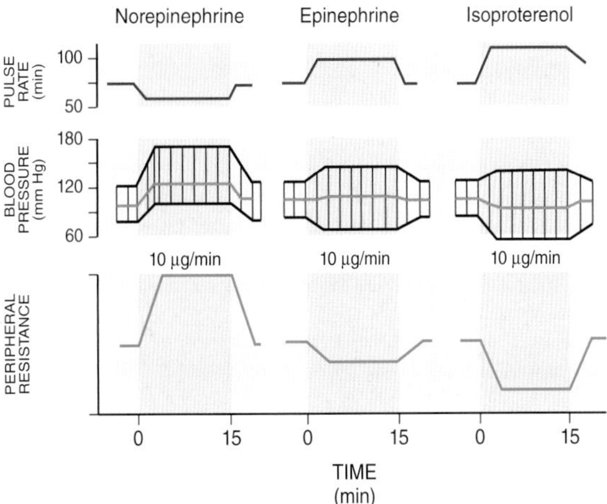

Figure 12–2 *Comparative effects of intravenous infusion of NE, EPI, and INE.* (Reproduced with permission from Allwood MJ, Cobbold AF, Ginsberg J. Peripheral vascular effects of noradrenaline, isopropyl-noradrenaline, and dopamine. *Br Med Bull.* **1963**;*19*:132–136. With permission from Oxford University Press.)

TABLE 12–2 ■ COMPARATIVE EFFECTS OF INFUSIONS OF EPINEPHRINE AND NOREPINEPHRINE IN HUMAN BEINGS[a]

EFFECT	EPI	NE
Cardiac		
Heart rate	+	–[b]
Stroke volume	++	++
Cardiac output	+++	0, –
Arrhythmias	++++	++++
Coronary blood flow	++	++
Blood pressure		
Systolic arterial	+++	+++
Mean arterial	+	++
Diastolic arterial	+, 0, –	++
Mean pulmonary	++	++
Peripheral circulation		
Total peripheral resistance	–	++
Cerebral blood flow	+	0, –
Muscle blood flow	+++	0, –
Cutaneous blood flow	–	–
Renal blood flow	–	–
Splanchnic blood flow	+++	0,+
Metabolic effects		
Oxygen consumption	++	0, +
Blood glucose	+++	0, +
Blood lactic acid	+++	0, +
Eosinopenic response	+	0
CNS		
Respiration	+	+
Subjective sensations	+	+

+, increase; 0, no change; –, decrease. Data from Goldenberg M, et al. *Arch Intern Med.* **1950**;86:823.

[a]0.1–0.4 μg/kg per minute.

[b]After atropine.

offset by decreased blood flow during systole because of more forceful contraction of the surrounding myocardium and an increase in mechanical compression of the coronary vessels. The increased flow during diastole is further enhanced if aortic blood pressure is elevated by EPI; as a consequence, total coronary flow may be increased. The second factor is a metabolic dilator effect that results from the increased strength of contraction and myocardial O_2 consumption due to the direct effects of EPI on cardiac myocytes. This vasodilation is mediated in part by adenosine released from cardiac myocytes, which tends to override a direct vasoconstrictor effect of EPI that results from activation of α receptors in coronary vessels.

Cardiac Effects. Epinephrine is a powerful cardiac stimulant. It acts directly on the predominant β_1 receptors of the myocardium and of the cells of the pacemaker and conducting tissues; β_2, β_3, and α receptors also are present in the heart, although there are considerable species differences. The heart rate increases, and the rhythm often is altered. Cardiac systole is shorter and more powerful, cardiac output is enhanced, and the work of the heart and its oxygen consumption are markedly increased. Cardiac efficiency (work done relative to oxygen consumption) is lessened. *Direct responses to EPI include increases in contractile force, accelerated rate of rise of isometric tension, enhanced rate of relaxation, decreased time to peak tension, increased excitability, acceleration of the rate of spontaneous beating, and induction of automaticity in specialized regions of the heart.*

In accelerating the heart, EPI preferentially shortens systole so that the duration of diastole usually is not reduced. Indeed, activation of β receptors increases the rate of relaxation of ventricular muscle. EPI speeds the heart by accelerating the slow depolarization of SA nodal cells that takes place during diastole, that is, during phase 4 of the action potential (Chapter 30). Consequently, the transmembrane potential of the pacemaker cells rises more rapidly to the threshold level of action potential initiation. The amplitude of the action potential and the maximal rate of depolarization (phase 0) also are increased. A shift in the location of the pacemaker within the SA node often occurs, owing to activation of latent pacemaker cells. In Purkinje fibers, EPI also accelerates diastolic depolarization and may activate latent pacemaker cells. These changes do not occur in atrial and ventricular muscle fibers, where EPI has little effect on the stable, phase 4 membrane potential after repolarization. If large doses of EPI are given, premature ventricular contractions occur and may herald more serious ventricular arrhythmias. This rarely is seen with conventional doses in humans, but ventricular extrasystoles, tachycardia, or even fibrillation may be precipitated by release of endogenous EPI when the heart has been sensitized to this action of EPI by certain anesthetics or by myocardial ischemia. The mechanism of induction of these cardiac arrhythmias is not clear.

Some effects of EPI on cardiac tissues are largely secondary to the increase in heart rate and are small or inconsistent when the heart rate is kept constant. For example, the effect of EPI on repolarization of atrial muscle, Purkinje fibers, or ventricular muscle is small if the heart rate is unchanged. When the heart rate is increased, the duration of the action potential is consistently shortened, and the refractory period is correspondingly decreased.

Conduction through the Purkinje system depends on the level of membrane potential at the time of excitation. Excessive reduction of this potential results in conduction disturbances, ranging from slowed conduction to complete block. EPI often increases the membrane potential and improves conduction in Purkinje fibers that have been excessively depolarized.

Epinephrine normally shortens the refractory period of the human AV node by direct effects on the heart, although doses of EPI that slow the heart through reflex vagal discharge may indirectly tend to prolong it. EPI also decreases the grade of AV block that occurs as a result of disease, drugs, or vagal stimulation. Supraventricular arrhythmias are apt to occur from the combination of EPI and cholinergic stimulation. Depression of sinus rate and AV conduction by vagal discharge probably plays a part in EPI-induced ventricular arrhythmias because various drugs that block the vagal effect confer some protection. The actions of EPI in enhancing cardiac automaticity and in causing arrhythmias are effectively antagonized by β receptor antagonists such as propranolol. However, α_1 receptors exist in most regions of the heart, and their activation prolongs the refractory period and strengthens myocardial contractions.

Cardiac arrhythmias have been seen in patients after inadvertent intravenous administration of conventional subcutaneous doses of EPI. Premature ventricular contractions can appear, which may be followed by multifocal ventricular tachycardia or ventricular fibrillation. Pulmonary edema also may occur.

Epinephrine decreases the amplitude of the T wave of the ECG in normal persons. In animals given relatively larger doses, additional effects are seen on the T wave and the ST segment. After decreasing in amplitude, the T wave may become biphasic, and the ST segment can deviate either above or below the isoelectric line. Such ST segment changes are similar to those seen in patients with angina pectoris during spontaneous or EPI-induced attacks of pain. These electrical changes therefore have been attributed to myocardial ischemia. Also, EPI as well as other catecholamines may cause myocardial cell death, particularly after intravenous infusions. Acute toxicity is associated with contraction band necrosis and other pathological changes. Recent interest has focused on the possibility that prolonged sympathetic stimulation of the heart, such as in congestive cardiomyopathy, may promote apoptosis of cardiomyocytes.

Effects on Smooth Muscles. The effects of EPI on the smooth muscles of different organs and systems depend on the type of adrenergic receptor in the muscle (Table 8–1). In general, EPI relaxes *GI smooth muscle* due to activation of both α and β receptors. Intestinal tone and the frequency and amplitude of spontaneous contractions are reduced. The stomach usually is relaxed and the pyloric and ileocecal sphincters are contracted, but these effects depend on the preexisting tone of the muscle. If tone already is high, EPI causes relaxation; if low, contraction.

The responses of *uterine muscle* to EPI vary with species, phase of the sexual cycle, state of gestation, and dose given. During the last month of pregnancy and at parturition, EPI inhibits uterine tone and contractions. Effects of adrenergic agents and other drugs on the uterus are discussed further in this chapter and in Chapter 44. *EPI relaxes the detrusor muscle of the bladder as a result of activation of β receptors and contracts the trigone and sphincter muscles owing to its α agonist activity.* This can result in hesitancy in urination and may contribute to retention of urine in the bladder. Activation of smooth muscle contraction in the prostate promotes urinary retention.

Respiratory Effects. *Epinephrine has a powerful bronchodilator action,* most evident when bronchial muscle is contracted because of disease, as in bronchial asthma, or in response to drugs or various autacoids. The beneficial effects of EPI in asthma also may arise from inhibition of antigen-induced release of inflammatory mediators from mast cells and to a lesser extent from diminution of bronchial secretions and congestion within the mucosa. *Inhibition of mast cell secretion is mediated by β_2 receptors, while the effects on the mucosa are mediated by α receptors;* however, other drugs, such as glucocorticoids and leukotriene receptor antagonists, have much more profound anti-inflammatory effects in asthma (Chapters 40 and 46).

Effects on the CNS. Because EPI is a polar compound, it penetrates poorly into the CNS and thus is not a powerful CNS stimulant. While the drug may cause restlessness, apprehension, headache, and tremor in many persons, these effects in part may be secondary to the effects of EPI on the cardiovascular system, skeletal muscles, and intermediary metabolism; that is, they may be the result of somatic manifestations of anxiety.

Metabolic Effects. Epinephrine elevates the concentrations of glucose and lactate in blood. *EPI inhibits secretion of insulin through an interaction with α_2 receptors, whereas activation of β_2 receptors enhances insulin secretions; the predominant effect of EPI is inhibition. Glucagon secretion is enhanced via activation of β receptors of the α cells of pancreatic islets.* EPI also decreases the uptake of glucose by peripheral tissues, at least in part not only because of its effects on the secretion of insulin, but also possibly due to direct effects on skeletal muscle. Glycosuria rarely occurs. The effect of EPI to stimulate glycogenolysis in most tissues and in most species involves β receptors. EPI raises the concentration of free fatty acids in blood by stimulating β receptors in adipocytes. The result is activation of triglyceride lipase, which accelerates the triglyceride breakdown to free fatty acids and glycerol. The calorigenic action of EPI (increase in metabolism) is reflected in humans by an increase of 20%–30% in O_2 consumption after conventional doses, an effect due mainly to enhanced breakdown of triglycerides in brown adipose tissue, providing an increase in oxidizable substrate (Chapter 8).

Miscellaneous Effects. Epinephrine reduces circulating plasma volume by loss of protein-free fluid to the extracellular space, thereby increasing hematocrit and plasma protein concentration. However, conventional doses of EPI do not significantly alter plasma volume or packed red cell volume under normal conditions, although such doses may have variable effects in the presence of shock, hemorrhage, hypotension, or anesthesia. EPI rapidly increases the number of circulating polymorphonuclear leukocytes, likely due to β receptor–mediated demargination of these cells. EPI accelerates blood coagulation and promotes fibrinolysis.

The effects of EPI on secretory glands are not marked; in most glands, secretion usually is inhibited, partly owing to the reduced blood flow caused by vasoconstriction. EPI stimulates lacrimation and scanty mucus secretion from salivary glands. Sweating and pilomotor activity are minimal after systemic administration of EPI, but occur after intradermal injection of very dilute solutions of either EPI or NE. Such effects are inhibited by α receptor antagonists.

Mydriasis occurs with physiological sympathetic stimulation but not when EPI is instilled into the conjunctival sac of normal eyes. However, EPI usually lowers intraocular pressure, possibly the result of reduced production of aqueous humor due to vasoconstriction and enhanced outflow (Chapter 69).

Although EPI does not directly excite *skeletal muscle, it facilitates neuromuscular transmission*, particularly that following prolonged rapid stimulation of motor nerves. In apparent contrast to the effects of α receptor activation at presynaptic nerve terminals in the autonomic nervous system (α_2 receptors), stimulation of α receptors causes a more rapid increase in transmitter release from the somatic motor neuron, perhaps as a result of enhanced influx of Ca^{2+}. These responses likely are mediated by α_1 receptors. These actions may explain in part the ability of EPI (given intra-arterially) to briefly increase strength of the injected limb of patients with myasthenia gravis. EPI also acts directly on white, fast-twitch muscle fibers to prolong the active state, thereby increasing peak tension. Of greater physiological and clinical importance is the capacity of EPI and selective β_2 agonists to increase physiological tremor, at least in part due to β receptor–mediated enhancement of discharge of muscle spindles.

Epinephrine promotes a fall in plasma K^+, largely due to stimulation of K^+ uptake into cells, particularly skeletal muscle, due to activation of β_2 receptors. This is associated with decreased renal K^+ excretion. These receptors have been exploited in the management of hyperkalemic familial periodic paralysis, which is characterized by episodic flaccid paralysis, hyperkalemia, and depolarization of skeletal muscle. The β_2-selective agonist albuterol apparently is able to ameliorate the impairment in the ability of the muscle to accumulate and retain K^+.

The administration of large or repeated doses of EPI or other sympathomimetic amines to experimental animals damages arterial walls and myocardium, even inducing necrosis in the heart that is indistinguishable from myocardial infarction. The mechanism of this injury is not yet clear, but α and β receptor antagonists and Ca^{2+} channel blockers may afford substantial protection against the damage. Similar lesions occur in many patients with pheochromocytoma or after prolonged infusions of NE.

ADME

Epinephrine is not effective after oral administration because it is rapidly conjugated and oxidized in the GI mucosa and liver. Absorption from subcutaneous tissues occurs relatively slowly because of local vasoconstriction. Absorption is more rapid after intramuscular injection. In emergencies, it may be necessary to administer EPI intravenously. When relatively concentrated solutions are nebulized and inhaled, the actions of the drug largely are restricted to the respiratory tract; however, systemic reactions such as arrhythmias may occur, particularly if larger amounts are used.

Epinephrine is rapidly inactivated in the liver by COMT and MAO (see Figure 8–9). Although only small amounts appear in the urine of normal persons, the urine of patients with pheochromocytoma may contain relatively large amounts of EPI, NE, and their metabolites.

Epinephrine is available in a variety of formulations geared for different clinical indications and routes of administration, including self-administration for anaphylactic reactions. EPI is unstable in alkaline solution; when exposed to air or light, it turns pink from oxidation to adrenochrome and then brown from formation of polymers. Injectable EPI is available in solutions of 1, 0.5, and 0.1 mg/mL. A subcutaneous dose ranges from 0.3 to 0.5 mg. The intravenous route is used cautiously if an immediate and reliable effect is mandatory. If the solution is given by vein, it must be adequately diluted and injected very slowly. The dose is seldom as much as 0.25 mg, except for cardiac arrest, when larger doses may be required.

Toxicity, Adverse Effects, and Contraindications

Epinephrine may cause restlessness, throbbing headache, tremor, and palpitations. The effects rapidly subside with rest, quiet, recumbency, and reassurance. More serious reactions include cerebral hemorrhage and cardiac arrhythmias. The use of large doses or the accidental, rapid intravenous injection of EPI may result in cerebral hemorrhage from the sharp rise in blood pressure. Ventricular arrhythmias may follow the administration of EPI. Angina may be induced by EPI in patients with coronary artery disease. *The use of EPI generally is contraindicated in patients who are receiving nonselective β receptor antagonists because its unopposed actions on vascular α_1 receptors may lead to severe hypertension and cerebral hemorrhage.*

Therapeutic Uses

A major use of EPI is to provide rapid, emergency relief of hypersensitivity reactions, including anaphylaxis, to drugs and other allergens. EPI also is used to prolong the action of local anesthetics, presumably by decreasing local blood flow and reducing systemic absorption. (Chapter 22). Its cardiac effects may be of use in restoring cardiac rhythm in patients with cardiac arrest due to various causes. It also is used as a topical hemostatic agent on bleeding surfaces, such as in the mouth or in bleeding peptic ulcers during endoscopy of the stomach and duodenum. Systemic absorption of the drug can occur with dental application. Inhalation of EPI may be useful in the treatment of postintubation and infectious croup.

Norepinephrine

Norepinephrine (levarterenol, *l*-noradrenaline, *l*-β-[3,4-dihydroxyphenyl]-α-aminoethanol) is a major chemical mediator liberated by mammalian *postganglionic sympathetic nerves*. It differs from EPI only by lacking the methyl substitution in the amino group (Table 12–1). NE constitutes 10%–20% of the catecholamine content of human adrenal medulla and as much as 97% in some pheochromocytomas, which may not express the enzyme phenylethanolamine-*N*-methyltransferase.

Pharmacological Properties

The pharmacological actions of NE and EPI are compared in Table 12–2. Both drugs are direct agonists on effector cells, and their actions differ mainly in the ratio of their effectiveness in stimulating α and β_2 receptors. *They are approximately equipotent in stimulating β_1 receptors. NE is a potent α agonist and has relatively little action on β_2 receptors*; however, it is somewhat less potent than EPI on the α receptors of most organs.

Cardiovascular Effects

In response to intravenous infusion of NE in humans (Figure 12–2), *systolic and diastolic pressures, and usually pulse pressure, are increased. Cardiac output is unchanged or decreased, and total peripheral resistance is raised. Compensatory vagal reflex activity slows the heart, overcoming a direct cardioaccelerator action, and stroke volume is increased. The peripheral vascular resistance increases in most vascular beds, and renal blood flow is reduced. NE constricts mesenteric vessels and reduces splanchnic and hepatic blood flow. Coronary flow usually is increased, probably owing both to indirectly induced coronary dilation, as with EPI, and to elevated blood pressure.* Although generally a poor β_2 receptor agonist, NE may increase coronary blood flow directly by stimulating β_2 receptors on coronary vessels. Patients with Prinzmetal variant angina may be supersensitive to the α adrenergic vasoconstrictor effects of NE.

Unlike EPI, NE in small doses does not cause vasodilation or lower blood pressure because the blood vessels of skeletal muscle constrict rather than dilate; α adrenergic receptor antagonists therefore abolish the pressor effects but do not cause significant reversal (i.e., hypotension).

Other Effects

Other responses to NE are not prominent in humans. The drug causes hyperglycemia and other metabolic effects similar to those produced by EPI, but these are observed only when large doses are given because NE is not as effective a "hormone" as EPI. Intradermal injection of suitable doses causes sweating that is not blocked by atropine.

ADME

Norepinephrine, like EPI, is ineffective when given orally and is absorbed poorly from sites of subcutaneous injection. It is rapidly inactivated in the body by the same enzymes that methylate (COMT) and oxidatively deaminate EPI (MAO). Small amounts normally are found in the urine. The excretion rate may be greatly increased in patients with pheochromocytoma.

Toxicity, Adverse Effects, and Precautions

The untoward effects of NE are similar to those of EPI, although there typically is greater elevation of blood pressure with NE. Excessive doses can cause severe hypertension.

Care must be taken that necrosis and sloughing do not occur at the site of intravenous injection owing to extravasation of the drug. The infusion should be made high in the limb, preferably through a long plastic cannula extending centrally. Impaired circulation at injection sites, with or without extravasation of NE, may be relieved by infiltrating the area with phentolamine, an α receptor antagonist. Blood pressure must be determined frequently during the infusion, particularly during adjustment of the rate of the infusion. Reduced blood flow to organs such as kidney and intestines is a constant danger with the use of NE.

Therapeutic Uses

Norepinephrine is used as a vasoconstrictor to raise or support blood pressure under certain intensive care conditions (discussed further in this chapter).

Droxidopa, a Synthetic Prodrug of Norepinephrine

Droxidopa (L-threo-3,4,-dihydroxyphenylserine) is a synthetic prodrug that is converted by AAAD into NE. It is FDA-approved for the treatment of orthostatic dizziness and light-headiness in adults with symptomatic neurogenic orthostatic hypotension associated with primary autonomic failure and impaired compensatory autonomic reflexes (Keating, 2014). The pharmacological effects of droxidopa are thought to be mediated through NE rather than through the parent drug or other metabolites. Droxidopa can cross the blood-brain barrier, presumably as the substrate of an amino acid transporter.

Dopamine

Dopamine (3,4-dihydroxyphenylethylamine) (Table 12–1) is the immediate metabolic precursor of NE and EPI; it is a central neurotransmitter particularly important in the regulation of movement (Chapters 14, 16, and 18) and possesses important intrinsic pharmacological properties. In the periphery, it is synthesized in epithelial cells of the proximal tubule and is thought to exert local diuretic and natriuretic effects. DA is a substrate for both MAO and COMT and thus is ineffective when administered orally. Classification of DA receptors is described in Chapter 13.

Pharmacological Properties Cardiovascular Effects

The cardiovascular effects of DA are mediated by several distinct types of receptors that vary in their affinity for DA (Chapter 13). At low concentrations, the primary interaction of DA is with vascular D_1 receptors, especially in the renal, mesenteric, and coronary beds. By activating adenylyl cyclase and raising intracellular concentrations of cAMP, D_1 receptor stimulation leads to vasodilation. Infusion of low doses of DA causes an increase in glomerular filtration rate, renal blood flow, and Na^+ excretion. Activation of D_1 receptors on renal tubular cells decreases Na^+ transport by cAMP-dependent and cAMP-independent mechanisms. Increasing cAMP production in the proximal tubular cells and the medullary part of the thick ascending limb of the loop of Henle inhibits the Na^+-H^+ exchanger and the Na^+,K^+-ATPase pump. The renal tubular actions of DA that cause natriuresis may be augmented by the increase in renal blood flow and the small increase in the glomerular filtration rate that follows its administration. The resulting increase in hydrostatic pressure in the peritubular capillaries and reduction in oncotic pressure may contribute to diminished reabsorption of Na^+ by the proximal tubular cells. As a consequence, DA has pharmacologically appropriate effects in the management of states of low cardiac output associated with compromised renal function, such as severe congestive heart failure.

At higher concentrations, DA exerts a positive inotropic effect on the myocardium, acting on β_1 adrenergic receptors. DA also causes the release of NE from nerve terminals, which contributes to its effects on the heart. Tachycardia is less prominent during infusion of DA than of INE (discussed further in the chapter). DA usually increases systolic blood pressure and pulse pressure and either has no effect on diastolic blood pressure or increases it slightly. Total peripheral resistance usually is unchanged when low or intermediate doses of DA are given, probably because of the ability of DA to reduce regional arterial resistance in some vascular beds, such as mesenteric and renal, while causing only minor increases in others. At high concentrations, DA activates vascular α_1 receptors, leading to more general vasoconstriction.

CNS Effects

Although there are specific DA receptors in the CNS, injected DA usually has no central effects because it does not readily cross the blood-brain barrier.

Precautions, Adverse Reactions, and Contraindications

Before DA is administered to patients in shock, hypovolemia should be corrected by transfusion of whole blood, plasma, or other appropriate fluid. Untoward effects due to overdosage generally are attributable to excessive sympathomimetic activity (although this also may be the response to worsening shock). Nausea, vomiting, tachycardia, anginal pain, arrhythmias, headache, hypertension, and peripheral vasoconstriction may be encountered during DA infusion. Extravasation of large amounts of DA during infusion may cause ischemic necrosis and sloughing. Rarely, gangrene of the fingers or toes has followed prolonged infusion of the drug. DA should be avoided or used at a much reduced dosage if the patient has received a MAO inhibitor. Careful adjustment of dosage also is necessary in patients who are taking tricyclic antidepressants.

Therapeutic Uses

Dopamine is used in the treatment of severe congestive heart failure, particularly in patients with oliguria and low or normal peripheral vascular resistance. The drug also may improve physiological parameters in the treatment of cardiogenic and septic shock. While DA may acutely improve cardiac and renal function in severely ill patients with chronic heart disease or renal failure, there is relatively little evidence supporting long-term benefit in clinical outcome (Marik and Iglesias, 1999).

Dopamine hydrochloride is used only intravenously, preferably into a large vein to prevent perivascular infiltration; extravasation may cause necrosis and sloughing of the surrounding tissue. The use of a calibrated infusion pump to control the rate of flow is necessary. The drug is administered at a rate of 2–5 μg/kg per min; this rate may be increased gradually up to 20–50 μg/kg per min or more as the clinical situation dictates. During the infusion, patients require clinical assessment of myocardial function, perfusion of vital organs such as the brain, and the production of urine. Reduction in urine flow, tachycardia, or the development of arrhythmias may be indications to slow or terminate the infusion. The duration of action of DA is brief, and hence the rate of administration can be used to control the intensity of effect.

Fenoldopam and Dopexamine. *Fenoldopam*, a benzazepine derivative, is a rapidly acting vasodilator used for not more than 48 h for control of severe hypertension (e.g., malignant hypertension with end-organ damage) in hospitalized patients. Fenoldopam is an agonist for peripheral D_1 receptors and binds with moderate affinity to α_2 adrenergic receptors; it has no significant affinity for D_2 receptors or α_1 or β adrenergic receptors. Fenoldopam is a racemic mixture; the R-isomer is the active component. It dilates a variety of blood vessels, including coronary arteries, afferent and efferent arterioles in the kidney, and mesenteric arteries (Murphy et al., 2001). Fenoldopam must be administered using a calibrated infusion pump; the usual dose rate ranges from 0.01 to 1.6 μg/kg per min.

Less than 6% of an orally administered dose is absorbed because of extensive first-pass formation of sulfate, methyl, and glucuronide conjugates. The elimination $t_{1/2}$ of intravenously infused fenoldopam is about 10 min. Adverse effects are related to the vasodilation and include headache, flushing, dizziness, and tachycardia or bradycardia.

Dopexamine is a synthetic analogue related to DA with intrinsic activity at DA D_1 and D_2 receptors as well as at β_2 receptors; it may have other effects, such as inhibition of catecholamine uptake (Fitton and Benfield, 1990). It has favorable hemodynamic actions in patients with severe congestive heart failure, sepsis, and shock. In patients with low cardiac output, dopexamine infusion significantly increases stroke volume with a decrease in systemic vascular resistance. Tachycardia and hypotension can occur, but usually only at high infusion rates. Dopexamine is not currently available in the U.S.

β Adrenergic Receptor Agonists

β Adrenergic receptor agonists play a major role only in the treatment of bronchoconstriction in patients with asthma (reversible airway obstruction) or COPD. Minor uses include management of preterm labor, treatment of complete heart block in shock, and short-term treatment of cardiac decompensation after surgery or in patients with congestive heart failure or myocardial infarction. The development of β_2-selective agonists has resulted in drugs with even more valuable characteristics, including adequate oral bioavailability, lack of α adrenergic activity and relative lack of β_1 adrenergic activity, and thus diminished likelihood of adverse cardiovascular effects.

β Receptor agonists may be used to stimulate the rate and force of cardiac contraction. The chronotropic effect is useful in the emergency treatment of arrhythmias such as torsades de pointes, bradycardia, or heart block (Chapter 30), whereas the inotropic effect is useful when it is desirable to augment myocardial contractility.

Isoproterenol

Isoproterenol (INE, isopropyl norepinephrine, isoprenaline, isopropylarterenol, isopropyl noradrenaline, *d,l*-β-[3,4-dihydroxyphenyl]-α-isopropylaminoethanol) (Table 12–1) is a potent, nonselective β receptor agonist with very low affinity for α receptors. Consequently, INE has powerful effects on all β receptors and almost no action at α receptors.

Pharmacological Actions

The major cardiovascular effects of INE (compared with EPI and NE) are illustrated in Figure 12–2. *Intravenous infusion of INE lowers peripheral vascular resistance,* primarily in skeletal muscle but also in renal and mesenteric vascular beds. *Diastolic pressure falls. Systolic blood pressure may remain unchanged or rise, although mean arterial pressure typically falls. Cardiac output is increased because of the positive inotropic and chronotropic effects of the drug in the face of diminished peripheral vascular resistance.* The cardiac effects of INE may lead to palpitations, sinus tachycardia, and more serious arrhythmias; large doses of INE cause myocardial necrosis in experimental animals.

Isoproterenol relaxes almost all varieties of smooth muscle when the tone is high, an action that is most pronounced on bronchial and GI smooth muscle. INE prevents or relieves bronchoconstriction. Its effect in asthma may be due in part to an additional action to inhibit antigen-induced release of histamine and other mediators of inflammation, an action shared by β_2-selective stimulants.

ADME

Isoproterenol is readily absorbed when given parenterally or as an aerosol. *It is metabolized by COMT, primarily in the liver but also by other tissues.* INE is a relatively poor substrate for MAO and NET (SLC6A2) and is not taken up by sympathetic neurons to the same extent as are EPI and NE. The duration of action of INE therefore may be longer than that of EPI, but it still is relatively brief.

Therapeutic Uses

Isoproterenol may be used in emergencies to stimulate heart rate in patients with bradycardia or heart block, particularly in anticipation of inserting an artificial cardiac pacemaker or in patients with the ventricular arrhythmia torsades de pointes. In disorders such as asthma and shock, INE largely has been replaced by other sympathomimetic drugs (see further in this chapter and in Chapter 40).

Adverse Effects

Palpitations, tachycardia, headache, and flushing are common. Cardiac ischemia and arrhythmias may occur, particularly in patients with underlying coronary artery disease.

Dobutamine

Dobutamine resembles DA structurally but possesses a bulky aromatic substituent on the amino group (Table 12–1). The pharmacological effects of dobutamine are due to direct interactions with α and β receptors; its actions do not appear to result from release of NE from sympathetic nerve endings, and they are not exerted by dopaminergic receptors.

Dobutamine possesses a center of asymmetry; both enantiomeric forms are present in the racemate used clinically. The (–) isomer of dobutamine is a potent α_1 agonist and can cause marked pressor responses. In contrast, (+)-dobutamine is a potent α_1 receptor antagonist, which can block the effects of (–)-dobutamine. Both isomers are full agonists at β receptors; the (+) isomer is a more potent β agonist than the (–) isomer by about 10-fold.

Cardiovascular Effects

The cardiovascular effects of racemic dobutamine represent a composite of the distinct pharmacological properties of the (–) and (+) stereoisomers. Compared to INE, dobutamine has relatively more prominent inotropic than chronotropic effects on the heart. Although not completely understood, this useful selectivity may arise because peripheral resistance is relatively unchanged. Alternatively, cardiac α_1 receptors may contribute to the inotropic effect. At equivalent inotropic doses, dobutamine enhances automaticity of the sinus node to a lesser extent than does INE; however, enhancement of AV and intraventricular conduction is similar for both drugs.

In animals, infusion of dobutamine increases cardiac contractility and cardiac output without markedly changing total peripheral resistance; the relatively constant peripheral resistance presumably reflects counterbalancing of α_1 receptor–mediated vasoconstriction and β_2 receptor–mediated vasodilation. Heart rate increases only modestly when dobutamine is administered at less than 20 μg/kg per min. After administration of β receptor antagonists, infusion of dobutamine fails to increase cardiac output, but total peripheral resistance increases, confirming that dobutamine has modest direct effects on α adrenergic receptors in the vasculature.

ADME

Dobutamine has a $t_{1/2}$ of about 2 min; the major metabolites are conjugates of dobutamine and 3-*O*-methyldobutamine. The onset of effect is rapid. Steady-state concentrations generally are achieved within 10 min of initiation of the infusion by calibrated infusion pump. The rate of infusion required to increase cardiac output typically is between 2.5 and 10 μg/kg per min, although higher infusion rates occasionally are required. The rate and duration of the infusion are determined by the clinical and hemodynamic responses of the patient.

Therapeutic Uses

Dobutamine is indicated for the short-term treatment of cardiac decompensation that may occur after cardiac surgery or in patients with congestive heart failure or acute myocardial infarction. Dobutamine increases cardiac output and stroke volume in such patients, usually without a marked increase in heart rate. Alterations in blood pressure or peripheral resistance usually are minor, although some patients may have marked increases in blood pressure or heart rate. An infusion of dobutamine in combination with echocardiography is useful in the noninvasive assessment of patients with coronary artery disease.

Adverse Effects

Blood pressure and heart rate may increase significantly during dobutamine administration requiring reduction of infusion rate. Patients with a history of hypertension may exhibit an exaggerated pressor response more frequently. Because dobutamine facilitates AV conduction, patients with atrial fibrillation are at risk of marked increases in ventricular response rates; digoxin or other measures may be required to prevent this from occurring. Some patients may develop ventricular ectopic activity. Dobutamine may increase the size of a myocardial infarct by increasing myocardial O_2 demand, a property common to inotropic agents. The efficacy of dobutamine over a period of more than a few days is uncertain; there is evidence for the development of tolerance.

β_2-Selective Adrenergic Receptor Agonists

Some of the major adverse effects of β receptor agonists in the treatment of asthma or COPD are caused by stimulation of β_1 receptors in the heart. β_2-Selective agents have been developed to avoid these adverse effects. This selectivity, however, is not absolute and is lost at high concentrations of these drugs. Moreover, up to 40% of the β receptors in the human heart are β_2 receptors, activation of which can also cause cardiac stimulation (Brodde and Michel, 1999).

A second strategy that has increased the usefulness of several β_2-selective agonists in the treatment of asthma and COPD has been structural modification that results in lower rates of metabolism and enhanced oral bioavailability. Modifications have included placing the hydroxyl groups at positions 3 and 5 of the phenyl ring or substituting another moiety for the hydroxyl group at position 3. This has yielded drugs such as metaproterenol, terbutaline, and albuterol, which are not substrates for COMT. Bulky substituents on the amino group of catecholamines contribute to potency at β receptors with decreased activity at α receptors and decreased metabolism by MAO.

A final strategy to enhance preferential activation of pulmonary β_2 receptors is the administration by inhalation of small doses of the drug in aerosol form. This approach typically leads to effective activation of β_2 receptors in the bronchi but very low systemic drug concentrations. Consequently, there is less potential to activate cardiac β_1 or β_2 receptors or to stimulate β_2 receptors in skeletal muscle, which can cause tremor and thereby limit oral therapy.

Subcutaneous injection also causes prompt bronchodilation; for an orally administered agent, the peak effect may be delayed for several hours. Administration of β receptor agonists by aerosol (Chapter 40) typically leads to a very rapid therapeutic response, generally within minutes, although some agonists such as *salmeterol* have a delayed onset of action. Aerosol therapy depends on the delivery of drug to the distal airways. This, in turn, depends on the size of the particles in the aerosol and respiratory parameters such as inspiratory flow rate, tidal volume, breath-holding time, and airway diameter. Only about 10% of an inhaled dose actually enters the lungs; much of the remainder is swallowed and ultimately may be absorbed. Successful aerosol therapy requires that each patient master the technique of drug administration. In some patients, particularly children and the elderly, spacer devices may enhance the efficacy of inhalation therapy.

In the treatment of asthma and COPD, β receptor agonists are used to activate pulmonary receptors that relax bronchial smooth muscle and decrease airway resistance. β Receptor agonists also may suppress the release of leukotrienes and histamine from mast cells in lung tissue, enhance mucociliary function, decrease microvascular permeability, and possibly inhibit phospholipase A_2. Airway inflammation also contributes airway hyperresponsiveness; consequently, the use of anti-inflammatory drugs such as inhaled steroids has primary importance. Most authorities recommend that long-acting β agonists should not be used without concomitant anti-inflammatory therapy in the treatment of asthma (see Chapter 40; Drazen and O'Byrne, 2009; Fanta, 2009).

Short-Acting β_2 Adrenergic Agonists

Metaproterenol. Metaproterenol (called orciprenaline in Europe), along with *terbutaline* and *fenoterol*, belongs to the structural class of resorcinol bronchodilators that have hydroxyl groups at positions 3 and 5 of the phenyl ring (rather than at positions 3 and 4 as in catechols) (Table 12–1).

Consequently, metaproterenol is resistant to methylation by COMT, and a substantial fraction (40%) is absorbed in active form after oral administration. It is excreted primarily as glucuronic acid conjugates. Metaproterenol is considered to be β_2 selective, although it probably is less selective than albuterol or terbutaline and hence is more prone to cause cardiac stimulation. Effects occur within minutes of inhalation and persist for several hours. After oral administration, onset of action is slower, but effects last 3–4 h. Metaproterenol is used for the long-term treatment of obstructive airway diseases and asthma and for treatment of acute bronchospasm (Chapter 40). Side effects are similar to the short- and intermediate-acting sympathomimetic bronchodilators.

Albuterol. Albuterol is a selective β_2 receptor agonist with pharmacological properties and therapeutic indications similar to those of terbutaline. It can be administered by inhalation or orally for the symptomatic relief of bronchospasm.

When administered by inhalation, it produces significant bronchodilation within 15 min, and effects persist for 3–4 h. The cardiovascular effects of albuterol are much weaker than those of INE when doses that produce comparable bronchodilation are administered by inhalation. Oral albuterol has the potential to delay preterm labor. Although rare, CNS and respiratory side effects are sometimes observed.

Albuterol has been made available in a metered-dose inhaler free of CFCs (chlorofluorocarbons). The alternate propellant, HFA (hydrofluoroalkane), is inert in the human airway, but unlike CFCs, it does not deplete stratospheric ozone.

Levalbuterol. Levalbuterol is the *R*-enantiomer of albuterol, a racemate used to treat asthma and COPD. Although originally available only as a solution for a nebulizer, it is now available as a CFC-free metered-dose inhaler. Levalbuterol is β_2 selective and acts like other β_2 adrenergic agonists. In general, levalbuterol has similar pharmacokinetic and pharmacodynamics properties as albuterol.

Pirbuterol. Pirbuterol is a relatively selective β_2 agonist. Its structure differs from that of albuterol by the substitution of a pyridine ring for the benzene ring. Pirbuterol acetate is available for inhalation therapy; dosing is typically every 4–6 h. Pirbuterol is the only preparation available in a breath-activated metered-dose inhaler, a device meant to optimize medication delivery by releasing a spray of medication only on the patient's initiation of inspiration.

Terbutaline. Terbutaline is a β_2-selective bronchodilator. It contains a resorcinol ring and thus is not a substrate for COMT methylation. It is effective when taken orally or subcutaneously or by inhalation (not marketed for inhalation in the U.S.). Effects are observed rapidly after inhalation or parenteral administration; after inhalation, its action may persist 3–6 h. With oral administration, the onset of effect may be delayed 1–2 h. Terbutaline is used for the long-term treatment of obstructive airway diseases and for treatment of acute bronchospasm; it also is available for parenteral use for the emergency treatment of status asthmaticus (Chapter 40).

Isoetharine. Isoetharine is an older β_2-selective drug. Its selectivity for β_2 receptors does not approach that of some newer agents. Although resistant to metabolism by MAO, it is a catecholamine and thus is a good substrate for COMT. Consequently, it is used only by inhalation for the treatment of acute episodes of bronchoconstriction. Isoetharine is no longer marketed in the U.S.

Fenoterol. Fenoterol is a β_2-selective receptor agonist. After inhalation, it has a prompt onset of action, and its effect typically is sustained for 4–6 h. A possible association of fenoterol use with increased deaths from asthma, although controversial (Suissa and Ernst, 1997), has led to its withdrawal from the market. The dysrhythmias and cardiac effects associated with fenoterol are likely due to effects on β_1 adrenergic receptors.

Procaterol. Procaterol is a β_2-selective receptor agonist. After inhalation, it has a prompt onset of action that is sustained for about 5 h. Procaterol is not available in the U.S.

Long-Acting β_2 Adrenergic Agonists (LABAs)

Salmeterol

Mechanism of Action. Salmeterol is a lipophilic β_2-selective agonist with a prolonged duration of action (>12 h) and a selectivity for β_2 receptors about 50-fold greater than that of albuterol. Salmeterol provides symptomatic relief and improves lung function and quality of life in patients with COPD. It is as effective as the cholinergic antagonist ipratropium, more effective than theophylline, and has additive effects when used in combination with inhaled ipratropium or oral theophylline. Salmeterol also may have anti-inflammatory activity.

ADME. The onset of action of inhaled salmeterol is relatively slow, so it is not suitable monotherapy for acute attacks of bronchospasm. Salmeterol is metabolized by CYP3A4 to α-hydroxy-salmeterol, which is eliminated primarily in the feces.

Clinical Use, Precautions, and Adverse Effects. Salmeterol and formoterol are the agents of choice for nocturnal asthma in patients who remain symptomatic despite anti-inflammatory agents and other standard management.

Salmeterol generally is well tolerated but has the potential to increase heart rate and plasma glucose concentration, to produce tremors, and to decrease plasma K^+ concentration through effects on extrapulmonary β_2 receptors. Salmeterol should not be used more than twice daily (morning and evening) and should not be used to treat acute asthma symptoms, which should be treated with a short-acting β_2 agonist (e.g., *albuterol*) when breakthrough symptoms occur despite twice-daily use of salmeterol (Redington, 2001).

Patients with moderate or severe persistent asthma or COPD benefit from the use of LABAs like salmeterol in combination with an inhaled corticosteroid. For that reason, salmeterol is available in a single formulate combination with the corticosteroid fluticasone. These benefits must be counterbalanced against data, oft-criticized, showing that the addition of a LABA to "usual therapy" was associated with an increased risk of fatal or near-fatal asthmatic attacks, as compared with usual therapy alone. On the other hand, there is a lack of reports of increased asthma mortality among patients taking both a LABA and an inhaled corticosteroid (Fanta, 2009). Nevertheless, the FDA has placed a **black-box warning** in the labeling information for *salmeterol, formoterol,* and *arformoterol.* Expert panels (Fanta, 2009) recommend the use of LABAs only for patients in whom inhaled corticosteroids alone either failed to achieve good asthma control or for initial therapy.

Formoterol. Formoterol is a long-acting β_2-selective receptor agonist. Significant bronchodilation, which may persist for up to 12 h, occurs within minutes of inhalation of a therapeutic dose. It is highly lipophilic and has high affinity for β_2 receptors. Its major advantage over many other β_2-selective agonists is this prolonged duration of action, which may be particularly advantageous in settings such as nocturnal asthma. Formoterol's sustained action is due to its insertion into the lipid bilayer of the plasma membrane, from which it gradually diffuses to provide prolonged stimulation of β_2 receptors. It is FDA-approved for treatment of asthma and bronchospasm, prophylaxis of exercise-induced bronchospasm, and COPD. It can be used concomitantly with short-acting β_2 agonists, glucocorticoids (inhaled or systemic), and theophylline (Goldsmith and Keating, 2004). Formoterol is also available as a single formulaic combination with the glucocorticoids mometasone or budesonide for treatment of COPD.

Arformoterol. Arformoterol, an enantiomer of formoterol, is a selective LABA that has twice the potency of racemic formoterol. It is FDA-approved for the long-term treatment of bronchoconstriction in patients with COPD, including chronic bronchitis and emphysema (Matera and Cazzola, 2007). It was the first LABA developed as inhalational therapy for use with a nebulizer (Abdelghany, 2007).

Systemic exposure to arformoterol is due to pulmonary absorption, with plasma levels reaching a peak in 0.25–1 h. It is primarily metabolized by direct conjugation to glucuronide or sulfate conjugates and secondarily by O-demethylation by CYP2D6 and CYP2C19. It does not inhibit any of the common CYPs (Fanta, 2009).

Very Long-Acting β_2 Adrenergic Agonists (VLABAs)

Very long-acting β_2 adrenergic agonists have been developed primarily for treating COPD. These drugs are not recommended for treating asthma.

Indacaterol, the first once-daily LABA approved for COPD, is a potent β_2 agonist with high intrinsic efficacy. It has a fast onset of action, appears well tolerated, and is effective in COPD with little tachyphylaxis on continued use. In contrast to salmeterol, indacaterol does not antagonize the bronchorelaxant effect of short-acting β_2 adrenergic agonists.

Olodaterol is also a once-daily, long-acting β_2 agonist approved for use in COPD. It is also offered in combination with tiotropium bromide, an antagonist at M_3 muscarinic receptors.

Vilanterol is a VLABA approved for use in combination with fluticasone. Vilanterol is available in Europe in combination with the long-acting muscarinic antagonist umeclidinium.

Other β_2-Selective Agonists

Ritodrine. Ritodrine is a β_2-selective agonist that was developed specifically for use as a uterine relaxant. Its pharmacological properties closely resemble those of the other agents in this group. The pharmacokinetic properties of ritodrine are complex and incompletely defined, especially in pregnant women. Ritodrine is rapidly but incompletely (30%) absorbed following oral administration: The drug may be administered intravenously to selected patients to arrest premature labor. β_2-Selective agonists may not have clinically significant benefits on perinatal mortality and may actually increase maternal morbidity. Ritodrine is not available in the U.S. See Chapter 44 for the pharmacology of tocolytic agents.

Adverse Effects of β_2-Selective Agonists

The major adverse effects of β receptor agonists occur as a result of excessive activation of β receptors. Patients with underlying cardiovascular disease are particularly at risk for significant reactions. However, the likelihood of adverse effects can be greatly decreased in patients with lung disease by administering the drug by inhalation rather than orally or parenterally.

Tremor is a relatively common adverse effect of the β_2-selective receptor agonists. Tolerance generally develops to this effect; it is not clear whether tolerance reflects desensitization of the β_2 receptors of skeletal muscle or adaptation within the CNS. This adverse effect can be minimized by starting oral therapy with a low dose of drug and progressively increasing the dose as tolerance to the tremor develops. Feelings of restlessness, apprehension, and anxiety may limit therapy with these drugs, particularly oral or parenteral administration.

Tachycardia is a common adverse effect of systemically administered β receptor agonists. Stimulation of heart rate occurs primarily by means of β_1 receptors. It is uncertain to what extent the increase in heart rate also is due to activation of cardiac β_2 receptors or to reflex effects that stem from β_2 receptor–mediated peripheral vasodilation. During a severe asthma attack, heart rate actually may decrease during therapy with a β agonist, presumably because of improvement in pulmonary function with consequent reduction in endogenous cardiac sympathetic stimulation. In patients without cardiac disease, β agonists rarely cause significant arrhythmias or myocardial ischemia; however, patients with underlying coronary artery disease or preexisting arrhythmias are at greater risk. The risk of adverse cardiovascular effects also is increased in patients who are receiving MAO inhibitors. In general, at least 2 weeks should elapse between the use of MAO inhibitors and administration of β_2 agonists or other sympathomimetics.

When given parenterally, these drugs also may increase the concentrations of glucose, lactate, and free fatty acids in plasma and decrease the concentration of K^+. The decrease in K^+ concentration may be especially important in patients with cardiac disease, particularly those taking digoxin and diuretics. In some diabetic patients, hyperglycemia may be worsened by these drugs, and higher doses of insulin may be required. Side effects of LABAs and VLABAs include nasopharyngitis and increase in incidence of pneumonia. As a result of these side effects, postmarketing safety studies are under way.

Large doses of β receptor agonists cause myocardial necrosis in laboratory animals.

β_3 Adrenergic Receptor Agonists

The existence of the β_3 adrenergic receptor subtype was first proposed in the 1970s but was not confirmed until the receptor was cloned in 1989 (Emorine et al., 1989). The β_3 receptor couples to the G_s-cAMP pathway and has a much stronger affinity for NE than EPI. The β_3 receptor displays much lower affinities for classic β antagonists (such as propranolol or atenolol) than do β_1 and β_2 receptors. In humans, the β_3 receptor is expressed in brown adipose tissue, gallbladder, and ileum and to a lesser extent in white adipose tissue and the detrusor muscle of the bladder; there is little expression elsewhere (Berkowitz et al., 1995). To date, the major therapeutic target that has emerged from this field has been the development of β_3 receptor agonists for use in urinary incontinence (Michel, 2016).

Mirabegron is a β_3 adrenergic receptor agonist approved for use against incontinence. Activation of this receptor in the bladder leads to detrusor muscle relaxation and increased bladder capacity. This action prevents voiding and provides relief for those with an overactive bladder and urinary incontinence. Side effects include increased blood pressure, increased incidence of urinary tract infection, and headache. Mirabegron is also a moderate CYP2D6 inhibitor, so care must be taken when prescribing with other drugs metabolized by CYP2D6, such as digoxin, metoprolol, and desipramine.

α Adrenergic Receptor Agonists

α_1-Selective Adrenergic Receptor Agonists

The major effects of a number of sympathomimetic drugs are due to activation of α adrenergic receptors in vascular smooth muscle. As a result, peripheral vascular resistance is increased, and blood pressure is maintained or elevated. The clinical utility of these drugs is limited to the treatment of some patients with hypotension, including orthostatic hypotension, or shock. *Phenylephrine* and *methoxamine* (discontinued in the U.S.) are direct-acting vasoconstrictors and are selective activators of α_1 receptors. *Mephentermine* and *metaraminol* act both directly and indirectly. Midodrine is a prodrug that is converted, after oral administration, to *desglymidodrine*, a direct-acting α_1 agonist.

Phenylephrine

Phenylephrine is an α_1-selective agonist; it activates β receptors only at much higher concentrations. The pharmacological effects of phenylephrine are similar to those of methoxamine. The drug causes marked arterial vasoconstriction during intravenous infusion. Phenylephrine also is used as a nasal decongestant and as a mydriatic in various nasal and ophthalmic formulations (see Chapter 69).

Metaraminol

Metaraminol exerts *direct effects* on vascular α adrenergic receptors and acts *indirectly* by stimulating the release of NE. The drug has been used in the treatment of hypotensive states or off-label to relieve attacks of paroxysmal atrial tachycardia, particularly those associated with hypotension (see Chapter 30).

Midodrine

Midodrine is an orally effective α_1 receptor agonist. It is a prodrug, converted to an active metabolite, *desglymidodrine*, which achieves peak concentrations about 1 h after a dose of midodrine. The $t_{1/2}$ of desglymidodrine is about 3 h; its duration of action is about 4–6 h. Midodrine-induced rises in blood pressure are associated with contraction of both arterial and venous smooth muscle. This is advantageous in the treatment of patients with autonomic insufficiency and postural hypotension (McClellan et al., 1998). A frequent complication in these patients is supine hypertension. This can be minimized by administering the drug during periods when the patient will remain upright, avoiding dosing within 4 h of bedtime, and elevating the head of the bed. Very cautious use of a short-acting antihypertensive drug at bedtime may be useful in some patients. Typical dosing, achieved by careful titration of blood pressure responses, varies between 2.5 and 10 mg three times daily.

α_2-Selective Adrenergic Receptor Agonists

α_2-Selective adrenergic agonists are used primarily for the treatment of systemic hypertension. Their efficacy as antihypertensive agents is somewhat surprising, because many blood vessels contain postsynaptic α_2 adrenergic receptors that promote vasoconstriction (Chapter 8). Clonidine, an α_2-agonist, was developed as a vasoconstricting nasal decongestant; its lowers blood pressure by activating α_2 receptors in the CNS, thereby suppressing sympathetic outflow from the brain.

The α_2 agonists also reduce intraocular pressure by decreasing the production of aqueous humor. Two derivatives of clonidine, apraclonidine and brimonidine, applied topically to the eye, decrease intraocular pressure with little or no effect on systemic blood pressure.

Clonidine

Clonidine is an imidazoline derivative and an α_2 adrenergic agonist.

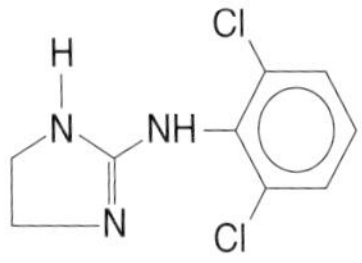

CLONIDINE

Mechanisms of Action and Pharmacological Effects. Intravenous infusion of clonidine causes an acute rise in blood pressure because of activation of postsynaptic α_2 receptors in vascular smooth muscle. This transient vasoconstriction (not usually seen with oral administration) is followed by a more prolonged hypotensive response that results from decreased sympathetic outflow from the CNS. The effect appears to result, at least in part, from activation of α_2 receptors in the lower brainstem region. Clonidine also stimulates parasympathetic outflow, which may contribute to the slowing of heart rate. In addition, some of the antihypertensive effects of clonidine may be mediated by activation of presynaptic α_2 receptors that suppress the release of NE, ATP, and NPY from postganglionic sympathetic nerves. Clonidine decreases the plasma concentration of NE and reduces its excretion in the urine.

Does Clonidine Act Via Imidazoline I_1 Receptors?

Studies in knockout animals demonstrated the requirement for a functional α_2 receptor for the hypotensive effect of clonidine. Clonidine and its congeners, as imidazolines, also bind to imidazoline receptors, of which there are three subtypes (I_1, I_2, and I_3) that are widely distributed in the body, including the CNS. Activation of the I_1 receptor appears to reduce sympathetic outflow from the CNS. Whether activation of the CNS I_1 imidazoline receptor also plays a role in the hypotensive effects of clonidine and its congeners is a topic of ongoing research. The current hypothesis is that I_1 receptors are upstream from the hypotensive α_2 receptors in the CNS and work in tandem with them, such that activation of the I_1 receptors results in catecholamine release onto the α_2 receptors (Lowry and Brown, 2014; Nikolic and Agbaba 2012), thereby reducing sympathetic outflow and reducing blood pressure.

Clonidine decreases discharges in sympathetic preganglionic fibers in the splanchnic nerve and in postganglionic fibers of cardiac nerves. These effects are blocked by α_2-selective antagonists such as yohimbine. *Clonidine also stimulates parasympathetic outflow, which may contribute to the slowing of heart rate as a consequence of increased vagal tone and diminished sympathetic drive.* In addition, some of the antihypertensive effects of clonidine may be mediated by activation of presynaptic α_2 receptors that suppress the release of NE, ATP, and NPY from postganglionic sympathetic nerves. Clonidine decreases the plasma concentration of NE and reduces its excretion in the urine.

ADME. Clonidine is well absorbed after oral administration, with bioavailability about 100%. Peak concentration in plasma and the maximal hypotensive effect are observed 1–3 h after an oral dose. The elimination $t_{1/2}$ is 6–24 h (mean about 12 h). About half of an administered dose can be recovered unchanged in the urine; the $t_{1/2}$ of the drug may increase with renal failure. A transdermal delivery patch permits continuous administration of clonidine as an alternative to oral therapy. The drug is released at an approximately constant rate for a week; 3–4 days are required to reach steady-state concentrations in plasma. When the patch is removed, plasma concentrations remain stable for about 8 h and then decline gradually over a period of several days; this decrease is associated with a rise in blood pressure.

Therapeutic Uses. Clonidine is used mainly in the treatment of hypertension (see Chapter 27). Clonidine also has apparent efficacy in the off-label treatment of a range of other disorders: in reducing diarrhea in some diabetic patients with autonomic neuropathy; in treating and preparing addicted subjects for withdrawal from narcotics, alcohol, and tobacco (see Chapter 24) by ameliorating some of the adverse sympathetic nervous activity associated with withdrawal and decreasing craving for the drug; and in reducing the incidence of menopausal hot flashes (transdermal application). Acute administration of clonidine has been used in the differential diagnosis of patients with hypertension and suspected pheochromocytoma. Among the other off-label uses of clonidine are atrial fibrillation, ADHD, constitutional growth delay in children, cyclosporine-associated nephrotoxicity, Tourette syndrome, hyperhidrosis, mania, posthepatic neuralgia, psychosis, restless leg syndrome, ulcerative colitis, and allergy-induced inflammatory reactions in patients with extrinsic asthma.

Adverse Effects. The major adverse effects of clonidine are dry mouth and sedation, which may diminish in intensity after several weeks of therapy. Sexual dysfunction also may occur. Marked bradycardia is observed in some patients. These effects of clonidine frequently are related to dose, and their incidence may be lower with transdermal administration of clonidine. About 15%–20% of patients develop contact dermatitis when using the transdermal system. Withdrawal reactions follow abrupt discontinuation of long-term therapy with clonidine in some hypertensive patients (see Chapter 28).

Apraclonidine

Apraclonidine is a relatively selective α_2 receptor agonist that is used topically to reduce intraocular pressure with minimal systemic effects. This agent does not cross the blood-brain barrier and is more useful than clonidine for ophthalmic therapy. Apraclonidine is useful as short-term adjunctive therapy in patients with glaucoma whose intraocular pressure is not well controlled by other pharmacological agents. The drug also is used to control or prevent elevations in intraocular pressure that occur in patients after laser trabeculoplasty or iridotomy (see Chapter 69).

Brimonidine

Brimonidine is a clonidine derivative and α_2-selective agonist that is administered ocularly to lower intraocular pressure in patients with ocular hypertension or open-angle glaucoma. Unlike apraclonidine, brimonidine can cross the blood-brain barrier and can produce hypotension and sedation, although these CNS effects are slight compared to those of clonidine.

Guanfacine

Guanfacine is an α_2 receptor agonist that is more selective than clonidine for α_2 receptors. Like clonidine, guanfacine lowers blood pressure by activation of brainstem receptors with resultant suppression of sympathetic activity. A sustained-release form is FDA-approved for treatment of ADHD in children aged 6–17 years.

Clinical Use. The drug is well absorbed after oral administration. About 50% of guanfacine appears unchanged in the urine; the rest is metabolized. The $t_{1/2}$ for elimination ranges from 12 to 24 h. Guanfacine and clonidine appear to have similar efficacy for the treatment of hypertension and a similar pattern of adverse effects. A withdrawal syndrome may occur after the abrupt discontinuation, but it is less frequent and milder than the syndrome that follows clonidine withdrawal; this difference may relate to the longer $t_{1/2}$ of guanfacine.

Guanabenz

Guanabenz is a centrally acting α_2-agonist that decreases blood pressure by a mechanism similar to those of clonidine and guanfacine. Guanabenz has a $t_{1/2}$ of 4–6 h and is extensively metabolized by the liver. Dosage adjustment may be necessary in patients with hepatic cirrhosis. The adverse effects caused by guanabenz (e.g., dry mouth and sedation) are similar to those seen with clonidine.

Methyldopa

Methyldopa (α-methyl-3,4-dihydroxyphenylalanine) is a centrally acting antihypertensive agent. It is metabolized to α-methylnorepinephrine in the brain, and this compound is thought to activate central α_2 receptors and lower blood pressure in a manner similar to that of clonidine (see Chapter 27).

Tizanidine

Tizanidine is a muscle relaxant used for the treatment of spasticity associated with cerebral and spinal disorders. It is also an α_2-agonist with some properties similar to those of clonidine.

Moxonidine

Moxonidine is a mixed α_2 receptor and imidazole I_1 receptor agonist. It acts to reduce sympathetic outflow from the CNS and thereby reduces blood pressure. Moxonidine also has analgesic activity, interacts synergistically with opioid agonists, and is used in treating neuropathic pain.

Miscellaneous Sympathomimetic Agonists

Amphetamine

Amphetamine, racemic β phenylisopropylamine (Table 12–1), has powerful CNS stimulant actions in addition to the peripheral α and β actions common to indirect-acting sympathomimetic drugs. Unlike EPI, it is effective after oral administration, and its effects last for several hours.

Cardiovascular System

Amphetamine given orally raises both systolic and diastolic blood pressure. Heart rate often is reflexly slowed; with large doses, cardiac arrhythmias may occur. Cardiac output is not enhanced by therapeutic doses, and cerebral blood flow does not change much. The *l*-isomer is slightly more potent than the *d*-isomer in its cardiovascular actions.

Other Smooth Muscles

In general, smooth muscles respond to amphetamine as they do to other sympathomimetic amines. The contractile effect on the sphincter of the urinary bladder is particularly marked, and for this reason amphetamine has been used in treating enuresis and incontinence. Pain and difficulty in micturition occasionally occur. The GI effects of amphetamine are unpredictable. If enteric activity is pronounced, amphetamine may cause relaxation and delay the movement of intestinal contents; if the gut already is relaxed, the opposite effect may occur. The response of the human uterus varies, but there usually is an increase in tone.

CNS

Amphetamine is one of the most potent sympathomimetic amines in stimulating the CNS. It stimulates the medullary respiratory center, lessens the degree of central depression caused by various drugs, and produces other signs of CNS stimulation. In eliciting CNS excitatory effects, the *d*-isomer (dextroamphetamine) is three to four times more potent than the *l*-isomer. The psychic effects depend on the dose and the mental state and personality of the individual. The main results of an oral dose of 10–30 mg include wakefulness, alertness, and a decreased sense of fatigue; elevation of mood, with increased initiative, self-confidence, and ability to concentrate; often, elation and euphoria; and increase in motor and speech activities. Performance of simple mental tasks is improved, but, although more work may be accomplished, the number of errors may increase. Physical performance (e.g., in athletes) is improved, and the drug often is abused for this purpose. These effects are variable and may be reversed by overdosage or repeated usage. Prolonged use or large doses are nearly always followed by depression and fatigue. Many individuals given amphetamine experience headache, palpitation, dizziness, vasomotor disturbances, agitation, confusion, dysphoria, apprehension, delirium, or fatigue.

Fatigue and Sleep. In general, amphetamine prolongs the duration of adequate performance before fatigue appears, and the effects of fatigue are at least partly reversed, most strikingly when performance has been reduced by fatigue and lack of sleep. Such improvement may be partly due to alteration of unfavorable attitudes toward the task. However, amphetamine reduces the frequency of attention lapses that impair performance after prolonged sleep deprivation and thus improves execution of tasks requiring sustained attention. The need for sleep may be postponed, but it cannot be avoided indefinitely. When the drug is discontinued after long use, the pattern of sleep may take as long as 2 months to return to normal.

Analgesia. Amphetamine and some other sympathomimetic amines have a small analgesic effect that is not sufficiently pronounced to be therapeutically useful. However, amphetamine can enhance the analgesia produced by opiates.

Respiration. Amphetamine stimulates the respiratory center, increasing the rate and depth of respiration. In normal individuals, usual doses of the drug do not appreciably increase respiratory rate or minute volume. Nevertheless, when respiration is depressed by centrally acting drugs, amphetamine may stimulate respiration.

Appetite. Amphetamine and similar drugs have been used for the treatment of obesity, although the wisdom of this use is at best questionable. Weight loss in obese humans treated with amphetamine is almost entirely due to reduced food intake and only in small measure to increased metabolism. The site of action probably is in the lateral hypothalamic feeding center; injection of amphetamine into this area, but not into the ventromedial region, suppresses food intake. Neurochemical mechanisms of action are unclear but may involve increased release of NE or DA. In humans, tolerance to the appetite suppression develops rapidly. Hence, continuous weight reduction usually is not observed in obese individuals without dietary restriction.

Mechanisms of Action in the CNS

Amphetamine exerts most or all of its effects in the CNS by releasing biogenic amines from their storage sites in nerve terminals. The neuronal DAT and the VMAT2 appear to be two of the principal targets of amphetamine's action (Fleckenstein, 2007; Sitte and Freissmuth, 2015). These mechanisms include amphetamine-induced exchange diffusion, reverse transport, channel-like transport phenomena, and effects resulting from the weakly basic properties of amphetamine. Amphetamine analogues affect monoamine transporters through phosphorylation, transporter trafficking, and the production of reactive oxygen and nitrogen species. These mechanisms may have potential implications for neurotoxicity as well as dopaminergic neurodegenerative diseases (discussed further in the chapter).

The alerting effect of amphetamine, its anorectic effect, and at least a component of its locomotor-stimulating action presumably are mediated by release of NE from central noradrenergic neurons. These effects can be prevented in experimental animals by inhibiting tyrosine hydroxylase and thus catecholamine synthesis. Some aspects of locomotor activity and the stereotyped behavior induced by amphetamine probably are a consequence of the release of DA from dopaminergic nerve terminals, particularly in the neostriatum. Higher doses are required to produce these behavioral effects, and this correlates with the higher concentrations of amphetamine required to release DA from brain slices or synaptosomes in vitro. With still higher doses of amphetamine, disturbances of perception and overt psychotic behavior occur. These effects may be due to release of 5HT from serotonergic neurons and of DA in the mesolimbic system. In addition, amphetamine may exert direct effects on CNS receptors for

5HT (Chapter 13).

Toxicity and Adverse Effects

The acute toxic effects of amphetamine usually are extensions of its therapeutic actions and as a rule result from overdosage. CNS effects commonly include restlessness, dizziness, tremor, hyperactive reflexes, talkativeness, tenseness, irritability, weakness, insomnia, fever, and sometimes euphoria. Confusion, aggressiveness, changes in libido, anxiety, delirium, paranoid hallucinations, panic states, and suicidal or homicidal tendencies occur, especially in mentally ill patients. However, these psychotic effects can be elicited in any individual if sufficient quantities of amphetamine are ingested for a prolonged period. Fatigue and depression usually follow central stimulation. Cardiovascular effects are common and include headache, chilliness, pallor or flushing, palpitation, cardiac arrhythmias, anginal pain, hypertension or hypotension, and circulatory collapse. Excessive sweating occurs. GI symptoms include dry mouth, metallic taste, anorexia, nausea, vomiting, diarrhea, and abdominal cramps. Fatal poisoning usually terminates in convulsions and coma, and cerebral hemorrhages are the main pathological findings.

The toxic dose of amphetamine varies widely. Toxic manifestations occasionally occur as an idiosyncratic reaction after as little as 2 mg but are rare with doses less than 15 mg. Severe reactions have occurred with 30 mg, yet doses of 400–500 mg are not uniformly fatal. Larger doses can be tolerated after chronic use of the drug. Treatment of acute amphetamine intoxication may include acidification of the urine by administration of ammonium chloride; this enhances the rate of elimination. Sedatives may be required for the CNS symptoms. Severe hypertension may require administration of sodium nitroprusside or an α adrenergic receptor antagonist.

Chronic intoxication with amphetamine causes symptoms similar to those of acute overdosage, but abnormal mental conditions are more common. Weight loss may be marked. A psychotic reaction with vivid hallucinations and paranoid delusions, often mistaken for schizophrenia, is the most common serious effect. Recovery usually is rapid after withdrawal of the drug, but occasionally the condition becomes chronic. In these persons, amphetamine may act as a precipitating factor hastening the onset of incipient schizophrenia.

The abuse of amphetamine as a means of overcoming sleepiness and of increasing energy and alertness should be discouraged. The drug should be used only under medical supervision. The amphetamines are schedule II drugs under federal regulations. The additional contraindications and precautions for the use of amphetamine generally are similar to those described for EPI. Amphetamine use is inadvisable in patients with anorexia, insomnia, asthenia, psychopathic personality, or a history of homicidal or suicidal tendencies.

Dependence and Tolerance

Psychological dependence often occurs when amphetamine or dextroamphetamine is used chronically, as discussed in Chapter 24. Tolerance almost invariably develops to the anorexigenic effect of amphetamines and often is seen also in the need for increasing doses to maintain improvement of mood in psychiatric patients. Tolerance is striking in individuals who are dependent on the drug; a daily intake of 1.7 g without apparent ill effects has been reported. Development of tolerance is not invariable, and cases of narcolepsy have been treated for years without requiring an increase in the initially effective dose.

Therapeutic Uses

Amphetamine is used chiefly for its CNS effects. Dextroamphetamine, with greater CNS action and less peripheral action, is FDA-approved for the treatment of narcolepsy and ADHD (see discussion later in this chapter).

Methamphetamine

Methamphetamine is closely related chemically to amphetamine and ephedrine (Table 12–1). The drug acts centrally to release DA and other biogenic amines and to inhibit neuronal and VMATs as well as MAO. Small doses have prominent central stimulant effects without significant peripheral actions; somewhat larger doses produce a sustained rise in systolic and diastolic blood pressures, due mainly to cardiac stimulation. Cardiac output is increased, although the heart rate may be reflexly slowed. Venous constriction causes peripheral venous pressure to increase. These factors tend to increase the venous return and thus cardiac output; pulmonary arterial pressure is raised.

Methamphetamine is a schedule II drug under federal regulations and has high potential for abuse (Chapter 24). It is widely abused as a cheap, accessible recreational drug. Illegal production of methamphetamine in clandestine laboratories throughout the U.S. is common. It is used principally for its central effects, which are more pronounced than those of amphetamine and are accompanied by less-prominent peripheral actions (see Therapeutic Uses of Sympathomimetic Drugs).

Methylphenidate

Methylphenidate is a piperidine derivative that is structurally related to amphetamine. Methylphenidate is a mild CNS stimulant with more prominent effects on mental than on motor activities. However, large doses produce signs of generalized CNS stimulation that may lead to convulsions.

The effects of methylphenidate resemble those of the amphetamines. Methylphenidate also shares the abuse potential of the amphetamines and is listed as a schedule II controlled substance in the U.S. Methylphenidate is effective in the treatment of narcolepsy and ADHD (described in the material that follows). Methylphenidate is readily absorbed after oral administration, reaching a peak C_p in about 2 h. The drug is a racemate; its more potent (+) enantiomer has a $t_{1/2}$ of about 6 h; the less-potent (–) enantiomer has a $t_{1/2}$ of approximately 4 h. Concentrations in the brain exceed those in plasma. The main urinary metabolite is a deesterified product, ritalinic acid, which accounts for 80% of the dose. The use of methylphenidate is contraindicated in patients with glaucoma.

Dexmethylphenidate

Dexmethylphenidate is the *d*-threo enantiomer of racemic methylphenidate. It is FDA-approved for the treatment of ADHD and is listed as a schedule II controlled substance in the U.S.

Pemoline

Pemoline is structurally dissimilar to methylphenidate but elicits similar changes in CNS function with minimal effects on the cardiovascular system. It is employed in treating ADHD. It can be given once daily because of its long $t_{1/2}$. Clinical improvement may require treatment for 3–4 weeks. Use of pemoline has been associated with severe hepatic failure. The drug was discontinued in the U.S. in 2006.

Lisdexamphetamine

Lisdexamphetamine is a therapeutically inactive prodrug that is converted primarily in the blood to lysine and D-amphetamine, the active component (Childress and Berry, 2012). It is approved for the treatment of ADHD in children, adolescents, and adults. The drug produces mild-to-moderate side effects, including decreased appetite, dizziness, dry mouth, fatigue, headache, insomnia, irritability, nasal congestion, nasal pharyngitis, upper respiratory infection, vomiting, and decreased weight.

Ephedrine

Ephedrine is an agonist at both α and β receptors; in addition, it enhances release of NE from sympathetic neurons and thus is a mixed-acting sympathomimetic (see Table 12–1 and Figure 12–1). Only *l*-ephedrine and racemic ephedrine are used clinically.

ADME and Pharmacological Actions

Ephedrine is effective after oral administration; effects may persist for several hours. Ephedrine is eliminated in the urine largely as unchanged drug, with a $t_{1/2}$ of 3–6 h. The drug stimulates heart rate and cardiac output and variably increases peripheral resistance; as a result, ephedrine usually increases blood pressure. Stimulation of the α receptors of smooth muscle cells in the bladder base may increase the resistance to the outflow of urine. Activation of β receptors in the lungs promotes bronchodilation. Ephedrine is a potent CNS stimulant.

Therapeutic Uses and Untoward Effects

The use of ephedrine as a bronchodilator in asthmatic patients is less common with the availability of β_2-selective agonists. Ephedrine has been used to promote urinary continence. Indeed, the drug may cause urinary retention, particularly in men with BPH. Ephedrine also has been used to treat the hypotension that may occur with spinal anesthesia.

Untoward effects of ephedrine include hypertension and insomnia. Tachyphylaxis may occur with repetitive dosing. Usual or higher-than-recommended doses may cause important adverse effects in susceptible individuals, especially in patients with underlying cardiovascular disease that might be unrecognized. Large amounts of herbal preparations containing ephedrine (ma huang, ephedra) are utilized around the world. There can be considerable variability in the content of ephedrine in these preparations, which may result in inadvertent consumption of higher-than-usual doses of ephedrine and its isomers, leading to significant toxicity and death. Thus, the FDA has banned the sale of dietary supplements containing ephedra. In addition, the Combat Methamphetamine Epidemic Act of 2005 regulates the sale of ephedrine, phenylpropanolamine, and pseudoephedrine, which can be used as precursors in the illicit manufacture of amphetamine and methamphetamine.

Other Sympathomimetic Agents

Several sympathomimetic drugs (e.g., propylhexedrine, naphazoline, oxymetazoline, and xylometazoline) are used primarily as vasoconstrictors for local application to the nasal mucous membrane or the eye.

Phenylephrine, pseudoephedrine (a stereoisomer of ephedrine), and phenylpropanolamine are the sympathomimetic drugs that have been used most commonly in oral preparations for the relief of nasal congestion. *Pseudoephedrine* is available without a prescription in a variety of solid and liquid dosage forms. *Phenylpropanolamine* shares the pharmacological properties of ephedrine and is approximately equal in potency except that it causes less CNS stimulation. Due to concern about the possibility that phenylpropanolamine increases the risk of hemorrhagic stroke, the drug is no longer licensed for marketing in the U.S.

Therapeutic Uses of Sympathomimetic Drugs

Shock

Shock is a clinical syndrome characterized by inadequate perfusion of tissues; it usually is associated with hypotension and ultimately with the failure of organ systems. Shock is an immediately life-threatening impairment of delivery of O_2 and nutrients to the organs of the body. Causes of shock include hypovolemia; cardiac failure; obstruction to cardiac output (due to pulmonary embolism, pericardial tamponade, or aortic dissection); and peripheral circulatory dysfunction (sepsis or anaphylaxis). Recent research on shock has focused on the accompanying increased permeability of the GI mucosa to pancreatic proteases, and on the role of these degradative enzymes on microvascular inflammation and multiorgan failure (Delano et al., 2013; Schmid-Schoenbein and Hugli, 2005). The treatment of shock consists of specific efforts to reverse the underlying pathogenesis as well as nonspecific measures aimed at correcting hemodynamic abnormalities. The accompanying fall in blood pressure generally leads to marked activation of the sympathetic nervous system. This, in turn, causes peripheral vasoconstriction and an increase in the rate and force of cardiac contraction. In the initial stages of shock, these mechanisms may maintain blood pressure and cerebral blood flow, although blood flow to the kidneys, skin, and other organs may be decreased, leading to impaired production of urine and metabolic acidosis.

The initial therapy of shock involves basic life support measures. It is essential to maintain blood volume, which often requires monitoring of hemodynamic parameters. Specific therapy (e.g., antibiotics for patients in septic shock) should be initiated immediately. If these measures do not lead to an adequate therapeutic response, it may be necessary to use vasoactive drugs in an effort to improve abnormalities in blood pressure and flow. Many of these pharmacological approaches, while apparently clinically reasonable, are of uncertain efficacy. Adrenergic receptor agonists may be used in an attempt to increase myocardial contractility or to modify peripheral vascular resistance. In general terms, β receptor agonists increase heart rate and force of contraction, α receptor agonists increase peripheral vascular resistance, and DA promotes dilation of renal and splanchnic vascular beds, in addition to activating β and α receptors (Breslow and Ligier, 1991).

Cardiogenic shock due to myocardial infarction has a poor prognosis; therapy is aimed at improving peripheral blood flow. Medical intervention is designed to optimize cardiac filling pressure (preload), myocardial contractility, and peripheral resistance (afterload). Preload may be increased by administration of intravenous fluids or reduced with drugs such as diuretics and nitrates. A number of sympathomimetic amines have been used to increase the force of contraction of the heart. Some of these drugs have disadvantages: INE is a powerful chronotropic agent and can greatly increase myocardial O_2 demand; NE intensifies peripheral vasoconstriction; and EPI increases heart rate and may predispose the heart to dangerous arrhythmias. DA is an effective inotropic agent that causes less increase in heart rate than does INE. DA also promotes renal arterial dilation; this may be useful in preserving renal function. When given in high doses (>10–20 μg/kg per min), DA activates α receptors, causing peripheral and renal vasoconstriction. Dobutamine has complex pharmacological actions that are mediated by its stereoisomers; the clinical effects of the drug are to increase myocardial contractility with little increase in heart rate or peripheral resistance.

In some patients in shock, hypotension is so severe that vasoconstricting drugs are required to maintain a blood pressure that is adequate for CNS perfusion. The α agonists such as NE, phenylephrine, metaraminol, mephentermine, midodrine, ephedrine, EPI, DA, and methoxamine all have been used for this purpose. This approach may be advantageous in patients with hypotension due to failure of the sympathetic nervous system (e.g., after spinal anesthesia or injury). However, in patients with other forms of shock, such as cardiogenic shock, reflex vasoconstriction generally is intense, and α receptor agonists may further compromise blood flow to organs such as the kidneys and gut and adversely increase the work of the heart. Indeed, vasodilating drugs such as nitroprusside are more likely to improve blood flow and decrease cardiac work in such patients by decreasing afterload if a minimally adequate blood pressure can be maintained.

The hemodynamic abnormalities in septic shock are complex and poorly understood. Most patients with septic shock initially have low or barely normal peripheral vascular resistance, possibly owing to excessive effects of endogenously produced NO as well as normal or increased cardiac output. If the syndrome progresses, myocardial depression, increased peripheral resistance, and impaired tissue oxygenation occur. The primary treatment of septic shock is antibiotics. Therapy with drugs such as DA or dobutamine is guided by hemodynamic monitoring.

Hypotension

Drugs with predominantly α agonist activity can be used to raise blood pressure in patients with decreased peripheral resistance in conditions such as spinal anesthesia or intoxication with antihypertensive medications. However, hypotension per se is not an indication for treatment with these agents unless there is inadequate perfusion of organs such as the brain, heart, or kidneys. Furthermore, adequate replacement of fluid or blood may be more appropriate than drug therapy for many patients with hypotension.

Patients with orthostatic hypotension (excessive fall in blood pressure with standing) often represent a pharmacological challenge. There are diverse causes for this disorder, including the Shy-Drager syndrome and idiopathic autonomic failure. Therapeutic approaches include physical maneuvers and a variety of drugs (fludrocortisone, prostaglandin synthesis inhibitors, somatostatin analogues, caffeine, vasopressin analogues, and DA antagonists). A number of sympathomimetic drugs also have been used in treating this disorder. The ideal agent would enhance venous constriction prominently and produce relatively little arterial constriction to avoid supine hypertension. No such agent currently is available. Drugs used in this disorder to activate α_1 receptors include both direct- and indirect-acting agents. Midodrine shows promise in treating this challenging disorder.

Hypertension

Centrally acting α_2 receptor agonists such as clonidine are useful in the treatment of hypertension. Drug therapy of hypertension is discussed in Chapter 28.

Cardiac Arrhythmias

Cardiopulmonary resuscitation in patients with cardiac arrest due to ventricular fibrillation, electromechanical dissociation, or asystole may be facilitated by drug treatment. EPI is an important therapeutic agent in patients with cardiac arrest; EPI and other α agonists increase diastolic pressure and improve coronary blood flow. The α agonists also help to preserve cerebral blood flow during resuscitation. Cerebral blood vessels are relatively insensitive to the vasoconstricting effects of catecholamines, and perfusion pressure is increased. Consequently, during external cardiac massage, EPI facilitates distribution of the limited cardiac output to the cerebral and coronary circulations. The optimal dose of EPI in patients with cardiac arrest is unclear. Once a cardiac rhythm has been restored, it may be necessary to treat arrhythmias, hypotension, or shock.

In patients with paroxysmal supraventricular tachycardias, particularly those associated with mild hypotension, careful infusion of an α agonist (e.g., phenylephrine) to raise blood pressure to about 160 mm Hg may end the arrhythmia by increasing vagal tone. However, this method of treatment has been replaced largely by Ca^{2+} channel blockers with clinically significant effects on the AV node, β antagonists, adenosine, and electrical cardioversion (Chapter 30). A β agonist such as INE may be used as adjunctive or temporizing therapy with atropine in patients with marked bradycardia who are compromised hemodynamically; if long-term therapy is required, a cardiac pacemaker usually is the treatment of choice.

Congestive Heart Failure

At first glance, sympathetic stimulation of β receptors in the heart would appear to be an important compensatory mechanism for maintenance of cardiac function in patients with congestive heart failure. However, the failing heart does not respond well to excess sympathetic stimulation. While β agonists may increase cardiac output in acute emergency settings such as shock, long-term therapy with β agonists as inotropic agents is not efficacious. Indeed, interest has grown in the use of β receptor antagonists in the treatment of patients with congestive heart failure, a topic covered in detail in Chapter 29.

Local Vascular Effects

Epinephrine is used in surgical procedures in the nose, throat, and larynx to shrink the mucosa and improve visualization by limiting hemorrhage. Simultaneous injection of EPI with local anesthetics retards their absorption and increases the duration of anesthesia (Chapter 22). Injection of α agonists into the penis may be useful in reversing priapism, a complication of the use of α receptor antagonists or PDE 5 inhibitors (e.g., sildenafil) in the treatment of erectile dysfunction. Both phenylephrine and oxymetazoline are efficacious vasoconstrictors when applied locally during sinus surgery.

Nasal Decongestion

α Receptor agonists are used as nasal decongestants in patients with allergic or vasomotor rhinitis and in acute rhinitis in patients with upper respiratory infections. These drugs probably decrease resistance to airflow by decreasing the volume of the nasal mucosa; this may occur by activation of α receptors in venous capacitance vessels in nasal tissues that have erectile characteristics. The receptors that mediate this effect appear to be α_1 receptors. α_2 Receptors may mediate contraction of arterioles that supply nutrition to the nasal mucosa. Intense constriction of these vessels may cause structural damage to the mucosa. A major limitation of therapy with nasal decongestants is loss of efficacy, "rebound" hyperemia, and worsening of symptoms with chronic use or when the drug is stopped. Although mechanisms are uncertain, possibilities include receptor desensitization and damage to the mucosa. Agonists that are selective for α_1 receptors may be less likely to induce mucosal damage.

The α agonists may be administered either orally or topically. Sympathomimetic decongestants should be used with great caution in patients with hypertension and in men with prostatic enlargement; these agents are contraindicated in patients who are taking MAO inhibitors. Topical decongestants are particularly useful in acute rhinitis because of their more selective site of action, but they are apt to be used excessively by patients, leading to rebound congestion. Oral decongestants are much less likely to cause rebound congestion but carry a greater risk of inducing adverse systemic effects. Patients with uncontrolled hypertension or ischemic heart disease generally should avoid the oral consumption of OTC products or herbal preparations containing sympathomimetic drugs.

Asthma

Use of β adrenergic agonists in the treatment of asthma and COPD is discussed in Chapter 40.

Allergic Reactions

Epinephrine is the drug of choice to reverse the manifestations of serious acute hypersensitivity reactions (e.g., from food, bee sting, or drug allergy). A subcutaneous injection of EPI rapidly relieves itching, hives, and swelling of lips, eyelids, and tongue. In some patients, careful intravenous infusion of EPI may be required to ensure prompt pharmacological effects. This treatment may be life-saving when edema of the glottis threatens airway patency or when there is hypotension or shock in patients with anaphylaxis. In addition to its cardiovascular effects, EPI is thought to activate β receptors that suppress the release from mast cells of mediators such as histamine and leukotrienes. Although glucocorticoids and antihistamines frequently are administered to patients with severe hypersensitivity reactions, EPI remains the mainstay. EPI autoinjectors are employed widely for the emergency self-treatment of anaphylaxis.

Ophthalmic Uses

Ophthalmic uses are discussed in Chapter 69.

Narcolepsy and Sleep/Wake Imbalance

Hypocretin neurons activate wake-promoting pathways in the CNS. A deficiency of hypocretin, likely due to autoimmune destruction of hypocretin neurons, produces narcolepsy, a condition of hypersomnia, including excessive daytime sleepiness and attacks of sleep that may occur suddenly under conditions that are not normally conducive to sleep. Hypocretin agonists will likely be available in the future. At present, treatment relies on the fact that monoamine pathways promote wakefulness; thus, current treatments utilize CNS stimulants, including those that enhance transmission in monoamine pathways (Black et al., 2015).

The CNS stimulants modafinil (a mixture of *R*- and *S*-enantiomers) and armodafinil (the *R*-enantiomer of modafinil) are first-line agents for narcolepsy. In the U.S., modafinil is a schedule IV controlled substance. Its mechanism of action in narcolepsy is unclear. Methylphenidate and amphetamines are also used. Therapy with amphetamines is complicated by the risk of abuse and the likelihood of the development of tolerance. Depression, irritability, and paranoia also may occur. Amphetamines may disturb nocturnal sleep, which increases the difficulty of avoiding daytime attacks of sleep in these patients. Armodafinil is also indicated to improve wakefulness in shift workers and to combat excessive sleepiness in patients with obstructive sleep apnea-hypopnea syndrome. See previous sections for more details on these agents. Some patients respond to tricyclic antidepressants (Chapter 15) or MAO inhibitors (Chapter 8).

Sodium γ-hydroxybutyrate (Na^+-oxybate) is FDA-approved for treating the sleep/wake imbalance and cataplexy of narcolepsy. The mechanism of action of oxybate is unknown but likely relates to its structural similarity to glutamate and GABA and to actions on NE and DA neurons mediated by $GABA_B$ receptors. Oxybate is a schedule III controlled substance, available through a special program with the manufacturer. Oxybate carries an FDA black-box warning about severe CNS depressants and must be used with great caution (see FDA, 2012).

Weight Reduction

Amphetamine promotes weight loss by suppressing appetite rather than by increasing energy expenditure. Other anorexic drugs include methamphetamine, dextroamphetamine (and a prodrug form, lisdexamfetamine), phentermine, benzphetamine, phendimetrazine, phenmetrazine, diethylpropion, mazindol, phenylpropanolamine, and sibutramine (a mixed adrenergic/serotonergic drug). Phenmetrazine, mazindol, and phenylpropanolamine have been discontinued in the U.S. Available evidence does not support the isolated use of these drugs in the absence of a more comprehensive program that stresses exercise and modification of diet under medical supervision.

The β_3 receptor agonists have remarkable antiobesity and antidiabetic effects in rodents.

Mirabegron (see previous discussion) has some promising effects in humans (Cypess et al., 2015). Use of β_3 agonists in the treatment of obesity remains a possibility for the future (Arch, 2011).

Attention-Deficit/Hyperactivity Disorder

The ADHD syndrome, usually first evident in childhood, is characterized by excessive motor activity, difficulty in sustaining attention, and impulsiveness. Children with this disorder frequently are troubled by difficulties in school, impaired interpersonal relationships, and excitability. Academic underachievement is an important characteristic. A substantial number of children with this syndrome have characteristics that persist into adulthood. Behavioral therapy may be helpful in some patients.

Catecholamines may be involved in the control of attention at the level of the cerebral cortex. A variety of stimulant drugs have been utilized in the treatment of ADHD, and they are particularly indicated in moderate-to-severe cases. Dextroamphetamine has been demonstrated to be more effective than placebo. Methylphenidate is effective in children with ADHD and is the most common intervention (Swanson and Volkow, 2003). Treatment may start with a dose of 5 mg of methylphenidate in the morning and at lunch; the dose is increased gradually over a period of weeks depending on the response as judged by parents, teachers, and the clinician. The total daily dose generally should not exceed 60 mg; because of its short duration of action, most children require two or three doses of methylphenidate each day. The timing of doses is adjusted individually in accordance with rapidity of onset of effect and duration of action.

Methylphenidate, dextroamphetamine, and amphetamine probably have similar efficacy in ADHD and are the preferred drugs in this disorder. Sustained-release preparations of dextroamphetamine, methylphenidate, dexmethylphenidate, and amphetamine, Adderall may be used once daily in children and adults. Lisdexamfetamine can be administered once daily, and a transdermal formulation of methylphenidate is marketed for daytime use. Potential adverse effects of these medications include insomnia, abdominal pain, anorexia, and weight loss, which may be associated with suppression of growth in children. Minor symptoms may be transient or may respond to adjustment of dosage or administration of the drug with meals. Other drugs that have been utilized include tricyclic antidepressants, antipsychotic agents, and clonidine. A sustained-release formulation of guanfacine, an α_{2A} receptor agonist, has recently been approved for use in children (ages 6–17 years) in treating ADHD (May and Kratochvil, 2010).

Adrenergic Receptor Antagonists

Many types of drugs interfere with the function of the sympathetic nervous system and thus have profound effects on the physiology of sympathetically innervated organs. Several of these drugs are important in clinical medicine, particularly for the treatment of cardiovascular diseases.

The remainder of this chapter focuses on the pharmacology of adrenergic receptor *antagonists*, drugs that inhibit the interaction of NE, epinephrine, and other sympathomimetic drugs with *α* and *β* receptors (Figure 12–3). Most of these agents are competitive antagonists; an important exception is phenoxybenzamine, an irreversible antagonist that binds covalently to *α* receptors.

There are important structural differences amongst the various types of adrenergic receptors, differences that have permitted development of compounds with substantially different affinities for the various receptors. Thus, it is possible to interfere selectively with responses that result from stimulation of the sympathetic nervous system. The selectivity is relative,

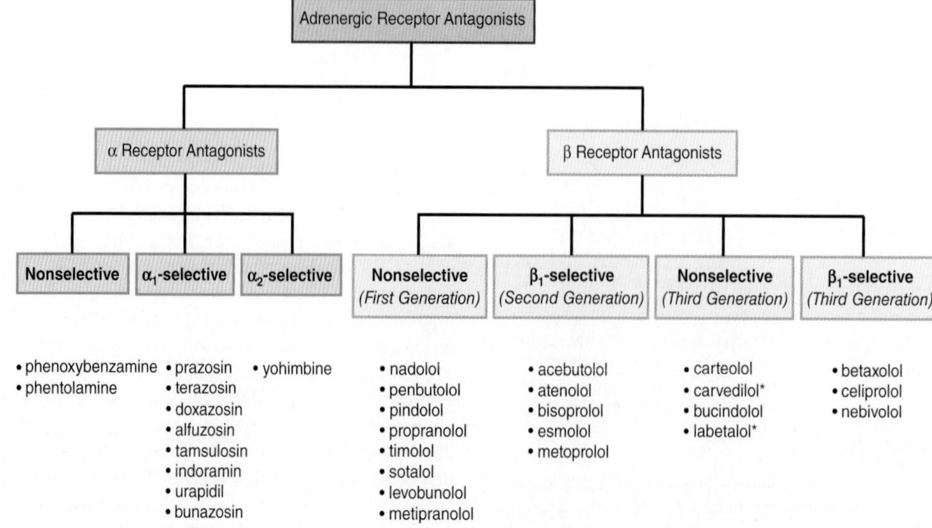

Figure 12-3 *Classification of adrenergic receptor antagonists.* Drugs marked by an asterisk (*) also block α_1 receptors.

not absolute. Nonetheless, selective antagonists of β_1 receptors block *most* actions of epinephrine and NE on the heart, while having less effect on β_2 receptors in bronchial smooth muscle and no effect on responses mediated by α_1 or α_2 receptors.

Detailed knowledge of the autonomic nervous system and the sites of action of drugs that act on adrenergic receptors is essential for understanding the pharmacological properties and therapeutic uses of this important class of drugs. Additional background material is presented in Chapter 8. Agents that block DA receptors are considered in Chapter 13.

α Adrenergic Receptor Antagonists

The α adrenergic receptors mediate many of the important actions of endogenous catecholamines. The α_1 receptors mediate contraction of arterial, venous, and visceral smooth muscle, while the α_2 receptors are involved in suppressing sympathetic output, increasing vagal tone, facilitating platelet aggregation, inhibiting the release of NE and acetylcholine from nerve endings, and regulating metabolic effects (e.g., suppression of insulin secretion and inhibition of lipolysis). The α_2 receptors also mediate contraction of some arteries and veins.

Some of the most important effects of α receptor antagonists observed clinically are on the cardiovascular system. Actions in both the CNS and the periphery are involved; the outcome depends on the cardiovascular status of the patient at the time of drug administration and the relative selectivity of the agent for α_1 and α_2 receptors.

The α receptor antagonists have a wide spectrum of pharmacological specificities and are chemically heterogeneous. Some of these drugs have markedly different affinities for α_1 and α_2 receptors. For example, *prazosin* is much more potent in blocking α_1 than α_2 receptors (i.e., α_1 selective), whereas *yohimbine* is α_2 selective; *phentolamine* has similar affinities for both of these receptor subtypes. More recently, agents that discriminate among the various subtypes of a particular receptor have become available; for example, *tamsulosin* has higher potency at α_{1A} than at α_{1B} receptors. Prior editions of this textbook contain information about the chemistry of α receptor antagonists.

Catecholamines increase the output of glucose from the liver; in humans, this effect is mediated predominantly by β receptors, although α receptors may contribute. The α receptor antagonists therefore may reduce glucose release. Receptors of the α_{2A} subtype facilitate platelet aggregation; the effect of blockade of platelet α_2 receptors in vivo is not clear. Activation of α_2 receptors in the pancreatic islets suppresses insulin secretion; conversely, blockade of pancreatic α_2 receptors may facilitate insulin release (Chapter 47).

α_1 Adrenergic Receptor Antagonists

General Pharmacological Properties

Blockade of α_1 adrenergic receptors inhibits vasoconstriction induced by endogenous catecholamines; vasodilation may occur in both arteriolar resistance vessels and veins. The result is a fall in blood pressure due to decreased peripheral resistance.

The magnitude of such effects depends on the activity of the sympathetic nervous system at the time the antagonist is administered and thus is less in supine than in upright subjects and is particularly marked if there is hypovolemia. For most α receptor antagonists, the fall in blood pressure is opposed by *baroreceptor reflexes* that cause increases in heart rate and cardiac output, as well as fluid retention. These *reflexes* are exaggerated if the antagonist also blocks α_2 receptors on peripheral sympathetic nerve endings, leading to enhanced release of NE and increased stimulation of postsynaptic β_1 receptors in the heart and on juxtaglomerular cells (Chapter 8) (Starke et al., 1989). Although stimulation of α_1 receptors in the heart may cause an increased force of contraction, the importance of blockade at this site in humans is uncertain.

Blockade of α_1 receptors also inhibits vasoconstriction and the increase in blood pressure produced by the administration of a sympathomimetic amine. The pattern of effects depends on the adrenergic agonist that is administered: Pressor responses to phenylephrine can be completely suppressed; those to NE are only incompletely blocked because of residual stimulation of cardiac β_1 receptors; and pressor responses to EPI may be transformed to vasodepressor effects because of residual stimulation of β_2 receptors in the vasculature with resultant vasodilation.

Blockade of α_1 receptors can alleviate some of the symptoms of BPH. The symptoms of BPH include a resistance to urine outflow. This results from mechanical pressure on the urethra due to an increase in smooth muscle mass and an α adrenergic receptor–mediated increase in smooth muscle tone in the prostate and neck of the bladder. Antagonism of α_1 receptors permits relaxation of the smooth muscle and decreases the resistance to the outflow of urine. The prostate and lower urinary tract tissues exhibit a high proportion of α_{1A} receptors (Michel and Vrydag, 2006).

Available Agents

Prazosin. Due in part to its greater α_1 receptor selectivity, this class of α receptor antagonists exhibits greater clinical utility and has largely replaced the nonselective haloalkylamine (e.g., phenoxybenzamine) and imidazoline (e.g., phentolamine) α receptor antagonists.

Prazosin is the prototypical α_1-selective antagonist. The affinity of prazosin for α_1 adrenergic receptors is about 1000-fold greater than that for α_2 adrenergic receptors. Prazosin has similar potencies at α_{1A}, α_{1B}, and α_{1D} subtypes. Interestingly, the drug also is a relatively potent inhibitor of cyclic nucleotide PDEs, and it originally was synthesized for this purpose. *Prazosin* and the related α receptor antagonists *doxazosin* and *tamsulosin* frequently are used for the treatment of hypertension (Chapter 28).

Pharmacological Effects. The major effects of prazosin result from its blockade of α_1 receptors in arterioles and veins. This leads to a fall in peripheral vascular resistance and in venous return to the heart. Unlike other vasodilating drugs, administration of prazosin usually does not increase heart rate. Because prazosin has little or no α_2 receptor–blocking effect, it probably does not promote the release of NE from sympathetic nerve endings in the heart. Prazosin decreases cardiac preload and has little effect on cardiac output and rate, in contrast to vasodilators such as hydralazine that have minimal dilatory effects on veins. Although the combination of reduced preload and selective α_1 receptor blockade might be sufficient to account for the relative absence of reflex tachycardia, prazosin also may act in the CNS to suppress sympathetic outflow. Prazosin appears to depress baroreflex function in hypertensive patients. Prazosin and related drugs in this class decrease LDLs and triglycerides and increase concentrations of HDLs.

ADME. *Prazosin* is well absorbed after oral administration, and bioavailability is about 50%–70%. Peak concentrations of prazosin in plasma generally are reached 1–3 h after an oral dose. The drug is tightly bound to plasma proteins (primarily α_1-acid glycoprotein), and only 5% of the drug is free in the circulation; diseases that modify the concentration of this protein (e.g., inflammatory processes) may change the free fraction. Prazosin is extensively metabolized in the liver, and little unchanged drug is excreted by the kidneys. The plasma $t_{1/2}$ is about 3 h (may be prolonged to 6–8 h in congestive heart failure). The duration of action is approximately 7–10 h in the treatment of hypertension.

The initial dose should be 1 mg, usually given at bedtime so that the patient will remain recumbent for at least several hours to reduce the risk of syncopal reactions that may follow the first dose of prazosin. The dose is titrated upward depending on the blood pressure. A maximal effect generally is observed with a total daily dose of 20 mg in patients with hypertension. In the off-label treatment of BPH, doses from 1 to 5 mg twice daily typically are used.

Terazosin. *Terazosin*, a close structural analogue of prazosin, is less potent than prazosin but retains high specificity for α_1 receptors; terazosin does not discriminate among α_{1A}, α_{1B}, and α_{1D} receptors. The major distinction between the two drugs is in their pharmacokinetic properties.

Terazosin is more soluble in water than is prazosin, and its bioavailability is high (>90%). The $t_{1/2}$ of elimination of terazosin is about 12 h, and its duration of action usually extends beyond 18 h. Consequently, the drug may be taken once daily to treat hypertension and BPH in most patients. Terazosin has been found more effective than finasteride in treatment of BPH (Lepor et al., 1996). *Terazosin* and *doxazosin* induce apoptosis in prostate smooth muscle cells. This apoptosis may lessen the symptoms associated with chronic BPH by limiting cell proliferation. The apoptotic effect of terazosin and doxazosin appears to be related to the quinazoline moiety rather than α_1 receptor antagonism; tamsulosin, a nonquinazoline α_1 receptor antagonist, does not produce apoptosis (Kyprianou, 2003). Only about 10% of terazosin is excreted unchanged in the urine. An initial first dose of 1 mg is recommended. Doses are slowly titrated upward depending on the therapeutic response. Doses of 10 mg/d may be required for maximal effect in BPH.

Doxazosin. *Doxazosin* is another congener of prazosin and a highly selective antagonist at α_1 receptors. It is nonselective among α_1 receptor subtypes and differs from prazosin in its pharmacokinetic profile.

The $t_{1/2}$ of doxazosin is about 20 h, and its duration of action may extend to 36 h. The bioavailability and extent of metabolism of doxazosin and prazosin are similar. Most doxazosin metabolites are eliminated in the feces. The hemodynamic effects of doxazosin appear to be similar to those of prazosin. Doxazosin should be given initially as a 1-mg dose in the treatment of hypertension or BPH. Doxazosin also may have beneficial actions in the long-term management of BPH related to apoptosis that are independent of α_1 receptor antagonism. Doxazosin is typically administered once daily. An extended-release formulation marketed for BPH is not recommended for the treatment of hypertension.

Alfuzosin. *Alfuzosin* is a quinazoline-based α_1 receptor antagonist with similar affinity at all of the α_1 receptor subtypes. It has been used extensively in treating BPH; it is not approved for treatment of hypertension. Alfuzosin has a $t_{1/2}$ of 3–5 h. Alfuzosin is a substrate of CYP3A4, and the concomitant administration of CPY3A4 inhibitors (e.g., ketoconazole, clarithromycin, itraconazole, ritonavir) is contraindicated. Alfuzosin should be avoided in patients at risk for prolonged QT syndrome. The recommended dosage is one 10-mg extended-release tablet daily to be taken after the same meal each day.

Tamsulosin. *Tamsulosin*, a benzenesulfonamide, is an α_1 receptor antagonist with some selectivity for α_{1A} (and α_{1D}) subtypes compared to the α_{1B} subtype (Kenny et al., 1996). This selectivity may favor blockade of α_{1A} receptors in prostate. Tamsulosin is efficacious in the treatment of BPH with little effect on blood pressure (Beduschi et al., 1998); tamsulosin is not approved for the treatment of hypertension. Tamsulosin is well absorbed and has a $t_{1/2}$ of 5–10 h. It is extensively metabolized by CYPs. Tamsulosin may be administered at a 0.4-mg starting dose; a dose of 0.8 mg ultimately will be more efficacious in some patients. Abnormal ejaculation is an adverse effect of tamsulosin, experienced by about 18% of patients receiving the higher dose.

Silodosin. *Silodosin* exhibits selectivity for the α_{1A}, over the α_{1B}, adrenergic receptor. The drug is metabolized by several pathways; the main metabolite is a glucuronide formed by UGT2B7; coadministration with inhibitors of this enzyme (e.g., probenecid, valproic acid, fluconazole) increases systemic exposure to silodosin. The drug is approved for the treatment of BPH and has lesser effects on blood pressure than the non–α_1-subtype selective antagonists. Nevertheless, dizziness and orthostatic hypotension can occur. The chief side effect of silodosin is retrograde ejaculation (in 28% of those treated). Silodosin is available as 4-mg and 8-mg capsules.

Adverse Effects

A major potential adverse effect of prazosin and its congeners is the first-dose effect; marked postural hypotension and syncope sometimes are seen 30–90 min after an initial dose of prazosin and 2–6 h after an initial dose of doxazosin.

Syncopal episodes also have occurred with a rapid increase in dosage or with the addition of a second antihypertensive drug to the regimen of a patient who already is taking a large dose of prazosin. The risk of the first-dose phenomenon is minimized by limiting the initial dose (e.g., 1 mg at bedtime), by increasing the dosage slowly, and by introducing additional antihypertensive drugs cautiously.

Because orthostatic hypotension may be a problem during long-term treatment with prazosin or its congeners, it is essential to check standing as well as recumbent blood pressure. Nonspecific adverse effects such as headache, dizziness, and asthenia rarely limit treatment with prazosin.

Therapeutic Uses

Hypertension. Prazosin and its congeners have been used successfully in the treatment of essential hypertension (Chapter 28). Pleotropic effects of these drugs improve lipid profiles and glucose-insulin metabolism in patients with hypertension who are at risk for atherosclerotic disease (Deano and Sorrentino, 2012). Catecholamines are also powerful stimulators of vascular smooth muscle hypertrophy, acting by α_1 receptors. To what extent these effects of α_1 antagonists have clinical significance in diminishing the risk of atherosclerosis is not known.

Congestive Heart Failure. α Receptor antagonists have been used in the treatment of congestive heart failure but are not the drugs of choice. Short-term effects of α receptor blockade in these patients are due to dilation of both arteries and veins, resulting in a reduction of preload and afterload, which increases cardiac output and reduces pulmonary congestion. In contrast to results obtained with inhibitors of angiotensin-converting enzyme or a combination of hydralazine and an organic nitrate, prazosin has not been found to prolong life in patients with congestive heart failure.

Benign Prostatic Hyperplasia. In a significant percentage of older men, BPH produces symptomatic urethral obstruction that leads to weak stream, increased urinary frequency, and nocturia. These symptoms are due to a combination of mechanical pressure on the urethra due to the increase in smooth muscle mass and the α_1 receptor–mediated increase in smooth muscle tone in the prostate and neck of the bladder (Kyprianou, 2003). α_1 Receptors in the trigone muscle of the bladder and urethra contribute to the resistance to outflow of urine. *Prazosin* reduces this resistance in some patients with impaired bladder emptying caused by prostatic obstruction or parasympathetic decentralization from spinal injury.

Finasteride and *dutasteride*, two drugs that inhibit conversion of testosterone to dihydrotestosterone (Chapter 45) and can reduce prostate volume in some patients, are approved as monotherapy and in combination with α receptor antagonists. α_1-Selective antagonists have efficacy in BPH owing to relaxation of smooth muscle in the bladder neck, prostate capsule, and prostatic urethra. α_1-Selective antagonists rapidly improve urinary flow, whereas the actions of finasteride are typically delayed for months. Combination therapy with doxazosin and finasteride reduces the risk of overall clinical progression of BPH significantly more than treatment with either drug alone (McConnell et al., 2003). Tamsulosin at the recommended dose of 0.4 mg daily and silodosin at 0.8 mg are less likely to cause orthostatic hypotension than are the other drugs. The predominant α_1 subtype expressed in the human prostate is the α_{1A} receptor (Michel and Vrydag, 2006). Developments in this area will provide the basis for the selection of α receptor antagonists with specificity for the relevant subtype of α_1 receptor. However, the possibility remains that some of the symptoms of BPH are due to α_1 receptors in other sites, such as bladder, spinal cord, or brain.

Other Disorders. Some studies indicated that prazosin can decrease the incidence of digital vasospasm in patients with Raynaud disease; however, its relative efficacy as compared with Ca^{2+} channel blockers is not known. Prazosin may have some benefit in patients with other vasospastic disorders. Prazosin may be useful for the treatment of patients with mitral or aortic valvular insufficiency, presumably by reducing afterload.

α_2 Adrenergic Receptor Antagonists

Activation of presynaptic α_2 receptors inhibits the release of NE and other cotransmitters from peripheral sympathetic nerve endings. Activation of α_2 receptors in the pontomedullary region of the CNS inhibits sympathetic nervous system activity and leads to a fall in blood pressure; these receptors are a site of action for drugs such as clonidine. *Blockade of α_2 receptors with selective antagonists such as yohimbine thus can increase sympathetic outflow and potentiate the release of NE from nerve endings, leading to activation of α_1 and β_1 receptors in the heart and peripheral vasculature with a consequent rise in blood pressure.* Antagonists that also block α_1 receptors give rise to similar effects on sympathetic outflow and release of NE, but the net increase in blood pressure is prevented by inhibition of vasoconstriction.

Although certain vascular beds contain α_2 receptors that promote contraction of smooth muscle, it is thought that these receptors are preferentially stimulated by circulating catecholamines, whereas α_1 receptors are activated by NE released from sympathetic nerve fibers. In other vascular beds, α_2 receptors reportedly promote vasodilation by stimulating the release of NO from endothelial cells. The physiological role of vascular α_2 receptors in the regulation of blood flow within various vascular beds is uncertain. The α_2 receptors contribute to smooth muscle contraction in the human saphenous vein, whereas α_1 receptors are more prominent in dorsal hand veins. The effects of α_2 receptor antagonists on the cardiovascular system are dominated by actions in the CNS and on sympathetic nerve endings.

Yohimbine

Yohimbine is a competitive antagonist that is selective for α_2 receptors. The compound is an indolealkylamine alkaloid and is found in the bark of the tree *Pausinystalia yohimbe* and in *Rauwolfia* root; its structure resembles that of *reserpine*. Yohimbine readily enters the CNS, where it acts to increase blood pressure and heart rate; it also enhances motor activity and produces tremors. These actions are opposite to those of clonidine, an α_2 agonist. Yohimbine also antagonizes effects of 5HT. In the past, it was used extensively to treat male sexual dysfunction (Tam et al., 2001). However, the efficacies of PDE5 inhibitors (e.g., *sildenafil*, *vardenafil*, and *tadalafil*) and *apomorphine* (off-label) have been much more conclusively demonstrated in oral treatment of erectile dysfunction. Some studies suggested that yohimbine may be useful for diabetic neuropathy and in the treatment of postural hypotension. In the U.S., yohimbine can be legally sold as a dietary supplement; however, labeling claims that it will arouse or increase sexual desire or improve sexual performance are prohibited. Yohimbine is approved in veterinary medicine for the reversal of xylazine anesthesia.

Nonselective α Adrenergic Antagonists

Phenoxybenzamine and Phentolamine

Phenoxybenzamine and *phentolamine* are nonselective α receptor antagonists. Phenoxybenzamine, a haloalkylamine compound, produces an irreversible antagonism, while phentolamine, an imidazaline, produces a competitive antagonism.

Phenoxybenzamine and *phentolamine* cause a progressive decrease in peripheral resistance due to antagonism of α receptors in the vasculature and an increase in cardiac output that is due in part to reflex sympathetic nerve stimulation. The cardiac stimulation is accentuated by enhanced release of NE from cardiac sympathetic nerve due to antagonism of presynaptic α_2 receptors by these nonselective α blockers. Postural hypotension is a prominent feature with these drugs, and this, accompanied by reflex tachycardia that can precipitate cardiac arrhythmias, severely limits the use of these drugs to treat essential hypertension. The α_1-selective antagonists, such as *prazosin*, have replaced the "classical" α-blockers in the management of essential hypertension. Phenoxybenzamine and phentolamine are still marketed for several specialized uses.

Therapeutic Uses. Phenoxybenzamine is used in the treatment of pheochromocytomas, tumors of the adrenal medulla and sympathetic neurons that secrete enormous quantities of catecholamines into the circulation. The usual result is hypertension, which may be episodic and severe. The vast majority of pheochromocytomas are treated surgically; phenoxybenzamine is often used in preparing the patient for surgery. The drug controls episodes of severe hypertension and minimizes other adverse effects of catecholamines, such as contraction of plasma volume and injury of the myocardium. A conservative approach is to initiate treatment with phenoxybenzamine (at a dosage of 10 mg twice daily) 1–3 weeks before the operation. The dose is increased every other day until the desired effect on blood pressure is achieved. The usual daily dose of phenoxybenzamine in patients with pheochromocytoma is 40–120 mg given in two or three divided portions. Prolonged treatment with phenoxybenzamine may be necessary in patients with inoperable or malignant pheochromocytoma. In some patients, particularly those with malignant disease, administration of *metyrosine*, a competitive inhibitor of tyrosine hydroxylase (the rate-limiting enzyme in the synthesis of catecholamines), may be a useful adjunct (Chapter 8). β Receptor antagonists also are used to treat pheochromocytoma, *but only after the administration of an α receptor antagonist* (described later in the chapter).

Phentolamine can also be used in short-term control of hypertension in patients with pheochromocytoma. Rapid infusions of phentolamine may cause severe hypotension, so the drug should be administered cautiously. Phentolamine also may be useful to relieve pseudo-obstruction of the bowel in patients with pheochromocytoma.

Phentolamine has been used locally to prevent dermal necrosis after the inadvertent extravasation of an α receptor agonist. The drug also may be useful for the treatment of hypertensive crises that follow the abrupt withdrawal of clonidine or that may result from the ingestion of tyramine-containing foods during the use of nonselective MAO inhibitors. Although excessive activation of α receptors is important in the development of severe hypertension in these settings, there is little information about the safety and efficacy of phentolamine compared with those of other antihypertensive agents in the treatment of such patients. Buccally or orally administered phentolamine may have efficacy in some men with sexual dysfunction.

Phentolamine is FDA-approved for reversing or limiting the duration of soft tissue anesthesia. Sympathomimetics are frequently administered with local anesthetics to slow the removal of the anesthetic by causing vasoconstriction. When the need for anesthesia is over, phentolamine can help reverse it by antagonizing the α receptor–induced vasoconstriction.

Phenoxybenzamine has been used off-label to control the manifestations of autonomic hyperreflexia in patients with spinal cord transection.

Toxicity and Adverse Effects. Hypotension is the major adverse effect of phenoxybenzamine and phentolamine. In addition, reflex cardiac stimulation may cause alarming tachycardia, cardiac arrhythmias, and ischemic cardiac events, including myocardial infarction. Reversible inhibition of ejaculation may occur due to impaired smooth muscle contraction in the vas deferens and ejaculatory ducts. Phentolamine stimulates GI smooth muscle, an effect antagonized by atropine, and also enhances gastric acid secretion due in part to histamine release. Thus, phentolamine should be used with caution in patients with a history of peptic ulcer. Phenoxybenzamine is mutagenic in the Ames test, and repeated administration of this drug to experimental animals causes peritoneal sarcomas and lung tumors.

Additional α Adrenergic Receptor Antagonists

Ergot Alkaloids

The ergot alkaloids were the first adrenergic receptor antagonists to be discovered. Ergot alkaloids exhibit a complex variety of pharmacological properties. To varying degrees, these agents act as partial agonists or antagonists at α receptors, DA receptors, and serotonin receptors. Additional information about the ergot alkaloids can be found in Chapter 13.

Indoramin

Indoramin is a selective, competitive α_1-selective receptor antagonist that also antagonizes H_1 and 5HT receptors. Indoramin lowers blood pressure with minimal tachycardia. The drug is not available in the U.S.; outside the U.S., indoramin is used for the treatment of hypertension and BPH and in the prophylaxis of migraine. The drug also decreases the incidence of attacks of Raynaud phenomenon. Some of the adverse effects of indoramin include sedation, dry mouth, and failure of ejaculation.

Ketanserin

Although developed as a 5HT receptor antagonist, ketanserin also blocks α_1 receptors. Ketanserin (not available in the U.S.) is discussed in Chapter 13.

Urapidil

Urapidil is a selective α_1 receptor antagonist that has a chemical structure distinct from those of prazosin and related compounds; the drug is not commercially available in the U.S. Blockade of peripheral α_1 receptors appears to be primarily responsible for the hypotension produced by urapidil, although it has actions in the CNS as well.

Bunazosin

Bunazosin is an α_1-selective antagonist of the quinazoline class that has been shown to lower blood pressure in patients with hypertension. Bunazosin is not available in the U.S.

Neuroleptic Agents

Chlorpromazine, haloperidol, and other neuroleptic drugs of the phenothiazine and butyrophenone types produce significant blockade of both α and D_2 receptors in humans.

β Adrenergic Receptor Antagonists

HISTORICAL PERSPECTIVE

Ahlquist's hypothesis that the effects of catecholamines were mediated by activation of distinct α and β receptors provided the initial impetus for the synthesis and pharmacological evaluation of β receptor antagonists (Chapter 8). The first such selective agent was dichloroisoproterenol, a partial agonist. Sir James Black and his colleagues initiated a program in the late 1950s to develop additional β blockers, with the resulting synthesis and characterization of propranolol.

Overview

Competitive antagonists of β adrenergic receptors, or β blockers, have received enormous clinical attention because of their efficacy in the treatment of hypertension, ischemic heart disease, congestive heart failure, and certain arrhythmias.

The myriad β antagonists can be distinguished by the following properties:

- Relative affinity for β_1 and β_2 receptors
- Intrinsic sympathomimetic activity
- Blockade of α receptors
- Differences in lipid solubility (CNS penetration)
- Capacity to induce vasodilation
- Pharmacokinetic parameters

Propranolol is a competitive β receptor antagonist and remains the prototype to which other β antagonists are compared. Propranolol is *a nonselective β adrenergic receptor antagonist* with equal affinity for β_1 and β_2 adrenergic receptors. Agents such as metoprolol, atenolol, acebutolol, bisoprolol, and esmolol have somewhat greater affinity for β_1 than for β_2 receptors; these are examples of *β_1-selective antagonists*, even though the selectivity is not absolute. Propranolol is a pure antagonist, and it has no capacity to activate β receptors. Several β blockers (e.g., pindolol and acebutolol) activate β receptors partially in the absence of catecholamines; however, the intrinsic activities of these drugs are less than that of a full agonist such as INE. These partial agonists have *intrinsic sympathomimetic activity*; this slight residual activity may prevent profound bradycardia or negative inotropy in a resting heart. The potential clinical advantage of this property, however, is unclear and may be disadvantageous in the context of secondary prevention of myocardial infarction. Other β receptor antagonists have the property of *inverse agonism* (Chapter 3); these drugs can decrease basal activity of β receptor signaling by shifting the equilibrium of spontaneously active receptors toward an inactive state (see Chapters 3 and 8).

Several β receptor antagonists also have local anesthetic or membrane-stabilizing activity, independent of β blockade. Such drugs include propranolol, acebutolol, and carvedilol. Pindolol, metoprolol, betaxolol, and labetalol have slight membrane-stabilizing effects. Although most β receptor antagonists do not block α adrenergic receptors, labetalol, carvedilol, and bucindolol block both α_1 and β adrenergic receptors. In addition to carvedilol, labetalol, and bucindolol, other β receptor antagonists have vasodilating properties due to mechanisms discussed in the following material. These include celiprolol, nebivolol, nipradilol, carteolol, betaxolol, bopindolol, and bevantolol (Toda, 2003).

Pharmacological Properties

The pharmacological properties of β receptor antagonists can be deduced and explained largely from knowledge of the responses elicited by the receptors in the various tissues and the activity of the sympathetic nerves that innervate these tissues (Table 8–1). For example, β receptor blockade has relatively little effect on the normal heart of an individual at rest but has profound effects when sympathetic control of the heart is dominant, as during exercise or stress.

The β adrenergic receptor antagonists are classified as non subtype-selective ("first generation"), β_1 selective ("second generation"), and non subtype- or subtype-selective *with additional cardiovascular actions* ("third generation"). These last drugs have additional cardiovascular properties (especially vasodilation) that seem unrelated to β blockade. Table 12–3 summarizes pharmacological and pharmacokinetic properties of β receptor antagonists.

Cardiovascular System. The major therapeutic effects of β receptor antagonists are on the cardiovascular system. It is important to distinguish these effects in normal subjects from those in subjects with cardiovascular disease such as hypertension or myocardial ischemia.

Catecholamines have positive chronotropic and inotropic actions. Conversely, β receptor antagonists slow the heart rate and decrease myocardial contractility, *if there are sympathetic stimuli to antagonize.* When tonic stimulation of β receptors is low, this effect is correspondingly modest. However, when the sympathetic nervous system is activated, as during exercise or stress, β receptor antagonists attenuate the expected rise in heart rate.

Short-term administration of β receptor antagonists decreases cardiac output; peripheral resistance increases in proportion to maintain blood pressure as a result of blockade of vascular β_2 receptors and compensatory reflexes, such as increased sympathetic nervous system activity, leading to activation of vascular α receptors. However, with long-term use of β antagonists, total peripheral resistance returns to initial values (Mimran and Ducailar, 1988) *or decreases in patients with hypertension* (Man in't Veld et al., 1988). With β antagonists that also are α_1 receptor antagonists, such as labetalol, carvedilol, and bucindolol, cardiac output is maintained with a greater fall in peripheral resistance. This also is seen with β receptor antagonists that are direct vasodilators.

The β receptor antagonists have significant effects on cardiac rhythm and automaticity. Although it had been thought that these effects were due exclusively to blockade of β_1 receptors, β_2 receptors likely also regulate heart rate in humans (Altschuld and Billman, 2000; Brodde and Michel, 1999). The β_3 receptors also have been identified in normal myocardial tissue (Moniotte et al., 2001). Signal transduction for β_3 receptors is complex and includes not only G_s but also G_i/G_o; stimulation of cardiac β_3 receptors inhibits cardiac contraction and relaxation. The physiological role of β_3 receptors in the heart remains to be established (Morimoto et al., 2004). β Receptor antagonists reduce the sinus rate, decrease the spontaneous rate of depolarization of ectopic pacemakers, slow conduction in the atria and in the AV node, and increase the functional refractory period of the AV node.

Although high concentrations of many β blockers exert a membrane-stabilizing activity, it is doubtful that this is significant at usual therapeutic doses. However, this effect may be important when there is overdosage. *d*-Propranolol may suppress ventricular arrhythmias independently of β receptor blockade.

The cardiovascular effects of β receptor antagonists are most evident during dynamic exercise. In the presence of β receptor blockade, exercise-induced increases in heart rate and myocardial contractility are attenuated. However, the exercise-induced increase in cardiac output is less affected because of an increase in stroke volume. The effects of β receptor antagonists on exercise are somewhat analogous to the changes that occur with normal aging. In healthy elderly persons, catecholamine-induced increases in heart rate are smaller than in younger individuals; however, the increase in cardiac output in older people may be preserved because of an increase in stroke volume during exercise. β Blockers tend to decrease work capacity, as assessed by their effects on intense short-term or more

TABLE 12–3 ■ PHARMACOLOGICAL/PHARMACOKINETIC PROPERTIES OF β ADRENERGIC RECEPTOR BLOCKING AGENTS

DRUG	MEMBRANE STABILIZING ACTIVITY	INTRINSIC AGONIST ACTIVITY	LIPID SOLUBILITY	EXTENT OF ABSORPTION (%)	ORAL AVAILABILITY (%)	PLASMA $t_{1/2}$ (HOURS)	PROTEIN BINDING (%)
Classical nonselective β blockers: First generation							
Nadolol	0	0	Low	30	30–50	20–24	30
Penbutolol	0	+	High	~100	~100	~5	80–98
Pindolol	+	+++	Low	>95	~100	3–4	40
Propranolol	++	0	High	<90	30	3–5	90
Timolol	0	0	Low to moderate	90	75	4	<10
β_1 Selective blockers: Second generation							
Acebutolol	+	+	Low	90	20–60	3–4	26
Atenolol	0	0	Low	90	50–60	6–7	6–16
Bisoprolol	0	0	Low	≤90	80	9–12	~30
Esmolol	0	0	Low	NA	NA	0.15	55
Metoprolol	+[a]	0	Moderate	~100	40–50	3–7	12
Nonselective β blockers with additional actions: Third generation							
Carteolol	0	++	Low	85	85	6	23–30
Carvedilol	++	0	Moderate	>90	~30	7–10	98
Labetalol	+	+	Low	>90	~33	3–4	~50
β_1 selective blockers with additional actions: Third generation							
Betaxolol	+	0	Moderate	>90	~80	15	50
Celiprolol	0	+	Low	~74	30–70	5	4–5
Nebivolol	0	0	Low	NA	NA	11–30	98

[a]Detectable only at doses much greater than required for β blockade.

prolonged steady-state exertion. Exercise performance may be impaired to a lesser extent by β_1 selective agents than by nonselective antagonists. Blockade of β_2 receptors blunts the increase in blood flow to active skeletal muscle during submaximal exercise and also may attenuate catecholamine-induced activation of glucose metabolism and lipolysis.

Coronary artery blood flow increases during exercise or stress to meet the metabolic demands of the heart. By increasing heart rate, contractility, and systolic pressure, catecholamines increase myocardial O_2 demand. However, in patients with coronary artery disease, fixed narrowing of these vessels attenuates the expected increase in flow, leading to myocardial ischemia. β Receptor antagonists decrease the effects of catecholamines on the determinants of myocardial O_2 consumption. However, these agents may tend to increase the requirement for O_2 by increasing end-diastolic pressure and systolic ejection period. Usually, the net effect is to improve the relationship between cardiac O_2 supply and demand; exercise tolerance generally is improved in patients with angina, whose capacity to exercise is limited by the development of chest pain (Chapter 27).

Antihypertensive Activity. β Receptor antagonists generally do not reduce blood pressure in patients with normal blood pressure. However, these drugs lower blood pressure in patients with hypertension, but the mechanisms responsible for this important clinical effect are not fully understood. The release of *renin* from the juxtaglomerular cells is stimulated by the sympathetic nervous system by means of β_1 receptors, and this effect is blocked by β receptor antagonists (see Chapter 26). Some investigators have found that the antihypertensive effect of β blockade is most marked in patients with elevated concentrations of plasma renin, compared to patients with low or normal concentrations of renin. However, β receptor antagonists are effective even in patients with low plasma renin.

Presynaptic β receptors enhance the release of NE from sympathetic neurons, and diminished release of NE from β blockade is a possible response. Although β blockers would not be expected to decrease the contractility of vascular smooth muscle, long-term administration of these drugs to hypertensive patients ultimately leads to a fall in peripheral vascular resistance (Man in't Veld et al., 1988). The mechanism for this effect is not known, but this delayed fall in peripheral vascular resistance in the face of a persistent reduction of cardiac output appears to account for much of the antihypertensive effect of these drugs.

Some β receptor antagonists have additional effects that may contribute to their capacity to lower blood pressure. These drugs all produce peripheral vasodilation; at least six properties have been proposed to contribute to this effect, including production of NO, activation of β_2 receptors, blockade of α_1 receptors, blockade of Ca^{2+} entry, opening of K^+ channels, and antioxidant activity (see Table 12–4 and Figure 12–4). These mechanisms appear to contribute to the antihypertensive effects by enhancing hypotension, increasing peripheral blood flow, and decreasing afterload. *Celiprolol* and *nebivolol* also have been observed to produce vasodilation and thereby reduce preload.

Nonselective β receptor antagonists inhibit the vasodilation caused by INE and augment the pressor response to EPI. This is particularly significant in patients with pheochromocytoma, in whom β receptor antagonists should be used only after adequate α receptor blockade has been established. This avoids uncompensated α receptor–mediated vasoconstriction caused by EPI secreted from the tumor.

Pulmonary System. Nonselective β receptor antagonists such as propranolol block β_2 receptors in bronchial smooth muscle. This usually has little effect on pulmonary function in normal individuals. However, *in patients with COPD, such blockade can lead to life-threatening*

SECTION II NEUROPHARMACOLOGY

TABLE 12–4 ■ THIRD-GENERATION β RECEPTOR ANTAGONISTS WITH PUTATIVE ADDITIONAL MECHANISMS OF VASODILATION

NITRIC OXIDE PRODUCTION	$β_2$ RECEPTOR AGONISM	$α_1$ RECEPTOR ANTAGONISM	Ca^{2+} ENTRY BLOCKADE	K^+ CHANNEL OPENING	ANTIOXIDANT ACTIVITY
Celiprolol[a]	Celiprolol[a]	Carvedilol	Carvedilol	Tilisolol[a]	Carvedilol
Nebivolol	Carteolol	Bucindolol[a]	Betaxolol		
Carteolol	Bopindolol[a]	Bevantolol[a]	Bevantolol[a]		
Bopindolol[a]		Nipradilol[a]			
Nipradilol[a]		Labetalol			

[a]Not currently available in the U.S., where most are under investigation for use.

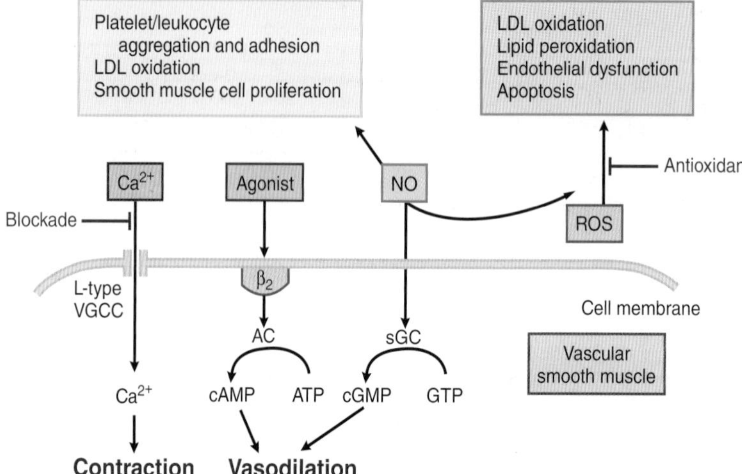

Figure 12-4 *Mechanisms underlying actions of vasodilating β blockers in blood vessels.* AC: adenylyl cyclase; sGC: soluble guanylyl cyclase; NO: nitric oxide; ROS: reactive oxygen species; VGCC: voltage-gated Ca^{2+} channel. (Modified with permission from Toda N. Vasodilating β adrenoceptor blockers as cardiovascular therapeutics. *Pharmacol Ther*, **2003**, 100:215–234. Copyright © Elsevier.)

bronchoconstriction. Although $β_1$-selective antagonists or antagonists with intrinsic sympathomimetic activity are less likely than propranolol to increase airway resistance in patients with asthma, these drugs should be used only with great caution, if at all, in patients with bronchospastic diseases. Drugs such as celiprolol, with $β_1$ receptor selectivity and $β_2$ receptor partial agonism, are of potential promise, although clinical experience is limited.

Metabolic Effects. The β receptor antagonists modify the metabolism of carbohydrates and lipids. Catecholamines promote glycogenolysis and mobilize glucose in response to hypoglycemia. Nonselective β blockers may delay recovery from hypoglycemia in type 1 (insulin-dependent) diabetes mellitus, but infrequently in type 2 diabetes mellitus. In addition to blocking glycogenolysis, β receptor antagonists can interfere with the counterregulatory effects of catecholamines secreted during hypoglycemia by blunting the perception of symptoms such as tremor, tachycardia, and nervousness. Thus, β adrenergic receptor antagonists should be used with great caution in patients with labile diabetes and frequent hypoglycemic reactions. If such a drug is indicated, a $β_1$-selective antagonist is preferred because these drugs are less likely to delay recovery from hypoglycemia (DiBari et al., 2003).

The β receptors mediate activation of hormone-sensitive lipase in fat cells, leading to release of free fatty acids into the circulation. This increased flux of fatty acids is an important source of energy for exercising muscle. β Receptor antagonists can attenuate the release of free fatty acids from adipose tissue. Nonselective β receptor antagonists consistently reduce HDL cholesterol, increase LDL cholesterol, and increase triglycerides. In contrast, $β_1$-selective antagonists, including celiprolol, carteolol, nebivolol, carvedilol, and bevantolol, reportedly improve the serum lipid profile of dyslipidemic patients. While drugs such as propranolol and atenolol increase triglycerides, plasma triglycerides are reduced with chronic celiprolol, carvedilol, and carteolol (Toda, 2003).

In contrast to classical β blockers, which decrease insulin sensitivity, the vasodilating β receptor antagonists (e.g., celiprolol, nipradilol, carteolol, carvedilol, and dilevalol) increase insulin sensitivity in patients with insulin resistance. Together with their cardioprotective effects, improvement in insulin sensitivity from vasodilating β receptor antagonists may partially counterbalance the hazard from worsened lipid abnormalities associated with diabetes.

When β blockers are required, $β_1$-selective or vasodilating β receptor antagonists are preferred. In addition, it may be necessary to use β receptor antagonists in conjunction with other drugs, (e.g., HMG CoA reductase inhibitors) to ameliorate adverse metabolic effects (Dunne et al., 2001).

The β receptor agonists decrease the plasma concentration of K^+ by promoting its uptake, predominantly into skeletal muscle. At rest, an infusion of EPI causes a decrease in the plasma concentration of K^+. The marked increase in the concentration of EPI that occurs with stress (such as myocardial infarction) may cause hypokalemia, which could predispose to cardiac arrhythmias. The hypokalemic effect of EPI is blocked by an experimental antagonist, ICI 118551, which has a high affinity for $β_2$ and, to a lesser degree, $β_3$ receptors. Exercise causes an increase in the efflux of K^+ from skeletal muscle. Catecholamines tend to buffer the rise in K^+ by increasing its influx into muscle. β Blockers negate this buffering effect.

Other Effects. The β receptor antagonists block catecholamine-induced tremor. They also block inhibition of mast cell degranulation by catecholamines.

Adverse Effects and Precautions

Cardiovascular System. β Receptor blockade may cause or exacerbate heart failure in patients with compensated heart failure, acute myocardial infarction, or cardiomegaly. It is not known whether β receptor antagonists that possess intrinsic sympathomimetic activity or peripheral vasodilating properties are safer in these settings. Nonetheless, there is convincing evidence that chronic administration of β receptor antagonists is efficacious in prolonging life in the therapy of heart failure in selected patients (discussed in Chapter 29).

Bradycardia is a normal response to β receptor blockade; however, in patients with partial or complete AV conduction defects, β antagonists may cause life-threatening *bradyarrhythmias*. Particular caution is indicated in patients who are taking other drugs, such as verapamil or various antiarrhythmic agents, which may impair sinus node function or AV conduction.

Some patients complain of cold extremities while taking β receptor antagonists. Symptoms of peripheral vascular disease may occasionally worsen, or Raynaud phenomenon may develop.

Abrupt discontinuation of β receptor antagonists after long-term treatment can exacerbate angina and may increase the risk of sudden death. There is enhanced sensitivity to β receptor agonists in patients who have undergone long-term treatment with certain β receptor antagonists after the blocker is withdrawn abruptly. This increased sensitivity is evident several days after stopping a β receptor antagonist and may persist for at least 1 week. Such enhanced sensitivity can be attenuated by tapering the dose of the β blocker for several weeks before discontinuation. Supersensitivity to INE also has been observed after abrupt discontinuation of metoprolol, but not of pindolol. This enhanced β responsiveness may result from upregulation of β receptors. The number of β receptors on circulating lymphocytes is increased in subjects who have received propranolol for long periods; pindolol has the opposite effect. For discontinuation of β blockers, it is prudent to decrease the dose gradually and to restrict exercise during this period.

Pulmonary Function. A major adverse effect of β receptor antagonists is caused by blockade of $β_2$ receptors in bronchial smooth muscle. These receptors are particularly important for promoting bronchodilation in patients with bronchospastic disease, and $β_2$ blockade may cause a life-threatening increase in airway resistance in such patients. Drugs with selectivity for $β_1$ receptors or those with intrinsic sympathomimetic activity at $β_2$ receptors seem less likely to induce bronchospasm. β Blocker drugs should be avoided if at all possible in patients with asthma. However, in selected patients with COPD and cardiovascular disease, the advantages of using $β_1$ receptor antagonists may outweigh the risk of worsening pulmonary function (Salpeter et al., 2005).

CNS. The adverse effects of β receptor antagonists that are referable to the CNS may include fatigue, sleep disturbances (including insomnia and nightmares), and depression. Interest has focused on the relationship between the incidence of the adverse effects of β receptor antagonists and their lipophilicity; however, no clear correlation has emerged.

Metabolism. β Adrenergic blockade may blunt recognition of hypoglycemia by patients; it also may delay recovery from insulin-induced hypoglycemia. β Receptor antagonists should be used with great caution in patients with diabetes who are prone to hypoglycemic reactions; $β_1$-selective agents may be preferable for these patients. The benefits of β receptor antagonists in type 1 diabetes with myocardial infarction may outweigh the risk in selected patients (Thompson, 2013).

Sexual Function and Reproduction. The incidence of sexual dysfunction in men with hypertension who are treated with β receptor antagonists is not clearly defined. Although experience with the use of β adrenergic receptor antagonists in pregnancy is increasing, information about the safety of these drugs during pregnancy still is limited.

Overdosage. The manifestations of poisoning with β receptor antagonists depend on the pharmacological properties of the ingested drug, particularly its $β_1$ selectivity, intrinsic sympathomimetic activity, and membrane-stabilizing properties. Hypotension, bradycardia, prolonged AV conduction times, and widened QRS complexes are common manifestations of overdosage. Seizures and depression may occur. Hypoglycemia and bronchospasm can occur. Significant bradycardia should be treated initially with atropine, but a cardiac pacemaker often is required. Large doses of INE or an α receptor agonist may be necessary to treat hypotension. Glucagon, acting through its own G protein–coupled receptor and independently of the β adrenergic receptor, has positive chronotropic and inotropic effects on the heart, and the drug has been useful in some patients who have an overdose of a β receptor antagonist.

Drug Interactions. Aluminum salts, cholestyramine, and colestipol may decrease the absorption of β blockers. Drugs such as phenytoin, rifampin, and phenobarbital, as well as smoking, induce hepatic biotransformation enzymes and may decrease plasma concentrations of β receptor antagonists that are metabolized extensively (e.g., propranolol). Cimetidine and hydralazine may increase the bioavailability of agents such as propranolol and metoprolol by affecting hepatic blood flow. β Receptor antagonists can impair the clearance of lidocaine.

Additive effects on blood pressure by β blockers and other antihypertensive agents often are employed to clinical advantage. However, the antihypertensive effects of β receptor antagonists can be opposed by indomethacin and other nonsteroidal anti-inflammatory drugs (see Chapter 38).

Therapeutic Uses

Cardiovascular Diseases. The β receptor antagonists are used extensively in the treatment of hypertension, angina and acute coronary syndromes, and congestive heart failure (Chapters 27–29). These drugs also are used frequently in the treatment of supraventricular and ventricular arrhythmias (Chapter 30). β Receptor antagonists are used in the treatment of hypertrophic obstructive cardiomyopathy, relieving angina, palpitations, and syncope in patients with this disorder. Efficacy probably is related to partial relief of the pressure gradient along the outflow tract. β Blockers also may attenuate catecholamine-induced cardiomyopathy in pheochromocytoma.

β Blockers are used frequently in the medical management of acute dissecting aortic aneurysm; their usefulness comes from reduction in the force of myocardial contraction and the rate of development of such force. Nitroprusside is an alternative, but when given in the absence of β receptor blockade, it causes an undesirable reflex tachycardia. Chronic treatment with β antagonists may be efficacious in slowing the progression of aortic dilation and its complications in patients with Marfan syndrome, although surgical aortic repair is still warranted as aortic diameter expands; losartan, an ACEI, is showing promise as a more effective treatment (Hiratzka et al., 2010).

Glaucoma. The β receptor antagonists are used in the treatment of chronic open-angle glaucoma (see Chapter 69). These agents decrease the production of aqueous humor, which appears to be the mechanism for their clinical effectiveness.

Other Uses. Many of the signs and symptoms of hyperthyroidism are reminiscent of the manifestations of increased sympathetic nervous system activity. β Receptor antagonists control many of the cardiovascular signs and symptoms of hyperthyroidism and are useful adjuncts to more definitive therapy. In addition, propranolol inhibits the peripheral conversion of thyroxine to triiodothyronine, an effect that may be independent of β receptor blockade (see Chapter 43).

Propranolol, timolol, and metoprolol are effective for the prophylaxis of migraine; these drugs are not useful for treatment of acute attacks of migraine.

Propranolol and other β blockers are effective in controlling acute panic symptoms in individuals who are required to perform in public or in other anxiety-provoking situations. Tachycardia, muscle tremors, and other evidence of increased sympathetic activity are reduced.

β Blockers may be of some value in the treatment of patients undergoing withdrawal from alcohol or those with akathisia. Propranolol and nadolol are efficacious in the primary prevention of variceal bleeding in patients with portal hypertension caused by cirrhosis of the liver (Bosch, 1998).

Clinical Selection of a β Receptor Antagonist

The various β receptor antagonists that are used for the treatment of hypertension and angina appear to have similar efficacies. Selection of the most appropriate drug for an individual patient should be based on pharmacokinetic and pharmacodynamic differences among the drugs, cost, and whether there are concurrent medical problems. β_1-Selective antagonists are preferable in patients with bronchospasm, diabetes, peripheral vascular disease, or Raynaud phenomenon. Although no clinical advantage of β receptor antagonists with intrinsic sympathomimetic activity has been clearly established, such drugs may be preferable in patients with bradycardia. In addition, third-generation β antagonists that block α_1 receptors, stimulate β_2 receptors, enhance NO production, block Ca^{2+} entry, open K^+ channels, or possess antioxidant properties may offer therapeutic advantages.

Nonselective β Adrenergic Receptor Antagonists

Propranolol

Propranolol (Table 12–5) interacts with β_1 and β_2 receptors with equal affinity, lacks intrinsic sympathomimetic activity, and does not block α receptors.

ADME. Propranolol is highly lipophilic and almost completely absorbed after oral administration. Much of the drug is metabolized by the liver during its first passage through the portal circulation; only about 25% reaches the systemic circulation. In addition, there is great interindividual variation in the presystemic clearance of propranolol by the liver; this contributes to enormous variability in plasma concentrations (~20-fold) after oral administration of the drug and to the wide dosage range for clinical efficacy. The degree of hepatic extraction of propranolol declines as the dose is increased. The bioavailability of propranolol may be increased by the concomitant ingestion of food and during long-term administration of the drug.

Propranolol readily enters the CNS. Approximately 90% of the drug in the circulation is bound to plasma proteins. It is extensively metabolized, with most metabolites appearing in the urine. One product of hepatic metabolism is 4-hydroxypropranolol, which has some β adrenergic antagonist activity.

Analysis of the distribution of propranolol, its clearance by the liver, and its activity is complicated by the stereospecificity of these processes (Walle et al., 1988). The (–) enantiomers of propranolol and other β-blockers are the active forms. The (–) enantiomer of propranolol appears to be cleared more slowly from the body than is the inactive enantiomer. The clearance of propranolol may vary with hepatic blood flow and liver disease and also may change during the administration of other drugs that affect hepatic metabolism.

Despite its short $t_{1/2}$ in plasma (~4 h), twice-daily administration suffices to produce the antihypertensive effect in some patients. Sustained-release formulations of propranolol maintain therapeutic concentrations of propranolol in plasma throughout a 24-h period. For the treatment of hypertension and angina, the initial oral dose of propranolol generally is 40–80 mg per day. The dose may then be titrated upward until the optimal response is obtained. For the treatment of angina, the dose may be increased at intervals of less than 1 week, as indicated clinically. In hypertension, the full blood pressure response may not develop for several weeks. Typically, doses are less than 320 mg/d. If propranolol is taken twice daily for hypertension, blood pressure should be measured just prior to a dose to ensure that the duration of effect is sufficiently prolonged. Adequacy of β adrenergic blockade can be assessed by measuring suppression of exercise-induced tachycardia (Table 12–5).

Propranolol may be administered intravenously for the management of life-threatening arrhythmias or to patients under anesthesia. Under these circumstances, the usual dose is 1–3 mg, administered slowly (<1 mg/min) with careful and frequent monitoring of blood pressure, ECG, and cardiac function. If an adequate response is not obtained, a second dose may be given after several minutes. If bradycardia is excessive, atropine should be administered to increase heart rate. A change to oral therapy should be initiated as soon as possible.

Nadolol

Nadolol is a long-acting antagonist with equal affinity for β_1 and β_2 receptors. It is devoid of both membrane-stabilizing and intrinsic sympathomimetic activity. A distinguishing characteristic of nadolol is its relatively long $t_{1/2}$. It can be used to treat hypertension and angina pectoris. Unlabeled uses have included migraine prophylaxis, parkinsonian tremors, and variceal bleeding in portal hypertension.

ADME. Nadolol is very soluble in water and is incompletely absorbed from the gut; its bioavailability is about 35%. Interindividual variability is less than with propranolol. The low lipid solubility of nadolol may result in lower concentrations of the drug in the brain. Nadolol is not extensively metabolized and is largely excreted intact in the urine. The $t_{1/2}$ of the drug in plasma is about 20 h; consequently, it generally is administered once daily. Nadolol may accumulate in patients with renal failure, and dosage should be reduced in such individuals.

Timolol

Timolol is a potent, nonselective β receptor antagonist with no intrinsic sympathomimetic or membrane-stabilizing activity. It is used for hypertension, congestive heart failure, acute myocardial infarction, and migraine prophylaxis. In ophthalmology, timolol has been used in the treatment of open-angle glaucoma and intraocular hypertension. The drug appears to reduce aqueous humor production through blockade of β receptors on the ciliary epithelium.

ADME. Timolol is well absorbed from the GI tract. It is metabolized extensively by CYP2D6 in the liver. Only a small amount of unchanged drug appears in the urine. The $t_{1/2}$ in plasma is about 4 h. The ocular formulation of timolol may be absorbed systemically (Chapter 69) and produce adverse effects in susceptible patients, such as those with asthma or congestive heart failure. The systemic administration of cimetidine with topical ocular timolol increases the degree of β blockade, resulting in a reduction of resting heart rate, intraocular pressure, and exercise tolerance (Ishii et al., 2000). For ophthalmic use, timolol is available combined with other medications (e.g., with dorzolamide or travoprost). Timolol also provides benefits to patients with coronary heart disease: In the acute period after myocardial infarction, timolol produced a 39% reduction in mortality in the Norwegian Multicenter Study.

Pindolol

Pindolol is a nonselective β receptor antagonist *with intrinsic sympathomimetic activity*. It has low membrane-stabilizing activity and low lipid solubility. It is used to treat angina pectoris and hypertension. β-Blockers with slight partial agonist activity may be preferred as antihypertensive agents in individuals with diminished cardiac reserve or a propensity for bradycardia. Nonetheless, the clinical significance of partial agonism has not been substantially demonstrated in controlled trials but may be of importance in individual patients.

ADME. Pindolol is almost completely absorbed after oral administration; the drug has a moderately high bioavailability and plasma $t_{1/2}$ of about 4 h. Approximately 50% of pindolol ultimately is metabolized in the liver; the remainder is excreted unchanged in the urine. Clearance is reduced in patients with renal failure.

β_1-Selective Adrenergic Receptor Antagonists

Metoprolol

Metoprolol is a β_1-selective receptor antagonist that is devoid of intrinsic sympathomimetic activity and membrane-stabilizing activity.

ADME. Metoprolol is almost completely absorbed after oral administration, but bioavailability is relatively low (~40%) due to first-pass metabolism. Plasma concentrations of the drug vary widely (up to 17-fold), possibly due to genetically determined differences in the rate of metabolism in the liver by CYP2D6. Only 10% of the administered drug is recovered unchanged in the urine. The $t_{1/2}$ of metoprolol is 3–4 h, but can increase to 7–8 h in CYP2D6 poor metabolizers who have a 5-fold higher risk for developing adverse effects (Wuttke et al., 2002). An extended-release formulation is available for once-daily administration.

Therapeutic Uses. Metoprolol has been used to treat essential hypertension, angina pectoris, tachycardia, heart failure, and vasovagal syncope and as secondary prevention after myocardial infarction, an adjunct in treatment of hyperthyroidism, and for migraine prophylaxis. For the treatment of hypertension, the usual initial dose is 100 mg/d. The drug sometimes is effective when given once daily, although it frequently is used in two divided doses. Dosage may be increased at weekly intervals until optimal reduction of blood pressure is achieved. Metoprolol generally is used in two divided doses for the treatment of stable angina. For the initial treatment of patients with acute myocardial infarction, an intravenous formulation of metoprolol tartrate is available; oral dosing is initiated as soon as the clinical situation permits. Metoprolol generally is contraindicated for the treatment of acute myocardial infarction in patients with heart rates of less than 45 beats per min, heart block greater than first-degree (PR interval ≥ 0.24 sec), systolic blood pressure less than 100 mm Hg, or moderate-to-severe heart failure.

Atenolol

Atenolol is a β_1-selective antagonist that is devoid of intrinsic sympathomimetic and membrane-stabilizing activity. Atenolol is very hydrophilic and appears to penetrate the CNS only to a limited extent.

ADME. Atenolol is available in 25-, 50-, and 100-mg oral tablets (initial dose is 50 mg/d). It is incompletely absorbed (~50%) and is excreted largely unchanged in the urine, with elimination $t_{1/2}$ of 5–8 h. The drug accumulates in patients with renal failure, and dosage should be adjusted for patients whose creatinine clearance is less than 35 mL/min.

Therapeutic Uses. Atenolol can be used to treat hypertension, coronary heart disease, arrhythmias, and angina pectoris and to treat or reduce the risk of heart complications following myocardial infarction. Recent meta-analysis and clinical trials demonstrated a lack of benefit compared with placebo or other antihypertensive agents for reduction of stroke, cardiovascular and all-cause, in spite of similar blood pressure reduction compared to other antihypertensive agents (Ripley and Saseen, 2014). Compared with other active treatments, atenolol was associated with increased risk of all-cause mortality, cardiovascular mortality, and stroke and had a neutral effect on myocardial infarction. Atenolol is also used to treat Graves disease until antithyroid medication can take effect. The initial dose of atenolol for the treatment of hypertension usually is 50 mg/d, given once daily. If an adequate therapeutic response is not evident within several weeks, the daily dose may be increased to 100 mg. Atenolol has been shown to be efficacious, in combination with a diuretic, in elderly patients with isolated systolic hypertension. Atenolol causes fewer CNS side effects (depression, nightmares) than most β-blockers and few bronchospastic reactions due to its pharmacological and pharmacokinetic profile (Varon, 2008).

Esmolol

Esmolol is a β_1-selective antagonist with a rapid onset and a very short duration of action. It has little if any intrinsic sympathomimetic activity and lacks membrane-stabilizing actions. Esmolol is administered intravenously and is used when β blockade of short duration is desired or in critically ill patients in whom adverse effects of bradycardia, heart failure, or hypotension may necessitate rapid withdrawal of the drug. It is a class II antiarrhythmic agent (Chapter 30).

ADME. Esmolol is given by slow intravenous injection. Because esmolol is used in urgent settings where immediate onset of β blockade is warranted, a partial loading dose (500 μg/kg over 1 min) typically is administered, followed by a continuous infusion of the drug (maintenance dose of 50 μg/kg/min for 4 min). If an adequate therapeutic effect is not observed within 5 min, the same loading dose is repeated, followed by a maintenance infusion at a higher rate. This may need to be repeated until the desired end point (e.g., lowered heart rate or blood pressure) is approached. The drug is hydrolyzed rapidly by esterases in erythrocytes and has a $t_{1/2}$ of about 8 min. The $t_{1/2}$ of the carboxylic acid metabolite of esmolol is far longer (~4 h) and will accumulate during prolonged infusion of esmolol. However, this metabolite has very low potency as a β receptor antagonist (1/500 of the potency of esmolol); it is excreted in the urine.

Therapeutic Uses. Esmolol is commonly used in patients during surgery to prevent or treat tachycardia and in the treatment of supraventricular tachycardia. The onset and cessation of β receptor blockade with esmolol are rapid; peak hemodynamic effects occur within 6–10 min of administration of a loading dose, and there is substantial diminution of β-blockade within 20 min of stopping an infusion. Esmolol is particularly useful in severe postoperative hypertension and is a suitable agent in situations where cardiac output, heart rate, and blood pressure are increased. The American Heart Association/American College of Cardiology guidelines recommend against using esmolol in patients already on β blocker therapy, bradycardic patients, and patients with decompensated heart failure, as the drug may compromise their myocardial function (Varon, 2008). Esmolol is generally tolerated well, but it is associated with an increased risk of hypotension that is rapidly reversible (Garnock-Jones, 2012).

Acebutolol

Acebutolol is a β_1-selective antagonist with some intrinsic sympathomimetic and membrane-stabilizing activity.

ADME. Acebutolol is administered orally (starting dose 200 mg twice daily titrated up to 1200 mg/d). It is well absorbed and undergoes significant first-pass metabolism to an active metabolite, diacetolol, which accounts for most of the drug's activity. Overall bioavailability is 35%–50%. The elimination $t_{1/2}$ of acebutolol typically is about 3 h, but the $t_{1/2}$ of diacetolol is 8–12 h; it is excreted largely in the urine. Acebutolol has lipophilic properties and crosses the blood-brain barrier. It has no negative impact on serum lipids (cholesterol, triglycerides, or HDL).

Therapeutic Uses. Acebutol has been used to treat hypertension, ventricular and atrial cardiac arrhythmias, acute myocardial infarction in high-risk patients, and Smith-Magenis syndrome. The initial dose of acebutolol in hypertension usually is 400 mg/d; it may be given as a single dose, but two divided doses may be required for adequate control of blood pressure. Optimal responses usually occur with doses of 400–800 mg per day (range 200–1200 mg).

Bisoprolol

Bisoprolol is a highly selective β_1 receptor antagonist that lacks intrinsic sympathomimetic or membrane-stabilizing activity (McGavin and Keating, 2002). It has a higher degree of β_1-selective activity than atenolol, metoprolol, or betaxolol but less than nebivolol. It is approved for the treatment of hypertension.

Bisoprolol generally is well tolerated; side effects include dizziness, bradycardia, hypotension, and fatigue. Bisoprolol is well absorbed following oral administration, with bioavailability of about 90%. It is eliminated by renal excretion (50%) and liver metabolism to pharmacologically inactive metabolites (50%). Bisoprolol has a plasma $t_{1/2}$ of approximately 11–17 h. Bisoprolol can be considered a standard treatment option when selecting a β-blocker for use in combination with ACEIs and diuretics in patients with stable, moderate-to-severe chronic heart failure and in treating hypertension (McGavin and Keating, 2002; Simon et al., 2003). It has also been used to treat arrhythmias and ischemic heart disease. Bisoprolol was associated with a 34% mortality benefit in the CIBIS-II (Cardiac Insufficiency Bisoprolol Study-II).

Betaxolol

Betaxolol is a selective β_1 receptor antagonist with no partial agonist activity and slight membrane-stabilizing properties. Betaxolol is used to treat hypertension, angina pectoris, and glaucoma. The drug is well absorbed with high bioavailability; its elimination $t_{1/2}$ varies from 14 to 22 h. It is usually well tolerated; side effects are mild and transient.

β Adrenergic Receptor Antagonists With Additional Cardiovascular Effects ("Third-Generation" β-Blockers)

In addition to the classical nonselective and β_1 selective adrenergic receptor antagonists, there are drugs that possess vasodilating actions (Toda, 2003). These effects are produced through a variety of mechanisms, including the following:

- *α_1 adrenergic receptor blockade* (labetalol, carvedilol, bucindolol, bevantolol, nipradilol)
- *increased production of NO* (celiprolol, nebivolol, carteolol, bopindolol, nipradolol)
- *β_2 agonist properties* (celiprolol, carteolol, bopindolol)
- *Ca^{2+} entry blockade* (carvedilol, betaxolol, bevantolol)
- *opening of K^+ channels* (tilisolol)
- *antioxidant action* (carvedilol)

These actions are summarized in Table 12–4 and Figure 12–4. Some third-generation β receptor antagonists are not yet available in the U.S. but have undergone clinical trials and are available elsewhere.

Labetalol

Labetalol is representative of a class of drugs that act as competitive antagonists at both α_1 and β receptors. Labetalol has two optical centers, and the formulation used clinically contains equal amounts of the four diastereomers. The pharmacological properties of the drug are complex because each isomer displays different relative activities. The properties of the mixture include selective blockade of α_1 receptors (as compared with the α_2 subtype), blockade of β_1 and β_2 receptors, partial agonist activity at β_2 receptors, and inhibition of neuronal uptake of NE (cocaine-like effect) (Chapter 8). The potency of the mixture for β receptor blockade is 5- to 10-fold that for α_1 receptor blockade.

The pharmacological effects of labetalol have become clearer since the four isomers were separated and tested individually.

- *The R,R isomer* is about four times more potent as a β receptor antagonist than is racemic labetalol and accounts for much of the β blockade produced by the mixture of isomers. As an α_1 antagonist, this isomer is less than 20% as potent as the racemic mixture. The *R,R* isomer has some intrinsic sympathomimetic activity at β_2 adrenergic receptors; this may contribute to vasodilation.
- *The R,S isomer* is almost devoid of both α and β blocking effects.
- *The S,R isomer* has almost no β-blocking activity, yet is about five times more potent as an α_1 blocker than is racemic labetalol.
- *The S,S isomer* is devoid of β blocking activity and has a potency similar to that of racemic labetalol as an α_1 receptor antagonist.

The actions of labetalol on both α_1 and β receptors contribute to the fall in blood pressure observed in patients with hypertension. α_1 Receptor blockade leads to relaxation of arterial smooth muscle and vasodilation, particularly when the patient is upright. The β_1 blockade also contributes to a fall in blood pressure, in part by blocking reflex sympathetic stimulation of the heart. In addition, the intrinsic sympathomimetic activity of labetalol at β_2 receptors may contribute to vasodilation, and the drug may have some direct vasodilating capacity.

Labetalol is available in oral form for therapy of chronic hypertension and as an intravenous formulation for use in hypertensive emergencies. Labetalol has been associated with hepatic injury in a limited number of patients. Labetalol has been recommended as treatment of acute severe hypertension (hypertensive emergency). Its hypotensive action begins within 2–5 min after intravenous administration, reaching its peak at 5–15 min and lasting about 2–4 h. Heart rate is either maintained or slightly reduced, and cardiac output is maintained. Labetalol reduces systemic vascular resistance without reducing total peripheral blood flow. Cerebral, renal, and coronary blood flow is maintained. It can be used in the setting of pregnancy-induced hypertensive crisis because little placental transfer occurs due to the poor lipid solubility of labetalol.

ADME. Although labetalol is completely absorbed from the gut, there is extensive first-pass clearance; bioavailability is about 20%–40% but may be increased by food intake. The drug is rapidly metabolized in the liver; very little unchanged drug is found in the urine. The rate of metabolism of labetalol is sensitive to changes in hepatic blood flow. The elimination $t_{1/2}$ of the drug is about 8 h. The $t_{1/2}$ of the *R,R* isomer of labetalol is approximately 15 h.

Carvedilol

Carvedilol is a third-generation β receptor antagonist that has a unique pharmacological profile. *It blocks β_1, β_2, and α_1 receptors similarly to labetalol but also has antioxidant and anti-inflammatory properties* (Dandona et al., 2007). The antioxidant and anti-inflammatory properties may be beneficial in treating congestive heart failure. The drug has membrane-stabilizing activity but lacks intrinsic sympathomimetic activity.

Carvedilol reduces arterial blood pressure by decreasing vascular resistance and maintaining cardiac output while decreasing sympathetic vascular tone (DiNicolantonio et al., 2015; Zepeda et al., 2012). The hemodynamic effect exerted by carvedilol is similar to that of ACEIs and superior to that of traditional β blockers. Carvedilol is renoprotective and has favorable effects in patients with diabetes or metabolic syndrome. The drug is FDA-approved for use in hypertension, congestive heart failure, and left ventricular dysfunction following myocardial infarction.

Carvedilol possesses two distinct antioxidant properties: It is a chemical antioxidant that can bind to and scavenge ROS, and it can suppress the biosynthesis of ROS and oxygen radicals. Carvedilol is extremely lipophilic and protects cell membranes from lipid peroxidation. It prevents LDL oxidation, which in turn induces the uptake of LDL into the coronary vasculature. Carvedilol also inhibits ROS-mediated loss of myocardial contractility, stress-induced hypertrophy, apoptosis, and the accumulation and activation of neutrophils. *At high doses, carvedilol exerts Ca^{2+} channel-blocking activity.* Carvedilol does not increase β receptor density and does not show a high level of inverse agonist activity (Cheng et al., 2001; Dandona et al., 2007; Keating and Jarvis, 2003).

Carvedilol has been tested in numerous controlled trials (Cleland, 2003; Poole-Wilson et al., 2003). These trials showed that carvedilol improves ventricular function and reduces mortality and morbidity in patients with mild-to-severe congestive heart failure. Several experts recommend it as the standard treatment option in this setting. In addition, carvedilol combined with conventional therapy reduces mortality and attenuates myocardial infarction. In patients with chronic heart failure, carvedilol reduces cardiac sympathetic drive, but it is not clear if blockade of α_1 receptor–mediated vasodilation is maintained over long periods of time.

ADME. Carvedilol is rapidly absorbed following oral administration, with peak plasma concentrations occurring in 1–2 h. It is highly lipophilic and more than 95% protein bound. Hepatic CYPs 2D6 and 2C9 metabolized carvedilol, yielding a $t_{1/2}$ of 7–10 h. Stereoselective first-pass metabolism results in more rapid clearance of S(−)-carvedilol than R(+)-carvedilol. No significant changes in the pharmacokinetics of carvedilol are seen in elderly patients with hypertension, and no change in dosage is needed in patients with moderate-to-severe renal insufficiency (Cleland, 2003; Keating and Jarvis, 2003). Because of carvedilol's extensive oxidative metabolism by the liver, its pharmacokinetics can be profoundly affected by drugs that induce or inhibit oxidation. These include the inducer rifampin and inhibitors such as cimetidine, quinidine, fluoxetine, and paroxetine.

Bucindolol

Bucindolol is a third-generation *nonselective β adrenergic antagonist with weak α_1 adrenergic blocking properties.*

Bucindolol increases left ventricular systolic ejection fraction and decreases peripheral resistance, thereby reducing afterload. It increases plasma HDL cholesterol but does not affect plasma triglycerides. A large comprehensive clinical trial, the BEST (*β* Blocker Evaluation of Survival

Trial), was terminated early because of a lack of a demonstrable survival benefit with bucindolol versus placebo. Further analysis has demonstrated that polymorphisms in β_1 and α_{2c} receptors predict the effect of bucindolol to prevent new-onset atrial fibrillation and ventricular arrhythmias (Cooper-DeHoff and Johnson, 2016; O'Connor et al., 2012).

Celiprolol

Celiprolol is a third-generation cardioselective β receptor antagonist. It has low lipid solubility and possesses weak vasodilating and bronchodilating effects attributed to *partial selective β_2-agonist* activity and possibly papaverine-like relaxant effects on smooth muscle (including bronchial). It also has been reported to *antagonize peripheral α_2 adrenergic receptor activity, to promote NO production, and to inhibit oxidative stress.* There is evidence for intrinsic sympathomimetic activity at the β_2 receptor. Celiprolol is devoid of membrane-stabilizing activity. Weak α_2 antagonistic properties are present but are not considered clinically significant at therapeutic doses (Toda, 2003).

Celiprolol reduces heart rate and blood pressure and can increase the functional refractory period of the AV node. Oral bioavailability ranges from 30% to 70%, and peak plasma levels are seen at 2–4 h. It is excreted largely unchanged in the urine and feces. The predominant mode of excretion is renal. Celiprolol is used for treatment of hypertension and angina (Witchitz et al., 2000).

Nebivolol

Nebivolol is a third-generation, long-acting, and highly selective β_1 adrenergic receptor antagonist that stimulates NO-mediated vasodilation via β_3 receptor agonism (Fongemia and Felix-Getzik, 2015). Nebivolol is devoid of intrinsic sympathomimetic effects as well as membrane-stabilizing activity and α_1 receptor blocking properties.

Therapeutic Uses. Nebivolol is approved for treatment of hypertension and has potential utility in the treatment of heart failure with reduced ejection traction. The drug lowers blood pressure by reducing peripheral vascular resistance and significantly increases stroke volume with preservation of cardiac output and maintains systemic flow and blood flow to target organs. Nebivolol also reduces oxidative stress and may have favorable effects on both carbohydrate and lipid metabolism. These benefits are also observed in the presence of metabolic syndrome, which often copresents with hypertension (Ignarro, 2008).

ADME. Nebivolol is administered as the racemate containing equal amounts of the *d*- and *l*-enantiomers. The *d*-isomer is the active β blocking component; the *l*-isomer is responsible for enhancing production of NO.

Nebivolol undergoes extensive first-pass metabolism, primarily by CYP2D6, yielding a mean terminal $t_{1/2}$ of about 10 h. Active metabolites (e.g., 4-OH nebivolol) contribute to the β-blocking effect of nebivolol. Polymorphisms in the CYP2D6 gene affect nebivolol's metabolism but not its efficacy due to the production of active hydroxylated metabolites (Lefebvre et al., 2007).

Nebivolol is lipophilic, and concomitant administration of chlorthalidone, hydrochlorothiazide, theophylline, or digoxin with nebivolol may reduce its extent of absorption. The NO-dependent vasodilating action of nebivolol and its high β_1 adrenergic receptor selectivity likely contribute to the drug's efficacy and comparative tolerability as an antihypertensive agent (e.g., less fatigue and sexual dysfunction) (Moen and Wagstaff, 2006).

Bibliography

Abdelghany O. Arformoterol: the first nebulized long-acting beta$_2$-adrenergic agonist. *Formulary,* **2007**, *42*:99–109.

Altschuld RA, Billman GE. β_2-Adrenoceptors and ventricular fibrillation. *Pharmacol Ther,* **2000**, *88*:1–14.

Allwood MJ, et al. Peripheral vascular effects of noradrenaline, isopropylnoradrenaline, and dopamine. *Br Med Bull,* **1963**, *19*:132–136.

Arch JRS. Challenges in β_3-adrenoceptor agonist drug development. *Ther Adv Endocrinol Metab,* **2011**, *2*:59–64.

Beduschi MC, et al. α-Blockade therapy for benign prostatic hyperplasia: from a nonselective to a more selective α_{1A}-adrenergic antagonist. *Urology,* **1998**, *51*:861–872.

Berkowitz DE, et al. Distribution of beta 3-adrenoceptor mRNA in human tissues. *Eur J Pharmacol,* **1995**, *289*:223–228.

Black SW, et al. Challenges in the development of therapeutics for narcolepsy. *Prog Neurobiol,* **2015**, *pii*:S0301-0082(15)30023-X. doi:10.1016/j.pneurobio.2015.12.002.

Bosch J. Medical treatment of portal hypertension. *Digestion,* **1998**, *59*:547–555.

Breslow MJ, Ligier B. Hyperadrenergic states. *Crit Care Med,* **1991**, *19*:1566–1579.

Brodde OE, Michel MC. Adrenergic and muscarinic receptors in the human heart. *Pharmacol Rev,* **1999**, *51*:651–690.

Cheng J, et al. Carvedilol: molecular and cellular basis for its multifaceted therapeutic potential. *Cardiovasc Drug Rev,* **2001**, *19*:152–171.

Childress AC and Berry, SA. Pharmacotherapy of attention-deficit hyperactivity in adolescents. *Drugs,* **2012**, *72*:309–325.

Cleland JG. β-Blockers for heart failure: why, which, when, and where. *Med Clin North Am,* **2003**, *87*:339–371.

Cooper-DeHoff RM, Johnson JJ. Hypertension pharmacogenomics: in search of personalized treatment approaches. *Nat Rev Nephrol,* **2016**, *12*:110–122.

Cypess AM, et al. Activation of human brown adipose tissue by a β_3-adrenergic receptor agonist. *Cell Metab,* **2015**, *21*:33–38.

Dandona P, et al. Antioxidant activity of carvedilol in cardiovascular disease. *J Hypertension,* **2007**, *25*:731–741.

Deano R, Sorrentino M. Lipid effects of antihypertensive medications. *Curr Atheroscler Rep,* **2012**, *14*:70–77.

Delano FA, et al. Pancreatic digestive enzyme blockade in the intestine increases survival after experimental shock. *Sci Transl Med,* **2013**, *5*:169ra11.

DiBari M, et al. β-Blockers after acute myocardial infarction in elderly patients with diabetes mellitus: time to reassess. *Drugs Aging,* **2003**, *20*:13–22.

DiNicolantonio JJ, et al. β-Blockers in hypertension diabetes, heart failure and acute myocardial infarction. A review of the literature. *Open Heart,* **2015**, *2*:e000230.

Drazen JM, O'Byrne PM. Risks of long acting beta-agonists in achieving asthma control. *N Engl J Med,* **2009**, *360*:1671–1672.

Dunne F, et al. β-Blockers in the management of hypertension in patients with type 2 diabetes mellitus: is there a role? *Drugs,* **2001**, *61*:428–435.

Emorine LJ, et al. Molecular characterization of the human B_3 adrenergic receptor. *Science,* **1989**, *245*:1118–1121.

Fanta CH. Asthma. *N Engl J Med,* **2009**, *360*:1002–1014.

FDA. Full prescribing information, sodium oxybate. Revised **December 2012**. Available at: http://www.accessdata.fda.gov/drugsatfda_docs/label/2012/021196s013lbl.pdf. Accessed November 29, 2016.

Fitton A, Benfield P. Dopexamine hydrochloride. A review of its pharmacodynamic and pharmacokinetic properties and therapeutic potential in acute cardiac insufficiency. *Drugs,* **1990**, *39*:308–330.

Fleckenstein A. New insights into the mechanism of actions of amphetamines. *Annu Rev Pharmacol,* **2007**, *47*:691–698.

Fongemie J, Felix-Getzik E. A review of nebivolol pharmacology and clinical evidence. *Drugs,* **2015**, *75*:1349–1371. doi:1011007/s40265-015-0435-5.

Garnock-Jones KP. Esmolol. A review of its use in the short-term treatment of tachyarrhythmias and the short-term control of tachycardia and hypertension. *Drugs,* **2012**, *72*:109–132.

Goldsmith DR, Keating GM. Budesonide/fomoterol: a review of its use in asthma. *Drugs,* **2004**, *64*:1597–1618.

Hiratzka LF, et al. Guidelines for the diagnosis and management of patients with thoracic aortic disease. *Circulation,* **2010**, *121*:e266–e369. Available at: doi.org/10.1161/CIR.0b013e3181d4739e. Accessed June 26, 2017.

Ignarro LJ. Different pharmacological properties of two enantiomers in a unique β-blocker, nebivolol. *Cardiovasc Ther,* **2008**, *26*:115–134.

Ishii Y, et al. Drug interaction between cimetidine and timolol ophthalmic solution: effect on heart rate and intraocular pressure in healthy Japanese volunteers. *J Clin Pharmacol,* **2000**, *40*:193–199.

Keating GM. Droxidopa: a review of its use in symptomatic neurogenic

TABLE 12–5 ■ SUMMARY OF ADRENERGIC AGONISTS AND ANTAGONISTS

SUB-CLASS	DRUGS	PROMINENT PRINCIPAL PHARMACOLOGICAL ACTIONS	THERAPEUTIC APPLICATIONS	UNTOWARD EFFECTS	COMMENTS
Direct-acting nonselective agonists					
	Epinephrine (α_1, α_2, β_1, β_2, β_3)	↑ Heart rate; ↑ blood pressure; ↑ contractility; slight ↓ in PVR; ↑ cardiac output; vasoconstriction (viscera); vasodilation (skeletal muscle); ↑ blood glucose and lactate	Open-angle glaucoma With local anesthetics to prolong action Anaphylactic shock Complete heart block or cardiac arrest Bronchodilator in asthma	Palpitation Cardiac arrhythmias Cerebral hemorrhage Headache Tremor Restlessness	Not given orally Life saving in anaphylaxis or cardiac arrest
	Norepinephrine (α_1, α_2, β_1 >> β_2)	↑ Systolic and diastolic blood pressure; vasoconstriction; ↑ PVR; direct ↑ in heart rate and contraction; reflex ↓ in heart rate	Hypotension	Similar to EPI Hypertension	Not absorbed orally
β Receptor agonists					
Nonselective ($\beta_1 + \beta_2$)	Isoproterenol	↓ PVR; ↑ cardiac output; bronchodilation	Bronchodilator in asthma Complete heart block or cardiac arrest Shock	Palpitations Tachycardia Tachyarrhythmias Headache Flushed skin Cardiac ischemia in patients with coronary artery disease	Intravenous administration Administered by inhalation in asthma
β_1 Selective	Dobutamine	↑ Contractility; some ↑ heart rate; ↑ AV conduction	Short-term treatment of cardiac decompensation after surgery or patients with congestive heart failure or myocardial infarction	↑ Blood pressure and heart rate	Intravenous only Use with caution in patients with hypertension or cardiac arrhythmias
β_2 Selective (intermediate acting)	Albuterol Bitolterol Fenoterol Isoetharine Levalbuterol Metaproterenol Pirbuterol Procaterol Terbutaline	Relaxation of bronchial smooth muscle Relaxation of uterine smooth muscle Activation of other β_2 receptors after systemic administration	Bronchodilators for treatment of asthma and COPD Short-/intermediate-acting drugs for acute bronchospasm	Skeletal muscle tremor Tachycardia and other cardiac effects seen after systemic administration (much less with inhalational use)	Use with caution in patients with cardiovascular disease (reduced by inhalational administration) Minimal side effects

(*Continued*)

TABLE 12–5 ■ SUMMARY OF ADRENERGIC AGONISTS AND ANTAGONISTS (*CONTINUED*)

SUB-CLASS	DRUGS	PROMINENT PRINCIPAL PHARMACOLOGICAL ACTIONS	THERAPEUTIC APPLICATIONS	UNTOWARD EFFECTS	COMMENTS
(Long acting)	Formoterol Salmeterol Arformoterol Carniterol Indacaterol Ritodrine	Relaxation of bronchial smooth muscle Relaxation of uterine smooth muscle	Bronchodilators for treatment of COPD Best choice for prophylaxis due to long action Ritodrine, to stop premature labor	Contraindicated in asthma	Long action, favored for prophylaxis
α Receptor agonists					
α_1 Selective	Methoxamine Phenylephrine Mephentermine Metaraminol Midodrine	Vasoconstriction	Nasal congestion (used topically) Postural hypotension	Hypertension Reflex bradycardia Dry mouth, sedation, rebound hypertension on abrupt withdrawal	Mephentermine and metaraminol also act indirectly to release NE Midodrine, a prodrug activated in vivo
α_2 Selective	Clonidine Apraclonidine Guanfacine Guanabenz Brimonidine α-Methyldopa	↓ Sympathetic outflow from brain to periphery resulting in ↓ PVR and blood pressure ↓ Nerve-evoked release of sympathetic transmitters ↓ Production of aqueous humor	Adjunctive therapy in shock Hypertension To reduce sympathetic response to withdrawal from narcotics, alcohol, and tobacco Glaucoma		Apraclonidine and brimonidine used topically for glaucoma and ocular hypertension Methyldopa is converted in CNS to α-methyl NE, an effective α_2 agonist
Indirect acting	Amphetamine Methamphetamine Methylphenidate (releases NE peripherally; NE, DA, 5HT centrally)	CNS stimulation ↑ Blood pressure Myocardial stimulation	Treatment of ADHD Narcolepsy Obesity (rarely)	Restlessness Tremor Insomnia Anxiety Tachycardia Hypertension Cardiac arrhythmias	Schedule II drugs Marked tolerance occurs Chronic use leads to dependence Can result in hemorrhagic stroke in patients with underlying disease Long-term use can cause paranoid schizophrenia
Mixed acting	Dopamine (α_1; α_2, β_1, D_1; releases NE)	Vasodilation (coronary, renal mesenteric beds) ↑ Glomerular filtration rate and natriuresis ↑ Heart rate and contractility ↑ Systolic blood pressure	Cardiogenic shock Congestive heart failure Treatment of acute renal failure	High doses lead to vasoconstriction Restlessness	Important for its ability to maintain renal blood flow Administered intravenously
	Ephedrine (α_1, α_2, β_1, β_2; releases NE)	Similar to epinephrine but longer lasting CNS stimulation	Bronchodilator for treatment of asthma Nasal congestion Treatment of hypotension and shock	Tremor Insomnia Anxiety Tachycardia Hypertension	Administered by all routes Not commonly used

α Blockers					
Nonselective (classical α blockers)	PBZ Phentolamine Tolazoline	↓ PVR and blood pressure Venodilation	Treatment of catecholamine excess (e.g., pheochromocytoma)	Postural hypotension Failure of ejaculation	Cardiac stimulation due to initiation of reflexes and to enhanced release of NE via α_2 receptor blockade PBZ produces long-lasting α receptor blockade, can block neuronal and extraneuronal uptake of amines
α_1 Selective	Prazosin Terazosin Doxazosin Trimazosin Alfuzosin Tamsulosin Silodosin	↓ PVR and blood pressure Relax smooth muscles in neck of urinary bladder and in prostate	Primary hypertension Increase urine flow in BPH	Postural hypotension when therapy instituted	Prazosin and related quinazolines are selective for α_1 receptors Tamsulosin exhibits some selectivity for α_{1A} receptors
β Blockers					
Nonselective (first generation)	Nadolol Penbutolol Pindolol Propranolol Timolol	↓ Heart rate ↓ Contractility ↓ Cardiac output Slow conduction in atria and AV node ↑ Refractory period, AV node Bronchoconstriction Prolonged hypoglycemia ↓ Plasma free fatty acids ↓ HDL cholesterol ↑ LDL cholesterol and triglycerides Hypokalemia	Angina pectoris Hypertension Cardiac arrhythmias Congestive heart failure Pheochromocytoma Glaucoma Hypertrophic obstructive cardiomyopathy Hyperthyroidism Migraine prophylaxis Acute panic symptoms Substance abuse withdrawal Variceal bleeding in portal hypertension	Bradycardia Negative inotropy ↓ Cardiac output Bradyarrhythmias ↓ AV conduction Bronchoconstriction Fatigue Sleep disturbances (insomnia, nightmares) Prolongation of hypoglycemia Sexual dysfunction in men Drug interactions	Effects depend on sympathoadrenal tone Bronchoconstriction (do not use in asthma and COPD) Hypoglycemia (of concern in hypoglycemics and diabetics) Membrane-stabilizing effect (propranolol, and betaxolol) ISA (strong for pindolol; weak for penbutolol, carteolol, and betaxolol)
β_1 Selective (second generation)	Acebutolol Atenolol Bisoprolol Betaxolol Esmolol Metoprolol	Similar to above but with less adverse effect on bronchial constriction	Similar to above	Similar to above	Effects depend on sympathoadrenal tone Bronchoconstriction effect is less than for non-specific agents but use only with great caution in asthma and COPD
Nonselective (third-generation) vasodilators	Carteolol Carvedilol Bucindolol Labetalol	See text. These agents affect multiple receptor types and signaling pathways. They are used to treat hypertension; carvedilol is also used to treat heart failure. Effects and applications generally resemble those of other β blockers with some α blocking properties: • α_1 adrenergic receptor blockade (labetalol, carvedilol, bucindolol) • increased production of NO (celiprolol, nebivolol, carteolol) • β_2 agonist properties (celiprolol, carteolol) • Ca^{2+} entry blockade (carvedilol) • antioxidant action (carvedilol)			Vasodilation seen in third-generation drugs; multiple mechanisms (see Figure 12–4) Weak ISA for labetalol Receptor polymorphisms affect response to bucindolol's anti-arrhythmic properties
β_1 Selective (third-generation) vasodilators	Celiprolol Nebivolol				

orthostatic hypotension. *Adis Drug Evaluation*, **2014**, *10*:1007/S40265-019-0342. *Drugs*, **2015**, *75*:197–206.

Keating GM, Jarvis B. Carvedilol: a review of its use in chronic heart failure. *Drugs*, **2003**, *63*:1697–1741.

Kenny B, et al. Evaluation of the pharmacological selectivity profile of α_1 adrenoceptor antagonists at prostatic α_1 adrenoceptors: binding, functional and in vivo studies. *Br J Pharmacol*, **1996**, *118*:871–878.

Kyprianou N. Doxazosin and terazosin suppress prostate growth by inducing apoptosis. Clinical significance. *J Urol*, **2003**, *169*:1520–1525.

Lefebvre J, et al. The influence of CYP2D6 phenotype on the clinical response of nebivolol in patients with essential hypertension. *Br J Clin Pharmacol*, **2007**, *63*:575–582.

LePor H, et al. The efficacy of terazosin, finasteride, or both in benign prostatic hyperplasia. *N Eng J Med*, **1996**, *335*:533–539.

Lowry JA, Brown JT. Significance of the imidazoline receptors in toxicology. *J Clin Toxicol*, **2014**, *52*:454–469.

Man in't Veld AJ, et al. Do β blockers really increase peripheral vascular resistance? Review of the literature and new observations under basal conditions. *Am J Hypertens*, **1988**, *1*:91–96.

Marik PE, Iglesias J. Low-dose dopamine does not prevent acute renal failure in patients with septic shock and oliguria. NORASEPT II Study Investigators. *Am J Med*, **1999**, *107*:387–390.

Matera MG, Cazzola M. Ultra-long acting β_2-adrenoceptor agonist. An emerging therapeutic option for asthma and COPD. *Drugs*, **2007**, *67*:503–515.

May, DE, Kratochvil, CJ. Attention deficit hyperactivity disorder: recent advances in paediatric pharmacotherapy. *Drugs*, **2010**, *70*:15–40.

McClellan KJ, et al. Midodrine. A review of its therapeutic use in the management of orthostatic hypotension. *Drugs Aging*, **1998**, *12*:76–86.

McConnell JD, et al. The long-term effect of doxazosin, finasteride, and combination therapy on the clinical progression of benign prostatic hyperplasia. *N Engl J Med*, **2003**, *349*:2387–2398.

McGavin JK, Keating GM. Bisoprolol. A review of its use in chronic heart failure. *Drugs*, **2002**, *62*:2677–2696.

Michel MC. How β_3-adrenoceptor-selective is mirabegron? *Br J Pharmacol*, **2016**, *173*:429–430.

Michel MC, Vrydag W. α_1-, α_2- and β-Adrenoceptors in the urinary bladder urethra and prostate. *Br J Pharmacolol*, **2006**, *147*:S88–S119.

Mimran A, Ducailar G. Systemic and regional haemodynamic profile of diuretics and α- and β-blockers. A review comparing acute and chronic effects. *Drugs*, **1988**, *35*(suppl 6):60–69.

Moen MD, Wagstaff AJ. Nebivolol: a review of its use in the management of hypertension and chronic heart failure. *Drugs*, **2006**, *66*:1389–1409.

Moniotte S, et al. Upregulation of β_3-adrenoceptors and altered contractile response to inotropic amines in human failing myocardium. *Circulation*, **2001**, *103*:1649–1655.

Morimoto A, et al. Endogenous β_3-adrenoceptor activation contributes to left ventricular and cardiomyocyte dysfunction in heart failure. *Am J Physiol Heart Circ Physiol*, **2004**, *286*:H2425–H2433.

Murphy MB, et al. Fenoldopam: a selective peripheral dopamine receptor agonist for the treatment of severe hypertension. *N Engl J Med*, **2001**, *345*:1548–1557.

Nikolic K, Agbaba D. Imidazoline antihypertensive drugs: selective I(1)-imidazoline receptors activation. *Cardiovasc Ther*, **2012**, *30*:209–216.

O'Connor CM, et al. Combinatorial pharmacogenetic interactions of bucindolol and β1, α2C adrenergic receptor polymorphisms. *PLoS One*, **2012**, *7*:e44324. Available at: doi.org/10.1371/journal.pone.0044324. Accessed June 27, 2017.

Poole-Wilson PA, et al. Comparison of carvedilol and metoprolol on clinical outcomes in patients with chronic heart failure in the Carvedilol Or Metoprolol European Trial (COMET): randomised controlled trial. *Lancet*, **2003**, *362*:7–13.

Redington AE. Step one for asthma treatment: β_2-agonists or inhaled corticosteroids? *Drugs*, **2001**, *61*:1231–1238.

Ripley TL, Saseen JJ. β Blockers: a review of their pharmacological and physiological diversity. *Ann Pharmacother*, **2014**, *48*:723–733.

Salpeter SR, et al. Cardioselective beta-blockers for chronic obstructive pulmonary disease. *Cochrane Database Syst Rev*, **2005**, (*4*):CD003566.

Schmid-Schoenbein G, Hugli T. A new hypothesis for microvascular inflammation in shock and multiorgan failure: self-digestion by pancreatic enzymes. *Microcirculation*, **2005**, *12*:71–82.

Simon T, et al. Bisoprolol dose-response relationship in patients with congestive heart failure: a subgroups analysis in the cardiac insufficiency bisoprolol study (CIBIS II). *Eur Heart J*, **2003**, *24*:552–559.

Sitte HH, Freissmuth M. Amphetamines, new psychoactive drugs, and the monoamine transporter cycle. *Trends Pharmacol Sci*, **2015**, *36*: 41–50.

Starke K, et al. Modulation of neurotransmitter release by presynaptic autoreceptors. *Physiol Rev*, **1989**, *69*:864–989.

Suissa S, Ernst P. Optical illusions from visual data analysis: example of the New Zealand asthma mortality epidemic. *J Clin Epidemiol*, **1997**, *50*:1079–1088.

Swanson JM, Volkow ND. Serum and brain concentrations of methylphenidate: implications for use and abuse. *Neurosci Biobehav Rev*, **2003**, *27*:615–621.

Tam SW, et al. Yohimbine: a clinical review. *Pharmacol Ther*, **2001**, *91*: 215–243.

Thompson PL. Should β-blockers still be routine after myocardial infarction? *Curr Opin Cardiol*, **2013**, *28*:399–404.

Toda N. Vasodilating β-adrenoceptor blockers as cardiovascular therapeutics. *Pharmacol Ther*, **2003**, *100*:215–234.

Varon J. Treatment of acute severe hypertension: current and newer agents. *Drugs*, **2008**, *68*:283–297.

Walle T, et al. Stereoselective delivery and actions of β receptor antagonists. *Biochem Pharmacol*, **1988**, *37*:115–124.

Witchitz S, et al. Treatment of heart failure with celiprolol, a cardioselective β blocker with β-2 agonist vasodilator properties. The CELICARD Group. *Am J Cardiol*, **2000**, *85*:1467–1471.

Wuttke H, et al. Increased frequency of cytochrome P450 2D6 poor metabolizers among patients with metoprolol-associated adverse effects. *Clin Pharmacol Ther*, **2002**, *72*:429–437.

Zependa RJ, et al. Carvedilol and nebivolol on oxidative stress-related parameters and endothelial function in patients with essential hypertension. *Basic Clin Pharmacol Toxicol*, **2012**, *111*:309–316.

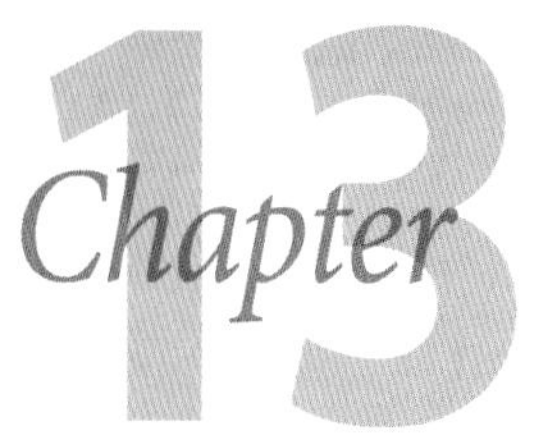

5-Hydroxytryptamine (Serotonin) and Dopamine

David R. Sibley, Lisa A. Hazelwood, and Susan G. Amara

第十三章　5-羟色胺（血清素）和多巴胺

中文导读

本章主要介绍：导论；5-羟色胺，包括其合成与代谢、脑中的血清素能投射途径、5-羟色胺受体；5-羟色胺在生理系统中的作用，包括血小板、心血管系统、胃肠道、炎症、中枢神经系统、睡眠-觉醒周期、攻击和冲动、食欲与肥胖；影响5-羟色胺信号的药物，包括5-羟色胺1B/1D受体激动药（曲普坦），麦角生物碱，5-羟色胺受体部分激动药、SSRIs和MSAAs，以及5-羟色胺水平的临床调控与5-羟色胺综合征；多巴胺，包括其合成与代谢、多巴胺受体、多巴胺转运蛋白；多巴胺在生理系统中的作用，包括心脏与血管、肾脏、垂体、儿茶酚胺释放、中枢神经系统；影响多巴胺信号的药物，包括多巴胺受体激动药和拮抗药。

Abbreviations

AADC: aromatic L-amino acid decarboxylase
AC: adenylyl cyclase
ACh: acetylcholine
ADD: attention-deficit disorder
ADHD: attention-deficit/hyperactivity disorder
ALDH: aldehyde dehydrogenase
BBB: blood-brain barrier
CNS: central nervous system
COMT: catechol-*O*-methyl transferase
CSF: cerebrospinal fluid
DA: dopamine
DAG: diacylglycerol
DAT: dopamine transporter
L-dopa: 3,4-dihydroxyphenylalanine
DOPAC: 3,4-dihydroxyphenylacetic acid
ENT: equilibrative nucleoside transporter
EPI: epinephrine
EPS: extrapyramidal symptoms
FDA: Food and Drug Administration
FSIAD: female sexual interest/arousal disorder
GABA: γ-aminobutyric acid
GI: gastrointestinal
GPCR: G protein–coupled receptor
GSK-3: glycogen synthase kinase 3
5-HIAA: 5-hydroxyindole acetic acid
HSDD: hypoactive sexual desire disorder
5HT: 5-hydroxytryptamine, serotonin
HVA: homovanillic acid
LAT1: L-type amino acid transporter 1
LSD: lysergic acid diethylamide
MAO: monoamine oxidase
MPP^+: 1-methyl-4-phenylpyridinium
MPTP: 1-methyl-4-phenyl-1,2,3,6-tetrahydropyridine
MSAA: multifunctional serotonin agonist and antagonist
NE: norepinephrine
NET: norepinephrine transporter
NMDA: *N*-methyl-D-aspartate
NO: nitric oxide
NSS: neurotransmitter–sodium symporter
OCT: organic cation transporter
6-OHDA: 6-hydroxydopamine
PCPA: para-chlorophenylalanine
PD: Parkinson disease
PFC: prefrontal cortex
PH: phenylalanine hydroxylase
PKC: protein kinase C
PL_: phospholipase _, as in PLC
RLS: restless leg syndrome
SERT: serotonin transporter
SNRI: serotonin-norepinephrine reuptake inhibitor
SSRI: selective serotonin reuptake inhibitor
TAAR1: trace amine-associated receptor 1
TCA: tricyclic antidepressant
TH: tyrosine hydroxylase
TPH: tryptophan hydroxylase
VMAT2: vesicular monoamine transporter
VNTR: variable number of tandem repeats

Introduction

5-Hydroxytryptamine (5HT, serotonin) and DA are neurotransmitters in the CNS and also have prominent peripheral actions. 5HT is found in high concentrations in enterochromaffin cells throughout the GI tract, in storage granules in platelets, and throughout the CNS. The highest concentrations of DA are found in the brain; DA stores are also present peripherally in the adrenal medulla, in the plexuses of the GI, and in the enteric nervous system. Fourteen 5HT receptor subtypes and five DA receptor subtypes have been delineated by structural and pharmacological analyses. The identification of individual receptor subtypes has allowed for the development of subtype-selective drugs and the elucidation of actions of these neurotransmitters at a molecular level. Increasingly, therapeutic goals are being achieved by using drugs that selectively target one or more of the subtypes of 5HT or DA receptors, or that act on a combination of both 5HT and DA receptors.

5-Hydroxytryptamine

In the 1930s, Erspamer began to study the distribution of enterochromaffin cells, which were stained with a reagent for indoles. The highest concentrations of these cells were found in GI mucosa, followed by platelets and the CNS. Soon thereafter, Page and colleagues isolated and chemically characterized a vasoconstrictor substance released from platelets in clotting blood. This substance, named serotonin, was shown to be identical to the indole isolated by Erspamer. Subsequent discovery of the biosynthetic and degradative pathways for 5HT and clinical presentation of patients with carcinoid tumors of intestinal enterochromaffin cells spurred interest in 5HT. In the mid-1950s, the discovery that the pronounced behavioral effects of reserpine are accompanied by a profound decrease in brain 5HT led to the proposal that serotonin may function as a neurotransmitter in the mammalian CNS. Numerous synthetic or naturally occurring congeners of 5HT have pharmacological activity (see Figure 13–1 for chemical structures). Many of the *N*- and *O*-methylated indoleamines, such as *N,N*-dimethyltryptamine, are hallucinogens. Another close relative of 5HT, melatonin (5-methoxy-*N*-acetyltryptamine), is formed by sequential *N*-acetylation and *O*-methylation (Figure 13–1). Melatonin, not to be confused with the pigment melanin, is the principal indoleamine in the pineal gland, where it serves a role in regulating circadian rhythms and shows promise in the treatment of jet lag and other sleep disturbances, such as insomnia. In that regard, melatonin could be thought of as a pigment of the imagination.

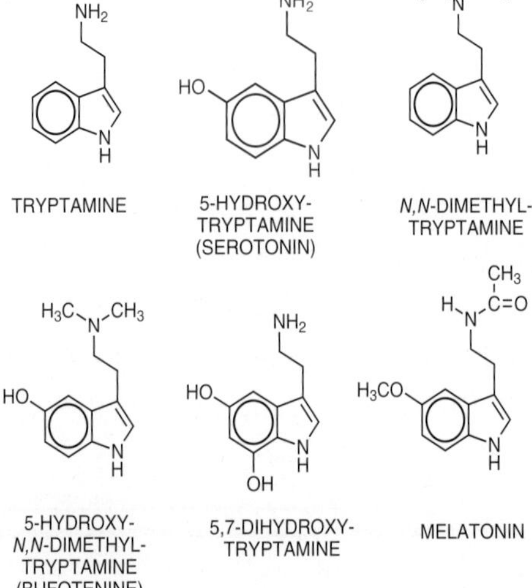

Figure 13–1 *Structures of representative indolealkylamines.*

Synthesis and Metabolism of 5HT

Synthesis of 5HT is by a two-step pathway from the essential amino acid tryptophan (Figure 13–2). Tryptophan is actively transported into the brain by LAT1, a heteromeric carrier protein that also transports other large neutral and branched-chain amino acids and some drugs. Levels of tryptophan in the brain are influenced not only by its plasma concentration but also by the plasma concentrations of other amino acids that compete for the transporter. TPH, a mixed-function oxidase that requires molecular O_2 and a reduced pteridine cofactor for activity, is the rate-limiting enzyme in the synthetic pathway. TPH2, a brain-specific isoform of TPH, is entirely responsible for the synthesis of brain 5HT. Brain TPH is not generally saturated with substrate; consequently, the concentration of tryptophan in the brain influences the synthesis of 5HT.

L-5-hydroxytryptophan is converted to 5HT by AADC; AADC is widely distributed and has broad substrate specificity. The synthesized product, 5HT, is accumulated in secretory granules by VMAT2, which can be selectively inhibited by reserpine, thus depleting vesicular stores of monoamine transmitters. Based on its ability to deplete NE or DA, reserpine was once used an antihypertensive and antipsychotic agent. Stored vesicular 5HT is released by exocytosis from serotonergic neurons in response to an action potential. In the nervous system, the action of released 5HT is terminated via neuronal uptake by a specific SERT, localized in the membrane of serotonergic axon terminals and in the membranes of platelets. This uptake system is the means by which platelets acquire 5HT because they lack the enzymes required for 5HT synthesis. SERT is distinct from VMAT2, which concentrates amines in intracellular storage vesicles and is a nonspecific amine carrier. SERT, the 5HT transporter or reuptake system is specific (see discussion that follows) and can be inhibited by SSRIs that are used to treat depression and other mood disorders.

The principal route of metabolism of 5HT involves oxidative deamination by MAO; the aldehyde intermediate thus formed is converted to 5-HIAA by aldehyde dehydrogenase (see Figure 13–2). An alternative route, reduction of the acetaldehyde to an alcohol, 5-hydroxytryptophol, is normally insignificant. 5-HIAA is actively transported out of the brain by a process that is sensitive to the nonspecific transport inhibitor probenecid. 5-HIAA from brain and peripheral sites of 5HT storage and metabolism is excreted in the urine along with small amounts of 5-hydroxytryptophol sulfate or glucuronide conjugates.

Of the two isoforms of MAO (see Chapter 8), MAO-A preferentially metabolizes 5HT and NE. Selective MAO-A inhibitors increase stores of 5HT and NE and are first-generation antidepressant agents (Chapter 15) MAO-B prefers β-phenylethylamine and benzylamine as substrates; low-dose selegiline is a relatively selective inhibitor of MAO-B. DA and tryptamine are metabolized equally well by both isoforms. Neurons contain both isoforms of MAO, localized primarily in the outer membrane of mitochondria. MAO-B is the principal isoform in platelets, which contain large amounts of 5HT.

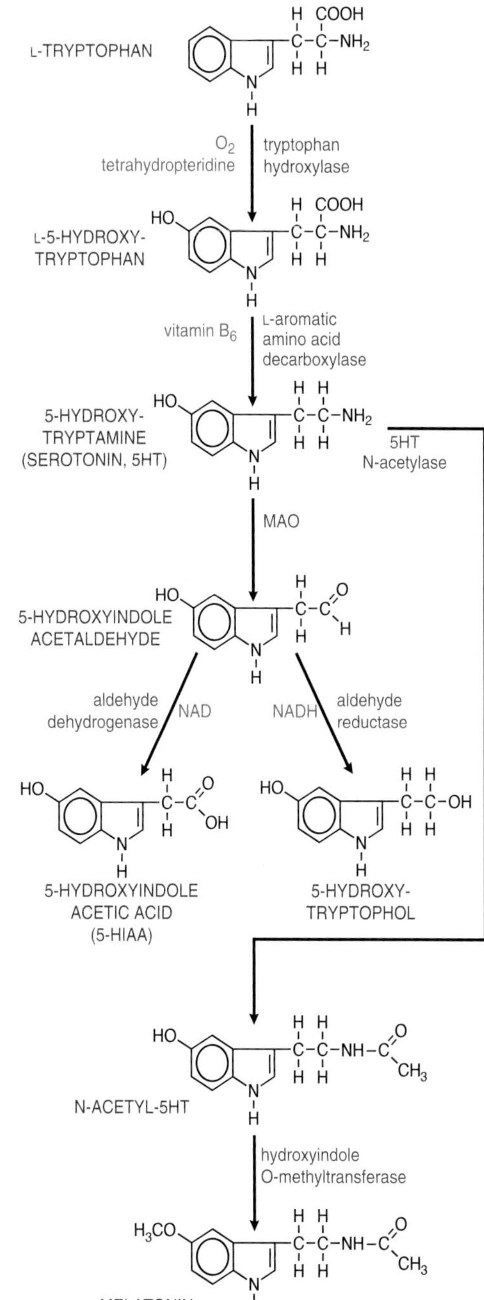

Figure 13–2 *Synthesis and inactivation of serotonin.* Enzymes are identified in red lettering, and cofactors are shown in *blue*.

Serotonergic Projection Pathways in the Brain

In the CNS, 5HT is almost entirely synthesized by cells located in the raphe nuclei in the brainstem. These neurons exhibit extensive projections throughout the brain and spinal cord. These projections are so extensive that it has been hypothesized that every neuron in the brain may be in synaptic contact with a serotonergic projection fiber (Figure 13–3).

A model of a serotonergic synapse is depicted in Figure 13–4. 5HT released from the nerve terminal activates cell-specific postsynaptic receptors, leading to signal transduction. Presynaptic 5HT receptors also exist on the nerve terminal where they can act to modulate 5HT release. Reuptake of 5HT by the 5HT transporter is the primary mechanism for termination of 5HT action and allows for either vesicular repackaging of transmitter or metabolism.

The 5HT Receptors

Multiple 5HT receptor subtypes mediate serotonin's diverse array of physiologic effects and comprise the largest known neurotransmitter-receptor family (Hoyer et al., 1994). The 5HT receptor subtypes are expressed in distinct but often overlapping patterns and are coupled to different transmembrane signaling mechanisms (Table 13–1). All of the 5HT receptor subtypes are GPCRs, with the exception of the $5HT_3$ receptor, which is a ligand-gated ion channel (see Figures 3–11 and 11–1).

The $5HT_1$ Receptor Subfamily

- The $5HT_1$ receptor family comprises five members, all of which preferentially couple to $G_{i/o}$ and inhibit adenylyl cyclase. $5HT_1$ receptors are also known to modulate K^+ and Ca^{2+} channels.
- The $5HT_{1A}$ and $5HT_{1B/1D}$ receptors all act as autoreceptors, either on the cell bodies ($5HT_{1A}$) or on the axon terminals ($5HT_{1B/1D}$)

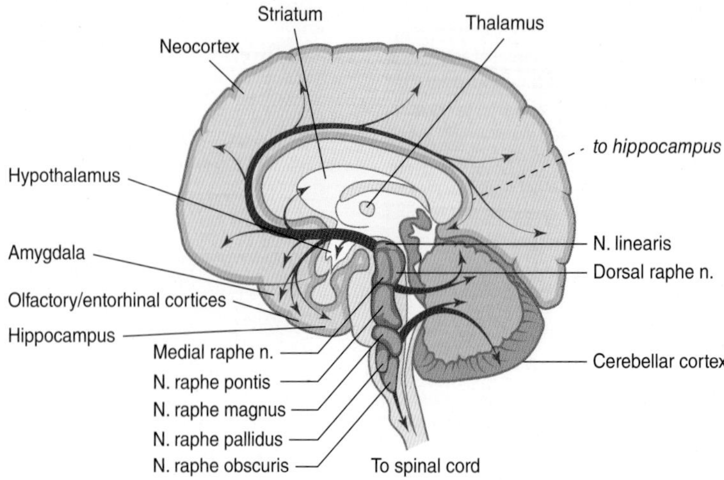

Figure 13–3 *Serotonergic pathways in the brain.* Serotonin is produced by several discrete brainstem nuclei, shown here in rostral and caudal clusters. The rostral nuclei, which include the nucleus, dorsal raphe, medial raphe, and raphe pontis, innervate most of the brain, including the cerebellum. The caudal nuclei, which comprise the raphe magnus, raphe pallidus, and raphe obscuris, have more limited projections that terminate in the cerebellum, brainstem, and spinal cord. Together, the rostral and caudal nuclei innervate most of the CNS. (Modified with permission from Nestler EJ et al., eds. *Molecular Neuropharmacology*. McGraw-Hill, New York, **2015**.)

(Figure 13–5). Antimigraine triptan drugs are $5HT_{1B/1D}$ antagonists (see further discussion).

- In early literature, the $5HT_{2C}$ receptor (see next section) was referred to as the $5HT_{1C}$ receptor. To avoid confusion, the name $5HT_{1C}$ is no longer in use (Hoyer et al., 1994).
- The $5HT_{1D}$ receptors, abundantly expressed in the substantia nigra and basal ganglia, also regulate the firing rate of DA-containing cells and the release of DA at axonal terminals.
- The precise physiological roles of the $5HT_{1E}$ and $5HT_{1F}$ receptors are unclear at present.

The $5HT_2$ Receptor Subfamily

- The three subtypes of $5HT_2$ receptors couple to G_q/G_{11} proteins and activate PLC-DAG/IP_3-Ca^{2+}-PKC pathways (Table 13–1). $5HT_{2A}$ and $5HT_{2C}$ receptors also activate phospholipase A_2, promoting the release of arachidonic acid.
- The $5HT_{2A}$ receptors are broadly distributed in the CNS, primarily in serotonergic terminal areas. High densities are found in several brain structures, including prefrontal, parietal, and somatosensory cortex, as well as in blood platelets and smooth muscle cells. Many antipsychotic drugs inhibit $5HT_{2A}$ receptors.
- The $5HT_{2C}$ receptor is the only GPCR that is regulated by RNA editing. Multiple $5HT_{2C}$ receptor isoforms are generated by RNA editing; extensively edited isoforms have modified G protein–coupling efficiencies (Burns et al., 1997). The $5HT_{2C}$ receptor has been implicated in the control of CSF production and in feeding behavior and mood.

$5HT_3$ Receptors

- The $5HT_3$ receptor is the only monoamine neurotransmitter receptor that functions as a ligand-gated ion channel.
- The functional $5HT_3$ receptor forms pentameric complexes consisting of three distinct subunits; activation of these ligand-gated channels elicits a rapidly desensitizing depolarization, mediated by the gating of cations.
- The $5HT_3$ receptors are located on parasympathetic terminals in the GI tract, including vagal and splanchnic afferents. In the CNS, a high density of $5HT_3$ receptors occurs in the solitary tract nucleus and the area postrema. $5HT_3$ receptors in both the GI tract and the CNS participate in the emetic response, providing a basis for the antiemetic property of the FDA-approved $5HT_3$ receptor antagonists, including ondansetron and dolasetron.

$5HT_4$ Receptors

- The $5HT_4$ receptor subtype couples to G_s to activate AC and increase cAMP production.
- In the CNS, $5HT_4$ receptors are found on neurons of the superior and inferior colliculi and in the hippocampus. In the GI tract, $5HT_4$ receptors are located on neurons of the myenteric plexus and on smooth muscle and secretory cells. Stimulation of the $5HT_4$ receptor is thought to evoke secretion and to facilitate the peristaltic reflex. The latter effect may explain the utility of prokinetic benzamides in GI disorders (see Chapter 50)
- Effects of pharmacological manipulation of $5HT_4$ receptors on memory and feeding in animal models suggest possible clinical applications in the future.

$5HT_5$ Receptors

- The $5HT_5$ subfamily couples to $G_{i/o}$ to inhibit AC.
- Humans only express a functional $5HT_{5A}$ receptor, while rodents express both $5HT_{5A}$ and $5HT_{5B}$ receptors. The human $5HT_{5B}$ gene is interrupted by a stop codon leading to a nonfunctional protein product.
- The $5HT_{5A}$ receptor is expressed widely in the CNS, and its function is linked to circadian rhythms and cognition.

$5HT_6$ Receptors

- The $5HT_6$ receptors couple to G_s to activate AC and increase intracellular cAMP.
- The $5HT_6$ receptor is almost exclusively found in the CNS; its abundance in cortical, limbic, and extrapyramidal regions suggests that it is important for motor control and cognition.
- Recent studies have focused on $5HT_6$ receptor agonists as a therapeutic modality for cognitive decline in patients with Alzheimer disease.

$5HT_7$ Receptors

- The $5HT_7$ receptor couples to G_s to activate AC and increase intracellular cAMP. It is widely distributed throughout the CNS.
- Blockade of the $5HT_7$ receptor has recently been investigated as a putative therapeutic mechanism to treat depression. $5HT_7$ receptors may also play a role in the relaxation of smooth muscle in the GI tract and the vasculature.

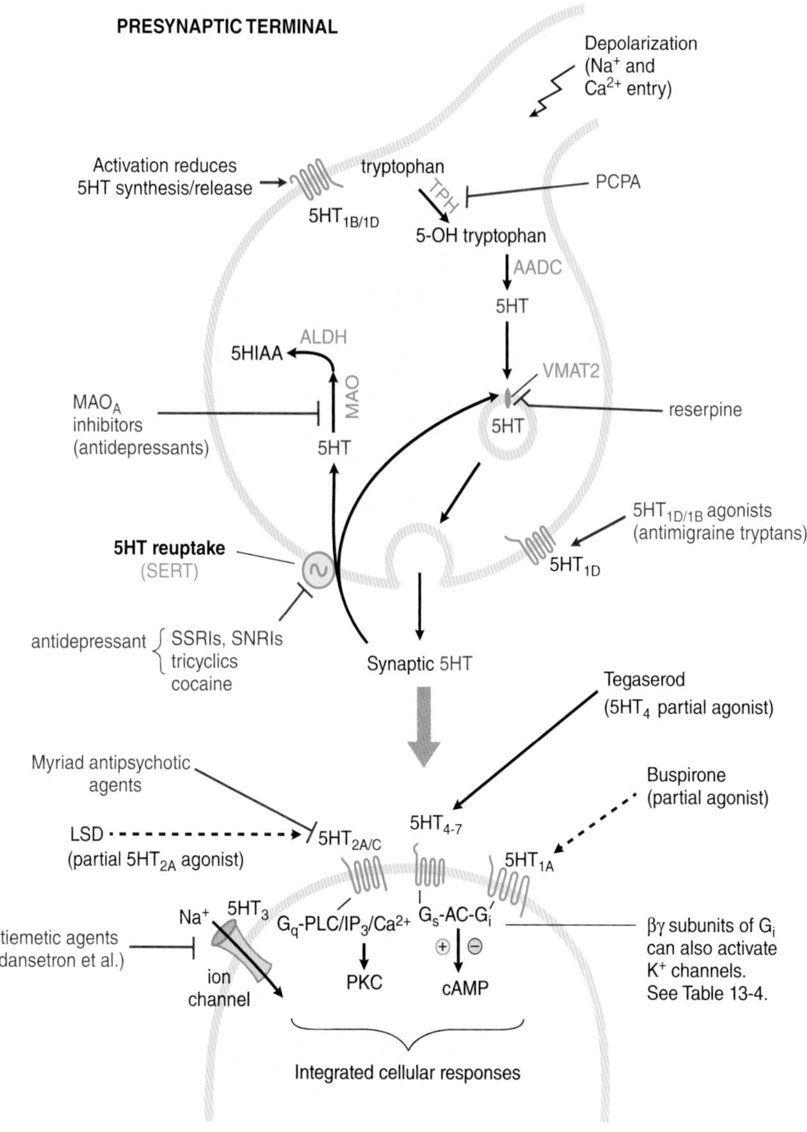

Figure 13–4 *A serotonergic synapse.* Presynaptic and postsynaptic molecular entities involved in the synthesis, release, signaling, and reuptake of serotonin are shown. MAO is shown extracellularly and in mitochondria within serotonergic nerve terminals.

The 5HT Transporter

- The actions of 5HT are primarily terminated by SERT, the transport protein responsible for the reuptake of 5HT into serotonergic neurons.
- Encoded by a single gene, SERT possesses 12 membrane-spanning domains and is a member of the NSS family that includes the carriers for DA, NE, GABA, and glycine. SERT is expressed prominently in central serotonin neurons that originate in the raphe nucleus, but is also found in platelets, placenta, lung, gut, enteric nervous system, and adrenal gland.
- SERT couples the transport of serotonin to the movement of Na^+ into the cell.
- SSRIs such as fluoxetine, paroxetine, citalopram, and sertraline bind to the SERT and inhibit serotonin transport. TCAs and a newer class of SNRIs that includes venlafaxine and duloxetine, block SERT, the NE transporter, or both with varying degrees of selectivity.
- SSRIs and SNRIs are prescribed for major depressive disorder, obsessive-compulsive disorder, panic disorder, generalized anxiety disorder, fibromyalgia and neuropathic pain.

Actions of 5HT in Physiological Systems

Platelets

Platelets differ from other formed elements of blood in expressing mechanisms for uptake, storage, and exocytotic release of 5HT. 5HT is not synthesized in platelets but is taken up from the circulation and stored in secretory granules by active transport, similar to the uptake and storage of serotonin by serotonergic nerve terminals. When platelets make contact with injured endothelium (see Chapter 32), they release substances that promote platelet aggregation; secondarily, they release 5HT (see Figure 13–6). 5HT binds to platelet $5HT_{2A}$ receptors and elicits a weak aggregation response that is markedly augmented by the presence

TABLE 13–1 ■ SEROTONIN RECEPTOR SUBTYPES[a]

SUBTYPE	SIGNALING EFFECTOR	LOCALIZATION	FUNCTION	AGONISTS	ANTAGONISTS
$5HT_{1A}$	↓ AC	Raphe nuclei, cortex, hippocampus	Somatodendritic autoreceptor	8-OH-DPAT, buspirone	WAY 100135
$5HT_{1B}$	↓ AC	Subiculum, globus pallidus, substantia nigra	Presynaptic autoreceptor	Sumatriptan, CP94253	GR-55562
$5HT_{1D}$	↓ AC	Cranial vessels, globus pallidus, substantia nigra	Presynaptic autoreceptor, vasoconstriction	Sumatriptan	SB 714786
$5HT_{1E}$	↓ AC	Cortex, striatum	—	—	—
$5HT_{1F}$	↓ AC	Dorsal raphe, hippocampus, periphery	—	LY334370	—
$5HT_{2A}$	↑ PLC, PLA_2	Platelets, smooth muscle, cerebral cortex	Aggregation, contraction, neuronal excitation	α-CH_3-5HT, DOI, MCPP	Ketanserin, LY53857
$5HT_{2B}$	↑ PLC	Stomach fundus	Smooth muscle contraction	α-CH_3-5HT, DOI	LY53857
$5HT_{2C}$	↑ PLC, PLA_2	Choroid plexus, substantia nigra, basal ganglia	CSF production, neuronal excitation	α-CH_3-5HT, DOI	LY53857, mesulergine
$5HT_3$	Cations	Parasympathetic nerves, solitary tract, area postrema, GI tract	Neuronal excitation	2-CH_3-5HT, quipazine	Ondansetron, tropisetron
$5HT_4$	↑ AC	Hippocampus, striatum, GI tract	Neuronal excitation	Renzapride	GR 113808
$5HT_{5A}$	↓ AC	Cortex, hippocampus	Unknown	—	SB-699551
$5HT_{5B}$	Unknown	—	Pseudogene in humans	—	—
$5HT_6$	↑ AC	Hippocampus, striatum, nucleus accumbens	Neuronal excitation	WAY-181187	SB-271046
$5HT_7$	↑ AC	Hypothalamus, hippocampus, GI tract	Smooth muscle relaxation	5-CT, LP-12	SB-269970

[a]For further information on the pharmacological properties of the 5HT subtypes, see IUPHAR/BPS Guide to Pharmacology: http://www.guidetopharmacology.org/index.jsp.
Abbreviations: 5-CT, 5-carboxamino-tryptamine; DOI, 1-(2,5-dimethoxy-4-iodophenyl) isopropylamine; 8-OH-DPAT, 8-hydroxy-(2-*N*,*N*-dipropylamino)-tetraline; MCPP, metachlorphenylpiperazine; others are manufacturers' designations.

of collagen. If the damaged blood vessel is injured to a depth where vascular smooth muscle is exposed, 5HT exerts a direct vasoconstrictor effect, thereby contributing to hemostasis, which is enhanced by locally released autocoids (thromboxane A_2 [TxA_2], kinins, and vasoactive peptides). Conversely, 5HT may interact with endothelial cells to stimulate production of NO and antagonize its own vasoconstrictor action, as well as the vasoconstriction produced by other locally released agents.

Cardiovascular System

The classical response of blood vessels to 5HT is contraction, particularly in the splanchnic, renal, pulmonary, and cerebral vasculatures. 5HT also induces a variety of responses in the heart that are the result of activation of multiple 5HT receptor subtypes, stimulation or inhibition of autonomic nerve activity, or dominance of reflex responses to 5HT. Thus, 5HT has positive inotropic and chronotropic actions on the heart that may be blunted by simultaneous stimulation of afferent nerves from baroreceptors and chemoreceptors. Activation of $5HT_3$ receptors on vagus nerve endings elicits the Bezold-Jarisch reflex, causing extreme bradycardia and hypotension. The local response of arterial blood vessels to 5HT also may be inhibitory, the result of the stimulation of endothelial NO production and prostaglandin synthesis and blockade of NE release from sympathetic nerves. Conversely, 5HT amplifies the local constrictor actions of NE, angII, and histamine, which reinforce the hemostatic response to 5HT.

Gastrointestinal Tract

Enterochromaffin cells in the gastric mucosa are the site of the synthesis and most of the storage of 5HT in the body and are the source of circulating 5HT. Motility of gastric and intestinal smooth muscle may be either enhanced or inhibited via signaling mediated by at least five subtypes of 5HT receptors (Table 13–2).

Mechanical stretching augments basal release of enteric 5HT, such as that caused by food and by efferent vagal stimulation. Released 5HT enters the portal vein and is metabolized by hepatic MAO-A. 5HT that survives hepatic oxidation may be captured by platelets or rapidly removed by the endothelium of lung capillaries and inactivated. 5HT released from enterochromaffin cells also acts locally to regulate GI function. $5HT_3$ receptors in the GI tract and the CNS participate in the emetic response, providing a basis for the antiemetic property of $5HT_3$ receptor antagonists (see Figure 50–5 and Table 50–6). A large series of selective $5HT_3$ receptor antagonists, the "setrons," including ondansetron, dolasetron, granisetron, and palonosetron, are used in the treatment of various GI disturbances. All $5HT_3$ receptor antagonists are highly efficacious in the treatment of nausea, and alosetron and cilansetron are licensed for treating irritable bowel syndrome.

Inflammation

Acting via the $5HT_{2A}$ receptor, 5HT exerts a pro-inflammatory influence in acute inflammatory states, including models of airway inflammation and asthma (Nau et al., 2015). These preclinical findings agree with reports of higher expression of $5HT_{2A}$ receptors in peripheral blood mononuclear cells in patients with a history of asthma as compared to healthy volunteers (Ahangari et al., 2015). This research builds on several decades of analysis linking levels of plasma 5HT to incidents of asthma in human patients (Lechin et al., 2002). While this correlation between the $5HT_{2A}$ receptor and human inflammatory disease is still preliminary, the findings are compelling and merit additional investigation into the untapped role of 5HT and the $5HT_{2A}$ receptor in airway inflammation.

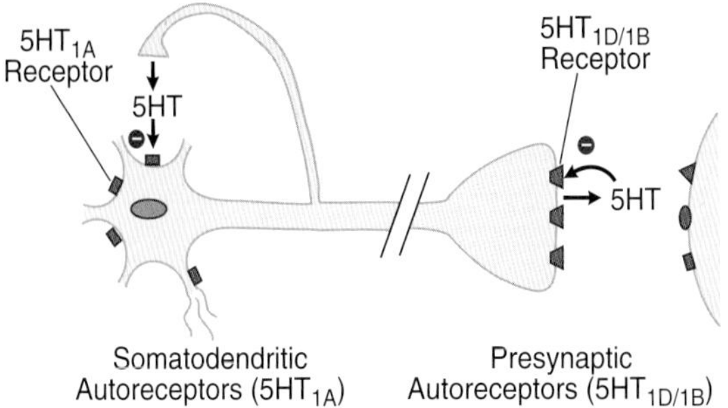

Figure 13–5 *Two classes of 5HT autoreceptors with differential localizations.* Somatodendritic $5HT_{1A}$ autoreceptors decrease raphe cell firing when activated by 5HT released from axon collaterals of the same or adjacent neurons. The receptor subtype of the presynaptic autoreceptor on axon terminals in the forebrain has different pharmacological properties and has been classified as $5HT_{1D}$ (in humans) or $5HT_{1B}$ (in rodents). This receptor modulates the release of 5HT. Postsynaptic $5HT_1$ receptors are also indicated.

CNS

All 5HT receptor subtypes are expressed in the brain, where 5HT influences a multitude of functions, including sleep, cognition, sensory perception, motor activity, temperature regulation, nociception, mood, appetite, sexual behavior, and hormone secretion. The principal cell bodies of 5HT neurons are located in raphe nuclei of the brainstem and project throughout the brain and spinal cord (Figure 13–3). In addition to release at discrete synapses, serotonin release seems to occur at sites of axonal varicosities that do not form distinct synaptic contacts. 5HT released at nonsynaptic varicosities is thought to diffuse to outlying targets, rather than acting on discrete synaptic targets, perhaps acting as a neuromodulator as well as a neurotransmitter (see Chapter 14).

Sleep-Wake Cycle

Control of the sleep-wake cycle is one of the first behaviors in which a role for 5HT was identified. Depletion of 5HT with *p*-chlorophenylalanine, a tryptophan hydroxylase inhibitor, elicits insomnia that is reversed by the 5HT precursor, 5-hydroxytryptophan. Conversely, treatment with L-tryptophan or with nonselective 5HT agonists accelerates sleep onset and prolongs total sleep time. 5HT antagonists reportedly can increase and decrease slow-wave sleep, probably reflecting interacting or opposing roles for subtypes of 5HT receptors. One relatively consistent finding in humans and in laboratory animals is an increase in slow-wave sleep following administration of a selective $5HT_{2A/2C}$ receptor antagonist such as ritanserin.

Aggression and Impulsivity

Serotonin serves a critical role in aggression and impulsivity. Human studies reveal a correlation between low CSF 5-HIAA and violent impulsivity and aggression. Gene knockout mice lacking the $5HT_{1B}$ receptor exhibit extreme aggression, suggesting either a role for $5HT_{1B}$ receptors in the development of neuronal pathways important in aggression or a direct role in the mediation of aggressive behavior. A human genetic study identified a point mutation in the gene encoding MAO-A that was associated with extreme aggressiveness and mental retardation (Brunner et al., 1993); this has been confirmed in knockout mice lacking MAO-A (Cases et al., 1995).

Appetite and Obesity

Lorcaserin is a $5HT_{2C}$ receptor agonist approved for weight loss. The drug is thought to decrease food consumption and promote satiety by selectively activating $5HT_{2C}$ receptors on anorexigenic proopiomelanocortin neurons in the arcuate nucleus of the hypothalamus. Halogenated amphetamines, which are known to promote the release of 5HT and block its reuptake, are valuable experimental tools; two of them, fenfluramine and dexfenfluramine, were used clinically to reduce appetite; the once-popular diet drug regimen, "fen-phen," combined fenfluramine and phentermine. Fenfluramine and dexfenfluramine were withdrawn from the U.S. market in the late 1990s after reports of life-threatening heart valve disease and pulmonary hypertension associated with their use. This toxicity was the result of $5HT_{2B}$ receptor activation (Hutcheson et al., 2011).

Drugs Affecting 5HT Signaling

Direct-acting 5HT receptor agonists have widely different chemical structures and diverse pharmacological properties and are used in the pharmacotherapy of a number of disorders (Table 13–3), including anxiety,

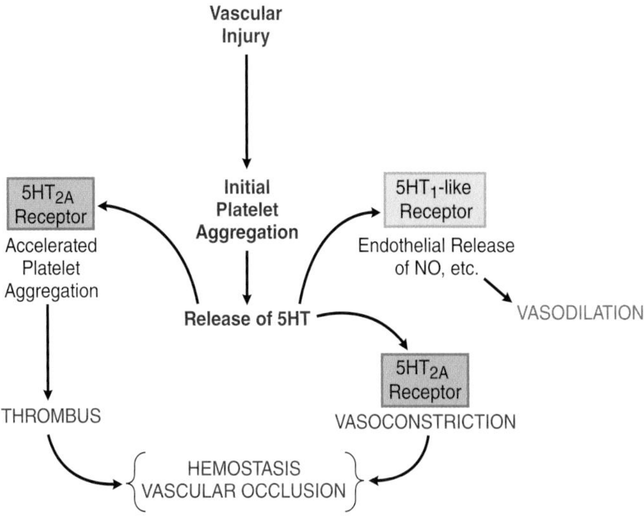

Figure 13–6 *The local influences of platelet 5HT.* The release of 5HT stored in platelets is triggered by aggregation. The local actions of 5HT include feedback actions on platelets (shape change and accelerated aggregation) mediated by interaction with platelet $5HT_{2A}$ receptors, stimulation of NO production mediated by $5HT_1$-like receptors on vascular endothelium, and contraction of vascular smooth muscle mediated by $5HT_{2A}$ receptors. These influences act in concert with many other mediators to promote thrombus formation and hemostasis. See Chapter 32 for details of adhesion and aggregation of platelets and factors contributing to thrombus formation and blood clotting.

TABLE 13–2 ■ ACTIONS OF 5HT IN THE GASTROINTESTINAL TRACT

SITE	RESPONSE	RECEPTOR
Enterochromaffin cells	Release of 5HT	$5HT_3$
	Inhibition of 5HT release	$5HT_4$
Enteric ganglion cells (presynaptic)	Release of ACh	$5HT_4$
	Inhibition of ACh release	$5HT_{1P}$[a] $5HT_{1A}$
Enteric ganglion cells (postsynaptic)	Fast depolarization	$5HT_3$
	Slow depolarization	$5HT_{1P}$[a]
Smooth muscle, intestinal	Contraction	$5HT_{2A}$
Smooth muscle, stomach fundus	Contraction	$5HT_{2B}$
Smooth muscle, esophagus	Contraction	$5HT_4$

[a]$5HT_{1P}$ is an operationally defined serotoninergic response in the gut that does not correspond to any known monoamine receptor subtype. 5HT and certain 5HT derivatives are potent and selective agonists. The $5HT_{1P}$ response may be due to receptor heteromerization resulting in a novel pharmacology.

depression, nausea, disorders of GI motility, and migraine. 5HT is a key mediator in the pathogenesis of migraine. Consistent with the 5HT hypothesis of migraine, 5HT receptor agonists are a mainstay for acute treatment of migraine headaches. The efficacy of antimigraine drugs varies with the absence or presence of aura, duration of the headache, its severity and intensity, and as yet undefined environmental and genetic factors.

$5HT_{1B/1D}$ Receptor Agonists: The Triptans

The triptans are indole derivatives that are effective, acute antimigraine agents. Their capacity to decrease the nausea and vomiting of migraine is an important advance in the treatment of the condition. Available compounds include almotriptan, eletriptan, frovatriptan, naratriptan, rizatriptan, sumatriptan, and zolmitriptan. Sumatriptan for migraine headaches is also marketed in a fixed-dose combination with naproxen. The triptans are effective in the acute treatment of migraine (with or without aura) but are not intended for use in prophylaxis of migraine. Treatment with triptans should begin as soon as possible after onset of a migraine attack. Oral dosage forms of the triptans are the most convenient to use, but they may not be practical in patients experiencing migraine-associated nausea and vomiting.

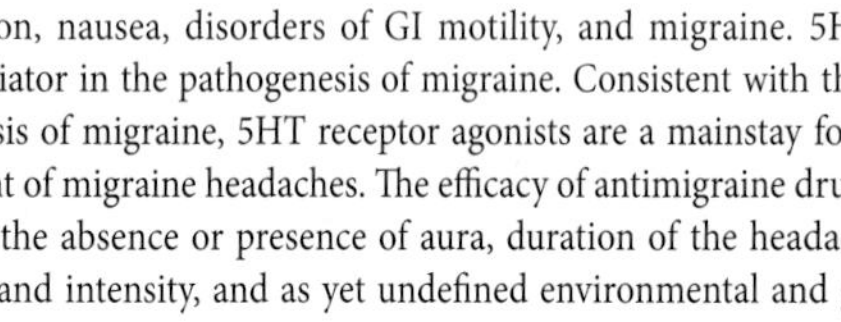

$H_3CNHSO_2CH_2$ — $CH_2CH_2N(CH_3)_2$

Sumatriptan

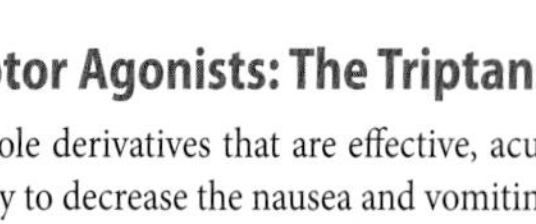

HO — CH_2CH_2NH

Serotonin

Migraine

Migraine headache afflicts 10%–20% of the population. Although migraine is a specific neurological syndrome, the manifestations vary widely. The principal types are migraine without aura (common migraine); migraine with aura (classic migraine, which includes subclasses of migraine with typical aura, migraine with prolonged aura, migraine aura without headache, and migraine with acute-onset aura), and several rarer types. Premonitory aura may begin as long as 24 h before the onset of pain and often is accompanied by photophobia, hyperacusis, polyuria, and diarrhea and by disturbances of mood and appetite. A migraine attack may last for hours or days and be followed by prolonged pain-free intervals. The frequency of migraine attacks is extremely variable. Therapy of migraine headaches is complicated by the variable responses among and within individual patients and by the lack of a firm understanding of the pathophysiology of the syndrome. The efficacy of antimigraine drugs varies with the absence or presence of aura, duration of the headache, its severity and intensity, and possibly undefined environmental and genetic factors.

The pathogenesis of migraine headache is complex, involving both neural and vascular elements. Evidence suggesting that 5HT is a key mediator in the pathogenesis of migraine includes the following:

- Plasma and platelet concentrations of 5HT vary with the different phases of the migraine attack.
- Urinary concentrations of 5HT and its metabolites are elevated during most migraine attacks.
- Migraine may be precipitated by agents (e.g., reserpine and fenfluramine) that release 5HT from intracellular storage sites.

Consistent with the 5HT hypothesis, 5HT receptor agonists have become a mainstay for *acute* treatment of migraine headaches. Treatments for the *prevention* of migraines, such as β adrenergic antagonists and newer antiepileptic drugs, have mechanisms of action that are, presumably, unrelated to 5HT (Mehrotra et al., 2008).

Mechanism of Action

The pharmacological effects of the triptans appear to be limited to the $5HT_1$ family of receptors, providing evidence that this receptor subclass plays an important role in the acute relief of a migraine attack. The triptans interact potently with $5HT_{1B}$ and $5HT_{1D}$ receptors and have a low or no affinity for other subtypes of 5HT receptors or for α_1 and α_2 adrenergic, β adrenergic, dopaminergic, muscarinic cholinergic, and benzodiazepine receptors. Clinically effective doses of the triptans correlate well with their affinities for both $5HT_{1B}$ and $5HT_{1D}$ receptors, supporting the hypothesis that $5HT_{1B}$ and $5HT_{1D}$ receptors are the most likely receptors involved in the mechanism of action of acute antimigraine drugs.

The mechanism of the efficacy of $5HT_{1B/1D}$ agonists in migraine is not resolved. One hypothesis of migraine suggests that unknown events lead to the abnormal dilation of carotid arteriovenous anastomoses in the head and shunting of carotid arterial blood flow, producing cerebral ischemia and hypoxia perceived as migraine pain; activation of $5HT_{1B/1D}$ receptors may cause constriction of intracranial blood vessels, including arteriovenous anastomoses, closing the shunts and restoring blood flow to the brain. An alternative hypothesis proposes that both $5HT_{1B}$ and $5HT_{1D}$ receptors serve as presynaptic autoreceptors that block the release of neurotransmitter or pro-inflammatory neuropeptides at nerve terminals in the perivascular space, which could account for the efficacy of agonists at those receptors in the acute treatment of migraine.

ADME

When given subcutaneously, sumatriptan reaches its peak plasma concentration in about 12 min, and an autoinjector with 6 mg of sumatriptan is available. Following oral administration of a tablet, sumatriptan has a bioavailability of about 15% and reaches a peak plasma concentration within 1–2 h; oral disintegrating tablets take advantage of sublingual absorption and produce more rapid effects; a nasal spray formulation of sumatriptan has an onset of action of about 15 min. A sumatriptan-naproxen combination tablet is available. An iontophoretic transdermal sumatriptan patch was recently withdrawn from the market. The other, newer triptans (see Drug Facts table) have higher oral bioavailabilities, and reach C_{Pmax} values within 1–3 h after ingestion of a tablet. The agents differ in their affinities for the $5HT_{1B}$ and $5HT_{1D}$ receptors, their half-lives and metabolic routes

TABLE 13–3 ■ SEROTONERGIC DRUGS: PRIMARY ACTIONS AND CLINICAL INDICATIONS

RECEPTOR	ACTION	DRUG EXAMPLES	CLINICAL DISORDER
$5HT_{1A}$	Partial agonist	Buspirone, ipsaperone	Anxiety, depression
$5HT_{1D}$	Agonist	Sumatriptan	Migraine
$5HT_{2A/2C}$	Antagonist	Methysergide, risperidone, ketanserin	Migraine, depression, schizophrenia
$5HT_3$	Antagonist	Ondansetron	Chemotherapy-induced emesis
$5HT_4$	Agonist	Cisapride	GI disorders
SERT (5HT transporter)	Inhibitor	Fluoxetine, sertraline	Depression, obsessive-compulsive disorder, panic disorder, social phobia, posttraumatic stress disorder

(usually CYP3A4 or MAO-A), and their reliance on the kidney for excretion. These differences, detailed in the Drug Facts table at the end of this chapter, define the likely drug interactions and precautions with age and reduced hepatic and renal function.

Clinical Use

The triptans are effective in the acute treatment of migraine (with or without aura) but are not intended for prophylaxis of migraine. Treatment with triptans should begin as soon as possible after onset of a migraine attack. Oral dosage forms of the triptans are the most convenient to use but may not be practical in patients experiencing migraine-associated nausea and vomiting, for whom injectable and nasal spray formulations are useful. Approximately 70% of individuals report significant headache relief from a 6-mg subcutaneous dose of sumatriptan, a dose that may be repeated once within a 24-h period if the first dose does not relieve the headache. The recommended oral dose of sumatriptan is 25–100 mg, repeatable after 2 h up to a total dose of 200 mg over a 24-h period. When administered by nasal spray, from 5 to 20 mg of sumatriptan is recommended, repeatable after 2 h up to a maximum dose of 40 mg over a 24-h period. The other triptans have distinct dosing requirements as summarized on their FDA-approved package inserts. A recent meta-analysis concluded that eletriptan is the most likely triptan to produce a favorable outcome at the 2-h and 24-h times after administration (Thorlund et al., 2014). The safety of treating more than three or four headaches over a 30-day period with triptans has not been established. No triptan should be used concurrently with (or within 24 h of) an ergot derivative (described in the next section) or another triptan.

Adverse Effects and Contraindications

In general, only minor side effects are seen with the triptans in the acute treatment of migraine. After subcutaneous injection of sumatriptan, patients often experience irritation at the site of injection (transient mild pain, stinging, or burning sensations). The most common side effect of sumatriptan nasal spray is a bitter taste. Triptans can cause paresthesias; asthenia and fatigue; flushing; feelings of pressure, tightness, or pain in the chest, neck, and jaw; drowsiness; dizziness; nausea; and sweating. In the extreme, these agents can cause serotonin syndrome, a consequence of a generalized excess of 5HT at 5HT receptors, especially when used in combination with SSRIs, SNRIs, TCAs, and MAO inhibitors.

Rare but serious cardiac events have been associated with the administration of $5HT_1$ agonists, including coronary artery vasospasm, transient myocardial ischemia, atrial and ventricular arrhythmias, and myocardial infarction, predominantly in patients with risk factors for coronary artery disease. The triptans are contraindicated in patients with a history of ischemic or vasospastic coronary artery disease (including history of stroke or transient ischemic attacks), cerebrovascular or peripheral vascular disease, hemiplegic or basilar migraines, other significant cardiovascular diseases, or ischemic bowel diseases. Because triptans may cause an acute, usually small, increase in blood pressure, they also are contraindicated in patients with uncontrolled hypertension. Naratriptan is contraindicated in patients with severe renal or hepatic impairment; rizatriptan should be used with caution in such patients. Eletriptan is contraindicated in hepatic disease. Almotriptan, rizatriptan, sumatriptan, and zolmitriptan are contraindicated in patients who have taken a MAO inhibitor within the preceding 2 weeks, and all triptans are contraindicated in patients with near-term prior exposure to ergot alkaloids, other triptans or 5HT agonists, SSRIs, and SNRIs. The triptans are classified as *pregnancy category C* (i.e., there are no adequate and well-controlled studies in pregnant women; use during pregnancy only if the potential benefit justifies a potential risk to the fetus) and should also be used with caution in nursing mothers; evidence of safety in pregnancy is best with sumatriptan. Källén and Reis (2016) have reviewed drugs for managing pain, including migraine, during pregnancy.

The Ergot Alkaloids

Ergot is the product of a fungus (*Claviceps purpurea*) that grows on rye and other grains. The elucidation of the constituents of ergot and their complex actions was an important chapter in the evolution of modern pharmacology, even though the very complexity of their actions limits their therapeutic uses. The pharmacological effects of the ergot alkaloids are varied and complex; in general, the effects result from their actions as partial agonists or antagonists at serotonergic, dopaminergic, and adrenergic receptors. All ergot alkaloids can all be considered to be derivatives of the tetracyclic compound 6-methylergoline (Table 13–4).

The natural alkaloids of therapeutic interest are amide derivatives of *d*-lysergic acid. Numerous semisynthetic derivatives of the ergot alkaloids have been prepared by catalytic hydrogenation of the natural alkaloids (e.g., dihydroergotamine). The synthetic derivative, bromocriptine (2-bromo-α-ergocryptine), is used to control the secretion of prolactin, a property derived from its DA agonist effect. Other products of this series include LSD, a potent hallucinogen, and methysergide, a serotonin antagonist. LSD interacts with most brain 5HT receptors as an agonist/partial agonist and elicits sensory distortions (especially visual) and hallucinations at doses as low as 1 μg/kg. Current hypotheses of the mechanism of action of LSD and other hallucinogens focus on $5HT_{2A}$ receptor-mediated disruption of thalamic gating with sensory overload of the cortex (Nichols, 2016). Of note, positron emission tomography imaging studies revealed that administration of the hallucinogen psilocybin (the active component of "shrooms") mimics the pattern of brain activation found in schizophrenic patients experiencing hallucinations. This action of psilocybin is blocked by pretreatment with a $5HT_{2A/2C}$ antagonist. These and other studies have suggested that stimulation of the $5HT_{2A}$ receptor can lead to hallucinations (Nichols, 2016).

Ergots in the Treatment of Migraine

The multiple pharmacological effects of ergot alkaloids have complicated the determination of their precise mechanism of action in the acute treatment of migraine. The actions of ergot alkaloids at $5HT_{1B/1D}$ receptors

TABLE 13–4 ■ NATURAL AND SEMISYNTHETIC ERGOT ALKALOIDS

A. AMINE ALKALOIDS AND CONGENERS			B. AMINO ACID ALKALOIDS		
ALKALOID	**X**	**Y**	**ALKALOID**[b]	**R(2′)**	**R′(5′)**
d-Lysergic acid	$-COOH$	$-H$	Ergotamine	$-CH_3$	$-CH_2-$phenyl
d-Isolysergic acid	$-H$	$-COOH$	Ergosine	$-CH_3$	$-CH_2CH(CH_3)_2$
d-Lysergic acid diethylamide (LSD)	$-C(=O)-N(CH_2CH_3)_2$	$-H$	Ergostine	$-CH_2CH_3$	$-CH_2-$phenyl
Ergonovine (ergometrine)	$-C(=O)-NH-CH(CH_3)CH_2OH$	$-H$	Ergotoxine group:		
			Ergocornine	$-CH(CH_3)_2$	$-CH(CH_3)_2$
			Ergocristine	$-CH(CH_3)_2$	$-CH_2-$phenyl
Methylergonovine	$-C(=O)-NH-CH(CH_2CH_3)(CH_2OH)$	$-H$	α-Ergocryptine	$-CH(CH_3)_2$	$-CH_2CH(CH_3)_2$
			β-Ergocryptine	$-CH(CH_3)_2$	$-CH(CH_3)CH_2CH_3$
Methysergide[a]	$-C(=O)-NH-CH(CH_2CH_3)(CH_2OH)$	$-H$	Bromocriptine[c]	$-CH(CH_3)_2$	$-CH_2CH(CH_3)_2$

[a]Contains methyl substitution at N1. [b]Dihydro derivatives contain hydrogen atoms at C9 and C10. [c]Contains bromine atom at C2.

likely mediate their *acute* antimigraine effects. The use of ergot alkaloids for migraine should be restricted to patients having frequent, moderate migraine or infrequent, severe migraine attacks. Ergot preparations should be administered as soon as possible after the onset of a headache. GI absorption of ergot alkaloids is erratic, perhaps contributing to the large variation in patient response to these drugs. Methysergide (1-methyl-*d*-lysergic acid butanolamide) is an ergot derivative but has very weak vasoconstrictor and oxytocic activity. It interacts with $5HT_1$ receptors, but its therapeutic effects appear primarily to reflect blockade of $5HT_{2A}$ and $5HT_{2C}$ receptors. Methysergide is used for the prophylactic treatment of migraine and other vascular headaches. A potentially serious complication of prolonged treatment is inflammatory fibrosis, giving rise to various syndromes that include pleuropulmonary fibrosis and coronary and endocardial fibrosis. Usually, the fibrosis regresses after drug withdrawal, although persistent cardiac valvular damage has been reported.

Use of Ergot Alkaloids in Postpartum Hemorrhage

All of the natural ergot alkaloids markedly increase the motor activity of the uterus; however, ergonovine and its semisynthetic derivative methylergonovine have primarily been used as uterine-stimulating agents in obstetrics. As the dose is increased, contractions become more forceful and prolonged, resting tone is dramatically increased, and sustained contracture can result. This characteristic is compatible with their use postpartum or after abortion to control bleeding and maintain uterine contraction. Oxytocin (see Chapter 44) is now the more prevalent agent in controlling postpartum hemorrhage.

Serotonin Receptor Partial Agonists, SSRIs, and MSAAs

Anxiolytic and Antidepressant Agents

Buspirone, gepirone, and ipsapirone are selective partial agonists at $5HT_{1A}$ receptors. Buspirone has been effective in the treatment of anxiety (see Chapter 15). Buspirone mimics the antianxiety properties of benzodiazepines but does not interact with $GABA_A$ receptors or display the sedative and anticonvulsant properties of benzodiazepines. The effects of 5HT–active drugs in anxiety and depressive disorders, like the effects of SSRIs, strongly suggest a role for 5HT in the neurochemical mediation of these disorders. Inhibition of neuronal reuptake of 5HT via the 5HT transporter prolongs the dwell time of 5HT in the synapse. SSRIs, such as fluoxetine, potentiate and prolong the action of 5HT released by neuronal activity. When coadministered with L-5-hydroxytryptophan, SSRIs elicit profound activation of serotonergic responses. However, the capacity to enhance serotonergic neurotransmission alone does not explain the antidepressant effectiveness: Uptake inhibition occurs immediately, whereas weeks of treatment are required to achieve clinical efficacy. This has led to the proposal that long-term homeostatic adaptations in brain function underlie the therapeutic effects of this class of antidepressants. SSRIs (citalopram, escitalopram, fluoxetine, fluvoxamine, paroxetine, and sertraline) are the most widely used treatment of major depressive disorder (see Chapter 15). Vilazadone is an SSRI and a partial agonist at the $5HT_{1A}$ receptor; it is FDA approved in adults for treatment of depression.

5HT and Sexual Dysfunction

One of the most common side effects of SSRIs and SNRIs is sexual dysfunction, such as anorgasmia, erectile dysfunction, diminished libido, and sexual anhedonia. Poor sexual function is one of the most common reasons that patients discontinue taking these medications. The mechanism by which SSRIs/SNRIs cause sexual side effects is not well understood. In contrast, the serotonergic drug flibanserin has recently been approved to treat hypoactive sexual desire disorder (HSDD) in premenopausal women. This disorder is also referred to as female sexual interest/arousal disorder (FSIAD). Flibanserin can increase the number of satisfying sexual events in some, but not all, women with this disorder. Flibanserin is a potent agonist of the $5HT_{1A}$ receptor and a moderately potent antagonist of the $5HT_2$ receptor subfamily; the drug is classified as a MSAA. Flibanserin is also a weak blocker of the D_4 DA receptor. Administration of flibanserin can decrease 5HT levels in the cortex while increasing DA and NE levels. This redistribution of monoamine levels has been speculated to be the mechanism of the observed response of increased sexual function.

Clinical Manipulation of 5HT Levels: Serotonin Syndrome

Excessive elevation of 5HT levels in the body can cause *serotonin syndrome*, a constellation of symptoms sometimes observed in patients starting new or increased antidepressant therapy or combining an SSRI with an NE reuptake inhibitor or a triptan (for migraine). Symptoms may include restlessness, confusion, shivering, tachycardia, diarrhea, muscle twitches/rigidity, fever, seizures, loss of consciousness, and even death. Serotonin syndrome and its treatment are discussed in Chapter 15.

Dopamine

Dopamine consists of a catechol moiety linked to an ethyl amine, leading to its classification as a catecholamine (Figure 13–7). DA is a polar molecule that does not readily cross the BBB. It is closely related to melanin, a pigment that is formed by oxidation of DA, tyrosine, or L-dopa. Melanin exists in the skin and cuticle and gives the substantia nigra brain region its namesake dark color. Both DA and L-dopa are readily oxidized by nonenzymatic pathways to form cytotoxic reactive oxygen species and quinones. DA- and dopa-quinones form adducts with α-synuclein, a major constituent of Lewy bodies in PD (Chapter 22).

HISTORICAL PERSPECTIVE

Dopamine was first synthesized in 1910. Later that year, Henry Dale characterized the biological properties of DA in the periphery and described it as a weak, adrenaline-like substance. In the 1930s, DA was recognized as a transitional compound in the synthesis of NE and EPI but was believed to be little more than a biosynthetic intermediate. Not until the early 1950s were stores of DA identified in tissues, suggesting that DA had a signaling function of its own. Soon thereafter, Hornykiewicz discovered the DA deficit in Parkinsonian brains, fueling interest in the role of DA in neurological diseases and disorders (Hornykiewicz, 2002).

Synthesis and Metabolism

The biosynthesis and metabolism of DA are summarized in Figure 13–8. Phenylalanine and tyrosine are the precursors of DA. For the most part,

Catechol Dopamine

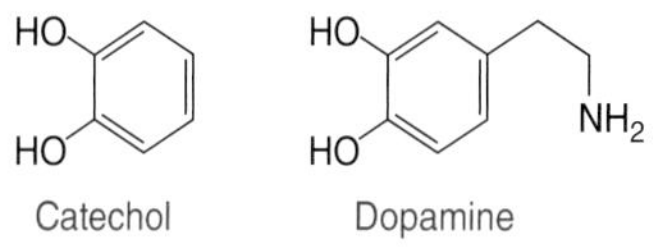

Figure 13–7 *The catechol nucleus of catecholamines.*

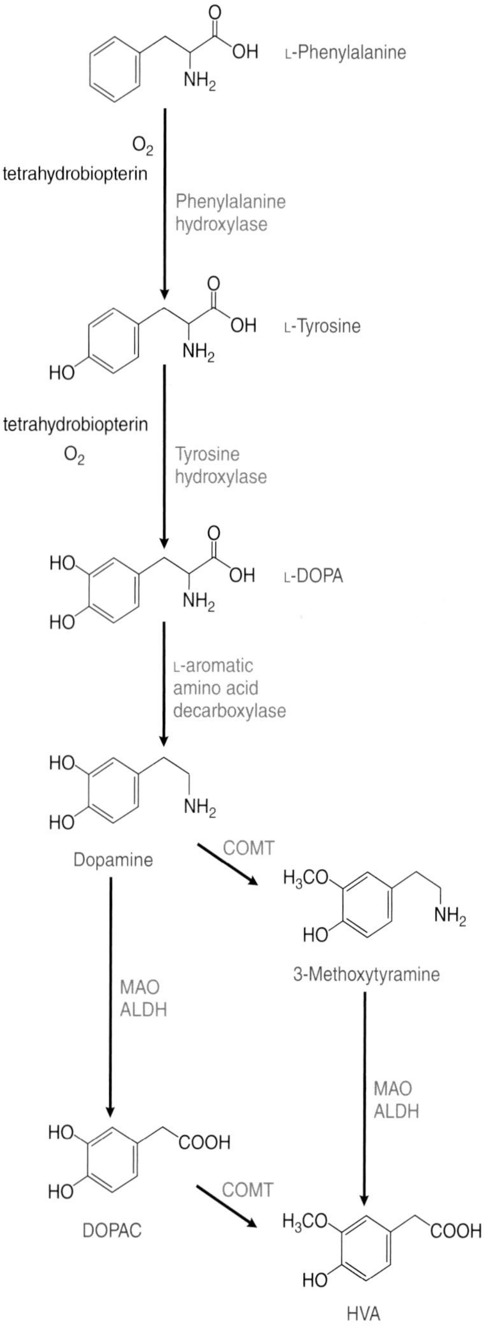

L-Phenylalanine
O_2 tetrahydrobiopterin Phenylalanine hydroxylase
L-Tyrosine
tetrahydrobiopterin O_2 Tyrosine hydroxylase
L-DOPA
L-aromatic amino acid decarboxylase
Dopamine
COMT
3-Methoxytyramine
MAO ALDH
MAO ALDH
DOPAC
COMT
HVA

Figure 13–8 *Synthesis and inactivation of DA.* Enzymes are identified in blue lettering, and cofactors are shown in black letters.

mammals convert dietary phenylalanine to tyrosine by phenylalanine hydroxylase. Diminished levels of phenylalanine hydroxylase lead to high levels of phenylalanine, producing a condition known as phenylketonuria, which must be controlled by dietary restrictions to avoid intellectual impairment. Tyrosine crosses readily into the brain through uptake; normal brain levels of tyrosine are typically saturating. Conversion of tyrosine to L-dopa by the tyrosine hydroxylase is the rate-limiting step in the synthesis of DA (as in NE synthesis; see Chapter 8). Once generated, L-dopa is rapidly converted to DA by AADC, the same enzyme that generates 5HT from L-5-hydroxytryptophan. Unlike DA, L-dopa readily crosses the BBB and is converted to DA in the brain, which explains its utility in therapy for PD (see Chapter 18).

Metabolism of DA occurs primarily by MAO in both pre- and postsynaptic elements. MAO acts on DA to generate an inactive aldehyde derivative by oxidative deamination; the aldehyde is subsequently metabolized by aldehyde dehydrogenase to form DOPAC. DOPAC can be further metabolized by COMT to form HVA. In humans, HVA is the principal metabolite of DA. DOPAC, HVA, and DA are excreted in the urine, where they are readily measured. Levels of DOPAC and HVA are reliable indicators of DA turnover; ratios of these metabolites to DA in CSF serve as accurate representations of brain dopaminergic activity. In addition to metabolizing DOPAC, COMT acts on DA to generate 3-methoxytyramine, which is subsequently converted to HVA by MAO. MAO_B-selective inhibitors, such as selegiline and rasagiline, can increase DA levels and are currently used to treat PD (see Chapter 18). COMT in the periphery also metabolizes L-dopa to 3-*O*-methyldopa, which then competes with L-dopa for uptake into the CNS (see Figure 18–4). Consequently, L-dopa given in the treatment of PD must be coadministered with peripheral COMT inhibitors, such as entacapone and tolcapone, to preserve L-dopa and allow sufficient entry into the CNS.

Figure 13–9 summarizes the neurochemical events that underlie DA neurotransmission. In dopaminergic neurons, synthesized DA is packaged into secretory vesicles by VMAT2. Drugs such as reserpine, which inhibit VMAT and deplete DA levels, were once used to treat psychosis. This packaging allows DA to be stored in readily releasable quanta and protects the transmitter from further anabolism or catabolism. By contrast, in adrenergic and noradrenergic cells, DA is not packaged; instead, it is converted to NE by DA β-hydroxylase and, in adrenergic cells, methylated to EPI in cells expressing phenylethanolamine *N*-methyltransferase (Chapter 8).

Synaptically released DA activates postsynaptic receptor subtypes, the expression of which is cell specific, leading to signal transduction via G protein–mediated pathways, although in some cases G protein–independent signaling is possible (see further discussion). DA receptor subtypes are also the targets of many therapeutically employed drugs and pharmacological tool compounds. Specific receptor subtypes of the D_2-like category can also be expressed on the presynaptic nerve terminal, where they regulate the release of DA. Reuptake of released DA by the DA transporter is the primary mechanism for termination of DA action and allows for either vesicular repackaging of transmitter or metabolism.

The DA transporter, DAT, localizes to dendrites, axons, and soma of mesencephalic DA neurons and is also found peripherally in the stomach, pancreas, and lymphocytes. Psychostimulants, such as cocaine, amphetamine, and methamphetamine, induce euphoria and hyperactivity by

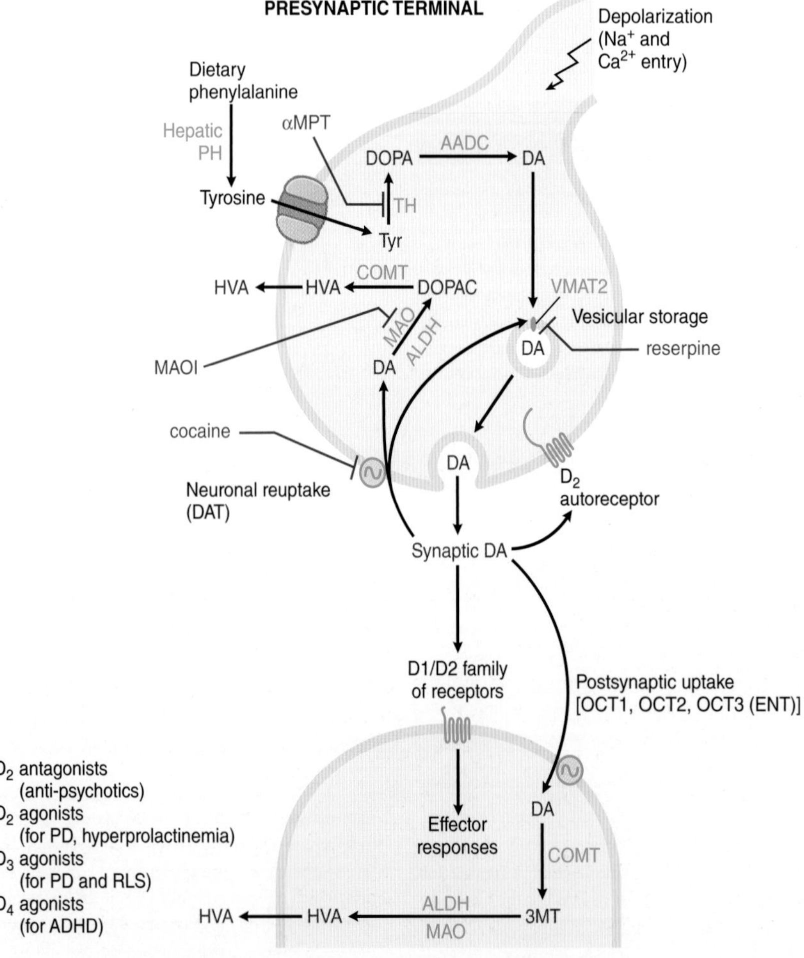

Figure 13–9 *A dopaminergic synapse.* Dopamine is synthesized from tyrosine in the nerve terminal by the sequential actions of TH and AADC. DA is sequestered by VMAT2 in storage granules and released by exocytosis. Synaptic DA activates presynaptic autoreceptors and postsynaptic D1 and D2 receptors. Synaptic DA may be taken up into the neuron via the DA transporter (DAT) or removed by postsynaptic uptake via OCT transporters. Cytosolic DA is subject to degradation by MAO/ALDH in the neuron, and by COMT in non-neuronal cells; the final metabolic product is HVA. See structures in Figure 13–8.

increasing extracellular DA. Cocaine potentiates DA signaling by acting as a nontransported antagonist of the plasma membrane DAT. However, the actions of amphetamines are more complex; amphetamines are competitive substrates for both the DATs and the VMATs. Amphetamines enter the cell through the DAT, where they displace DA from vesicular stores, causing an accumulation of DA within the neuronal cytoplasm. This resulting increase in cytosolic DA drives the release of DA by a nonvesicular mechanism that involves efflux through the DAT (Sitte et al., 2015). Newer studies also support the idea that amphetamines have additional targets within DA neurons that activate cellular signaling pathways, including G_s-dependent pathways coupled to increases in cAMP and $G_{12/13}$-dependent pathways coupled to the activation of the small GTPase, RhoA (Wheeler et al., 2015). The trace amine-associated receptor TAAR1, a predominantly intracellular GPCR, is activated by amphetamines, DA, and a variety of drugs and trace amines and has been proposed to mediate some of the intracellular actions of amphetamines (Miller, 2011).

The DA transporter can also serve as a molecular entryway for some neurotoxins, including 6-OHDA and MPP^+, the neurotoxic metabolite of MPTP. Following uptake into dopaminergic neurons, MPP^+ and 6-OHDA facilitate intra- and extracellular DA release and generate reactive oxygen species such as superoxide radicals (O_2^-) that cause neuronal death. This selective dopaminergic degeneration mimics PD and serves as an animal model for this disorder.

Dopamine Receptors

Early investigations found that DA increases cAMP levels in both the brain and retina, presumably by activating a DA-sensitive AC enzyme. Subsequent studies revealed the existence of DA receptors not linked to AC activation, suggesting multiple DA receptor subtypes. These were initially categorized as D_1 and D_2 receptors and could be distinguished on the basis of pharmacological properties and physiological function (Kebabian et al., 1979). Molecular biological studies have identified not only genes encoding the biochemically defined D_1 and D_2 receptor subtypes but also genes for additional DA receptors. We now recognize that there are five distinct DA receptors in mammals that are organized into two D_1-like and D_2-like subfamilies. The D_1-like subfamily consists of the D_1 and D_5 receptors; the D_2, D_3, and D_4 subtypes comprise the D_2-like subfamily. Receptors in the D_1-like subfamily (D_1 and D_5) couple to G_s or G_{olf} proteins to activate AC and increase cAMP levels; the D_2-like receptors (D_2, D_3, and D_4) couple to G_i or G_o proteins, which inhibit AC and diminish cyclic cAMP production. Activation of $G_{i/o}$ proteins can also directly modulate the activity of certain K^+ and Ca^{2+} channels (Figure 13–10). Signaling of D_2 receptors through β-arrestin–mediated pathways has also been postulated (see following discussion).

Pharmacological agents targeting DA receptors are used in the treatment of numerous neuropsychiatric disorders, including PD, schizophrenia, bipolar disorder, Huntington disease, ADHD, and Tourette syndrome. Like many GPCRs, DA receptors may form homo- and hetero-oligomers and also oligomerize with other GPCRs as well as ligand-gated ion channels (Fuxe et al., 2015). In most cases, the physiological significance of receptor oligomerization remains unclear. For recent in-depth reviews on DA receptor signaling, see the work of Beaulieu and Gainetdinov (2011) and Beaulieu et al. (2015).

The D_1 Receptor

- The D_1 receptor is the most highly expressed of the DA receptors; highest levels of D_1 receptor protein are found within the CNS, but it is also located in the kidney, retina, and cardiovascular system.
- The neostriatum expresses the highest levels of D_1 receptor in the CNS but does not express any detectable $G\alpha_s$. In this region, the D_1 receptor appears to couple to G_{olf} to increase levels of cAMP and its downstream effectors.
- The gene for the human D_1 receptor lacks introns.
- In addition to activating G proteins, the D_1 receptor can form hetero-oligomers with ionotropic NMDA glutamate receptors (Chapter 14) to modulate glutamatergic signaling.

The D_2 Receptor

- The D_2 receptor is the second most highly expressed DA receptor and consists of short (D_{2S}) and long (D_{2L}) isoforms that arise from alternative messenger RNA splicing. The D_{2S} isoform is missing 29 amino acids in the third intracellular loop that are present in the D_{2L} variant.
- The D_{2S} and D_{2L} receptors are pharmacologically identical; both couple to G_i or G_o to decrease cAMP production. The D_{2L} receptor is more prevalent and postulated to function postsynaptically. In contrast, the D_{2S} isoform functions as a putative presynaptic autoreceptor that regulates DA synthesis and release.
- The D_2 receptors can signal through $G_{\beta\gamma}$ subunits to regulate a variety of functions, including inwardly rectifying K^+ channels, N-type Ca^{2+} channels, and L-type Ca^{2+} channels.
- The D_2 receptor can signal through recruitment of the scaffolding protein, β-arrestin, thereby coupling to downstream signaling through the protein kinases PKB and GSK-3 (Beaulieu and Gainetdinov, 2011; Beaulieu et al., 2015).

The D_3 Receptor

- The D_3 receptor is less abundant than the D_2 receptor and is mainly expressed in the limbic regions of the brain. The highest levels of the D_3 receptor are found in the islands of Calleja, nucleus accumbens, substantia nigra pars compacta, and ventral tegmental area.
- The D_3 receptor signals through pertussis toxin–sensitive $G_{i/o}$ proteins, although not as effectively as the D_2 receptor.
- The D_3 receptor's tertiary structure has been determined by X-ray crystallography (Chien et al., 2010).

The D_4 Receptor

- The D_4 receptor is expressed in the retina, hypothalamus, PFC, amygdala, and hippocampus.

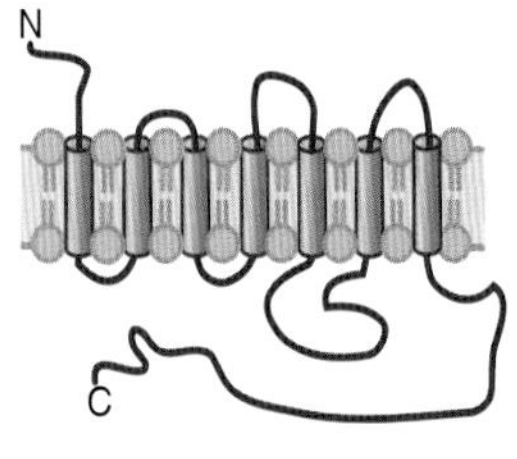

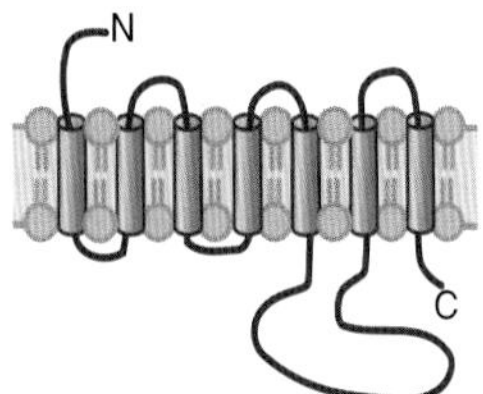

Figure 13–10 *The two subfamilies of DA receptors and their major signaling pathways.*

- The D_4 receptor is highly polymorphic, containing a VNTR encoding sequences within the third intracellular loop. In humans, the four-repeat variant is the most common. Association between a seven-repeat VNTR variant of the D_4 receptor and ADHD has been suggested.
- The D_4 receptor couples to $G_{i/o}$ to inhibit AC activity and depress intracellular cAMP levels.

The D_5 Receptor

- The D_5 receptor is most highly expressed in the hippocampus, but also is found in the substantia nigra, hypothalamus, striatum, cerebral cortex, nucleus accumbens, and olfactory tubercle.
- The D_5 receptor gene, like the D_1 receptor gene, is intronless.
- The D_5 receptor activates G_s and G_{olf} to increase cAMP production and can also modulate Na^+ currents and N-, P-, and L-type Ca^{2+} currents via PKA-dependent pathways. The D_5 receptor can also directly interact with $GABA_A$ receptors to decrease Cl^- flux.

The Dopamine Transporter

- DAT (SLC6A3) clears extracellular DA released during neurotransmission and is a major target for both therapeutic and addictive psychostimulant drugs.
- Like SERT, the DAT is a member of the Neurotransmitter Sodium Symporter (NSS) family (see *Transporters and Pharmacodynamics: Drug Action in the Brain*, in Chapter 5), which couples neurotransmitter transport across the plasma membrane to the movement of Na^+ ions into the cell.
- The DAT has 12 membrane-spanning domains; a recent high-resolution X-ray structure of a *Drosophila* DAT has been determined (Penmatsa et al., 2015).
- The DAT protein is abundantly expressed in mesostriatal, mesolimbic, and mesocortical DA pathways, where it can be found on cell bodies, dendrites, and axons of DA neurons (Ciliax et al., 1999). However, the DAT is not readily detected within synapses, suggesting that rather than regulating synaptic neurotransmitter concentrations, it is poised to regulate spillover and diffusion of DA away from sites of release.
- The DAT is the therapeutic target of methylphenidate and amphetamine, the two major drugs used to treat attention-deficit disorders. The DAT inhibitor bupropion is used to treat depression and to support smoking cessation.

Actions of Dopamine in Physiological Systems

Heart and Vasculature

At low concentrations, circulating DA primarily stimulates vascular D_1 receptors (see discussion that follows), causing vasodilation and reducing cardiac load. The net result is a decrease in blood pressure and an increase in cardiac contractility. As circulating DA concentrations rise, DA is able to activate β adrenergic receptors to further increase cardiac contractility. At very high concentrations, circulating DA activates α adrenergic receptors in the vasculature, thereby causing vasoconstriction; thus, high concentrations of DA increase blood pressure. Clinically, DA administration is used to treat severe congestive heart failure, sepsis, or cardiogenic shock. It is only administered intravenously and is not considered a long-term treatment.

Kidney

Dopamine is a paracrine/autocrine transmitter in the kidney and binds to receptors of both the D_1 and D_2 subfamilies. Renal DA primarily serves to increase natriuresis, although it can also increase renal blood flow and glomerular filtration. Under basal sodium conditions, DA regulates Na^+ excretion by inhibiting the activity of various Na^+ transporters, including the apical Na^+-H^+ exchanger and the basolateral Na^+,K^+-ATPase. Activation of D_1 receptors increases renin secretion, whereas DA, acting on D_3 receptors, reduces renin secretion. Abnormalities in the DA system and its receptors have been implicated in human hypertension.

Pituitary Gland

Dopamine is the primary regulator of prolactin secretion from the pituitary gland. DA released from the hypothalamus into the hypophyseal portal blood supply acts on lactotroph D_2 receptors to decrease prolactin secretion (see Chapter 42). The ergot-based DA agonists bromocriptine and cabergoline are used in the treatment of hyperprolactinemia. Both have high affinity for D_2 receptors, with lower affinity for D_1, 5HT, and adrenergic receptors; both activate D_2 receptors in the pituitary to reduce prolactin secretion. The risk of valvular heart disease in ergot therapy is not associated with the lower doses used in treating hyperprolactinemia. The use of bromocriptine and cabergoline in the management of hyperprolactinemia is described in Chapter 42.

Catecholamine Release

Both D_1 and D_2 receptors modulate the release of NE and EPI. The D_2 receptor provides tonic inhibition of EPI release from chromaffin cells of the adrenal medulla and of NE release from sympathetic nerve terminals. In contrast, activation of the D_1 receptor promotes the release of catecholamines from the adrenal medulla.

CNS

There are three major groups of DA projections in the brain (Figure 13–11): mesocorticomesolimbic (originating in the ventral tegmental area), nigrostriatal (originating in the substantia nigra pars compacta), and tuberoinfundibular (originating in the hypothalamus). The physiological processes under dopaminergic control include reward, emotion, cognition, memory, and motor activity. Dysregulation of the dopaminergic system is critical in a number of disease states, including PD, Tourette syndrome, bipolar depression, schizophrenia, ADHD, and addiction/substance abuse.

The mesolimbic pathway is associated with reward and, less so, with learned behaviors. Dysfunction in this pathway is associated with addic-

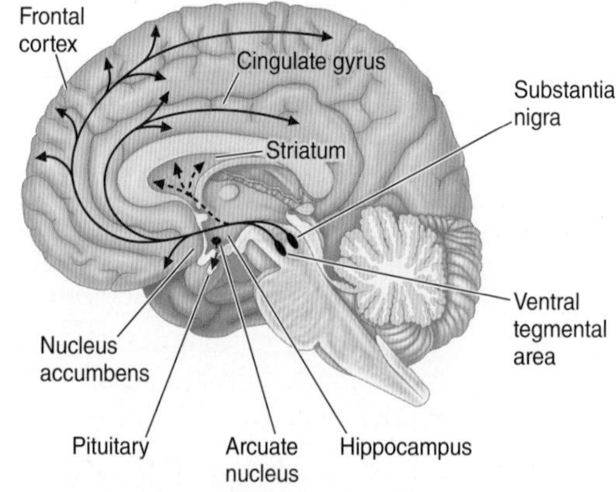

Figure 13–11 Major dopaminergic projections in the CNS.

- The nigrostriatal (or mesostriatal) pathway. Neurons in the substantia nigra compacta project to the dorsal striatum (*upward dashed blue arrows*); this is the pathway that degenerates in Parkinson disease.
- The mesocortico/mesolimbic pathway. Neurons in the ventral tegmental area project to the ventral striatum (nucleus accumbens), olfactory bulb, amygdala, hippocampus, orbital and medial prefrontal cortex, and cingulate gyrus (*solid blue arrows*).
- The tuberoinfundibular pathway. Neurons in the arcuate nucleus of the hypothalamus project by the tuberoinfundibular pathway in the hypothalamus, from which DA is delivered to the anterior pituitary (*red arrows*).

tion, schizophrenia, and psychoses (including bipolar depression) and learning deficits. The mesocortical projections are important for "higher-order" cognitive functions, including motivation, reward, emotion, and impulse control; they are also implicated in psychoses, including schizophrenia, and in ADHD. The nigrostriatal pathway is a key regulator of movement (see Chapter 18). Impairments in this pathway are involved in PD and underlie detrimental motor side effects associated with dopaminergic therapy, including tardive dyskinesia. As noted previously, DA released in the tuberoinfundibular pathway is carried by the hypophyseal blood supply to the pituitary, where it regulates prolactin secretion.

Dopaminergic neurons are strongly influenced by excitatory glutamate and inhibitory GABA input. In general, glutamate inputs enable burst-like firing of dopaminergic neurons, resulting in high concentrations of synaptic DA. GABA inhibition of DA neurons causes a tonic, basal level of DA release into the synapse. DA release also modulates GABA and glutamate neurons, thus providing an additional level of interaction between DA and other neurotransmitters.

Motor Control and Parkinson Disease

In the early 1980s, several young people in California developed rapid-onset Parkinsonism. All of the affected individuals had injected a synthetic analogue of meperidine that was contaminated with MPTP. MPTP is metabolized by MAO-B to the neurotoxin MPP^+. Because of the high specificity of MPP^+ for the DA transporter, neuronal death is largely restricted to the substantia nigra and ventral tegmental area, resulting in a phenotype remarkably similar to PD. 6-OHDA is similar to MPTP in both mechanism of action and utility in animal models. Administration of MPTP or 6-OHDA to animals results in tremor, grossly diminished locomotor activity, and rigidity. As with PD, these motor deficits are alleviated with L-dopa therapy or dopaminergic agonists.

Other pharmacological agents that act on the DAT are known to potentiate locomotor activity via dopaminergic actions, including cocaine and amphetamine. The accumulation of extracellular DA increases stimulation of DA receptors and results in heightened locomotor activity. Mice lacking DAT are hyperactive and do not display increased locomotion in response to cocaine or amphetamine treatment.

Reward: Implications for Addiction

In general, drugs of abuse increase DA levels in the nucleus accumbens, an area critical for rewarded behaviors. This role for mesolimbic DA in addiction has led to numerous studies of abused drugs in DA receptor "knockout" mice in which the genes expressing specific receptors have been disrupted. Studies of D_1 receptor knockout mice showed a reduction in the rewarding properties of ethanol, suggesting that the rewarding and reinforcing properties of ethanol are dependent, at least in part, on the D_1 receptor. D_2 receptor knockout mice also display reduced preference for ethanol consumption. Morphine lacks rewarding properties in D_2 knockout mice when measured by conditioned place-preference or self-administration paradigms. However, mice lacking the D_2 receptor exhibit enhanced self-administration of high doses of cocaine. These data suggest a complex and drug-specific role for the D_2 receptor in rewarding and reinforcing behaviors. The D_3 receptor, highly expressed in the limbic system, has also been implicated in the rewarding properties of several drugs of abuse. However, D_3 knockout mice display drug-associated place preference similar to wild-type mice following amphetamine or morphine administration. Recently developed D_3 receptor-preferring ligands implicate a role for the D_3 receptor in motivation for drug seeking and in drug relapse, rather than in the direct reinforcing effects of the drugs (Heidbreder and Newman, 2010).

Cognition and Memory

Seminal work by Goldman-Rakic, Arnsten, and their colleagues (Vijayraghavan et al., 2007) showed that an optimum level of D_1 receptor activity in the PFC is required for optimum performance in learning and memory tasks. Either too little or too much D_1 receptor stimulation impairs PFC function in rats, monkeys, and humans. Thus, low doses of D_1 agonists improve working memory and attention, whereas high levels of DA release, such as during stress, impair PFC function. These observations have led to the "inverted U" hypothesis of the relationship between D_1 receptor stimulation and normal physiological functioning of the PFC (see Figure 4–2A). Interestingly, suboptimal levels of D_1 receptor stimulation have been suggested to underlie age-associated learning deficits and to contribute to the decreased cognition observed in various pathophysiological states, especially schizophrenia. Unsurprisingly, the D_1 receptor provides an attractive drug target for the treatment of a number of neuropsychiatric disorders.

Drugs Affecting Dopamine Signaling

Dopamine Receptor Agonists

Dopamine receptor agonists are mainly used in the treatment of PD, RLS, and hyperprolactinemia. One of the primary limitations to the therapeutic use of dopaminergic agonists is the lack of receptor subtype selectivity. Recent advances in receptor-ligand structure-function relationships have enabled the development of drugs that can distinguish between D_1-like and D_2-like receptor subfamilies and, in some cases, show a preference for individual receptor subtypes. Many of these compounds have already proven to be useful experimental tools (Table 13–5), and this remains an active area of research.

Parkinson Disease

Dopamine does not cross the BBB; thus, the principal pharmacotherapy for PD is to administer the precursor to DA, L-dopa, which crosses the BBB and is converted to DA in the brain. Commonly, L-dopa is formulated with a decarboxylase inhibitor to prevent the peripheral conversion of L-dopa to DA, which can result in adverse side effects. While the response to L-dopa by patients with PD is usually quite favorable, longer-term treatment can result in a loss of effectiveness and the emergence of dyskinetic syndromes referred to as L-dopa–induced dyskinesias. These limitations to the therapeutic effects of L-dopa have generated interest in developing alternative therapies for PD, with the intent of either delaying the use of L-dopa or alleviating its side effects. DA receptor agonists can be used in conjunction with lower doses of L-dopa in a combined therapy approach or as monotherapy. Two general classes of dopaminergic agonists have been used in the treatment of PD: ergots and nonergots. The detailed use of these drugs in the management of PD is described in Chapter 18.

Ergot derivatives (see Table 13–4) act on several different neurotransmitter systems, including DA, 5HT, and adrenergic receptors. Bromocriptine and pergolide have been used for the treatment of PD; however, their use is associated with risk for serious cardiac complications, specifically, the promotion of valvular heart disease due to $5HT_{2B}$ serotonin receptor stimulation (Hutcheson et al., 2011). Bromocriptine is a potent D_2 receptor agonist and a weak D_1 antagonist. Pergolide is a partial agonist of D_1

TABLE 13–5 ■ EXPERIMENTAL TOOLS AT DA RECEPTORS

RECEPTOR	AGONIST	ANTAGONIST
D_1-like[a]	SKF-81297 SKF-83959	SCH-23390 SCH-39166
D_2-like[b]	Quinpirole	Sulpiride
D_2	Sumanirole	L-741626 ML321
D_3	PD128907	SB-277011 SB-269652
D_4	PD168077	L-745870

[a]These compounds are selective for D_1-like versus D_2-like receptors. There are no useful tool compounds that can differentiate D_1 from D_5 receptors.
[b]These compounds are selective for D_2-like versus D_1-like receptors.

receptors and a strong D_2 family agonist with high affinity for both D_2 and D_3 receptor subtypes. Ergot derivatives are commonly reported to cause unpleasant side effects, including nausea, dizziness, and hallucinations. Pergolide was removed from the U.S. market as therapy for PD after it was associated with an increased risk for valvular heart disease. Bromocriptine remains on the market primarily for the treatment of hyperprolactinemia or prolactin-secreting adenomas, where lower (D_2-selective) doses can be employed to avoid cardiac complications.

Several nonergot alkaloids are also employed in the management of PD. Apomorphine is a pan-DA receptor agonist most commonly used in the acute treatment of sudden "off" periods (bradykinesia, freezing) that can occur after long-term L-dopa treatment. Pramipexole and ropinirole are widely used in the treatment of PD, are agonists at all D_2-like receptors, but have the highest affinities for the D_3 receptor subtype. However, these agents are less effective than L-dopa in the early stages of PD treatment, and both are associated with the development of impulse control disorders, such as compulsive gambling or hypersexuality; notably, fewer drug-induced dyskinesias are observed. The mechanisms underlying the impulse control disorders are currently unknown. Rotigotine is a DA agonist with preference for the D_2-like subfamily and is offered in a transdermal patch that is approved for the treatment of PD.

Hyperprolactinemia

Despite the contraindications for PD, ergot-based DA agonists are still used in the treatment of hyperprolactinemia. Like bromocriptine, cabergoline is a strong agonist at D_2 receptors and has lower affinity for D_1, 5HT, and α adrenergic receptors. The therapeutic utility of bromocriptine and cabergoline in hyperprolactinemia is derived from their properties as DA receptor agonists: They activate D_2 receptors in the pituitary to reduce prolactin secretion. The risk of valvular heart disease from ergot therapy is associated with higher doses of drug (necessary for PD treatment) but not with the lower doses used in treating hyperprolactinemia. The use of bromocriptine and cabergoline in the management of hyperprolactinemia is described in Chapter 42.

Restless Leg Syndrome

Restless leg syndrome is a neurological deficit characterized by abnormal sensations in the legs that are alleviated by movement. Decreased DA receptor expression and mild dopaminergic hypofunction are noted in patients with RLS. Rotigotine, ropinirole, and pramipexole are FDA-approved as pharmacotherapies for both PD and RLS.

Dopamine Receptor Antagonists

Just as enhancing DA neurotransmission can be clinically important, so can inhibiting dopaminergic signaling be useful in certain disease states. As with the DA receptor agonists, a lack of subtype-specific antagonists has limited the therapeutic utility of this group of ligands. Recent advances in elucidating GPCR structures and modeling ligand binding have advanced drug design, and subtype-selective antagonists are beginning to emerge as experimental tools (Table 13–5). Some receptor subtype-selective antagonists are in early stages of preclinical testing for therapeutic utility.

Schizophrenia

Dopamine receptor antagonists of the D_2-like subfamily are a mainstay in the pharmacotherapy of schizophrenia. While many neurotransmitter systems likely contribute to the complex pathology of schizophrenia (Chapter 16), modulating DA signaling is considered the basis of treatment. The DA hypothesis of schizophrenia has its origins in the characteristics of the drugs used to treat this disorder: All antipsychotic compounds used clinically have high affinity for DA receptors, especially with the D_2 receptor subtype. Moreover, psychostimulants that increase extracellular DA levels can induce or worsen psychotic symptoms in schizophrenic patients. The advent of neuroimaging techniques for visualization of DA in human brain regions has led to new insights in the role of specific DA systems. DA hyperfunction in subcortical regions, most notably the striatum, has been associated with the positive symptoms of schizophrenia, which respond well to antipsychotic treatment. In contrast, the PFC of schizophrenic patients exhibits dopaminergic hypofunction, which has been associated with the more treatment-refractory negative/cognitive symptoms. The drugs currently used to treat schizophrenia are classified as either typical (also referred to as first-generation) or atypical (second-generation) antipsychotics. This nomenclature stems from the fewer EPSs, or parkinsonian-like side effects, observed with atypical antipsychotics.

Typical Antipsychotics. The first antipsychotic drug used to treat schizophrenia was chlorpromazine. Its antipsychotic properties were attributed to its antagonism of DA receptors, especially the D_2 receptor. More D_2-selective ligands (e.g., haloperidol) were developed to improve the antipsychotic properties (see Chapter 16). Notably, drugs that are completely selective for the D_2 receptor subtype, without overlapping with affinity for the D_3 or D_4 receptor subtypes, are currently unavailable. While all typical antipsychotics markedly improve positive symptoms (hallucinations, etc.), they are not very beneficial in the treatment of negative or cognitive symptoms of this disease.

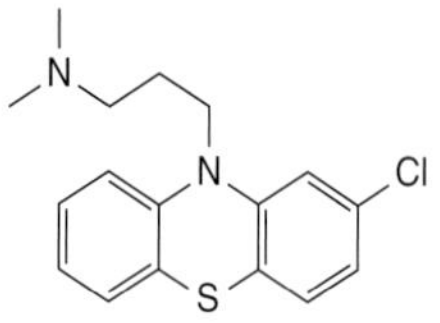

CHLORPROMAZINE

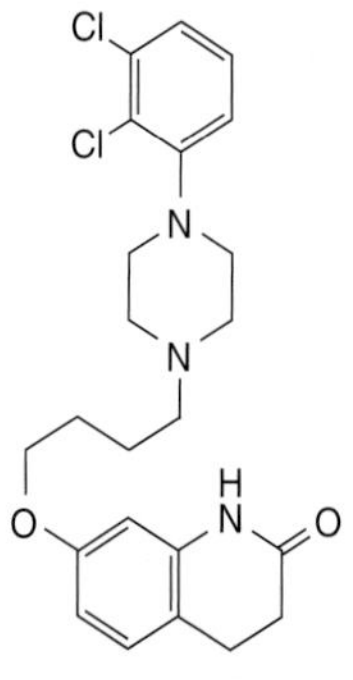

ARIPIPRAZOLE

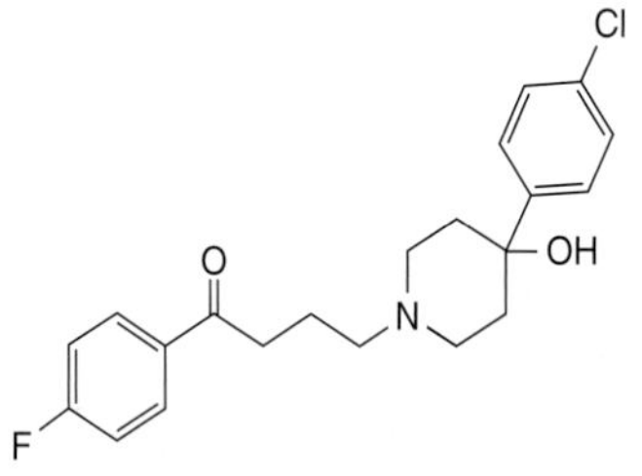

HALOPERIDOL

Atypical Antipsychotics. This class of antipsychotic drugs originated with clozapine and is distinguished by lower EPSs than typical antipsychotics. Atypical agents are also less likely to stimulate prolactin production. The lack of extrapyramidal side effects has been partly attributed to a much lower affinity for the D_2 receptor compared to typical antipsychotics. Most atypical antipsychotics are also high-affinity antagonists or inverse agonists at the $5HT_{2A}$ receptor. While the precise role of $5HT_{2A}$ receptor blockade in the atypical effects of antipsychotics remains unclear, dual DA–5HT receptor blockade has contributed to the development of antipsychotics for several decades (see Chapter 16).

Partial D_2-Like Receptor Agonists. Aripiprazole has even fewer side effects than earlier atypical antipsychotics. Aripiprazole diverges from the traditional atypical profile in several ways: First, it has higher affinity for D_2 receptors than for $5HT_{2A}$ receptors; second, it is a partial agonist at D_2 receptors. As a partial agonist, aripiprazole may diminish subcortical (striatal) DA hyperfunction by competing with DA for receptor binding, while simultaneously enhancing dopaminergic neurotransmission in the PFC by acting as an agonist. The dual mechanism afforded by a partial agonist may thus treat both the positive and negative symptoms associated with schizophrenia. Aripiprazole also exhibits functional selectivity at the D_2 receptor in that it exhibits higher efficacy for β-arrestin–mediated signaling than for G protein–mediated signaling. How this property may contribute to the unique effects of aripiprazole is not yet clear.

Recently, a derivative of aripiprazole, brexpiprazole, has been approved for the treatment of schizophrenia and as an adjunctive treatment of depression. The pharmacological properties of brexpiprazole are similar to those of aripiprazole except that brexpiprazole has lower D_2 receptor agonist efficacy and high partial agonist effects at the $5HT_{1A}$ receptor; perhaps this latter property underlies its effectiveness in treating depression.

Another partial agonist of the D_2 receptor, cariprazine, has recently been approved for treating schizophrenia and bipolar disorder. Interestingly, cariprazine is also a partial agonist at the D_3 receptor and actually exhibits higher affinity for the D_3 versus the D_2 receptor. In some studies, cariprazine has been shown to exhibit procognitive effects, suggesting that it may be useful for treating negative as well as positive symptoms of schizophrenia.

D_3 Receptor Antagonists and Drug Addiction

Although much work remains to determine their clinical utility, D_3-selective antagonists show promise in the treatment of addiction (Heidbreder and Newman, 2010; Newman et al., 2012). This interest stems from the high expression of the D_3 receptor in the limbic system, the

Drug Facts for Your Personal Formulary: *Serotonergic Ligands*

Drugs	Therapeutic Uses	Clinical Pharmacology and Tips
$5HT_3$ Receptor Antagonists • Antiemetic agents • Additional detail in Chapters 50 and 51		
Ondansetron Dolasetron Granisetron Palonosetron	• Antiemetics • Treatment of nausea	• Associated with asymptomatic electrocardiogram changes, including prolongation of PT and QTc intervals
Cilansetron Alosetron	• Antiemetics • Treatment of nausea • Irritable bowel syndrome	• Most useful in irritable bowel syndrome when diarrhea is the principal symptom
$5HT_{2C}$ Receptor Agonists • Weight loss		
Lorcarserin	• Promotes weight loss through decreased food consumption and increased satiety	• Hallucinogenic at supraclinical doses, likely caused by $5HT_{2A}$ agonist activity that can occur with higher doses • Hallucinogenic properties resulted in a class IV schedule designation
The Triptans: $5HT_{1B/1D}$ Receptor Agonists • Migraine		
Almotriptan[a] Eletriptan Frovatriptan Naratriptan Rizatriptan Sumatriptan[b] Zolmitriptan	• Acute treatment of migraine	• Most effective in acute settings; should be used as soon as possible after onset of attack • Usually dosed orally; onset, 1–3 h • Use with caution in patients with cardiovascular issues; contraindicated in patients with ischemic heart disease and coronary artery vasospasm • Drug interactions: CYP3A4 inhibitors ↑ C_p and $t_{1/2}$ of eletriptan, naratriptan; MAO inhibitors ↑levels of almo-, riza-, suma-, and zolmitriptan. • Side effects: dizziness, somnolence, neck and chest pain • May cause fetal harm; not recommended during pregnancy and nursing; reduce dose in renal and hepatic impairment; do not administer within 24 h of other triptans, ergots, SSRIs/SNRIs • Beware serotonin syndrome, especially in combination with SSRIs and SNRIs
The Ergot Alkaloids • Interact with multiple 5HT receptor isoforms • Broad therapeutic utility		
LSD	• No longer employed clinically • Potent hallucinogen	• Positron emission tomographic imaging reveals similar activation patterns between schizophrenic patients experiencing hallucinations and LSD-induced hallucinations • $5HT_{2A}$ receptor activation is believed to mediate the hallucinogenic effect of LSD
Methysergide	• Acute treatment of migraine • Treatment of vascular headaches	• Restricted to use in patients with frequent, moderate, or infrequent, severe migraine attacks • Erratic drug absorption • Potential for inflammatory fibrosis with prolonged use, including pleuropulmonary and endocardial fibrosis
Ergonovine Methylergonovine	• Prevention of postpartum hemorrhage	• Increasing dose results in prolonged duration and increased force of uterine contraction • Sustained contracture can result at high doses
$5HT_{1A}$ Receptor Partial Agonists and SSRIs • Anxiolytics and antidepressants • Additional detail in Chapter 15		
Buspirone	Treatment of anxiety	• Mimics antianxiety effects of benzodiazepines but does not interact with $GABA_A$ receptors • Partial agonist of the $5HT_{1A}$ receptor
Fluoxetine Fluvoxamine Paroxetine Citalopram Escitalopram Sertraline Vilazodone	• Antidepressants • Also used to treat anxiety, panic disorder, obsessive-compulsive disorder, fibromyalgia, and neuropathic pain	• Selectively inhibit the serotonin transporter (SSRIs) • Most widely used treatments for major depressive disorder • Sexual dysfunction is a common side effect with SSRIs • Precaution: serotonin syndrome
MSAAs • Treatment of sexual dysfunction • Activity at multiple receptor isoforms		
Flibanserin	• Treatment of HSDD/FSIAD in premenopausal women	• Potent $5HT_{1A}$ receptor agonist and $5HT_2$ receptor family antagonist • Exerts both agonist and antagonist activity at 5HT receptors ⟹ MSAA designation (multifunctional serotonin agonist and antagonist)

Drug Facts for Your Personal Formulary: *Serotonergic Ligands (continued)*

Drugs	Therapeutic Uses	Clinical Pharmacology and Tips
Dopamine Receptor Agonists • Little to no subtype specificity		
Dopamine	• Congestive heart failure • Sepsis • Cardiogenic shock	• Only used acutely via intravenous administration
Bromocriptine Cabergoline	• PD (see Chapter 22) • Hyperprolactinemia	• Ergot derivatives with D_2 agonist activity and D_1 antagonist activity • Limited utility due to high potential for cardiac valvulopathies via $5HT_{2B}$ stimulation • Bromocriptine and cabergoline can be used at low doses to treat hyperprolactinemia
Apomorphine Pramipexole Ropinirole Rotigotine	• PD (see Chapter 22 for more details) • RLS	• Nonergot alkaloids with broader DA receptor agonist activity • Less efficacious than L-dopa in PD; often used as adjunct therapy in advanced PD • Use in early PD can lead to poor impulse control • Pramipexole, ropinirole, and rotigotine are used to treat RLS
Dopamine Receptor Antagonists • Antipsychotics • Emerging subtype specificity of ligands (Additional detail in Chapter 16)		
Chlorpromazine Haloperidol	• Schizophrenia (see Chapter 16)	• Classified as typical antipsychotics • Agents block D_2 receptors but are not completely selective • Improvements are most notable in positive symptoms of schizophrenia
Clozapine	• Schizophrenia (see Chapter 16)	• Classified as atypical antipsychotics • Mixed $5HT_{2A}$–D_2 receptor blockade • Fewer extrapyramidal side effects than typical antipsychotics
Aripiprazole Brexpiprazole Cariprazine	• Schizophrenia (see Chapter 16)	• D_2 partial agonists with varied profiles at 5HT receptors • Improved side effect profile over many other antipsychotics
DAT Ligands • High potential for abuse • Interact with the dopamine transporter		
Bupropion	• Depression • Smoking cessation	• Also inhibits NET • ↑ risk of suicidal ideation in pediatric/young adult patients taking this medication
Cocaine	• Rarely used therapeutically	• Schedule II classification • Limited clinical utility as a topical anesthetic in eye and nasal surgeries
Methylphenidate Methamphetamine Amphetamine	• ADHD, ADD • Narcolepsy • Obesity	• Can worsen psychosis; use with extreme caution in patients with bipolar disorder • Schedule II drug classification due to psychostimulant properties if misused

[a]Fewest side effects.
[b]Has best evidence for safety in pregnancy.

reward center of the brain, and from animal studies of highly D_3-selective antagonists that suggest a role for the D_3 receptor in the motivation to abuse drugs and in the potential for drug-abuse relapse.

Acknowledgment: *Elaine Sanders-Bush and Steven E. Mayer contributed to this chapter in recent editions of this book. We have retained some of their text in the current edition.*

Bibliography

Ahangari G, et al. Investigation of 5HT2A gene expression in PBMCs of patients with allergic asthma. *Inflamm Allergy Drug Targets*, **2015**, *14*:60–64.

Beaulieu JM, Gainetdinov RR. The physiology, signaling, and pharmacology of dopamine receptors. *Pharmacol Rev*, **2011**, *63*:182–217.

Beaulieu JM, et al. Dopamine receptors—IUPHAR review 13. *Br J Pharmacol*, **2015**, *172*:1–23.

Brunner HG, et al. Abnormal behavior associated with a point mutation in the structural gene for monoamine oxidase A. *Science*, **1993**, *262*:578–580.

Burns CM, et al. Regulation of serotonin-2C receptor G-protein coupling by RNA editing. *Nature*, **1997**, *387*:303–308.

Cases O, et al. Aggressive behavior and altered amounts of brain serotonin and norepinephrine in mice lacking MAOA. *Science*, **1995**, *268*:1763–1766.

Chien EY, et al. Structure of the human dopamine D_3 receptor in complex with a D_2/D_3 selective antagonist. *Science*, **2010**, *330*:1091–1095.

Ciliax BJ, et al. Immunocytochemical localization of the dopamine transporter in human brain. *J Comp Neurol*, **1999**, *409*:38–56.

Fuxe K, et al. Dopamine heteroreceptor complexes as therapeutic targets in Parkinson's disease. *Expert Opin Ther Targets*, **2015**, *19*:377–398.

Heidbreder CA, Newman AH. Current perspectives on selective dopamine D(3) receptor antagonists as pharmacotherapeutics for addictions and related disorders. *Ann N Y Acad Sci*, **2010**, *1187*:4–34.

Hornykiewicz O. L-Dopa: from a biologically inactive amino acid to a successful therapeutic agent. *Amino Acids*, **2002**, *23*:65–70.

Hoyer D, et al. International Union of Pharmacology classification of receptors for 5-hydroxytryptamine (serotonin). *Pharmacol Rev*, **1994**, *46*:157–203.

Hutcheson JD, et al. Serotonin receptors and heart valve disease—it was meant 2B. *Pharmacol Ther*, **2011**, *132*:146–157.

Källén B, Reis M. Ongoing pharmacological management of chronic pain in pregnancy. *Drugs*, **2016**, *76*:915–924.

Kebabian JW, et al. Multiple receptors for dopamine. *Nature*, **1979**, *277*:93–96.

Lechin F, et al. Severe asthma and plasma serotonin. *Allergy*, **2002**, *57*:258–259.

Mehrotra S, et al. Current and prospective pharmacological targets in relation to antimigraine action. *N-S Arch Pharmacol*, **2008**, *378*:371–394.

Miller GM. The emerging role of trace amine-associated receptor 1 in the functional regulation of monoamine transporters and dopaminergic activity. *J Neurochem*, **2011**, *116*:164–176.

Nau F Jr, et al. Serotonin 5HT(2) receptor activation prevents allergic asthma in a mouse model. *Am J Physiol,* **2015**, *308*:L191–L198.

Newman AH, et al. Medication discovery for addiction: translating the dopamine D_3 receptor hypothesis. *Biochem Pharmacol,* **2012**, *84*:882–890.

Nichols DE. Psychedelics. *Pharmacol Rev,* **2016**, *68*:264–355.

Penmatsa A, et al. X-ray structures of *Drosophila* dopamine transporter in complex with nisoxetine and reboxetine. *Nat Struct Mol Biol,* **2015**, *22*:506–508.

Sitte H, et al. Amphetamines, new psychoactive drugs and the monoamine transporter cycle. *Trends Pharmacol Sci,* **2015**, *36*:41–50.

Thorlund K, et al. Comparative efficacy of triptans for the abortive treatment of migraine: a multiple treatment comparison meta-analysis. *Cephalalgia,* **2014**, *34*:258–267.

Vijayraghavan S, et al. Inverted-U dopamine D_1 receptor actions on prefrontal neurons engaged in working memory. *Nat Neurosci,* **2007**, *10*:376–384.

Wheeler DS, et al. Amphetamine activates Rho GTPase signaling to mediate dopamine transporter internalization and acute behavioral effects of amphetamine. *Proc Natl Acad Sci U S A,* **2015**, *112*:E7138–E7147.

Neurotransmission in the Central Nervous System

R. Benjamin Free, Janet Clark, Susan Amara, and David R. Sibley

第十四章　中枢神经系统的神经传递

中文导读

本章主要介绍：大脑的细胞组织结构，包括神经元和支持细胞；血脑屏障；神经兴奋性和离子通道；中枢神经系统的化学通信，包括中枢神经递质的鉴定、细胞信号传导与突触传递；中枢神经递质，包括氨基酸、乙酰胆碱、单胺类、微量胺类、肽类、嘌呤类、神经调节脂质、气体；调节物质，包括神经营养因子、神经甾体、细胞因子。

Abbreviations

AC: adenylyl cyclase
ACh: acetylcholine
ACTH: corticotropin (formerly adrenocorticotropic hormone)
ADHD: attention-deficit/hyperactivity disorder
AMPA: α-amino-3-hydroxy-5-methyl-4-isoxazole propionic acid
AP: action potential
BBB: blood-brain barrier
BDNF: brain-derived neurotrophic factor
cAMP: cyclic adenosine monophosphate
CFTR channel: cystic fibrosis transmembrane conductance regulated channel
CGRP: calcitonin gene–related peptide
CLC: chloride channel
CLIP: corticotropin-like intermediate lobe peptide
CNG channel: cyclic nucleotide–gated channel
CNS: central nervous system
CO: carbon monoxide
COX: cyclooxygenase
CSF: cerebrospinal fluid
CYP: cytochrome P450
DA: dopamine
DAG: diacylglycerol
DAT: dopamine transporter
DHEAS: dehydroepiandrosterone sulfate
EAAT: excitatory amino acid transporter
EPAC: exchange protein activated by cyclic AMP
EPI: epinephrine
ERK: extracellular signal-regulated kinase
GABA: γ-aminobutyric acid
GABA-T: GABA transaminase
GAD: glutamic acid decarboxylase
GAT: GABA transporter
GHB: γ-hydroxybutyric acid
GluR: AMPA/kainate type of glutamate receptor
GLYT: glycine transporter
GPCR: G protein–coupled receptor
GRK: G protein–coupled receptor kinase
HCN channel: hyperpolarization-activated, cyclic nucleotide–gated channel
HP loops: hairpin loop
5HT: serotonin
IL: interleukin
IFN: interferon
IP_3: inositol 1,4,5-trisphosphate
IPSP: inhibitory postsynaptic potential
IUPHAR/BPS: International Union of Basic and Clinical Pharmacology/British Pharmacological Society
KA: kainic acid
LOX: lipoxygenase
γ-LPH: γ-lipotrophic hormone
LTD: long-term depression
LTP: long-term potentiation
MAO: monoamine oxidase
MAPK: mitogen-activated protein kinase
mGluR: metabotropic glutamate receptor
MSH: melanocyte-stimulating hormone
mtPTP: mitochondrial permeability transition pore
NCX: Na^+/Ca^{2+} exchanger
NE: norepinephrine
NET: norepinephrine transporter
NGF: nerve growth factor
NMDA: *N*-methyl-D-aspartate
NMDA-R: NMDA receptor
NO: nitric oxide
NOS: nitric oxide synthase
NT: neurotrophin
O_2^-: superoxide radical
OCT: organic cation transporter
PC: phosphatidylcholine
PCP: phencyclidine
PDE: phosphodiesterase
PE: phosphatidylethanolamine
PEA: phenethylamine
PI3K: phosphoinositide 3-kinase
PIP_2: phosphatidylinositol 4,5-bisphosphate
PK_: protein kinase _, as in PKA, PKC
PL_: phospholipase _, as in PLA, PLD
POMC: pro-opiomelanocortin
SERT: serotonin transporter
SLC: solute carrier
TAAR: trace amine–associated receptor
TARPs: transmembrane AMPA receptor regulatory proteins
TAS2: taste receptor 2
THC: delta-9-tetrahydrocannabinol
TNF-α: tumor necrosis factor alpha
TRP channel: transient receptor potential channel
VAChT: vesicular acetylcholine transporter
VGAT: vesicular GABA and glycine transporter
VGLUT: vesicular glutamate transporter
VMAT: vesicular monoamine transporter
VSCC: voltage-sensitive Ca^{2+} channel

The brain is a complex assembly of interacting cells that regulate many of life's activities in a dynamic fashion, generally through the communication process of chemical neurotransmission. Because the CNS drives so many physiological responses, it stands to reason that centrally-acting drugs are invaluable for a plethora of conditions. CNS-acting drugs are used not only to treat anxiety, depression, mania, and schizophrenia, but also to target diverse pathophysiological conditions, such as pain, fever, movement disorders, insomnia, eating disorders, nausea, vomiting, and migraine. However, as the CNS dictates such diverse physiology, the recreational use of some CNS-acting drugs can lead to physical dependence (Chapter 24) with enormous societal impacts. The sheer breadth of physiological and pathological activities mediated by drug molecules acting in the CNS makes this class of therapeutics both wide-ranging and immeasurably important.

The identification of CNS targets, as well as the development of drug molecules for those targets, presents extraordinary scientific challenges. While years of investigation have begun to dissect the cellular and molecular bases for many aspects of neuronal signaling, complete understanding of the functions of the human brain remains in its infancy. Complicating the effort is the fact that a CNS-active drug may act at multiple sites with disparate and even opposing effects. Furthermore, many CNS disorders likely involve multiple brain regions and pathways, which can frustrate efforts focusing on a single therapeutic agent.

The pharmacology of CNS-acting drugs is primarily driven by two broad and overlapping goals:

- to develop/use drugs as probe compounds to both elucidate and manipulate the normal CNS; and

- to develop drugs to correct pathophysiological changes in the abnormal CNS.

Modern advances in molecular biology, neurophysiology, structural biology, epigenetics, biomarkers, immunity, and an array of other fields have facilitated both our understanding of the brain and the development of an ever-expanding repertoire of drugs that can selectively treat diseases of the CNS.

This chapter introduces fundamental principles and guidelines for the comprehensive study of drugs that affect the CNS. Specific therapeutic approaches to neurological and psychiatric disorders are discussed in subsequent chapters. For further detail, see specialized texts (Brady et al., 2012; Kandel et al., 2013; Nestler et al., 2015; Sibley, 2007). Detailed information on nearly all specific receptors and ion channels can be found at the official databases of the IUPHAR/BPS Guide to Pharmacology (http://www.guidetopharmacology.org).

Cellular Organization of the Brain

The CNS is made up of several types of specialized cells that are physiologically integrated to form complex functional brain tissue. The primary communicating cell is the neuron, which is strongly influenced and sustained by a variety of important supporting cells. Specific connections between neurons, both within and across the macrodivisions of the brain, are essential for neurological function. Through patterns of neuronal circuitry, individual neurons form functional ensembles to regulate the flow of information within and between the regions of the brain. Under these guidelines, present understanding of the cellular organization of the CNS can be viewed from the perspective of the size, shape, location, and interconnections between neurons (Shepherd, 2004; Squire, 2013).

Neurons

Neurons are the highly polarized signaling cells of the brain and are subclassified into types based on a large number of factors, including function (sensory, motor, or interneuron); location; morphology; neurotransmitter phenotype; or the class(es) of receptor expressed. Neurons are electrically active cells that express a variety of ion channels and ion transport proteins that allow them to conduct nerve impulses or action potentials that ultimately trigger release of neurotransmitters during chemical neurotransmission. Neurons also exhibit the cytological characteristics of highly active secretory cells: large nuclei, large amounts of smooth and rough endoplasmic reticulum, and frequent clusters of specialized smooth endoplasmic reticulum (Golgi complex), in which secretory products of the cell are packaged into membrane-bound organelles for transport from the perikaryon to the axon or dendrites (Figure 14–1). The sites of interneuronal communication in the CNS are termed *synapses*. Although synapses are functionally analogous to "junctions" in the somatic motor and autonomic nervous systems, central synapses contain an array of specific proteins that comprise the active zone for transmitter release and response. Like peripheral junctions, central synapses are denoted by accumulations of tiny (50- to 150-nm) *synaptic vesicles*. The proteins of these vesicles have specific roles in neurotransmitter storage, vesicle docking, and secretion and reaccumulation of neurotransmitter (see Figures 8–3 through Figures 8–6). The release of these neurotransmitters and their action on the neighboring cells via specific receptors, through mechanisms discussed in the material that follows, underlie the ability of these specialized cells to communicate with each other to dictate complex physiological actions.

Support Cells

A diverse cast of support cells outnumbers neurons in the CNS. These include neuroglia, vascular elements, the CSF-forming cells found within the intracerebral ventricular system, and the meninges that cover the surface of the brain and comprise the CSF-containing envelope. *Neuroglia* (sometimes referred to simply as *glia*) are the most abundant support cells. They are nonneuronal cells that maintain important brain functions, such as holding neurons in place, supplying oxygen and nutrients to neurons,

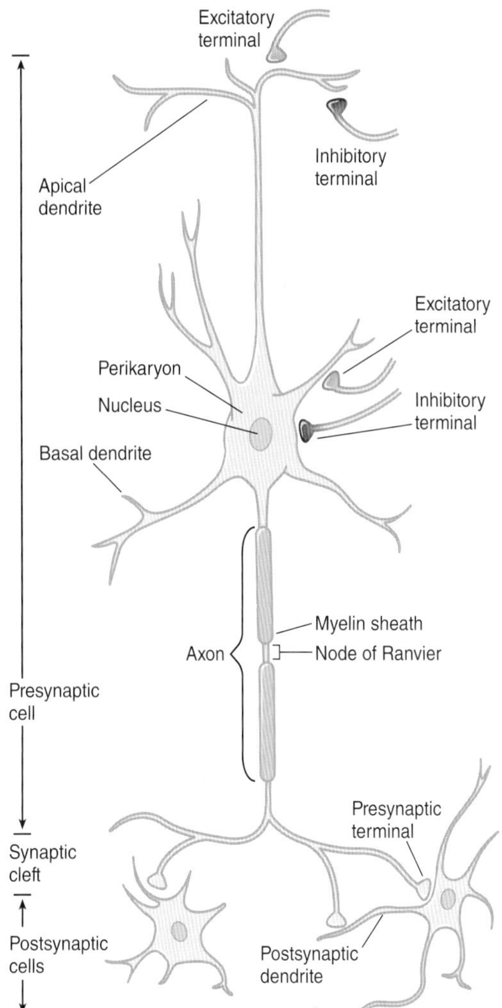

Figure 14–1 *Principal features of a neuron.* Dendrites, including apical dendrites, receive synapses from presynaptic terminals. The cell body (~50 μm in diameter) contains the nucleus and is the site of transcription and translation. The axon (0.2 to 20 μm wide, 100 μm to 2 m in length) carries information from the perikaryon to the presynaptic terminals, which form synapses (up to 1000) with the dendrites of other neurons. Axosomatic synapses also occur. Many CNS-active pharmacological agents act at the presynaptic and postsynaptic membranes of the synaptic clefts and at areas of transmitter storage near the synapses. (Adapted with permission from Kandel ER, et al., eds. *Principles of Neural Science*. 4th ed. McGraw-Hill, New York, **2000**, p. 22.)

insulating signaling between neurons, and destroying potential pathogens. Traditionally, it was thought that neuroglia acted only in a supporting role; however, newer studies have demonstrated that they may also be involved in some signaling processes.

Neuroglia are classified as either *micro-* or *macroglia*. In the CNS, the macroglia consist of astrocytes, oligodendroglia, ependymal cells, and radial glia. Astrocytes (cells interposed between the vasculature and the neurons) are the most abundant of these and often surround individual compartments of synaptic complexes. They play a variety of metabolic support roles, including furnishing energy intermediates, anchoring neurons to their blood supply, and regulating the external environment of the neuron by active removal of neurotransmitters and excess ions following release. The oligodendroglia produce myelin, the multilayer, compacted membranes that electrically insulate segments of axons and permit nondecremental propagation of action potentials. Ependymal

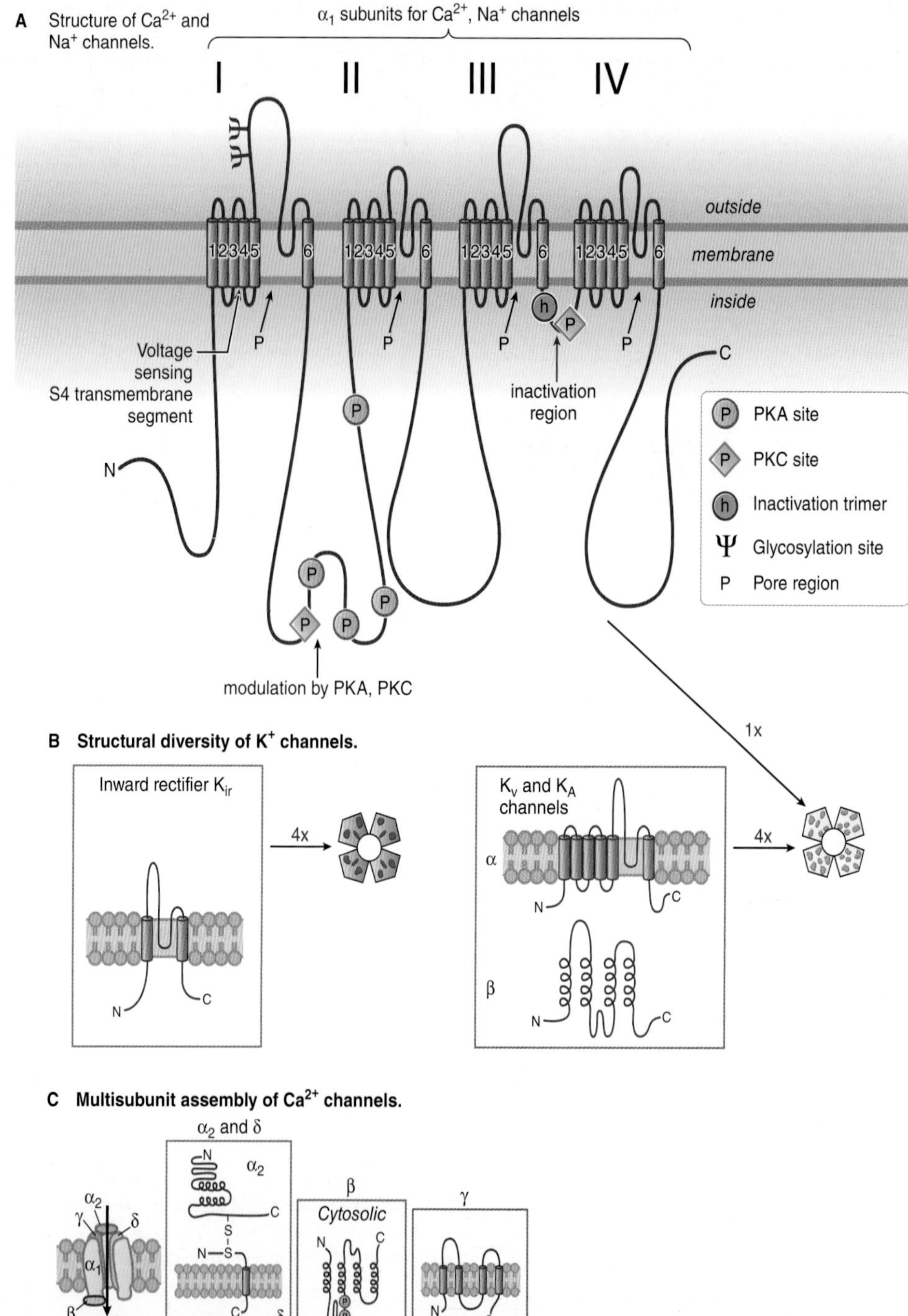

Figure 14–2 *Voltage-sensitive Na^+, Ca^{2+}, and K^+ channels.* Voltage-dependent channels provide for rapid changes in ion permeability along axons and within dendrites and for excitation-secretion coupling that releases neurotransmitters from presynaptic sites. The transmembrane Na^+ gradient (~140 mM outside vs. ~ 14 mM inside the cell) means that increases in permeability to Na^+ causes *depolarization.* In contrast, the K^+ gradient (~4 mM outside the cell vs. ~ 120 mM inside) is such that increased permeability to K^+ results in *hyperpolarization.* Changes in the concentration of intracellular Ca^{2+} (extracellular free Ca^{2+}: 1.25 mM; intracellular Ca^{2+}: resting ~ 100 nM, rising to ~ 1 μM when Ca^{2+} entry is stimulated) affects multiple processes in the cell and are critical in the release of neurotransmitters. **A.** *Structure of Ca^{2+} and Na^+ channels.* The α subunit in both Ca^{2+} and Na^+ channels consists of four sub-subunits or segments (labeled **I** through **IV**), each with six TM hydrophobic domains (blue cylinders). The hydrophobic regions that connect TM5 and TM6 in each segment associate to form the pore of the channel. Segment 4 in each domain includes the voltage sensor. (Adapted with permission from Catterall W. *Neuron* **2000**, *26*:13–25. © Elsevier.) **B.** *Structural diversity of K^+ channels. Inward rectifier, K_{ir}.* The basic subunit of the inwardly rectifying K^+ channel protein K_{ir} has the general configuration of TM5 and TM6 of a segment of the α subunit shown in panel **A.** Four of these subunits assemble to create the pore. *Voltage-sensitive K^+ channel, K_v.* The α subunits of the voltage-sensitive K^+ channel K_v and the rapidly activating K^+ channel K_A share a putative hexaspanning structure resembling in overall configuration a single segment of the Na^+ and Ca^{2+} channel structure, with six TM domains. Four of these assemble to form the pore. Regulatory β subunits (cytosolic) can alter K_v channel functions. **C.** *Multisubunit assembly of Ca^{2+} channels.* Ca^{2+} channels variably require several auxiliary small proteins (α_2, β, γ, and δ); α_2 and δ subunits are linked by a disulfide bond. Likewise, regulatory subunits also exist for Na^+ channels.

cells line the spinal cord and ventricular system and are involved in the creation of CSF, while radial cells act as neuroprogenitors and scaffolds. *Microglia* consist of specialized immune cells found within the CNS. Although the brain is immunologically protected by the BBB (see discussion that follows), these microglia act as macrophages to protect the neurons and are therefore mediators of immune response in the CNS. Microglia respond to neuronal damage and inflammation, and many diseases are associated with deficient microglia. In some instances, such as in chronic neuroinflammation, the balance between the numbers of microglia and astrocytes can determine whether there will be resulting cell damage or protection. Thus, in addition to neurons, support cells such as glia are key players in facilitating most aspects of neuronal function and CNS signaling.

Blood-Brain Barrier

The *BBB* is an important boundary separating the periphery (capillaries carrying blood) from the CNS. This barrier consists of endothelial cells, astrocytes, and pericytes on a noncellular basement membrane. The BBB prevents or diminishes unencumbered access to the brain by circulating blood components. In terms of CNS therapeutics, the BBB represents a substantial obstacle to overcome for drug delivery to the site of action. An exception exists for lipophilic molecules, which diffuse fairly freely across the BBB and accumulate in the brain. In addition to its relative impermeability to small charged molecules such as neurotransmitters, the BBB can be viewed as a combination of the partitioning of solute across the vasculature (which governs passage by definable properties such as molecular weight, charge, and lipophilicity) and the presence or absence of energy-dependent transport systems (see Chapter 5). However, the cells within the barrier also have the capacity to actively transport molecules such as glucose and amino acids that are critical for brain function (see Chapter 5). One of these transport systems that is selective for large amino acids catalyzes the movement of L-dopa across the BBB and thus contributes to the therapeutic utility of L-dopa in the treatment of Parkinson disease. Furthermore, for some compounds, including neurotransmitter metabolites such as homovanillic acid and 5-hydroxyindoleacetic acid, the acid transport system of the choroid plexus provides an important route for clearance from the brain.

Substances that rarely gain access to the brain from the bloodstream can often reach the brain when injected directly into the CSF, and, under certain therapeutic conditions, bypassing the barrier may be beneficial to permit the entry of chemotherapeutic agents. Other clinical manifestations, such as cerebral ischemia and inflammation, can also modify the BBB, thereby increasing access to substances that ordinarily would not enter the brain. The barrier is nonexistent in the peripheral nervous system and is much less prominent in the hypothalamus and several small, specialized organs (the circumventricular organs) lining the third and fourth ventricles of the brain: the median eminence, area postrema, pineal gland, subfornical organ, and subcommissural organ. Although their structure and anatomical positioning may make these areas more accessible for physiological and pharmacological modulation, overall the BBB remains a constant consideration for pharmacological access to the CNS. For a pharmacologist's view of the BBB, see The Blood-Brain Barrier: A Pharmacological View in Chapter 5.

Neuronal Excitability and Ion Channels

As noted, neurons, the primary signaling cells of the brain, release neurotransmitters in response to a rapid rise and fall in membrane potential known as an action potential. Voltage-dependent ion channels within the plasma membrane open when the membrane potential increases to a threshold value, thus regulating the electrical excitability of neurons. Action potentials are the signals by which the brain and neurons receive and transmit information to one another through pathways determined by their connectivity.

We now understand in considerable detail how three major cations, Na^+, K^+, and Ca^{2+}, as well as Cl^- anion, are regulated via their flow through highly discriminative ion channels (Figures 14–2 and 14–3). The relatively high extracellular concentration of Na^+ (~140 mM) compared to its intracellular concentration (~14 mM) means that increases in permeability to Na^+ cause cellular depolarization, ultimately leading to the generation of an action potential. In contrast, the intracellular concentration of K^+ is relatively high (~120 mM, vs. 4 mM outside the cell), and increased permeability to K^+ results in hyperpolarization. Changes in the concentration of intracellular Ca^{2+} (100 nM to 1 μM) affects multiple processes in the cell and are critical in the release of neurotransmitters. Under basal conditions, cellular homeostatic mechanisms (Na^+,K^+-ATPase; Na^+,Ca^{2+} exchanger; Ca^{2+}-ATPases; etc.) and the sequestration of releasable Ca^{2+} in storage vesicles maintain the concentrations of these ions. Electrical excitability thus generates the action potential through changes in the distribution of charged ions across the neuronal cell membrane.

The Cl^- channels are a superfamily of ion channels that are important for maintaining resting potential and are also responsible for the IPSPs that dampen neuronal excitability. In most neurons, the Cl^- gradient across the plasma membrane is inwardly driven (~116 mM outside vs. 20 mM inside the cell), and, as a result, inactivation of these channels leads to hyperexcitability. There are several families of both voltage-gated and ligand-gated Cl^- channels (Figure 14–3). Ligand-gated Cl^- channels are linked to inhibitory transmitters, including GABA and glycine (discussed in detail in material that follows). A class of secondary active transporters, the cation-chloride cotransporters, plays an essential role in establishing the electrochemical Cl^- gradient that is required for the hyperpolarizing postsynaptic inhibition mediated by both GABA receptors and glycine

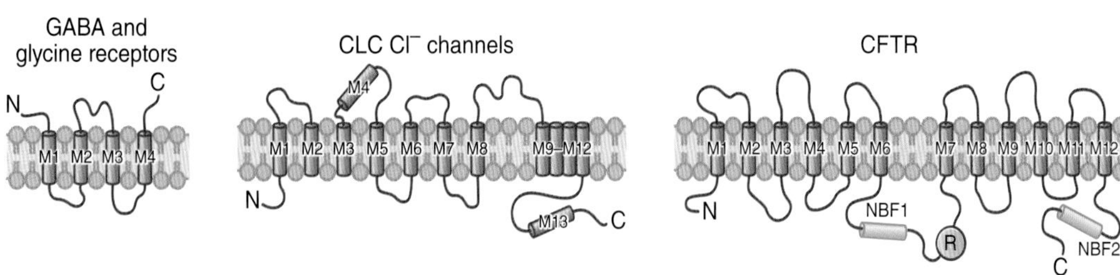

Figure 14–3 *Three families of Cl^- channels.* Due to the Cl^- gradient across the plasma membrane (~116 mM outside vs. 20 mM inside the cell), activation of Cl^- channels causes an IPSP that dampens neuronal excitability; inactivation of these channels can lead to hyperexcitability. There are three distinct types of Cl^- channel: *Ligand-gated channels* are linked to inhibitory transmitters, including GABA and glycine. *CLC Cl^- channels, of which nine subtypes have been cloned, affect Cl flux, membrane potential, and the pH of intracellular vesicles. CFTR channels bind ATP and are regulated by phosphorylation of serine residues.* M, transmembrane domains; NBF, nucleotide-binding fold; R, regulatory (phosphorylation) domain. (Reproduced with permission from Jentsch J. Chloride channels: a molecular perspective. *Curr Opin Neurobiol*, **1996**, 6:303–310. Copyright Elsevier.)

receptors. In addition, during brain development, changes in the expression of neuronal cation-chloride cotransporter isoforms can result in shifts in the direction of the chloride gradient such that activation of a ligand-gated chloride channel becomes excitatory.

The CLC family of chloride channels comprises plasma membrane channels that affect Cl^- flux and membrane potential as well as channels that function as Cl^-/H^+ antiporters. CLC members can also influence the pH of intracellular vesicles. *CFTR channels* are gated by ATP and increase the conductance of certain anions. Overall, these channels are responsible for a variety of important neurophysiological roles, including regulation of membrane potential, volume homeostasis, and regulation of pH on internal extracellular compartments.

The *CNG channels* are nonselective cation channels that regulate ion flux in neurons. CNG channels are activated as a result of cyclic nucleotide binding, and their primary function involves sensory transduction, especially in the retina and olfactory neurons. Because CNG channels are nonselective and also allow alkali ions to flow, they can result in either depolarization or hyperpolarization. These channels consist of four subunits assembled around a central pore and are subclassified into α (four genes) and β (two genes) subunits. HCN channels are another type of cyclic nucleotide-gated channel; they are nonselective, ligand-gated, cation channels that are encoded by four genes and are widely expressed in the heart and throughout the CNS. These channels open with hyperpolarization and close with depolarization; the binding of cyclic AMP or cyclic GMP to the channels shifts their activation curves to more hyperpolarized potentials. These channels play essential roles in cardiac pacemaker cells and in rhythmic and oscillatory activity in the CNS.

The *TRP channels* are a large family of about 28 ion channels that are nonselectively permeable to cations, including Na^+, Ca^{2+}, and Mg^{2+}. They are broadly grouped into six receptor subfamilies possessing six transmembrane domains containing the cation-permeable pore. These channels can have diverse modes of activation and permeation. TRP channels respond to multiple stimuli and function in sensory physiology, including thermosensation, osmosensation, and taste. Importantly, some TRP channels are also mediators of pain as they function as detectors of thermal and chemical stimuli that activate sensory neurons. Spices such as garlic, chili powder, and wasabi activate certain subtypes. Others respond to such diverse chemicals as menthol, peppermint, and camphor. Mutations in TRP channels have been associated with neurodegenerative diseases as well as cancer. The diversity of their physiology has led to their investigation as important drug targets, particularly for the treatment of chronic pain, for which they play a central role in nociception associated with inflammation and neuropathy. In recent years, TRP channels have become novel and important targets for drug development (Nilius and Szallasi, 2014).

Chemical Communication in the CNS

A central concept of neuropsychopharmacology is that drugs that improve the functional status of patients with neurological or psychiatric diseases typically act by enhancing or blunting neurotransmission in the CNS. Therapeutic targets include *ion channels* (discussed previously), which mediate changes in excitability induced by neurotransmitters; *neurotransmitter receptors*, which physiologically respond to activation by neurotransmitters; and *transport proteins*, which reaccumulate released transmitter.

Identification of Central Neurotransmitters

Neurotransmitters are endogenous chemicals in the brain that act to enable signaling across a chemical synapse. They carry, boost, and modulate signals between neurons or other cell types and act on a variety of targets to elicit a host of biological functions. An essential step in understanding the functional properties of neurotransmitters within the context of the circuitry of the brain is to identify substances that are transmitters at specific interneuronal connections. The precise number of transmitters is unknown, but more than 100 chemical messengers have been identified to date. The criteria for identification of central transmitters is similar to that used to establish the transmitters of the autonomic nervous system (see Chapter 8):

- *The transmitter must be present in the presynaptic terminals of the synapse and in the neurons from which those presynaptic terminals arise.*
- *The transmitter must be released from the presynaptic nerve concomitantly with nerve activity, and in high enough quantity to have an effect.*
- *The effects of experimental application of the putative transmitter should mimic the effects of stimulating the presynaptic pathway.*
- *If available, specific pharmacological agonists and antagonists should stimulate and block, respectively, the measured functions of the putative transmitter.*
- *There should be a mechanism present (either reuptake or enzymatic degradation) that terminates the actions of the transmitter.*

Many nerve terminals contain multiple transmitter substances and coexisting substances (presumed to be released together) that either act jointly on the postsynaptic membrane or act presynaptically to affect release of transmitter from the presynaptic terminal. In these cases, the milieu of concurrently released signaling molecules makes mimicking or fully antagonizing the action of a given transmitter substance with a single drug compound difficult. This has emphasized complexity in identifying signaling molecules that has been partially overcome using defined in vitro cell culture systems, which can then be extrapolated back to the CNS.

Cell Signaling and Synaptic Transmission

Cellular signaling links neurotransmitter receptor activation to downstream biological effects. A number of mechanisms have been identified that can be broadly classified into two main types of signaling, fast and slow neurotransmission. The most commonly seen postreceptor events are fast transmission resulting from rapid changes in ion flux through ion channels. Slow neurotransmission is primarily the role of a second major group of receptors, the GPCRs, which interact with heterotrimeric GTP-binding proteins (Figure 3–10). There are additional and distinct mechanisms of signaling for growth factor receptors (Table 3–1; Figure 3–12) and for the nuclear receptors that transduce steroid hormone signaling (Figures 3–14 and 6–13). Because the majority of cell-to-cell communication in the CNS involves chemical transmission, neurons require specialized cellular functions to mediate these actions (Figure 14–4):

- *Neurotransmitter synthesis.* Small-molecule neurotransmitters are synthesized in nerve terminals, whereas others, such as peptides, are synthesized in cell bodies and transported to nerve terminals.
- *Neurotransmitter storage.* Synaptic vesicles store transmitters, often in association with various proteins and frequently with ATP.
- *Neurotransmitter release.* Release of stored transmitter from the storage vesicle into the synaptic cleft occurs by exocytosis. Depolarization of the presynaptic neuron results in a complex initiation of stimulus-secretion coupling, which involves vesicle docking at the plasma membrane, the formation of membrane fusion/release complexes, and the Ca^{2+}-dependent release of vesicular contents. Recycling of the transmitter storage vesicle generally follows. For details, see Figures 8–4 through 8–6.
- *Neurotransmitter recognition.* Neurotransmitters diffuse from sites of release and bind selectively to receptor proteins to initiate intracellular signal transduction events within the postsynaptic cell.
- *Termination of action.* A variety of mechanisms terminate the action of synaptically released transmitters, including diffusion from the synapse, enzymatic inactivation (for ACh and peptides), and uptake into neurons or glial cells by specific transporters.

Fast Neurotransmission

Responses to activation of receptors consisting of an ion channel as part of its structure tend to be rapid (milliseconds) because the effects are direct and generally do not require multiple steps leading to second-messenger generation and activation of a signaling pathway. In fast neurotransmission (also called directly gated transmission), neurotransmitters bind

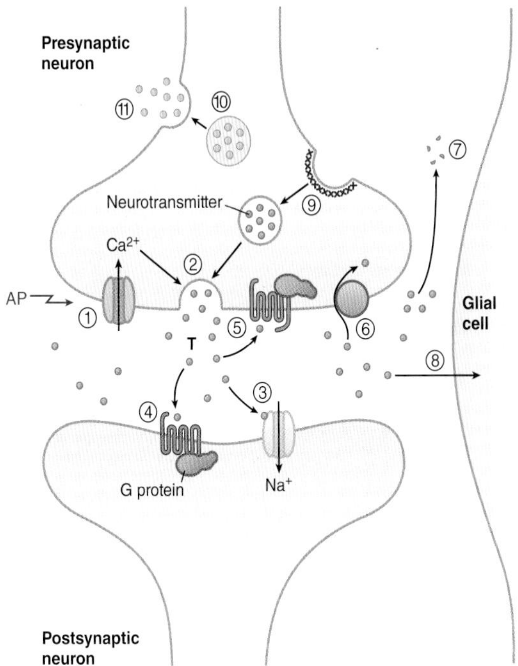

Figure 14–4 *Transmitter release, action, and inactivation.* Depolarization opens voltage-dependent Ca^{2+} channels in the presynaptic nerve terminal (1). The influx of Ca^{2+} during an action potential (AP) triggers (2) the exocytosis of small synaptic vesicles that store neurotransmitter (**T**). Released neurotransmitter interacts with receptors in the postsynaptic membranes that either couple directly with ion channels (3) or act through second messengers, such as GPCRs (4). Neurotransmitter receptors in the presynaptic nerve terminal membrane (5) can inhibit or enhance subsequent exocytosis. Released neurotransmitter is inactivated by reuptake into the nerve terminal by (6) a transport protein coupled to the Na^+ gradient (e.g., for DA, NE, or GABA); by (7) degradation (ACh, peptides); or by (8) uptake and metabolism by glial cells (glutamate). The synaptic vesicle membrane is recycled by (9) clathrin-mediated endocytosis. Neuropeptides and proteins are sometimes stored in (10) larger, dense core granules within the nerve terminal. These dense core granules can be released from sites (11) distinct from active zones after repetitive stimulation.

directly to ligand-gated ion channels on the postsynaptic membrane to rapidly open the channel and change the permeability of the postsynaptic site, leading to depolarization or hyperpolarization. Depolarization results in continuation of the nerve impulse, while hyperpolarization leads to diminished signaling (see Figure 11–5). Ligand-gated ion channels mediating fast transmission (also called ionotropic receptors) consist of multiple subunits, each usually having four transmembrane domains that associate to form pentameric receptors (Figure 14–5). Receptors with this structure include the receptors for the amino acids GABA, glycine, glutamate, and aspartate; the serotonin $5HT_3$ receptor; and the nicotinic ACh receptor. The nicotinic ACh receptor provides a good example of receptor structure and how subunit composition varies with anatomic location and affects function (Figure 14–6).

Slow Neurotransmission

Slower transmission (although still relatively fast, often on a time scale of seconds) is mediated by neurotransmitters that do not bind to ion channels but to receptors with a very different architecture called metabotropic receptors. Upon activation, these receptors generate second messengers. This major group of receptors consists of the membrane heptaspanning GPCRs (Figure 3–9). There are more than 825 human GPCRs, which can be classified into five major families: rhodopsin (class A); secretin (class B); adhesion; glutamate (class C); and frizzled. The GPCRs in the CNS are largely in the rhodopsin family. These receptors have sites for N-linked glycosylation on the extracellular amino tail and sometimes on the second extracellular loop. There are also multiple potential sites for phosphorylation on the third intracellular loop and the carboxyl tail, and some members of this class are palmitoylated on the carboxyl tail. Phosphorylation can regulate GPCR-G protein–effector coupling and provide docking sites for arrestins and other scaffolding proteins (see Chapter 3).

The GPCRs are associated with a broad spectrum of physiological effects, including activation of K^+ channels, activation of PLC-IP_3-Ca^{2+} pathways and regulation of adenylyl cyclase activity and downstream systems affected by cyclic AMP (multiple isoforms of PKA, EPAC, HCN, CNG, and PDE). These effects are typically mediated through the activation of specific G proteins, each a heterotrimer of α, β, and γ subunits where the β and γ units are constitutively associated. The GTP-binding α subunits can modulate the activities of numerous effectors (e.g., adenylyl cyclase, PLC). The βγ subunits are also active in mediating signaling, especially in the regulation of ion channels. Table 14–1 shows examples of the variety of physiological functions mediated by G proteins. G protein activation-inactivation signaling dynamics are described in Chapter 3. Notably, GPCRs can also signal to downstream pathways through other intermediary proteins, such as the β arrestins (Shukla et al., 2011). Drugs targeting GPCRs represent a core of modern medicine and make up as much as 40% of all pharmaceuticals.

Termination of Neurotransmitter Action

Mechanisms to terminate the actions of released neurotransmitters are essential for maintaining the balance of neuronal signaling. There are two primary mechanisms for terminating the signaling of released transmitters. One is the conversion of the transmitter into an inactive compound via an enzymatic reaction. The best example of enzymatic inactivation is for the transmitter ACh, which, after activating the receptor, is hydrolyzed by acetylcholinesterase to choline and acetate. A second mechanism involves the clearance of the neurotransmitter by transport proteins present on presynaptic neurons, neighboring glial cells, and other neurons so that it can no longer act on the target receptors. In addition to these, slow diffusion of the transmitter away from the synapse and subsequent degradation also play a role for both conventional neurotransmitters and neuropeptides.

Neurons and glial cells express specific transporter proteins, such as those for the monoamines NE (NET), serotonin (SERT) and DA (DAT), which remove NE, 5HT, and DA, respectively, from the extracellular space by transporting it back into the presynaptic neuron (see Chapters 5, 8, and 13). These plasma membrane carriers serve as a major mechanism for limiting the extent and duration of neurotransmitter signaling. To accomplish this task, they couple the movement of neurotransmitters to the influx of Na^+, which provides a strong thermodynamic driving force for inward transport. The carriers for NE, 5HT, DA, GABA, and glycine have 12 hydrophobic membrane-spanning domains with their amino and carboxy termini located within the cytoplasm (Figure 14–8). These transporters are generally glycosylated along the large (second) extracellular loop and possess sites of phosphorylation and binding to intracellular regulatory proteins, primarily on their amino and carboxy tails.

A second family of plasma membrane neurotransmitter transporters mediates the clearance of glutamate and aspartate released during synaptic transmission. In humans, five subtypes of glutamate transporters (referred to as EAATs 1–5) clear glutamate into neurons and glial cells. The two glial carriers, EAATs 1 and 2, are responsible for the bulk of glutamate transport activity in the CNS and are critical for limiting the excitotoxic actions of glutamate described further in this chapter. These transporters have eight transmembrane domains (TM1–8) and two reentrant hairpin loops (HP1 and HP2) that appear to serve as intracellular and extracellular gates during the transport process (Figure 14–9). EAATs are members of the solute carrier family (SLC1A 1–3, 6, and 7) and are powered by Na^+ and other cations running down their electrochemical gradients.

There are also at least three distinct gene families of vesicular neurotransmitter transporters that sequester the neurotransmitters within synaptic

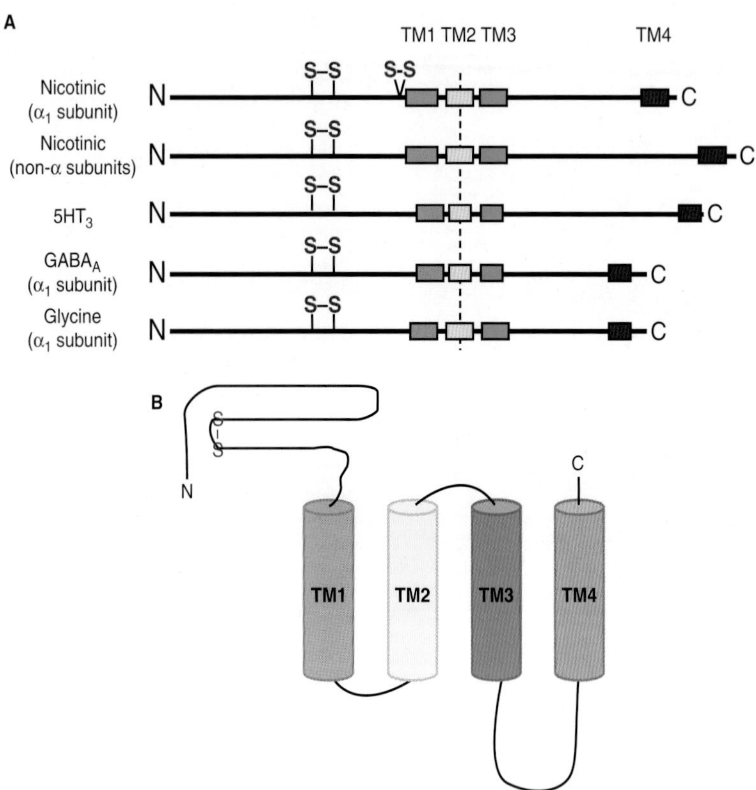

Figure 14–5 *Pentameric ligand-gated ion channels.* The subunits of these channels, which mediate fast synaptic transmission, are embedded in the plasma membrane to form a roughly cylindrical structure with a central pore. In response to binding of transmitter, the receptor proteins change conformation; the channel gate opens, and ions diffuse along their concentration gradient across the membrane through a hydrophilic opening in the otherwise-hydrophobic membrane. **A.** *Subunit organization.* For each subunit of these pentameric receptors, the amino terminal region of ~ 210 amino acids is extracellular. It is followed by four hydrophobic regions that span the membrane (TM1–TM4); a small carboxyl terminus is on the extracellular surface. The TM2 region is α helical, and TM2 regions from each subunit line the internal pore of the pentameric receptor. Two disulfide loops at positions 128–142 and 192–193 are found in the α subunit of the nicotinic receptor. The 128–142 motif is conserved in the family of pentameric receptors; the vicinal cysteines at 192–193 occur only in α subunit of the nicotinic receptor. **B.** *Schematic rendering of a nicotinic ACh non–α subunit.* Five such subunits form a pentameric receptor. See Figure 14–6 for an example.

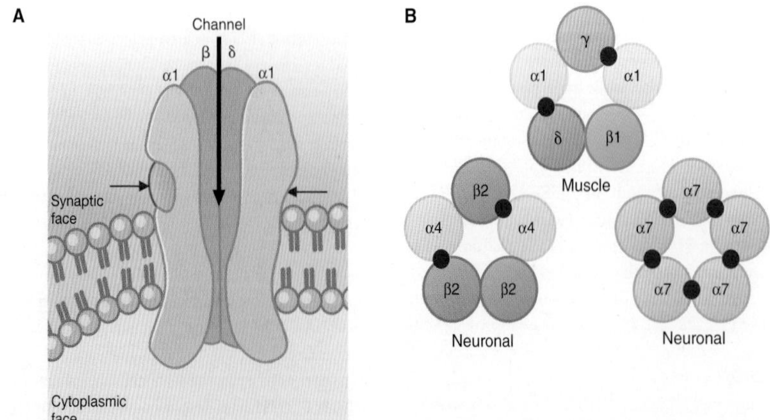

Figure 14–6 *Subunit arrangement: the nicotinic ACh receptor.* **A.** *Longitudinal view of receptor schematic with the γ subunit removed.* The remaining subunits, two copies of α, one of β, and one of δ, are shown to surround an internal channel with an outer vestibule and its constriction located deep in the membrane bilayer region. Spans of α helices with slightly bowed structures form the perimeter of the channel and come from the TM2 region of the linear sequence (Figure 14–5). ACh-binding sites, indicated by red arrows, occur at the αγ and αδ (not visible) interfaces. **B.** *Nicotinic receptor subunit arrangements.* Agonist-binding sites (red circles) occur at α subunit–containing interfaces. At least 17 functional receptor isoforms have been observed in vivo, with different ligand specificity, relative Ca^{2+}/Na^{+} permeability, and physiological function determined by their subunit composition. The only isoform found at the neuromuscular junction is shown for comparison. The neuronal receptor isoforms found at autonomic ganglia and in the CNS are homomeric or heteromeric pentamers of α (α2–α10) and β (β2–β4) subunits.

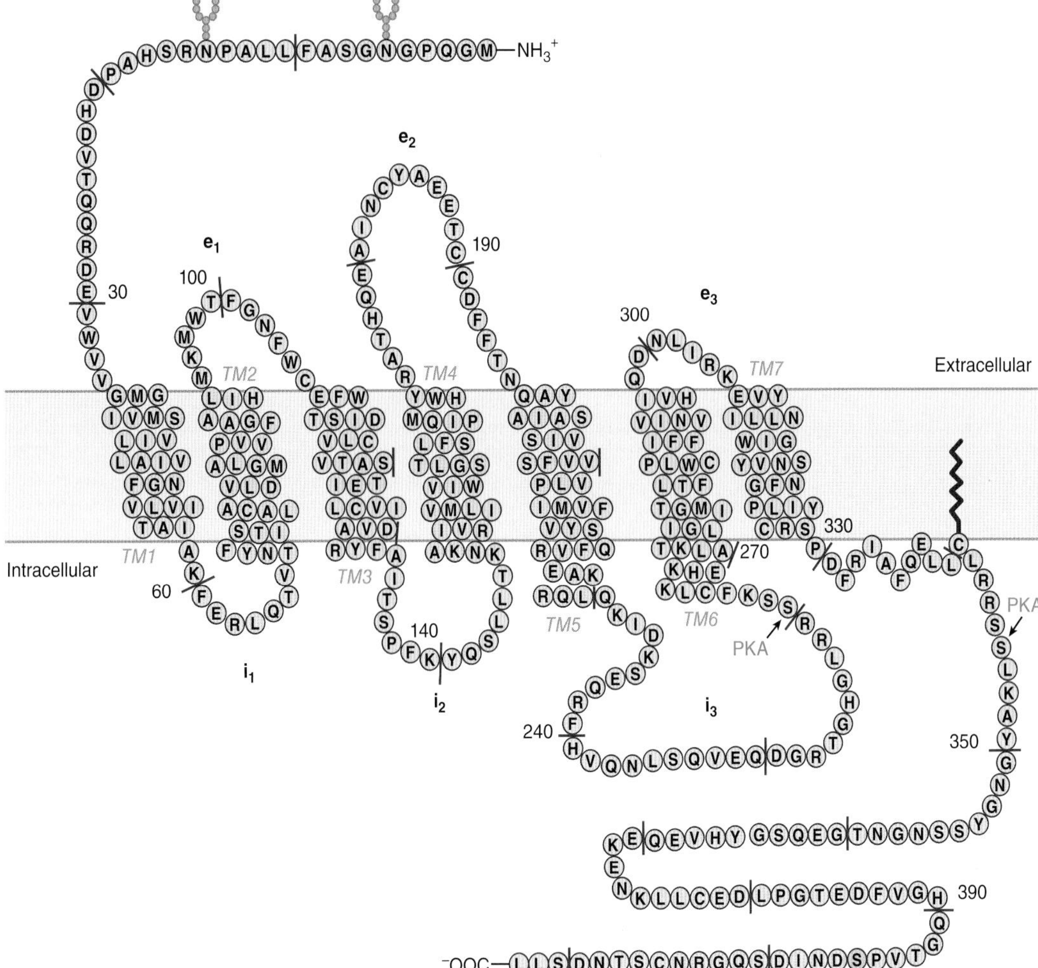

Figure 14–7 *The β adrenergic receptor as a model for GPCRs.* This two-dimensional model illustrates features common to most GPCRs. Red lines mark segments with 10 amino acids. The amino terminus (N) is extracellular, and the carboxyl terminus (C) is intracellular; in between are seven hydrophobic TM domains and alternating intracellular and extracellular loops (e_{1-3} and i_{1-3}). Glycosylation sites are found near the N terminus; consensus sites for phosphorylation by PKA (arrows) are found in the i_3 loop and the carboxyl terminal tail. An aspartate residue in TM3 (asp^{113}) interacts with the nitrogen of catecholamine agonists while two serines (ser^{204}, ser^{207}) in TM5 interact with the hydroxyl groups on the phenyl ring of catecholamine agonists. A cysteine residue (cys^{341}) is a substrate for palmitoylation. Interaction of the palmitoyl group with membrane lipids reduces the flexibility of the carboxyl tail. (Reproduced with permission from Rasmussen SGF et al. Crystal structure of the human β2 adrenergic G-protein-coupled receptor. *Nature*, **2007**, *450*:383. Copyright © 2007.)

vesicles for storage and, ultimately, for release during neuronal signaling. These include VMAT1, VMAT2, and VAChT (see Chapter 8), a vesicular carrier for both GABA and glycine (VGAT), and three vesicular glutamate carriers, VGLUT1, VGLUT2, and VGLUT3. These transporters ensure that vesicles fill rapidly during neurotransmission and provide a means for reducing cytoplasmic concentrations of neurotransmitter in areas where rates of reuptake are high. The driving force for vesicular uptake of neurotransmitter by these transporters is a proton electrochemical gradient across the membrane of the storage vesicle (vesicle interior more acidic than the cytosol).

The monoamine transporters DAT, NET, and SERT are well-established targets for therapeutic antidepressants and for addictive drugs, including cocaine and amphetamines. Selective inhibitors of these carriers can increase the duration and spatial extent of the actions of neurotransmitters. Inhibitors of the uptake of NE or 5HT are used to treat depression and other behavioral disorders, as described in Chapters 15 and 16. The psychostimulants methylphenidate and amphetamine are the major drugs used to treat ADHD in children and in adults. Although the two drugs have stimulant actions in healthy individuals, in patients with ADHD they reduce hyperactivity and increase attention by inhibiting DAT and NET and enhancing DA and NE neurotransmission. Transporters are discussed in further detail in Chapters 5, 8, and 13.

Central Neurotransmitters

Neurotransmitters can be classified by chemical structure into various categories, including *amino acids, ACh, monoamines, neuropeptides, purines, lipids,* and even *gases.* This section describes each category and examines some prominent members.

Amino Acids

The CNS contains high concentrations of certain amino acids, notably glutamate and GABA, that potently alter neuronal firing. They are ubiquitously distributed within the brain and produce rapid and readily reversible effects on neurons. The dicarboxylic amino acids glutamate and aspartate produce excitation, while the monocarboxylic amino acids GABA, glycine, β-alanine, and taurine cause inhibition. Following the emergence of selective agonists and antagonists, the identification of pharmacologically distinct amino acid receptor subtypes became possible

TABLE 14–1 ■ HETEROTRIMERIC G PROTEIN SUBUNITS

FAMILY	α SUBUNITS	SIGNALS TRANSDUCED
Family members		
G_s family		
G_s	α_s	Activation of AC
G_{olf}	α_{olf}	Activation of AC
G_i family		
G_{i}/G_o	α_i, α_o	Inhibition of AC
G_z	α_z	Inhibition of AC
G_{gust}	α_{gust}	Activation of PDE6
G_t	α_t	Activation of PDE6
G_q family		
G_q	α_q, α_{11}, α_{14}, α_{15}, α_{16}	Activation of PLC
$G_{12/13}$ family		
$G_{12/13}$	α_{12}, α_{13}	Activation of Rho GTPases
βγ Subunits[a] (acting as a heterodimer)		
G_β	β1, β2, β3, β4, β5	↓ AC, ↑ Ca^{2+} and K^+ channels, ↑ PI3K, ↑ PLC_β, ↑AC2 and AC4, ↑ Ras-dependent MAPK activation, ↑ recruitment of GRK2 and GRK3
G_γ	γ1, γ2, γ3, γ4, γ5, γ7, γ8, γ9, γ10, γ11, γ12, γ13	

[a]Khan and colleagues (2013) have reviewed the expanding roles of the βγ subunits.

(see discussion that follows). Figure 14–10 shows these amino acid transmitters and their drug congeners.

Gamma-Aminobutyric Acid

GABA is the main inhibitory neurotransmitter in the CNS. GABA is synthesized in the brain from the Krebs cycle intermediate α-ketoglutarate, which is transaminated to glutamate by GABA-T. GABA is subsequently formed from glutamate by the enzyme GAD; the presence of GAD in a neuron therefore delineates a neuron that uses GABA as a transmitter. Interestingly, intraneuronal GABA is also inactivated by GABA-T which converts it to succinic semialdehyde, but only in the presence of adequate α-ketoglutarate. This GABA shunt or cycle serves to maintain levels of GABA; thus, GABA-T is both a synthetic and a degradative enzyme (Brady et al., 2012). There is a vesicular GABA transporter (VGAT, SLC32A1, a member of the amino acid/polyamine transporter family) that is involved in storing GABA in vesicles for subsequent release into the synaptic cleft. The action of GABA is primarily terminated by reuptake by one of four different GATs present on both neurons and glia. GABA acts by binding to and activating specific ionotropic or metabotropic receptors on both pre- and postsynaptic membranes. *$GABA_A$ receptors* (the most prominent GABA receptor subtype) are ionotropic, ligand-gated Cl^- channels. The *$GABA_B$ receptors* are metabotropic GPCRs. One subtype formerly known as the *$GABA_C$ receptor* is now classified as a type of $GABA_A$ receptor.

The *$GABA_A$ receptors* have been extensively characterized as important drug targets and are the site of action of many neuroactive drugs, notably benzodiazepines (such as valium), barbiturates, ethanol, anesthetic steroids, and volatile anesthetics, among others. These drugs are used to treat various neuropsychiatric disorders, including epilepsy, Huntington disease, addictions, sleep disorders, and more. As ligand-gated ion channels, $GABA_A$ receptors are pentamers of subunits that each contain four transmembrane domains and assemble around a central anion-specific pore (Figures 14–5 and 14–6). The major forms of the $GABA_A$ receptor contain at least three different types of subunits: α, β, and γ, with a likely stoichiometry of 2α, 2β, and 1γ. The IUPHAR/BPS recognizes 19 unique subunits that are known to form at least 11 native $GABA_A$ receptors that can be pharmacologically differentiated. The particular combination of α and γ subunits can affect the efficacy of benzodiazepine binding and channel modulation. Many drugs, such as those noted, act as positive allosteric modulators of the $GABA_A$ receptor, that is, act at sites distinct from the GABA-binding site to positively modulate the function of the receptor (Figure 14–11). The interaction of these drugs with the $GABA_A$ receptor and their therapeutic use are discussed further in Chapter 17.

The *$GABA_B$ receptors* are metabotropic GPCRs that function as obligate heterodimers of two subunits named $GABA_{B1}$ and $GABA_{B2.}$ $GABA_B$ receptors are widespread in the CNS and regulate both pre- and postsynaptic activity. These receptors interact with G_i to inhibit adenylyl cyclase, activate K^+ channels, and reduce Ca^{2+} conductance and interact with G_q to enhance PLC activity. Presynaptic $GABA_B$ receptors function as autoreceptors, inhibiting GABA release, and may play the same role on neurons releasing other transmitters. A number of $GABA_B$ agonists have been identified, including baclofen (Figure 14–10), which is a skeletal muscle relaxant, and the psychoactive drug GHB, which is sometimes used to treat narcolepsy but is also used recreationally as an intoxicant.

Glycine

Glycine is an amino acid normally incorporated into proteins that can also act as an inhibitory neurotransmitter, particularly in the spinal cord and brainstem. Glycine is synthesized primarily from serine by serine hydroxymethyltransferase (SHMT). Glycine is imported into synaptic vesicles by a vesicular transport system identical to that used by GABA (VGAT). The action of glycine in the synaptic cleft is terminated by reuptake through specific transporters (GLYT1 and GLYT2) located on presynaptic nerve terminals and glia cells. These transporters can be distinguished pharmacologically and present attractive therapeutic targets for the modulation of glycine levels.

Actions of glycine are an active area of research, especially considering that there are glycine-binding sites on NMDA receptors. Glycine acts as a coagonist at NMDA receptors, such that both glutamate and glycine must be present for activation to occur (see discussion that follows). In addition to the NMDA receptor site, there are specific ionotropic glycine receptors that contain many of the structural features described for other ligand-gated ion channels (pentamers of subunits containing four transmembrane domains). These function as hyperpolarizing Cl^- channels and are prominent in the brainstem and spinal cord. Multiple subunits (currently four known α subunits and a single β subunit) can assemble into a variety of glycine receptor subtypes. Taurine and β-alanine are agonists of glycine receptors; strychnine, a potent convulsant, is a selective antagonist (Figure 14–10).

Glutamate

Glutamate and aspartate are dicarboxylate amino acid neurotransmitters with excitatory actions in the CNS. Both amino acids are found in high concentrations in the brain and have powerful excitatory effects on neurons in virtually every region of the CNS. Glutamate is the most abundant excitatory neurotransmitter and the principal fast excitatory neurotransmitter. Glutamate acts though receptors that are classified as either *ligand-gated ion channels (ionotropic)* or *metabotropic GPCRs* (Table 14–2). A well-characterized phenomenon involving glutamate transmission is the induction of LTP and its converse, LTD. These phenomena are known for strengthening and changing synapses and have long been hypothesized to be an important mechanism in learning and memory.

Ionotropic glutamate receptors are ligand-gated ion channels that were historically divided into three classes, each named for its preferred synthetic ligand (Figure 14–10): NMDA receptors, AMPA receptors, and KA receptors. With the discovery of an increasing number of subunits comprising these receptor categories, this classification has recently been refined (see Table 14–2).

The *NMDA receptors* consist of heteromers that are made up of multiple subunit combinations (termed GluN*x*) with the minimal receptor being a dimer of the GluN1 subunit and a GluN2 subunit. However, more complex heteromeric complexes are generated incorporating multiple

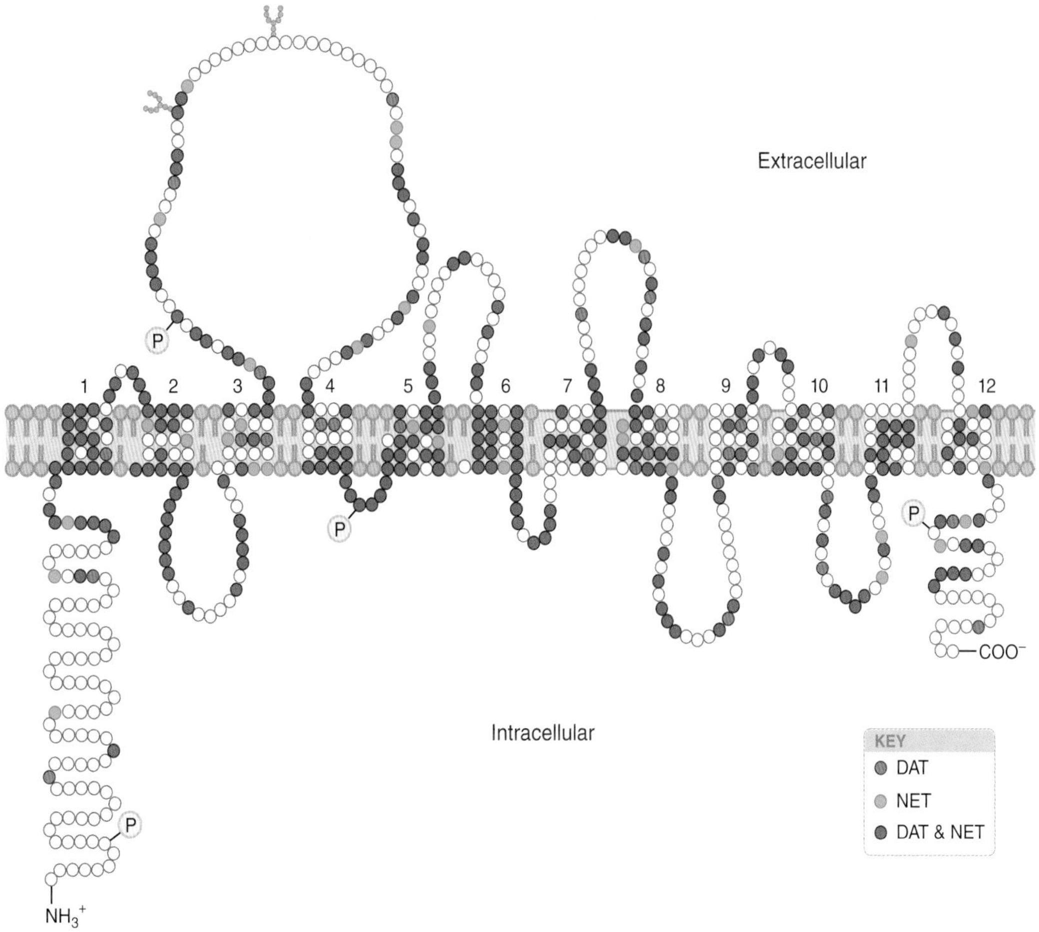

Extracellular

Intracellular

KEY
DAT
NET
DAT & NET

Figure 14–8 *Structure of the rat 5HT transport protein.* Both the N terminus (NH_3^+) and C terminus (COO^-) are intracellular. These proteins typically have 12 hydrophobic, membrane-spanning domains with intervening extracellular and intracellular loops. The second extracellular loop is the largest and contains several potential glycosylation sites (indicated with tree-like symbols). Amino acid residues that are homologous to those in the DAT and the NET are colored, as noted. The most highly conserved regions of these transporters are located in the transmembrane domains; the most divergent areas occur in the N and C termini. (Used with permission from Dr. Beth J. Hoffman, Vertex Pharmaceuticals, San Diego, CA.)

subunits. The NMDA receptors have relatively high permeability to Ca^{2+} and are blocked by Mg^{2+} in a voltage-dependent manner. These receptors are unique in that their activation requires the simultaneous binding of two different agonists: In addition to glutamate, glycine binding appears necessary for activation (Figure 14–12). While NMDA receptors are involved in normal synaptic transmission, their activation is more closely associated with the induction of various forms of synaptic plasticity rather than fast point-to-point signaling in the brain. Aspartate is also a selective NMDA receptor agonist. Other NMDA receptor ligands include open-channel blockers such as PCP ("angel dust"); antagonists include 5,7-dichlorokynurenic acid, which acts at an allosteric glycine-binding site, and ifenprodil, which selectively inhibits NMDA receptors containing GluN2B subunits. The activity of NMDA receptors is sensitive to pH and to modulation by a variety of endogenous agents, including Zn^{2+}, some neurosteroids, arachidonic acid, redox reagents, and polyamines such as spermine.

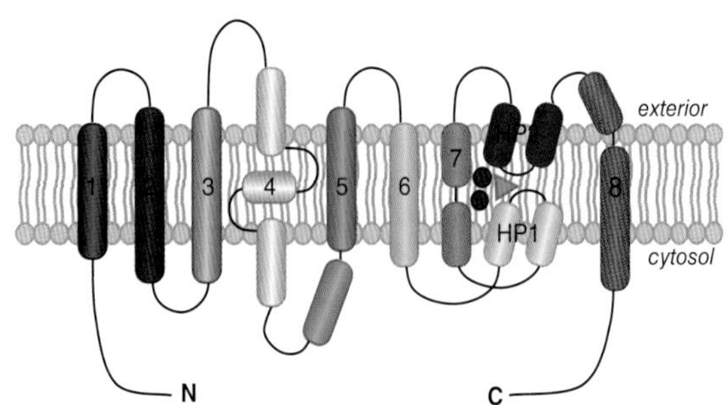

Figure 14–9 *General model of the mammalian EAATs.* The EAAT family includes the plasma membrane transporters EAAT1 to EAAT5. In this schematic model, transmembrane domains (colored oblongs) are labeled 1–8. Approximate binding sites occupied by Na^+ (blue dots) and substrate (green triangle) are formed by the nonhelical segments at the tips of two hairpin loops, HP1 and HP2.

The *AMPA receptors* exist predominantly as heterotetramers and contain multiple subunits (termed GluA*x*) as indicated in Table 14–2. In addition, there are TARPs that, together with a variety of scaffolding and regulatory proteins, modulate channel properties and alter the trafficking of receptors to and from perisynaptic and postsynaptic regions. AMPA receptors open and close rapidly, making them well suited to mediate the vast majority of excitatory synaptic transmission in the brain. Like NMDA receptors, AMPA receptors are involved in synaptic plasticity. They can be selectively antagonized by NBQX and CNQX, and similar antagonists are being explored as neuroprotective drugs for the treatment of stroke.

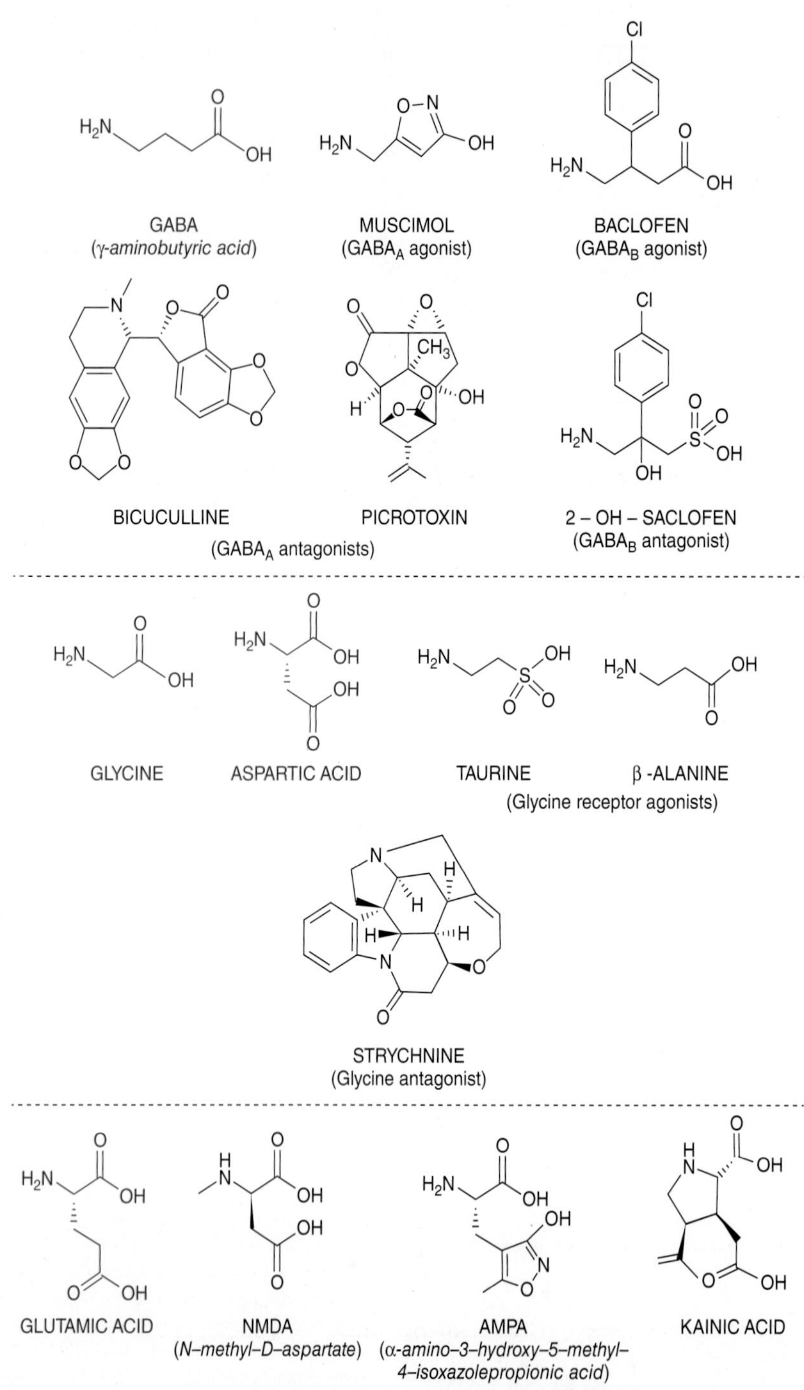

Figure 14–10 *Amino acid transmitters (red) and congeners (black).*

The *KA receptors* are composed of a distinct array of subunits (termed GluK*x*) that assemble as homo- or heterotetramers to form functional receptors. An important difference between KA and AMPA receptors is that KA receptors require extracellular Na^+ and Cl^- for activation. KA receptors differ functionally from AMPA and NMDA receptors in other important ways. KA receptors do not reside predominantly within postsynaptic signaling complexes and are positioned to modulate neuronal excitability and synaptic transmission by altering the likelihood that the postsynaptic cell will fire in response to subsequent stimulation. Presynaptic KA receptors have also been implicated in modulating GABA release through presynaptic mechanisms.

Glutamate-mediated excitotoxicity may underlie the damage that occurs when ischemia or hypoglycemia in the brain leads to a massive release and impaired reuptake of glutamate, resulting in excess stimulation of glutamate receptors and subsequent cell death. The cascade of events leading to neuronal death is thought to be triggered by excessive activation of NMDA or AMPA/KA receptors, allowing significant influx of Ca^{2+} into neurons (Figure 14–13). NMDA receptor

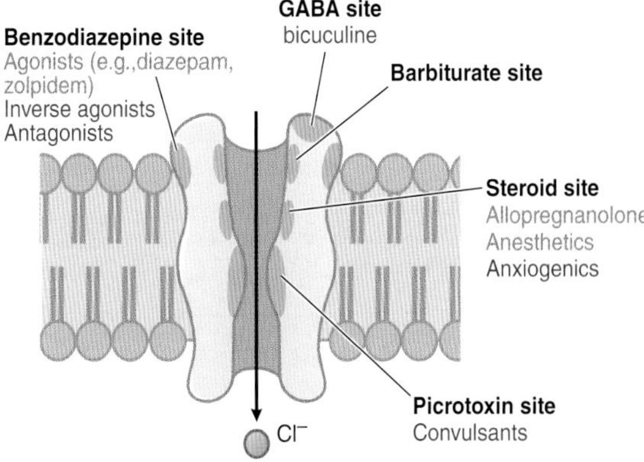

Figure 14–11 *Pharmacologic binding sites on the $GABA_A$ receptor.* GABA binds at the orthosteric site on the $GABA_A$ receptor. Other sites noted are allosteric sites at which agonists and antagonists may promote (green) or inhibit (red) receptor function. The $GABA_A$ receptor is a member of the Cys-loop family (Figure 11–1) but has a larger number of cavities in the transmembrane region and is susceptible to fewer natural toxins than several other family members. Miller and Smart (2010) have reviewed the features of this receptor and other Cys-loop receptors that contribute to orthosteric and allosteric modulation of receptor function. Hibbs and colleagues (Hibbs and Gouax, 2011; Morales-Perez et al, 2016) have recently provided structural data that suggest the mechanisms of activation, desensitization, and ion permeation in a Cys-loop receptor. Yamaura and colleagues (2016) have described a rapid screening procedure for putative allosteric modulators of the $GABA_A$ receptor.(Modified with permission from Nestler EJ et al., eds. *Molecular Neuropharmacology*. 3rd ed. McGraw-Hill, New York, **2015**.)

antagonists can attenuate neuronal cell death induced by activation of these receptors. Glutamate receptors have become targets for diverse therapeutic interventions. For example, disordered glutamatergic transmission may play a role in the etiology of chronic neurodegenerative diseases (Chapter 18).

The *mGluRs* are GPCRs structurally defined by the presence of a large glutamate-binding N-terminal (extracellular) domain of about 560 amino acids. There are eight unique mGluRs organized into three subgroups (Table 14–2). mGluRs bind glutamate and function to "fine-tune" excitatory and inhibitory transmission by presynaptic, postsynaptic, and glial mechanisms, including the modulation of release and signaling of other neurotransmitters, among which are GABA, purines, DA, 5HT, and neuropeptides. Group I mGluRs couple to G_q, while groups II and III couple to G_i/G_o. mGluRs are located in a variety of brain regions and sometimes are linked to opposing functional responses. In general, group I receptors increase neuronal excitability, whereas both group II and group III suppress excitability. mGluRs play roles in the modulation of other receptors, function in synaptic plasticity, and are linked to several neurological diseases. They have recently become important drug targets, as subtype-selective agents are being discovered and investigated as potential therapies for various neuropsychiatric disorders.

Acetylcholine

Acetylcholine is present throughout the nervous system and functions as a neurotransmitter. It was the first neurotransmitter discovered and plays a primary role in the autonomic nervous system in ganglionic transmission as well as the peripheral nervous system, where it is the main neurotransmitter at the neuromuscular junction in vertebrates. ACh is synthesized by choline acetyltransferase and stored in the nerve endings. Following release and receptor activation, it is degraded by acetylcholinesterase (see Chapters 8–11). The effects of ACh result from interaction with two broad classes of receptors: ionotropic ligand-gated ion channels termed nicotinic receptors and metabotropic GPCRs called muscarinic receptors. In the CNS, ACh is found primarily in interneurons. The degeneration of particular cholinergic pathways is a hallmark of Alzheimer disease.

Nicotinic ACh receptors are found in skeletal muscle (see Figures 11–1 and 11–2) as well as in autonomic ganglia, the adrenal gland, and the CNS. Their activation by ACh results in a rapid increase in the influx of Na^+, depolarization, and the influx of Ca^{2+}. Nicotinic receptors are pentamers consisting of various combinations of 17 known subunits that can

TABLE 14–2 ■ CLASSIFICATION OF GLUTAMATE RECEPTORS

FAMILY	SUBTYPE	AGONISTS	ANTAGONISTS	
Ionotropic				
NMDA	GluN1, GluN2A, GluN2B, GluN2C, GluN2D, GluN3A, GluN3B	NMDA, aspartate	D-AP5, 2R-CPPene, MK-801, ketamine, phenycylidine, D-aspartate	
AMPA	GluA1, GluA2, GluA3, GluA4	AMPA, kainate, (s)-5-fluorowillardiine	CNQX, NBQX, GYK153655	
Kainate	GluK1, GluK2, GluK3, GluK4, GluK5	Kainate, ATPA, LY-339,434, SYM-2081, 5-iodowillardiine	CNQX, LY294486	
Metabotropic				
				SIGNALING
Group I	$mGlu_1$, $mGlu_5$	3,5-DHPG, quisqualate	AIDA S-(+)-CBPG	Activation of PLC (Gq)
Group II	$mGlu_2$, $mGlu_3$	APDC, MGS0028 DCG-IV, LY354740	EGLU PCCG-4	Inhibition of AC (Gi/Go)
Group III	$mGlu_4$, $mGlu_6$, $mGlu_7$, $mGlu_8$	L-AP4, (RS)-PPG	CPPG, MPPG, MSOP, LY341495	Inhibition of AC (Gi/Go)

AIDA, 1-aminoindan-1,5-dicarboxylic acid; AMPA, α-amino-3-hydroxy-5-methyl-4-isoxazolepropionic acid; L-AP4, L-2-amino-4-phosphonobutiric acid; ATPA, 2-amino-3(3-hydroxy-5-tert-butylisoxa-zol-4-yl)propanoic acid; CBPG, (S)-(+)-2-(3-carboxybicyclo(1.1.1)pentyl)-glycine; CNQX, 6-cyano-7-nitroquinoxaline-2,3-dione; D-AP5, D-2-amino-5-phosphonovaleric acid; DCG-IV, (2S,2'R,3'R)-2-(2',3'-Dicarboxycyclopropyl)glycine; (S)-3,4-DCPG, (S)-3,4-dicarboxyphenylglycine; 3,5-DHPG, 3,5-dihydroxyphenylglycine; EGLU, (2S)-α-ethylglutamic acid; MPPG, (RS)-α-methyl-4-phosphonophenylglycine; MSOP, (RS)-α-methylserine-O-phosphate; NBQX, 1,2,3,4-tetrahydro-6-nitro-2,3-dioxo-benzo[f]quinoxaline-7-sulfonamide; NMDA, *N*-methyl-D-aspartate; PCCG-4, phenylcarboxycyclopropylglycine; (RS)-PPG, (RS)-4-phosphonophenylglycine.

Glutamate is the principal agonist at both ionotropic and metabotropic receptors for glutamate and aspartate.

SECTION II NEUROPHARMACOLOGY

Glycine site
Glycine
D-Serine
D-Cycloserine
5-7 dichlorokyurenate
Glutamate site
NMDA
D-aminophosphonopentanoate
Na+
Ca++
S
S
Redox-sensitive site
exterior
H+ site
Polyamine site
spermine
naphthyl acetyl spermine
Mg++
plasma membrane
Zn++
PCP site
phencyclidine
ketamine
MK801
cytosol
P P
Modulation by protein kinases

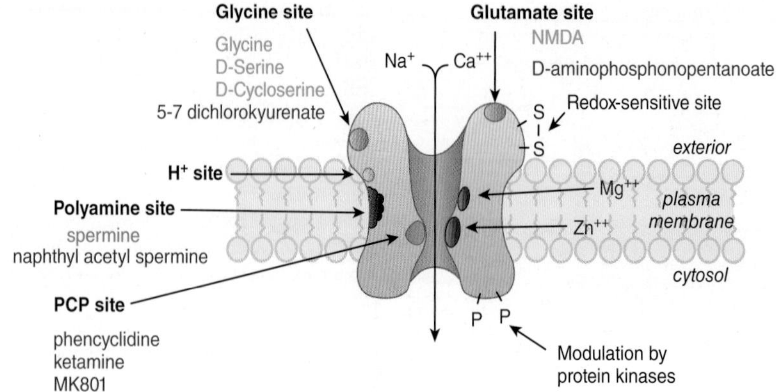

Figure 14–12 *Pharmacologic binding sites on the NMDA receptor.* Agents that promote receptor function are shown in ◐. Those that inhibit receptor function appear in ◐. Binding of both glutamate and glycine is necessary for activation.

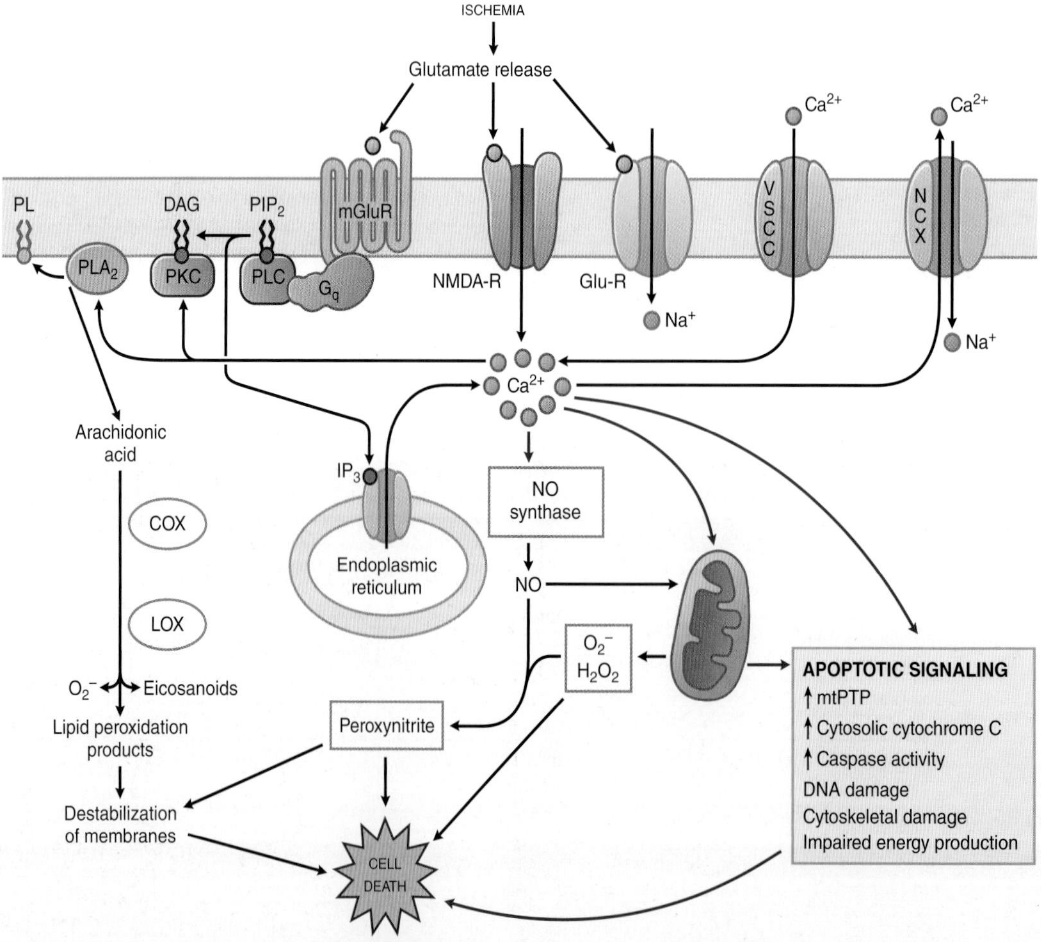

ISCHEMIA
Glutamate release
Ca2+
Ca2+
PL
DAG
PIP2
mGluR
PLA2
PKC
PLC
Gq
NMDA-R
Glu-R
VSCC
NCX
Na+
Na+
Ca2+
Arachidonic acid
IP3
COX
LOX
Endoplasmic reticulum
NO synthase
NO
O2−
H2O2
O2−
Eicosanoids
Lipid peroxidation products
Peroxynitrite
Destabilization of membranes
CELL DEATH
APOPTOTIC SIGNALING
↑mtPTP
↑Cytosolic cytochrome C
↑Caspase activity
DNA damage
Cytoskeletal damage
Impaired energy production

Figure 14–13 *Mechanisms contributing to glutamate-induced cytotoxicity/neuronal injury during ischemia-reperfusion–induced glutamate release.* Several pathways contribute to excitotoxic neuronal injury in ischemia, with excess cytosolic Ca^{2+} playing a precipitating role. (Reproduced with permission from Dugan LL, Kim-Han JS. Hypoxic-ischemic brain injury and oxidative stress. In: Siegel GS, et al., eds. *Basic Neurochemistry: Molecular, Cellular, and Medical Aspects.* 7th ed. Elsevier Academic Press, Burlington, MA, **2006**, 564. © 2006, American Society for Neurochemistry.) (See also Brady et al., 2012.)

TABLE 14-3 ■ SUBTYPES OF MUSCARINIC RECEPTORS IN THE CNS

SUBTYPE	TRANSDUCER EFFECTOR	AGONISTS (EXAMPLES)	ANTAGONISTS (EXAMPLES)
M_1	G_q Activation of PLC	Acetylcholine, carbachol, oxotremorine, pilocarpine, McN-A-343	Pirenzepine, telenzepine, 4-DAMP, xanomeline
M_2	G_i/G_o Inhibition of AC	Acetylcholine, carbachol, oxotremorine	AF-DX 116, AF-DX 384, AQ-RA 741, tolterodine, (S)-(+)-dimethindene maleate, methoctramine
M_3	G_q Activation of PLC	Acetylcholine, carbachol, oxotremorine, pilocarpine, cevimeline	Darifenacin, 4-DAMP, DAU 5884, J-104129, tropicamide, tolterodine
M_4	G_i/G_o Inhibition of AC	Acetylcholine, carbachol oxotremorine	AF-DX384, 4-DAMP, PD 102807, xanomeline
M_5	G_q Activation of PLC	Acetylcholine, carbachol, oxotremorine, pilocarpine	4-DAMP, xanomeline, VU-0488130 (ML381)

Acetylcholine is the endogenous transmitter for all muscarinic receptors. Nonselective antagonists include atropine, scopolamine, and ipratropium. 4-DAMP, 1,1-dimethyl-4-diphenylacetoxypiperidinium iodide.

form the ion channel (Figure 14–6). In the CNS, nicotinic receptors are assembled as combinations of α(2–7) and β(2–4) subunits. While pairwise combinations of α and β (e.g., α3β4 and α4β2), and in at least one case a homomeric α7 are sufficient to form a functional receptor in vitro, far more complex isoforms have been identified in vivo. The subunit composition strongly influences the biophysical and pharmacological properties of the receptor. Comprehensive listings of nicotinic receptor subunit combinations identified from recombinant expression systems, or in vivo, can be found in the work of Millar and Gotti (2009). Nicotinic cholinergic receptors have high therapeutic value, not only in the treatment of smoking cessation (they are the primary receptors for nicotine; see Chapter 11) but also for other neurological pathologies.

Muscarinic ACh receptors are GPCRs consisting of five subtypes, all of which are expressed in the brain. M_1, M_3, and M_5 couple to G_q, while the M_2 and M_4 receptors couple to G_i (Table 14–3). Chapter 9 presents detailed information on the physiology and pharmacology of muscarinic receptors.

Monoamines

Monoamines are neurotransmitters whose structure contains an amino group connected to an aromatic ring by a two-carbon chain. All are derived from aromatic amino acids and regulate neurotransmission that underlies cognitive processes, including emotion. Drugs that affect monoamine receptors and signaling are used to treat a variety of conditions, such as depression, schizophrenia, and anxiety, as well as movement disorders like Parkinson disease. Monoamines include DA, NE, EPI, histamine, 5HT, and the trace amines. Each system is anatomically distinct and serves separate, functional roles within its field of innervation.

Dopamine

Dopamine, NE, and EPI are catecholamine neurotransmitters (see Chapters 8 and 13). Notably, in contrast to the periphery, DA is the predominant catecholamine in the CNS. Its synthesis, degradation, and pharmacology are discussed in Chapter 13. There are several distinct pathways mediating DA signaling, including ones that play a role in motivation and reward (most drugs of abuse increase DA signaling), motor control, and the release of various hormones. These effects are mediated by five distinct GPCRs grouped into two subfamilies: D1-like receptors (D_1 and D_5) that stimulate adenylyl cyclase activity via coupling to G_s or G_{olf}, and D2-like receptors (D_2, D_3, and D_4) that couple to G_i/G_o to inhibit adenylyl cyclase activity and modulate various voltage-gated ion channels. DA receptor subtypes are discussed extensively in Chapter 13. DA-containing pathways and receptors have been implicated in the pathophysiology of schizophrenia and Parkinson disease and in the side effects following the pharmacotherapy of these disorders (see Chapters 16 and 18). There are three major DA-containing pathways in the CNS: the nigrostriatal, the mesocortical/mesolimbic, and the tuberoinfundibular, depicted in Figure 13–11.

Norepinephrine

NE is an endogenous neurotransmitter for the α and β adrenergic receptor subtypes that are present in the CNS; all are GPCRs (Table 14–4; see also Chapter 8). β adrenergic receptors couple to G_s to activate adenylyl cyclase. The α_1 adrenergic receptors couple to G_q, resulting in stimulation of the PLC-IP_3/DAG-Ca^{2+}-PKC pathway, and are associated predominantly with neurons. The interaction of NE with α_1 adrenergic receptors on noradrenergic target neurons causes a decrease in K^+ conductance, resulting in *depolarizing responses*. The α_2 adrenergic receptors are found on glial and vascular elements, as well as on neurons. They are prominent

TABLE 14-4 ■ ADRENERGIC RECEPTORS IN THE CNS

FAMILY	SUBTYPES	TRANSDUCER	AGONIST	ANTAGONIST
α_1 Adrenergic	α_{1A} α_{1B} α_{1D}	$G_{q/11}$	Epinephrine, phenylephrine, oxymetazoline, dabuzalgron (α_{1A}) A61603 (α_{1B})	Prazosin, doxazosin, terazosin, tamsulosin, alfuzosin, S(+)-niguldipine (α_{1A}), L-765314 (α_{1B}), BMY-7378 (α_{1D})
α_2 Adrenergic	α_{2A} α_{2B} α_{2C}	G_i/G_o	Epinephrine, norepinephrine, dexmedetomidine, clonidine, guanfacine	Yohimbine, rauwolscine
β Adrenergic	β_1 β_2 β_3	G_s	Epinephrine, norepinephrine, prenalterol (β_1), fenoterol (β_2), salbutamol (β_2), mirabegron (β_3), BRL37344 (β_3)	Carvedilol, bupranolol, levobunolol, metoprolol, propranolol, betaxolol (β_1), ICI118554 (β_2), SR 59230A (β_3)

on noradrenergic neurons, where they couple to G_i, inhibit adenylyl cyclase, and mediate a *hyperpolarizing response* due to enhancement of an inwardly rectifying K^+ channel (via the $\beta\gamma$ heterodimer). The α_2 adrenergic receptors are also located presynaptically, where they function as inhibitory autoreceptors to diminish the release of NE. The antihypertensive effects of clonidine may result from stimulation of such autoreceptors.

There are relatively large amounts of NE within the hypothalamus and in certain parts of the limbic system, such as the central nucleus of the amygdala and the dentate gyrus of the hippocampus. NE also is present in significant amounts in most brain regions. Mapping studies indicated that noradrenergic neurons of the locus ceruleus innervate specific target cells in a large number of cortical, subcortical, and spinomedullary fields.

Epinephrine

Most EPI in the brain is contained in vascular elements. Neurons in the CNS that contain EPI were recognized only after the development of sensitive enzymatic assays and immunocytochemical staining techniques for phenylethanolamine-*N*-methyltransferase, the enzyme that converts NE into EPI. EPI-containing neurons are found in the medullary reticular formation and make restricted connections to pontine and diencephalic nuclei, eventually coursing as far rostrally as the paraventricular nucleus of the thalamus. Their physiological properties have not been unequivocally identified.

Histamine

Histamine is a monoamine neurotransmitter in the CNS in addition to its well-known physiological function in immune and digestive responses in the periphery. Histaminergic neurons are located in the ventral posterior hypothalamus, where they give rise to long ascending and descending tracts that are typical of patterns characteristic of other monoaminergic systems. The histaminergic system is thought to affect arousal, body temperature, and vascular dynamics. The biosynthesis of histamine is described in Chapter 39. Histamine signals through four GPCR subtypes (H_1–H_4) that regulate either adenylyl cyclase or PLC (Figure 14–14). Interestingly, unlike other monoamine and amino acid transmitters, histamine does not appear to be a substrate for a unique reuptake transporter following its release, however, there are reports of its transport by NET and OCT3. Termination of its action likely involves its degradation by histamine-*N*-methyltransferase, a widely expressed cytosolic enzyme; diamine oxidase, which can oxidatively deaminate histamine, is lacking in the CNS. The histamine receptors, structure, signaling, functioning, and current understandings are reviewed in Chapter 39 and by Panula and colleagues (2015).

The *H_1 receptors* are widely distributed in the brain, where high densities are found in regions linked to neuroendocrine, behavioral, and nutritional state control. H_1 receptor activation excites neurons in most brain regions, and genetic knockout of the H_1 receptor results in behavioral abnormalities, consistent with the receptor's being a major player in cortical control of the sleep/wake cycle. This is evident in the well-known sedative actions of first-generation H_1 receptor blockers that are used in the treatment of allergies. The development of H_1 antagonists with low CNS penetration has reduced the incidence of sedation in the treatment of allergy-related disorders (see the table, Drug Facts for Your Personal Formulary: *H_1 Antagonists*, in Chapter 39), although, in some conditions the sedative effect of first-generation antihistamines can be beneficial in inducing sleep.

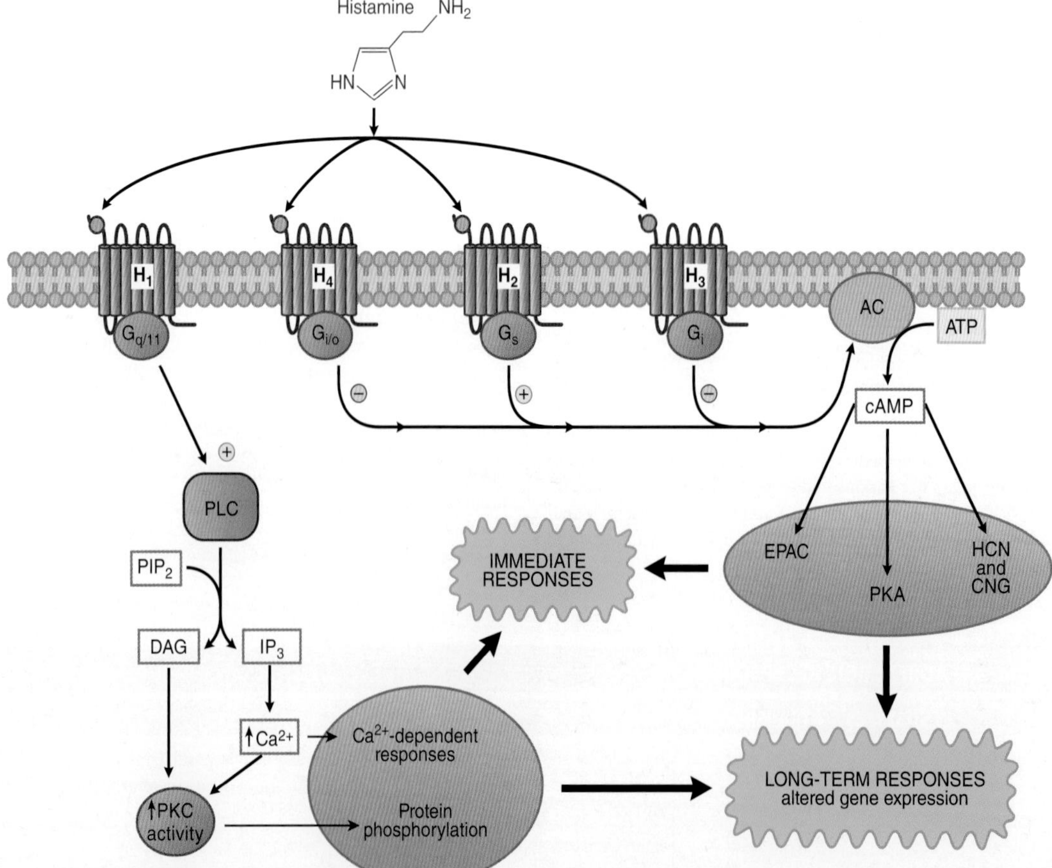

Figure 14–14 *Signal transduction pathways for histamine receptors.* Histamine can couple to a variety of G protein–linked signal transduction pathways via four different receptors. H_1 receptors activate phosphatidylinositol turnover via $G_{q/11}$. The other receptors couple either positively (H_2 receptor) or negatively (H_3 and H_4 receptor) to adenylyl cyclase activity via G_s and $G_{i/o}$, respectively. Signaling pathways affected by histamine provide both immediate and long-term regulation of cell function.

The H_2 *receptors* activate adenylyl cyclase and are primarily involved in gastric acid secretion and smooth muscle relaxation. H_2 receptor antagonists are a mainstay of treatment of dyspepsia and GI ulcers (see Chapter 49). H_2 receptors are also highly expressed in the brain, where they regulate neuronal physiology and plasticity. Mice lacking H_2 receptors show cognitive defects and impaired hippocampal LTP along with abnormalities in nociception. Difficulties in studying H_2 receptor signaling in the CNS are attributed to the fact that H_2 receptor ligands generally exhibit poor BBB penetration. However, there have been several clinical trials investigating H_2 receptor antagonists for treating supraspinal nociception; these trials have met with mixed results.

The H_3 *receptors* are also present in the CNS and can act as autoreceptors on histaminergic neurons to inhibit histamine synthesis and release. These receptors act to inhibit adenylyl cyclase and to modulate N-type voltage-gated Ca^{2+} channels. While it is known that H_3 receptors function as autoreceptors, they are not confined to histaminergic neurons and have been found to regulate serotonergic, cholinergic, noradrenergic, and dopaminergic neurotransmitter release. Exploiting the ability to modulate other neurotransmitters, the H_3 receptor has become a therapeutic target for treating conditions such as obesity, movement disorders, schizophrenia, ADHD, and wakefulness. A wide array of compounds have been developed that interact with the H_3 receptor, which have proved to be useful pharmacological tools both in vitro and in vivo. One compound, pitolisant, an inverse agonist at the H_3 receptor, has been granted orphan drug status for the treatment of narcolepsy and is currently in clinical trials for schizophrenia and Parkinson disease.

The H_4 *receptors* are expressed on cells of hematopoietic origin (eosinophils, T cells, mast cells, basophils, and dendritic cells) and are involved in eosinophil shape and mast cell chemotaxis. While some evidence has suggested that H_4 receptors are expressed in the CNS, this remains controversial and in need of further research. H_4 receptors have recently been demonstrated on microglia where they may indirectly affect neurons. Regardless, the vast majority of information about this subtype is related to allergy, asthma, and the antipruritic properties of H_4 antagonists.

Serotonin

The synthesis and degradation of 5HT are discussed in Chapter 13. There are diverse pathways mediating serotonin signaling that play a role in modulating mood, depression, anxiety, phobia, and GI effects. All but one of the serotonin receptors are GPCRs and are targets for both therapeutic and recreational (hallucinogenic) drugs. These effects are mediated by 13 distinct GPCRs and 1 ligand-gated ion channel, which exhibit characteristic ligand-binding profiles, couple to different intracellular signaling systems, and exhibit subtype-specific distribution within the CNS. The 5HT receptors and their pharmacology are discussed in detail in Chapter 13.

Trace Amines

Trace amines, while discovered long ago, have only recently been appreciated as neurotransmitters. As the name implies, they are detected at trace levels (they have very short half-lives due to rapid metabolism by MAO). However, at least some trace amines act as neuromodulators/neurotransmitters at specific trace amine receptors. Trace amines are structurally related to catecholamines and consist of the PEAs (*N*-methylphenethylamine [an endogenous amphetamine isomer], phenylethanolamine, tyramine, tryptamine, *N*-methyltyramine, octopamine, synephrine, and 3-methoxytyramine). These trace amines are thought to act through GPCRs that were originally termed "trace amine receptors" but are now called TAARs because not all members have very high affinity for trace amines. The first receptor was identified in 2001 (Borowsky et al., 2001), and to date six TAAR genes (*TAAR1*, *TAAR2*, *TAAR5*, *TAAR6*, *TAAR8*, and *TAAR9*) have been identified in humans along with several potential pseudogenes. Multiple TAAR-related receptor genes have been identified in other species; several display prominent expression in the olfactory epithelium and are regarded as putative olfactory receptors for volatile amines. Only one TAAR (TAAR1) has been recognized by IUPHAR as a trace amine receptor; it has been given the abbreviation TA_1. TA_1 has the highest affinity for the trace amines tyramine, β-phenylephrine, and octopamine. Emerging evidence suggests that TA_1 may modulate monoaminergic activity in the CNS. In addition to trace amines, TAARs can be activated by amphetamine-like psychostimulants and endogenous thyronamines such as thyronamine and 3-iodothyronamine.

Peptides

Neuropeptides typically behave as modulators in the CNS rather than causing direct excitation or inhibition. A growing number of neuropeptides have been described (Table 14–5) and are involved in a wide array of brain functions, ranging from analgesia to social behaviors, learning, and

TABLE 14–5 ■ EXAMPLES OF NEUROPEPTIDES

Calcitonin Family	**Pituitary Hormones**
Calcitonin	Corticotropin (formerly adrenocorticotropic hormone; ACTH)
Calcitonin gene-related peptide (CGRP)	α-Melanocyte-stimulating hormone (α-MSH)
Hypothalamic Hormones	Growth hormone (GH)
Oxytocin, vasopressin	Follicle-stimulating hormone (FSH)
Hypothalamic Releasing and Inhibitory Hormones	β-Lipotropin (β-LPH), luteinizing hormone (LH)
Corticotropin-releasing factor (CRF or CRH)	**Tachykinins**
Gonadotropin-releasing hormone (GnRH)	Neurokinins A and B
Growth hormone-releasing hormone (GHRH)	Neuropeptide K, substance P
Somatostatin (SST)	**VIP-Glucagon Family**
Thyrotropin-releasing hormone (TRH)	Glucagon, glucagon-like peptide (GLP-1)
Neuropeptide Y Family	Pituitary adenylyl cyclase–activating peptide (PACAP)
Neuropeptide Y (NPY)	Vasoactive intestinal polypeptide (VIP)
Neuropeptide YY (PYY)	**Other Peptides**
Pancreatic polypeptide (PP)	Agouti-related peptide (ARP)
Opioid Peptides	Bombesin, bradykinin (BK)
β-Endorphin (also pituitary hormone)	Cholecystokinin (CCK)
Dynorphin peptides	Cocaine/amphetamine-regulated transcript (CART)
Leu-enkephalin	Galanin, ghrelin
Met-enkephalin	Melanin-concentrating hormone (MCH)
	Neurotensin, nerve growth factor (NGF)
	Orexins, orphanin FQ (nociceptin)
	Hemopressin (CB_1 inverse agonist)

Source: Modified with permission from Nestler EJ, et al., eds. *Molecular Neuropharmacology*. 2nd ed. McGraw-Hill, New York, **2009**.

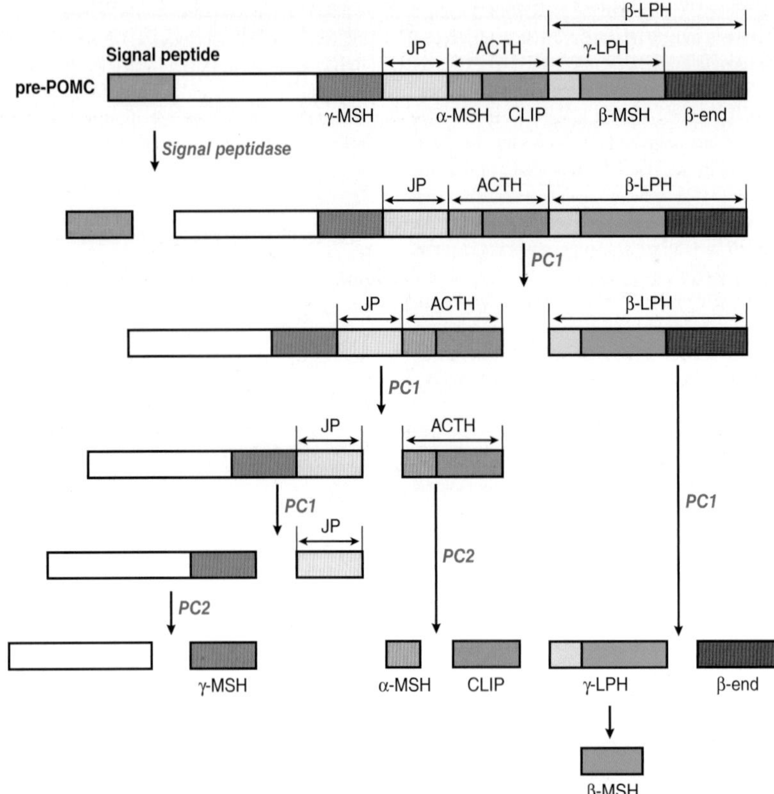

Figure 14–15 *Proteolytic processing of POMC.* After removal of the signal peptide from pre-POMC, the remaining propeptide undergoes endoproteolysis by prohormone convertases 1 and 2 (PC1 and PC2) at dibasic residues. PC1 liberates the bioactive peptides ACTH, β-endorphin (β-end), and γ-LPH. PC2 cleaves ACTH into CLIP and α-MSH and also releases γ-MSH from the N-terminal portion of the propeptide. The JP (joining peptide) is the region between ACTH and γ-MSH. β-MSH is formed by cleavage of γ-LPH. Some of the resulting peptides are amidated or acetylated before they become fully active.

memory. In contrast to the biogenic amines or amino acids, peptide synthesis requires transcription of DNA to mRNA and translation of mRNA into protein. This takes place primarily in perikarya, and the resulting peptide is then transported to nerve terminals. Single genes can therefore, through transcriptional and posttranslational modifications, give rise to multiple neuropeptides. For example, proteolytic processing of POMC gives rise to, among other peptides, ACTH; α-, γ-, and β-MSHs; and β-endorphin (Figure 14–15). In addition, alternative splicing of RNA transcripts in different tissues may result in distinct mRNA species (e.g., calcitonin and CGRP). Furthermore, while some CNS peptides function independently, most are thought to act in concert with coexisting neurotransmitters. They are often packaged into vesicles and released along with other neurotransmitters to modulate their actions. While classical neurotransmitters generally signal to neurons by depolarizing or hyperpolarizing, neuropeptides have more diverse mechanisms of action and can also affect gene expression. Their action is not terminated by rapid reuptake into the presynaptic cell; rather, they are enzymatically inactivated by extracellular peptidases. As a result, their effects on neuronal signaling can be prolonged.

Neuropeptide Receptors

Most neuropeptide receptors are GPCRs, with the extracellular domains of the receptors playing primary roles in peptide-receptor interaction. As with other transmitter systems, there are often multiple receptor subtypes for the same peptide transmitter (Table 14–6). Neuropeptide receptors can exhibit different affinities for nascent neuropeptides and peptide analogues. Because peptides are typically inefficient as drugs, particularly at CNS targets due to difficulties permeating the BBB, major efforts have been made to develop small-molecule drugs that are effective as either agonists or antagonists at peptide receptors. Through a combination of structural biology, chemistry, high-throughput screening, and drug development, there are now small-molecule ligands for many neuropeptide receptors. Some of these compounds are listed in Table 14–6. Notably, natural products have not typically been good sources of drugs that affect peptidergic transmission. One exception is the plant alkaloid morphine, which acts selectively at opioid receptor subtypes (see Chapter 20).

Purines

Adenosine, ATP, UDP, and UTP have roles as extracellular signaling molecules. ATP is also a component of many neurotransmitter storage vesicles and is released along with transmitters. Intracellular nucleotides may reach the exterior cell surface by other means; for example, for example, extracellular adenosine can result from cellular release and metabolism of ATP. Released nucleotides can be hydrolyzed extracellularly by ectonucleotidases. Extracellular nucleotides and adenosine can act on a family of diverse purinergic receptors, which have been implicated in a variety of functions, including memory and learning, locomotor behavior, and feeding.

Purinergic Receptors

Purinergic receptors are divided into three classes: adenosine receptors (also called P1), P2Y, and P2X (Table 14–7). *Adenosine receptors* are GPCRs that consist of four subtypes (A_1, A_{2A}, A_{2B}, and A_3) activated endogenously by adenosine. A_1 and A_3 couple to G_i; A_2 receptors couple to G_s. Activation of A_1 receptors is associated with inhibition of adenylyl cyclase, activation of K^+ currents, and in some instances, activation of PLC; stimulation of A_2 receptors activates adenylyl cyclase. In the CNS, both A_1 and A_{2A} receptors are involved in regulating the release of other neurotransmitters, such as glutamate and DA, making the A_{2A} receptor a potential therapeutic target for disorders, including Parkinson disease.

TABLE 14–6 ■ PEPTIDE TRANSMITTERS AND RECEPTORS

FAMILY	SUBTYPE	TRANSDUCER	AGONISTS	ANTAGONISTS
Opioid	δ κ μ NOP	G_i/G_o	β-Endorphin, dynorphin, DPDPE (δ), salvinorin A(κ), hydromorphone (μ), fentanyl (μ), codeine (μ), methadone (μ), DAMGO (μ), etorphine Ro64-6198 (NOP)	Naltrexone, naloxone, SB612111
Somatostatin	sst_1, sst_2 sst_3, sst_4 sst_5	G_i	SST-14, SST-18, pasireotide, cortistatin, BIM23059, BIM23066, BIM23313, CGP23996, octreotide ($sst_{2,3,5}$)	SRA880 (sst_1), D-Tyr8-CYN154806 (sst_2), NVPACQ090 (sst_3)
Neurotensin	NTS_1 NTS_2	$G_{q/11}$	EISAI-1, JMV431, JMV449 (NTS_1), levocabastine (NTS_2)	SR142948A, meclinertant (NTS_1)
Orexin	OX_1 OX_2	$G_{q/11}$, G_s, G_i	Orexin-A, Orexin-B	Suvorexant, filorexant, SB-649868, almorexant, SB-410220, JNJ 10397049
Tachykinin	NK_1 NK_2 NK_3	$G_{q/11}$	Neurokinin A, neurokinin B, substance P, GR 73632 (NK_1), GR 64349 (NK_2), senktide	Aprepitant (NK_1), GR 159897 (NK_2), SB218795 (NK_3)
Cholecystokinin	CCK_1 CCK_2	$G_{q/11}$ (CCK_1), G_s	Cholecystokinin-8, CCK-33, CCK-58, gastrin, A-71623 (CCK_1)	Proglumide, FK-480, lintitript, PD-149164, devazepide (CCK_1), CL988 (CCK_2)
Neuropeptide Y	Y_1 Y_2 Y_4 Y_5	G_i/G_o	Neuropeptide Y, BWX 46	BIBO 3304 (Y_1), BIIE0246 (Y_2), UR-AK49, CGP 71683A GW438014A (Y_5)
Neuropeptide FF	NPFF1 NPFF2	$G_{q/11}$, G_i/G_o	Neuropeptide FF, RFRP-3 (NPFF1)	RF9

The *P2Y receptors* are also GPCRs and are activated by ATP, ADP, UTP, UDP, and UDP-glucose. There are eight known subtypes of P2Y receptors that couple to a variety of G proteins (Table 14–7). The $P2Y_{14}$ receptor is expressed in the CNS, where it is stimulated by UDP-glucose and may play a role in neuroimmune functions. The $P2Y_{12}$ receptor is important clinically: Inhibition of this receptor in platelets inhibits platelet aggregation.

In contrast to the other two families, ATP-sensitive *P2X receptors* are ligand-gated cation channels that are expressed throughout the CNS on both presynaptic and postsynaptic nerve terminals and on glial cells. P2X receptors are found on nociceptive sensory neurons, where they primarily gate Na^+, K^+, and Ca^+ and are implicated in mediating sensory transduction. There are seven subtypes of P2X receptors with varying sensitivities to their endogenous agonist ATP (Table 14–7). Functional P2X receptors have a trimeric topology, existing as either homopolymers or heteropolymers with other P2X receptors, as confirmed by X-ray crystallography of a $P2X_4$ receptor (Kawate et al., 2009). The study of compounds that are selective for some P2X subtypes suggests that targeting these receptors may be useful in the therapy of neuropathic and inflammatory pain, thrombosis, arthritis, and depression.

Neuromodulatory Lipids

Cannabinoids

In the 1960s, THC (Figure 14–16) was identified as a psychoactive substance in marijuana. This led to the discovery and cloning of the two cannabinoid receptors and the identification of endogenous compounds that modulate them. The two receptor subtypes (CB_1 and CB_2) are GPCRs that couple to G_i/G_o to inhibit adenylyl cyclase and, in some cell types, inhibit voltage-gated Ca^+ channels or stimulate K^+ channels. The receptors share relatively low overall homology and are found in differing locations, although both are found in the CNS. CB_1 receptors are found in high levels throughout the brain, whereas CB_2 receptors are prominent in immune cells. Within the CNS, CB_2 receptors are expressed less than CB_1 receptors and are thought to occur primarily on microglia. Several orphan GPCRs (GPCRs with no known endogenous agonist) have been implicated as being cannabinoid-like, and as such, more cannabinoid receptor subtypes may exist. The finding of endogenous cannabinoids responsible for signaling to these receptors, along with a host of clinical data from marijuana use, has fueled interest in this signaling system and has greatly expanded our understanding of its physiology.

The *ECS* (endogenous cannabinoid system) consists of the cannabinoid receptors, endogenous cannabinoids, and the enzymes that synthesize and degrade endocannabinoids. The endocannabinoids are lipid molecules and include anandamide (*N*-arachidonoylethanolamine) and 2-arachidonoylglycerol (2-AG), as well as other compounds that have been putatively identified to serve as endogenous endocannabinoids, including *O*-arachidonoylethanolamine (virodhamine), *N*-dihomo-γ-linolenoylethanolamine, *N*-docosatetraenoic-ethanolamine, oleamide, 2-arachidonyl-glyceryl-ether (2-AGE), N-arachidonoyl-dopamine (NADA), and *N*-oleoyl-dopamine. The actions of endocannabinoids are terminated by their uptake into cells, followed by hydrolysis. Two enzymes known to break down anandamide and 2-AG are fatty acid amide hydrolase (FAAH) and monoacylglycerol lipase (MGL), respectively. Although a few studies suggested the existence of a specific transport system for endocannabinoids, no molecular entity that mediates such a carrier-mediated process has been identified. Obviously, drugs that inhibit the transport or degradation of endocannabinoids would prolong their physiological actions.

There is now strong evidence that the ECS functions as a retrograde signaling messenger system, generally serving to inhibit the presynaptic release of neurotransmitters (Figure 14–17). Depending on the cell type, this action can last from seconds to hours, resulting in a large influence on neuronal circuit function. Endocannabinoids thus function as neuromodulators and have been linked to a variety of neuronal processes, including pain sensation, stress response, anxiety, appetite, and motor learning. The ECS has been targeted pharmacologically in a variety of ways, including

TABLE 14–7 ■ CHARACTERISTICS OF PURINERGIC RECEPTORS

CLASS	RECEPTOR							
Adenosine (P1)[a]	**A_1**	**A_{2A}**	**A_{2B}**	**A_3**				
Transducer	$G_{i/o}$	G_S	G_S	$G_{i/o}$				
Agonists	CPA	CGS21680	BAY 60-6583	1B-MECA				
Antagonists	CPX	SCH58261	MRS1754	VUF5574				
P2X (ionotropic)	**$P2X_1$**	**$P2X_2$**	**$P2X_3$**	**$P2X_4$**	**$P2X_5$**	**$P2X_6$**	**$P2X_7$**	
Substrate specificity	ATP	ATP	ATP	ATP>CTP	ATP	ATP	ATP	
Antagonist	NF449, TNP-ATP	NF770	TNP-ATP	5-BDBD, paroxetine	PPADS, suramin		AZ10606120	
P2Y (metabotropic)	**$P2Y_1$**	**$P2Y_2$**	**$P2Y_4$**	**$P2Y_6$**	**$P2Y_{11}$**	**$P2Y_{12}$**	**$P2Y_{13}$**	**$P2Y_{14}$**
Transducer	$G_{q/11}$	$G_{q/11}$	$G_{q/11}$	$G_{q/11}$	G_s, $G_{q/11}$	$G_{i/o}$	$G_{i/o}$	$G_{i/o}$
Substrate specificity	ADP>ATP	ATP>UTP	UTP>ATP	UDP>>UTP>ADP	ATP=UTP	ADP	ADP>>ATP	UDP-glucose[b]
Agonists	MRS2365	MRS2698, PSB1114	MRS4062	MRS2957	AR-C67085	2MeSADP	2MeSADP	MRS2690
Antagonists	MRS2279	ARC118925X		MRS2578	NF157	ticagrelor, clopidogrel	MRS2211, cangrelor	PPTN

CPA, N6-cyclopentyladenosine; CPX, 8-cyclopentyl-l,3-dipropylxanthine; 1B-MECA, N6-(3-iodobenzyl)-adenosine-5α-*N*-methylcarboxamide; NECA, l-(6-amino-9H-purin-9-yl)-l-deoxy-*N*-ethyl-β-D-ribofuronamide; PPADS, pyridoxalphosphate-6-azophenyl-2′,4′-disulfonic acid; TNP-ATP, 2′,3′-O-(2,4,6-trinitrophenyl)adenosine-5′-triphosphate. For further details, consult information about the three classes of purinergic receptors at http://www.guidetopharmacology.org.

[a]NECA is a nonselective agonist of P1 receptors.

[b]$P2Y_{14}$ binds UDP-glucose, UDP-galactose, or UDP-acetylglucosamine.

Anandamide

2-Arachidonylglycerol

Rimonabant

Δ^9-Tetrahydrocannabinol

Figure 14–16 *Cannabinoid receptor ligands.* Anandamide and 2-arachidonylglycerol are endogenous agonists. Rimonabant is a synthetic CB receptor antagonist. Δ^9-tetrahydrocannabinol is a CB agonist derived from marijuana.

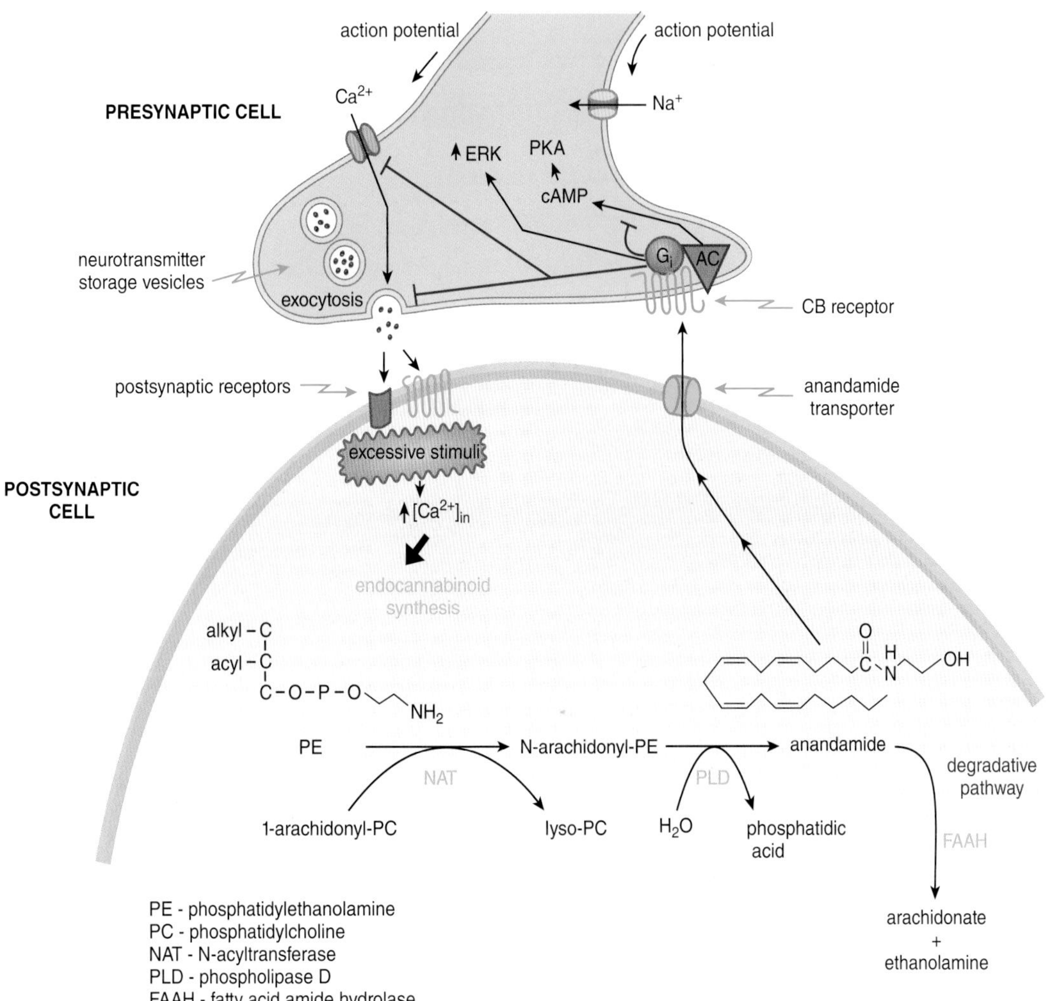

Figure 14–17 *Anandamide synthesis and signaling in the CNS.* Endocannabinoids, synthesized on demand in stimulated postsynaptic cells, appear to function as a negative feedback system to limit further presynaptic transmitter release.

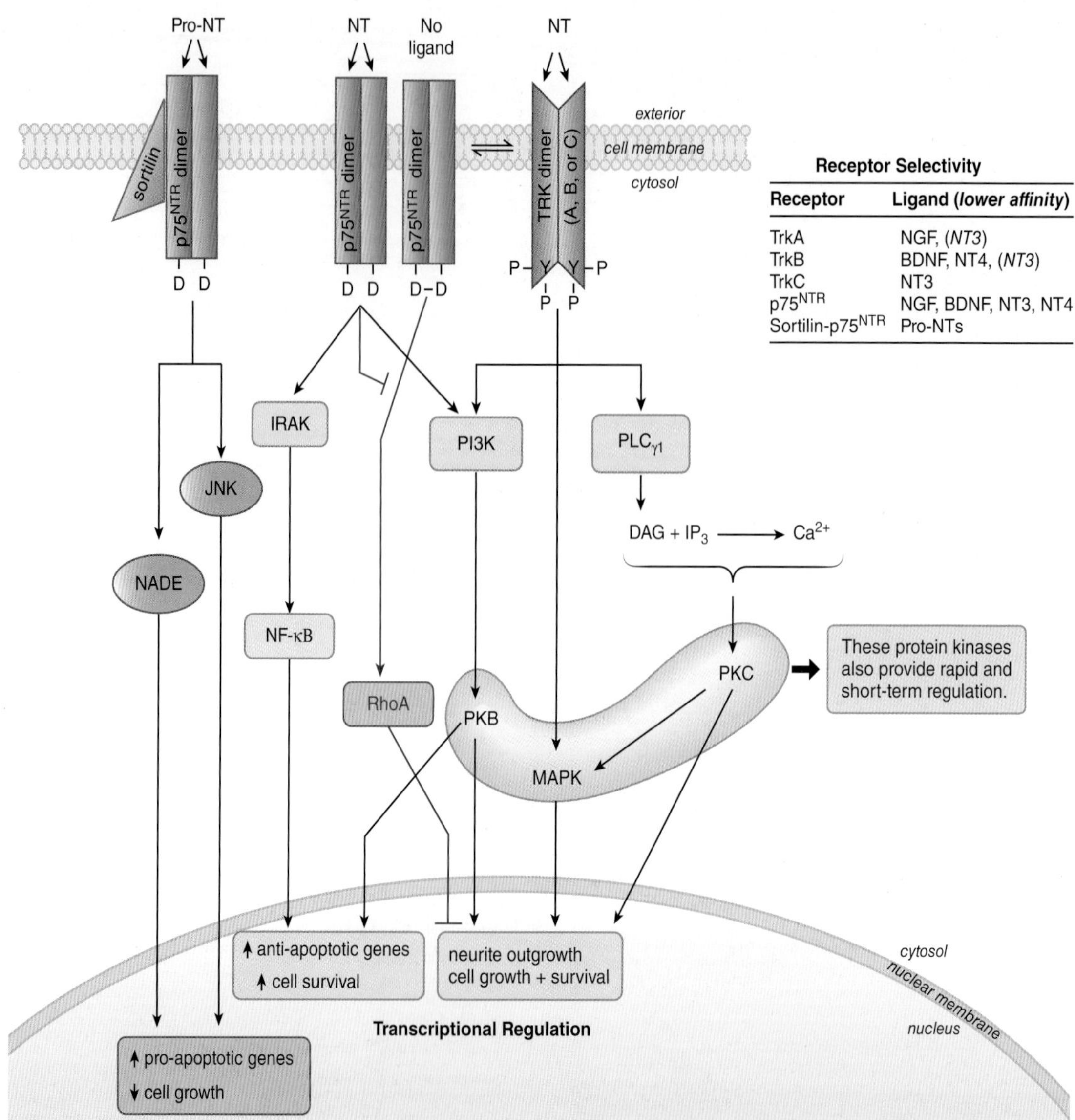

Figure 14–18 *Neurotrophic factor signaling in the CNS.* This schematic is a simplification of NT signaling pathways, which are complex and incompletely understood, with differential expression of NT receptors and NTs in different areas of the nervous system and a host of interacting systems that can affect signaling (Skaper, 2012; Bothwell, 2016). Pro-NTs and NTs interact with membrane receptor dimers of TRK receptors A, B, and C and of p75^{NTR} (a "death receptor" and member of the TNF receptor superfamily) with the specificities indicated by the table at the upper right. Ligand-receptor interactions stimulate signaling pathways that regulate transcription. Formation of an NT-TRK receptor dimer activates intracellular TRK receptor tyrosine kinase activities on the cytosolic tail of the receptor. Tyrosine phosphorylation (Y-P) provides binding sites for the adaptor proteins that lead to activation of the PI3K, MAPK, and PLCγ_1-PKC pathways (green boxes), which promote transcriptional regulation in support of neurite extension, cell growth, antiapoptosis, and cell survival. Unliganded p75^{NTR} may also modulate the activity of TRK receptor signaling. Unliganded p75^{NTR} dimers have a basal activity that results in activation of the RhoA pathway, leading to pro-apoptotic signaling (red boxes). NT binding to p75^{NTR} does not initiate intracellular signaling via activation of a receptor tyrosine kinase. Rather, NT binding to p75^{NTR} alters binding of various modulatory factors and causes proteolytic cleavages in the death domain region (DD); these perturbations of p75^{NTR} result in activation of the IRAK/NF-κB and PI3K pathways and inhibition of the RhoA pathway. The net result is neurite extension, cell growth, antiapoptosis, and cell survival. Pro-NT binding to p75^{NTR} in the presence of an accessory protein, sortilin, activates cellular events that permit binding/dimerization of death domain proteins (D), facilitating the activation of the NADE and JNK pathways, leading to inhibition of cell growth and an acceleration of pro-apoptotic events. A host of other signaling proteins can interact along the pathways sketched here. In addition, Trk receptors use signaling endosomes. Following activation near innervated tissues that produce NTs, Trk-NT complexes are endocytosed, and some receptors are recycled to the membrane, while others are destroyed in lysosomes. But, some other receptor-NT complexes (e.g., TrkA-NGF) are stable within the endosome and travel retrogradely along the neuron to the cell body as a signaling endosome. The cytoplasmic tail of an NT-p75^{NTR} complex may be cleaved and release into the cytosol, promoting signaling. IRAK, interleukin-associated kinase; JNK, c-Jun N-terminal kinase; NADE, p75NTR-associated death executor; NF-κB, nuclear factor kappa B; NT, neutrophin; NTR, neutrophin receptor; Trk, tropomyosin receptor kinase (tyrosine receptor kinase).

compounds that act on the enzymes responsible for breaking down (FAAH inhibitors) or synthesizing endocannabinoids, compounds that target the transport mechanism (AM404, *N*-arachidonoylaminophenol), or drugs that directly stimulate or inhibit the CB receptors.

Marijuana is known to stimulate appetite via activation of the CB_1 receptor; thus, efforts have been undertaken to develop CB_1 antagonists for the treatment of obesity. Rimonabant, an inverse agonist of the CB_1 receptor, was initially approved in Europe as an anorectic, but subsequently was withdrawn due to adverse effects, including increased suicidality and depression. It currently remains unclear whether CB_1 receptor antagonism will prove useful for the treatment of appetitive or addictive disorders. However, CB_1 receptor agonists have a wide variety of effects that make them attractive candidates for drug discovery efforts. They stimulate appetite in patients with AIDS, reduce seizure frequency in epilepsy, decrease intraocular pressure in patients with glaucoma, treat nausea caused by cancer chemotherapy (dronabinol; see Table 50–4 and Figure 50–5), and reduce pain (nabilone). This wide range of potential therapeutic benefits has driven the medical marijuana movement such that, in some states, marijuana can be legally used as a therapeutic under a doctor's prescription.

Other Lipid Mediators

Arachidonic acid, normally stored within the cell membrane as a glycerol ester, can be liberated during phospholipid hydrolysis (by pathways involving phospholipases A_2, C, and D). Arachidonic acid can be converted to highly reactive modulators by three major enzymatic pathways (see Chapter 37: *cyclooxygenases* (leading to prostaglandins and thromboxane), *lipoxygenases* (leading to the leukotrienes and other transient catabolites of eicosatetraenoic acid), and *CYPs* (which are inducible and also expressed at low levels in brain). Arachidonic acid metabolites have been implicated as diffusible modulators in the CNS, possibly involved with the formation of LTP and other forms of neuronal plasticity.

Gases

Nitric Oxide and Carbon Monoxide

Both constitutive and inducible forms of NOS are expressed in the brain. The application of inhibitors of NOS (e.g., methylarginine) and of NO donors (such as nitroprusside) suggests the involvement of NO in a host of CNS phenomena, including LTP, activation of soluble guanylyl cyclase, neurotransmitter release, and enhancement of glutamate (NMDA)–mediated neurotoxicity. CO, generated in neurons or glia, is another diffusible gas that may act as an intracellular messenger stimulating soluble guanylyl cyclase through nonsynaptic actions. NO synthesis and signaling are presented in Chapter 3.

Regulatory Substances

Neurotrophins

The NTs constitute a family of proteins that include NGF, BDNF, NT-3, and NT-4/5, which regulate neuronal proliferation, differentiation, survival, migration, dendritic arborization, synaptogenesis, and activity-dependent forms of synaptic plasticity in the developing and mature CNS. NTs are synthesized as pro-NT precursors and processed to smaller, active NTs of about 13–26 kDa. Biological effects of NTs and pro-NTs are mediated by the Trk family of tyrosine kinase receptors and the p75 NT receptor through activation of complex signaling mechanisms summarized by Figure 14–18.

The function of BDNF has been most prominently studied; it modulates the establishment of neuronal circuits that regulate complex behaviors. Transcription and translation of the *Bdnf* gene are exquisitely regulated in the CNS with at least eight distinct promotors that initiate transcription of multiple distinct mRNA transcripts, each containing a full-length BDNF transcript after alternative splicing (Aid et al., 2007). In addition, *Bdnf* transcripts populate two different pools of mRNAs that are localized to distinct subcellular compartments in neurons (Timmusk et al., 1993). Finally, BDNF is initially synthesized as a precursor protein (preproBDNF) and, on cleavage of the signal peptide, is sorted into constitutive or regulated secretory vesicles. Conversion of the proBDNF to mature BDNF (mBDNF) occurs prior to release, and mBDNF is thought to be the main biologically active form, although proBDNF has biological activity at the sortilin-$p75^{NTR}$ complex (Bothwell, 2016). There is strong evidence that BDNF plays a role in synaptic plasticity and cognitive function (Greenberg et al., 2009; Lu et al., 2008). As a consequence, dysregulation of BDNF function or expression is implicated in the pathophysiology of age-related neurodegenerative diseases (Pang and Lu, 2004) and susceptibility to neuropsychiatric disorders such as anxiety and depression. Efforts to deliver NTs or modulate regulation of NT expression are being pursued as treatments for these CNS disorders. Despite these efforts, NTs are not yet used routinely in the clinic.

Neurosteroids

Neuroactive steroids that are synthesized in neuronal tissue are known as neurosteroids. Synthesis of neurosteroids occurs de novo from cholesterol or from circulating hormones (Reddy and Estes, 2016) by several key steroidogenic enzymes that are expressed throughout the vertebrate brain (Do Rego et al., 2009). Based on structural features, the neurosteroids can be categorized into three subtypes:

- pregnane neurosteroids such as allopregnanolone;
- androstane neurosteroids such as androstanediol; and
- sulfated neurosteroids such as DHEAS (Rahmani et al., 2015).

Neurosteroids can mediate an array of biological activities in the CNS through modulation of nuclear hormone receptors or through modulation of membrane receptor activity. More specifically, neurosteroids can allosterically modulate $GABA_A$ receptor complexes; glutamate receptors, including NMDA, AMPA, and KA; nicotinic and muscarinic ACh receptors; as well as sigma and glycine receptors (Do Rego et al., 2009). While little is known regarding the regulation of neurosteroid synthesis in the brain, in vivo studies indicate that these molecules can regulate a variety of neurophysiological and behavioral processes, including cognition, stress, sleep, and arousal (Engel and Grant, 2001; Reddy and Estes, 2016). Neurosteroids are not currently used in the clinic, but there is evidence to suggest their utility for the treatment of psychiatric disorders, including cognitive deficits and negative symptoms in schizophrenia, anxiety and mood disorders, as well as mood-stabilizing agents in bipolar disorder (Vallee, 2016).

Cytokines

Cytokines are low-molecular-weight proteins that are secreted by many different cell types to modulate key cellular functions. The primary immune effector cells in the CNS are glia, microglia, and astrocytes. These cells can express and release a variety of cytokines, including the IL-1β and IL-6, TNF-α, and IFN-γ. Constitutive expression of cytokines is required for normal physiological functioning in the brain, particularly regarding the molecular and cellular mechanisms involved in neurite outgrowth, neurogenesis, neuronal survival, synaptic pruning during brain development, the strength of synaptic transmission, and synaptic plasticity. While glial cells are typically thought of as neuroprotective, overexpression or sustained stimulation can cause an elevation of pro-inflammatory cytokines in the brain, resulting in neuroinflammation, an innate immune response mediated by protein complexes known as inflammasomes (Singhal et al., 2014). Acute neuroinflammation involves the release of cytokines and chemokines, is the first line of defense against pathogens in the CNS, and is not likely to cause neuronal damage. Sustained chronic neuroinflammation accompanied by sustained brain exposure to pro-inflammatory cytokines is, however, a factor in the pathogenesis of neurodegenerative and psychiatric illnesses leading to cognitive and memory deficits and behavioral abnormalities (Furtado and Katzman, 2015; Heneka et al., 2015).

Acknowledgment: *Floyd E. Bloom and Perry B. Molinoff contributed to this chapter in recent editions of this book. We have retained some of their text in the current edition.*

Bibliography

Aid T, et al. Mouse and rat BDNF gene structure and expression revisited. *J Neurosci Res*, **2007**, *85*:525–535.

Borowsky B. et al. Trace amines: identification of a family of mammalian G protein-coupled receptors. *Proc Natl Acad Sci USA*, **2001**, 98: 8966–8971.

Bothwell M. Recent advances in understanding neurotrophin signaling. *F1000Research* **2016** 5:F1000 Faculty Rev-1885. doi:10.12688/f1000research.8434.1. Accessed March 7, 2017.

Brady ST, et al. *Basic Neurochemistry: Principles of Molecular, Cellular, and Medical Neurobiology*. AElsevier/Academic Press, Boston, **2012.**

Catterall WA. From ionic currents to molecular mechanisms: the structure and function of voltage-gated sodium channels. *Neuron*, **2000**, *26*:13–25.

Do Rego JL, et al. Neurosteroid biosynthesis: enzymatic pathways and neuroendocrine regulation by neurotransmitters and neuropeptides. *Front Neuroendocrinol*, **2009**, *30*:259–301.

Engel SR, Grant KA. Neurosteroids and behavior. *Int Rev Neurobiol*, **2001**, *46*:321–348.

Furtado M, Katzman MA. Examining the role of neuroinflammation in major depression. *Psychiatry Res*, **2015**, *229*(1–2):27–36.

Greenberg ME, et al. New insights in the biology of BDNF synthesis and release: implications in CNS function. *J Neurosci*, **2009**, *29*:12764–12767.

Heneka MT, et al. Neuroinflammation in Alzheimer's disease. *Lancet Neurol*, **2015**, *14*:388–405.

Hibbs RE, Gouaux E. Principles of activation and permeation in an anion-selective Cys-loop receptor. *Nature*, **2011**, 474:54–60.

Jentsch TJ. Chloride channels: a molecular perspective. *Curr Opin Neurobiol*, **1996**, *6*:303–310.

Kandel ER, et al. *Principles of Neural Science*. 5th ed. McGraw-Hill, Health Professions Division, New York, **2013**.

Kawate T, et al. Crystal structure of the ATP-gated P2X(4) ion channel in the closed state. *Nature*, **2009**, *460*:592–598.

Khan SM. The expanding roles of Gbg subunits in G protein–coupled receptor signaling and drug action. *Pharmacol Rev*, **2013**, *65*:545–577.

Lu Y, et al. BDNF: a key regulator for protein synthesis-dependent LTP and long-term memory? *Neurobiol Learn Mem*, **2008**, *89*:312–323.

Miller PS, Smart TG. Binding, activation, and modulation of Cys loop receptors. Trends Pharmacol Sci, **2010**, 31:161–174.

Millar NS, Gotti C. Diversity of vertebrate nicotinic acetylcholine receptors. *Neuropharmacology*, **2009**, 56:237–246.

Morales-Perez CL, Noviello CM, Hibbs RE. X-ray structure of the human a4ß2 nicotinic receptor. *Nature*, **2016**, 538:411–415.

Nestler EJ, et al. *Molecular Neuropharmacology: A Foundation for Clinical Neuroscience*. McGraw-Hill Companies, Inc., New York, **2015.**

Nilius B, Szallasi A. Transient receptor potential channels as drug targets: from the science of basic research to the art of medicine. *Pharmacol Rev*, **2014**, *66*:676–814.

Pang PT, Lu B. Regulation of late-phase LTP and long-term memory in normal and aging hippocampus: role of secreted proteins tPA and BDNF. *Ageing Res Rev*, **2004**, *3*:407–430.

Panula P, et al. International Union of Basic and Clinical Pharmacology. XCVIII. Histamine receptors. *Pharmacol Rev*, **2015**, *67*:601–655.

Rahmani B, et al. Neurosteroids; potential underpinning roles in maintaining homeostasis. *Gen Comp Endocrinol*, **2015**, *225*:242–250.

Reddy DS, Estes WA. Clinical potential of neurosteroids for CNS disorders. *Trends Pharmacol Sci*, **2016**, *37*:543–561.

Shepherd GM. *The Synaptic Organization of the Brain*. Oxford University Press, Oxford, U.K., **2004**.

Shukla AK, et al. Emerging paradigms of beta-arrestin-dependent seven transmembrane receptor signaling. *Trends Biochem Sci*, **2011**, *36*:457–469.

Sibley DR. *Handbook of Contemporary Neuropharmacology*. Wiley, Hoboken, NJ, **2007.**

Singhal G, et al. Inflammasomes in neuroinflammation and changes in brain function: a focused review. *Front Neurosci*, **2014**, *8*:315.

Skaper SD. The neurotrophin family of neurotrophic factors: an overview. *Methods Mol Biol*, **2012**, *846*:1–12.

Squire LR. *Fundamental Neuroscience*. Elsevier/Academic Press, Boston, **2013.**

Timmusk T, et al. Multiple promoters direct tissue-specific expression of the rat BDNF gene. *Neuron*, **1993**, *10*:475–489.

Vallee M. Neurosteroids and potential therapeutics: Focus on pregnenolone. *J Steroid Biochem Mol Biol*, **2016**, *160*:78–87.

Yamaura K, et al. Discovery of allosteric modulators for $GABA_A$ receptors by ligand-directed chemistry. *Nat Chem Biol*, **2016**, 12:822–830.

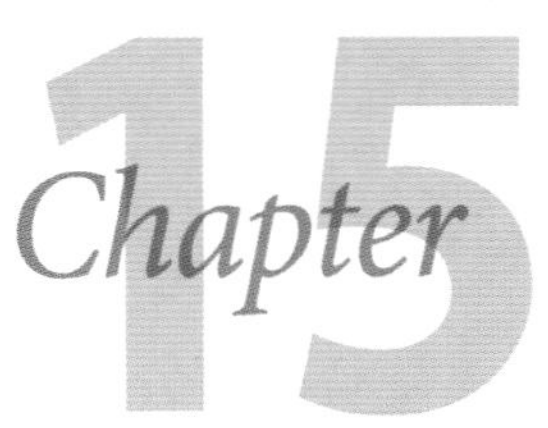

Drug Therapy of Depression and Anxiety Disorders

James M. O'Donnell, Robert R. Bies, and Richard C. Shelton

第十五章　抑郁症和焦虑症的药物治疗

中文导读

本章主要介绍：抑郁症和焦虑症的特征，包括抑郁症和焦虑症的症状；抑郁症和焦虑症的药物治疗，包括抗抑郁药的临床考虑、抗抑郁药和抗焦虑药的分类、药物代谢动力学、不良反应和药物相互作用；抗焦虑药，包括其临床考虑。

Depression and anxiety disorders are the most common mental illnesses, each affecting in excess of 15% of the population at some point in the life span. With the advent of more selective and safer drugs, the use of antidepressants and anxiolytics has moved from the exclusive domain of psychiatry to other medical specialties, including primary care. *The relative safety of the majority of commonly used antidepressants and anxiolytics notwithstanding, their optimal use requires a clear understanding of their mechanisms of action, pharmacokinetics, adverse effects, potential drug interactions, and the differential diagnosis of psychiatric illnesses* (Thronson and Pagalilauan, 2014).

Both depression and anxiety can affect an individual patient simultaneously; some of the drugs discussed here are effective in treating both types of disorders, suggesting common underlying mechanisms of pathophysiology and response to pharmacotherapy. In large measure, our current understanding of pathophysiological mechanisms underlying depression and anxiety has been inferred from the mechanisms of action of psychopharmacological compounds, notably their actions on neurotransmission involving serotonin (5HT), NE, and GABA (see Chapter 14). While depression and anxiety disorders comprise a wide range of symptoms, including changes in mood, behavior, somatic function, and cognition, some progress has been made in developing animal models that respond with some sensitivity and selectivity to antidepressant or anxiolytic drugs (Cryan and Holmes, 2005; Xu et al., 2012). The last half-century has seen notable advances in the discovery and development of drugs for treating depression and anxiety (Hillhouse and Porter, 2015).

Characterization of Depressive and Anxiety Disorders

Symptoms of Depression

Depression is classified as major depression (i.e., unipolar depression), persistent depressive disorder (dysthymia), or bipolar I and II disorders (i.e., manic-depressive illness). Bipolar depression and its treatment are discussed in Chapter 16. Lifetime risk of unipolar major depression is approximately 15%. Females are affected with major depression twice as frequently as males (Kessler et al., 1994). Depressive episodes are characterized by sad mood, pessimistic worry, diminished interest in normal

Abbreviations

ACh: acetylcholine
ADHD: attention-deficit/hyperactivity disorder
α_2 AR: α_2 adrenergic receptor
BDNF: brain-derived neurotrophic factor
CNS: central nervous system
C_p: plasma concentration
CREB: cyclic AMP response element binding protein
CYP: cytochrome P450
DA: dopamine
DAT: dopamine transporter
EEG: electroencephalogram
FDA: Food and Drug Administration
GABA: γ-aminobutyric acid
GI: gastrointestinal
GPCR: G protein–coupled receptor
5HT: serotonin (5-hydroxytryptamine)
IP_3: inositol 1,4,5-trisphosphate
MAO: monoamine oxidase
MAOI: monoamine oxidase inhibitor
MDMA: methylenedioxymethamphetamine (Ecstasy)
NE: norepinephrine
NET: NE transporter
NMDA: *N*-methyl-D-aspartate
PTSD: posttraumatic stress disorder
SERT: 5HT transporter
SNRI: serotonin-norepinephrine reuptake inhibitor
SSRI: selective serotonin reuptake inhibitor
TCA: tricyclic antidepressant
VMAT2: vesicular monoamine transporter

activities, mental slowing and poor concentration, insomnia or increased sleep, significant weight loss or gain due to altered eating and activity patterns, psychomotor agitation or retardation, feelings of guilt and worthlessness, decreased energy and libido, and suicidal ideation. In depressive episodes, these symptoms occur most days for a period of at least 2 weeks. In some cases, the primary complaint of patients involves somatic pain or other physical symptoms and can present a diagnostic challenge for primary care physicians. Depressive symptoms also can occur secondary to other illnesses, such as hypothyroidism, Parkinson disease, and inflammatory conditions. Further, depression often complicates the management of other medical conditions (e.g., severe trauma, cancer, diabetes, and cardiovascular disease, especially myocardial infarction) (Andrews and Nemeroff, 1994).

Depression is underdiagnosed and undertreated (Johansson et al., 2013; Suominen et al., 1998). Given that approximately 10%–15% of those with severe depression attempt suicide at some time (Chen and Dilsaver, 1996), it is important that symptoms of depression be recognized and treated in a timely manner. Furthermore, the response to treatment must be assessed and decisions made regarding continued treatment with the initial drug, dose adjustment, adjunctive therapy, or alternative medication.

Symptoms of Anxiety

Anxiety is a normal human emotion that serves an adaptive function from a psychobiological perspective. Anxiety disorders encompass a constellation of symptoms and include generalized anxiety disorder, obsessive-compulsive disorder, panic disorder, acute stress disorder, PTSD, separation anxiety disorder, social phobia, and specific phobias (Atack, 2003). In general, symptoms of anxiety that lead to pharmacological treatment are those that interfere significantly with normal function. In the psychiatric setting, feelings of fear or dread that are unfocused (e.g., generalized anxiety disorder) or out of scale with the perceived threat (e.g., specific phobias) often require treatment. All of these conditions, with the exception of specific phobias, can be treated with antidepressant medications, particularly SSRIs. Drug treatment includes acute drug administration to manage episodes of anxiety and chronic treatment to manage unrelieved and continuing anxiety disorders. Symptoms of anxiety also are often associated with depression and other medical conditions.

Pharmacotherapy for Depression and Anxiety

In general, antidepressants enhance serotonergic or noradrenergic transmission. Sites of interaction of antidepressant drugs with noradrenergic and serotonergic neurons are depicted in Figure 15–1. Table 15–1 summarizes the actions of the most widely used antidepressants. The most commonly used medications, often referred to as second-generation antidepressants, are the SSRIs and the SNRIs, which have less toxicity and improved safety compared to the first-generation drugs, which include MAOIs and TCAs (Millan, 2006; Rush et al., 2006).

In monoamine systems, neurotransmitter reuptake occurs via presynaptic high-affinity transporter proteins; inhibition of these transporters enhances neurotransmission, presumably by slowing clearance of the transmitter and prolonging its dwell time in the synapse (Shelton and Lester, 2006). Reuptake inhibitors block the neuronal SERT, the neuronal NET, or both. Similarly, TCAs and MAOIs enhance monoaminergic neurotransmission—the TCAs by inhibiting 5HT and NE reuptake via SERT or NET and the MAOIs by inhibiting monoamine metabolism and thereby increasing the levels of neurotransmitter in storage granules available for later release.

Long-term effects of antidepressant drugs evoke regulatory mechanisms that might contribute to the effectiveness of therapy (Shelton, 2000). These responses include altered adrenergic or serotonergic receptor density or sensitivity, altered receptor–G protein coupling and cyclic nucleotide signaling, induction of neurotrophic factors, and increased neurogenesis in the hippocampus (Schmidt and Duman, 2007). Persistent antidepressant effects depend on the continued inhibition of SERT or NET or enhanced serotonergic or noradrenergic neurotransmission achieved by an alternative pharmacological mechanism (Delgado et al., 1991; Heninger et al., 1996). Compelling evidence suggests that sustained signaling via NE or 5HT increases the expression of specific downstream gene products, particularly BDNF, which appears to influence dendritic spine formation, synaptogenesis, and neurogenesis (Duman and Duman, 2015).

Genome-wide association studies have suggested novel pathways that might be exploited for the discovery of antidepressants (Cannon and Keller, 2006; Lin and Lane, 2015). One promising avenue of investigation is the targeting of NMDA glutamatergic receptors with ketamine; this results in a rapid and somewhat persistent antidepressant effect in patients (Abdallah et al., 2015). Other approaches involve enhancing neurogenesis (Pascual-Brazo et al., 2014) or cyclic nucleotide signaling (O'Donnell and Zhang, 2004), which may be impaired in depressed patients (Fujita et al, 2012).

Clinical Considerations With Antidepressant Drugs

The response to antidepressant drug treatment generally has a "therapeutic lag" lasting 3–4 weeks before a measurable therapeutic effect becomes evident; however, symptoms respond differentially, with sleep disturbances improving sooner and mood and cognitive deficits later (Katz et al., 2004). While some of the lag is pharmacokinetic in nature, it is likely that a component is related to delayed postsynaptic changes. After the successful initial treatment phase, a 6- to 12-month maintenance treatment phase is typical, after which the drug is gradually withdrawn. If a patient is chronically depressed (i.e., has been depressed for more than 2 years), lifelong treatment with an antidepressant is advisable. Approximately two-thirds of patients show a marked decrease in depressive symptoms with an initial course of treatment, with one-third showing complete remission (Rush et al., 2006).

Antidepressants are not recommended as monotherapy for bipolar disorder. These drugs, notably TCAs, SNRIs, and, to a lesser extent, SSRIs, can induce a switch from a depressed episode to a manic or hypomanic episode in some patients (Gijsman et al., 2004; Goldberg and Truman, 2003).

A controversial issue regarding the use of all antidepressants is their relationship to suicide (Mann et al., 2006). Data establishing a clear link between antidepressant treatment and suicide are lacking. However, the FDA has issued a "black-box" warning regarding the use of SSRIs and a number of other antidepressants in children and adolescents due to the possibility of an association between antidepressant treatment and suicide (Isacsson and Rich, 2014). For seriously depressed patients, the risk of not being on an effective antidepressant drug outweighs the risk of being treated with one (Gibbons et al., 2007). However, it is important to monitor patients closely, particularly during initial treatment.

Classes of Antidepressant and Antianxiety Agents

Selective Serotonin Reuptake Inhibitors

The SSRIs are effective in treating major depression. SSRIs also are anxiolytics with demonstrated efficacy in the treatment of generalized anxiety, panic, social anxiety, and obsessive-compulsive disorders (Rush et al., 2006). Sertraline and paroxetine are approved for the treatment of PTSD. SSRIs also are used for treatment of premenstrual dysphoric syndrome and for preventing vasovagal symptoms in postmenopausal women.

The reuptake of 5HT into presynaptic terminals is mediated by SERT; neuronal uptake is the primary process by which neurotransmission via 5HT is terminated (see Figure 15–1). SSRIs block reuptake and enhance and prolong serotonergic neurotransmission. SSRIs used clinically are relatively selective for inhibition of SERT over NET (Table 15–2).

Treatment with an SSRI causes stimulation of $5HT_{1A}$ and $5HT_7$ autoreceptors on cell bodies in the raphe nucleus and of $5HT_{1D}$ autoreceptors on serotonergic terminals; this reduces 5HT synthesis and release. With repeated treatment with SSRIs, there is a gradual downregulation and desensitization of these autoreceptor mechanisms. In addition, downregulation of postsynaptic $5HT_{2A}$ receptors may contribute to antidepressant efficacy directly or by influencing the function of noradrenergic and other neurons via serotonergic heteroreceptors. Other postsynaptic 5HT receptors likely remain responsive to increased synaptic concentrations of 5HT and contribute to the therapeutic effects of the SSRIs.

Later-developing effects of SSRI treatment also may be important in mediating ultimate therapeutic responses. These include sustained increases in cyclic AMP signaling and phosphorylation of the nuclear transcription factor CREB, as well as increases in the expression of trophic

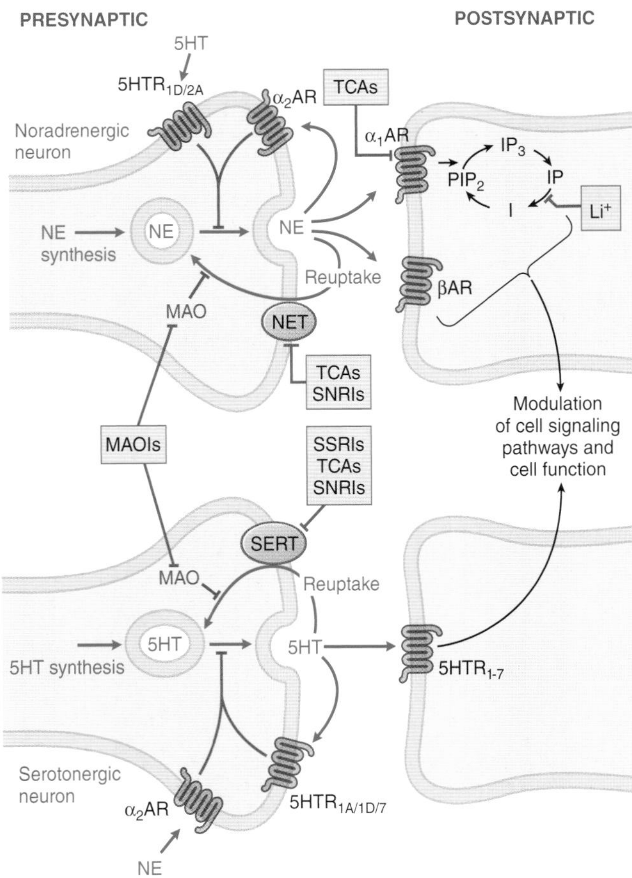

Figure 15–1 *Sites of action of antidepressants at noradrenergic (top) and serotonergic (bottom) nerve terminals.* SSRIs, SNRIs, and TCAs increase noradrenergic or serotonergic neurotransmission by blocking the NE or 5HT transporter (NET or SERT) at presynaptic terminals. MAOIs inhibit the catabolism of NE and 5HT. Trazodone and related drugs have direct effects on 5HT receptors (5HTRs) that contribute to their clinical effects. Chronic treatment with a number of antidepressants desensitizes presynaptic autoreceptors and heteroreceptors, producing long-lasting changes in monoaminergic neurotransmission. Postreceptor effects of antidepressant treatment, including modulation of GPCR signaling and activation of protein kinases and ion channels, are involved in the mediation of the long-term effects of antidepressant drugs. Li^+ inhibits IP breakdown and thereby enhances its accumulation and sequelae (Ca^{++} mobilization, PKC activation, depletion of cellular I). Li^+ may also alter release of neurotransmitters by a variety of putative mechanisms (see Chapter 16: Hypotheses for the Mechanism of Action of Lithium and Relationship to Anticonvulsants). Note that NE and 5HT may also affect each other's neurons by activating presynaptic receptors that couple to signaling pathways that reduce transmitter release. I, inositol; IP, inositol monophosphate; IP3, inositol 1,4,5-trisphosphate; PIP2, phosphatidylinositol 4,5-bisphosphate.

TABLE 15–1 ■ PROFILES OF REPRESENTATIVE ANTIDEPRESSANTS

CLASS Agent	DOSE[a] mg/d	BIOGENIC AMINE	SIDE EFFECTS									
			AGITATION	SEIZURES	SEDATION	HYPO-TENSION	ANTI-ACh EFFECTS	GI EFFECTS	WEIGHT GAIN	SEXUAL EFFECTS	CARDIAC EFFECTS	
NE reuptake inhibitors: 3° amine tricyclics												Imipramine
Amitriptyline	100–200	NE, 5HT	0	2+	3+	3+	3+	0/+	2+	2+	3+	
Clomipramine	100–200	NE, 5HT	0	3+	2+	2+	3+	+	2+	3+	3+	
Doxepin	100–200	NE, 5HT	0	2+	3+	2+	2+	0/+	2+	2+	3+	
Imipramine	100–200	NE, 5HT	0/+	2+	2+	2+	2+	0/+	2+	2+	3+	
(+)-Trimipramine	75–200	NE, 5HT	0	2+	3+	2+	3+	0/+	2+	2+	3+	
NE reuptake inhibitors: 2° amine tricyclics												Desipramine
Amoxapine	200–300	NE, DA	0	2+	+	2+	+	0/+	+	2+	2+	
Desipramine	100–200	NE	+	+	0/+	+	+	0/+	+	2+	2+	
Maprotiline	100–150	NE	0/+	3+	2+	2+	2+	0/+	+	2+	2+	
Nortriptyline	75–150	NE	0	+	+	+	+	0/+	+	2+	2+	
Protriptyline	15–40	NE	2+	2+	0/+	+	2+	0/+	+	2+	3+	
SSRIs												Fluoxetine
(±)-Citalopram	20–40	5HT	0/+	0	0/+	0	0	3+	0	3+	0	
(+)-Escitalopram	10–20	5HT	0/+	0	0/+	0	0	3+	0	3+	0	
(±)-Fluoxetine	20–80	5HT	+	0/+	0/+	0	0	3+	0/+	3+	0/+	
Fluvoxamine	100–200	5HT	0	0	0/+	0	0	3+	0	3+	0	
(−)-Paroxetine	20–40	5HT	+	0	0/+	0	0/+	3+	0	3+	0	
(+)-Sertraline	100–150	5HT	+	0	0/+	0	0	3+	0	3+	0	
(±)-Venlafaxine	75–225	5HT, NE	0/+	0	0	0	0	3+	0	3+	0/+	
Atypical antidepressants												Bupropion
(−)-Atomoxetine	40–80[b]	NE	0	0	0	0	0	0/+	0	0	0	
Bupropion	200–300	DA, ?NE	3+	4+	0	0	0	2+	0	0	0	
(+)-Duloxetine	80–100	NE, 5HT	+	0	0/+	0/+	0	0/+	0/+	0/+	0/+	
(±)-Mirtazapine	15–45	5HT, NE	0	0	4+	0/+	0	0/+	0/+	0	0	
Nefazodone	200–400	5HT	0	0	3+	0	0	2+	0/+	0/+	0/+	
Trazodone	150–200	5HT	0	0	3+	0	0	2+	+	+	0/+	
MAO inhibitors												Selegiline
Phenelzine	30–60	NE, 5HT, DA	0/+	0	+	+	0	0/+	+	3+	0	
Tranylcypromine	20–30	NE, 5HT, DA	2+	0	0	+	0	0/+	+	2+	0	
(−)-Selegiline	10	DA, ?NE, ?5HT	0	0	0	0	0	0	0	+	0	

0, negligible; 0/+, minimal; +, mild; 2+, moderate; 3+, moderately severe; 4+, severe. Other significant side effects for individual drugs are described in the text. Selegiline transdermal patch approved for depression.
[a]Higher and lower doses are sometimes used, depending on patient's needs and response to the drug; see the literature and FDA recommendations.
[b]Children, 0.5–1 mg/kg, up to 70 kg; see black-box warning.

factors such as BDNF and increases of neurogenesis from progenitor cells in the hippocampus and subventricular zone (Licznerski and Duman, 2013; Santarelli et al., 2003). Repeated treatment with SSRIs reduces the expression of SERT, resulting in reduced clearance of released 5HT and increased serotonergic neurotransmission (Benmansour et al., 1999).

Serotonin-Norepinephrine Reuptake Inhibitors

Five medications with a nontricyclic structure that inhibit the reuptake of both 5HT and NE have been approved for use in the U.S. for treatment of depression, anxiety disorders, pain, or other specific conditions: venlafaxine and its demethylated metabolite desvenlafaxine; duloxetine; milnacipran, and levomilnacipran.

The SNRIs inhibit both SERT and NET (see Table 15–2) and cause enhanced serotonergic or noradrenergic neurotransmission. Similar to the action of SSRIs, the initial inhibition of SERT induces activation of $5HT_{1A}$ and $5HT_{1D}$ autoreceptors, resulting in a decrease in serotonergic neurotransmission by a negative-feedback mechanism until these serotonergic autoreceptors are desensitized. Then, the enhanced 5HT concentration in the synapse can interact with postsynaptic 5HT receptors. The noradrenergic action of these drugs may contribute to downstream gene expression changes affecting BDNF, Trk-B (tyrosine receptor kinase B), and other neurotrophic factors and their signaling pathways (Shelton, 2000). Repeated treatment with SNRIs reduces the expression of SERT or NET, resulting in reduced neurotransmitter clearance and increased serotonergic or noradrenergic neurotransmission (Zhao et al., 2009).

The SNRIs were developed with the rationale that they might improve overall treatment response compared to SSRIs (Entsuah et al., 2001). The remission rate for venlafaxine appears slightly better than for SSRIs in head-to-head trials. Duloxetine, in addition to being approved for use in the treatment of depression and anxiety, is used for treatment of fibromyalgia and neuropathic pain associated with peripheral neuropathy (Finnerup et al., 2015). Off-label uses include stress urinary incontinence (duloxetine), autism, binge-eating disorders, hot flashes, pain syndromes, premenstrual dysphoric disorders, and PTSD (venlafaxine).

TABLE 15–2 ■ SELECTIVITY OF ANTIDEPRESSANTS AT THE HUMAN BIOGENIC AMINE TRANSPORTERS

DRUG	SELECTIVITY	DRUG	SELECTIVITY
NE SELECTIVE	**NET vs. SERT**	**5HT SELECTIVE**	**SERT vs. NET**
Oxaprotiline	800	*S*-Citalopram	7127
Maprotiline	532	*R,S*-Citalopram	3643
Viloxazine	109	Sertraline	1390
Nomifensine	64	Fluvoxamine	591
Desipramine	22	Paroxetine	400
Protriptyline	14	Fluoxetine	305
Atomoxetine	12	Clomipramine	123
Reboxetine	8.3	Venlafaxine	116
Nortriptyline	4.2	Zimelidine	60
Amoxapine	3.6	Trazodone	52
Doxepin	2.3	Imipramine	26
DA SELECTIVE	**DAT vs. NET**	Amitriptyline	8.0
Bupropion	1000	Duloxetine	7.0
		Dothiepin	5.5
		Milnacipran	1.6

Selectivity is defined as ratio of the relevant K_i values (SERT/NET, NET/SERT, NET/DAT). Bupropion is selective for the DAT relative to the NET and SERT.
Data from Frazer, 1997; Owens et al., 1997; and Leonard and Richelson, 2000.

Serotonin Receptor Antagonists

Several antagonists of the $5HT_2$ family of receptors are effective antidepressants. These include two close structural analogues, trazodone and nefazodone, as well as mirtazapine and mianserin (not marketed in the U.S.).

The efficacy of trazodone may be somewhat more limited than that of the SSRIs; however, low doses of trazodone (50–200 mg) have been used widely, both alone and concurrently with SSRIs or SNRIs, to treat insomnia. Both mianserin and mirtazapine are quite sedating and are treatments of choice for some depressed patients with insomnia. Trazodone blocks $5HT_2$ and α_1 adrenergic receptors. Trazodone also inhibits SERT but is markedly less potent for this action relative to its blockade of $5HT_{2A}$ receptors. Similarly, the most potent pharmacological action of nefazodone also is the blockade of the $5HT_2$ receptors. Both mirtazapine and mianserin potently block histamine H_1 receptors. They also have some affinity for α_2 adrenergic receptors. Their affinities for $5HT_{2A}$, $5HT_{2C}$, and $5HT_3$ receptors are high, although less so than for histamine H_1 receptors. Both of these drugs increase the antidepressant response when combined with SSRIs compared to the action of the SSRIs alone. Vortioxetine is a potent SERT inhibitor and binds to a number of serotonergic receptors, resulting in complex mechanisms of action (Bang-Andersen et al., 2011). Vortioxetine is a partial agonist at $5HT_{1A}$ and $5HT_{1B}$ receptors and an antagonist at $5HT_{1D}$, $5HT_3$, and $5HT_7$ receptors.

Bupropion

Bupropion has the backbone of β-phenethylamine; it is discussed separately because it appears to act via multiple mechanisms that differ somewhat from the mechanisms of SSRIs and SNRIs (Foley et al., 2006; Gobbi et al., 2003). It enhances both noradrenergic and dopaminergic neurotransmission via inhibition of reuptake by NET and DAT (although its effects on DAT are not potent in animal studies) (see Table 15–2). Bupropion's mechanism of action also may involve the presynaptic release of NE and DA and effects on VMAT2 (see Figure 8–6). The hydroxybupropion metabolite may contribute to the therapeutic effects of the parent compound: This metabolite appears to have a similar pharmacology and is present at substantial levels. Bupropion is indicated for the treatment of depression, prevention of seasonal depressive disorder, and as a smoking cessation treatment (Carroll et al., 2014). Bupropion has effects on sleep EEGs that are opposite those of most antidepressant drugs. Bupropion may improve symptoms of ADHD and has been used off label for neuropathic pain and weight loss. Clinically, bupropion is widely used in combination with SSRIs with the intent of obtaining a greater antidepressant response; however, there are limited clinical data providing strong support for this practice.

Atypical Antipsychotics

In addition to their use in schizophrenia, bipolar depression, and major depression with psychotic disorders, atypical antipsychotics have gained further, off-label use for major depression without psychotic features (Jarema, 2007). The combination of aripiprazole or quetiapine with SSRIs and SNRIs and a combination of olanzapine and the SSRI fluoxetine have been FDA-approved for treatment-resistant major depression (i.e., following an inadequate response to at least two different antidepressants).

The olanzapine-fluoxetine combination is available in fixed-dose combinations of 3, 6, or 12 mg of olanzapine and 25 or 50 mg of fluoxetine. Quetiapine may have either primary antidepressant actions on its own or adjunctive benefit for treatment-resistant depression; it is used off label for insomnia. The mechanism of action and adverse effects of the atypical antipsychotics are described in Chapter 16. The major risks of these agents are weight gain and metabolic syndrome, a greater problem for quetiapine and olanzapine than for aripiprazole.

Tricyclic Antidepressants

While TCAs have long-established efficacy, they exhibit serious side effects and generally are not used as first-line drugs for the treatment of depression (Hollister, 1981). TCAs and first-generation antipsychotics are synergistic for the treatment of psychotic depression. Tertiary amine TCAs (e.g., doxepin, amitriptyline) have been used for many years in relatively low doses for treating insomnia. In addition, because of the roles of NE and 5HT in nociception, these drugs are commonly used to treat a variety of pain conditions (Finnerup et al., 2015).

The pharmacological action of TCAs is antagonism of SERT and NET (see Table 15–2). In addition to inhibiting NET somewhat selectively (desipramine, nortriptyline, protriptyline, amoxapine) or both SERT and NET (imipramine, amitriptyline), these drugs block other receptors (H_1 histamine, $5HT_2$, α_1 adrenergic, and muscarinic cholinergic receptors). Given the comparable activities of clomipramine and SSRIs (see Tables 15–2 and 15–4; see also Decloedt and Stein, 2010), it is tempting to suggest that some combination of these additional pharmacological actions contributes to the therapeutic effects of TCAs and possibly SNRIs. One TCA, amoxapine, also is a DA receptor antagonist; its use, unlike that of other TCAs, poses some risk for the development of extrapyramidal side effects such as tardive dyskinesia.

Monoamine Oxidase Inhibitors

Monoamine oxidases A and B are widely distributed mitochondrial enzymes. MAO activities in the GI tract and liver, mainly MAO_A, protect the body from biogenic amines in the diet. In presynaptic nerve terminals, MAO metabolizes monoamine neurotransmitters via oxidative deamination. MAO_A preferentially metabolizes 5HT and NE and can metabolize DA; MAO_B is effective against 5HT and DA (see Chapters 8 and 13; see also Nestler et al., 2015). MAOIs have efficacy equivalent to that of the TCAs but are rarely used because of their toxicity and major interactions with some drugs (e.g., sympathomimetics and some opioids) and foods (those containing high amounts of tyramine) (Hollister, 1981). The MAOIs approved in the U.S. for treatment of depression include tranylcypromine, phenelzine, and isocarboxazid. These agents irreversibly inhibit both MAO_A and MAO_B, thereby inhibiting the body's capacity to metabolize not only endogenous monoamines such an NE and 5HT but also exogenous biogenic amines such as tyramine. Global inhibition of MAOs increases the bioavailability of dietary tyramine; tyramine-induced NE release can cause marked increases in blood pressure (hypertensive crisis) (see Chapter 8).

This potential to exacerbate the effects of indirectly acting sympathomimetic amines seems to relate mainly to inhibition of MAO_A. Selegiline is an irreversible MAO inhibitor but with specificity for MAO_B at low doses, thereby sparing MAO_A activity in the GI tract and elsewhere, and is less likely to cause this interaction (although at higher doses, selegiline will also inhibit MAO_A). Selegiline is available as a transdermal patch for the treatment of depression; transdermal delivery may reduce the risk for diet-associated hypertensive reactions. Some MAOIs are reversible competitive inhibitors of MAO_A. These agents such as moclobemide and eprobemide, permit tyramine to compete for MAO_A and thus exhibit reduced capacity to potentiate the effects of dietary tyramine; these agents are used elsewhere but are not approved for use in the U.S. (Finberg, 2014).

Pharmacokinetics

The metabolism of most antidepressants is mediated by hepatic CYPs (Table 15–3) (Probst-Schendzielorz et al., 2015). Some antidepressants inhibit the clearance of other drugs by the CYP system, and this possibility of drug interactions should be a significant factor in considering the choice of agents. Likewise, dose considerations have to include awareness of hepatic function (Mauri et al., 2014). While there are genetic polymorphisms that influence antidepressant metabolism, CYP genotyping has not yet been shown to have a practical influence on choice of drug treatment in clinical settings (Dubovsky, 2015).

Selective Serotonin Reuptake Inhibitors

All of the SSRIs are orally active and possess elimination half-lives consistent with once-daily dosing (Hiemke and Hartter, 2000). In the case of fluoxetine, the combined action of the parent and the demethylated metabolite norfluoxetine allows for a once-weekly formulation. CYP2D6 is involved in the metabolism of most SSRIs, and the SSRIs are at least moderately potent inhibitors of this isoenzyme. This creates a significant potential for drug interaction for postmenopausal women taking the breast cancer drug and estrogen antagonist tamoxifen (see Chapter 68). Because venlafaxine and desvenlafaxine are weak inhibitors of CYP2D6, these antidepressants are not contraindicated in this clinical situation. However, care should be used in combining SSRIs with drugs that are metabolized by CYPs. SSRIs such as escitalopram and citalopram that exhibit an age-dependent decrease in CYP2C19 metabolism should be dosed with care in elderly patients.

Serotonin-Norepinephrine Reuptake Inhibitors

Both immediate-release and extended-release (tablet or capsule) preparations of venlafaxine result in steady-state levels of drug in plasma within

TABLE 15–3 ■ DISPOSITION OF ANTIDEPRESSANTS

DRUG	ELIMINATION $t_{1/2}$ (h) OF PARENT DRUG ($t_{1/2}$ *of active metabolite*)	TYPICAL C_P (ng/mL)	PREDOMINANT CYP INVOLVED IN METABOLISM
Tricyclic antidepressants			
Amitriptyline	16 *(30)*	100–250	2D6, 2C19, 3A3/4, 1A2
Amoxapine	8 *(30)*	200–500	
Clomipramine	32 *(70)*	150–500	
Desipramine	30	125–300	
Doxepin	18 *(30)*	150–250	
Imipramine	12 *(30)*	175–300	
Maprotiline	48	200–400	
Nortriptyline	31	60–150	
Protriptyline	80	100–250	
Trimipramine	16 *(30)*	100–300	
Selective serotonin reuptake inhibitors			
R,S-Citalopram	36	75–150	3A4, 2C19
S-Citalopram	30	40–80	3A4, 2C19
Fluoxetine	53 *(240)*	100–500	2D6, 2C9
Fluvoxamine	18	100–200	2D6, 1A2, 3A4, 2C9
Paroxetine	17	30–100	2D6
Sertraline	23 *(66)*	25–50	2D6
Serotonin-norepinephrine reuptake inhibitors			
Duloxetine	11	—	2D6
Venlafaxine	5 *(11)*	—	2D6, 3A4
Other antidepressants			
Atomoxetine	5–20; child, 3	—	2D6, 3A3/4
Bupropion	11	75–100	2B6
Mirtazapine	16	—	2D6
Nefazodone	2–4	—	3A3/4
Reboxetine	12	—	—
Trazodone	6	800–1600	2D6

Values shown are elimination $t_{1/2}$ values for a number of clinically used antidepressant drugs; numbers in parentheses are $t_{1/2}$ values of active metabolites. Fluoxetine (2D6), fluvoxamine (1A2, 2C8, 3A3/4), paroxetine (2D6), and nefazodone (3A3/4) are potent inhibitors of CYPs; sertraline (2D6), citalopram (2C19), and venlafaxine are less-potent inhibitors. Plasma concentrations are those observed at typical clinical doses.
Information sources: FDA-approved package inserts and Appendix II of this book.

3 days. The elimination half-lives for the parent venlafaxine and its active and major metabolite desmethylvenlafaxine are 5 and 11 h, respectively. Desmethylvenlafaxine is eliminated by hepatic metabolism and by renal excretion. Venlafaxine dose reductions are suggested for patients with renal or hepatic impairment. Duloxetine has a $t_{1/2}$ of 12 h. Duloxetine is not recommended for those with end-stage renal disease or hepatic insufficiency.

Serotonin Receptor Antagonists

Mirtazapine has an elimination $t_{1/2}$ of 16–30 h. Thus, dose changes are suggested no more often than 1–2 weeks. The recommended initial dosing of mirtazapine is 15 mg/d, with a maximal recommended dose of 45 mg/d. Clearance of mirtazapine is decreased in the elderly and in patients with moderate-to-severe renal or hepatic impairment. Pharmacokinetics and adverse effects of mirtazapine may have an enantiomer-selective component (Brockmöller et al., 2007). Steady-state trazodone is observed within 3 days following a dosing regimen. Trazodone typically is started at 150 mg/d in divided doses, with 50-mg increments every 3–4 days. The maximally recommended dose is 400 mg/d for outpatients and 600 mg/d for inpatients. Nefazodone has a $t_{1/2}$ of only 2–4 h; its major metabolite hydroxynefazodone has a $t_{1/2}$ of 1.5–4 h.

Bupropion

Bupropion elimination has a $t_{1/2}$ of 21 h and involves both hepatic and renal routes. Patients with severe hepatic cirrhosis should receive a maximum dose of 150 mg every other day; consideration for a decreased dose should also be made in cases of renal impairment.

Tricyclic Antidepressants

The TCAs, or their active metabolites, have plasma half-lives of 8–80 h; this makes once-daily dosing possible for most of the compounds (Rudorfer and Potter, 1999). Steady-state concentrations occur within several days to several weeks of beginning treatment, as a function of the $t_{1/2}$. TCAs are largely eliminated by hepatic CYPs (see Table 15–3). Dosage adjustments of TCAs are typically made according to a patient's clinical response, not based on plasma levels. Nonetheless, monitoring the plasma exposure has an important relationship to treatment response: There is a relatively narrow therapeutic window. About 7% of patients metabolize TCAs slowly due to a variant CYP2D6 isoenzyme, causing a 30-fold difference in plasma concentrations among different patients given the same TCA dose. To avoid toxicity in "slow metabolizers," plasma levels should be monitored and doses adjusted downward.

Monoamine Oxidase Inhibitors

The MAOIs are metabolized by acetylation. A significant portion of the population (50% of the Caucasian population and an even higher percentage among Asians) are "slow acetylators" (see Table 7–2 and Figure 60–4) and will exhibit elevated plasma levels. The nonselective MAOIs used in the treatment of depression are irreversible inhibitors; thus, it takes up to 2 weeks for MAO activity to recover, even though the parent drug is excreted within 24 h (Livingston and Livingston, 1996). Recovery of normal enzyme function is dependent on synthesis and transport of new MAO to monoaminergic nerve terminals.

Adverse Effects

Selective Serotonin Reuptake Inhibitors

The SSRIs have no major cardiovascular side effects. The SSRIs are generally free of antimuscarinic side effects (dry mouth, urinary retention, confusion) and do not block α adrenergic receptors; most SSRIs, with the exception of paroxetine, do not block histamine receptors and usually are not sedating (Table 15–4).

Adverse side effects of SSRIs from excessive stimulation of brain $5HT_2$ receptors may result in insomnia, increased anxiety, irritability, and decreased libido, effectively worsening prominent depressive symptoms. Excess activity at spinal $5HT_2$ receptors causes sexual side effects, including erectile dysfunction, anorgasmia, and ejaculatory delay (Clayton et al., 2014). These effects may be more prominent with paroxetine (Vaswani et al., 2003). Aspects of sexual dysfunction can be treated in both men and women with the phosphodiesterase 5 inhibitor sildenafil (Nurnberg, 2001; Nurnberg et al., 2008; see also Chapter 45). Stimulation of $5HT_3$ receptors in the CNS and periphery contributes to GI effects, which are usually limited to nausea but may include diarrhea and emesis. Some patients experience an increase in anxiety, especially with the initial dosing of SSRIs. With continued treatment, some patients also report a dullness of intellectual abilities and concentration. In general, there is not a strong relationship between SSRI serum concentrations and therapeutic efficacy. Thus, dosage adjustments are based more on evaluation of clinical response and management of side effects.

Sudden withdrawal of antidepressants can precipitate a discontinuation syndrome (Harvey and Slabbert, 2014). For SSRIs or SNRIs, the symptoms of withdrawal may include dizziness, headache, nervousness, nausea, and insomnia. This withdrawal syndrome appears most intense for paroxetine and venlafaxine due to their relatively short half-lives and, in the case of paroxetine, lack of active metabolites. Conversely, the active metabolite of fluoxetine, norfluoxetine, has such a long $t_{1/2}$ (1–2 weeks) that few patients experience any withdrawal symptoms with discontinuation of fluoxetine.

TABLE 15–4 ■ POTENCIES OF SELECTED ANTIDEPRESSANTS AT MUSCARINIC, HISTAMINE H_1, AND α_1 ADRENERGIC RECEPTORS

	RECEPTOR TYPE		
DRUG	MUSCARINIC CHOLINERGIC	HISTAMINE H_1	α_1 ADRENERGIC
Amitriptyline	18	1.1	27
Amoxapine	1000	25	50
Atomoxetine	≥1000	≥1000	≥1000
Bupropion	40,000	6700	4550
R,S-Citalopram	1800	380	1550
S-Citalopram	1240	1970	3870
Clomipramine	37	31.2	39
Desipramine	196	110	130
Doxepin	83.3	0.24	24
Duloxetine	3000	2300	8300
Fluoxetine	2000	6250	5900
Fluvoxamine	24,000	>100,000	7700
Imipramine	91	11.0	91
Maprotiline	560	2.0	91
Mirtazapine	670	0.1	500
Nefazodone	11,000	21	25.6
Nortriptyline	149	10	58.8
Paroxetine	108	22,000	>100,000
Protriptyline	25	25	130
Reboxetine	6700	312	11,900
Sertraline	625	24,000	370
Trazodone	>100,000	345	35.7
Trimipramine	59	0.3	23.8
Venlafaxine	>100,000	>100,000	>100,000

Values are experimentally determined potencies (K_i values, nM) for binding to receptors that contribute to common side effects of clinically used antidepressant drugs: muscarinic cholinergic receptors (e.g., dry mouth, urinary retention, confusion); histamine H_1 receptors (sedation); and α_1 adrenergic receptors (orthostatic hypotension, sedation).
Data from Leonard and Richelson, 2000.

Unlike the other SSRIs, paroxetine is associated with an increased risk of congenital cardiac malformations when administered in the first trimester of pregnancy (Gadot and Koren, 2015). Venlafaxine also is associated with an increased risk of perinatal complications.

Serotonin-Norepinephrine Reuptake Inhibitors

The SNRIs have a side-effect profile similar to that of the SSRIs, including nausea, constipation, insomnia, headaches, and sexual dysfunction. The immediate-release formulation of venlafaxine can induce sustained diastolic hypertension (diastolic blood pressure > 90 mm Hg at consecutive weekly visits) in 10%–15% of patients at higher doses; this risk is reduced with the extended-release form. This effect of venlafaxine may not be associated simply with inhibition of NET because duloxetine does not share this side effect.

Serotonin Receptor Antagonists

Regarding the serotonin receptor antagonists, the main side effects of mirtazapine, seen in more than 10% of the patients, are somnolence, increased appetite, and weight gain. A rare side effect of mirtazapine is agranulocytosis. Trazodone use is associated with priapism in rare instances. Nefazodone was voluntarily withdrawn from the market in several countries after rare cases of liver failure were associated with its use. In the U.S., nefazodone is marketed with a black-box warning regarding hepatotoxicity.

Bupropion

Typical side effects associated with bupropion include anxiety, mild tachycardia and hypertension, irritability, and tremor. Other side effects include headache, nausea, dry mouth, constipation, appetite suppression, insomnia, and, rarely, aggression, impulsivity, and agitation. Seizures are dependent on dose and C_p, with seizures occurring rarely within the recommended dose range. Bupropion should be avoided in patients with seizure disorders as well as those with bulimia due to an increased risk of seizures (Horne et al., 1988; Noe et al., 2011). At doses higher than that recommended for depression (450 mg/d), the risk of seizures increases significantly. The use of extended-release formulations often blunts the maximum concentration observed after dosing and minimizes the chance of reaching drug levels associated with an increased risk of seizures.

Tricyclic Antidepressants

The TCAs are potent antagonists at histamine H_1 receptors, and this antagonism contributes to the sedative effects of TCAs (see Table 15–4). Antagonism of muscarinic ACh receptors contributes to cognitive dulling as well as a range of adverse effects mediated by the parasympathetic nervous system (blurred vision, dry mouth, tachycardia, constipation, difficulty urinating). Some tolerance does occur for these anticholinergic effects. Antagonism of α_1 adrenergic receptors contributes to orthostatic hypotension and sedation. Weight gain is another side effect of this class of antidepressants.

The TCAs have quinidine-like effects on cardiac conduction that can be life threatening with overdose and limit the use of TCAs in patients with heart disease. This is the primary reason that only a limited supply should be available to the patient at any given time. Like other antidepressant drugs, TCAs also lower the seizure threshold.

Monoamine Oxidase Inhibitors

Hypertensive crisis resulting from food or drug interactions is one of the life-threatening toxicities associated with use of the MAOIs (Rapaport, 2007). Foods containing tyramine are a contributing factor. MAO_A within the intestinal wall and MAO_A and MAO_B in the liver normally degrade dietary tyramine. When MAO_A is inhibited, tyramine can enter the systemic circulation and be taken up into adrenergic nerve endings, where it causes release of catecholamines from storage vesicles. The released catecholamines stimulate postsynaptic receptors in the periphery, increasing blood pressure to dangerous levels. The concurrent use of MAOIs and medications that contain sympathomimetic compounds also results in a potentially life-threatening elevation of blood pressure. In comparison to tranylcypromine and isocarboxazid, the selegiline (selective for MAO_B) transdermal patch is better tolerated and safer, as are the reversible, competitive inhibitors moclobemide and eprobemide. Another serious, life-threatening issue with chronic administration of MAOIs is hepatotoxicity.

Drug Interactions

Many of these drugs are metabolized by hepatic CYPs, especially CYP2D6. Thus, other agents that are substrates or inhibitors of CYP2D6 can increase plasma concentrations of the primary drug. The combination of other classes of antidepressant agents with MAOIs is inadvisable and can lead to *serotonin syndrome*, a serious triad of abnormalities consisting of cognitive, autonomic, and somatic effects due to excess serotonin. Symptoms of the serotonin syndrome include hyperthermia, muscle rigidity, myoclonus, tremors, autonomic instability, confusion, irritability, and agitation; this can progress toward coma and death.

Selective Serotonin Reuptake Inhibitors

Paroxetine and, to a lesser degree, fluoxetine are potent inhibitors of CYP2D6 (Hiemke and Hartter, 2000). The other SSRIs, outside of fluvoxamine, are at least moderate inhibitors of CYP2D6. This inhibition can result in disproportionate increases in plasma concentrations of drugs metabolized by CYP2D6 when doses of these drugs are increased. Fluvoxamine directly inhibits CYP1A2 and CYP2C19; fluoxetine and fluvoxamine also inhibit CYP3A4. A prominent interaction is the increase in TCA exposure that may be observed during coadministration of TCAs and SSRIs.

The MAOIs enhance the effects of SSRIs due to inhibition of 5HT metabolism. Administration of these drugs together can produce synergistic increases in extracellular brain 5HT, leading to the serotonin syndrome (see previous discussion). Other drugs that may induce the serotonin syndrome include substituted amphetamines such as MDMA (Ecstasy), which directly releases 5HT from nerve terminals.

The SSRIs should not be started until at least 14 days following discontinuation of treatment with an MAOI; this allows for synthesis of the new MAO. For all SSRIs but fluoxetine, at least 14 days should pass prior to beginning treatment with an MAOI following the end of treatment with an SSRI. Because the active metabolite norfluoxetine has a $t_{1/2}$ of 1–2 weeks, at least 5 weeks should pass between stopping fluoxetine and beginning an MAOI.

Serotonin-Norepinephrine Reuptake Inhibitors

While a 14-day period is recommended between ending MAOI therapy and starting venlafaxine treatment, an interval of 7 days is considered safe. Duloxetine has a similar interval for initiation following MAOI therapy; conversely, only a 5-day waiting period is needed before beginning MAOI treatment after ending duloxetine. Failure to observe these required waiting periods can result in the serotonin syndrome.

Serotonin Receptor Antagonists

Trazodone dosing may need to be lowered when given together with drugs that inhibit CYP3A4. Mirtazapine is metabolized by CYPs 2D6, 1A2, and 3A4 and may interact with drugs that share these CYP pathways, requiring mutual dose reductions. Trazodone and nefazodone are weak inhibitors of 5HT uptake and should not be administered with MAOIs due to concerns about serotonin syndrome.

Bupropion

The major route of metabolism for bupropion is CYP2B6. Bupropion and its metabolite hydroxybupropion can inhibit CYP2D6, the CYP responsible for metabolism of several SSRIs (Table 15–3) as well as some β blockers and haloperidol, among others. Thus, the potential for interactions of bupropion with SSRIs and other drugs metabolized by CYP2D6 should be kept in mind until the safety of the combination is firmly established.

Tricyclic Antidepressants

Drugs that inhibit CYP2D6, such as bupropion and SSRIs, may increase plasma exposures of TCAs. TCAs can potentiate the actions of sympathomimetic amines and should not be used concurrently with MAOIs or within 14 days of stopping MAOIs. A *number of other drugs have similar side-effect profiles as TCAs, and concurrent use risks enhanced side effects* (see previous discussion in Adverse Effects); this includes phenothiazine antipsychotic agents, type 1C antiarrhythmic agents, and other drugs with antimuscarinic, antihistaminic, and α adrenergic antagonistic effects.

Monoamine Oxidase Inhibitors

Serotonin syndrome is the most serious drug interaction for the MAOIs (see Adverse Effects). The most common cause of serotonin syndrome in patients taking MAOIs is the accidental coadministration of a 5HT reuptake-inhibiting antidepressant or tryptophan. Other serious drug interactions include those with meperidine and tramadol. MAOIs also interact with sympathomimetics such as pseudoephedrine, phenylephrine, oxymetazoline, phenylpropanolamine, and amphetamine; these are commonly found in cold and allergy medication and diet aids and should be avoided by patients taking MAOIs. Likewise, patients on MAOIs must avoid foods containing high levels of tyramine: soy products, dried meats and sausages, dried fruits, home-brewed and tap beers, red wine, pickled or fermented foods, and aged cheeses (FDA, 2010).

ANXIOLYTIC DRUGS

Primary treatments for anxiety-related disorders include the SSRIs, SNRIs, benzodiazepines, buspirone, and β adrenergic antagonists (Atack, 2003). The SSRIs and the SNRI venlafaxine are well tolerated with a reasonable side-effect profile; in addition to their documented antidepressant activity, they have anxiolytic activity with chronic treatment. The benzodiazepines are effective anxiolytics as both acute and chronic treatment. There is concern regarding their use because of their potential for dependence and abuse as well as negative effects on cognition and memory. Buspirone, like the SSRIs, is effective following chronic treatment. It acts, at least in part, via the serotonergic system, where it is a partial agonist at $5HT_{1A}$ receptors. Buspirone also has antagonistic effects at DA D_2 receptors, but the relationship between this effect and its clinical actions is uncertain. β Adrenergic antagonists, particularly those with higher lipophilicity (e.g., propranolol and nadolol), are occasionally used for performance anxiety such as fear of public speaking; their use is limited due to significant side effects, such as hypotension.

Antihistamines and sedative-hypnotic agents have been tried as anxiolytics but are generally not recommended because of their side-effect profiles and the availability of superior drugs. Hydroxyzine, which produces short-term sedation, is used in patients who cannot use other types of anxiolytics (e.g., those with a history of drug or alcohol abuse where benzodiazepines would be avoided). Chloral hydrate has been used for situational anxiety, but there is a narrow dose range where anxiolytic effects are observed in the absence of significant sedation; therefore, the use of chloral hydrate is not recommended.

Clinical Considerations With Anxiolytic Drugs

The choice of pharmacological treatment of anxiety is dictated by the specific anxiety-related disorders and the clinical need for acute anxiolytic effects (Millan, 2003). Among the commonly used anxiolytics, only the benzodiazepines and β adrenergic antagonists are effective acutely; the use of β adrenergic antagonists is generally limited to treatment of situational anxiety. Chronic treatment with SSRIs, SNRIs, and buspirone is required to produce and sustain anxiolytic effects. When an immediate anxiolytic effect is desired, benzodiazepines are typically selected.

Benzodiazepines, such as alprazolam, chlordiazepoxide, clonazepam, clorazepate, diazepam, lorazepam, and oxazepam, are effective in the treatment of generalized anxiety disorder, panic disorder, and situational anxiety. In addition to their anxiolytic effects, benzodiazepines produce sedative, hypnotic, anesthetic, anticonvulsant, and muscle relaxant effects. The benzodiazepines also impair cognitive performance and memory, adversely affect motor control, and potentiate the effects of other sedatives, including alcohol. The anxiolytic effects of this class of drugs are mediated by allosteric interactions with the pentameric benzodiazepine-$GABA_A$ receptor complex, in particular $GABA_A$ receptors comprising α2, α3, and α5 subunits (Chapters 14 and 19). The primary effect of the anxiolytic benzodiazepines is to enhance the inhibitory effects of the neurotransmitter GABA.

One area of concern regarding the use of benzodiazepines in the treatment of anxiety is the potential for habituation, dependence, and abuse. Patients with certain personality disorders or a history of drug or alcohol abuse are particularly susceptible. However, the risk of dependence must be balanced with the need for treatment because benzodiazepines are effective in both short- and long-term treatment of patients with sustained or recurring bouts of anxiety. Further, premature discontinuation of benzodiazepines, in the absence of other pharmacological treatment, results in a high rate of relapse. Withdrawal of benzodiazepines after chronic treatment, particularly with benzodiazepines with short durations of action, can include increased anxiety and seizures. For this reason, it is important that discontinuation be carried out in a gradual manner.

Benzodiazepines cause many adverse effects, including sedation, mild memory impairments, decreased alertness, and slowed reaction time (which may lead to accidents). Memory problems can include visual-spatial deficits but will manifest clinically in a variety of ways, including difficulty in word finding. Occasionally, paradoxical reactions can occur with benzodiazepines, such as increases in anxiety, sometimes reaching panic attack proportions. Other pathological reactions can include irritability, aggression, or behavioral disinhibition. Amnesic reactions (i.e., loss of memory for particular periods) can also occur. Benzodiazepines should not be used in pregnant women; there have been rare reports of craniofacial defects. In addition, benzodiazepines taken prior to delivery may result in sedated, underresponsive newborns and prolonged withdrawal reactions. In the elderly, benzodiazepines increase the risk for falls and must be used cautiously. These drugs are safer than classical sedative-hypnotics in overdosage and typically are fatal only if combined with other CNS depressants.

Benzodiazepines have some abuse potential, although their capacity for abuse is considerably below that of other classical sedative-hypnotic agents. When these agents are abused, it is generally in a multidrug abuse pattern, frequently connected with failed attempts to control anxiety. Tolerance to the anxiolytic effects develops with chronic administration, with the result that some patients escalate the dose of benzodiazepines over time. Ideally, benzodiazepines should be used for short periods of time and in conjunction with other medications (e.g., SSRIs) or evidence-based psychotherapies (e.g., cognitive behavioral therapy for anxiety disorders).

The SSRIs and the SNRI venlafaxine are first-line treatments for most types of anxiety disorders, except when an acute drug effect is desired; fluvoxamine is approved only for obsessive-compulsive disorder. As for their antidepressant actions, the anxiolytic effects of these drugs become manifest following chronic treatment. Other drugs with actions on serotonergic neurotransmission, including trazodone, nefazodone, and mirtazapine, also are used in the treatment of anxiety disorders. Details regarding the pharmacology of these classes were presented previously in this chapter.

Both SSRIs and SNRIs are beneficial in specific anxiety conditions, such as generalized anxiety disorder, social phobias, obsessive-compulsive disorder, and panic disorder. These effects appear to be related to the capacity of serotonin to regulate the activity of brain structures, such as the amygdala and locus coeruleus, that are thought to be involved in the genesis of anxiety. Interestingly, the SSRIs and SNRIs often will produce some increases in anxiety in the short term that dissipate with time. Therefore, the maxim "start low and go slow" is indicated with anxious patients; however, many patients with anxiety disorders ultimately will require doses that are about the same as those required for the treatment of depression. Anxious patients appear to be particularly prone to severe discontinuation reactions with certain medications such as venlafaxine and paroxetine; therefore, slow off-tapering is required.

Buspirone is used in the treatment of generalized anxiety disorder (Goodman, 2004). Like the SSRIs, buspirone requires chronic treatment for effectiveness. Also, like the SSRIs, buspirone lacks many of the other pharmacological effects of the benzodiazepines: It is not an anticonvulsant, muscle relaxant, or sedative, and it does not impair psychomotor performance or result in dependence. Buspirone is primarily effective in the treatment of generalized anxiety disorder, but not for other anxiety disorders. In fact, patients with panic disorder often note an increase in anxiety acutely following initiation of buspirone treatment; this may be the result of the fact that buspirone causes increased firing rates of the locus coeruleus, which is thought to underlie part of the pathophysiology of panic disorder.

Acknowledgment: *Ross J. Baldessarini contributed to this chapter in recent editions of this book. We have retained some of his text in the current edition.*

Drug Facts for Your Personal Formulary: *Depression and Anxiety Disorders*

Drugs	Therapeutic Uses	Clinical Pharmacology and Tips
Selective Serotonin Reuptake Inhibitors		
Citalopram Escitalopram Fluoxetine Fluvoxamine Paroxetine Sertraline Vilazodone	• Anxiety and depression disorders • Obsessive-compulsive disorder, PTSD • SERT selective; little effect on NET • Vilazodone also acts as $5HT_{1A}$ partial agonist	• Side effects include GI disturbances • May cause sexual dysfunctions • May increase risk of suicidal thoughts or behavior • Serotonin syndrome with MAOIs • Some CYP interactions • Vilazodone is not associated with sexual dysfunction or weight gain
Serotonin-Norepinephrine Reuptake Inhibitors		
Venlafaxine Desvenlafaxine Duloxetine Milnacipran Levomilnacipran	• Anxiety and depression, ADHD, autism, fibromyalgia, PTSD, menopause symptoms • Inhibitors of SERT and NET	• Side effects include nausea and dizziness • May increase risk of suicidal thoughts or behavior • May cause sexual dysfunctions • Duloxetine and milnacipran contraindicated in uncontrolled narrow-angle or angle-closure glaucoma
Tricyclic Antidepressants		
Amitriptyline Clomipramine Doxepin Imipramine Trimipramine Nortriptyline Maprotiline Protriptyline Desipramine Amoxapine	• Block SERT, NET, α_1, H_1, and M_1 receptors • Major depression	• Generally replaced by newer antidepressants with fewer side effects • Numerous side effects: orthostatic hypertension, weight gain, GI disturbances, sexual dysfunction, seizures, irregular heart beats • Should not be used within 14 days of taking MAOIs • Suicidal thoughts or behavior
Atypical Antipsychotics		
Aripiprazole Brexpiprazole Lurasidone Olanzapine Quetiapine Risperidone	• Resistant major depression and psychotic disorders • Schizophrenia • Bipolar depression	• See Chapter 16 for details • Metabolic syndrome and weight gain
Monoamine Oxidase Inhibitors		
Isocarboxazid Phenelzine Selegiline Tranylcypromine	• Inhibit MAO_A and MAO_B to prevent NE, DA, and 5HT breakdown • Major depression disorders resistant to other antidepressants	• Many side effects, including weight gain and sexual dysfunction; replaced by newer antidepressants • Suicidal thoughts • Slow elimination • May cause hypertensive crisis if taken with tyramine-containing foods/beverages • Selegiline at lower doses is selective for MAO_B (found in serotonergic neurons) • Selegiline, as a transdermal patch, is approved for treatment of depression
Atypical Antidepressants		
Bupropion Trazodone Nefazodone Mirtazapine Mianserin (not marketed in the U.S.) Vortioxetine	• Depression • Smoking cessation (bupropion) • Insomnia (low-dose trazodone)	• Bupropion is a DAT inhibitor used to help quit smoking; no weight gain side effect • Mirtazapine, trazodone, and nefazodone are $5HT_2$ receptor antagonists • Mirtazapine and trazodone may cause drowsiness and should be taken at bedtime • Risk of hepatic failure with nefazodone • Vortioxetine: SERT inhibitor, $5HT_{1A}$ agonist, and $5HT_3$ antagonist • Suicidal thoughts or behavior • Do not use within 14 days of taking MAOI

Bibliography

Abdallah CG, et al. Ketamine as a promising prototype for a new generation of rapid-acting antidepressants. *Ann N Y Acad Sci*, **2015**, *1344*:66–77.

Andrews JM, Nemeroff CB. Contemporary management of depression. *Am J Med*, **1994**, *97*:24S–32S.

Atack JR. Anxioselective compounds acting at the GABA(A) receptor benzodiazepine binding site. *Curr Drug Targets CNS Neurol Disord*, **2003**, *2*:213–232.

Bang-Andersen B, et al. Discovery of 1-[2-(2,4-dimethylphenyl-sulfanyl) phenyl]piperazine (Lu AA21004): a novel multimodal compound for the treatment of major depressive disorder. *J Med Chem*, **2011**, *54*:3206–3221.

Benmansour S, et al. Effects of chronic antidepressant treatments on serotonin transporter function, density, and mRNA level. *J Neurosci*, **1999**, *19*:10494–10501.

Brockmöller J, et al. Pharmacokinetics of mirtazapine: enantioselective effects of the CYP2D6 ultra rapid metabolizer genotype and correlation with adverse effects. *Clin Pharmacol Ther*, **2007**, *81*:699–707.

Cannon TD, Keller MC. Endophenotypes in the genetic analyses of mental disorders. *Annu Rev Clin Psychol*, **2006**, *2*:267–290.

Carroll FI, et al. Bupropion and bupropion analogs as treatments for CNS disorders. *Adv Pharmacol*, **2014**, *69*:177–216.

Chen YW, Dilsaver SC. Lifetime rates of suicide attempts among subjects with bipolar and unipolar disorders relative to subjects with other axis I disorders. *Biol Psychiatry*, **1996**, *39*:896–899.

Clayton AH, et al. Antidepressants and sexual dysfunction: mechanisms and clinical implications. *Postgrad Med*, **2014**, *126*:91–99.

Cryan JF, Holmes, A. The ascent of mouse: advances in modelling human depression and anxiety. *Nat Rev*, **2005**, *4*:775–790.

Decloedt EH, Stein DJ. Current trends in drug treatment of obsessive-compulsive disorder. *Neuropsychiatr Dis Treat*, **2010**, *6*:233–242.

Delgado PL, et al. Rapid serotonin depletion as a provocative challenge test for patients with major depression: relevance to antidepressant action and the neurobiology of depression. *Psychopharmacol Bull*, **1991**, *27*:321–330.

Dubovsky SL. The usefulness of genotyping cytochrome P450 enzymes in the treatment of depression. *Expert Opin Drug Metab Toxicol*, **2015**, *11*:369–379.

Duman CH, Duman RS. Spine synapse remodeling in the pathophysiology and treatment of depression. *Neurosci Lett*, **2015**, *601*:20–29.

Entsuah AR, et al. Response and remission rates in different subpopulations with major depressive disorder administered venlafaxine, selective serotonin reuptake inhibitors, or placebo. *J Clin Psychiatry*, **2001**, *62*:869–877.

FDA. Avoid food-drug interactions. Publication no. (FDA) CDER 10-1933, **2010**, pp. 21–22. Available at: http://www.fda.gov/drugs. Accessed March 17, 2016.

Finberg JP. Update on the pharmacology of selective inhibitors of MAO-A and MAO-B: focus on modulation of CNS monoamine neurotransmitter release. *Pharmacol Ther*, **2014**, *143*:133–152.

Finnerup NB, et al. Pharmacotherapy for neuropathic pain in adults: a systematic review and meta-analysis. *Lancet Neurol*, **2015**, *14*:162–173.

Foley KF, et al. Bupropion: pharmacology and therapeutic applications. *Expert Rev Neurother*, **2006**, *6*:1249–1265.

Frazer A. Pharmacology of antidepressants. *J Clin Psychopharmacol*, **1997**, *17*(suppl 1):2S–18S.

Fujita M, et al. Downregulation of brain phosphodiesterase type IV measured with 11C-(R)-rolipram positron emission tomography in major depressive disorder. *Biol Psychiatry*, **2012**, *72*:548–554.

Gadot Y, Koren G. The use of antidepressants in pregnancy: focus on maternal risks. *J Obstet Gynaecol Can*, **2015**, *37*:56–63.

Gibbons RD, et al. Early evidence on the effects of regulators' suicidality warnings on SSRI prescriptions and suicide in children and adolescents. *Am J Psychiatry*, **2007**, *164*:1356–1363.

Gijsman HJ, et al. Antidepressants for bipolar depression: a systematic review of randomized, controlled trials. *Am J Psychiatry*, **2004**, *161*:1537–1547.

Gobbi G, et al. Neurochemical and psychotropic effects of bupropion in healthy male subjects. *J Clin Psychopharmacol*, **2003**, *23*:233–239.

Goldberg JF, Truman CJ. Antidepressant-induced mania: an overview of current controversies. *Bipolar Disord*, **2003**, *5*:407–420.

Goodman WK. Selecting pharmacotherapy for generalized anxiety disorder. *J Clin Psychiatry*, **2004**, *65*(suppl 13):8–13.

Harvey BH, Slabbert FN. New insights on the antidepressant discontinuation syndrome. *Hum Psychopharmacol*, **2014**, *29*:503–516.

Heninger GR, et al. The revised monoamine theory of depression: a modulatory role for monoamines, based on new findings from monoamine depletion experiments in humans. *Pharmacopsychiatry*, **1996**, *29*:2–11.

Hiemke C, Hartter S. Pharmacokinetics of selective serotonin reuptake inhibitors. *Pharmacol Ther*, **2000**, *85*:11–28.

Hillhouse TM, Porter JH. A brief history of the development of antidepressant drugs: from monoamines to glutamate. *Exp Clin Psychopharmacol*, **2015**, *23*:1–21.

Hollister LE. Current antidepressant drugs: their clinical use. *Drugs*, **1981**, *22*:129–152.

Horne RL, et al. Treatment of bulimia with bupropion: a multicenter controlled trial. *J Clin Psychiatry*, **1988**, *49*:262–266.

Isacsson G, Rich CL. Antidepressant drugs and the risk of suicide in children and adolescents. *Paediatr Drugs*, **2014**, *16*:115–122.

Jarema M. Atypical antipsychotics in the treatment of mood disorders. *Curr Opin Psychiatry*, **2007**, *20*:23–29.

Johansson R, et al. Depression, anxiety and their comorbidity in the Swedish general population: point prevalence and the effect on health-related quality of life. *Peer J*, **2013**, *1*:e98. doi:10.7717/peerj.98. Accessed March 16, 2016.

Katz MM, et al. Onset and early behavioral effects of pharmacologically different antidepressants and placebo in depression. *Neuropsychopharmacology*, **2004**, *29*:566–579.

Kessler RC, et al. Lifetime and 12-month prevalence of *DSM-III-R* psychiatric disorders in the United States. Results from the National Comorbidity Survey. *Arch Gen Psychiatry*, **1994**, *51*:8–19.

Leonard BE, Richelson E. Synaptic effects of anitdepressants. In: Buckley PF, Waddington JL, eds. *Schizophrenia and Mood Disorders: The New Drug Therapies in Clinical Practice*. Butterworth-Heinemann, Boston, **2000**, 67–84.

Licznerski P, Duman RS. Remodeling of axo-spinous synapses in the pathophysiology and treatment of depression. *Neuroscience*, **2013**, *251*:33–50.

Lin E, Lane HY. Genome-wide association studies in pharmacogenomics of antidepressants. *Pharmacogenomics*, **2015**, *6*:555–566.

Livingston MG, Livingston HM. Monoamine oxidase inhibitors. An update on drug interactions. *Drug Saf*, **1996**, *14*:219–227.

Mann JJ, et al. ACNP Task Force report on SSRIs and suicidal behavior in youth. *Neuropsychopharmacology*, **2006**, *31*:473–492.

Mauri MC, et al. Pharmacokinetics of antidepressants in patients with hepatic impairment. *Clin Pharmacokinet*, **2014**, *53*:1069–1081.

Millan MJ. The neurobiology and control of anxious states. *Prog Neurobiol*, **2003**, *70*:83–244.

Millan MJ. Multi-target strategies for the improved treatment of depressive states: conceptual foundations and neuronal substrates, drug discovery and therapeutic application. *Pharmacol Ther*, **2006**, *110*:135–370.

Nestler EJ, et al. *Molecular Neuropharmacology*. 3rd ed. McGraw-Hill, New York, **2015**.

Noe KH, et al. Treatment of depression in patients with epilepsy. *Curr Treat Options Neurol*, **2011**, *13*:371–379.

Nurnberg HG. Managing treatment-emergent sexual dysfunction associated with serotonergic antidepressants: before and after sildenafil. *J Psychiatr Pract*, **2001**, *7*:92–108.

Nurnberg HG, et al. Sildenafil treatment of women with antidepressant-associated sexual dysfunction: a randomized controlled trial. *JAMA*, **2008**, *300*:395–404.

O'Donnell JM, Zhang HT. Antidepressant effects of inhibitors of cAMP phosphodiesterase (PDE4). *Trends Pharmacol Sci*, **2004**, *25*:158–163.

Owens MJ, et al. Neurotransmitter receptor and transporter binding profile of antidepressants and their metabolites. *J Pharmacol Exp Ther*, **1997**, *283*:1305–1322.

Pascual-Brazo J, et al. Neurogenesis as a new target for the development of antidepressant drugs. *Curr Pharm Des*, **2014**, *20*:3763–3775.

Probst-Schendzielorz K, et al. Effect of cytochrome P450 polymorphism on the action and metabolism of selective serotonin reuptake inhibitors. *Expert Opin Drug Metab Toxicol*, **2015**, *11*:1219–1232.

Rapaport MH. Dietary restrictions and drug interactions with monoamine oxidase inhibitors: the state of the art. *J Clin Psychiatry*, **2007**, *68*(suppl 8):42–46.

Rudorfer MV, Potter WZ. Metabolism of tricyclic antidepressants. *Cell Mol Neurobiol*, **1999**, *19*:373–409.

Rush AJ, et al. Acute and longer-term outcomes in depressed outpatients requiring one or several treatment steps: a STAR*D report. *Am J Psychiatry*, **2006**, *163*:1905–1917.

Santarelli L, et al. Requirement of hippocampal neurogenesis for the behavioral effects of antidepressants. *Science*, **2003**, *301*:805–809.

Schmidt HD, Duman RS. The role of neurotrophic factors in adult hippocampal neurogenesis, antidepressant treatments and animal models of depressive-like behavior. *Behav Pharmacol*, **2007**, *18*:391–418.

Shelton RC. Cellular mechanisms in the vulnerability to depression and response to antidepressants. *Psychiatr Clin North Am*, **2000**, *23*:713–729.

Shelton RC, Lester N. SSRIs and newer antidepressants. In: Stein DJ, Kupfer DJ, Schatzburg AF, eds. *APA Textbook of Mood Disorders*. APA Press, Washington, DC, **2006**, Chapter 16.

Suominen KH, et al. Inadequate treatment for major depression both before and after attempted suicide. *Am J Psychiatry*, **1998**, *155*:1778–1780.

Thronson LR, Pagalilauan GL. Psychopharmacology. *Med Clin North Am*, **2014**, *98*:927–958.

Vaswani M, et al. Role of selective serotonin reuptake inhibitors in psychiatric disorders: a comprehensive review. *Prog Neuropsychopharmacol Biol Psychiatry*, **2003**, *27*:85–102.

Xu Y, et al. Animal models of depression and neuroplasticity: assessing drug action in relation to behavior and neurogenesis. *Methods Mol Biol*, **2012**, *829*:103–124.

Zhao Z, et al. Association of changes in norepinephrine and serotonin transporter expression with the long-term behavioral effects of antidepressant drugs. *Neuropsychopharmacology*, **2009**, *34*:1467–1481.

Pharmacotherapy of Psychosis and Mania

Jonathan M. Meyer

第十六章　精神病和躁狂症的药物治疗

中文导读

本章主要介绍：精神病的治疗，包括多巴胺假说、相关病理生理学综述、精神病病理学和药物治疗的总体目标回顾、短期治疗、长期治疗、抗精神病药药理学、其他治疗的应用、不良反应和药物相互作用、主要可用药物；躁狂症的治疗，包括抗躁狂药的药理特性、锂的应用；躁狂症的临床总结。

Treatment of Psychosis

Psychosis is a symptom of mental illnesses characterized by a distorted or nonexistent sense of reality. Psychotic disorders have different etiologies, each of which demands a unique treatment approach. Common psychotic disorders include mood disorders (major depression or mania) with psychotic features, substance-induced psychosis, dementia with psychotic features, delirium with psychotic features, brief psychotic disorder, delusional disorder, schizoaffective disorder, and schizophrenia.

Schizophrenia has a worldwide prevalence of 1% and is considered the prototypic disorder for understanding the phenomenology of psychosis and the impact of antipsychotic treatment, but patients with schizophrenia exhibit features that extend beyond those seen in other psychotic illnesses. Hallucinations, delusions, disorganized speech, and disorganized or agitated behavior are psychotic symptoms found individually, and occasionally together, in all psychotic disorders and are typically responsive to pharmacotherapy. In addition to *positive symptoms*, schizophrenia patients also suffer from *negative symptoms* (apathy, avolition, alogia) and *cognitive deficits*, with the latter the most disabling aspect of the disorder (Young and Geyer, 2015).

The Dopamine Hypothesis

The syntheses of chlorpromazine (1950) and haloperidol (1958) allowed Carlsson to deduce that postsynaptic DA receptor antagonism was their common mechanism. Carlsson's discovery informed the development of numerous *typical* or first-generation antipsychotic drugs that were found to act specifically at D_2 receptors (Seeman, 2013). The discovery of clozapine's unique clinical features and binding profile stimulated development of second-generation antipsychotics that potently antagonize the $5HT_{2A}$ receptor while possessing less affinity for D_2 receptors than typical antipsychotic agents, resulting in antipsychotic efficacy with lower potential for extrapyramidal side effects. Subsequent research led to the development of agents with D_2 partial agonist properties that act

Abbreviations

ACEI: angiotensin-converting enzyme inhibitor
AUC: area under the curve
CBC: complete blood cell count
CNS: central nervous system
COX-2: cyclooxygenase 2
CV: cardiovascular
DA: dopamine
DAAO: D-amino acid oxidase
DAT: DA transporter
DM: diabetes mellitus
ECG: electrocardiogram
ECT: electroconvulsive therapy
eGFR: estimated glomerular filtration rate
EM: extensive metabolizer
ENaC: epithelial sodium channel
EPS: extrapyramidal symptom
FDA: Food and Drug Administration
G-CSF: granulocyte colony-stimulating factor
GFR: glomerular filtration rate
GlyT: glycine transporter
GSK: glycogen synthase kinase
5HT: serotonin
I_{kr}: inwardly rectifying K^+ channels
IM: intramuscular
LAI: long-acting injectable
MAO: monoamine oxidase
mGlu: metabotropic glutamate
NDI: nephrogenic diabetes insipidus
NE: norepinephrine
NMDA: *N*-methyl-D-aspartate
NMS: neuroleptic malignant syndrome
ODT: oral dissolving tablet
PDP: Parkinson disease psychosis
PET: positron emission tomography
PGP: P-glycoprotein
PK_: protein kinase _, as in PKA, PKC
PP2A: protein phosphatase 2A
SCD: sudden cardiac death
T_4: levorotatory thyroxine
TD: tardive dyskinesia
TH: tyrosine hydroxylase
TSH: thyrotropin (previously thyroid-stimulating hormone)
VMAT2: vesicular monoamine transporter 2

as modulators of dopaminergic neurotransmission (Meyer and Leckband, 2013).

The DA model of antipsychotic action has limitations: It does not explain the psychotomimetic effects of LSD (e.g., a potent $5HT_{2A}$ receptor agonist) or the effects of phencyclidine and ketamine, antagonists of the NMDA glutamate receptor. However, phencyclidine and ketamine indirectly act to stimulate DA availability by decreasing the glutamate-mediated tonic inhibition of DA release in the mesolimbic DA pathway (Howes et al., 2015). Exploration of nondopaminergic antipsychotic mechanisms led to approval of pimavanserin, a potent $5HT_{2A}$ inverse agonist for treatment of Parkinson disease psychosis (PDP). Phase 3 trials of glutamate modulators have not been successful. Except for pimavanserin, all approved antipsychotic agents share a common mechanism of action: direct modulation of D_2 receptor activity (Figure 16–1).

Mechanism of Action of D_2 Receptors

Dopamine D_2 receptors share common properties with D_3 and D_4 receptors in that each is linked to inhibitory G protein G_i, and receptor stimulation results in decreased cyclic AMP production and thus a reduction in intracellular cyclic AMP (Figure 16–1), whereas agonists at D_1 and D_5 receptors stimulate the G_s–adenylyl cyclase–cyclic AMP pathway (Seeman, 2013). Antipsychotic actions at D_2 receptors are also mediated through non-G protein, particularly via modulation of the activity of GSK-3β through a β-arrestin-2/PKB/PP2A signaling complex (see Chapter 3). Atypical antipsychotics antagonize D_2 receptor/β-arrestin-2 interactions more than G protein–dependent signaling, but typical antipsychotics inhibit both pathways with similar efficacy (Urs et al., 2012).

Review of Relevant Pathophysiology

Not all psychosis is schizophrenia, and the pathophysiology relevant to effective schizophrenia treatment may not apply to other psychotic disorders. The effectiveness of dopamine D_2 antagonists for the positive symptoms of psychosis seen in most psychotic disorders suggests a common etiology related to excessive dopaminergic neurotransmission in mesolimbic DA pathways (i.e., the associative striatum) (Kuepper et al., 2012).

Delirium, Dementia, and Parkinson Disease Psychosis

The psychoses related to delirium and dementia, particularly dementia of the Alzheimer type, may share a common etiology: deficiency in muscarinic cholinergic neurotransmission due to medications, age- or disease-related neuronal loss (Koppel and Greenwald, 2014; Salahudeen et al., 2014). Delerium may have precipitants besides medication, such as infection, electrolyte imbalance, metabolic derangement, all of which require specific treatment, in addition to removal of anticholinergic medications (Khan et al., 2012). The development of PDP is due to Lewy body associated loss of serotonin raphe neurons and subsequent upregulation of cortical $5HT_{2A}$ receptors. The specific treatment for PDP is pimavanserin, a selective $5HT_{2A}$ inverse agonist devoid of DA receptor activity (Cummings et al., 2014).

Schizophrenia

Schizophrenia is a neurodevelopmental disorder with complex genetics and incompletely understood pathophysiology. In addition to environmental exposures such as fetal second-trimester infectious or nutritional insults, birth complications, and substance abuse in the late teen or early adult years, over 150 genes appear to contribute to schizophrenia risk. Implicated are genes that regulate neuronal migration, synaptogenesis, cellular adhesion, and neurite outgrowth (*neuregulin 1, disrupted-in-schizophrenia-1*); synaptic DA availability (*Val [108/158]Met polymorphism of catechol-O-methyltransferase*, which increases DA catabolism); glutamate and DA neurotransmission (*dystrobrevin binding protein 1* or *dysbindin*); and nicotinic activity (*α7-receptor polymorphisms*) (Escudero and Johnstone, 2014). Patients with schizophrenia also have increased rates of genome-wide DNA microduplications, termed *copy number variants*, and *epigenetic* changes, including disruptions in DNA methylation patterns in various brain regions (Gavin and Floreani, 2014). This genetic variability is consistent with the heterogeneity of the clinical disease and suggests that any one specific mechanism is unlikely to account for large amounts of disease risk.

Review of Psychosis Pathology and the General Goals of Pharmacotherapy

Common to all psychotic disorders are positive symptoms, which may include hallucinatory behavior, disturbed thinking, and behavioral dyscontrol. Common to effective schizophrenia treatments is an impact on dopaminergic neurotransmission (Figure 16–1).

Short-Term Antipsychotic Treatment

For many psychotic disorders, the symptoms are transient, and antipsychotic drugs are only administered during and shortly after periods of

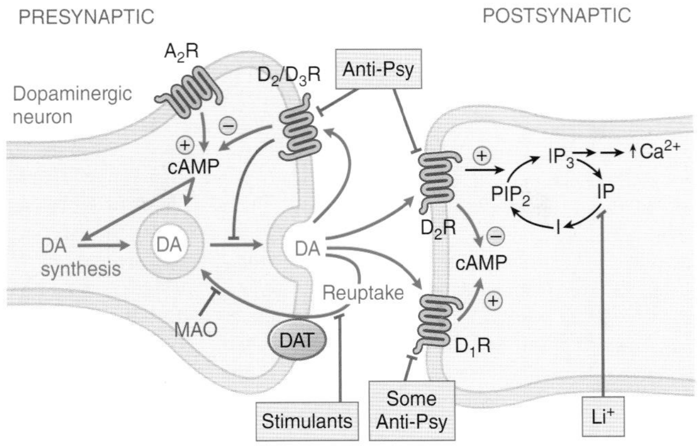

Figure 16–1 *Sites of action of antipsychotic agents and Li^+.* Following exocytotic release, DA interacts with postsynaptic receptors (R) of D_1 and D_2 types and presynaptic D_2 and D_3 autoreceptors. Termination of DA action occurs primarily by active transport of DA into presynaptic terminals via the DAT, with secondary deamination by mitochondrial MAO. Stimulation of postsynaptic D_1 receptors activates the G_s–adenylyl cyclase–cAMP pathway. D_2 receptors couple through G_i to inhibit adenylyl cyclase and through G_q to activate the PLC-IP_3-Ca^{2+} pathway. Activation of the G_i pathway can also activate K^+ channels, leading to hyperpolarization. Li^+ inhibits IP breakdown and thereby enhances its accumulation and sequelae (Ca^{2+} mobilization, PKC activation, depletion of cellular I). Li^+ may also alter release of neurotransmitter by a variety of putative mechanisms (see text). D_2-like autoreceptors suppress synthesis of DA by diminishing phosphorylation of rate-limiting TH, and by limiting DA release. In contrast, presynaptic A_2Rs) activate the adenylyl cyclase–cAMP–PKA pathway and thence TH activity. All antipsychotic agents act at D_2 receptors and autoreceptors; some also block D_1 receptors (Table 16–2). Stimulant agents inhibit DA reuptake by DAT, thereby prolonging the dwell time of synaptic DA. Initially in antipsychotic treatment, DA neurons release more DA, but following repeated treatment, they enter a state of physiological depolarization inactivation, with diminished production and release of DA, in addition to continued receptor blockade. ——|, inhibition or blockade; ⊕, elevation of activity; ⊖, reduction of activity; cAMP, cyclic AMP; IP, inositol phosphate; IP3, inositol 1,4,5-trisphosphate; PIP2, phosphatidylinositol 4,5-bisphosphate.

symptom exacerbation. Patients with delirium, dementia, major depressive disorder or mania with psychotic features, substance-induced psychoses, and brief psychotic disorder will typically receive short-term antipsychotic treatment that is discontinued after resolution of psychotic symptoms, although the duration may vary considerably based on the etiology. Bipolar patients in particular may have antipsychotic treatment extended for several months after resolution of mania and psychosis because antipsychotic medications are effective in reducing mania relapse. Chronic psychotic symptoms in patients with dementia may also be amenable to drug therapy, but potential benefits must be balanced with the documented risk of mortality and cerebrovascular events associated with the use of antipsychotic medications in this patient population (Maust et al., 2015).

Long-Term Antipsychotic Treatment

Delusional disorder, schizophrenia, schizoaffective disorder, and PDP are chronic diseases that require long-term antipsychotic treatment. For schizophrenia and schizoaffective disorder in particular, the goal of antipsychotic treatment is to maximize functional recovery by decreasing the severity of positive symptoms and their behavioral influence and possibly improving negative symptoms and remediating cognitive dysfunction, although the impact on the last two symptom domains is modest at best. Continuous antipsychotic treatment reduces 1-year relapse rates from 80% among unmedicated patients to about 15% (Zipursky et al., 2014). Poor adherence to antipsychotic treatment increases relapse risk and is often related to adverse drug events, cognitive dysfunction, substance use, and limited illness insight (Remington et al., 2014).

Regardless of the underlying pathology, the immediate goal of antipsychotic treatment is a decrease in acute symptoms that induce patient distress, particularly behavioral symptoms (e.g., hostility, agitation) that may present a danger to the patient or others. The dosing, route of administration, and choice of antipsychotic depend on the underlying disease state, clinical acuity, drug-drug interactions with concomitant medications, and patient sensitivity to short- or long-term adverse effects. With the exception of pimavanserin for PDP, and clozapine's superior efficacy in treatment-refractory schizophrenia, neither the clinical presentation nor biomarkers predicts the likelihood of response to a specific antipsychotic class or agent. As a result, avoidance of adverse effects based on patient and drug characteristics and exploitation of certain medication properties (e.g., sedation related to histamine H_1 or muscarinic antagonism) are the principal determinants for choosing initial antipsychotic therapy (Leucht et al., 2013).

Short-Term Treatment

Delirium, Dementia, and Parkinson Disease Psychosis

Psychotic symptoms of delirium or dementia are generally treated with low medication doses, although doses may have to be repeated at frequent intervals initially to achieve adequate behavioral control. Despite widespread clinical use, no antipsychotic has received approval for dementia-related psychosis. Moreover, all antipsychotic drugs carry warnings that they may increase mortality in this setting (Maust et al., 2015). Because anticholinergic drug effects may worsen delirium and dementia, high-potency typical antipsychotic drugs (e.g., haloperidol) or atypical antipsychotic agents with limited antimuscarinic properties (e.g., risperidone) are often the drugs of choice (Khan et al., 2012).

The doses for patients with dementia are one-fourth of adult schizophrenia doses (e.g., risperidone 0.5–1.5 mg/d), as EPSs, orthostasis, and sedation are particularly problematic in this patient population (Chapter 18). In acute psychosis, significant antipsychotic benefits are usually seen within 60–120 min after drug administration. Delirious or demented patients may be reluctant or unable to swallow tablets, but ODT preparations or liquid concentrate forms are available. Intramuscular administration of ziprasidone or olanzapine represents an option for treating agitated and minimally cooperative patients and presents less risk for drug-induced parkinsonism than haloperidol. An inhaled form of loxapine 10 mg is available in the U.S., with a median T_{max} of less than 2 min. Following rapid distribution, levels drop 75% over the next 10 min and then follow typical kinetics with a $t_{1/2}$ of 7.6 h. Inhaled loxapine can be administered only in healthcare facilities that can provide advanced airway management in the rare event of acute bronchospasm. Pimavanserin for PDP has a $t_{1/2}$

of 57 h, and clinical effects are seen over 2-6 weeks. (See Use in Pediatric Populations and Use in Geriatric Populations later in the chapter.)

Mania

All atypical antipsychotics medications with the exception of clozapine, iloperidone, brexpiprazole, and lurasidone, have indications for acute mania, and doses are titrated rapidly close to or at the maximum FDA-approved dose over the first 24–72 h of treatment. Typical antipsychotic drugs are also effective in acute mania, but often are eschewed due to the risk for EPSs. Clinical response (decreased psychomotor agitation and irritability, increased sleep, and reduced or absent delusions and hallucinations) usually occurs within 7 days but may be apparent as early as day 2. Patients with mania may need to continue on antipsychotic treatment for many months after the resolution of psychotic and manic symptoms, typically in combination with a mood stabilizer such as lithium or valproic acid preparations (e.g., divalproex) (Malhi et al., 2012). Oral aripiprazole and olanzapine have indications as monotherapy for bipolar disorder maintenance treatment, but the use of olanzapine has decreased dramatically due to concerns over adverse metabolic effects (e.g., weight gain, hyperlipidemia, hyperglycemia). LAI risperidone also has indications for maintenance monotherapy (and adjunctively with lithium or valproate) in patients with bipolar I disorder.

Combining an antipsychotic agent with a mood stabilizer often improves control of manic symptoms and further reduces the risk of relapse. Weight gain from the additive effects of antipsychotic agents and mood stabilizers presents a significant clinical problem. Antipsychotic agents with greater weight-gain liabilities (e.g., olanzapine, clozapine) should be avoided unless patients are refractory to preferred treatments.

The recommended duration of treatment after resolution of bipolar mania varies considerably, but as symptoms permit, a gradual drug taper should be attempted after 6 months of treatment, to lessen weight gain when combined with a mood stabilizer (Yatham et al., 2016).

Major Depression

Patients with major depressive disorder with psychotic features require lower-than-average doses of antipsychotic drugs, given in combination with an antidepressant. Extended antipsychotic treatment is not usually required, but certain atypical antipsychotic agents provide adjunctive antidepressant benefit (Farahani and Correll, 2012). Most antipsychotic drugs show limited antidepressant benefit when used as monotherapy, with the exception of amisulpride, loxapine, lurasidone, and quetiapine. Some atypical antipsychotic agents are effective as adjunct therapy in treatment-resistant unipolar depression. The primary mechanisms of action include $5HT_{2C}$ antagonism (olanzapine and quetiapine's metabolite, norquetiapine), which facilitates DA and NE release, and DA D_3 partial agonism (aripiprazole, brexpiprazole, craiprazine), which may result in stimulation of reward centers. Quetiapine at doses of 300 mg/d is effective for bipolar depression, as is lurasidone in the dosage range of 20–120 mg/d administered with an evening meal of at least 350 kcal. One of lurasidone's postulated antidepressant mechanisms is potent $5HT_7$ antagonism (Turner et al., 2014; Wright et al., 2013).

Schizophrenia

The immediate goals of acute antipsychotic treatment are the reduction of agitated, disorganized, or hostile behavior, decreasing the impact of hallucinations, improvement in the organization of thought, and the reduction of social withdrawal. Doses used acutely may be higher than those required for maintenance treatment of stable patients. Aside from clozapine, which is uniquely efficacious in refractory schizophrenia, atypical antipsychotics are not more effective than typical agents but offer a better neurological side-effect profile than typical antipsychotic drugs. Excessive D_2 blockade, as is often the case with the use of high-potency typical agents (e.g., haloperidol), not only increases risk for neurological effects (e.g., muscular rigidity, bradykinesia, tremor, akathisia) but also slows mentation (bradyphrenia) and interferes with central reward pathways, resulting in patient complaints of anhedonia (loss of capacity to experience pleasure). Low-potency typical agents such as chlorpromazine are not commonly used due to the high affinities for H_1, M_1, and α_1 receptors that result in undesirable effects (sedation, anticholinergic properties, orthostasis). Concerns regarding QT_c prolongation further limit their clinical usefulness. In acute psychosis, sedation may be desirable, but the use of a sedating antipsychotic drug may interfere with cognitive function and assessment.

Because schizophrenia requires long-term treatment, antipsychotic agents with greater metabolic liabilities, especially weight gain (discussed further in this chapter), should be avoided as first-line therapies. Ziprasidone, aripiprazole, iloperidone, brexpiprazole, cariprazine, and lurasidone are the most weight and metabolically benign atypical agents (De Hert et al., 2012; Rummel-Kluge et al., 2010). Ziprasidone is available in acute intramuscular form, thus permitting continuation of the same drug treatment initiated parenterally in the emergency room. Patients with schizophrenia have a 2-fold higher prevalence of metabolic syndrome and type 2 DM and 2-fold greater CV-related mortality rates than the general population (Torniainen et al., 2015). For this reason, consensus guidelines recommend baseline determination of serum glucose, lipids, weight, blood pressure, and personal and family histories of metabolic and CV disease.

With the low EPS risk among atypical antipsychotic agents, prophylactic use of antiparkinsonian medications (e.g., benztropine, trihexyphenidyl) is not necessary. Drug-induced parkinsonism can occur at higher dosages or among elderly patients exposed to antipsychotic agents that have higher D_2 affinity; recommended doses are about 50% of those used in younger patients with schizophrenia. (See also Use in Pediatric Populations and Use in Geriatric Populations further in the chapter.)

Long-Term Treatment

The need for long-term treatment poses issues almost exclusively to the chronic psychotic illnesses, schizophrenia and schizoaffective disorder. However, long-term antipsychotic treatment is sometimes used for manic patients, for ongoing psychosis in patients with dementia, for PDP, and for adjunctive use in treatment-resistant depression. Safety concerns combined with limited long-term efficacy data have dampened enthusiasm for extended antipsychotic drug use in patients with dementia (Maust et al., 2015). Justification for ongoing use, based on documentation of patient response to tapering of antipsychotic medication, is often mandated in long-term care settings.

Antipsychotic Agents

The choice of antipsychotic agents for long-term schizophrenia treatment is based primarily on avoidance of adverse effects, prior history of patient response, and the need for a long-acting injectable formulation due to adherence issues. While concerns over EPSs and TD have abated with the introduction of the atypical antipsychotic agents, there has been increased concern over metabolic effects of antipsychotic treatment: weight gain, dyslipidemia (particularly hypertriglyceridemia), and an adverse impact on glucose-insulin homeostasis (Rummel-Kluge et al., 2010). Clozapine and olanzapine have the highest metabolic risk and are only used as last resort. Olanzapine is often used prior to clozapine after failure of more metabolically benign agents such as aripiprazole, ziprasidone, asenapine, iloperidone, and lurasidone.

Acutely psychotic patients usually respond within hours after drug administration, but weeks may be required to achieve maximal drug response, especially for negative symptoms. Analyses of symptom response in clinical trials indicate that the majority of response to any antipsychotic treatment in acute schizophrenia is seen by week 4 (Jager et al., 2010). Failure of response after 2 weeks should prompt clinical reassessment, including determination of medication adherence, before a decision is made to increase the dose or consider switching to another agent (Kinon et al., 2010). Patients with first-episode schizophrenia often respond to lower doses, and chronic patients may require doses that exceed recommended ranges. While the acute behavioral impact of treatment is seen within hours to days, long-term studies indicate improvement may not plateau for 6 months, underscoring the importance of ongoing antipsychotic treatment in functional recovery for patients with schizophrenia.

Usual dosages for acute and maintenance treatment are noted in Table 16–1. Dosing should be adjusted based on clinically observable signs of antipsychotic benefit and adverse effects. For example, higher

TABLE 16–1 ■ DRUGS FOR PSYCHOSIS AND SCHIZOPHRENIA: DOSING AND METABOLIC RISK PROFILE

GENERIC NAME *Dosage Forms*	ORAL DOSAGE (mg/d)				METABOLIC SIDE EFFECTS		
	ACUTE PSYCHOSIS		MAINTENANCE				
	1ST EPISODE	CHRONIC	1ST EPISODE	CHRONIC	WEIGHT GAIN	LIPIDS	GLUCOSE
Phenothiazines							
Chlorpromazine ***O, S, IM***	200–600	400–800	150–600	250–750	+++	+++	++
Perphenazine ***O, S, IM***	12–50	24–48	12–48	24–60	+/–	–	–
Trifluoperazine ***O, S, IM***	5–30	10–40	2.5–20	10–30	+/–	–	–
Fluphenazine ***O, S, IM***	2.5–15	5–20	2.5–10	5–15	+/–	–	–
decanoate ***Depot IM***	12.5–25 mg/wk (maximum 3 doses)		12.5–75 mg/2 wk		+/–	–	–
Selected other first-generation agents							
Loxapine ***O, S, IM, Inhaled***	15–50	30–60	15–50	30–60	+	–	–
Thiothixene ***O, S***	5–30	10–40	2.5–20	10–30	+/–	–	–
Haloperidol ***O, S, IM***	2.5–10	5–20	2.5–10	5–15	+/–	–	–
decanoate ***Depot IM***	100–200 mg/wk (max 3 loading doses)		100–400 mg/month		+/–	–	–
Second-generation agents							
Aripiprazole ***O***	10–20	15–30	10–20	15–30	+/–	–	–
monohydrate/lauroxil ***Depot IM***	Not for acute use		see note ***a***	see note ***a***	+/–	–	–
Amisulpride ***O, S***[b]	200–800	400–1200	200–800	400–1200	+/–	–	–
Asenapine ***ODT***	10	10–20	10	10–20	+/–	–	–
Brexpiprazole ***O***	2–4	4	2–4	4	+/–	–	–
Cariprazine ***O***	3–6	3–6	3–6	3–6	+/–	–	–
Clozapine ***O, S, ODT***	200–600	400–900	200–600	300–900	++++	+++	+++
Iloperidone ***O***		12–24[c]		8–16	+	+/–	+/–
Lurasidone ***O***[d]	40–160	80–160	40–160	80–160	+	+/–	+/–
Olanzapine ***O, ODT, IM***	7.5–20	10–30	7.5–15	15–30	++++	+++	+++
pamoate ***Depot IM***[e]	Not for acute use		300–405	300–405	++++	+++	+++
Paliperidone	6–9	6–12	3–9	6–15	+	+/–	+/–
palmitate ***O Depot IM***[f]	See note *f* on dosing				+	+/–	+/–
Quetiapine ***O***	200–600	400–900	200–600	300–900	+	+	+/–
Risperidone ***O, S, ODT***	2–4	3–6	2–6	3–8	+	+/–	+/–
microspheres ***Depot IM***	Not for acute use		25–50 mg/2 wk		+	+/–	+/–
Sertindole ***O***[b]	4–16	12–20	12–20	12–32	+/–	–	–
Ziprasidone ***O, IM***[g]	120–160	120–200	80–160	120–200	+/–	–	–

Dosage Forms: IM, acute intramuscular; ODT, orally dissolving tablet; O, tablet; S, solution.

[a]Aripiprazole monohydrate dose: 300-400 mg IM/4 wks, with 14 days oral overlap. Aripiprazole lauroxil dose: 662-882 mg/4 wks or 882 mg/6 wks (equiv. to 662 mg/4 wks) with 21 days oral overlap. Dosages need to be adjusted for patients who are CYP2D6 poor metabolizers or those who are exposed to CYP2D6 or CYP3A4 inhibitors.

[b]Not available in the U.S.

[c]Due to orthostasis risk, dose titration of iloperidone is 1 mg twice daily on day 1, increasing to 2, 4, 6, 8, 10, and 12 mg twice daily on days 2–7 (as needed).

[d]Dose must be given with 350 kcal food to facilitate absorption. Administration with evening meal improves tolerability.

[e]Due to cases of postinjection delirium/sedation syndrome, patients must be observed after the injection for at least 3 h in a registered facility with ready access to emergency response services.

[f]Exists in two forms: 1-month and 3-month doses. In acute schizophrenia, deltoid intramuscular loading of 1-month form using doses of 234 mg at day 1 and 156 mg at day 8 to provide paliperidone levels equivalent to 6 mg oral paliperidone during the first week and peaking on day 15 at a level comparable to 12 mg oral paliperidone. No oral antipsychotic needed in first week. Maintenance intramuscular doses can be given every 4 weeks after day 8. Maintenance dose options for 1-month form: 39 to 234 mg every 4 weeks. Failure to give initiation doses (except for those switching from depot) will result in subtherapeutic levels for months. The 3-month form is only for those on 1-month dosing for at least 4 months. The 3-month dose is 3.5 times the stable monthly dose, administered every 12 weeks.

[g]Oral dose must be given with 500 kcal food to facilitate absorption.

TABLE 16–2 ■ POTENCIES OF ANTIPSYCHOTIC AGENTS AT NEUROTRANSMITTER RECEPTORS[a]

	DOPAMINE	SEROTONIN	MUSCARINIC	ADRENERGIC		HISTAMINE
	D_2	$5HT_{2A}$	M_1	A_{1A}	A_{1B}	H_1
First-generation agents						
Haloperidol	1.2	57	>10,000	12	7.6	1700
Fluphenazine	0.8	3.2	1100	6.5	13	14
Thiothixene	0.7	50	>10,000	12	35	8
Perphenazine	0.8	5.6	1500	10	—	8.0
Loxapine	11	4.4	120	42	53	4.9
Molindone[b]	20	>5000	>10,000	2600	—	2100
Thioridazine	8.0	28	13	3.2	2.4	16
Chlorpromazine	3.6	3.6	32	0.3	0.8	3.1
Second-generation agents						
Lurasidone	1.0	0.5	>1000	48	—	>1000
Aripiprazole	1.6[c]	8.7	6800	26	34	28
Brexpiprazole	0.4[c]	0.5	>1000	—	0.2	19
Cariprazine	0.6[c]	19	>1000	130	>1000	23
Asenapine	1.4	0.1	>10,000	1.2	3.9	1.0
Ziprasidone	6.8	0.6	>10,000	18	9.0	63
Sertindole[b]	2.7	0.4	>5000	1.8	—	130
Zotepine[b]	8.0	2.7	330	6.0	5.0	3.2
Risperidone	3.2	0.2	>10,000	5.0	9.0	20
Paliperidone	4.2	0.7	>10,000	2.5	0.7	19
Iloperidone	6.3	5.6	4900	0.3	—	12
Amisulpride[b]	2.2	8300	>10,000	>10,000	>10,000	>10,000
Olanzapine	31	3.7	2.5	110	260	2.2
Quetiapine	380	640	37	22	39	6.9
Clozapine	160	5.4	6.2	1.6	7.0	1.1

[a]Data are averaged K_i values (nM) from published sources determined by competition with radioligands for binding to the indicated cloned human receptors. Data derived from receptor binding to human or rat brain tissue were used when cloned human receptor data were lacking.
[b]Not available in the U.S.
[c]Partial agonist at D_2 receptor.
[d]Pimavanserin is a novel agent only indicated for PDP. Ki values: 5HT2A = 0.087 nM; 5HT2C = 0.44 nM. Affinity for DA, M1, H1 and other receptors > 300 nM
Source: PDSP K_i Database: https://kidbdev.med.unc.edu/databases/pdsp.php (Accessed June 1, 2015).

TABLE 16–3 ■ KINETIC PROPERTIES OF DEPOT ANTIPSYCHOTICS

PREPARATION	DILUENT	DOSAGE	T_{max} (days)	STEADY-STATE HALF-LIFE (days)
First-generation antipsychotics				
Fluphenazine decanoate	Sesame oil	12.5–100 mg/2 wk	0.3–1.5	14
Haloperidol decanoate	Sesame oil	25–400 mg/4 wk	3–9	21
Perphenazine decanoate[a]	Sesame oil	25–400 mg/4 wk	7	65
Zuclopenthixol decanoate[a]	Coconut oil (fractionated)	100–800 mg/4 wk	7	19
Atypical antipsychotics				
Aripiprazole monohydrate[b]	Water	300–400 mg/4 wk	6.5–7.1	30–46
Aripiprazole lauroxil[b]	Water	441–882 mg/4 wk	44–50	29–35
Olanzapine pamoate[c]	Water	150–300 mg/2 wk *or*, 300–405 mg/4 wk	7	30
Paliperidone palmitate monthly	Water	39–234 mg/4 wk	13	25–49
Paliperidone palmitate 3 months[d]	Water	273–819 mg/12 wk	30–33	84–95 (deltoid) 118–139 (gluteal)
Risperidone microspheres	Water	12.5–50 mg/2 wk	21	3–6

[a]Not available in the U.S.
[b]Dosages need to be adjusted for patients who are CYP2D6 poor metabolizers or those who are exposed to CYP2D6 or CYP3A4 inhibitors.
[c]Due to cases of postinjection delirium/sedation syndrome, patients must be observed after the injection for at least 3 h in a registered facility with ready access to emergency response services.
[d]Only indicated for patients who have been on paliperidone palmitate monthly injectable for at least 4 months.

EPS risk is noted for risperidone doses that exceed 6 mg/d in nonelderly adult patients with schizophrenia. However, in the absence of EPSs, increasing the dose from 6 to 8 mg would be a reasonable approach in a patient with ongoing positive symptoms. Certain antipsychotic adverse effects, including weight gain, sedation, orthostasis, and EPSs, can be predicted based on potencies at neurotransmitter receptors (Table 16–2). The detection of dyslipidemia or hyperglycemia is based on laboratory monitoring (Table 16–1). Dose reduction often resolves hyperprolactinemia, EPSs, orthostasis, and sedation, but metabolic abnormalities improve only with discontinuation of the offending agent and a switch to a more metabolically benign medication. The decision to switch patients with stable schizophrenia and metabolic dysfunction solely for metabolic benefit must be individualized based on patient preferences, severity of the metabolic disturbance, likelihood of metabolic improvement with antipsychotic switching, and history of response to prior agents. Patients with refractory schizophrenia on clozapine are not good candidates for switching because they are resistant to other medications (see the definition of refractory schizophrenia further in this section).

Psychotic Relapse

There are many reasons for psychotic relapse or inadequate response to antipsychotic treatment in patients with schizophrenia; reasons include substance use, psychosocial stressors, inherent refractory illness, and poor medication adherence. The common problem of medication nonadherence among patients with schizophrenia has led to the development of LAI antipsychotic medications, often referred to as depot antipsychotics (Meyer, 2013). There are currently eight LAI forms available in the U.S.: decanoate esters of fluphenazine and haloperidol, risperidone-impregnated microspheres, 1-month and 3-month formulations of paliperidone palmitate, aripiprazole monohydrate, aripiprazole lauroxil, and olanzapine pamoate (Table 16–3). Patients receiving LAI antipsychotic medications show consistently lower relapse rates compared to patients receiving comparable oral forms and may have fewer adverse effects due to lower peak plasma levels.

Refractory Illness

Lack of response to adequate antipsychotic drug doses for adequate periods of time may indicate treatment-refractory illness. Use of antipsychotic plasma levels can help separate those who are nonadherent or are kinetic failures from those who are not responding to adequate medication exposure (Meyer, 2014). In treatment-refractory schizophrenia, response rates are 0% for typical antipsychotic agents, less than 10% for newer agents, but consistently about 60% for clozapine. Various studies have found correlations between trough plasma clozapine levels greater than 327–504 ng/mL and likelihood of clinical response (Rostami-Hodjegan et al., 2004). When therapeutic serum concentrations are reached, response to clozapine occurs within 8 weeks. Clozapine can have numerous adverse effects: risk of agranulocytosis (requires hematological monitoring), high metabolic burden, dose-dependent lowering of the seizure threshold, orthostasis, sedation, anticholinergic effects (especially constipation), and sialorrhea.

Electroconvulsive therapy also has proven efficacy for refractory schizophrenia.

Pharmacology of Antipsychotic Agents

Chemistry

Most early agents were derived from phenothiazine or butyrophenone structures. Presently, antipsychotic agents include many different chemical structures with a range of activities at different neurotransmitter receptors (e.g., $5HT_{2A}$ antagonism, $5HT_{1A}$ partial agonism). As a result, structure-function relationships that were relied on in the past have become less important, while receptor binding and functional assays are more clinically relevant. Aripiprazole represents a good example of how an examination of the structure provides little insight into its mechanism, which is based on partial agonism at D_2 DA receptors (discussed further in this chapter). Detailed knowledge of receptor affinities (Table 16–2) and the functional effect at specific receptors (e.g., full, partial, or inverse agonism or antagonism) can provide important insight into the therapeutic and adverse effects of antipsychotic agents. Nevertheless, there are limits. For example, it is not known which properties are responsible for clozapine's unique effectiveness in refractory schizophrenia, although many hypotheses exist. Other notable antipsychotic properties not fully explained by receptor parameters include the reduced seizure threshold, the effects of antipsychotic agents on glucose and lipid metabolism, and the increased risk for cerebrovascular events and mortality among patients with dementia (see Adverse Effects and Drug Interactions further in the chapter).

ARIPIPRAZOLE

CLOZAPINE

Mechanism of Action

With the exception of pimavanserin for PDP, no clinically available effective antipsychotic is devoid of D_2-modulating activity (Howes et al., 2015). This reduction in dopaminergic neurotransmission is presently achieved through one of two mechanisms: D_2 antagonism or partial D_2 agonism (aripiprazole, brexpiprazole, and cariprazine). The mechanism of action for partial agonist antipsychotics relies on intrinsic activity at D_2 receptors that is a fraction of the efficacy of DA (i.e., 20%–25% of DA's activity), as depicted in Figure 16–2 for aripiprazole. (Recall that a partial agonist will also occupy the receptor and antagonize the binding of full agonists; see Chapter 3). Unlike other antipsychotic agents, in which striatal D_2 occupancy (i.e., reduction in postsynaptic D_2 signal) greater than 78% increases risk for EPSs, partial agonist antipsychotics require significantly higher D_2 occupancy levels (80%–95%) (Sparshatt et al., 2010). However, the intrinsic dopaminergic agonism generates a sufficient postsynaptic signal to remain below the EPS threshold, although reports do exist, primarily in antipsychotic-naïve, younger patients.

Clozapine was not suspected to possess antipsychotic activity until experimental human use in the mid-1960s revealed it to be an effective treatment of schizophrenia, particularly in patients who had failed other antipsychotic medications, and with virtually absent EPS risk. Clozapine possesses weaker D_2 antagonism than existing antipsychotic agents, combined with potent $5HT_{2A}$ antagonism that facilitates DA release in mesocortical and nigrostriatal pathways. Clozapine, and its active metabolite *N*-desmethylclozapine, also possesses activity at numerous other receptors, including antagonism and agonism at various muscarinic receptor subtypes and antagonism at DA D_4 receptors (other D_4 antagonists that do not also have D_2 antagonism lack antipsychotic activity; Meyer and Leckband, 2013).

A search for the basis of clozapine's unique efficacy in refractory schizophrenia has recently pointed toward activity at glutamatergic sites, especially the NMDA receptor. The evolving NMDA hypofunction hypothesis of schizophrenia led to clinical development of metabotropic glutamate $mGlu_2$ and $mGlu_3$ agonists and inhibitors of the type 1 glycine transporter. At present, however, it is unclear whether glutamate agonists that lack direct D_2 antagonist properties will be effective for schizophrenia treatment; agents with the mechanisms indicated have failed phase III studies (Howes et al., 2015).

Patients with schizophrenia also exhibit specific neurophysiological and cognitive abnormalities, including deficiencies in sensorimotor gating

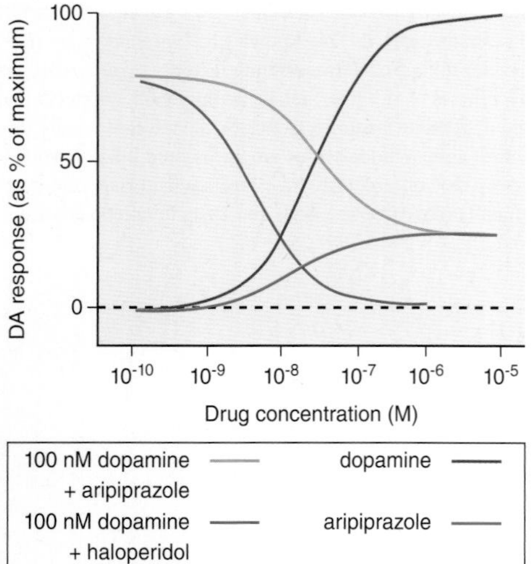

Figure 16–2 *Partial agonist activity of aripiprazole at D_2 receptors.* Aripiprazole is a partial D_2 agonist and thus also an antagonist. In this stylized representation, aripiprazole inhibits the effects of DA and reduces stimulation at the D_2 receptor only to the extent of its own capacity as an agonist (orange tracing); in the absence of DA, its partial agonist effects are apparent (green line), becoming maximal at about 25% of the maximal effect of DA alone (purple line). Haloperidol, an antagonist without agonist activity, completely antagonizes D_2 receptor activation by 100 nM DA (red tracing). Here, receptor activation is measured as inhibition of forskolin-induced cAMP accumulation in cultured cells transfected with human D_{2L} DNA. (Data from Burris KD, et al. Aripiprazole, a novel antipsychotic, is a high-affinity partial agonist at human dopamine D2 receptors. *J Pharmacol Exp Ther*, **2002**, *302*: 381–389.)

as assessed by prepulse inhibition (PPI) of the acoustic startle reflex. PPI is the automatic suppression of startle magnitude that occurs when the louder acoustic stimulus is preceded 30–500 milliseconds by a weaker prepulse (Javitt and Freedman 2015; Powell et al., 2012). In patients with schizophrenia, PPI is increased more robustly with atypical than typical antipsychotic agents, and in animal models, atypical antipsychotic agents are also more effective at opposing PPI disruption by NMDA antagonists.

Increased understanding of the pharmacological basis for neurophysiological deficits provides another means for developing antipsychotic treatments that are specifically effective for schizophrenia and may not necessarily apply to other forms of psychosis. Numerous agents have also been examined for remediating the cognitive deficits of schizophrenia, typically utilizing nicotinic and muscarinic agonism, but none has been approved (Prickaerts et al., 2012).

Dopamine Receptor Occupancy and Behavioral Effects

Dopaminergic projections from the midbrain terminate on septal nuclei, the olfactory tubercle and basal forebrain, the amygdala, and other structures within the temporal and prefrontal cerebral lobes and the hippocampus. Excessive dopaminergic neurotransmission in the associative striatum is central to the positive symptoms of psychosis. The behavioral effects and the time course of antipsychotic response parallel the decrease in postsynaptic D_2 activity in this region (Kuepper et al., 2012). Receptor occupancy predicts clinical efficacy, EPSs, and plasma level–clinical response relationships. Occupancy of greater than 78% of D_2 receptors in the basal ganglia is associated with a risk of EPSs across all DA antagonist antipsychotic agents, while occupancies in the range of 60%–75% are associated with antipsychotic efficacy (Figure 16–3). With the exception of the D_2 partial agonists, all atypical antipsychotic drugs at low doses have much greater occupancy of $5HT_{2A}$ receptors (e.g., 75%–99%) than typical agents (Table 16–3). Given the large variations in drug metabolism, plasma levels of antipsychotic agents (rather than doses) are the best predictors of D_2 occupancy.

The Role of Nondopamine Receptors for Atypical Antipsychotic Agents. The concept of atypicality was initially based on clozapine's absence of EPSs combined with potent $5HT_2$ receptor antagonism. $5HT_{2A}$ antagonism exerts its greatest effect on prefrontal and basal ganglia DA release, decreasing EPS risk in the context of nigrostriatal D_2 antagonism. The $5HT_{2C}$ antagonists stimulate midbrain noradrenergic outflow (Dremencov et al., 2006). Thus, $5HT_{2C}$ antagonist atypical agents exhibit a spectrum of antidepressant properties, although pure $5HT_{2C}$ agents are not, by themselves, effective antidepressants (Dremencov et al., 2006). Most atypical antipsychotics are partial agonists at $5HT_{1A}$ receptors, resulting in hyperpolarization of cortical pyramidal cells and clinically relevant anxiolytic effects. Pimavanserin is an inverse agonist at $5HT_{2A}$ receptors; its effectiveness in PDP may reflect on the unique pathology of PDP.

PIMAVANSERIN

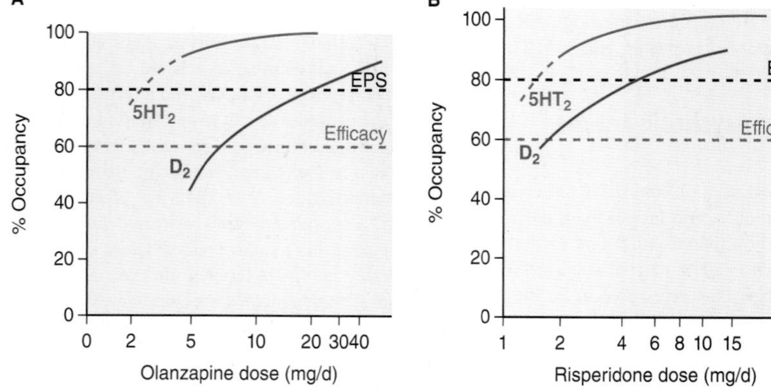

Figure 16–3 *Receptor occupancy and clinical response for antipsychotic agents.* Typically, in D_2 receptor occupancy by the drug more than 60% provides antipsychotic effects, receptor occupancy greater than 80% causes EPSs. Atypical agents combine weak D_2 receptor blockade with more potent $5HT_{2A}$ antagonism/inverse agonism. Inverse agonism at $5HT_2$ receptor subtypes may contribute to the reduced EPS risk of olanzapine (**A**) and risperidone (**B**) and efficacy at lower D_2 receptor occupancy (olanzapine, **A**). Aripiprazole is a partial D_2 agonist that can achieve only 75% functional blockade (see Figure 16–2).

TABLE 16–4 ■ DRUG DISPOSITION AND EFFECTS OF CYP INHIBITION AND INDUCTION ON ORAL ANTIPSYCHOTIC LEVELS

	T_{max}; Oral Tablet Bioavailability	METABOLISM	EFFECT OF CYP INHIBITION	EFFECT OF CYP INDUCTION
Commonly used atypical antipsychotics				
Aripiprazole	Bioavailability: 87% T_{max} 3–5 h	CYPs 2D6 and 3A4 produce active metabolite, dehydroaripiprazole. $t_{1/2}$: aripiprazole, 75h; dehydroaripiprazole, 94 h, Metabolite = 40% of AUC at steady state	In 2D6 PM: ↑ AUC of aripiprazole up to 80%, 30% ↓ AUC of metabolite. $t_{1/2}$: 146 h in PMs. Strong CYP2D6 inhibitors (e.g., ketoconazole) can double AUC of parent drug. Ketoconazole (a strong 3A4 inhibitor) increased the AUCs of aripiprazole and its active metabolite by 63% and 77%, respectively.	3A4 induction ↓ max concentration and AUC of aripiprazole and metabolite by 70%.
Asenapine	Bioavailability: Sublingual: 35% Oral: <2% T_{max} 1 h	Primarily glucuronidation (UGT 1A4); limited oxidation via CYP 1A2 and to lesser extent 2D6 and 3A4. No active metabolites. $t_{1/2}$: 24 h	Fluvoxamine, (25 mg twice daily for 8 days) ↑ C_{max} by 13% and AUC 29%. Paroxetine ↓ AUC and C_{max} (13%) Asenapine can double paroxetine exposure.	Smoking: no effect on clearance or other kinetic parameters. Carbamazepine, can ↓ C_{max} and AUC (16%).
Brexpiprazole	Bioavailability: 95% T_{max}: 4 h	CYPs 2D6 and 3A4 convert brexpiprazole to inactive metabolite (DM-3411). $t_{1/2}$: 91 h	Strong 2D6 or 3A4 inhibitor: ↑ $AUC_{0\text{-}24\,h}$ by 2-fold. Strong 3A4 inhibitor with 2D6 inhibitor (or with 2D6 PM): ↑ $AUC_{0\text{-}24\,h}$ by ~5 fold. ↓ dose by 50% with strong 2D6 or 3A4 inhibitor. ↓ dose by 75% with combined 2D6/3A4 inhibitors.	Inducers of CYP3A4 ↓ exposure AUC by ~70%. Do not use brexpiprazole with inducers.
Cariprazine	Bioavailability: 65% T_{max}: 3–6 h	CYP3A4 converts cariprazine to active metabolites DCAR and DDCAR. At steady state on 6 mg/d: cariprazine 28%, DCAR 9%, and DDCAR 63%. CYP2D6 is a minor pathway. Parent drug and DDCAR show good brain penetration; after oral cariprazine, brain-to-plasma ratios for both are ~9.8 $t_{1/2}$: 31.6–68.4 h; DCAR, 29.7–39.5 h; DDCAR, 314–446 h ≥50% of DDCAR present 1 week after discontinuation.	Ketoconazole 400 mg/d + cariprazine 0.5 mg/kg: ↑ AUCs of cariprazine (4×) and DDCAR (1.5), and ↑ DCAR AUC (~33%). Reduce dose by 50% with strong 3A4 inhibitors. No impact from 2D6 inhibitors.	Not studied. Impact unknown. Not recommended with 3A4 inducers.
Clozapine	Bioavailability: 60%–70% T_{max} 2.5 h	Multiple CYPs (mainly 1A2, 2C19, 3A4) produce active desmethyl metabolite $t_{1/2}$: 12 h (up to 66 h with chronic dosing)	Fluvoxamine ↑ serum levels 5- to 10-fold. 2D6 inhibition may double *Cp*.	Loss of smoking-related 1A2 induction ⇒ 50% ↑ in clozapine serum levels. Carbamazepine decreases clozapine levels on average by 50%.

(*Continued*)

TABLE 16–4 ■ DRUG DISPOSITION AND EFFECTS OF CYP INHIBITION AND INDUCTION ON ORAL ANTIPSYCHOTIC LEVELS (*CONTINUED*)

	T_{max}; Oral Tablet Bioavailability	METABOLISM	EFFECT OF CYP INHIBITION	EFFECT OF CYP INDUCTION
Iloperidone	Bioavailability: well absorbed, no food effect on AUC T_{max} 2–4 h	2D6/3A4 produce active metabolites P88 & P95 Exposure to P88 and P95 can be significant P88 $t_{1/2}$: EM, 26 h; PM, 37 h P95 $t_{1/2}$: EM, 23h; PM, 31 h $t_{1/2}$: 18 h (CYP 2D6 EMs), 33 h (CYP 2D6 PMs)	Ketoconazole, fluoxetine, and paroxetine can ↑ AUC of iloperidone and metabolites by 50% to 300%, with similar effects on C_{max} at steady-state.	Impact of 3A4 inducers not documented.
Lurasidone	Bioavailability: 9%–19% Mean C_{max} and AUC increased 3-fold and 2-fold, respectively, when administered with food T_{max} 1–3 h	CYP 3A4 $t_{1/2}$: 18–36 h	DO NOT USE with strong 3A4 inhibitors (e.g., ketoconazole), which increase C_{max} 6.9-fold and AUC 9-fold. Moderate 3A4 inhibitors (diltiazem) increase C_{max} 2.1-fold and AUC 2.2-fold.	DO NOT USE with strong 3A4 inducers. Concurrent rifampin can decrease C_{max} to a seventh of prior levels and AUC by 80%.
Olanzapine	Bioavailability: 60% T_{max} 6 h	Direct glucuronidation or 1A2-mediated oxidation to *N*-desmethylolanzapine (inactive) $t_{1/2}$: 30 (21–54) h	Increase in olanzapine C_{max} following fluvoxamine is 54% in female nonsmokers and 77% in male smokers. Mean increases in olanzapine AUC are 52% and 108%, respectively.	Carbamazepine use increases clearance by 50%. Smokers have lower Cp and increased clearance.
Paliperidone	Bioavailability: 28% T_{max} 24 h	59% excreted unchanged in urine, 32% excreted as metabolites. Phase 2 metabolism accounts for no more than 10%.	Unlikely to have much of an effect	Carbamazepine use decreased steady-state C_{max} and AUC by 37%.
Quetiapine	Bioavailability: 9% T_{max} 1.5 h	3A4 mediated sulfoxidation to inactive metabolite $t_{1/2}$: 6 h (CNS half-life longer by neuroimaging)	Ketoconazole (200 mg once daily for 4 days) reduced oral clearance of quetiapine by 84%, ⇒ 335% increase in C_{max}.	Phenytoin increases clearance 5-fold.
Risperidone	Bioavailability: 66% in 2D6 EMs T_{max}: 1 h for risperidone, 3 h for 9-OH risperidone (paliperidone)	2D6 converts risperidone to, 9-OH risperidone (active). $t_{1/2}$: 3–4 h; 20–24 h (9-OH risperidone) In 2D6 PMs, half-lives are: risperidone, 20 h; 9-OH risperidone, 30 h.	SSRIs can increase plasma levels. Fluoxetine: ↑ [risperidole] ~2.6 fold Paroxetine: ↑ [risperidole] ~3–9 fold	Risperidone (6 mg/day for 3 weeks), followed by Carbamazepine (3 weeks), ⇒ 50% decrease in concentration (risperidone + 9-OH risperidone).

Ziprasidone	Bioavailability: 60% when given with food A 500-kcal meal (of any composition) ↑ AUC of a 20-mg, 40-mg, and 80-mg capsule by 48%, 87% and 101%, respectively. T_{max} 6–8 h	Aldehyde oxidase (66%), CYP3A4 (34%) $t_{1/2}$: 7.5 h	35%–40% increase in ziprasidone AUC by concomitantly administered ketoconazole.	35% decrease in ziprasidone AUC by carbamazepine.
Typical antipsychotics				
Haloperidol	Bioavailability: 60% T_{max} 2–6 h	Multiple CYP pathways, particularly 2D6, 3A4. Most metabolites inactive, except reduced haloperidol formed by ketone reductase and transformed to haloperidol via CYP2D6. Therapeutic serum levels not well defined; 5–20 ng/mL used as a target for dosing. $t_{1/2}$: 24 h (12–36 h)[a]	In CYP2D6 PM: $t_{1/2}$ prolonged, [reduced haloperidol] increased significantly. Individuals with only one functional 2D6 gene experience 2-fold greater trough serum levels; those with no functioning alleles 3- to 4-fold higher.	Carbamazepine or phenytoin ↑ haloperidol clearance ~32%, with variable decrease in plasma levels (mean 47%). Discontinuation of carbamazepine results in 2.2- to 3.0-fold ↑ in serum levels.
Chlorpromazine	Bioavailability: 20–32% T_{max} 1–4 h	CYP2D6, over 10 identified human metabolites, most inactive. Chlorpromazine is a 2D6 inhibitor and induces its own metabolism. Levels drop ~30% during weeks 1–3 of treatment. $t_{1/2}$: 24 h (8–35 h with chronic dosing)	Case report of fluoxetine-chlorpromazine interaction, but no serum level data on extent of effect.	3A4/PGP inducers (e.g., phenobarbital, carbamazepine) ↓ chlorpromazine levels by ~35%. Carbamazepine discontinuation increases serum levels (~50%).

[a]May have multiphasic elimination with much longer terminal half-life.

Tolerance and Physical Dependence

As defined in Chapter 24, antipsychotic drugs are not addicting; however, tolerance to the α adrenergic, antihistaminic, and anticholinergic effects of antipsychotic agents usually develops over days or weeks. Loss of efficacy with prolonged treatment is not known to occur with antipsychotic agents; however, tolerance to antipsychotic drugs and cross-tolerance among the agents are demonstrable in behavioral and biochemical experiments in animals. One correlate of tolerance in striatal dopaminergic systems is the development of receptor supersensitivity (mediated by upregulation of supersensitive DA receptors), referred to as D_2^{High} receptors (Seeman, 2013). These changes may underlie the clinical phenomenon of withdrawal-emergent dyskinesias and may contribute to the pathophysiology of TD. These effects may also partly explain the ability of certain patients with chronic schizophrenia to tolerate high doses of potent DA antagonists with limited EPSs.

ADME

Absorption for most of these agents following oral administration is quite high, and concurrent administration of anticholinergic antiparkinsonian agents does not appreciably diminish intestinal absorption. Most ODTs and liquid preparations provide similar pharmacokinetics because there is little mucosal absorption and effects depend on swallowed drug. Asenapine is the only exception: it is available only as an ODT preparation administered sublingually; and absorption occurs via the oral mucosa with bioavailability of 35%. If asenapine is swallowed, the first-pass effect is greater than 98% and the drug is essentially not bioavailable. Intramuscular administration avoids much of the first-pass enteric metabolism and provides measurable concentrations in plasma within 15–30 min.

The pharmacokinetic constants and metabolic pathways for many atypical and typical antipsychotic drugs are listed in Table 16–4. Most antipsychotic drugs are highly lipophilic and accumulate in the brain, lung, and other tissues with a rich blood supply. Most antipsychotic agents are highly protein bound, primarily to acid glycoprotein, and do not significantly displace other medications bound to prealbumin or albumin. Antipsychotic agents also enter the fetal circulation and breast milk. Despite half-lives that may be short, the biological effects of single doses of most antipsychotic medications usually persist for at least 24 h, permitting once-daily dosing after the patient has adjusted to initial side effects. Due to accumulation in tissue stores, both parent compound and metabolites of LAI medications can been detected several months after discontinuation, a useful property for those who may miss injections (see Table 16–3).

Other Therapeutic Uses

Antipsychotic agents are also utilized in several nonpsychotic neurological disorders and as antiemetics.

Anxiety Disorders

Double-blind, placebo-controlled trials have shown the benefit of adjunctive treatment with antipsychotic drugs for obsessive-compulsive disorder, with a recent meta-analysis showing significant efficacy for risperidone but not for quetiapine and olanzapine (Dold et al., 2013). For generalized anxiety disorder, clinical trials demonstrated efficacy for quetiapine as monotherapy and for adjunctive low-dose risperidone. Recent data do not support routine use of risperidone for posttraumatic stress disorder (Krystal et al., 2011).

Tourette Disorder

The ability of antipsychotic drugs to suppress tics in patients with Tourette disorder relates to reduced D_2 neurotransmission in basal ganglia sites. Aripiprazole is the only antipsychotic that is FDA-approved for the treatment of Tourette disorder; this agent is considered a first-line agent for this purpose, starting at doses of 2 mg/d and increasing if needed to a maximum of 10 mg/d for those weighing less than 50 kg or 20 mg/d if weighing 50 kg or more (Mogwitz et al., 2013).

In prior decades, low-dose, high-potency typical antipsychotic agents (e.g., haloperidol, pimozide) were treatments of choice, but these nonpsychotic patients are extremely sensitive to the impact of DA blockade on cognitive processing speed and on reward centers. Moreover, safety concerns regarding pimozide's QT_c prolongation and increased risk for ventricular arrhythmias have largely ended its clinical use.

Huntington Disease

Huntington disease is another neuropsychiatric condition that, like tic disorders, is associated with basal ganglia pathology. DA blockade can suppress the severity of choreoathetotic movements but is not strongly endorsed due to the risks associated with excessive DA antagonism that outweigh the marginal benefit. Inhibition of the vesicular monoamine transporter 2 (VMAT2) with tetrabenazine compounds has replaced DA receptor blockade in the management of chorea (Chapter 18).

Autism

Autism is a disease whose neuropathology is incompletely understood, but in some patients is associated with explosive behavioral outbursts and aggressive or self-injurious behaviors that may be stereotypical. Risperidone and aripiprazole have FDA approval for irritability associated with autism in child and adolescent patients ages 5–16, with common use for disruptive behavior problems in autism and forms of mental retardation. Initial risperidone daily doses are 0.25 mg for patients weighing less than 20 kg and 0.5 mg for others, with a target dose of 0.5 mg/d in those weighing less than 20 kg and 1.0 mg/d for other patients, with a range of 0.5–3.0 mg/d. For aripiprazole, the starting dose is 2 mg/d, with a target range of 5–10 mg/d and maximum daily dose of 15 mg.

Antiemetic Use

Most antipsychotic drugs protect against the nausea- and emesis-inducing effects of DA agonists such as apomorphine that act at central DA receptors in the chemoreceptor trigger zone of the medulla. Drugs or other stimuli that cause emesis by an action on the nodose ganglion, or locally on the GI tract, are not antagonized by antipsychotic drugs, but potent piperazines and butyrophenones are sometimes effective against nausea caused by vestibular stimulation. The commonly used antiemetic phenothiazines are weak DA antagonists (e.g., prochlorperazine) without antipsychotic activity but can occasionally be associated with EPSs or akathisia. Emesis and antiemetic agents are discussed at length in Chapter 50.

Adverse Effects and Drug Interactions

Adverse Effects Predicted by Monoamine Receptor Affinities

Dopamine D_2 Receptors. With the exception of pimavanserin and the D_2 partial agonists (aripiprazole, brexpiprazole, cariprazine), all other antipsychotic agents possess D_2 antagonist properties, the strength of which determines the likelihood for EPSs, long-term TD risk, akathisia, NMS, and hyperprolactinemia.

Extrapyramidal Symptoms. The manifestations of EPSs are described in Table 16–5, along with the usual treatment approach. Acute dystonic reactions occur in the early hours and days of treatment, with highest risk among younger patients (peak incidence ages 10–19), especially antipsychotic, naïve individuals, in response to abrupt decreases in nigrostriatal D_2 neurotransmission. The dystonia typically involves head and neck muscles and the tongue and, in its severest form, the oculogyric crisis, extraocular muscles, and is frightening to the patient.

Parkinsonism resembling its idiopathic form may occur; it will respond to dose reduction or switching to an antipsychotic with weaker D_2 antagonism. If this is neither possible nor desirable, antiparkinsonian medication may be employed. Elderly patients are at greatest risk.

Muscarinic cholinergic receptors modulate nigrostriatal DA release, with blockade increasing synaptic DA availability. Important issues in the use of anticholinergics include the negative impact on cognition and memory; peripheral antimuscarinic adverse effects (e.g., urinary retention, dry mouth, cycloplegia, etc.); exacerbation of TD; and risk of cholinergic rebound following abrupt anticholinergic withdrawal. For parenteral administration, diphenhydramine (25–50 mg IM) and benztropine (1–2 mg IM) are the agents most commonly used. The

TABLE 16–5 ■ NEUROLOGICAL SIDE EFFECTS OF ANTIPSYCHOTIC DRUGS

REACTION	FEATURES	TIME OF ONSET AND RISK INFO	PROPOSED MECHANISM	TREATMENT
Acute dystonia	Spasm of muscles of tongue, face, neck, back	Time: 1–5 days. Young, antipsychotic, naïve patients at highest risk	Acute DA antagonism	Antiparkinsonian agents are diagnostic and curative[a]
Akathisia	Subjective and objective restlessness; *not* anxiety or "agitation"	Time: 5–60 days	Unknown	Reduce dose or change drug; clonazepam, propranolol more effective than antiparkinsonian agents[b]
Parkinsonism	Bradykinesia, rigidity, variable tremor, mask facies, shuffling gait	Time: 5–30 days. Elderly at greatest risk	DA antagonism	Dose reduction; change medication; antiparkinsonian agents[c]
Neuroleptic malignant syndrome	Extreme rigidity, fever, unstable blood pressure, myoglobinemia; can be fatal	Time: weeks–months. Can persist for days after stopping antipsychotic	DA antagonism	Stop antipsychotic immediately; supportive care; dantrolene and bromocriptine[d]
Perioral tremor ("rabbit syndrome")	Perioral tremor (may be a late variant of parkinsonism)	Time: months or years of treatment	Unknown	Antiparkinsonian agents often help[c]
Tardive dyskinesia	Orofacial dyskinesia; rarely widespread choreoathetosis or dystonia	Time: months or years of treatment. Elderly at 5-fold greater risk. Risk proportional to potency of D_2 blockade	Postsynaptic DA receptor supersensitivity, upregulation	May be reversible with early recognition and drug discontinuation VMAT2 inhibitors valbenazine and deutetrabenazine are FDA-approved for TD

[a]Treatment: diphenhydramine 25–50 mg IM or benztropine 1–2 mg IM. Due to long antipsychotic $t_{1/2}$, may need to repeat or follow with oral medication.
[b]Propranolol often effective in relatively low doses (20–80 mg/d in divided doses). β_1-selective adrenergic receptor antagonists are less effective. Nonlipophilic β adrenergic antagonists have limited CNS penetration and are of no benefit (e.g., atenolol).
[c]Use of amantadine avoids anticholinergic effects of benztropine or diphenhydramine.
[d]Despite the response to dantrolene, there is no evidence of abnormal Ca^{2+} transport in skeletal muscle; with persistent antipsychotic effects (e.g., long-acting injectable agents) prolonged bromocriptine may be necessary in large doses (10–40 mg/d). Antiparkinsonian agents are not effective.

antihistamine diphenhydramine also possesses anticholinergic properties. Benztropine combines a benzhydryl group with a tropane group to create a compound that is more anticholinergic than trihexyphenidyl but less antihistaminic than diphenhydramine. The clinical effect of a single dose lasts 5 h, thereby requiring two or three daily doses. Dosing usually starts at 0.5–1 mg twice daily, with a daily maximum of 6 mg, although slightly higher doses are used in rare circumstances. The piperidine compound trihexyphenidyl was one of the first synthetic anticholinergic agents available; it also inhibits the presynaptic DA reuptake transporter, which creates a higher risk of abuse than for the antihistamines or benztropine. Trihexyphenidyl has good GI absorption, achieving peak plasma levels in 1–2 h, with a serum $t_{1/2}$ of about 10–12 h generally necessitating multiple-daily dosing to achieve satisfactory clinical results. The total daily dosage range is 5–15 mg, given two or three times a day as divided doses. Biperiden is another drug in this class.

Amantadine, originally marketed as an antiviral agent for influenza A, is an alternative medication for antipsychotic-induced parkinsonism and avoids the adverse CNS and peripheral effects of anticholinergic medications (Ogino et al., 2014). Its mechanism of action is unclear but appears to involve presynaptic DA reuptake blockade, facilitation of DA release, postsynaptic DA agonism, and receptor modulation. Amantadine is well absorbed after oral administration, with peak levels achieved 1–4 h after ingestion; clearance is renal, with more than 90% recovered unmetabolized in the urine. The plasma $t_{1/2}$ is 12–18 h in healthy young adults but is longer in those with renal impairment, necessitating a 50% dose reduction. Starting dosage is 100 mg orally once daily in healthy adults, which may be increased to 100 mg twice daily. A dose of 100 mg twice daily yields peak plasma levels of 0.5–0.8 μg/mL and trough levels of 0.3 μg/mL. Toxicity is seen at serum levels between 1 and 5 μg/mL.

Tardive Dyskinesia. Tardive dyskinesia results from increased nigrostriatal dopaminergic activity as a consequence of postsynaptic receptor supersensitivity and upregulation from chronically high levels of postsynaptic D_2 blockade (and possible direct toxic effects of high-potency DA antagonists). TD occurs more frequently in older patients, and the risk may be somewhat greater in patients with mood disorders than in those with schizophrenia. Its prevalence averages 15%–25% in young adults treated with typical antipsychotic agents for more than a year; the risk is a third to a fifth of that with atypical agents.

Tardive dyskinesia is characterized by stereotyped, repetitive, painless, involuntary, quick choreiform (tic-like) movements of the face, eyelids (blinks or spasm), mouth (grimaces), tongue, extremities, or trunk, with varying degrees of slower athetosis (twisting movements); tardive dystonia and tardive akathisia are rare now that the use of high-dose, high-potency typical antipsychotic medications has abated. The movements disappear during sleep (as do many other extrapyramidal syndromes), vary in intensity over time, and are dependent on the level of arousal or emotional distress, sometimes reappearing during acute psychiatric illnesses following prolonged disappearance. The dyskinetic movements can be suppressed partially by use of a potent DA antagonist, but such interventions over time may worsen the severity, as this was part of the initial pharmacological insult. Switching patients from potent D_2 antagonists to weaker agents, especially clozapine, can be effective. When possible, drug discontinuation may be beneficial but is effective in less than 33% of cases.

The VMAT2 inhibitors valbenazine and deuterated-tetrabenazine (deutetrabenazine) were FDA-approved for TD in 2017. Both are derivatives of tetrabenazine and share mechanism and many of the adverse effects of tetrabenazine. Velbenazine is active and is metabolized to an active metabolite, dihydotetrabenazine. The clearance of valbenazine and its active metabolite involve CYPs 2D6 and 3A4. Thus, exposure to the parent drug and its active metabolite will be increased in CYP2D6 poor metabolizers, in the presence of strong inhibitors of 2D6 (e.g., paroxetine) or 3A4 (e.g., ketoconazole), or in patients with moderate-to-severe hepatic impairment. Use of valbenazine in the presence of strong inducers of 3A4 (e.g., rifampin) is not recommended; concomitant use of MAOIs should be avoided. Valbenazine inhibits P-glycoprotein and will increase digoxin exposure. Deutetrabenazine is also approved for treating the chorea of Huntington disease and is described in Chapter 18, as is tetrabenazine.

Akathisia. Unlike antipsychotic-induced parkinsonism and acute dystonia, the phenomenology and treatment of akathisia suggest involvement of structures outside the nigrostriatal pathway. Despite the association with D_2 blockade, akathisia does not have as robust a response to antiparkinsonian drugs, so other treatment strategies are often employed acutely, including high-potency benzodiazepines (e.g., clonazepam) and nonselective β blockers with good CNS penetration (e.g., propranolol). Over time, one should consider dose reduction or switching to another antipsychotic agent. That clonazepam and propranolol have significant cortical activity and are ineffective for other forms of EPSs points to an extrastriatal origin for akathisia symptoms.

Neuroleptic Malignant Syndrome. The rare NMS resembles a severe form of parkinsonism, with signs of autonomic instability (hyperthermia and labile pulse, blood pressure, and respiration rate), stupor, elevation of creatine kinase in serum, and sometimes myoglobinemia with potential nephrotoxicity. At its most severe, this syndrome may persist for more than a week after the offending agent is discontinued and is associated with mortality. This reaction has been associated with myriad antipsychotic agents, but its prevalence may be greater with relatively high doses of potent agents. Aside from cessation of antipsychotic treatment and provision of supportive care, including aggressive cooling measures, specific pharmacological treatment is unsatisfactory, although administration of dantrolene and the dopaminergic agonist bromocriptine may be helpful. While dantrolene also is used to manage the syndrome of malignant hyperthermia induced by general anesthetics, the neuroleptic-induced form of hyperthermia probably is not associated with a defect in Ca^{2+} metabolism in skeletal muscle. There are anecdotal reports of NMS with atypical antipsychotic agents, but this syndrome is now rarely seen in its full presentation (Gurrera et al., 2011).

Hyperprolactinemia. Hyperprolactinemia results from blockade of the pituitary actions of the tuberoinfundibular dopaminergic neurons; these neurons project from the arcuate nucleus of the hypothalamus to the median eminence, where they deliver DA to the anterior pituitary via the hypophyseoportal vessels. D_2 receptors on lactotropes in the anterior pituitary mediate the tonic prolactin-inhibiting action of DA. Correlations between the D_2 potency of antipsychotic drugs and prolactin elevations are excellent. With the exception of risperidone and paliperidone, atypical antipsychotic agents show limited effects (asenapine, iloperidone, olanzapine, quetiapine, ziprasidone) to almost no effects (clozapine, aripiprazole, brexpiprazole, cariprazine) on prolactin secretion.

Hyperprolactinemia can directly induce breast engorgement and galactorrhea and can cause amenorrhea in women and sexual dysfunction or infertility in women and men. Dose reduction can be tried to decrease serum prolactin levels, but caution must be exercised to keep treatment within the antipsychotic therapeutic range. When switching from offending antipsychotic agents is not feasible, bromocriptine can be employed. The hyperprolactinemia from antipsychotic drugs is rapidly reversed when the drugs are discontinued.

Histamine H_1 Receptors. Central antagonism of H_1 receptors is associated with two major adverse effects: sedation and weight gain via appetite stimulation (Kim et al., 2007), and certain antipsychotic agents cause these adverse effects.

Sedation. Examples of sedating antipsychotic drugs include low-potency typical agents such as chlorpromazine and the atypical agents clozapine and quetiapine. The sedating effect is predicted by their high H_1 receptor affinities (Table 16–2). Some tolerance to the sedative properties will develop, a helpful fact to remember when considering switching a patient to a nonsedating agent. Rapid discontinuation of sedating antihistaminic antipsychotic drugs is inevitably followed by significant complaints of rebound insomnia and sleep disturbance. If discontinuation of sedating antipsychotic treatment is deemed necessary, except for emergency cessation of clozapine for agranulocytosis, the medication should be tapered slowly over 4–12 weeks, and the clinician should be prepared to utilize a sedative at the end of the taper. Generous dosing of another antihistamine (hydroxyzine) or the anticholinergic antihistamine diphenhydramine are reasonable replacements. Sedation may be useful during acute psychosis, but excessive sedation can interfere with patient evaluation, may prolong emergency room and psychiatric hospital stays unnecessarily, and is poorly tolerated among elderly patients with dementia and delirium; thus, appropriate caution must be exercised with the choice of agent and the dose.

Weight Gain. Weight gain is a significant problem during long-term use of antipsychotic drugs and represents a major barrier to medication adherence, as well as a significant threat to the physical and emotional health of the patient. Weight gain has effectively replaced concerns over EPS as the adverse effect causing the most consternation among patients and clinicians alike. Appetite stimulation is the primary mechanism involved, with little evidence to suggest that decreased activity (due to sedation) is a main contributor to antipsychotic-related weight gain. Laboratory studies indicated that medications with significant H_1 antagonism induce appetite stimulation through effects at hypothalamic sites (Kim et al., 2007). The low-potency phenothiazine chlorpromazine and the atypical antipsychotic drugs olanzapine and clozapine are the agents of highest risk, but some weight gain occurs with nearly all antipsychotic drugs.

Acutely psychotic patients may lose weight; in placebo-controlled acute schizophrenia trials, the placebo cohort inevitably loses weight. Younger and antipsychotic drug-naïve patients are much more sensitive to the weight gain from all antipsychotic agents, including those that appear roughly weight neutral in adult studies, leading some to conjecture that DA blockade may also play a small additive role in weight gain (Correll et al., 2014). Antagonism at $5HT_{2C}$ receptors may play an additive role in promoting weight gain for medications that possess high H_1 affinities (e.g., clozapine, olanzapine) but appears to have no effect in the absence of significant H_1 blockade, as seen with ziprasidone, an antipsychotic with low weight gain risk but an extremely high $5HT_{2C}$ affinity.

Switching to more weight-neutral medications can achieve significant results; however, when changing medications is not feasible or unsuccessful, behavioral strategies must be employed, and should be considered for all chronically mentally ill patients given the prevalence of obesity in this patient population. There is also compelling data for the use of metformin to moderate the antipsychotic-induced weight gain from olanzapine and clozapine, particularly when commencing the antipsychotic (Praharaj et al., 2011).

Muscarinic M_1 Receptors. Muscarinic antagonism is responsible for the central and peripheral anticholinergic effects of medications. The muscarinic receptor affinity and clinically relevant anticholinergic effects of the atypical antipsychotics are limited, whereas clozapine and low-potency phenothiazines have significant anticholinergic adverse effects (Table 16–2). Quetiapine has modest muscarinic affinity; its active metabolite norquetiapine is likely responsible for anticholinergic effects. Clozapine is particularly associated with significant constipation, perhaps due to anticholinergic properties, and possibly effects at sigma receptors. Routine use of stool softeners and repeated inquiry into bowel habits are necessary to prevent serious intestinal obstruction from undetected constipation. Medications with significant anticholinergic properties should be particularly avoided in elderly patients, especially those with dementia or delirium.

Adrenergic α_1 Receptors. α_1 Adrenergic antagonism is associated with risk of orthostatic hypotension and can be particularly problematic for elderly patients who have poor vasomotor tone. The extent to which antipsychotic agents cause this effect in clinical practice is dependent on the doses employed and the rapidity of titration. Compared to high-potency typical agents, low-potency typical agents generally have greater affinities for α_1 receptors and pose greater risk for orthostasis. Among newer medications, iloperidone carries a warning regarding minimization of orthostasis risk through slower titration. Clozapine can be associated with significant orthostasis, even when titrated slowly. Because clozapine-treated patients have few other antipsychotic options, the potent mineralocorticoid fludrocortisone is sometimes tried (0.1–0.3 mg/d) as a volume expander.

Adverse Effects Not Predicted by Monoamine Receptor Affinities

Adverse Metabolic Effects. Metabolic effects are the area of greatest concern during long-term antipsychotic treatment, paralleling the overall concern for the high prevalence of prediabetic conditions, type 2 DM, and 2-fold greater CV mortality among patients with schizophrenia (Correll et al., 2014). Aside from weight gain, the two predominant metabolic adverse side effects seen with antipsychotic drugs are dyslipidemia, primarily elevated serum triglycerides, and impairments in glycemic control.

Low-potency phenothiazines elevate serum triglyceride values, an effect that is not seen with high-potency phenothiazines. Among atypical antipsychotic drugs, significant increases in fasting triglyceride levels are noted during clozapine and olanzapine exposure and, to a lesser extent, with quetiapine. Effects on total cholesterol and cholesterol fractions are significantly less but show expected associations related to agents of highest risk: clozapine, olanzapine, and quetiapine (Rummel-Kluge et al., 2010). Weight gain in general may induce deleterious lipid changes; the evidence indicates that antipsychotic-induced hypertriglyceridemia is a weight-independent adverse event that occurs within weeks of starting an offending medication and resolves within 6 weeks after medication discontinuation. In individuals not exposed to antipsychotic drugs, elevated fasting triglycerides are a direct consequence of insulin resistance because insulin-dependent lipases in fat cells are normally inhibited by insulin. As insulin resistance worsens, inappropriately high levels of lipolysis lead to the release of excess amounts of free fatty acids, which are transformed into triglyceride particles (Meyer and Stahl, 2009). Elevated fasting triglyceride levels thus become a sensitive marker of insulin resistance, leading to the hypothesis that the triglyceride increases seen during antipsychotic treatment are the result of derangements in glucose-insulin homeostasis.

The ability of antipsychotic drugs to induce hyperglycemia was first noted during low-potency phenothiazine treatment; indeed, chlorpromazine was occasionally exploited for this specific property as adjunctive presurgical treatment of insulinoma. As atypical antipsychotic drugs found widespread use, numerous case series documented the association of new-onset diabetes and diabetic ketoacidosis associated with treatment with atypical antipsychotic drugs, with most of cases observed during clozapine and olanzapine therapy (Meyer and Stahl, 2009). The mechanism by which antipsychotic drugs disrupt glucose-insulin homeostasis is not known, but in vivo animal experiments document immediate dose-dependent effects of clozapine and olanzapine on whole-body and hepatic insulin sensitivity (Meyer and Stahl, 2009).

There may also be inherent disease-related mechanisms that increase risk for metabolic disorders among patients with schizophrenia (Meyer and Stahl, 2009), but the medication itself is the primary risk factor, and all atypical antipsychotic drugs in the U.S. include a hyperglycemia warning on the drug label, although there is limited evidence that the newer medications asenapine, iloperidone, aripiprazole, brexpiprazole, cariprazine, and ziprasidone cause hyperglycemia. Use of metabolically more benign agents is recommended for the initial treatment of all patients for whom long-term treatment is expected. Clinicians should obtain baseline metabolic data, including a fasting glucose or hemoglobin A_{1c}, a fasting lipid panel, and weight and establish a plan for ongoing monitoring of these metabolic parameters. As with weight gain, the changes in fasting glucose and lipids should prompt reevaluation of ongoing treatment, institution of measures to improve metabolic health (diet, exercise, nutritional counseling), and consideration of switching antipsychotic agents.

Adverse Cardiac Effects. Multiple ion channels are involved in the depolarization and repolarization of cardiac ventricular cells (Chapters 29 and 30). Some antipsychotic agents can interfere with the functioning of these channels, making the risk of ventricular arrhythmias and SCD a concern with the use of these drugs. While most of the older antipsychotic agents (e.g., thioridazine) significantly inhibited inwardly rectifying K^+ channels (I_{kr}) in cardiac myocytes, this effect is much less pronounced for newer agents (Leucht et al., 2013). Chapters 29 and 30. Antagonism of voltage-gated Na^+ channels causes QRS widening and an increase in the PR interval, with increased risk for ventricular arrhythmia. Thioridazine can inhibit Na^+ channels at high dosages, but other antipsychotic medications do not (Nielsen et al., 2011). Myocyte repolarization is mediated in part by K^+ current through two channels: the rapid I_{kr} and the slow I_{ks} channels. The α subunit of the I_{kr} channel, $K_v11.1$, is encoded by *hERG*, the human-ether-à-go-go related gene that codes for Kv11.1, the α subunit of the K^+ channel that mediates the repolarizing I_{Kr} current of the cardiac action potential. Polymorphisms of *hERG* are involved in the congenital long QT syndrome associated with syncope and SCD. Antagonism of I_{kr} channels is responsible for most cases of drug-induced QT prolongation and is the suspected mechanism for the majority of antipsychotic-induced SCDs (Nielsen et al., 2011).

Aside from individual agents, for which anecdotal and pharmacosurveillance data indicate risk for torsade de pointes (e.g., thioridazine, pimozide), most of the commonly used newer antipsychotic agents are not associated with a known increased risk for ventricular arrhythmias, including ziprasidone in overdose up to 12,000 mg. One exception is sertindole, an agent not available in the U.S. that was withdrawn in 1998 based on anecdotal reports of torsade de pointes, but reintroduced in Europe in 2006 with strict ECG monitoring guidelines (Nielsen et al., 2011). Although in vitro data revealed sertindole's affinity for I_{kr}, several epidemiological studies published over the past decade were unable to confirm an increased risk of sudden death due to sertindole exposure, thereby providing justification for its reintroduction.

Currently, no data suggest a benefit of routine ECG monitoring for prevention of SCD among patients using antipsychotic drugs. Nonetheless, all antipsychotic medications marketed in the U.S. (with the exception of lurasidone) carry a class label warning regarding QT_c prolongation. A specific black-box warning exists for thioridazine, pimozide, intramuscular droperidol, and haloperidol (intravenous formulation but not oral or intramuscular) concerning torsade de pointes and subsequent fatal ventricular arrhythmias (discussed next and in Chapter 30).

Other Adverse Effects. In the U.S., there is a class label warning for seizure risk on all antipsychotic agents (except pimavanserin), with reported incidences well below 1%. Among commonly used newer antipsychotic drugs, only clozapine has a dose-dependent seizure risk, with a prevalence of 3%–5%. The structurally related olanzapine had an incidence of 0.9% in premarketing studies. Patients with seizure disorder who commence antipsychotic treatment must receive adequate prophylaxis, with consideration given to avoiding carbamazepine and phenytoin due to their capacity to induce CYPs and P-glycoprotein. Carbamazepine is also contraindicated during clozapine treatment due to its bone marrow effects. Valproate derivatives (e.g., divalproex sodium) are used for clozapine-associated seizures as they best cover the spectrum of generalized and myoclonic seizures (Meltzer, 2012).

Clozapine causes a host of other adverse effects, the most concerning of which is agranulocytosis, with an incidence of slightly under 1%; the highest risk occurs during the initial 6 months of treatment, peaking at months 2–3 and diminishing rapidly thereafter (Meltzer, 2012). The mechanism is immune mediated, and patients who have verifiable clozapine-related agranulocytosis are usually not rechallenged. An extensive algorithm guiding clinical response to agranulocytosis and lesser forms of neutropenia is available from manufacturer websites and must be followed, along with mandated CBC monitoring.

Other adverse effects include pigmentary retinopathy (thioridazine at daily doses ≥ 800 mg/d), photosensitivity (low-potency phenothiazines), and elevations of alkaline phosphatase and, rarely, hepatic transaminases (phenothiazines).

Increased Mortality in Patients With Dementia. Perhaps the least-understood adverse effect is the increased risk for cerebrovascular events and all-cause mortality among elderly patients with dementia exposed to antipsychotic medications (~1.7-fold increased mortality risk for drug vs. placebo) (Maust et al., 2015). Mortality is due to heart failure, sudden death, or pneumonia. The underlying etiology for antipsychotic-related cerebrovascular and mortality risk is unknown, but the finding of virtually equivalent mortality risk for typical agents compared to atypical antipsychotic drugs (including aripiprazole) suggests an impact of reduced D_2 signaling regardless of individual antipsychotic mechanisms.

Overdose with typical antipsychotic agents is of particular concern with *low*-potency agents (e.g., chlorpromazine) due to the risk of torsades de pointes, sedation, anticholinergic effects, and orthostasis. Patients who overdose on *high*-potency typical antipsychotic drugs (e.g., haloperidol) and the substituted benzamides are at greater risk for EPSs (due to the high D_2 affinity) and for ECG changes. Overdose experience with newer agents indicates a much lower risk for torsade de pointes ventricular arrhythmias compared to older antipsychotic medications; however, combinations of antipsychotic agents with other medications can lead to fatality, primarily through respiratory depression.

Drug-Drug Interactions

Antipsychotic agents are not significant inhibitors of CYPs, with a few notable exceptions: chlorpromazine, perphenazine, and thioridazine inhibit CYP2D6. The plasma half-lives of a number of these agents are altered by induction or inhibition of hepatic CYPs and by genetic polymorphisms that alter specific CYP activities (Table 16–4). While antipsychotic drugs are highly protein bound, there is no evidence of significant displacement of other protein-bound medications, so dosage adjustment is not required for anticonvulsants, warfarin, or other agents with narrow therapeutic indices.

With respect to drug-drug interactions, it is important to consider the effects of environmental exposures (smoking, nutraceuticals, grapefruit juice) and changes in these behaviors. Changes in smoking status can be especially problematic for clozapine-treated patients and will alter serum levels by 50% or more (Rostami-Hodjegan et al., 2004) due to the capacity of aromatic hydrocarbons in tobacco smoke to induce CYP1A2, the major metabolizer of clozapine. Thus, hospitalization of a smoker in a smoke-free environment results in decreased CYP1A2 activity and an elevation of clozapine plasma levels, with potentially toxic results. Conversely, a patient discharged from a nonsmoking ward who resumes smoking will experience an increase in CYP1A2 activity and a 50% decrease in plasma clozapine levels. Monitoring of plasma clozapine concentrations, anticipation of changes in smoking habits, and dosage adjustment can minimize development of subtherapeutic or supratherapeutic levels.

Use in Pediatric Populations

Aripiprazole, olanzapine, quetiapine, risperidone, lurasidone, and paliperidone have indications for adolescent schizophrenia (ages 13–17). Aripiprazole, quetiapine, and risperidone are approved in child and adolescent bipolar disorder (acute mania) for ages 10–17; risperidone and aripiprazole are also FDA-approved for irritability associated with autism in child and adolescent patients ages 5–16. As discussed in the sections on adverse effects, antipsychotic drug-naïve patients and younger patients are more susceptible than other patients to EPSs and weight gain (Correll et al., 2014; Peruzzolo et al., 2013). Use of the minimum effective dose can minimize EPS risk, and use of agents with lower weight gain liability is critical. The greater impact of risperidone and paliperidone on serum prolactin must be monitored by clinical inquiry. Delayed sexual maturation was not seen in adolescents in clinical trials with risperidone; nonetheless, the physician must be alert for such changes and for issues such as amenorrhea in girls and gynecomastia in boys and girls.

Use in Geriatric Populations

The increased sensitivity to EPSs, orthostasis, sedation, and anticholinergic effects are important for the geriatric population and often dictate the choice of antipsychotic medication. Avoidance of drug-drug interactions is also important, as older patients on numerous concomitant medications have multiple opportunities for interactions. Dose adjustment can offset known drug-drug interactions, but clinicians must be attentive to changes in concurrent medications and the potential pharmacokinetic consequences. Vigilance must also be maintained for the additive pharmacodynamic effects of α_1 adrenergic, antihistaminic, and anticholinergic properties of other agents.

Elderly patients have an increased risk for TD and parkinsonism, with TD rates about 5-fold higher than those seen with younger patients. With typical antipsychotics, the reported annual TD incidence among elderly patients is 20%–25% compared to 4%–5% for younger patients. With atypical antipsychotics, the annual TD rate in elderly patients is much lower (2%–3%). Increased risk for cerebrovascular events and all-cause mortality is also seen in elderly patients with dementia (see Increased Mortality in Patients With Dementia). Compared to younger patients, antipsychotic-induced weight gain is lower in elderly patients.

Use During Pregnancy and Lactation

Human data from large database studies do not show increased rates of major congenital malformations after first trimester exposure (Huybrechts et al., 2016). Nonetheless, the use of any medication during pregnancy must be balanced by concerns over fetal impact, especially first-trimester exposure, and the mental health of the mother. As antipsychotic drugs are designed to cross the blood-brain barrier, all have high rates of placental passage. Placental passage ratios are estimated to be highest for olanzapine (72%), followed by haloperidol (42%), risperidone (49%), and quetiapine (24%). Neonates exposed to olanzapine, the atypical agent with highest placental passage ratio, exhibit a trend toward greater neonatal intensive care unit admission. Use in nursing mothers raises a separate set of concerns due to the reduced capacity of the newborn to metabolize xenobiotics, thus presenting a significant risk for antipsychotic drug toxicity. Available data do not provide adequate guidance on choice of agent.

Major Drugs Available in the Class

Atypical antipsychotic drugs have largely replaced older agents, primarily due to their more favorable EPS profile. The older, typical agents are widely used when a higher level of D_2 antagonism is required. Table 16–1 describes the acute and maintenance doses for adult schizophrenia treatment based on consensus recommendations. There are numerous LAI formulations of typical antipsychotics (Table 16–3), but in the U.S., the only available LAI typical agents are fluphenazine and haloperidol (as decanoate esters) (Meyer, 2013), suitable for weekly injections. There are now six LAI atypical antipsychotics approved, including a 3-month form of LAI paliperidone. Pimavanserin is the only medication indicated for PDP, and does not worsen motor symptoms due to the lack of DA antagonism (Cummings et al., 2014).

Treatment of Mania

Mania is a period of elevated, expansive, or irritable mood with coexisting symptoms of increased energy and goal-directed activity and decreased need for sleep. Mania represents one pole of bipolar disorder (American Psychiatric Association, 2013). As with psychosis, mania may be induced by medications (e.g., DA agonists, antidepressants, stimulants) or substances of abuse, primarily cocaine and amphetamines, although periods of substance-induced mania should not be relied on solely to make a diagnosis of bipolar disorder. Nonetheless, there is recognition that patients who develop antidepressant-induced mania do have a bipolar diathesis even with no prior independent history of mania and should be followed carefully, especially if antidepressant treatment is again considered during periods of major depression.

Mania is distinguished from its less-severe form, hypomania, by the fact that hypomania, by definition, does not result in functional impairment or hospitalization and is not associated with psychotic symptoms. Patients who experience periods of hypomania and major depression have bipolar II disorder; those with mania at any time, bipolar I; and those with hypomania but less-severe forms of depression, cyclothymia (American Psychiatric Association, 2013). The prevalence of bipolar I disorder is roughly 1% of the population, and the prevalence of all forms of bipolar disorder is 3%–5%.

Genetics studies of bipolar disorder have yielded several loci of interest associated with disease risk and predictors of treatment response, but the data are not yet at the phase of clinical application. Unlike schizophrenia, for which the biological understanding of monoamine neurotransmission has permitted synthesis of numerous effective compounds, no medication

TABLE 16–6 ■ COMPARATIVE EFFICACY AND TARGET SERUM LEVELS FOR MOOD STABILIZERS

	ACUTE MANIA	PROPHYLAXIS	BIPOLAR DEPRESSION
Lithium	+++ 1.0–1.5 mEq/L[a]	+++ 0.6–1.0 mEq/L	++ 0.6–1.0 mEq/L
Valproate	++++ 100–120 μg/mL[b]	+++ 60–100 μg/mL	—
Carbamazepine	+ 6–12 μg/mL	++ 6–12 μg/mL	+/– 6–12 μg/mL
Lamotrigine	–	++	++

[a]Lithium can be loaded with individual 10-mg/kg doses of an extended-release preparation administered at 4 PM, 6 PM, and 8 PM (Kook et al., 1985). Treatment should continue on day 2 with lithium carbonate given once nightly to minimize the risk of polyuria and renal insufficiency.
[b]Divalproex can be loaded at 30 mg/kg over 24 h, administered as a single dose or separated into two doses.

has yet been designed to treat the full spectrum of bipolar disorder based on biological hypotheses of the illness. Lithium carbonate was introduced fortuitously in 1949 for the treatment of mania and approved for this purpose in the U.S. in 1970. While many classes of agents demonstrate efficacy in acute mania, including Li^+, antipsychotic drugs, and certain anticonvulsants, no medication has surpassed lithium's efficacy for prophylaxis of future manic and depressive phases of bipolar disorder, and no other medication has demonstrated lithium's reduction in suicidality among bipolar patients (Geddes and Miklowitz, 2013).

Pharmacological Properties of Agents for Mania

Antipsychotic Agents

The chemistry and pharmacology of antipsychotic medications are addressed earlier in this chapter. When used for acute mania, the dosages are often at the high end of approved maximum dosing. Clozapine can be beneficial in patients with refractory mania as adjunctive therapy and as monotherapy (Geddes and Miklowitz, 2013). Certain antipsychotics have efficacy for adjunctive use (olanzapine) or as monotherapy (quetiapine, lurasidone) for bipolar depression, typically at much lower dosages than for acute mania.

Anticonvulsants

The pharmacology and chemistry of the anticonvulsants with significant use in treating acute mania (valproic acid compounds, carbamazepine) and for bipolar maintenance (lamotrigine) are covered extensively in Chapter 17. The therapeutic serum levels for the commonly used mood-stabilizing anticonvulsants and for Li^+ are listed in Table 16–6.

Lithium

Lithium is the lightest of the alkali metals (group Ia). Salts of Li^+ share some characteristics with those of Na^+ and K^+. Li^+ is readily assayed in biological fluids and can be detected in brain tissue by magnetic resonance spectroscopy. Traces of the ion occur normally in animal tissues, but it has no known physiological role. Lithium carbonate and lithium citrate are used therapeutically in the U.S.

Therapeutic concentrations of Li^+ have almost no discernible psychotropic effects in individuals without psychiatric symptoms. There are numerous molecular and cellular actions of Li^+, some of which overlap with identified properties of other mood-stabilizing agents (particularly valproate) and are discussed next. An important characteristic of Li^+ is that, unlike Na^+ and K^+, Li^+ develops a relatively small gradient across biological membranes. Although it can replace Na^+ in supporting a single action potential in a nerve cell, it is not a substrate for the Na^+ pump and therefore cannot maintain membrane potentials. It is uncertain whether therapeutic concentrations of Li^+ (0.5–1.0 mEq/L) affect the transport of other monovalent or divalent cations by nerve cells.

Hypotheses for the Mechanism of Action of Lithium and Relationship to Anticonvulsants

Plausible hypotheses for the mechanism of action focus on lithium's impact on monoamines implicated in the pathophysiology of mood disorders and on second-messenger and other intracellular molecular mechanisms involved in signal transduction, gene regulation, and cell survival. Li^+ has limited effects on catecholamine-sensitive adenylyl cyclase activity or on the binding of ligands to monoamine receptors in brain tissue, although it can influence response of 5HT autoreceptors to agonists (Grandjean and Aubry, 2009b). 5HT release from presynaptic terminals is regulated by $5HT_{1A}$ autoreceptors located on the cell body and $5HT_{1B}$ receptors on the nerve terminal. In vitro electrophysiological studies suggest that Li^+ facilitates 5HT release. Li^+ augments effects of antidepressants, and in animal models of depression, lithium's activity appears to be mediated through desensitizing actions at $5HT_{1B}$ sites; Li^+ also antagonizes mouse behaviors induced by administration of selective $5HT_{1B}$ agonists (Grandjean and Aubry, 2009b).

Li^+ inhibits inositol monophosphatase and interferes with the cycling of the PI pathway (Figure 16–1) (Grandjean and Aubry, 2009b). One result is an enhancement of IP_3 accumulation when the G_q-PLC-IP_3-Ca^{2+} pathway is activated. As a result, IP_3 signaling and consequent mobilization of Ca^{2+} from intracellular stores may also be enhanced acutely, along with the sequelae of those effects; Ca^{2+} mobilization, PKC activation, depletion of cellular inositol; another result is a decrease in available inositol for resynthesis/reincorporation into membrane PI phosphates. The uncompetitive inhibition of IP phosphatase by Li^+ occurs within the range of therapeutic Li^+ concentrations. A genome-wide association study implicated diacylglycerol kinase in the etiology of bipolar disorder, strengthening the association between Li^+ actions and PI metabolism. Further support for the rôle of inositol signaling in mania rests on the finding that valproate and its derivatives decrease intracellular inositol concentrations. Unlike Li^+, valproate decreases inositol through inhibition of *myo*-inositol-1-phosphate synthase. In cultured cell systems, carbamazepine appears to act via inositol depletion. Perhaps such a mechanism contributes to carbamazepine's mood-stabilizing properties (Rapoport et al., 2009).

Treatment with Li^+ ultimately leads to decreased activity of several protein kinases in brain tissue, including PKC, particularly isoforms α and β (Einat, 2014). Among other proposed antimanic or mood-stabilizing agents, this effect is also shared with valproate (particularly for PKC) but not with carbamazepine. Long-term treatment of rats with lithium carbonate or valproate decreases cytoplasm-to-membrane translocation of PKC and reduces PKC stimulation–induced release of 5HT from cerebral cortical and hippocampal tissue. Excessive PKC activation can disrupt prefrontal cortical regulation of behavior, but pretreatment of monkeys and rats with lithium carbonate or valproate blocks the impairment in working memory induced by activation of PKC in a manner also seen with the PKC inhibitor chelerythrine (Einat, 2014). A major substrate for cerebral PKC is the MARCKS protein, which is implicated in synaptic and neuronal plasticity. The expression of MARCKS protein is reduced by treatment with both Li^+ and valproate but not by carbamazepine, antipsychotic medications, or antidepressants (Wang et al., 2001). This proposed mechanism of PKC inhibition has been the basis for therapeutic trials of tamoxifen, a selective estrogen receptor modulator that is also a potent centrally active PKC inhibitor. In acutely manic patients with bipolar I, tamoxifen has shown evidence of efficacy as adjunctive treatment (Einat,

2014). The impact of Li^+ or valproate on PKC activity may secondarily alter the activity of tyrosine hydroxylase. Li^+ may alter the release of neurotransmitters and hormones by a variety of putative mechanisms, and its acute effects may differ from its longterm effects (Sharp et al., 1991; Millienne-Petiot et al, 2017; Can et al, 2016; Fortin et al, 2016).

Both Li^+ and valproate treatment also inhibit the activity of GSK-3β (Williams et al., 2002). GSK-3 inhibition increases hippocampal levels of β-catenin, a function implicated in mood stabilization. In animal models, Li^+ induces molecular and behavioral effects comparable to that seen when one GSK-3β gene locus is inactivated (Urs et al., 2012). These lithium-sensitive behaviors are related to the impact of GSK-3β inhibition on the β-arrestin-2/PKB/PP2A signaling complex. Li^+ disrupts β-arrestin-2/PKB/PP2A complex formation by directly inhibiting GSK-3β.

Another proposed common mechanism for the actions of Li^+ and valproate relates to reduction in arachidonic acid turnover in brain membrane phospholipids. Rats fed Li^+ in amounts that achieve therapeutic CNS drug levels have reduced turnover of PI (↓83%) and phosphatidylcholine (↓73%); chronic intraperitoneal valproate achieves reductions of 34% and 36%, respectively. Li^+ also decreases gene expression of phospholipase A_2 and levels of COX-2 and its products (Rapoport et al., 2009).

ADME

Li^+ is almost completely absorbed from the GI tract. Peak plasma concentrations occur 2–4 h after an oral dose. Slow-release preparations of lithium carbonate minimize peak-to-trough ratios and permit once-daily dosing. Li^+ initially distributes to the extracellular fluid, does not bind appreciably to plasma proteins, and gradually accumulates in tissues, with a volume of distribution of 0.7–0.9 L/kg. The concentration gradient across plasma membranes is much smaller than those for Na^+ and K^+. Passage through the blood-brain barrier is slow, and when a steady state is achieved, the concentration of Li^+ in the cerebrospinal fluid and in brain tissue is about 40%–50% of the concentration in plasma. The kinetics of Li^+ can be monitored in human brain with magnetic resonance spectroscopy (Grandjean and Aubry, 2009b).

Approximately 95% of a single dose of Li^+ is eliminated in the urine, with a $t_{1/2}$ of about 24 h (varies with age and can be ~12 h in the young and ~36 h in the elderly [secondary to reduced GFR]). The $t_{1/2}$ generally supports once-daily dosing, which improves adherence and decreases risk for renal insufficiency by at least 20% (Castro et al., 2016). With repeated administration, Li^+ levels and excretion increase until a steady state is achieved (after four to five half-lives). When Li^+ is stopped, there is a rapid phase of renal excretion followed by a slow 10- to 14-day phase. Although the pharmacokinetics of Li^+ vary considerably among subjects, the volume of distribution and clearance are relatively stable in an individual patient.

Less than 1% of ingested Li^+ leaves the human body in the feces; 4%–5% is secreted in sweat (Grandjean and Aubry, 2009c). Li^+ is secreted in saliva in concentrations about twice those in plasma, while its concentration in tears is about equal to that in plasma. Li^+ is secreted in human milk, but serum levels in breast-fed infants are about 20% that of maternal levels and are not associated with notable behavioral effects (Diav-Citrin et al., 2014).

Li^+ competes with Na^+ for tubular reabsorption, and Li^+ retention can be increased by Na^+ loss related to diuretic use or diarrhea and other GI illness. Heavy sweating leads to a preferential secretion of Li^+ over Na^+; the repletion of excessive sweating using free water without electrolytes can cause hyponatremia and promote Li^+ retention (Grandjean and Aubry, 2009b).

Serum-Level Monitoring and Dose

Because of the low therapeutic index for Li^+, regular determination of serum concentrations is crucial. Concentrations considered to be effective and acceptably safe are between 0.6 and 1.5 mEq/L. The range of 1.0–1.5 mEq/L is favored for treatment of acutely manic patients. Somewhat lower values (0.6–1.0 mEq/L) are considered adequate and are safer for long-term prophylaxis. Serum concentrations of Li^+ have been found to follow a clear dose-effect relationship between 0.4 and 1.0 mEq/L, but with a corresponding dose-dependent rise in polyuria and tremor as indices of adverse effects (Grandjean and Aubry, 2009b, 2009c). Nonetheless, patients who maintain trough levels of 0.8–1.0 mEq/L experience decreased relapse risk compared to those maintained at lower serum concentrations. There are patients who may do well with serum levels of 0.5–0.8 mEq/L, but there are no current clinical or biological predictors to permit a priori identification of these individuals. Individualization of serum levels is often necessary to obtain a favorable risk-benefit relationship.

By convention, the serum Li^+ concentration is measured from samples obtained 10–12 h after the last oral dose of the day. When the peaks are reached, intoxication may result, even when concentrations in morning samples of plasma at the daily nadir are in the acceptable range of 0.6–1 mEq/L. Single daily doses generate relatively large oscillations of plasma Li^+ concentration but lower mean trough levels than with multiple-daily dosing; moreover, single-nightly dosing means that peak serum levels occur during sleep, so complaints of CNS adverse effects are minimized (Grandjean and Aubry, 2009c). While relatively uncommon, GI complaints are a compelling reason for using delayed-release Li^+ preparations, also given once daily.

Therapeutic Uses

Drug Treatment of Bipolar Disorder. Treatment with Li^+ ideally is conducted in patients with normal cardiac and renal function. Occasionally, patients with severe systemic illnesses are treated with Li^+, provided that the indications are compelling, but the need for diuretics, nonsteroidal anti-inflammatory agents, or other medications that pose potential kinetic problems often precludes Li^+ use in those with multiple medical problems. Treatment of acute mania and the prevention of recurrences of bipolar illness in adults or adolescents are uses approved by the FDA. Li^+ is the mood stabilizer with the most robust data on suicide reduction in bipolar patients; Li^+ is also efficacious for augmentation in unipolar depressive patients who respond inadequately to antidepressant therapy (Grandjean and Aubry, 2009a).

Pharmacotherapy of Mania. The modern treatment of the manic, depressive, and mixed-mood phases of bipolar disorder was revolutionized by the introduction of Li^+ in 1949, initially for acute mania only and later for prevention of recurrences of mania. While Li^+, valproate, and carbamazepine have efficacy in acute mania, in clinical practice these are usually combined with atypical antipsychotic drugs, even in manic patients without psychotic features, due to their complementary modes of action. Li^+, carbamazepine, and valproic acid preparations are effective only with daily dosing that maintains adequate serum levels (requires monitoring of serum levels). Patients with mania are often irritable and poorly cooperative with medication administration and phlebotomy; thus, atypical antipsychotic drugs may be the sole initial therapy, and they have proven efficacy as monotherapy. Moreover, acute intramuscular forms of olanzapine and ziprasidone can be used to achieve rapid control of psychosis and agitation. Benzodiazepines are often used adjunctively for agitation and sleep induction.

Li^+ is effective in acute mania and can be loaded in those with normal renal function using three individual 10-mg/kg doses of a sustained-release preparation administered at 2-h intervals. The sustained-release form is used to minimize GI adverse effects (e.g., nausea, diarrhea); treatment may then be continued with Li^+ carbonate. Acutely manic patients may require higher dosages to achieve therapeutic serum levels, and downward adjustment may be necessary once the patient is euthymic. Efficacy following loading can be achieved within 5 days. When adherence with oral capsules or tablets is an issue, the liquid Li^+ citrate can be used.

The anticonvulsant sodium valproate also provides antimanic effects, with therapeutic benefit seen within 3–5 days (Cipriani et al., 2013). The most common form of valproate in use is divalproex sodium due to lower incidence of GI and other adverse effects. Divalproex is initiated at 30 mg/kg given as single or divided doses and titrated to effect based on the desired serum level. Serum concentrations of 90–120 μg/mL show the best response in clinical studies (Cipriani et al., 2013). With immediate-release forms of valproic acid and divalproex sodium, 12-h troughs are used to guide treatment. With the extended-release divalproex preparation, the true trough occurs 24 h after dosing. Obtaining serum levels at night may be difficult in outpatient settings, so 12-h troughs are commonly used, bearing in mind that 12-h trough levels are 18%–25% higher than the 24-h trough (Reed and Dutta, 2006).

Carbamazepine is effective for acute mania, but immediate-release forms of carbamazepine cannot be loaded or rapidly titrated over 24 h due to the development of adverse effects such as dizziness or ataxia, even within the therapeutic range (6–12 μg/mL) (Geddes and Miklowitz, 2013). An extended-release form of carbamazepine is effective as monotherapy with once-daily dosing. Carbamazepine response rates are lower than those for valproate compounds or for Li^+, with mean rates of 45%–60% cited in the literature (Geddes and Miklowitz, 2013). Nevertheless, certain individuals respond to carbamazepine after failing Li^+ and valproate. Initial doses are 400 mg/d in two divided doses. Titration proceeds by 200-mg increments every 24–48 h based on clinical response and serum trough levels, not to exceed 1600 mg/d.

The FDA has warned that serious and potentially fatal skin reactions (e.g., Stevens-Johnson syndrome and toxic epidermal necrolysis) may occur with the administration of carbamazepine in patients positive for the *HLA-B*1502* allele. Thus, the FDA recommends genetic screening for patients of Asian ancestry (among whom the prevalence of this allele exceeds 15%) before initiation of carbamazepine therapy and using alternative therapies in patients positive for the allele. See Chapter 17 for more information on carbamazepine.

Lamotrigine has no role in acute mania due to the slow, extended titration necessary to minimize risk of Stevens-Johnson syndrome and is used for bipolar maintenance (Rapoport et al., 2009; Selle et al., 2014).

Prophylactic Treatment of Bipolar Disorder. The choice of ongoing prophylaxis is determined by the need for continued antipsychotic drug use and for use of a mood-stabilizing agent. Both aripiprazole and olanzapine are effective as monotherapy for mania prophylaxis, but olanzapine use is eschewed out of concern for metabolic effects, and aripiprazole shows no benefit for prevention of depressive relapse. LAI risperidone is approved for bipolar maintenance treatment as monotherapy or adjunctively with Li^+ or valproate. If LAI risperidone is used as monotherapy, coverage with an oral antipsychotic is necessary for the first 4 weeks after the initial injection. When antipsychotic drugs have been employed as adjunctive agents, the optimal duration of treatment is unclear; recent data indicate no greater benefit beyond 6 months after remission from an acute manic episode (Yatham et al., 2016).

Overriding concerns guiding bipolar treatment are the high recurrence rate and the high risk of suicide. Individuals who experience mania have an 80%–90% lifetime risk of subsequent manic episodes. As with schizophrenia, lack of insight, poor psychosocial support, and substance abuse all interfere with treatment adherence. While the anticonvulsants lamotrigine, carbamazepine, and divalproex have data supporting their use in bipolar prophylaxis, only lithium has consistently been shown to reduce the risk of suicide compared to other treatments, specifically when compared to valproate acid derivatives (Goodwin et al., 2003).

A recent large trial comparing Li^+ and valproate found no significant differences in time to relapse between the two agents (Cipriani et al., 2013). Lamotrigine has proven effective for bipolar patients whose most recent mood episode was manic or depressed, with greater effect on depressive relapse (Selle et al., 2014). The ability to provide prophylaxis for future depressive episodes combined with data in acute bipolar depression has made lamotrigine a useful choice for bipolar treatment, given that patients with bipolar I and II spend large amounts of time in depressive phases (Selle et al., 2014).

Bipolar disorder is a lifetime illness with high recurrence rates. Individuals who experience an episode of mania should be educated about the probable need for ongoing treatment. Stopping mood stabilizer therapy can be considered in patients who have experienced only one lifetime manic episode, particularly when there may have been a pharmacological precipitant (e.g., substance or antidepressant use), and who have been euthymic for extended periods. For patients with bipolar II, the impact of hypomania is relatively limited, so the decision to recommend prolonged maintenance treatment with a mood stabilizer is based on clinical response and risk:benefit ratio. Discontinuation of maintenance Li^+ treatment in patients with bipolar I carries a high risk of early recurrence and of suicidal behavior over a period of several months, even if the treatment had been successful for several years. Recurrence is much more rapid than is predicted by the natural history of untreated bipolar disorder, in which cycle lengths average about 1 year. This risk may be moderated by slow, gradual removal of Li^+; rapid discontinuation should be avoided unless dictated by medical emergencies.

Other Uses of Lithium. Li^+ is effective as adjunct therapy in treatment-resistant major depression (Grandjean and Aubry, 2009a). Clinical data also support Li^+ use as monotherapy for unipolar depression. Meta-analyses indicated that lithium's benefit on suicide reduction extends to patients with unipolar mood disorder (Baldessarini and Tondo, 2000). While maintenance Li^+ levels of 0.6–1.0 mEq/L are used for bipolar prophylaxis, a lower range (0.4–0.8 mEq/L) is recommended for antidepressant augmentation.

Based on its neuroprotective properties, Li^+ treatment has been suggested for conditions associated with excitotoxic and apoptotic cell death, such as stroke and spinal cord injury, and in neurodegenerative disorders, including dementia of the Alzheimer type, Parkinson disease, Huntington disease, amyotrophic lateral sclerosis, progressive supranuclear palsy, and spinocerebellar ataxia type I (Chiu et al., 2013).

Drug Interactions. Thiazide diuretics cause significant reductions in Li^+ clearance that result in toxic levels. The K^+-sparing diuretics have more modest effects on the excretion of Li^+, with concomitantly smaller increases in serum levels. Loop diuretics such as furosemide seem to have limited impact on Li^+ levels (Grandjean and Aubry, 2009b). Administration of osmotic diuretics or acetazolamide increases renal excretion of Li^+ but not sufficiently for the management of acute Li^+ intoxication. Through alteration of renal perfusion, some nonsteroidal anti-inflammatory agents can facilitate renal proximal tubular resorption of Li^+ and thereby increase serum concentrations (Grandjean and Aubry, 2009b). This interaction appears to be particularly prominent with indomethacin, but also may occur with ibuprofen, naproxen, and COX-2 inhibitors and possibly less so with sulindac and aspirin. ACEIs, particularly lisinopril, also cause Li^+ retention, with isolated reports of toxicity among stable Li^+-treated patients switched from fosinopril to lisinopril (Meyer et al., 2005).

Amiloride blocks entry of Li^+ into renal distal tubule ENaCs and has been used to safely manage NDI associated with Li^+ therapy (Bedford et al., 2008). The development of NDI is related to accumulation of Li^+ in distal tubular cells and subsequent inhibition of GSK-3β, leading to vasopressin insensitivity and downregulation of aquaporin-2 channels. The use of amiloride for this purpose requires electrolyte monitoring and Li^+ dosage adjustments to prevent toxicity (Bedford et al., 2008).

Adverse Effects of Lithium

CNS Effects. The most common effect of Li^+ in the therapeutic dose range is fine postural hand tremor, indistinguishable from essential tremor. Severity and risk for tremor are dose dependent, with incidence ranging from 15% to 70%. In addition to the avoidance of caffeine and other agents that increase tremor amplitude, therapeutic options include dose reduction (bearing in mind the increased relapse risk with lower serum Li^+ levels) and β adrenergic blockade (Grandjean and Aubry, 2009c); the approach to valproate-induced tremor is identical. At peak serum (and CNS) levels of Li^+, patients may complain of incoordination, ataxia, or slurred speech, all of which can be avoided by dosing Li^+ at bedtime. Patients may also complain of mental fatigue or cognitive dulling at higher serum Li^+ levels, but this should be carefully assessed to determine whether this reflects a true side effect or a desire to regain the mental high from hypomania.

Seizures have been reported in nonepileptic patients with therapeutic plasma concentrations of Li^+. Li^+ treatment has also been associated with increased risk of post-ECT confusion and is generally tapered off prior to a course of ECT (Grandjean and Aubry, 2009c). In some instances, addition of Li^+ to existing antipsychotics may increase the sensitivity to D_2 blockade, resulting in EPSs.

Li$^+$ treatment results in significant weight gain, a problem that is magnified by concurrent use of antipsychotic drugs. Mean weight change at 1 year in prospective Li$^+$ trials ranges from − 1 kg to + 4 kg, but the proportion of individuals who gain more than 5% of baseline weight is 13%–62%. Although the mechanism is unclear, central appetite stimulation at hypothalamic sites is the most plausible explanation (Grandjean and Aubry, 2009c).

Renal Effects. The kidney's ability to concentrate urine decreases during Li$^+$ therapy, and about 60% of individuals exposed to Li$^+$ experience some form of polyuria and compensatory polydipsia. The mechanism of polyuria is related to the fact that Li$^+$ has 1.5- to 2.0-fold greater affinity than Na$^+$ for ENaC present on the apical (i.e., luminal) surfaces of distal tubular cells. Once in the cell, Li$^+$ is a poor substrate for the Na$^+$-K$^+$-ATPase present on the basal membrane, leading to accumulation of Li$^+$ in these distal tubular cells (Grunfeld and Rossier, 2009). High intracellular Li$^+$ concentrations inhibit GSK-3β, leading to vasopressin insensitivity, downregulation of aquaporin-2 channels, and NDI. Mean 24-h urinary volumes of 3 L/d are common among long-term Li$^+$ users. Li$^+$ discontinuation or a switch to single-daily dosing may reverse the impact on renal concentrating ability in patients with less than 5 years of Li$^+$ exposure. Patients exposed to multiple-daily dosing are at greater risk for renal effects. Renal function should be monitored with semiannual serum blood urea nitrogen and creatinine levels and calculation of eGFR using standard formulas (Morriss and Benjamin, 2008). Spot urine osmolality measurements are used to determine the extent and development of problems with NDI and polyuria. Reassessment of Li$^+$ treatment should be considered when the eGFR is less than 60 mL/min on several periodic measurements, daily urinary volume exceeds 4 L, or serum creatinine continues to rise on three separate occasions (Morriss and Benjamin, 2008). With modern monitoring principles, no patient should develop chronic kidney disease to the extent of requiring renal dialysis (Aiff et al., 2014).

Thyroid and Endocrine Effects. A small number of patients on Li$^+$ develop a benign, diffuse, nontender thyroid enlargement suggestive of compromised thyroid function; many of these patients will have normal thyroid function. Measurable effects of Li$^+$ on thyroid indices are seen in a fraction of patients: 7%–10% develop overt hypothyroidism, and 23% have subclinical disease, with women at three to nine times greater risk (Grandjean and Aubry, 2009c). Ongoing monitoring of TSH and free T_4 is recommended throughout the course of Li$^+$ treatment. The development of hypothyroidism is easily treated through exogenous replacement and is not a reason to discontinue Li$^+$ therapy. Rare reports of hyperthyroidism during Li$^+$ treatment also exist (Persad et al., 1993). Hypercalcemia related to hyperparathyroidism has been reported in about ~10% of Li$^+$-treated patients. Routine monitoring of serum Ca^{2+} should be included with measurements of electrolytes, thyroid indices, renal function, and serum Li$^+$ levels (Shapiro and Davis, 2015).

ECG Effects. The prolonged use of Li$^+$ causes benign and reversible T-wave flattening in about 20% of patients. At therapeutic concentrations, there are rare reports of Li$^+$-induced effects on cardiac conduction and pacemaker automaticity, effects that become pronounced during overdose and lead to sinus bradycardia, A-V block, and possible CV compromise (Grandjean and Aubry, 2009c). Routine ECG monitoring may be considered in older patients, particularly those with a history of arrhythmia or coronary heart disease.

Skin Effects. Allergic reactions such as dermatitis, folliculitis, and vasculitis can occur with Li$^+$ administration. Worsening of acne vulgaris, psoriasis, and other dermatological conditions is a common problem that is usually treatable by topical measures but in a small number may improve only on discontinuation of Li$^+$ (Grandjean and Aubry, 2009c). Some patients on Li$^+$ (and valproate) may experience alopecia.

Pregnancy and Lactation. The use of Li$^+$ in early pregnancy may be associated with an increase in the incidence of CV anomalies of the newborn, especially Ebstein malformation. The risk of Ebstein anomaly (about 1 per 20,000 live births in controls) may rise several-fold with first-trimester Li$^+$ exposure; recent estimates indicate a risk of up to 1 per 2500 (Diav-Citrin et al., 2014). In balancing the risk versus benefit of using Li$^+$ in pregnancy, it is important to evaluate the risk of inadequate prophylaxis for the patient with bipolar disorder patient and subsequent risk that mania poses for the patient and fetus. If there is a compelling need for Li$^+$, screening ultrasonography for CV anomalies is recommended. In patients who choose to forgo medication exposure during the first trimester, potentially safer treatments for acute mania include antipsychotic drugs or ECT.

In pregnancy, maternal polyuria may be exacerbated by Li$^+$. Concomitant use of Li$^+$ with medications that waste Na$^+$ or a low-Na$^+$ diet during pregnancy can contribute to maternal and neonatal Li$^+$ intoxication. Li$^+$ freely crosses the placenta, and fetal or neonatal Li$^+$ toxicity may develop when maternal blood levels are within the therapeutic range (Grandjean and Aubry, 2009c). Fetal Li$^+$ exposure is associated with neonatal goiter, CNS depression, hypotonia ("floppy baby" syndrome), and cardiac murmur. Most experts recommend withholding Li$^+$ therapy for 24–48 h before delivery, and this is considered standard practice to avoid the potentially toxic increases in maternal and fetal serum Li$^+$ levels associated with postpartum diuresis. The physical and CNS sequelae of late-term neonatal Li$^+$ exposure are reversible once Li$^+$ exposure has ceased, and no long-term neurobehavioral consequences are observed (Diav-Citrin et al., 2014).

Other Effects. A benign, sustained increase in circulating polymorphonuclear leukocytes (12,000–15,000 cells/mm^3) commonly occurs, related to Li$^+$-induced increases in urinary levels of G-CSF and augmented production of G-CSF by peripheral blood mononuclear cells (Focosi et al., 2009). Li$^+$ also directly stimulates the proliferation of pluripotent stem cells. Some patients may complain of a metallic taste, making food less palatable.

Acute Toxicity and Overdose. The occurrence of toxicity is related to the serum concentration of Li$^+$ and its rate of rise following administration. Acute intoxication is characterized by vomiting, profuse diarrhea, coarse tremor, ataxia, coma, and convulsions. Symptoms of milder toxicity are most likely to occur at the absorptive peak of Li$^+$ and include nausea, vomiting, abdominal pain, diarrhea, sedation, and fine tremor. The more serious effects involve the nervous system and include mental confusion, hyperreflexia, gross tremor, dysarthria, seizures, and cranial nerve and focal neurological signs, progressing to coma and death. Sometimes both cognitive and motor neurological damage may be irreversible, with persistent cerebellar tremor the most common (El-Mallakh, 1986). Other toxic effects are cardiac arrhythmias, hypotension, and albuminuria.

Treatment of Lithium Intoxication. There is no specific antidote for Li$^+$ intoxication, and treatment is supportive, including intubation if indicated and continuous cardiac monitoring. Levels greater than 1.5 mEq/L are considered toxic, but inpatient medical admission is usually not indicated (in the absence of symptoms) until levels exceed 2 mEq/L. Care must be taken to ensure that the patient is not Na$^+$ and water depleted (Grandjean and Aubry, 2009c). Dialysis is the most effective means of removing Li$^+$ and is necessary in severe poisonings, that is, in patients exhibiting symptoms of toxicity or patients with serum Li$^+$ concentrations of 3 mEq/L or greater in acute overdoses. Complete recovery occurs with an average maximal level of 2.5 mEq/L; permanent neurological symptoms result from mean levels of 3.2 mEq/L; death occurs with mean maximal levels of 4.2 mEq/L (El-Mallakh, 1986).

Use in Pediatric Populations. Li$^+$ is FDA-approved for child/adolescent bipolar disorder for ages 12 years or older (Peruzzolo et al., 2013). Aripiprazole, quetiapine, and risperidone are FDA approved for acute mania in children and adolescents aged 10–17 years. Children and adolescents have higher volumes of body water and higher eGFR than adults. The resulting shorter $t_{1/2}$ of Li$^+$ demands dosing increases on a milligram/kilogram basis, and multiple-daily dosing is often required. In children ages 6–12 years, a dose of 30 mg/kg/d given in three divided doses will produce a Li$^+$ concentration of 0.6–1.2 mEq/L in 5 days, although dosing is always guided by serum levels and clinical response (Peruzzolo et al., 2013). Use in children under 12 represents an off-label use for Li$^+$, and caregivers should be alert to signs of toxicity. As with adults, ongoing monitoring of renal and thyroid function is important, along with clinical inquiry into extent of polyuria.

A limited number of controlled studies suggested that valproate has efficacy comparable to that of Li^+ for mania in children or adolescents (Peruzzolo et al., 2013). As with Li^+, weight gain and tremor can be problematic; moreover, there are reports of hyperammonemia in children with urea cycle disorders. Ongoing monitoring of platelets and liver function tests, in addition to serum drug levels, is recommended.

Use in Geriatric Populations. The majority of older patients on Li^+ therapy are those maintained for years on the medication. Elderly patients frequently take numerous medications for other illnesses, and the potential for drug-drug interactions is substantial. Age-related reductions in total body water and creatinine clearance reduce the safety margin for Li^+ treatment in older patients. Targeting lower maintenance serum levels (0.6–0.8 mEq/L) may reduce the risk of toxicity. As eGFR drops below 50 mL/min, strong consideration must be given to use of alternative agents, despite lithium's therapeutic advantages (Morriss and Benjamin, 2008). Li^+ toxicity occurs more frequently in elderly patients, in part as the result of concurrent use of loop diuretics and ACEIs (Grandjean and Aubry, 2009c). Anticonvulsants, especially extended-release divalproex, are a reasonable alternative to Li^+. Elderly patients who are drug naïve may be more sensitive to the CNS adverse effects of all types of medications used for acute mania, especially parkinsonism and TD from D_2 antagonism, confusion from antipsychotic medications with antimuscarinic properties, and ataxia or sedation from Li^+ or anticonvulsants.

Clinical Summary: Treatment of Mania

Despite decades of data substantiating the superior efficacy of Li^+ in patients with bipolar disorder, including suicide reduction, Li^+ remains underutilized. Long-term studies spanning 10 or more years demonstrated that while polyuria may be relatively common, significant declines in renal function to the point of stage 4 chronic kidney disease are rare during Li^+ treatment. Many agents are effective for acute mania, but long-term treatment requires careful consideration of extent and severity of prior depressive episodes, past history of treatment response, concurrent medical illness and medication use, patient preference, and concerns over particular adverse effects (e.g., weight gain). Combining mood stabilizers and antipsychotic agents shows greater benefit for acute mania than monotherapy of either agent class but may be associated with increased long-term weight gain. A realistic discussion with patients regarding long-term side effects for various treatments and clinical outcomes is paramount to improve adherence.

Serum-level monitoring is necessary for Li^+, valproate acid compounds, and carbamazepine. Lamotrigine may be particularly useful in patients with type II bipolar disorder, for which mania prophylaxis is not a concern. The clinical data make a compelling argument for Li^+ as the treatment of choice in bipolar I disorder. Ongoing research into lithium's mechanism of action may yield new agents without lithium's adverse effect profile, as well as genetic predictors of Li^+ response.

Acknowledgment: *Ross J. Baldessarini and Frank I. Tarazi contributed to this chapter in recent editions of this book. We have retained some of their text in the current edition.*

Drug Facts for Your Personal Formulary: *Antipsychotic and Mood-Stabilizing Agents*

Drugs	Therapeutic Uses	Clinical Pharmacology and Tips
First-Generation Antipsychotics • Low-potency D_2 antagonists		
Chlorpromazine	• Schizophrenia • Acute mania	• High M_1, H_1, and $α_1$ adrenergic affinities increase rates of anticholinergic side effects, sedation and weight gain, and hypotension, respectively • Less QT_c prolongation at high plasma levels than thioridazine • High risk of metabolic adverse effects • Photosensitivity
First-Generation Antipsychotics • Medium- and high-potency D_2 antagonists		
Haloperidol	• Schizophrenia • Acute mania	• Higher rates of EPSs, akathisia, hyperprolactinemia • Limited anticholinergic side effects, sedation, weight gain, and hypotension • Avoid intravenous use due to QT_c prolongation • Chlorpromazine 100 mg oral equivalence: 2 mg
Fluphenazine	• Schizophrenia • Acute mania	• Higher rates of EPSs, akathisia, hyperprolactinemia • Limited anticholinergic side effects, sedation, weight gain, and hypotension • Chlorpromazine 100 mg oral equivalence: 2 mg
Trifluoperazine	• Schizophrenia • Acute mania	• Higher rates of EPSs, akathisia, hyperprolactinemia • Limited anticholinergic side effects, sedation, weight gain, and hypotension • Chlorpromazine 100 mg oral equivalence: 5 mg
Thiothixene	• Schizophrenia • Acute mania	• Higher rates of EPSs, akathisia, hyperprolactinemia • Limited anticholinergic side effects, sedation, weight gain, and hypotension • Chlorpromazine 100 mg oral equivalence: 5 mg
Perphenazine	• Schizophrenia • Acute mania	• Modest rates of EPSs, akathisia • Limited anticholinergic side effects, sedation, weight gain, and hypotension • Chlorpromazine 100 mg oral equivalence: 10 mg
Loxapine	• Schizophrenia • Acute mania	• Modest rates of EPS, akathisia • Limited anticholinergic side effects, sedation, weight gain, and hypotension • Chlorpromazine 100 mg oral equivalence: 10 mg

Drug Facts for Your Personal Formulary: *Antipsychotic and Mood-Stabilizing Agents (continued)*

Drugs	Therapeutic Uses	Clinical Pharmacology and Tips
Second-Generation Antipsychotics • $5HT_{2A}$ and D_2 antagonists		
Asenapine	• Schizophrenia • Acute mania	• Only available in ODT formulation due to 98% first-pass effect if swallowed • Administer sublingually: avoid water for 10 min to achieve maximum oral-buccal absorption (avoiding water for 2 min achieves 80% of maximum absorption) • Low risk of metabolic adverse effects
Clozapine	• Refractory schizophrenia • Refractory mania	• Must register patient and prescriber due to mandatory hematological monitoring • High M_1, H_1, and α_1 adrenergic affinity increases rates of anticholinergic side effects, sedation and weight gain, and hypotension, respectively • High risk of metabolic adverse effects • Significant constipation; avoid other anticholinergic agents, manage aggressively • Sialorrhea; manage with locally administered agents (sublingual atropine 1% drops or ipratropium 0.06% spray)
Iloperidone	• Schizophrenia	• High α_1 adrenergic affinity; titrate to minimize orthostasis • Low risk of metabolic adverse effects
Lurasidone	• Schizophrenia • Bipolar depression (monotherapy and adjunct)	• Low risk for anticholinergic side effects, sedation and weight gain, and hypotension, respectively • Low risk of metabolic adverse effects • Absorption increased 100% by administration with 350 kcal food
Olanzapine	• Schizophrenia • Acute mania • Bipolar depression (in combination with fluoxetine)	• High risk of metabolic adverse effects • Anticholinergic effects at high dosages
Paliperidone	• Schizophrenia	• Moderate risk of metabolic adverse effects • High rates of hyperprolactinemia
Quetiapine	• Schizophrenia • Acute mania • Bipolar depression (monotherapy) • Unipolar depression (adjunct)	• High risk of metabolic adverse effects at full therapeutic dosages for schizophrenia • High H_1 and α_1 adrenergic affinities increase rates of sedation and hypotension, respectively • Low rates of EPSs, akathisia, and hyperprolactinemia
Risperidone	• Schizophrenia • Acute mania	• Moderate risk of metabolic adverse effects • High rates of hyperprolactinemia
Sertindole	• Schizophrenia	• Not available in the U.S. • Restricted use in Europe, with extensive monitoring for QT_c prolongation • Low risk of metabolic adverse effects
Ziprasidone	• Schizophrenia • Acute mania	• Low risk of metabolic adverse effects • Absorption increased 100% by administration with 500 kcal food • Improved tolerability at starting doses > 80 mg/d with food
Second-Generation Antipsychotics • D_2 partial agonists		
Aripiprazole	• Schizophrenia • Acute mania • Unipolar depression (adjunct)	• Low risk of metabolic adverse effects • Lowers serum prolactin • Akathisia noted in depression trials—can be lessened with starting dose of 2.0–2.5 mg at bedtime
Brexpiprazole	• Schizophrenia • Unipolar depression (adjunct)	• Low risk of metabolic adverse effects • Lowers serum prolactin
Cariprazine	• Schizophrenia • Acute mania	• Low risk of metabolic adverse effects • Lowers serum prolactin
Second-Generation Antipsychotics • D_2 and D_3 antagonists		
Amisulpride	• Schizophrenia • Unipolar depression (adjunct, at low dosages)	• Higher rates of EPSs • Higher rates of hyperprolactinemia • Low risk of metabolic adverse effects
$5HT_{2A}$ Inverse Agonist Without D_2 Binding		
Pimavanserin	Parkinson disease psychosis (PDP)	• Potent $5HT_{2A}$ inverse agonist with no D2 affinity • Monotherapy efficacy data for psychosis available only for PDP • Only one dose available: 34 mg once daily, with or without food • ↓ dose by 50% with concurrent strong 3A4 inhibitors; may lose efficacy with strong 3A4 inducers • Clinical effects may not be seen for 2-6 weeks

Drug Facts for Your Personal Formulary: *Antipsychotic and Mood-Stabilizing Agents (continued)*

Drugs	Therapeutic Uses	Clinical Pharmacology and Tips
Mood Stabilizers • Acute mania and/or bipolar maintenance		
Lithium	• Acute mania • Bipolar maintenance • Unipolar depression (adjunct)	• Reduces suicidality more than other treatments • Renally cleared • Higher risk for weight gain • Monitor TSH, renal function tests, levels • May cause tremor, hair loss • Therapeutic serum level: acute mania 1.0–1.5 mEq/mL • Therapeutic serum level: maintenance 0.6–1.0 mEq/mL
Valproate (divalproex)	• Acute mania • Bipolar maintenance	• Can be loaded in acute mania: 30 mg/kg over 24 h • Highly protein bound • Higher risk for weight gain • May cause thrombocytopenia, leukopenia, hyperammonemia, tremor, hair loss • Monitor CBC, liver function tests, levels • Therapeutic serum level: acute mania 100–120 µg/mL • Therapeutic serum level: maintenance 60–100 µg/mL
Carbamazepine	• Acute mania • Bipolar maintenance	• Less effective than lithium and valproic acid • Highly protein bound • HLA testing for those from east Asia to identify high risk of Stevens-Johnson syndrome • May cause hyponatremia, leukopenia • Strong inducer of CYP3A4 and P-glycoprotein • Avoid rapid titration to minimize risk of sedation, ataxia • Therapeutic serum level 6–12 µg/mL
Lamotrigine	• Bipolar maintenance	• Prolonged titration to minimize risk of Stevens-Johnson syndrome • 50% dosage reduction required if patient on valproic acid or divalproex

Bibliography

Aiff H, et al. The impact of modern treatment principles may have eliminated lithium-induced renal failure. *J Psychopharmacol*, **2014**, *28*:151–154.

American Psychiatric Association. (2013). *Diagnostic and Statistical Manual of Mental Disorders*. 5th ed. American Psychiatric Press, Washington, DC.

Baldessarini RJ, Tondo L. Does lithium treatment still work? Evidence of stable responses over three decades. *Arch Gen Psychiatry*, **2000**, *57*:187–190.

Bedford JJ, et al. Lithium-induced nephrogenic diabetes insipidus: renal effects of amiloride. *Clin J Am Soc Nephrol*, **2008**, *3*:1324–1331.

Burris KD, et al. Aripiprazole, a novel antipsychotic, is a high-affinity partial agonist at human dopamine D_2 receptors. *J Pharmacol Exp Ther*, **2002**, *302*:381–389.

Can A, et al. Chronic lithium treatment rectifies maladaptive dopamine release in the nucleus accumbens. *J Neurochem*, **2016**, *139*:576–585.

Castro VM, et al. Stratifying risk for renal insufficiency among lithium-treated patients: an electronic health record study. *Neuropsychopharmacol*, **2016**, *41*:1138–1143.

Chiu CT, et al. Therapeutic potential of mood stabilizers lithium and valproic acid: beyond bipolar disorder. *Pharmacol Rev*, **2013**, *65*:105–142.

Cipriani A, et al. Valproic acid, valproate and divalproex in the maintenance treatment of bipolar disorder. *Cochrane Database Syst Rev*, **2013**, *10*:CD003196.

Correll CU, et al. Cardiometabolic risk in patients with first-episode schizophrenia spectrum disorders: baseline results from the RAISE-ETP study. *JAMA Psychiatry*, **2014**, *71*:1350–1363.

Cummings J, et al. Pimavanserin for patients with Parkinson's disease psychosis: a randomised, placebo-controlled phase 3 trial. *Lancet*, **2014**, *383*:533–540.

De Hert M, et al. Body weight and metabolic adverse effects of asenapine, iloperidone, lurasidone and paliperidone in the treatment of schizophrenia and bipolar disorder: a systematic review and exploratory meta-analysis. *CNS Drugs*, **2012**, *26*:733–759.

Diav-Citrin O, et al. Pregnancy outcome following in utero exposure to lithium: a prospective, comparative, observational study. *Am J Psychiatry*, **2014**, *171*:785–794.

Dold M, et al. Antipsychotic augmentation of serotonin reuptake inhibitors in treatment-resistant obsessive-compulsive disorder: a meta-analysis of double-blind, randomized, placebo-controlled trials. *Int J Neuropsychopharmacol*, **2013**, *16*:557–574.

Dremencov E, et al. Modulation of dopamine transmission by 5-HT2C and 5-HT3 receptors: a role in the antidepressant response. *Current Drug Targets*, **2006**, *7*:165–175.

Einat H. Partial effects of the protein kinase C inhibitor chelerythrine in a battery of tests for manic-like behavior in black Swiss mice. *Pharmacol Rep*, **2014**, *66*:722–725.

El-Mallakh RS. Acute lithium neurotoxicity. *Psychiatr Dev*, **1986**, *4*:311–328.

Escudero I, Johnstone M. Genetics of schizophrenia. *Curr Psychiatry Rep*, **2014**, *16*:502.

Farahani A, Correll CU. Are antipsychotics or antidepressants needed for psychotic depression? A systematic review and meta-analysis of trials comparing antidepressant or antipsychotic monotherapy with combination treatment. *J Clin Psychiatry*, **2012**, *73*:486–496.

Focosi D, et al. Lithium and hematology: established and proposed uses. *J Leukocyte Biol*, **2009**, *85*:20–28.

Fortin SM, et al. The Aversive Agent Lithium Chloride Suppresses Phasic Dopamine Release Through Central GLP-1 Receptors. *Neuropsychopharmacol*, **2016**, *41*:906–915.

Gavin DP, Floreani C. Epigenetics of schizophrenia: an open and shut case. *Int Rev Neurobiol*, **2014**, *115*:155–201.

Geddes JR, Miklowitz DJ. Treatment of bipolar disorder. *Lancet*, **2013**, *381*:1672–1682.

Goodwin FK, et al. Suicide risk in bipolar disorder during treatment with lithium and divalproex. *JAMA*, **2003**, *290*:1467–1473.

Grandjean EM, Aubry JM. Lithium: updated human knowledge using an evidence-based approach: part I: clinical efficacy in bipolar disorder. *CNS Drugs*, **2009a**, *23*:225–240.

Grandjean EM, Aubry JM. Lithium: updated human knowledge using an evidence-based approach. Part II: clinical pharmacology and therapeutic monitoring. *CNS Drugs*, **2009b**, *23*:331–349.

Grandjean EM, Aubry JM. Lithium: updated human knowledge using an evidence-based approach: part III: clinical safety. *CNS Drugs*, **2009c**, *23*:397–418.

Grunfeld JP, Rossier BC. Lithium nephrotoxicity revisited. *Nat Rev Nephrol*, **2009**, *5*:270–276.

Gurrera RJ, et al. An international consensus study of neuroleptic malignant syndrome diagnostic criteria using the Delphi method. *J Clin Psychiatry*, **2011**, *72*:1222–1228.

Howes O, et al. Glutamate and dopamine in schizophrenia: an update for the 21st century. *J Psychopharmacol*, **2015**, *29*:97–115.

Huybrechts KF, et al. Antipsychotic use in pregnancy and the risk for congenital malformations. *JAMA Psychiatry*, **2016**, *73*:938–946.

Jager M, et al. Time course of antipsychotic treatment response in schizophrenia: results from a naturalistic study in 280 patients. *Schizophr Res*, **2010**, *118*:183–188.

Javitt DC, Freedman R. Sensory processing dysfunction in the personal experience and neuronal machinery of schizophrenia. *Am J Psychiatry*, **2015**, *172*:17–31.

Khan BA, et al. Delirium in hospitalized patients: implications of current evidence on clinical practice and future avenues for research—a systematic evidence review. *J Hosp Med*, **2012**, *7*:580–589.

Kim SF, et al. From the cover: antipsychotic drug-induced weight gain mediated by histamine H_1 receptor-linked activation of hypothalamic AMP-kinase. *Proc Natl Acad Sci U S A*, **2007**, *104*:3456–3459.

Kinon BJ, et al. Early response to antipsychotic drug therapy as a clinical marker of subsequent response in the treatment of schizophrenia. *Neuropsychopharmacology*, **2010**, *35*:581–590.

Kook KA, et al. Accuracy and safety of a priori lithium loading. *J Clin Psychiatry*, **1985**, *46*:49–51.

Koppel J, Greenwald BS. Optimal treatment of Alzheimer's disease psychosis: challenges and solutions. *Neuropsychiatr Dis Treat*, **2014**, *10*:2253–2262.

Krystal JH, et al. Adjunctive risperidone treatment for antidepressant-resistant symptoms of chronic military service-related PTSD: a randomized trial. *JAMA*, **2011**, *306*:493–502.

Kuepper R, et al. The dopamine dysfunction in schizophrenia revisited: new insights into topography and course. *Handb Exp Pharmacol*, **2012**, *212*:1–26.

Leucht S, et al. Comparative efficacy and tolerability of 15 antipsychotic drugs in schizophrenia: a multiple-treatments meta-analysis. *Lancet*, **2013**, *382*:951–962.

Malhi GS, et al. Mania: diagnosis and treatment recommendations. *Curr Psychiatry Rep*, **2012**, *14*:676–686.

Maust DT, et al. Antipsychotics, other psychotropics, and the risk of death in patients with dementia: number needed to harm. *JAMA Psychiatry*, **2015**, *72*:438–445.

Meltzer HY. Clozapine: balancing safety with superior antipsychotic efficacy. *Clin Schizophr Relat Psychoses*, **2012**, *6*:134–144.

Meyer JM. Understanding depot antipsychotics: an illustrated guide to kinetics. *CNS Spectr*, **2013**, *18*:55–68.

Meyer JM. A rational approach to employing high plasma levels of antipsychotics for violence associated with schizophrenia: case vignettes. *CNS Spectr*, **2014**, *19*:432–438.

Meyer JM, et al. Lithium toxicity after switch from fosinopril to lisinopril. *Int Clin Psychopharmacol*, **2005**, *20*:115–118.

Meyer JM, Leckband SG. A history of clozapine and concepts of atypicality. In: Domino EF, ed. *History of Psychopharmacology*. Vol. 2. Domemtech/NPP Books, Arlington, MA, **2013**, 95–106.

Meyer JM, Stahl SM. The metabolic syndrome and schizophrenia. *Acta Psychiatr Scand*, **2009**, *119*:4–14.

Millienne-Petiot M, et al. The effects of reduced dopamine transporter function and chronic lithium on motivation, probabilistic learning, and neurochemistry in mice: Modeling bipolar mania. *Neuropharmacology*, **2017**, 113, part A: 260–270.

Mogwitz S, et al. Clinical pharmacology of dopamine-modulating agents in Tourette's syndrome. *Int Rev Neurobiol*, **2013**, *112*:281–349.

Morriss R, Benjamin B. Lithium and eGFR: a new routinely available tool for the prevention of chronic kidney disease. *Br J Psychiatry*, **2008**, *193*:93–95.

Nielsen J, et al. Assessing QT prolongation of antipsychotic drugs. *CNS Drugs*, **2011**, *25*:473–490.

Ogino S, et al. Benefits and limits of anticholinergic use in schizophrenia: focusing on its effect on cognitive function. *Psychiatry Clin Neurosci*, **2014**, *68*:37–49.

Persad E, et al. Hyperthyroidism after treatment with lithium. *Can J Psychiatry* **1993**, *38*:599–602.

Peruzzolo TL, et al. Pharmacotherapy of bipolar disorder in children and adolescents: an update. *Rev Bras Psiquiatr*, **2013**, *35*:393–405.

Powell SB, et al. Genetic models of sensorimotor gating: relevance to neuropsychiatric disorders. *Curr Topics Behav Neurosci*, **2012**, *12*:251–318.

Praharaj SK, et al. Metformin for olanzapine-induced weight gain: a systematic review and meta-analysis. *Br J Clin Pharmacol*, **2011**, *71*:377–382.

Prickaerts J, et al. EVP-6124, a novel and selective alpha7 nicotinic acetylcholine receptor partial agonist, improves memory performance by potentiating the acetylcholine response of alpha7 nicotinic acetylcholine receptors. *Neuropharmacology*, **2012**, *62*:1099–1110.

Rapoport SI, et al. Bipolar disorder and mechanisms of action of mood stabilizers. *Brain Res Rev*, **2009**, *61*:185–209.

Reed RC, Dutta S. Does it really matter when a blood sample for valproic acid concentration is taken following once-daily administration of divalproex-ER? *Ther Drug Monitor*, **2006**, *28*:413–418.

Remington G, et al. The neurobiology of relapse in schizophrenia. *Schizophr Res*, **2014**, *152*:381–390.

Rostami-Hodjegan A, et al. Influence of dose, cigarette smoking, age, sex, and metabolic activity on plasma clozapine concentrations: a predictive model and nomograms to aid clozapine dose adjustment and to assess compliance in individual patients. *J Clin Psychopharmacol*, **2004**, *24*:70–78.

Rummel-Kluge C, et al. Head-to-head comparisons of metabolic side effects of second generation antipsychotics in the treatment of schizophrenia: a systematic review and meta-analysis. *Schizophr Res*, **2010**, *123*:225–233.

Salahudeen MS, et al. Impact of anticholinergic discontinuation on cognitive outcomes in older people: a systematic review. *Drugs Aging* **2014**, *31*:185–192.

Seeman P. Schizophrenia and dopamine receptors. *Eur Neuropsychopharmacol*, **2013**, *23*:999–1009.

Selle V, et al. Treatments for acute bipolar depression: meta-analyses of placebo-controlled, monotherapy trials of anticonvulsants, lithium and antipsychotics. *Pharmacopsychiatry*, **2014**, *47*:43–52.

Shapiro HI, Davis KA. Hypercalcemia and "primary" hyperparathyroidism during lithium therapy. *Am J Psychiatry*, **2015**, *172*:12–15.

Sharp T, et al. Effect of Short- and Long-Term Administration of Lithium on the Release of Endogenous 5-HT in the Hippocampus of the Rat *In Vivo* and *In Vitro*. *Neuropharmacology*, **1991**, *30*: 971–984.

Sparshatt A, et al. A systematic review of aripiprazole—dose, plasma concentration, receptor occupancy, and response: implications for therapeutic drug monitoring. *J Clin Psychiatry*, **2010**, *71*:1447–1456.

Torniainen M, et al. Antipsychotic treatment and mortality in schizophrenia. *Schizophr Bull*, **2015**, *41*:656–663. doi:10.1093/schbul/sbu164.

Turner P, et al. A systematic review and meta-analysis of the evidence base for add-on treatment for patients with major depressive disorder who have not responded to antidepressant treatment: a European perspective. *J Psychopharmacol*, **2014**, *28*:85–98.

Urs NM, et al. Deletion of GSK-3beta in D2R-expressing neurons reveals distinct roles for beta-arrestin signaling in antipsychotic and lithium action. *Proc Natl Acad Sci USA*, **2012**, *109*:20732–20737.

Wang L, et al. Transcriptional down-regulation of MARCKS gene expression in immortalized hippocampal cells by lithium. *J Neurochem*, **2001**, *79*:816–825.

Williams RS, et al. A common mechanism of action for three mood-stabilizing drugs. *Nature* **2002**, *417*:292–295.

Wright BM, et al. Augmentation with atypical antipsychotics for depression: a review of evidence-based support from the medical literature. *Pharmacotherapy*, **2013**, *33*:344–359.

Yatham LN et al. Optimal duration of risperidone or olanzapine adjunctive therapy to mood stabilizer following remission of a manic episode: A CANMAT randomized double-blind trial. *Molec Psychiatry*, **2016**, *21*:1050–1056.

Young JW, Geyer MA. Developing treatments for cognitive deficits in schizophrenia: the challenge of translation. *J Psychopharmacol*, **2015**, *29*:178–196.

Zipursky RB, et al. Risk of symptom recurrence with medication discontinuation in first-episode psychosis: a systematic review. *Schizophr Res*, **2014**, *152*:408–414.

Pharmacotherapy of the Epilepsies

Misty D. Smith, Cameron S. Metcalf, and Karen S. Wilcox

第十七章　癫痫的药物治疗

中文导读

本章主要介绍：癫痫和抗癫痫治疗；常见术语和癫痫分类；癫痫的性质、发病机制和抗麻醉药，包括局灶性癫痫、全身发作性癫痫——失神发作、癫痫的遗传学；抗癫痫药物概述，包括孤独症谱系障碍（ASD）发展史及其治疗；乙内酰脲类抗癫痫药，如苯妥英；苯二氮䓬类抗癫痫药；巴比妥类抗癫痫药，包括苯巴比妥和普利米酮；亚氨基芪类抗癫痫药，包括卡马西平、奥卡西平和醋酸艾司利卡西平；琥珀酰亚胺类抗癫痫药，如乙琥胺；其他抗癫痫药，包括乙酰唑胺、依佐加滨、非氨酯、加巴喷丁和普加巴林、拉科酰胺、拉莫三嗪、左乙拉西坦和布立西坦、紫杉醇、卢非酰胺、司替戊醇、替加宾、托吡酯、丙戊酸、维加巴特林、唑尼沙胺；癫痫治疗的一般原则和药物选择，包括治疗时长、局灶性和局灶性至双侧强直-阵挛性发作、失神发作、肌阵挛性发作、高热惊厥、婴幼儿癫痫发作、癫痫持续状态和其他惊厥急症、抗癫痫治疗与妊娠。

Abbreviations

AMPA: α-amino-3-hydroxy 5-methyl-4-isoxazolepropionic acid
ASD: antiseizure drug
CSF: cerebrospinal fluid
DS: depolarization shift
EEG: electroencephalogram
ETSP: Epilepsy Therapy Screening Project
GABA: γ-aminobutyric acid
JME: juvenile myoclonic epilepsy
NMDA: *N*-methyl-D-aspartate receptor
PEMA: phenylethylmalonamide
SV2A: synaptic vesicle glycoprotein 2A

Epilepsy and Antiseizure Therapy

The epilepsies are common and frequently devastating disorders, affecting about 2.5 million people in the U.S. alone. More than 40 distinct forms of epilepsy have been identified. Seizures often cause transient impairment of awareness, leaving the individual at risk of bodily harm and often interfering with education and employment. Current therapy is symptomatic: available ASDs inhibit seizures; neither effective prophylaxis nor cure is available. Adherence to prescribed treatment regimens is a major problem because of the need for long-term therapy together with unwanted effects of many drugs.

The mechanisms of action of ASDs fall into these major categories (see also Porter et al., 2012):

1. Modulation of cation channels (Na^+, K^+, Ca^{2+}). This can include prolongation of the inactivated state of voltage-gated Na^+ channels, positive modulation of K^+ channels, and inhibition of Ca^{2+} channels.
2. Enhancement of GABA neurotransmission through actions on $GABA_A$ receptors, modulation of GABA metabolism, and inhibition of GABA reuptake into the synaptic terminal.
3. Modulation of synaptic release through actions on the synaptic vesicle protein SV2A or Ca^{2+} channels containing the α2δ subunit.
4. Diminishing synaptic excitation mediated by ionotropic glutamate receptors (e.g., AMPA receptors).

Beyond these broad classifications, many ASDs act through mechanisms distinct from the primary known mode of action. Furthermore, ASDs with similar mechanistic categories may have disparate clinical uses.

Much effort is devoted to elucidating the genetic causes and the cellular and molecular mechanisms by which a neural circuit becomes prone to seizure activity, with the goal of providing molecular targets for both symptomatic and preventive therapies.

Terminology and Seizure Classification

The term *seizure* refers to a transient alteration of behavior due to the disordered, synchronous, and rhythmic firing of populations of brain neurons. The term *epilepsy* refers to a disorder of brain function characterized by the periodic and unpredictable occurrence of seizures. Seizures can be provoked (i.e., by chemical agents or electrical stimulation) or unprovoked; the condition of epilepsy denotes the occurrence of spontaneous, unprovoked seizures. While agents in current clinical use inhibit seizures, whether any of these prevent the development of epilepsy (epileptogenesis) is uncertain.

This chapter employs the revised classification for seizures. Thus, seizures previously classified as *partial* seizures are referred to as *focal* seizures, whereas *generalized* seizures, those that involve both hemispheres widely from the outset, will still be referred to as generalized seizures (Fisher et al., 2017). In addition, the International League Against Epilepsy (ILAE) has added a classification for seizures with *unknown onset*, which includes such seizure types as tonic-clonic, atonic, and epileptic spasms.

From a network perspective, seizures arise from cortical, thalamocortical, limbic, or even brainstem circuits. The behavioral manifestations of a seizure are determined by the functions normally served by the brain region at which the seizure arises. For example, a seizure involving motor cortex is associated with clonic jerking of the body part controlled by this region of cortex. Thus, this type of focal seizure is associated with preservation of awareness. Focal seizures may also be associated with impairments of awareness. The majority of such focal seizures originate from the temporal lobe. Generalized seizures are now distinguished by the involvement of the motor system or those that lack motor involvement, for example, typical and atypical absence, eyelid myoclonic. The type of seizure is one determinant of the drug selected for therapy. Detailed information pertaining to seizure classifications is presented in Table 17–1.

Apart from this seizure classification, an additional classification specifies epilepsy syndromes, which refer to a cluster of symptoms frequently occurring together and include seizure types, etiology, age of onset, and other factors (Fisher RJ et al., 2017). More than 50 distinct epilepsy syndromes have been identified and categorized into focal versus generalized epilepsies. The focal epilepsies may consist of any of the focal seizure types (Table 17–1) and account for roughly 60% of all epilepsies. The etiology commonly consists of a cortical lesion, such as a tumor, developmental malformation, or damage due to trauma or stroke. Such lesions often are evident on brain MRI. Alternatively, the etiology may be genetic. The generalized epilepsies are characterized most commonly by one or more of the generalized seizure types listed in Table 17–1 and account for about 40% of all epilepsies; the etiology is usually genetic. The most common generalized epilepsy is referred to as juvenile myoclonic epilepsy (JME), accounting for about 10% of all epilepsy syndromes. The age of onset is in the early teens, and the condition is characterized by myoclonic, tonic-clonic, and often absence seizures. Like most of the generalized-onset epilepsies, JME is a complex genetic disorder that is probably due to inheritance of multiple susceptibility genes; there is a familial clustering of cases, but the pattern of inheritance is not Mendelian. The classification of epileptic syndromes guides clinical assessment and management and, in some instances, selection of ASDs.

TABLE 17–1 ■ CLASSIFICATION OF EPILEPTIC SEIZURES

SEIZURE TYPE	FEATURES	CONVENTIONAL ANTISEIZURE DRUGS	RECENTLY DEVELOPED ANTISEIZURE DRUGS
Focal seizures			
Focal Aware	Diverse manifestations determined by the region of cortex activated by the seizure (e.g., if motor cortex representing left thumb, clonic jerking of left thumb results; if somatosensory cortex representing left thumb, paresthesia of left thumb results), lasting approximating 20–60 sec. *Key feature is preservation of awareness.*	Carbamazepine, phenytoin, valproate	Brivaracetam, eslicarbazepine, ezogabine, gabapentin, lacosamide, lamotrigine, levetiracetam, perampanel, rufinamide, tiagabine, topiramate, zonisamide
Focal with Impaired Awareness	Impaired consciousness lasting 30 sec to 2 min, often associated with purposeless movements such as lip smacking or hand wringing.		
Focal to Bilateral Tonic-Clonic	Simple or complex focal seizure evolves into a tonic-clonic seizure with loss of awareness and sustained contractions (tonic) of muscles throughout the body, followed by periods of muscle contraction alternating with periods of relaxation (clonic), typically lasting 1–2 min.	Carbamazepine, phenobarbital, phenytoin, primidone, valproate	
Generalized seizures			
Generalized Absence	Abrupt onset of impaired consciousness associated with staring and cessation of ongoing activities, typically lasting less than 30 sec.	Ethosuximide, valproate, clonazepam	Lamotrigine
Generalized Myoclonic	A brief (perhaps a second), shock-like contraction of muscles that may be restricted to part of one extremity or may be generalized.	Valproate, clonazepam	Levetiracetam
Generalized Tonic-Clonic	As described above for partial with secondarily generalized tonic-clonic seizure except that it is not preceded by a partial seizure.	Carbamazepine, phenobarbital, phenytoin, primidone, valproate	Lamotrigine, levetiracetam, topiramate

Nature and Mechanisms of Seizures and Antiseizure Drugs

Focal Epilepsies

More than a century ago, John Hughlings Jackson, the father of modern concepts of epilepsy, proposed that seizures were caused by "occasional, sudden, excessive, rapid and local discharges of gray matter," and that a generalized seizure resulted when normal brain tissue was invaded by the seizure activity initiated in the abnormal focus. This insightful proposal provided a framework for thinking about mechanisms of focal epilepsy. The advent of the EEG in the 1930s permitted the recording of electrical activity from the scalp of humans with epilepsy and demonstrated that the epilepsies are disorders of neuronal excitability.

The pivotal role of synapses in mediating communication amongst neurons in the mammalian brain suggested that defective synaptic function might lead to a seizure. That is, a reduction of inhibitory synaptic activity or enhancement of excitatory synaptic activity might be expected to trigger a seizure. Pharmacological studies of seizures support this notion. The neurotransmitters mediating the bulk of synaptic transmission in the mammalian brain are amino acids, with GABA and glutamate the principal inhibitory and excitatory neurotransmitters, respectively (Chapter 14). Pharmacological studies disclosed that *antagonists* of the $GABA_A$ receptor or *agonists* of different glutamate-receptor subtypes (NMDA, AMPA, or kainic acid) trigger seizures in experimental animals in vivo. Conversely, pharmacological agents that enhance GABA-mediated synaptic inhibition suppress seizures in diverse models. Glutamate-receptor antagonists also inhibit seizures in diverse models, including seizures evoked by electroshock and chemical convulsants (e.g., pentylenetetrazol).

These findings suggest pharmacological regulation of synaptic function can regulate the propensity for seizures and provide a framework for electrophysiological analyses aimed at elucidating the role of both synaptic and nonsynaptic mechanisms in seizures and epilepsy. Technical progress has fostered the progressive refinement of the analysis of seizure mechanisms from the EEG to populations of neurons (field potentials) to individual neurons to individual synapses and individual ion channels on individual neurons. Beginning in the mid-1960s, cellular electrophysiological studies of epilepsy focused on elucidating the mechanisms underlying the DS, the intracellular correlate of the "interictal spike" (Figure 17–1). The interictal (or between-seizures) spike is a sharp waveform recorded in the EEG of patients with epilepsy; it is asymptomatic, as it is not accompanied by overt change in the patient's behavior. However, the location of the interictal spike helps localize the brain region from which seizure activity originates in a given patient. The DS consists of a large depolarization of the neuronal membrane associated with a burst of action potentials. In most cortical neurons, the DS is generated by a large excitatory synaptic current that can be enhanced by activation of voltage-gated intrinsic membrane currents. Although the mechanisms generating the DS and whether the interictal spike triggers a seizure, inhibits a seizure, or is an epiphenomenon remains unclear, the study of the mechanisms underlying DS generation set the stage for inquiry into the cellular mechanisms of a seizure.

During the 1980s, various in vitro models of seizures were developed in isolated brain slice preparations in which many synaptic connections are preserved. Electrographic events with features similar to those recorded during seizures in vivo have been produced in hippocampal slices by multiple methods, including altering ionic constituents of media bathing the brain slices (McNamara, 1994), such as low Ca^{2+}, zero Mg^{2+}, or elevated K^+. The accessibility and experimental control provided by these in vitro

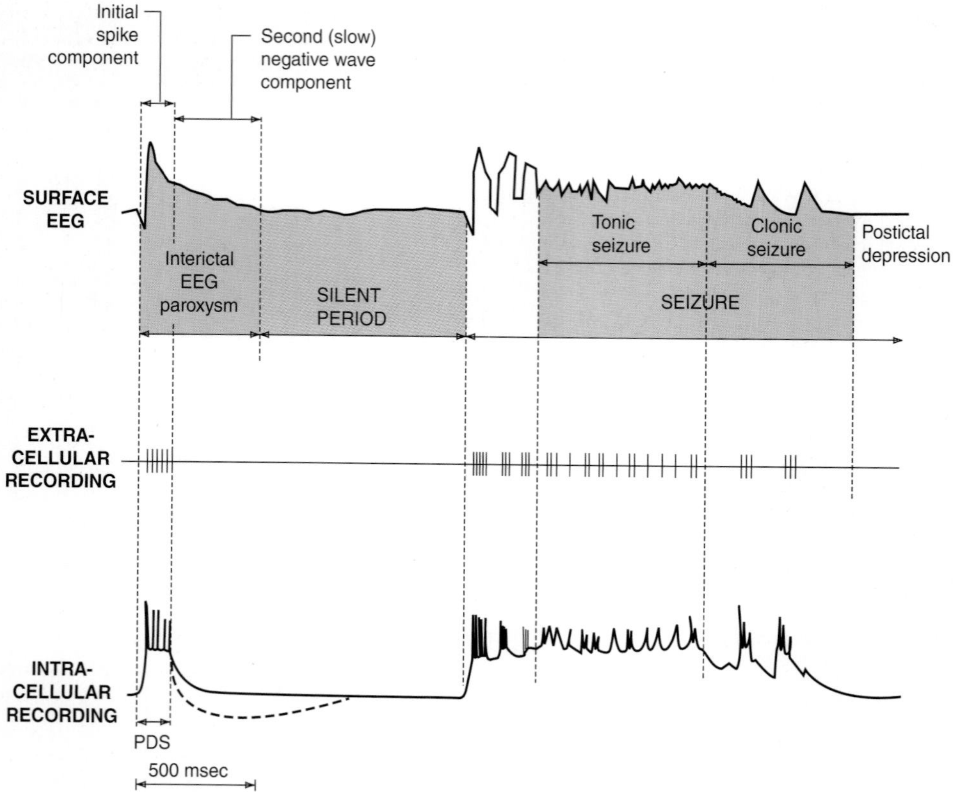

Figure 17–1 *Cortical EEG, extracellular, and intracellular recordings in a seizure focus induced by local application of a convulsant agent to mammalian cortex.* The extracellular recording was made through a high-pass filter. High-frequency firing of the neuron is evident in both extracellular and intracellular recording during the paroxysmal depolarization shift (PDS). (Modified with permission from Ayala GF *et al.* Genesis of epileptic interictal spikes. New knowledge of cortical feedback systems suggests a neurophysiological explanation of brief paroxysms. *Brain Res*, **1973**, *52*:1–17. © Elsevier.)

preparations has permitted mechanistic investigations into the induction of seizures. Data from in vitro models confirmed the importance of synaptic function for initiating a seizure, demonstrating that subtle reductions (e.g., 20%) of inhibitory synaptic function could lead to epileptiform activity and that activation of excitatory synapses could be pivotal in seizure initiation. Other important factors include the volume of the extracellular space and intrinsic properties of a neuron, such as voltage-gated ion channels (e.g., K^+, Na^+, and Ca^{2+} channels) (Traynelis and Dingledine, 1988). Identification of these diverse synaptic and nonsynaptic factors controlling seizures in vitro provides potential pharmacological targets for regulating seizure susceptibility in vivo.

Some common forms of focal epilepsy arise months to years after cortical injury sustained as a consequence of stroke, trauma, infection, or other factors. Effective prophylaxis administered to patients at high risk would be highly desirable in the clinical setting. However, no effective antiepileptogenic agent has been identified. The drugs described in this chapter provide symptomatic therapy; that is, the drugs inhibit seizures in patients with epilepsy.

Understanding the mechanisms of epileptogenesis in cellular and molecular terms should provide a framework for development of novel therapeutic approaches. The availability of animal models provides an opportunity to investigate the underlying mechanisms and have also enabled the discovery of numerous ASDs that are proven safe and efficacious in humans.

One model, termed *kindling*, is induced by periodic administration of brief, low-intensity electrical stimulation of the amygdala or other limbic structures that evoke a brief electrical seizure recorded on the EEG without behavioral change. Repeated (e.g., 10–20) stimulations result in progressive intensification of seizures, culminating in tonic-clonic seizures that, once established, persist for the life of the animal. Additional models are produced by induction of continuous seizures that last for hours ("status epilepticus"). The inciting agent used in these models is typically either a chemoconvulsant, such as kainic acid or pilocarpine, or sustained electrical stimulation. The episode of status epilepticus is followed weeks later by the onset of spontaneous seizures, an intriguing parallel to the scenario of complicated febrile seizures in young children preceding the emergence of spontaneous seizures years later. In contrast to the limited or absent neuronal loss characteristic of the kindling model, overt destruction of hippocampal neurons occurs in models of status epilepticus, reflecting aspects of hippocampal sclerosis observed in humans with severe limbic seizures. Indeed, the discovery that complicated febrile seizures precede and presumably are the cause of hippocampal sclerosis in young children (VanLandingham et al., 1998) establishes yet another commonality between these preclinical models and the human condition.

Several questions arise with respect to these models. What transpires during the latent period between status epilepticus and emergence of spontaneous seizures that causes the epilepsy? Might an antiepileptogenic agent that was effective in one of these models demonstrate disease-modifying effects in other models and perhaps in patients?

Important insights into the mechanisms of action of drugs that are effective against focal seizures have emerged (Rogawski and Löscher, 2004), insights largely from electrophysiological studies of relatively simple in vitro models, such as neurons isolated from the mammalian CNS and maintained in primary culture. The experimental control and accessibility provided by these models—together with careful attention to clinically relevant concentrations of the drugs—led to clarification of their mechanisms. Although it is difficult to prove unequivocally that a given drug effect observed in vitro is both necessary and sufficient to inhibit a seizure in an animal or humans in vivo, there is an excellent likelihood that the putative mechanisms identified (Table 17–2) do in fact underlie the clinically relevant antiseizure effects. Electrophysiological analyses of individual neurons during a focal seizure demonstrate that the neurons undergo depolarization and fire action potentials at high frequencies (Figure 17–1). This pattern of neuronal firing is characteristic of a seizure and is uncommon during physiological neuronal activity. Thus, selective inhibition of this pattern of firing would be expected to reduce seizures with minimal adverse effects on neurons. Carbamazepine, lamotrigine, phenytoin, lacosamide, and valproate inhibit high-frequency firing at concentrations known to be effective at limiting seizures in humans (Rogawski and Löscher, 2004). Inhibition of the high-frequency firing is thought to be mediated by reducing the ability of Na^+ channels to recover from inactivation (Figure 17–2). The rationale is as follows:

1. Depolarization-triggered opening of the Na^+ channels in the axonal membrane of a neuron is required for an action potential.
2. After opening, the channels spontaneously close, a process termed *inactivation*.
3. This inactivation period is thought to cause the refractory period, a short time after an action potential during which it is not possible to evoke another action potential.
4. On recovery from inactivation, the Na^+ channels are again poised to participate in another action potential.
5. Inactivation has little or no effect on low-frequency firing because firing at a slow rate permits sufficient time for Na^+ channels to recover from inactivation.
6. Reducing the rate of recovery of Na^+ channels from inactivation could limit the ability of a neuron to fire at high frequencies, an effect that

TABLE 17–2 ■ PROPOSED MECHANISMS OF ACTION OF ANTISEIZURE DRUGS

MOLECULAR TARGET AND ACTIVITY	DRUG	CONSEQUENCES OF ACTION
Na^+ channel modulators that: *Enhance fast inactivation*	PHT, CBZ, LTG, FBM, OxCBZ, TPM, VPA, ESL, RUF	• Block action potential propagation • Stabilize neuronal membranes • ↓ Neurotransmitter release, focal firing, and seizure spread
Enhance slow inactivation	LCM	• ↑ Spike frequency adaptation • ↓ Action potential bursts, focal firing, and seizure spread • Stabilize neuronal membrane
Ca^{2+} channel blockers	ESM, VPA, LTG	• ↓ Neurotransmitter release (N- and P- types) • ↓ Slow-depolarization (T-type) and spike-wave discharges
$\alpha 2\delta$ Ligands	GBP, PGB	• Modulate neurotransmitter release
$GABA_A$ receptor allosteric modulators	BZDs, PB, FBM, PRM, TPM, CBZ, OxCBZ, STP, CLB	• ↑ Membrane hyperpolarization and seizure threshold • ↓ Focal firing BZDs—attenuate spike-wave discharges PB, CBZ, OxCBZ—aggravate spike-wave discharges
GABA uptake inhibitors/GABA-transaminase inhibitors	TGB, VGB	• ↑ Extrasynaptic GABA levels and membrane hyperpolarization • ↓ Focal firing • Aggravate spike-wave discharges
NMDA receptor antagonists	FBM	• ↓ Slow excitatory neurotransmission • ↓ Excitatory amino acid neurotoxicity • Delay epileptogenesis
AMPA/kainate receptor antagonists	PB, TPM, PER	• ↓ Fast excitatory neurotransmission and focal firing
Enhancers of HCN channel activity	LTG	• Buffers large hyperpolarizing and depolarizing inputs • Suppresses action potential initiation by dendritic inputs
Positive allosteric modulator of KCNQ2-5	EZG	• suppresses bursts of action potentials • hyperpolarizes membrane potentials
SV2A protein ligand	LEV, BRV	• Unknown; may decrease transmitter release
Inhibitors of brain carbonic anhydrase	ACZ, TPM, ZNS	• ↑ HCN-mediated currents • ↓ NMDA-mediated currents • ↑ GABA-mediated inhibition

ACZ, acetazolamide; BRV, brivaracetam; BZDs, benzodiazepines; CBZ, carbamazepine; CLB, clobazam; ESL, eslicarbazepine; EZG, ezogabine; FBM, felbamate; GBP, gabapentin; LEV, levetiracetam; LCM, lacosamide; LTG, lamotrigine; OxCBZ, oxcarbazepine; PER, perampanel; PB, phenobarbital; PGB, pregabalin; PHT, phenytoin; PRM, primidone; RUF, rufinamide; STP, stiripentol; TGB, tiagabine; TPM, topiramate; VGB, vigabatrin; VPA, valproate; ZNA, zonisamide.

Source: Modified with permission from Leppik IE, et al. Basic research in epilepsy and aging. *Epilepsy Res*, **2006**, *68*(suppl 1):21. Copyright © Elsevier.

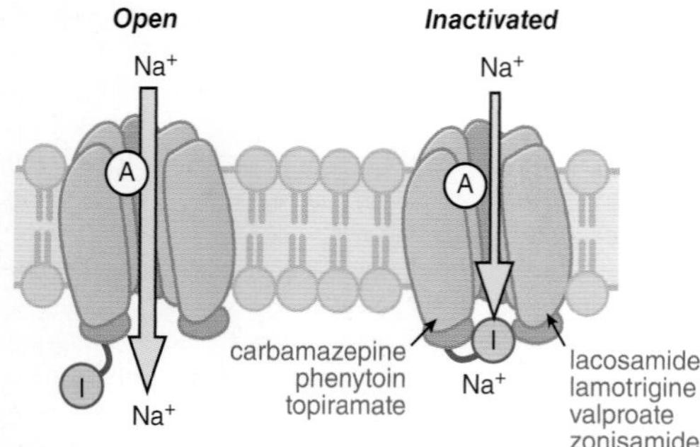

Figure 17–2 *Antiseizure drug-enhanced Na+ channel inactivation.* Some antiseizure drugs (noted in blue text) prolong the inactivation of the Na+ channels, thereby reducing the ability of neurons to fire at high frequencies. The inactivated channel itself appears to remain open but is blocked by the inactivation gate, **I**. Activation gate, **A**.

likely underlies the effects of carbamazepine, lamotrigine, lacosamide, phenytoin, topiramate, valproate, and zonisamide against focal seizures.

Insights into mechanisms of seizures suggest that enhancing GABA-mediated synaptic inhibition would reduce neuronal excitability and raise the seizure threshold. Several drugs are thought to inhibit seizures by regulating GABA-mediated synaptic inhibition through an action at distinct sites of the synapse (Rogawski and Löscher, 2004). The principal postsynaptic receptor of synaptically released GABA is termed the $GABA_A$ receptor (Chapter 14). Activation of the $GABA_A$ receptor inhibits the postsynaptic cell by increasing the inflow of Cl^- ions into the cell, which tends to hyperpolarize the neuron. Clinically relevant concentrations of benzodiazepines and barbiturates enhance $GABA_A$ receptor–mediated inhibition through distinct actions on the $GABA_A$ receptor (Figure 17–3), and this enhanced inhibition probably underlies the effectiveness of these compounds against focal and tonic-clonic seizures in humans. At higher concentrations, such as might be used for status epilepticus, these drugs also can inhibit high-frequency firing of action potentials. A second mechanism of enhancing GABA-mediated synaptic inhibition is thought to underlie the antiseizure mechanism of tiagabine; tiagabine inhibits the GABA transporter GAT-1, reducing neuronal and glial uptake of GABA (Rogawski and Löscher, 2004), prolonging its dwell time in the synaptic cleft where it activates $GABA_A$ receptors. Finally, ASDs can decrease GABA metabolism GABA transaminase (i.e., valproate, vigabatrin) resulting in increased GABA concentrations (Ben-Menachem, 2011; Cai et al., 2012; Larsson et al., 1986) and increased signaling via the $GABA_A$ receptor.

Generalized-Onset Epilepsies: Absence Seizures

In contrast to focal seizures, which arise from localized regions of the brain, generalized-onset seizures arise from the reciprocal firing of the thalamus and cerebral cortex (Huguenard and McCormick, 2007). Amongst the diverse forms of generalized seizures, absence seizures have been studied most intensively. The striking synchrony in appearance of generalized seizure discharges in widespread areas of neocortex led to the idea that a structure in the thalamus or brainstem (the "centrencephalon") synchronized these seizure discharges. Focus on the thalamus emerged from the demonstration that low-frequency stimulation of midline thalamic structures triggered EEG rhythms in the cortex similar to spike-and-wave discharges characteristic of absence seizures. Intracerebral electrode recordings from humans subsequently demonstrated the presence of thalamic and neocortical involvement in the spike-and-wave discharge of absence seizures. Many of the structural and functional properties of the thalamus and neocortex that led to the generalized spike-and-wave discharges have been elucidated (Huguenard and McCormick, 2007).

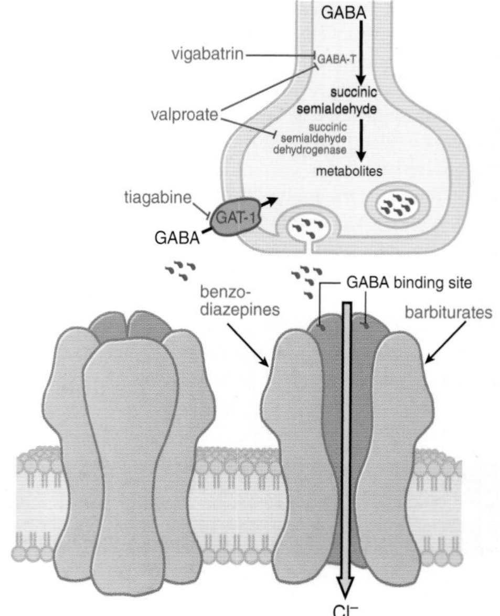

Figure 17–3 *Some antiseizure drugs enhance GABA synaptic transmission.* In the presence of GABA, the $GABA_A$ receptor (structure on bottom left) is opened, allowing an influx of Cl^-, which in turn increases membrane polarization. Some ASDs (shown in blue text) act by reducing the metabolism of GABA. Others act at the $GABA_A$ receptor, enhancing Cl^- influx in response to GABA or by prolonging its synaptic dwell time by inhibiting its reuptake by GAT-1. Gabapentin acts presynaptically to promote GABA release; its molecular target is currently under investigation. ⸱, GABA molecules. GABA-T, GABA transaminase; GAT-1, neuronal GABA transporter (SLC6A1).

The EEG hallmark of an absence seizure is generalized spike-and-wave discharges at a frequency of 3 Hz (3/s). These bilaterally synchronous spike-and-wave discharges, recorded locally from electrodes in both the thalamus and the neocortex, represent oscillations between the thalamus and neocortex. A comparison of EEG and intracellular recordings reveals that the EEG spikes are associated with the firing of action potentials and the following slow wave with prolonged inhibition. These reverberatory, low-frequency rhythms are made possible by a combination of factors, including reciprocal excitatory synaptic connections between the neocortex and thalamus as well as intrinsic properties of neurons in the thalamus (Huguenard and McCormick, 2007).

One intrinsic property of thalamic neurons that is involved in the generation of the 3-Hz spike-and-wave discharges is the low threshold ("T-type") Ca^{2+} current. T-type Ca^{2+} channels are activated at a much more negative membrane potential (hence, "low threshold") than most other voltage-gated Ca^{2+} channels expressed in the brain. T-type currents are much larger in many thalamic neurons than in neurons outside the thalamus. Indeed, bursts of action potentials in thalamic neurons are mediated by activation of the T-type currents. T-type currents amplify thalamic membrane potential oscillations, with one oscillation being the 3-Hz spike-and-wave discharge of the absence seizure. Importantly, the principal mechanism by which anti–absence seizure drugs (ethosuximide, valproate) are thought to act is by inhibition of the T-type Ca^{2+} channels (Figure 17–4) (Rogawski and Löscher, 2004). Thus, inhibiting voltage-gated ion channels is a common mechanism of action among ASDs, with anti–focal seizure drugs inhibiting voltage-activated Na^+ channels and anti–absence seizure drugs inhibiting voltage-activated Ca^{2+} channels.

Genetics of the Epilepsies

Genetic causes contribute to a wide diversity of human epilepsies. Genetic causes are solely responsible for rare forms inherited in an autosomal

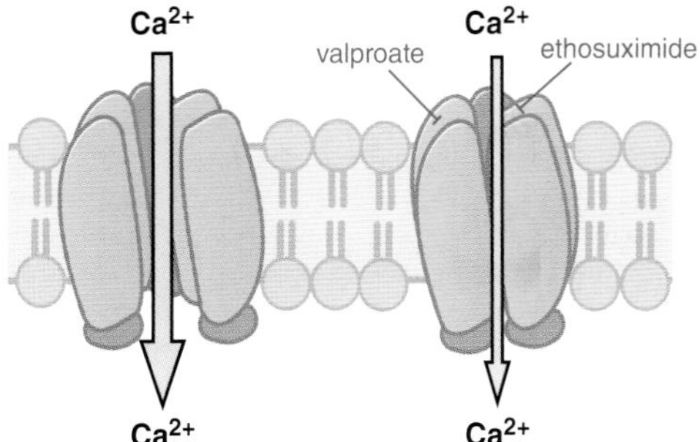

Figure 17–4 *Antiseizure drug-induced reduction of current through T-type Ca^{2+} channels.* Some antiseizure drugs (e.g., valproate and ethosuximide) reduce the flow of Ca^{2+} through T-type Ca^{2+} channels, thereby reducing the pacemaker current that underlies the thalamic rhythm in spikes and waves seen in generalized absence seizures.

dominant or autosomal recessive manner. Genetic causes also are mainly responsible for more common forms such as Dravet syndrome, JME, or childhood absence epilepsy, the majority of which are likely due to inheritance of two or more susceptibility genes. Genetic determinants also may contribute some degree of risk to epilepsies caused by injury of the cerebral cortex.

Mutations in more than 70 genes are known to contribute to epilepsy. Not surprisingly, many of the identified epilepsy-conferring mutations are in genes that encode voltage- or ligand-gated ion channels (Reid et al., 2009). However, mutations have also been identified in signaling pathways, transporters, and even synaptic vesicle proteins (EpiPM Consortium, 2015). Furthermore, many of the mutations arise de novo, thus complicating efforts in diagnoses. The genotype-phenotype correlations of these genetic syndromes are complex; the same mutation in one channel can be associated with divergent clinical syndromes, ranging from simple febrile seizures to intractable seizures with intellectual decline. Conversely, clinically indistinguishable epilepsy syndromes have been associated with mutation of distinct genes. The implication of genes encoding ion channels in familial epilepsy is particularly interesting because episodic disorders involving other organs also result from mutations of these genes. For example, episodic disorders of the heart (cardiac arrhythmias), skeletal muscle (periodic paralyses), cerebellum (episodic ataxia), vasculature (familial hemiplegic migraine), and other organs all have been linked to mutations in genes encoding components of voltage-gated ion channels (Ptacek and Fu, 2001).

The cellular electrophysiological consequences of these mutations can inform our understanding of the mechanisms of seizures and the actions of ASDs and allow for the determination of precise therapies for patients with specific mutations. For example, generalized epilepsy with febrile seizures is caused, in some cases, by a point mutation in the β subunit of a voltage-gated Na^+ channel (*SCN1B*). Several ASDs act on Na^+ channels to promote their inactivation; the phenotype of the mutated Na^+ channel appears to involve defective inactivation (Wallace et al., 1998).

Spontaneous mutations in *SCN1A* (encoding the α subunit of the major voltage-gated Na^+ channel in neurons) that result in truncations and presumed loss of Na^+ channel function have been identified in a subset of infants with a catastrophic severe myoclonic epilepsy of infancy or Dravet syndrome. That these loss-of-function mutations in Na^+ channels result in seizures is somewhat surprising. However, seizures may arise as a consequence of the cell types that express these channels within neural circuits that underlie seizure initiation. Interestingly, patients with these mutations are generally found to be refractory to ASDs that block Na^+ channels.

Antiseizure Drugs: General Considerations

History of ASD Development

The first ASD was bromide, which was used in the late 19th century. Phenobarbital was the first synthetic organic agent recognized as having antiseizure activity. Its usefulness, however, was limited to generalized tonic-clonic seizures and, to a lesser degree, focal seizures. It had no effect on absence seizures. Merritt and Putnam developed the electroshock seizure test in experimental animals to screen chemical agents for antiseizure effectiveness; in the course of screening a variety of drugs, they discovered that diphenylhydantoin (later renamed phenytoin) suppressed seizures in the absence of sedative effects. The maximal electroshock seizure test is extremely valuable because drugs that are effective against the tonic hind limb extension induced by corneal electroshock generally have proven to be effective against focal and generalized tonic-clonic seizures in humans. In contrast, seizures induced by the chemoconvulsant pentylenetetrazol are most useful in the identification of ASDs that are effective against myoclonic seizures in humans. These screening tests and other phenotypically or etiologically relevant acute and chronic animal models are used in developing new ASDs.

The chemical structures of most of the drugs introduced before 1965 were closely related to phenobarbital. These included the hydantoins and the succinimides. Between 1965 and 1990, the chemically distinct structures of the benzodiazepines, an iminostilbene (carbamazepine), and a branched-chain carboxylic acid (valproate) were introduced, followed in the 1990s by a phenyltriazine (lamotrigine), a cyclic analogue of GABA (gabapentin), a sulfamate-substituted monosaccharide (topiramate), a nipecotic acid derivative (tiagabine), and a pyrrolidine derivative (levetiracetam). Since the 1970s, the National Institutes of Health has spurred development of ASDs via sponsorship of the Epilepsy Therapy Screening Program (ETSP), an ongoing partnership between government, private industry, and the University of Utah.

Therapeutic Aspects

The ideal ASD would suppress all seizures without causing any unwanted effects. Unfortunately, the drugs used currently not only fail to control seizure activity in approximately one-third of patients, but frequently cause unwanted adverse effects that range in severity from minimal impairment of the CNS to death from aplastic anemia or hepatic failure. In 2009, all manufacturers of ASDs were required by the FDA to update their product labeling to include a warning about an increased risk of suicidal thoughts or actions and to develop information targeted at helping patients understand this risk. The risk applies to all ASDs used for any indication. Details are available online at the FDA website.

The clinician who treats patients with epilepsy is faced with the task of selecting the appropriate drug or combination of drugs that best controls seizures in an individual patient at an acceptable level of untoward effects. As a general rule, complete control of seizures can be achieved in up to 50% of patients, while another 25% can be improved significantly. The degree of success varies as a function of seizure type, cause, and other factors.

To minimize toxicity, treatment with a single drug is preferred. If seizures are not controlled with the initial agent at adequate plasma concentrations, substitution of a second drug is preferred to the concurrent administration of another agent. However, multiple-drug therapy may be required, especially when two or more types of seizure occur in the same patient. With each concurrent add-on ASD, the likelihood of seizure freedom decreases (Kwan and Brodie, 2000).

Measurement of drug concentrations in plasma facilitates optimizing antiseizure medication, especially when therapy is initiated, after dosage adjustments, in the event of therapeutic failure, when toxic effects appear, or when multiple-drug therapy is instituted. However, clinical effects of some drugs do not correlate well with their concentrations in plasma, and recommended concentrations are only guidelines for therapy. *The ultimate therapeutic regimen must be determined by clinical assessment of effect and toxicity.*

The individual agents are introduced in the next sections, followed by a discussion of some general principles of the drug therapy of the epilepsies.

Hydantoins

Phenytoin

Phenytoin is effective against all types of focal and tonic-clonic seizures but not absence seizures. Oral phenytoin is indicated for the control of focal-to-bilateral tonic-clonic seizures and the prevention and treatment of seizures occurring during or following neurosurgery. Parenteral phenytoin is indicated for the control of generalized tonic-clonic status epilepticus and the treatment of seizures occurring during neurosurgery. Parenteral phenytoin should only be used when oral phenytoin administration is not possible.

Pharmacological Effects in the CNS

Phenytoin exerts antiseizure activity without causing general depression of the CNS. In toxic doses, it may produce excitatory signs and at lethal levels a type of decerebrate rigidity.

Mechanism of Action

Phenytoin limits the repetitive firing of action potentials evoked by a sustained depolarization of mouse spinal cord neurons maintained in vitro (McLean and Macdonald, 1986a). This effect is mediated by slowing of the rate of recovery of voltage-activated Na^+ channels from inactivation, an action that is both voltage (greater effect if membrane is depolarized) and use dependent. At therapeutic concentrations, the effects on Na^+ channels are selective, and no changes of spontaneous activity or responses to iontophoretically applied GABA or glutamate are detected. At concentrations 5- to 10-fold higher, multiple effects of phenytoin are evident, including reduction of spontaneous activity and enhancement of responses to GABA; these effects may underlie some of the unwanted toxicity associated with high levels of phenytoin.

ADME and Drug Interactions

Phenytoin is available in two types of oral formulations that differ in their pharmacokinetics: rapid-release and extended-release forms. Once-daily dosing is possible only with the extended-release formulations, and due to differences in dissolution and other formulation-dependent factors, the plasma phenytoin level may change when converting from one formulation to another. Confusion also can arise because different formulations can include either phenytoin or phenytoin sodium. Therefore, comparable doses can be approximated by considering "phenytoin equivalents," but serum-level monitoring is also necessary to ensure therapeutic safety. When changing routes of administration from oral to intramuscular (or vice versa), appropriate dose adjustments and blood level monitoring are recommended.

The pharmacokinetic characteristics of phenytoin are influenced markedly by its binding to serum proteins, by the nonlinearity of its elimination kinetics, and by its metabolism by hepatic CYPs (Table 17–3). Phenytoin is extensively bound (~90%) to serum proteins, mainly albumin. Small variations in the percentage of phenytoin that is bound dramatically affect the absolute amount of free (active) drug. Some agents can compete with phenytoin for binding sites on plasma proteins and increase free phenytoin at the time the new drug is added to the regimen. However, the effect on free phenytoin is only short-lived and usually does not cause clinical complications unless inhibition of phenytoin metabolism also occurs. For example, valproate competes for protein-binding sites and inhibits phenytoin metabolism, resulting in marked and sustained increases in free phenytoin. Measurement of free rather than total phenytoin permits direct assessment of this potential problem in patient management.

The rate of elimination of phenytoin varies as a function of its concentration (i.e., the rate is nonlinear). The plasma $t_{1/2}$ of phenytoin ranges between 6 and 24 h at plasma concentrations below 10 μg/mL. At low blood levels, metabolism follows first-order kinetics; as blood levels rise, the maximal limit of the liver to metabolize phenytoin is approached, and C_p increases disproportionately as dosage is increased, even with small adjustments for levels near the therapeutic range.

The majority (95%) of phenytoin is metabolized by CYP2C9 and to a lesser extent by CYP2C19 (Table 17–3). The principal metabolite, a parahydroxyphenyl derivative, is inactive. Because its metabolism is saturable, other drugs that are metabolized by these CYP enzymes can inhibit the metabolism of phenytoin and increase its plasma concentration. Conversely, the degradation rate of other drugs that serve as substrates for these enzymes can be inhibited by phenytoin; one such drug is warfarin, and addition of phenytoin to a patient receiving warfarin can lead to bleeding disorders (Chapter 32).

An alternative mechanism of drug interactions arises from phenytoin's ability to induce various CYPs (see discussion that follows and Chapter 6). Of particular note in this regard are oral contraceptives, which are metabolized by CYP3A4; treatment with phenytoin can enhance the metabolism of oral contraceptives and lead to unplanned pregnancy. The potential teratogenic effects of phenytoin underscore the importance of attention to this interaction. Carbamazepine, oxcarbazepine, phenobarbital, and primidone also induce CYP3A4 and likewise might increase degradation of oral contraceptives.

Concurrent administration of any drug metabolized by CYP2C9 can increase the plasma concentration of phenytoin by decreasing its rate of metabolism (Table 17–3). Conversely, the degradation rate of other drugs that are substrates for these enzymes can be inhibited by phenytoin. Carbamazepine, which may enhance the metabolism of phenytoin, causes a well-documented *decrease* in phenytoin concentration. Phenytoin can also induce expression of a number of different CYPs, leading to increased degradation of coadministered drugs, such as oral contraceptives. Conversely, phenytoin reduces the concentration of carbamazepine.

The low water solubility of phenytoin hindered its intravenous use and led to production of fosphenytoin, a water-soluble prodrug. Fosphenytoin is converted into phenytoin by phosphatases in liver and red blood cells with a $t_{1/2}$ of 8–15 min. Fosphenytoin is extensively bound (95%–99%) to human plasma proteins, primarily albumin. This binding is saturable and fosphenytoin displaces phenytoin from protein-binding sites. Fosphenytoin is useful for adults with focal or generalized seizures when either intravenous or intramuscular route of administration is indicated.

Adverse Effects and Toxicity

The toxic effects of phenytoin depend on the route of administration, the duration of exposure, and the dosage. When fosphenytoin, the water-soluble prodrug, is administered intravenously at an excessive rate in the emergency treatment of status epilepticus, the most notable toxic signs are cardiac arrhythmias with or without hypotension and CNS depression. Although cardiac toxicity occurs more frequently in older patients and in those with known cardiac disease, it also can develop in young, healthy patients. Because of the risk of adverse cardiovascular reactions with rapid administration, IV administartion should not exceed 50 mg per minute in adults. In pediatric patients, the drug should be administered at a rate not exceeding 1–3 mg/kg/min or 50 mg/min, whichever is slower. Acute oral overdosage results primarily in signs referable to the cerebellum and vestibular system; high doses have been associated with marked cerebellar atrophy.

Toxic effects associated with chronic treatment also are primarily dose-related cerebellar-vestibular effects but also include other CNS effects, behavioral changes, increased frequency of seizures, GI symptoms, gingival hyperplasia, osteomalacia, and megaloblastic anemia. Hirsutism is an annoying untoward effect in young females. Usually, these phenomena can be diminished by proper adjustment of dosage. Serious adverse effects, including those on the skin, bone marrow, and liver, probably are manifestations of drug allergy. Although rare, they necessitate withdrawal of the drug. Moderate transient elevation of the plasma concentrations of hepatic transaminases sometimes can also occur.

Gingival hyperplasia occurs in about 20% of all patients during chronic administration and can be minimized by good oral hygiene. Related to

TABLE 17–3 ■ INTERACTIONS OF ANTI-SEIZURE DRUGS WITH HEPATIC MICROSOMAL ENZYMES

	INDUCES		INHIBITS		METABOLIZED BY	
DRUG	CYP	UGT	CYP	UGT	CYP	UGT
Brivaracatam	No	No	No	No	2C19/2C9	No
Carbamazepine	1A2/2C9/ 3A4	Yes	No	No	1A2/2C8/3A4	No
Clobazam	No	No	No	No	3A4	No
Clonazepam	No	No	No	No	3A4	No
Eslicarbazepine	3A4	No	No	No	No	Yes
Ethosuximide	No	No	No	No	3A4	No
Ezogabine	No	No	No	No	No	Yes
Felbamate	3A4	No	2C19	No	3A4/2E1	?
Gabapentin	No	No	No	No	No	No
Lacosamide	No	No	No	No	2C19	?
Lamotrigine	No	No	No	No	No	UGT1A4
Levetiracetam	No	No	No	No	No	No
Oxcarbazepine	3A4/5	UGT1A4	2C19	Weak	No	Yes
Perampanel	No	No	Weak	Weak	3A4/3A5	Yes
Phenobarbital	2C9/3A4/ 1A2	Yes	No	No	2C9/19/2E1	Yes
Phenytoin	2C9/3A4/ 1A2	Yes	2C9	No	2C9/19	No
Pregabalin	No	No	No	No	No	No
Primidone	2C/3A	Yes	Yes	No	2C9/19	No
Rufinamide	3A4 (weak)	No	2E1 (weak)	No	No	No
Stiripentol	No	No	1A2/3A4/ 2C19/2D6	No	No	No
Tiagabine	No	No	No	No	3A4	No
Topiramate	3A4 (>200 mg/day)	No	2C19	No	Yes	No
Valproate	No	No	2C9/3A4?	Yes	2C9/2C19/2A6/2B6	UGT1A3/2B7
Vigabatrin	No	No	No	No	No	No
Zonisamide	No	No	No	No	3A4	No

CYP, cytochrome P450; UGT, uridine diphosphate-glucuronosyltransferase. (Data modified from Johannessen and Johannessen, 2010 and Wheles and Vasquez, 2010, *Epilepsy Currents,* 10:1–6 and Cawello, 2015, *Clin Pharmacokinetic, 54*: 904–914.)

this, phenytoin can also produce coarsening of facial features. Inhibition of release of ADH has been observed. Hyperglycemia and glycosuria appear to be due to inhibition of insulin secretion. Osteomalacia, with hypocalcemia and elevated alkaline phosphatase activity, has been attributed to both altered metabolism of vitamin D and the attendant inhibition of intestinal absorption of Ca^{2+}. Phenytoin also increases the metabolism of vitamin K and reduces the concentration of vitamin K–dependent proteins that are important for normal Ca^{2+} metabolism in bone. This may explain why the osteomalacia is not always ameliorated by the administration of vitamin D.

Hypersensitivity reactions include morbilliform rash in 2%–5% of patients and occasionally more serious skin reactions, including Stevens-Johnson syndrome and toxic epidermal necrolysis. Drug-induced systemic lupus erythematosus; potentially fatal hepatic necrosis; hematological reactions, including neutropenia and leukopenia; red cell aplasia; agranulocytosis; and mild thrombocytopenia also have been reported. Hypoprothrombinemia and hemorrhage have occurred in the newborns of mothers who received phenytoin during pregnancy; vitamin K is effective treatment or prophylaxis.

Plasma Drug Concentrations

A good correlation usually is observed between the total concentration of phenytoin in plasma and its clinical effect. Thus, control of seizures generally is obtained with total concentrations above 10 μg/mL, while toxic effects such as nystagmus develop at total concentrations around 20 μg/mL. Control of seizures generally is obtained with free phenytoin concentrations of 0.75–1.25 μg/mL.

Therapeutic Uses

Epilepsy. Phenytoin is one of the more widely used ASDs; it is effective against focal and generalized tonic-clonic, focal-to-bilateral tonic-clonic, tonic-clonic of unknown onset (tonic-clonic), but not generalized absence seizures. The use of phenytoin and other agents in the therapy of epilepsies is discussed further at the end of this chapter. Phenytoin preparations differ significantly in bioavailability and rate of absorption. In general, patients should consistently be treated with the same drug from a single manufacturer. However, if it becomes necessary to temporarily switch between products, care should be taken to select a therapeutically equivalent product, and patients should be monitored for loss of seizure control or onset of new toxicities.

Other Uses. Trigeminal and related neuralgias occasionally respond to phenytoin, but carbamazepine may be preferable. The use of phenytoin in the treatment of cardiac arrhythmias is discussed in Chapter 30.

Benzodiazepines

The benzodiazepines are used primarily as sedative-antianxiety drugs; their pharmacology is described in Chapters 15 and 19. Discussion here is limited to their use in the therapy of the epilepsies. A large number of benzodiazepines have broad antiseizure properties. Clonazepam is FDA-approved alone or as an adjunctive treatment of Lennox-Gestaut syndrome, akinetic, and myoclonic seizures. It may also benefit patients with absence seizures which are inadequately responding to succinimides. Clorazepate is approved as an adjunct therapy for the management of focal seizures. Midazolam was designated an orphan drug in 2006 for intermittent treatment of bouts of increased seizure activity in refractory patients with epilepsy who are on stable regimens of ASDs. More recently, midazolam was granted orphan drug designation in 2009 as a rescue treatment of seizures in patients who require control of intermittent bouts of increased seizure activity (i.e., acute repetitive seizure clusters), in 2012 for the treatment of nerve agent-induced seizures, and in 2016 for the treatment of status epilepticus and seizures induced by organophosporous poisoning. Diazepam and lorazepam have well-defined roles in the management of status epilepticus. Unlike other marketed 1,4-benzodiazepines, clobazam is a 1,5-benzodiazepine that is less lipophilic and less acidic and may be better tolerated than traditional 1,4-benzodiazepines (see benzodiazepine structure in Chapter 19). Clobazam is used in a variety of seizure phenotypes and is approved in the U.S. for the treatment of Lennox-Gastaut syndrome in patients aged 2 years or older.

Antiseizure Properties

In animal models, inhibition of pentylenetetrazol-induced seizures by the benzodiazepines is much more prominent than is their modification of the maximal electroshock seizure pattern. Clonazepam is unusually potent in antagonizing the effects of pentylenetetrazol, but it is almost without action on seizures induced by maximal electroshock. Benzodiazepines, including clonazepam, suppress the spread of kindled seizures and generalized seizures produced by stimulation of the amygdala, but do not abolish the abnormal discharge at the site of stimulation.

Mechanism of Action

The antiseizure actions of the benzodiazepines result in large part from their capacity to enhance GABA-mediated synaptic inhibition. Molecular cloning and study of recombinant receptors have demonstrated that the benzodiazepine receptor is an integral part of the $GABA_A$ receptor (see Figures 14–11 and 17–3). At therapeutically relevant concentrations, benzodiazepines act at subsets of $GABA_A$ receptors and increase the frequency, but not duration, of openings at GABA-activated Cl^- channels (Twyman et al., 1989). At higher concentrations, diazepam and many other benzodiazepines can reduce sustained high-frequency firing of neurons, similar to the effects of phenytoin, carbamazepine, and valproate. Although these concentrations correspond to concentrations achieved in patients during treatment of status epilepticus with diazepam, they are considerably higher than those associated with antiseizure or anxiolytic effects in ambulatory patients. Clobazam potentiates GABA-mediated neurotransmission in the same fashion as other benzodiazepines at $GABA_A$ receptors.

ADME

Benzodiazepines are well absorbed after oral administration, and concentrations in plasma are usually maximal within 1–4 h. After intravenous administration, they redistribute in a manner typical of that for highly lipid-soluble agents. Central effects develop promptly, but wane rapidly as the drugs move to other tissues. Diazepam is redistributed especially rapidly, with a $t_{1/2}$ of redistribution of about 1 h. The extent of binding of benzodiazepines to plasma proteins correlates with lipid solubility, ranging from about 99% for diazepam to about 85% for clonazepam.

Table 19–1 shows the scheme for metabolism of benzodiazepines, the major metabolite of diazepam, *N*-desmethyl-diazepam, is somewhat less active than the parent drug and may behave as a partial agonist. This metabolite also is produced by the rapid decarboxylation of clorazepate following its ingestion. Both diazepam and *N*-desmethyl-diazepam are slowly hydroxylated to other active metabolites, such as oxazepam. The $t_{1/2}$ of diazepam in plasma is ~43 h (see Table 19–2); that of *N*-desmethyl-diazepam is about 60 h. Clonazepam is metabolized principally by reduction of the nitro group to produce inactive 7-amino derivatives. Less than 1% of the drug is recovered unchanged in the urine. The $t_{1/2}$ of clonazepam in plasma is about 23 h. Lorazepam is metabolized chiefly by conjugation with glucuronic acid; its $t_{1/2}$ in plasma is about 14 h. Clobazam has a $t_{1/2}$ of 18 h and is effective at doses between 0.5 and 1 mg/kg daily, with limited development of tolerance. The active metabolite of clobazam is norclobazam.

Plasma Drug Concentrations

Because tolerance affects the relationship between drug concentration and drug antiseizure effect, plasma concentrations of benzodiazepines are of limited value.

Therapeutic Uses

Clonazepam is useful in the therapy of absence seizures as well as myoclonic seizures in children. However, tolerance to its antiseizure effects usually develops after 1–6 months of administration, after which some patients will no longer respond to clonazepam at any dosage. The initial dose of clonazepam for adults should not exceed 1.5 mg per day and for children 0.01–0.03 mg/kg per day. The dose-dependent side effects are reduced if two or three divided doses are given each day. The dose may be increased every 3 days in amounts of 0.25–0.5 mg per day in children and 0.5–1 mg per day in adults. The maximal recommended dose is 20 mg per day for adults and 0.2 mg/kg per day for children. Clonazepam intranasal spray is designated as an orphan drug for recurrent acute repetitive seizures.

While diazepam is an effective agent for treatment of status epilepticus, the effective duration of action of this lipid soluble agent is shortened by its rapid redistribution. Thus, lorazepam is more frequently used; it is less lipid soluble, is more effectively confined to the vascular compartment, and has a longer effective half-life after a single dose. Diazepam is not useful as an oral agent for the treatment of seizure disorders. Clorazepate is effective in combination with certain other drugs in the treatment of focal seizures. The maximal initial dose of clorazepate is 22.5 mg/d in three portions for adults and children older than 12 years and 15 mg/d in two divided doses in children 9–12 years of age. Clorazepate is not recommended for children under the age of 9. Clobazam is used in a variety of seizure phenotypes and is FDA-approved for the treatment of Lennox-Gastaut syndrome in patients aged 2 years or older. In patients weighing more than 30 kg, clobazam is initiated orally at 5 mg every 12 h and then titrated up to a maximum of 40 mg/d if tolerated. Dose escalation must be done gradually, not exceeding more than once per week.

Adverse Effects

The principal side effects of long-term oral therapy with clonazepam are drowsiness and lethargy. According to FDA-approved labeling, up to 30% of patients show a loss of anticonvulsant activity with continued administration of clonazepam, often within 3 months. In some cases, dose adjustment may reestablish efficacy. Muscular incoordination and ataxia are less frequent. Although these symptoms usually can be kept to tolerable levels by reducing the dosage or the rate at which it is increased, they sometimes force drug discontinuation.

Other side effects include hypotonia, dysarthria, and dizziness. Behavioral disturbances, especially in children, can be troublesome; these include aggression, hyperactivity, irritability, and difficulty in concentration. Both anorexia and hyperphagia have been reported. Increased salivary and bronchial secretions may cause difficulties in children. Seizures are sometimes exacerbated, and status epilepticus may be precipitated if the drug is discontinued abruptly. Other aspects of the toxicity of the benzodiazepines are discussed in Chapter 19. Cardiovascular and respiratory depression may occur after the intravenous administration of diazepam, clonazepam, or lorazepam, particularly if other ASDs or central depressants have been administered previously.

Antiseizure Barbiturates

While most barbiturates have antiseizure properties, only some barbiturates, such as phenobarbital, exert maximal antiseizure effects at doses below those that cause hypnosis. This therapeutic index determines a barbiturate's clinical utility as an antiseizure therapeutic drug. The pharmacology of the barbiturates as a class is described in Chapter 19; discussion in this chapter is limited to phenobarbital and primidone.

Phenobarbital

Phenobarbital was the first effective organic antiseizure agent. It has relatively low toxicity, is inexpensive, and is still one of the more effective and widely used antiseizure drugs.

Mechanism of Action

The mechanism by which phenobarbital inhibits seizures likely involves potentiation of synaptic inhibition through an action on the $GABA_A$ receptor. Phenobarbital enhances responses to iontophoretically applied GABA in mouse cortical and spinal neurons, effects that are observed at therapeutically relevant concentrations of phenobarbital; in patch-clamp studies, phenobarbital increases the $GABA_A$ receptor–mediated current by increasing the duration of bursts of $GABA_A$ receptor–mediated currents without changing the frequency of bursts (Twyman et al., 1989). At levels exceeding therapeutic concentrations, phenobarbital also limits sustained repetitive firing; this may underlie some of the antiseizure effects of higher concentrations of phenobarbital achieved during therapy of status epilepticus.

ADME

Oral absorption of phenobarbital is complete but somewhat slow; peak concentrations in plasma occur several hours after a single dose. It is 40%–60% bound to plasma proteins and bound to a similar extent in tissues, including brain. Up to 25% of a dose is eliminated by pH-dependent renal excretion of the unchanged drug; the remainder is inactivated by hepatic microsomal enzymes, principally CYP2C9, with minor metabolism by CYP2C19 and CYP2E1. Phenobarbital induces UGT enzymes as well as the CYP2C and CYP3A subfamilies. Drugs metabolized by these enzymes can be more rapidly degraded when coadministered with phenobarbital; importantly, oral contraceptives are metabolized by CYP3A4. The terminal $t_{1/2}$ of phenobarbital varies widely, 50–140 h in adults and 40–70 h in children younger than 5 years of age, often longer in neonates. Phenobarbital's duration of effect usually exceeds 6–12 h in nontolerant patients.

Plasma Drug Concentrations

During long-term therapy in adults, the plasma concentration of phenobarbital averages 10 μg/mL per daily dose of 1 mg/kg; in children, the value is 5–7 μg/mL per 1 mg/kg. Although a precise relationship between therapeutic results and concentration of drug in plasma does not exist, plasma concentrations of 10–35 μg/mL are usually recommended for control of seizures. The relationship between plasma concentration of phenobarbital and adverse effects varies with the development of tolerance. Sedation, nystagmus, and ataxia usually are absent at concentrations below 30 μg/mL during long-term therapy, but adverse effects may be apparent for several days at lower concentrations when therapy is initiated or whenever the dosage is increased. Concentrations more than 60 μg/mL may be associated with marked intoxication in the nontolerant individual. Because significant behavioral toxicity may be present despite the absence of overt signs of toxicity, the tendency to maintain patients, particularly children, on excessively high doses of phenobarbital should be resisted. The plasma phenobarbital concentration should be increased above 30–40 μg/mL only if the increment is adequately tolerated and only if it contributes significantly to control of seizures.

Therapeutic Uses

Phenobarbital is an effective agent for generalized tonic-clonic, focal-to-bilateral tonic-clonic, tonic-clonic of unknown onset (generalized tonic-clonic), and focal seizures. Its efficacy, low toxicity, and low cost make it an important agent for these types of epilepsy. However, its sedative effects and its tendency to disturb behavior in children have reduced its use as a primary agent. It is not effective for absence seizures.

Adverse Effects, Drug Interactions, and Toxicity

Sedation, the most frequent undesired effect of phenobarbital, is apparent to some extent in all patients on initiation of therapy, but tolerance develops during chronic medication. Nystagmus and ataxia occur at excessive dosage. Phenobarbital can produce irritability and hyperactivity in children and agitation and confusion in the elderly. Scarlatiniform or morbilliform rash, possibly with other manifestations of drug allergy, occurs in 1%–2% of patients. Exfoliative dermatitis is rare. Hypoprothrombinemia with hemorrhage has been observed in the newborns of mothers who have received phenobarbital during pregnancy; vitamin K is effective for treatment or prophylaxis. As with phenytoin, megaloblastic anemia that responds to folate and osteomalacia that responds to high doses of vitamin D occur during chronic phenobarbital therapy of epilepsy. Other adverse effects of phenobarbital are discussed in Chapter 19.

Interactions between phenobarbital and other drugs usually involve induction of the hepatic CYPs by phenobarbital. The interaction between phenytoin and phenobarbital is variable. Concentrations of phenobarbital in plasma may be elevated by as much as 40% during concurrent administration of valproate.

Primidone

Although primidone is indicated in the U.S. for patients with focal or generalized epilepsy, it has largely been replaced by carbamazepine and other newer ASDs that possess lower incidence of sedation.

Mechanism of Action

The exact mechanism of primidone's antiseizure effects is not fully understood. It is metabolized to two active metabolites: phenobarbital and phenylethylmalonamide (PEMA). Primidone and its two metabolites each have antiseizure effects on focal and generalized tonic-clonic seizures.

ADME

Primidone is completely absorbed and generally reaches peak plasma concentration within about 3 h of oral administration. Primidone is 30% protein bound in plasma and is rapidly metabolized to both phenobarbital and PEMA. Both primidone and phenobarbital undergo extensive conjugation prior to excretion. Primidone's $t_{1/2}$ is about 6–8 h. In contrast, the terminal $t_{1/2}$ of phenobarbital varies with age, with values ranging in adults from 50 to 140 h and in children less than 5 years of age from 40 to 70 h. Because of both slow accumulation and clearance, phenobarbital reaches therapeutic concentrations approximately two to three times higher than that of primidone. In fact, care should be taken and plasma closely monitored during titration of primidone doses because primidone may reach steady-state levels rapidly (1–2 days), whereas the metabolites phenobarbital and PEMA each attain steady state more slowly (20 days and 3–4 days, respectively).

Therapeutic Uses

Doses of 10–20 mg/kg/d reach clinically relevant steady-state plasma concentrations (8–12 μg/mL), although interpatient variability is common. In addition to its early use in patients with focal-onset or generalized epilepsy, primidone is still considered to be a first-line therapy for essential tremor with the β blocker propranolol.

Adverse Effects

The dose-dependent adverse effects of primidone are similar to those of phenobarbital, except that pronounced drowsiness is observed early after primidone administration. Common adverse effects include ataxia and vertigo, both of which diminish and may disappear with continued therapy. Primidone is contraindicated in patients with either porphyria or hypersensitivity to phenobarbital.

Iminostilbenes

Carbamazepine

Carbamazepine is considered to be a primary drug for the treatment of generalized tonic-clonic, focal-to-bilateral tonic-clonic, tonic-clonic of unknown onset (generalized tonic-clonic), and focal seizures. It is also used for the treatment of trigeminal neuralgia.

Carbamazepine is related chemically to the tricyclic antidepressants. It is a derivative of iminostilbene with a carbamyl group at the 5 position; this moiety is essential for potent antiseizure activity.

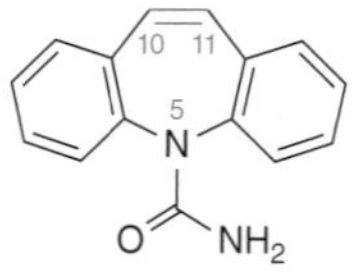

CARBAMAZEPINE

Mechanism of Action

Like phenytoin, carbamazepine limits the repetitive firing of action potentials evoked by a sustained depolarization of mouse spinal cord or cortical neurons maintained in vitro (McLean and Macdonald, 1986a). This appears to be mediated by slowing of the rate of recovery of voltage-activated Na^+ channels from inactivation. These effects of carbamazepine are evident at concentrations in the range of therapeutic drug levels in CSF in humans and are relatively selective, producing no effects on spontaneous activity or on responses to iontophoretically applied GABA or glutamate. The carbamazepine metabolite 10,11-epoxycarbamazepine also limits sustained repetitive firing at therapeutically relevant concentrations, suggesting that this metabolite may contribute to the antiseizure efficacy of carbamazepine.

ADME

The pharmacokinetics of carbamazepine are complex. They are influenced by its limited aqueous solubility and by the capacity of many ASDs, including carbamazepine itself, to increase conversion to active metabolites by hepatic enzymes (Table 17–3). Carbamazepine is absorbed slowly and erratically after oral administration. Peak concentrations in plasma usually are observed 4–8 h after oral ingestion, but may be delayed by as much as 24 h, especially following the administration of a large dose. Once absorbed, the drug distributes rapidly into all tissues. Approximately 75% of carbamazepine binds to plasma proteins; concentrations in the CSF appear to correspond to the concentration of free drug in plasma. The predominant pathway of metabolism in humans involves conversion to the 10,11-epoxide, a metabolite as active as the parent compound; its concentrations in plasma and brain may reach 50% of those of carbamazepine, especially during the concurrent administration of phenytoin or phenobarbital. The 10,11-epoxide is metabolized further to inactive compounds that are excreted in the urine principally as glucuronides. Carbamazepine also is inactivated by conjugation and hydroxylation. Hepatic CYP3A4 is primarily responsible for the agent's biotransformation. Carbamazepine induces CYP2C, CYP3A, and UGT, thus enhancing the metabolism of drugs degraded by these enzymes. Of particular importance in this regard are oral contraceptives, which are also metabolized by CYP3A4.

Plasma Drug Concentrations

There is no simple relationship between the dose of carbamazepine and concentrations of the drug in plasma. Therapeutic concentrations are reported to be 6–12 μg/mL, although considerable variation occurs. Side effects referable to the CNS are frequent at concentrations above 9 μg/mL.

Therapeutic Uses

Carbamazepine is useful in patients with generalized tonic-clonic and both focal aware and focal with impaired awareness seizures (Table 17–1). When it is used, renal and hepatic function and hematological parameters should be monitored. The therapeutic use of carbamazepine is discussed further at the end of this chapter.

Carbamazepine can produce therapeutic responses in patients with bipolar disorder, including some for whom lithium carbonate is not effective. Further, carbamazepine has antidiuretic effects that are sometimes associated with increased concentrations of antidiuretic hormone (ADH) in plasma via mechanisms that are not clearly understood.

Carbamazepine is the primary agent for treatment of trigeminal and glossopharyngeal neuralgias. It is also effective for lightning-type ("tabetic") pain associated with bodily wasting. Carbamazepine is also used in the treatment of bipolar affective disorders, as discussed further in Chapter 16.

Adverse Effects, Drug Interactions, and Toxicity

Acute intoxication with carbamazepine can result in stupor or coma, hyperirritability, convulsions, and respiratory depression. During long-term therapy, the more frequent untoward effects of the drug include drowsiness, vertigo, ataxia, diplopia, and blurred vision. The frequency of seizures may increase, especially with overdose. Other adverse effects include nausea; vomiting; serious hematological toxicity (aplastic anemia, agranulocytosis); and hypersensitivity reactions (dangerous skin reactions, eosinophilia, lymphadenopathy, splenomegaly). A late complication of therapy with carbamazepine is retention of water, with decreased osmolality and concentration of Na^+ in plasma, especially in elderly patients with cardiac disease.

Some tolerance develops to the neurotoxic effects of carbamazepine, and they can be minimized by gradual increase in dosage or adjustment of maintenance dosage. Various hepatic or pancreatic abnormalities have been reported during therapy with carbamazepine, most commonly a transient elevation of hepatic transaminases in plasma in 5%–10% of patients. A transient, mild leukopenia occurs in about 10% of patients during initiation of therapy and usually resolves within the first 4 months of continued treatment; transient thrombocytopenia also has been noted. In about 2% of patients, a persistent leukopenia may develop that requires withdrawal of the drug. The initial concern that aplastic anemia might be a frequent complication of long-term therapy with carbamazepine has not materialized. In most cases, the administration of multiple drugs or the presence of another underlying disease has made it difficult to establish a causal relationship. The prevalence of aplastic anemia appears to be about 1 in 200,000 patients. It is not clear whether monitoring of hematological function can help to avert the development of irreversible aplastic anemia. Carbamazepine is not known to be carcinogenic in humans. Possible teratogenic effects are discussed later in the chapter.

Phenobarbital, phenytoin, and valproate may increase the metabolism of carbamazepine by inducing CYP3A4; carbamazepine may enhance the biotransformation of phenytoin. Concurrent administration of carbamazepine may lower concentrations of valproate, lamotrigine, tiagabine, and topiramate. Carbamazepine reduces both the plasma concentration and the therapeutic effect of haloperidol. The metabolism of carbamazepine may be inhibited by propoxyphene, erythromycin, cimetidine, fluoxetine, and isoniazid.

Oxcarbazepine

Oxcarbazepine is FDA-approved for monotherapy or adjunct therapy for focal seizures in adults, as monotherapy for focal seizures in children ages 4–16, and as adjunctive therapy in children aged 2–16 years. Oxcarbazepine

(10,11-dihydro-10-oxocarbamazepine) is a keto analogue of carbamazepine and is a prodrug that is rapidly converted to its metabolite, eslicarbazepine. Eslicarbazepine is then extensively converted to its S(+) enantiomer, the active metabolite S-licarbazepine. Oxcarbazepine is inactivated by glucuronide conjugation, is eliminated by renal excretion, and has a short $t_{1/2}$ of only about 1–2 h.

Oxcarbazepine has a mechanism of action similar to that of carbamazepine but is a less-potent enzyme inducer than carbamazepine. Substitution of oxcarbazepine for carbamazepine is associated with increased levels of phenytoin and valproate, presumably because of reduced induction of hepatic enzymes. Oxcarbazepine does not induce the hepatic enzymes involved in its own degradation. Although oxcarbazepine does not appear to reduce the anticoagulant effect of warfarin, it does induce CYP3A and thus reduces plasma levels of steroid oral contraceptives. Fewer hypersensitivity reactions have been associated with oxcarbazepine, and cross-reactivity with carbamazepine does not always occur. Although most adverse effects are similar to that with carbamazepine, hyponatremia may occur more commonly with oxcarbazepine than with carbamazepine.

Eslicarbazepine Acetate

Eslicarbazepine acetate is a prodrug approved in the U.S. as a monotherapy and adjunctive treatment of focal-onset seizures. Eslicarbazepine is converted to its active metabolite S-licarbazepine faster than its prodrug, oxcarbazepine; eslicarbazepine has a similar mechanism of action as oxcarbazepine because both are prodrugs that produce the same active metabolite, S-licarbazepine. Eslicarbazepine competitively inhibits fast voltage-gated sodium channels, stabilizing the inactivated state and the sodium-dependent release of neurotransmitters. Eslicarbazepine has a $t_{1/2}$ similar to that of carbamazepine, about 8–12 h, after which it is excreted as a glucuronide. Eslicarbazepine acetate in adults may be initiated at 400–1200 mg/d. Higher doses require careful titration based on patient response. Reduction in dosing is necessary in patients with renal impairment.

Succinimides

Ethosuximide

Ethosuximide is a primary agent for the treatment of generalized absence seizures.

Mechanism of Action

Ethosuximide reduces low threshold T-type Ca^{2+} currents in thalamic neurons (Coulter et al., 1989), and inhibition of T-type currents likely is the mechanism by which ethosuximide inhibits absence seizures. The thalamus plays an important role in generation of 3-Hz spike-and-wave rhythms typical of absence seizures (Huguenard and McCormick, 2007). Neurons in the thalamus exhibit large-amplitude T-type currents that underlie bursts of action potentials and likely play an important role in thalamic oscillatory activity, such as 3-Hz spike-and-wave activity. Ethosuximide reduces this current without modifying the voltage dependence of steady-state inactivation or the time course of recovery from inactivation. Ethosuximide does not inhibit sustained repetitive firing or enhance GABA responses at clinically relevant concentrations.

ADME

Absorption of ethosuximide appears to be complete, with peak C_p occurring within about 3 h after a single oral dose. Ethosuximide is not significantly bound to plasma proteins; during long-term therapy, its concentration in the CSF is similar to that in plasma. The apparent volume of distribution averages 0.7 L/kg.

Approximately 25% of the drug is excreted unchanged in the urine. The remainder is metabolized by hepatic microsomal enzymes, but whether CYPs are responsible is unknown. The major metabolite, the hydroxyethyl derivative, accounts for about 40% of ethosuximide metabolism, is inactive, and is excreted as such and as the glucuronide in the urine. The plasma $t_{1/2}$ of ethosuximide averages between 40 and 50 h in adults and about 30 h in children.

Plasma Drug Concentrations

During long-term therapy, the plasma concentration of ethosuximide averages about 2 μg/mL per daily dose of 1 mg/kg. A plasma concentration of 40–100 μg/mL usually is required for satisfactory control of absence seizures.

Therapeutic Uses

Ethosuximide is effective against absence seizures, but not tonic-clonic seizures. An initial daily dose of 250 mg in children (3–6 years old) and 500 mg in older children, and adult dosage is increased by 250-mg increments at weekly intervals until seizures are adequately controlled or toxicity intervenes. Divided dosage is required occasionally to prevent nausea or drowsiness associated with once-daily dosing. The usual maintenance dose is 20 mg/kg/d. Increased caution is required if the daily dose exceeds 1500 mg in adults or 750–1000 mg in children. The therapeutic use of ethosuximide is discussed further at the end of the chapter.

Adverse Effects and Toxicity

The most common dose-related side effects are GI complaints (nausea, vomiting, and anorexia) and CNS effects (drowsiness, lethargy, euphoria, dizziness, headache, and hiccough). Some tolerance to these effects develops. Parkinson-like symptoms and photophobia have been reported. Restlessness, agitation, anxiety, aggressiveness, inability to concentrate, and other behavioral effects have occurred primarily in patients with a prior history of psychiatric disturbance.

Urticaria and other skin reactions, including Stevens-Johnson syndrome, systemic lupus erythematosus, eosinophilia, leukopenia, thrombocytopenia, pancytopenia, and aplastic anemia, also have been attributed to the drug. The leukopenia may be transient despite continuation of the drug, but several deaths have resulted from bone marrow depression. Renal and hepatic toxicity have not been reported.

Other Antiseizure Drugs

Acetazolamide

Acetazolamide, the prototype for the carbonic anhydrase inhibitors, is discussed in Chapter 25. Its antiseizure actions have been discussed in previous editions of this textbook. Although it is sometimes effective against absence seizures, its usefulness is limited by the rapid development of tolerance. Adverse effects are minimal when it is used in moderate dosage for limited periods.

Ezogabine

Mechanisms of Action

Ezogabine is a first-in-class K^+ channel opener, known as retigabine in the E.U. Ezogabine enhances transmembrane K^+ currents mediated by the KCNQ family of ion channels (i.e., Kv7.2–Kv7.5). Through its activation of the KCNQ channels, ezogabine may stabilize the resting membrane potential and reduce neuronal excitability. In vitro studies suggested that ezogabine may also enhance GABA-mediated currents.

ADME

Dosing in adults is typically initiated at 300 mg per day and gradually titrated to 600–1200 mg/d over several weeks. Ezogabine is rapidly absorbed after oral administration, and absorption is not affected by food. Ezogabine is approximately 80% protein bound in plasma. Ezogabine is metabolized by glucuronidation and acetylation and has a $t_{1/2}$ of 7–11 h; it and its metabolites are excreted in the urine. Thus, ezogabine generally requires dosing thrice daily. Concomitant administration of phenytoin or carbamazepine may reduce plasma concentrations of ezogabine; consequently, an increase in ezogabine dosage should be considered when adding phenytoin or carbamazepine.

Therapeutic Use

Ezogabine was approved in the U.S. as adjunctive treatment of focal-onset seizures in patients aged 18 years and older with inadequate response to alternative ASDs and for whom the benefits outweigh the risk of retinal abnormalities and potential visual acuity deficits. However, the FDA issued a warning for ezogabine citing safety concerns, including blue discoloration and retinal abnormalities. In response, the manufacturer announced that production of ezogabine would cease in June, 2017.

Adverse Effects and Toxicity

The most common adverse effects associated with ezogabine include dizziness, somnolence, fatigue, confusion, and blurred vision. Vertigo, diplopia, memory impairment, gait disturbance, aphasia, dysarthria, and balance problems also may occur. Serious side effects include skin discoloration, QT prolongation, and neuropsychiatric symptoms, including suicidal thoughts and behavior, psychosis, and hallucinations. Due to the presence of Kv7.2–Kv7.5 in the bladder uroepithelium, ezogabine is also associated with urinary retention. Blue pigmentation of skin and lips occurs in as many as one-third of patients maintained on long-term ezogabine therapy. Chronic treatment with ezogabine may cause retinal abnormalities, independent of changes in skin coloration. The FDA has changed the labeling of ezogabine to warn about the risks serious adverse effects, all of which may be permanent. Ezogabine should thus be discontinued if clinical benefit is not achieved after careful titration; however, the discontinuation of ezogabine should be done gradually, while under the care of a physician. In additon, the FDA recommends that all patients taking ezogabine should have baseline and periodic (every 6 months) systemic visual monitoring by an opthalmic professional, which includes both visual acuity and dilated fundus photography.

Felbamate

Felbamate is not indicated as a first-line therapy for any type of seizure activity. Rather, felbamate is FDA-approved for focal seizures in patients who have inadequately responded to alternative ASDs and in patients for whom the severity of their epilepsy outweighs the substantial risk of drug-induced aplastic anemia or liver failure. The potential for such serious and life-threatening adverse effects has limited the clinical utility of felbamate.

Mechanisms of Action

Clinically relevant concentrations of felbamate inhibit NMDA-evoked responses and potentiate GABA-evoked responses in whole-cell, voltage-clamp recordings of cultured rat hippocampal neurons (Rho et al., 1994). This dual action on excitatory and inhibitory transmitter responses may contribute to the wide spectrum of action of the drug in seizure models; however, the mechanism(s) by which felbamate exerts its anticonvulsant activity remain unknown.

Therapeutic Use

Despite the potential serious adverse effects, felbamate is used at doses ranging from 1 to 4 g/d. Clinical studies demonstrate the efficacy of felbamate in patients with poorly controlled focal and secondarily generalized seizures (Sachdeo et al., 1992) and in patients with Lennox-Gastaut syndrome (Felbamate Study Group in Lennox-Gastaut Syndrome, 1993). The clinical efficacy of this unique compound, which inhibits responses to NMDA while potentiating GABAergic neurotransmission, underscores the potential therapeutic value of identifying additional ASDs with novel mechanisms of action.

Gabapentin and Pregabalin

Gabapentin and pregabalin are ASDs that consist of a GABA molecule covalently bound to a lipophilic cyclohexane ring or isobutane, respectively. Gabapentin was designed to be a centrally active GABA agonist, with its high lipid solubility aimed at facilitating its transfer across the blood-brain barrier; the actual mechanism of action is notably different (see below).

Mechanisms of Action

Gabapentin inhibits tonic hind limb extension in the electroshock seizure model. Interestingly, gabapentin also inhibits clonic seizures induced by pentylenetetrazol. Its efficacy in both of these tests parallels that of valproate and distinguishes it from phenytoin and carbamazepine. Despite their design as GABA agonists, neither gabapentin nor pregabalin mimics GABA when iontophoretically applied to neurons in primary culture. Rather, these compounds bind with high affinity to a protein in cortical membranes with an amino acid sequence identical to that of the Ca^{2+} channel subunit α2δ-1 (Gee et al., 1996). This interaction with the α2δ-1 protein may mediate the anticonvulsant effects of gabapentin, but whether and how the binding of gabapentin to the α2δ-1 subunit regulates neuronal excitability remains unclear. Pregabalin binding is reduced but not eliminated in mice carrying a mutation in the α2δ-1 protein (Field et al., 2006). Analgesic efficacy of pregabalin is eliminated in these mice; whether the anticonvulsant effects of pregabalin are also eliminated was not reported.

ADME

Gabapentin and pregabalin are absorbed after oral administration and are not metabolized in humans. These compounds are not bound to plasma proteins and are excreted unchanged, mainly in the urine. Their half-lives, when used as monotherapy, approximate 6 h. These compounds have no known interactions with other ASDs.

Therapeutic Uses

Gabapentin and pregabalin are effective for focal onset seizures, with and without progression to bilateral tonic-clonic seizures, when used in addition to other ASDs. Gabapentin is also indicated for the management of the neuropathic pain associated with postherpetic neuralgia in adults. Pregabalin is FDA-approved as an adjunctive therapy for adults with focal onset seizures. It is also indicated for the management of fibromyalgia and the neuropathic pain associated diabetic peripheral neuropathy, postherpetic neuralgia, or spinal cord injury.

In double-blind, placebo-controlled trials of adults with refractory focal seizures, addition of gabapentin or pregabalin to other ASDs is superior to placebo (French et al., 2003; Sivenius et al., 1991). Gabapentin monotherapy (900 or 1800 mg/d) is equivalent to carbamazepine (600 mg/d) for newly diagnosed focal or generalized epilepsy (Chadwick et al., 1998).

Gabapentin usually is effective in doses of 900–1800 mg daily in three doses, although 3600 mg may be required in some patients to achieve reasonable seizure control. Therapy usually is begun with a low dose (300 mg once on the first day), which is increased in daily increments of 300 mg until an effective dose is reached. In comparison, pregabalin is generally initiated at 50 mg three times a day (150 mg/day) and increase within 1 week to 300 mg/day based on efficacy and tolerability. Since both gabapentin and pregabalin are eliminated by renal excretion, appropriate dose adjustments are necessary in patients with reduced renal function.

Adverse Effects

Overall, gabapentin is well tolerated, with the most common adverse effects of somnolence, dizziness, ataxia, and fatigue. These effects usually are mild to moderate in severity but resolve within 2 weeks of onset during continued treatment. Gabapentin and pregabalin are both listed in pregnancy category C.

Lacosamide

Lacosamide is a stereoselective enantiomer of the amino acid, L-serine. This functionalized amino acid is FDA approved as adjunctive therapy for focal-onset seizures in patients older than 17 years. The FDA assigned lacosamide a Controlled Substance Act (CSA) schedule V designation, meaning it has a low potential for abuse.

Mechanisms of Action

Lacosamide is the first ASD to enhance (prolong) the slow inactivation of voltage-gated Na^+ channels and to limit sustained repetitive firing, the neuronal firing pattern characteristic of focal seizures. Lacosamide also binds collapsin response mediator protein-2 (CRMP-2), a phosphoprotein involved in neuronal differentiation and axon outgrowth, but the contribution of CRMP-2 to lacosamide's antiseizure efficacy remains unclear. Lacosamide was extensively evaluated by the ETSP and found to be highly effective in numerous preclinical animal models of seizures and epilepsy, including maximal electroshock, hippocampal kindling, Frings and 6-Hz models, giving lacosamide a unique preclinical profile compared to other Na^+ channel blockers.

ADME

Peak lacosamide plasma concentrations occur about 1–4 h after oral administration, and food consumption does not affect the absorption. Lacosamide has a $t_{1/2}$ of 12–16 h; 95% is excreted in the urine, about half of which is the unchanged parent compound. The major metabolite, O-desmethyl-lacosamide, is inactive.

Therapeutic Uses

Lacosamide is approved for both monotherapy and add-on therapy for focal-onset seizures in patients 17 years and older. As a monotherapy for the treatment of focal seizures, the initial recommended dose is 50–100 mg twice daily and, depending on patient response, may be increased at weekly intervals by 50 mg twice daily to a recommended maintenance dose of 100 mg to 200 mg twice daily, or 200–400 mg/d. The pharmacological profile is advantageous for hospitalized patients because it is available in an intravenous formulation, has minimal hepatic metabolism, and has no adverse respiratory effects. In addition, double-blind, placebo-controlled studies of adults with refractory focal seizures suggest that addition of lacosamide to other ASDs is superior to the addition of placebo.

Adverse Effects

Lacosamide is generally well tolerated. Although it has been associated with a brief (6-ms) prolongation of the PR interval, well-controlled studies in healthy patients suggested lacosamide does not prolong the QT interval. However, patients who are taking concomitant agents that prolong the PR internal should have a baseline electrocardiogram before starting lacosamide and be closely monitored due to a risk of AV block or bradycardia. Patients with renal impairment or hepatic impairment who are taking inhibitors of CYP3A4 or CYP2C9 may experience a significant increase in lacosamide exposure. No major adverse effects have been reported, although minor adverse effects include headache, dizziness, double vision, nausea, vomiting, fatigue, tremor, loss of balance, and somnolence. Like most currently available ASDs, lacosamide may contribute to suicidal ideations and suicide. As a consequence, the FDA has mandated a black-box warning for this agent.

Lamotrigine

Lamotrigine is a phenyltriazine derivative initially developed as an antifolate agent, based on the incorrect idea that reducing folate would effectively combat seizures. Structure-activity studies have since indicated that its effectiveness as an ASD is unrelated to its antifolate properties (Macdonald and Greenfield, 1997).

Mechanisms of Action

Lamotrigine suppresses tonic hind limb extension in the maximal electroshock model and focal and secondarily generalized seizures in the kindling model, but does not inhibit clonic motor seizures induced by pentylenetetrazol. Lamotrigine blocks sustained repetitive firing of mouse spinal cord neurons and delays the recovery from inactivation of recombinant Na^+ channels, mechanisms similar to those of phenytoin and carbamazepine (Xie et al., 1995). This may well explain lamotrigine's actions on focal and secondarily generalized seizures. However, as mentioned below, lamotrigine is effective against a broader spectrum of seizures than are phenytoin and carbamazepine, suggesting that lamotrigine may have actions in addition to regulating recovery from inactivation of Na^+ channels. One possibility, supported by basic research, is that lamotrigine inhibits synaptic release of glutamate by acting at Na^+ channels themselves.

ADME

Lamotrigine is completely absorbed from the GI tract. The drug is metabolized primarily by glucuronidation, yielding a plasma $t_{1/2}$ of a single dose of 24–30 h. Administration of phenytoin, carbamazepine, or phenobarbital reduces the $t_{1/2}$ and plasma concentrations of lamotrigine. Conversely, addition of valproate markedly increases plasma concentrations of lamotrigine, likely by inhibiting glucuronidation. Addition of lamotrigine to valproate produces a reduction of valproate concentrations by about 25% over a few weeks. Concurrent use of lamotrigine and carbamazepine is associated with increases of the 10,11-epoxide of carbamazepine and clinical toxicity in some patients.

Therapeutic Use

Lamotrigine is useful for monotherapy and add-on therapy of focal and secondarily generalized tonic-clonic seizures in adults and Lennox-Gastaut syndrome in both children and adults. Lennox-Gastaut syndrome is a disorder of childhood characterized by multiple seizure types, mental retardation, and refractoriness to antiseizure medication.

Lamotrigine monotherapy in newly diagnosed focal or generalized tonic-clonic seizures is equivalent to monotherapy with carbamazepine or phenytoin (Brodie et al., 1995; Steiner et al., 1999). Addition of lamotrigine to existing ASDs is effective against tonic-clonic seizures and drop attacks in children with the Lennox-Gastaut syndrome (Motte et al., 1997). Lamotrigine is also superior to placebo in children with newly diagnosed absence epilepsy (Frank et al., 1999).

Patients who are already taking a CYP-inducing ASD (e.g., carbamazepine, phenytoin, phenobarbital, or primidone, but not valproate) should be given lamotrigine initially at 50 mg/d for 2 weeks. The dose is increased to 50 mg twice per day for 2 weeks and then increased in increments of 100 mg/d each week up to a maintenance dose of 300–500 mg/d divided into two doses. For patients taking valproate in addition to an enzyme-inducing ASD, the initial dose should be 25 mg every other day for 2 weeks, followed by an increase to 25 mg/d for 2 weeks; the dose then can be increased by 25–50 mg/d every 1–2 weeks up to a maintenance dose of 100–150 mg/d divided into two doses.

Adverse Effects

The most common adverse effects are dizziness, ataxia, blurred or double vision, nausea, vomiting, and rash when lamotrigine is added to another ASD. A few cases of Stevens-Johnson syndrome and disseminated intravascular coagulation have been reported. The incidence of serious rash in pediatric patients (~0.8%) is higher than in the adult population (0.3%).

Levetiracetam and Brivaracetam

Levetiracetam is a pyrrolidine, the racemically pure S-enantiomer of α-ethyl-2-oxo-1-pyrrolidineacetamide, and is FDA-approved for adjunctive therapy for myoclonic, focal-onset, and generalized onset tonic-clonic seizures in adults and children as young as 4 years old. Brivaracetam, an analogue of levetiracetam, was FDA-approved in 2016 as an adjunctive therapy for focal-onset seizures in patients aged 16 years and older with epilepsy.

Mechanism of Action

Levetiracetam exhibits a novel pharmacological profile: It inhibits focal and secondarily generalized tonic-clonic seizures in the kindling model, yet is ineffective against maximum electroshock- and pentylenetetrazol-induced seizures, findings consistent with clinical effectiveness against focal and secondarily generalized tonic-clonic seizures. The mechanism by which levetiracetam exerts these antiseizure effects is not fully understood. However, the correlation between binding affinity of levetiracetam and its analogues and their potency toward audiogenic seizures suggests that the synaptic vesicle protein SV2A mediates the anticonvulsant effects of levetiracetam (Rogawski and Bazil, 2008). SV2A is an integral transmembrane glycoprotein; expression of human SV2A in hexose transport-deficient yeast shows that SV2A can function as a galactose transporter (Madeo et al, 2014). The neuronal function of the SV2A protein is not fully understood, but binding of levetiracetam to SV2A might affect neuronal excitability by modifying the release of glutamate and GABA through an action on vesicular function. In mice, a missense mutation in SV2A is reportedly associated with disruption of action-potential invoked GABA release in limbic regions (Ohno and Tokudome, 2017). Other workers have suggested that SV2A may play a role in vesicle recycling following exocytosis of neurotransmitter (Bartolome, et al., 2017). In addition, levetiracetam inhibits N-type Ca^{2+} channels and Ca^{2+} release from intracellular stores.

Brivaracetam binds with high affinity to SV2A and inhibits neuronal voltage-gated Na^+ channels (Kenda et al., 2004; Zona et al., 2010); preclinical studies suggested a broad spectrum of anticonvulsant protection (Matagne et al., 2008).

ADME

Levetiracetam is rapidly and almost completely absorbed after oral administration and is not bound to plasma proteins. The plasma $t_{1/2}$ is 6–8 h, but may be longer in elderly patients. Ninety-five percent of the drug and its inactive metabolite are excreted in the urine, 65% of which is unchanged drug; 24% of the drug is metabolized by hydrolysis of the acetamide group. Because levetiracetam neither induces nor is a high-affinity substrate for CYPs or glucuronidation enzymes, it is devoid of known interactions with other ASDs, oral contraceptives, or anticoagulants.

Brivaracetam is rapidly absorbed and well tolerated, with an elimination $t_{1/2}$ of approximately 7–8 h.

Therapeutic Use

Levetiracetam is marketed for the adjunctive treatment of focal seizures in adults and children, for primary onset tonic-clonic seizures, and for myoclonic seizures of JME. It is available in tablet (10, 25, 50, 75, or 100 mg), oral solution (10 mg/mL), or injectable form (50 mg/5 mL). Adult dosing is initiated at 500–1000 mg/d and increased every 2–4 weeks by 1000 mg to a maximum dose of 3000 mg/d. The drug is administered twice daily. In adults with either refractory focal seizures or uncontrolled generalized tonic-clonic seizures associated with idiopathic generalized epilepsy, addition of levetiracetam to other antiseizure medications is superior to placebo. Levetiracetam also has efficacy as adjunctive therapy for refractory generalized myoclonic seizures (Andermann et al., 2005). Insufficient evidence is available about its use as monotherapy for focal or generalized epilepsy.

The recommended starting dose for brivaracetam is 50 mg twice daily, which may be adjusted to either 25 mg twice daily or 100 mg twice daily, based on patient response and tolerability.

Adverse Effects

Both levetiracetam and brivaracetam are well tolerated. The most frequently reported adverse effects associated with levetiracetam are somnolence, asthenia, ataxia, and dizziness. Behavioral and mood changes are serious, but less common. For brivaracetam, the most common adverse effects are similarly mild and include somnolence, sedation, dizziness, and GI upset. In patients with hepatic insufficiency, dose adjustment may be required with brivaracetam to 25 mg twice daily and a maximal dosage of 75 mg twice daily. Hypersensitivity reactions may occur.

Perampanel

Mechanisms of Action

Perampanel is a first-in class selective, noncompetitive antagonist of the AMPA-type ionotropic glutamate receptor (Bialer and White, 2010; Stephen and Brodie, 2011). Unlike NMDA antagonists, which shorten the duration of repetitive discharges, AMPA receptor antagonists prevent repetitive neuronal firing. Preclinical studies demonstrated a broad spectrum of activity in both acute and chronic seizure models, indicating that perampanel reduces fast excitatory signaling critical to the seizure generation (Tortorella et al., 1997) and spread (Namba et al., 1994; Rogawski and Donevan, 1999). Perampanel seems to have a greater inhibitory effect on seizure propagation than on seizure initiation (Hanada et al., 2011).

ADME and Drug Interactions

Perampanel is absorbed well after oral administration with a plasma $t_{1/2}$ of about 105 h, permitting once-daily administration. The drug is 95% bound to plasma protein, mainly albumin, and is metabolized by hepatic oxidation and glucuronidation. A linear relationship between perampanel dose and plasma concentration has been reported over the dose range of 2–12 mg/d.

Primary metabolism is mediated by hepatic CYP3A; thus, specific drug interactions and dose adjustments need to be considered. For example, perampanel may decrease the effectiveness of progesterone-containing hormone contraceptives, carbamazepine, clobazam, lamotrigine, and valproate, but it may increase the level of oxcarbazepine. Furthermore, serum perampanel may be decreased when taken with carbamazepine, oxcarbazepine, and topiramate.

Therapeutic Use

Perampanel is FDA-approved as an adjunctive therapy for the treatment of focal-onset seizures in patients 12 years and older with or without secondarily generalized seizures. The recommended oral starting dose is 2 mg once daily, titrated to a maximal dose of 4–12 mg/d at bedtime.

Adverse Effects

Common adverse effects include somnolence, anxiety, confusion, imbalance, double vision, dizziness, GI distress or nausea, and weight gain. Rare, but serious, adverse behavioral reactions, including hostility, aggression, and suicidal thoughts and behaviors, independent of clinical history of psychiatric disorder, have also been reported.

Rufinamide

Rufinamide, a triazole derivative, is structurally unrelated to other marketed ASDs. It is FDA-approved for adjunctive treatment of seizures related to Lennox-Gastaut syndrome in children more than 4 years old and adults.

Mechanism of Action

Rufinamide prolongs slow inactivation of voltage-gated Na^+ channels and limits sustained repetitive firing, the firing pattern characteristic of focal seizures. The complete mechanism of action of rufinamide remains unclear.

ADME

Rufinamide is well absorbed orally, binds minimally to plasma proteins, and reaches peak plasma concentrations about 4–6 h after oral administration. The $t_{1/2}$ is 6–10 h. Rufinamide is metabolized independent of CYPs and then excreted in the urine.

Therapeutic Use

Rufinamide has been shown to be effective against all seizure phenotypes in Lennox-Gastaut syndrome. In adults, 400–800 mg/d rufinamide is initially administered in two equal doses. Doses are then titrated upward every other day by 10 mg/kg to a maximum of the lesser of 45 mg/kg/d or 3200 mg/d. Children are initiated at 10 mg/kg/d divided into two equal daily doses, increasing to a maximum of the lesser of 45 mg/kg/d or 3200 mg/d.

Adverse Effects

Common adverse effects include headache, dizziness, somnolence, fatigue, and nausea.

Stiripentol

Stiripentol is an aromatic alcohol, structurally unrelated to any other ASDs. Stiripentol was granted orphan drug status for the treatment of Dravet syndrome in 2008 but has not received FDA approval due its complex pharmacokinetic and pharmacodynamic interactions with other drugs.

Mechanisms of Action

Although the exact nature of its antiseizure mechanism is not clear, stiripentol may increase CNS levels of the inhibitory transmitter GABA by inhibition of synaptosomal uptake of GABA or by inhibition of GABA transaminase. In model systems, stiripentol also enhances $GABA_A$ receptor–mediated neurotransmission and increases the mean open duration of $GABA_A$ receptor chloride channels in a barbiturate-like fashion (Fisher, 2011; Quilichini et al., 2006).

ADME and Drug Interactions

Stiripentol is quickly absorbed, reaching a peak C_p in about 1.5 h; the drug is highly bound to plasma proteins. Stiripentol's elimination kinetics are nonlinear, with a $t_{1/2}$ ranging from 4 to 13 h. Plasma clearance decreases markedly at high doses and after repeated administration, probably due to inhibition or saturation of the CYPs responsible for stiripentol metabolism. Metabolites are excreted in the urine.

Stiripentol has diverse pharmacokinetic and pharmacodynamic interactions with concomitantly administered drugs. It is a potent inhibitor of CYPs 3A4, 1A2, and 2C19. Thus, adjunctively administered ASDs, such as carbamazepine, valproate, phenytoin, phenobarbital, and benzodiazepines, may require dose adjustments due to the potent inhibition of CYPs involved in their hepatic metabolism. Concomitant stiripentol can increase clobazam and valproate concentrations by 2- to 3-fold, and dose reduction of either or both ASDs may be necessary to avoid toxicity.

Therapeutic Use

Stiripentol is used clinically in conjunction with clobazam and valproate as an adjunctive therapy for refractory generalized tonic-clonic seizures in patients with severe myoclonic epilepsy in infancy (Dravet syndrome) whose seizures are not adequately controlled with clobazam and valproate (Aneja and Sharma, 2013; Plosker, 2012). Adjunctive stiripentol in children with Dravet syndrome who fail to respond to valproate and clobazam have a 71% response rate (Chiron et al., 2000; Nabbout and Chiron, 2012). Stiripentol also reduces the frequency and severity of tonic-clonic seizures as well as status epilepticus in infants and children with a variety of epilepsy syndromes (Inoue et al., 2009; Perez et al., 1999; Rey et al., 1999).

Use of stiripentol is replete with potential drug interactions (see the section on ADME) that must be considered. Initiation of adjunctive therapy with stiripentol should be undertaken gradually, with frequent plasma monitoring for both the parent ASDs and their active metabolites. Plasma monitoring is important to inform reductions in concomitant ASDs as needed, based on patient response.

Adverse Effects

The most commonly reported adverse effects in patients on stiripentol include anorexia, weight loss, insomnia, drowsiness, ataxia, hypotonia, and dystonia.

Tiagabine

Tiagabine is a derivative of nipecotic acid and is FDA-approved as adjunct therapy for focal seizures in adults.

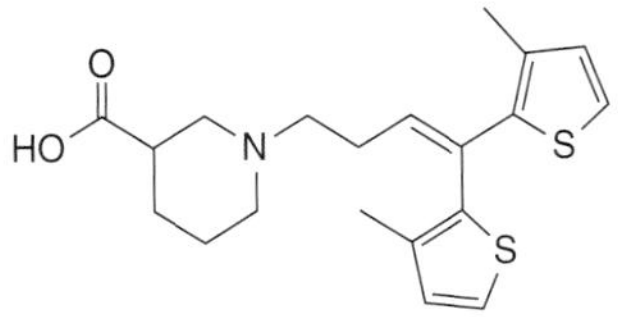

TIAGABINE
(nipecotic acid in black)

Mechanism of Action

Tiagabine inhibits the GABA transporter GAT-1 and thereby reduces GABA uptake into neurons and glia and prolongs the dwell time of GABA in the synaptic space. In CA1 neurons of the hippocampus, tiagabine increases the duration of inhibitory synaptic currents, findings consistent with prolonging the effect of GABA at inhibitory synapses through reducing its reuptake by GAT-1. Tiagabine inhibits maximum electroshock seizures and both limbic and secondarily generalized tonic-clonic seizures in the kindling model, results suggestive of clinical efficacy against focal and tonic-clonic seizures.

ADME

Tiagabine is rapidly absorbed after oral administration, extensively bound to serum proteins, and metabolized mainly in the liver, predominantly by CYP3A. Its $t_{1/2}$ of about 8 h is shortened by 2–3 h when coadministered with CYP-inducing drugs such as phenobarbital, phenytoin, or carbamazepine.

Therapeutic Use

Tiagabine is efficacious as add-on therapy for refractory focal seizures with or without secondary generalization. Its efficacy as monotherapy for newly diagnosed or refractory focal and generalized epilepsy has not been established.

Adverse Effects and Precautions

The principal adverse effects include dizziness, somnolence, and tremor; they are mild to moderate in severity and appear shortly after initiation of therapy. Tiagabine and other drugs that enhance effects of synaptically released GABA can facilitate spike-and-wave discharges in animal models of absence seizures. Case reports suggest that tiagabine treatment of patients with a history of spike-and-wave discharges causes exacerbations of their EEG abnormalities. Thus, tiagabine may be contraindicated in patients with generalized absence epilepsy. Paradoxically, tiagabine has been associated with the occurrence of seizures in patients without epilepsy; thus, off-label use of the drug is discouraged.

Topiramate

Topiramate is a sulfamate-substituted monosaccharide that is FDA-approved as initial monotherapy (in patients at least 10 years old) and as adjunctive therapy (for patients as young as 2 years) for focal-onset or primary generalized tonic-clonic seizures, for Lennox-Gastaut syndrome in patients 2 years of age and older, and for migraine headache prophylaxis in adults.

Mechanisms of Action

Topiramate reduces voltage-gated Na^+ currents in cerebellar granule cells and may act on the inactivated state of the channel similarly to phenytoin. In addition, topiramate activates a hyperpolarizing K^+ current, enhances postsynaptic $GABA_A$ receptor currents, and limits activation of the AMPA-kainate subtype(s) of glutamate receptors. The drug is a weak inhibitor of carbonic anhydrase. Topiramate inhibits maximal electroshock and pentylenetetrazol-induced seizures as well as focal and secondarily generalized tonic-clonic seizures in the kindling model, findings predictive of a broad spectrum of antiseizure actions clinically.

ADME

Topiramate is rapidly absorbed after oral administration, exhibits little (10%–20%) binding to plasma proteins, and is excreted largely unchanged in the urine. A small fraction undergoes metabolism by hydroxylation, hydrolysis, and glucuronidation, with no single metabolite accounting for more than 5% of an oral dose. Its $t_{1/2}$ is about 1 day. Reduced estradiol plasma concentrations occur with concurrent topiramate, suggesting the need for higher doses of oral contraceptives when coadministered with topiramate.

Therapeutic Use

Topiramate is equivalent to valproate and carbamazepine in children and adults with newly diagnosed focal and primary generalized epilepsy (Privitera et al., 2003). The agent is effective as monotherapy for refractory focal epilepsy (Sachdeo et al., 1997) and refractory generalized tonic-clonic seizures (Biton et al., 1999). Topiramate is significantly more effective than placebo against both drop attacks and tonic-clonic seizures in patients with Lennox-Gastaut syndrome (Sachdeo et al., 1999).

Adverse Effects

Topiramate is well tolerated. The most common adverse effects are somnolence, fatigue, weight loss, and nervousness. It may precipitate renal calculi (kidney stones), probably due to inhibition of carbonic anhydrase. Topiramate has been associated with cognitive impairment, and patients may complain about a change in the taste of carbonated beverages.

Valproate

The antiseizure properties of valproic acid were discovered serendipitously when it was employed as a vehicle for other compounds that were being screened for antiseizure activity. Valproate (*n*-dipropylacetic acid) is a simple branched-chain carboxylic acid. Certain other branched-chain carboxylic acids have potencies similar to that of valproic acid in antagonizing pentylenetetrazol-induced seizures. However, increasing the number of carbon atoms to nine introduces marked sedative properties. Straight-chain carboxylic acids have little or no activity.

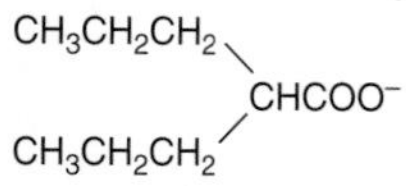

$$\begin{array}{l} CH_3CH_2CH_2 \diagdown \\ \qquad\qquad\qquad CHCOO^- \\ CH_3CH_2CH_2 \diagup \end{array}$$

VALPROATE

Pharmacological Effects

Valproate is strikingly different from phenytoin or ethosuximide in that it is effective in inhibiting seizures in a variety of models. Like phenytoin and carbamazepine, valproate inhibits tonic hind limb extension in maximal electroshock seizures and kindled seizures at nontoxic doses. Like ethosuximide, valproate at subtoxic doses inhibits clonic motor seizures induced by pentylenetetrazol. Its efficacy in diverse models parallels its efficacy against absence as well as focal and generalized tonic-clonic seizures in humans.

Mechanisms of Action

Valproate produces effects on isolated neurons similar to those of phenytoin and ethosuximide. At therapeutically relevant concentrations, valproate inhibits sustained repetitive firing induced by depolarization of mouse cortical or spinal cord neurons (McLean and Macdonald, 1986b). The action is similar to that of phenytoin and carbamazepine (Table 17–2) and appears to be mediated by a prolonged recovery of voltage-activated Na^+ channels from inactivation. Valproate does not modify neuronal responses to iontophoretically applied GABA. In neurons isolated from the nodose ganglion, valproate also produces small reductions of T-type Ca^{2+} currents (Kelly et al., 1990) at clinically relevant concentrations that are slightly higher than those that limit sustained repetitive firing; this effect on T-type currents is similar to that of ethosuximide in thalamic neurons (Coulter et al., 1989). Together, these actions of limiting sustained repetitive firing and reducing T-type currents may contribute to the effectiveness of valproate against focal and tonic-clonic seizures and absence seizures, respectively.

In model systems, valproate can increase brain content of GABA, stimulate GABA synthesis (by glutamate decarboxylase), and inhibit GABA degradation (by GABA transaminase and succinic semialdehyde dehydrogenase). Such data notwithstanding, it has been difficult to relate the increased GABA levels to the antiseizure activity of valproate. Valproate is also a potent inhibitor of histone deacetylase. Thus, some of its antiseizure activity may be due to its ability to modulate gene expression through this mechanism.

ADME

Valproate is absorbed rapidly and completely after oral administration. Peak C_p occurs in 1 to 4 h, although this can be delayed for several hours if the drug is administered in enteric-coated tablets or is ingested with meals. Its extent of binding to plasma proteins is usually about 90%, but the fraction bound is reduced as the total concentration of valproate is increased through the therapeutic range. Although concentrations of valproate in CSF suggest equilibration with free drug in the blood, there is evidence for carrier-mediated transport of valproate both into and out of the CSF.

Valproate undergoes hepatic metabolism (95%), with less than 5% excreted unchanged in urine. Its hepatic metabolism occurs mainly by UGTs and β-oxidation. Valproate is a substrate for CYPs 2C9 and 2C19, but these enzymes account for a relatively minor portion of its elimination. Some of the drug's metabolites, notably 2-propyl-2-pentenoic acid and 2-propyl-4-pentenoic acid, are nearly as potent antiseizure agents as the parent compound; however, only the former accumulates in plasma and brain to a potentially significant extent. The $t_{1/2}$ of valproate is about 15 h but is reduced in patients taking other antiseizure drugs.

Plasma Drug Concentrations

Valproate plasma concentrations associated with therapeutic effects are about 30–100 μg/mL. However, there is a poor correlation between the plasma concentration and efficacy. There appears to be a threshold at about 30–50 μg/mL, the concentration at which binding sites on plasma albumin begin to become saturated.

Therapeutic Uses

Valproate is a broad-spectrum ASD effective in the treatment of absence, myoclonic, focal, and tonic-clonic seizures. The initial daily dose usually is 15 mg/kg, increased at weekly intervals by 5–10 mg/kg/d to a maximum daily dose of 60 mg/kg. Divided doses should be given when the total daily dose exceeds 250 mg. The therapeutic uses of valproate in epilepsy are discussed further at the end of this chapter.

Adverse Effects and Drug Interactions

The most frequent side effects are transient GI symptoms, including anorexia, nausea, and vomiting (~16%). Effects on the CNS include sedation, ataxia, and tremor; these symptoms occur infrequently and usually respond to a decrease in dosage. Rash, alopecia, and stimulation of appetite have been observed occasionally; weight gain has been seen with chronic valproate treatment in some patients. Elevation of hepatic transaminases in plasma is observed in up to 40% of patients and often occurs asymptomatically during the first several months of therapy.

A rare but frequently fatal complication is fulminant hepatitis. Children below 2 years of age with other medical conditions who were given multiple ASDs were especially likely to suffer fatal hepatic injury; there were no deaths reported for patients over the age of 10 years who received only valproate (Dreifuss et al., 1989). Acute pancreatitis and hyperammonemia have been frequently associated with the use of valproate. This agent can also produce teratogenic effects, such as neural tube defects.

Valproate inhibits the metabolism of drugs that are substrates for CYP2C9, including phenytoin and phenobarbital. Valproate also inhibits UGTs and thus inhibits the metabolism of lamotrigine and lorazepam. The high molar concentrations of valproate used clinically result in valproate's displacing phenytoin and other drugs from albumin. With respect to phenytoin in particular, valproate's inhibition of that drug's metabolism is exacerbated by displacement of phenytoin from albumin. The concurrent administration of valproate and clonazepam is associated with the development of absence status epilepticus; however, this complication appears to be rare.

Vigabatrin

Vigabatrin is FDA-approved as adjunct therapy of refractory focal seizures with impaired awareness in adults. In addition, vigabatrin is designated as an orphan drug for treatment of infantile spasms (described in the Therapeutic Use section that follows).

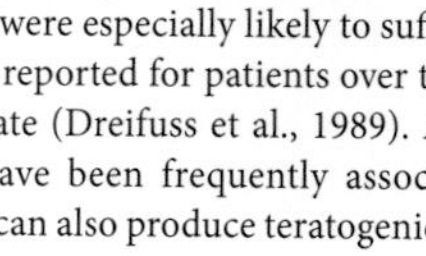

OH, H, O, CH_2, NH_2

VIGABATRIN

Mechanism of Action

Vigabatrin, a structural analogue of GABA, irreversibly inhibits the major degradative enzyme for GABA, GABA transaminase, thereby leading to increased concentrations of GABA in the brain. This effect is hypothesized to result in increased extracellular GABA at its receptors and enhanced GABAergic transmission.

ADME

An oral dose is well absorbed, reaching a maximal C_p within 1 h; the presence of food prolongs absorption but does not reduce the area under the curve. Vigabatrin is excreted unmetabolized by the kidney, and the dose must be reduced for patients with renal impairment. Although vigabatrin has a $t_{1/2}$ of only 6–8 h, the pharmacodynamic effects are prolonged and do not correlate well with plasma $t_{1/2}$ or the C_p. Such kinetics would be expected due to the irreversible nature of the drug's inhibition of GABA transaminase and a recovery period that reflects the rate of enzyme resynthesis rather than the rate of drug elimination. Vigabatrin induces CYP2C9.

Therapeutic Use

Adult dosing is generally initiated orally at 500 mg twice daily and then increased in 500-mg increments weekly to 1.5 g twice daily.

A 2-week, randomized, single masked clinical trial of vigabatrin for infantile spasms in children younger than 2 years revealed time- and dose-dependent increases in responders, evident as freedom from spasms for 7 consecutive days. Children in whom infantile spasms were caused by tuberous sclerosis were particularly responsive to vigabatrin. As with other ASDs, vigabatrin should be withdrawn slowly, not stopped abruptly.

Toxicity, Adverse Effects, and Precautions

Due to progressive and permanent bilateral vision loss (FDA box warning), vigabatrin must be reserved for patients who have failed several alternative therapies. A patient's vision must be professionally monitored at the beginning of therapy and regularly throughout and after a therapeutic course. Due to this serious toxicity, vigabatrin is available only through SHARE (1-888-45-SHARE), a restricted distribution program.

The most common side effects (>10% patients) include weight gain, concentric visual field constriction, fatigue, somnolence, dizziness, hyperactivity, and seizures. Data in animal models suggest that vigabatrin may harm a developing fetus, and the drug is classified in pregnancy category C. Vigabatrin is excreted in the milk of nursing mothers.

Zonisamide

Zonisamide is FDA-approved as adjunctive therapy of focal seizures in adults 12 years or older.

Mechanism of Action

Zonisamide inhibits the sustained, repetitive firing of spinal cord neurons, presumably by prolonging the inactivated state of voltage-gated Na^+ channels in a manner similar to actions of phenytoin and carbamazepine and by preventing neurotransmitter release. In addition, zonisamide inhibits T-type Ca^{2+} currents and reduces the influx of calcium. Zonisamide can also inhibit carbonic anhydrase and scavenge free radicals; whether and how these actions may contribute to the drug's neuroprotective effects are unknown.

ADME

Zonisamide is almost completely absorbed after oral administration, has a long $t_{1/2}$ (~60 h), is about 40% bound to plasma protein, and has linear kinetics at doses ranging from 100 to 400 mg. Approximately 85% of an oral dose is excreted in the urine, principally as unmetabolized zonisamide and a glucuronide of sulfamoylacetyl phenol, the product of metabolism by CYP3A4. Thus, phenobarbital, phenytoin, and carbamazepine will decrease the plasma concentration/dose ratio of zonisamide, whereas lamotrigine will increase this ratio. Zonisamide has little effect on the plasma concentrations of other ASDs.

Therapeutic Use

The addition of zonisamide to other drugs is superior to placebo. There is insufficient evidence for zonisamide's efficacy as monotherapy for newly diagnosed or refractory epilepsy.

Toxicity

Overall, zonisamide is well tolerated. The most common adverse effects include somnolence, dizziness, cognitive impairment, ataxia, anorexia, nervousness, and fatigue. Potentially serious skin rashes are rare but may occur. Approximately 1% of individuals develop renal calculi during treatment, which may relate to inhibition of carbonic anhydrase by zonisamide. As a carbonic anhydrase inhibitor, zonisamide may also cause metabolic acidosis. Thus, patients with predisposing conditions (e.g., renal disease, severe respiratory disorders, diarrhea, surgery, ketogenic diet) may be at greater risk for metabolic acidosis while taking zonisamide, a risk that appears to be more frequent and severe in younger patients. Measurement of serum bicarbonate prior to initiating therapy and periodically thereafter, even in the absence of symptoms, is recommended. Last, spontaneous abortions and congenital abnormalities have been reported at twice the rate (7%) of the healthy, control population (2%–3%) in female patients of childbearing age receiving polytherapy including zonisamide.

General Principles and Choice of Drugs for Therapy of the Epilepsies

Early diagnosis and treatment of seizure disorders with a single appropriate agent offers the best prospect of achieving prolonged seizure-free periods with the lowest risk of toxicity. An attempt should be made to determine the cause of the epilepsy with the hope of discovering a correctable lesion, either structural or metabolic. The drugs commonly used for distinct seizure types are listed in Table 17–1. The cost/benefit ratio of the efficacy and the adverse effects of a given drug should be considered in determining which drug is optimal for a given patient.

The first decision to make is whether and when to initiate treatment (French and Pedley, 2008). For example, it may not be necessary to initiate therapy after an isolated tonic-clonic seizure in a healthy young adult who lacks a family history of epilepsy and who has a normal neurological exam, a normal EEG, and a normal brain MRI scan. The odds of seizure recurrence in the next year (15%) are similar to the risk of a drug reaction sufficiently severe to warrant discontinuation of medication (Bazil and Pedley, 1998). On the other hand, a similar seizure occurring in an individual with a positive family history of epilepsy, an abnormal neurological exam, an abnormal EEG, and an abnormal MRI carries a risk of recurrence approximating 60%, odds that favor initiation of therapy.

Unless extenuating circumstances such as status epilepticus exist, only monotherapy should be initiated. Initial dosing should target a C_{pss} within the lower portion of the range associated with clinical efficacy to minimize dose-related adverse effects. Dosage is increased at appropriate intervals as required for control of seizures or as limited by toxicity, with monitoring of plasma drug concentrations. Compliance with a properly selected, single drug in maximal tolerated dosage results in complete control of seizures in about 50% of patients. If a seizure occurs despite optimal drug levels, the physician should assess the presence of potential precipitating factors such as sleep deprivation, a concurrent febrile illness, or drugs (e.g., large amounts of caffeine or over-the-counter medications that can lower the seizure threshold).

If compliance has been confirmed yet seizures persist, substitute another drug. Unless serious adverse effects of the drug dictate otherwise, always reduce dosage gradually to minimize risk of seizure recurrence. In the case of focal seizures in adults, the diversity of available drugs permits selection of a second drug that acts by a different mechanism (see Table 17–2). Among previously untreated patients, 47% became seizure free with the first drug and an additional 14% became seizure free with a second or third drug (Kwan and Brodie, 2000).

If therapy with a second single drug also is inadequate, combination therapy is warranted. This decision should not be taken lightly because most patients obtain optimal seizure control with the fewest adverse effects when taking a single drug. Nonetheless, some patients will not be controlled adequately without the simultaneous use of two or more ASDs. The chances of complete control with this approach are not high; according to Kwan and Brodie (2000), epilepsy is controlled by treatment with two drugs in only 3% of patients. It seems wise to select two drugs that act by distinct mechanisms (e.g., one that promotes Na^+ channel inactivation and another that enhances GABA-mediated synaptic inhibition). Side effects of each drug and the potential drug interactions also should be considered. As specified in Table 17–3, many of these drugs induce expression of CYPs and thereby affect the metabolism of themselves or other drugs.

Essential to optimal management of epilepsy is the filling out of a seizure chart by the patient or a relative. Frequent visits to the physician may be necessary early in the period of treatment because hematological and other possible side effects may require a change in medication. Long-term follow-up with neurological examinations and possibly EEG and neuroimaging studies is appropriate. *Most crucial for successful management is patient adherence to the drug regimen; noncompliance is the most frequent cause for failure of therapy with ASDs.*

Measurement of plasma drug concentration at appropriate intervals facilitates the initial adjustment of dosage to minimize dose-related adverse effects without sacrificing seizure control. Periodic monitoring during maintenance therapy can also detect noncompliance. Knowledge of plasma drug concentrations can be especially helpful during multidrug therapy. If toxicity occurs, monitoring helps to identify the particular drug(s) responsible and can guide adjustment of dosage.

Duration of Therapy

Once initiated, ASDs are typically continued for at least 2 years. Tapering and discontinuing therapy should be considered if the patient is seizure free after 2 years; tapering should be done slowly over several months.

Factors associated with high risk for recurrent seizures following discontinuation of therapy include EEG abnormalities, known structural lesions, abnormalities on neurological exam, and history of frequent seizures or medically refractory seizures prior to control. Conversely, factors associated with low risk for recurrent seizures include idiopathic epilepsy, normal EEG, onset in childhood, and seizures easily controlled with a single drug. The risk of recurrent seizures ranges from 12% to 66% (French and Pedley, 2008). Typically, 80% of recurrences will occur within 4 months of discontinuing therapy. The clinician and patient must weigh the risk of recurrent seizure and the associated potential deleterious consequences (e.g., loss of driving privileges) against the implications of continuing medication, including cost, unwanted effects, implications of diagnosis of epilepsy, and so on.

Focal and Focal-to-Bilateral Tonic-Clonic Seizures

The efficacy and toxicity of carbamazepine, phenobarbital, and phenytoin for treatment of focal and secondarily generalized tonic-clonic seizures in adults have been examined (Mattson et al., 1985). Carbamazepine and phenytoin were the most effective agents. The choice between carbamazepine and phenytoin required assessment of toxic effects of each drug. Decreased libido and impotence were associated with all three drugs (carbamazepine 13%, phenobarbital 16%, and phenytoin 11%). In direct comparison with valproate, carbamazepine provided superior control of complex focal seizures (Mattson et al., 1992). With respect to adverse effects, carbamazepine was more commonly associated with skin rash, but valproate was more commonly associated with tremor and weight gain. Overall, carbamazepine and phenytoin are preferable for treatment of focal seizures, but phenobarbital and valproate are also efficacious.

Control of secondarily generalized tonic-clonic seizures does not differ significantly with carbamazepine, phenobarbital, or phenytoin (Mattson et al., 1985). Valproate was as effective as carbamazepine for control of secondarily generalized tonic-clonic seizures (Mattson et al., 1992). Because secondarily generalized tonic-clonic seizures usually coexist with focal seizures, these data indicate that among drugs introduced before 1990, carbamazepine and phenytoin are the first-line drugs for these conditions.

One key issue confronting the treating physician is choosing the optimal drug for initiating treatment in new-onset epilepsy. At first glance, this issue may appear unimportant because about 50% of newly diagnosed patients become seizure free with the first drug, whether old or new drugs are used (Kwan and Brodie, 2000). However, responsive patients typically receive the initial drug for several years, underscoring the importance of proper drug selection. Phenytoin, carbamazepine, and phenobarbital induce hepatic CYPs, thereby complicating use of multiple ASDs as well as affecting metabolism of oral contraceptives, warfarin, and many other drugs. Phenytoin, carbamazepine, and phenobarbital also enhance metabolism of endogenous compounds, including gonadal steroids and vitamin D, potentially affecting reproductive function and bone density. By contrast, most of the newer drugs have little, if any effect, on the CYPs. Factors arguing against use of recently introduced drugs include higher costs and less clinical experience with the compounds.

Ideally, a prospective study would systematically compare newly introduced ASDs with drugs available before 1990 in a study design adjusting dose as needed and observing responses for extended periods of time (e.g., 2 years or more), in much the same manner as that used when comparing the older ASDs with one another as described previously (Mattson et al., 1985). Unfortunately, such a study has not been performed. Many studies have compared a new ASD with an older ASD, but study design did not permit declaring a clearly superior drug; moreover, differences in study design and patient populations preclude comparing a new drug with multiple older drugs or with other new drugs.

The use of recently introduced ASDs for newly diagnosed epilepsy was analyzed by subcommittees of the American Academy of Neurology and the American Epilepsy Society (French et al., 2004a, 2004b); the authors concluded that available evidence supported the use of gabapentin, lamotrigine, and topiramate for newly diagnosed focal or mixed seizure disorders. None of these drugs, however, has been approved by the FDA for either of these indications. Insufficient evidence is available on the remaining newly introduced drugs to permit meaningful assessment of their effectiveness for this indication.

Generalized Absence Seizures

Ethosuximide and valproate are considered equally effective in the treatment of generalized absence seizures (Mikati and Browne, 1988). Between 50% and 75% of newly diagnosed patients are free of seizures following therapy with either drug. If tonic-clonic seizures are present or emerge during therapy, valproate is the agent of first choice. Available evidence also indicates that lamotrigine is effective for newly diagnosed absence epilepsy, but lamotrigine is not approved for this indication by the FDA (Ben-Menachem, 2011).

Myoclonic Seizures

Valproate is the drug of choice for myoclonic seizures in the syndrome of JME, in which myoclonic seizures often coexist with tonic-clonic and absence seizures. Levetiracetam also has demonstrated efficacy as adjunctive therapy for refractory generalized myoclonic seizures.

Febrile Convulsions

Between 2% and 4% of children experience a convulsion associated with a febrile illness; 25%–33% of these children will have another febrile convulsion. Only 2%–3% become epileptic in later years, a 6-fold increase in risk compared with the general population. Several factors are associated with an increased risk of developing epilepsy: preexisting neurological disorder or developmental delay, a family history of epilepsy, or a complicated febrile seizure (i.e., the febrile seizure lasted > 15 min, was one sided, or was followed by a second seizure in the same day). If all of these risk factors are present, the risk of developing epilepsy is about 10%.

The increased risk of developing epilepsy or other neurological sequelae led many physicians to prescribe ASDs prophylactically after a febrile seizure. Uncertainties regarding the efficacy of prophylaxis for reducing epilepsy combined with substantial side effects of phenobarbital prophylaxis (Farwell et al., 1990) argue against the use of chronic therapy for prophylactic purposes (Freeman, 1992). For children at high risk of developing recurrent febrile seizures and epilepsy, rectally administered diazepam at the time of fever may prevent recurrent seizures and avoid side effects of chronic therapy.

Seizures in Infants and Young Children

Infantile spasms with *hypsarrhythmia* (abnormal interictal high-amplitude slow waves and multifocal asynchronous spikes on EEG) are refractory to the usual ASD. Corticotropin or glucocorticoids are commonly used; repository corticotropin is designated as an orphan drug for this purpose. Vigabatrin (γ-vinyl GABA) is efficacious in comparison to placebo (Appleton et al., 1999); however, constriction of visual fields has been reported in a high percentage of patients treated with vigabatrin (Miller et al., 1999). To emphasize the potential for progressive and permanent vision loss, the FDA has instituted a black-box warning for vigabatrin, which is marketed under a restrictive distribution program. Vigabatrin has orphan drug status for the treatment of infantile spasms in the U.S. and is FDA-approved as adjunctive therapy for adults with refractory focal seizures with impaired awareness. Ganaxolone also has been designated as an orphan drug for the treatment of infantile spasms and completed a phase II clinical trial for uncontrolled focal-onset seizures in adults in 2009.

The Lennox-Gastaut syndrome is a severe form of epilepsy that usually begins in childhood and is characterized by cognitive impairments and multiple types of seizures, including tonic-clonic, tonic, atonic, myoclonic, and atypical absence seizures. Addition of lamotrigine to other ASDs improves seizure control in comparison to placebo in this treatment-resistant form of epilepsy (Motte et al., 1997). Felbamate also is effective for seizures in this syndrome, but the occasional occurrence of aplastic anemia and hepatic failure have limited its use (French et al., 1999). Topiramate is effective for Lennox-Gastaut syndrome (Sachdeo et al., 1999), and clobazam is approved for the adjunctive treatment in Lennox-Gastaut.

Status Epilepticus and Other Convulsive Emergencies

Status epilepticus is a neurological emergency. Mortality for adults approximates 20% (Lowenstein and Alldredge, 1998). The goal of treatment is rapid termination of behavioral and electrical seizure activity; the longer the episode of status epilepticus goes untreated, the more difficult it is to control and the greater the risk of permanent brain damage. Critical to the management are a clear plan, prompt treatment with effective drugs in adequate doses, and attention to hypoventilation and hypotension. Because hypoventilation may result from high doses of drugs used for treatment, it may be necessary to assist respiration temporarily.

To assess the optimal initial drug regimen, four intravenous treatments have been compared: diazepam followed by phenytoin; lorazepam; phenobarbital; and phenytoin alone (Treiman et al., 1998). The treatments had similar efficacies, with success rates ranging from 44% to 65%. Lorazepam alone was significantly better than phenytoin alone. No significant differences were found with respect to recurrences or adverse reactions. The more recent RAMPART trial indicated that midazolam (intramuscular) is as effective as intravenous lorazepam and was not associated with respiratory distress or seizure recurrence. Thus, emergency treatment with midazolam (intramuscular) may prove to be the preferred treatment prior to arrival to the hospital.

Antiseizure Therapy and Pregnancy

Use of ASDs has diverse implications of great importance for the health of women. Issues include interactions with oral contraceptives, potential teratogenic effects, and effects on vitamin K metabolism in pregnant women (Pack, 2006). Guidelines for the care of women with epilepsy have been published by the American Academy of Neurology (Morrell, 1998).

The effectiveness of oral contraceptives appears to be reduced by concomitant use of ASDs. The failure rate of oral contraceptives is 3.1/100 years in women receiving ASDs compared to a rate of 0.7/100 years in nonepileptic controls. One attractive explanation of the increased failure rate is the increased rate of oral contraceptive metabolism caused by ASDs that induce hepatic enzymes (Table 17–2); particular caution is needed with ASDs that induce CYP3A4.

Teratogenicity

Epidemiological evidence suggests that ASDs have teratogenic effects (Pack, 2006). These teratogenic effects add to the deleterious consequences of oral contraceptive failure. Infants of epileptic mothers are at 2-fold greater risk of major congenital malformations than offspring of nonepileptic mothers (4%–8% compared to 2%–4%). These malformations include congenital heart defects, neural tube defects, cleft lip, cleft palate, and others. Inferring causality from the associations found in large epidemiological studies with many uncontrolled variables can be hazardous, but a causal role for ASDs is suggested by association of congenital defects with higher concentrations of a drug or with polytherapy compared to monotherapy. Phenytoin, carbamazepine, valproate, lamotrigine, and phenobarbital all have been associated with teratogenic effects. Newer ASDs have teratogenic effects in animals, but whether such effects occur in humans is yet uncertain.

One consideration for a woman with epilepsy who wishes to become pregnant is a trial free of ASDs; monotherapy with careful attention to drug levels is another alternative. Polytherapy with toxic levels should be avoided. Folate supplementation (0.4 mg/d) has been recommended by the U.S. Public Health Service for all women of childbearing age to reduce the likelihood of neural tube defects, and this is appropriate for epileptic women as well.

The ASDs that induce CYPs have been associated with vitamin K deficiency in the newborn, which can result in a coagulopathy and intracerebral hemorrhage. Treatment with vitamin K_1, 10 mg/d during the last month of gestation, has been recommended for prophylaxis.

Acknowledgment: *James O. McNamara contributed to this chapter in recent editions of this book. We have retained some of his text in the current edition.*

Bibliography

Andermann E, et al. Seizure control with levetiracetam in juvenile myoclonic epilepsies. *Epilepsia*, **2005**, *46*(suppl 8):205.

Aneja S, Sharma S. Newer anti-epileptic drugs. *Indian Pedatr*, **2013**, *50*: 1033–1040.

Appleton RE, et al. Randomised, placebo-controlled study of vigabatrin as first-line treatment of infantile spasms. *Epilepsia*, **1999**, *40*:1627–1633.

Bartholome O, et al. Puzzling out synaptic vesicle 2 family members functions. *Front Mol Neurosci*, **2017**, *10*:148(1–15).

Bazil CW, Pedley TA. Advances in the medical treatment of epilepsy. *Annu Rev Med*, **1998**, *49*:135–162.

Ben-Menachem E. Mechanism of action of vigabatrin: correcting misperceptions. *Acta Neurol Scand Suppl*, **2011**, *192*:5–15.

Bialer M, White HS. Key factors in the discovery and development of new antiepileptic drugs. *Nat Rev Drug Disc*, **2010**, *9*:68–82.

Biton V, et al. A randomized, placebo-controlled study of topiramate in primary generalized tonic-clonic seizures: Topiramate YTC Study Group. *Neurology*, **1999**, *52*:1330–1337.

Brodie MJ, et al. Double-blind comparison of lamotrigine and carbamazepine in newly diagnosed epilepsy. UK Lamotrigine/Carbamazepine Monotherapy Trial Group. *Lancet*, **1995**, *345*:476–479.

Cai K, et al. The impact of gabapentin administration of brain GABA and glutamate concentrations: a 7T ^{1}H-MRS study. *Neuropsychopharmacology*, **2012**, *37*:2764–2771.

Chadwick DW, et al. A double-blind trial of gabapentin monotherapy for newly diagnosed partial seizures: International Gabapentin Monotherapy Study Group 945–77. *Neurology*, **1998**, *51*:1282–1288.

Drug Facts for Your Personal Formulary: *Antiseizure Agents*

Drugs	Therapeutic Uses (Seizure Types)	Clinical Pharmacology and Tips
Sodium Channel Modulators • Enhance fast inactivation		
Phenytoin	*Focal* • Aware • With impaired awareness *Generalized* • Tonic-clonic	• Once-daily dosing only available with extended-release formulation • Intravenous use with fosphenytoin • Nonlinear pharmacokinetics • May interfere with drugs metabolized by CYP2C9/19 • Induces CYPs (e.g., CYP3A4) • *Side effects*: gingival hyperplasia, facial coarsening; hypersensitivity (rare)
Carbamazepine	*Focal* • Aware • With impaired awareness • Focal to bilateral tonic-clonic *Generalized* • Tonic-clonic	• Induces CYP enzymes (e.g., CYP2C, CYP3A) and UGT • Active metabolite (10,11-epoxide) • *Side effects*: drowsiness, vertigo, ataxia, blurred vision, increased seizure frequency
Eslicarbazepine	*Focal* • Aware • With impaired awareness	
Lamotrigine	*Focal* • Aware • With impaired awareness *Generalized* • Absence • Tonic-clonic	• Reduced half-life in the presence of phenytoin, carbamazepine, or phenobarbital • Increased concentration in the presence of valproate • Also used in Lennox-Gastaut syndrome
Oxcarbazepine	*Focal* • Aware • With impaired awareness	• Prodrug, metabolized to eslicarbazepine • Short half-life • Less-potent enzyme induction (vs. carbamazepine) • *Side effects:* lower incidence of hypersensitivity reactions (vs. carbamazepine)
Rufinamide	*Focal* • Aware • With impaired awareness	• Can be used in Lennox-Gastaut syndrome
Sodium Channel Modulators • Enhance slow inactivation		
Lacosamide	*Focal* • Aware • With impaired awareness	
Calcium Channel Blockers • Block T-type calcium channels		
Ethosuximide	*Generalized* • Absence	• *Side effects*: gastrointestinal complaints, drowsiness, lethargy, dizziness, headache, hypersensitivity/skin reactions • Titration can reduce side-effect occurrence
Zonisamide	*Focal* • Aware • With impaired awareness	• *Side effects*: somnolence, ataxia, anorexia, fatigue
Calcium Channel Modulators • α2δ ligands		
Gabapentin	*Focal* • Aware • With impaired awareness	• *Side effects*: somnolence, dizziness, ataxia, fatigue
Pregabalin	*Focal* • Aware • With impaired awareness	• *Side effects: dizziness, somnolence* • Linear pharmacokinetics • Low potential for drug-drug interactions
GABA-Enhancing Drugs • $GABA_A$ receptor allosteric modulators (benzodiazepines, barbiturates)		
Clonazepam	*Generalized* • Absence • Myoclonic	• *Side effects*: drowsiness, lethargy, behavioral disturbances • Abrupt withdrawal can facilitate seizures • Tolerance to antiseizure effects
Clobazam	*Lennox-Gastaut syndrome* *Generalized* • Atonic • Tonic • Myoclonic	• *N*-Desmethyl-clobazam, clobazam's active metabolite, is increased in patients with poor CYP2C19 metabolism • *Side effects:* somnolence, sedation • Tapered withdrawal recommended

Drug Facts for Your Personal Formulary: *Antiseizure Agents (continued)*

Drugs	Therapeutic Uses (Seizure Types)	Clinical Pharmacology and Tips
GABA-Enhancing Drugs • GABA$_A$ receptor allosteric modulators (benzodiazepines, barbiturates) (continued)		
Diazepam	*Status epilepticus*	• Short duration of action • *Side effects*: drowsiness, lethargy, behavioral disturbances • Abrupt withdrawal can facilitate seizures • Tolerance to antiseizure effects
Phenobarbital	*Focal* • Focal to bilateral tonic-clonic *Generalized* • Tonic-clonic	• Induces CYPs (e.g., CYP3A4) and UGT • *Side effects*: sedation, nystagmus, ataxia; irritability and hyperactivity (children); agitation and confusion (elderly); allergy, hypersensitivity (rare)
Primidone	*Focal* • Focal to bilateral tonic-clonic *Generalized* • Tonic-clonic	• Induces CYP enzymes (e.g., CYP3A4) • Not commonly used
GABA-Enhancing Drugs • GABA uptake/GABA transaminase inhibitors		
Tiagabine	*Focal* • Aware • With impaired awareness	• Metabolized by CYP3A • *Side effects*: dizziness, somnolence, tremor
Stiripentol	*Generalized* • Tonic-clonic (Dravet syndrome)	• Used in Dravet syndrome • Inhibits CYP3A4/2C19
Vigabatrin	*Focal* • With impaired awareness	• Used in infantile spasms, especially when caused by tuberous sclerosis • *Side effects:* can cause progressive and bilateral vision loss
Glutamate Receptor Antagonists • AMPA receptor antagonists		
Perampanel	*Focal* • Aware • With impaired awareness	• Metabolized by CYP3A • *Side effects*: anxiety, confusion, imbalance, visual disturbance, aggressive behavior, suicidal thoughts
Potassium Channel Modulators • KCNQ2-5–positive allosteric modulator		
Ezogabine	*Focal* • Aware • With impaired awareness	• *Side effects*: blue pigmentation of skin and lips, dizziness, somnolence, fatigue, vertigo, tremor, attention disruption, memory impairment, retinal abnormalities, urinary retention, QT prolongation (rare)
Synaptic Vesicle 2A Modulators		
Levetiracetam	*Focal* • Aware • With impaired awareness *Generalized* • Myoclonic • Tonic-clonic	• *Side effects*: somnolence, asthenia, ataxia, dizziness, mood changes
Brivaracetam	*Focal* • Aware • With impaired awareness	
Mixed Mechanisms of Action		
Topiramate	*Focal* • Aware • With impaired awareness *Generalized* • Tonic-clonic	• Used in Lennox-Gastaut syndrome • *Side effects*: somnolence, fatigue, cognitive impairment
Valproate	*Focal* • Aware • With impaired awareness • Focal to bilateral tonic-clonic *Generalized* • Absence • Myoclonic • Tonic-clonic	• *Side effects*: transient gastrointestinal symptoms, sedation, ataxia, tremor, hepatitis (rare) • Inhibits CYP2C9, UGT

Chiron C, et al. Stiripentol in severe myoclonic epilepsy in infancy: a randomized placebo-controlled syndrome-dedicated trial, STICLO study group. *Lancet*, **2000**, *356*:1638–1642.

Coulter DA, et al. Characterization of ethosuximide reduction of low-threshold calcium current in thalamic neurons. *Ann Neurol*, **1989**, *25*:582–593.

Dreifuss FE, et al. Valproic acid hepatic fatalities. II. U.S. experience since 1984. *Neurology*, **1989**, *39*:201–207.

EpiPM Consortium. A roadmap for precision medicine in the epilepsies. *Lancet Neurol*, **2015**, *14*:1219–1228

Farwell JR, et al. Phenobarbital for febrile seizures—effects on intelligence and on seizure recurrence. *N Engl J Med*, **1990**, *322*:364–369.

Felbamate Study Group in Lennox-Gastaut Syndrome. Efficacy of felbamate in childhood epileptic encephalopathy (Lennox-Gastaut Syndrome). *N Engl J Med*, **1993**, *328*:29–33.

Field MJ, et al. Identification of the α_2-δ-1 subunit of voltage-dependent calcium channels as a molecular target for pain mediating the analgesic actions of pregabalin. *Proc Natl Acad Sci USA*, **2006**, *103*: 17537–17542.

Fisher JL. The effects of stiripentol on GABA(A) receptors. *Epilepsia*, **2011**, *52*(suppl 2):76–78.

Fisher RJ, et al. Operational classification of seizure types by the International League Against Epilepsy. *Epilepsia*, **2017**, *58*:522–530.

Frank LM, et al. Lamictal (lamotrigine) monotherapy for typical absence seizure in children. *Epilepsia*, **1999**, *40*:973–979.

Freeman JM. The best medicine for febrile seizures. *N Engl J Med*, **1992**, *327*:1161–1163.

French JA, et al. Efficacy and tolerability of new antiepilepitic drugs. I. Treatment of new-onset epilepsy: report of the TTA and QSS subcommittees of the American Academy of Neurology and American Epilepsy Society. *Neurology*, **2004a**, *62*:1252–1260.

French JA, et al. Efficacy and tolerability of the new antiepileptic drugs. II. Treatment of refractory epilepsy: report of the TTA and QSS subcommittees of the American Academy of Neurology and the American Epilepsy Society. *Neurology*, **2004b**, *62*:1261–1273.

French JA, et al. Dose-response trial of pregabalin adjunctive therapy in patiens with partial seizures. *Neurology*, **2003**, *60*:1631–1637.

French JA, Pedley TA. Initial management of epilepsy. *N Engl J Med*, **2008**, *359*:166–176.

French J, et al. Practice advisory: the use of felbamate in the treatment of patients with intractable epilepsy. Report of the Quality Standards Subcommittee of the American Academy of Neurology and the American Epilepsy Society. *Neurology*, **1999**, *52*:1540–1545.

Gee NS, et al. The novel anticonvulsant drug, gabapentin (Neurontin) binds to the 2 subunit of a calcium channel. *J Biol Chem*, **1996**, *271*:5768–5776.

Hanada T, et al. Perampanel: a novel, orally active, noncompetitive AMPA-receptor antagonist that reduces seizure activity in rodent models of epilepsy. *Epilepsia*, **2011**, *52*:1331–1340.

Huguenard JR, McCormick DA. Thalamic synchrony and dynamic regulation of global forebrain oscillations. *Trends Neurosci*, **2007**, *30*:350–356.

Inoue Y, et al. Stiripentol open study in Japanese patients with Dravet syndrome. *Epilepsia*, **2009**, *50*:2362–2368.

Kelly KM, et al. Valproic acid selectively reduces the low-threshold (T) calcium current in rat nodose neurons. *Neurosci Lett*, **1990**, *116*:233–238.

Kenda BM, et al. Discovery of 4-substituted pyrrolidone butanamides as new agents with significant antiepileptic activity. *J Med Chem*, **2004**, *47*:530–549.

Kwan P, Brodie MJ. Early identification of refractory epilepsy. *N Engl J Med*, **2000**, *342*:314–319.

Larsson OM, et al. Mutual inhibition kinetic analysis of gamma-aminobutyric acid, taurine, and beta-alanine high-affinity transport into neurons and astrocytes: evidence for similarity between the taurine and beta-alanine carriers in both cell types. *J Neurochem*, **1986**, *47*:426–432.

Lowenstein DH, Alldredge BK. Status epilepticus. *N Engl J Med*, **1998**, *338*:970–976.

Macdonald RL, Greenfield LJ Jr. Mechanisms of action of new antiepileptic drugs. *Curr Opin Neurol*, **1997**, *10*:121–128.

Madeo M, et al. The human synaptic vesicle protein, SV2A, functions as a galactose transporter in Saccharomyces cerevisiae. *J Biol Chem*, **2014**, *289*:33066–33071.

Matagne A, et al. Anti-convulsive and anti-epileptic properties of brivaracetam (ucb 34714), a high-affinity ligand for the synaptic vesicle protein, SV2A. *Br J Pharmacol*, **2008**, *154*:1662–1671.

Mattson RH, et al. A comparison of valproate with carbamazepine for the treatment of complex partial seizures and secondarily generalized tonic-clonic seizures in adults. The Department of Veterans Affairs Epilepsy Cooperative Study No. 264 Group. *N Engl J Med*, **1992**, *327*:765–771.

Mattson RH, et al. Comparison of carbamazepine, phenobarbital, phenytoin, and primidone in partial and secondarily generalized tonic-clonic seizures. *N Engl J Med*, **1985**, *313*:145–151.

McLean MJ, Macdonald RL. Carbamazepine and 10,11-epoxycarbamazepine produce use- and voltage-dependent limitation of rapidly firing action potentials of mouse central neurons in cell culture. *J Pharmacol Exp Ther*, **1986a**, *238*:727–738.

McLean MJ, Macdonald RL. Sodium valproate, but not ethosuximide, produces use- and voltage-dependent limitation of high-frequency repetitive firing of action potentials of mouse central neurons in cell culture. *J Pharmacol Exp Ther*, **1986b**, *237*:1001–1011.

McNamara JO. Cellular and molecular basis of epilepsy. *J Neurosci*, **1994**, *14*:3413–3425.

Mikati MA, Browne TR. Comparative efficacy of antiepileptic drugs. *Clin Neuropharmacol*, **1988**, *11*:130–140.

Miller NR, et al. Visual dysfunction in patients receiving vigabatrin: clinical and electrophysiologic findings. *Neurology*, **1999**, *53*:2082–2087.

Morrell MJ. Guidelines for the care of women with epilepsy. *Neurology*, **1998**, *51*:S21–S27.

Motte J, et al. Lamotrigine for generalized seizures associated with the Lennox-Gastaut syndrome. Lamictal Lennox-Gastaut Study Group. *N Engl J Med*, **1997**, *337*:1807–1812.

Nabbout R, Chiron C. Stiripentol: an example of antiepileptic drug development in childhood epilepsies. *Eur J Pediatr Neurol*, **2012**, *16*: S13–S17.

Namba T, et al. Antiepileptogenic and anticonvulsant effects of NBQX, a selective AMPA receptor antagonist, in the rat kindling model of epilepsy. *Brain Res*, **1994**, *638*:36–44.

Ohno Y, Tokudome K. Therapeutic role of synaptic vesicle glycoprotein 2A (SV2A) in modulating epileptogenesis. *CNS Neurol Disord Drug Targets*, **2017**, DOI: 10.2174/1871527316666170404115027. Accessed July 14, 2017.

Pack AM. Therapy insight: clinical management of pregnant women with epilepsy. *Nat Clin Prac Neurol*, **2006**, *2*:190–200.

Perez J, et al. Stiripentol: efficacy and tolerability in children with epilepsy. *Epilepsia*, **1999**, *40*:1618–1626.

Plosker GL. Stiripentol: in severe myoclonic epilepsy of infancy (Dravet syndrome). *CNS Drugs*, **2012**, *26*:993–1001.

Porter RJ, et al. Mechanisms of action of antiseizure drugs. *Handb Clin Neurol*, **2012**, *108*:663–681.

Privitera MD, et al. Topiramate, carbamazepine and valproate monotherapy: double-blind comparison in newly diagnosed epilepsy. *Acta Neurol Scand*, **2003**, *107*:165–175.

Ptacek LJ, Fu YH. Channelopathies: episodic disorders of the nervous system. *Epilepsia*, **2001**, *42*(suppl 5):35–43.

Quilichini PP, et al. Stiripentol, a putative antiepileptic drug, enhances the duration of opening of GABA-A receptor channels. *Epilepsia*, **2006**, *47*:704–716.

Reid CA, et al. Mechanisms of human inherited epilepsies. *Prog Neurobiol*, **2009**, *87*:41–57.

Rey E, et al. Stiripentol potentiates clobazam in childhood epilepsy: a pharmacological study. *Epilepsia*, **1999**, *40*:112–113.

Rho JM, et al. Mechanism of action of the anticonvulsant felbamate: opposing effects on *N*-methyl-D-aspartate and $GABA_A$ receptors. *Ann Neurol*, **1994**, *35*:229–234.

Rogawski MA, Bazil CW. New molecular targets for antiepileptic drugs: alpha(2)delta, SV2A, and K_v7/KCNQ/M potassium channels. *Curr Neurol Neurosci Rep*, **2008**, *8*:345–352.

Rogawski MA, Donevan SD. AMPA receptors in epilepsy and as targets for antiepileptic drugs. *Adv Neurol*, **1999**, *79*:947–963.

Rogawski MA, Löscher W. The neurobiology of antiepileptic drugs. *Nat Rev Neurosci*, **2004**, *5*:553–564.

Sachdeo RC, et al. A double-blind, randomized trial of topiramate in Lennox-Gastaut syndrome: Topiramate YL Study Group. *Neurology*, **1999**, *52*:1882–1887.

Sachdeo RC, et al. Felbamate monotherapy: controlled trial in patients with partial onset seizures. *Ann Neurol*, **1992**, *32*:386–392.

Sachdeo RC, et al. Tiagabine therapy for complex partial seizures: a dose-frequency study. The Tiagabine Study Group. *Arch Neurol*, **1997**, *54*:595–601.

Sivenius J, et al. Double-blind study of gabapentin in the treatment of partial seizures. *Epilepsia*, **1991**, *32*:539–542.

Steiner TJ, et al. Lamotrigine mono-therapy in newly diagnosed untreated epilepsy: a double-blind comparison with phenytoin. *Epilepsia*, **1999**, *40*:601–607.

Stephen LJ, Brodie MJ. Pharmacotherapy of epilepsy: newly approved and developmental agents. *CNS Drugs*, **2011**, *25*:89–107.

Tortorella A, et al. A crucial role of the alpha-amino-3-hydroxy-5-methylisoxazole-4-propionic acid subtype of glutamate receptors in piriform and perirhinal cortex for the initiation and propagation of limbic motor seizures. *J Pharmacol Exp Ther*, **1997**, *280*:1401–1405.

Traynelis SF, Dingledine R. Potassium-induced spontaneous electrographic seizures in the rat hippocampal slice. *J Neurophysiol*, **1988**, *59*:259–276.

Treiman DM, et al. A comparison of four treatments for generalized convulsive status epilepticus. Veterans Affairs Status Epilepticus Cooperative Study Group. *N Engl J Med*, **1998**, *339*:792–798.

Twyman RE, et al. Differential regulation of γ-aminobutyric acid receptor channels by diazepam and phenobarbital. *Ann Neurol*, **1989**, *25*:213–220.

VanLandingham KE, et al. Magnetic resonance imaging evidence of hippocampal injury after prolonged focal febrile convulsions. *Ann Neurol*, **1998**, *43*:413–426.

Wallace RH, et al. Febrile seizures and generalized epilepsy associated with a mutation in the Na^+-channel β1 subunit gene *SCN1B*. *Nat Genet*, **1998**, *19*:366–370.

Xie X, et al. Interaction of the antiepileptic drug lamotrigine with recombinant rat brain type IIA Na^+ channels and with native Na^+ channels in rat hippocampal neurons. *Pflugers Arch*, **1995**, *430*:437–446.

Zona C1, et al. Brivaracetam (ucb 34714) inhibits Na(+) current in rat cortical neurons in culture. *Epilepsy Res*, **2010**, *88*:46–54.

Chapter 18 Treatment of Central Nervous System Degenerative Disorders

Erik D. Roberson

第十八章　中枢神经系统退行性疾病的治疗

中文导读

本章主要介绍：神经退行性疾病导论；神经退行性疾病的共同特征，包括蛋白质病、选择易损性、遗传与环境、治疗方法；帕金森病，包括临床概述、病理生理学和治疗；阿尔茨海默病，包括临床概述、诊断、遗传学、病理生理学、神经化学和治疗；亨廷顿病，包括病理学与病理生理学、遗传学和治疗；肌萎缩侧索硬化（ALS），包括病因学、治疗方法、ALS的对症治疗——痉挛。

Abbreviations

AADC: aromatic L-amino acid decarboxylase
Aβ: amyloid β
ACh: acetylcholine
AChE: acetylcholinesterase
AD: Alzheimer disease
ALDH: aldehyde dehydrogenase
ALS: amyotrophic lateral sclerosis
apoE: apolipoprotein E
APP: amyloid precursor protein
BuChE: butyrylcholinesterase
CNS: central nervous system
COMT: catechol-*O*-methyltransferase
DA: dopamine
DAT: DA transporter
DβH: dopamine-β-hydroxylase
DOPAC: 3,4-dihydroxyphenylacetic acid
GABA: γ-aminobutyric acid
Glu: glutamatergic
GPe: globus pallidus extern
GPi: globus pallidus interna
HD: Huntington disease
5HT: serotonin
HVA: homovanillic acid
MAO: monamine oxidase
MCI: mild cognitive impairment
MPTP: *N*-methyl-4-phenyl-1,2,3,6-tetrahydropyridine
3MT: 3-methoxyltyramine
NE: norepinephrine
NET: NE transporter
NMDA: *N*-methyl-D-aspartate
3-OMD: 3-*O*-methyl dopa
PD: Parkinson disease
PDD: Parkinson disease dementia
PET: positron emission tomography
PH: phenylalanine hydroxylase
REM: rapid eye movement
SNpc: substantia nigra pars compacta
SNpr: substantia nigra pars reticulate
SOD: superoxide dismutase
SSRI: selective serotonin reuptake inhibitor
STN: subthalamic nucleus
TAR: transactivation response element
TDP-43: TAR DNA-binding protein 43
TH: tyrosine hydrolase
VA/VL: ventroanterior and ventrolateral
VMAT2: vesicular monoamine transporter 2

Introduction to Neurodegenerative Disorders

Neurodegenerative disorders are characterized by progressive and irreversible loss of neurons from specific regions of the brain. Prototypical neurodegenerative disorders include PD and HD, where loss of neurons from structures of the basal ganglia results in abnormalities in the control of movement; AD, where the loss of hippocampal and cortical neurons leads to impairment of memory and cognitive ability; and ALS, where muscular weakness results from the degeneration of spinal, bulbar, and cortical motor neurons. Currently available therapies for neurodegenerative disorders alleviate the disease symptoms but do not alter the underlying neurodegenerative process.

Common Features of Neurodegenerative Disorders

Proteinopathies

Each of the major neurodegenerative disorders is characterized by accumulation of particular proteins in cellular aggregates: *α-synuclein* in PD; Aβ and the *microtubule-associated protein tau* in AD; *TDP-43* in most cases of ALS; and *huntingtin* in HD (Prusiner, 2013). The reason for accumulation of these proteins is unknown, and it is also unclear in most cases whether it is the large cellular aggregates or smaller soluble species of the proteins that most strongly drive pathogenesis.

Selective Vulnerability

A striking feature of neurodegenerative disorders is the exquisite specificity of the disease processes for particular types of neurons. For example, in PD there is extensive destruction of the dopaminergic neurons of the substantia nigra, whereas neurons in the cortex and many other areas of the brain are unaffected. In contrast, neural injury in AD is most severe in the hippocampus and neocortex, and even within the cortex, the loss of neurons is not uniform but varies dramatically in different brain networks. In HD, the mutant gene responsible for the disorder is expressed throughout the brain and in many other organs, yet the pathological changes are most prominent in the neostriatum. In ALS, there is loss of spinal motor neurons and the cortical neurons that provide their descending input. The diversity of these patterns of neural degeneration suggests that the process of neural injury results from the interaction of intrinsic properties of different neural circuits, genetics, and environmental influences. The intrinsic factors may include susceptibility to excitotoxic injury, regional variation in capacity for oxidative metabolism, and the production of toxic free radicals as by-products of cellular metabolism.

Genetics and Environment

Each of the major neurodegenerative disorders may be familial in nature. *HD is exclusively familial*; it is transmitted by autosomal dominant inheritance of an expanded repeat in the *huntingtin* gene. Nevertheless, environmental factors importantly influence the age of onset and rate of progression of HD symptoms. PD, AD, and ALS are usually sporadic, but for each there are well-recognized genetic forms. For example, there are both dominant (*α-synuclein, LRRK2*) and recessive (*parkin, DJ-1, PINK1*) gene mutations that may give rise to PD (Kumar et al., 2012; Singleton et al., 2013). In AD, mutations in the genes coding for APP and the *presenilins* (involved in APP processing) lead to inherited forms of the disease. About 10% of ALS cases are familial, most commonly due to mutations in the *C9ORF72* gene (Renton et al., 2014).

There are also genetic risk factors that influence the probability of disease onset and modify the phenotype. For example, the apoE genotype constitutes an important risk factor for AD. Three distinct isoforms of this protein exist, and individuals with even one copy of the high-risk allele, ε4, having several-fold higher risk of developing AD than those with the most common allele, ε3.

Environmental factors, including infectious agents, environmental toxins, and acquired brain injury, have been proposed in the etiology of neurodegenerative disorders. Traumatic brain injury has been suggested as a trigger for neurodegenerative disorders. At least one toxin, MPTP, can induce a condition closely resembling PD. More recently, evidence has linked pesticide exposure with PD. Exposure of soldiers to neurotoxic chemicals has been implicated in ALS (as part of "Gulf War syndrome").

Approaches to Therapy

Certain themes are apparent in the pharmacological approaches described in this chapter. Many of the existing therapies are *neurochemical*, aiming to replace or compensate for damage to specific neurotransmitter systems that are selectively impaired. For example, dopaminergic therapy is a mainstay of PD therapy, and the primary agents used in AD aim to boost acetylcholinergic transmission. The goal of much current research is to identify therapies that are *neuroprotective* and can modify the underlying neurodegenerative process.

One target of neuroprotective therapies is *excitotoxicity, neural injury* that results from the presence of excess glutamate in the brain. *Glutamate* is used as a neurotransmitter to mediate most excitatory synaptic transmission in the mammalian brain. The presence of excessive amounts of glutamate can lead to excitotoxic cell death (see Figure 14–13). The destructive effects of glutamate are mediated by glutamate receptors, particularly those of the NMDA type (see Table 14–2). Excitotoxic injury contributes to the neuronal death that occurs in acute processes such as stroke and head trauma. The role of excitotoxicity is less certain in the chronic neurodegenerative disorders; nevertheless, *glutamate antagonists* have been developed as neuroprotective therapies for neurodegeneration, with two such agents (*memantine* and *riluzole*, described later in the chapter) currently in clinical use.

Aging is the most important risk factor for all of the neurodegenerative diseases, and a likely contributor to the effect of age is the progressive impairment in the capacity of neurons for oxidative metabolism with consequent production of reactive compounds such as hydrogen peroxide and oxygen radicals. These reactive species can lead to DNA damage, peroxidation of membrane lipids, and neuronal death. This has led to pursuit of drugs that can enhance cellular metabolism (such as the mitochondrial cofactor coenzyme Q_{10}) and antioxidant strategies as treatments to prevent or retard degenerative diseases.

The discovery of specific proteins that accumulate and aggregate in each of the neurodegenerative disorders has opened the door to new therapeutic approaches. To date, there are no approved therapies that directly target the disease proteins (e.g., α-synuclein, Aβ, tau, TDP-43). However, there is intensive research to bring disease-modifying treatments that do directly target these proteins, such as passive immunotherapy with antibodies, into clinical care.

Parkinson Disease

Clinical Overview

Parkinsonism is a clinical syndrome with four cardinal features:

- Bradykinesia (slowness and poverty of movement)
- Muscular rigidity
- Resting tremor (which usually abates during voluntary movement)
- Impairment of postural balance, leading to disturbances of gait and to falling

The most common form of parkinsonism is idiopathic PD, first described by James Parkinson in 1817 as *paralysis agitans*, or the "shaking palsy." *The pathological hallmark of PD is the loss of the pigmented, dopaminergic neurons of the substantia nigra pars compacta, with the appearance of intracellular inclusions known as Lewy bodies.* The principal component of the Lewy bodies is aggregated α-synuclein (Goedert et al., 2013). A loss of 70%–80% of the DA-containing neurons accompanies symptomatic PD.

Without treatment, PD progresses over 5–10 years to a rigid, akinetic state in which patients are incapable of caring for themselves (Suchowersky et al., 2006). Death frequently results from complications of immobility, including aspiration pneumonia or pulmonary embolism. The availability of effective pharmacological treatment has radically altered the prognosis of PD; in most cases, good functional mobility can be maintained for many years. Life expectancy of adequately treated patients is increased substantially, but overall mortality remains higher than that of the general population.

While DA neuron loss is the most well-recognized feature of the disease, the disorder affects a wide range of other brain structures, including the brainstem, hippocampus, and cerebral cortex (Langston, 2006). There is increasing awareness of the "nonmotor" features of PD, which likely arise from pathology outside the DA system (Zesiewicz et al., 2010). Some nonmotor features may present before the characteristic motor symptoms: anosmia, or loss of the sense of smell; REM behavior disorder, a disorder of sleep with marked agitation and motion during periods of REM sleep; and disturbances of autonomic nervous system function, particularly constipation. Other nonmotor features are seen later in the disease and include depression, anxiety, and dementia.

Several disorders other than idiopathic PD also may produce parkinsonism, including some relatively rare neurodegenerative disorders, stroke, and intoxication with DA receptor antagonists. Drugs that may cause parkinsonism include antipsychotics such as haloperidol and chlorpromazine (see Chapter 16) and antiemetics such as prochlorperazine and metoclopramide (see Chapter 50). The distinction between idiopathic PD and other causes of parkinsonism is important because parkinsonism arising from other causes usually is refractory to all forms of treatment.

Pathophysiology

The dopaminergic deficit in PD arises from a loss of the neurons in the substantia nigra pars compacta that provide innervation to the striatum (caudate and putamen). The current understanding of the pathophysiology of PD is based on the finding that the striatal DA content is reduced in excess of 80%, with a parallel loss of neurons from the substantia nigra, suggesting that replacement of DA could restore function. We now have a model of the function of the basal ganglia that, while incomplete, is still useful.

Dopamine Synthesis, Metabolism, and Receptors

Dopamine, a catecholamine, is synthesized in the terminals of dopaminergic neurons from tyrosine and stored, released, reaccumulated, and metabolized by processes described in Chapter 13 and summarized in Figure 18–1. The actions of DA in the brain are mediated by the DA receptor, of which there are two broad classes, D1 and D2, with five distinct subtypes, D_1-D_5. All the DA receptors are GPCRs. Receptors of the **D1 group** (D_1 and D_5 subtypes) couple to G_s and thence to activation of the cyclic AMP pathway. The **D2 group** (D_2, D_3, and D_4 receptors) couple to G_i to reduce the adenylyl cyclase activity and voltage-gated Ca^{2+} currents while activating K^+ currents. Each of the five DA receptors has a distinct anatomical pattern of expression in the brain. D_1 and D_2 proteins are abundant in the striatum and are the most important receptor sites with regard to the causes and treatment of PD. The D_4 and D_5 proteins are largely extrastriatal, whereas D_3 expression is low in the caudate and putamen but more abundant in the nucleus accumbens and olfactory tubercle.

Neural Mechanism of Parkinsonism: A Model of Basal Ganglia Function

Considerable effort has been devoted to understanding how the loss of dopaminergic input to the neurons of the neostriatum gives rise to the clinical features of PD (Hornykiewicz, 1973). The basal ganglia can be viewed as a modulatory side loop that regulates the flow of information from the cerebral cortex to the motor neurons of the spinal cord (Albin et al., 1989) (Figure 18–2).

The neostriatum is the principal input structure of the basal ganglia and receives excitatory glutamatergic input from many areas of the cortex. Most neurons within the striatum are projection neurons that innervate other basal ganglia structures. A small but important subgroup of striatal neurons consists of interneurons that connect neurons within the striatum but do not project beyond its borders. ACh and neuropeptides are used as transmitters by these striatal interneurons.

The outflow of the striatum proceeds along two distinct routes, termed the *direct* and *indirect pathways* (Calabresi et al., 2014). The direct pathway is formed by neurons in the striatum that project directly to the output stages of the basal ganglia, the SNpr and the GPi; these, in turn, relay to the VA and VL thalamus, which provides excitatory input to the cortex. The neurotransmitter in both links of the direct pathway is GABA, which is inhibitory, so that *the net effect of stimulation of the direct pathway at the level of the striatum is to increase the excitatory outflow from the thalamus to the cortex.*

The indirect pathway is composed of striatal neurons that project to the GPe. This structure, in turn, innervates the STN, which provides outflow to the SNpr and GPi output stage. The first two links—the projections from striatum to GPe and GPe to STN—use the inhibitory transmitter

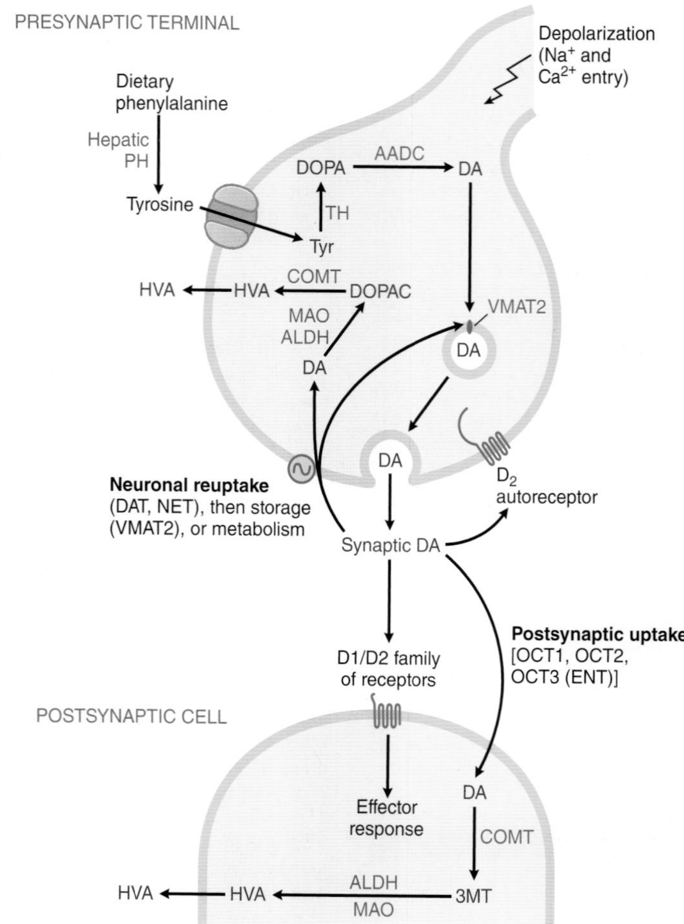

Figure 18–1 *Dopaminergic nerve terminal.* Dopamine is synthesized from tyrosine in the nerve terminal by the sequential actions of TH and AADC. DA is sequestered by VMAT2 in storage granules and released by exocytosis. Synaptic DA activates presynaptic autoreceptors and postsynaptic D1 and D2 receptors. Synaptic DA may be taken up into the neuron via the DA and NE transporters (DAT, NET) or removed by postsynaptic uptake via the organic cation transporter, OCT3 (see Chapter 5). Cytosolic DA is subject to degradation by MAO and ALDH in the neuron and by COMT and MAO/ALDH in nonneuronal cells; the final metabolic product is HVA. See structures in Figure 18–4.

GABA; however, the final link—the projection from STN to SNpr and GPi—is an excitatory glutamatergic pathway. Thus, *the net effect of stimulating the indirect pathway at the level of the striatum is to reduce the excitatory outflow from the thalamus to the cerebral cortex.* The key feature of this model of basal ganglia function, which accounts for the symptoms observed in PD as a result of loss of dopaminergic neurons, is the differential effect of DA on the direct and indirect pathways (Figure 18–3).

The dopaminergic neurons of the SNpc innervate all parts of the striatum; however, the target striatal neurons express distinct types of DA receptors. The striatal neurons giving rise to the direct pathway express primarily the *excitatory* D_1 DA receptor protein, whereas the striatal neurons forming the indirect pathway express primarily the *inhibitory* D_2 type. *Thus, DA released in the striatum tends to increase the activity of the direct pathway and reduce the activity of the indirect pathway, whereas the depletion that occurs in PD has the opposite effect. The net effect of the reduced dopaminergic input in PD is to increase markedly the inhibitory outflow from the SNpr and GPi to the thalamus and reduce excitation of the motor cortex.* There are several limitations of this model of basal ganglia function. The anatomical connections are considerably more complex, and many of the pathways involved use several neurotransmitters. Limitations notwithstanding, the model is useful and has important implications for the rational design and use of pharmacological agents in PD.

Treatment of Parkinson Disease

Levodopa

Levodopa (also called L-DOPA or L-3,4-dihydroxyphenylalanine), the metabolic precursor of DA, is the single most effective agent in the treatment of PD (Cotzias et al., 1969; Fahn et al., 2004). The effects of levodopa result from its decarboxylation to DA. When administered orally, levodopa is absorbed rapidly from the small bowel by the transport system for aromatic amino acids. Concentrations of the drug in plasma usually peak between 0.5 and 2 h after an oral dose. The $t_{1/2}$ in plasma is short (1–3 h). The rate and extent of absorption of levodopa depend on the rate of gastric emptying, the pH of gastric juice, and the length of time the drug is exposed to the degradative enzymes of the gastric and intestinal mucosa. Administration of levodopa with high-protein meals delays absorption and reduces peak plasma concentrations. *Entry of the drug into the CNS across the blood-brain barrier is mediated by a membrane transporter for aromatic amino acids.* In the brain, levodopa is converted to DA by decarboxylation primarily within the presynaptic terminals of dopaminergic neurons in the striatum. The DA produced is responsible for the therapeutic effectiveness of the drug in PD; after release, it is either transported back into dopaminergic terminals by the presynaptic uptake mechanism or metabolized by the actions of MAO and COMT (Figure 18–4).

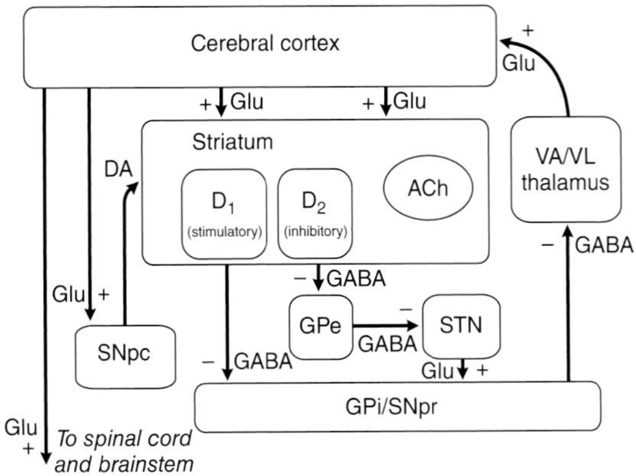

Figure 18–2 *Schematic wiring diagram of the basal ganglia.* The striatum is the principal input structure of the basal ganglia and receives excitatory glutamatergic input from many areas of cerebral cortex. The striatum contains projection neurons expressing predominantly D_1 or D_2 DA receptors, as well as interneurons that use ACh as a neurotransmitter. Outflow from the striatum proceeds along two routes. The direct pathway, from the striatum to the SNpr and GPi, uses the inhibitory transmitter GABA. The indirect pathway, from the striatum through the GPe and the STN to the SNpr and GPi, consists of two inhibitory GABA-ergic links and one excitatory Glu projection. The SNpc provides dopaminergic innervation to the striatal neurons, giving rise to both the direct and the indirect pathways, and it regulates the relative activity of these two paths. The SNpr and GPi are the output structures of the basal ganglia and provide feedback to the cerebral cortex through the VA/VL nuclei of the thalamus.

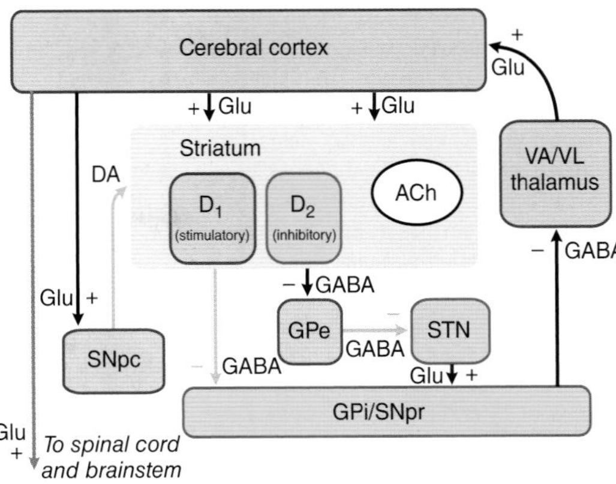

Figure 18–3 *The basal ganglia in PD.* The primary defect is destruction of the dopaminergic neurons of the SNpc. The striatal neurons that form the direct pathway from the striatum to the SNpr and GPi express primarily the *excitatory* D_1 DA receptor, whereas the striatal neurons that project to the GPe and form the indirect pathway express the *inhibitory* D_2 DA receptor. Thus, loss of the dopaminergic input to the striatum has a differential effect on the two outflow pathways; the direct pathway to the SNpr and GPi is less active (structures in purple), whereas the activity in the indirect pathway is increased (structures in red). The net effect is that neurons in the SNpr and GPi become more active. This leads to increased inhibition of the VA/VL thalamus and reduced excitatory input to the cortex. Light blue lines indicate primary pathways with reduced activity. (See Abbreviations list for definitions of anatomical abbreviations.)

In clinical practice, levodopa is almost always administered in combination with a peripherally acting inhibitor of AADC, such as *carbidopa* (used in the U.S.) or *benserazide* (available outside the U.S.), drugs that do not penetrate well into the CNS. If levodopa is administered alone, the drug is largely decarboxylated by enzymes in the intestinal mucosa and other peripheral sites so that relatively little unchanged drug reaches the cerebral circulation, and probably less than 1% penetrates the CNS. In addition, DA release into the circulation by peripheral conversion of levodopa produces undesirable effects, particularly nausea. Inhibition of peripheral decarboxylase markedly increases the fraction of administered levodopa that remains unmetabolized and available to cross the blood-brain barrier (Figure 18–5), and reduces the incidence of GI side effects and drug-induced orthostatic hypotension.

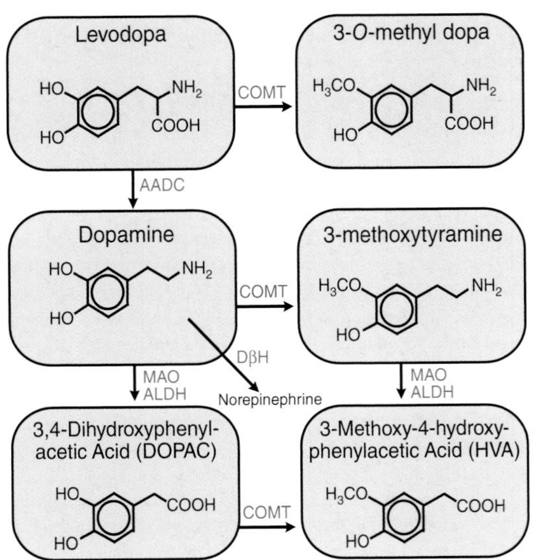

Figure 18–4 *Metabolism of levodopa (L-DOPA).*

A daily dose of 75 mg carbidopa is generally sufficient to prevent the development of nausea. For this reason, the most commonly prescribed form of carbidopa/levodopa is the 25/100 form, containing 25 mg carbidopa and 100 mg levodopa. With this formulation, dosage schedules of three or more tablets daily provide acceptable inhibition of decarboxylase in most individuals.

Levodopa therapy can have a dramatic effect on all the signs and symptoms of PD. Early in the course of the disease, the degree of improvement in tremor, rigidity, and bradykinesia produced by carbidopa/levodopa may be nearly complete. With long-term levodopa therapy, the "buffering" capacity is lost, and the patient's motor state may fluctuate dramatically with each dose of levodopa, producing the *motor complications* of levodopa (Pahwa et al., 2006).

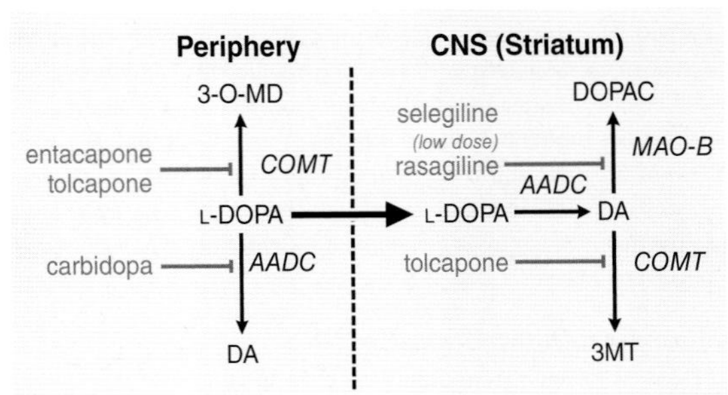

Figure 18–5 *Pharmacological preservation of levodopa (L-dopa) and striatal DA.* The principal site of action of inhibitors of COMT (e.g., tolcapone and entacapone) is in the peripheral circulation. They block the *O*-methylation of L-dopa and increase the fraction of the drug available for delivery to the brain. Tolcapone also has effects in the CNS. Inhibitors of MAO-B, such as low-dose selegiline and rasagiline, will act within the CNS to reduce oxidative deamination of DA, thereby enhancing vesicular stores.

A common problem is the development of the "wearing off" phenomenon: Each dose of levodopa effectively improves mobility for a period of time, perhaps 1–2 h, but rigidity and akinesia return rapidly at the end of the dosing interval. Increasing the dose and frequency of administration can improve this situation, but this often is limited by the development of dyskinesias, excessive and abnormal involuntary movements. In the later stages of PD, patients may fluctuate rapidly between being "off," having no beneficial effects from their medications, and being "on" but with disabling dyskinesias (the *on/off phenomenon*). A sustained-release formulation consisting of carbidopa/levodopa in an erodable wax matrix is helpful in some cases, but absorption of this older sustained-release formulation is not entirely predictable.

Recently, two new formulations of levodopa intended to address wearing off have been approved. RYTARY carbidopa-levodopa extended-release capsules contain both immediate- and extended-release beads that provide reduced off time in patients with motor fluctuations (Hauser et al., 2013). DUOPA carbidopa-levodopa intestinal gel is administered through a gastrostomy tube into the jejunum using a pump and can have a dramatic effect on reducing "off" time (Olanow et al., 2014).

Does levodopa alter the course of the underlying disease or merely modify the symptoms? While the answer to this question is not entirely certain, a randomized trial has provided evidence that levodopa does not have an adverse effect on the course of the underlying disease, but has also confirmed that high doses of levodopa are associated with early onset of dyskinesias. Most practitioners have adopted a pragmatic approach, using levodopa only when the symptoms of PD cause functional impairment and other treatments are inadequate or not well tolerated.

A frequent and troubling adverse effect is the induction of hallucinations and confusion, especially in elderly patients or in patients with preexisting cognitive dysfunction. Conventional antipsychotic agents, such as the phenothiazines, are effective against levodopa-induced psychosis but may cause marked worsening of parkinsonism, probably through actions at the D_2 DA receptor, and should not be used in PD. An alternative approach has been to use "atypical" antipsychotic agents (see Chapter 16). The two drugs that are most effective and best tolerated in patients with advanced PD are clozapine and quetiapine. Both of these drugs, and others in the class, are associated with an increased rate of death due to stroke and other causes when used in the elderly. This risk needs to be weighed carefully against the risks created by hallucinations and psychosis.

Levodopa (and the DA agonists, described in the next section) may also lead to the development of "impulse control disorders" (Weintraub et al., 2015). These include compulsive behaviors, gambling, and hypersexuality and can be destructive socially. PD also appears to be associated with an increased risk of suicidality, but whether this is associated with the disease or a specific treatment is uncertain. Vigilance for signs of depression and suicidality should be practiced in all patients with PD.

Administration of levodopa with nonspecific inhibitors of MAO accentuates the actions of levodopa and may precipitate life-threatening hypertensive crisis and hyperpyrexia; nonspecific MAO inhibitors always should be discontinued at least 14 days before levodopa is administered (note that this prohibition does not include the MAO-B subtype-specific inhibitors selegiline and rasagiline). Abrupt withdrawal of levodopa or other dopaminergic medications may precipitate the *neuroleptic malignant syndrome* of confusion, rigidity, and hyperthermia, a potentially lethal adverse effect.

Dopamine Receptor Agonists

The DA receptor agonists in clinical use have durations of action substantially longer than that of levodopa; they are often used in the management of dose-related fluctuations in motor state and may be helpful in preventing motor complications (Parkinson Study Group, 2000). DA receptor agonists are proposed to have the potential to modify the course of PD by reducing endogenous release of DA as well as the need for exogenous levodopa, thereby reducing free-radical formation.

Two orally administered DA receptor agonists are commonly used for treatment of PD: *ropinirole* and *pramipexole*. Both are well absorbed orally and have similar therapeutic actions. There is also a transdermal formulation of the DA agonist *rotigotine* available. Ropinirole and pramipexole have selective activity at D2 class sites (specifically at the D_2 and D_3 receptor). Rotigotine acts at D2 sites and also has activity at D1 class sites. Like levodopa, these DA agonists can relieve the clinical symptoms of PD. The duration of action of the DA agonists (8–24 h) often is longer than that of levodopa (6–8 h), and they are particularly effective in the treatment of patients who have developed on/off phenomena. Both ropinirole and pramipexole are also available in once-daily sustained-release formulations, which are more convenient and may reduce adverse effects related to intermittent dosing. The transdermal delivery of rotigotine produces stable plasma drug levels over 24 h.

Pramipexole, ropinirole, and rotigotine may produce hallucinosis or confusion, similar to that observed with levodopa, and may cause nausea and orthostatic hypotension. They should be initiated at low dose and titrated slowly to minimize these effects. The DA agonists, as well as levodopa itself, are also associated with fatigue and somnolence. Patients should be warned about the potential for sleepiness, especially while driving. Many practitioners prefer a DA agonist as initial therapy in younger patients to reduce the occurrence of motor complications. In older patients or those with substantial comorbidity, levodopa/carbidopa is generally better tolerated.

Apomorphine. Apomorphine is a dopaminergic agonist that can be administered by subcutaneous injection. It has high affinity for D_4 receptors; moderate affinity for D_2, D_3, D_5, and adrenergic α_{1D}, α_{2B}, and α_{2C} receptors; and low affinity for D_1 receptors. Apomorphine is FDA-approved as a "rescue therapy" for the acute intermittent treatment of "off" episodes in patients with a fluctuating response to dopaminergic therapy.

Apomorphine has the same side effects as the oral DA agonists. Apomorphine is highly emetogenic and requires pre- and posttreatment antiemetic therapy. Oral trimethobenzamide, at a dose of 300 mg, three times daily, should be started 3 days prior to the initial dose of apomorphine and continued at least during the first 2 months of therapy. Profound hypotension and loss of consciousness have occurred when apomorphine was administered with ondansetron; hence, the concomitant use of apomorphine with antiemetic drugs of the $5HT_3$ antagonist class is contraindicated. Other potentially serious side effects of apomorphine include QT prolongation, injection site reactions, and the development of a pattern of abuse characterized by increasingly frequent dosing leading to hallucinations, dyskinesia, and abnormal behavior.

Because of these potential adverse effects, use of apomorphine is appropriate only when other measures, such as oral DA agonists or COMT inhibitors, have failed to control the off episodes. Apomorphine therapy should be initiated with a 2-mg test dose in a setting where the patient can be monitored carefully. If tolerated, it can be titrated slowly up to a maximum dosage of 6 mg. For effective control of symptoms, patients may require three or more injections daily.

Catechol-O-Methyltransferase Inhibitors

Orally administered levodopa is largely converted by AADC to DA (see Figure 18–5), which causes nausea and hypotension. Addition of an AADC inhibitor such as carbidopa reduces the formation of DA but increases the fraction of levodopa that is methylated by COMT. COMT inhibitors block this peripheral conversion of levodopa to 3-*O*-methyl DOPA, increasing both the plasma $t_{1/2}$ of levodopa and the fraction of each dose that reaches the CNS.

The COMT inhibitors *tolcapone* and *entacapone* reduce significantly the "wearing off" symptoms in patients treated with levodopa/carbidopa (Parkinson Study Group, 1997). The two drugs differ in their pharmacokinetic properties and adverse effects: Tolcapone has a relatively long duration of action and appears to act by inhibition of both central and peripheral COMT. Entacapone has a short duration of action (2 h) and principally inhibits peripheral COMT. Common adverse effects of both agents include nausea, orthostatic hypotension, vivid dreams, confusion, and hallucinations. An important adverse effect associated with tolcapone is hepatotoxicity. At least three fatal cases of fulminant hepatic failure in patients taking tolcapone have been observed, leading to addition of a black-box warning to the label. Tolcapone should be used only in patients who have not responded to other therapies and with appropriate monitoring for hepatic injury.

Entacapone has not been associated with hepatotoxicity. Entacapone also is available in fixed-dose combinations with levodopa/carbidopa.

Selective MAO-B Inhibitors

Two isoenzymes of MAO oxidize catecholamines: MAO-A and MAO-B. MAO-B is the predominant form in the striatum and is responsible for most of the oxidative metabolism of DA in the brain. Selective MAO-B inhibitors are used for the treatment of PD: *selegiline* and *rasagiline*. These agents selectively and irreversibly inactivate MAO-B. Both agents exert modest beneficial effects on the symptoms of PD. The basis of this efficacy is, presumably, inhibition of breakdown of DA in the striatum.

Selective MAO-B inhibitors do not substantially inhibit the peripheral metabolism of catecholamines and can be taken safely with levodopa. These agents also do not exhibit the "cheese effect," the potentially lethal potentiation of catecholamine action observed when patients on nonspecific MAO inhibitors ingest indirectly acting sympathomimetic amines such as the tyramine found in certain cheeses and wine.

Selegiline is generally well tolerated in younger patients for symptomatic treatment of early or mild PD. In patients with more advanced PD or underlying cognitive impairment, selegiline may accentuate the adverse motor and cognitive effects of levodopa therapy. Metabolites of selegiline include amphetamine and methamphetamine, which may cause anxiety, insomnia, and other adverse symptoms. Selegiline is available in an orally disintegrating tablet as well as a transdermal patch. Both of these delivery routes are intended to reduce hepatic first-pass metabolism and limit the formation of the amphetamine metabolites.

Unlike selegiline, rasagiline does not give rise to undesirable amphetamine metabolites. Rasagiline monotherapy is effective in early PD. Adjunctive therapy with rasagiline significantly reduces levodopa-related wearing off symptoms in advanced PD (Olanow et al., 2008). Although selective MAO-B inhibitors are generally well tolerated, drug interactions can be troublesome. Similar to the nonspecific MAO inhibitors, selegiline can lead to the development of stupor, rigidity, agitation, and hyperthermia when administered with the analgesic meperidine. Although the mechanics of this interaction are uncertain, selegiline or rasagiline should not be given in combination with meperidine. Tramadol, methadone, propoxyphene dextromethorphan, St. John's wort, and cyclobenzaprine are also contraindicated with MAO-B inhibitors. Although development of the *serotonin syndrome* has been reported with coadministration of MAO-B inhibitors and antidepressants (tricyclic or serotonin reuptake inhibitors), this appears to be rare, and many patients are treated with this combination without difficulty. If concurrent treatment with MAO-B inhibitors and antidepressants is undertaken, close monitoring and use of low doses of the antidepressant are advisable (Panisset et al., 2014).

Muscarinic Receptor Antagonists

Antimuscarinic drugs currently used in the treatment of PD include *trihexyphenidyl* and *benztropine mesylate*, as well as the antihistaminic *diphenhydramine hydrochloride*, which also interacts at central muscarinic receptors. The biological basis for the therapeutic actions of muscarinic antagonists is not completely understood. They may act within the neostriatum through the receptors that normally mediate the response to intrinsic cholinergic innervation of this structure, which arises primarily from cholinergic striatal interneurons.

These drugs have relatively modest antiparkinsonian activity and are used only in the treatment of early PD or as an adjunct to dopamimetic therapy. Adverse effects result from their anticholinergic properties. Most troublesome are sedation and mental confusion. All anticholinergic drugs must be used with caution in patients with narrow-angle glaucoma (see Chapter 69), and in general anticholinergics are not well tolerated in the elderly. The pharmacology and signaling mechanisms of muscarinic receptors are thoroughly covered in Chapter 9.

Amantadine

Amantadine, an antiviral agent used for the prophylaxis and treatment of influenza A (see Chapter 62), has antiparkinsonian activity. Amantadine appears to alter DA release in the striatum, has anticholinergic properties, and blocks NMDA glutamate receptors. It is used as initial therapy of mild PD. It also may be helpful as an adjunct in patients on levodopa with dose-related fluctuations and dyskinesias. Amantadine is usually administered at a dose of 100 mg, twice per day, and is well tolerated. Dizziness, lethargy, anticholinergic effects, and sleep disturbance, as well as nausea and vomiting, side effects are mild and reversible.

Clinical Summary

Pharmacological treatment of PD should be tailored to the individual patient (Connolly and Lang, 2014). Drug therapy is not obligatory in early PD; many patients can be managed for a time with exercise and lifestyle interventions. For patients with mild symptoms, MAO-B inhibitors, amantadine, or (in younger patients) anticholinergics are reasonable choices. In most patients, treatment with a dopaminergic drug, either levodopa or a DA agonist, is eventually required. Many practitioners prefer a DA agonist as initial therapy in younger patients in an effort to reduce the occurrence of motor complications, although the evidence supporting this practice is inconclusive. In older patients or those with substantial comorbidity, levodopa/carbidopa is generally better tolerated.

Alzheimer Disease

Clinical Overview

The brain region most vulnerable to neuronal dysfunction and cell loss in AD is the medial temporal lobe, including entorhinal cortex and hippocampus. The proteins that accumulate in AD are Aβ and tau (Giacobini and Gold, 2013). AD has three major stages:

1. A "preclinical" stage during which accumulation of Aβ and tau begins, before any symptoms appear.
2. An MCI stage with episodic memory loss (repeated questions, misplaced items, etc.) that is not severe enough to impair daily function.
3. A dementia stage with progressive loss of functional abilities.

Death usually ensues within 6–12 years of onset, most often from a complication of immobility such as pneumonia or pulmonary embolism.

Diagnosis

Alzheimer disease remains a clinical diagnosis, based on the presence of memory impairment and other cognitive impairments that are insidious, progressive, and not well explained by another disorder. In recent years, there has been steady progress toward inclusion of biomarkers in the diagnostic criteria. This includes both *fluid biomarkers*, such as changes in Aβ and tau in the cerebrospinal fluid, and *imaging biomarkers*, such as hippocampal atrophy on structural magnetic resonance imaging and cortical hypometabolism on fluorodeoxyglucose PET scans. One of the most exciting advances is the ability to detect, using amyloid PET scans, Aβ deposition in patients. Three agents, *florbetapir*, *flutemetamol*, and *florbetaben*, are FDA-approved for determining whether individuals with cognitive impairment have Aβ deposition, which would suggest AD as a possible etiology. Similar agents for PET imaging of tau deposition are currently in development.

Genetics

Mutations in three genes have been identified as causes of autosomal dominant, early onset AD: *APP*, which encodes Aβ precursor protein, and *PSEN1* and *PSEN2*, encoding presenilin 1 and 2, respectively. All three genes are involved in the production of Aβ peptides. Aβ is generated by sequential proteolytic cleavage of APP by two enzymes, β-secretase and γ-secretase; the presenilins form the catalytic core of γ-secretase. The genetic evidence, combined with the fact that Aβ accumulates in the brain in the form of soluble oligomers and amyloid plaques and is toxic when applied to neurons, forms the basis for the amyloid hypothesis of AD pathogenesis. Many genes have been identified as having alleles that increase AD risk. By far the most important of these is *APOE*, which encodes the lipid carrier protein apoE. Individuals inheriting the ε4 allele of *APOE* have a 3-fold or more higher risk of developing AD. While these individuals make up less than one-fourth of the population, they account for more than half of all AD cases.

Pathophysiology

The pathological hallmarks of AD are amyloid plaques, which are extracellular accumulations of Aβ, and intracellular neurofibrillary tangles composed of the microtubule-associated protein tau. The development of amyloid plaques occurs earlier, and tangle burden accrues over time in a manner that correlates more closely with the development of cognitive impairment. In autosomal dominant AD, Aβ accumulates due to mutations that cause its overproduction. Aggregation of Aβ is an important event in AD pathogenesis. While plaques consist of highly ordered fibrils of Aβ, it appears that soluble Aβ oligomers, perhaps as small as dimers, are more highly pathogenic. Tau also aggregates to form the paired helical filaments that make up neurofibrillary tangles. Posttranslational modifications of tau, including phosphorylation, proteolysis, and other changes, increase tau's propensity to aggregate. Mechanisms by which Aβ and tau induce neuronal dysfunction and death may include direct impairment of synaptic transmission and plasticity, excitotoxicity, oxidative stress, and neuroinflammation.

Neurochemistry

The most striking neurochemical disturbance in AD is a *deficiency of ACh*. The anatomical basis of the cholinergic deficit is atrophy and degeneration of subcortical cholinergic neurons. The selective deficiency of ACh in AD and the observation that central cholinergic antagonists (e.g., atropine) can induce a confusional state resembling the dementia of AD have given rise to the "cholinergic hypothesis" that a deficiency of ACh is critical in the genesis of the symptoms of AD. AD, however, is complex and also involves multiple neurotransmitter systems, including glutamate, 5HT, and neuropeptides, and there is destruction of not only cholinergic neurons but also the cortical and hippocampal targets that receive cholinergic input.

Treatment

At present, no disease-modifying therapy for AD is available; current treatment is aimed at alleviating symptoms (Roberson and Mucke, 2006; Selkoe, 2013).

Treatment of Cognitive Symptoms

Augmentation of the cholinergic transmission is currently the mainstay of AD treatment. Three drugs, *donepezil, rivastigmine*, and *galantamine*, are widely used for this purpose (Table 18–1). All three are reversible antagonists of cholinesterases (see Chapter 10). Cholinesterase inhibitors are the usual first-line therapy for symptomatic treatment of cognitive impairments in mild or moderate AD. They are also widely used to treat other neurodegenerative diseases with cholinergic deficits, including dementia with Lewy bodies and vascular dementia. Their effect is generally modest, usually producing no dramatic improvement in symptoms but rather a 6- to 12-month delay in progression, after which clinical deterioration resumes. The drugs are usually well tolerated, with the most common side effects being GI distress, muscle cramping, and abnormal dreams. They should be used with caution in patients with bradycardia or syncope.

Memantine. Memantine is a noncompetitive antagonist of the NMDA-type glutamate receptor. It is used as either an adjunct or an alternative to cholinesterase inhibitors in AD, generally in later stages of dementia, as there is less evidence for its efficacy earlier. Memantine delays clinical deterioration in patients with moderate-to-severe AD dementia. Adverse effects of memantine include mild headache or dizziness. The drug is excreted by the kidneys, and dosage should be reduced in patients with severe renal impairment.

Treatment of Behavioral Symptoms

In addition to cognitive decline, behavioral and psychiatric symptoms in dementia (BPSD) are common, particularly in middle stages of the disease. These symptoms include irritability and agitation, paranoia and delusional thinking, wandering, anxiety, and depression. Treatment can be difficult, and nonpharmacological approaches should generally be first line.

A variety of pharmacological options are also available. Both cholinesterase inhibitors and memantine reduce some BPSD. However, their effects are modest, and they do not treat some of the most troublesome symptoms, such as agitation. *Citalopram*, an SSRI (see Chapter 15), showed efficacy for agitation in a randomized clinical trial. Atypical antipsychotics, such as risperidone, olanzapine, and quetiapine (see Chapter 16) are perhaps even more efficacious for agitation and psychosis in AD, but their use is often limited by adverse effects, including parkinsonism, sedation, and falls. In addition, the use of atypical antipsychotics in elderly patients with dementia-related psychosis has been associated with a higher risk of stroke and overall mortality, leading to an FDA black-box warning (Schneider et al., 2005). Benzodiazepines (see Chapter 15) can be used for occasional control of acute agitation but are not recommended for long-term management because of their adverse effects on cognition and other risks in the elderly population. The typical antipsychotic haloperidol (see Chapter 16) may be useful for aggression, but sedation and extrapyramidal symptoms limit its use to control of acute episodes.

TABLE 18–1 ■ CHOLINESTERASE INHIBITORS USED FOR THE TREATMENT OF ALZHEIMER DISEASE

	DONEPEZIL	RIVASTIGMINE	GALANTAMINE
Enzymes inhibited[a]	AChE	AChE, BuChE	AChE
Mechanism	Noncompetitive	Noncompetitive	Competitive
Typical maintenance dose[b]	10 mg once daily	9.5 mg/24 h (transdermal) 3–6 mg twice daily (oral)	8–12 mg twice daily (immediate release) 16–24 mg/d (extended release)
FDA-approved indications	Mild-severe AD	Mild-moderate AD Mild-moderate PDD	Mild-moderate AD
Metabolism[c]	CYP2D6, CYP3A4	Esterases	CYP2D6, CYP3A4

[a]AChE is the major cholinesterase in the brain; BuChE is a serum and hepatic cholinesterase that is upregulated in AD brain.
[b]Typical starting doses are one-half of the maintenance dose and are given for the first month of therapy.
[c]Drugs metabolized by CYP2D6 and CYP3A4 are subject to increased serum levels when coadministered with drugs known to inhibit these enzymes, such as ketoconazole and paroxetine.

Clinical Summary

The typical patient with AD presenting in early stages of disease should probably be treated with a cholinesterase inhibitor. Patients and families should be counseled that a realistic goal of therapy is to induce a temporary reprieve from progression, or at least a reduction in the rate of decline, rather than long-term recovery of cognition. As the disease progresses, memantine can be added to the regimen. Behavioral symptoms are often treated with a serotonergic antidepressant or, if they are severe enough to warrant the risk of higher mortality, an atypical antipsychotic. Eliminating drugs likely to aggravate cognitive impairments, particularly anticholinergics, benzodiazepines, and other sedative/hypnotics, from the patient's regimen is another important aspect of AD pharmacotherapy.

Huntington Disease

Huntington disease is a dominantly inherited disorder characterized by the gradual onset of motor incoordination and cognitive decline in midlife (Bates et al., 2015). Symptoms develop insidiously, as a movement disorder manifest by brief, jerk-like movements of the extremities, trunk, face, and neck (chorea), as personality changes, or both. Fine-motor incoordination and impairment of rapid eye movements are early features. As the disorder progresses, the involuntary movements become more severe, dysarthria and dysphagia develop, and balance is impaired. The cognitive disorder manifests first as slowness of mental processing and difficulty in organizing complex tasks. Memory is impaired, but affected persons rarely lose their memory of family, friends, and the immediate situation. Such persons often become irritable, anxious, and depressed. The outcome of HD is invariably fatal; over a course of 15–30 years, the affected person becomes totally disabled and unable to communicate, requiring full-time care; death ensues from the complications of immobility.

Pathology and Pathophysiology

Huntington disease is characterized by prominent neuronal loss in the striatum (caudate/putamen) of the brain. Atrophy of these structures proceeds in an orderly fashion, first affecting the tail of the caudate nucleus and then proceeding anteriorly from mediodorsal to VL. Other areas of the brain also are affected. Interneurons and afferent terminals are largely spared, whereas the striatal projection neurons (the medium spiny neurons) are severely affected. This leads to large decreases in striatal GABA concentrations, whereas somatostatin and DA concentrations are relatively preserved.

Selective vulnerability also appears to underlie the development of chorea. In most adult-onset cases, the medium spiny neurons that project to the GPi and SNpr (the indirect pathway) appear to be affected earlier than those projecting to the GPe (the direct pathway; see Figure 18–2). *The disproportionate impairment of the indirect pathway increases excitatory drive to the neocortex, producing involuntary choreiform movements* (Figure 18–6). In some individuals, rigidity rather than chorea is the predominant clinical feature; this is especially common in juvenile-onset cases. Here, the striatal neurons giving rise to both the direct and indirect pathways are impaired to a comparable degree.

Genetics

Huntington disease is an autosomal dominant disorder with nearly complete penetrance. The average age of onset is between 35 and 45 years, but the range varies from as early as age 2 to as late as the middle 80s. Although the disease is inherited equally from mother and father, more than 80% of those developing symptoms before age 20 inherit the defect from the father. Known homozygotes for HD show clinical characteristics identical to the typical HD heterozygote, indicating that the unaffected chromosome does not attenuate the disease symptomatology.

A region near the end of the short arm of chromosome 4 contains a polymorphic $(CAG)_n$ trinucleotide repeat that is significantly expanded in all individuals with HD. The expansion of this trinucleotide repeat is the genetic alteration responsible for HD. The range of CAG repeat length in normal individuals is between 9 and 34 triplets, with a median repeat length on normal chromosomes of 19. The repeat length in HD varies from

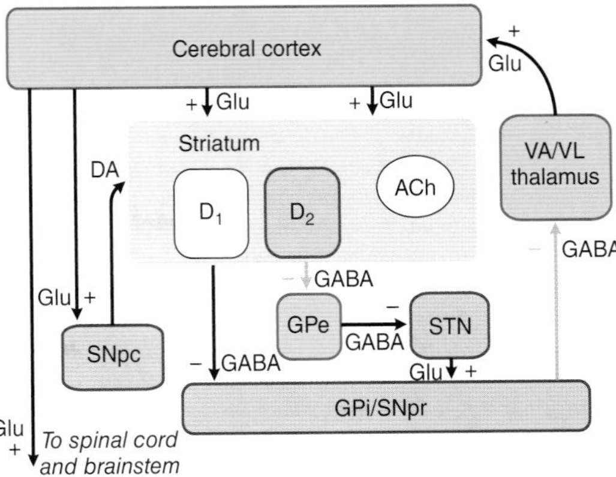

Figure 18–6 *The basal ganglia in Huntington disease.* HD is characterized by loss of neurons from the striatum. The neurons that project from the striatum to the GPe and form the indirect pathway are affected earlier in the course of the disease than those that project to the GPi. This leads to a loss of inhibition of the GPe. The increased activity in this structure, in turn, inhibits the STN, SNpr, and GPi, resulting in a loss of inhibition to the VA/VL thalamus and increased thalamocortical excitatory drive. Structures in purple have reduced activity in HD, whereas structures in red have increased activity. Light blue lines indicate primary pathways of reduced activity. (See Abbreviations list for definitions of anatomical abbreviations.)

40 to over 100. Repeat length is correlated inversely with age of onset of HD. The younger the age of onset, the higher the probability of a large repeat number. The mechanism by which the expanded trinucleotide repeat leads to the clinical and pathological features of HD is unknown. The HD mutation lies within a large gene (10 kb) designated *HTT* (previously *IT15*) that encodes *huntingtin*, a protein of about 348,000 Da. The trinucleotide repeat, which encodes the amino acid glutamine, occurs at the 5′ end of HTT. Huntingtin does not resemble any other known protein.

Treatment

Symptomatic Treatment

None of the currently available medications slows the progression of the disease (Ross et al., 2014).

Tetrabenazine is used for the treatment of chorea associated with HD. Tetrabenazine and the related drug reserpine are inhibitors of VMAT2 and cause presynaptic depletion of catecholamines. Tetrabenazine is a reversible inhibitor; inhibition by reserpine is irreversible and may lead to long-lasting effects. Both drugs may cause hypotension and depression with suicidality; the shorter duration of effect of tetrabenazine simplifies clinical management. The recommended starting dose of tetrabenazine is 12.5 mg daily. Most patients can be managed with doses of 50 mg a day or less; however, tetrabenazine is extensively metabolized by CYP2D6. Genotyping for CYP2D6 may be needed to optimize therapy and is recommended for patients who require more than 50 mg daily. As might be expected with a drug that depletes DA stores, tetrabenazine can also cause parkinsonism. The recently approved deuterated tetrabenazine, *deutetrabenazine*, takes advantage of the stronger bonds that deuterium forms with carbon (the kinetic-isotope effect). The active deuterated dehydrometabolites are VMAT2 inhibitors with longer half-lives than the corresponding products of tetrabenazine metabolism. Deutetrabenazine has therapeutic uses and an adverse effect profile similar to those of tetrabenazine.

Symptomatic treatment is needed for patients who are depressed, irritable, paranoid, excessively anxious, or psychotic. Depression can be treated effectively with standard antidepressant drugs with the caveat that drugs with substantial anticholinergic profiles can exacerbate chorea. Fluoxetine (see Chapter 15) is effective treatment of both the depression and the irritability manifest in symptomatic HD. Carbamazepine (see

Chapter 17) also has been found to be effective for the depression. Paranoia, delusional states, and psychosis are treated with antipsychotic drugs, usually at lower doses than those used in primary psychiatric disorders (see Chapter 16). These agents also reduce cognitive function and impair mobility and thus should be used in the lowest doses possible and should be discontinued when the psychiatric symptoms resolve. In individuals with predominantly rigid HD, clozapine, quetiapine (see Chapter 16), or carbamazepine may be more effective for treatment of paranoia and psychosis.

Many patients with HD exhibit worsening of involuntary movements as a result of anxiety or stress. In these situations, judicious use of sedative or anxiolytic benzodiazepines can be helpful. In juvenile-onset cases where rigidity rather than chorea predominates, DA agonists have had variable success in the improvement of rigidity. These individuals also occasionally develop myoclonus and seizures that can be responsive to clonazepam, valproate, and other anticonvulsants (see Chapter 17).

Amyotrophic Lateral Sclerosis

Amyotrophic lateral sclerosis (ALS or Lou Gehrig disease) is a disorder of the motor neurons of the ventral horn of the spinal cord (lower motor neurons) and the cortical neurons that provide their afferent input (upper motor neurons) (Gordon, 2013). The disorder is characterized by rapidly progressive weakness, muscle atrophy and fasciculations, spasticity, dysarthria, dysphagia, and respiratory compromise. Many patients with ALS exhibit behavioral changes and cognitive dysfunction, and there is clinical, genetic, and neuropathological overlap between ALS and frontotemporal dementia spectrum disorders. ALS usually is progressive and fatal. Most patients die of respiratory compromise and pneumonia after 2–3 years, although some survive for many years.

Etiology

About 10% of ALS cases are familial (FALS), usually with an autosomal dominant pattern of inheritance. The most common genetic cause is a hexanucleotide repeat expansion in *C9ORF72*, which is responsible for up to 40% of FALS and around 5% of sporadic cases (Rohrer et al., 2015). Another 10% of FALS cases are due to mutations in the Cu/Zn SOD1. Mutations in the *TARDBP* gene encoding TDP-43 and in the *FUS/TLS* gene have been identified as causes of FALS. Both TDP-43 and FUS/TLS bind DNA and RNA and regulate transcription and alternative splicing. About 90% of ALS cases are sporadic. Of these, a few are caused by de novo mutations in *C9ORF72* (up to 7%), *SOD1*, *TDP-43*, *FUS/TLS*, or other genes, but for the majority of sporadic cases, the etiology remains unclear. The underlying pathophysiology remains under investigation, including roles for abnormal RNA processing, glutamate excitotoxicity, oxidative stress, and mitochondrial dysfunction.

Treatments

Riluzole

Riluzole (2-amino-6-[trifluoromethoxy] benzothiazole) is an agent with complex actions in the nervous system. Riluzole is absorbed orally and is highly protein bound. It undergoes extensive metabolism in the liver by CYP-mediated hydroxylation and glucuronidation. Its $t_{1/2}$ is about 12 h. In vitro studies showed that riluzole has both presynaptic and postsynaptic effects. It not only inhibits glutamate release, but also blocks postsynaptic NMDA- and kainate-type glutamate receptors and inhibits voltage-dependent Na^+ channels. The recommended dose is 50 mg twice daily, taken 1 h before or 2 h after a meal. Riluzole usually is well tolerated, although nausea or diarrhea may occur. Rarely, riluzole may produce hepatic injury with elevations of serum transaminases, and periodic monitoring of these is recommended. Meta-analyses of the available clinical trials indicated that riluzole extends survival by 2–3 months. Although the magnitude of the effect of riluzole on ALS is small, it represents a significant therapeutic milestone in the treatment of a disease refractory to all previous treatments (Miller et al., 2007).

Edaravone

Edaravone

Edaravone was approved by the FDA in 2017 for treatment of ALS, the first new drug approved for this indication since 1995. It is a small molecule with free radical scavenging properties that may reduce oxidative stress, although the exact mechanism of action is unknown. Edaravone has been used in Japan for acute stroke since 2001 and was approved by the FDA for ALS under an orphan drug designation. A phase 3 study showed no benefit, but after posthoc subgroup analyses suggested an effect in early ALS, a subsequent trial enrolling only early stage patients showed a smaller functional decline over 6 months in patients treated with edaravone. It is administered intravenously, with the first round daily for 14 days, followed by a 14 day holiday, then in subsequent cycles, 10 out of every 14 days followed by a 14-day holiday. The drug is metabolized to a glucuronide and a sulfate and excreted primarily in the urine as the glucuronide, yielding a terminal $t_{1/2}$ of 4.5-6 h. At clinical doses, edaravone is not expected to inhibit major CYPs, UGTs, or drug transporters, or to induce CYPs 1A2, 2B6, or 3A4; nor should inhibitors of these enzymes have substantial effects on the pharmacokinetics of edaravone. The infusion contains sodium bisulfite, which can cause hypersensitivity reactions. Other adverse effects include bruising, gait disorder, and headache.

Symptomatic Therapy of ALS: Spasticity

Spasticity is an important component of the clinical features of ALS and the feature most amenable to present forms of treatment. *Spasticity* is defined as an increase in muscle tone characterized by an initial resistance to passive movement of a joint, followed by a sudden relaxation (the so-called clasped-knife phenomenon). Spasticity results from loss of descending inputs to the spinal motor neurons, and the character of the spasticity depends on which nervous system pathways are affected.

Baclofen

The best agent for the symptomatic treatment of spasticity in ALS is baclofen, a $GABA_B$ receptor agonist (see Figure 14–10). Initial doses of 5–10 mg/d are recommended, which can be increased to as much as 200 mg/d, if necessary. Alternatively, baclofen can be delivered directly into the space around the spinal cord using a surgically implanted pump and an intrathecal catheter. This approach minimizes the adverse effects of the drug, especially sedation, but it carries the risk of potentially life-threatening CNS depression.

Tizanidine

Tizanidine is an agonist of α_2 adrenergic receptors in the CNS. It reduces muscle spasticity, probably by increasing presynaptic inhibition of motor neurons. Tizanidine is primarily used in the treatment of spasticity in multiple sclerosis or after stroke, but it also may be effective in patients with ALS. Treatment should be initiated at a low dose of 2–4 mg at bedtime and titrated upward gradually. Drowsiness, asthenia, and dizziness may limit the dose that can be administered.

Other Agents

Benzodiazepines (see Chapter 19) such as *clonazepam* are effective antispasticity agents, but they may contribute to respiratory depression in patients with advanced ALS.

Dantrolene, approved in the U.S. for the treatment of muscle spasm, *is not used* in ALS because it can exacerbate muscular weakness. Dantrolene acts directly on skeletal muscle fibers, impairing Ca^{2+} release from the sarcoplasmic reticulum. It is effective in treating spasticity associated with stroke or spinal cord injury and in treating malignant hyperthermia (see Chapter 11). Dantrolene may cause hepatotoxicity, so it is important to monitor liver-associated enzymes before and during therapy with the drug.

Acknowledgment: *David G. Standaert contributed to this chapter in recent editions of this book. We have retained some of his text in the current edition.*

Drug Facts for Your Personal Formulary: *Drugs for Neurodegenerative Disease*

Drugs	Therapeutic Uses	Clinical Pharmacology and Tips
Anti-Parkinson: L-DOPA (DA precursor); Carbidopa (inhibits AADC, reduces peripheral conversion of L-DOPA to DA)		
Carbidopa/levodopa	• Most effective symptomatic therapy for PD	• Therapeutic window narrows after several years of treatment: wearing off, dyskinesias, on/off phenomenon • Available as immediate-release tablets and orally disintegrated tablets
Carbidopa/levodopa sustained release	• Patients with PD with motor fluctuations on regular carbidopa/levodopa	• Bioavailability of immediate-release form, 75%
Carbidopa-levodopa extended-release capsules (RYTARY)	• Patients with PD with motor fluctuations on regular carbidopa/levodopa	• Mixture of immediate- and extended-release beads
Carbidopa-levodopa intestinal gel (DUOPA)	• Patients with PD with motor fluctuations on regular carbidopa/levodopa	• Requires placement of gastrostomy tube with jejunal extension • Useful for wearing off issues
Anti-Parkinson: DA agonists (longer acting than L-DOPA; can produce psychosis, impulse control disorder, sleepiness)		
Ropinirole	• PD • Restless legs syndrome	• Selective D2 receptor class agonist • Available in immediate release (3 times daily) and sustained release (once daily)
Pramipexole	• PD • Restless legs syndrome	• Selective D2 receptor class agonist • Available in immediate release (3 times daily) and sustained release (once daily)
Rotigotine	• PD • Restless legs syndrome	• D2 and D1 receptor class agonist • Transdermal formulation
Apomorphine	• Rescue therapy for acute intermittent treatment of off episodes	• Subcutaneous formulation • Emetogenic, requires concurrent antiemetic • Contraindicated with $5HT_3$ antagonists
Anti-Parkinson: COMT Inhibitors (reduce peripheral conversion of levodopa, increasing $t_{1/2}$ and CNS dose)		
Entacapone	• Adjunctive PD therapy given with each dose of levodopa, for wearing off	• Short $t_{1/2}$, inhibits peripheral COMT
Tolcapone	• Adjunctive PD therapy given with each dose of levodopa, for wearing off	• Long $t_{1/2}$, inhibits central and peripheral COMT • May be hepatotoxic; use only in patients not responding satisfactorily to other treatments; monitor liver function
Carbidopa/levodopa/entacapone	• PD, especially for wearing off on levodopa alone	• Fixed-dose combination formulation
Anti-Parkinson: MAO-B Inhibitors (reduce oxidative metabolism of dopamine in the CNS)		
Rasagiline	• PD, either as initial monotherapy or adjunct to levodopa	• Adjunct to reduce wearing off • Many drug interactions • Should not be given with meperidine • When administered with CYP1A2 inhibitors, C_p of rasagiline may double • Risk of serotonin syndrome
Selegiline	• PD, as adjunctive therapy in patients with deteriorating response to levodopa	• Generates amphetamine metabolites, which can cause anxiety and insomnia • MAO-B selectivity lost at doses > 30–40 mg/d • Many drug interactions • Should not be given with meperidine • Risk of serotonin syndrome • Available in immediate release, orally disintegrating tablet, or transdermal patch
Anti-Parkinson: Other		
Amantadine	• Early, mild PD • Levodopa-induced dyskinesias • Influenza	• Unclear mechanism of antiparkinsonian effects • Effective against dyskinesia
Trihexyphenidyl	• PD, as adjunctive therapy	• Muscarinic receptor antagonist • Anticholinergic side effects
Benztropine	• PD, as adjunctive therapy	• Muscarinic receptor antagonist

Drug Facts for Your Personal Formulary: *Drugs for Neurodegenerative Disease (continued)*

Drugs	Therapeutic Uses	Clinical Pharmacology and Tips
Anti-Alzheimer: Acetylcholinesterase Inhibitors (boost cholinergic neurotransmission; first line treatment)		
Donepezil	• Mild, moderate, severe AD dementia	• GI symptoms: main dose-limiting side effect • Bradycardia/syncope less common
Rivastigmine	• Mild-moderate AD dementia • Mild-moderate PD dementia	• Transdermal formulation available, with lower risk of GI side effects • Also inhibits BuChE
Galantamine	• Mild-moderate AD dementia	• GI symptoms: main dose-limiting side effect • Bradycardia/syncope less common than GI side effects
Anti-Alzheimer: Low-Affinity Uncompetitive NMDA Antagonist		
Memantine	• Moderate, severe AD dementia	• Reduces excitotoxicity through use-dependent blockade of NMDA receptors
Anti-Huntington		
Tetrabenazine Deutetrabenazine	• Chorea in HD	• Reversible VMAT2 inhibitor: depletes presynaptic catecholamines • Adverse effects: hypotension, depression with suicidality • Adjust dose for CYP2D6 status; 2D6 inhibitors (e.g., paroxetine, fluoxetine, quinidine, bupropion) ↑ exposure ~3 fold • Contraindications: concurrent or recent MAO inhibitor or reserpine
Anti-ALS		
Riluzole	Extends survival in ALS up to 3 months	• Uncertain mechanism of action: inhibits glutamate release, blocks sodium channels and glutamate receptors
Edaravone	Reduces progression in early stages of ALS	• Intensive intravenous administration regimen
Anti-Spastic Agents Baclofen	• $GABA_B$ receptor agonist	• Sedation and CNS depression
Tizanidine	• α_2 adrenergic receptor agonist	• Causes drowsiness; treatment is initiated with low dose and titrated upward
Benzodiazepines (e.g., clonazepam)	• See Chapter 19	• May contribute to respiratory depression
Dantrolene	• *Not used in ALS*, but for treating muscle spasm in stroke or spinal injury and for treating malignant hyperthermia	• May cause hepatotoxicity

Bibliography

Albin RL, et al. The functional anatomy of basal ganglia disorders. *Trends Neurosci*, **1989**, *12*:366–375.

Bates GP, et al. Huntington disease. *Nat Rev Dis Primers*, **2015**, *1*:15005.

Calabresi P, et al. Direct and indirect pathways of basal ganglia: a critical reappraisal. *Nat Neurosci*, **2014**, *17*(8):1022–1030.

Connolly BS, Lang AE. Pharmacological treatment of Parkinson disease: a review. *JAMA*, **2014**, *311*(16):1670–1683.

Cotzias GC, et al. Modification of Parkinsonism: chronic treatment with L-dopa. *N Engl J Med*, **1969**, *280*:337–345.

Fahn S, et al. Levodopa and the progression of Parkinson's disease. *N Engl J Med*, **2004**, *351*:2498–2508.

Giacobini E, Gold G. Alzheimer disease therapy—moving from amyloid-β to tau. *Nat Rev Neurol*, **2013**, *9*:677–686.

Goedert M, et al. 100 years of Lewy pathology. *Nat Rev Neurol*, **2013**, *9*(1):13–24.

Gordon PH. Amyotrophic lateral sclerosis: an update for 2013 clinical features, pathophysiology, management and therapeutic trials. *Aging Dis*, **2013**, *4*(5):295–310.

Hauser RA, et al. Extended-release carbidopa-levodopa (IPX066) compared with immediate-release carbidopa-levodopa in patients with Parkinson's disease and motor fluctuations: a phase 3 randomised, double-blind trial. *Lancet Neurol*, **2013**, *12*(4):346–356.

Hornykiewicz O. Dopamine in the basal ganglia: its role and therapeutic indications (including the clinical use of L-dopa). *Br Med Bull*, **1973**, *29*:172–178.

Kumar KR, et al. Genetics of Parkinson disease and other movement disorders. *Curr Opin Neurol*, **2012**, *25*(4):466–474.

Langston JW. The Parkinson's complex: parkinsonism is just the tip of the iceberg. *Ann Neurol*, **2006**, *59*:591–596.

Miller RG, et al. Riluzole for amyotrophic lateral sclerosis (ALS)/motor neuron disease (MND). *Cochrane Database Syst Rev*, **2007**, (1):CD001447.

Olanow CW, et al. Continuous intrajejunal infusion of levodopa-carbidopa intestinal gel for patients with advanced Parkinson's disease: a randomised, controlled, double-blind, double-dummy study. *Lancet Neurol*, **2014**, *13*(2):141–149.

Olanow CW, et al. A randomized, double-blind, placebo-controlled, delayed start study to assess rasagiline as a disease modifying therapy in Parkinson's disease (the ADAGIO study): rationale, design, and baseline characteristics. *Mov Disord*, **2008**, *23*:2194–2201.

Pahwa R, et al. Practice parameter: treatment of Parkinson disease with motor fluctuations and dyskinesia (an evidence-based review): report of the Quality Standards Subcommittee of the American Academy of Neurology. *Neurology*, **2006**, *66*(7):983–995.

Panisset M, et al. Serotonin toxicity association with concomitant antidepressants and rasagiline treatment: retrospective study (STACCATO). *Pharmacotherapy*, **2014**, *34*(12):1250–1258.

Parkinson Study Group. Entacapone improves motor fluctuations in levodopa-treated Parkinson's disease patients. *Ann Neurol*, **1997**, *42*:747–755 (published erratum appears in *Ann Neurol*, **1998**, *44*:292).

Parkinson Study Group. Pramipexole vs. levodopa as initial treatment for Parkinson's disease: a randomized, controlled trial. *JAMA*, **2000**, *284*:1931–1938.

Prusiner SB. Biology and genetics of prions causing neurodegeneration. *Annu Rev Genet*, **2013**, *47*:601–623.

Renton AE, et al. State of play in amyotrophic lateral sclerosis genetics. *Nat Neurosci*, **2014**, *17*:17–23.

Roberson ED, Mucke L. 100 years and counting: prospects for defeating Alzheimer's disease. *Science*, **2006**, *314*:781–784.

Rohrer JD, et al. C9orf72 expansions in frontotemporal dementia and amyotrophic lateral sclerosis. *Lancet Neurol*, **2015**, *14*:291–301.

Ross CA, et al. Huntington disease: natural history, biomarkers and prospects for therapeutics. *Nat Rev Neurol*, **2014**, *10*:204–216.

Selkoe DJ. The therapeutics of Alzheimer's disease: where we stand and where we are heading. *Ann Neurol*, **2013**, *74*:328–336.

Schneider LS, et al. Risk of death with atypical antipsychotic drug treatment for dementia: meta-analysis of randomized placebo-controlled trials. *JAMA*, **2005**, *294*:1934–1943.

Singleton AB, et al. The genetics of Parkinson's disease: progress and therapeutic implications. *Mov Disord*, **2013**, *28*(1):14–23.

Suchowersky O, et al. Practice parameter: diagnosis and prognosis of new onset Parkinson disease (an evidence-based review): report of the Quality Standards Subcommittee of the American Academy of Neurology. *Neurology*, **2006**, *66*:968–975.

Weintraub D, et al. Clinical spectrum of impulse control disorders in Parkinson's disease. *Mov Disord*, **2015**, *30*(2):121–127.

Zesiewicz TA, et al. Practice parameter: treatment of nonmotor symptoms of Parkinson disease: report of the Quality Standards Subcommittee of the American Academy of Neurology. *Neurology*, **2010**, *74*:924–931.

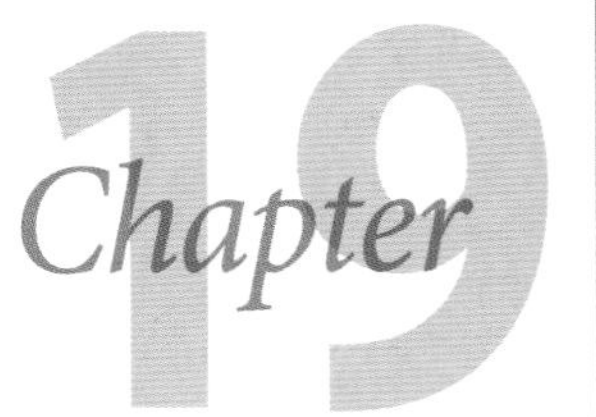

Hypnotics and Sedatives

S. John Mihic, Jody Mayfield, and R. Adron Harris

第十九章　催眠药和镇静药

中文导读

本章主要介绍：苯二氮䓬类药物，包括苯二氮䓬类药物的分子靶标和药理特性；新型苯二氮䓬类受体激动药，包括扎来普隆、唑吡坦和右佐匹克隆；长期苯二氮䓬类药物治疗后的患者管理；苯二氮䓬类受体拮抗药氟马西尼；褪黑素类似物，包括拉米替隆和他司美琼；巴比妥类药物；其他镇静催眠药，包括水合氯醛、甲丙氨酯和其他药物；非处方催眠药；新兴药物，包括苏沃雷生、多塞平、普瑞巴林、利他林和阿戈美拉汀；失眠症的管理，包括失眠症的类别、失眠症治疗指南。

Abbreviations

ACh: acetylcholine
ALA: δ-aminolevulinic acid
AMPA: α-amino-3-hydroxy-5-methyl-4-isoxazole propionic acid
COPD: chronic obstructive pulmonary disease
CNS: central nervous system
CYP: cytochrome P450
EEG: electroencephalogram
FDA: Food and Drug Administration
GABA: γ-aminobutyric acid
GI: gastrointestinal
GPCR: G protein–coupled receptor
IM: intramuscular
IV: intravenous
MT: melatonin
OL: off-label use
OSA: obstructive sleep apnea
OTC: over the counter
REM: rapid eye movement
SSRI: selective serotonin reuptake inhibitor

A *sedative* drug decreases activity, moderates excitement, and calms the recipient, whereas a *hypnotic* drug produces drowsiness and facilitates the onset and maintenance of a state of sleep that resembles natural sleep in its electroencephalographic characteristics and from which the recipient can be aroused easily. Sedation is a side effect of many drugs that are not considered general CNS depressants (e.g., antihistamines and antipsychotic agents). Although these and other agents can intensify the effects of CNS depressants, they usually produce their desired therapeutic effects at concentrations lower than those causing substantial CNS depression. For example, benzodiazepine sedative-hypnotics do not produce generalized CNS depression. Although coma may occur at very high doses, neither surgical anesthesia nor fatal intoxication is produced by benzodiazepines unless other drugs with CNS-depressant actions are concomitantly administered; an important exception is *midazolam*, which has been associated with decreased tidal volume and respiratory rate. Moreover, specific antagonists of benzodiazepines exist, such as *flumazenil*, which is used to treat cases of benzodiazepine overdose. This constellation of properties sets the benzodiazepine receptor agonists apart from other sedative-hypnotic drugs and imparts a measure of safety, such that benzodiazepines and the newer benzodiazepine receptor agonists (the "Z compounds") have largely displaced older agents for the treatment of insomnia and anxiety.

The CNS depressants discussed in this chapter include benzodiazepines, the Z compounds, barbiturates, as well as several sedative-hypnotic agents of diverse chemical structure. The sedative-hypnotic drugs that do not specifically target the benzodiazepine receptor belong to a group of older, less-safe, sedative-hypnotic drugs that depress the CNS in a dose-dependent fashion, progressively producing a spectrum of responses from mild sedation to coma and death. These older sedative-hypnotic compounds share these properties with a large number of chemicals, including general anesthetics (see Chapter 21) and alcohols, most notably ethanol (see Chapter 23). The newer sedative-hypnotic agents, such as benzodiazepines and Z drugs, are safer in this regard.

HISTORICAL PERSPECTIVE

Humans have long sought sleep unburdened by worry and, to this end, have consumed many potions. In the mid-19th century, bromide was introduced specifically as a sedative-hypnotic. Chloral hydrate, paraldehyde, urethane, and sulfonal were used before the introduction of barbiturates (barbital, 1903; phenobarbital, 1912), of which about 50 were distributed commercially. Barbiturates were so dominant that fewer than a dozen other sedative-hypnotics were marketed successfully before 1960.

The partial separation of sedative-hypnotic-anesthetic properties from anticonvulsant properties characteristic of phenobarbital led to searches for agents with more selective effects on CNS functions. As a result, relatively nonsedating anticonvulsants, notably phenytoin and trimethadione, were developed in the late 1930s and early 1940s (Chapter 17). The advent of chlorpromazine and meprobamate in the early 1950s, with their taming effects in animals, and the development of increasingly sophisticated methods for evaluating the behavioral effects of drugs, set the stage in the 1950s for the synthesis of chlordiazepoxide, the introduction of which into clinical medicine in 1961 ushered in the era of benzodiazepines. Most of the benzodiazepines in the marketplace were selected for high anxiolytic potency in relation to their depression of CNS function. However, all benzodiazepines possess sedative-hypnotic properties to varying degrees; these properties are exploited extensively clinically, especially to facilitate sleep. Mainly because of their remarkably low capacity to produce fatal CNS depression, the benzodiazepines displaced the barbiturates as sedative-hypnotic agents.

Benzodiazepines

All benzodiazepines in clinical use promote the binding of the major inhibitory neurotransmitter GABA to the $GABA_A$ receptor, a pentameric ligand-gated, anion-conducting channel. Considerable heterogeneity exists among human $GABA_A$ receptors; this heterogeneity is thought to contribute to the myriad effects of these agents in vivo. Because receptor subunit composition appears to govern the interaction of various allosteric modulators with these channels, there has been a surge in efforts to find agents displaying different combinations of benzodiazepine-like properties that may reflect selective actions on one or more subtypes of $GABA_A$ receptors. A number of distinct mechanisms of action, reflecting involvement of specific subunits of the $GABA_A$ receptor, likely contribute to distinct effects of various benzodiazepines—the sedative-hypnotic, muscle-relaxant, anxiolytic, amnesic, and anticonvulsant effects.

Although the benzodiazepines exert qualitatively similar clinical effects, quantitative differences in their pharmacodynamic spectra and pharmacokinetic properties have led to varying patterns of therapeutic application. While only the benzodiazepines used primarily for hypnosis are discussed in detail, this chapter describes the general properties of the group and important differences amongst individual agents (Figure 19–1) (see also Chapters 15 and 17).

The Molecular Target for Benzodiazepines

Benzodiazepines act at $GABA_A$ receptors by binding directly to a specific site that is distinct from the GABA binding site.

The $GABA_A$ Receptor

The $GABA_A$ receptor is the major inhibitory receptor in the CNS. It is a transmembrane protein composed of five subunits that co-assemble

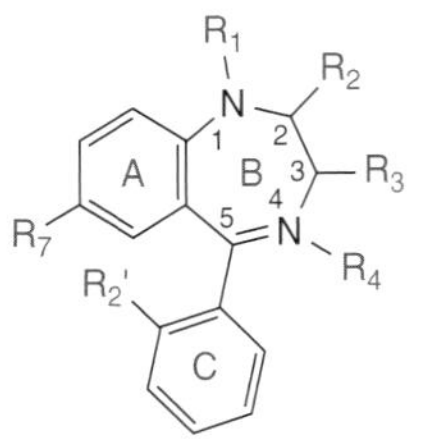

Figure 19–1 *Basic structure of benzodiazepines. Benzodiazepine* refers to the portion of this structure comprising the benzene ring (A) fused to a seven-member diazepine ring (B). Because all the important benzodiazepines contain a 5-aryl substituent (ring C) and a 1,4-diazepine ring, the term has come to mean the 5-aryl-1,4-benzodiazepines. Numerous modifications in the structure of the ring systems and substituents have yielded compounds with similar activities, including the benzodiazepine receptor antagonist flumazenil, in which ring C is replaced with a keto function at position 5 and a methyl substituent is added at position 4. A number of nonbenzodiazepine compounds (e.g., β-carbolines, zolpidem, eszopiclone) plus classic benzodiazepines and flumazenil bind to the benzodiazepine receptor, an allosteric site on the ionotropic $GABA_A$ receptor, a pentameric structure that forms a GABA-stimulated Cl^- channel.

around a central anion-conducting channel. Each subunit is composed of a large extracellular amino terminus, four transmembrane segments (M1-M4) and a short carboxy terminus. The M2 segment of each subunit contributes to the formation of the central anion-conducting pore. GABA binds at the interfaces of α and β classes of subunits, while benzodiazepines bind at α/γ interfaces. The five subunits come from 19 isoforms, so the number of possible pentameric combinations is large. The number of pentamers actually expressed in nature is uncertain, but likely numbers in the dozens. The $GABA_A$ receptor shares subunit organization with a number of other cys-loop ligand-gated ion channels and with the ACh binding protein (Figure 11–1).

The $GABA_A$ receptor pentamer contains a single benzodiazepine binding site, as well as other allosteric sites at which a variety of sedative-hypnotic-anesthetic agents exert modulatory effects on $GABA_A$ receptor function (Figure 14–11). The exact functional properties of the pentameric receptor depend on the subunit composition and arrangement of the individual subunits, and this heterogeneity likely contributes to the pharmacological diversity of benzodiazepine effects observed in behavioral, biochemical, and functional studies and to the selective effects of the Z compounds.

Effects of Benzodiazepines on $GABA_A$ Receptor–Mediated Events

Benzodiazepines are allosteric modulators of $GABA_A$ receptor function (Sieghart, 2015). They increase the affinity of the $GABA_A$ receptor for GABA and thereby enhance GABA-induced Cl^- currents. Thus, in terms of channel kinetics, benzodiazepines increase the frequency of opening of the $GABA_A$ receptor Cl^- channel in the presence of GABA (Nestler et al., 2015; Sigel and Steinmann, 2012). Inverse agonists do just the opposite, reducing GABA binding and the frequency of channel opening. Benzodiazepine antagonists (e.g., flumazenil) competitively block benzodiazepine binding and effect but do not independently alter channel function (Nestler et al., 2015; Sigel and Steinmann, 2012).

In pharmacodynamic terms, agonists at the benzodiazepine binding site shift the GABA concentration-response curve to the left, whereas inverse agonists shift the curve to the right. Both these effects are blocked by antagonists (e.g., flumazenil) that bind at the benzodiazepine binding site. Application of a benzodiazepine site antagonist, in the absence of either an agonist or antagonist at this same site, results in no change in $GABA_A$ receptor function. The behavioral and electrophysiological effects of benzodiazepines can also be reduced or prevented by prior treatment with antagonists of GABA binding (e.g., bicuculline).

The remarkable safety profile of the benzodiazepines likely relates to the fact that their effects in vivo depend on the presynaptic release of GABA; in the absence of GABA, benzodiazepines have no effects on $GABA_A$ receptor function.

The behavioral and sedative effects of benzodiazepines can be ascribed in part to potentiation of GABAergic pathways that serve to regulate the firing of monoamine-containing neurons known to promote behavioral arousal and to be important mediators of the inhibitory effects of fear and punishment on behavior. Inhibitory effects on muscular hypertonia or the spread of seizure activity can be attributed to potentiation of inhibitory GABAergic circuits at various levels of the neuraxis. The magnitude of the effects produced by benzodiazepines varies widely depending on such factors as the types of inhibitory circuits that are operating, the sources and intensity of excitatory input, and the manner in which experimental manipulations are performed and assessed. Accordingly, benzodiazepines markedly prolong the period after brief activation of recurrent GABAergic pathways during which neither spontaneous nor applied excitatory stimuli can evoke neuronal discharge; this effect is reversed by the $GABA_A$ receptor antagonist *bicuculline* (see Figure 14–10).

Benzodiazepines Versus Barbiturates at the $GABA_A$ Receptor

The two classes of agents, barbiturates and benzodiazepines, differ in their potencies: Barbiturates act to enhance $GABA_A$ receptor function at low micromolar concentrations; benzodiazepines bind with nanomolar affinity. Both benzodiazepines and barbiturates bind to allosteric sites on the $GABA_A$ receptor pentamer and thereby enhance GABA-stimulated Cl^- channel function. However, barbiturates also have an additional effect: Higher concentrations of barbiturates directly activate $GABA_A$ receptors. Furthermore, when tested using equieffective concentrations of GABA, maximally effective concentrations of barbiturates produce greater enhancement of $GABA_A$ receptor function than do benzodiazepines. This direct effect possibly contributes to the profound CNS depression that barbiturates can cause. The lack of direct channel activation by benzodiazepines and their dependence on the presynaptic release of GABA at the $GABA_A$ receptor likely contribute to the safety of these agents as compared to barbiturates.

Pharmacological Properties of Benzodiazepines

The therapeutic effects of the benzodiazepines result from their actions on the CNS. The most prominent of these effects are sedation, hypnosis, decreased anxiety, muscle relaxation, anterograde amnesia, and anticonvulsant activity. Only two effects of these drugs result from peripheral actions: coronary vasodilation, seen after intravenous administration of therapeutic doses of certain benzodiazepines, and neuromuscular blockade, seen only with very high doses.

CNS Effects

While benzodiazepines depress activity at all levels of the neuraxis, some structures are affected preferentially. The benzodiazepines do not produce the same magnitudes of neuronal depression produced by barbiturates and volatile anesthetics, likely because they have weaker enhancing effects at $GABA_A$ receptors than those compounds, even at saturating concentrations. All the benzodiazepines have similar pharmacological profiles. Nevertheless, the drugs differ in selectivity, and the clinical usefulness of individual benzodiazepines thus varies considerably. The vast majority of effects of benzodiazepine site agonists and inverse agonists can be reversed or prevented by flumazenil, which competes with agonists and inverse agonists at a common binding site at the $GABA_A$ receptor. As the dose of a benzodiazepine is increased, sedation progresses to hypnosis and then to stupor. Although the clinical literature often refers to the "anesthetic" effects and uses of certain benzodiazepines, these drugs do not cause a true general anesthesia; awareness usually persists, and a failure to respond to a noxious stimulus sufficient to allow surgery cannot be achieved. Nonetheless, at "preanesthetic" doses, there is amnesia for events occurring subsequent to administration of the drug. Although many attempts have been made to separate the anxiolytic actions of benzodiazepines from their sedative-hypnotic effects, distinguishing between these behaviors is problematic. Accurate measurements of anxiety and sedation are difficult in humans, and the validity of animal models for measuring anxiety and sedation is uncertain.

Although analgesic effects of benzodiazepines have been observed in experimental animals, only transient analgesia is apparent in humans after intravenous administration. Such effects actually may involve the production of amnesia. Unlike barbiturates, benzodiazepines do not cause hyperalgesia.

Tolerance. Although most patients who chronically ingest benzodiazepines report that drowsiness wanes over a few days, tolerance to the impairment seen in some measures of psychomotor performance (e.g., visual tracking) is not usually observed. Whether tolerance develops to the anxiolytic effects of benzodiazepines remains debatable. Many patients use a fairly constant maintenance dose; increases or decreases in dosage appear to correspond with changes in their perceived problems or stresses. Conversely, other patients either do not reduce their dosages when stress is relieved or steadily escalate dosing. Such behavior may be associated with the development of drug dependence (see Chapter 24).

Some benzodiazepines induce muscle hypotonia without interfering with normal locomotion and can decrease rigidity in patients with cerebral palsy. *Clonazepam* in nonsedating doses causes muscle relaxation, but *diazepam* and most other benzodiazepines do not. Tolerance occurs to the muscle relaxant and ataxic effects of these drugs.

Experimentally, benzodiazepines inhibit seizure activity induced by either pentylenetetrazol or picrotoxin, but suppress strychnine- and maximal electroshock-induced seizures only at doses that also severely impair locomotor activity. *Clonazepam, nitrazepam*, and *nordazepam* have greater selective anticonvulsant activity than do most other benzodiazepines. Benzodiazepines also suppress photic seizures in baboons and ethanol withdrawal seizures in humans. However, the development of tolerance to the anticonvulsant effects has limited the usefulness of benzodiazepines in the treatment of recurrent seizure disorders in humans (see Chapter 17).

Effects on the Electroencephalogram and Sleep Stages. The effects of benzodiazepines on the waking EEG resemble those of other sedative-hypnotic drugs. Alpha rhythm activity is decreased, but there is an increase in low-voltage fast activity. Tolerance also occurs to these effects. With respect to sleep, some differences in the patterns of effects exerted by the various benzodiazepines have been noted, but benzodiazepine users usually report a sense of deep or refreshing sleep. Benzodiazepines decrease sleep latency, especially when first used, and diminish the number of awakenings and the time spent in stage 0 (a stage of wakefulness). They also produce an increased arousal threshold from sleep. Time in stage 1 (descending drowsiness) usually is decreased, and there is a prominent decrease in the time spent in slow-wave sleep (stages 3 and 4). Most benzodiazepines increase the latency from onset of spindle sleep to the first burst of REM sleep. The time spent in REM sleep is usually shortened, but the number of cycles of REM sleep is typically increased, mostly late in the sleep time. *Zolpidem* and *zaleplon* suppress REM sleep less extensively than benzodiazepines and thus may be superior to benzodiazepines for use as hypnotics (Dujardin et al., 1998).

Despite the shortening of durations of stage 4 and REM sleep, benzodiazepine administration typically increases total sleep time, largely by increasing the time spent in stage 2, which is the major fraction of non-REM sleep. This effect is greatest in subjects with the shortest baseline total sleep time. In addition, despite the increased number of REM cycles, the number of shifts to lighter sleep stages (1 and 0) and the amount of body movement are diminished with benzodiazepine use. Nocturnal peaks in the secretion of growth hormone, prolactin, and luteinizing hormone are not affected. During chronic nocturnal use of benzodiazepines, the effects on the various stages of sleep usually decline within a few nights. When such use is discontinued, the pattern of drug-induced changes in sleep parameters may "rebound," and an increase in the amount and density of REM sleep may be especially prominent. If the dosage has not been excessive, patients usually will note only a shortening of sleep time rather than an exacerbation of insomnia.

Systemic Effects

Respiration. Hypnotic doses of benzodiazepines are without effect on respiration in normal subjects, but special care must be taken in the treatment of children and individuals with impaired hepatic or pulmonary function. At higher doses, such as those used for preanesthetic medication or for endoscopy, benzodiazepines slightly depress alveolar ventilation and cause respiratory acidosis as the result of a decrease in hypoxic rather than hypercapnic drive; these effects are exaggerated in patients with COPD, and alveolar hypoxia and CO_2 narcosis may result. These drugs can cause apnea during anesthesia or when given with opioids. Patients severely intoxicated with benzodiazepines only require respiratory assistance when they also have ingested another CNS depressant drug, most commonly ethanol.

Hypnotic doses of benzodiazepines may worsen sleep-related breathing disorders by adversely affecting control of the upper airway muscles or by decreasing the ventilatory response to CO_2. The latter effect may cause hypoventilation and hypoxemia in some patients with severe COPD. In patients with OSA, hypnotic doses of benzodiazepines may decrease muscle tone in the upper airway and exaggerate the impact of apneic episodes on alveolar hypoxia, pulmonary hypertension, and cardiac ventricular load. Benzodiazepines may promote the appearance of episodes of apnea during REM sleep (associated with decreases in O_2 saturation) in patients recovering from a myocardial infarction; however, no impact of these drugs on survival of patients with cardiac disease has been reported.

Cardiovascular System. The cardiovascular effects of benzodiazepines are minor in normal subjects except in cases of severe intoxication (see previous discussion for adverse effects in patients with obstructive sleep disorders or cardiac disease). At preanesthetic doses, all benzodiazepines decrease blood pressure and increase heart rate. With *midazolam*, the effects appear to be secondary to a decrease in peripheral resistance; however, with *diazepam*, the effects are secondary to a decrease in left ventricular work and cardiac output. *Diazepam* increases coronary flow, possibly by an action to increase interstitial concentrations of adenosine, and the accumulation of this cardiodepressant metabolite also may explain the negative inotropic effects of the drug. In large doses, *midazolam* considerably decreases cerebral blood flow and O_2 assimilation.

GI Tract. Benzodiazepines are thought by some gastroenterologists to improve a variety of "anxiety-related" GI disorders. There is a paucity of evidence for direct actions. Although diazepam markedly decreases nocturnal gastric secretion in humans, other drug classes are considerably more effective in acid-peptic disorders (see Chapter 49).

ADME

All benzodiazepines are absorbed completely except *clorazepate*. Clorazepate is decarboxylated rapidly in gastric juice to *N*-desmethyldiazepam (nordazepam), which subsequently is absorbed completely. Drugs active at the benzodiazepine receptor may be divided into four categories based on their elimination $t_{1/2}$:

- Ultrashort-acting benzodiazepines
- Short-acting agents ($t_{1/2}$ < 6 h), including midazolam, triazolam, the nonbenzodiazepine zolpidem ($t_{1/2}$ ~2 h), and eszopiclone ($t_{1/2}$, 5–6 h)
- Intermediate-acting agents ($t_{1/2}$, 6–24 h), including estazolam and temazepam
- Long-acting agents ($t_{1/2}$ > 24 h), including flurazepam, diazepam, and quazepam

Flurazepam itself has a short $t_{1/2}$ (~2.3 h), but a major active metabolite, *N*-des-alkyl-flurazepam, is long lived ($t_{1/2}$, 47–100 h); such features complicate the classification of certain benzodiazepines.

The benzodiazepines and their active metabolites bind to plasma proteins. The extent of binding correlates strongly with the oil:water partition coefficient and ranges from about 70% for alprazolam to nearly 99% for diazepam. The concentration in the cerebrospinal fluid is approximately equal to the concentration of free drug in plasma. Uptake of benzodiazepines occurs rapidly into the brain and other highly perfused organs after intravenous administration (or oral administration of a rapidly absorbed compound); rapid uptake is followed by a phase of redistribution into tissues that are less well perfused but capacious, especially muscle and fat (see Table 2–2 and Figure 2–4). Redistribution is most rapid for benzodiazepines with the highest oil:water partition coefficients. The kinetics of redistribution of diazepam and other lipophilic benzodiazepines are complicated by enterohepatic circulation. These drugs cross the placental barrier and are also secreted into breast milk.

Most benzodiazepines are metabolized extensively by hepatic CYPs, particularly CYP 3A4 and 2C19. Some benzodiazepines, such as *oxazepam*, are not metabolized by CYPs but are conjugated directly by phase 2 enzymes. Erythromycin, clarithromycin, ritonavir, itraconazole, ketoconazole, nefazodone, and grapefruit juice are examples of CYP3A4 inhibitors (see Chapter 6) that can affect the rate of metabolism of benzodiazepines. Benzodiazepines do not significantly induce hepatic CYPs, so their chronic administration does not usually affect metabolism of benzodiazepines or other drugs. Cimetidine and oral contraceptives inhibit *N*-dealkylation and 3-hydroxylation of benzodiazepines. Ethanol, isoniazid, and phenytoin are less effective in this regard. These phase 1 reactions usually are reduced to a greater extent in elderly patients and in patients with chronic liver disease than are those reactions involving conjugation.

The active metabolites of some benzodiazepines are biotransformed more slowly than are the parent compounds; thus, the durations of action of many benzodiazepines bear little relationship to the $t_{1/2}$ of elimination of the parent drug. Conversely, the rate of biotransformation of drugs that are inactivated by the initial metabolic reaction is an important determinant of their durations of action; examples include oxazepam, lorazepam, temazepam, triazolam, and midazolam.

Benzodiazepine metabolism can seem daunting but can be organized around a few basic principles. Metabolism of the benzodiazepines occurs in three major stages. These stages and the relationships between the drugs and their metabolites are shown in Table 19–1.

For benzodiazepines that bear a substituent at position 1 (or 2) of the diazepine ring, the *first phase* of metabolism involves modification or removal of the substituent. The eventual products are *N*-desalkylated compounds that are biologically active. Exceptions are triazolam, alprazolam, estazolam, and midazolam, which contain either a fused triazolo or an imidazolo ring and are α-hydroxylated.

The *second phase* of metabolism involves hydroxylation at position 3 and also usually yields an active derivative (e.g., oxazepam from nordazepam). The rates of these reactions are usually much slower than the first stage ($t_{1/2}$ > 40–50 h), such that appreciable accumulation of hydroxylated products with intact substituents at position 1 does not occur. (There are two significant exceptions to this rule: First, small amounts of temazepine accumulate during the chronic administration of diazepam; and second, following the replacement of S with O in quazepam, most of the resulting 2-oxoquazepam is hydroxylated slowly at position 3 without removal of the *N*-alkyl group. However, only small amounts of the 3-hydroxyl

TABLE 19–1 ■ STAGES AND RELATIONSHIPS AMONG SOME OF THE DIAZEPINES[a]

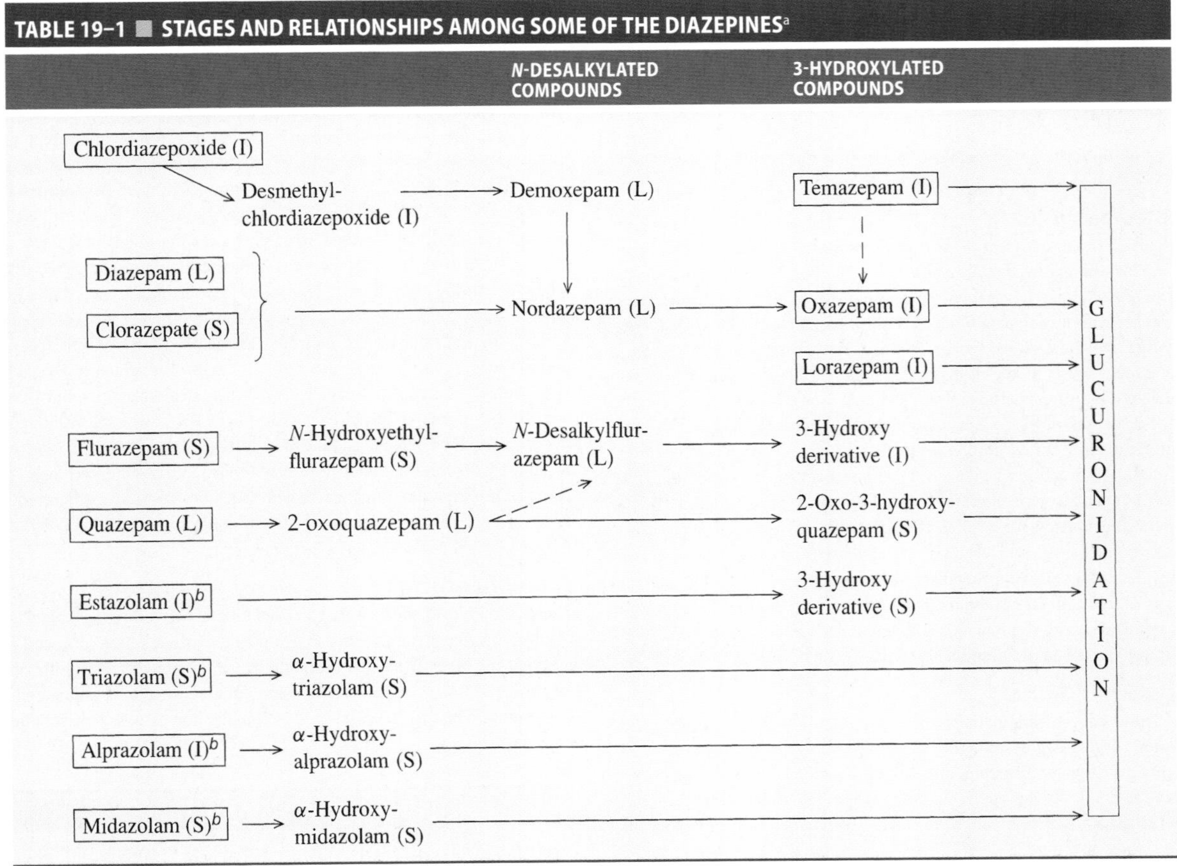

[a]Compounds enclosed in boxes are marketed in the U.S. The approximate half-lives of the various compounds are denoted in parentheses; S (short-acting), $t_{1/2}$ <6 h; I (intermediate-acting), $t_{1/2}$ = 6-24 h; L (long-acting), $t_{1/2}$ = >24 h. All compounds except clorazepate are biologically active; the activity of 3-hydroxydesalkylflurazepam has not been determined. Clonazepam (not shown) is an *N*-desalkyl compound, and it is metabolized primarily by reduction of the 7-NO_2 group to the corresponding amine (inactive), followed by acetylation; its $t_{1/2}$ is 20-40 h. [b]See text for discussion of other pathways of metabolism.

derivative accumulate during chronic administration of quazepam because this compound is conjugated at an unusually rapid rate. In contrast, the *N*-desalkylflurazepam that is formed by the "minor" metabolic pathway does accumulate during quazepam administration, and it contributes significantly to the overall clinical effect.)

The *third major phase* of metabolism is the conjugation of the 3-hydroxyl compounds, principally with glucuronic acid; the $t_{1/2}$ values of these reactions usually are about 6–12 h, and the products invariably are inactive. Conjugation is the only major route of metabolism for oxazepam and lorazepam and is the preferred pathway for temazepam because of the slower conversion of this compound to oxazepam. Triazolam and alprazolam are metabolized principally by initial hydroxylation of the methyl group on the fused triazolo ring; the absence of a chlorine residue in ring C of alprazolam slows this reaction significantly. The products, sometimes referred to as *α-hydroxylated compounds,* are quite active but are metabolized rapidly, primarily by conjugation with glucuronic acid, such that there is no appreciable accumulation of active metabolites. The fused triazolo ring in estazolam lacks a methyl group and is hydroxylated to only a limited extent; the major route of metabolism involves the formation of the 3-hydroxyl derivative. The corresponding hydroxyl derivatives of triazolam and alprazolam also are formed to a significant extent. Compared with compounds without the triazolo ring, the rate of this reaction for all three drugs is unusually swift, and the 3-hydroxyl compounds are rapidly conjugated or oxidized further to benzophenone derivatives before excretion.

Midazolam is metabolized rapidly, primarily by hydroxylation of the methyl group on the fused imidazo ring; only small amounts of 3-hydroxyl compounds are formed. The α-hydroxylated compound, which has appreciable biological activity, is eliminated with a $t_{1/2}$ of 1 h after conjugation with glucuronic acid. Variable and sometimes substantial accumulation of this metabolite has been noted during intravenous infusion (Oldenhof et al., 1988).

The aromatic rings (A and C) of the benzodiazepines are hydroxylated only to a small extent. The only important metabolism at these sites is reduction of the 7-nitro substituents of clonazepam, nitrazepam, and flunitrazepam; the $t_{1/2}$ of these reactions are usually 20–40 h. The resulting amines are inactive and are acetylated to varying degrees before excretion.

Therapeutic Uses

Table 19–2 summarizes the therapeutic uses and routes of administration of benzodiazepines that are marketed in the U.S. Most benzodiazepines can be used interchangeably. For example, diazepam can be used to treat alcohol withdrawal symptoms, and most benzodiazepines work as hypnotics. Benzodiazepines that are useful as anticonvulsants have a long $t_{1/2}$, and rapid entry into the brain is required for efficacy in treatment of status epilepticus. Antianxiety agents, in contrast, should have a long $t_{1/2}$ despite the drawback of the risk of neuropsychological deficits caused by drug accumulation. For a hypnotic sleep medication, one would want to have a rapid onset of action when taken at bedtime, a sufficiently sustained action to maintain sleep throughout the night, and no residual action by the following morning. In practice, there are some disadvantages to the use of agents that have a relatively rapid rate of disappearance, such as triazolam, including the early morning insomnia experienced by some patients and a greater likelihood of rebound insomnia on drug discontinuation. With careful selection of dosage, flurazepam and other benzodiazepines with slower rates of elimination than triazolam's can be used effectively.

Untoward Effects

At peak concentrations in plasma, hypnotic doses of benzodiazepines cause varying degrees of light-headedness, lassitude, increased reaction time, motor incoordination, impairment of mental and motor functions, confusion, and anterograde amnesia. Cognition appears to be affected less than motor performance. *All of these effects can greatly impair driving and other psychomotor skills, especially if combined with ethanol.* When the drug is given at the intended time of sleep, persistence of these effects into the following waking hours is adverse. These dose-related residual effects can be insidious because most subjects underestimate the degree of their impairment. Residual daytime sleepiness also may occur, even though successful drug therapy can reduce the daytime sleepiness resulting from chronic insomnia. The intensity and incidence of CNS toxicity generally increase with age (Monane, 1992). Other common side effects of benzodiazepines are weakness, headache, blurred vision, vertigo, nausea and vomiting, epigastric distress, and diarrhea; joint pains, chest pains, and incontinence are much rarer. Anticonvulsant benzodiazepines sometimes increase the frequency of seizures in patients with epilepsy.

A wide variety of serious allergic, hepatotoxic, and hematologic reactions to the benzodiazepines may occur, but the incidence is low; these reactions have been associated with the use of *flurazepam, triazolam,* and *temazepam.* Large doses taken just before or during labor may cause hypothermia, hypotonia, and mild respiratory depression in the neonate. Abuse by the pregnant mother can result in a withdrawal syndrome in the newborn.

Adverse Psychological Effects

Benzodiazepines may at times cause paradoxical effects. *Flurazepam* occasionally increases the incidence of nightmares—especially during the first week of use—and sometimes causes garrulousness, anxiety, irritability, tachycardia, and sweating. Amnesia, euphoria, restlessness, hallucinations, sleep-walking, sleep-talking, other complex behaviors, and hypomanic behavior have been reported to occur during use of various benzodiazepines. Bizarre uninhibited behavior may occur in some users, hostility and rage in others; collectively, these are sometimes referred to as *disinhibition* or *dyscontrol reactions.* Paranoia, depression, and suicidal ideation also occasionally may accompany the use of these agents. Such paradoxical or disinhibition reactions are rare and appear to be dose related. Because of reports of an increased incidence of confusion and abnormal behaviors, triazolam has been banned in the U.K. The FDA declared triazolam to be safe and effective in low doses of 0.125–0.25 mg.

Chronic benzodiazepine use poses a risk for development of dependence and abuse (Woods et al., 1992). Mild dependence may develop in many patients who have taken therapeutic doses of benzodiazepines on a regular basis for prolonged periods, but not to the same extent as seen with older sedatives and other recognized drugs of abuse (Chapter 24; Uhlenhuth et al., 1999). Withdrawal symptoms may include temporary intensification of the problems that originally prompted their use (e.g., insomnia or anxiety). Dysphoria, irritability, sweating, unpleasant dreams, tremors, anorexia, and faintness or dizziness also may occur, especially when withdrawal of the benzodiazepine occurs abruptly. Hence, it is prudent to taper the dosage gradually when therapy is to be discontinued. Despite their adverse effects, benzodiazepines are relatively safe drugs, and fatalities are rare unless other drugs are taken concomitantly. Ethanol is a common contributor to deaths involving benzodiazepines, but true coma is uncommon in the absence of another CNS depressant. Although overdosage with a benzodiazepine rarely causes severe cardiovascular or respiratory depression, therapeutic doses of benzodiazepines can further compromise respiration in patients with COPD or OSA. Benzodiazepine abuse of a different sort includes the use of *flunitrazepam* (Rohypnol; not licensed for use in the U.S.) as a "date rape drug."

Drug Interactions

Except for additive effects with other sedative or hypnotic drugs, reports of clinically important pharmacodynamic interactions between benzodiazepines and other drugs have been infrequent. Ethanol increases both the rate of absorption of benzodiazepines and the associated CNS depression. Valproate and benzodiazepines used in combination may cause psychotic episodes.

Novel Benzodiazepine Receptor Agonists

Hypnotics in this class are commonly referred to as "Z compounds." They include zolpidem, zaleplon, zopiclone (not marketed in the U.S.), and eszopiclone, which is the S(+) enantiomer of zopiclone (Huedo-Medina et al., 2012). Although the Z compounds are structurally unrelated to each other and to benzodiazepines, their therapeutic efficacy as hypnotics is due to

TABLE 19–2 ■ THERAPEUTIC USES OF BENZODIAZEPINES

COMPOUND	ROUTES OF ADMINISTRATION	THERAPEUTIC USES[a]	COMMENTS	$t_{1/2}$ (h)[b]	USUAL SEDATIVE-HYPNOTIC DOSE, mg[c]
Alprazolam	Oral	Anxiety disorders, agoraphobia (OL)	Withdrawal symptoms may be especially severe	12 ± 2	—
Chlordiazepoxide	Oral, IM, IV	Anxiety disorders, management of alcohol withdrawal, preanesthetic medication (OL)	Long-acting and self-tapering because of active metabolites	10 ± 3.4	50–100, 1–41× daily[d] (1 daily for sleep)
Clobazam	Oral	Adjunctive treatment of seizures associated with Lennox-Gastaut syndrome (U.S. approved use), other types of epilepsies, anxiety disorders	Active metabolite $t_{1/2}$ 71–82 h; tolerance develops to anticonvulsant effects; not recommended in patients with severe hepatic impairment; decrease dose and titrate in CYP2C19 poor metabolizers	36–42	—
Clonazepam	Oral	Seizure disorders, panic disorder, adjunctive treatment in acute mania and certain movement disorders (OL)	Tolerance develops to anticonvulsant effects	23 ± 5	0.25–0.5 (hypnotic)
Clorazepate	Oral	Anxiety disorders, seizure disorders, management of alcohol withdrawal	Prodrug; activity due to formation of nordazepam during absorption	2.0 ± 0.9	3.75–20, 2–4× daily[d]
Diazepam	Oral, IM, IV, rectal	Anxiety disorders, alcohol withdrawal, status epilepticus, skeletal muscle relaxation, preanesthetic medication, Meniere disease (OL)	Prototypical benzodiazepine	43 ± 13	5–10, every 4 h
Estazolam	Oral	Insomnia	Contains triazolo ring; adverse effects may be similar to those of triazolam	10–24	1–2
Flurazepam	Oral	Insomnia	Active metabolites accumulate with chronic use	74 ± 24	15–30
Lorazepam	Oral, IM, IV	Anxiety disorders, alcohol withdrawal, preanesthetic medication, seizure disorders	Metabolized solely by conjugation	14 ± 5	1–4
Midazolam	Oral, IV, IM	Preanesthetic and intraoperative medication, anxiety disorders (agitation, alcohol withdrawal, seizure disorders, OL)	Rapidly inactivated	1.9 ± 0.6	1–5[e]
Oxazepam	Oral	Anxiety disorders, alcohol withdrawal	Metabolized solely by conjugation	8.0 ± 2.4	15–30, 3–4× daily[d]
Quazepam	Oral	Insomnia	Active metabolites accumulate with chronic use	39	7.5–15
Temazepam	Oral	Insomnia	Metabolized mainly by conjugation	11 ± 6	7.5–30
Triazolam	Oral	Insomnia	Rapidly inactivated; may cause disturbing daytime side effects	2.9 ± 1.0	0.125–0.5

[a]The therapeutic uses are examples to emphasize that most benzodiazepines can be used interchangeably. In general, the therapeutic uses of a given benzodiazepine are related to its $t_{1/2}$ and may not match the marketed indications. The issue is addressed more extensively in the text.
[b]Half-life of active metabolite may differ. See Appendix II for additional information.
[c]For additional dosage information, see Chapter 21 (anesthesia), Chapter 15 (anxiety), and Chapter 17 (seizure disorders).
[d]Approved as a sedative-hypnotic only for management of alcohol withdrawal; doses in a nontolerant individual would be smaller.
[e]Recommended doses vary considerably depending on specific use, condition of patient, and concomitant administration of other drugs.

agonist effects at the benzodiazepine site of the $GABA_A$ receptor (Hanson et al., 2008). Compared to benzodiazepines, Z compounds are less effective as anticonvulsants or muscle relaxants, which may be related to their relative selectivity for $GABA_A$ receptors containing the α_1 subunit. Over the last decade, Z compounds have largely replaced benzodiazepines in the treatment of insomnia. Z compounds were initially promoted as having less potential for dependence and abuse than traditional benzodiazepines. However, based on postmarketing clinical experience with zopiclone and zolpidem, tolerance and physical dependence can be expected during long-term use of Z compounds, especially with higher doses. The Z drugs are classified as schedule IV drugs in the U.S. The clinical presentation of overdose with Z compounds is similar to that of benzodiazepine overdose and can be treated with the benzodiazepine antagonist flumazenil.

Zaleplon

Zaleplon is a member of the pyrazolopyrimidine class. Zaleplon preferentially binds to the benzodiazepine binding site on $GABA_A$ receptors containing the α_1 receptor subunit. It is absorbed rapidly and reaches peak plasma concentrations in about 1 h. Its bioavailability is about 30% because of presystemic metabolism. Zaleplon is metabolized largely by aldehyde oxidase and to a lesser extent by CYP3A4. Its $t_{1/2}$ is short, about 1 h. Zalepon's oxidative metabolites are converted to glucuronides and eliminated in urine. Less than 1% of zaleplon is excreted unchanged; none of zaleplon's metabolites is pharmacologically active. Zaleplon is usually administered in 5-, 10-, or 20-mg doses (Dooley and Plosker, 2000). Zaleplon-treated subjects with either chronic or transient insomnia experience shorter periods of sleep onset latency.

Zolpidem

Zolpidem is an imidazopyridine sedative-hypnotic. The actions of zolpidem are due to agonist effects at the benzodiazepine receptor site on $GABA_A$ receptors and generally resemble those of benzodiazepines. The drug has little effect on the stages of sleep in normal human subjects. It is effective in shortening sleep latency and prolonging total sleep time in patients with insomnia. After discontinuation of zolpidem, the beneficial effects on sleep reportedly persist for up to 1 week, but mild rebound insomnia on the first night of withdrawal may occur. Zolpidem is approved only for the short-term treatment of insomnia; however, tolerance and physical dependence are rare (Morselli, 1993). At therapeutic doses (5–10 mg), zolpidem infrequently produces residual daytime sedation or amnesia; the incidence of other adverse effects also is low. As with the benzodiazepines, large overdoses of zolpidem do not produce severe respiratory depression unless other agents (e.g., ethanol) also are ingested. Hypnotic doses increase the hypoxia and hypercarbia of patients with OSA.

Zolpidem is absorbed readily from the GI tract; first-pass hepatic metabolism results in an oral bioavailability of about 70% (lower when the drug is ingested with food). Zolpidem is eliminated almost entirely by conversion to inactive products in the liver, largely through oxidation of the methyl groups on the phenyl and imidazopyridine rings to the corresponding carboxylic acids. Its plasma $t_{1/2}$ is about 2 h in normal individuals, but this value may increase 2-fold or more in those with cirrhosis and also tends to be greater in older patients, requiring adjustment of dosage. Although little or no unchanged zolpidem is found in the urine, elimination of the drug is slower in patients with chronic renal insufficiency; the increased elimination time largely is due to an increase in its apparent volume of distribution.

Zaleplon and Zolpidem Compared

Zaleplon and zolpidem are effective in relieving sleep-onset insomnia. Both drugs are FDA-approved for use up to 7–10 days at a time. Zaleplon and zolpidem have sustained hypnotic efficacy without occurrence of rebound insomnia on abrupt discontinuation. Zolpidem has a $t_{1/2}$ of about 2 h, which is sufficient to cover most of a typical 8-h sleep period, and is presently approved for bedtime use only. Zaleplon has a shorter $t_{1/2}$ of about 1 h, which offers the possibility for safe dosing later in the night, within 4 h of the anticipated rising time. Zaleplon and zolpidem differ in residual side effects; late-night administration of zolpidem has been associated with morning sedation, delayed reaction time, and anterograde amnesia, whereas zaleplon does not differ from placebo.

Eszopiclone

Eszopiclone is the active S(+) enantiomer of zopiclone. It exerts its sleep-promoting effects by enhancing $GABA_A$ receptor function via the benzodiazepine binding site. Eszopiclone is used for the long-term (~12 months) treatment of insomnia, for sleep maintenance, and to decrease the latency to onset of sleep (Melton et al., 2005; Rosenberg et al., 2005). It is available in 1-, 2-, or 3-mg tablets. In clinical studies, no tolerance was observed, and no signs of serious withdrawal, such as seizures or rebound insomnia, were seen on discontinuation of the drug; however, there are such reports for *zopiclone*, the racemate used outside the U.S. Mild withdrawal consisting of abnormal dreams, anxiety, nausea, and upset stomach can occur (≤2%). A minor reported adverse effect of eszopiclone is a bitter taste. Eszopiclone is absorbed rapidly after oral administration, with a bioavailability of about 80%, and shows wide distribution throughout the body. It is 50%–60% bound to plasma proteins, is metabolized by CYPs 3A4 and 2E1, and has a $t_{1/2}$ of about 6 h.

Management of Patients After Long-Term Benzodiazepine Therapy

If a benzodiazepine has been used regularly for more than 2 weeks, its use should be tapered rather than discontinued abruptly. In some patients taking hypnotics with a short $t_{1/2}$, it is easier to switch first to a hypnotic with a long $t_{1/2}$ and then to taper. The onset of withdrawal symptoms from medications with a long $t_{1/2}$ may be delayed. Consequently, the patient should be warned about the symptoms associated with withdrawal effects.

Flumazenil: A Benzodiazepine Receptor Antagonist

Flumazenil is an imidazobenzodiazepine that binds with high affinity to the benzodiazepine binding site on the $GABA_A$ receptor, where it competitively antagonizes the binding and allosteric effects of benzodiazepines and other ligands (Hoffman and Warren, 1993). Flumazenil antagonizes both the electrophysiological and behavioral effects of agonist and inverse-agonist benzodiazepines and β-carbolines.

Flumazenil is available only for intravenous administration. Administration of a series of small injections is preferred to a single bolus injection. A total of 1 mg flumazenil given over 1–3 min usually is sufficient to abolish the effects of therapeutic doses of benzodiazepines. Additional courses of treatment with flumazenil may be needed within 20–30 min should sedation reappear. The duration of clinical effects usually is only 30–60 min. Although absorbed rapidly after oral administration, less than 25% of the drug reaches the systemic circulation owing to extensive first-pass hepatic metabolism. Flumazenil is eliminated almost entirely by hepatic metabolism to inactive products with a $t_{1/2}$ of about 1 h. Oral doses are apt to cause headache and dizziness.

The primary indications for the use of flumazenil are the management of suspected benzodiazepine overdose and the reversal of sedative effects produced by benzodiazepines administered during general anesthesia and diagnostic or therapeutic procedures. Flumazenil is not effective in single-drug overdoses with either barbiturates or tricyclic antidepressants. The administration of flumazenil in these settings may be associated with the onset of seizures, especially in patients poisoned with tricyclic antidepressants. Seizures or other withdrawal signs may be precipitated in patients taking benzodiazepines for protracted periods and in whom tolerance or dependence may have developed.

Melatonin Congeners

Melatonin is a circadian signaling molecule. In some fish and amphibians, melatonin modulates skin coloration through an action on melanin-containing pigment granules in melanophores. In humans, melatonin, not to be confused with the pigment melanin, is the principal indoleamine in the pineal gland, where it may be said to constitute a pigment of the imagination. The synthesis of melatonin in the pineal gland (by *N*-acetylation and *O*-methylation of serotonin; see Figure 13–2) is influenced by external factors, including environmental light. In mammals, melatonin induces pigment lightening in skin cells and suppresses ovarian functions; it also serves a role in regulating biological rhythms and has been studied as a treatment of jet lag and other sleep disturbances. Melatonin analogues have recently been approved for the treatment of insomnia.

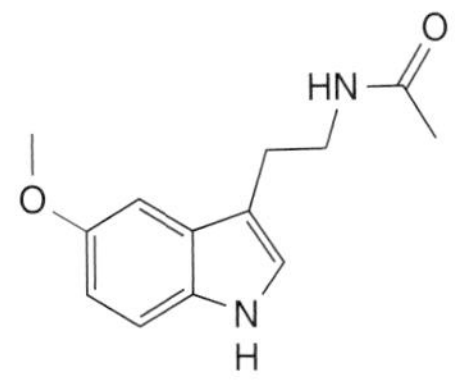

MELATONIN 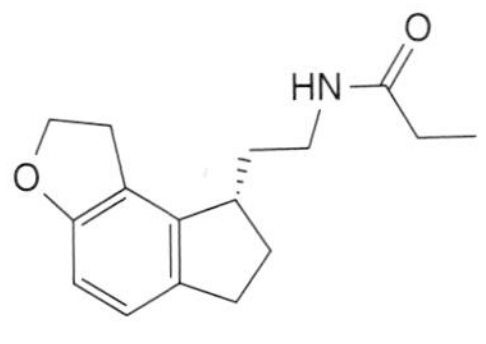 RAMELTEON

Ramelteon

Ramelteon is a synthetic tricyclic analogue of melatonin, approved in the U.S. for the treatment of insomnia, specifically difficulties of sleep onset (Spadoni et al., 2011).

Mechanism of Action

Melatonin levels in the suprachiasmatic nucleus rise and fall in a circadian fashion, with concentrations increasing in the evening as an individual prepares for sleep and then reaching a plateau and ultimately decreasing as the night progresses. Two GPCRs for melatonin, MT_1 and MT_2, in the suprachiasmatic nucleus, each play a different role in sleep. Binding of agonists such as melatonin to MT_1 receptors promotes the onset of sleep; melatonin binding to MT_2 receptors shifts the timing of the circadian system. Ramelteon binds to both MT_1 and MT_2 receptors with high affinity, but, unlike melatonin, it does not bind appreciably to quinone reductase 2, the structurally unrelated MT_3 receptor. Ramelteon is not known to bind to any other classes of receptors, such as nicotinic ACh, neuropeptide, dopamine, and opiate receptors, or the benzodiazepine binding site on $GABA_A$ receptors.

Clinical Pharmacology

Prescribing guidelines suggest that an 8-mg tablet be taken about 30 min before bedtime. Ramelteon is rapidly absorbed from the GI tract. Because of the significant first-pass metabolism that occurs after oral administration, ramelteon bioavailability is less than 2%. The drug is largely metabolized by hepatic CYPs 1A2, 2C, and 3A4, with a $t_{1/2}$ of about 2 h in humans. Of the four metabolites, M-II, acts as an agonist at MT_1 and MT_2 receptors and may contribute to the sleep-promoting effects of ramelteon.

Ramelteon is efficacious in combating both transient and chronic insomnia, with no tolerance occurring in its reduction of sleep onset latency even after 6 months of drug administration (Mayer et al., 2009). It is generally well tolerated by patients and does not impair next-day cognitive function. Sleep latency was consistently found to be shorter in patients given ramelteon compared to placebo controls. No evidence of rebound insomnia or withdrawal effects were noted on ramelteon withdrawal. Unlike most agents mentioned in this chapter, ramelteon is not a controlled substance.

Tasimelteon

Tasimelteon is a selective agonist for MT_1 and MT_2 receptors. It has been approved in the U.S. for treatment of non–24-h sleep-wake syndrome in totally blind patients experiencing circadian rhythm disorder (Johnsa and Neville, 2014).

Barbiturates

The barbiturates were once used extensively as sedative-hypnotic drugs. Except for a few specialized uses, they have been largely replaced by the much safer benzodiazepines and Z compounds. Table 19–3 lists the common barbiturates and their pharmacological properties.

Barbiturates are derivatives of this parent structure:

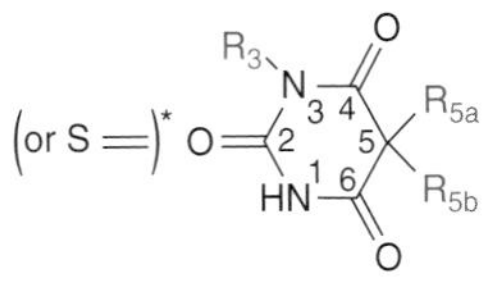

(or S =)* O; R_3; R_{5a}; R_{5b}; HN

*O except in thiopental, where it is replaced by S.

Barbituric acid is 2,4,6-trioxohexahydropyrimidine. This compound lacks central depressant activity, but the presence of alkyl or aryl groups at position 5 confers sedative-hypnotic and sometimes other activities. Barbiturates in which the oxygen at C2 is replaced by sulfur are called *thiobarbiturates.* These compounds are more lipid soluble than the corresponding *oxybarbiturates.* In general, structural changes that increase lipid solubility decrease duration of action, decrease latency to onset of activity, accelerate metabolic degradation, and increase hypnotic potency.

Pharmacological Properties

The barbiturates reversibly depress the activity of all excitable tissues. The CNS is particularly sensitive, and even when barbiturates are given in anesthetic concentrations, direct effects on peripheral excitable tissues are weak. However, serious deficits in cardiovascular and other peripheral functions occur in acute barbiturate intoxication.

ADME

For sedative-hypnotic use, the barbiturates usually are administered orally (see Table 19–2). Na^+ salts are absorbed more rapidly than the corresponding free acids, especially from liquid formulations. The onset of action varies from 10 to 60 min and is delayed by the presence of food. Intramuscular injections of solutions of the Na^+ salts should be placed deeply into large muscles to avoid the pain and possible necrosis that can result at more superficial sites. The intravenous route usually is reserved for the management of status epilepticus (phenobarbital sodium) or for the induction or maintenance of general anesthesia (e.g., thiopental or methohexital).

Barbiturates distribute widely in the body and readily cross the placenta. The highly lipid-soluble barbiturates such as *thiopental* and *methohexital,* used to induce anesthesia, undergo rapid redistribution after intravenous injection. Redistribution into less-vascular tissues, especially muscle and fat, leads to a decline in the concentration of barbiturate in the plasma and brain. With thiopental and methohexital, this results in the awakening of patients within 5–15 min of the injection of the usual anesthetic doses (see Figures 2–4 and 21–2).

Except for the less lipid-soluble *aprobarbital* and *phenobarbital,* nearly complete metabolism or conjugation of barbiturates in the liver precedes their renal excretion. The oxidation of radicals at C5 is the most important biotransformation that terminates biological activity. In some instances (e.g., phenobarbital), *N*-glycosylation is an important metabolic pathway. Other biotransformations include *N*-hydroxylation, desulfuration of thiobarbiturates to oxybarbiturates, opening of the barbituric acid ring, and *N*-dealkylation of *N*-alkyl barbiturates to active metabolites (e.g., mephobarbital to phenobarbital). About 25% of phenobarbital and nearly all of aprobarbital are excreted unchanged in the urine. Their renal excretion can be increased greatly by osmotic diuresis or alkalinization of the urine.

The metabolic elimination of barbiturates is more rapid in young people than in the elderly and infants, and half-lives are increased during pregnancy partly because of the expanded volume of distribution. Chronic liver disease, especially cirrhosis, often increases the $t_{1/2}$ of the biotransformable barbiturates. Repeated administration, especially of phenobarbital, shortens the $t_{1/2}$ of barbiturates that are metabolized as a result of the induction of microsomal enzymes.

The barbiturates commonly used as hypnotics in the U.S. have $t_{1/2}$ *values such that the drugs are not fully eliminated in 24 h* (see Table 19–3). *Thus, these barbiturates will accumulate during repeated administration unless*

TABLE 19–3 ■ THERAPEUTIC USES OF BARBITURATES

COMPOUND	ROUTES OF ADMINISTRATION	THERAPEUTIC USES	COMMENTS	$t_{1/2}$ (h)
Amobarbital	IM, IV	Insomnia, preoperative sedation, emergency management of seizures	Only Na^+ salt for injection is sold in the U.S.	10–40
Butabarbital	Oral	Insomnia, preoperative sedation, daytime sedation	Redistribution shortens duration of action of single dose to 8 h	35–50
Mephobarbital (not licensed for use in the U.S.)	Oral	Seizure disorders, daytime sedation	Second-line anticonvulsant	10–70
Methohexital	IV	Induction and maintenance of anesthesia	Only Na^+ salt available; single dose provides 5–7 min of anesthesia	3–5
Pentobarbital	Oral, IM, IV, rectal (only injectable form is marketed in the U.S.)	Insomnia, preoperative and procedural sedation, emergency management of seizures	Administer only Na^+ salt parenterally	15–50
Phenobarbital	Oral, IM, IV	Seizure disorders, status epilepticus, daytime sedation (hyperbilirubinemia, OL use)	First-line anticonvulsant; only Na^+ salt administered parenterally	80–120
Secobarbital	Oral	Insomnia, preoperative sedation	Only Na^+ salt available	15–40
Thiopental (not currently produced or marketed in the U.S.)	IV	Induction/maintenance of anesthesia, preoperative sedation, emergency management of seizures, intracranial pressure	Only Na^+ salt available; single dose provides brief period of anesthesia	8–10 ($t_{1/2}$ of anesthetic effects is short due to redistribution; see Figures 2–4 and 21–2)

appropriate adjustments in dosage are made. Furthermore, the persistence of the drug in plasma during the day favors the development of tolerance and abuse.

CNS Effects

Actions on the $GABA_A$ Receptor

Enhancement of inhibition occurs primarily at synapses where neurotransmission is mediated by GABA acting at $GABA_A$ receptors. Barbiturates bind to a distinct allosteric site on the $GABA_A$ receptor (Figure 14–11); binding leads to an increase in the mean open time of the GABA-activated Cl^- channel, with no effect on frequency. At higher concentrations, barbiturates directly activate channel opening, even in the absence of GABA (Nestler et al., 2015). Barbiturates also reportedly inhibit excitatory AMPA/kainate receptors (Marszalec and Narahashi, 1993) and inhibit glutamate release via an effect on voltage-activated Ca^{2+} channels. These multiple actions, especially the direct gating effect on the $GABA_A$ channel, may explain the potent CNS depressant effects of barbiturates as compared to benzodiazepines.

Effects in the CNS

Barbiturates enhance GABA-mediated inhibitory transmission throughout the CNS; nonanesthetic doses preferentially suppress polysynaptic responses. Facilitation is diminished, and inhibition usually is enhanced. The site of inhibition is either postsynaptic, as at *cortical and cerebellar pyramidal cells* and in the *cuneate nucleus, substantia nigra,* and *thalamic relay neurons,* or presynaptic, as in the *spinal cord.*

Barbiturates can produce all degrees of depression of the CNS, ranging from mild sedation to general anesthesia (see Chapter 21). Certain barbiturates, particularly those containing a 5-phenyl substituent (e.g., phenobarbital and mephobarbital), have selective anticonvulsant activity (see Chapter 17). The antianxiety properties of the barbiturates are inferior to those exerted by the benzodiazepines.

Except for the anticonvulsant activities of phenobarbital and its congeners, the barbiturates possess a low degree of selectivity and a low therapeutic index. Pain perception and reaction are relatively unimpaired until the moment of unconsciousness, and in small doses, barbiturates increase reactions to painful stimuli. Hence, they cannot be relied on to produce sedation or sleep in the presence of even moderate pain.

Effects on Stages of Sleep

Hypnotic doses of barbiturates increase the total sleep time and alter the stages of sleep in a dose-dependent manner. Like the benzodiazepines, barbiturates decrease sleep latency, the number of awakenings, and the durations of REM and slow-wave sleep. During repetitive nightly administration, some tolerance to the effects on sleep occurs within a few days, and the effect on total sleep time may be reduced by as much as 50% after 2 weeks of use. Discontinuation leads to rebound increases in all the sleep parameters initially decreased by barbiturates.

Tolerance, Abuse, and Dependence

With chronic administration of gradually increasing doses, pharmacodynamic tolerance continues to develop over a period of weeks to months, depending on the dosage schedule, whereas pharmacokinetic tolerance reaches its peak in a few days to a week. Tolerance to the euphoric, sedative, and hypnotic effects occurs more readily and is greater than that to the anticonvulsant and lethal effects; thus, as tolerance increases, the therapeutic index decreases. Pharmacodynamic tolerance to barbiturates confers cross-tolerance to all general CNS depressant drugs, including ethanol. Like other CNS depressant drugs, barbiturates are abused, and some individuals develop physical dependence (see Chapter 24).

Effects on Peripheral Nerve Structures

Barbiturates selectively depress transmission in autonomic ganglia and reduce nicotinic excitation by choline esters. This effect may account, at least in part, for the fall in blood pressure produced by intravenous oxybarbiturates and by severe barbiturate intoxication. At skeletal neuromuscular junctions, the blocking effects of both *tubocurarine* and *decamethonium* are enhanced during barbiturate anesthesia. These actions probably result from the capacity of barbiturates at hypnotic or anesthetic concentrations to inhibit current flow through nicotinic ACh receptors. Several distinct mechanisms appear to be involved, and little stereoselectivity is evident.

Systemic Effects

Respiration

Barbiturates depress both the respiratory drive and the mechanisms responsible for the rhythmic character of respiration. The neurogenic drive is essentially eliminated by a dose three times greater than that used normally to induce sleep. Such doses also suppress the hypoxic drive and, to a lesser extent, the chemoreceptor drive. However, the margin between the lighter planes of surgical anesthesia and dangerous respiratory depression is sufficient to permit the ultrashort-acting barbiturates to be used, with suitable precautions, as anesthetic agents.

The barbiturates only slightly depress protective reflexes until the degree of intoxication is sufficient to produce severe respiratory depression. Coughing, sneezing, hiccoughing, and laryngospasm may occur when barbiturates are employed as intravenous anesthetic agents.

Cardiovascular System

When given orally in sedative or hypnotic doses, barbiturates do not produce significant overt cardiovascular effects. In general, the effects of thiopental anesthesia on the cardiovascular system are benign in comparison with those of the volatile anesthetic agents; there usually is either no change or a fall in mean arterial pressure (see Chapter 21). Barbiturates can blunt cardiovascular reflexes by partial inhibition of ganglionic transmission, most evident in patients with congestive heart failure or hypovolemic shock. Because barbiturates also impair reflex cardiovascular adjustments to inflation of the lung, positive-pressure respiration should be used cautiously and only when necessary to maintain adequate pulmonary ventilation in patients who are anesthetized or intoxicated with a barbiturate.

Other cardiovascular changes often noted when thiopental and other intravenous thiobarbiturates are administered after conventional preanesthetic medication include decreased renal and cerebral blood flow with a marked fall in CSF pressure. Although cardiac arrhythmias are observed only infrequently, intravenous anesthesia with barbiturates can increase the incidence of ventricular arrhythmias, especially when epinephrine and halothane also are present. Anesthetic concentrations of barbiturates depress the function of Na^+ channels and at least two types of K^+ channels. However, direct depression of cardiac contractility occurs only when doses several times those required to cause anesthesia are administered.

GI Tract

The oxybarbiturates tend to decrease the tone of the GI musculature and the amplitude of rhythmic contractions; the locus of action is partly peripheral and partly central. A hypnotic dose does not significantly delay gastric emptying in humans. The relief of various GI symptoms by sedative doses is probably largely due to the central depressant action.

Liver

The effects vary with the duration of exposure to the barbiturate. *Acutely*, the barbiturates interact with several CYPs and inhibit the biotransformation of a number of other drugs and endogenous substrates, such as steroids; other substrates may reciprocally inhibit barbiturate biotransformations (see Chapter 6).

Chronic administration of barbiturates markedly increases the protein and lipid content of the hepatic smooth endoplasmic reticulum, as well as the activities of glucuronyl transferase and CYPs 1A2, 2C9, 2C19, and 3A4. The induction of these enzymes increases the metabolism of a number of drugs (including barbiturates) and endogenous substances, including steroid hormones, cholesterol, bile salts, and vitamins K and D. The self-induced increase in barbiturate metabolism partly accounts for tolerance to barbiturates. The inducing effect is not limited to the microsomal enzymes; for example, there are increases in ALA synthetase, a mitochondrial enzyme, and aldehyde dehydrogenase, a cytosolic enzyme. The effect of barbiturates on ALA synthetase can cause dangerous disease exacerbations in persons with intermittent porphyria.

Kidney

Severe oliguria or anuria may occur in acute barbiturate poisoning largely as a result of the marked hypotension.

Therapeutic Uses

The major uses of individual barbiturates are listed in Table 19–3. As with the benzodiazepines, the selection of a particular barbiturate for a given therapeutic indication is based primarily on pharmacokinetic considerations. Benzodiazepines and other compounds have largely replaced barbiturates as sedatives.

Untoward Effects

Aftereffects

Drowsiness may last for only a few hours after a hypnotic dose of barbiturate, but residual CNS depression sometimes is evident the following day, and subtle distortions of mood and impairment of judgment and fine motor skills may be demonstrable. Residual effects also may take the form of vertigo, nausea, vomiting, or diarrhea or sometimes may be manifested as overt excitement.

Paradoxical Excitement

In some persons, barbiturates produce excitement rather than depression, and the patient may appear to be inebriated. This type of idiosyncrasy is relatively common among geriatric and debilitated patients and occurs most frequently with phenobarbital and *N*-methylbarbiturates. Barbiturates may cause restlessness, excitement, and even delirium when given in the presence of pain and may worsen a patient's perception of pain.

Hypersensitivity

Allergic reactions occur, especially in persons with asthma, urticaria, angioedema, or similar conditions. Hypersensitivity reactions include localized swellings, particularly of the eyelids, cheeks, or lips, and erythematous dermatitis. Rarely, exfoliative dermatitis may be caused by phenobarbital and can prove fatal; the skin eruption may be associated with fever, delirium, and marked degenerative changes in the liver and other parenchymatous organs.

Other

Because barbiturates enhance porphyrin synthesis, they are absolutely contraindicated in patients with acute intermittent porphyria or porphyria variegata. Hypnotic doses in the presence of pulmonary insufficiency are contraindicated. Rapid intravenous injection of a barbiturate may cause cardiovascular collapse before anesthesia ensues. Blood pressure can fall to shock levels; even slow intravenous injection of barbiturates often produces apnea and occasionally laryngospasm, coughing, and other respiratory difficulties.

Drug Interactions

Barbiturates combine with other CNS depressants to cause severe depression; interactions with ethanol and with first-generation antihistamines are common. Isoniazid, methylphenidate, and monoamine oxidase inhibitors also increase the CNS depressant effects of barbiturates.

Barbiturates competitively inhibit the metabolism of certain other drugs; however, the greatest number of drug interactions results from induction of hepatic CYPs (as described previously) and the accelerated disappearance of many drugs and endogenous substances from the body. Hepatic enzyme induction enhances metabolism of endogenous steroid hormones, which may cause endocrine disturbances, and enhances metabolism of oral contraceptives, which may increase the likelihood of unwanted pregnancy. Barbiturates also induce the hepatic generation of toxic metabolites of chlorocarbons (chloroform, trichloroethylene, carbon tetrachloride) and consequently promote lipid peroxidation, which facilitates periportal necrosis of the liver caused by these agents.

Barbiturate Poisoning

The incidence of barbiturate poisoning has declined markedly, largely as a result of their decreased use as sedative-hypnotic agents. Most of the cases are the result of attempts at suicide, but some are from accidental poisonings in children or drug abusers. The lethal dose of barbiturate varies, but severe poisoning is likely to occur when more than 10 times the full hypnotic dose has been ingested at once. The lethal dose becomes lower if alcohol or other depressant drugs are present. In severe intoxication, the patient is comatose; respiration is affected early. Breathing may be either slow or rapid and shallow. Eventually, blood pressure falls because the effect of the drug and of hypoxia on medullary vasomotor centers; depression of cardiac contractility and sympathetic ganglia also contributes. Pulmonary complications (e.g., atelectasis, edema, and bronchopneumonia) and renal failure are likely to be the fatal complications of severe barbiturate poisoning.

The treatment of acute barbiturate intoxication is based on general supportive measures, which are applicable in most respects to poisoning by any CNS depressant. The use of CNS stimulants is contraindicated. If renal and cardiac functions are satisfactory and the patient is hydrated, forced diuresis and alkalinization of the urine will hasten the excretion of phenobarbital. See Chapter 4, Drug Toxicity and Poisoning.

Miscellaneous Sedative-Hypnotic Drugs

Many drugs with diverse structures have been used for their sedative-hypnotic properties, including *ramelteon, chloral hydrate, meprobamate,* and paraldehyde (no longer licensed in the U.S.). With the exception of ramelteon and meprobamate, the pharmacological actions of these drugs generally resemble those of the barbiturates:

- They all are general CNS depressants that can produce profound hypnosis with little or no analgesia.
- Their effects on the stages of sleep are similar to those of the barbiturates.
- Their therapeutic indices are low, and acute intoxication, which produces respiratory depression and hypotension, is managed similarly to barbiturate poisoning.
- Their chronic use can result in tolerance and physical dependence.
- The syndrome after chronic use can be severe and life threatening.

Chloral Hydrate

Chloral hydrate may be used to treat patients with paradoxical reactions to benzodiazepines. Chloral hydrate is reduced rapidly to the active compound trichloroethanol (CCl_3CH_2OH), largely by hepatic alcohol dehydrogenase. Its pharmacological effects probably are caused by trichloroethanol, which can exert barbiturate-like effects on $GABA_A$ receptor channels in vitro. Chloral hydrate is regulated as a schedule IV controlled substance.

In the U.S., chloral hydrate is best known as a literary poison, the "knockout drops" added to a strong alcoholic beverage to produce a "Mickey Finn" or "Mickey," a cocktail given to an unwitting imbiber to render the person malleable or unconscious, most famously Sam Spade in Dashiell Hammett's 1930 novel, *The Maltese Falcon*. Now that detectives drink wine rather than whiskey, this off-label use of chloral hydrate has waned.

Meprobamate

Meprobamate, a *bis*-carbamate ester, was introduced as an antianxiety agent, and this remains its only approved use in the U.S. However, it also became popular as a sedative-hypnotic agent. The pharmacological properties of meprobamate resemble those of the benzodiazepines in a number of ways. Meprobamate can release suppressed behaviors in experimental animals at doses that cause little impairment of locomotor activity, and although it can cause CNS depression, it cannot produce anesthesia. Large doses of meprobamate cause severe respiratory depression, hypotension, shock, and heart failure. Meprobamate appears to have a mild analgesic effect in patients with musculoskeletal pain, and it enhances the analgesic effects of other drugs.

Meprobamate is well absorbed when administered orally. Nevertheless, an important aspect of intoxication with meprobamate is the formation of gastric bezoars consisting of undissolved meprobamate tablets; treatment may require endoscopy, with mechanical removal of the bezoar. Most of the drug is metabolized in the liver by side-chain hydroxylation and glucuronidation; the kinetics of elimination may depend on dose. The $t_{1/2}$ of meprobamate may be prolonged during its chronic administration. The major unwanted effects of the usual sedative doses of meprobamate are drowsiness and ataxia; larger doses impair learning and motor coordination and prolong reaction time. Meprobamate enhances the CNS depression produced by other drugs. After long-term medication, abrupt discontinuation evokes a withdrawal syndrome usually characterized by anxiety, insomnia, tremors, and, frequently, hallucinations; generalized seizures occur in about 10% of cases.

Carisoprodol, a skeletal muscle relaxant whose active metabolite is meprobamate, also has abuse potential and has become a popular "street drug." Meprobamate and carisoprodol are designated as schedule IV controlled substances.

Other Agents

Etomidate is used in the U.S. and other countries as an intravenous anesthetic, often in combination with fentanyl. It is advantageous because it lacks pulmonary and vascular depressant activity, although it has a negative inotropic effect on the heart. Its pharmacology and anesthetic uses are described in Chapter 21.

Clomethiazole has sedative, muscle relaxant, and anticonvulsant properties. Given alone, its effects on respiration are slight, and the therapeutic index is high. However, deaths from adverse interactions with ethanol are relatively frequent.

Propofol is a rapidly acting and highly lipophilic diisopropylphenol used in the induction and maintenance of general anesthesia (see Chapter 21), as well as in the maintenance of long-term sedation. Propofol has found use in intensive care sedation in adults (McKeage and Perry, 2003), for sedation during GI endoscopy procedures, and during transvaginal oocyte retrieval.

Nonprescription Hypnotic Drugs

The antihistamines *diphenhydramine* and *doxylamine* are FDA-approved as ingredients in OTC nonprescription sleep aids. With elimination $t_{1/2}$ of about 9–10 h, these antihistamines can be associated with prominent residual sleepiness the morning after when taken as a sleep aid the night before.

New and Emerging Agents

Suvorexant

Suvorexant, an inhibitor of orexin 1 and 2 receptors, was approved by the FDA in late 2014 for the treatment of insomnia (Winrow and Renger, 2014). Orexins, produced by neurons in the lateral hypothalamus and projecting broadly throughout the CNS, play a major role in regulation of the sleep cycle. These neurons are quiescent during sleep but are active during wakefulness; thus, orexins promote wakefulness, while antagonists at orexin receptors enhance REM and non-REM sleep. Suvorexant decreases sleep onset latency and is superior to placebo in sleep maintenance. One 10-mg dose should be taken within 30 min of going to bed if at least 7 h remain until the projected time of awakening. The most common adverse reaction is daytime somnolence, and there is a possibility of the worsening of depression or suicidal ideation. Surorexant is a schedule IV controlled substance. A number of other orexin receptor antagonists are currently in clinical trials.

Doxepin

Doxepin, a tricyclic antidepressant, enhances subjective measures of sleep quality and is indicated for the treatment of difficulties with sleep maintenance (Yeung et al., 2015). It acts presumably via antagonism of H_1 receptor function when administered in low doses. Doxepin should be taken in initial doses of 6 mg (3 mg in the elderly) within 30 min of bedtime. Abnormal thinking and behavior have been observed following its use, and it can worsen suicidal ideation and depression. Doxepin was approved by the FDA in 2010 for the treatment of sleep maintenance insomnia.

Pregabalin

Pregabalin, an anxiolytic agent that binds to Ca^{2+} channel $\alpha_2\delta$ subunits, has proved useful in clinical trials (Holsboer-Trachsler and Prieto, 2013); pregabalin slightly decreased sleep onset latency and increased the proportion of time spent in slow-wave sleep. Pregabalin appears to be an effective treatment of the insomnia seen in patients suffering from a generalized anxiety disorder. Pregabalin is designated as a schedule V controlled substance.

Ritanserin

Ritanserin and other $5HT_{2A/2C}$ receptor antagonists show an ability to promote slow-wave sleep in patients with chronic primary insomnia or generalized anxiety disorder (Monti, 2010). Ritanserin is not licensed for use in the U.S.

Agomelatine

Agomelatine, a melatonin receptor agonist and a $5HT_{2C}$ receptor antagonist, is prescribed for the treatment of depression and may aid in ameliorating sleep disturbances often associated with depression. Agomelatine is not licensed for use in the U.S.

Management of Insomnia

Insomnia is one of the most common complaints in general medical practice. A number of pharmacological agents are available for the treatment of insomnia. The "perfect" hypnotic would allow sleep to occur with normal sleep architecture. It would not cause next-day effects, either of rebound anxiety or of continued sedation. It would not interact with other medications. It could be used chronically without causing dependence or rebound insomnia on discontinuation. Controversy in the management of insomnia revolves around two issues:

- Pharmacological versus nonpharmacological treatment
- Use of short-acting versus long-acting hypnotics

The side effects of hypnotic medications must be weighed against the sequelae of chronic insomnia, which include a 4-fold increase in serious accidents (Balter and Uhlenhuth, 1992). Regular moderate exercise or even small amounts of exercise often are effective in promoting sleep. In addition to appropriate pharmacological treatment, the management of insomnia should correct identifiable causes, address inadequate sleep hygiene, eliminate performance anxiety related to falling asleep, provide entrainment of the biological clock so that maximum sleepiness occurs at the hour of attempted sleep, and suppress the use of alcohol and OTC sleep medications.

Categories of Insomnia

- *Transient insomnia* lasts less than 3 days and usually is caused by a brief environmental or situational stressor. If hypnotics are prescribed, they should be used at the lowest dose and for only 2–3 nights. Note that benzodiazepines given acutely before important life events, such as examinations, may result in impaired performance.
- *Short-term insomnia* lasts from 3 days to 3 weeks and usually is caused by a personal stressor such as illness, grief, or job problems. Hypnotics may be used adjunctively for 7–10 nights and are best used intermittently during this time, with the patient skipping a dose after 1–2 nights of good sleep.
- *Long-term insomnia* lasts for more than 3 weeks; a specific stressor may not be identifiable.

Insomnia Accompanying Major Psychiatric Illnesses

The insomnia caused by major psychiatric illnesses often responds to specific pharmacological treatment of that illness. For example, in major depressive episodes with insomnia, SSRIs, which may cause insomnia as a side effect, usually will result in improved sleep because they treat the depressive syndrome. In a patient whose depression is responding to an SSRI but has persistent insomnia as a side effect of the medication, judicious use of evening trazodone may improve sleep, as well as augment the antidepressant effect of the reuptake inhibitor. However, the patient should be monitored for priapism, orthostatic hypotension, and arrhythmias.

Adequate control of anxiety disorders often produces adequate resolution of the accompanying insomnia. Sedative use in patients with anxiety disorders is decreasing because of a growing appreciation of the effectiveness of other agents, such as β adrenergic receptor antagonists (Chapter 12) for performance anxiety and SSRIs for obsessive-compulsive disorder and perhaps generalized anxiety disorder. The profound insomnia in patients with acute psychosis owing to schizophrenia or mania usually responds to dopamine receptor antagonists (see Chapters 13 and 16). Benzodiazepines often are used adjunctively in this situation to reduce agitation and improve sleep.

Insomnia Accompanying Other Medical Illnesses

For long-term insomnia owing to other medical illnesses, adequate treatment of the underlying disorder, such as congestive heart failure, asthma, or COPD, may resolve the insomnia. Adequate pain management in conditions of chronic pain will treat both the pain and the insomnia and may make hypnotics unnecessary. *Adequate attention to sleep hygiene, including reduced caffeine intake, avoidance of alcohol, adequate exercise, and regular sleep and wake times, often will reduce the insomnia.*

Conditioned (Learned) Insomnia

In those who have no major psychiatric or other medical illness and in whom attention to sleep hygiene is ineffective, attention should be directed to conditioned (learned) insomnia. These patients have associated the bedroom with activities consistent with wakefulness rather than sleep. In such patients, all other activities associated with waking, even such quiescent activities as reading and watching television, should be done outside the bedroom.

Sleep-State Misperception

Some patients complain of poor sleep but have been shown to have no objective polysomnographic evidence of insomnia. They are difficult to treat.

Long-Term Insomnia

Nonpharmacological treatments are important for all patients with long-term insomnia. These include education about sleep hygiene, relaxation training, and behavioral modification approaches, such as sleep restriction and stimulus-control therapies.

Long-term hypnotic use leads to a decrease in effectiveness and may produce rebound insomnia on discontinuance. Almost all hypnotics change sleep architecture. The barbiturates reduce REM sleep; the benzodiazepines reduce slow-wave non-REM sleep and, to a lesser extent, REM sleep. While the significance of these findings is not clear, there is an emerging consensus that slow-wave sleep is particularly important for physical restorative processes. REM sleep may aid in the consolidation of learning. The blockade of slow-wave sleep by benzodiazepines may partly account for their diminishing effectiveness over the long term, and it also may explain their effectiveness in blocking sleep terrors, a disorder of arousal from slow-wave sleep.

Long-acting benzodiazepines can cause next-day confusion, whereas shorter-acting agents can produce rebound next-day anxiety. Paradoxically, the acute amnestic effects of benzodiazepines may be responsible for the patient's subsequent report of restful sleep. Anterograde amnesia may be more common with triazolam. Hypnotics should not be given to patients with sleep apnea, especially the obstructive type, because these agents decrease upper airway muscle tone while also decreasing the arousal response to hypoxia.

Insomnia in Older Patients

The elderly, like the very young, tend to sleep in a *polyphasic* (multiple sleep episodes per day) pattern rather than the *monophasic* pattern characteristic of younger adults. This pattern makes assessment of adequate sleep time difficult.

Changes in the pharmacokinetic profiles of hypnotic agents occur in the elderly because of reduced body water, reduced renal function, and increased body fat, leading to a longer $t_{1/2}$ for benzodiazepines. A dose that produces pleasant sleep and adequate daytime wakefulness during week 1 may produce daytime confusion and amnesia by week 3 as the drug level continues to rise, particularly with long-acting hypnotics. For example, the benzodiazepine diazepam is highly lipid soluble and is excreted by the kidney. Because of the increase in body fat and the decrease in renal excretion that typically occur from age 20 to 80, the $t_{1/2}$ of the drug may increase 4-fold over this span.

Injudicious use of hypnotics in the elderly can produce daytime cognitive impairment and thereby impair overall quality of life. Once an older patient has been taking benzodiazepines for an extended period, whether for daytime anxiety or for nighttime sedation, terminating the drug can be a long, involved process. Attempts at drug withdrawal may not be successful, and it may be necessary to leave the patient on the medication, with adequate attention to daytime side effects.

Prescribing Guidelines for Managing Insomnia

Hypnotics that act at $GABA_A$ receptors—benzodiazepine hypnotics and the newer agents zolpidem, zopiclone, and zaleplon—are preferred to barbiturates; the $GABA_A$ receptor agents have a higher therapeutic index, smaller effects on sleep architecture, and less abuse potential. Compounds with a shorter $t_{1/2}$ are favored in patients with sleep-onset insomnia but without significant daytime anxiety who need to function at full effectiveness during the day. These compounds also are appropriate for the elderly because of a decreased risk of falls and respiratory depression. However, the patient and physician should be aware that early morning awakening, rebound daytime anxiety, and amnestic episodes also may occur. These undesirable side effects are more common at higher doses of the benzodiazepines.

Benzodiazepines with longer $t_{1/2}$ values are favored for patients who have significant daytime anxiety. These benzodiazepines also are appropriate for patients receiving treatment of major depressive episodes because the short-acting agents can worsen early morning awakening. However, longer-acting benzodiazepines can be associated with next-day cognitive impairment or delayed daytime cognitive impairment (after 2–4 weeks of treatment) as a result of drug accumulation with repeated administration.

Older agents—barbiturates, chloral hydrate, and meprobamate—should be avoided for the management of insomnia. They have high abuse potential and are dangerous in overdose.

Drug Facts for Your Personal Formulary: *Sedative-Hypnotic Agents*

Drug	Therapeutic Uses	Clinical Pharmacology and Tips
Benzodiazepines-synergistic with other CNS depressants, esp. ethanol; see Table 19–2.		
Alprazolam	Anxiety disorders, agoraphobia	Withdrawal symptoms may be especially severe
Chlordiazepoxide	Anxiety disorders, alcohol withdrawal, preanesthetic medication	Long-acting and self-tapering because of active metabolites
Clobazam	Adjunctive treatment of seizures associated with Lennox-Gastaut syndrome, other epilepsy and anxiety disorders	Active metabolite has long half-life Decrease dose and titrate in CYP2C19 poor metabolizers Tolerance develops to anticonvulsant effects
Clonazepam	Seizure disorders, adjunctive treatment in acute mania and certain movement disorders	Tolerance develops to anticonvulsant effects
Clorazepate	Anxiety disorders, seizure disorders	Prodrug; activity due to formation of nordazepam during absorption
Diazepam	Anxiety disorders, alcohol withdrawal, status epilepticus, skeletal muscle relaxation, preanesthetic medication	Prototypical benzodiazepine
Estazolam	Insomnia	Contains triazolo ring; adverse effects may be similar to those of triazolam
Flurazepam	Insomnia	Active metabolites accumulate with chronic use
Lorazepam	Anxiety disorders, alcohol withdrawal, preanesthetic medication	Metabolized solely by conjugation
Midazolam	Preanesthetic and intraoperative medication	Rapidly inactivated
Oxazepam	Anxiety disorders, alcohol withdrawal	Metabolized solely by conjugation
Quazepam	Insomnia	Active metabolites accumulate with chronic use
Temazepam	Insomnia	Metabolized mainly by conjugation
Triazolam	Insomnia	Rapidly inactivated; may cause disturbing daytime side effects
"Z" Compounds-nonbenzodiazepines with agonist effects at the benzodiazepine site of $GABA_A$ receptors; have largely replaced benzodiazepines for treating insomnia.		
Zaleplon	Insomnia	Very short elimination half-life
Zolpidem	Insomnia	Short-term (2–6 week) treatment of insomnia
Eszopiclone	Insomnia	S(+) enantiomer of zopiclone
Benzodiazepine Antagonist		
Flumenazil	Benzodiazepine overdose (benzodiazepine and β-carboline antagonist	Headache, dizziness; do not use in tricyclic antidepressant poisoning (seizures!)

Drug Facts for Your Personal Formulary: *Sedative-Hypnotic Agents (continued)*

Drug	Therapeutic Uses	Clinical Pharmacology and Tips
Miscellaneous and Emerging Agents		
Ramelteon	Insomnia	Melatonin receptor agonist; significant first-pass effect
Tasimelteon	Circadian rhythm disorder in blind patients	Melatonin receptor agonist
Suvorexant	Insomnia	Orexin receptor antagonist; needs at least 7 h after 10-mg dose before awakening
Doxepin	Depression, insomnia	Tricyclic antidepressant; sedating effects likely occur through H_1 receptor antagonism; beware of abnormal behavior, suicide ideation, depression; use half dose in the elderly
Propofol	Induction/maintenance of anesthesia, procedural sedation	Rapid recovery
Pregabalin (β-isobutyl–GABA)	Nerve/muscle pain, fibromyalgia, seizures	Schedule V substance, abuse potential; some concern for suicide ideation and angioedema
Barbiturates-synergistic with other CNS depressants, esp. ethanol; induce CYPs; respiratory depressants; see Table 19–3.		
Amobarbital	Insomnia, preoperative sedation, emergency management of seizures	• IM and IV • Short-acting (3-8 h)
Butabarbital	Insomnia, preoperative sedation, daytime sedation	• Oral • Fast onset of action • Short-acting (3-8 h)
Mephobarbital (not licensed for use in U.S.)	Seizure disorders, daytime sedation	• Oral • Short-acting (3-8 h)
Methohexital	Induction and maintenance of anesthesia	• IV • Ultra short-acting (5-15 min)
Pentobarbital	Insomnia, preoperative and procedural sedation, emergency management of seizures	• Oral, IM, IV, or rectal • Administer Na^+ salt parenterally • Short-acting (3-8 h)
Phenobarbital	Seizure disorders, status epilepticus, daytime sedation	• Oral, IM, IV • First-line anticonvulsant (see chapter 17); administer Na^+ salt parenterally • Long-acting (days)
Secobarbital	Insomnia, preoperative sedation	• Oral • Short-acting (3-8 h)
Thiopental	Induction and maintenance of anesthesia, preoperative sedation, emergency management of seizures, intracranial hypertension	• IV single dose provides brief period of anesthesia • Ultra short-acting (5-15 min)

Bibliography

Balter MB, Uhlenhuth EH. New epidemiologic findings about insomnia and its treatment. *J Clin Psychiatry,* **1992**, *53*(suppl):34–39.

Dooley M, Plosker GL. Zaleplon: a review of its use in the treatment of insomnia. *Drugs,* **2000**, *60*:413–445.

Dujardin K, et al. Comparison of the effects of zolpidem and flunitrazepam on sleep structure and daytime cognitive functions: a study of untreated insomniacs. *Pharmacopsychiatry,* **1998**, *31*:14–18.

Hanson SM, et al. Structural requirements for eszopiclone and zolpidem binding to the gamma-aminobutyric acid type-A ($GABA_A$) receptor are different. *J Med Chem,* **2008**, *51*:7243–7252.

Hoffman EJ, Warren EW. Flumazenil: a benzodiazepine antagonist. *Clin Pharmacol,* **1993**, *12*:641–656.

Holsboer-Trachsler E, Prieto R. Effects of pregabalin on sleep in generalized anxiety disorder. *Int J Neuropsychopharmacol,* **2013**, *16*:925–936.

Huedo-Medina TB, et al. Effectiveness of non-benzodiazepine hypnotics in treatment of adult insomnia: meta-analysis of data submitted to the Food and Drug Administration. *BMJ,* **2012**, *345*:e8343.

Johnsa JD, Neville MW. Tasimelteon: a melatonin receptor agonist for non-24-hour sleep-wake disorder. *Ann Pharmacother,* **2014**, *48*:1636–1641.

Marszalec W, Narahashi T. Use-dependent pentobarbital block of kainate and quisqualate currents. *Brain Res,* **1993**, *608*:7–15.

Mayer G, et al. Efficacy and safety of 6-month nightly ramelteon administration in adults with chronic primary insomnia. *Sleep,* **2009**, *32*:351–360.

McKeage K, Perry CM. Propofol: a review of its use in intensive care sedation of adults. *CNS Drugs,* **2003**, *17*:235–272.

Melton ST, et al. Eszopiclone for insomnia. *Ann Pharmacother,* **2005**, *39*:1659–1666.

Monane M. Insomnia in the elderly. *J Clin Psychiatry,* **1992**, *53*(suppl):23–28.

Monti JM. Serotonin 5-HT(2A) receptor antagonists in the treatment of insomnia: present status and future prospects. *Drugs Today (Barc),* **2010**, *46*:183–193.

Morselli PL. Zolpidem side effects. *Lancet,* **1993**, *342*:868–869.

Nestler EJ, et al. *Molecular Neuropharmacology.* 3rd ed. McGraw-Hill, New York, **2015**.

Oldenhof H, et al. Clinical pharmacokinetics of midazolam in intensive care patients, a wide interpatient variability? *Clin Pharmacol Ther,*

1988, *43*:263–269.

Rosenberg R, et al. An assessment of the efficacy and safety of eszopiclone in the treatment of transient insomnia in healthy adults. *Sleep Med,* **2005**, *6*:15–22.

Sieghart W. Allosteric modulation of $GABA_A$ receptors via multiple drug-binding sites. *Adv Pharmacol,* **2015**, *72*:53–96.

Sigel E, Steinmann ME. Structure, function, and modulation of $GABA_A$ receptors. *J Biol Chem,* **2012**, *287*:40224–40231.

Spadoni G, et al. Melatonin receptor agonists: new options for insomnia and depression treatment. *CNS Neurosci Ther,* **2011**, *17*:733–741.

Uhlenhuth EH, et al. International study of expert judgment on therapeutic use of benzodiazepines and other psychotherapeutic medications: IV. Therapeutic dose dependence and abuse liability of benzodiazepines in the long-term treatment of anxiety disorders. *J Clin Psychopharmacol,* **1999**, *19*(suppl 2):23S–29S.

Winrow CJ, Renger JJ. Discovery and development of orexin receptor antagonists as therapeutics for insomnia. *Br J Pharmacol,* **2014**, *171*:283–293.

Woods JH, et al. Benzodiazepines: use, abuse, and consequences. *Pharmacol Rev,* **1992**, *44*:151–347.

Yeung WF, et al. Doxepin for insomnia: a systematic review of randomized placebo-controlled trials. *Sleep Med Rev,* **2015**, *19*:75–83.

Opioids, Analgesia, and Pain Management

Tony Yaksh and Mark Wallace

第二十章　阿片类药物、镇痛药和疼痛管理

PAIN

ENDOGENOUS OPIOID PEPTIDES
- Pro-opiomelanocortin
- Proenkephalin
- Prodynorphin
- Endomorphins

OPIOID RECEPTORS
- Classes of Receptors
- Opioid Receptor Distribution
- Opioid Receptor Ligands
- Opioid Receptor Structure
- Opioid Receptor Signaling
- Regulation of Postactivation Opiate Receptor Trafficking; Biased Opioid Agonism

EFFECTS OF ACUTE AND CHRONIC OPIATE RECEPTOR ACTIVATION
- Desensitization
- Tolerance
- Dependence
- Addiction

MECHANISMS OF TOLERANCE/DEPENDENCE/WITHDRAWAL
- Receptor Disposition
- Adaptation of Intracellular Signaling Mechanisms
- System-Level Counteradaptation
- Differential Tolerance Development and Fractional Occupancy Requirements

EFFECTS OF CLINICALLY USED OPIOIDS
- Analgesia
- Mood Alterations and Rewarding Properties
- Respiratory Effects
- Opioid-Induced Hyperalgesia
- Sedation
- Neuroendocrine Effects

CLINICALLY EMPLOYED OPIOID DRUGS
- Morphine and Structurally Related Agonists
- Other Morphinans
- Piperidine and Phenylpiperidine Analgesics
- Fentanyl and Congeners
- Methadone
- Other Opioid Agonists
- Opioid Partial Agonists
- Opioid Antagonists

CENTRALLY ACTIVE ANTITUSSIVES
- Dextromethorphan
- Other Antitussives

ROUTES OF ANALGESIC DRUG ADMINISTRATION
- Patient-Controlled Analgesia
- Spinal Delivery
- Rectal Administration
- Oral Transmucosal Administration
- Transnasal Administration
- Transdermal Administration

THERAPEUTIC CONSIDERATIONS IN PAIN CONTROL
- Acute Pain States
- Chronic Pain States
- Guidelines for Opiate Dosing

VARIABLES MODIFYING THE THERAPEUTIC USE OF OPIATES
- Patient Variability
- Pain
- Opioid Tolerance
- Patient Physical State and Genetic Variables
- Routes of Administration
- Dose Selection and Titration
- Opioid Rotation
- Combination Therapy

NONANALGESIC THERAPEUTIC USES OF OPIOIDS
- Dyspnea
- Anesthetic Adjuvants

ACUTE OPIOID TOXICITY
- Symptoms and Diagnosis
- Treatment

NOVEL NONOPIOID TREATMENTS FOR PAIN
- Ziconotide

中文导读

本章主要介绍：疼痛；内源性阿片肽，包括阿片-促黑素细胞皮质素原、前脑啡肽原、强啡肽原和内吗啡肽；阿片受体，包括受体类别、阿片受体分布、阿片受体配体、阿片受体结构、阿片受体信号、阿片受体激活后迁移的调节、阿片受体偏向激动剂；急性和慢性阿片受体激活作用，包括脱敏、耐受、依赖和成瘾；耐受、依赖、戒断的机制，包括受体移位、胞内信号传导机制的适应、系统水平的逆适应、不同耐受的形成和部分占领的需求；临床用阿片类药物的作用，包括镇痛、情绪改变与奖赏特性、呼吸作用、阿片类药物引起的痛觉过敏、镇静和神经内分泌作用；临床使用的阿片类药物，包括吗啡及其结构相关的激动药、其他吗啡类药物、哌啶和苯基哌啶镇痛药、芬太尼及其类似物、美沙酮、其他阿片类激动药、阿片类部分激动药和阿片类拮抗药；中枢性镇咳药，包括右美沙芬和其他镇咳药；镇痛药的给药途径，包括患者自控镇痛、脊柱输送、直肠给药、口腔黏膜给药、经鼻给药和透皮给药；疼痛控制中的治疗注意事项，包括急性疼痛状态、慢性疼痛状态和阿片类药物剂量指南；影响阿片类药物镇痛治疗的因素，包括患者差异、疼痛、阿片类药物耐受、患者的身体状态和遗传变异、给药途径、剂量选择和滴定、阿片类药物轮替和联合治疗；阿片类药物的非镇痛治疗用途，包括呼吸困难和麻醉佐剂；急性阿片类药物中毒，包括症状、诊断和治疗；新型非阿片类镇痛药物齐考诺肽。

Pain

Pain is a component of virtually all clinical pathologies, and management of pain is a primary clinical imperative. Opioids are a mainstay of acute pain treatment, but in recent years, the efficacy and safety of long-term use of opioids to treat chronic pain has been questioned as instances of addiction and death from their misuse have mounted. Opioids are certainly no longer first-line treatment of chronic pain, and a more conservative approach may involve other drug classes, such as NSAIDs, anticonvulsants, and antidepressants.

The term *opiate* refers to compounds structurally related to products found in opium, a word derived from *opos*, the Greek word for "juice," natural opiates being derived from the resin of the opium poppy, *Papaver somniferum*. Opiates include the natural plant alkaloids, such as morphine, codeine, thebaine, and many semisynthetic derivatives. An *opioid* is any agent that has the functional and pharmacological properties of an opiate. Endogenous opioids are naturally occurring ligands for opioid receptors found in animals. The term *endorphin* not only is used synonymously with *endogenous opioid peptides* but also refers to a specific endogenous opioid, *β-endorphin*. The term *narcotic* was derived from the Greek word *narkotikos*, for "benumbing" or "stupor." Although the term ***narcotic*** originally referred to any drug that induced narcosis or sleep, the word has become associated with opioids and is often used in a legal context to refer to substances with abuse or addictive potential.

Endogenous Opioid Peptides

A biological molecule found within the brain that acts through an opioid receptor is an endogenous opioid. The opioid peptide precursors are a protean family defined by the prohormone from which they are derived (Figure 20–1). Several distinct families of endogenous opioid peptides have been identified: principally the *enkephalins, endorphins,* and *dynorphins* (Table 20–1) (Höllt, 1986). These families have several common properties:

- Each derives from a distinct precursor protein, pre-POMC, *preproenkephalin*, and *preprodynorphin*, respectively, each encoded by a corresponding gene.
- Each precursor is subject to complex cleavages by distinct trypsin-like enzymes and to a variety of posttranslational modifications resulting in the synthesis of multiple peptides, some of which are active as opioids.
- Most opioid peptides with activity at a receptor share the common amino-terminal sequence of *Tyr-Gly-Gly-Phe-(Met or Leu),* followed by various C-terminal extensions yielding peptides of 5–31 residues; the endomorphins, with different terminal sequences, are exceptions.
- Not all cells that make a given opioid prohormone precursor store and release the same mixture of opioid peptides; this results from differential post-translational processing secondary to variations in the cellular complement of peptidases that produce and degrade the active opioid fragments.

Abbreviations

AAG: α_1-acid glycoprotein
AC: adenylyl cyclase
ACE: angiotensin-converting enzyme
ACh: acetylcholine
ACTH: corticotropin; formerly adrenocorticotropic hormone
ADH: antidiuretic hormone
ADME: absorption, distribution, metabolism, excretion
AT_1: angiotensin II receptor, type 1
ATC: around the clock
BBB: blood-brain barrier
CaMK: Ca^{2+}/calmodulin-dependent protein kinase
CDC: Centers for Disease Control and Prevention
CLIP: corticotropin-like intermediate lobe peptide
CNS: central nervous system
COPD: chronic obstructive pulmonary disease
COX: cyclooxygenase
CRH: corticotropin-releasing hormone
CSF: cerebrospinal fluid
CYP: cytochrome P450
DA: dopamine
DAMGO: [D-Ala^2,MePhe^4,Gly(ol)^5]enkephalin
DHEA: dehydroepiandrosterone
DOR: δ opioid receptor
DYN: dynorphin
EEG: electroencephalogram
β-END: β-endorphin
L-ENK: Leu-enkephalin
ER/LA: extended-release/long-acting (a)
FDA: Food and Drug Administration
FSH: follicle-stimulating hormone
GABA: γ-aminobutyric acid
GI: gastrointestinal
GIRK: G protein–activated inwardly rectifying K^+ channel
GnRH: gonadotropin-releasing hormone
GPCR: G protein-coupled receptor
GRK: GPCR kinase
HPA: hypothalamic-pituitary-adrenal
5HT: serotonin
IM: intramuscular
IP_3: inositol triphosphate
IV: intravenous
JNK: c-Jun *N*-terminal kinase
KOR: κ opioid receptor
LH: luteinizing hormone
LPH: lipotropin
6-MAM: 6-monoacetylmorphine
MAO: monoamine oxidase
MAP: mitogen-activated protein
M-ENK: Met-enkephalin
MME: morphine milligram equivalent
MOR: μ opioid receptor
MSH: melanocyte-stimulating hormone
NAc: nucleus accumbens
NE: norepinephrine
α-NEO: α neoendorphin
NF-κB: nuclear factor kappa B
NMDA: *N*-methyl-D-aspartate
NOP: nociceptin/orphanin FQ (N/OFQ) receptor
NSAID: nonsteroidal anti-inflammatory drug
PAG: periaqueductal gray
PCA: patient-controlled anesthesia
PDMP: prescription drug monitoring program
PFC: prefrontal cortex
PI3K: phosphoinositide 3 kinase
PK: protein kinase
PLC: phospholipase C
POMC: pro-opiomelanocortin
pre-proDYN: pre-prodynorphin
pre-ProENK: pre-proenkephalin
SNRI: serotonin-norepinephrine reuptake inhibitor
SSRI: selective serotonin reuptake inhibitor
TM: transmembrane
VP: ventral pallidum
VTA: ventral tegmental area

- Processing of these peptides is altered by physiological demands, leading to the release of a different mix of post-translationally derived peptides by a given cell under different conditions.
- Opioid peptides are found in plasma and reflect release from secretory systems such as the pituitary and the adrenals and thus do not reflect neuraxial release. Conversely, levels of these peptides in brain/spinal cord and in CSF arise from neuraxial systems and not from peripheral systems.

Pro-opiomelanocortin

The major opioid peptide derived from *POMC* is *the potent opioid agonist β-endorphin.* The *POMC* sequence also is processed into a variety of nonopioid peptides, including ACTH, α-MSH, and β-LPH. Although β-endorphin contains the sequence for met-enkephalin at its amino terminus, it is not typically converted to this peptide.

Proenkephalin

The *prohormone* contains multiple copies of *met-enkephalin,* as well as a single copy of *leu-enkephalin. Proenkephalin peptides* are present in areas of the CNS believed to be related to the processing of pain information (e.g., spinal cord dorsal horn, the spinal trigeminal nucleus, and the PAG); to the modulation of affective behavior (e.g., amygdala, hippocampus, locus ceruleus, and frontal cerebral cortex); to the modulation of motor control (e.g., caudate nucleus and globus pallidus); to the regulation of the autonomic nervous system (e.g., medulla oblongata); and to neuroendocrinological functions (e.g., median eminence). Peptides from proenkephalin also are found in chromaffin cells of the adrenal medulla and in nerve plexuses and exocrine glands of the stomach and intestine. Circulating proenkephalin products are considered to be largely derived from these sites.

Prodynorphin

Prodynorphin contains three peptides of differing lengths that all begin with the leu-enkephalin sequence: *dynorphin A,* rimorphin *(dynorphin B), and neoendorphin. Nociceptin peptide* or *orphanin FQ* (now termed N/OFQ) shares structural similarity with dynorphin A. The peptides derived from prodynorphin are distributed widely in neurons and to a lesser extent in astrocytes throughout the brain and spinal cord and are frequently found coexpressed with other opioid peptide precursors.

Endomorphins

The endomorphin peptides belong to a novel family of peptides that include *endomorphin 1* (*Tyr-Pro-Trp-Phe-NH_2*) and *endomorphin 2* (*Tyr-Pro-Phe-Phe-NH_2*). Endomorphins have an atypical structure and display selectivity toward the MOR.

HISTORICAL PERSPECTIVE

The first undisputed reference to opium is found in the writings of Theophrastus in the 3rd century BC. Arab physicians were well versed in the uses of opium. Arab traders introduced the opium concoction to the Orient, where it was employed mainly for the control of dysentery. Paracelsus named the product laudanum. By 1680, the utility of laudanum was so well appreciated that Thomas *Sydenham*, a 17th-century pioneer in English medicine noted that, "Among the remedies which it has pleased Almighty God to give to man to relieve his sufferings, none is so universal and so efficacious as opium," thereby, in his own way, connecting religion and opiates almost 200 years ahead of Marx.

Opium contains more than 20 distinct alkaloids. In 1806, Frederich Sertürner, a pharmacist's assistant, reported the isolation by crystallization of a pure substance in opium that he named morphine, after Morpheus, the Greek god of dreams (Booth, 1999). By the middle of the 19th century, the use of pure alkaloids in place of crude opium preparations began to spread throughout the medical world, an event that coincided with the development of the hypodermic syringe and hollow needle, permitting direct delivery of water-soluble formulations "under the skin" into the body.

In addition to the remarkable salutary benefits of opioids, the side effects and addictive potential of these drugs have been known for centuries. In the U.S. Civil War, the administration of "soldier's joy" often led to "soldier's disease," the opiate addiction brought about by medication of chronic pain states arising from war wounds. These problems stimulated a search for potent synthetic opioid analgesics free of addictive potential and other side effects. The early discovery of the synthetic product heroin by C.R. Alder Wright in 1874 was followed by its widespread utilization as a purportedly nonaddictive cough suppressant and sedative. Unfortunately, heroin and all subsequent synthetic opioids that have been introduced into clinical use share the liabilities of classical opioids, including their addictive properties. However, this search for new opioid agonists led to the synthesis of opioid antagonists and compounds with mixed agonist-antagonist properties, which expanded therapeutic options and provided important tools for exploring mechanisms of opioid actions.

Until the early 1970s, the effects of morphine, heroin, and other opioids as antinociceptive and addictive agents were well described, but mechanisms mediating the interaction of the opioid alkaloids with biological systems were unknown. Goldstein began a search for stereoselective binding sites in the CNS using radioligands (Goldstein et al., 1971), and Pert convincingly employed radioligands to demonstrate opiate-binding sites and an effect of Na^+ that distinguished agonist from antagonist binding (Pert et al., 1973). In vivo and in vitro physiological studies of the pharmacology of opiate agonists, their antagonists, and cross-tolerance led to the hypothesis of three separate receptors: mu (μ), kappa (κ), and sigma (σ) (Martin et al., 1976). Efforts to isolate endogenous opioids led to the discovery of the molecules (see discussion that follows) that acted on a distinct receptor, the delta (δ) receptor. The μ, κ, and δ receptors, but not the σ receptor, shared the common property of being sensitive to blockade from agonist by agents such as naloxone. In concert with identification of these opioid receptors, Kostelitz and associates (Hughes et al., 1975) identified an endogenous opiate-like factor that they called *enkephalin* ("from the head"). Soon afterward, two more classes of endogenous opioid peptides were isolated, the endorphins and dynorphins (Akil et al., 1984).

In the early work by Martin, the σ receptor was thought to represent a site that accounted for paradoxical excitatory effects of opiates; this site is now thought to be the phencyclidine-binding site and is not, strictly speaking, an opiate receptor or an opiate site. Thus, three distinct receptors are now the basis of opioid pharmacology. The three-receptor hypothesis has been confirmed by cloning (Waldhoer et al., 2004). In 2000, the Committee on Receptor Nomenclature and Drug Classification of the International Union of Pharmacology adopted the terms MOP, DOP, and KOP receptors (**m**u **o**pioid **p**eptide receptor, etc.). This text uses MOR, DOR, and KOR to refer to both peptide and nonpeptide MORs, DORs, and KORs.

Attempts over at least half a century to dissociate the powerful analgesic effects of opioids from their undesirable effects have failed (Corbett et al., 2006). However, with our advancing understanding of biased agonism, prospects are looking up.

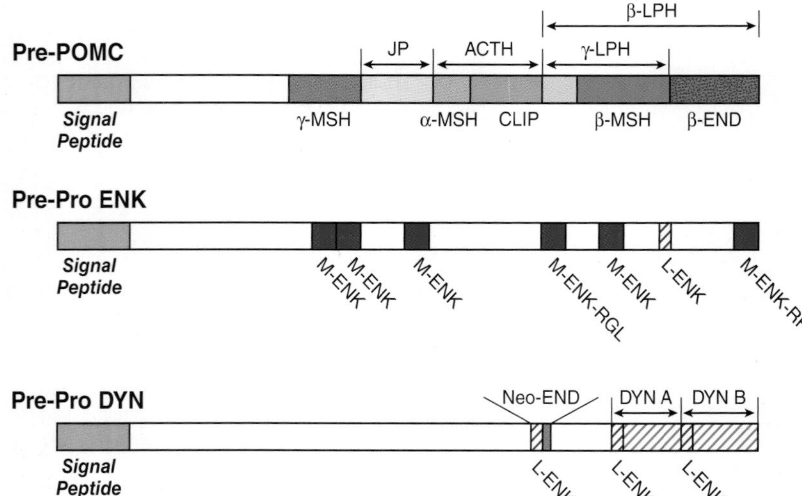

Figure 20–1 *Opioid peptide precursors.* Opioid peptides derive from precursor proteins that may also contain nonopioid peptides. *Pre-POMC* is a good example. Proteolytic processing of a pre-pro form by a signal peptidase removes the signal peptide; then, various prohormone convertases (endoproteases) attack at dibasic sequences, yielding α-, β-, and γ-MSH, ACTH, CLIP, β- and γ-LPH, and β-END. In similar manners, *Pre-ProENK* yields L-ENK and M-ENK and two relatives of M-ENK, M-ENK-RGL (Arg-Gly-Leu), and M-ENK-RF (Arg-Phe); and Pre-ProDYN yields α neoendorphin (α-NEO) and DYN A and DYN B, each of which contains an L-ENK sequence (Tyr-Gly-Gly-Phe-Leu) at its amino terminus. Figure 14–15 shows the processing of pre-POMC in greater detail. JF, joining peptide.

TABLE 20–1 ■ ENDOGENOUS OPIOID PEPTIDES

OPIOID LIGANDS	RECEPTOR SPECIFICITY μ	δ	κ
Met-enkephalin (**Tyr-Gly-Gly-Phe-Met**)	++	+++	
Leu-enkephalin (**Tyr-Gly-Gly-Phe-Leu**)	++	+++	
β-Endorphin (**Tyr-Gly-Gly-Phe-Met**-Thr-Ser-Glu-Lys-Ser-Gln-Thr-Pro-Leu-Val-Thr-Leu-Phe-Lys-Asn-Ala-Ile-Ile-Lys-Asn-Ala-Tyr-Lys-Lys-Gly-Glu)	+++	+++	
Dynorphin A (**Tyr-Gly-Gly-Phe-Leu**-Arg-Arg-Ile-Arg-Pro-Lys-Leu-Lys-Trp-Asp-Asn-Gln)	++		+++
Dynorphin B (**Tyr-Gly-Gly-Phe-Leu**-Arg-Arg-Gln-Phe-Lys-Val-Val-Thr)	+	+	+++
α-Neoendorphin (**Tyr-Gly-Gly-Phe-Leu**-Arg-Lys-Tyr-Pro-Lys)	+	+	+++
Endomorphin 1 (Tyr-Pro-Trp-Phe-NH_2)	+++		

+, agonist; + < ++ < +++ in potency.
Reproduced with permission from Raynor K, et al. Pharmacological characterization of the cloned kappa-, delta-, and mu-opioid receptors. *Mol Pharmacol*, **1994**, *45*:330–334.

TABLE 20–2 ■ OPIOID AGONISTS

OPIOID LIGANDS	RECEPTOR TYPES μ	δ	κ
Etorphine	+++	+++	+++
Fentanyl	+++		
Hydromorphone	+++		+
Levorphanol	+++		
Methadone	+++		
Morphine[a]	+++		+
Sufentanil	+++	+	+
DAMGO[a] ([D-Ala²,MePhe⁴,Gly(ol)⁵] enkephalin)	+++		
Bremazocine[c]	+	+	+++
Buprenorphine	P		– –
Butorphanol[c]	P		+++
Nalbuphine	– –		++
DPDPE[b] ([D-Pen2,5]-Enkephalin])	+++		
U50,488[c]		++	

+, agonist; –, antagonist; P, partial agonist. In potency: + < ++ < +++
[a]Protoypical μ-preferring. [b]Prototypical δ-preferring. [c]Prototypical κ-preferring.
Source: Modified with permission from Raynor K et al. Pharmacological characterization of the cloned kappa-, delta-, and mu-opioid receptors. *Mol Pharmacol*, **1994**;*45*:330–334.

Opioid Receptors

Classes of Receptors

The three classes of opiate receptors—MOR, DOR, and KOR—share extensive sequence homologies (55%–58%) and belong to the rhodopsin family of GPCRs (see Figure 3–9). Opioid receptors appear early in vertebrate evolution (Stevens, 2009). Human opiate receptors have been mapped to chromosome 1p355–33 (DOR), chromosome 8q11.23–21 (KOR), and chromosome 6q25–26 (MOR) (Dreborg et al., 2008). Low-stringency hybridization procedures have identified no opioid receptor types other than these three cloned opioid receptors.

An opiate receptor-like protein (ORL_1 or NOP; chromosome 20q13.33) was cloned based on its structural homology (48%–49% identity) to other members of the opioid receptor family; it is G protein coupled, has an endogenous ligand (nociceptin [orphanin FQ]) but does not display an opioid pharmacology. As noted, a sigma (σ) receptor was early identified and was thought to represent a site that accounted for the paradoxical excitatory effects of opiates; agonist binding to the σ receptor is not antagonized by naloxone, and the receptor is not classified as an opiate receptor (Waldhoer et al., 2004).

Opioid Receptor Distribution

As defined by the distribution of receptor protein, message, ligand binding, and the pharmacological effects initiated by opiate molecules, all of the opioid receptors are widely distributed in the periphery and neuraxis on neuronal cell soma and terminals. Less well appreciated is the presence of opioid-binding sites on a variety of nonneuronal cells, including macrophage cell types (peripheral and central microglia) and astrocytes (Dannals, 2013; Yaksh, 1987), and in the enteric nervous system of the GI tract (Galligan and Akbarali, 2014).

Opioid Receptor Ligands

Opioid receptor ligands may be broadly defined by their functional properties as agonists and antagonists at the particular receptor.

Agonists

Highly selective agonists have been developed for the three binding sites (e.g., DAMGO for MOR; DPDPE for DOR; and U-50,488 for KOR) (Table 20–2). Virtually all of the clinically useful agonists are targeted at the μ receptor. Ligands that bind specifically but have limited intrinsic activity are referred to as partial agonists; for MOR, one such ligand is *buprenorphine*.

Antagonists

Commonly used opiate antagonists, such as *naloxone* or *naltrexone*, are pan antagonists with affinity for all known opioid receptors. Antagonists for specific opiate receptors have been developed for research (Table 20–3) and include cyclic analogues of somatostatin, such as CTOP (D-Phe-Cys-Tyr-D-Trp-Orn-Thr-Pen-Thr-NH2) as an MOR antagonist, a derivative of naloxone called *naltrindole* as a DOR antagonist, and a bivalent derivative of naltrexone called nor-BNI as a KOR antagonist.

Opioid Receptor Structure

Each of the opiate receptors consists of an extracellular N-terminus, seven TM helices, three extra- and intracellular loops, and an intracellular C-terminus characteristic of the GPCRs (Figure 20–2). The opioid receptors also possess two conserved cysteine residues in the first and second extracellular loops, which form a disulfide bridge. Though there is significant complexity in opiate-receptor interactions (Kane et al., 2006), several general principles define binding and selectivity.

- All opioid receptors display a binding pocket formed by TM_3-TM_7.
- The pocket in the respective receptor is partially covered by the extracellular loops, which, together with the extracellular termini of the TM segments, provide a gate-conferring selectivity, allowing ligands, particularly peptides, to be differentially accessible to the different receptor types. Thus, alkaloids (e.g., morphine) bind in the core of

TABLE 20–3 ■ OPIOID ANTAGONISTS

OPIOID LIGANDS	RECEPTOR TYPES		
	μ	δ	κ
Naloxone[a]	– – –	–	– –
Naltrexone[a]	– – –	–	– – –
CTOP[b]	– – –		
Diprenorphine	– – –	– –	– – –
β-Funaltrexamine[b,c]	– – –	–	++
Naloxonazine	– – –	–	–
nor-Binaltorphimine (nor-BNI)	–	–	– – –
Naltrindole[d]	–	– – –	–
Naloxone benzoylhydrazone	– – –	–	–

+, agonist; –, antagonist. – < – – < – – – in potency. CTOP, (D-Phe-Cys-Tyr-D-Trp-Orn-Thr-Pen-Thr-NH_2).
[a]Universal ligand.
[b]Prototypical μ preferring.
[c]Irreversible ligand.
[d]Prototypical δ preferring.
Reproduced with permission from Raynor K, et al. Pharmacological characterization of the cloned kappa-, delta-, and mu-opioid receptors. *Mol Pharmacol*, **1994**, *45*:330–334.

the TM portion of the receptor, whereas large peptidyl ligands bind at the extracellular loops. As noted, it is the extracellular loops that show the greatest structural diversity across receptors.

- Selectivity has been attributed to extracellular loops: first and third for the MOR, second for the KOR, and third for the DOR. Alkaloid antagonists are thought to bind more deeply in the pocket, sterically hindering conformational changes and leading to a functional antagonism.
- In the membrane, opiate receptors can form both homo- and heterodimers, thereby altering the pharmacological properties of the receptors. Thus, the diversity of responses is increased beyond those of the basic MOR, DOR, and KOR monomers.
- Hetero- and homodimerization of opiate receptors and their postactivation trafficking are important in understanding the selectivity of several ligands and the physiological responses to them. The development of tolerance to opioids may involve mechanisms of receptor trafficking.
- Splice variants exist for the opioid receptors. For example, the gene for the human MOR has at least two promoters, multiple exons, with many exons generating at least 11 splice variants that encode multiple morphine-binding isoforms, varying largely at their carboxy termini. This alternative splicing is likely crucial to receptor and response diversity (Pan, 2005; Xu et al., 2017).

Opioid Receptor Signaling

The MOR, DOR, and KOR couple to pertussis toxin–sensitive, G_i/G_o proteins. On receptor activation, the G_i/G_o coupling results in a number of intracellular events that are mediated by α and βγ subunits of these G proteins (see Figure 20–3), including the following:

- Inhibition of AC activity
- Reduced opening of voltage-gated Ca^{2+} channels (reduces neurotransmitter release from presynaptic terminals)
- Stimulation of K^+ current through several channels, including GIRKs (hyperpolarizes and inhibits postsynaptic neurons)
- Activation of PKC and PLCβ (Shang and Filizola, 2015)

Regulation of Postactivation Opiate Receptor Trafficking; Biased Opioid Agonism

The MORs and DORs undergo rapid agonist-mediated internalization. MORs recycle to the membrane after internalization; DORs are degraded on internalization (Zhang et al., 2015). KORs do not internalize after prolonged agonist exposure (Williams et al., 2013).

Internalization of the MORs and DORs apparently occurs via partially distinct endocytic pathways, suggesting receptor-specific interactions with different mediators of intracellular trafficking. These processes may be induced differentially as a function of the structure of the ligand. For example, certain agonists, such as etorphine and enkephalins, cause rapid

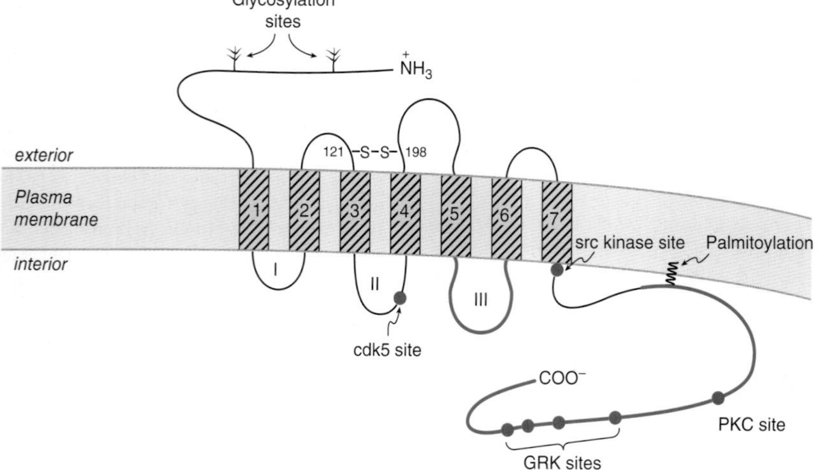

Figure 20–2 *General structure of an opioid receptor.* This schematic is based on the DOR (Gendron et al., 2016). The receptor has the characteristics of a GPCR: long external amino terminus with glycosylation sites, seven TM regions, a long intracellular carboxy tail, and phosphorylation sites in the areas where arrestins interact (portions of intracellular loop III and the carboxy tail, noted in green). The differential interaction of arrestins 1 and 2 with the phosphorylated sites may be a factor in the differential responses to different agonists (see Figure 20–4). An unusual feature is the extracellular disulfide linkage between Cys[121] and Cys[198]. Na^+ affects receptor constitutive activity and ligand specificity of DOR, effects that have been localized to an allosteric site for Na^+ in the core of the seven-TM bundle of DOR; changing Asn[131] in the Na^+ site to Ala or Val alters the effect of naltrindole from DOR antagonist to a β-arrestin–biased agonist. The Na^+-interacting residues seem to function as an "efficacy switch" (Fenalti et al., 2014).

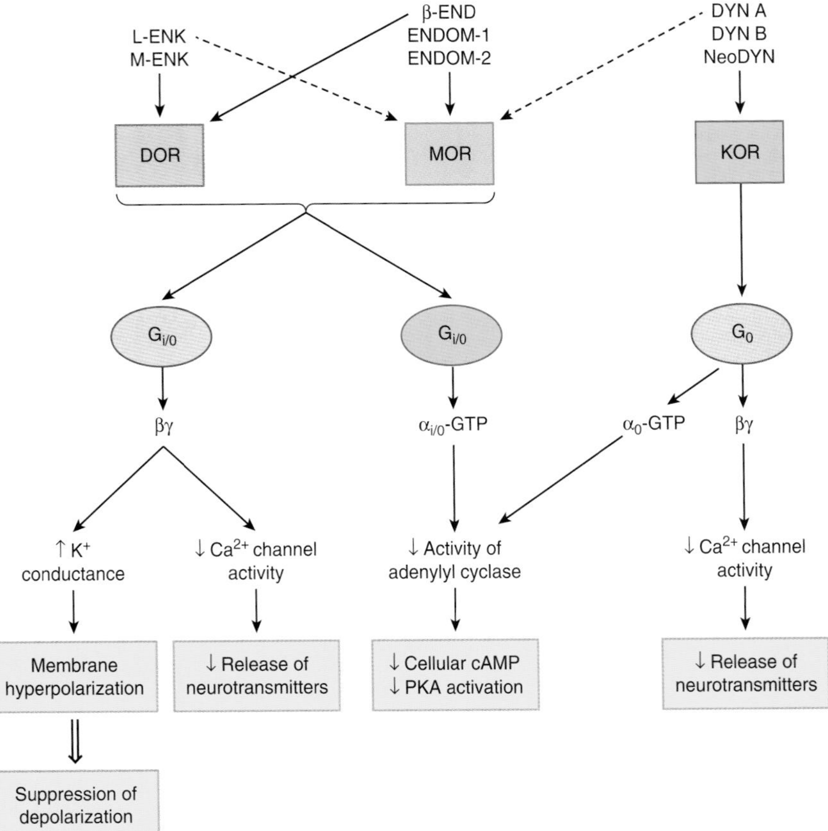

Figure 20–3 *Receptor specificity of endogenous opioids and effects of receptor activation on neurons.*

internalization of the receptor, whereas morphine does not cause MOR internalization, even though it decreases AC activity equally well. In addition, a truncated receptor with normal G protein coupling recycles constitutively from the membrane to the cytosol, suggesting that activation of signal transduction and internalization are controlled by distinct molecular mechanisms (von Zastrow et al., 2003). These studies support the assertion that different ligands induce different conformational changes in the receptor that result in divergent intracellular signaling, and they may provide an explanation for differences in the spectrum of effects of various opioids and point to novel therapeutics (Violin et al., 2014). Figure 20–4 shows some of the receptor-effector-signaling pathways that may contribute to biased opioid agonism and the complexity of immediate and long-term responses (desensitization, tolerance, dependence, withdrawal).

As noted, more than a single type of opioid receptor may be expressed on a cell. Functional data suggest opioid receptors may interact, forming homo- and heterodimers, and that such complexes may alter receptor signaling and trafficking and contribute to tolerance to morphine and possibly to disease states (Massotte, 2015; Zhang et al., 2015). The intracellular loops and amino tail of opioid receptors have numerous known and potential sites of phosphorylation by several cellular protein kinases that can alter the receptor's signaling and interaction with intracellular scaffolds and signaling pathways (Figures 20–2 and 20–4).

Effects of Acute and Chronic Opiate Receptor Activation

In addition to the intended relief from pain, agonist occupancy of opiate receptors over both short- and long-term intervals leads to the loss of effect, with distinguishable properties relating to the development of tolerance and dependence.

Desensitization

In the face of a transient activation (minutes to hours), acute tolerance or desensitization occurs that is specific for that receptor and disappears with a time course parallel to the clearance of the agonist. Short-term desensitization probably involves phosphorylation of the receptors resulting in an uncoupling of the receptor from its G protein or internalization of the receptor (Williams et al., 2013).

Tolerance

Tolerance to opioids refers to a decrease in the apparent effectiveness of the opioid agonist with continuous or repeated agonist administration (over days to weeks), that, following removal of the agonist, disappears over several weeks. This tolerance is reflected by a reduction in the maximum achievable effect or a right shift in the dose-response curve. This phenomenon can be manifested at the level of the intracellular cascade (e.g., reduced inhibition of AC) and at the organ system level (e.g., loss of sedative and analgesic effects) (Christie, 2008).

This loss of effect with persistent exposure to an opiate agonist has several key properties:

- Different physiological responses can develop tolerance at markedly different rates. Thus, at the organ system level, some end points show little or no tolerance development (pupillary miosis); some show moderate tolerance (constipation, emesis, analgesia, sedation); and some show rapid tolerance (euphoria). Accordingly, the chronic heroin abuser will continue to show pinpoint pupils and will require a rapid increase in dosing to achieve the drug-related euphoria.

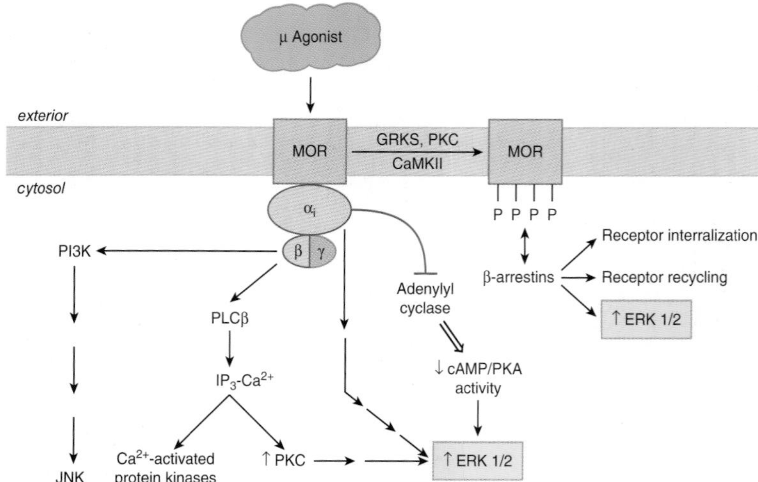

A. *Cell signaling pathways that may be differentially regulated opioid agonists.* Responses to opioid agonists may be biased toward β-arrestin signaling or toward G-protein signaling. ERK1/2 may be activated by either pathway, but possibly in distinct subcellular compartments with different sequelae. Activation of PI3K and PLCβ may lead to activation of additional protein kinases with numerous downstream effects. In addition to initiating signaling (e.g., ERK1/2), β-arrestins interact with phosphorylated receptors with consequences for desensitization and receptor trafficking. The differentiated state of the responding cell can affect what responses are possible, as can the properties of the agonist. Panel B shows some of the variables that can contribute to biased signaling in response to mu opioid agonists.

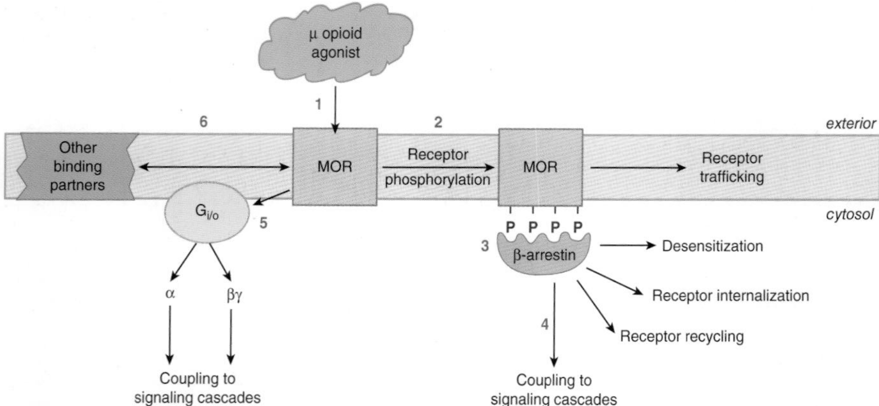

B. *Putative factors affecting the variable consequences of MOR activation.* The panoply of interactions that result from ligand binding to MOR is complex. As a consequence, biased activation of MOR may differentially affect multiple downstream pathways. A few possibilities are shown here, noted by number on the figure:

1. *Mu* agonists bind to MOR, a membrane GPCR. Biased responses could result from agonist preference for one of several forms of MOR that may result from alternative splicing. Biased responses could also result from interactions of *mu* agonists with MOR that stabilize conformations of the receptor that are agonist-specific and differ in their capacity to produce sequelae. In response to agonist, MOR interacts with a G-protein and is subject to phosphorylation, events that may also reflect a receptor isoform and the particular conformation stabilized by the agonist.

2. MOR has over a dozen phosphorylation sites accessible to various protein kinases. The pattern of phosphorylation may be determined by the receptor conformation that the agonist induces, mobilizing distinct protein kinases (e.g., GRKs, PKC, ERK1/2, CaMKII), or the receptor may fail to be phosphorylated. These protein kinases exist in multiple isoforms, lending additional variability/selectivity to the process. There are seven GRK isoforms (not uniformly expressed in all cells), and GRK-mediated phosphorylation may also be specific to agonist and receptor form (i.e., dependent on agonist-induced receptor conformation and heterogeneities [splice variants] in receptor structure).

3. MOR phosphorylation, largely by GRKs, facilitates β-arrestin binding, promotes uncoupling of MOR from G-proteins, and affects desensitization, receptor trafficking, and possibly tolerance. Two isoforms of β-arrestin can interact with phospho-MOR. These interactions appear to be agonist-specific (see **Panel C**). Interaction of phospho-MOR with β-arrestins initiates processes of receptor desensitization, internalization, and recycling. There is a strong correlation between MOR phosphorylation, recruitment of β-arrestin 2, and MOR internalization. The β-arrestin/phospho-MOR complex is recognized by clathrin. Phospho-MOR can be internalized to different fates depending on its participation in a clathrin-dependent or a clathrin-independent process.

4. The phospho-MOR/β-arrestin complexes can initiate cell signaling independently of G-proteins.

5. Agonist-liganded MOR interacts with the $G_{i/o}$ family to alter cell signaling pathways. The components of $G_{i/o}$ provide large possibilities for diversity of signaling (four α subunits; five β and twelve γ isoforms) and regulate proteins in the membrane and in various subcellular compartments (Khan et al, 2013).

6. Agonist-specific homo- and hetero-dimerization of receptor and its interaction with other proteins may also play roles in biased agonism.

Thus, a variety of ultimate responses are possible following the binding of a mu agonist to MOR. **Panel C** gives two examples.

Figure 20–4 *Biased Signaling via Opioid Receptors.*

Response		Morphine	Etorphine
G protein activation		+ + +	+ + +
MOR phosphorylation		+	+ + +
β-arrestin recruitment	β-arrestin 1	–	+ + +
	β-arrestin 2	+	+ + +
MOR internalization		+/–	+ + +
PKC_ε activation		+ + +	–
MOR desensitization** (assessed as Ca^{2+}release)		+ + +	–
ERK 1/2 activation		+ + +	+ + +

* Responses assembled from literature data, mostly from cultured cell systems. See papers by Raehal et al. (2011) and Zheng et al. (2011).
** Result depends on response measured.

C. *Biased agonism: disparate effects of two MOR agonists*.*

Figure 20–4 (*Continued*).

- In general, opiate agonists of a given class will typically show a reduced response in a system rendered tolerant to another agent of that class (e.g., cross-tolerance between the MOR agonists, such as morphine and fentanyl). For reasons that are not clear, this cross-tolerance is neither absolute nor complete. This lack of complete cross-tolerance between agonists forms the basis for the clinical strategy of "opioid rotation" in pain therapy (Smith and Peppin, 2014).

Dependence

Dependence represents a state of adaptation manifested by a withdrawal syndrome produced by cessation of drug exposure (e.g., by drug abstinence) or administration of an antagonist (e.g., naloxone). Dependence is specific to the drug class and receptor involved. At the organ system level, opiate withdrawal is manifested by significant somatomotor and autonomic outflow (reflected by agitation, hyperalgesia, hyperthermia, hypertension, diarrhea, pupillary dilation, and release of virtually all pituitary and adrenomedullary hormones) and by affective symptoms (dysphoria, anxiety, and depression). The state of withdrawal is highly aversive and motivates the drug recipient to make robust efforts to avoid withdrawal, that is, to consume more of the drug. Consistent with the phenomenon of cross-tolerance, drugs interacting with the same opiate receptor will suppress the withdrawal observed in organisms tolerant to another drug acting on the same receptor (e.g., morphine and methadone).

Addiction

Addiction is a behavioral pattern characterized by compulsive use of a drug. The positive, rewarding effects of opiates are considered to be the driving component for initiating the recreational use of opiates. This positive reward property is subject to the development of tolerance. Given the aversive nature of withdrawal symptoms, avoidance and alleviation of withdrawal symptoms may become a primary motivation for compulsive drug taking (Kreek and Koob, 1998). When the drive to acquire the drug leads to drug-seeking behaviors that occur in spite of the physical, emotional, or societal damage suffered by the drug seeker, then the obsession or compulsion to acquire and use the drug is considered to reflect an addicted state. In animals, this may be manifest by willingness to tolerate stressful conditions to acquire drug delivery. Importantly, *drug dependence is not synonymous with drug addiction*. Tolerance and dependence are physiological responses seen in all patients but are not predictors of addiction (see Chapter 24). For example, cancer pain often requires prolonged treatment with high doses of opioids, leading to tolerance and dependence. Yet, such patients are not considered to be either addicts or abusers of the drug.

Mechanisms of Tolerance/Dependence/Withdrawal

The mechanisms underlying chronic tolerance and dependence/withdrawal are controversial. Several types of events may contribute.

Receptor Disposition

Acute desensitization or receptor internalization may play a role in the initiation of chronic tolerance but is not sufficient to explain the persistent changes observed. For instance, morphine, unlike other μ agonists, does not promote significant MOR internalization, receptor phosphorylation, or desensitization. Receptor desensitization and downregulation are agonist specific. Endocytosis and sequestration of receptors do not invariably lead to receptor degradation but can also result in receptor dephosphorylation and recycling to the surface of the cell. Accordingly, opioid tolerance may not be related to receptor desensitization but rather to a lack of desensitization. Agonists that cause rapid internalization of opioid receptors also rapidly desensitize signaling, but sensitivity can be at least partially restored by recycling of "reactivated" opioid receptors.

Adaptation of Intracellular Signaling Mechanisms

Assessment of the coupling of MOR to cellular effects, such as inhibition of AC, activation of inwardly rectifying K^+ channels, inhibition of Ca^{2+} currents, and inhibition of neurotransmitter release demonstrates functional uncoupling of receptor occupancy from effector function. Importantly, chronic application of opioids initiates adaptive counterregulatory change. A common example of such cellular counterregulatory processes is the rebound increase in cellular cyclic AMP levels produced by "superactivation" of AC and upregulation of the amount of enzyme as a result of long-term exposure to an opiate followed by its abrupt withdrawal (Williams et al., 2013).

System-Level Counteradaptation

The loss of antinociceptive effect with chronic opiate exposure may reflect an enhanced excitability of the regulated link. Thus, tolerance to the analgesic action of chronically administered μ opiates may result from an activation of *bulbospinal* pathways that increases the excitability of spinal dorsal horn pain transmission linkages. With chronic opiate exposure, opiate receptor occupancy will lead to the activation of PKC, which can phosphorylate and enhance the activation of local NMDA glutamate receptors. These receptors are considered to play an important role as an excitatory link in enhanced pain processing (see Chapter 14). Blockade of these receptors can at least partially attenuate the loss of analgesic efficacy with continued opiate exposure. Such system-level counteradaptation mechanisms may apply to specific systems (e.g., pain modulation) but not necessarily to others (e.g., sedation or miosis) (Christie, 2008). These changes may be mechanistically important in the phenomenon called opioid-induced hyperalgesia, by which higher doses of opiates may lead to a paradoxical increase in pain processing (Fletcher and Martinez, 2014).

Differential Tolerance Development and Fractional Occupancy Requirements

An interesting problem in explaining tolerance relates to the differential rates of the development of tolerance. It is unclear why responses such as miosis show no tolerance over extended exposure (indeed, miosis is considered symptomatic in drug overdose of highly tolerant patients), whereas analgesia and sedation are likely to show a reduction. One possibility is that tolerance represents a functional uncoupling of some fraction of the receptor population and that different physiological end points may require activation of different fractions of their coupled receptors to produce a given physiological effect.

Effects of Clinically Used Opioids

Opiates, depending on their receptor specificities, produce a variety of effects consistent with the roles played by the organ systems with which the receptors are associated. Although the primary clinical use of opioids is for their pain-relieving properties, opioids produce a host of other effects. This is not surprising in view of the wide distribution of opioid receptors in brain, spinal cord, and the periphery. Within the nervous system, these effects range from analgesia to effects on motivation and higher-order affect (euphoria), arousal, and a number of autonomic, hormonal, and motor processes. In the periphery, opiates can influence a variety of visceromotor systems, including those related to GI motility and smooth muscle tone.

Analgesia

Morphine-like drugs produce *analgesia*, *drowsiness*, and *euphoria* (changes in mood and mental clouding). When therapeutic doses of morphine are given to patients with pain, patients report the pain to be less intense or entirely gone. In addition to relief of distress, some patients may experience euphoria. Analgesia often occurs without loss of consciousness, although drowsiness commonly occurs. Morphine at these doses does not have anticonvulsant activity and usually does not cause slurred speech, emotional lability, or significant impairment of motor coordination. When an analgesic dose of morphine is administered to normal, pain-free individuals, the patients may report the drug experience to be frankly unpleasant. They may experience drowsiness, difficulty in mentation, apathy, and lessened physical activity. As the dose is increased, the subjective, analgesic, and toxic effects, including respiratory depression, become more pronounced. The relief of pain by morphine-like opioids is selective in that other sensory modalities, such as light touch, proprioception, and the sense of moderate temperatures, are unaffected. Low doses of morphine can produce reductions in the affective response but not the perceived intensity of the pain experience; higher, clinically effective doses reduce both perceived intensity and affective responses to the pain (Price et al., 1985). Continuous dull pain (as generated by tissue injury and inflammation) is relieved more effectively than sharp intermittent (incident) pain, such as that associated with the movement of an inflamed joint. With sufficient amounts of opioid, it is possible to relieve even the severe piercing pain associated with, for example, acute renal or biliary colic.

Pain States and Mechanisms

Any meaningful discussion of the action of analgesic agents must include the appreciation that all pain is not the same, and that a number of variables contribute to the patient's pain report and therefore to the effect of the analgesic. Heuristically, one may think mechanistically of pain as several distinct sets of events, described in the next sections (Yaksh et al., 2015).

Acute Nociception. Acute activation of small, high-threshold sensory afferents (Aδ and C fibers) generates transient, stimulus-dependent input into the spinal cord, which in turn leads to activation of dorsal horn neurons that project contralaterally to the thalamus and thence to the somatosensory cortex. A parallel spinofugal projection runs through the medial thalamus and thence to portions of the limbic cortex, such as the anterior cingulate. The output produced by acutely activating these ascending systems is sufficient to evoke pain reports. Examples of such stimuli include a hot coffee cup, a needlestick, or an incision.

Tissue Injury. Following tissue injury or local inflammation (e.g., local skin burn, toothache, rheumatoid joint), an ongoing pain state arises that is characterized by burning, throbbing, or aching, and an abnormal pain response termed *hyperalgesia*, which can be evoked by otherwise innocuous or mildly aversive stimuli (tepid bathwater on a sunburn; moderate extension of an injured joint). This pain typically reflects the effects of active factors such as prostaglandins, bradykinin, cytokines, serine proteases, and H^+ ions, among many mediators. Such mediators are released locally into the injury site and have the capacity, through eponymous receptors on the terminals of small, high-threshold afferents (Aδ and C fibers), to activate these sensory afferents and to reduce the stimulus intensity required for their activation (e.g., peripheral sensitization). In addition, the ongoing afferent traffic initiated by the tissue injury and inflammation leads to activation of spinal facilitatory cascades, yielding a greater output to the brain for any given afferent input. This facilitation is thought to underlie hyperalgesic states (e.g., central sensitization). Such tissue injury/inflammation-evoked pain is often referred to as *nociceptive* pain (Figure 20–5) (Sorkin and Wallace, 1999). Examples of such states would be burn, postincision, abrasion of the skin, musculoskeletal injury, or inflammation of the joint.

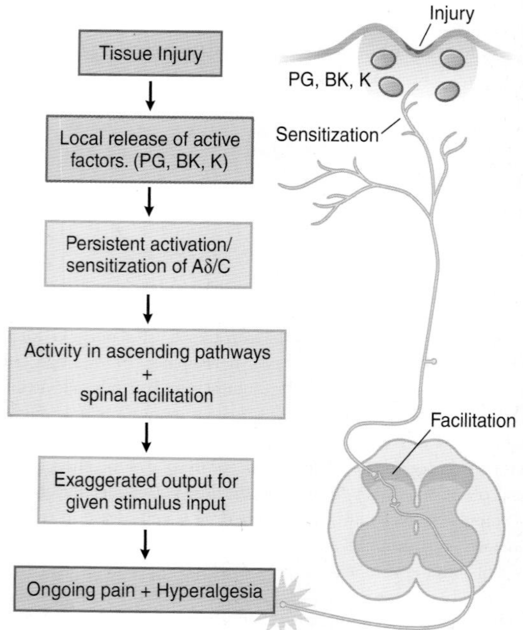

Figure 20–5 *Mechanisms of tissue injury-evoked nociception.* BK, bradykinin; K, potassium; PG, prostaglandins.

Nerve Injury. Injury to a peripheral nerve yields complex anatomical and biochemical changes in the nerve and spinal cord that induce *spontaneous dysesthesias* (shooting, burning pain) and *allodynia* (hurt from a light touch). This nerve injury pain state may not depend on the activation of small afferents but may be initiated by low-threshold sensory afferents (e.g., Aβ fibers). Such nerve injuries result in the development of ectopic activity arising from neuromas formed by nerve injury and the dorsal root ganglia of the injured axons as well as changes in dorsal horn sensory processing. Such changes include activation of nonneuronal (glial) cells and loss of constitutive inhibitory circuits, such that low-threshold afferent input carried by Aβ fibers evokes a pain state (West et al., 2015). Examples of such nerve injury–inducing events include mononeuropathies secondary to nerve trauma or compression (carpal tunnel syndrome) and the postherpetic state (shingles). Polyneuropathies such as those occurring in diabetes or after chemotherapy (as for cancer) can also lead to ongoing dysesthesias and evoked hyperpathias. These pain states are said to be neuropathic (Figure 20–6). Many clinical pain syndromes, such as found in cancer, typically represent a combination of these inflammatory and neuropathic mechanisms. Although nociceptive pain usually is responsive to opioid analgesics, neuropathic pain is typically considered to respond less well to opioid analgesics. There is a growing perception that, in the face of chronic tissue injury or inflammation (e.g., arthritis), there can be a transition from an inflammatory to a neuropathic pain phenotype. Such a transition has important implications for analgesic drug efficacy.

Sensory Versus Affective Dimensions. Information generated by a high-intensity peripheral stimulus initiates activity in pathways activating higher-order systems that reflect the aversive magnitude of the stimulus. Painful stimuli have the certain ability to generate strong emotional components that reflect a distinction between pain as a specific sensation subserved by distinct neurophysiological structures (the *sensory discriminative* dimension) and pain such as suffering (the original sensation plus the reactions evoked by the sensation: the *affective motivational* dimension of the pain experience) (Melzack and Casey, 1968). Opiates have potent effects on both components of the pain experience.

Mechanisms of Opioid-Induced Analgesia

The analgesic actions of opiates after systemic delivery represent actions in the brain, spinal cord, and in some instances the periphery.

Supraspinal Actions. Microinjections of morphine into a number of highly circumscribed brain regions will produce a potent analgesia that is reversible by naloxone, an MOR antagonist. The best characterized of these sites is the mesencephalic PAG region. Several mechanisms exist whereby opiates with an action limited to the PAG may act to alter nociceptive transmission. These are summarized in Figure 20–7. MOR agonists block release of the inhibitory transmitter GABA from tonically active PAG systems that regulate activity in projections to the medulla. PAG projections to the medulla activate medullospinal release of NE and 5HT at the level of the spinal dorsal horn. This release can attenuate dorsal horn excitability (Yaksh, 1997). Interestingly, this PAG organization can also serve to increase excitability of dorsal raphe and locus coeruleus, from which ascending serotonergic and noradrenergic projections to the limbic forebrain, respectively, originate. Aside from direct supraspinal effects on forebrain structures, these limbic projections provide a mechanism for the effects of opiates on emotional tone (the role of forebrain 5HT and NE in mediating emotional tone is discussed in Chapter 15).

Spinal Opiate Action. A local action of opiates in the spinal cord will selectively depress the discharge of spinal dorsal horn neurons evoked by small (high-threshold) but not large (low-threshold) afferent nerve fibers. Intrathecal administration of opioids in animals ranging from mice to humans will reliably attenuate the response of the organism to a variety of somatic and visceral stimuli that otherwise evoke pain states. Specific opiate receptors are largely limited to the *substantia gelatinosa* of the superficial dorsal horn, the region in which small, high-threshold sensory afferents show their principal termination. A significant proportion of these opiate receptors are associated with small peptidergic primary afferent C fibers; the remainder are on local dorsal horn neurons.

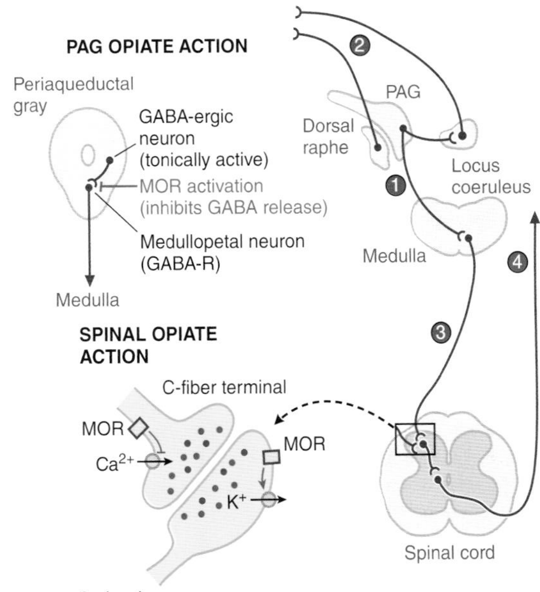

Figure 20–7 *Mechanisms of opiate action in producing analgesia.* **Top left:** Schematic of organization of opiate action in the PAG. **Top right:** Opiate-sensitive pathways in the PAG. Opiate actions via MOR block the release of GABA from tonically active systems that otherwise regulate the projections to the medulla (1), leading to an activation of PAG outflow that results in activation of forebrain (2) and spinal (3) monoamine receptors that regulate spinal cord projections (4), which provide sensory input to higher centers and mood. **Bottom left:** Schematic of primary afferent synapse with second-order dorsal horn spinal neuron, showing pre- and postsynaptic opiate receptors coupled to Ca^{2+} and K^+ channels, respectively. Opiate receptor binding is highly expressed in the superficial spinal dorsal horn (substantia gelatinosa). These receptors are located presynaptically on the terminals of small primary afferents (C fibers) and postsynaptically on second-order neurons. Presynaptically, activation of MOR blocks the opening of the voltage-sensitive Ca^{2+} channel, which otherwise initiates transmitter release. Postsynaptically, MOR activation enhances opening of K^+ channels, leading to hyperpolarization. Thus, an opiate agonist acting at these sites jointly serves to attenuate the afferent-evoked excitation of the second-order neuron.

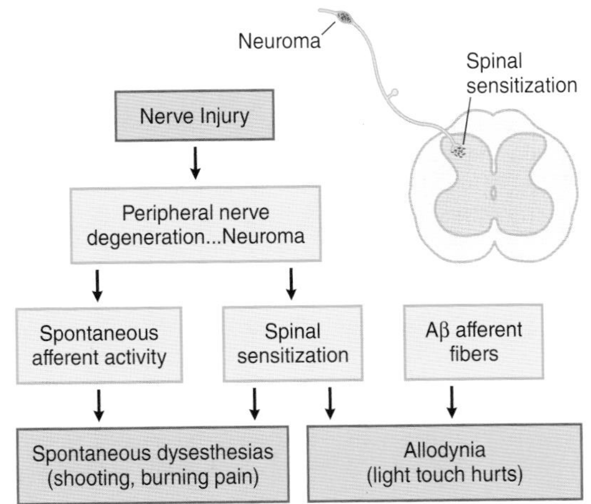

Figure 20–6 *Mechanisms of nerve injury–evoked nociception.*

Spinal opiates act on opiate receptors located presynaptically on small, high-threshold primary afferents to *prevent the opening of voltage-sensitive Ca^{2+} channels*, thereby preventing transmitter release from those afferents. A postsynaptic action is demonstrated by the ability of opiates to block excitation of dorsal horn neurons directly evoked by glutamate, reflecting a direct activation of dorsal horn projection neurons partly by *hyperpolarizing the neurons through the activation of K^+ channels*, such that the membrane potential more closely approximates the equilibrium potential for K^+. The joint capacity of spinal opiates to reduce the release of excitatory neurotransmitters from C fibers and to decrease the excitability of dorsal horn neurons is believed to account for the powerful and selective effect of opiates on spinal nociceptive processing. A variety of opiates delivered spinally (intrathecally or epidurally) can induce powerful analgesia that is reversed by low doses of systemic naloxone (Yaksh, 1997).

Peripheral Action. Direct application of high concentrations of opiates to a peripheral nerve can, in fact, produce a local anesthetic-like action, but this effect is not reversed by naloxone and is believed to reflect a "nonspecific" action. Conversely, at peripheral sites under conditions of inflammation where there is an increased terminal sensitivity leading to an exaggerated pain response (e.g., hyperalgesia), direct injection of opiates produces a local action that can exert a normalizing effect on the exaggerated thresholds. Whether the effects are uniquely on the peripheral afferent terminal or whether the opiate acts on inflammatory cells that release products that sensitize the nerve terminal, or both, is not known (Stein and Machelska, 2011).

Mood Alterations and Rewarding Properties

The mechanisms by which opioids produce euphoria, tranquility, and other alterations of mood (including rewarding properties) are complex and not entirely understood. Neural systems that mediate opioid reinforcement overlap with, but are distinct from, those involved in physical dependence and analgesia (Koob and Le Moal, 2008). Behavioral and pharmacological data point to a pivotal role of the mesocorticolimbic dopamine system that projects to the *NAc* in drug-induced reward and motivation (Figure 20–8). Increased dopamine release in this region is considered to underlie a positive reward state. In the NAc, MORs are present postsynaptically on GABAergic neurons. The reinforcing effects of opiates are thought to be mediated partly via inhibition of local GABAergic neuronal activity, which otherwise acts to inhibit DA outflow.

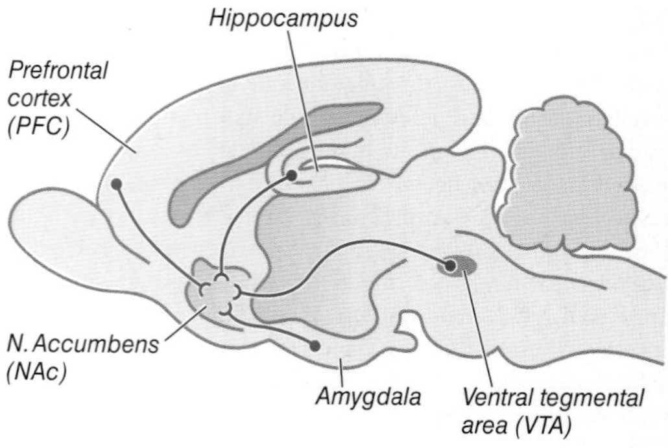

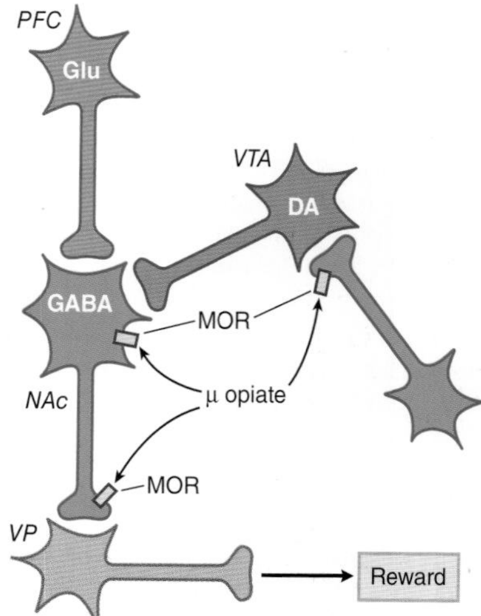

Figure 20–8 *Pathways underlying rewarding properties of opiates.* **Upper panel:** This sagittal section of rat brain shows DA and GABA inputs from the VTA and PFC, respectively, into the NAc. **Lower panel:** Neurons are labeled with their primary neurotransmitters. At a cellular level, MOR agonists reduce excitability and transmitter release at the sites indicated by inhibiting Ca^{2+} influx and enhancing K^+ current (see Figure 20–7). Thus, opiate-induced inhibition in the VTA on GABAergic interneurons or in the NAc reduce GABA-mediated inhibition and increase outflow from the ventral pallidum (VP), which appears to correlate with a positive reinforcing state (enhanced reward).

Respiratory Effects

Although effects of opiates on respiration are readily demonstrated, clinically significant respiratory depression rarely occurs with standard analgesic doses in the absence of other contributing variables (discussed in the next sections). It should be stressed, however, that *respiratory depression represents the primary cause of morbidity secondary to opiate therapy*. In humans, death from opiate poisoning is nearly always due to respiratory arrest or obstruction. Opiates depress all phases of respiratory activity (rate, minute volume, and tidal exchange) and produce irregular and aperiodic breathing. The diminished respiratory volume is due primarily to a slower rate of breathing; with toxic amounts of opioids, the rate may fall to 3–4 breaths/min. Thus, to avoid apnea due to a decrease in respiratory drive coinciding with an increased airway resistance, opioids must be used with caution in patients with asthma, COPD, cor pulmonale, decreased respiratory reserve, preexisting respiratory depression, hypoxia, or hypercapnia. Although respiratory depression is not considered to be a favorable therapeutic effect of opiates, their ability to suppress respiratory drive is used as therapeutic advantage to treat dyspnea resulting, for example, in patients with COPD, where air hunger leads to extreme agitation, discomfort, and gasping; opiates will suppress the gasping and decease the panic of the patient. Similarly, opiates find use in patients who require artificial ventilation (Clemens and Klaschik, 2007).

Mechanisms Underlying Respiratory Depression

Morphine-like opioids depress respiration through MOR by several mechanisms:

- direct depressant effect on rhythm generation;
- depression of the ventilatory response to increased CO_2; and
- an effect on carotid and aortic body chemosensors that reduces ventilatory responses that are normally driven by hypoxia.

Respiratory rate and tidal volume depend on intrinsic rhythm generators located in the ventrolateral medulla. These systems generate a "respiratory" rhythm that is driven by afferent input reflecting the partial pressure of arterial O_2 as measured by chemosensors in the carotid and aortic bodies and CO_2 as measured by chemosensors in the brainstem. Morphine-like opioids depress respiration through MORs in part by a direct depressant effect on rhythm generation, with changes in respiratory pattern and rate observed at lower doses than changes in tidal volume. A key property of opiate effects on respiration is the depression of the ventilatory response to increased CO_2. This effect is mediated by opiate depression of the excitability of brainstem chemosensory neurons. In addition to the effects on the CO_2 response, opiates will depress ventilation otherwise driven by hypoxia though an effect on carotid and aortic body chemosensors. Importantly, with opiates, hypoxic stimulation of chemoreceptors still may be effective when opioids have decreased the responsiveness to CO_2, and inhalation of O_2 may remove the residual drive resulting from the elevated PO_2 and produce apnea (Pattinson, 2008). In addition to the effect on respiratory rhythm and chemosensitivity, opiates can have mechanical effects on airway function by increasing chest wall rigidity and diminishing upper airway patency (Lalley, 2008).

Factors Exacerbating Opiate-Induced Respiratory Depression

A number of factors can increase the risk of opiate-related respiratory depression even at therapeutic doses:

- *Other medications.* The combination of opiates with other depressant medications, such as general anesthetics, tranquilizers, alcohol, or sedative-hypnotics, produces additive depression of respiratory activity.
- *Sleep.* Natural sleep produces a decrease in the sensitivity of the medullary center to CO_2, and the depressant effects of morphine and sleep are at least additive. Obstructive sleep apnea is considered to be an important risk factor for increasing the likelihood of fatal respiratory depression.
- *Age.* Newborns can show significant respiratory depression and desaturation; this may be evident in lower Apgar scores if opioids are administered parenterally to women within 2–4 h of delivery because of transplacental passage of opioids. Elderly patients are at greater risk of depression because of reduced lung elasticity, chest wall stiffening, and decreased vital capacity.
- *Disease.* Opiates may cause a greater depressant action in patients with chronic cardiopulmonary or renal diseases because they can manifest a desensitization of their response to increased CO_2.
- *COPD.* Enhanced depression can also be noted in patients with COPD and sleep apnea secondary to diminished hypoxic drive.
- *Relief of pain.* Because pain stimulates respiration, removal of the painful condition (as with the analgesia resulting from the therapeutic use of the opiate) will reduce the ventilatory drive and lead to apparent respiratory depression.

Comparative Respiratory Effects of Different Opiates

Numerous studies have compared morphine and morphine-like opioids with respect to their ratios of analgesic to respiratory-depressant activities, and most have found that when equianalgesic doses are used, there is no significant difference. Maximal respiratory depression occurs within 5–10 min of intravenous administration of morphine or within 30–90 min of intramuscular or subcutaneous administration. Maximal respiratory depressant effects occur more rapidly with more lipid-soluble agents. After therapeutic doses, respiratory minute volume may be reduced for as long as 4–5 h. Agents that have persistent kinetics, such as methadone, must be carefully monitored, particularly after dose incrementation. Respiratory depression produced by any opiate agonist can be readily reversed by delivery of an opiate antagonist. Opiate antagonist reversal in the somnolent patient is considered to be indicative of an opiate-mediated depression. It is important to remember that most opiate antagonists have a relatively short duration of action compared to an agonist such as morphine or methadone, and fatal "renarcotization" can occur if vigilance is not exercised.

Opioid-Induced Hyperalgesia

A paradoxical increase in pain states has been observed in response to acute (hours to days) and chronic opiate exposure. This increase may be reflected by unexplained increases in pain reports, increased levels of pain with increasing opiate dosages, or a diffuse sensitivity unassociated with the original pain (Lee et al., 2011). The mechanisms of this increased pain profile is not understood, although an enhanced excitability of central systems with chronic opiate exposure is considered relevant. Other avenues have pointed to the stimulatory effects of opioids on innate immune signaling through Toll-like receptor 4 activation, leading to central sensitization (Grace et al., 2014).

Sedation

Opiates can produce drowsiness and cognitive impairment. Such depression can augment respiratory impairment. These effects are most typically noted following initiation of opiate therapy or after dose incrementation. Importantly, these effects on arousal resolve over a few days. As with respiratory depression, the degree of drug effect can be enhanced by a variety of predisposing patient factors, including dementia, encephalopathies, brain tumors, and other depressant medications, including sleep aids, antihistamines, antidepressants, and anxiolytics (Cherny, 1996).

Neuroendocrine Effects

The regulation of the release of hormones and factors from the pituitary is under complex regulation by opiate receptors in the HPA axis. Broadly considered, morphine-like opioids reduce the release of a large number of HPA hormones (Armario, 2010).

Sex Hormones

In males, acute opiate therapy reduces plasma cortisol, testosterone, and gonadotrophins. Inhibition of adrenal function is reflected by reduced cortisol production and reduced adrenal androgens (DHEA). In females, morphine will also result in lower LH and FSH release. In both males and females, chronic therapy can result in endocrinopathies, including hypogonadotrophic hypogonadism. In men, this may result in decreased libido and, with extended exposure, reduced secondary sex characteristics. In women, these exposures are associated with menstrual cycle irregularities. These changes are reversible with removal of the opiate.

Prolactin. Prolactin release from the anterior pituitary is under inhibitory control by DA released from neurons of the arcuate nucleus. MOR agonists act presynaptically on these DA-releasing terminals to inhibit DA release and thereby increase plasma prolactin.

Antidiuretic Hormone and Oxytocin. The effects of opiates on ADH and oxytocin release are complex. These hormones are synthesized in the perikarya of the magnocellular neurons in the paraventricular and supraoptic nuclei of the hypothalamus and released from the posterior pituitary (Chapter 42). KOR agonists inhibit the release of oxytocin and ADH and cause prominent diuresis. Note, however, that agents such as morphine may yield a hypotension secondary to histamine release; this would, by itself, promote ADH release.

Miosis

The MOR agonists induce pupillary constriction (miosis) in the awake state and block pupillary reflex dilation during anesthesia. The parasympathetic outflow from the *Edinger Westphal nucleus* activates parasympathetic outflow through the ciliary ganglion to the pupil, producing constriction. This outflow is locally regulated by GABAergic interneurons. Opiates block this GABAergic interneuron-mediated inhibition, leading to increased parasympathetic outflow (Larson, 2008). At high doses of agonists, the miosis is marked, and pinpoint pupils are pathognomonic; however, marked mydriasis will occur with the onset of asphyxia. While some tolerance to the miotic effect develops, addicts with high circulating concentrations of opioids continue to have constricted pupils. Therapeutic doses of morphine increase accommodative power and lower intraocular tension in normal and glaucomatous eyes (Larson, 2008).

Seizures and Convulsions

In older children and adults, moderately higher doses of opiates produce EEG slowing. In the newborn, morphine can produce epileptiform activity and occasionally seizure activity (Young and da Silva, 2000). Several mechanisms are likely involved in these excitatory actions:

- *Inhibition of inhibitory interneurons.* Morphine-like drugs indirectly excite certain groups of neurons, such as hippocampal pyramidal cells, by inhibiting the inhibition otherwise exerted by GABAergic interneurons (McGinty, 1988).

- *Direct stimulatory effects.* Opiates may interact with receptors coupled through both inhibitory and stimulatory G proteins, with the inhibitory coupling but not the excitatory coupling showing tolerance with continued exposures (King et al., 2005).
- *Actions mediated by nonopioid receptors.* The metabolites of several opiates (morphine-3-glucuronide, normeperidine) have been implicated in seizure activity (Seifert and Kennedy, 2004; Smith, 2000).

A special case is the withdrawal syndrome from an opiate-dependent state in the adult and in the infant born to an opiate-dependent mother. Withdrawal in these circumstances, either by antagonists or abstinence, can lead to prominent EEG activation, tremor, and rigidity. Approaches to the management of such activation are controversial. Anticonvulsant agents may not always be effective in suppressing opioid-induced seizures (see Chapter 17).

Cough

Cough is a protective reflex evoked by airway stimulation. It involves rapid expression of air against a transiently closed glottis. The reflex is complex, involving the central and peripheral nervous systems as well as the smooth muscle of the bronchial tree. Morphine and related opioids depress the cough reflex at least in part by a direct effect on a cough center in the medulla; this cough suppression can be achieved without altering the protective glottal function (Chung and Pavord, 2008). There is no obligatory relationship between depression of respiration and depression of coughing, and effective antitussive agents are available that do not depress respiration (antitussives are discussed further in the chapter).

Nauseant and Emetic Effects

Nausea and vomiting produced by morphine-like drugs are side effects caused by direct stimulation of the chemoreceptor trigger zone for emesis in the *area postrema* of the medulla (see Figure 50–5). All clinically useful agonists produce some degree of nausea and vomiting. Nausea and vomiting are relatively uncommon in recumbent patients given therapeutic doses of morphine, but nausea occurs in about 40% and vomiting in 15% of ambulatory patients given analgesic doses. Morphine and related synthetic analgesics produce an increase in vestibular sensitivity. A component of nausea is likely also due to the gastric stasis that occurs postoperatively and that is exacerbated by analgesic doses of morphine. (Greenwood-Van Meerveld, 2007).

Cardiovascular System

In the supine patient, therapeutic doses of morphine-like opioids have no major effect on blood pressure or cardiac rate and rhythm. Such doses can, however, produce peripheral vasodilation, reduced peripheral resistance, and an inhibition of baroreceptor reflexes. Thus, when supine patients assume the head-up position, orthostatic hypotension and fainting may occur. The peripheral arteriolar and venous dilation produced by morphine involves several mechanisms:

- Morphine induces *release of histamine* from mast cells, leading to vasodilation; this effect is reversed by naloxone but only partially blocked by H_1 antagonists.
- Morphine *blunts reflex vasoconstriction* caused by increased Pco_2.

High doses of MOR agonists, such as fentanyl and sufentanil, used as anesthetic induction agents, have only modest effects on hemodynamic stability, in part because they do not cause release of histamine (Monk et al., 1988). Morphine may exert its therapeutic effect in the treatment of angina pectoris and acute myocardial infarction by decreasing preload, inotropy, and chronotropy, thus favorably altering determinants of myocardial O_2 consumption. Morphine also produces cardioprotective effects. Morphine can mimic the phenomenon of ischemic preconditioning, whereby a short ischemic episode paradoxically protects the heart against further ischemia. This effect appears to be mediated through receptors signaling through a mitochondrial ATP-sensitive K^+ channel in cardiac myocytes; the effect also is produced by other GPCRs signaling through G_i. Morphine-like opioids should be used with caution in patients who have decreased blood volume because these agents can aggravate hypovolemic shock. Morphine should be used with great care in patients with cor pulmonale; deaths after ordinary therapeutic doses have been reported. Concurrent use of certain CNS depressants (phenothiazines, ethanol, benzodiazepines) may increase the risk of morphine-induced hypotension. Cerebral circulation is not affected directly by therapeutic doses of opiates. However, opioid-induced respiratory depression and CO_2 retention can result in cerebral vasodilation and an increase in CSF pressure. This pressure increase does not occur when Pco_2 is maintained at normal levels by artificial ventilation.

Skeletal Muscle Tone

At therapeutic doses required for analgesia, opiates have little effect on motor tone or function. However, high doses of opioids, as used for anesthetic induction, produce muscular rigidity. Myoclonus, ranging from mild twitching to generalized spasm, is an occasional side effect that has been reported with all clinically used opiate agonists and is particularly prevalent in patients receiving high doses. The increased muscle tone is mediated by a central effect, although the mechanisms of its effects are not clear. High doses of spinal opiates can increase motor tone, possibly through an inhibition of inhibitory interneurons in the ventral horn of the spinal cord. Alternately, intracranial delivery can initiate rigidity in animal models, possibly reflecting increased extrapyramidal activity. Increased motor tone and rigidity are reversed by opiate antagonists.

GI Tract

Opiates have important effects on all aspects of GI function. Between 40% and 95% of patients treated with opioids develop constipation and changes in bowel function (Benyamin et al., 2008). Opioid receptors are densely distributed in enteric neurons between the myenteric and submucosal plexuses and on a variety of secretory cells. The importance of these peripheral systems in altering GI motility is emphasized by the therapeutic efficacy of peripherally limited opiate agonists such as loperamide as antidiarrheals and the utility of peripherally limited opiate antagonists such as methylnaltrexone to reverse the constipatory actions of systemic opiate agonists.

Esophagus. The esophageal sphincter is under control by brainstem reflexes that activate cholinergic motor neurons originating in the esophageal myenteric plexus. This system regulates passage of material from the esophagus to the stomach and prevents regurgitation; conversely, it allows relaxation in the act of emesis. Morphine inhibits lower esophageal sphincter relaxation induced by swallowing and by esophageal distension; the effect is believed to be centrally mediated because peripherally restricted opiates such as loperamide do not alter esophageal sphincter tone (Sidhu and Triadafilopoulos, 2008).

Stomach. Morphine increases tonic contracture of the antral musculature and upper duodenum and reduces resting tone in the musculature of the gastric reservoir, thereby prolonging gastric emptying time and increasing the likelihood of esophageal reflux. Passage of the gastric contents through the duodenum may be delayed by as much as 12 h, and the absorption of orally administered drugs is retarded. Morphine and other opioid agonists usually decrease secretion of hydrochloric acid. Activation of opioid receptors on parietal cells enhances secretion, but indirect effects, including increased secretion of somatostatin from the pancreas and reduced release of ACh appear to be dominant in most circumstances (Kromer, 1988).

Intestine. Morphine reduces propulsive activity in the small and large intestines and diminishes intestinal secretions. Opiate agonists suppress rhythmic inhibition of muscle tone, leading to concurrent increases in basal tone in the circular muscle of the small and large intestines. This results in enhanced high-amplitude phasic contractions, which are *nonpropulsive* (Wood and Galligan, 2004). The upper part of the small intestine, particularly the duodenum, is affected more than the ileum. A period of relative atony may follow the period of elevated basal tone. The reduced rate of passage of the intestinal contents, along with reduced intestinal secretion, leads to increased water absorption, increasing viscosity of the bowel contents, and constipation. The tone of the anal sphincter is augmented greatly, and reflex relaxation in response to rectal distension is reduced. Patients who take opioids chronically remain constipated. Intestinal secretion arises from activation of enterocytes by local cholinergic submucosal plexus secretomotor neurons. Opioids act though μ/δ receptors on these secretomotor neurons to inhibit their excitatory output to the enterocytes and thereby reduce intestinal secretion (Kromer, 1988).

Biliary Tract. Morphine constricts the sphincter of Oddi, and the pressure in the common bile duct may rise more than 10-fold within 15 min. Fluid pressure also may increase in the gallbladder and produce symptoms that may vary from epigastric distress to typical biliary colic. All opioids can cause biliary spasm. Some patients with biliary colic experience exacerbation rather than relief of pain when given opioids. Spasm of the sphincter of Oddi probably is responsible for elevations of plasma amylase and lipase that sometimes occur after morphine administration. Atropine only partially prevents morphine-induced biliary spasm, but opioid antagonists prevent or relieve it.

Ureter and Urinary Bladder

Morphine inhibits the urinary voiding reflex and increases the tone of the external sphincter with a resultant increase in the volume of the bladder. Tolerance develops to these effects of opioids on the bladder. Clinically, opiate-mediated inhibition of micturition can be of such clinical severity that catheterization sometimes is required after therapeutic doses of morphine, particularly with spinal drug administration. Importantly, the inhibition of systemic opiate effects on micturition is reversed by peripherally restricted antagonists (Rosow et al., 2007).

Uterus

Morphine may prolong labor. If the uterus has been made hyperactive by oxytocics, morphine tends to restore the contractions to normal.

Skin

Therapeutic doses of morphine cause dilation of cutaneous blood vessels. The skin of the face, neck, and upper thorax frequently becomes flushed. Pruritus commonly follows systemic administration of morphine. Itching is readily seen with morphine and meperidine but to a much lesser extent with fentanyl or sufentanil. The systemic action is sensitive to antihistamines (diphenhydramine) and correlates with the mast cell degranulating properties of the opiate. Neither the pruritus nor the degranulation is reversed by opiate antagonists (Barke and Hough, 1993). This pruritus also can be caused by epidural or intrathecal opiate administration through a centrally mediated, naloxone-reversible mechanism (Kumar and Singh, 2013).

Immune System

Opioids modulate immune function by direct effects on cells of the immune system and indirectly through centrally mediated neuronal mechanisms (Vallejo et al., 2004). The acute central immunomodulatory effects of opioids may be mediated by activation of the sympathetic nervous system; the chronic effects of opioids may involve modulation of the HPA axis. Direct effects on immune cells may involve unique variants of the classical neuronal opioid receptors, with MOR variants being most prominent. A proposed mechanism for the immune-suppressive effects of morphine on neutrophils is through NO-dependent inhibition of NF-κB activation, or via activation of MAP kinases. Convincing data suggest that several opiates, including morphine, may interact with Toll-like receptor 4 to activate a variety of immunocytes independent of an opiate receptor (Hutchinson et al., 2007). Overall, however, opioids are modestly immunosuppressive, and increased susceptibility to infection and tumor spread have been observed. In some situations, immune effects appear more prominent with acute administration than with chronic administration, which could have important implications for the care of the critically ill.

In addition to the effects of opiates on immune function, many opiate agonists evoke mast cell degranulation and histamine release. This action can cause bronchoconstriction and vasodilation. As a consequence, morphine has the potential to precipitate or exacerbate asthmatic attacks and should be avoided in patients with a history of asthma. The effect on mast cells is not prevented by opiate antagonists and appears to be independent of MORs. After potent opioids such as fentanyl, the incidence of mast cell degranulation is reduced compared to the effect of morphine. Through such mechanisms, opioid analgesics may evoke allergic phenomena that usually are manifested as urticaria, other types of skin rashes, and pruritus. The pruritus is often managed with antihistamines.

Temperature Regulation

Opioids alter the equilibrium point of the hypothalamic heat-regulatory mechanisms such that body temperature usually falls slightly. Agonists at the MOR (e.g., alfentanil and meperidine), acting in the CNS, result in slightly increased thresholds for sweating and significantly lower the threshold temperatures for evoking vasoconstriction and shivering.

Clinically Employed Opioid Drugs

Most of the clinically used opioid agonists presented in Table 20–4 are relatively selective for MORs. They produce analgesia, affect mood and rewarding behavior, and alter respiratory, cardiovascular, GI, and neuroendocrine function. KOR agonists, with few exceptions (e.g., butorphanol), are not typically employed for long-term therapy because they may produce dysphoric and psychotomimetic effects. DOR agonists, while analgesically active, have not found clinical utility, and NOP agonists lack analgesic effects. Opiates that are relatively receptor selective at lower doses may interact with additional receptor types when given at high doses, especially as doses are escalated to overcome tolerance.

The mixed agonist-antagonist agents frequently interact with more than one receptor type at usual clinical doses. A "ceiling effect" limiting the amount of analgesia attainable often is seen with these drugs, as is the case with buprenorphine, which is approved for the treatment of opioid dependence. Some mixed agonist-antagonist drugs, such as pentazocine and nalorphine (not available in the U.S.), can precipitate withdrawal in opioid-tolerant patients. For these reasons, except for the sanctioned use of buprenorphine to manage opioid addiction, the clinical use of mixed agonist-antagonist drugs is generally limited.

The dosing guidelines and duration of action for the numerous drugs that are part of opioid therapy are summarized in Table 20–4.

Morphine and Structurally Related Agonists

Sources of Opium

Two groups have recently reported the scalable biosynthesis of opiates in the laboratory using yeast (Galanie et al., 2015) or *Escherichia coli* (Nakagawa et al., 2016); thus, nonagricultural systems of opiate production may be at hand. Typically, however, morphine is obtained from opium or extracted from poppy straw. Opium is obtained from the unripe seed capsules of the poppy plant, *Papaver somniferum*. The milky juice is dried and powdered to make powdered opium. Powdered opium contains a number of alkaloids, only a few of which (morphine, codeine, and papaverine) have clinical utility. These opium alkaloids are divided into two distinct chemical classes, phenanthrenes and benzylisoquinolines. The principal phenanthrenes are morphine (10% of opium), codeine (0.5%), and thebaine (0.2%). The principal benzylisoquinolines are papaverine (1%) (a smooth muscle relaxant) and noscapine (6%).

Morphine and Its Congeners

Morphine remains the standard against which new analgesics are measured.

Chemistry. The structures of morphine and some of its surrogates and antagonists are shown in Figure 20–9. Many semisynthetic derivatives are made by relatively simple modifications of morphine or thebaine. Codeine is methylmorphine, the methyl substitution being on the phenolic hydroxyl group. Thebaine differs from morphine only in that both hydroxyl groups are methylated and that the ring has two double bonds (6,7; 8,14). Thebaine has little analgesic action but is a precursor of several important 14-OH compounds, such as oxycodone and naloxone. Certain derivatives of thebaine are more than 1000 times as potent as morphine (e.g., etorphine). Diacetylmorphine, or heroin, is made from morphine

TABLE 20–4 ■ DOSING DATA FOR CLINICALLY EMPLOYED OPIOID ANALGESICS

DRUG	APPROXIMATE EQUIANALGESIC ORAL DOSE	APPROXIMATE EQUIANALGESIC PARENTERAL DOSE	RECOMMENDED STARTING DOSE (Adults > 50 kg) ORAL	RECOMMENDED STARTING DOSE (Adults > 50 kg) PARENTERAL	RECOMMENDED STARTING DOSE (Children and Adults < 50 kg) ORAL	RECOMMENDED STARTING DOSE (Children and Adults < 50 kg) PARENTERAL
Opioid Agonists						
Morphine	30 mg/3–4 h	10 mg/3–4 h	15 mg/3–4 h	5 mg/3–4 h	0.3 mg/kg/3–4 h	0.1 mg/kg/3–4 h
Codeine	130 mg/3–4 h	75 mg/3–4 h	30 mg/3–4 h	30 mg/2 h (IM/SC)	0.5 mg/kg/3–4 h	Not recommended
Hydromophone	6 mg/3–4 h	1.5 mg/3–4 h	2 mg/3–4 h	0.5 mg/3–4 h	0.03 mg/kg/3–4 h	0.005 mg/kg/3–4 h
Hydrocodone (typically with acetaminophen)	30 mg/3–4 h	Not available	5 mg/3–4 h	Not available	0.1 mg/kg/3–4 h	Not available
Levorphanol	4 mg/6–8 h	2 mg/6–8 h	4 mg/6–8 h	2 mg/6–8 h	0.04 mg/kg/6–8 h	0.02 mg/kg/6–8 h
Meperidine	300 mg/2–3 h	100 mg/3 h	Not recommended	50 mg/3 h	Not recommended	0.75 mg/kg/2–3 h
Methadone	10 mg/6–8 h	10 mg/6–8 h	5 mg/12 h	Not recommended	0.1 mg/kg/12 h	Not recommended
Oxycodone	20 mg/3–4 h	Not available	5 mg/3–4 h	Not available	0.1 mg/kg/3–4 h	Not available
Oxymorphone	10 mg/3–4 h	1 mg/3–4 h	5 mg/3–4 h	1 mg/3–4 h	0.1 mg/kg/3–4 h	Not recommended
Tramadol	100 mg	100 mg	50–100 mg/6 h	50–100 mg/6 h	Not recommended	Not recommended
Fentanyl	Transdermal 72-h patch (25 μg/h) = morphine 50 mg/24 h					
Opioid Agonist-Antagonists or Partial Agonists						
Buprenorphine	Not available	0.3–0.4 mg/6–8 h	Not available	0.4 mg/6–8 h	Not available	0.004 mg/kg/6–8 h
Butorphanol	Not available	2 mg/3–4 h	Not available	2 mg/3–4 h	Not available	Not recommended
Nalbuphine	Not available	10 mg/3–4 h	Not available	10 mg/3–4 h	Not available	0.1 mg/kg/3–4 h

These data are merely guidelines. Clinical response must be the guide for each patient, with consideration to hepatic and renal function, disease, age, concurrent medications (their effects and dose limitations [acetaminophen, 3 g/d for adults]), and other factors that could modify pharmacokinetics and drug response. Recommended start doses are approximately but not precisely equianalgesic and are driven by doses available from manufacturers. Transdermal fentanyl is contraindicated for acute pain and in patients receiving < 60 mg oral morphine equivalent per day. Use Table 20–8 for converting morphine to methadone dosing.

For morphine, hydromorphone, and oxymorphone, rectal administration is an alternate route for patients unable to take oral medications, but equianalgesic doses may differ from oral and parenteral doses because of pharmacokinetic differences.

Doses listed for patients with body weight less than 50 kg cannot be used as initial starting doses in babies less than 6 months of age; consult the *Clinical Practice Guideline #1, Acute Pain Management: Operative or Medical Procedures and Trauma* (cited below), section on neonates, for recommendations.

Source: Modified and updated from Agency for Healthcare Policy and Research, 1992. Acute Pain Management Guideline Panel. AHCPR Clinical Practice Guidelines, No. 1: Acute Pain Management: Operative or Medical Procedures and Trauma [Rockville (MD): Agency for Health Care Policy and Research (AHCPR); 1992].

by acetylation at the 3 and 6 positions. Apomorphine, which also can be prepared from morphine, is a potent emetic and dopaminergic agonist at D2- and D1-type receptors, does not interact with opiate receptors, and displays no analgesic actions (see Chapters 13, 18, and 50). Hydromorphone, oxymorphone, hydrocodone, and oxycodone also are made by modifying the morphine molecule.

Structure-Activity Relationship of the Morphine-Like Opioids. In addition to morphine, codeine, and the semisynthetic derivatives of the natural opium alkaloids, a number of other structurally distinct chemical classes of drugs have pharmacological actions similar to those of morphine. Clinically useful compounds include the morphinans, benzomorphans, methadones, phenylpiperidines, and propionanilides. Although the two-dimensional representations of these chemically diverse compounds appear to be quite different, molecular models show common characteristics. Among the important properties of the opioids that can be altered by structural modification are their affinities for various types of opioid receptors, their activities as agonists versus antagonists, their lipid solubilities, and their resistance to metabolic breakdown. For example, blockade of the phenolic hydroxyl at position 3, as in codeine and heroin, drastically reduces binding to receptors; these compounds are converted in vivo to the potent analgesics morphine and 6-acetyl morphine, respectively.

ADME. ***Absorption.*** In general, the opioids are modestly well absorbed from the GI tract; absorption through the rectal mucosa is adequate, and a few agents (e.g., morphine, hydromorphone) are available in suppositories. The more lipophilic opioids are absorbed readily through the nasal or buccal mucosa. Those with the greatest lipid solubility also can be absorbed transdermally. Opioids, particularly morphine, have been widely used for spinal delivery to produce analgesia though a spinal action. These agents display useful transdural movement adequate to permit their use epidurally.

With most opioids, including morphine, the effect of a given dose is less after oral than after parenteral administration because of variable but significant first-pass metabolism in the liver. For example, the bioavailability of oral preparations of morphine is only about 25%. The shape of the time-effect curve also varies with the route of administration, so the duration of action often is somewhat longer with the oral route. If adjustment is made for variability of first-pass metabolism and clearance, adequate relief of pain can be achieved with oral administration of morphine. Satisfactory analgesia in patients with cancer is associated with a broad range of steady-state concentrations of morphine in plasma (16–364 ng/mL) (Neumann et al., 1982).

When morphine and most opioids are given intravenously, they act promptly. However, the more lipid-soluble compounds (e.g., fentanyl) act more rapidly than morphine after subcutaneous administration because of differences in the rates of absorption and entry into the CNS. Compared with more lipid-soluble opioids such as codeine, heroin, and methadone, morphine crosses the blood-brain barrier at a considerably lower rate.

Distribution and Metabolism. About one-third of morphine in the plasma is protein bound after a therapeutic dose. Morphine itself does

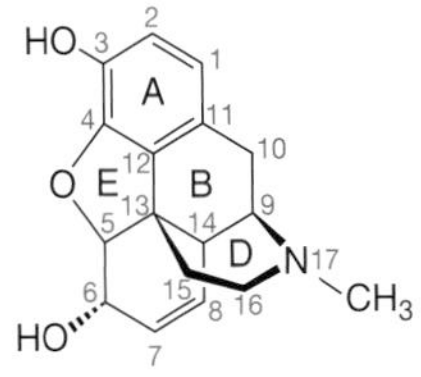

Nonproprietary name	Chemical radicals and position[a]			Other changes†
	3	6	17	
Morphine	—OH	—OH	—CH_3	—
Heroin	—$OCOCH_3$	—$OCOCH_3$	—CH_3	—
Hydromorphone	—OH	=O	—CH_3	(1)
Oxymorphone	—OH	=O	—CH_3	(1), (2)
Levorphanol	—OH	—H	—CH_3	(1), (3)
Levallorphan	—OH	—H	—$CH_2CH{=}CH_2$	(1), (3)
Codeine	—OCH_3	—OH	—CH_3	—
Hydrocodone	—OCH_3	=O	—CH_3	(1)
Oxycodone	—OCH_3	=O	—CH_3	(1), (2)
Nalmefene	—OH	=CH_2	—CH_2—cyclopropyl	(1), (2)
Nalorphine	—OH	—OH	—$CH_2CH{=}CH_2$	—
Naloxone	—OH	=O	—$CH_2CH{=}CH_2$	(1), (2)
Naltrexone	—OH	=O	—CH_2—cyclopropyl	(1), (2)
Buprenorphine	—OH	—OCH_3	—CH_2—cyclopropyl	(1), (4)
Butorphanol	—OH	—H	—CH_2—cyclobutyl	(1), (2), (3)
Nalbuphine	—OH	—OH	—CH_2—cyclobutyl	(1), (2)
Methylnaltrexone	—OH	=O	—(N)—CH_2—cyclopropyl, N—CH_3	(1), (2)

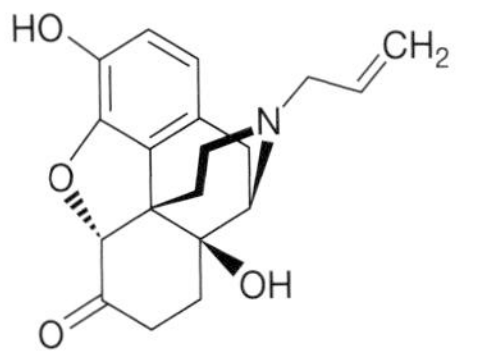

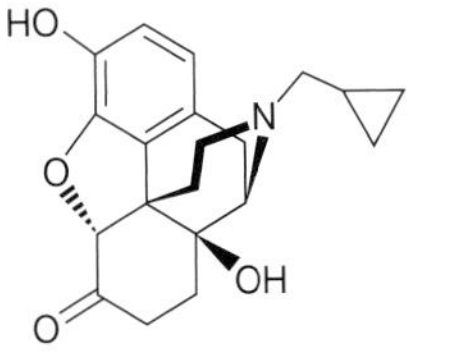

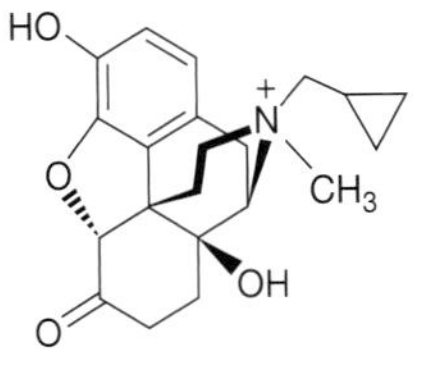

[a]The numbers 3, 6, and 17 refer to positions in the morphine molecule, as shown above. †Other changes in the morphine molecule are (1) Single instead of double bond between C7 and C8; (2) OH added to C14; (3) No oxygen between C4 and C5; (4) *Endo*etheno bridge between C6 and C14; 1-hydroxy-1,2,2-trimethylpropyl substitution on C7.

Figure 20–9 *Structures of morphine-related opiate agonists and antagonists.*

not persist in tissues, and 24 h after the last dose, tissue concentrations are low.

The major pathway for the metabolism of morphine is conjugation with glucuronic acid. The two major metabolites formed are morphine-6-glucuronide and morphine-3-glucuronide. Small amounts of morphine-3,6-diglucuronide also may be formed. Although the 3-and 6-glucuronides are polar, both still can cross the blood-brain barrier to exert significant clinical effects (Christrup, 1997).

Morphine-6-glucuronide has pharmacological actions indistinguishable from those of morphine. Morphine-6-glucuronide given systemically is approximately twice as potent as morphine in animal models and in humans (Osborne et al., 1992). With chronic administration, the 6-glucuronide accounts for a significant portion of morphine's analgesic actions. Indeed, with chronic oral dosing, the blood levels of morphine-6-glucuronide typically exceed those of morphine. Given its greater MOR potency and its higher concentration, morphine-6-glucuronide may be responsible for most of morphine's analgesic activity in patients receiving chronic oral morphine. Morphine-6-glucuronide is excreted by the kidney. In renal failure, the levels of morphine-6-glucuronide can accumulate, perhaps explaining morphine's potency and long duration in patients with compromised renal function. In adults, the $t_{1/2}$ of morphine is about 2 h; the $t_{1/2}$ of morphine-6-glucuronide is somewhat longer. Children achieve adult renal function values by 6 months of age. In elderly patients, lower doses of morphine are recommended based on a smaller volume of distribution and the general decline in renal function in the elderly (Owens, et al, 1983).

Morphine-3-glucuronide, another important metabolite, has little affinity for opioid receptors but may contribute to excitatory effects of morphine (Smith, 2000). *N*-Demethylation of morphine to normorphine is a minor metabolic pathway in humans. *N*-Dealkylation also is important in the metabolism of some congeners of morphine.

Excretion. Morphine is eliminated by glomerular filtration, primarily as morphine-3-glucuronide; 90% of the total excretion takes place during the first day. Very little morphine is excreted unchanged. Enterohepatic circulation of morphine and its glucuronides occurs, which accounts for the presence of small amounts of morphine in feces and urine for several days after the last dose.

Morphine Congeners. ***Codeine.*** Codeine is an important natural product found in the poppy resin. It displays a modest affinity for the μ receptor, but its analgesic actions are considered by many to arise at least in part by its hepatic metabolism to morphine (see further discussion). Thus, in contrast to morphine, codeine is about 60% as effective orally as parenterally as an analgesic and as a respiratory depressant. Codeine is commonly employed for the management of cough, frequently in combination dose forms with acetaminophen or aspirin. The drug has an exceptionally low affinity for opioid receptors, and while the analgesic effect of codeine is likely due to its conversion to morphine, codeine's antitussive actions may involve distinct receptors that bind codeine itself.

Once absorbed, codeine is metabolized by the liver. Codeine analogues such as levorphanol, oxycodone, and methadone have a high ratio of oral-to-parenteral potency. The greater oral efficacy of these drugs reflects lower first-pass metabolism in the liver. Codeine's metabolites are excreted chiefly as inactive forms in the urine. A small fraction (~10%) of administered codeine is *O*-demethylated to morphine, and free and conjugated morphine can be found in the urine after therapeutic doses of codeine. The $t_{1/2}$ of codeine in plasma is 2–4 h. CYP2D6 catalyzes the conversion of codeine to morphine. Genetic polymorphisms in CYP2D6 lead to the inability to convert codeine to morphine, thus making codeine ineffective as an analgesic for about 10% of the Caucasian population (Eichelbaum and Evert, 1996). Other polymorphisms (e.g., the CYP2D6*2x2 genotype) can lead to ultrarapid metabolism and thus increased sensitivity to codeine's effects due to higher than expected serum morphine levels. Other variations in metabolic efficiency among ethnic groups are apparent. For example, Chinese produce less morphine from codeine than do Caucasians and also are less sensitive to morphine's effects. The reduced sensitivity to morphine may be due to decreased production of morphine-6-glucuronide (Caraco et al., 1999). Thus, it is important to consider the possibility of metabolic enzyme polymorphism in any patient who experiences toxicity or does not receive adequate analgesia from codeine or other opioid prodrugs (e.g., hydrocodone and oxycodone) (Johansson and Ingelman-Sundberg, 2011).

Heroin. Heroin (diacetylmorphine) is rapidly hydrolyzed to 6-MAM, which in turn is hydrolyzed to morphine. Heroin and 6-MAM are more lipid soluble than morphine and enter the brain more readily. Evidence suggests that morphine and 6-MAM are responsible for the pharmacological actions of heroin. Heroin is excreted mainly in the urine, largely as free and conjugated morphine (Rook et al., 2006).

Hydromorphone. Hydromorphone is a semisynthetic hydrogenated ketone derivative of morphine. It displays all of the opioid actions of morphine. It is commonly used as an intravenous medication. The drug is formulated in parenteral, rectal, subcutaneous, and oral preparations and as a nebulized formulation and is given off label by epidural or intrathecal routes. Hydromorphone has a higher lipid solubility than morphine, resulting in more rapid onset than morphine, and is considered to be several times more potent than morphine. Hydromorphone is metabolized in the liver to hydromorphone-3-glucoronide.

Oxycodone. Oxycodone is a semisynthetic opioid synthesized from the alkaloid thebaine. The molecule undergoes hepatic metabolism to the more potent μ opioid oxymorphone. Oxycodone is available as single-ingredient medication in immediate-release and controlled-release formulations. Parenteral formulations of 10 mg/mL and 50 mg/mL are available in the U.K. for intravenous or intramuscular administration. Combination products are also available as immediate-release formulations with non-narcotic ingredients such as NSAIDs. At present, oxycodone is one of the most commonly abused pharmaceutical drugs in the U.S.

Hydrocodone. Hydrocodone is synthesized from codeine. It is used orally for relief of moderate-to-severe pain and is employed in a liquid formulation as a cough suppressant. It is approximately equipotent to oxycodone, with an onset of action of 10–30 min and duration of 4–6 h. Hepatic CYPs 2D6 and 3A4 convert hydrocodone to hydromorphone and norhydrocodone, respectively. Hydrocodone shows a serum half-life of about 4 h.

Oxymorphone. Oxymorphone, a semisynthetic alkaloid, is produced from thebaine. Oxymorphone is a potent MOR agonist with an onset of analgesia after parenteral dosing of about 5–10 min and a duration of action of 3–4 h. Oxymorphone is extensively metabolized in liver and excreted as the 3- and 6-glucuronides.

Adverse Effects and Precautions

Morphine and related opioids, aside from their effects as analgesics, produce a wide spectrum of effects reflecting the distribution of opiate receptors across organ systems. These effects include respiratory depression, nausea, vomiting, dizziness, mental clouding, dysphoria, pruritus, constipation, increased pressure in the biliary tract, urinary retention, hypotension, and, rarely, delirium. Increased sensitivity to pain may occur after analgesia has worn off, and removal of opiate receptor occupancy (abstinence, antagonism) may lead to a highly aversive state of withdrawal.

Factors Affecting Patient Response to Morphine and Congeners

Beyond those mentioned, a number of other factors may alter a patient's response to opioid analgesics.

- *Blood-Brain Barrier.* Morphine is hydrophilic, so proportionately less morphine normally crosses into the CNS than with more lipophilic opioids. In neonates or when the blood-brain barrier is compromised, lipophilic opioids may give more predictable clinical results than morphine.
- *Age.* In adults, the duration of the analgesia produced by morphine increases progressively with age; however, the degree of analgesia that is obtained with a given dose changes little.
- *Pain State.* The patient with severe pain may tolerate larger doses of morphine. However, as the pain subsides, the patient may exhibit sedation and even respiratory depression as the stimulatory effects of pain are diminished.
- *Opioid Metabolism.* All opioid analgesics are metabolized by the liver and should be used with caution in patients with hepatic disease. Renal disease also significantly alters the pharmacokinetics of morphine, codeine, dihydrocodeine, and meperidine. Although single doses of morphine are well tolerated, the active metabolite, morphine-6-glucuronide, may accumulate with continued dosing, and symptoms of opioid overdose may result. This metabolite also may accumulate during repeated administration of codeine to patients with impaired renal function. When repeated doses of meperidine are given to such patients, the accumulation of normeperidine may cause tremor and seizures. Similarly, the repeated administration of propoxyphene may lead to naloxone-insensitive cardiac toxicity caused by accumulation of the metabolite norpropoxyphene.
- *Sex.* There is a growing body of data that examines gender differences in the responses to pain and analgesics (Mogil, 2012). Females have the majority of chronic pain syndromes, and surveys examining sex differences in acute pain models report either no sex difference or greater sensitivity in females. Data on sex differences in opiate analgesia have thus far been inconsistent (Loyd and Murphy, 2014).
- *Respiratory Function.* Morphine and related opioids must be used cautiously in patients with compromised respiratory function (e.g., emphysema, kyphoscoliosis, severe obesity, or cor pulmonale). Although many patients with such conditions seem to be functioning within normal limits, they are already using compensatory mechanisms, such as increased

respiratory rate. Many have chronically elevated levels of plasma CO_2 and may be less sensitive to the stimulating actions of CO_2. The further imposition of the depressant effects of opioids can be disastrous.

- *Head Injury.* The respiratory-depressant effects of opioids and the related capacity to elevate intracranial pressure must be considered in the presence of head injury or an already-elevated intracranial pressure. While head injury per se does not constitute an absolute contraindication to the use of opioids, the possibility of exaggerated depression of respiration and the potential need to control ventilation of the patient must be considered. Finally, because opioids may produce mental clouding and side effects such as miosis and vomiting, which are important signs in following the clinical course of patients with head injuries, the advisability of their use must be weighed carefully against these risks.
- *Hypovolemia; Hypotension.* Reduced blood volume causes patients to be considerably more susceptible to the vasodilating effects of morphine and related drugs, and these agents must be used cautiously in patients with hypotension from any cause.
- *Asthma; Allergic Responses; Histamine Release.* Morphine causes histamine release, which can cause bronchoconstriction and vasodilation. Morphine can precipitate or exacerbate asthmatic attacks and should be avoided in patients with a history of asthma. Other receptor agonists associated with a lower incidence of histamine release, such as the fentanyl derivatives, may be better choices for such patients.

Aside from their capacity to release histamine, opioid analgesics may evoke allergic phenomena, but a true allergic response is uncommon. The effects usually are manifested as urticaria and fixed eruptions; contact dermatitis in nurses and pharmaceutical workers also occurs. Wheals at the site of injection of morphine, codeine, and related drugs are likely secondary to histamine release. Anaphylactoid reactions have been reported after intravenous administration of codeine and morphine, but such reactions are rare. In addicts who use intravenous heroin, such reactions may contribute to sudden death, episodes of pulmonary edema, and other complications.

Other Morphinans

Levorphanol

Levorphanol is an opioid agonist of the morphinan series (Figure 20–9). Levorphanol has affinity at the MORs, KORs, and DORs and is available for intravenous, intramuscular, and oral administration. The pharmacological effects of levorphanol closely parallel those of morphine. Compared to morphine, this agent is about seven times more potent and may produce less nausea and vomiting. Levorphanol is metabolized less rapidly than morphine and has a $t_{1/2}$ of 12–16 h; repeated administration at short intervals may thus lead to accumulation of the drug in plasma (Prommer, 2014). The D-isomer (dextrorphan) is devoid of analgesic action but has inhibitory effects at NMDA receptors.

Piperidine and Phenylpiperidine Analgesics

Meperidine, Diphenoxylate, Loperamide

The agents meperidine, diphenoxylate, and loperamide are MOR agonists with principal pharmacological effects on the CNS and neural elements in the bowel.

Meperidine. Meperidine is predominantly an MOR agonist that produces a pattern of effects similar but not identical to those already described for morphine (Latta et al., 2002).

CNS Actions. Meperidine is a potent agonist at MORs in the CNS, yielding strong analgesic actions. Meperidine causes pupillary constriction, increases the sensitivity of the labyrinthine apparatus, and has effects on the secretion of pituitary hormones similar to those of morphine. Meperidine sometimes causes CNS excitation, characterized by tremors, muscle twitches, and seizures. These effects are due largely to accumulation of a metabolite, normeperidine. Meperidine has well-known local anesthetic properties, particularly noted after epidural administration. As with morphine, respiratory depression is responsible for an accumulation of CO_2, which in turn leads to cerebrovascular dilation, increased cerebral blood flow, and elevation of CSF pressure.

Cardiovascular Effects. The effects of meperidine on the cardiovascular system generally resemble those of morphine, including the release of histamine following parenteral administration. Intramuscular administration of therapeutic doses of meperidine does not affect heart rate significantly, but intravenous administration frequently produces a marked increase in heart rate.

Actions on Smooth Muscle, GI Tract, and Uterus. Meperidine does not cause as much constipation as morphine, even when given over prolonged periods; this may be related to its greater ability to enter the CNS, thereby producing analgesia at lower systemic concentrations. As with other opioids, clinical doses of meperidine slow gastric emptying sufficiently to delay absorption of other drugs significantly. The uterus of a nonpregnant woman usually is mildly stimulated by meperidine. Administered before an oxytocic, meperidine does not exert any antagonistic effect. Therapeutic doses given during active labor do not delay the birth process; in fact, frequency, duration, and amplitude of uterine contraction may be increased.

ADME. Meperidine is absorbed by all routes of administration. The peak plasma concentration usually occurs at about 45 min, but the range is wide. After oral administration, only about 50% of the drug escapes first-pass metabolism to enter the circulation, and peak concentrations in plasma occur in 1–2 h. Meperidine is metabolized chiefly in the liver, with a $t_{1/2}$ of about 3 h. Metabolites are the *N*-demethyl product, normeperidine, and the hydrolysis product, meperidinate, both of which may be conjugated. In patients with cirrhosis, the bioavailability of meperidine is increased to as much as 80%, and the $t_{1/2}$ of both meperidine and the metabolite normeperidine ($t_{1/2}$ ~ 15–20 h) are prolonged. Only a small amount of meperidine is excreted unchanged.

Therapeutic Use. The major use of meperidine is for analgesia. The analgesic effects of meperidine are detectable about 15 min after oral administration, peak in 1–2 h, and subside gradually. The onset of analgesic effect is faster (within 10 min) after subcutaneous or intramuscular administration, and the effect reaches a peak in about 1 h, corresponding closely to peak concentrations in plasma. In clinical use, the duration of effective analgesia is about 1.5–3 h. Peak respiratory depression is observed within 1 h of intramuscular administration, and there is a return toward normal starting at about 2 h. In general, 75–100 mg meperidine hydrochloride given parenterally is approximately equivalent to 10 mg morphine. In terms of total analgesic effect, meperidine is about one-third as effective when given orally as when administered parenterally.

Single doses of meperidine can be effective in the treatment of postanesthetic shivering. Meperidine, 25–50 mg, is used frequently with antihistamines, corticosteroids, acetaminophen, or NSAIDs to prevent or ameliorate infusion-related rigors and shaking chills that accompany the intravenous administration of agents such as amphotericin B, aldesleukin (interleukin 2), trastuzumab, and alemtuzumab. Meperidine crosses the placental barrier, and even in reasonable analgesic doses causes a significant increase in the percentage of babies who show delayed respiration, decreased respiratory minute volume, or decreased O_2 saturation or who require resuscitation. Fetal and maternal respiratory depression induced by meperidine can be treated with naloxone. Meperidine produces less respiratory depression in the newborn than does an equianalgesic dose of morphine or methadone (Fishburne, 1982).

Untoward Effects, Precautions, and Contraindications. The overall incidence of untoward effects is similar to those observed after equianalgesic doses of morphine, except that constipation and urinary retention and nausea may be less common. Patients who experience nausea and vomiting with morphine may not do so with meperidine; the converse also may be true. In patients or addicts who are tolerant to the depressant effects of meperidine, large doses repeated at short intervals may produce an excitatory syndrome that includes hallucinations, tremors, muscle twitches, dilated pupils, hyperactive reflexes, and convulsions. These excitatory symptoms are due to the accumulation of the long-lived metabolite normeperidine, which has a $t_{1/2}$ of 15–20 h, compared to 3 h for meperidine. Decreased renal or hepatic function increases the likelihood of toxicity. As a result of these properties, meperidine is not recommended for the treatment of chronic pain because of concerns over metabolite toxicity. It should not be used for longer than 48 h or in doses greater than 600 mg/d.

Interactions With Other Drugs. Severe reactions may follow the administration of meperidine to patients being treated with MAO inhibitors. There are two basic types of interaction. The more prominent is an excitatory reaction ("serotonin syndrome") with delirium, hyperthermia, headache, hyper- or hypotension, rigidity, convulsions, coma, and death. This reaction may be due to the capacity of meperidine to block neuronal reuptake of 5HT, resulting in serotonergic overactivity. Dextromethorphan (an analogue of levorphanol used as a nonnarcotic cough suppressant) also inhibits neuronal 5HT uptake and must be avoided in these patients. In the second type of interaction, several MAO inhibitors are substrates or inhibitors of hepatic CYPs and reduce meperidine metabolism, creating a condition resembling acute narcotic overdose. Therefore, meperidine and its congeners are contraindicated in patients taking MAO inhibitors or within 14 days after discontinuation of an MAO inhibitor.

Chlorpromazine increases the respiratory-depressant effects of meperidine, as do tricyclic antidepressants (but not diazepam). Concurrent administration of drugs such as promethazine or chlorpromazine also may greatly enhance meperidine-induced sedation without slowing clearance of the drug. Treatment with phenobarbital or phenytoin increases systemic clearance and decreases oral bioavailability of meperidine. As with morphine, concomitant administration of amphetamine has been reported to enhance the analgesic effects of meperidine and its congeners while counteracting sedation.

Diphenoxylate. Diphenoxylate is a meperidine congener that has a definite constipating effect in humans. Its only approved use is in the treatment of diarrhea. Diphenoxylate is unusual in that even its salts are virtually insoluble in aqueous solution, thus reducing the probability of abuse by the parenteral route. Diphenoxylate hydrochloride is available only in combination with atropine sulfate. The recommended daily dosage of diphenoxylate for the treatment of diarrhea in adults is 20 mg in divided doses. Difenoxin a metabolite of diphenoxylate and is marketed in a fixed dose with atropine for the management of diarrhea.

Loperamide. Loperamide, like diphenoxylate, is a piperidine derivative. It slows GI motility by effects on the circular and longitudinal muscles of the intestine (Kromer, 1988). Part of its antidiarrheal effect may be due to a reduction of GI secretory processes (see Chapter 50). In controlling chronic diarrhea, loperamide is as effective as diphenoxylate and little tolerance develops to its constipating effect. Concentrations of drug in plasma peak about 4 h after ingestion. The apparent elimination $t_{1/2}$ is 7–14 h. Loperamide is poorly absorbed after oral administration and, in addition, apparently does not penetrate well into the brain due to the exporting activity of P-glycoprotein, which is widely expressed in the brain endothelium. The usual dosage is 4–8 mg/d; the daily dose should not exceed 16 mg (Regnard et al., 2011). The most common side effect is abdominal cramps. Loperamide is unlikely to be abused parenterally because of its low solubility; large doses of loperamide given to human volunteers do not elicit pleasurable effects typical of opioids.

Fentanyl and Congeners

Fentanyl

Fentanyl is a synthetic opioid related to the phenylpiperidines. The actions of fentanyl and its congeners sufentanil, remifentanil, and alfentanil are similar to those of other MOR agonists. Fentanyl and sufentanil are important drugs in anesthetic practice because of their relatively short time to peak analgesic effect, rapid termination of effect after small bolus doses, cardiovascular safety, and capacity to significantly reduce the dosing requirement for the volatile agents (see Chapter 21). In addition to a role in anesthesia, fentanyl is used in the management of severe pain states delivered by several routes of administration (Willens and Myslinski, 1993).

ADME. These agents are highly lipid soluble and rapidly cross the blood-brain barrier. This is reflected in the $t_{1/2}$ for equilibration between the plasma and CSF of about 5 min for fentanyl and sufentanil. The levels in plasma and CSF decline rapidly owing to redistribution of fentanyl from highly perfused tissue groups to other tissues, such as muscle and fat. As saturation of less well-perfused tissue occurs, the duration of effect of fentanyl and sufentanil approaches the length of their elimination $t_{1/2}$, 3–4 h. Fentanyl and sufentanil undergo hepatic metabolism and renal excretion. With the use of higher doses or prolonged infusions, the drugs accumulate, these clearance mechanisms become progressively saturated, and fentanyl and sufentanil become longer acting.

Pharmacological Effects. CNS. Fentanyl and its congeners are all extremely potent analgesics and typically exhibit a very short duration of action when given parenterally. As with other opioids, nausea, vomiting, and itching can be observed. Muscle rigidity, while possible after all narcotics, appears to be more common after the high doses used in anesthetic induction. Rigidity can be treated with depolarizing or nondepolarizing neuromuscular-blocking agents, while controlling the patient's ventilation, but care must be taken to make sure that the patient is not simply immobilized and aware. Respiratory depression is similar to that observed with other MOR agonists, but onset is more rapid. As with analgesia, respiratory depression after small doses is of shorter duration than with morphine but of similar duration after large doses or long infusions. Delayed respiratory depression also can be seen after the use of fentanyl or sufentanil, possibly owing to enterohepatic circulation.

Cardiovascular System. Fentanyl and its derivatives decrease heart rate through vagal activation and may modestly decrease blood pressure. However, these drugs do not release histamine, and direct depressant effects on the myocardium are minimal. For this reason, high doses of fentanyl or sufentanil are commonly used as the primary anesthetic for patients undergoing cardiovascular surgery or for patients with poor cardiac function.

Therapeutic Uses. Fentanyl citrate and sufentanil citrate have widespread popularity as anesthetic adjuvants (see Chapter 21), administered intravenously and epidurally. After systemic delivery, fentanyl is about 100 times more potent than morphine; sufentanil is about 1000 times more potent than morphine. The time to peak analgesic effect after intravenous administration of fentanyl and sufentanil (~5 min) is notably less than that for morphine and meperidine (~15 min). Recovery from analgesic effects also occurs more quickly. However, with larger doses or prolonged infusions, the effects of these drugs become more lasting, with durations of action becoming similar to those of longer-acting opioids.

The use of fentanyl in chronic pain treatment has become more widespread. Transdermal patches that provide sustained release of fentanyl for 48–72 h are available. However, factors promoting increased absorption (e.g., fever) can lead to relative overdosage and increased side effects. Transbuccal absorption by the use of buccal tablets and lollipop-like lozenges permits rapid absorption and has found use in the management of acute incident pain and for the relief of breakthrough cancer pain. As fentanyl is poorly absorbed in the GI tract, the optimal absorption is through buccal administration. Fentanyl should only be used in opioid-tolerant patients, defined as consuming more than 60 mg of oral morphine equivalent. Epidural use of fentanyl and sufentanil for postoperative or labor analgesia is popular. A combination of epidural opioids with local anesthetics permits reduction in the dosage of both components. Illicit use (self-administration by chewing) of fentanyl patches can be deadly, and practitioners must be aware of this potential and keep careful control of fentanyl stocks.

Remifentanil

The pharmacological properties of remifentanil are similar to those of fentanyl and sufentanil. Remifentanil produces similar incidences of nausea, vomiting, and dose-dependent muscle rigidity.

ADME. Remifentanil has a more rapid onset of analgesic action than fentanyl or sufentanil. Analgesic effects occur within 1–1.5 min following intravenous administration. Peak respiratory depression after bolus doses of remifentanil occurs after 5 min. Remifentanil is metabolized by plasma esterases, with a $t_{1/2}$ of 8–20 min; thus, elimination is independent of hepatic metabolism or renal excretion. Age and weight can affect clearance of remifentanil. After 3- to 5-h infusions of remifentanil, recovery of respiratory function can be seen within 3–5 min; full recovery from all effects of remifentanil occurs within 15 min. The primary metabolite, remifentanil acid, has 0.05%–0.025% of the potency of the parent compound and is excreted renally.

Therapeutic Uses. Remifentanil hydrochloride is useful for short, painful procedures that require intense analgesia and blunting of stress responses; the drug is routinely given by continuous intravenous infusion because of its short duration of action. When postprocedural analgesia is required, remifentanil alone is a poor choice. In this situation, either a longer-acting opioid or another analgesic modality should be combined with remifentanil for prolonged analgesia, or another opioid should be used. Remifentanil is not used intraspinally (epidural or intrathecal administration) because of its formulation with glycine, an inhibitory neurotransmitter in the dorsal horn of the spinal cord (Stroumpos et al., 2010).

Methadone

Methadone is a long-acting MOR agonist with pharmacological properties qualitatively similar to those of morphine. The analgesic activity of methadone, a racemate, is almost entirely the result of its content of L-methadone, which is 8–50 times more potent than the D-isomer. D-Methadone also lacks significant respiratory depressant action and addiction liability but possesses antitussive activity (Fredheim et al., 2008).

Propoxyphene is a methadone analogue that was used to treat mild-to-moderate pain. The FDA removed the drug (trade name: DARVON) from the U.S. market in 2010 due to reports of cardiac toxicity.

Pharmacological Effects

The outstanding properties of methadone are its analgesic activity, its efficacy by the oral route, its extended duration of action in suppressing withdrawal symptoms in physically dependent individuals, and its tendency to show persistent effects with repeated administration. Miotic and respiratory-depressant effects can be detected for more than 24 h after a single dose; on repeated administration, marked sedation is seen in some patients. Effects on cough, bowel motility, biliary tone, and the secretion of pituitary hormones are qualitatively similar to those of morphine.

ADME

Methadone is absorbed well from the GI tract and can be detected in plasma within 30 min of oral ingestion; it reaches peak concentrations at about 4 h. Peak concentrations occur in brain within 1–2 h of subcutaneous or intramuscular administration, and this correlates well with the intensity and duration of analgesia. Methadone also can be absorbed from the buccal mucosa. Methadone undergoes extensive biotransformation in the liver. The major metabolites, pyrrolidine and pyrroline, result from *N*-demethylation and cyclization and are excreted in the urine and the bile along with small amounts of unchanged drug. The amount of methadone excreted in the urine is increased when the urine is acidified. The $t_{1/2}$ of methadone is long, 15–40 h. Methadone appears to be firmly bound to protein in various tissues, including brain. After repeated administration, there is gradual accumulation in tissues. When administration is discontinued, low concentrations are maintained in plasma by slow release from extravascular binding sites; this process probably accounts for the relatively mild but protracted withdrawal syndrome.

Therapeutic Uses

The primary use of methadone hydrochloride is detoxification and maintenance treatment of opioid addiction within certified treatment programs. Outside treatment programs, methadone is used for the management of chronic pain. The onset of analgesia occurs 10–20 min after parenteral administration and 30–60 min after oral medication. The typical oral dose is 2.5–10 mg repeated every 8–12 h as needed depending on the severity of the pain and the response of the patient. Care must be taken when increasing the dosage because of the prolonged $t_{1/2}$ of the drug and its tendency to accumulate over a period of several days with repeated dosing. The peak respiratory depressant effects of methadone typically occur later and persist longer than peak analgesia, so it is necessary to exercise vigilance and strongly caution patients against self-medicating with CNS depressants, particularly during treatment initiation and dose titration. Methadone should not be used in labor. Despite its longer plasma $t_{1/2}$, the duration of the analgesic action of single doses is essentially the same as that of morphine. With repeated use, cumulative effects are seen, so either lower dosages or longer intervals between doses become possible.

Because of its oral bioavailability and long $t_{1/2}$, methadone has been widely implemented as a replacement modality to treat heroin addiction. Figure 24-3 compares the time courses of response to heroin and methadone, emphasizing the favorable pharmacokinetics of oral methadone in treating addiction. Methadone, like other opiates, will produce tolerance and dependence. Thus, addicts who receive daily subcutaneous or oral therapy develop partial tolerance to the nauseant, anorectic, miotic, sedative, respiratory-depressant, and cardiovascular effects of methadone. Many former heroin users treated with oral methadone show virtually no overt behavioral effects. Development of physical dependence during the long-term administration of methadone can be demonstrated following abrupt drug withdrawal or by administration of an opioid antagonist. Likewise, subcutaneous administration of methadone to former opioid addicts produces euphoria equal in duration to that caused by morphine, and its overall abuse potential is comparable with that of morphine.

Adverse Effects

Side effects are similar to those described for morphine. Rifampin and phenytoin accelerate the metabolism of methadone and can precipitate withdrawal symptoms. Unlike other opioids, methadone is associated with the prolonged QT syndrome and is additive with agents known to prolong the QT interval.

Other Opioid Agonists

Tramadol

Tramadol is a synthetic codeine analogue that is a weak MOR agonist. Part of its analgesic effect is produced by inhibition of uptake of NE and 5HT. In the treatment of mild-to-moderate pain, tramadol is as effective as morphine or meperidine. However, for the treatment of severe or chronic pain, tramadol is less effective. Tramadol is as effective as meperidine in the treatment of labor pain and may cause less neonatal respiratory depression (Grond and Sablotzki, 2004). Tramadol is also available as a fixed-dose combination with acetaminophen.

ADME. Tramadol is 68% bioavailable after a single oral dose. Its affinity for the MOR is only 1/6000 that of morphine. The primary *O*-demethylated metabolite of tramadol is two to four times more potent than the parent drug and may account for part of the analgesic effect. Tramadol is supplied as a racemate that is more effective than either enantiomer alone. The (+)-enantiomer binds to the receptor and inhibits 5HT uptake. The (−)-enantiomer inhibits NE uptake and stimulates α_2 adrenergic receptors. Tramadol undergoes extensive hepatic metabolism by a number of pathways, including CYPs 2D6 and 3A4, and by conjugation with subsequent renal excretion. The elimination $t_{1/2}$ is 6 h for tramadol and 7.5 h for its active metabolite. Analgesia begins within an hour of oral dosing and peaks within 2–3 h. The duration of analgesia is about 6 h. The maximum recommended daily dose is 400 mg (300 mg in patients > 75 years old and for extended-release formulations; 200 mg is given for patients with low creatinine clearance).

Adverse Effects. Side effects of tramadol include nausea, vomiting, dizziness, dry mouth, sedation, and headache. Respiratory depression appears to be less than with equianalgesic doses of morphine, and the degree of constipation is less than that seen after equivalent doses of codeine. Tramadol can cause seizures and possibly exacerbate seizures in patients with predisposing factors. Tramadol-induced respiratory depression is reversed by naloxone. Precipitation of withdrawal necessitates that tramadol be tapered prior to discontinuation. Tramadol should not be used in patients taking MAO inhibitors, SSRIs, or other drugs that lower the seizure threshold.

Tapentadol

Tapentadol is structurally and mechanistically similar to tramadol. It is a weak inhibitor of monoamine reuptake but has a significantly more potent activity at MORs, similar to oxycodone. Serotonin syndrome is a risk, especially when tapentadol is used concomitantly with SSRIs, SNRIs, tricyclic antidepressants, or MAO inhibitors that impair 5HT metabolism. Tapentadol is metabolized largely by glucuronidation. The drug is in pregnancy category C.

Opioid Partial Agonists

The drugs described in this section differ from clinically used MOR agonists. Drugs such as *nalbuphine* and *butorphanol* are competitive MOR antagonists but exert their analgesic actions by acting as agonists at KOR receptors. *Pentazocine* qualitatively resembles these drugs, but it may be a weaker MOR receptor antagonist or partial agonist while retaining its KOR agonist activity. *Buprenorphine* is a partial MOR agonist. The stimulus for the development of mixed agonist-antagonist drugs was a desire for analgesics with less respiratory depression and addictive potential. However, the clinical use of these compounds is often limited by undesirable side effects and limited analgesic effects.

Pentazocine

Pentazocine was synthesized as part of a deliberate effort to develop an effective analgesic with little or no abuse potential. It has agonistic actions and weak opioid antagonistic activity (Goldstein, 1985).

Pharmacological Actions and Side Effects. The pattern of CNS effects produced by pentazocine generally is similar to that of the morphine-like opioids, including analgesia, sedation, and respiratory depression. The analgesic effects of pentazocine are due to agonistic actions at KORs. Higher doses of pentazocine (60–90 mg) elicit dysphoric and psychotomimetic effects; these effects may be reversible by naloxone. The cardiovascular responses to pentazocine differ from those seen with typical receptor agonists in that high doses cause an increase in blood pressure and heart rate. Pentazocine acts as a weak antagonist or partial agonist at MORs. Pentazocine does not antagonize the respiratory depression produced by morphine. However, when given to patients who are dependent on morphine or other MOR agonists, pentazocine may precipitate withdrawal. Ceiling effects for analgesia and respiratory depression are observed at doses above 50–100 mg of pentazocine.

Pentazocine lactate injection is indicated for the relief of mild-to-moderate pain and is also used as a preoperative medication and as a supplement to anesthesia. Pentazocine tablets for oral use are only available in fixed-dose combinations with acetaminophen or naloxone. Combination of pentazocine with naloxone reduces the potential misuse of tablets as a source of injectable pentazocine by producing undesirable effects in subjects dependent on opioids. An oral dose of about 50 mg pentazocine results in analgesia equivalent to that produced by a 60-mg oral dose of codeine.

Nalbuphine

Nalbuphine is a KOR agonist–MOR antagonist opioid with effects that qualitatively resemble those of pentazocine; however, nalbuphine produces fewer dysphoric side effects than pentazocine (Schmidt et al., 1985).

Pharmacological Actions and Side Effects. An intramuscular dose of 10 mg nalbuphine is equianalgesic to 10 mg morphine, with similar onset and duration of analgesic and subjective effects. Nalbuphine depresses respiration as much as equianalgesic doses of morphine; however, nalbuphine exhibits a ceiling effect such that increases in dosage beyond 30 mg produce no further respiratory depression or analgesia. In contrast to pentazocine and butorphanol, 10 mg nalbuphine given to patients with stable coronary artery disease does not produce an increase in cardiac index, pulmonary arterial pressure, or cardiac work, and systemic blood pressure is not significantly altered; these indices also are relatively stable when nalbuphine is given to patients with acute myocardial infarction. Nalbuphine produces few side effects at doses of 10 mg or less; sedation, sweating, and headache are the most common. At much higher doses (70 mg), psychotomimetic side effects (e.g., dysphoria, racing thoughts, and distortions of body image) can occur. Nalbuphine is metabolized in the liver and has a plasma $t_{1/2}$ of 2–3 h. Nalbuphine is 20%–25% as potent when administered orally as when given intramuscularly. Prolonged administration of nalbuphine can produce physical dependence. The withdrawal syndrome is similar in intensity to that seen with pentazocine.

Therapeutic Use. Nalbuphine is used to produce analgesia. Because it is an agonist-antagonist, administration to patients who have been receiving morphine-like opioids may create difficulties unless a brief drug-free interval is interposed. The usual adult dose is 10 mg parenterally every 3–6 h; this may be increased to 20 mg in nontolerant individuals. A caveat: Agents that act through the KORs are reportedly more effective in women than in men (Fillingim and Gear, 2004).

Butorphanol

Butorphanol is a morphinan congener with a profile of actions similar to those of pentazocine and nalbuphine: KOR agonist and MOR antagonist.

Pharmacological Actions and Side Effects. In postoperative patients, a parenteral dose of 2–3 mg butorphanol produces analgesia and respiratory depression approximately equal to that produced by 10 mg morphine or 80–100 mg meperidine. The plasma $t_{1/2}$ of butorphanol is about 3 h. Like pentazocine, analgesic doses of butorphanol produce an increase in pulmonary arterial pressure and in the work of the heart; systemic arterial pressure is slightly decreased. The major side effects of butorphanol are drowsiness, weakness, sweating, feelings of floating, and nausea. While the incidence of psychotomimetic side effects is lower than that with equianalgesic doses of pentazocine, they are qualitatively similar. Nasal administration is associated with drowsiness and dizziness. Physical dependence can occur.

Therapeutic Use. Butorphanol is used for the relief of acute pain (e.g., postoperative) and, because of its potential for antagonizing MOR agonists, should not be used in combination. Because of its side effects on the heart, it is less useful than morphine or meperidine in patients with congestive heart failure or myocardial infarction. The usual dose is 1–4 mg of the tartrate given intramuscularly, or 0.5–2 mg given intravenously, every 3–4 h. A nasal formulation is available and has proven to be effective in pain relief, including migraine pain (Gillis et al., 1995).

Buprenorphine

Buprenorphine is a highly lipophilic MOR partial agonist that is derived from thebaine and is 25–50 times more potent than morphine. As a partial MOR agonist, buprenorphine has limited intrinsic activity and accordingly can display antagonism when used in conjunction with a full agonist such as morphine. These properties have led it to have utility in managing opiate abuse and withdrawal (Elkader and Sproule, 2005).

ADME. Buprenorphine is well absorbed by most routes and produces analgesia and other CNS effects that are qualitatively similar to those of morphine. The $t_{1/2}$ for dissociation from the receptor is 166 min for buprenorphine, as opposed to 7 min for fentanyl. Therefore, plasma levels of buprenorphine may not parallel clinical effects. Cardiovascular and other side effects (e.g., sedation, nausea, vomiting, dizziness, sweating, and headache) appear to be similar to those of morphine-like opioids. Administered sublingually, buprenorphine (0.4–0.8 mg) produces satisfactory analgesia in postoperative patients. Concentrations in blood peak within 5 min of intramuscular injection and within 1–2 h of oral or sublingual administration. While the plasma $t_{1/2}$ in plasma is about 3 h, this value bears little relationship to the rate of disappearance of effects. Buprenorphine is metabolized to norbuprenorphine by CYP3A4 and should not be taken with known inhibitors of CYP3A4 (e.g., azole antifungals, macrolide antibiotics, and HIV protease inhibitors) or drugs that induce CYP3A4 activity (e.g., certain anticonvulsants and rifampin). Both *N*-dealkylated and conjugated metabolites are detected in the urine, but most of the drug is excreted unchanged in the feces. When buprenorphine is discontinued, a withdrawal syndrome develops that is delayed in onset for 2–14 days and persists for 1–2 weeks.

Therapeutic Use. Buprenorphine injection and transdermal film are indicated for use as an analgesic. Sublingual/buccal formulations of buprenorphine alone and in fixed-dose combinations with naloxone are used for treatment of opioid dependence; the partial agonist properties of buprenorphine limit its utility in the treatment of addicts who require high maintenance doses of opioids; in the U.S., this use is limited by the Drug Addiction Treatment Act. The usual intramuscular or intravenous dose for analgesia is 0.3 mg given every 6 h.

About 0.3 mg IM buprenorphine is equianalgesic with 10 mg IM morphine. Some of the subjective and respiratory-depressant effects are unequivocally slower in onset and last longer than those of morphine. Buprenorphine is a partial MOR agonist; thus, it may cause symptoms of abstinence in patients who have been receiving MOR agonists for several weeks. It antagonizes the respiratory depression produced by anesthetic doses of fentanyl about as well as naloxone without completely reversing opioid pain relief. The respiratory depression and other effects of buprenorphine can be prevented by prior administration of naloxone, but they are not readily reversed by high doses of naloxone once the effects have been produced, probably due to slow dissociation of buprenorphine from opioid receptors.

Opioid Antagonists

A variety of agents bind competitively to one or more of the opioid receptors, display little or no intrinsic activity, and robustly antagonize the effects of receptor agonists. Relatively minor changes in the structure of an opioid can convert a drug that is primarily an agonist into one with antagonistic actions at one or more types of opioid receptors. Simple substitutions transform morphine to *nalorphine*, levorphanol to *levallorphan,* and oxymorphone to *naloxone* or naltrexone. In some cases, congeners are produced that are competitive antagonists at MOR but that also have agonistic actions at KORs; *nalorphine* and *levallorphan* have such properties. Other congeners, especially *naloxone* and *naltrexone*, appear to be devoid of agonistic actions and interact with all types of opioid receptors, albeit with somewhat different affinities. *Nalmefene* (not marketed in the U.S.) is a relatively pure MOR antagonist that is more potent than naloxone. The majority of these agents are relatively lipid soluble and have excellent CNS penetration after systemic delivery (Barnett et al., 2014). A recognition for antagonism limited to peripheral sites, as for example to manage opiate-induced constipation, led to the development of agents that have poor CNS bioavailability, such as *methylnaltrexone* (Becker et al., 2007).

Pharmacological Properties

Opioid antagonists have obvious therapeutic utility in the treatment of opioid overdose. Under ordinary circumstances, these opioid antagonists produce few effects in the absence of an exogenous agonist. However, under certain conditions (e.g., shock), when the endogenous opioid systems are activated, the administration of an opioid antagonist alone may have positive effects on hemodynamic changes.

Effects in the Absence of Opioid Agonist. Subcutaneous doses of naloxone up to 12 mg produce no discernible effects in humans, and 24 mg causes only slight drowsiness. Naltrexone also is a relatively pure antagonist but with higher oral efficacy and a longer duration of action. The effects of opiate receptor antagonists are usually both subtle and limited, likely reflecting the low levels of tonic activity and organizational complexity of the opioid systems in various physiologic systems. Opiate antagonism in humans is associated with variable effects, ranging from no effect to mild hyperalgesia. A number of studies have suggested that agents such as naloxone may attenuate the analgesic effects of placebo medications and acupuncture.

Endogenous opioid peptides participate in the regulation of pituitary secretion apparently by exerting tonic inhibitory effects on the release of certain hypothalamic hormones (see Chapter 42). Thus, the administration of naloxone or naltrexone increases the secretion of GnRH and CRH and elevates the plasma concentrations of LH, FSH, and ACTH, as well as the steroid hormones produced by their target organs. Naloxone stimulates the release of prolactin in women. Endogenous opioid peptides probably have some role in the regulation of feeding or energy metabolism; however, naltrexone does not accelerate weight loss in very obese subjects, even though short-term administration of opioid antagonists reduces food intake in lean and obese individuals. Long-term administration of antagonists increases the density of opioid receptors in the brain and causes a temporary exaggeration of responses to the subsequent administration of opioid agonists.

Effects in the Presence of Opioid Agonists. Antagonistic Effects. Small doses (0.4–0.8 mg) of naloxone given intramuscularly or intravenously prevent or *promptly* reverse the effects of receptor agonists. In patients with respiratory depression, an increase in respiratory rate is seen within 1–2 min. Sedative effects are reversed, and blood pressure, if depressed, returns to normal. Higher doses of naloxone are required to antagonize the respiratory-depressant effects of buprenorphine; 1 mg naloxone intravenously completely blocks the effects of 25 mg heroin. Naloxone reverses the psychotomimetic and dysphoric effects of agonist-antagonist agents such as pentazocine, but much higher doses (10–15 mg) are required. The duration of antagonistic effects depends on the dose but usually is 1–4 h. Antagonism of opioid effects by naloxone often is accompanied by an "overshoot" phenomenon. For example, respiratory rates depressed by opioids transiently become higher than before the period of depression. Rebound release of catecholamines may cause hypertension, tachycardia, and ventricular arrhythmias. Pulmonary edema also has been reported after naloxone administration.

Effects in Opioid-Dependent Patients. In subjects who are dependent on morphine-like opioids, small subcutaneous doses of naloxone (0.5 mg) precipitate a moderate-to-severe withdrawal syndrome that is similar to that seen after abrupt withdrawal of opioids, except that the syndrome appears within minutes of administration and subsides in about 2 h. The severity and duration of the syndrome are related to the dose of the antagonist and to the degree and type of dependence. Higher doses of naloxone will precipitate a withdrawal syndrome in patients dependent on pentazocine, butorphanol, or nalbuphine. In dependent patients, peripheral side effects of opioids, notably reduced GI motility and constipation, can be reversed by methylnaltrexone, with subcutaneous doses (0.15 mg/kg) producing reliable bowel movements and no evidence of centrally mediated withdrawal signs (Thomas et al., 2008). Naloxone produces an *overshoot phenomenon* suggestive of early acute physical dependence 6–24 h after even a single dose of an MOR agonist.

ADME

Although absorbed readily from the GI tract, naloxone is almost completely metabolized by the liver (primarily by conjugation with glucuronic acid) before reaching the systemic circulation and thus must be administered parenterally. The $t_{1/2}$ of naloxone is about 1 h, but its clinically effective duration of action can be even less.

Compared with naloxone, naltrexone has more efficacy by the oral route, and its duration of action approaches 24 h after moderate oral doses. Peak concentrations in plasma are reached within 1–2 h and then decline with an apparent $t_{1/2}$ of about 3 h. Naltrexone is metabolized to 6-naltrexol, which is a weaker antagonist with longer $t_{1/2}$, about 13 h. Naltrexone is much more potent than naloxone, and 100-mg oral doses given to patients addicted to opioids produce concentrations in tissues sufficient to block the euphorigenic effects of 25-mg IV doses of heroin for 48 h. Methylnaltrexone is similar to naltrexone; it is converted to methyl-6-naltrexol isomers and eliminated primarily via active renal secretion. The $t_{1/2}$ of methylnaltrexone is about 8 h.

Therapeutic Uses

Treatment of Opioid Overdoses. Opioid antagonists, particularly naloxone, have an established use in the treatment of opioid-induced toxicity, especially respiratory depression. Its specificity is such that reversal by naloxone is virtually diagnostic for the contribution of an opiate to the depression. Naloxone acts rapidly to reverse the respiratory depression associated with even high doses of opioids. It should be titrated cautiously as it will precipitate withdrawal in dependent subjects and cause undesirable cardiovascular side effects (hypertension/tachycardia). The duration of action of naloxone is relatively short, and it often must be given repeatedly or by continuous infusion to prevent renarcotization. In the home setting, 0.4 mg of naloxone can be administered via autoinjector every 2–3 min while awaiting emergency medical assistance. Opioid antagonists also have been employed effectively to decrease neonatal respiratory depression secondary to the intravenous or intramuscular administration of opioids to the mother. In the neonate, the initial dose is 10 μg/kg given intravenously, intramuscularly, or subcutaneously.

Management of Constipation. The peripherally limited antagonists methylnaltrexone and naloxegol have important roles in the management of the constipation and the reduced GI motility present in the patient undergoing chronic opioid therapy (as for chronic pain or methadone maintenance). The use of the type 2 chloride channel activator lubiprostone and other strategies for the management of opioid-induced constipation are described in Chapter 50. An important application of the peripherally restricted opiate receptor antagonists is their use in managing ileus (disruption of normal propulsive activity in the GI tract) secondary to abdominal surgery. Treatment with such agents facilitates recovery of normal bowel function and leaves the analgesic (CNS) activity of the postoperative opiate intact (Vaughan-Shaw et al., 2012).

Alvimopan. Alvimopan is an MOR antagonist with quaternary amino group that restricts the distribution of the drug to the periphery. The drug has a high affinity for MOR of 0.4 nM. Following oral administration, a deamidated metabolite of alvimopam slowly and variably appears in the bloodstream and is attributed to activity of the intestinal microbiome. This metabolite is also an MOR antagonist (Ki = 0.8 nM). The parent drug appears to enter an enterohepatic cycle coupled to deamidation in the GI tract; both parent drug and metabolite have terminal half-lives of 10–18 h. The drug, as the deamidated metabolite, is excreted in the feces and urine. Alvimopan is FDA-approved for treatment of postoperative ileus in patients with less than 7 days of opioid exposure immediately prior to beginning alvimopan (usually 12 mg administered just prior to surgery and 12 mg twice daily for 7 days). This agent carries a black-box warning about increased incidence of myocardial infarction with prolonged use and thus is available only for short-term use (15 doses) through a restricted program.

Management of Abuse Syndromes. There has been interest in the use of opiate antagonists such as naltrexone and nalmefene (not available in the U.S.) as adjuvants in treating a variety of nonopioid dependency syndromes, such as alcoholism (see Chapters 23 and 24), where an opiate antagonist may decrease the rate of relapse (Anton, 2008). Interestingly, patients with a single-nucleotide polymorphism in the MOR gene have significantly lower relapse rates to alcoholism when treated with naltrexone (Haile et al., 2008). Naltrexone is FDA-approved for treatment of alcohol dependence, to block the effects of exogenously administered opioids, and for the prevention of relapse to opioid dependence following detoxification. Naltrexone in combination with bupropion is also FDA-approved as an adjunct for weight management in patients with obesity.

Centrally Active Antitussives

Cough is a useful physiological mechanism that serves to clear the respiratory passages of foreign material and excess secretions; it should not be suppressed indiscriminately. There are, however, situations in which cough does not serve any useful purpose but may, instead, annoy the patient, prevent rest and sleep, or hinder adherence to otherwise-beneficial medication regimens (e.g., ACE inhibitor–induced cough). In such situations, the physician should try to substitute a drug with a different side-effect profile (e.g., an AT_1 antagonist in place of an ACE inhibitor) or add an antitussive agent that will reduce the frequency or intensity of the coughing. A number of drugs reduce cough as a result of their central actions, including opioid analgesics, of which codeine and hydrocodone are most commonly used. Cough suppression often occurs with lower doses of opioids than those needed for analgesia. A 10- or 20-mg oral dose of codeine, although ineffective for analgesia, produces a demonstrable antitussive effect, and higher doses produce even more suppression of chronic cough. A few other antitussive agents are noted next.

Dextromethorphan

Dextromethorphan (D-3-methoxy-*N*-methylmorphinan) is the D-isomer of the codeine analogue methorphan; however, unlike the L-isomer, it has no analgesic or addictive properties and does not act through opioid receptors. Rather, the drug acts centrally to elevate the threshold for coughing. Its effectiveness in patients with pathological cough has been demonstrated in controlled studies; its potency is nearly equal to that of codeine, but dextromethorphan produces fewer subjective and GI side effects. In therapeutic dosages, the drug does not inhibit ciliary activity, and its antitussive effects persist for 5–6 h. Its toxicity is low, but extremely high doses may produce CNS depression. The average adult dosage of dextromethorphan hydrobromide is 10–20 mg every 4 h or 30 mg every 6–8 h, not to exceed 120 mg daily. The drug is marketed for over-the-counter sale in liquids, syrups, capsules, soluble strips, lozenges, and freezer pops or in combinations with antihistamines, bronchodilators, expectorants, and decongestants. An extended-release dextromethorphan suspension is approved for twice-daily administration.

Although dextromethorphan is known to function as an NMDA receptor antagonist, the dextromethorphan binding sites are not limited to the known distribution of NMDA receptors. Naloxone antagonizes the antitussive effects of codeine but not those of dextromethorphan. Thus, the mechanisms by which dextromethorphan exerts its antitussive effects still are not clear. Pharmacological cough suppression can apparently be achieved by a variety of mechanisms.

Other Antitussives

Pholcodine [3-*O*-(2-morpholinoethyl) morphine] is used clinically in many countries outside the U.S. Although structurally related to the opioids, pholcodine has no opioid-like actions. Pholcodine is at least as effective as codeine as an antitussive; it has a long $t_{1/2}$ and can be given once or twice daily.

Benzonatate is a long-chain polyglycol derivative chemically related to procaine and believed to exert its antitussive action on stretch or cough receptors in the lung, as well as by a central mechanism. It is available in oral capsules. The dosage is 100 mg three times daily; doses as high as 600 mg daily have been used safely.

Routes of Analgesic Drug Administration

In addition to the traditional oral and parenteral formulations for opioids, many other methods of administration have been developed in an effort to improve therapeutic efficacy while minimizing side effects.

Patient-Controlled Analgesia

With PCA, the patient has limited control of the dosing of opioid from an infusion pump programmed within tightly mandated parameters. PCA can be used for intravenous, subcutaneous, epidural, or intrathecal administration of opioids. This technique avoids delays inherent in administration by a caregiver and generally permits better alignment between pain control and individual differences in pain perception and responsiveness to opioids. The PCA technique also gives the patient a greater sense of control over the pain. With shorter-acting opioids, serious toxicity or excessive use rarely occurs; however, caution is warranted due to the potential for serious medication errors associated with this delivery method. PCA is suitable for adults and children capable of understanding the principles involved. It is generally conceded that PCA is preferred over intramuscular injections for postoperative pain control.

Spinal Delivery

Administration of opioids into the epidural or intrathecal spaces provides more direct access to the first pain-processing synapse in the dorsal horn of the spinal cord. This permits the use of doses substantially lower than those required for oral or parenteral administration (Table 20–5). In postoperative pain management, sustained-release epidural injections are accomplished through the incorporation of morphine into a liposomal formulation, providing up to 48 h of pain relief (Hartrick and Hartrick, 2008). The management of chronic pain with spinal opiates has been addressed by the use of chronically implanted intrathecal catheters connected to subcutaneously implanted refillable pumps (Yaksh et al., 2017).

Epidural and intrathecal opioids have their own dose-dependent side effects, such as pruritus, nausea, vomiting, respiratory depression, and urinary retention. *Hydrophilic opioids* such as morphine have longer residence times in the CSF. As a consequence, after intrathecal or epidural morphine, respiratory depression can be delayed for as long as 24 h after a bolus dose. Given their more rapid clearance, the risk of *delayed* respiratory depression is reduced, *but not eliminated,* with *opioids that are more lipophilic*.

Extreme vigilance and appropriate monitoring are required for all opioid-naïve patients receiving intraspinal narcotics. Use of intraspinal opioids in the opioid-naïve patient is reserved for postoperative pain control in an inpatient monitored setting. Epidural administration of opioids has become popular in the management of postoperative pain and for providing analgesia during labor and delivery. Lower systemic opioid levels are achieved with epidural opioids, leading to less placental transfer and less potential for respiratory depression of the newborn. Many opioids and other adjuvants are commonly used for neuraxial administration in adults and children; however, the majority of agents employed have not undergone appropriate preclinical safety evaluation and approval for these clinical indications; thus, such uses are "off label." Thus, at this time, those agents approved for spinal delivery are certain preservative-free formulations of morphine sulfate and sufentanil. It is important to remember that the spinal route of delivery represents a novel environment wherein the neuraxis may be exposed to exceedingly high concentrations of an agent for an extended period of time and safety by another route (e.g., oral, intravenous) may not translate to safety after spinal delivery (Yaksh and Allen, 2004).

Patients on chronic spinal opioid therapy are less likely to experience respiratory depression. Selected patients who fail conservative therapies for chronic pain may receive intraspinal opioids chronically through an implanted programmable pump. Analogous to the relationship between systemic opioids and NSAIDs, intraspinal narcotics often are combined with other agents that include local anesthetics, N-type Ca^{2+} channel blockers (e.g., ziconotide), α_2 adrenergic agonists, and $GABA_B$ agonists. This permits synergy between drugs with different mechanisms, allowing the use of lower concentrations of both agents, minimizing side effects and the opioid-induced complications (Yaksh et al., 2017).

Use of intraspinal opioids in the opioid-naïve patient is reserved for postoperative pain control in an inpatient monitored setting. Epidural administration of opioids has become popular in the management of postoperative pain and for providing analgesia during labor and delivery. Lower systemic opioid levels are achieved with epidural opioids, leading to less placental transfer and less potential for respiratory depression of the newborn. Agents approved for spinal delivery are *specific preservative-free formulations* of morphine sulfate. A hydromorphone formulation is currently in clinical trials. The spinal route of delivery represents a novel environment wherein the neuraxis may be exposed to exceedingly high concentrations of an agent for an extended period of time. Safety as defined by another route of administration (e.g., oral, intravenous) may not translate temporally or dose-wise to safety after spinal delivery.

An important side effect associated with continued infusion of high concentrations of several opiates is formation of a space-occupying mass (a granuloma) at the catheter tip in the intrathecal space. These granulomas arise from meningeal mast cell degranulation and are the result of meningeal-derived fibroblast proliferation though an effect independent of an opioid receptor (Eddinger et al., 2016). The consequence of the spinal cord compression and neurologic sequelae may require discontinuation of spinal delivery and, in the extreme case, surgical removal of the mass (Deer, 2017).

Rectal Administration

The rectal route is an alternative for patients with difficulty swallowing or other oral pathology and who prefer a less invasive route than parenteral administration. This route is not well tolerated by most children. Onset of action is within 10 min. In the U.S., only morphine, hydromorphone, and opium (in combination with belladonna) are available in rectal suppository formulations.

Oral Transmucosal Administration

Opioids can be absorbed through the oral mucosa more rapidly than through the stomach. Bioavailability is greater owing to avoidance of first-pass metabolism, and lipophilic opioids are absorbed better by this

TABLE 20–5 ■ EPIDURAL OR INTRATHECAL OPIOIDS FOR THE TREATMENT OF ACUTE (BOLUS) OR CHRONIC (INFUSION) PAIN

DRUG	SINGLE DOSE (mg)[a]	INFUSION RATE (mg/h)[b]	ONSET (min)	DURATION OF EFFECT OF SINGLE DOSE (h)[c]
Epidural				
Morphine	1–6	0.1–1.0	30	6–24
Meperidine	20–150	5–20	5	4–8
Methadone	1–10	0.3–0.5	10	6–10
Hydromorphone	1–2	0.1–0.2	15	10–16
Fentanyl	0.025–0.1	0.025–0.10	5	2–4
Sufentanil	0.01–0.06	0.01–0.05	5	2–4
Alfentanil	0.5–1	0.2	15	1–3
Subarachnoid (Intrathecal)				
Morphine	0.1–0.3		15	8–24+
Fentanyl	0.005–0.025		5	3–6

[a]Low doses may be effective when administered to the elderly or when injected in the thoracic region.
[b]If combining with a local anesthetic, consider using 0.0625% bupivacaine.
[c]Duration of analgesia varies widely; higher doses produce longer duration. With the exception of epidural/intrathecal morphine or epidural sufentanil, all other spinal opioid use is considered to be off label.
Source: Adapted and updated from Ready LB, Edwards WT, eds. *Management of Acute Pain: A Practical Guide*. International Association for Study of Pain, Seattle, **1992**.

route than are hydrophilic compounds such as morphine. A variety of formulations of fentanyl are available for oral transmucosal use: Suspensions of fentanyl in a dissolvable sugar-based lollipop or rapidly dissolving buccal tablet, a buccal fentanyl "film," and a sublingual fentanyl tablet are approved for the treatment of cancer pain. In this setting, transmucosal fentanyl relieves pain within 15 min, and patients easily can titrate the appropriate dose.

Transnasal Administration

Butorphanol, a KOR agonist/MOR antagonist, has been employed intranasally. A transnasal, pectin-based, metered fentanyl spray is FDA-approved for the treatment of breakthrough cancer pain. Administration is well tolerated, and pain relief occurs within 10 min of delivery.

Transdermal Administration

Transdermal fentanyl patches are approved for use in sustained pain. The opioid permeates the skin, and a "depot" is established in the *stratum corneum* layer (see Figure 70–1). However, fever and external heat sources (heating pads, hot baths) can increase absorption of fentanyl and potentially lead to an overdose.

This modality is well suited for cancer pain treatment because of its ease of use, prolonged duration of action, and stable blood levels. It may take up to 12 h to develop analgesia and up to 16 h to observe full clinical effect. Plasma levels stabilize after two sequential patch applications, and the kinetics do not appear to change with repeated applications (Portenoy et al., 1993). However, there may be substantial variability in plasma levels after a given dose. The plasma $t_{1/2}$ after patch removal is about 17 h. If excessive sedation or respiratory depression occurs, antagonist infusions may need to be maintained for an extended period. Dermatological side effects from the patches, such as rash and itching, usually are mild. Opiate-addicted patients have been known to chew the patches and receive an overdose, sometimes with fatal outcomes, following rapid and efficient buccal and sublingual absorption.

Therapeutic Considerations in Pain Control

Given its profound impact on patient physiology and quality of life, the management of pain must be an important element in any therapeutic intervention. Failure to adequately manage pain can have important negative consequences on physiological function, such as autonomic hyperreactivity (increased blood pressure, heart rate, suppression of GI motility, reduced secretions); and reduced mobility, leading to deconditioning, muscle wasting, joint stiffening, and decalcification; and can contribute to deleterious changes in the psychological state (depression, helplessness syndromes, anxiety). By many hospital-accrediting organizations, and by law in many states, appropriate pain assessment and adequate pain management are considered to be standard of care, with pain considered the "fifth vital sign."

Acute Pain States

In acute pain states, opioids will reduce the intensity of pain. However, physical signs (such as abdominal rigidity with an acute abdomen) generally will remain. Relief of pain can facilitate history taking and examination in the emergency room and the patient's ability to tolerate diagnostic procedures. In most cases, analgesics should not be withheld for fear of obscuring the progression of underlying disease.

Chronic Pain States

The problems that arise in the relief of pain associated with chronic conditions are more complex. Repeated daily administration of opioid analgesics eventually will produce tolerance and some degree of physical dependence. The degree will depend on the particular drug, the frequency of administration, the quantity administered, the genetic predisposition, and the psychosocial status of the patient. The decision to control any chronic symptom, especially pain, by the repeated administration of an opioid must be made carefully. When pain is due to chronic nonmalignant disease, conservative measures using nonopioid drugs should be tried before resorting to the opioids. Such measures include the use of NSAIDs, local nerve blocks, antidepressant drugs, electrical stimulation, acupuncture, hypnosis, and behavioral modification. In end-of-life care, the analgesia, tranquility, and even euphoria afforded by the use of opioids can make the final days of life far less distressing for patient and family. Although physical dependence and tolerance may develop, this possibility should not prevent physicians from fulfilling their primary obligation to ease the patient's discomfort. The physician should not wait until the pain becomes agonizing; no patient should ever wish for death because of a physician's reluctance to use adequate amounts of effective opioids. This sometimes may entail the regular use of opioid analgesics in substantial doses. Such patients, while they may be physically dependent, are not "addicts" even though they may need large doses on a regular basis. As noted, physical dependence is not equivalent to addiction.

Guidelines for Opiate Dosing

The World Health Organization provides a three-step ladder as a guide to treat both cancer pain and chronic noncancer pain (Table 20–6). The three-step ladder encourages the use of more conservative therapies before initiating opioid therapy. Weaker opioids can be supplanted by stronger opioids in cases of moderate and severe pain. Antidepressants such as duloxetine and amitriptyline that are used in the treatment of chronic neuropathic pain have limited intrinsic analgesic actions in acute pain; however, antidepressants may enhance morphine-induced analgesia. In the presence of severe pain, the opioids should be considered sooner rather than later.

There has been a growing concern over the appropriate use of opiates in pain management. Since the last edition of this textbook, there has been increasing scrutiny of the use of opioids to treat chronic pain due to the high correlation between prescription opioids and opioid abuse. Drug overdose has become the leading cause of accidental death in the U.S., driven by opioid addiction (NIDA, 2017; Rudd et al., 2016). These circumstances have led to several changes in the use of opioids in the U.S.:

- the rescheduling of hydrocodone to schedule II
- an FDA mandate that all ER/LA opioids fall under the Risk Evaluation and Mitigation Strategy, a classification reserved for "high-risk pharmaceuticals"

TABLE 20–6 ■ WORLD HEALTH ORGANIZATION ANALGESIC LADDER

Step 1 Mild-to-Moderate Pain Nonopioid ± adjuvant agent • Acetaminophen or an NSAID should be used, unless contraindicated. Adjuvant agents are those that enhance analgesic efficacy, treat concurrent symptoms that exacerbate pain, or provide independent analgesic activity for specific types of pain.
Step 2 Mild-to-Moderate Pain or Pain Uncontrolled After Step 1 Short-acting opioid as required ± nonopioid ATC ± adjuvant agent • Morphine, oxycodone, or hydromorphone should be added to acetaminophen or an NSAID for maximum flexibility of opioid dose.
Step 3 Moderate-to-Severe Pain or Pain Uncontrolled After Step 2 Sustained-release/long-acting opioid ATC or continuous infusion + short-acting opioid as required ± nonopioid ± adjuvant agent • Sustained-release oxycodone, morphine, oxymorphone, or transdermal fentanyl is indicated.

Source: Adapted from http://www.who.int/cancer/palliative/painladder/en/.

- the FDA's relabeling of all ER/LA opioids with a black-box warning that highlights the risks of addiction, abuse, misuse, overdose, and death; the risk of fatal respiratory depression on initiation or increase of dose; the necessity of swallowing, not chewing, an oral opioid formulation; the danger of accidental consumption, especially by children; for pregnant women who require opioids, possible requirement for treatment of neonatal opioid withdrawal syndrome and danger of life-threatening fetal opioid withdrawal syndrome with prolonged maternal use; and any adverse interactions with ethanol
- an updating by the FDA of postmarketing surveillance requirements for opioid analgesics, especially for ER/LA opioid analgesics
- the release by the CDC of new chronic opioid treatment guidelines (Dowell et al., 2016), as summarized by Table 20–7

The CDC guidelines were in response to an increasing number of deaths related to opioid overdose (of both prescription and illicit opioids), which exceeded 33,000 in 2015. The new guidelines are intended for primary care physicians who prescribe opioids to treat chronic pain. The guidelines stress the primary use of nonopioid pharmacotherapy, avoidance of ER/LA opioids in favor of immediate-release agents, and frequent and persistent follow-up by the prescribing physician. Methadone dosing is considered separately in Table 20–8. Suggestions for the oral and parenteral dosing of commonly used opioids (see Table 20–2) must be appreciated as representing only guidelines. Such guidelines are typically based on the use of these agents in the management of acute (e.g., postoperative) pain in opioid-naïve patients. A number of factors contribute to the dosing requirement (see the discussion that follows).

Variables Modifying the Therapeutic Use of Opiates

Patient Variability

There is substantial individual variability in the response to opioids. Thus, a standard intramuscular dose of 10 mg morphine sulfate will relieve severe pain adequately in two of three patients but will not suffice in one of three patients. Similarly, the minimal effective analgesic concentration for opioids, such as morphine, meperidine (pethidine), alfentanil, and sufentanil, varies among patients by factors of 5–10. Adjustments must be made based on clinical response. Appropriate therapeutics typically involve undertaking a treatment strategy that most efficiently addresses the pain state, minimizes the potential for undesired drug effects, and accounts for the variables described next that can influence an individual patient's response to opiate analgesia.

TABLE 20–7 ■ SUMMARY OF CDC RECOMMENDATIONS FOR PRESCRIBING OPIOIDS FOR CHRONIC PAIN

Determining When to Initiate or Continue Opioids for Chronic Pain

- Nonpharmacological therapy and nonopioid pharmacologic therapy are preferred for chronic pain. Consider opioid therapy only if expected benefits for both pain and function are anticipated to outweigh risks to the patient. If opioids are used, combine them with nonpharmacological therapy and nonopioid pharmacotherapy, as appropriate.
- Before starting opioid therapy for chronic pain, establish treatment goals with the patient, including realistic goals for pain and function. Consider how therapy will be discontinued if benefits do not outweigh risks. Continue opioid therapy only if there is clinically meaningful improvement in pain and function that outweighs risks to patient safety.
- Before starting and periodically during opioid therapy, discuss with patient the known risks and realistic benefits of opioid therapy and patient and clinician responsibilities for managing therapy.

Opioid Selection, Dosage, Duration, Follow-Up, and Discontinuation

- When starting opioid therapy for chronic pain, prescribe immediate-release opioids instead of ER/LA opioids.
- When opioids are started, prescribe the lowest effective dosage. Use caution when prescribing opioids at any dosage. Reassess evidence of individual benefits and risks when increasing dosage to ≥ 50 MME/d. Avoid increasing dosage to ≥ 90 MME/d or carefully justify a decision to exceed this limit.
- Long-term opioid use often begins with treatment of acute pain. When opioids are used for acute pain, prescribe the lowest effective dose of immediate-release opioids and in no greater quantity than needed for the expected duration of pain severe enough to require opioids. Three days or less will often be sufficient; more than 7 days will rarely be needed.
- Reevaluate benefits and harms of opioids with the patient within 1 to 4 weeks of starting opioid therapy for chronic pain or of dose escalation and thereafter every 3 months or more frequently. If benefits do not outweigh harms of continued opioid therapy, optimize other therapies and work with the patient to taper opioids to lower dosages or to taper and discontinue opioids.

Assessing Risk and Addressing Harms of Opioid Use

- Incorporate into the management plan strategies to mitigate risk, including considering offering naloxone when factors that increase risk for opioid overdose, such as history of overdose, history of substance use disorder, higher opioid dosages (≥50 MME/d), or concurrent benzodiazepine use are present.
- Review the patient's history of controlled substance prescriptions using state PDMP data to determine whether the patient is receiving opioid dosages or dangerous combinations that carry high risk for overdose. Review PDMP data when starting opioid therapy for chronic pain and periodically during opioid therapy for chronic pain, ranging from every prescription to every 3 months.
- When prescribing opioids for chronic pain, use urine drug testing before starting opioid therapy and consider urine drug testing at least annually to assess for prescribed medications and other controlled prescription drugs and illicit drugs.
- Avoid prescribing opioid pain medication and benzodiazepines concurrently whenever possible.
- Offer or arrange evidence-based treatment (usually medication-assisted treatment with buprenorphine or methadone in combination with behavioral therapies) for a patient with opioid use disorder.

Note: Excluding active cancer, palliative, and end-of-life care.

Source: Adapted from Dowell D, et al. CDC guideline for prescribing opioids for chronic pain—United States, 2016. *MMWR Recomm Rep* **2016**, 65(RR-1):1–49. doi: http://dx.doi.org/10.15585/mmwr.rr6501e1. Accessed May 4, 2017.

TABLE 20-8 ■ MORPHINE MILLIGRAM EQUIVALENT (MME) DOSES FOR COMMONLY PRESCRIBED OPIOIDS

OPIOID	CONVERSION FACTOR[a]
Codeine	0.15
Fentanyl transdermal (in μg/h)	2.4
Hydrocodone	1
Hydromorphone	4
Methadone	
1–20 mg/d	4
21–40 mg/d	8
41–60 mg/d	10
≥61–80 mg/d	12
Morphine	1
Oxycodone	1.5
Oxymorphone	3

[a]Multiply the dose for each opioid by the conversion factor to determine the dose in MMEs. For example, tablets containing hydrocodone 5 mg and acetaminophen 300 mg taken four times a day would contain a total of 20 mg of hydrocodone daily, equivalent to 20 MME daily; extended-release tablets containing oxycodone 10 mg taken twice a day would contain a total of 20 mg of oxycodone daily, equivalent to 30 MME daily. Note the following precautions: (1) All doses are in milligrams/day except for fentanyl, which is micrograms/hour. (2) Equianalgesic dose conversions are only estimates and cannot account for individual variability in genetics and pharmacokinetics. (3) Do not use the calculated dose in MMEs to determine the doses to use when converting one opioid to another; when converting opioids, the new opioid is typically dosed at substantially lower than the calculated MME dose to avoid accidental overdose due to incomplete cross-tolerance and individual variability in opioid pharmacokinetics. (4) Use particular caution with methadone dose conversions because the conversion factor increases at higher doses. (5) Use particular caution with fentanyl because it is dosed in micrograms/hour instead of milligrams/day, and its absorption is affected by heat and other factors.

Source: Dowell D, et al. CDC guideline for prescribing opioids for chronic pain—United States, 2016. *MMWR Recomm Rep* **2016**, *65*(No. RR-1):1–49. doi:http://dx.doi.org/10.15585/mmwr.rr6501e1. Accessed May 4, 2017.

Adapted by the CDC from Von Korff M, et al. *Clin J Pain*, **2008**, *24*:521–527 and Washington State Interagency Guideline on Prescribing Opioids for Pain (http://www.agencymeddirectors.wa.gov/Files/2015AMDGOpioidGuideline.pdf).

Pain

Pain Intensity

Increased pain intensity may require titrating doses to produce acceptable analgesia with tolerable side effects.

Type of Pain State

Systems underlying a pain state may be broadly categorized as being mediated by events secondary to injury and inflammation and by injury to the sensory afferent or nervous system. Neuropathic conditions may be less efficaciously managed by opiates than pain secondary to tissue injury and inflammation. Such pain states are more efficiently managed by combination treatment modalities.

Acuity and Chronicity of Pain

In chronic pain states, the daily course of the pain may fluctuate, for example, being greater in the morning hours or on awakening. Arthritic states display flares that are associated with an exacerbated pain condition. Changes in the magnitude of pain occur during the daily routine, resulting in "breakthrough pain" during episodic events such as dressing changes (incident pain). These examples emphasize the need for individualized management of increased or decreased pain levels with baseline analgesic dosing supplemented with the use of short-acting "rescue" medications as required. In the face of ongoing severe pain, analgesics should be dosed in continuous or "around-the-clock" fashion rather than on an as-needed basis. This provides more consistent analgesic levels and avoids unnecessary suffering.

Opioid Tolerance

Chronic exposure to one opiate agonist typically leads to a reduction in the efficacy of other opiate agonists. The degree of tolerance can be remarkable. For example, 10 mg of an oral opioid (such as morphine) is considered a high dose for a treatment-naïve individual, whereas 100 mg IV may produce only minor sedation in a severely tolerant individual.

Patient Physical State and Genetic Variables

Codeine, hydrocodone, and oxycodone are weak analgesic prodrugs that are metabolized into the much more effective analgesic drugs morphine, hydromorphone, and oxymorphone, respectively, by CYP2D6 (Supernaw, 2001). CYP2D6 activity is genetically diminished in 7% of whites, 3% of blacks, and 1% of Asians (Eichelbaum and Evert, 1996), rendering oxycodone, hydrocodone, and codeine relatively ineffective analgesics in these "poor metabolizers" and potentially toxic for "ultrarapid" metabolizers.

The activity of CYP2D6 is inhibited by SSRIs, which may render opioids less effective as analgesics in some patients. Whereas diminished activity of the CYP2D6 isoenzyme will lead to less efficacy of prodrug opioids, the opposite occurs with methadone. Although methadone is primarily metabolized by CYP3A4, other CYPs participate, and genetic polymorphisms involving deficiencies in the CYPs 2B6 and 2D6 may lead to high methadone C_p values (Zhou et al., 2009).

Opioids are highly protein bound, and factors such as plasma pH may dramatically change binding. In addition, AAG is an acute-phase reactant protein that is elevated in cancer patients and has a high affinity for basic drugs such as methadone and meperidine. Morphine and meperidine should be avoided in patients with renal impairment because morphine-6-glucuronide (a metabolite of morphine) and normeperidine (a metabolite of meperidine) are excreted by the kidney and will accumulate and lead to toxicity. Other states that may increase the risk of adverse effects of the opioids include COPD, sleep apnea, dementia, benign prostatic hypertrophy, unstable gait, and pretreatment constipation.

Routes of Administration

Typically, one chooses the least invasive routes, such as oral, buccal, or transdermal delivery, to facilitate patient compliance. Intravenous routes are more useful in pre- and post-operative in-hospital pain management and during end-of-life care. Patients with chronic pain states where side effects from systemic drug exposure are intolerable may be candidates for chronic spinal drug delivery, requiring surgery for indwelling catheterization and pump placement.

Dose Selection and Titration

The conservative approach to initiating chronic opioid therapy suggests starting with low doses that may be incremented on the basis of the pharmacokinetics of the drug. In chronic pain states, the aim would be to use long-acting medications to permit once- or twice-daily dosing (e.g., controlled-release formulations or methadone). Such agents reach steady state slowly. Rapid incrementation is to be avoided, and rescue medication should be made available for breakthrough pain during initial dosing titration.

Opioid Rotation

Changing to a different opioid, when the patient fails to achieve benefit or side effects become limiting before analgesia is sufficient, is widely employed. Failure or intolerance of one opioid cannot necessarily predict the patient's response or acceptance to another (Quang-Cantagrel et al., 2000). Practically, opioid rotation involves incrementing the dose of a given opioid (e.g., morphine) to a level limited by side effects and insufficient analgesia and then substituting an alternate opioid medication at an equieffective dose. Agents typically involved in such rotation sequences are various oral opioids (e.g., morphine, methadone, dilaudid, oxycodone) and the fentanyl patch systems. Care must be taken to titrate the doses and monitor the patient closely during such drug transitions.

TABLE 20–9 ■ SUMMARY OF DRUG TARGET AND SITE OF ACTION OF COMMON DRUG CLASSES AND RELATIVE EFFICACY BY PAIN STATE

DRUG CLASS (example)	DRUG ACTION	SITE OF ACTION[a]	RELATIVE EFFICACY IN PAIN STATES[a]
NSAIDs (ibuprofen, aspirin, acetaminophen)	Nonspecific COX inhibitors	Peripheral and spinal	Tissue injury >> acute stimuli = nerve injury = 0 (Chapter 38)
COX-2 inhibitor (celecoxib)	COX-2–selective inhibitor	Peripheral and spinal	Tissue injury >> acute stimuli = nerve injury = 0 (Chapter 38)
Opioids (morphine)	μ receptor agonist	Supraspinal and spinal	Tissue injury = acute stimuli ≥ nerve injury > 0 (see this chapter)
Anticonvulsants (gabapentin)	Na^+ channel block, $\alpha_2\delta$ subunit of Ca^{2+} channel	Supraspinal and spinal	Nerve injury > tissue injury = acute stimuli = 0 (Chapter 17)
Tricyclic antidepressants (amitryptiline)	Inhibit uptake of 5HT/NE	Supraspinal and spinal	Nerve injury ≥ tissue injury >> acute stimuli = 0 (Chapters 15 and 19)

[a]As defined by studies in preclinical models.

Combination Therapy

In general, the use of combinations of drugs with the same pharmacological kinetic profile is not warranted (e.g., morphine plus methadone). The same holds if the drugs have overlapping targets and opposing effects (e.g., combining an MOR agonist with an agent having mixed agonist/antagonist properties). On the other hand, certain opiate combinations are useful. For example, in a chronic pain state with periodic incident or breakthrough pain, the patient might receive a slow-release formulation of morphine for baseline pain relief, and the acute incident (breakthrough) pain may be managed with a rapid-onset/short-lasting formulation such as buccal fentanyl. For inflammatory or nociceptive pain, opioids may be usefully combined with other analgesic agents, such as acetaminophen or other NSAIDs (Table 20–9). In some situations, NSAIDs can provide analgesia equal to that produced by 60 mg codeine. In the case of neuropathic pain, other drug classes may be useful alone or in combination with an opiate. For example, antidepressants that block amine reuptake, such as amitriptyline or duloxetine, and anticonvulsants such as gabapentin may enhance the analgesic effect and may be synergistic in some pain states.

Nonanalgesic Therapeutic Uses of Opioids

Dyspnea

Morphine is used to alleviate the dyspnea of acute left ventricular failure and pulmonary edema, and the patient's response to intravenous morphine may be dramatic. The mechanism underlying this pronounced relief is not clear. It may involve an alteration of the patient's reaction to impaired respiratory function and an indirect reduction of the work of the heart owing to reduced fear and apprehension. However, it is more probable that the major benefit is due to cardiovascular effects, such as decreased peripheral resistance secondary to histamine release and an increased capacity of the peripheral and splanchnic vascular compartments. Nitroglycerin, which also causes vasodilation, may be superior to morphine in this condition. In patients with normal blood gases but severe breathlessness owing to chronic obstruction of airflow ("pink puffers"), dihydrocodeine, 16 mg orally before exercise, reduces the feeling of breathlessness and increases exercise tolerance. Nonetheless, opioids generally are contraindicated in pulmonary edema unless severe pain is also present.

Anesthetic Adjuvants

High doses of opioids, notably fentanyl and sufentanil, are widely used as the primary anesthetic agents in many surgical procedures. They have powerful "MAC-sparing" effects; for example, they reduce the concentrations of volatile anesthetic otherwise required to produce an adequate anesthetic depth (see Chapter 21). Although respiration is so depressed that physical assistance is required, patients can retain consciousness. Therefore, when using an opioid as the primary anesthetic agent, it is used in conjunction with an agent that results in unconsciousness and produces amnesia, such as the benzodiazepines or lower concentrations of volatile anesthetics. High doses of opiate as employed in the operating room setting also result in prominent rigidity of the chest wall and masseters, requiring concurrent treatment with muscle relaxants to permit intubations and ventilation.

Acute Opioid Toxicity

Acute opioid toxicity may result from clinical overdosage, accidental overdosage, or attempts at suicide. Occasionally, a delayed type of toxicity may occur from the injection of an opioid into chilled skin areas or in patients with low blood pressure and shock. The drug is not fully absorbed; therefore, a subsequent dose may be given. When normal circulation is restored, an excessive amount may be absorbed suddenly. In nontolerant individuals, serious toxicity with methadone may follow the oral ingestion of 40–60 mg. In the case of morphine, a normal, pain-free adult is not likely to die after oral doses less than 120 mg or to have serious toxicity with less than 30 mg parenterally.

Symptoms and Diagnosis

The triad of coma, pinpoint pupils, and depressed respiration strongly suggests opioid poisoning. The patient who has taken an overdose of an opioid usually is stuporous or, if a large overdose has been taken, may be in a profound coma. The respiratory rate will be very low, or the patient may be apneic, and possibly cyanotic. If adequate oxygenation is restored early, the blood pressure will improve; if hypoxia persists untreated, there may be capillary damage, and measures to combat shock may be required. The pupils will be symmetrical and pinpoint in size; however, if hypoxia is severe, they may be dilated. Urine formation is depressed. Body temperature falls, and the skin becomes cold and clammy. The skeletal muscles are flaccid, the jaw is relaxed, and the tongue may fall back and block the airway. Frank convulsions occasionally may be noted in infants and children. When death occurs, it is nearly always from respiratory failure. Even if respiration is restored, death still may occur as a result of complications that develop during the period of coma, such as pneumonia or shock. Noncardiogenic pulmonary edema is seen commonly with opioid poisoning.

Treatment

The first step is to establish a patent airway and ventilate the patient. Opioid antagonists can produce dramatic reversal of the severe respiratory depression, and the antagonist naloxone is the treatment of choice. However, care should be taken to avoid precipitating withdrawal in dependent patients, who may be extremely sensitive to antagonists. The safest approach is to dilute the standard naloxone dose (0.4 mg) and slowly administer it intravenously, monitoring arousal and respiratory function. With care, it usually is possible to reverse the respiratory depression without precipitating a major withdrawal syndrome. If no response is seen with the first dose, additional doses can be given. Patients should be observed for rebound increases in sympathetic nervous system activity, which may result in cardiac arrhythmias and pulmonary edema. For reversing opioid poisoning in children, the initial dose of naloxone is 0.01 mg/kg. If no effect is seen after a total dose of 10 mg, one can reasonably question the role of an opiate in the diagnosis. Pulmonary edema sometimes associated with opioid overdosage may be countered by positive-pressure respiration. Tonic-clonic seizures, occasionally seen as part of the toxic syndrome with meperidine and tramadol, are ameliorated by treatment with naloxone.

The presence of general CNS depressants does not prevent the salutary effect of naloxone, and in cases of mixed intoxications, the situation will be improved largely owing to antagonism of the respiratory-depressant effects of the opioid (however, some evidence indicates that naloxone and naltrexone may also antagonize some of the depressant actions of sedative-hypnotics). One need not attempt to restore the patient to full consciousness. The duration of action of the available antagonists is shorter than that of many opioids; hence, patients can slip back into coma (e.g., renarcotization). This is particularly important when the overdosage is due to methadone. The depressant effects of these drugs may persist for 24–72 h, and fatalities have occurred as a result of premature discontinuation of naloxone. In cases of overdoses of these drugs, a continuous infusion of naloxone should be considered. Toxicity from overdose of pentazocine and other opioids with mixed actions may require higher doses of naloxone.

Novel Nonopioid Treatments for Pain

Myriad marine toxins target GPCRs, neurotransmitter transporters, and ion channels; a number (i.e., tetrodotoxin, saxitoxin, kainic acid, and various venoms from cone snails) have been useful to basic scientists (Sakai and Swanson 2014). One that has become an FDA-approved treatment of chronic pain is ziconotide.

Ziconotide

Ziconotide is a synthetic copy of a neuroactive cone snail toxin, a 25–amino acid basic polypeptide with three disulfide bridges. The molecule is hydrophilic and readily soluble in water and isotonic saline.

Mechanism of Action

Ziconotide binds to and blocks N-type Ca^{2+} channels on nociceptive afferents in the dorsal horn of the spinal cord. This leads to blockade of the release of excitatory neurotransmitter involved in nociception (Patel et al., 2017).

ADME

Ziconotide is administered intrathecally as a continuous infusion by a controlled microinfusion pump. The toxin's serum $t_{1/2}$ is 1.3 h; the $t_{1/2}$ in CSF is 4.6 h. The volume distribution in CSF approximates the total CSF volume, 140 mL. Ziconotide is stable in CSF but, following passage from the CSF into the systemic circulation, is metabolized by endo- and exopeptidases that are widely expressed in most tissues.

Therapeutic Use

Ziconotide is used to treat severe chronic pain in adults for whom intrathecal therapy is warranted and for whom other treatments have failed or are not suitable (allergy, etc.). The dosing should follow the FDA-approved schedule, titrating upward from 2.4 μg/d in increments of 2.4 μg no more than two or three times weekly to the maximum recommended intrathecal dose of 19.2 μg/d.

Adverse Effects and Precautions

Side effects include dizziness, nausea, confusion, nystagmus, anxiety, confusion, and blurred vision. Hallucinations and paranoia can occur; thus, ziconotide is contraindicated in patients with a preexisting history of psychosis. Inadvertent intravenous or epidural administration of ziconotide will cause hypotension. The analgesic effects of ziconotide appear to add with those of morphine; in laboratory experiments, intrathecal ziconotide potentiated the GI effects of morphine but not the respiratory depressant effects. Ziconotide is not an opiate, and its effects cannot be reversed by naloxone. Treatment of overdose is withdrawal of the agent and supportive care in a hospital. The agent is classified in pregnancy category C. The difficulties of long-term intrathecal delivery, the production of state-independent blockade, and the side-effect profile have been barriers to use of ziconotide (Patel et al., 2017).

Drug Facts for Your Personal Formulary: *Opioid Agonists and Antagonists*

Drug	Therapeutic Use	Clinical Pharmacology and Tips
Agonists: See Table 20-7 for CDC guidelines for prescribing opioids for chronic pain		
Morphine Hydromorphone Oxycodone Hydrocodone	• Potent μ agonists • Strong analgesic in moderate-to-severe pain states. • Morphine is a useful adjunct in pulmonary edema and general anesthesia.	• ↓ GI motility ⇒ constipation • Hydrocodone, oxycodone formulated with NSAIDs • Hydrocodone, oxycodone, and fentanyl are more potent than morphine • Among licit agents, LA/ER agents often preferred by abusers
Fentanyl	• Potent μ agonist • Administered orally (buccal tablet, sublingual tablet/spray, oral lozenge), intravenous (push/infusion), intramuscular, topical, topical iontophoretic, neuraxial	• Rapid onset, short duration of action • Slightly longer effective $t_{1/2}$ than sufentanil, alfentanil, and remifentanil
Sufentanil Alfentanil Remifentanil	• Similar to fentanyl • Rapid onset, short duration of action • Administered intravenously	• Sufentanil and alfentanil also given epidurally • Remifentanil: ultrashort acting
Meperidine	• Potent μ agonist • Rapid onset, intermediate duration of action	• Not for extended use due to accumulation of seizure-inducing metabolite
Methadone	• Potent MOR agonist • Rapid onset, long duration of action • Used in maintenance/rehab programs	• Long $t_{1/2}$, ~ 27 h ⇒ potential for accumulation with too frequent repeated delivery • Anticholinergic effects

Drug Facts for Your Personal Formulary: *Opioid Agonists and Antagonists (continued)*

Drug	Therapeutic Use	Clinical Pharmacology and Tips
Codeine	• Weak prodrug for morphine • Useful for mild-to-moderate pain • Less efficacious than morphine but will antagonize strong μ agonists • Administered orally	• Useful antitussive effects • Formulated with NSAIDs
Levorphanol	• Affinity at the MOR, KOR, and DOR • 5HT/NE reuptake inhibitor; NMDA receptor antagonist • Rapid onset, modest duration of analgesia • Administered orally	• Long elimination $t_{1/2}$, ~ 14h ⇒ potential for accumulation with too frequent repeated delivery • Adverse effects: delirium, hallucinations
Peripherally Restricted Agonist		
Loperamide	• Mu opioid agonist • Effective antidiarrheal • Administered orally	• Loperamide crosses BBB poorly, can be formulated with simethicone
Agonist Restricted by Coformulation		
Diphenoxylate	• Mu opioid agonist • Effective antidiarrheal • Administered orally	• Diphenoxylate will cross the BBB, so it is formulated with atropine, the anticholinergic effects of which (weakness, nausea) discourage abuse.
Partial Agonists; Agonist/Antagonist Combinations		
Buprenorphine	• Partial agonist at MOR; KOR antagonist • Mild-to-moderate pain (ceiling effect) • Administered by intramuscular, intravenous, sublingual, transdermal, buccal film • Coformulated with naloxone for use in abuse management	• Delivery to a patient on a full opiate agonist may initiate withdrawal (may be done therapeutically in management of heroin addiction)
Butorphanol Nalbuphine Pentazocine	• KOR agonist/MOR antagonist • Analgesia to mild-to-moderate pain	• Delivery to patient on a full opiate agonist may initiate withdrawal • Ceiling effect • Pentazocine is also formulated with naloxone.
Other Agonists		
Tramadol	• Weak μ agonist and a 5HT/NE uptake inhibitor • Analgesia for moderate pain • Available as a fixed-dose combination with acetaminophen	• Potential for seizures • Serotonin syndrome risk • As an adjunct to other opioids for chronic pain
Tapentadol	• Weak μ agonist and a 5HT/NE uptake inhibitor • Analgesia for moderate pain	• Serotonin syndrome risk
Central Antitussives		
Dextromethorphan	• ↓ Cough reflex; receptor mechanisms unclear • Administered orally • Available as an extended-release formulation	• Serotonin syndrome risk • Has no analgesic or addictive properties
Codeine	• See codeine listing, above	• See codeine listing, above
Antagonists		
Naloxone	• Antagonist at MOR/DOR/KOR • Rapid onset, moderately short acting • Rapidly reverses central and peripheral opiate effects • Used in treating opioid overdose • Autoinjector available for emergency administration	• $t_{1/2}$ ~ 64 min • Renarcotization may occur with long-lasting agonists as naloxone is metabolized • May induce moderate hyperalgesia • Known as NARCAN; used by emergency medical technicians to revive comatose opioid abusers
Naltrexone Nalmefene	• Antagonist at MOR/DOR/KOR • Rapid onset, longer acting than naloxone • Reverses central and peripheral opiate effects • Used in treating alcohol and opiate dependence	• Naltrexone: formulated with bupropion for managing obesity and with morphine for severe pain; contraindicated in hepatitis and liver failure (*Black-Box Warning:* excessive doses cause hepatocellular injury) • Start naltrexone only after 7–10 days of abstinence from opioids • Long-term use of naltrexone ⇒ hypersensitivity to opioids

Drug Facts for Your Personal Formulary: *Opioid Agonists and Antagonists (continued)*

Drug	Therapeutic Use	Clinical Pharmacology and Tips
Peripherally Restricted Antagonists		
Methylnaltrexone	• Antagonist at MOR/DOR/KOR • Reverses peripheral opiate effects (e.g., opiate-induced constipation) but not analgesia	• Does not cross BBB, thus not useful in treating addiction or reversing CNS effects of opioids
Alvimopan	• Antagonist at MOR/DOR/KOR • Penetrates poorly into CNS • FDA approved for ileus	• Reverses peripheral opiate effects

Bibliography

Akil H, et al. Endogenous opioids: biology and function. *Annu Rev Neurosci,* **1984**, *7*:223–255.

Anton RF. Naltrexone for the management of alcohol dependence. *N Engl J Med,* **2008**, *359*:715–721.

Armario A. Activation of the hypothalamic-pituitary-adrenal axis by addictive drugs: different pathways, common outcome. *Trends Pharmacol Sci,* **2010**, *31*:318–325.

Barke KE, Hough LB. Opiates, mast cells and histamine release. *Life Sci,* **1993**, *53*:1391–1399.

Barnett V, et al. Opioid antagonists. *J Pain Symptom Manage,* **2014**, *47*:341–352.

Becker G, et al. Peripherally acting opioid antagonists in the treatment of opiate-related constipation: a systematic review. *J Pain Symptom Manage,* **2007**, *34*:547–565.

Benyamin R, et al. Opioid complications and side effects. *Pain Physician,* **2008**, *11*:S105–S120.

Booth M. *Opium: A History.* Macmillan, New York, **1999**.

Caraco Y, et al. Impact of ethnic origin and quinidine coadministration on codeine's disposition and pharmacodynamic effects. *J Pharmacol Exp Ther,* **1999**, *290*:413–422.

Cherny NI. Opioid analgesics: comparative features and prescribing guidelines. *Drugs,* **1996**, *51*:713–737.

Christie MJ. Cellular neuroadaptations to chronic opioids: tolerance, withdrawal and addiction. *Br J Pharmacol,* **2008**, *154*:384–396.

Chung KF, Pavord ID. Prevalence, pathogenesis, and causes of chronic cough. *Lancet,* **2008**, *371*:1364–1374.

Clemens KE, Klaschik E. Symptomatic therapy of dyspnea with strong opioids and its effect on ventilation in palliative care patients. *J Pain Symptom Manage,* **2007**, *33*:473–481.

Corbett AD, et al. 75 years of opioid research: the exciting but vain quest for the Holy Grail. *Brit J Pharmacol,* **2006**, *147*, S153–S162.

Dannals RF. Positron emission tomography radioligands for the opioid system. *J Labelled Comp Radiopharm,* **2013**, *56*:187–195.

Deer TR, et al. The polyanalgesic consensus conference (PACC): recommendations for intrathecal drug delivery: guidance for improving safety and mitigating risks. *Neuromodulation,* **2017**, *20*:155–176.

Dowell D, et al. CDC Guideline for prescribing opioids for chronic pain—United States, 2016. *MMWR Recomm Rep,* **2016**, *65*:1–49. doi:http://dx.doi.org/10.15585/mmwr.rr6501e1. Accessed April 30, 2017.

Dreborg S, et al. Evolution of vertebrate opioid receptors. *Proc Natl Acad Sci U S A,* **2008**, *105*:15487–15492.

Eddinger KA, et al. Intrathecal catheterization and drug delivery in Guinea pigs: a small-animal model for morphine-evoked granuloma formation. *Anesthesiology,* **2016**, *12*:378–394.

Eichelbaum M, Evert B. Influence of pharmacogenetics on drug disposition and response. *Clin Exp Pharmacol Physiol,* **1996**, *23*:983–985.

Elkader A, Sproule B. Buprenorphine: clinical pharmacokinetics in the treatment of opioid dependence. *Clin Pharmacokinet,* **2005**, *44*:661–680.

Fenalti G, et al. Molecular control of δ-opioid receptor signaling. *Nature,* **2014**, *506*:191–196.

Fillingim RB, Gear RW. Sex differences in opioid analgesia: clinical and experimental findings. *Eur J Pain,* **2004**, *8*:413–425.

Fishburne JI. Systemic analgesia during labor. *Clin Perinatol,* **1982**, *9*:29–53.

Fletcher D, Martinez V. Opioid-induced hyperalgesia in patients after surgery: a systematic review and a meta-analysis. *Br J Anaesth,* **2014**, *112*:991–1004.

Fredheim OM, et al. Clinical pharmacology of methadone for pain. *Acta Anaesthesiol Scand,* **2008**, *52*:879–889.

Galanie S, et al. Complete biosynthesis of opioids in yeast. *Science,* **2015**, *349*:1095–1100.

Galligan JJ, Akbarali HI. Molecular physiology of enteric opioid receptors. *Am J Gastroenterol Suppl,* **2014**, *2*:17–21.

Gendron L, et al. Molecular pharmacology of δ-opioid receptors. *Pharmacol Rev,* **2016**, *68*:631–700.

Gillis JC, et al. Transnasal butorphanol. A review of its pharmacodynamic and pharmacokinetic properties, and therapeutic potential in acute pain management. *Drugs,* **1995**, *50*:157–175.

Gintzler AR, Chakrabarti S. Post-opioid receptor adaptations to chronic morphine; altered functionality and associations of signaling molecules. *Life Sci,* **2006**, *79*:717–722.

Goldstein A, et al. Stereospecific and nonspecific interactions of the morphine congener levorphanol in subcellular fractions of mouse brain. *Proc Natl Acad Sci U S A,* **1971**, *68*:1742–1747.

Goldstein G. Pentazocine. *Drug Alcohol Depend,* **1985**, *14*:313–323.

Grace PM, et al. Pathological pain and the neuroimmune interface. *Nat Rev Immunol,* **2014**, *14*:217–231.

Greenwood-Van Meerveld B. Emerging drugs for postoperative ileus. *Expert Opin Emerg Drugs,* **2007**, *12*:619–626.

Grond S, Sablotzki A. Clinical pharmacology of tramadol. *Clin Pharmacokinet,* **2004**, *43*:879–923.

Haile CN, et al. Pharmacogenetic treatments for drug addiction: alcohol and opiates. *Am J Drug Alcohol Abuse,* **2008**, *34*:355–381.

Höllt V. Opioid peptide processing and receptor selectivity. *Annu Rev Pharmacol Toxicol,* **1986**, *26*:59–77.

Hughes J, et al. Identification of two related pentapeptides from the brain with potent opiate agonist activity. *Nature,* **1975**, *258*:577–580.

Hutchinson MR, et al. Opioid-induced glial activation: mechanisms of activation and implications for opioid analgesia, dependence, and reward. *Scientific World J,* **2007**, *7*:98–111.

Johansson I, Ingelman-Sundberg M. Genetic polymorphism and toxicology—with emphasis on cytochrome P450. *Toxicol Sci,* **2011**, *120*:1–13.

Kane BE, et al. Molecular recognition of opioid receptor ligands. *AAPS J,* **2006**, *8*:E126–E137.

Khan SM, et al. The expanding roles of Gβγ subunits in G Protein–coupled receptor signaling and drug action. *Pharmacol Rev,* **2013**, *65*:545–577.

Koob GF, Le Moal M. Neurobiological mechanisms for opponent motivational processes in addiction. *Philos Trans R Soc Lond B Biol Sci,* **2008**, *363*:3113–3123.

Kreek MJ, Koob GF. Drug dependence: stress and dysregulation of brain reward pathways. *Drug Alcohol Depend*, **1998**, *51*:23–47.

Kromer W. Endogenous and exogenous opioids in the control of gastrointestinal motility and secretion. *Pharmacol Rev*, **1988**, *40*:121–162.

Kumar K, Singh SI. Neuraxial opioid-induced pruritus: an update. *J Anaesthesiol Clin Pharmacol*, **2013**, *29*:303–307.

Lalley PM. Opioidergic and dopaminergic modulation of respiration. *Respir Physiol Neurobiol*, **2008**, *164*:160–167.

Larson MD. Mechanism of opioid-induced pupillary effects. *Clin Neurophysiol*, **2008**, *119*:1358–1364.

Latta KS, et al. Meperidine: a critical review. *Am J Ther*, **2002**, *9*:53–68.

Lee M, et al. A comprehensive review of opioid-induced hyperalgesia. *Pain Physician*, **2011**, *14*:145–161.

Loyd DR, Murphy AZ. The neuroanatomy of sexual dimorphism in opioid analgesia. *Exp Neurol*, **2014**, *259*:57–63.

Martin WR, et al. The effects of morphine- and nalorphine-like drugs in the non-dependent and morphine-dependent chronic spinal dog. *J Pharmacol Exp Ther*, **1976**, *197*:517–532.

Massotte D. In vivo opioid receptor heteromerization: where do we stand? *Br J Pharmacol*, **2015**, *172*:420–434.

McGinty JF. What we know and still need to learn about opioids in the hippocampus. *NIDA Res Monogr*, **1988**, *82*:1–11.

Melzack R, Casey KL. Sensory, motivational, and central control determinants of chronic pain: A new conceptual model. In: The Skin Senses, [ed. D.L.Kenshalo] pp. 423–443. Springfield, Illinois. Thomas, 1968.

Mogil JS. Sex differences in pain and pain inhibition: multiple explanations of a controversial phenomenon *Nat Rev Neurosci*, **2012**, *13*:859–866.

Monk JP, et al. Sufentanil. A review of its pharmacological properties and therapeutic use. *Drugs*, **1988**, *36*:286–313.

Nakagawa A, et al. Total biosynthesis of opiates by stepwise fermentation using engineered *Escherichia coli*. *Nat Commun*, **2016**, *7*:10390. doi:10.1038/ncomms10390.

Neumann PB, et al. Plasma morphine concentrations during chronic oral administration in patients with cancer pain. *Pain*, **1982**, *13*:247–252.

NIDA. Overdose death rates. Revised January **2017**. https://www.drugabuse.gov/related-topics/trends-statistics/overdose-death-rates. Accessed April 30, 2017.

Osborne, R, et al. The analgesic activity of morphine-6-glucuronide. *Brit J Clin Pharmacol*, **1992**, *34*:130–138.

Owen JA, et al. Age-related morphine kinetics. *Clin Pharmacol Ther*, **1983**, *34*:364–368.

Pan YX. Diversity and complexity of the mu opioid receptor gene: alternative pre-mRNA splicing and promoters. *DNA Cell Biol*, **2005**, *24*:736–750.

Patel R, et al. Calcium channel modulation as a target in chronic pain control. *Br J Pharmacol*, **2017**. doi:10.1111/bph.13789.

Pattinson KT. Opioids and the control of respiration. *Br J Anaesth*, **2008**, *100*:747–758.

Pert CB, et al. Opiate agonists and antagonists discriminated by receptor binding in brain. *Science*, **1973**, *182*:1359–1361.

Portenoy RK, et al. Transdermal fentanyl for cancer pain. Repeated dose pharmacokinetics. *Anesthesiology*, **1993**, *78*:36–43.

Price DD, et al. A psychophysical analysis of morphine analgesia. *Pain*, **1985**, *22*:261–269.

Prommer E. Levorphanol: revisiting an underutilized analgesic. *Palliat Care*, **2014**, *8*:7–10.

Quang-Cantagrel ND, et al. Opioid substitution to improve the effectiveness of chronic non-cancer pain control: a chart review. *Anesth Analg*, **2000**, *90*:933–937.

Regnard C, et al. Loperamide. *J Pain Symptom Manage*, **2011**, *42*:319–323.

Rook EJ, et al. Pharmacokinetics and pharmacokinetic variability of heroin and its metabolites: review of the literature. *Curr Clin Pharmacol*, **2006**, *1*:109–118.

Rosow CE, et al. Reversal of opioid-induced bladder dysfunction by intravenous naloxone and methylnaltrexone. *Clin Pharmacol Ther*, **2007**, *82*:48–53.

Rudd RA, et al. Increases in drug and opioid-involved overdose deaths—United States, 2010–2015. *MMWR Morb Mortal Wkly Rep*, **2016**, 65:1445–1452. doi:http://dx.doi.org/10.15585/mmwr.mm655051e1. Accessed April 30, 2017.

Sakai R, Swanson GT. Recent progress in neuroactive marine natural products. *Nat Prod Rep*, **2014**, *31*:273–309.

Schmidt WK, et al. Nalbuphine. *Drug Alcohol Depend*, **1985**, *14*:339–362.

Seifert CF, Kennedy S. Meperidine is alive and well in the new millennium: evaluation of meperidine usage patterns and frequency of adverse drug reactions. *Pharmacotherapy*, **2004**, *24*:776–783.

Shang Y, Filizola M. Opioid receptors: structural and mechanistic insights into pharmacology and signaling. *Eur J Pharmacol*, **2015**, *763*:206–213.

Sidhu AS, Triadafilopoulos G. Neuro-regulation of lower esophageal sphincter function as treatment for gastroesophageal reflux disease. *World J Gastroenterol*, **2008**, *14*:985–990.

Smith HS, Peppin JF. Toward a systematic approach to opioid rotation. *J Pain Res*, **2014**, *7*:589–608.

Smith MT. Neuroexcitatory effects of morphine and hydromorphone: evidence implicating the 3-glucuronide metabolites. *Clin Exp Pharmacol Physiol*, **2000**, *27*:524–528.

Sorkin LS, Wallace MS. Acute pain mechanisms. *Surg Clin North Am*, **1999**, *79*:213–229.

Stein C, Machelska H. Modulation of peripheral sensory neurons by the immune system: implications for pain therapy. *Pharmacol Rev*, **2011**, *63*:860–881.

Stevens CW. The evolution of vertebrate opioid receptors. *Front Biosci*, **2009**, *14*:1247–1269.

Stroumpos C, et al. Remifentanil, a different opioid: potential clinical applications and safety aspects. *Expert Opin Drug Saf*, **2010**, *9*:355–364.

Supernaw RB. CYP2D6 and the efficacy of codeine and codeine-like drugs. *Am J Pain Manage*, **2001**, *11*:30–31.

Thomas J, et al. Methylnaltrexone for opioid-induced constipation in advanced illness. *N Engl J Med*, **2008**, *358*: 2332–2343.

Vallejo R, et al. Opioid therapy and immunosuppression: a review. *Am J Ther*, **2004**, *11*:354–365.

Van Rijn RM, et al. Novel pharmaco-types and trafficking-types induced by opioid receptor heteromerization. *Curr Opin Pharmacol*, **2010**, *10*: 73–79.

Vaughan-Shaw PG, et al. A meta-analysis of the effectiveness of the opioid receptor antagonist alvimopan in reducing hospital length of stay and time to GI recovery in patients enrolled in a standardized accelerated recovery program after abdominal surgery. *Dis Colon Rectum*, **2012**, *55*:611–620.

Violin JD, et al. Biased ligands at G-protein-coupled receptors: promise and progress. *Trends Pharmacol Sci*, **2014**, *35*:308–316.

von Zastrow M, et al. Regulated endocytosis of opioid receptors: cellular mechanisms and proposed roles in physiological adaptation to opiate drugs. *Curr Opin Neurobiol*, **2003**, *13*:348–353.

Waldhoer M, et al. Opioid receptors. *Annu Rev Biochem*, **2004**, *73*: 953–990.

West SJ, et al. Circuitry and plasticity of the dorsal horn - Toward a better understanding of neuropathic pain. *Neuroscience*, **2015**, *300*:254–275.

Williams JT, et al. Regulation of μ-opioid receptors: desensitization, phosphorylation, internalization, and tolerance. *Pharmacol Rev*, **2013**, *65*:223–254.

Willens JS, Myslinski NR. Pharmacodynamics, pharmacokinetics, and clinical uses of fentanyl, sufentanil, and alfentanil. *Heart Lung*, **1993**, *22*:239–251.

Wood JD, Galligan JJ. Function of opioids in the enteric nervous system. *Neurogastroenterol Motil*, **2004**, 16(suppl 2):17–28.

Xu J, et al. Alternatively spliced mu opioid receptor C termini impact the diverse actions of morphine. *J Clin Invest*, **2017**, *127*:1561–1573.

Yaksh TL, et al. The search for novel analgesics: targets and mechanisms. *F1000Prime Rep*, **2015**, 7:56. doi:10.12703/P7-56. Accessed April 5, 2017.

Yaksh TL. Opioid receptor systems and the endorphins: a review of their spinal organization. *J Neurosurg*, **1987**, *67*:157–176.

Yaksh TL. Pharmacology and mechanisms of opioid analgesic activity. *Acta Anaesthesiol Scand*, **1997**, *41*:94–111.

Yaksh TL, et al. Current and future issues in the development of spinal agents for the management of pain. *Curr Neuropharmacol*, **2017**, *15*: 232–259.

Yaksh TL, Allen JW. Preclinical insights into the implementation of intrathecal midazolam: a cautionary tale. *Anesth Analg*, **2004**, 98: 1509–1511.

Young GB, da Silva OP. Effects of morphine on the electroencephalograms of neonates: A prospective, observational study. *Clin Neurophysiol*, **2000**, *111*:1955–1960.

Zhang X, et al. Opioid receptor trafficking and interaction in nociceptors. *Brit J Pharmacol*, **2015**, *172*:364–374.

Zhou S-F et al. Polymorphism of human cytochrome P450 enzymes and its clinical impact. *Drug Metab Rev*, **2009**, *41*:289–295.

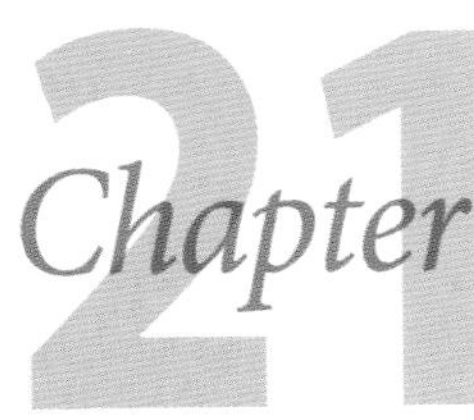

General Anesthetics and Therapeutic Gases

Hemal H. Patel, Matthew L. Pearn, Piyush M. Patel, and David M. Roth

第二十一章　全身麻醉药和治疗性气体

GENERAL PRINCIPLES OF SURGICAL ANESTHESIA
- Hemodynamic Effects of General Anesthesia
- Respiratory Effects of General Anesthesia
- Hypothermia
- Nausea and Vomiting
- Other Emergent and Postoperative Phenomena

ACTIONS AND MECHANISMS OF GENERAL ANESTHETICS
- The Anesthetic State
- Mechanisms of Anesthesia
- Anatomic Sites of Anesthetic Action

PARENTERAL ANESTHETICS
- Pharmacokinetic Principles
- Specific Parenteral Agents

INHALATIONAL ANESTHETICS
- Pharmacokinetic Principles
- Specific Inhalational Agents

ANESTHETIC ADJUNCTS
- Benzodiazepines
- α_2 Adrenergic Agonists
- Analgesics
- Neuromuscular Blocking Agents

ANESTHETIC TOXICITY AND CYTOPROTECTION

THERAPEUTIC GASES
- Oxygen
- Carbon Dioxide
- Nitric Oxide
- Helium
- Hydrogen Sulfide

中文导读

本章主要介绍：外科麻醉的一般原则，包括全身麻醉对血流动力学和呼吸的影响、低体温、恶心和呕吐，其他急症和术后现象；全身麻醉药的作用和机制，包括麻醉状态、麻醉机制和麻醉作用的解剖部位；肠胃外麻醉药，包括药物代谢动力学原理和特定的肠胃外麻醉药；吸入麻醉药，包括药物代谢动力学原理和特定的吸入麻醉药；麻醉辅助用药，包括苯二氮䓬类、α_2-肾上腺素受体激动药、镇痛药和神经肌肉阻滞药；麻醉药的毒性和细胞保护作用；治疗性气体，包括氧气、二氧化碳、一氧化氮、氦气和硫化氢。

Abbreviations

ACh: acetylcholine
AChE: acetylcholinesterase
ADME: absorption, distribution, metabolism, excretion
CBF: cerebral blood flow
CL: clearance
CMR: cerebral metabolic rate
$CMRo_2$: cerebral metabolic rate of O_2 consumption
CNS: central nervous system
CO: cardiac output
DA: dopamine
ED_{50}: median effective dose
EEG: electroencephalogram
FDA: Food and Drug Administration
Fio_2: inspired O_2 fraction
GABA: γ-aminobutyric acid
GFR: glomerular filtration rate
GPCR: G protein–coupled receptor
Hb: hemoglobin
HR: heart rate
5HT: 5-hydroxytryptamine: serotonin
ICP: intracranial pressure
IV: intravenous
LD_{50}: median lethal dose
MAC: minimum alveolar concentration
MAP: mean arterial pressure
MI: myocardial infarction
NE: norepinephrine
NK1: neurokinin 1
NMDA: *N*-methyl-D-aspartate
NSAID: nonsteroidal anti-inflammatory drug
$Paco_2$: arterial CO_2 tension
Po_2: partial pressure of O_2
PRIS: propofol infusion syndrome
RBF: renal blood flow
RR: respiratory rate
RT: room temperature
$t_{1/2}\beta$: β-phase (tissue elimination) half-life
TREK channel: mechanosensitive K^+ channel
$\dot{V}_E$: minute ventilation
VLPO: ventrolateral preoptic
V_{ss}: volume of distribution at steady state

General anesthetics depress the CNS to a sufficient degree to permit the performance of surgery and unpleasant procedures. General anesthetics have low therapeutic indices and thus require great care in administration. The selection of specific drugs and routes of administration to produce general anesthesia is based on the pharmacokinetic properties and on the secondary effects of the various drugs. The practitioner should consider the context of the proposed diagnostic or surgical procedure and the individual patient's characteristics and associated medical conditions when choosing appropriate anesthetic agents.

General Principles of Surgical Anesthesia

The administration of general anesthesia is driven by three general objectives:

1. *Minimizing the potentially deleterious direct and indirect effects of anesthetic agents and techniques.*
2. *Sustaining physiologic homeostasis during surgical procedures* that may involve major blood loss, tissue ischemia, reperfusion of ischemic tissue, fluid shifts, exposure to a cold environment, and impaired coagulation.
3. *Improving postoperative outcomes* by choosing techniques that block or treat components of the surgical stress response that may lead to short- or long-term sequelae.

Hemodynamic Effects of General Anesthesia

The most prominent physiological effect of anesthesia induction is a decrease in systemic arterial blood pressure. The causes include direct vasodilation, myocardial depression, or both; a blunting of baroreceptor control; and a generalized decrease in central sympathetic tone. Agents vary in the magnitude of their specific effects, but in all cases the hypotensive response is enhanced by underlying volume depletion or preexisting myocardial dysfunction.

Respiratory Effects of General Anesthesia

Nearly all general anesthetics reduce or eliminate both ventilatory drive and the reflexes that maintain airway patency. Therefore, ventilation generally must be assisted or controlled for at least some period during surgery. The gag reflex is lost, and the stimulus to cough is blunted. Lower esophageal sphincter tone also is reduced, so both passive and active regurgitation may occur. Endotracheal intubation has been a major reason for a decline in the number of aspiration deaths during general anesthesia. Muscle relaxation is valuable during the induction of general anesthesia where it facilitates management of the airway, including endotracheal intubation. Neuromuscular blocking agents commonly are used to effect such relaxation (see Chapter 11). Alternatives to an endotracheal tube include a face mask and a laryngeal mask, an inflatable mask placed in the oropharynx forming a seal around the glottis. Airway management techniques are based on the anesthetic procedure, the need for neuromuscular relaxation, and the physical characteristics of the patient.

Hypothermia

Patients commonly develop hypothermia (body temperature < 36°C) during surgery. The reasons include low ambient temperature, exposed body cavities, cold intravenous fluids, altered thermoregulatory control, and reduced metabolic rate. Metabolic rate and total body O_2 consumption decrease with general anesthesia by about 30%, reducing heat generation. Hypothermia may lead to an increase in perioperative morbidity. Prevention of hypothermia is a major goal of anesthetic care.

Nausea and Vomiting

Nausea and vomiting continue to be significant problems following general anesthesia and are caused by an action of anesthetics on the chemoreceptor trigger zone and the brainstem vomiting center, which are modulated by 5HT, histamine, ACh, DA, and NK1. The $5HT_3$ receptor antagonists ondansetron, dolasetron, and palonosetron (see Chapters 13 and 50) are effective in suppressing nausea and vomiting. Common preventive strategies include anesthetic induction with propofol; the combined use of droperidol, metoclopramide, and dexamethasone; and avoidance of nitrous oxide (N_2O). A new subclass of antiemetic drugs includes NK1 antagonists (e.g., aprepitant, rolapitant).

Other Emergent and Postoperative Phenomena

Hypertension and tachycardia are common during emergence from anesthesia as the sympathetic nervous system regains its tone and is enhanced by pain. Myocardial ischemia can appear or worsen during emergence in patients with coronary artery disease. Emergence excitement occurs in 5%–30% of patients and is characterized by tachycardia, restlessness, crying, moaning, and thrashing. Neurologic signs, including delirium, spasticity, hyperreflexia, and Babinski sign, are often manifest in the patient emerging from anesthesia. Postanesthesia shivering occurs frequently because of core hypothermia. A small dose of meperidine (12.5 mg) lowers the shivering trigger temperature and effectively stops the activity. The incidence of all of these emergence phenomena is greatly reduced with opioids and α_2 adrenergic agonists (dexmedetomidine).

Airway obstruction may occur during the postoperative period because of residual anesthetic effects. Pulmonary function is reduced following all types of anesthesia and surgery, and hypoxemia may occur. In the immediate postoperative period, pulmonary function reduction can be compounded by the respiratory suppression associated with opioids used for pain control. Regional anesthetic techniques are an important part of a perioperative approach that employs local anesthetic wound infiltration; epidural, spinal, and plexus blocks; and nonsteroidal anti-inflammatory drugs, opioids, α_2 adrenergic receptor agonists, and NMDA receptor antagonists.

Actions and Mechanisms of General Anesthetics

The Anesthetic State

The components of the anesthetic state include

- *Amnesia*
- *Analgesia*
- *Unconsciousness*
- *Immobility* in response to noxious stimulation
- *Attenuation of autonomic responses* to noxious stimulation

The potency of general anesthetic agents is measured by determining the concentration of general anesthetic that prevents movement in response to surgical stimulation. For inhalational anesthetics, anesthetic potency is measured in *MAC units*, with 1 MAC defined as the minimum alveolar concentration that prevents movement in response to surgical stimulation in 50% of subjects. The strengths of MAC as a measurement are the following:

- Alveolar concentrations can be monitored continuously by measuring end-tidal anesthetic concentration using infrared spectroscopy or mass spectrometry.
- MAC provides a direct correlate of the free concentration of the anesthetic at its site(s) of action in the CNS.
- MAC is a simple-to-measure end point that reflects an important clinical goal.

End points other than immobilization also can be used to measure anesthetic potency. For example, the ability to respond to verbal commands (MAC_{awake}) and the ability to form memories also have been correlated with alveolar anesthetic concentration. Verbal response and memory formation are suppressed at a fraction of MAC. The ratio of the anesthetic concentrations required to produce amnesia and immobility vary significantly among different inhalational anesthetic agents.

Generally, the potency of intravenous agents is defined as the free plasma concentration (at equilibrium) that produces loss of response to surgical incision (or other end points) in 50% of subjects.

Mechanisms of Anesthesia

The molecular and cellular mechanisms by which general anesthetics produce their effects have remained one of the great mysteries of pharmacology. The leading unitary theory was that anesthesia is produced by perturbation of the physical properties of cell membranes. This thinking was based largely on the observation that the anesthetic potency of a gas correlated with its solubility in olive oil. This correlation is referred to as the Meyer-Overton rule. Clear exceptions to the Meyer-Overton rule (Franks, 2006) suggest protein targets that may account for anesthetic effect. Increasing evidence supports the hypothesis that different anesthetic agents produce specific components of anesthesia by actions at different molecular targets. Given these insights, the unitary theory of anesthesia has been largely discarded.

Molecular Mechanisms of General Anesthetics

Most intravenous general anesthetics act predominantly through $GABA_A$ receptors and perhaps through some interactions with other ligand-gated ion channels such as NMDA receptors and two-pore K^+ channels. Chloride channels gated by the inhibitory $GABA_A$ receptors (see Figures 14–5 and 14–11) are sensitive to a wide variety of anesthetics, including the halogenated inhalational agents, many intravenous agents (propofol, barbiturates, and etomidate), and neurosteroids. At clinical concentrations, general anesthetics increase the sensitivity of the $GABA_A$ receptor to GABA, thereby enhancing inhibitory neurotransmission and depressing nervous system activity. The action of anesthetics on the $GABA_A$ receptor probably is mediated by binding of the anesthetics to specific sites on the $GABA_A$ receptor protein (but they do not compete with GABA for its binding site). The capacity of propofol and etomidate to inhibit the response to noxious stimuli is mediated by a specific site on the β_3 subunit of the $GABA_A$ receptor, whereas the sedative effects of these anesthetics are mediated by on the β_2 subunit.

Structurally related to the $GABA_A$ receptors are other ligand-gated ion channels, including *glycine receptors* and neuronal *nicotinic ACh receptors* (see Figure 14–5). Glycine-gated Cl^- channels (glycine receptors) may play a role in mediating inhibition by anesthetics of responses to noxious stimuli. Inhalational anesthetics enhance the capacity of glycine to activate glycine receptors, which play an important role in inhibitory neurotransmission in the spinal cord and brainstem. Propofol, neurosteroids, and barbiturates also potentiate glycine-activated currents, whereas etomidate and ketamine do not. Subanesthetic concentrations of the inhalational anesthetics inhibit some classes of neuronal nicotinic ACh receptors, which seem to mediate other components of anesthesia such as analgesia or amnesia.

Ketamine, nitrous oxide, cyclopropane, and xenon are the only general anesthetics that do not have significant effects on $GABA_A$ or glycine receptors. These agents inhibit a different type of ligand-gated ion channel, the NMDA receptor (see Figure 14–12 and Table 14–2). NMDA receptors are glutamate-gated cation channels that are somewhat selective for Ca^{2+} and are involved in long-term modulation of synaptic responses (long-term potentiation) and glutamate-mediated neurotoxicity.

Halogenated inhalational anesthetics activate some members of a class of K^+ channels known as *two-pore domain channels*; other two-pore domain channel family members are activated by xenon, N_2O, and cyclopropane. These channels are located in both presynaptic and postsynaptic sites. The postsynaptic channels may be the molecular locus through which these agents hyperpolarize neurons.

Cellular Mechanisms of Anesthesia

General anesthetics produce two important physiologic effects at the cellular level:

1. Inhalational anesthetics can hyperpolarize neurons. Neuronal hyperpolarization may affect pacemaker activity and pattern-generating circuits.
2. Both inhalational and intravenous anesthetics have substantial effects on synaptic transmission and much smaller effects on action potential generation or propagation.

Inhalational anesthetics inhibit excitatory synapses and enhance inhibitory synapses in various preparations. The inhalational anesthetics inhibit neurotransmitter release. Inhalational anesthetics also can act postsynaptically, altering the response to released neurotransmitter. These actions are thought to be due to specific interactions of anesthetic agents with neurotransmitter receptors.

Intravenous anesthetics produce a narrower range of physiological effects. Their predominant actions are at the synapse, where they have profound and relatively specific effects on the postsynaptic response to released neurotransmitter. Most of the intravenous agents act predominantly by enhancing inhibitory neurotransmission, whereas ketamine predominantly inhibits excitatory neurotransmission at glutamatergic synapses.

Anatomic Sites of Anesthetic Action

In principle, general anesthetics could interrupt nervous system function at myriad levels, including peripheral sensory neurons, the spinal cord, the brainstem, and the cerebral cortex. Most anesthetics cause, with some exceptions, a global reduction in CMR and in CBF. A consistent feature of general anesthesia is a suppression of metabolism in the thalamus (Alkire et al., 2008), which serves as a major relay by which sensory input from the periphery ascends to the cortex. Suppression of thalamic activity may serve as a switch between the awake and anesthetized states (Franks, 2008). General anesthesia also suppresses activity in specific regions of the cortex, including the mesial parietal cortex, posterior cingulate cortex, precuneus, and inferior parietal cortex.

Similarities between natural sleep and the anesthetized state suggest that anesthetics might also modulate endogenous sleep-regulating pathways, which include VLPO and tuberomammillary nuclei. VLPO projects inhibitory GABAergic fibers to ascending arousal nuclei, which in turn project to the cortex, forebrain, and subcortical areas; release histamine, 5HT, orexin, NE, and ACh; and mediate wakefulness. Intravenous and inhalational agents with activity at $GABA_A$ receptors can increase the inhibitory effects of VLPO, thereby suppressing consciousness. Dexmedetomidine, an α_2 adrenergic agonist, also increases VLPO-mediated inhibition by suppressing the inhibitory effect of locus ceruleus neurons on VLPO. Finally, both intravenous and inhalational anesthetics depress hippocampal neurotransmission, a probable locus for their amnestic effects.

Parenteral Anesthetics

Parenteral anesthetics are the most common drugs used for anesthetic induction of adults. Their lipophilicity, coupled with the relatively high perfusion of the brain and spinal cord, results in rapid onset and short duration after a single bolus dose. These drugs ultimately accumulate in fatty tissue. Each of these anesthetics has its own unique properties and side effects (Tables 21–1 and 21–2). Propofol is advantageous for procedures where rapid return to a preoperative mental status is desirable. Etomidate usually is reserved for patients at risk for hypotension or myocardial ischemia. Ketamine is best suited for patients with asthma or for children undergoing short, painful procedures. Thiopental has a long-established track record of safety; however, clinical use is limited currently by availability.

Pharmacokinetic Principles

Parenteral anesthetics are small, hydrophobic, substituted aromatic or heterocyclic compounds (Figure 21–1). Hydrophobicity is the key factor governing their pharmacokinetics. After a single intravenous bolus, these drugs preferentially partition into the highly perfused and lipophilic tissues of the brain and spinal cord, where they produce anesthesia within a single circulation time. Subsequently, blood levels fall rapidly, resulting in drug redistribution out of the CNS back into the blood. The anesthetic then diffuses into less-perfused tissues, such as muscle and viscera, and at a slower rate into the poorly perfused but very hydrophobic adipose tissue. Termination of anesthesia after single boluses of parenteral anesthetics primarily reflects redistribution out of the CNS rather than metabolism (see Figure 2-4).

After redistribution, anesthetic blood levels fall according to a complex interaction between the metabolic rate and the amount and lipophilicity of the drug stored in the peripheral compartments. Thus, parenteral anesthetic half-lives are "context sensitive," and the degree to which a $t_{1/2}$ is contextual varies greatly from drug to drug, as might be predicted based on their differing hydrophobicities and metabolic clearances (Figure 21–2; Table 21–1). For example, after a single bolus of thiopental, patients usually emerge from anesthesia within 10 min; however, a patient may require more than a day to awaken from a prolonged thiopental infusion. Most individual variability in sensitivity to parenteral anesthetics can be accounted for by pharmacokinetic factors. For example, in patients with lower cardiac output, the relative perfusion of the brain and the fraction of anesthetic dose delivered to the brain are higher; thus, patients in septic shock or with cardiomyopathy usually require lower doses of parenteral anesthetics. The elderly also typically require a smaller parenteral anesthetic dose, primarily because of a smaller initial volume of distribution.

Specific Parenteral Agents

Propofol, Fospropofol

Propofol is the most commonly used parenteral anesthetic in the U.S. Fospropofol is a prodrug form that is converted to propofol in vivo. The clinical pharmacological properties of propofol are summarized in Table 21–1.

The active ingredient in propofol, 2,6-diisopropylphenol, is an oil at room temperature and insoluble in aqueous solutions. Propofol is formulated for intravenous administration as a 1% (10-mg/mL) emulsion in 10% soybean oil, 2.25% glycerol, and 1.2% purified egg phosphatide. In the U.S., disodium EDTA (0.05 mg/mL) or sodium metabisulfite (0.25 mg/mL) is added to inhibit bacterial growth. Propofol should be administered

TABLE 21–1 ■ PHARMACOLOGICAL PROPERTIES OF PARENTERAL ANESTHETICS

DRUG	IV INDUCTION DOSE (mg/kg)	MINIMAL HYPNOTIC LEVEL (μg/mL)	INDUCTION DOSE DURATION (min)	$t_{1/2}\beta$ (h)	*CL* (mL/min/kg)	PROTEIN BINDING (%)	V_{ss} (L/kg)
Propofol	1.5–2.5	1.1	4–8	1.8	30	98	2.3
Etomidate	0.2–0.4	0.3	4–8	2.9	17.9	76	2.5
Ketamine	1.0–4.5	1	5–10	2.5	19.1	27	3.1
Thiopental	3–5	15.6	5–8	12.1	3.4	85	2.3
Methohexital	1.0–1.5	10	4–7	3.9	10.9	85	2.2

TABLE 21–2 ■ SOME PHARMACOLOGICAL EFFECTS OF PARENTERAL ANESTHETICS[a]

DRUG	CBF	$CMRo_2$	ICP	MAP	HR	CO	RR	$\dot{V}_E$
Propofol	−−−	−−−	−−−	−−	+	−	−−	−−−
Etomidate	−−−	−−−	−−−	0	0	0	−	−
Ketamine	++	0	++	+	++	+	0	0
Thiopental	−−−	−−−	−−−	−	+	−	−	−−

[a]Typical effects of a single induction dose in humans; see text for references. Qualitative scale from − − − to +++ signifies slight, moderate, or large decrease or increase, respectively; 0 indicates no significant change.

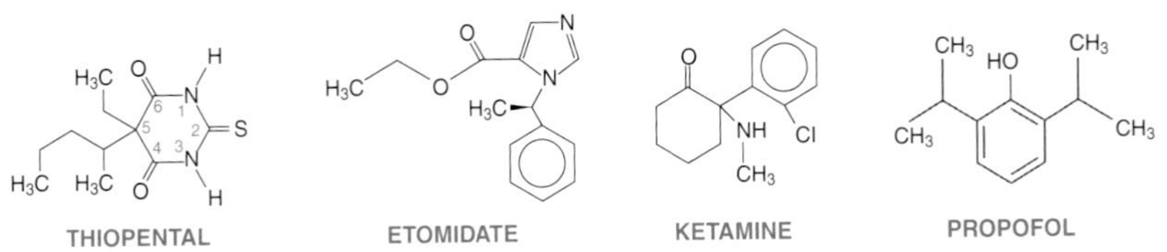

THIOPENTAL ETOMIDATE KETAMINE PROPOFOL

Figure 21–1 *Structures of some parenteral anesthetics.*

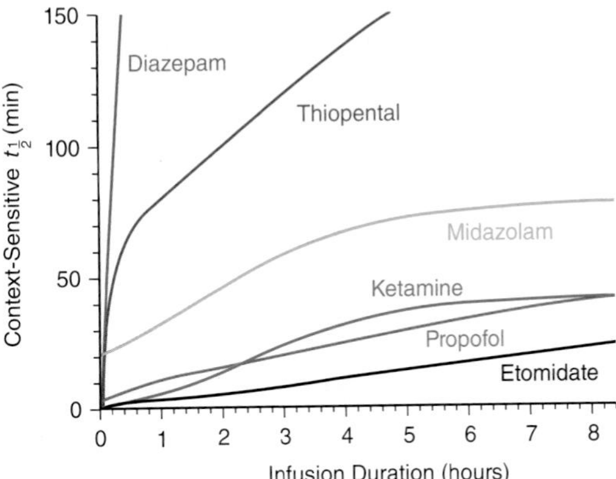

Figure 21–2 *Context-sensitive half-time of general anesthetics.* The duration of action of single intravenous doses of anesthetic/hypnotic drugs is similarly short for all and is determined by redistribution of the drugs away from their active sites (see Figure 2–4). However, after prolonged infusions, drug half-lives and durations of action are dependent on a complex interaction between the rate of redistribution of the drug, the amount of drug accumulated in fat, and the drug's metabolic rate. This phenomenon has been termed the *context-sensitive half-time*; that is, the $t_{1/2}$ of a drug can be estimated only if one knows the context—the total dose and over what time period it has been given. Note that the half-times of some drugs such as etomidate, propofol, and ketamine increase only modestly with prolonged infusions; others (e.g., diazepam and thiopental) increase dramatically. (Reproduced with permission from Reves JG, Glass PSA, Lubarsky DA, et al. Intravenous anesthetics. In: Miller RD, et al., eds. *Miller's Anesthesia*. 7th ed. Churchill Livingstone, Philadelphia, **2010**, 718. Copyright © Elsevier.)

within 4 h of its removal from sterile packaging; unused drug should be discarded. The lipid emulsion formulation of propofol is associated with significant pain on injection and hyperlipidemia.

A new aqueous formulation of propofol, fospropofol, which is not associated with these adverse effects, is available for use for sedation in patients undergoing diagnostic procedures (Fechner et al., 2008). Fospropofol, which itself is inactive, is a phosphate ester prodrug of propofol that is hydrolyzed by endothelial alkaline phosphatases to yield propofol, phosphate, and formaldehyde. The formaldehyde is rapidly converted to formic acid, which then is metabolized by tetrahydrofolate dehydrogenase to CO_2 and water.

Clinical Use and ADME. The induction dose of propofol in a healthy adult is 2–2.5 mg/kg. Dosages should be reduced in the elderly and in the presence of other sedatives and increased in young children. Because of its reasonably short elimination $t_{1/2}$, propofol often is used for maintenance of anesthesia as well as for induction. For short procedures, small boluses (10%–50% of the induction dose) every 5 min or as needed are effective. An infusion of propofol produces a more stable drug level (100–300 μg/kg/min) and is better suited for longer-term anesthetic maintenance. Sedating doses of propofol are 20%–50% of those required for general anesthesia.

Propofol has a context-sensitive $t_{1/2}$ of about 10 min with an infusion lasting 3 h and about 30 min for infusions lasting up to 8 h (see Figure 21–2). Propofol's shorter duration of action after infusion can be explained by its very high clearance, coupled with the slow diffusion of drug from the peripheral to the central compartment. Propofol is metabolized in the liver by conjugation to sulfate and glucuronide to less-active metabolites that are renally excreted. Propofol is highly protein bound, and its pharmacokinetics, like those of the barbiturates, may be affected by conditions that alter serum protein levels. Clearance of propofol is reduced in the elderly. In neonates, propofol clearance is also reduced. By contrast, in young children, a more rapid clearance in combination with a larger central volume may necessitate larger doses of propofol for induction and maintenance of anesthesia.

Fospropofol produces dose-dependent sedation and can be administered in otherwise-healthy individuals at 2–8 mg/kg intravenously (delivered either as a bolus or by a short infusion over 5–10 min). The optimum dose for sedation is about 6.5 mg/kg. This results in a loss of consciousness in about 10 min. The duration of the sedative effect is approximately 45 min.

Side Effects

Nervous System. The sedation and hypnotic actions of propofol are mediated by its action on $GABA_A$ receptors; agonism at these receptors results in an increased Cl^- conduction and hyperpolarization of neurons. Propofol suppresses the EEG, and, in sufficient doses, can produce burst suppression of the EEG. Propofol decreases the $CMRo_2$, CBF, and intracranial and intraocular pressures by about the same amount as thiopental. Propofol can be used in patients at risk for cerebral ischemia; however, no human outcome studies have been performed to determine its efficacy as a neuroprotectant.

Cardiovascular System. Propofol produces a dose-dependent decrease in blood pressure that is significantly greater than that produced by thiopental. The fall in blood pressure can be explained by both vasodilation and possibly mild depression of myocardial contractility. Propofol appears to blunt the baroreceptor reflex and reduce sympathetic nerve activity. Propofol should be used with caution in patients at risk for, or intolerant of, decreases in blood pressure.

Respiratory System. Propofol produces a slightly greater degree of respiratory depression than thiopental. Patients given propofol should be monitored to ensure adequate oxygenation and ventilation. Propofol appears to be less likely than barbiturates to provoke bronchospasm and may be the induction agent of choice in patients with asthma. The bronchodilator properties of propofol may be attenuated by the metabisulfite preservative in some propofol formulations.

Other Side Effects. Propofol has a significant antiemetic action. Propofol elicits pain on injection that can be reduced with lidocaine and the use of larger arm and antecubital veins. A rare but potentially fatal complication, *PRIS*, has been described primarily in prolonged, higher-dose infusions of propofol in young or head-injured patients (Kam and Cardone, 2007). PRIS is characterized by metabolic acidosis, hyperlipidemia, rhabdomyolysis, and liver enlargement.

Etomidate

Etomidate is a substituted imidazole that is supplied as the active d-isomer. Etomidate is poorly soluble in water and is formulated as a 2-mg/mL solution in 35% propylene glycol. Unlike thiopental, etomidate does not induce precipitation of neuromuscular blockers or other drugs frequently given during anesthetic induction.

Clinical Use and ADME. Etomidate is primarily used for anesthetic induction of patients at risk for hypotension. Induction doses of etomidate (see Table 21–1) are accompanied by a high incidence of pain on injection and myoclonic movements. Lidocaine effectively reduces the pain of injection, while myoclonic movements can be reduced by premedication with either benzodiazepines or opiates. Etomidate is pharmacokinetically suitable for off-label infusion for anesthetic maintenance (10 μg/kg/min) or sedation (5 μg/kg/min); however, long-term infusions are not recommended because of side effects.

An induction dose of etomidate has a rapid onset; redistribution limits the duration of action. Metabolism occurs in the liver, primarily to inactive compounds. Elimination is both renal (78%) and biliary (22%). Compared to thiopental, the duration of action of etomidate increases less with repeated doses (see Figure 21–2).

Side Effects

Nervous System. Etomidate produces hypnosis and has no analgesic effects. The effects of etomidate on CBF, metabolism, and intracranial and intraocular pressures are similar to those of thiopental (without dropping mean arterial blood pressure). Etomidate produces increased EEG activity in epileptogenic foci and has been associated with seizures.

Cardiovascular System. Cardiovascular stability after induction is a major advantage of etomidate over either propofol or barbiturates. Induction doses of etomidate typically produce a small increase in heart rate and little or no decrease in blood pressure or cardiac output. Etomidate has little effect on coronary perfusion pressure while reducing myocardial O_2 consumption.

Respiratory and Other Side Effects. The degree of respiratory depression due to etomidate appears to be less than that due to thiopental. Like methohexital, etomidate may induce hiccups; it does not significantly stimulate histamine release. Etomidate has been associated with nausea and vomiting. The drug also inhibits adrenal biosynthetic enzymes required for the production of cortisol and some other steroids. Although the hemodynamic profile of etomidate may be advantageous, potential negative effects on steroid synthesis raise concerns about its use in trauma and critically ill patients (van den Heuvel et al., 2013) and obviate etomidate use for long-term infusion. A rapidly metabolized and ultra-short-acting analogue, methoxycarbonyl-etomidate, retains the favorable pharmacological properties of etomidate but does not produce adrenocortical suppression after bolus dosing (Cotton and Claing, 2009).

Ketamine

Ketamine is an arylcyclohexylamine and congener of phencyclidine. Ketamine is supplied as a mixture of the R+ and S- isomers even though the S- isomers is more potent and has fewer side effects. Although more lipophilic than thiopental, ketamine is water soluble.

Clinical Use and ADME. Ketamine is useful for anesthetizing patients at risk for hypotension and bronchospasm and for certain pediatric procedures. However, significant side effects limit its routine use. Ketamine rapidly produces a hypnotic state quite distinct from that of other anesthetics. Patients have profound analgesia, unresponsiveness to commands, and amnesia but may have their eyes open, move their limbs involuntarily, and breathe spontaneously. This cataleptic state has been termed *dissociative anesthesia*. The administration of ketamine has been shown to reduce the development of tolerance to long-term opioid use. Ketamine typically is administered intravenously but also is effective by intramuscular, oral, and rectal routes. Ketamine does not elicit pain on injection or true excitatory behavior as described for methohexital, although involuntary movements produced by ketamine can be mistaken for anesthetic excitement. Low-dose ketamine has potential use in depression (Rasmussen et al., 2013).

The onset and duration of an induction dose of ketamine are determined by the same distribution/redistribution mechanisms operant for all the other parenteral anesthetics. Ketamine is metabolized to norketamine by hepatic CYPs (mainly by 3A4; less by 2B6 and 2D9). Norketamine, with ~20% of the activity of ketamine, is hydroxylated and excreted in urine and bile. Ketamine's large volume of distribution and rapid clearance make it suitable for continuous infusion (see Table 21–1 and Figure 21–2).

Side Effects

Nervous System. Ketamine has indirect sympathomimetic activity and produces distinct behavioral effects. The ketamine-induced cataleptic state is accompanied by nystagmus with pupillary dilation, salivation, lacrimation, and spontaneous limb movements with increased overall muscle tone. Patients are amnestic and unresponsive to painful stimuli. Ketamine produces profound analgesia, a distinct advantage over other parenteral anesthetics. Unlike other parenteral anesthetics, ketamine increases CBF and ICP with minimal alteration of cerebral metabolism. The effects of ketamine on CBF can be readily attenuated by the simultaneous administration of sedative-hypnotic agents.

Emergence delirium, characterized by hallucinations, vivid dreams, and delusions, is a frequent complication of ketamine that can result in serious patient dissatisfaction and can complicate postoperative management. Benzodiazepines reduce the incidence of emergence delirium.

Cardiovascular System. Unlike other anesthetics, induction doses of ketamine typically increase blood pressure, heart rate, and cardiac output. The cardiovascular effects are indirect and are most likely mediated by inhibition of both central and peripheral catecholamine reuptake. Ketamine has direct negative inotropic and vasodilating activity, but these effects usually are overwhelmed by the indirect sympathomimetic action. Thus, ketamine is a useful drug, along with etomidate, for patients at risk for hypotension during anesthesia. While not arrhythmogenic, ketamine increases myocardial O_2 consumption and is not an ideal drug for patients at risk for myocardial ischemia.

Respiratory System. The respiratory effects of ketamine are perhaps the best indication for its use. Induction doses of ketamine produce small and transient decreases in minute ventilation, but respiratory depression is less severe than with other parenteral anesthetics. Ketamine is a potent bronchodilator and is particularly well suited for anesthetizing patients at high risk for bronchospasm.

Barbiturates

Barbiturates are derivatives of barbituric acid with either an oxygen or a sulfur at the 2-position (see Figure 21–1 and Chapters 17 and 19). The three barbiturates most commonly used in clinical anesthesia are sodium *thiopental* (not currently marketed in the U.S.), *thiamylal* (currently licensed in the U.S. only for veterinary use), and *methohexital*. Sodium thiopental was used most frequently for inducing anesthesia.

Barbiturates are supplied as racemic mixtures despite enantioselectivity in their anesthetic potency. Barbiturates are formulated as the sodium salts with 6% sodium carbonate and reconstituted in water or isotonic saline to alkaline solutions, $10 < pH < 11$. *Mixing barbiturates with drugs in acidic solutions during anesthetic induction can result in precipitation of the barbiturate as the free acid; thus, standard practice is to delay the administration of other drugs until the barbiturate has cleared the intravenous tubing.*

The pharmacological properties and other therapeutic uses of the barbiturates are presented in Chapter 19. Table 19–3 lists the common barbiturates with their clinical pharmacological properties.

Clinical Use and ADME. Recommended intravenous dosing for parenteral barbiturates in a healthy young adult is given in Table 21–1. The availability of thiopental is limited currently by the lack of an FDA-licensed product and the prohibition of its import due to controversy over its use in administration of the death penalty by lethal injection.

The principal mechanism limiting anesthetic duration after single doses is redistribution of these hydrophobic drugs from the brain to other tissues. However, after multiple doses or infusions, the duration of action of the barbiturates varies considerably depending on their clearances. See Table 21–1 for pharmacokinetic parameters.

Methohexital differs from the other two intravenous barbiturates in its much more rapid clearance; thus, it accumulates less during prolonged infusions. Because of their slow elimination and large volumes of distribution, prolonged infusions or very large doses of thiopental and thiamylal can produce unconsciousness lasting several days. All three barbiturates are primarily eliminated by hepatic metabolism and subsequent renal excretion of inactive metabolites; a small fraction of thiopental undergoes desulfuration to the longer-acting hypnotic pentobarbital. Hepatic disease or other conditions that reduce serum protein concentrations will increase the initial free concentration and hypnotic effect of an induction dose.

Side Effects

Nervous System. Barbiturates suppress the EEG and can produce EEG burst suppression. They reduce the CMR, as measured by $CMRo_2$, in a dose-dependent manner. As a consequence of the decrease in $CMRo_2$, CBF and ICP are similarly reduced. Presumably, their CNS depressant activity contributes to their anticonvulsant effects (see Chapter 17). Methohexital can increase ictal activity, and seizures have been described in patients who received doses sufficient to produce burst suppression of the EEG, properties that make methohexital a good choice for anesthesia in patients who undergo electroconvulsive therapy.

Cardiovascular System. The anesthetic barbiturates produce dose-dependent decreases in blood pressure. The effect is due primarily to vasodilation, particularly venodilation, and to a lesser degree to a direct decrease in cardiac contractility. Typically, heart rate increases as a compensatory response to a lower blood pressure, although barbiturates also blunt the baroreceptor reflex. Thiopental maintains the ratio of myocardial O_2 supply to demand in patients with coronary artery disease within a normal blood pressure range. Hypotension can be severe in patients with an impaired ability to compensate for venodilation, such as those with hypovolemia, cardiomyopathy, valvular heart disease, coronary artery disease, cardiac tamponade, or β adrenergic blockade. None of the barbiturates has been shown to be arrhythmogenic.

Respiratory System. Barbiturates are respiratory depressants. Induction doses of thiopental decrease minute ventilation and tidal volume, with a smaller and inconsistent decrease in respiratory rate. Reflex responses to hypercarbia and hypoxia are diminished by anesthetic barbiturates; at higher doses or in the presence of other respiratory depressants such as opiates, apnea can result. Compared to propofol, barbiturates produce a higher incidence of wheezing in asthmatics, attributed to histamine release from mast cells during induction of anesthesia.

Other Side Effects. Short-term administration of barbiturates has no clinically significant effect on the hepatic, renal, or endocrine systems. True allergies to barbiturates are rare; however, direct drug-induced histamine release is occasionally seen. Barbiturates can induce fatal attacks of porphyria in patients with acute intermittent or variegate porphyria and are contraindicated in such patients. Methohexital can produce pain on injection to a greater degree than thiopental. Inadvertent intra-arterial injection of thiobarbiturates can induce a severe inflammatory and potentially necrotic reaction that can threaten limb survival. Methohexital, and to a lesser degree other barbiturates, can produce excitatory symptoms on induction, such as cough, hiccup, muscle tremors, twitching, and hypertonus.

Inhalational Anesthetics

A wide variety of gases and volatile liquids can produce anesthesia. The structures of the currently used inhalational anesthetics are shown in Figure 21–3. The inhalational anesthetics have therapeutic indices (LD_{50}/ED_{50}) that range from 2 to 4, making these among the most dangerous drugs in clinical use. The toxicity of these drugs is largely a function of their side effects, and each of the inhalational anesthetics has a unique side-effect profile. Hence, the selection of an inhalational anesthetic often is based on balancing a patient's pathophysiology with drug side-effect profiles.

Table 21–3 lists the widely varying physical properties of the inhalational agents in clinical use. Ideally, an inhalational agent would produce rapid induction of anesthesia and rapid recovery following discontinuation.

Pharmacokinetic Principles

Inhalational agents behave as gases rather than as liquids and thus require different pharmacokinetic constructs to be used in analyzing their uptake and distribution. Inhalational anesthetics distribute between tissues (or between blood and gas) such that equilibrium is achieved when the partial pressure of anesthetic gas is equal in the two tissues. When a person has breathed an inhalational anesthetic for a sufficiently long time that all tissues are equilibrated with the anesthetic, the partial pressure of the anesthetic in all tissues will be equal to the partial pressure of the anesthetic in inspired gas. While the partial pressure of the anesthetic may be equal in all tissues, the concentration of anesthetic in each tissue will be different. Indeed, anesthetic partition coefficients are defined as the ratio of anesthetic concentration in two tissues when the partial pressures of anesthetic are equal in the two tissues. Blood:gas, brain:blood, and fat:blood partition coefficients for the various inhalational agents are listed in Table 21–3. These partition coefficients show that inhalational anesthetics are more soluble in some tissues (e.g., fat) than they are in others (e.g., blood). In clinical practice, equilibrium is achieved when the partial pressure in inspired gas is equal to the partial pressure in end-tidal (alveolar) gas. For inhalational agents that are not very soluble in blood or any other tissue, equilibrium is achieved quickly, as illustrated for nitrous oxide in Figure 21–4. If an agent is more soluble in a tissue such as fat, equilibrium may take many hours to reach. This occurs because fat represents a huge anesthetic reservoir that will be filled slowly because of the modest blood flow to fat. Anesthesia is produced when anesthetic partial pressure in brain is equal to or greater than MAC. Because the brain is well perfused, anesthetic partial pressure in brain becomes equal to the partial pressure in alveolar gas (and in blood) over the course of several minutes. Therefore, anesthesia is achieved shortly after alveolar partial pressure reaches MAC.

Elimination of inhalational anesthetics is largely a reversal of uptake. For inhalational agents with high blood and tissue solubility, recovery will be a function of the duration of anesthetic administration. This occurs because the accumulated amounts of anesthetic in the fat reservoir will prevent blood (and therefore alveolar) partial pressures from falling

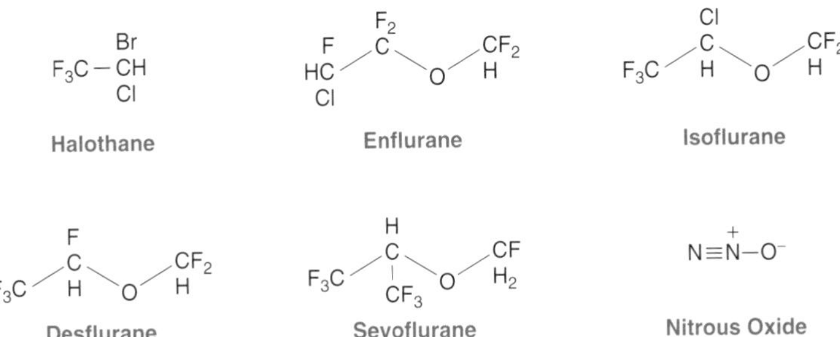

Figure 21–3 *Structures of inhalational general anesthetics.* Note that all inhalational general anesthetic agents except nitrous oxide and halothane are ethers, and that fluorine replaces chlorine in the development of the halogenated agents. All structural differences are associated with important differences in pharmacological properties.

TABLE 21–3 ■ PROPERTIES OF INHALATIONAL ANESTHETIC AGENTS

AGENT	MAC[a] (vol%)	MAC_{AWAKE}[b] (vol%)	VAPOR PRESSURE (mm Hg, 20°C)	PARTITION COEFFICIENT AT 37°C			% RECOVERED AS METABOLITES
				BLOOD/GAS	BRAIN/BLOOD (Brain/Gas)	FAT/BLOOD (Fat/Gas)	
Isoflurane[c]	1.05–1.28	0.4	238	1.43	2.6	45 (91)	0.17
Enflurane	1.68	0.4	175	1.91	1.4	36 (98)	2.4
Sevoflurane	1.4–3.3	0.6	157	0.63–0.69	1.7 (1.2)	48 (50)	3.5
Desflurane	5.2–9.2	2.4	669	0.424	1.3 (0.54)	27 (19)	<0.02
N_2O[c]	105	60.0	Gas	0.47	1.1	2.3	0.004
Xe	55–71	32.6	Gas	0.115	—	(1.9)	0

[a]MAC values are expressed as volume percent, the percentage of the atmosphere that is anesthetic. An MAC value greater than 100% means that hyperbaric conditions would be required.
[b]MAC_{AWAKE} is the concentration at which appropriate responses to commands are lost.
[c]EC_{50} for memory suppression (vol%): isoflurane, 0.24; N_2O, 52.5; values not available for other agents.

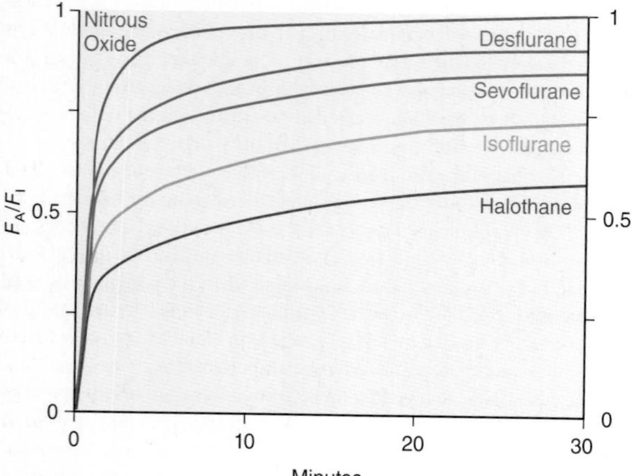

Figure 21–4 *Uptake of inhalational general anesthetics.* The rise in end-tidal alveolar F_A anesthetic concentration toward the inspired F_I concentration is most rapid with the least-soluble anesthetics (nitrous oxide and desflurane) and slowest with the most soluble anesthetic, halothane. All data are from human studies. (Reproduced with permission from Eger EI II. Inhaled anesthetics: uptake and distribution. In: Miller RD et al., eds. *Miller's Anesthesia.* 7th ed. Churchill Livingstone, Philadelphia, **2010**, 540. Copyright © Elsevier.)

rapidly. Patients will be arousable when alveolar partial pressure reaches MAC_{awake}, a partial pressure somewhat lower than MAC (see Table 21–3).

Specific Inhalational Agents

Isoflurane

Isoflurane is a volatile liquid at room temperature and is neither flammable nor explosive in mixtures of air or O_2. Isoflurane is a commonly used inhalational anesthetic worldwide.

Clinical Use and ADME. Isoflurane is typically used for maintenance of anesthesia *after induction* with other agents because of its pungent odor. Induction of anesthesia can be achieved in less than 10 min with an inhaled concentration of 1.5%–3% isoflurane in O_2; this concentration is reduced to 1%–2% (~1–2 MAC) for maintenance of anesthesia. The use of adjunct agents such as opioids or nitrous oxide reduces the concentration of isoflurane required for surgical anesthesia.

Isoflurane has a blood:gas partition coefficient substantially lower than that of enflurane. Consequently, induction with isoflurane and recovery from isoflurane are relatively faster. More than 99% of inhaled isoflurane is excreted unchanged by the lungs. Isoflurane does not appear to be a mutagen, teratogen, or carcinogen.

Side Effects

Cardiovascular System. Isoflurane produces a concentration-dependent decrease in arterial blood pressure; cardiac output is well maintained; hypotension is the result of decreased systemic vascular resistance. Isoflurane produces vasodilation in most vascular beds, with pronounced effects in skin and muscle, and is a potent coronary vasodilator, simultaneously producing increased coronary blood flow and decreased myocardial O_2 consumption. Isoflurane significantly attenuates baroreceptor function. Patients anesthetized with isoflurane generally have mildly elevated heart rates as a compensatory response to reduced blood pressure; however, rapid changes in isoflurane concentration can produce both transient tachycardia and hypertension due to isoflurane-induced sympathetic stimulation.

Respiratory System. Isoflurane produces concentration-dependent depression of ventilation. This drug is particularly effective at depressing the ventilatory response to hypercapnia and hypoxia. Although isoflurane is a bronchodilator, it also is an airway irritant and can stimulate airway reflexes during induction of anesthesia, producing coughing and laryngospasm.

Nervous System. Isoflurane dilates the cerebral vasculature, producing increased CBF (Drummond et al., 1983). There is a modest risk of an increase in ICP in patients with preexisting intracranial hypertension. Isoflurane reduces $CMRo_2$ in a dose-dependent manner.

Muscle. Isoflurane produces some relaxation of skeletal muscle by its central effects. It also enhances the effects of both depolarizing and nondepolarizing muscle relaxants. Like other halogenated inhalational anesthetics, isoflurane relaxes uterine smooth muscle and is not recommended for analgesia or anesthesia for labor and vaginal delivery.

Kidney. Isoflurane reduces renal blood flow and GFR, resulting in a small volume of concentrated urine.

Liver and GI Tract. Splanchnic and hepatic blood flows are reduced with increasing doses of isoflurane as systemic arterial pressure decreases. There are no reported incidences of hepatic toxicity.

Sevoflurane

Sevoflurane is a clear, colorless, volatile liquid at room temperature and must be stored in a sealed bottle. It is nonflammable and nonexplosive in mixtures of air or O_2. However, sevoflurane can undergo an exothermic reaction with desiccated CO_2 absorbent to produce airway burns or spontaneous ignition, explosion, and fire. *Sevoflurane must not be used with an anesthesia machine in which the CO_2 absorbent has been dried by prolonged gas flow through the absorbent. The reaction of sevoflurane with desiccated CO_2 absorbent also can produce CO, which can result in serious patient injury.*

Clinical Use and ADME. Sevoflurane is widely used for outpatient anesthesia because of its rapid recovery profile and because it is not irritating to the airway. Induction of anesthesia is rapidly achieved using inhaled concentrations of 2%–4% sevoflurane. Sevoflurane has properties that make it an ideal induction agent: pleasant smell, rapid onset, and lack of irritation to the airway. Thus, it has largely replaced halothane (not available in the U.S.) as the preferred agent for anesthetic induction in adult and pediatric patients.

The low solubility of sevoflurane in blood and other tissues provides for rapid induction of anesthesia and rapid changes in anesthetic depth following changes in delivered concentration. Approximately 5% of absorbed sevoflurane is metabolized by hepatic CYP2E1, with the predominant product being hexafluoroisopropanol. Hepatic metabolism of sevoflurane also produces inorganic fluoride. Interaction of sevoflurane with soda lime produces decomposition products that may be toxic, such as compound A, pentafluoroisopropenyl fluoromethyl ether (see kidney discussion under Side Effects).

Side Effects

Cardiovascular System. Sevoflurane produces concentration-dependent decreases in arterial blood pressure (due to systemic vasodilation) and cardiac output. Sevoflurane does not produce tachycardia and thus may be a preferable agent in patients prone to myocardial ischemia.

Respiratory System. Sevoflurane produces a concentration-dependent reduction in tidal volume and increase in respiratory rate in spontaneously breathing patients. The increased respiratory frequency does not compensate for reduced tidal volume, with the net effect being a reduction in minute ventilation and an increase in $PaCO_2$. Sevoflurane is not irritating to the airway and is a potent bronchodilator. As a result, sevoflurane is the most effective clinical bronchodilator of the inhalational anesthetics.

Nervous System. Sevoflurane produces effects on cerebral vascular resistance, $CMRO_2$, and CBF that are similar to those produced by isoflurane and desflurane. Sevoflurane can increase ICP in patients with poor intracranial compliance, the response to hypocapnia is preserved during sevoflurane anesthesia, and increases in ICP can be prevented by hyperventilation. In children, sevoflurane is associated with delirium on emergence from anesthesia. This delirium is short lived and without any reported adverse long-term sequelae.

Muscle. Sevoflurane produces skeletal muscle relaxation and enhances the effects of nondepolarizing and depolarizing neuromuscular blocking agents.

Kidney. Controversy has surrounded the potential nephrotoxicity of compound A, which is produced by interaction of sevoflurane with the CO_2 absorbent soda lime. Biochemical evidence of transient renal injury has been reported in human volunteers (Eger et al., 1997). Large clinical studies have shown no evidence of increased serum creatinine, blood urea nitrogen, or any other evidence of renal impairment following sevoflurane administration. *The FDA recommends that sevoflurane be administered with fresh gas flows of 1–2 L/min, with sevoflurane exposures not exceeding 2 MAC-hours to minimize exposure to compound A.*

Liver and GI Tract. Sevoflurane is not known to cause hepatotoxicity or alterations of hepatic function tests.

Desflurane

Desflurane is a highly volatile liquid at room temperature (vapor pressure = 669 mm Hg) and must be stored in tightly sealed bottles. Delivery of a precise concentration of desflurane requires the use of a specially heated vaporizer that delivers pure vapor that then is diluted appropriately with other gases (O_2, air, or N_2O). Desflurane is nonflammable and nonexplosive in mixtures of air or O_2.

Clinical Use and ADME. Desflurane is for outpatient surgery because of its rapid onset of action and rapid recovery time. The drug irritates the tracheobronchial tree and can provoke coughing, salivation, and bronchospasm. Anesthesia therefore usually is induced with an intravenous agent, with desflurane subsequently administered for maintenance of anesthesia. Maintenance of anesthesia usually requires inhaled concentrations of 6%–8% (~1 MAC). Lower concentrations of desflurane are required if it is coadministered with nitrous oxide or opioids.

Desflurane has a very low blood:gas partition coefficient (0.42) and also is not very soluble in fat or other peripheral tissues. Thus, the alveolar and blood concentrations rapidly rise to the level of inspired concentration, providing rapid induction of anesthesia and rapid changes in depth of anesthesia following changes in the inspired concentration. Emergence from desflurane anesthesia also is rapid. Desflurane is minimally metabolized; more than 99% of absorbed desflurane is eliminated unchanged through the lungs.

Side Effects

Cardiovascular System. Desflurane produces hypotension primarily by decreasing systemic vascular resistance. Cardiac output is well preserved, as is blood flow to the major organ beds (splanchnic, renal, cerebral, and coronary) (Eger, 1994). Transient tachycardia is often noted with abrupt increases in desflurane's delivered concentration, a result of this desflurane-induced stimulation of the sympathetic nervous system. The hypotensive effects of desflurane do not wane with increasing duration of administration.

Respiratory System. Desflurane causes a concentration-dependent increase in respiratory rate and a decrease in tidal volume. At low concentrations (<1 MAC), the net effect is to preserve minute ventilation. Desflurane concentrations greater than 1 MAC depress minute ventilation, resulting in elevated arterial CO_2 tension ($PaCO_2$). Desflurane is a bronchodilator. However, it also is a strong airway irritant and can cause coughing, breath-holding, laryngospasm, and excessive respiratory secretions. *Because of its irritant properties, desflurane is not used as the primary anesthetic for induction of anesthesia.*

Nervous System. Desflurane decreases cerebral vascular resistance and $CMRO_2$. Burst suppression of the EEG is achieved with ~2 MAC; at this level, $CMRO_2$ is reduced by ~50%. Under conditions of normocapnia and normotension, desflurane produces an increase in CBF and can increase ICP in patients with poor intracranial compliance. The vasoconstrictive response to hypocapnia is preserved during desflurane anesthesia, and increases in ICP thus can be prevented by hyperventilation.

Muscle, Kidney, Liver, and GI Tract. Desflurane produces direct skeletal muscle relaxation as well as enhances the effects of nondepolarizing and depolarizing neuromuscular blocking agents. Consistent with its minimal metabolic degradation, desflurane has no reported nephrotoxicity or hepatotoxicity.

Desflurane and Carbon Monoxide. Inhaled anesthetics are administered via a system that permits unidirectional flow of gas and rebreathing of exhaled gases. To prevent rebreathing of CO_2 (which can lead to hypercarbia), CO_2 absorbers are incorporated into the anesthesia delivery circuits. With almost complete desiccation of the CO_2 absorbents, substantial quantities of carbon monoxide can be produced. This effect is greatest with desflurane and can be prevented by the use of well-hydrated, fresh CO_2 absorbent.

Halothane

Halothane is a volatile liquid at room temperature and must be stored in a sealed container. Because halothane is a light-sensitive compound, it is marketed in amber bottles with thymol added as a preservative. Mixtures of halothane with O_2 or air are neither flammable nor explosive.

Clinical Use and ADME. Halothane has been used for maintenance of anesthesia. Concerns over hepatic toxicity have limited its use in developed countries. Halothane can produce fulminant hepatic necrosis (*halothane hepatitis*) in ~1 in 10,000 patients receiving halothane and "is referred to as halothane *hepatitis*" ("Summary," 1966). This syndrome (with a 50% fatality rate) is characterized by fever, anorexia, nausea, and vomiting, developing several days after anesthesia, and can be accompanied by a rash and peripheral eosinophilia. Halothane hepatitis may be the result of an immune response to hepatic proteins that become trifluoroacetylated as a consequence of halothane metabolism. Halothane has a low cost and is still widely used in developing countries. Due to its side-effect profile and the availability of safer agents with more favorable pharmacokinetic profiles, halothane is no longer marketed in the U.S. Those interested in further information on halothane should consult previous recent editions of this book.

Enflurane

Enflurane is a clear, colorless liquid at room temperature and has a mild, sweet odor. Like other inhalational anesthetics, it is volatile and must be stored in a sealed bottle. It is nonflammable and nonexplosive in mixtures of air or oxygen.

Clinical Use and ADME. Enflurane is primarily utilized for maintenance rather than induction of anesthesia. Surgical anesthesia can be induced with enflurane in less than 10 min with an inhaled concentration of 2%–4.5% in oxygen and maintained with concentrations from 0.5% to 3%. Enflurane concentrations required to produce anesthesia are reduced when it is coadministered with nitrous oxide or opioids. Concerns over enflurane's ability to decrease seizure threshold and potentially produce nephrotoxicity have limited its clinical utility in developed countries (Mazze et al., 1977).

Because of its relatively high blood:gas partition coefficient, induction of anesthesia and recovery from enflurane are relatively slow. Enflurane is metabolized to a modest extent, with 2%–8% of absorbed enflurane undergoing oxidative metabolism by hepatic CYP2E1. Fluoride ions are a by-product of enflurane metabolism, but plasma fluoride levels are low and nontoxic. Patients taking isoniazid exhibit enhanced metabolism of enflurane with consequent elevation of serum fluoride.

Side Effects. Enflurane causes a decrease in arterial blood pressure, the result of vasodilation and depression of myocardial contractility, with minimal effects on heart rate. The drug is an effective bronchodilator and produces a pattern of rapid shallow breathing. Due to its actions as a cerebral vasodilator, enflurane can increase ICP. It can produce seizure activity and should not be used in patients with seizure disorders. Enflurane relaxes skeletal and uterine muscle. As with other anesthetic gases, enflurane reduces renal blood flow, GFR, and urinary output.

Nitrous Oxide

Nitrous oxide is a colorless, odorless gas at room temperature. N_2O is sold in steel cylinders and must be delivered through calibrated flowmeters provided on all anesthesia machines. N_2O is neither flammable nor explosive, but it does support combustion as actively as oxygen does when it is present in proper concentration with a flammable anesthetic or material.

Clinical Use and ADME. N_2O is a weak anesthetic agent that has significant analgesic effects. Surgical anesthetic depth is only achieved under hyperbaric conditions. By contrast, analgesia is produced at concentrations as low as 20%. The analgesic property of N_2O is a function of the activation of opioidergic neurons in the periaqueductal gray matter and the adrenergic neurons in the locus ceruleus. N_2O is frequently used in concentrations of ~50% to provide analgesia and mild sedation in outpatient dentistry. N_2O cannot be used at concentrations above 80% because this limits the delivery of adequate O_2. Because of this limitation, N_2O is used primarily as an adjunct to other inhalational or intravenous anesthetics.

Nitrous oxide is very insoluble in blood and other tissues. This results in rapid equilibration between delivered and alveolar anesthetic concentrations and provides for rapid induction of anesthesia and rapid emergence following discontinuation of administration. The rapid uptake of N_2O from alveolar gas serves to concentrate coadministered halogenated anesthetics; this effect (the "second gas effect") speeds induction of anesthesia. On discontinuation of N_2O administration, N_2O gas can diffuse from blood to the alveoli, diluting O_2 in the lung. This can produce an effect called *diffusional hypoxia. To avoid hypoxia, 100% O_2 rather than air should be administered when N_2O is discontinued.* Almost all (99.9%) of the absorbed N_2O is eliminated unchanged by the lungs.

Side Effects

Cardiovascular System. Although N_2O produces a negative inotropic effect on heart muscle in vitro, depressant effects on cardiac function generally are not observed in patients because of the stimulatory effects of N_2O on the sympathetic nervous system. The cardiovascular effects of N_2O also are heavily influenced by the concomitant administration of other anesthetic agents. When N_2O is coadministered with halogenated inhalational anesthetics, one observes increases in heart rate, arterial blood pressure, and cardiac output. In contrast, when N_2O is coadministered with an opioid, one generally sees decreases in arterial blood pressure and cardiac output. N_2O also increases venous tone in both the peripheral and the pulmonary vasculature. The effects of N_2O on pulmonary vascular resistance can be exaggerated in patients with preexisting pulmonary hypertension; thus, the drug generally is not used in these patients.

Respiratory System. N_2O causes modest increases in respiratory rate and decreases in tidal volume in spontaneously breathing patients. Even modest concentrations of N_2O markedly depress the ventilatory response to hypoxia. Thus, it is prudent to monitor arterial O_2 saturation directly in patients receiving or recovering from N_2O.

Nervous System. N_2O can significantly increase CBF and ICP. This cerebral vasodilatory capacity of N_2O is significantly attenuated by the simultaneous administration of intravenous agents such as opiates and propofol. By contrast, the combination of N_2O and inhaled agents results in greater vasodilation than the administration of the inhaled agent alone at equivalent anesthetic depth.

Muscle. N_2O does not relax skeletal muscle and does not enhance the effects of neuromuscular blocking drugs.

Kidney, Liver, and GI Tract. N_2O is not known to have nephrotoxic or hepatotoxic effects.

Other Adverse Effects. A major problem with N_2O is that it will exchange with N_2 in any air-containing cavity in the body. Moreover, because of their differential blood:gas partition coefficients, N_2O will enter the cavity faster than N_2 escapes, thereby increasing the volume or pressure in this cavity. Examples of air collections that can be expanded by N_2O include a pneumothorax, an obstructed middle ear, an air embolus, an obstructed loop of bowel, an intraocular air bubble, a pulmonary bulla, and intracranial air. N_2O should be avoided in these clinical settings.

Nitrous oxide interacts with the cobalt of vitamin B_{12}, thereby preventing vitamin B_{12} from acting as a cofactor for methionine synthase (Sanders and Maze, 2007). Inactivation of methionine synthase can produce signs of vitamin B_{12} deficiency, including megaloblastic anemia and peripheral neuropathy, a particular concern in patients with malnutrition, vitamin B_{12} deficiency, or alcoholism. The clinical use of N_2O is controversial due to its potential metabolic effects related to increased homocysteine and changes in DNA and protein synthesis (Ko et al., 2014). For this reason, N_2O is not used as a chronic analgesic or as a sedative in critical care settings.

Xenon

Xenon, an inert gaseous element, is not approved for use in the U.S. and is unlikely to enjoy widespread use because it is a rare gas that cannot be manufactured and must be extracted from air; thus, xenon is expensive and available in limited quantities. Xenon, unlike other anesthetic agents, has minimal cardiorespiratory and other side effects.

Xenon exerts its analgesic and anesthetic effects at a number of receptor systems in the CNS. Of these, noncompetitive antagonism of the NMDA receptor and agonism at the TREK channel (a member of the two-pore K^+ channel family) are thought to be the central mechanisms of xenon action (Franks and Honore, 2004).

Xenon is extremely insoluble in blood and other tissues, providing for rapid induction and emergence from anesthesia. It is sufficiently potent to produce surgical anesthesia when administered with 30% oxygen. However, supplementation with an intravenous agent such as propofol appears to be required for clinical anesthesia. Xenon is well tolerated in patients of advanced age. No long-term side effects from xenon anesthesia have been reported.

Anesthetic Adjuncts

A general anesthetic is usually given with adjuncts to augment specific components of anesthesia, permitting lower doses of general anesthetics with fewer side effects.

Benzodiazepines

Benzodiazepines (see Chapters 15 and 19) can produce anesthesia similar to that of barbiturates; they are more commonly used for sedation rather than general anesthesia because prolonged amnesia and sedation

Drug Facts for Your Personal Formulary: *Pulmonary Hypertension Therapeutics*

Drug	Indication	Clinical Pharmacology and Tips
cGMP Signaling Modulators: PDE5 Inhibitors		
Sildenafil Tadalafil Vardenafil	• First-line therapy for moderate PAH (functional class II-III)	• Oral administration • Avoid nitrates and α adrenergic antagonists due to hypotension • Major side effects: epistaxis, headache, dyspepsia, vision or hearing loss (not sildenafil), flushing, insomnia, dyspnea, priapism • Vardenafil, currently not recommended due to limited evidence for efficacy in PAH
cGMP Signaling Modulators: sGC Stimulator		
Riociguat	• First-line therapy for moderate PAH (functional class II-III)	• Oral administration • Efficacy confirmed in PAH patients and CTEPH patients • Side effects: headache, dyspepsia, edema, nausea, dizziness, syncope
IP Receptor Agonists: Prostacyclin and Prostacyclin Analogs		
Epoprostenol	• First-line therapy for severe PAH (functional class IV)	• Administration by continuous IV infusion • Major side effects: jaw pain, hypotension, myalgia, flushing, nausea, vomiting, dizziness • Short half-life requires immediate medical attention to pump failure
Treprostinil	• Same as epoprostenol	• Available as IV, SC, inhaled and oral preps • Longer half-life than epoprostenol with similar side effects • Local adverse effects of SC dose may improve over time • Oral administration to be used as monotherapy only
Iloprost	• Alternative for epoprostenol in combination therapy for severe PAH (function class IV)	• Inhaled administration, at least 2 h apart • Side effects include flushing, hypotension, headache, nausea, throat irritation, cough, insomnia
Selexipag	• Alternative for eprostenol in combination therapy for severe PAH (functional class IV)	• Oral administration • Selective PGI_2 receptor agonist • Side effects include headache, jaw pain, nausea, diarrhea
Endothelin Receptor Antagonists: Oral administration, teratogenic		
Bosentan	• First-line therapy for moderate PAH (functional class II-III)	• Monitor liver function and hemoglobin levels • Metabolized by CYP2C9 and CYP3A4 • Side effects: liver impairment, palpitations, itching, edema, anemia, respiratory infections
Ambrisentan	• First-line therapy for moderate PAH (functional class II-III)	• Side effects: edema, nasal congestion, constipation, flushing, palpitations, abdominal pain • Cyclosporin coadministration increases drug levels • Low risk for liver toxicity
Macitentan	• First-line therapy for moderate PAH (functional class II-III)	• Metabolized by CYP3A4 • Side effects include nasopharyngitis, headache, anemia • Liver function and hemoglobin testing recommended prior to therapy
L-type Ca^{2+} Channel Blockers		
Nifedipine (long acting) Amlodipine Diltiazem	• Use only in PAH patients with positive vasodilator testing	• Oral administration • Side effects include edema, fatigue, hypotension • Diltiazem: significant negative chronotropic and inotropic effects; avoid in bradycardia

Abbreviations: PAH, Pulmonary Arterial Hypertension; ERA, Endothelin Receptor Antagonist; CTEPH, Chronic Thromboembolic Pulmonary Hypertension; IV, intravenous; SC, subcutaneous.

Bibliography

Abman SH. Inhaled nitric oxide for the treatment of pulmonary arterial hypertension. *Handb Exp Pharmacol,* **2013**, *218*:257–276.

Barst RJ, Beraprost Study Group. Beraprost therapy for pulmonary arterial hypertension. *J Am Coll Cardiol,* **2003**, *41*:2119–2125.

Barst RJ, Primary Pulmonary Hypertension Study Group. A comparison of continuous intravenous epoprostenol (prostacyclin) with conventional therapy for primary pulmonary hypertension. *N Engl J Med,* **1996**, *334*:296–301.

Benza RL, et al. An evaluation of long-term survival from time of diagnosis in pulmonary arterial hypertension from the REVEAL Registry. *Chest,* **2012**, *142*:448–456.

Budhiraja R. Endothelial dysfunction in pulmonary hypertension. *Circulation,* **2004**, *109*:159–165.

Bueno M, et al. Nitrite signaling in pulmonary hypertension: mechanisms of bioactivation, signaling, and therapeutics. *Antioxid Redox Signal,* **2013**, *18*:1797–1809.

Christman BW, et al. An imbalance between the excretion of thromboxane and prostacyclin metabolites in pulmonary hypertension. *N Engl J Med,* **1992**, *327*:70–75.

Cockrill BA, Waxman AB. Phosphodiesterase-5 inhibitors. *Handb Exp Pharmacol,* **2013**, *218*:229–255.

Craven KB, Zagotta WN. CNG and HCN channels: two peas, one pod. *Annu Rev Physiol,* **2006**, *68*:375–401.

Davenport AP, et al. Endothelin. *Pharmacol Rev,* **2016**, *68*:357–418.

Du L, et al. Signaling molecules in nonfamilial pulmonary hypertension. *N Engl J Med,* **2003**, *348*:500–509.

Fedullo P, et al. Chronic thromboembolic pulmonary hypertension. *Am J Respir Crit Care Med,* **2011**, *183*:1605–1613.

Frumkin LR. The pharmacological treatment of pulmonary arterial hypertension. *Pharmacol Rev,* **2012**, *64*:583–620.

Galiè N, Sildenafil Use in Pulmonary Arterial Hypertension Study Group. Sildenafil citrate therapy for pulmonary arterial hypertension. *N Engl J Med,* **2005**, *353*:2148–2157.

Galie, N, et al. Initial use of ambrisentan plus tadalafil in pulmonary arterial hypertension. *N Engl J Med,* **2015**, *373*:834-844.

Ghofrani HA, et al. Riociguat for the treatment of chronic thromboembolic pulmonary hypertension. *N Engl J Med,* **2013**, *369*:319–329.

Ghofrani HA, et al. Riociguat for the treatment of pulmonary arterial hypertension. *N Engl J Med,* **2013**, *369*:330–340.

Ghofrani HA, Humbert M. The role of combination therapy in managing pulmonary arterial hypertension. *Eur Respir Rev,* **2014**, *23*:469–475.

Giaid A, et al. Expression of endothelin-1 in the lungs of patients with pulmonary hypertension. *N Engl J Med,* **1993**, *328*:1732–1739.

Girgis RE, et al. Decreased exhaled nitric oxide in pulmonary arterial hypertension: response to bosentan therapy. *Am J Respir Crit Care Med,* **2005**, *172*:352–357.

Gomberg-Maitland M, et al. A dosing/cross-development study of the multikinase inhibitor sorafenib in patients with pulmonary arterial hypertension. *Clin Pharmacol Ther,* **2010**, *87*:303-310.

Griffiths MJ, Evans TW. Inhaled nitric oxide therapy in adults. *N Engl J Med,* **2005**, *353*:2683–2695.

Hemnes AR, et al. Peripheral blood signature of vasodilator-responsive pulmonary arterial hypertension. *Circulation,* **2015**, *131*:401–409.

Hoeper MM, et al. Imatinib mesylate as add-on therapy for pulmonary arterial hypertension: results of the randomized IMPRES study. *Circulation,* **2013**, *127*:1128–1138.

Humbert M, et al. Platelet-derived growth factor expression in primary pulmonary hypertension: comparison of HIV seropositive and HIV seronegative patients. *Eur Respir J,* **1998**, *11*:554–559.

Humbert M, Ghofrani H-A. The molecular targets of approved treatments for pulmonary arterial hypertension. *Thorax,* **2016**, *71*:73–83.

Ichinose F, et al. Inhaled nitric oxide: a selective pulmonary vasodilator: current uses and therapeutic potential. *Circulation,* **2004**, *109*: 3106–3111.

Jing ZC, et al. Efficacy and safety of oral treprostinil monotherapy for the treatment of pulmonary arterial hypertension: a randomized, controlled trial. *Circulation,* **2013**, *127*:624–633.

Kaufmann P, et al. Pharmacokinetics and tolerability of the novel oral prostacyclin IP receptor agonist selexipag. *Am J Cardiovasc Drugs,* **2015**, *15*:195–203.

Kawaguchi Y, et al. NOS2 polymorphisms associated with the susceptibility to pulmonary arterial hypertension with systemic sclerosis: contribution to the transcriptional activity. *Arthritis Res Ther,* **2006**, *8*:R104.

Kass DA, et al. Phosphodiesterase type 5: expanding roles in cardiovascular regulation. *Circ Res,* **2007**, *101*:1084–1095.

Kuhr FK, et al. New mechanisms of pulmonary arterial hypertension: role of Ca^{2+} signaling. *Am J Physiol Heart Circ Physiol,* **2012**, *302*: H1546–H1562.

Mandegar M, et al. Cellular and molecular mechanisms of pulmonary vascular remodeling: role in the development of pulmonary hypertension. *Microvasc Res,* **2004**, *68*:75–103.

McLaughlin VV, et al. ACCF/AHA 2009 expert consensus document on pulmonary hypertension. *J Am Coll Cardiol,* **2009**, *53*:1573–1619.

Moreno-Vinasco L, et al. Genomic assessment of a multikinase inhibitor, sorafenib, in a rodent model of pulmonary hypertension. *Physiol Genomics,* **2008**, *33*:278-291.

Morrell NW, et al. Cellular and molecular basis of pulmonary arterial hypertension. *J Am Coll Cardiol,* **2009**, *54*(suppl):S20–S31.

Muirhead GJ, et al. Comparative human pharmacokinetics and metabolism of single-dose oral and intravenous sildenafil. *Br J Clin Pharmacol,* **2002**, *53*(suppl 1):13S–20S.

O'Callaghan DS, et al. Endothelin receptor antagonists for the treatment of pulmonary arterial hypertension. *Expert Opin Pharmacother,* **2011**, *12*:1585–1596.

Olschewski H, et al. Prostacyclin and its analogues in the treatment of pulmonary hypertension. *Pharmacol Ther,* **2004**, *102*:139–153.

Olschewski H, et al. Aerosolized prostacyclin and iloprost in severe pulmonary hypertension. *Ann Intern Med,* **1996**, *124*:820–824.

Omori K, Kotera J. Overview of PDEs and their regulation. *Circ Res,* **2007**, *100*:309–327.

Pulido T, Seraphin Investigators. Macitentan and morbidity and mortality in pulmonary arterial hypertension. *N Engl J Med,* **2013**, *369*:809–818.

Ravipati G, et al. Type 5 phosphodiesterase inhibitors in the treatment of erectile dysfunction and cardiovascular disease. *Cardiol Rev,* **2007**, *15*:76–86.

Rich S, Brundage BH. High-dose calcium channel-blocking therapy for primary pulmonary hypertension: evidence for long-term reduction in pulmonary arterial pressure and regression of right ventricular hypertrophy. *Circulation,* **1987**, *76*:135–141.

Rossaint R, et al. Inhaled nitric oxide for the adult respiratory distress syndrome. *N Engl J Med,* **1993**, *328*:399–405.

Rubin LJ, et al. Bosentan therapy for pulmonary arterial hypertension. *N Engl J Med,* **2002**, *346*:896–903.

Rubin LJ, et al. Frosolono M, Handel F, Cato AE. Prostacyclin-induced acute pulmonary vasodilation in primary pulmonary hypertension. *Circulation,* **1982**, *66*:334–338.

Schermuly RT, et al. Reversal of experimental pulmonary hypertension by PDGF inhibition. *J Clin Invest,* **2005**, *115*:2811–2821.

Simonneau G, et al. Updated clinical classification of pulmonary hypertension. *J Am Coll Cardiol,* **2013**, *62*:D34–D41.

Simonneau G, et al. Selexipag: an oral, selective prostacyclin receptor agonist for the treatment of pulmonary arterial hypertension. *Eur Respir J,* **2012**, *40*:874–880.

Simonneau G, Treprostinil Study Group. Continuous subcutaneous infusion of treprostinil, a prostacyclin analogue, in patients with pulmonary arterial hypertension: a double-blind, randomized, placebo-controlled trial. *Am J Respir Crit Care Med,* **2002**, *165*: 800–804.

Sitbon O, Griphon Investigators. Selexipag for the treatment of pulmonary arterial hypertension. *N Engl J Med,* **2015**, *373*:2522–2533.

Sitbon O, et al. Long-term response to calcium channel blockers in idiopathic pulmonary arterial hypertension. *Circulation,* **2005**, *111*:3105–3111.

Sitbon O, et al. Upfront triple combination therapy in pulmonary arterial hypertension: a pilot study. *Eur Respir J,* **2014**, *43*:1691–1697.

Stasch JP, Evgenov OV. Soluble guanylate cyclase stimulators in pulmonary hypertension. *Handb Exp Pharmacol,* **2013**, *218*: 279–313.

Tapson VF, et al. Oral treprostinil for the treatment of pulmonary arterial hypertension in patients on background endothelin receptor antagonist and/or phosphodiesterase type 5 inhibitor therapy (the FREEDOM-C study): a randomized controlled trial. *Chest,* **2012**, *142*:1383–1390.

Yanagisawa M, et al. A novel potent vasoconstrictor peptide produced by vascular endothelial cells. *Nature,* **1988**, *332*:411–415.

Blood Coagulation and Anticoagulant, Fibrinolytic, and Antiplatelet Drugs

Kerstin Hogg and Jeffrey I. Weitz

第三十二章　凝血与抗凝血药、溶血栓药和抗血小板药

中文导读

本章主要介绍：止血的概述（血小板功能、血液凝固和纤维蛋白溶解），包括纤维蛋白原向纤维蛋白的转化；凝血因子的结构；无酶活性的蛋白辅助因子，包括启动辅助因子Ⅷ、Ⅴ；凝血酶原的激活，包括凝血机制的启动，纤维蛋白溶解，体外凝血，天然抗凝物的机制，肠外抗凝血药（肝素、LMWHs、磺达肝素），以及其他肠外抗凝血药；维生素K拮抗药，包括华法林；直接口服抗凝血药，包括直接口服凝血酶抑制药、直接口服因子Xa抑制药和直接口服抗凝血药逆转药；纤维蛋白溶解药，包括组织型纤溶酶原激活药；纤维蛋白溶解抑制药，包括ε-氨基己酸和氨甲环酸；抗血小板药，包括阿司匹林、双嘧达莫、$P2Y_{12}$受体拮抗药、凝血酶受体抑制药和糖蛋白Ⅱb/Ⅲa抑制药；维生素K的作用，包括维生素K的生理功能和药理作用、摄入不足、吸收不足和利用不足。

Abbreviations

ACT: activated clotting time
ADP: adenosine diphosphate
α_2-AP: α_2-antiplasmin
aPTT: activated partial thromboplastin time
CNS: central nervous system
COX: cyclooxygenase
CPR: cardiopulmonary resuscitation
CrCL: creatinine clearance
CYP: cytochrome P450
EDTA: ethylenediaminetetraacetic acid
EPCR: endothelial protein C receptor
GI: gastrointestinal
Gla: γ-carboxyglutamic acid
Glu: glutamic acid
GP: glycoprotein
INR: international normalized ratio
IP_3: inositol 1,4,5-trisphosphate
KGD: lysine-glycine-aspartate
LMWH: low-molecular-weight heparin
NO: nitric oxide
PAI: plasminogen activator inhibitor
PAR: protease-activated receptor
PGI_2: prostaglandin I_2 or prostacyclin
PLC: phospholipase C
PT: prothrombin time
RGD: arginine-glycine-aspartate
TF: tissue factor
TFPI: tissue factor pathway inhibitor
t-PA: tissue plasminogen activator
TxA_2: thromboxane A_2
u-PA: urokinase plasminogen activator
USP: U.S. Pharmacopeia
VKOR: vitamin K epoxide reductase
VKORC1: C1 subunit of vitamin K epoxide reductase
vWF: von Willebrand factor

Blood must remain fluid within the vasculature and yet clot quickly when exposed to subendothelial surfaces at sites of vascular injury. Under normal circumstances, a delicate balance between coagulation and fibrinolysis prevents both thrombosis and hemorrhage. Alteration of this balance in favor of coagulation results in thrombosis. Thrombi, composed of platelet aggregates, fibrin, and trapped red blood cells, can form in arteries or veins. Antithrombotic drugs used to treat thrombosis include antiplatelet drugs, which inhibit platelet activation or aggregation; anticoagulants, which attenuate fibrin formation; and fibrinolytic agents, which degrade fibrin. All antithrombotic drugs increase the risk of bleeding.

This chapter reviews the agents commonly used for controlling blood fluidity, including

- the parenteral anticoagulant heparin and its derivatives, which activate antithrombin, a natural inhibitor of coagulant proteases;
- the coumarin anticoagulants, which block multiple steps in the coagulation cascade;
- the direct oral anticoagulants, which inhibit factor Xa or thrombin;
- fibrinolytic agents, which degrade fibrin;
- antiplatelet agents, which attenuate platelet activation (aspirin, clopidogrel, prasugrel, ticagrelor, and vorapaxar) or aggregation (glycoprotein IIb/IIIa inhibitors); and
- vitamin K, which is required for the biosynthesis of key coagulation factors.

Overview of Hemostasis: Platelet Function, Blood Coagulation, and Fibrinolysis

Hemostasis is the cessation of blood loss from a damaged vessel. Platelets first adhere to macromolecules in the subendothelial regions of the injured blood vessel, where they become activated. Adherent platelets release substances that activate nearby platelets, thereby recruiting them to the site of injury. Activated platelets then aggregate to form the primary hemostatic plug.

Vessel wall injury also exposes tissue factor (*TF*), which initiates the coagulation system. Activated platelets enhance activation of the coagulation system by providing a surface onto which clotting factors assemble and by releasing stored clotting factors. This results in a burst of *thrombin* (*factor IIa*) generation. Thrombin converts soluble fibrinogen to fibrin, activates platelets, and feeds back to promote additional thrombin generation. The fibrin strands tie the platelet aggregates together to form a stable clot.

The processes of platelet activation and aggregation and blood coagulation are summarized in Figures 32–1 and 32–2 (see also the animation on the Goodman & Gilman site on *AccessMedicine.com*). Coagulation involves a series of zymogen activation reactions, as shown in Figure 32–2. At each stage, a precursor protein, or *zymogen*, is converted to an active protease by cleavage of one or more peptide bonds in the precursor molecule. The final protease generated is thrombin. Later, as wound healing occurs, the fibrin clot is degraded. The pathway of clot removal, fibrinolysis, is shown in Figure 32–3, along with sites of action of fibrinolytic agents.

Conversion of Fibrinogen to Fibrin

Fibrinogen, a 340,000-Da protein, is a dimer, each half of which consists of three pairs of polypeptide chains (designated Aα, Bβ, and γ). Disulfide bonds covalently link the chains and the two halves of the molecule. Thrombin converts fibrinogen to fibrin monomers by releasing fibrinopeptide A (a 16–amino acid fragment) and fibrinopeptide B (a 14–amino acid fragment) from the amino termini of the Aα and Bβ chains, respectively. Removal of the fibrinopeptides creates new amino termini, which form knobs that fit into preformed holes on other fibrin monomers to form a fibrin gel, which is the end point of in vitro tests of coagulation (see Coagulation In Vitro). Initially, the fibrin monomers are bound to each other noncovalently. Subsequently, factor XIII, a transglutaminase that is activated by thrombin, catalyzes interchain covalent cross-links between adjacent fibrin monomers, which strengthen the clot.

Structure of Coagulation Factors

In addition to factor XIII, the coagulation factors include factors II (prothrombin), VII, IX, X, XI, XII, high-molecular-weight kininogen and prekallikrein. A stretch of about 200 amino acid residues at the carboxyl termini of each of these zymogens exhibits homology to trypsin and contains the active site of the proteases. In addition, 9–12 Glu residues near the amino termini of factors II, VII, IX, and X are converted to Gla residues in a vitamin K–dependent posttranslational step. The Gla residues bind Ca^{2+} and are essential for the coagulant activities of these proteins by enabling their interaction with the anionic phospholipid membrane of activated platelets.

Nonenzymatic Protein Cofactors

TF, factor V, and factor VIII are critical cofactors in coagulation. A nonenzymatic lipoprotein cofactor, TF is not normally present on blood-contacting cells. TF is constitutively expressed on the surface of subendothelial smooth muscle cells and fibroblasts, which are exposed when the vessel wall is damaged. TF binds factor VIIa and enhances its catalytic efficiency. The TF/factor VIIa complex initiates coagulation by activating factors IX and X.

may result from anesthetizing doses. As adjuncts, benzodiazepines are used for anxiolysis, amnesia, and sedation prior to induction of anesthesia or for sedation during procedures not requiring general anesthesia. The benzodiazepine most frequently used in the perioperative period is midazolam, followed distantly by diazepam and lorazepam.

Midazolam is water soluble and typically is administered intravenously but also can be given orally, intramuscularly, or rectally; oral midazolam is particularly useful for sedation of young children. Midazolam produces minimal venous irritation (as opposed to diazepam and lorazepam, which are formulated in propylene glycol and are painful on injection, sometimes producing thrombophlebitis). Midazolam has the pharmacokinetic advantage, particularly over lorazepam, of being more rapid in onset and shorter in duration of effect. Sedative doses of midazolam (0.01–0.05 mg/kg IV) reach peak effect in about 2 min and provide sedation for approximately 30 min. Elderly patients tend to be more sensitive to and have a slower recovery from benzodiazepines. Midazolam is metabolized principally by hepatic CYP3A4, and drug interactions with inducers, inhibitors, and substrates of that CYP are predictable. Either for prolonged sedation or for general anesthetic maintenance, midazolam is more suitable than other benzodiazepines for infusion, although midazolam's duration of action ($t_{1/2}$) does significantly increase with prolonged infusions (see Figure 21–2). Benzodiazepines reduce CBF and cerebral metabolism, but at equianesthetic doses are less effective than barbiturates in this respect. Benzodiazepines modestly decrease blood pressure and respiratory drive, occasionally resulting in apnea.

α_2 Adrenergic Agonists

Dexmedetomidine is a selective α_2 adrenergic receptor agonist (Kamibayashi and Maze, 2000) used for short-term (<24 h) sedation of critically ill adults and for sedation prior to and during surgical or other medical procedures in nonintubated patients. Activation of the α_{2A} adrenergic receptor by dexmedetomidine produces both sedation and analgesia.

The recommended loading dose is 1 μg/kg given over 10 min, followed by infusion at a rate of 0.2–0.7 μg/kg/h. Reduced doses should be considered in patients with risk factors for severe hypotension. Dexmedetomidine is highly protein bound and is metabolized primarily in the liver; the glucuronide and methyl conjugates are excreted in the urine. Common side effects of dexmedetomidine include hypotension and bradycardia, attributed to decreased catecholamine release by activation peripherally and in the CNS of the α_{2A} receptor. Nausea and dry mouth also are common untoward reactions. At higher drug concentrations, the α_{2B} subtype is activated, resulting in hypertension and a further decrease in heart rate and cardiac output. Dexmedetomidine provides sedation and analgesia with minimal respiratory depression. However, dexmedetomidine does not appear to provide reliable amnesia, and additional agents may be needed.

Analgesics

Analgesics typically are administered with general anesthetics to reduce anesthetic requirements and minimize hemodynamic changes produced by painful stimuli. Nonsteroidal anti-inflammatory drugs, cyclooxygenase 2 inhibitors, and acetaminophen (see Chapter 38) sometimes provide adequate analgesia for minor surgical procedures. However, opioids are the primary analgesics used during the perioperative period because of the rapid and profound analgesia they produce. Fentanyl, sufentanil, alfentanil, remifentanil, meperidine, and morphine are the major parenteral opioids used in the perioperative period. The primary analgesic activity of each of these drugs is produced by agonist activity at μ opioid receptors (see Chapter 20).

The choice of a perioperative opioid is based primarily on duration of action because, at appropriate doses, all produce similar analgesia and side effects. Remifentanil has an ultrashort duration of action (<10 min), accumulates minimally with repeated doses, and is particularly well suited for procedures that are briefly painful. Single doses of fentanyl, sufentanil, and alfentanil all have similar intermediate durations of action (30, 20, and 15 min, respectively), but recovery after prolonged administration varies considerably. Fentanyl's duration of action lengthens the most with infusion, sufentanil's much less so, and alfentanil's the least.

The frequency and severity of nausea, vomiting, and pruritus after emergence from anesthesia are increased by all opioids to about the same degree. A useful side effect of meperidine is its capacity to reduce shivering, a common problem during emergence from anesthesia; other opioids are not as efficacious against shivering, perhaps due to less κ receptor agonism. Finally, opioids often are administered intrathecally and epidurally for management of acute and chronic pain (see Chapter 20). Neuraxial opioids with or without local anesthetics can provide profound analgesia for many surgical procedures; however, respiratory depression and pruritus usually limit their use to major operations.

Neuromuscular Blocking Agents

The practical aspects of the use of neuromuscular blockers as anesthetic adjuncts are briefly described here. The detailed pharmacology of this drug class is presented in Chapter 11.

Depolarizing (e.g., succinylcholine) and nondepolarizing (e.g., vecuronium) muscle relaxants often are administered during the induction of anesthesia to relax muscles of the jaw, neck, and airway and thereby facilitate laryngoscopy and endotracheal intubation. Nondepolarizing muscle relaxants are generally better tolerated. Barbiturates will precipitate when mixed with muscle relaxants and should be allowed to clear from the intravenous line prior to injection of a muscle relaxant. The action of nondepolarizing muscle relaxants usually is antagonized, once muscle paralysis is no longer desired, with an acetylcholinesterase inhibitor such as neostigmine or edrophonium (see Chapter 10), in combination with a muscarinic receptor antagonist (e.g., glycopyrrolate or atropine; see Chapter 9) to offset the muscarinic activation resulting from esterase inhibition. Sugammadex, a first-in-class selective relaxant binding agent specific for reversal of rocuronium muscle-relaxing effect, is approved in Europe and awaits FDA approval in the U.S. (Ledowski, 2015).

Anesthetic Toxicity and Cytoprotection

The conventional view of general anesthesia is that anesthetics produce a reversible loss of consciousness and that CNS function returns to basal levels on termination of anesthesia and recovery of anesthesia. Recent data, however, cast doubt on this notion. Exposure of rodents to anesthetic agents during the period of synaptogenesis results in widespread neurodegeneration in the developing brain (Jevtovic-Todorovic et al., 2003). This neuronal injury resulted in disturbed electrophysiologic function and cognitive dysfunction in adolescent and adult rodents exposed to anesthetics during the neonatal period. The cognitive deficits attendant with neonatal anesthetic exposure have been attributed to neuronal apoptosis; however, recently published data have cast doubt on this premise. There is convincing data that exposure to anesthetics in the neonatal period leads to actin cytoskeleton dysregulation and profound synaptic loss; this may contribute to later cognitive and behavioral dysfunction. A variety of agents, including isoflurane, propofol, midazolam, nitrous oxide, and thiopental, manifest this toxicity (Patel and Sun, 2009). The underlying mechanism(s) in animal models are unclear, and the threat to humans is still uncertain.

By contrast, anesthetics reduce ischemic injury to a variety of tissues, including the heart and brain. This protective effect is robust and results in better functional outcomes in comparison to ischemic injury that occurs in the unanesthetized awake subjects. In the brain, several mechanisms for anesthetic-mediated protection have been proposed, including suppression of excitotoxicity from excess glutamate release, reduction in inflammation, and increased prosurvival signaling (Head and Patel, 2007). In the heart, the molecular mechanisms attendant to anesthetic-mediated protection include activation of "classical" preconditioning pathways, including GPCRs, endothelial NO synthase, survival protein kinases, PKC, reactive oxygen species, ATP-dependent K^+ channels, and the mitochondrial permeable transition pore (Kunst and Klein, 2015).

Oxygen

Oxygen is essential to life. Hypoxia is a life-threatening condition in which O_2 delivery is inadequate to meet the metabolic demands of the tissues. Hypoxia may result from alterations in tissue perfusion, decreased O_2 tension in the blood, or decreased O_2 carrying capacity. In addition, hypoxia may result from restricted O_2 transport from the microvasculature to cells or impaired utilization within the cell. An inadequate supply of O_2 ultimately results in the cessation of aerobic metabolism and oxidative phosphorylation, depletion of high-energy compounds, cellular dysfunction, and death.

Normal Oxygenation

Oxygen makes up 21% of air, which at sea level represents a partial pressure of 21 kPa (158 mm Hg). While the fraction (percentage) of O_2 remains constant regardless of atmospheric pressure, the Po_2 decreases with lower atmospheric pressure. Ascent to elevated altitude reduces the uptake and delivery of O_2 to the tissues, whereas increases in atmospheric pressure (e.g., hyperbaric therapy or breathing at depth) raise the Po_2 in inspired air and increase gas uptake. As the air is delivered to the distal airways and alveoli, the Po_2 decreases by dilution with CO_2 and water vapor and by uptake into the blood.

Under ideal conditions, when ventilation and perfusion are well matched, the alveolar Po_2 will be about 14.6 kPa (110 mm Hg). The corresponding alveolar partial pressures of water and CO_2 are 6.2 kPa (47 mm Hg) and 5.3 kPa (40 mm Hg), respectively. Under normal conditions, there is complete equilibration of alveolar gas and lung capillary blood, and the Po_2 in end-capillary blood is typically within a fraction of a kilopascal of that in the alveoli. The Po_2 in arterial blood, however, is further reduced by venous admixture (shunt), the addition of mixed venous blood from the pulmonary artery, which has a Po_2 of about 5.3 kPa (40 mm Hg). Together, the diffusional barrier, ventilation-perfusion mismatches, and the shunt fraction are the major causes of the alveolar-to-arterial O_2 gradient, which is normally 1.3–1.6 kPa (10–12 mm Hg) when air is breathed and 4.0–6.6 kPa (30–50 mm Hg) when 100% O_2 is breathed. O_2 is delivered to the tissue capillary beds by the circulation and again follows a gradient out of the blood and into cells. Tissue extraction of O_2 typically reduces the Po_2 of venous blood by an additional 7.3 kPa (55 mm Hg). Although the Po_2 at the site of cellular O_2 utilization—the mitochondria—is not known, oxidative phosphorylation can continue at a Po_2 of only a few millimeters of mercury.

In the blood, O_2 is carried primarily in chemical combination with hemoglobin and is to a small extent dissolved in solution. The quantity of O_2 combined with hemoglobin depends on the Po_2, as illustrated by the sigmoidal oxyhemoglobin dissociation curve (Figure 21–5). Hemoglobin is about 98% saturated with O_2 when air is breathed under normal circumstances, and it binds 1.3 mL of O_2 per gram when fully saturated. The steep slope of this curve with falling Po_2 facilitates unloading of O_2 from hemoglobin at the tissue level and reloading when desaturated mixed venous blood arrives at the lung. Shifting of the curve to the right with increasing temperature, increasing Pco_2, and decreasing pH, as is found in metabolically active tissues, lowers the O_2 saturation for the same Po_2 and thus delivers additional O_2 where and when it is most needed. However, the flattening of the curve with higher Po_2 indicates that increasing blood Po_2 by inspiring O_2-enriched mixtures can increase the amount of O_2 carried by hemoglobin only minimally. Because of the low solubility of O_2 (0.226 mL/L per kPa or 0.03 mL/L per mm Hg at 37°C), breathing 100% O_2 can increase the amount of O_2 dissolved in blood by only 15 mL/L, less than one-third of normal metabolic demands. However, if the inspired Po_2 is increased to 3 atm (304 kPa) in a hyperbaric chamber, the amount of dissolved O_2 is sufficient to meet normal metabolic demands even in the absence of hemoglobin (Table 21–4).

Oxygen Deprivation. *Hypoxemia* generally implies a failure of the respiratory system to oxygenate arterial blood. Classically, there are five causes of hypoxemia:

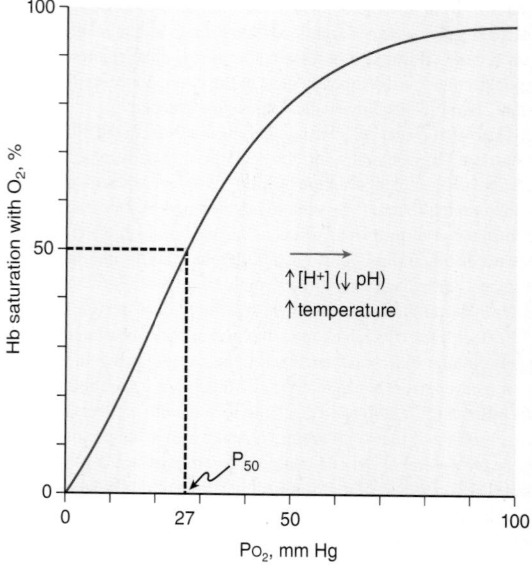

Figure 21–5 *Oxyhemoglobin dissociation curve for whole blood.* The relationship between Po_2 and Hb saturation is shown. The P_{50}, or the Po_2 resulting in 50% saturation, is indicated. An increase in temperature or a decrease in pH (as in working muscle) shifts this relationship to the right, reducing the hemoglobin saturation at the same Po_2 and thus aiding in the delivery of O_2 to the tissues.

- Low FIO_2
- Hypoventilation
- Ventilation-perfusion mismatch
- Shunt or venous admixture
- Increased diffusion barrier

The term *hypoxia* denotes insufficient oxygenation of the tissues. In addition to failure of the respiratory system to oxygenate the blood adequately, a number of other factors can contribute to hypoxia at the tissue level. These may be divided into categories of O_2 delivery and O_2 utilization. O_2 delivery decreases globally when cardiac output falls or locally when regional blood flow is compromised, such as from a vascular occlusion (e.g., stenosis, thrombosis, or microvascular occlusion) or increased downstream pressure (e.g., compartment syndrome, venous stasis, or venous hypertension). Decreased O_2 carrying capacity of the blood likewise will reduce O_2 delivery, such as occurs with anemia, carbon monoxide poisoning, or hemoglobinopathy. Finally, hypoxia may occur when transport of O_2 from the capillaries to the tissues is decreased (edema) or utilization of the O_2 by the cells is impaired (CN^- toxicity).

Effects of Hypoxia

Cellular and Metabolic Effects. At the molecular level, nonlethal hypoxia produces a marked alteration in gene expression, mediated in part by hypoxia inducible factor 1α (Guimarães-Camboa et al., 2015).

When the mitochondrial Po_2 falls below about 0.13 kPa (1 mm Hg), aerobic metabolism stops, and the less-efficient anaerobic pathways of glycolysis become responsible for the production of cellular energy. End products of anaerobic metabolism, such as lactic acid, are released into the circulation in measurable quantities. Energy-dependent ion pumps slow, and transmembrane ion gradients dissipate. Intracellular concentrations of Na^+, Ca^{2+}, and H^+ increase, finally leading to cell death. The time course of cellular demise depends on the relative metabolic demands, oxygen storage capacity, and anaerobic capacity of the individual organs. Restoration of perfusion and oxygenation prior to hypoxic cell death paradoxically can result in an accelerated form of cell injury (ischemia-reperfusion syndrome), which is thought to result from the generation of highly reactive oxygen free radicals.

TABLE 21–4 ■ THE CARRIAGE OF OXYGEN IN BLOOD[a]

ARTERIAL Po_2, kPa (mm Hg)	ARTERIAL O_2 CONTENT (mL O_2/L)			MIXED VENOUS Po_2 kPa (mm Hg)	MIXED VENOUS O_2 CONTENT (mL O_2/L)			EXAMPLES
	DISSOLVED	BOUND TO Hb	TOTAL		DISSOLVED	BOUND TO Hb	TOTAL	
4.0 (30)	0.9	109	109.9	2.7 (20)	0.6	59	59.6	High altitude; respiratory failure breathing air
12.0 (90)	2.7	192	194.7	5.5 (41)	1.2	144	145.2	Normal person breathing air
39.9 (300)	9.0	195	204	5.9 (44)	1.3	153	154.3	Normal person breathing 50% O_2
79.7 (600)	18	196	214	6.5 (49)	1.5	163	164.5	Normal person breathing 100% O_2
239 (1800)	54	196	250	20.0 (150)	4.5	196	200.5	Normal person breathing hyperbaric O_2

[a]This table illustrates the carriage of oxygen in the blood under a variety of circumstances. As arterial O_2 tension increases, the amount of dissolved O_2 increases in direct proportion to the Po_2, but the amount of oxygen bound to Hb reaches a maximum of 196 mL O_2 /L (100% saturation of Hb at 15 g/dL). Further increases in O_2 content require increases in dissolved oxygen. At 100% inspired O_2, dissolved O_2 still provides only a small fraction of total demand. Hyperbaric oxygen therapy is required to increase the amount of dissolved oxygen to supply all or a large part of metabolic requirements. Note that, during hyperbaric oxygen therapy, the hemoglobin in the mixed venous blood remains fully saturated with O_2. The figures in this table are approximate and are based on the assumptions of 15 g/dL Hb, 50 mL O_2/L whole-body oxygen extraction, and constant cardiac output. When severe anemia is present, arterial Po_2 remains the same, but arterial content is lower; oxygen extraction continues, resulting in lower O_2 content and tension in mixed venous blood. Similarly, as cardiac output falls significantly, the same oxygen extraction occurs from a smaller volume of blood and results in lower mixed venous oxygen content and tension.

Cell and Organ Survival. Ultimately, hypoxia results in the cessation of aerobic metabolism, exhaustion of high-energy intracellular stores, cellular dysfunction, and death. The time course of cellular demise depends on the tissue's relative metabolic requirements, O_2 and energy stores, and anaerobic capacity. Survival times (the time from the onset of circulatory arrest to significant organ dysfunction) range from 1–2 min in the cerebral cortex to around 5 min in the heart and 10 min in the kidneys and liver, with the potential for some degree of recovery if reperfused. Revival times (the duration of hypoxia beyond which recovery is no longer possible) are about four to five times longer.

Organ System Effects. Less-severe degrees of hypoxia have progressive physiological effects on different organ systems (Nunn, 2005).

Respiratory System. Hypoxia stimulates the carotid and aortic baroreceptors to cause increases in both the rate and the depth of ventilation. Minute volume almost doubles when normal individuals inspire gas with a Po_2 of 6.6 kPa (50 mm Hg). Dyspnea is not always experienced with simple hypoxia but occurs when the respiratory minute volume approaches half the maximal breathing capacity; this may occur with minimum exertion in patients in whom maximal breathing capacity is reduced by lung disease. In general, little warning precedes the loss of consciousness resulting from hypoxia.

Cardiovascular System. Hypoxia causes reflex activation of the sympathetic nervous system by both autonomic and humoral mechanisms, resulting in tachycardia and increased cardiac output. Peripheral vascular resistance, however, decreases primarily through local autoregulatory mechanisms, with the net result that blood pressure generally is maintained unless hypoxia is prolonged or severe. In contrast to the systemic circulation, hypoxia causes pulmonary vasoconstriction and hypertension, an extension of the normal regional vascular response that matches perfusion with ventilation to optimize gas exchange in the lung (hypoxic pulmonary vasoconstriction).

CNS. The CNS is least able to tolerate hypoxia. Hypoxia is manifest initially by decreased intellectual capacity and impaired judgment and psychomotor ability. This state progresses to confusion and restlessness and ultimately to stupor, coma, and death as the arterial Po_2 decreases below 4–5.3 kPa (30–40 mm Hg). Victims often are unaware of this progression.

Adaptation to Hypoxia

Long-term hypoxia results in adaptive physiological changes; these have been studied most thoroughly in persons exposed to high altitude. Adaptations include increased numbers of pulmonary alveoli, increased concentrations of hemoglobin in blood and myoglobin in muscle, and a decreased ventilatory response to hypoxia. Short-term exposure to high altitude produces similar adaptive changes. In susceptible individuals, however, acute exposure to high altitude may produce *acute mountain sickness*, a syndrome characterized by headache, nausea, dyspnea, sleep disturbances, and impaired judgment progressing to pulmonary and cerebral edema. Mountain sickness is treated with rest and analgesics when mild or supplemental O_2, descent to lower altitude, or an increase in ambient pressure when more severe. Acetazolamide (a carbonic anhydrase inhibitor) and dexamethasone also may be helpful. The syndrome usually can be avoided by a slow ascent to altitude, adequate hydration, and prophylactic use of acetazolamide or dexamethasone.

Examples of "normal" hypoxia are widespread, and the comparative physiology of hypoxic tolerance offers clues to the mechanisms involved. Aspects of fetal and newborn physiology are strongly reminiscent of adaptation mechanisms found in hypoxia-tolerant animals (Guimarães-Camboa et al., 2015; Mortola, 1999), including shifts in the oxyhemoglobin dissociation curve (fetal hemoglobin), reductions in metabolic rate and body temperature (hibernation-like mode), reductions in heart rate and circulatory redistribution (as in diving mammals), and redirection of energy utilization from growth to maintenance metabolism. These adaptations probably account for the relative tolerance of the fetus and neonate to both chronic (uterine insufficiency) and short-term hypoxia.

Oxygen Inhalation

Physiological Effects. O_2 inhalation is used primarily to reverse or prevent the development of hypoxia. However, when O_2 is breathed in excessive amounts or for prolonged periods, secondary physiological changes and toxic effects can occur.

Respiratory System. Inhalation of O_2 at 1 atm or above causes a small degree of respiratory depression in normal subjects, presumably as a result of loss of tonic chemoreceptor activity. However, ventilation typically increases within a few minutes of O_2 inhalation because of a paradoxical increase in the tension of CO_2 in tissues. This increase results from the increased concentration of oxyhemoglobin in venous blood, which causes less-efficient removal of carbon dioxide from the tissues. Expansion of poorly ventilated alveoli is maintained in part by the nitrogen content of alveolar gas; nitrogen is poorly soluble and thus remains in the air spaces while O_2 is absorbed. High O_2 concentrations delivered to poorly ventilated lung regions dilute the nitrogen content and can promote absorption atelectasis (partial or complete collapse of the lung), occasionally resulting in an increase in shunt and a paradoxical worsening of hypoxemia after a period of O_2 administration.

Cardiovascular System. Heart rate and cardiac output are slightly reduced when 100% O_2 is breathed; blood pressure changes little. Elevated pulmonary artery pressures in patients living at high altitude who have chronic hypoxic pulmonary hypertension may reverse with O_2 therapy or return to sea level. In neonates with congenital heart disease and left-to-right shunting of cardiac output, O_2 supplementation must be regulated carefully because of the risk of further reducing pulmonary vascular resistance and increasing pulmonary blood flow.

Metabolism. Inhalation of 100% O_2 does not produce detectable changes in O_2 consumption, CO_2 production, respiratory quotient, or glucose utilization.

Oxygen Administration

Oxygen is supplied as a compressed gas in steel cylinders; purity of 99% is *medical grade*. For safety, O_2 cylinders and piping are color coded (green in the U.S.), and some form of mechanical indexing of valve connections is used to prevent the connection of other gases to O_2 systems.

Oxygen is delivered by inhalation except during extracorporeal circulation, when it is dissolved directly into the circulating blood. A closed delivery system with an endotracheal tube produces an airtight seal to the patient's airway, and complete separation of inspired from expired gases can precisely control F_{IO_2}. In all other systems, such as nasal cannulas and face masks, the actual delivered F_{IO_2} will depend on the ventilatory pattern (i.e., rate, tidal volume, inspiratory-expiratory time ratio, and inspiratory flow) and delivery system characteristics.

Monitoring of Oxygenation. Monitoring and titration are required to meet the therapeutic goal of O_2 therapy and to avoid complications and side effects. Although cyanosis is a physical finding of substantial clinical importance, it is not an early, sensitive, or reliable index of oxygenation. Noninvasive monitoring of arterial O_2 saturation can be achieved using transcutaneous pulse oximetry, in which O_2 saturation is measured from the differential absorption of light by oxyhemoglobin and deoxyhemoglobin and the arterial saturation determined from the pulsatile component of this signal. Pulse oximetry measures hemoglobin saturation and not P_{O_2}. It is not sensitive to increases in P_{O_2} that exceed levels required to saturate the blood fully. Pulse oximetry is useful for monitoring the adequacy of oxygenation during procedures requiring sedation or anesthesia, rapid evaluation and monitoring of potentially compromised patients, and titrating O_2 therapy in situations where toxicity from O_2 or side effects of excess O_2 are of concern. A specific tool for measuring cerebral oxygenation is near-infrared spectroscopy (Guarracino, 2008).

Complications of Oxygen Therapy. In addition to the potential to promote absorption atelectasis and depress ventilation, high flows of dry O_2 can dry out and irritate mucosal surfaces of the airway and the eyes, as well as decrease mucociliary transport and clearance of secretions. Humidified O_2 thus should be used when prolonged therapy (>1 h) is required. Finally, any O_2-enriched atmosphere constitutes a fire hazard, and appropriate precautions must be taken. Hypoxemia can occur despite the administration of supplemental O_2. Therefore, it is essential that both O_2 saturation and adequacy of ventilation be assessed frequently.

Therapeutic Uses of Oxygen

Correction of Hypoxia. The primary therapeutic use of O_2 is to correct hypoxia. Hypoxia is most commonly a manifestation of an underlying disease, and administration of O_2 thus should be viewed as temporizing therapy. Efforts must be directed at correcting the cause of the hypoxia. Hypoxia resulting from most pulmonary diseases can be alleviated at least partially by administration of O_2, allowing time for definitive therapy to reverse the primary process.

Reduction of Partial Pressure of an Inert Gas. Because nitrogen constitutes some 79% of ambient air, it also is the predominant gas in most gas-filled spaces in the body. In situations such as bowel distension from obstruction or ileus, intravascular air embolism, or pneumothorax, it is desirable to reduce the volume of air-filled spaces. Because nitrogen is relatively insoluble, inhalation of high concentrations of O_2 (and thus low concentrations of nitrogen) rapidly lowers the total-body partial pressure of nitrogen and provides a substantial gradient for the removal of nitrogen from gas spaces. Administration of O_2 for air embolism is also beneficial because it helps to relieve localized hypoxia distal to the vascular obstruction. In the case of *decompression sickness*, or *bends*, lowering the inert gas tension in blood and tissues by O_2 inhalation prior to or during barometric decompression reduces the supersaturation that occurs after decompression so that bubbles do not form.

Hyperbaric Oxygen Therapy. O_2 can be administered at greater than atmospheric pressure in hyperbaric chambers (Thom, 2009). Clinical uses of hyperbaric O_2 therapy include the treatment of trauma, burns, radiation damage, infections, nonhealing ulcers, skin grafts, spasticity, and other neurological conditions. Hyperbaric O_2 may be useful in generalized hypoxia. In carbon monoxide poisoning, hemoglobin and myoglobin become unavailable for O_2 binding because of the high affinity of these proteins for carbon monoxide. High P_{O_2} facilitates competition of O_2 for hemoglobin binding sites as carbon monoxide is exchanged in the alveoli. In addition, hyperbaric O_2 increases the availability of dissolved O_2 in the blood (see Table 21–4). Adverse effects of hyperbaric O_2 therapy include middle ear barotrauma, CNS toxicity, seizures, lung toxicity, and aspiration pneumonia.

Hyperbaric O_2 therapy has two components: increased hydrostatic pressure and increased O_2 pressure. Both factors are necessary for the treatment of decompression sickness and air embolism. The hydrostatic pressure reduces bubble volume, and the absence of inspired nitrogen increases the gradient for elimination of nitrogen and reduces hypoxia in downstream tissues. Increased O_2 pressure at the tissue is the primary therapeutic goal for other indications for hyperbaric O_2. A small increase in P_{O_2} in ischemic areas enhances the bactericidal activity of leukocytes and increases angiogenesis. Repetitive brief exposures to hyperbaric O_2 may enhance therapy for chronic refractory osteomyelitis, osteoradionecrosis, crush injury, or the recovery of compromised skin and tissue grafts. Increased O_2 tension can be bacteriostatic and useful in the treatment of the spread of infection with *Clostridium perfringens* and clostridial myonecrosis (gas gangrene).

Oxygen Toxicity

Oxygen can have deleterious actions at the cellular level. O_2 toxicity may result from increased production of hydrogen peroxide and reactive intermediates such as superoxide anion, singlet oxygen, and hydroxyl radicals that attack and damage lipids, proteins, and other macromolecules, especially those in biological membranes. A number of factors limit the toxicity of oxygen-derived reactive agents, including enzymes such as superoxide dismutase, glutathione peroxidase, and catalase, which scavenge toxic oxygen by-products, and reducing agents such as iron, glutathione, and ascorbate. These factors, however, are insufficient to limit the destructive actions of oxygen when patients are exposed to high concentrations over an extended time period. Tissues show differential sensitivity to oxygen toxicity, which is likely the result of differences in both their production of reactive compounds and their protective mechanisms.

Respiratory Tract. The pulmonary system is usually the first to exhibit toxicity, a function of its continuous exposure to the highest O_2 tensions in the body. Subtle changes in pulmonary function can occur within 8–12 h of exposure to 100% O_2. Increases in capillary permeability, which will increase the alveolar/arterial O_2 gradient and ultimately lead to further hypoxemia, and decreased pulmonary function can be seen after only 18 h of exposure. Serious injury and death, however, require much longer exposures. Pulmonary damage is directly related to the inspired O_2 tension, and concentrations of less than 0.5 atm appear to be safe over long time periods. The capillary endothelium is the most sensitive tissue of the lung. Endothelial injury results in loss of surface area from interstitial edema and leaks into the alveoli.

Nervous System. Retinopathy of prematurity is an eye disease in premature infants involving abnormal vascularization of the developing retina that can result from O_2 toxicity or relative hypoxia. CNS problems are rare, and toxicity occurs only under hyperbaric conditions where exposure exceeds 200 kPa (2 atm). Symptoms include seizures and visual changes, which resolve when O_2 tension is returned to normal. In premature neonates and those who have sustained in utero asphyxia, hyperoxia and hypocapnia are associated with worse neurologic outcomes.

Carbon Dioxide

Carbon dioxide is produced by metabolism at approximately the same rate as O_2 is consumed. At rest, this value is about 3 mL/kg/min, but it may increase dramatically with exercise. CO_2 diffuses readily from the cells into the blood, where it is carried partly as bicarbonate ion (HCO_3^-), partly in chemical combination with hemoglobin and plasma proteins, and partly in solution at a partial pressure of about 6 kPa (46 mm Hg) in mixed venous blood. CO_2 is transported to the lung, where it is normally exhaled at the rate it is produced, leaving a partial pressure of about 5.2 kPa (40 mm Hg) in the alveoli and in arterial blood. An increase in Pco_2 results in respiratory acidosis and may be due to decreased ventilation or the inhalation of CO_2, whereas an increase in ventilation results in decreased Pco_2 and respiratory alkalosis. Because CO_2 is freely diffusible, the changes in blood Pco_2 and pH soon are reflected by intracellular changes in Pco_2 and pH and by widespread effects in the body, especially on respiration, circulation, and the CNS.

Respiration

Carbon dioxide is a rapid, potent stimulus to ventilation in direct proportion to the inspired CO_2. CO_2 stimulates breathing by acidifying central chemoreceptors and the peripheral carotid bodies. Elevated Pco_2 causes bronchodilation, whereas hypocarbia causes constriction of airway smooth muscle; these responses may play a role in matching pulmonary ventilation and perfusion.

Circulation

The circulatory effects of CO_2 result from the combination of its direct local effects and its centrally mediated effects on the autonomic nervous system. The direct effect of CO_2 on the heart, diminished contractility, results from pH changes and a decreased myofilament Ca^{2+} responsiveness. The direct effect on systemic blood vessels results in vasodilation. CO_2 causes widespread activation of the sympathetic nervous system. The results of sympathetic nervous system activation generally are opposite to the local effects of carbon dioxide. The sympathetic effects consist of increases in cardiac contractility, heart rate, and vasoconstriction (see Chapter 12). The balance of opposing local and sympathetic effects, therefore, determines the total circulatory response to CO_2. The net effect of CO_2 inhalation is an increase in cardiac output, heart rate, and blood pressure. In blood vessels, however, the direct vasodilating actions of CO_2 appear more important, and total peripheral resistance decreases when the Pco_2 is increased. CO_2 also is a potent coronary vasodilator. Cardiac arrhythmias associated with increased Pco_2 are due to the release of catecholamines.

Hypocarbia results in opposite effects: decreased blood pressure and vasoconstriction in skin, intestine, brain, kidney, and heart. These actions are exploited clinically in the use of hyperventilation to diminish intracranial hypertension.

CNS

Hypercarbia depresses the excitability of the cerebral cortex and increases the cutaneous pain threshold through a central action. This central depression has therapeutic importance. For example, in patients who are hypoventilating from narcotics or anesthetics, increasing Pco_2 may result in further CNS depression, which in turn may worsen the respiratory depression. This positive-feedback cycle can have lethal consequences.

Methods of Administration

Carbon dioxide is marketed in gray metal cylinders as the pure gas or as CO_2 mixed with O_2. It usually is administered at a concentration of 5%–10% in combination with O_2 by means of a face mask. Another method for the temporary administration of CO_2 is by rebreathing, such as from an anesthesia breathing circuit or from something as simple as a paper bag.

Therapeutic Uses

Carbon dioxide is used for insufflation during endoscopic procedures (e.g., laparoscopic surgery) because it is highly soluble and does not support combustion. CO_2 can be used to flood the surgical field during cardiac surgery. Because of its density, CO_2 displaces the air surrounding the open heart so that any gas bubbles trapped in the heart are CO_2 rather than insoluble N_2. It is used to adjust pH during cardiopulmonary bypass procedures when a patient is cooled.

Hypocarbia still has some uses in anesthesia; it constricts cerebral vessels, decreasing brain size slightly, and thus may facilitate the performance of neurosurgical operations. While short-term hypocarbia is effective for this purpose, sustained hypocarbia has been associated with worse outcomes in patients with head injury. Hypocarbia should be instituted with a clearly defined indication and normocarbia should be reestablished as soon the indication for hypocarbia no longer applies.

Nitric Oxide

Nitric oxide is a free-radical gas now known as a critical endogenous cell-signaling molecule with an increasing number of potential therapeutic applications.

Endogenous NO is produced from L-arginine by NO synthases (neural, inducible, and endothelial) (see Chapter 3). In the vasculature, basal production of NO by endothelial cells is a primary determinant of resting vascular tone. NO causes vasodilation of smooth muscle cells and inhibition of platelet aggregation and adhesion. Impaired NO production is implicated in atherosclerosis, hypertension, cerebral and coronary vasospasm, ischemia-reperfusion injury, and inflammation and in mediating central nociceptive pathways. NO is rapidly inactivated in the circulation by oxyhemoglobin and by the reaction of NO with the heme iron, leading to the formation of nitrosyl-hemoglobin. Small quantities of methemoglobin are also produced, and these are converted to the ferrous form of heme iron by cytochrome b5 reductase. The majority of inhaled NO is excreted in the urine in the form of nitrate.

Therapeutic Uses

Inhaled NO selectively dilates the pulmonary vasculature (Cooper, 1999) and has potential as a therapy for numerous diseases associated with increased pulmonary vascular resistance. Inhaled NO is FDA-approved for only one indication, persistent pulmonary hypertension of the newborn.

Diagnostic Uses

Inhaled NO can be used during cardiac catheterization to evaluate the pulmonary vasodilating capacity of patients with heart failure and infants with congenital heart disease. Inhaled NO also is used to determine the diffusion capacity (D_L) across the alveolar-capillary unit. NO is more effective than CO_2 in this regard because of its greater affinity for hemoglobin and its higher water solubility at body temperature. NO is produced from the nasal passages and from the lungs of normal human subjects and can be detected in exhaled gas. The measurement of fractional exhaled NO is a noninvasive marker for airway inflammation with utility in the assessment of respiratory tract diseases, including asthma, respiratory tract infection, and chronic lung disease.

Toxicity

Administered at low concentrations (0.1–50 ppm), inhaled NO appears to be safe and without significant side effects. Pulmonary toxicity can occur with levels higher than 50–100 ppm. NO is an atmospheric pollutant; the Occupational Safety and Health Administration places the 7-hour exposure limit at 50 ppm. Part of the toxicity of NO may be related to its further oxidation to NO_2 in the presence of high concentrations of O_2.

The development of methemoglobinemia is a significant complication of inhaled NO at higher concentrations, and rare deaths have been reported with overdoses of NO. Methemoglobin concentrations should be monitored intermittently during NO inhalation. Inhaled NO can inhibit platelet function and has been shown to increase bleeding time in some clinical studies, although bleeding complications have not been reported. In patients with impaired function of the left ventricle, NO has a potential to further impair left ventricular performance by dilating the pulmonary circulation and increasing the blood flow to the left ventricle, thereby increasing left atrial pressure and promoting pulmonary edema formation.

The most important requirements for safe NO inhalation therapy include the following:

- Continuous measurement of NO and NO_2 concentrations using either chemiluminescence or electrochemical analyzers
- Frequent calibration of monitoring equipment
- Intermittent analysis of blood methemoglobin levels
- The use of certified tanks of NO
- Administration of the lowest NO concentration required for therapeutic effect

Methods of Administration

Courses of treatment of patients with inhaled NO are highly varied, extending from 0.1 to 40 ppm in dose and for periods of a few hours to several weeks in duration. The determination of a dose-response relationship on a frequent basis should assist in the titration of the optimum dose of NO. Commercial NO systems are available that will accurately deliver inspired NO concentrations between 0.1 and 80 ppm and simultaneously measure NO and NO_2 concentrations.

Helium

Helium is an inert gas whose low density, low solubility, and high thermal conductivity provide the basis for its medical and diagnostic uses. Helium can be mixed with O_2 and administered by mask or endotracheal tube. Under hyperbaric conditions, it can be substituted for the bulk of other gases, resulting in a mixture of much lower density that is easier to breathe.

The primary uses of helium are in pulmonary function testing, the treatment of respiratory obstruction, laser airway surgery, as a label in imaging studies, and for diving at depth. Helium is also suited for determinations of residual lung volume, functional residual capacity, and related lung volumes. These measurements require a highly diffusible nontoxic gas that is insoluble and does not leave the lung by the bloodstream so that, by dilution, the lung volume can be measured. Helium can be added to O_2 to reduce turbulence due to airway obstruction because the density of helium is less than that of air, and the viscosity of helium is greater than that of air. Mixtures of helium and O_2 reduce the work of breathing. Helium has high thermal conductivity, making it useful during laser surgery on the airway. Laser-polarized helium is used as an inhalational contrast agent for pulmonary magnetic resonance imaging. Helium also has potential as a cytoprotective agent (Smit et al., 2015).

Hydrogen Sulfide

Hydrogen sulfide, which has a characteristic rotten egg smell, is a colorless, flammable, water-soluble gas that is primarily considered as a toxin due to its capacity to inhibit mitochondrial respiration through blockade of cytochrome c oxidase. Inhibition of respiration can be toxic; however, if depression of respiration occurs in a controlled manner, it may allow nonhibernating species exposed to inhaled H_2S to enter a state akin to suspended animation (i.e., a slowing of cellular activity to a point at which metabolic processes are inhibited but not terminal) and thereby increase tolerance to stress. H_2S activates ATP-dependent K^+ channels, has vasodilating properties, and serves as a free-radical scavenger. H_2S can protect against whole-body hypoxia, lethal hemorrhage, and ischemia-reperfusion injury in various organs, including the kidney, lung, liver, and heart. Currently, effort is under way for development of gas-releasing molecules that could deliver H_2S and other therapeutic gases to diseased tissue. H_2S in low quantities may have the potential to limit cell death (Lefer, 2007).

Acknowledgment: *Alex S. Evers, C. Michael Crowder, Jeffrey R. Balser, Brett A. Simon, Eric J. Moody, and Roger A. Johns contributed to this chapter in recent editions of this book. We have retained some of their text in the current edition.*

Drug Facts for Your Personal Formulary: *General Anesthetics and Therapeutic Gases*

Drugs	Therapeutic Uses	Clinical Pharmacology and Tips
Parenteral Anesthetics		
Propofol Etomidate Ketamine Thiopental	• Anesthetic induction • Rapid-onset and short-duration anesthetics used in procedures for rapid return to preoperative mental status	• Highly lipophilic ⇒ entry to brain and spinal cord, accumulation in fatty tissues • Propofol dosage: ↓ in elderly due to reduced clearance, ↑ in young children due to rapid clearance • PRIS: rare complication associated with prolonged and high-dose propofol infusion in young or head-injured patients • Etomidate: preferred for patients at risk of hypotension or MI; produces hypnosis, no analgesic effects; ↑ EEG activity, associated with seizures • Ketamine: suited for patients at risk for hypotension and asthma and for pediatric procedures; increases HR, BP, CO, CBF, and ICP; emergence delirium, hallucinations, vivid dreams limit use
Barbiturates Methohexital Thiopental	• Anesthetic induction	• Respiratory and EEG depressants • Methohexital: more rapid clearance than other barbiturates • Thiopental: action terminated by redistribution; good safety record; not available in the U.S. • Intra-arterial injection of thiobarbiturates ⇒ severe inflammatory and potentially necrotic reaction
Inhalational Anesthetics		
Isoflurane	• Maintenance of anesthesia • Commonly used inhalational anesthetic	• Highly volatile at RT; not flammable in air or O_2 • ↓ Ventilation and RBF; ↑ CBF • Induces hypotension and ↑ coronary blood flow, thus ↓ myocardial O_2 consumption • ↓ Baroreceptor function • Excreted unchanged by the lungs

Drug Facts for Your Personal Formulary: *General Anesthetics and Therapeutic Gases (continued)*

Drugs	Therapeutic Uses	Clinical Pharmacology and Tips
Inhalational Anesthetics		
Enflurane	• Maintenance of anesthesia	• Volatile at RT; store in tightly sealed bottles • Slow induction and recovery • ↓ Arterial BP due to vasodilation and ↓ myocardial contractility • Possible effects: ↑ ICP, seizure activity
Sevoflurane	• Preferred agent for anesthetic induction • Used for outpatient anesthesia (not irritating airway; induction and recovery are rapid)	• Reacts exothermically with desiccated CO_2 absorbent • Ideal induction agent (pleasant smell, rapid onset) • ↓ AP pressure and CO; potent bronchodilator • Preferred for patients with myocardial ischemia • Compound A, product of interaction of sevoflurane with the CO_2-absorbent soda lime, is nephrotoxic
Desflurane	• Used for outpatient surgery (rapid onset, rapid recovery)	• Highly volatile at RT; store in tightly sealed bottles • Nonflammable in mixtures of air or O_2 • An airway irritant
Halothane	• Maintenance of anesthesia	• Highly volatile at RT, light sensitive; store in tightly sealed amber bottles with thymol (preservative) • Possible hepatic toxicity has limited its use and is no longer available in the U.S.
Nitrous oxide (N_2O)	• Weak anesthetic agent used for its significant analgesic effects	• Colorless and odorless gas at RT; used as adjunct to other anesthetics. • Will expand volume of air-containing cavities; thus, avoid use in obstructions of ear and bowel, and in intraocular and intracranial air bubbles, etc. • To avoid diffusional hypoxia, administer 100% O_2 rather than air when discontinuing N_2O • Can increase CBF and ICP • Clinical use of N_2O is controversial due to potential metabolic effects related to increased homocysteine and changes in DNA and protein synthesis
Xenon	• Analgesic and anesthetic effects	• Rapid induction and emergence from anesthesia • In CNS: NMDA receptor antagonist, TREK channel agonist • Well tolerated in older patients
Anesthetic Adjuncts • Augment anesthetic effects of general anesthesia		
Benzodiazepines Midazolam, diazepam, lorazepam	Used for anxiolysis, amnesia, preanesthetic sedation, and sedation during procedures not requiring general anesthesia	• Midazolam most commonly used, followed distantly by diazepam and lorazepam (see Chapters 15 and 19)
α_2 Adrenergic agonists Dexmedetomidine	• Short-term (<24 h) sedation of critically ill adults • Sedation prior to and during surgical or medical procedures in nonintubated patients	• Activation of the α_{2A} adrenergic receptor by dexmedetomidine ⇒ sedation and analgesia • Side effects: hypotension and bradycardia due to decreased catecholamine release in the CNS; nausea and dry mouth
Analgesics *Opioids* Fentanyl, Sufentanil, Alfentanil, Remifentanil, Meperidine, Morphine	• To reduce anesthetic requirement and minimize hemodynamic changes due to painful stimuli	• Opioids are the primary analgesics during perioperative period; the choice of opioid is based on duration of action (see Chapter 20) • Opioids often are administered intrathecally and epidurally for management of acute and chronic pain
NSAIDs Acetaminophen		• NSAIDs and acetaminophen are used for minor surgical procedures to control postoperative pain
Neuromuscular Blocking Agents Succinylcholine (Depolarizing) Atracurium, Vecuronium, et al. (Nondepolarizing, Competitive)	• Skeletal muscle relaxant	• Action of nondepolarizing muscle relaxants usually is antagonized, once muscle paralysis is no longer desired, with an AChE inhibitor (e.g., neostigmine or edrophonium; see Chapter 10), in combination with a muscarinic receptor antagonist
THERAPEUTIC GASES		
Oxygen	• Used primarily to reverse or prevent the development of hypoxia	• Excessive O_2 ↓ ventilation • Monitoring and titration are required to avoid complications and side effects • HR and CO are slightly ↓ when 100% O_2 is breathed • High flows of dry O_2 can dry out and irritate mucosal surfaces of the airway and the eyes; humidified O_2 should be used with prolonged therapy (>1 h) • O_2-enriched atmosphere constitutes a fire hazard; take precautions

Drug Facts for Your Personal Formulary: *General Anesthetics and Therapeutic Gases (continued)*

Drugs	Therapeutic Uses	Clinical Pharmacology and Tips
THERAPEUTIC GASES		
Carbon dioxide	• Insufflation during endoscopic procedures • Flooding the surgical field during cardiac surgery • Adjusting pH during cardiopulmonary bypass	• CO_2 is highly soluble, noncombustible, denser than air. • ↑ P_{CO_2} ⇒respiratory acidosis • Effects on CV system: combination of direct CNS and reflex sympathetic effects; net effect: ↑ in CO, HR, and BP
Nitric oxide	• Inhaled NO is used to dilate pulmonary vasculature in persistent pulmonary hypertension of the newborn	• Cell-signaling molecule; induces vasodilation • Pulmonary toxicity can occur with levels > 50-100 ppm • Use lowest NO concentration required for therapeutic effect • Monitor blood methemoglobin levels intermittently during inhalation therapy
Helium	• Pulmonary function testing, treatment of respiratory obstruction, laser airway surgery • As a label in imaging studies	• Mixtures of He and O_2 reduce the work of breathing • Potential as a cytoprotective agent • For diving at depth
Hydrogen sulfide	• Potential therapeutic use for protection against effects of hypoxia	

Bibliography

Alkire MT, et al. Consciousness and anesthesia. *Science*, **2008**, *322*:876–880.

Cooper CE. Nitric oxide and iron proteins. *Biochim Biophys Acta*, **1999**, *1411*:290–309.

Cotton M, Claing A. G protein-coupled receptors stimulation and the control of cell migration. *Cell Signal*, **2009**, *21*:1045–1053.

Drummond JC, et al. Brain surface protrusion during enflurane, halothane, and isoflurane anesthesia in cats. *Anesthesiology*, **1983**, *59*:288–293.

Eger EI II. New inhaled anesthetics. *Anesthesiology*, **1994**, *80*:906–922.

Eger EI II, et al. Nephrotoxicity of sevoflurane versus desflurane anesthesia in volunteers. *Anesth Analg*, **1997**, *84*:160–168.

Fechner J, et al. Pharmacokinetics and pharmacodynamics of GPI 15715 or fospropofol (Aquavan injection)—a water-soluble propofol prodrug. *Handb Exp Pharmacol*, **2008**, 253–266.

Franks NP. Molecular targets underlying general anaesthesia. *Br J Pharmacol*, **2006**, 147(suppl 1):S72–S81.

Franks NP. General anaesthesia: from molecular targets to neuronal pathways of sleep and arousal. *Nat Rev Neurosci*, **2008**, *9*:370–386.

Franks NP, Honore E. The TREK K2P channels and their role in general anaesthesia and neuroprotection. *Trends Pharmacol Sci*, **2004**, *11*:601–608.

Guarracino F. Cerebral monitoring during cardiovascular surgery. *Curr Opin Anaesthesiol*, **2008**, *21*:50–54.

Guimarães-Camboa N, et al. HIF1α represses cell stress pathways to allow proliferation of hypoxic fetal cardiomyocytes. *Dev Cell*, **2015**, *33*:507–521.

Head BP, Patel P. Anesthetics and brain protection. *Curr Opin Anesthesiol*, **2007**, *20*:395–399.

Jevtovic-Todorovic V, et al. Prolonged exposure to inhalational anesthetic nitrous oxide kills neurons in adult rat brain. *Neuroscience*, **2003**, *122*:609–616.

Kam PC, Cardone D. Propofol infusion syndrome. *Anaesthesia*, **2007**, *62*:690–701.

Kamibayashi T, Maze M. Clinical uses of alpha2-adrenergic agonists. *Anesthesiology*, **2000**, *93*:1345–1349.

Ko H, et al. Nitrous oxide and perioperative outcomes. *J Anesthesia*, **2014**, *28*:420–428.

Kunst G, Klein AA. Peri-operative anaesthetic myocardial preconditioning and protection—cellular mechanisms and clinical relevance in cardiac anaesthesia. *Anaesthesia*, **2015**, *70*:467–482.

Ledowski T. Sugammadex: what do we know and what do we still need to know? A review of the recent (2013 to 2014) literature. *Anaesthes Intens Care*, **2015**, *43*:14–22.

Lefer DJ. A new gaseous signaling molecule emerges: cardioprotective role of hydrogen sulfide. *Proc Natl Acad Sci U S A*, **2007**, *104*:17907–17908.

Mazze RI, et al. Inorganic fluoride nephrotoxicity: prolonged enflurane and halothane anesthesia in volunteers. *Anesthesiology*, **1977**, *46*:265–271.

Mortola JP. How newborn mammals cope with hypoxia. *Respir Physiol*, **1999**, *116*:95–103.

Nunn JF. Hypoxia. In: *Nunn's Applied Respiratory Physiology*. Butterworth-Heineman, Oxford, UK, **2005**, 327–334.

Patel P, Sun L. Update on neonatal anesthetic neurotoxicity: insight into molecular mechanisms and relevance to humans. *Anesthesiology*, **2009**, *110*:703–708.

Rasmussen KG, et al. Serial infusions of low-dose ketamine for major depression. *J Psychopharmacol*, **2013**, *27*:444–450.

Sanders RD, Maze M. Alpha2-adrenoceptor agonists. *Curr Opin Invest Drugs*, **2007**, *8*:25–33.

Smit KF, et al. Noble gases as cardioprotectants—translatability and mechanism. *Br J Pharmacol*, **2015**, *172*:2062–2073.

Summary of the National Halothane Study. Possible association between halothane anesthesia and postoperative hepatic necrosis. *JAMA*, **1966**, *197*:775–788.

Thom SR. Oxidative stress is fundamental to hyperbaric oxygen therapy. *J Appl Physiol*, **2009**, *106*:988–995.

van den Heuvel I, et al. Pros and cons of etomidate—more discussion than evidence? *Curr Opin Anaesthesiol*, **2013**, *26*:404–408.

Local Anesthetics

William A. Catterall and Kenneth Mackie

第二十二章　局部麻醉药

中文导读

本章主要介绍：局部麻醉药的历史；化学与构-效关系；作用机制，包括细胞作用部位、钠离子通道上的局部麻醉药受体部位、作用的频率和电压依赖性、神经纤维的灵敏度差异、pH的影响、血管收缩药对药物作用时间的延长；局部麻醉药的不良反应，包括中枢神经系统、心血管系统、平滑肌、神经肌肉接头和突触神经元、过敏反应；代谢；毒性；局部麻醉药及相关药物，包括可卡因、利多卡因、布比卡因、适用于注射的局部麻醉药、主要用于黏膜和皮肤麻醉的药物、水溶性低的麻醉药、眼科用药、生物毒素（河豚毒素和石房蛤毒素）；局部麻醉药的临床用途，包括表面麻醉、浸润麻醉、区域阻滞麻醉、神经阻滞麻醉、静脉局部麻醉（Bier Block）、脊髓麻醉和硬膜外麻醉。

Abbreviations

ACh: acetylcholine
CSF: cerebrospinal fluid
CYP: cytochrome P450
EDTA: ethylenediaminetetraacetic acid
GI: gastrointestinal
IFM: isoleucine-phenylalanine-methionine
LA: local anesthetic
NE: norepinephrine
NET: norepinephrine transporter
PKA: protein kinase A, cyclic AMP-dependent protein kinase
PKC: protein kinase C
TRP: transient receptor potential
TRPV channel: TRP vanilloid subtype channel
TTX: tetrodotoxin

Local anesthetics bind reversibly to a specific receptor site within the pore of the Na^+ channels in nerves and block ion movement through this pore. When applied locally to nerve tissue in appropriate concentrations, local anesthetics can act on any part of the nervous system and on every type of nerve fiber, reversibly blocking the action potentials responsible for nerve conduction. Thus, a local anesthetic in contact with a nerve trunk can cause both sensory and motor paralysis in the area innervated. These effects of clinically relevant concentrations of local anesthetics are reversible with recovery of nerve function and no evidence of damage to nerve fibers or cells in most clinical applications.

History

The first local anesthetic, cocaine, was serendipitously discovered to have anesthetic properties in the late 19th century. Cocaine occurs in abundance in the leaves of the coca shrub (*Erythroxylon coca*). For centuries, Andean natives have chewed an alkali extract of these leaves for its stimulatory and euphoric actions. When, in 1860, Albert Niemann isolated cocaine, he tasted his newly isolated compound, noted that it numbed his tongue, and a new era began. Sigmund Freud studied cocaine's physiological actions, and Carl Koller introduced cocaine into clinical practice in 1884 as a topical anesthetic for ophthalmological surgery. Shortly thereafter, Halstead popularized its use in infiltration and conduction block anesthesia.

Chemistry and Structure-Activity Relationship

Cocaine is an ester of benzoic acid and the complex alcohol 2-carbomethoxy, 3-hydroxytropane (Figure 22–1). Because of its toxicity and addictive properties (Chapter 24), a search for synthetic substitutes for cocaine began in 1892 with the work of Einhorn and colleagues, resulting in the synthesis of procaine, which became the prototype for local anesthetics for nearly half a century. The most widely used agents today are lidocaine, bupivacaine, and tetracaine.

Typical local anesthetics contain hydrophilic and hydrophobic moieties that are separated by an intermediate ester or amide linkage. A broad range of compounds containing these minimal structural features can satisfy the requirements for action as local anesthetics. The hydrophilic group usually is a tertiary amine but also may be a secondary amine; the hydrophobic moiety must be aromatic. The nature of the linking group determines some of the pharmacological properties of these agents. For example, plasma esterases readily hydrolyze local anesthetics with an ester link.

The structure-activity relationship and the physicochemical properties of local anesthetics have been well reviewed (Courtney and Strichartz, 1987). Hydrophobicity increases both the potency and the duration of action of the local anesthetics; association of the drug at hydrophobic sites enhances the partitioning of the drug to its sites of action and decreases the rate of metabolism by plasma esterases and hepatic enzymes. In addition, the receptor site for these drugs on Na^+ channels is thought to be hydrophobic (see Mechanism of Action), so that receptor affinity for anesthetic agents is greater for the more hydrophobic drugs. Hydrophobicity also increases toxicity, so that the therapeutic index is decreased for more hydrophobic drugs.

Molecular size influences the rate of dissociation of local anesthetics from their receptor sites. Smaller drug molecules can escape from the receptor site more rapidly. This characteristic is important in rapidly firing cells, in which local anesthetics bind during action potentials and dissociate during the period of membrane repolarization. Rapid binding of local anesthetics during action potentials causes the frequency and voltage dependence of their action.

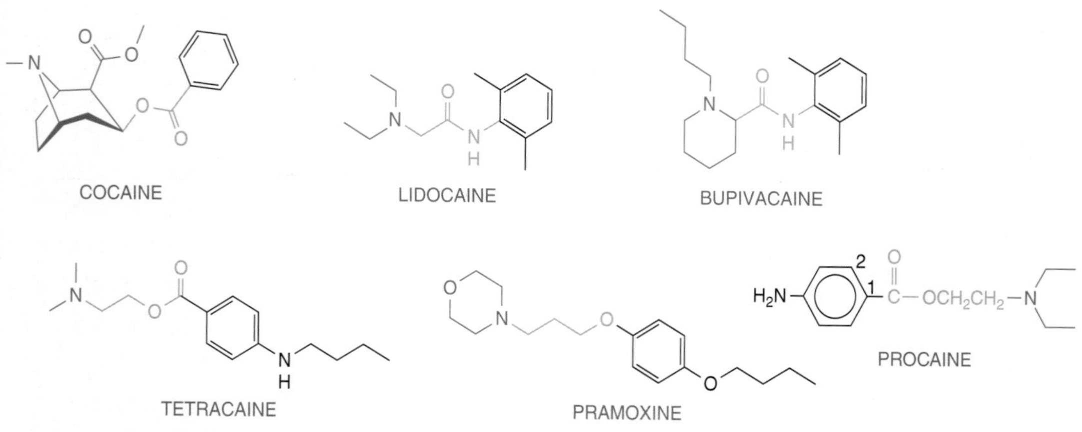

Figure 22–1 *Structural formulas of selected local anesthetics.* Most local anesthetics consist of a hydrophobic (aromatic) moiety (black), a linker region (orange), and a substituted amine (hydrophilic region, red). The structures at the top are grouped by the nature of the linker region. Procaine is a prototypic ester-type local anesthetic; esters generally are rapidly hydrolyzed by plasma esterases, contributing to the relatively short duration of action of drugs in this group. Lidocaine is a prototypic amide-type local anesthetic; these structures generally are more resistant to clearance and have longer durations of action. There are exceptions, including benzocaine (poorly water soluble; used only topically) and the structures with a ketone, an amidine, and an ether linkage. Chloroprocaine has a chlorine atom on C2 of the aromatic ring of procaine.

Mechanism of Action

Cellular Site of Action

Local anesthetics act at the cell membrane to prevent the generation and the conduction of nerve impulses. Conduction block can be demonstrated in squid giant axons from which the axoplasm has been removed.

Local anesthetics block conduction by decreasing or preventing the large transient increase in the permeability of excitable membranes to Na^+ that normally is produced by a slight depolarization of the membrane (Chapters 8, 11, and 14; Strichartz and Ritchie, 1987). This action of local anesthetics is due to their direct interaction with voltage-gated Na^+ channels. As the anesthetic action progressively develops in a nerve, the threshold for electrical excitability gradually increases, the rate of rise of the action potential declines, impulse conduction slows, and the safety factor for conduction decreases. These factors decrease the probability of propagation of the action potential, and nerve conduction eventually fails.

Local anesthetics can bind to other membrane proteins (Butterworth and Strichartz, 1990). In particular, they can block K^+ channels (Strichartz and Ritchie, 1987). However, because the interaction of local anesthetics with K^+ channels requires higher concentrations of drug, blockade of conduction is not accompanied by any large or consistent change in resting membrane potential.

Quaternary analogues of local anesthetics block conduction when applied internally to perfused giant axons of squid but are relatively ineffective when applied externally. These observations suggest that the site at which local anesthetics act, at least in their charged form, is accessible only from the inner surface of the membrane (Narahashi and Frazier, 1971; Strichartz and Ritchie, 1987). Therefore, local anesthetics applied externally first must cross the membrane before they can exert a blocking action.

The Local Anesthetic Receptor Site on Na^+ Channels

The major mechanism of action of these drugs involves their interaction with one or more specific binding sites within the Na^+ channel (Butterworth and Strichartz, 1990). The Na^+ channels of the mammalian brain are complexes of glycosylated proteins with an aggregate molecular size in excess of 300,000 Da; the individual subunits are designated α (260,000 Da) and β_1 to β_4 (33,000–38,000 Da). The large α subunit of the Na^+ channel contains four homologous domains (I–IV); each domain is thought to consist of six transmembrane segments in α-helical conformation (S1–S6; Figure 22–2) and an additional, membrane-reentrant pore (*P*) loop. The Na^+-selective transmembrane pore of the channel resides in the center of a nearly symmetrical structure formed by the four homologous domains. The voltage dependence of channel opening is hypothesized to reflect conformational changes that result from the movement of "gating charges" within the voltage sensor module of the sodium channel in response to changes in the transmembrane potential. The gating charges are located in the S4 transmembrane helices, which are hydrophobic and positively charged, containing lysine or arginine residues at every third position. These residues are thought to move perpendicular to the plane of the membrane under the influence of the transmembrane potential, initiating a series of conformational changes in all four domains, which leads to the open state of the channel (Figure 22–2) (Catterall, 2000; Yu et al., 2005).

The transmembrane pore of the Na^+ channel is surrounded by the S5 and S6 transmembrane helices and the short membrane-associated segments between them that form the *P* loop. Amino acid residues in these short segments are the most critical determinants of the ion conductance and selectivity of the channel.

After it opens, the Na^+ channel inactivates within a few milliseconds due to closure of an inactivation gate. This functional gate is formed by the short intracellular loop of protein that connects homologous domains III and IV. This loop folds over the intracellular mouth of the transmembrane pore during the process of inactivation and binds to an inactivation gate "receptor" formed by the intracellular mouth of the pore.

Amino acid residues important for local anesthetic binding are found in the S6 segments in domains I, III, and IV (Ragsdale et al., 1994; Yarov-Yarovoy et al., 2002). Hydrophobic amino acid residues near the center and the intracellular end of the S6 segment may interact directly with bound local anesthetics, locating the local anesthetic receptor site in the intracellular half of the transmembrane pore of the Na^+ channel, with part of its structure contributed by amino acids in the S6 segments of domains I, III, and IV (Figure 22–3). Ancestral Na^+ channels in bacteria comprise four identical subunits, each similar to one of the four domains of the mammalian Na^+ channel α subunit and containing a similar voltage sensor and pore-lining segment. The three-dimensional structure of an ancestral Na^+ channel (Payandeh et al., 2011) revealed the arrangement of its transmembrane segments and the amino acid residues in the local anesthetic binding site in the pore.

Frequency and Voltage Dependence

The degree of block produced by a given concentration of local anesthetic depends on how the nerve has been stimulated and on its resting membrane potential. Thus, a resting nerve is much less sensitive to a local anesthetic than one that is repetitively stimulated; higher frequency of stimulation and more positive membrane potential cause a greater degree of anesthetic block. These frequency- and voltage-dependent effects of local anesthetics occur because the charged form of the local anesthetic molecule gains access to its binding site within the pore primarily when the Na^+ channel is open and because the local anesthetic binds more tightly to and stabilizes the inactivated state of the Na^+ channel (Butterworth and Strichartz, 1990; Courtney and Strichartz, 1987; Hille, 1977). Remarkably, the conformation of the local anesthetic receptor site is changed considerably in the inactivated state (Payandeh et al., 2012; Figure 22–3D), revealing how preferential binding to inactivated Na^+ channels may occur.

Local anesthetics exhibit frequency and voltage dependence to different extents depending on their pK_a, lipid solubility, molecular size, and binding to different channel states. In general, the frequency dependence of local anesthetic action depends critically on the rate of dissociation from the receptor site in the pore of the Na^+ channel. A high frequency of stimulation is required for rapidly dissociating drugs so that drug binding during the action potential exceeds drug dissociation between action potentials. Dissociation of smaller and more hydrophobic drugs is more rapid, so a higher frequency of stimulation is required to yield frequency-dependent block. Frequency-dependent block of ion channels is also important for the actions of antiarrhythmic drugs (Chapter 30).

Differential Sensitivity of Nerve Fibers

For most patients, treatment with local anesthetics causes the sensation of pain to disappear first, followed by loss of the sensations of temperature, touch, deep pressure, and finally motor function (Table 22–1). Classical experiments with intact nerves showed that the δ wave in the compound action potential, which represents slowly conducting, small-diameter myelinated fibers, was reduced more rapidly and at lower concentrations of cocaine than was the α wave, which represents rapidly conducting, large-diameter fibers (Gasser and Erlanger, 1929). In general, autonomic fibers, small unmyelinated C fibers (mediating pain sensations), and small myelinated Aδ fibers (mediating pain and temperature sensations) are blocked before the larger myelinated Aγ, Aβ, and Aα fibers (mediating postural, touch, pressure, and motor information) (Raymond and Gissen, 1987). *The differential rate of block exhibited by fibers mediating different sensations is of considerable practical importance in the use of local anesthetics.*

The precise mechanisms responsible for this apparent specificity of local anesthetic action on pain fibers are not known, but several factors may contribute. The initial hypothesis was that sensitivity to local anesthetic block increases with decreasing fiber size, consistent with high sensitivity for pain sensation mediated by small fibers and low sensitivity for motor function mediated by large fibers (Gasser and Erlanger, 1929). However, when nerve fibers are dissected from nerves to allow direct measurement of action potential generation, no clear correlation of the concentration

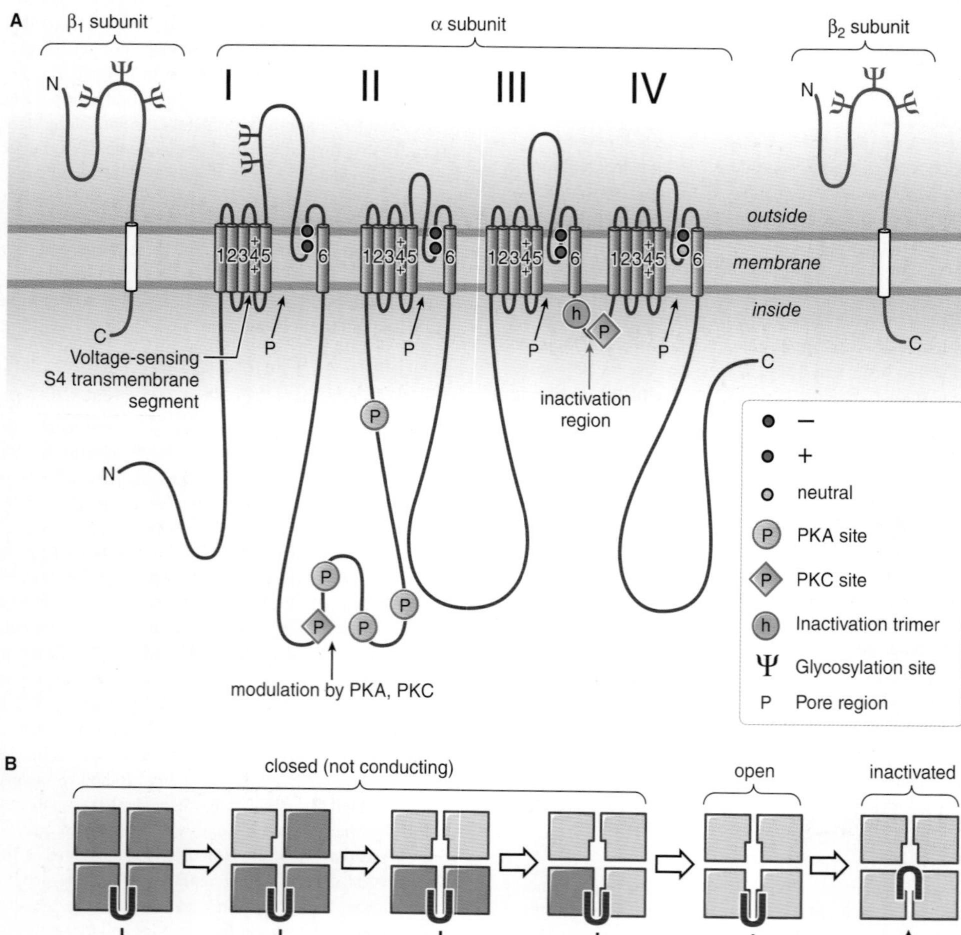

Figure 22–2 *Structure and function of voltage-gated Na⁺ channels.* **A.** A two-dimensional representation of the α (center), β_1 (left), and β_2 (right) subunits of the voltage-gated Na^+ channel from mammalian brain. The polypeptide chains are represented by continuous lines with length approximately proportional to the actual length of each segment of the channel protein. Cylinders represent regions of transmembrane α helices. ψ indicates sites of demonstrated *N*-linked glycosylation. Note the repeated structure of the four homologous domains (I–IV) of the α subunit. **Voltage Sensing**. The S4 transmembrane segments in each homologous domain of the α subunit serve as voltage sensors. (+) represents the positively charged amino acid residues at every third position within these segments. Electrical field (negative inside) exerts a force on these charged amino acid residues, pulling them toward the intracellular side of the membrane; depolarization allows them to move outward and initiate a conformational change that opens the pore. **Pore**. The S5 and S6 transmembrane segments and the short membrane-associated loop between them (*P* loop) form the walls of the pore in the center of an approximately symmetrical square array of the four homologous domains (see **B**). The amino acid residues indicated by circles in the *P* loop are critical for determining the conductance and ion selectivity of the Na^+ channel and its ability to bind the extracellular pore-blocking toxins TTX and saxitoxin. **Inactivation**. The short intracellular loop connecting homologous domains III and IV serves as the inactivation gate of the Na^+ channel. It is thought to fold into the intracellular mouth of the pore and occlude it within a few milliseconds after the channel opens. Three hydrophobic residues (IFM) at the position marked **h** appear to serve as an inactivation particle, entering the intracellular mouth of the pore and binding therein to an inactivation gate receptor there. **Modulation**. The gating of the Na^+ channel can be modulated by protein phosphorylation. Phosphorylation of the inactivation gate between homologous domains III and IV by PKC slows inactivation. Phosphorylation of sites in the intracellular loop between homologous domains I and II by either PKC or PKA reduces Na^+ channel activation. (Adapted with permission from Catterall WA. From ionic currents to molecular mechanisms: the structure and function of voltage-gated sodium channels. *Neuron*, **2000**, *26*:13–25. Copyright © Elsevier). **B.** The four homologous domains of the Na^+ channel α subunit are illustrated as a square array, as viewed looking down on the membrane. The sequence of conformational changes that the Na^+ channel undergoes during activation and inactivation is diagrammed. On depolarization, each of the four homologous domains sequentially undergoes a conformational change to an activated state. After all four domains have activated, the Na^+ channel can open. Within a few milliseconds after opening, the inactivation gate between domains III and IV closes over the intracellular mouth of the channel and occludes it, preventing further ion conductance (see Catterall, 2000).

dependence of local anesthetic block with fiber diameter is observed (Fink and Cairns, 1984; Franz and Perry, 1974; Huang et al., 1997). Therefore, it is unlikely that the fiber size per se determines the sensitivity to local anesthetic block under steady-state conditions. However, the spacing of nodes of Ranvier increases with the size of nerve fibers. Because a fixed number of nodes must be blocked to prevent conduction, small fibers with closely spaced nodes of Ranvier may be blocked more rapidly during treatment of intact nerves because the local anesthetic reaches a critical length of nerve more rapidly. Differences in tissue barriers and location of smaller C fibers and Aδ fibers in nerves also may influence the rate of local anesthetic action. Different combinations of Na^+ channel subtypes are also expressed in these nerve fibers, but all of these Na^+ channels have similar affinity for block by local anesthetics.

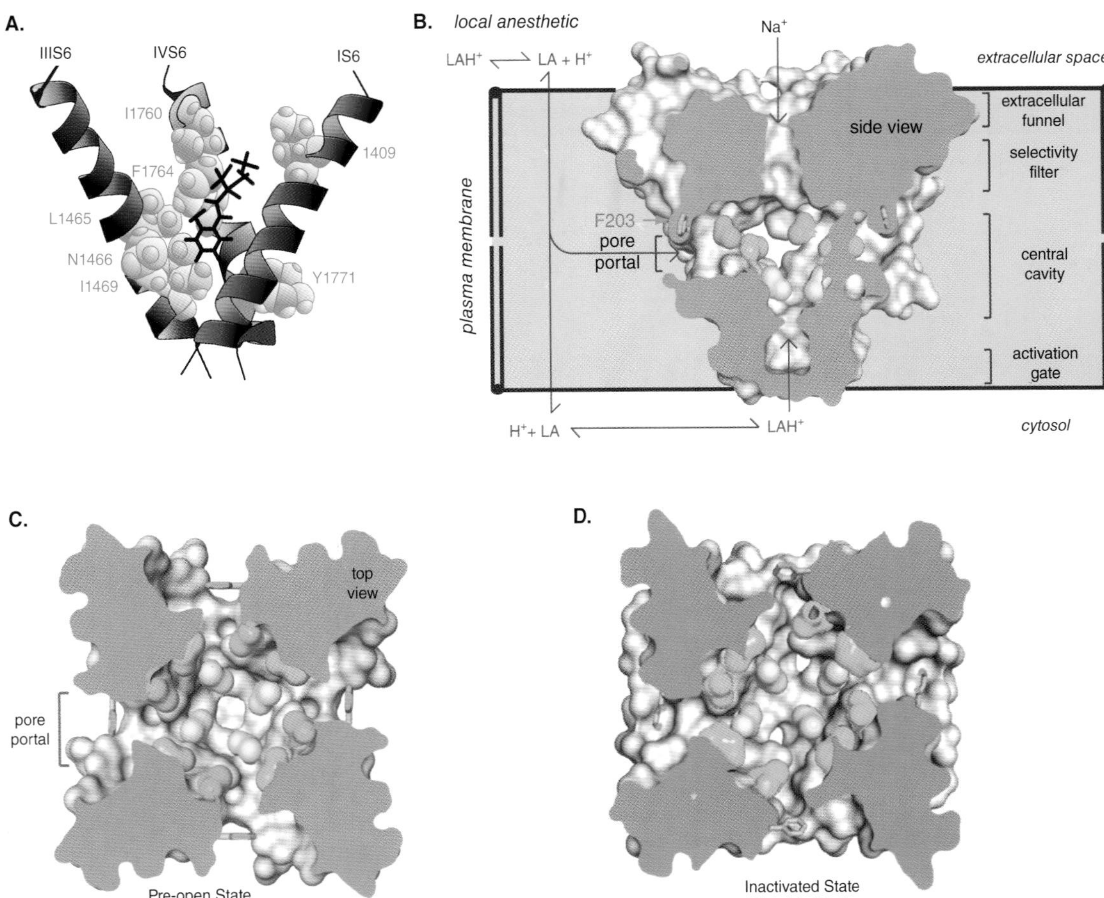

Figure 22–3 *A pharmacologist's view of the interaction of a local anesthetic with a voltage-gated Na^+ channel.* A voltage-gated Na^+ channel may be thought of as an antechamber (*extracellular funnel*) that feeds into a constricted area (*selectivity filter*), which opens onto a larger volume (*central cavity*) that has an exit door (*gate*). Functionally, the channel can exist in a cycle of multiple states, initiated by the local effects of an action potential on the S4 transmembrane segments of the α subunits of segments I–IV, shown in Figure 22–2A. These states are *resting/closed, intermediate/closed, open, inactivated.* LAs bind in the center of the region depicted by the light blue balls. LAs exist in charged and uncharged forms at physiological pH, in accordance with the Henderson-Hasselbalch relationship (Figure 2–2). The uncharged species, LA, can diffuse across the membrane, possibly interacting with the channel protein en route. Within the cell, LA equilibrates with H^+; the charged form, LAH^+, binds in the channel with greater affinity than does the uncharged species. The resting/closed conformation of the channel, in which the positive charges of the S4 segments are pulled toward the cell interior by the resting membrane potential, has a relatively low affinity for LA. The effect of an action potential is to initiate a conformational change in the selectivity funnel region of the channel, moving the positive charges outward and away from the pore interior. As a result, intermediate/closed, open, and inactivated states have a much higher affinity for LA. LAs prevent opening of the intermediate state, may block the channel in the open state, and extend the duration of the inactivated state. Ultimately, however, LA dissociates from its binding site (and the rate of LA's dissociation affects the extent of channel block), and the receptor returns to the resting state. Thus, stimulation of a nerve by an action potential enhances LA binding. With a low frequency of stimulation, LA has time to dissociate and the channels reliably return to their resting state (low affinity for LA). With a high frequency of stimulation, as in nociceptive sensory afferents after a wound, there is insufficient time for LA to fully dissociate; thus, the fraction of channels liganded by LA increases in the continued presence of LA, leading to greater and greater conduction blockade, as explained in the text. The marine neurotoxin TTX binds in the funnel with high affinity ($K_d = 10^{-10}$ nM), as does saxitoxin; both toxins block Na^+ channel activity.

Effect of pH

Local anesthetics tend to be only slightly soluble as unprotonated amines. Therefore, they generally are marketed as water-soluble salts, usually hydrochlorides. Because local anesthetics are weak bases (typical pK_a values range from 8 to 9), their hydrochloride salts are mildly acidic. This property increases the stability of the local anesthetic esters and the catecholamines added as vasoconstrictors. Under usual conditions of administration, the pH of the local anesthetic solution rapidly equilibrates to that of the extracellular fluids.

Although the unprotonated species of the local anesthetic is necessary for diffusion across cellular membranes, it is the cationic species that interacts preferentially with Na^+ channels. The results of experiments on anesthetized mammalian nonmyelinated fibers support this conclusion (Ritchie and Greengard, 1966). In these experiments, conduction could be blocked or unblocked merely by adjusting the pH of the bathing medium to 7.2 or 9.6, respectively, without altering the amount of anesthetic present. The primary role of the cationic form also was demonstrated by Narahashi and Frazier, who perfused the extracellular and axoplasmic surface of the giant squid axon with tertiary and quaternary amine local anesthetics and found that the quaternary amines were active only when perfused intracellularly (Narahashi and Frazier, 1971). However, the unprotonated molecular forms also possess some anesthetic activity (Butterworth and Strichartz, 1990). Recent reports indicated that quaternary local anesthetics such as QX-314 can gain access to the cytoplasmic surface of the nerve cell membrane via TRPV1 channels (reviewed

TABLE 22–1 ■ SUSCEPTIBILITY OF NERVE TYPES TO LOCAL ANESTHETICS

CLASSIFICATION	ANATOMIC LOCATION	MYELIN	DIAMETER (μm)	CONDUCTION VELOCITY (m/s)	FUNCTION	CLINICAL SENSITIVITY TO BLOCK
A fibers						
A α	Afferent to and efferent from muscles and joints	Yes	6–22	10–85	Motor and proprioception	+
A β						++
A γ	Efferent to muscle spindles	Yes	3–6	15–35	Muscle tone	++
A δ	Sensory roots and afferent peripheral nerves	Yes	1–4	5–25	Pain, temperature, touch	+++
B fibers	Preganglionic sympathetic	Yes	<3	3–15	Vasomotor, visceromotor, sudomotor, pilomotor	++++
C fibers						
Sympathetic	Postganglionic sympathetic	No	0.3–1.3	0.7–1.3	Vasomotor, visceromotor, sudomotor, pilomotor	++++
Dorsal root	Sensory roots and afferent peripheral nerves	No	0.4–1.2	0.1–2	Pain, temperature, touch	++++

Adapted with permission from Carpenter RL, Mackey DC. Local anesthetics. In: Barash PG, Cullen BF, Stoelting RK, eds. *Clinical Anesthesia*. 2nd ed. Lippincott, Philadelphia, **1992**, 509–541. http://lww.com.

by Butterworth and Oxford, 2009). TRP channels, and possibly other ion channels, appear to lose selectivity and permit permeation of molecules like QX-314 in the face of prolonged or intense activation.

Prolongation of Action by Vasoconstrictors

The duration of action of a local anesthetic is proportional to the time of contact with nerve. Consequently, maneuvers that keep the drug at the nerve prolong the period of anesthesia. For example, cocaine inhibits the neuronal membrane transporters for catecholamines, thereby potentiating the effect of NE at α adrenergic receptors in the vasculature, resulting in vasoconstriction and reduced cocaine absorption in vascular beds where α adrenergic effects predominate (Chapters 8 and 12). In clinical practice, a vasoconstrictor, usually epinephrine, is often added to local anesthetics. The vasoconstrictor performs a dual service. By decreasing the rate of absorption, it localizes the anesthetic at the desired site and allows the drug's elimination to keep pace with its entry into the systemic circulation, thereby reducing the drug's systemic toxicity. Note, however, that epinephrine dilates skeletal muscle vascular beds via actions at β_2 adrenergic receptors and therefore has the potential to increase systemic toxicity of anesthetic deposited in muscle tissue.

Some of the vasoconstrictor agents may be absorbed systemically, occasionally to an extent sufficient to cause untoward reactions (see the next section). There also may be delayed wound healing, tissue edema, or necrosis after local anesthesia. These effects seem to occur partly because sympathomimetic amines increase the O_2 consumption of the tissue; this, together with the vasoconstriction, leads to hypoxia and local tissue damage. Thus, the use of vasoconstrictors in local anesthetic preparations for anatomical regions with limited collateral circulation is avoided.

Undesired Effects of Local Anesthetics

In addition to blocking conduction in nerve axons in the peripheral nervous system, local anesthetics interfere with the function of all organs in which conduction or transmission of impulses occurs. Thus, these agents affect the CNS, autonomic ganglia, neuromuscular junctions, and all forms of muscle (for a review, see Covino, 1987; Garfield and Gugino, 1987; Gintant and Hoffman, 1987). The danger of such adverse reactions is proportional to the concentration of local anesthetic achieved in the circulation. In general, in local anesthetics with chiral centers, the *S*-enantiomer is less toxic than the *R*-enantiomer (McClure, 1996).

CNS

Following absorption, local anesthetics may cause CNS stimulation, producing restlessness and tremor that may progress to clonic convulsions. In general, the more potent the anesthetic, the more readily convulsions may be produced. Alterations of CNS activity are thus predictable from the local anesthetic agent in question and the blood concentration achieved. Central stimulation is followed by depression; death usually is caused by respiratory failure.

The apparent stimulation and subsequent depression produced by applying local anesthetics to the CNS presumably is due solely to depression of neuronal activity; a selective depression of inhibitory neurons likely accounts for the excitatory phase in vivo. Rapid systemic administration of local anesthetics may produce death with no or only transient signs of CNS stimulation. Under these conditions, the concentration of the drug probably rises so rapidly that all neurons are depressed simultaneously. Airway control, along with ventilatory and circulatory support, are essential features of treatment in the late stage of intoxication. Intravenously administered benzodiazepines are the drugs of choice for both the prevention and the arrest of convulsions. Neither propofol nor a rapidly acting barbiturate is preferred; both are more likely to produce cardiovascular depression than a benzodiazepine (Chapter 19).

Although drowsiness is the most frequent complaint that results from the CNS actions of local anesthetics, lidocaine may produce dysphoria or euphoria and muscle twitching. Moreover, lidocaine may produce a loss of consciousness that is preceded only by symptoms of sedation (Covino, 1987). Whereas other local anesthetics also show the effect, cocaine has a particularly prominent effect on mood and behavior. These effects of cocaine and its potential for abuse are discussed in Chapter 24.

Cardiovascular System

Following systemic absorption, local anesthetics act on the cardiovascular system. The primary site of action is the myocardium, where decreases in electrical excitability, conduction rate, and force of contraction occur. In addition, most local anesthetics cause arteriolar dilation. Untoward cardiovascular effects usually are seen only after high systemic concentrations are attained and CNS symptoms are evident. However, on rare occasions, lower doses of some local anesthetics will cause cardiovascular collapse and death, probably due to either an action on the pacemaker or the sudden onset of ventricular fibrillation. Ventricular tachycardia and fibrillation are relatively uncommon consequences of local anesthetics other than bupivacaine. The antiarrhythmic effects of local anesthetics such as lidocaine and procainamide are discussed in Chapter 30. Finally, it should be stressed that untoward cardiovascular effects of local anesthetic agents may result from their inadvertent intravascular administration, especially if epinephrine is also present.

Smooth Muscle

Local anesthetics depress contractions in the intact bowel and in strips of isolated intestine (Zipf and Dittmann, 1971). They also relax vascular and bronchial smooth muscle, although low concentrations initially may produce contraction (Covino, 1987). Spinal and epidural anesthesia, as well as instillation of local anesthetics into the peritoneal cavity, cause sympathetic nervous system paralysis, which can result in increased tone of GI musculature (described under Clinical Uses). Local anesthetics may increase the resting tone and decrease the contractions of isolated human uterine muscle; however, uterine contractions are seldom depressed directly during intrapartum regional anesthesia.

Neuromuscular Junction and Ganglia

Local anesthetics also affect transmission at the neuromuscular junction. At concentrations at which the muscle responds normally to direct electrical stimulation, procaine can block the response of skeletal muscle to maximal motor-nerve volleys and to ACh. Similar effects occur at autonomic ganglia. These effects are due to block of nicotinic ACh receptors by high concentrations of the local anesthetic (Charnet et al., 1990; Neher and Steinbach, 1978).

Hypersensitivity

Rare individuals are hypersensitive to local anesthetics. The reaction may manifest itself as an allergic dermatitis or a typical asthmatic attack (Covino, 1987). It is important to distinguish allergic reactions from toxic side effects and from the effects of coadministered vasoconstrictors. Hypersensitivity seems to occur more frequently with local anesthetics of the ester type and frequently extends to chemically related compounds. For example, individuals sensitive to procaine also may react to structurally similar compounds (e.g., tetracaine) through reaction to a common metabolite. Although allergic responses to agents of the amide type are uncommon, solutions of such agents may contain preservatives such as methylparaben that may provoke an allergic reaction (Covino, 1987). Local anesthetic preparations containing a vasoconstrictor also may elicit allergic responses due to the sulfite added as an antioxidant for the catecholamine/vasoconstrictor.

Metabolism

Local anesthetics of the ester type (e.g., tetracaine) are hydrolyzed and inactivated primarily by a plasma esterase, probably plasma cholinesterase. The liver also participates in hydrolysis of local anesthetics. Because spinal fluid contains little or no esterase, anesthesia produced by the intrathecal injection of an anesthetic agent will persist until the local anesthetic agent has been absorbed into the circulation. The amide-linked local anesthetics are, in general, degraded by the hepatic CYPs, with the initial reactions involving *N*-dealkylation and subsequent hydrolysis (Arthur, 1987). However, with prilocaine, the initial step is hydrolytic, forming *o*-toluidine metabolites that can cause methemoglobinemia. The extensive use of amide-linked local anesthetics in patients with severe hepatic disease requires caution.

Toxicity

The metabolic fate of local anesthetics is of great practical importance because toxicity can result from an imbalance between their rates of absorption and elimination. The rate of absorption of many local anesthetics into the systemic circulation can be considerably reduced by the incorporation of a vasoconstrictor agent in the anesthetic solution. However, the rate of degradation of local anesthetics varies greatly, and this is a major factor in determining the safety of a particular agent. Because toxicity is related to the concentration of free drug, binding of the anesthetic to proteins in the serum and to tissues reduces toxicity. For example, in intravenous regional anesthesia of an extremity, about half of the original anesthetic dose still is tissue bound 30 min after the restoration of normal blood flow (Arthur, 1987). Reversing the effects of local anesthetic systemic toxicity is a clinical challenge. One developing approach is promising and unusual: intravenous lipid emulsion therapy (Weinberg, 2012). Whether the lipids simply provide a favorable milieu of micelles into which lipophilic drugs can partition or the effect involves more complex biochemical pathways is not yet clear (Fettiplace et al., 2016).

Plasma binding sites serve to moderate local anesthetic levels on blood. The amide-linked local anesthetics bind extensively (55%–95%) to plasma proteins, particularly α_1-acid glycoprotein. Many factors increase (e.g., cancer, surgery, trauma, myocardial infarction, smoking, and uremia) or decrease (e.g., oral contraceptives) the level of this glycoprotein, thereby changing the amount of anesthetic delivered to the liver for metabolism and thus influencing systemic toxicity. Age-related changes in protein binding of local anesthetics also occur. The neonate is relatively deficient in plasma proteins that bind local anesthetics and thereby is more susceptible to toxicity. Plasma proteins are not the sole determinant of local anesthetic availability. Uptake by the lung also may play an important role in the distribution of amide-linked local anesthetics. Finally, reduced cardiac output slows delivery of the amide compounds to the liver, reducing their metabolism and prolonging their plasma half-lives.

Local Anesthetics and Related Agents

Cocaine

Chemistry

Cocaine, an ester of benzoic acid and methylecgonine, occurs in abundance in the leaves of the coca shrub. Ecgonine is an amino alcohol base closely related to tropine, the amino alcohol in atropine. It has the same fundamental structure as the synthetic local anesthetics (Figure 20–1).

Pharmacological Actions and Preparations

The clinically desired actions of cocaine are the blockade of nerve impulses as a consequence of its local anesthetic properties and local vasoconstriction secondary to inhibition of the NET (see Table 8–5). Toxicity and its potential for abuse have steadily decreased the clinical uses of cocaine. Its high toxicity is due to reduced catecholamine uptake in both the central and peripheral nervous systems and the resulting prolongation of transmitter dwell time in the synaptic cleft. Cocaine's euphoric properties are due primarily to inhibition of catecholamine uptake, particularly DA, in the CNS. Other local anesthetics do not block the uptake of NE and do not produce the sensitization to catecholamines, vasoconstriction, or mydriasis characteristic of cocaine. Currently, cocaine is used primarily for topical anesthesia of the upper respiratory tract, where its combination of both vasoconstrictor and local anesthetic properties provide anesthesia and shrinking of the mucosa. Cocaine hydrochloride is provided as a 1%, 4%, or 10% solution for topical application. For most applications, the 1% or 4% preparation is preferred to reduce toxicity. Because of its abuse potential, cocaine is listed as a schedule II controlled substance by the U.S. Drug Enforcement Agency.

Lidocaine

Lidocaine, an aminoethylamide (Figure 20–1), is the prototypical amide local anesthetic.

Pharmacological Actions and Preparations

Lidocaine produces faster, more intense, longer-lasting, and more extensive anesthesia than does an equal concentration of procaine. Lidocaine is an alternative choice for individuals sensitive to ester-type local anesthetics.

A lidocaine transdermal patch is used for relief of pain associated with postherpetic neuralgia. The combination of lidocaine (2.5%) and prilocaine (2.5%) under an occlusive dressing (EMLA, others) is used as an anesthetic prior to venipuncture, skin graft harvesting, and infiltration of anesthetics into genitalia. Lidocaine in combination with tetracaine in a formulation that generates a "peel" is approved for topical local analgesia prior to superficial dermatological procedures such as filler injections and laser-based treatments. Lidocaine in combination with tetracaine is also supplied in a formulation that generates heat on exposure to air, which is used prior to venous access and superficial dermatological procedures such as excision, electrodessication, and shave biopsy of skin lesions. The mild warming is intended to increase skin temperature by up to 5°C for the purpose of enhancing delivery of local anesthetic into the skin.

ADME

Lidocaine is absorbed rapidly after parenteral administration and from the GI and respiratory tracts. Although it is effective when used without any vasoconstrictor, epinephrine decreases the rate of absorption, thereby decreasing the probability of toxicity and prolonging the duration of action. In addition to preparations for injection, lidocaine is formulated for topical, ophthalmic, mucosal, and transdermal use.

Lidocaine is dealkylated in the liver by CYPs to monoethylglycine xylidide and glycine xylidide, which can be metabolized further to monoethylglycine and xylidide. Both monoethylglycine xylidide and glycine xylidide retain local anesthetic activity. In humans, about 75% of the xylidide is excreted in the urine as the further metabolite 4-hydroxy-2,6-dimethylaniline (Arthur, 1987).

Toxicity

The side effects of lidocaine seen with increasing dose include drowsiness, tinnitus, dysgeusia, dizziness, and twitching. As the dose increases, seizures, coma, and respiratory depression and arrest will occur. Clinically significant cardiovascular depression usually occurs at serum lidocaine levels that produce marked CNS effects. The metabolites monoethylglycine xylidide and glycine xylidide may contribute to some of these side effects.

Clinical Uses

Lidocaine has a wide range of clinical uses as a local anesthetic; it has utility in almost any application where a local anesthetic of intermediate duration is needed. Lidocaine also is used as an antiarrhythmic agent (Chapter 30).

Bupivacaine

Bupivacaine has a wide range of clinical uses as a local anesthetic; it has utility in almost any application where a local anesthetic of long duration is needed.

Pharmacological Actions and Preparations

Bupivacaine is a widely used amide local anesthetic; its structure is similar to that of lidocaine except that the amine-containing group is a butyl piperidine (Figure 20–1). Bupivacaine is a potent agent capable of producing prolonged anesthesia. Its long duration of action plus its tendency to provide more sensory than motor block has made it a popular drug for providing prolonged analgesia during labor or the postoperative period. By taking advantage of indwelling catheters and continuous infusions, bupivacaine can be used to provide several days of effective analgesia. Recently, a liposomal bupivacaine preparation has been FDA-approved. While safe and effective, its superiority over conventional bupivacaine and its ideal clinical applications remain to be determined (Uskova and O'Connor, 2015).

ADME

Bupivacaine is more slowly absorbed than lidocaine, so plasma levels increase more slowly following a bupivacaine nerve block or epidural. Conversely, bupivacaine levels fall more slowly following cessation of a continuous bupivacaine infusion than would be predicted from single-injection pharmacokinetics. Bupivacaine is primarily metabolized in the liver by CYP3A4 to pipecolylxylidine, which is then glucuronidated and excreted.

Toxicity

Bupivacaine is more cardiotoxic than equieffective doses of lidocaine. Clinically, this is manifested by severe ventricular arrhythmias and myocardial depression after inadvertent intravascular administration. Although lidocaine and bupivacaine both rapidly block cardiac Na^+ channels during systole, bupivacaine dissociates much more slowly than lidocaine during diastole, so a significant fraction of Na^+ channels at physiological heart rates remains blocked with bupivacaine at the end of diastole (Clarkson and Hondeghem, 1985). Thus, the block by bupivacaine is cumulative and substantially more than predicted by its local anesthetic potency. At least a portion of the cardiac toxicity of bupivacaine may be mediated centrally; direct injection of small quantities of bupivacaine into the medulla can produce malignant ventricular arrhythmias (Thomas et al., 1986). Bupivacaine-induced cardiac toxicity can be difficult to treat, and its severity is enhanced by coexisting acidosis, hypercarbia, and hypoxemia, emphasizing the importance of prompt airway control in resuscitation from bupivacaine overdose.

Local Anesthetics Suitable for Injection

The number of synthetic local anesthetics is so large that it is impractical to consider them all here. Some local anesthetic agents are too toxic to be given by injection. Their use is restricted to topical application to the eye (Chapter 69), the mucous membranes, or the skin (Chapter 70). Many local anesthetics are suitable, however, for infiltration or injection to produce nerve block; some of these also are useful for topical application. The discussion below presents the main categories of local anesthetics; agents are listed alphabetically.

Articaine

Articaine is approved in the U.S. for dental and periodontal procedures. Although it is an amide local anesthetic, it also contains an ester, whose hydrolysis terminates its action. Thus, articaine exhibits rapid onset (1–6 min) and duration of action of about 1 h.

Chloroprocaine

Chloroprocaine is a chlorinated derivative of procaine. Its major assets are its rapid onset and short duration of action and its reduced acute toxicity due to rapid metabolism (plasma $t_{1/2}$ ~ 25 sec). Enthusiasm for its use has been tempered by reports of prolonged sensory and motor block after epidural or subarachnoid administration of large doses. This toxicity appears to have been a consequence of low pH and the use of sodium metabisulfite as a preservative in earlier formulations. There are no reports of neurotoxicity with newer preparations of chloroprocaine that contain calcium EDTA as the preservative, although these preparations are not recommended for intrathecal administration. A higher-than-expected incidence of muscular back pain following epidural anesthesia with 2-chloroprocaine has also been reported (Stevens et al., 1993). This back pain is thought to be due to tetany in the paraspinus muscles, which may be a consequence of Ca^{2+} binding by the EDTA included as a preservative; the incidence of back pain appears to be related to the volume of drug injected and its use for skin infiltration.

Mepivacaine

Mepivacaine is an intermediate-acting amino amide with pharmacological properties resembling those of lidocaine. Mepivacaine, however, is more toxic to the neonate and thus is not used in obstetrical anesthesia. The increased toxicity of mepivacaine in the neonate is related to ion trapping of this agent because of the lower pH of neonatal blood and the pK_a of mepivacaine, rather than to its slower metabolism in the neonate. Mepivacaine appears to have a slightly higher therapeutic index in adults than does lidocaine. Its onset of action is similar to, and its duration slightly longer (~20%) than, that of lidocaine in the absence of a coadministered vasoconstrictor. Mepivacaine is not effective as a topical anesthetic.

Prilocaine

Prilocaine is an intermediate-acting amino amide. It has a pharmacological profile similar to that of lidocaine. The primary differences are that it causes little vasodilation and thus can be used without a vasoconstrictor; its increased volume of distribution reduces its CNS toxicity, making it suitable for intravenous regional blocks (described further in the chapter). The use of prilocaine is largely limited to dentistry because the drug is unique among the local anesthetics in its propensity to cause methemoglobinemia. This effect is a consequence of the metabolism of the aromatic ring to *o*-toluidine. Development of methemoglobinemia is dependent on the total dose administered, usually appearing after a dose of 8 mg/kg. If necessary, it can be treated by the intravenous administration of methylene blue (1–2 mg/kg).

Ropivacaine

The cardiac toxicity of bupivacaine stimulated interest in developing a less-toxic, long-lasting local anesthetic. One result of that search was the development of the amino ethylamide ropivacaine; the *S*-enantiomer was chosen because it has a lower toxicity than the *R*-isomer (McClure, 1996). Ropivacaine is slightly less potent than bupivacaine in producing anesthesia. Ropivacaine appears to be suitable for both epidural and regional anesthesia, with a duration of action similar to that of bupivacaine. Interestingly, it seems to be even more motor-sparing than bupivacaine.

Procaine

Procaine is no longer marketed in the U.S. as a single entity. It is an ingredient of some long-acting intramuscular formulations of penicillin.

Tetracaine

Tetracaine is a long-acting amino ester. It is significantly more potent and has a longer duration of action than procaine. Tetracaine may exhibit increased systemic toxicity because it is more slowly metabolized than the other commonly used ester local anesthetics. Currently, it is widely used in spinal anesthesia when a drug of long duration is needed. Tetracaine also is incorporated into several topical anesthetic preparations. With the introduction of bupivacaine, tetracaine is rarely used in peripheral nerve blocks because of the large doses often necessary, its slow onset, and its potential for toxicity.

Agents Used Primarily to Anesthetize Mucous Membranes and Skin

Some agents are useful as topical anesthetic agents on the skin or mucous membranes, although too irritating or too ineffective to be applied to the eye. These preparations are effective in the symptomatic relief of anal and genital pruritus, poison ivy rashes, and numerous other acute and chronic dermatoses. They sometimes are combined with a glucocorticoid or antihistamine and are available in a number of proprietary formulations.

Dibucaine

Dibucaine is a quinoline derivative. Its toxicity resulted in its removal from the U.S. market as an injectable preparation. It retains wide popularity outside the U.S. as a spinal anesthetic. It currently is available as an over-the-counter ointment for cutaneous use.

Dyclonine

Dyclonine hydrochloride is readily absorbed through the skin and mucous membranes. Its onset is rapid; its duration of action is short. Dyclonine is an active ingredient in a number of over-the-counter medications, including sore throat lozenges, a patch for cold sores, and a 0.75% solution.

Pramoxine

Pramoxine hydrochloride is a surface anesthetic agent that is not a benzoate ester. Its distinct chemical structure may help minimize the danger of cross-sensitivity reactions in patients allergic to other local anesthetics. Pramoxine produces satisfactory surface anesthesia and is reasonably well tolerated on the skin and mucous membranes. It is too irritating to be used on the eye or in the nose, but an otic solution containing chloroxylenol is marketed. Many preparations (currently 284 in the U.S.), including creams, lotions, sprays, gel, wipes, and foams, usually containing 1% pramoxine, are available for topical application.

Anesthetics With Low Aqueous Solubility

Some local anesthetics have low aqueous solubility and consequently are absorbed too slowly to cause classical local anesthetic toxicity. These compounds can be applied directly to wounds and ulcerated surfaces, where they remain localized for long periods of time, producing a sustained anesthetic action. Chemically, they are esters of para-aminobenzoic acid lacking the terminal amino group possessed by the previously described local anesthetics. The most important member of the series is benzocaine (ethyl aminobenzoate), which is incorporated into a large number of topical preparations. Benzocaine can cause methemoglobinemia (see the discussion of methemoglobinemia in the section on prilocaine); consequently, dosing recommendations must be followed carefully.

Agents for Ophthalmic Use

Anesthesia of the cornea and conjunctiva can be obtained readily by topical application of local anesthetics. However, most of the local anesthetics that have been described are too irritating for ophthalmological use. The two compounds used most frequently today are proparacaine and tetracaine. In addition to being less irritating during administration, proparacaine has the advantage of bearing little antigenic similarity to the other benzoate local anesthetics. Thus, it sometimes can be used in individuals sensitive to the amino ester local anesthetics.

For use in ophthalmology, these local anesthetics are instilled a single drop at a time. If anesthesia is incomplete, successive drops are applied until satisfactory conditions are obtained. The duration of anesthesia is determined chiefly by the vascularity of the tissue; thus, it is longest in normal cornea and shortest in inflamed conjunctiva. In the latter case, repeated instillations may be necessary to maintain adequate anesthesia. Long-term administration of topical anesthesia to the eye has been associated with retarded healing, pitting, and sloughing of the corneal epithelium and predisposition of the eye to inadvertent injury. Thus, these drugs should not be prescribed for self-administration. For issues of drug delivery, pharmacokinetics, and toxicity unique to drugs for ophthalmic use, see Chapter 69.

Biological Toxins: Tetrodotoxin and Saxitoxin

The two biological toxins, tetrodotoxin and saxitoxin, block the pore of the Na^+ channel. Tetrodotoxin is found in the gonads and other visceral tissues of some fish of the order Tetraodontiformes (to which the Japanese *fugu*, or puffer fish, belongs); it also occurs in the skin of some newts of the family Salamandridae and of the Costa Rican frog *Atelopus*. Saxitoxin is elaborated by the dinoflagellates *Gonyaulax catenella* and *G. tamarensis* and retained in the tissues of clams and other shellfish that eat these organisms. Given the right conditions of temperature and light, the *Gonyaulax* may multiply so rapidly as to discolor the ocean, causing the condition known as *red tide*. Shellfish feeding on *Gonyaulax* at this time become extremely toxic to humans and are responsible for periodic outbreaks of paralytic shellfish poisoning (Sakai and Swanson, 2014; Stommel and Watters, 2004). Although these toxins are chemically distinct, they have similar mechanisms of action. Both toxins, in nanomolar concentrations, specifically block the outer mouth of the pore of Na^+ channels in the membranes of excitable cells. As a result, the action potential is blocked. The receptor site for these toxins is formed by amino acid residues in the *P* loop of the Na^+ channel α subunit (Figure 22–2) in all four domains (Catterall, 2000; Terlau et al., 1991). Not all Na^+ channels are equally sensitive to tetrodotoxin; some Na^+ channels in cardiac myocytes and dorsal root ganglion neurons are resistant, and a tetrodotoxin-resistant Na^+ channel is expressed when skeletal muscle is denervated. Tetrodotoxin and saxitoxin are exceedingly potent; the minimal lethal dose of each in the mouse is about 8 μg/kg. Both toxins have caused fatal poisoning in humans due to paralysis of the respiratory muscles; therefore, the treatment of severe cases of poisoning requires support of respiration. Blockade of vasomotor nerves, together with a relaxation of vascular smooth muscle, seems to be responsible for the hypotension that is characteristic of tetrodotoxin poisoning. Early gastric lavage and pressor support also are indicated. If the patient survives paralytic shellfish poisoning for 24 h, the prognosis is good.

Clinical Uses of Local Anesthetics

Local anesthesia is the loss of sensation in a body part without the loss of consciousness or the impairment of central control of vital functions. It offers two major advantages over general anesthesia. First, physiological perturbations associated with general anesthesia are avoided. Second, neurophysiological responses to pain and stress can be modified beneficially. However, local anesthetics have the potential to produce deleterious side effects. Proper choice of a local anesthetic and care in its use are the primary determinants in avoiding these problems.

There is a poor relationship between the amount of local anesthetic injected and peak plasma levels in adults. Furthermore, peak plasma levels vary widely depending on the area of injection. They are highest with interpleural or intercostal blocks and lowest with subcutaneous infiltration. Thus, recommended maximum doses serve only as general guidelines. This discussion summarizes the pharmacological and physiological consequences of the use of local anesthetics categorized by method of administration. A more comprehensive discussion of their use and administration is presented in textbooks on regional anesthesia (Cousins et al., 2008).

Topical Anesthesia

Anesthesia of mucous membranes of the nose, mouth, throat, tracheobronchial tree, esophagus, and genitourinary tract can be produced by direct application of aqueous solutions of salts of many local anesthetics or by suspension of the poorly soluble local anesthetics. Tetracaine (2%), lidocaine (2%–10%), and cocaine (1%–4%) typically are used. Cocaine is used only in the nose, nasopharynx, mouth, throat, and ear, where it uniquely produces vasoconstriction as well as anesthesia. The shrinking of mucous membranes decreases operative bleeding while improving surgical visualization. Comparable vasoconstriction can be achieved with other local anesthetics by the addition of a low concentration of a vasoconstrictor such as phenylephrine (0.005%). Epinephrine, topically applied, has no significant local effect and does not prolong the duration of action of local anesthetics applied to mucous membranes because of poor penetration. *Maximal safe total dosages* for topical anesthesia in a healthy 70-kg adult are 300 mg for lidocaine, 150 mg for cocaine, and 50 mg for tetracaine.

Peak anesthetic effect following topical application of cocaine or lidocaine occurs within 2–5 min (3–8 min with tetracaine), and anesthesia lasts for 30–45 min (30–60 min with tetracaine). Anesthesia is entirely superficial; it does not extend to submucosal structures. This technique does not alleviate joint pain or discomfort from subdermal inflammation or injury.

Local anesthetics are absorbed rapidly into the circulation following topical application to mucous membranes or denuded skin. Thus, topical anesthesia always carries the risk of systemic toxic reactions. Systemic toxicity has occurred even following the use of local anesthetics to control discomfort associated with severe diaper rash in infants. Absorption is particularly rapid when local anesthetics are applied to the tracheobronchial tree. Concentrations in blood after instillation of local anesthetics into the airway are nearly the same as those following intravenous injection. Surface anesthetics for the skin and cornea have been described earlier in the chapter.

Eutectic mixtures of local anesthetics lidocaine (2.5%)/prilocaine (2.5%) (EMLA) and lidocaine (7%)/tetracaine (7%) (Pliagis) bridge the gap between topical and infiltration anesthesia. The efficacy of each of these combinations lies in the fact that the mixture has a melting point less than that of either compound alone, existing at room temperature as an oil that can penetrate intact skin. These creams produce anesthesia to a maximum depth of 5 mm and are applied as a cream on intact skin under an occlusive dressing in advance (~30–60 min) of any procedure. These mixtures are effective for procedures involving skin and superficial subcutaneous structures (e.g., venipuncture and skin graft harvesting). Beware: the component local anesthetics will be absorbed into the systemic circulation, potentially producing toxic effects. Guidelines are available to calculate the maximum amount of cream that can be applied and area of skin covered. These mixtures must not be used on mucous membranes or abraded skin, as rapid absorption across these surfaces may result in systemic toxicity.

Infiltration Anesthesia

Infiltration anesthesia is the injection of local anesthetic directly into tissue without taking into consideration the course of cutaneous nerves. Infiltration anesthesia can be so superficial as to include only the skin. It also can include deeper structures, including intra-abdominal organs, when these too are infiltrated.

The duration of infiltration anesthesia can be approximately doubled by the addition of epinephrine (5 μg/mL) to the injection solution; epinephrine also decreases peak concentrations of local anesthetics in blood. *Epinephrine-containing solutions are generally not injected into tissues supplied by end arteries—for example, fingers and toes, ears, the nose, and the penis—because of a concern that the resulting vasoconstriction may cause gangrene.* Similarly, epinephrine should be avoided in solutions injected intracutaneously. Because epinephrine also is absorbed into the circulation, its use should be avoided in those for whom adrenergic stimulation is undesirable.

The local anesthetics most frequently used for infiltration anesthesia are lidocaine (0.5%–1%) and bupivacaine (0.125%–0.25%). When used without epinephrine, up to 4.5 mg/kg of lidocaine or 2 mg/kg of bupivacaine can be employed in adults. When epinephrine is added, these amounts can be increased by one-third. Tumescent anesthesia is a special case of infiltration anesthesia for which large doses and volumes of lidocaine and epinephrine are administered (Lozinski and Huq, 2013).

Infiltration anesthesia and other regional anesthetic techniques have the advantage of providing satisfactory anesthesia without disrupting normal bodily functions. The chief disadvantage of infiltration anesthesia is that relatively large amounts of drug must be used to anesthetize relatively small areas. This is no problem with minor surgery. When major surgery is performed, however, the amount of local anesthetic that is required makes systemic toxic reactions likely. The amount of anesthetic required to anesthetize an area can be reduced significantly and the duration of anesthesia increased markedly by specifically blocking the nerves that innervate the area of interest. This can be done at one of several levels: subcutaneously, at major nerves, or at the level of the spinal roots.

Field Block Anesthesia

Field block anesthesia is produced by subcutaneous injection of a solution of local anesthetic to anesthetize the region distal to the injection. For example, subcutaneous infiltration of the proximal portion of the volar surface of the forearm results in an extensive area of cutaneous anesthesia that starts 2–3 cm distal to the site of injection. The same principle can be applied with particular benefit to the scalp, the anterior abdominal wall, and the lower extremity.

The drugs, concentrations, and doses recommended are the same as for infiltration anesthesia. The advantage of field block anesthesia is that less drug can be used to provide a greater area of anesthesia than when infiltration anesthesia is used. Knowledge of the relevant neuroanatomy obviously is essential for successful field block anesthesia.

Nerve Block Anesthesia

Injection of a solution of a local anesthetic into or about individual peripheral nerves or nerve plexuses produces even greater areas of anesthesia than do the techniques already described. Blockade of mixed peripheral nerves and nerve plexuses also usually anesthetizes somatic motor nerves, producing skeletal muscle relaxation, which is essential for some surgical procedures. The areas of sensory and motor block usually start several centimeters distal to the site of injection. Brachial plexus blocks are particularly useful for procedures on the upper extremity and shoulder. Intercostal nerve blocks are effective for anesthesia and relaxation of the anterior abdominal wall. Cervical plexus block is appropriate for surgery of the neck. Sciatic and femoral nerve blocks are useful for surgery distal to the knee. Other useful nerve blocks prior to surgical procedures include blocks of individual nerves at the wrist and at the ankle, blocks of individual nerves such as the median or ulnar at the elbow, and blocks of sensory cranial nerves.

There are four major determinants of the onset of sensory anesthesia following injection near a nerve: (1) proximity of the injection to the nerve; (2) concentration and volume of drug; (3) degree of ionization of the drug; and (4) time.

Local anesthetic is never intentionally injected into the nerve; this would be painful and could cause nerve damage. Instead, the anesthetic agent is deposited as close to the nerve as possible. Thus, the local anesthetic must diffuse from the site of injection into the nerve on which it acts. The rate of diffusion is determined chiefly by the concentration of the drug, its degree of ionization (ionized local anesthetic diffuses more slowly), its hydrophobicity, and the physical characteristics of the tissue surrounding the nerve. Higher concentrations of local anesthetic will provide a more rapid onset of peripheral nerve block. The utility of higher concentrations, however, is limited by systemic toxicity and by direct neural toxicity of concentrated local anesthetic solutions. For a given concentration, local anesthetics with lower pK_a values tend to have a more rapid onset of action because more drug is uncharged at neutral pH. For example, the onset of action of lidocaine occurs in about 3 min; 35% of lidocaine is in the basic form at pH 7.4. In contrast, the onset of action of bupivacaine requires about 15 min; only 5%–10% of bupivacaine is uncharged at this pH. Increased hydrophobicity might be expected to speed onset by increased penetration into nerve tissue. However, it also will increase binding in tissue lipids. Furthermore, the more hydrophobic local anesthetics also are more potent (and toxic) and thus must be used at lower concentrations, decreasing the concentration gradient for diffusion. Tissue factors also play a role in determining the rate of onset of anesthetic effects. The amount of connective tissue that must be penetrated can be significant in a nerve plexus compared to isolated nerves and can slow or even prevent adequate diffusion of local anesthetic to the nerve fibers.

Duration of nerve block anesthesia depends on the physical characteristics of the local anesthetic used and the presence or absence of vasoconstrictors. Especially important physical characteristics are lipid solubility and protein binding. Local anesthetics can be broadly divided into three categories:

- those with a short (20- to 45-min) duration of action in mixed peripheral nerves, such as procaine;
- those with an intermediate (60- to 120-min) duration of action, such as lidocaine and mepivacaine; and
- those with a long (400- to 450-min) duration of action, such as bupivacaine, ropivacaine, and tetracaine.

Block duration of the intermediate-acting local anesthetics such as lidocaine can be prolonged by the addition of epinephrine (5 μg/mL). The degree of block prolongation in peripheral nerves following the addition of epinephrine appears to be related to the intrinsic vasodilating properties of the local anesthetic and thus is most pronounced with lidocaine.

The types of nerve fibers that are blocked when a local anesthetic is injected about a mixed peripheral nerve depend on the concentration of drug used, nerve fiber size, internodal distance, and frequency and pattern of nerve impulse transmission (see the previous sections on Frequency and Voltage Dependence and Differential Sensitivity of Nerve Fibers). Anatomical factors are similarly important. A mixed peripheral nerve or nerve trunk consists of individual nerves surrounded by an investing epineurium. The vascular supply usually is centrally located. When a local anesthetic is deposited about a peripheral nerve, it diffuses from the outer surface toward the core along a concentration gradient. Consequently, nerves in the outer mantle of the mixed nerve are blocked first. These fibers usually are distributed to more proximal anatomical structures than are those situated near the core of the mixed nerve and often are motor. If the volume and concentration of local anesthetic solution deposited about the nerve are adequate, the local anesthetic eventually will diffuse inward in amounts adequate to block even the most centrally located fibers. Lesser amounts of drug will block only nerves in the mantle and the smaller and more sensitive central fibers. Furthermore, because removal of local anesthetics occurs primarily in the core of a mixed nerve or nerve trunk, where the vascular supply is located, the duration of blockade of centrally located nerves is shorter than that of more peripherally situated fibers.

The choice of local anesthetic and the amount and concentration administered are determined by the nerves and the types of fibers to be blocked, the required duration of anesthesia, and the size and health of the patient. For blocks of 2–4 h, lidocaine (1%–1.5%) can be used in the amounts recommended previously (see Infiltration Anesthesia). Mepivacaine (up to 7 mg/kg of a 1%–2% solution) provides anesthesia that lasts about as long as that from lidocaine. Bupivacaine (2–3 mg/kg of a 0.25%–0.375% solution) can be used when a longer duration of action is required. Addition of 5 μg/mL epinephrine slows systemic absorption and therefore prolongs duration and lowers the plasma concentration of the intermediate-acting local anesthetics.

Peak plasma concentrations of local anesthetics depend on the amount injected, the physical characteristics of the local anesthetic, whether epinephrine is used, the rate of blood flow to the site of injection, and the surface area exposed to local anesthetic. This is of particular importance in the safe application of nerve block anesthesia because the potential for systemic reactions is related to peak free serum concentrations. For example, peak concentrations of lidocaine in blood following injection of 400 mg without epinephrine for intercostal nerve blocks average 7 μg/mL; the same amount of lidocaine used for block of the brachial plexus results in peak concentrations in blood of about 3 μg/mL (Covino and Vassallo, 1976). Therefore, the amount of local anesthetic that can be injected must be adjusted according to the anatomical site of the nerve(s) to be blocked to minimize untoward effects. Addition of epinephrine can decrease peak plasma concentrations by 20%–30%. Multiple nerve blocks (e.g., intercostal block) or blocks performed in vascular regions require reduction in the amount of anesthetic that can be given safely because the surface area for absorption or the rate of absorption is increased.

Intravenous Regional Anesthesia (Bier Block)

The Bier block technique relies on using the vasculature to bring the local anesthetic solution to the nerve trunks and endings. In this technique, an extremity is exsanguinated with an Esmarch (elastic) bandage, and a proximally located tourniquet is inflated to 100–150 mm Hg above the systolic blood pressure. The Esmarch bandage is removed, and the local anesthetic is injected into a previously cannulated vein. Typically, complete anesthesia of the limb ensues within 5–10 min. Pain from the tourniquet and the potential for ischemic nerve injury limit tourniquet inflation to 2 h or less. However, the tourniquet should remain inflated for at least 15–30 min to prevent toxic amounts of local anesthetic from entering the circulation following deflation. Lidocaine, 40–50 mL (0.5 mL/kg in children) of a 0.5% solution without epinephrine, is the drug of choice for this technique. For intravenous regional anesthesia in adults using a 0.5% solution without epinephrine, the dose administered should not exceed 4 mg/kg. A few clinicians prefer prilocaine (0.5%) over lidocaine because of its higher therapeutic index.

The attractiveness of the Bier block lies in its simplicity. Its primary disadvantages are that it can be used only for a few anatomical regions, sensation (pain) returns quickly after tourniquet deflation, and premature release or failure of the tourniquet can produce toxic levels of local anesthetic (e.g., 50 mL of 0.5% lidocaine contains 250 mg of lidocaine). For the last reason and because its longer duration of action offers no advantage, the more cardiotoxic agent bupivacaine is not recommended for this technique. Intravenous regional anesthesia is used most often for surgery of the forearm and hand but can be adapted for the foot and distal leg.

Spinal Anesthesia

Spinal anesthesia follows the injection of local anesthetic into the CSF in the lumbar space. For a number of reasons, including the ability to produce anesthesia of a considerable fraction of the body with a dose of local anesthetic that produces negligible plasma levels, spinal anesthesia remains one of the most popular forms of anesthesia. In most adults, the spinal cord terminates above the second lumbar vertebra; between that point and the termination of the thecal sac in the sacrum, the lumbar and sacral roots are bathed in CSF. Thus, in this region there is a relatively large volume of CSF within which to inject drug, thereby minimizing the potential for direct nerve trauma.

The following is a brief discussion of the physiological effects of spinal anesthesia relating to the pharmacology of the local anesthetics. See more specialized texts (Cousins et al., 2008) for additional details.

Physiological Effects of Spinal Anesthesia

Most of the physiological side effects of spinal anesthesia are a consequence of the sympathetic blockade produced by local anesthetic block of the sympathetic fibers in the spinal nerve roots. A thorough understanding of these physiological effects is necessary for the safe and successful application of spinal anesthesia. Although some effects may be deleterious and require treatment, others can be beneficial for the patient or can improve operating conditions.

Most sympathetic fibers leave the spinal cord between T1 and L2 (see Figure 8–1). Although local anesthetic is injected below these levels in the lumbar portion of the dural sac, cephalad spread of the local anesthetic occurs with all but the smallest volumes injected. This cephalad spread is of considerable importance in the practice of spinal anesthesia and potentially is under the control of numerous variables, of which patient position and baricity (density of the drug relative to the density of the CSF) are the most important (Greene, 1983). The degree of sympathetic block is related to the height of sensory anesthesia; often, the level of sympathetic blockade is several spinal segments higher because the preganglionic sympathetic fibers are more sensitive to low concentrations of local anesthetic. The effects of sympathetic blockade involve both the actions (now partially unopposed) of the parasympathetic nervous system and the response of the unblocked portion of the sympathetic nervous system. Thus, as the level of sympathetic block ascends, the actions of the parasympathetic nervous system are increasingly dominant, and the compensatory mechanisms of the unblocked sympathetic nervous system are diminished. As most sympathetic nerve fibers leave the cord at T1 or below, few additional effects of sympathetic blockade are seen with cervical levels of spinal anesthesia. The consequences of sympathetic blockade will vary among patients as a function of age, physical conditioning, and disease state. Interestingly, sympathetic blockade during spinal anesthesia appears to be minimal in healthy children.

Clinically, the most important effects of sympathetic blockade during spinal anesthesia are on the cardiovascular system. At all but the lowest levels of spinal blockade, some vasodilation will occur. Vasodilation is more marked on the venous than on the arterial side of the circulation, resulting in blood pooling in the venous capacitance vessels. This reduction in circulating blood volume is well tolerated at low levels of spinal anesthesia in healthy patients. With an increasing level of block, this effect becomes more marked, and venous return becomes gravity dependent. If venous return decreases too much, cardiac output and organ perfusion decline precipitously. Venous return can be increased by a modest (10°–15°) head-down tilt or by elevating the legs.

At high levels of spinal blockade, the cardiac accelerator fibers, which exit the spinal cord at T1–T4, will be blocked. This is detrimental in patients dependent on elevated sympathetic tone to maintain cardiac output (e.g., during congestive heart failure or hypovolemia), and it also removes one of the compensatory mechanisms available to maintain organ perfusion during vasodilation. Thus, as the level of spinal block ascends, the rate of cardiovascular compromise can accelerate if not carefully observed and treated. Sudden asystole also can occur, presumably because of loss of sympathetic innervation in the continued presence of parasympathetic activity at the sinoatrial node (Caplan et al., 1988). In the usual clinical situation, blood pressure serves as a surrogate marker for cardiac output and organ perfusion. Treatment of hypotension usually is warranted when the blood pressure decreases to about 30% of *resting* values.

Therapy is aimed at maintaining brain and cardiac perfusion and oxygenation. To achieve these goals, administration of oxygen, fluid infusion, manipulation of patient position, and the administration of vasoactive drugs are all options. In practice, patients typically are administered a bolus (500–1000 mL) of fluid prior to the administration of spinal anesthesia in an attempt to prevent some of the deleterious effects of spinal blockade. Because the usual cause of hypotension is decreased venous return, possibly complicated by decreased heart rate, drugs with preferential venoconstrictive and chronotropic properties are preferred. For this reason, ephedrine, 5–10 mg intravenously, often is the drug of choice. In addition to the use of ephedrine to treat deleterious effects of sympathetic blockade, direct-acting α_1 adrenergic receptor agonists such as phenylephrine (Chapter 12) can be administered by either bolus or continuous infusion.

A beneficial effect of spinal anesthesia partially mediated by the sympathetic nervous system is on the intestine. Sympathetic fibers originating from T5 to L1 inhibit peristalsis; thus, their blockade produces a small, contracted intestine. This, together with flaccid abdominal musculature, produces excellent operating conditions for some types of bowel surgery. The consequences of spinal anesthesia on the respiratory system are mostly mediated by effects on the skeletal musculature. Paralysis of the intercostal muscles will reduce a patient's ability to cough and clear secretions, which may produce dyspnea in patients with bronchitis or emphysema. Respiratory arrest during spinal anesthesia seldom occurs due to paralysis of the phrenic nerves or to toxic levels of local anesthetic in the CSF of the fourth ventricle; it is much more likely to be due to medullary ischemia secondary to hypotension.

Pharmacology

Currently in the U.S., the drugs most commonly used in spinal anesthesia are lidocaine, tetracaine, and bupivacaine. The choice of local anesthetic is primarily determined by the desired duration of anesthesia. General guidelines are to use lidocaine for short procedures, bupivacaine for intermediate-to-long procedures, and tetracaine for long procedures. As mentioned, the factors contributing to the distribution of local anesthetics in the CSF have received much attention because of their importance in determining the height of block. The most important pharmacological factors include the amount, and possibly the volume, of drug injected and its baricity. The speed of injection of the local anesthesia solution also may affect the height of the block, just as the position of the patient can influence the rate of distribution of the anesthetic agent and the height of blockade achieved (described in the next section). For a given preparation of local anesthetic, administration of increasing amounts leads to a fairly predictable increase in the level of block attained. For example, 100 mg of lidocaine, 20 mg of bupivacaine, or 12 mg of tetracaine usually will result in a T4 sensory block. More complete tables of these relationships can be found in standard anesthesiology texts.

Epinephrine often is added to spinal anesthetics to increase the duration or intensity of block. Epinephrine's effect on duration of block is dependent on the technique used to measure duration. A commonly used measure of block duration is the length of time it takes for the block to recede by two dermatomes from the maximum height of the block, while a second is the duration of block at some specified level, typically L1. In most studies, addition of 200 μg of epinephrine to tetracaine solutions prolongs the duration of block by both measures. However, addition of epinephrine to lidocaine or bupivacaine does not affect the first measure of duration but does prolong the block at lower levels. In different clinical situations, one or the other measure of anesthesia duration may be more relevant, and this must be kept in mind when deciding whether to add epinephrine to spinal local anesthetics.

The mechanism of action of vasoconstrictors in prolonging spinal anesthesia is uncertain. It has been hypothesized that these agents decrease spinal cord blood flow, decreasing clearance of local anesthetic from the CSF, but this has not been convincingly demonstrated. Epinephrine and other α adrenergic agonists have been shown to decrease nociceptive transmission in the spinal cord, and studies in genetically modified mice suggested that α_{2A} adrenergic receptors play a principal role in this response (Stone et al., 1997). Such actions may contribute to the beneficial effects of epinephrine, clonidine, and dexmedetomidine when these agents are added to spinal local anesthetics.

Drug Baricity and Patient Position

The baricity of the local anesthetic injected will determine the direction of migration within the dural sac. Hyperbaric solutions will tend to settle in the dependent portions of the sac, while hypobaric solutions will tend to migrate in the opposite direction. Isobaric solutions usually will stay in the vicinity where they were injected, diffusing slowly in all directions. Consideration of the patient position during and after the performance of the block and the choice of a local anesthetic of the appropriate baricity is crucial for a successful block during some surgical procedures.

Lidocaine and bupivacaine are marketed in both isobaric and hyperbaric preparations and, if desired, can be diluted with sterile, preservative-free water to make them hypobaric.

Complications

Persistent neurological deficits following spinal anesthesia are extremely rare. Thorough evaluation of a suspected deficit should be performed in collaboration with a neurologist. Neurological sequelae can be both immediate and late. Possible causes include introduction of foreign substances (such as disinfectants, ultrasound gel, or talc) into the subarachnoid space, infection, hematoma, or direct mechanical trauma. Aside from drainage of an abscess or hematoma, treatment usually is ineffective; thus, avoidance and careful attention to detail while performing spinal anesthesia are necessary.

High concentrations of local anesthetic can cause irreversible block. After administration, local anesthetic solutions are diluted rapidly, quickly reaching nontoxic concentrations. However, there are several reports of transient or longer-lasting neurological deficits following lidocaine spinal anesthesia, particularly with 5% lidocaine HCl (i.e., ~ 180 mM) in 7.5% glucose (Zaric and Pace, 2009).

Spinal anesthesia sometimes is regarded as contraindicated in patients with preexisting disease of the spinal cord. No experimental evidence exists to support this hypothesis. Nonetheless, it is prudent to avoid spinal anesthesia in patients with progressive diseases of the spinal cord. However, spinal anesthesia may be useful in patients with a fixed, chronic spinal cord injury.

A more common sequela following any lumbar puncture, including spinal anesthesia, is a postural headache with classic features. The incidence of headache decreases with increasing age of the patient and decreasing needle diameter. Headache following lumbar puncture must be thoroughly evaluated to exclude serious complications such as meningitis. Treatment usually is conservative, with bed rest and analgesics. If this approach fails, an epidural blood patch with the injection of autologous blood can be performed; this procedure is usually successful in alleviating postdural puncture headaches, although a second blood patch may be necessary. If two epidural blood patches are ineffective in relieving the headache, the diagnosis of postdural puncture headache should be reconsidered. Intravenous caffeine (500 mg as the benzoate salt administered over 4 h) also has been advocated for the treatment of postdural puncture headache; however, the efficacy of caffeine is less than that of a blood patch, and relief usually is transient.

Evaluation of Spinal Anesthesia

Spinal anesthesia is a safe and effective technique, especially during surgery involving the lower abdomen, the lower extremities, and the perineum. It often is combined with intravenous medication to provide sedation and amnesia. The physiological perturbations associated with low spinal anesthesia often have less potential harm than those associated with general anesthesia. The same does not apply for high spinal anesthesia. The sympathetic blockade that accompanies levels of spinal anesthesia adequate for mid- or upper abdominal surgery, coupled with the difficulty in achieving visceral analgesia, is such that equally satisfactory and safer operating conditions can be realized by combining the spinal anesthetic with a "light" general anesthetic or by the administration of a general anesthetic and a neuromuscular blocking agent.

Epidural Anesthesia

Epidural anesthesia is administered by injecting local anesthetic into the epidural space—the space bounded by the ligamentum flavum posteriorly, the spinal periosteum laterally, and the dura anteriorly. Epidural anesthesia can be performed in the sacral hiatus (caudal anesthesia) or in the lumbar, thoracic, or cervical regions of the spine. Its current popularity arises from the development of catheters that can be placed into the epidural space, allowing either continuous infusions or repeated bolus administration of local anesthetics. The primary site of action of epidurally administered local anesthetics is on the spinal nerve roots. However, epidurally administered local anesthetics also may act on the spinal cord and on the paravertebral nerves.

The selection of drugs available for epidural anesthesia is similar to that for major nerve blocks. As for spinal anesthesia, the choice of drugs to be used during epidural anesthesia is dictated primarily by the duration of anesthesia desired. However, when an epidural catheter is placed, short-acting drugs can be administered repeatedly, providing more control over the duration of block. Bupivacaine, 0.5%–0.75%, is used when a long duration of surgical block is desired. Due to enhanced cardiotoxicity in pregnant patients, the 0.75% solution is not approved for obstetrical use. Lower concentrations—0.25%, 0.125%, or 0.0625%—of bupivacaine, often with 2 μg/mL of fentanyl added, frequently are used to provide analgesia during labor. They also are useful preparations for providing postoperative analgesia in certain clinical situations. Lidocaine 2% is the most frequently used intermediate-acting epidural local anesthetic. Chloroprocaine, 2% or 3%, provides rapid onset and a very short duration of anesthetic action. However, its use in epidural anesthesia has been clouded by controversy regarding its potential ability to cause neurological complications if the drug is accidentally injected into the subarachnoid space (discussed previously). The addition of epinephrine frequently prolongs the duration of action and reduces the toxicity of epidurally administered local anesthetics. Addition of epinephrine also makes inadvertent intravascular injection easier to detect and modifies the effect of sympathetic blockade during epidural anesthesia.

For each anesthetic agent, a relationship exists between the volume of local anesthetic injected epidurally and the segmental level of anesthesia achieved. For example, in 20- to 40-year-old, healthy, nonpregnant patients, each 1–1.5 mL of 2% lidocaine will give an additional segment of anesthesia. The amount needed decreases with increasing age and during pregnancy and in children. The concentration of local anesthetic used determines the type of nerve fibers blocked. The highest concentrations are used when sympathetic, somatic sensory, and somatic motor blockade are required. Intermediate concentrations allow somatic sensory anesthesia without muscle relaxation. Low concentrations will block only preganglionic sympathetic fibers. As an example, with bupivacaine these effects might be achieved with concentrations of 0.5%, 0.25%, and 0.0625%, respectively. The total amounts of drug that can be injected with safety at one time are approximately those mentioned in the sections Nerve Block Anesthesia and Infiltration Anesthesia. Performance of epidural anesthesia requires a greater degree of skill than does spinal anesthesia. The technique of epidural anesthesia and the volumes, concentrations, and types of drugs used are described in detail in standard texts on regional anesthesia (Cousins et al., 2008).

A significant difference between epidural and spinal anesthesia is that the dose of local anesthetic used can produce high concentrations in blood following absorption from the epidural space. Peak concentrations of lidocaine in blood following injection of 400 mg (without epinephrine) into the lumbar epidural space average 3–4 μg/mL; peak concentrations of bupivacaine in blood average 1 μg/mL after the lumbar epidural injection of 150 mg. Addition of epinephrine (5 μg/mL) decreases peak plasma concentrations by about 25%. Peak blood concentrations are a function of the total dose of drug administered rather than the concentration or volume of solution following epidural injection (Covino and Vassallo, 1976). The risk of inadvertent intravascular injection is increased in epidural anesthesia, as the epidural space contains a rich venous plexus.

Another major difference between epidural and spinal anesthesia is that there is no zone of differential sympathetic blockade with epidural anesthesia; thus, the level of sympathetic block is close to the level of sensory block. Because epidural anesthesia does not result in the zones of differential sympathetic blockade observed during spinal anesthesia, cardiovascular responses to epidural anesthesia might be expected to be less prominent. In practice, this is not the case; the potential advantage of epidural anesthesia is offset by the cardiovascular responses to the high concentration of anesthetic in blood that occurs during epidural anesthesia. This is most apparent when epinephrine is added to the epidural injection. The resulting concentration of epinephrine in blood is sufficient to produce significant β_2 adrenergic receptor–mediated vasodilation. As a consequence, blood pressure decreases, even though cardiac output increases due to the positive inotropic and chronotropic effects of epinephrine

(Chapter 12). The result is peripheral hyperperfusion and hypotension. Differences in cardiovascular responses to equal levels of spinal and epidural anesthesia also are observed when a local anesthetic such as lidocaine is used without epinephrine. This may be a consequence of the direct effects of high concentrations of lidocaine on vascular smooth muscle and the heart. The magnitude of the differences in responses to equal sensory levels of spinal and epidural anesthesia varies, however, with the local anesthetic used for the epidural injection (assuming no epinephrine is used). For example, local anesthetics such as bupivacaine, which are highly lipid soluble, are distributed less into the circulation than are less lipid-soluble agents such as lidocaine.

High concentrations of local anesthetics in blood during epidural anesthesia are of particular concern when this technique is used to control pain during labor and delivery. Local anesthetics cross the placenta, enter the fetal circulation, and at high concentrations may cause depression of the neonate. The extent to which they do so is determined by dosage, acid-base status, level of protein binding in both maternal and fetal blood, placental blood flow, and solubility of the agent in fetal tissue. These concerns have been lessened by the trend toward using more dilute solutions of bupivacaine for labor analgesia.

Epidural and Intrathecal Opiate Analgesia

Small quantities of opioid injected intrathecally or epidurally produce segmental analgesia (Yaksh and Rudy, 1976). This observation led to the clinical use of spinal and epidural opioids during surgical procedures and for the relief of postoperative and chronic pain (Cousins and Mather, 1984). As with local anesthesia, analgesia is confined to sensory nerves that enter the spinal cord dorsal horn in the vicinity of the injection. Presynaptic opioid receptors inhibit the release of substance P and other neurotransmitters from primary afferents, while postsynaptic opioid receptors decrease the activity of certain dorsal horn neurons in the spinothalamic tracts (Willcockson et al., 1986; see also Chapters 8 and 20). Because conduction in autonomic, sensory, and motor nerves is not affected by the opioids, blood pressure, motor function, and nonnociceptive sensory perception typically are not influenced by spinal opioids. The volume-evoked micturition reflex is inhibited, as manifested by urinary retention. Other side effects include pruritus, nausea, and vomiting in susceptible individuals. Delayed respiratory depression and sedation, presumably from cephalad spread of opioid within the CSF, occur infrequently with the doses of opioids currently used.

Spinally administered opioids by themselves do not provide satisfactory anesthesia for surgical procedures. Thus, opioids have found the greatest use in the treatment of postoperative and chronic pain, providing excellent analgesia following thoracic, abdominal, pelvic, or lower extremity surgery without the side effects associated with high doses of systemically administered opioids. For postoperative analgesia, spinally administered morphine, 0.2–0.5 mg, usually will provide 8–16 h of analgesia. Placement of an epidural catheter and repeated boluses or an infusion of opioid permits an increased duration of analgesia. Morphine, 2–6 mg every 6 h, commonly is used for bolus injections, while fentanyl, 20–50 μg/h, often combined with bupivacaine at 5–20 mg/h, is used for infusions. For cancer pain, repeated doses of epidural opioids can provide analgesia of several months' duration. The dose of epidural morphine is far less than the dose of systemically administered morphine that would be required to provide similar analgesia, thus reducing the complications that usually accompany the administration of high doses of systemic opioids, particularly sedation and constipation. Unfortunately, as with systemic opioids, tolerance will develop to the analgesic effects of epidural opioids, but this usually can be managed by increasing the dose.

Drug Facts for Your Personal Formulary: *Local Anesthetics*

Drugs	Therapeutic Uses or Duration	Clinical Pharmacology and Tips
Topical Anesthesia		
Lidocaine	• Superficial anesthesia of mucous membranes	• 2%–10% solution • ~30 min duration • Maximal healthy adult dose, ~4 mg/kg
Cocaine	• Superficial anesthesia of mucous membranes of nose, mouth, ear	• 1%–4% solution • ~30 min duration • Maximal healthy adult dose, ~1–3 mg/kg (maximum 400 mg); pediatric dose, < 1 mg/kg • Vasoconstriction + anesthesia
Eutectic mixtures, oil, or cream: Lidocaine (2.5%)/prilocaine (2.5%) (EMLA) or Lidocaine (7%)/tetracaine (7%) (PLIAGIS)	• Superficial anesthesia of cutaneous structures	• Effective to ~5-mm depth • Requires 30–60 min of contact to establish effective anesthesia • Should not be used on mucous membranes or abraded skin due to rapid absorption • Consult package insert for maximum dose
Infiltration Anesthesia		
Lidocaine	• Superficial anesthesia of cutaneous structures • Addition of dilute sodium bicarbonate (10:1—lidocaine: 8.4% sodium bicarbonate, ~0.75 mg/mL sodium bicarbonate) can lessen pain on injection	• 0.5%–1.0% solution • Maximal healthy adult dose, ~4 mg/kg • Addition of epinephrine (5 μg/mL) increases duration of action and maximal safe lidocaine dose
Bupivacaine	• Superficial anesthesia of cutaneous structures	• 0.125%–0.25% solution • Maximal healthy adult dose, ~2 mg/kg • Addition of epinephrine (5 μg/mL) increases duration of action and maximal safe bupivacaine dose
Nerve Block Anesthesia • Use with epinephrine-containing test dose • Risk of intravenous injection		
Articaine	• 1 h duration	• For dental and periodontal procedures • 4% solution, typically with epinephrine • Contains both an amide and ester, so degraded in both plasma and liver

Drug Facts for Your Personal Formulary: *Local Anesthetics (continued)*

Drugs	Therapeutic Uses or Duration	Clinical Pharmacology and Tips
Nerve Block Anesthesia • Use with epinephrine-containing test dose • Risk of intravenous injection		
Lidocaine, mepivacaine	• 1–2 h duration • Addition of epinephrine prolongs duration and increases maximal safe level of drug • Identification of blocked nerves (nerve stimulation or ultrasound) may increase safety and success of block	Safe doses depend on vascularity of tissue, generally: • Lidocaine: 1%–1.5%, maximal healthy adult dose, ~4 mg/kg • Mepivacaine: 1%–2%, maximal healthy adult dose, ~7 mg/kg (maximum 400 mg)
Bupivacaine, ropivacaine	• 6-8 h duration • Longer duration of sensory block with bupivacaine than with ropivacaine • Addition of epinephrine prolongs duration and increases maximal safe level of drug	Safe doses depend on vascularity of tissue, generally: • Bupivacaine: 0.25%–0.375%, maximal healthy adult dose, ~2–3 mg/kg (maximum 400 mg) • Ropivacaine: 0.5%–0.75%, maximal healthy adult dose, ~3–4 mg/kg (maximum 200 mg) • Infusions through a catheter placed adjacent to the nerve can provide sustained analgesia • Identification of blocked nerves (nerve stimulation or ultrasound) may increase safety and success of block
Epidural Anesthesia • Use with epinephrine-containing test dose • Risk of intravenous injection • Spread of block dependent on dose and volume injected • Epidural catheter allows repeated dosing • Consider coagulation status of patient		
Chloroprocaine	• Short duration • Epinephrine prolongs action	• 2%–3% solution • Possible increased incidence of postprocedure back pain
Lidocaine	• Intermediate duration • Epinephrine prolongs action	• 2% solution • Maximal healthy adult dose, ~4 mg/kg
Bupivacaine	• Long duration	• 0.5% solution • Maximal healthy adult dose, ~2–3 mg/kg
Ropivacaine	• Long duration	• 0.5%–1.0% solution • Maximal healthy adult dose, ~2–3 mg/kg • May have less toxicity than equiefficacious dose of bupivacaine
Spinal Anesthesia • Dose and baricity of anesthetic strongly influence spread • Addition of opioids can prolong analgesia • Consider coagulation status of patient		
Lidocaine	• Short duration (60–90 min)	• ~25–50 mg for perineal and lower extremity surgery • Association of spinal lidocaine with transient neurological symptoms
Tetracaine	• Long duration (210–240 min)	• Duration increased by epinephrine • ~5 mg for perineal surgery • ~10 mg for lower extremity surgery
Bupivacaine	• Long duration (210–240 min)	• ~10 mg for perineal and lower extremity surgery • 15–20 mg for abdominal surgery

Bibliography

Arthur GR. Pharmacokinetics. In: Strichartz GR, ed. *Local Anesthetics. Handbook of Experimental Pharmacology*, vol. 81. Springer-Verlag, Berlin, **1987**, 165–186.

Butterworth J, Oxford G. Local anesthetics: a new hydrophilic pathway for drug-receptor reaction. *Anesthesiology*, **2009**, *111*:12–14.

Butterworth JF IV, Strichartz GR. Molecular mechanisms of local anesthesia: a review. *Anesthesiology*, **1990**, *72*:711–734.

Caplan RA, et al. Unexpected cardiac arrest during spinal anesthesia: a closed claims analysis of predisposing factors. *Anesthesiology*, **1988**, *68*:5–11.

Carpenter RL, Mackey DC. Local anesthetics. In: Barash PG, Cullen BF, Stoelting RK, eds. *Clinical Anesthesia*. 2nd ed. Lippincott, Philadelphia, **1992**, 509–541.

Catterall WA. From ionic currents to molecular mechanisms: the structure and function of voltage-gated sodium channels. *Neuron*, **2000**, *26*:13–25.

Charnet P, et al. An open-channel blocker interacts with adjacent turns of α-helices in the nicotinic acetylcholine receptor. *Neuron*, **1990**, *4*:87–95.

Clarkson CW, Hondeghem LM. Mechanism for bupivacaine depression of cardiac conduction: fast block of sodium channels during the action potential with slow recovery from block during diastole. *Anesthesiology*, **1985**,*62*:396–405.

Courtney KR, Strichartz GR. Structural elements which determine local anesthetic activity. In: Strichartz GR, ed. *Local Anesthetics. Handbook of Experimental Pharmacology*, vol. 81. Springer-Verlag, Berlin, **1987**, 53–94.

Cousins MJ, Bridenbaugh PO, Carr DB, Horlocker TT, eds. *Neural Blockade in Clinical Anesthesia and Management of Pain*. 4th ed. Lippincott-Raven, Philadelphia, **2008**.

Cousins MJ, Mather LE. Intrathecal and epidural administration of opioids. *Anesthesiology*, **1984**, *61*:276–310.

Covino BG. Toxicity and systemic effects of local anesthetic agents. In: Strichartz GR, ed. *Local Anesthetics. Handbook of Experimental Pharmacology*, vol. 81. Springer-Verlag, Berlin, **1987**, 187–212.

Covino BG, Vassallo HG. *Local Anesthetics: Mechanisms of Action and Clinical Use*. Grune & Stratton, New York, **1976**.

Fettiplace MR, et al. Insulin signaling in bupivacaine-induced cardiac toxicity: sensitization during recovery and potentiation by lipid emulsion. *Anesthesiology*, **2016**, *124*: 428–442.

Fink BR, Cairns AM. Differential slowing and block of conduction by lidocaine in individual afferent myelinated and unmyelinated axons. *Anesthesiology*, **1984**, *60*:111–120.

Franz DN, Perry RS. Mechanisms for differential block among single myelinated and nonmyelinated axons by procaine. *J Physiol*, **1974**, *236*:193–210.

Garfield JM, Gugino L. Central effects of local anesthetics. In: Strichartz GR, ed. *Local Anesthetics. Handbook of Experimental Pharmacology*, vol. 81. Springer-Verlag, Berlin, **1987**, 253–284.

Gasser HS, Erlanger J. The role of fiber size in the establishment of a nerve block by pressure or cocaine. *Am J Physiol*, **1929**, *88*:581–591.

Gintant GA, Hoffman BF. The role of local anesthetic effects in the actions of antiarrhythmic drugs. In: Strichartz GR, ed. *Local Anesthetics. Handbook of Experimental Pharmacology*, vol. 81. Springer-Verlag, Berlin, **1987**, 213–251.

Greene NM. Uptake and elimination of local anesthetics during spinal anesthesia. *Anesth Analg*, **1983**, *62*:1013–1024.

Hille B. Local anesthetics: hydrophilic and hydrophobic pathways for the drug-receptor reaction. *J Gen Physiol*, **1977**, *69*:497–515.

Huang JH, et al. Susceptibility to lidocaine of impulses in different somatosensory fibers of rat sciatic nerve. *J Pharmacol Exp Ther*, **1997**, *292*:802–11.

Lozinski A, Huq NS. Tumescent liposuction. *Clin Plast Surg*, **2013**, *40*:593–613.

McClure JH. Ropivacaine. *Br J Anaesth*, **1996**, *76*:300–307.

Narahashi T, Frazier DT. Site of action and active form of local anesthetics. *Neurosci Res (NY)*, **1971**, *4*:65–99.

Neher E, Steinbach JH. Local anesthetics transiently block currents through single acetylcholine-receptor channels. *J Physiol*, **1978**, *277*:153–176.

Payandeh J, et al. The crystal structure of a voltage-gated sodium channel. *Nature*, **2011**, *475*:353–358.

Payandeh J, et al. Crystal structure of a voltage-gated sodium channel in two potentially inactivated states. *Nature*, **2012**, *486*:135–139.

Ragsdale DR, et al. Molecular determinants of state-dependent block of Na^+ channels by local anesthetics. *Science*, **1994**, *265*:1724–1728.

Raymond SA, Gissen AJ. Mechanism of differential nerve block. In: Strichartz GR, ed. *Local Anesthetics. Handbook of Experimental Pharmacology*, vol. 81. Springer-Verlag, Berlin, **1987**, 95–164.

Ritchie JM, Greengard P. On the mode of action of local anesthetics. *Annu Rev Pharmacol*, **1966**, *6*:405–430.

Sakai R, Swanson GT. Recent progress in neuroactive marine natural products. *Nat Prod Rep*, **2014**, *31*:273–309.

Stevens RA, et al. Back pain after epidural anesthesia with chloroprocaine. *Anesthesiology*, **1993**, *78*:492–497.

Stommel EW, Watters MR. Marine neurotoxins: ingestible toxins. *Curr Treat Options Neurol*, **2004**, *6*:105–114.

Stone LS, et al. The α_{2a} adrenergic receptor subtype mediates spinal analgesia evoked by α_2 agonists and is necessary for spinal adrenergic-opioid synergy. *J Neurosci*, **1997**, *17*:7157–7165.

Strichartz GR, Ritchie JM. The action of local anesthetics on ion channels of excitable tissues. In: Strichartz GR, ed. *Local Anesthetics. Handbook of Experimental Pharmacology*, vol. 81. Springer-Verlag, Berlin, **1987**, 21–53.

Terlau H, et al. Mapping the site of block by tetrodotoxin and saxitoxin of sodium channel II. *FEBS Lett*, **1991**, *293*:93–96.

Thomas RD, et al. Cardiovascular toxicity of local anesthetics: an alternative hypothesis. *Anesth Analg*, **1986**, *65*:444–450.

Uskova A, O'Connor JE. Liposomal bupivacaine for regional anesthesia. *Curr Opin Anaesthesiol*, **2015**, *28*:593–597.

Weinberg GL. Lipid emulsion infusion: resuscitation for local anesthetic and other drug overdose. *Anesthesiology*, **2012**, *117*:180–187.

Willcockson WS, et al. Actions of opioid on primate spinothalamic tract neurons. *J Neurosci*, **1986**, *6*:2509–2520.

Yaksh TL, Rudy TA. Analgesia mediated by a direct spinal action of narcotics. *Science*, **1976**, *192*:1357–1358.

Yarov-Yarovoy V, et al. Role of amino acid residues in transmembrane segments IS6 and IIS6 of the sodium channel α subunit in voltage-dependent gating and drug block. *J Biol Chem*, **2002**, *277*: 35393–35401.

Yu F, et al. Overview of molecular relationships in the voltage-gated ion channel super-family. *Pharmacol Rev*, **2005**, *57*:387–395.

Zaric D, Pace NL. Transient neurological symptoms (TNS) following spinal anesthesia with lidocaine versus other local anesthetics. *Cochrane Database Syst Rev*, **2009**, *2*:CD003006.

Zipf HF, Dittmann EC. General pharmacological effects of local anesthetics. In: Lechat P, ed. *Local Anesthetics*, vol. 1. *International Encyclopedia of Pharmacology and Therapeutics*, Sect. 8. Pergamon Press, Oxford, UK, **1971**, 191–238.

Ethanol

S. John Mihic, George F. Koob, Jody Mayfield, and R. Adron Harris

第二十三章　醇

中文导读

本章主要介绍：人类对酒精的消耗，包括简史和观点；乙醇的消耗；乙醇和甲醇的药理性质；乙醇对生理系统的影响，包括莎士比亚的智慧、中枢神经系统、神经内分泌系统、性功能、骨骼、体温、利尿和心血管系统；卒中，包括肺、骨骼肌、胃肠道与消化系统、癌症、血液学与免疫学影响，神经免疫机制；致畸作用——胎儿酒精谱系障碍；乙醇的临床用途；药物相互作用；酒精使用障碍与其他疾病的共病现象，包括精神疾病和创伤后应激障碍；酒精使用障碍、遗传学与遗传药理学；酒精使用障碍的药物治疗，包括双硫仑、纳曲酮、阿坎酸和其他药物。

Abbreviations

ACh: acetylcholine
ADH: alcohol dehydrogenase
ALDH: aldehyde dehydrogenase
ARBD: alcohol-related birth defect
ARND: alcohol-related neurodevelopmental disorder
AUD: alcohol use disorder
BEC: blood ethanol concentration
CHD: coronary heart disease
CYP: cytochrome P450
FAS: fetal alcohol syndrome
FASD: fetal alcohol spectrum disorder
GABA: γ-aminobutyric acid
HDL: high-density lipoprotein
5HT: serotonin
IHD: ischemic heart disease
LDL: low-density lipoprotein
LPS: lipopolysaccharide
nAChR: nicotinic acetylcholine receptor
NF-κB: nuclear factor kappa B
NMDA: *N*-methyl-D-aspartate
PTSD: post-traumatic stress disorder
SNP: single nucleotide polymorphism
SSRI: selective serotonin reuptake inhibitor
TLR: toll-like receptor

Ethanol (CH_3CH_2OH), or beverage alcohol, is a two-carbon alcohol that directly affects many different types of neurochemical systems and signaling cascades and has rewarding and addictive properties. It is the oldest recreational drug and likely contributes to more morbidity, mortality, and public health costs than all illicit drugs combined. The current *Diagnostic and Statistical Manual of Mental Disorders* (*DSM-5*) integrates alcohol abuse and alcohol dependence into a single disorder called *alcohol use disorder* (AUD), with mild, moderate, and severe subclassifications (American Psychiatric Association, 2013). This chapter presents an overview of the effects of ethanol on various physiological systems, then focuses on the mechanisms of ethanol's effects in the CNS as the basis for understanding the rewards, disease processes, and treatments for ethanol-related conditions.

Human Consumption of Ethanol: A Brief History and Perspective

The use of alcoholic beverages has been documented as far back as 10,000 BC. By about 3000 BC, the Greeks, Romans, and inhabitants of Babylon were incorporating ethanol into religious festivals, while also using it for pleasure and in medicinal practice. Over the last 2000 years, alcoholic beverages have been identified in most cultures, including pre-Columbian America about AD 200 and the Islamic world in the 8th century.

The dangers of heavy consumption of alcohol have long been recognized by almost all cultures, with most stressing the importance of moderation; yet, problems with ethanol are as ancient as the use of this beverage itself. The increase in ethanol consumption in the 1800s, along with industrialization and the need for a more dependable work force, contributed to the development of more widespread organized efforts to discourage drunkenness, including a constitutional ban on the sale of alcoholic beverages in the U.S. from 1920 to 1933.

Today, AUD is one of the most prevalent psychiatric disorders worldwide. In the U.S. among adults 18 years and older, AUD is associated with other substance use and psychiatric disorders; despite its prevalence and comorbidity, AUD often goes untreated (Grant et al., 2015). The highest quantities of ethanol intake per occasion are usually observed in the late teens to early 20s (CDC, 2012). Older adults drink more often but consume fewer total drinks each month (White et al., 2015). In the U.S., the per capita consumption of all alcoholic beverages for persons aged 14 and older is equivalent to 2.3 gallons (8.7 L) of absolute alcohol per year (NIAAA, 2015). Among drinkers, as many as half have experienced an alcohol-related problem, such as missing school or work, alcohol-related amnesia (blackouts), or operating a motor vehicle after consuming alcohol (Schuckit, 2009). Roughly one-third of men (36%) and one-quarter of women (23%) meet criteria for a mild, moderate, or severe AUD in their lifetimes (Grant et al, 2015). The CDC estimated that annually in the U.S. the excessive consumption of ethanol contributes to 10% of deaths of working adults 20–64 years old and to one-third of fatal traffic accidents and cost $249 billion in 2010 (CDC, 2014).

Ethanol Consumption

Compared with other drugs, surprisingly large amounts of ethanol are required for physiological effects. Ethanol is consumed in gram quantities. In contrast, most other drugs with affinities for specific proteins are taken in milligram or microgram doses. The alcohol content of beverages typically ranges from 4% to 6% (volume/volume) for beer, 10% to 15% for wine, and 40% and higher for distilled spirits (the proof of an alcoholic beverage is twice its percentage of alcohol; e.g., 40% alcohol is 80 proof). A 12-oz bottle of beer (355 mL), a 5-oz glass of wine (148 mL), and a 1.5-oz "shot" of 40% liquor (44 mL) each contain about 14 g ethanol (the density of ethanol is 0.79 g/mL at 25°C), and constitute what is defined as a "standard drink" in the U.S.

Because the ratio of ethanol in end-expiratory alveolar air and blood is relatively consistent, BECs in humans are readily estimated by the measurement of ethanol levels in expired air; the partition coefficient for ethanol between blood and alveolar air is about 2100:1. The legally allowed BEC for operating a motor vehicle is 80 mg% (80 mg ethanol per 100 mL blood; 0.08% w/v) in the United States, which is equivalent to a concentration of 17 mM ethanol in blood. The consumption of one standard drink (a 12-oz bottle of beer, a 5-oz glass of wine, or a 1.5-oz shot of 40% liquor) by a 70-kg person would produce a BEC of about 30 mg%. However, it is important to note that this is an estimation because the BEC is determined by several factors, including the rate of drinking, gender, body weight and water percentage, as well as the rates of metabolism and stomach emptying (see Acute Ethanol Intoxication further in the chapter).

Pharmacological Properties of Ethanol and Methanol

Ethanol

Absorption and Gastric Metabolism

After oral administration, ethanol is absorbed rapidly into the bloodstream from the stomach and small intestine and distributes into total body water (~0.65 L/kg body weight). Due to high surface area, absorption occurs more rapidly from the small intestine than from the stomach; delays in gastric emptying (e.g., due to the presence of food) slow ethanol absorption. Peak blood levels occur about 30 min after ingestion of ethanol when the stomach is empty. Because of first-pass metabolism by gastric and liver ADH, oral ingestion of ethanol leads to lower BECs than would be obtained if the same dose were administered intravenously. The rate of gastric metabolism of ethanol is lower in women than in men (Schuckit, 2006). Other factors also affect absorption and metabolism; for example, aspirin (1 g) inhibits gastric ADH and increases the bioavailability of ethanol in men.

Liver Metabolism

Only small amounts of ethanol are excreted in urine, sweat, and breath. The main enzymes involved in ethanol metabolism are ADH and ALDH, followed by catalase and CYP2E1. CYPs 1A2 and 3A4 may also participate. Ethanol is metabolized primarily by sequential hepatic oxidation, first to acetaldehyde by ADH and then to acetic acid by ALDH (Figure 23–1). Each metabolic step requires NAD^+; thus, oxidation of 1 mol ethanol (46 g) to 1 mol acetic acid requires 2 mol NAD^+ (approximately 1.3 kg). This greatly exceeds the supply of NAD^+ in the liver; thus, the bioavailability of NAD^+ limits ethanol metabolism to about 8 g/h (10 mL/h, 170 mmol/h) in a 70-kg adult. Ethanol metabolism proceeds via zero-order kinetics at BECs greater than 10 mg% and by first-order kinetics at BECs less than 10 mg%.

In addition to limiting the rate of ethanol metabolism, the large increase in the hepatic NADH:NAD^+ ratio resulting from ethanol oxidation has profound consequences. The function of NAD^+-requiring enzymes is impaired, resulting in accumulation of lactate, reduced activity of the tricarboxylic acid cycle, and accumulation of acetyl-CoA (which is produced from ethanol-derived acetic acid; Figure 23–1). The combination of increased NADH and elevated acetyl-CoA supports fatty acid synthesis and the storage and accumulation of triacylglycerides; ketone bodies then accrue, exacerbating lactic acidosis.

Although ADH is responsible for the majority of ethanol metabolism, CYP2E1 accounts for about 10%. This constituent of the microsomal ethanol-oxidizing system can be altered by acute or chronic ethanol consumption. Competition between ethanol and other drugs (e.g., phenytoin and warfarin) that are metabolized by CYP2E1 is observed after acute consumption of ethanol. CYP2E1 is also induced by chronic consumption of ethanol, resulting in increased clearance of its substrates and increased susceptibility to certain toxins (e.g., CCl_4, which CYP2E1 metabolizes and thereby activates to the highly reactive trichloromethyl radical). Ethanol metabolism by the CYP2E1 pathway elevates $NADP^+$ and limits the availability of NADPH for the regeneration of reduced glutathione, thereby enhancing oxidative stress.

The mechanisms underlying hepatic disease resulting from heavy ethanol use probably reflect a complex combination of these metabolic factors, CYP2E1 induction (and enhanced activation of toxins and production of H_2O_2 and oxygen radicals), and possibly enhanced release of endotoxin as a consequence of ethanol's effect on gram-negative flora in the GI tract. The often-poor nutritional status of alcoholics (malabsorption and lack of vitamins A and D and thiamine), suppression of immune function, and a variety of other generalized effects likely compound the more direct adverse effects of excessive ethanol consumption. An overview of ethanol metabolism and how it can lead to tissue injury is found in the work of Molina et al. (2014).

Genetic Variation in Ethanol Metabolism

Genetic variations in metabolic enzymes for ethanol can alter its metabolism and susceptibility to its effects, thus influencing the risk for developing AUD and other pathology. Linkage analyses indicated that genes clustered in the *ADH* region affect risk for alcohol dependence (Edenberg et al., 2006). SNPs across the *ADH* region show strong evidence of association in and around the *ADH4* gene. In addition, a SNP in the *ADH1B* gene (*ADH1B*2*) is found in high frequencies in East Asians that may protect against AUD. This genetic variation produces faster metabolism of ethanol and a transient higher blood level of acetaldehyde, which are associated with a lower risk for heavy drinking and other ethanol-related problems, but a higher risk for esophageal cancer if one drinks. The *ALDH2*2* polymorphism (see discussion that follows) also leads to an increased incidence of esophageal cancer in those who consume alcohol. Another polymorphism (*ADH1B*3*) is protective in African Americans and is associated with lower risk of heavy drinking and ethanol-related problems.

Polymorphisms in the *ALDH2* gene are implicated in the development of AUD (Chen et al., 2014). ALDH2 is the most efficient ALDH isozyme in humans for the metabolism of ethanol-derived acetaldehyde. Low

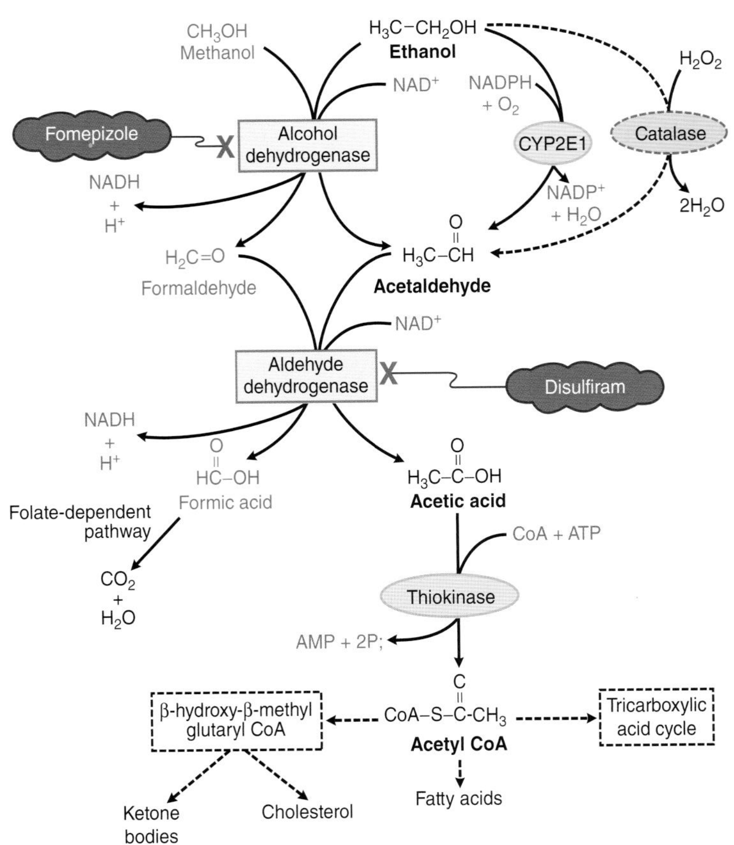

Figure 23–1 *Metabolism of ethanol and methanol.*

levels of acetaldehyde are rewarding and stimulating, while high blood levels produce adverse reactions such as vomiting, diarrhea, and unstable blood pressure; thus, genetic variation in ALDH activity could affect the rewarding or aversive properties of ethanol. A mutation in the *ALDH2* gene (*ALDH2**2*) produces an enzyme that is incapable of metabolizing ethanol. Approximately 10% of Asians are homozygous for *ALDH2**2* and develop severe adverse reactions after the consumption of one drink or less. Similar adverse reactions occur if ethanol is consumed with the ALDH inhibitor disulfiram. Approximately 30%–40% of Asians are heterozygous for *ALDH2**2*, and these individuals experience facial flushing and enhanced sensitivity to alcohol but do not necessarily report an overall adverse response to the drug. Thus, several polymorphisms may decrease an individual's risk for developing AUD and other diseases that may be related to the toxic effects of aldehydes. The section Alcohol Use Disorder, Genetics, and Pharmacogenetics provides additional evidence for genetic determinants in AUD.

Methanol

Methanol (CH_3OH), also known as methyl or wood alcohol, is an important industrial reagent and solvent found in products such as paint removers, shellac, and antifreeze. Methanol is added to industrial use ethanol to make it unsafe for human consumption. Ingestion of as little as 10 mg of methanol produces toxicity ranging from blindness to death. The toxic effects of methanol take about 12 or more hours to manifest themselves and are dependent on methanol metabolism to formaldehyde and formic acid (Figure 23–1). Methanol poisoning consists of headache, GI distress, and pain (partially related to pancreatic necrosis), difficulty breathing, restlessness, and blurred vision. The visual disturbances occur from injury to ganglion cells of the retina and the optic nerve by formic acid, which produces inflammation, atrophy, and potential bilateral blindness. Severe metabolic acidosis can develop due to the accumulation of formic acid, and respiratory depression may be severe, resulting in coma or death.

ADME and Treatment of Poisoning

Methanol is rapidly absorbed via oral administration, inhalation, and through the skin, with the last two routes most relevant in industrial settings. Absorption of methanol taken orally typically occurs within 30–60 min. Methanol is metabolized by ADH to formaldehyde, which is then metabolized to formic acid by ALDH. Competition between methanol and ethanol for ADH is the basis for using ethanol to treat methanol poisoning because ethanol slows the rate of formic acid production, lessening the toxicity associated with accidental methanol consumption.

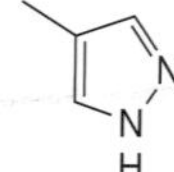

FOMEPIZOLE

Fomepizole (4-methylpyrazole), an ADH inhibitor (Figure 23–1), is also used to treat methanol or ethylene glycol poisoning, applied either alone or in combination with hemodialysis. Plasma levels of 0.8 mg/L are effective in inhibiting ADH. Fomepizole should not be used with ethanol because it prolongs the half-life of ethanol. Treatment of methanol poisoning also consists of treating patients with sodium bicarbonate to combat acidosis.

Effects of Ethanol on Physiological Systems

The Wisdom of Shakespeare

William Shakespeare described the acute pharmacological effects of imbibing ethanol in the Porter scene (act 2, scene 3) of *Macbeth*. The Porter, awakened from an alcohol-induced sleep by Macduff, explains three effects of alcohol and then wrestles with a fourth effect that combines the contradictory aspects of soaring overconfidence with physical impairment:

> **Porter:** … and drink, sir, is a great provoker of three things.
>
> **Macduff:** What three things does drink especially provoke?
>
> **Porter:** Marry, sir, nose-painting [*cutaneous vasodilation*], sleep [*CNS depression*], and urine [*a consequence of the inhibition of antidiuretic hormone (vasopressin) secretion, exacerbated by volume loading*]. Lechery, sir, it provokes and unprovokes: it provokes the desire but it takes away the performance. Therefore much drink may be said to be an equivocator with lechery: it makes him and it mars him; it sets him on and it takes him off; it persuades him and disheartens him, makes him stand to and not stand to [the imagination desires what the corpus cavernosum cannot deliver]; in conclusion, equivocates him in a sleep, and, giving him the lie, leaves him.

More recent research has added details to Shakespeare's enumeration—see the bracketed additions to the Porter's words in the preceding paragraph and the following sections on organ systems—but the most noticeable consequences of the recreational use of ethanol still are well summarized by the gregarious and garrulous Porter, whose delighted and devilish demeanor demonstrates a frequently observed influence of modest concentrations of ethanol on the CNS. The sections that follow detail ethanol's effects on physiological systems.

CNS

Ethanol is primarily a CNS depressant. Ingestion of moderate amounts of ethanol, like that of other sedative/hypnotics such as barbiturates and benzodiazepines, can have anxiolytic actions and produce behavioral disinhibition. Individual signs of intoxication vary from expansive and vivacious effects to uncontrolled mood swings and emotional outbursts that may have violent components. With more severe intoxication, CNS function becomes progressively more impaired, ultimately to the point of general anesthesia. Due to respiratory depression, there is little margin between the concentrations yielding the anesthetic and lethal effects of ethanol.

Acute Ethanol Intoxication

Many factors influence the BEC, including body weight, body composition, and the rate of absorption from the GI tract. In women with smaller body size and a lower body water percentage and, consequently, a lower volume of distribution for ethanol, BECs may be about 30%–50% higher than in men for the same quantity consumed.

Signs of intoxication typical of CNS depression are observed in most people after two or three drinks, with the most prominent effects seen at times of peak BEC, about 30–60 min following consumption on an empty stomach. These symptoms include an initial stimulatory effect (perhaps due to inhibition of CNS inhibitory systems), giddiness, muscle relaxation, and impaired judgment. Higher blood levels (~80 mg/dL or ~17 mM) are associated with slurred speech, incoordination, unsteady gait, and impaired attention; levels between 80 and 200 mg/dL are associated with more intense mood lability and greater cognitive deficits, potentially accompanied by aggressiveness, and anterograde amnesia (an "alcoholic blackout," i.e., loss of memory of events that transpired while intoxicated). BECs greater than 200 mg/dL can produce nystagmus and sedation, while levels of 300 mg/dL and higher produce failing vital signs, coma, and death. All of these symptoms are likely to be exacerbated and occur at a lower BEC if ethanol is taken along with other CNS depressants (e.g., benzodiazepines or barbiturates) or with any drug or medication that promotes sedation and incoordination (e.g., antihistamines).

The treatment of acute ethanol intoxication is based on the severity of respiratory and CNS depression. If respiratory depression is not severe, careful observation is the primary treatment. Patients with evidence of respiratory depression should be intubated to protect the airway and to provide ventilatory assistance; stomach lavage can also be considered if absorption is not yet complete. Because it is freely miscible with water, ethanol can be removed from the blood by hemodialysis. The usual protocol involves observing the patient in the emergency room for 4–6 h while the ingested ethanol is metabolized. The symptoms associated with diabetic coma, drug intoxication, cardiovascular accidents, and skull fractures are similar and may be confused with profound alcohol intoxication. Testing for breath odor in a case of suspected intoxication can be misleading because there can be other causes of breath odor similar to that of alcohol (e.g., diabetic ketoacidosis or other metabolic acidosis). Determining blood ethanol levels is necessary to confirm the absence or presence of alcohol intoxication, and diabetes or other underlying conditions should also be considered in patients with positive BECs.

Putative Mechanisms of Ethanol Action in the CNS

Ethanol produces distinct neuroadaptations that depend on acute versus chronic exposure. Ethanol perturbs the balance between excitatory and inhibitory transmission in the brain by either enhancing inhibitory or antagonizing excitatory neurotransmission (Table 23–1). The exact molecular sites responsible for ethanol action in vivo have yet to be resolved, although many ion channels have been implicated, including the ligand-gated NMDA and $GABA_A$ receptor-operated channels, as well as the large conductance Ca^+- and voltage-activated K^+ channel.

Advances in X-ray crystal structures of open and closed states of ion channels combined with structural modeling and site-directed mutagenesis have elucidated selective binding pockets for ethanol in different channel proteins (Howard et al., 2014; Trudell et al., 2014). Ethanol also alters ion channel function indirectly via receptor phosphorylation and trafficking mechanisms (Trudell et al., 2014). Mutant mouse models and genetic association studies in animals and humans further demonstrate a role for ligand-gated ion channels in alcohol dependence. To define the key sites of ethanol action, a combination of functional, structural, behavioral, and genomic approaches will be required.

Addiction, Tolerance, and Dependence

Alcohol use disorder is the chronically relapsing and compulsive use of alcohol, comprising three interacting stages that progressively worsen over time: binge-intoxication, withdrawal-negative affect, and preoccupation-anticipation ("craving"). The neurocircuitry of the basal ganglia is thought to mediate the neurobiological basis of the binge-intoxication stage, including the facilitation of incentive salience, a form of motivational salience associated with reward. The basal ganglia are associated with key functions, including voluntary motor control and procedural learning related to routine behaviors or habits. Release of dopamine and opioid peptides in the ventral striatum (nucleus accumbens) is associated with the reinforcing actions of alcohol (Volkow et al., 2007). Endocannabinoid signaling may also contribute to the motivational and reinforcing properties of ethanol, and ethanol drinking alters endocannabinoid levels and cannabinoid receptor 1 expression in brain nuclei associated with addiction pathways (Pava and Woodward, 2012). Alcohol use facilitates incentive salience by imparting motivational properties to previously neutral stimuli. Activation of the ventral striatum leads to recruitment of basal ganglia–globus pallidus–thalamic–cortical loops that engage the dorsal striatum habit formation, hypothesized to be the beginning of compulsive-like responding for drugs.

Tolerance rapidly develops to the rewarding effects of alcohol and is defined as a reduced behavioral or physiological response to the same dose of drug, or the requirement of a higher dose to obtain the same effect (see Chapter 24). The major forms of tolerance are *acute* and *chronic*. Acute functional tolerance, also known as the Mellanby effect, occurs within hours of alcohol administration and is due to CNS adaptations to its effects. This is demonstrated by comparing behavioral impairment at the same BECs on the ascending limb of the absorption phase of the BEC–time curve and on the descending limb of the curve, as metabolism reduces the BEC. Behavioral impairment and subjective feelings of intoxication are much greater at a given BEC on the ascending than on the descending limb. Chronic tolerance also develops in the long-term heavy drinker. In contrast to acute tolerance, chronic tolerance has both pharmacodynamic and pharmacokinetic elements, the latter due to induction of alcohol-metabolizing enzymes. In general, the maximum pharmacokinetic tolerance attained would be a doubling of the normal metabolic rate.

Dependence is defined by a withdrawal syndrome observed several hours to days after alcohol consumption is terminated. The symptoms and severity are determined by the amount and duration of drinking and include major motivational changes, sleep disruption, autonomic nervous system (sympathetic) activation, tremors, and, in severe cases, seizures. In addition, two or more days after withdrawal, some individuals experience *delirium tremens*, characterized by hallucinations, delirium, tachycardia, and a potentially fatal fever. Individuals with AUD also show evidence of negative emotional states during acute withdrawal that persist into protracted abstinence; such states include symptoms related to anxiety, dysphoria, and depression. Persistent depression/anxiety-like symptoms may be relevant in the treatment considerations for AUD.

Two processes are thought to form the neurobiological basis for the withdrawal–negative affect stage: a decrease in functioning in reward systems in the ventral striatum and recruitment of the stress systems in the extended amygdala. As dependence develops, brain stress systems, involving corticotropin-releasing factor, norepinephrine, and dynorphin, are recruited (Koob, 2014), producing a powerful motivation for reengaging in drug seeking.

The preoccupation-anticipation ("craving") stage involves dysregulation of prefrontal cortex circuits, causing loss of executive control. The completion of complex tasks in the AUD brain may involve two opposing systems. A "go" system, consisting of the anterior cingulate cortex and dorsolateral prefrontal cortex, engages habits via the basal ganglia, while the "stop" system, consisting of the ventrolateral prefrontal cortex and orbitofrontal cortex, inhibits the basal ganglia incentive salience system and the extended amygdala stress system (Koob, 2015). Individuals with AUD present with impairments in decision-making, spatial information, and behavioral inhibition, all of which drive craving. Craving can be divided into "reward" craving (drug seeking induced by drugs or stimuli linked to drugs) and "relief" craving (drug seeking induced by an acute stressor or a state of stress) (Heinz et al., 2003). Thus, deficits in prefrontal cortical control of basal ganglia and extended amygdala function may represent a key mechanism to explain individual differences in the predisposition to and perpetuation of addiction. Residual dysregulation of the neurocircuits mediating incentive salience and stress responsivity help perpetuate compulsive drug taking and relapse.

TABLE 23–1 ■ ETHANOL TARGETS ION CHANNELS

LIGAND- AND VOLTAGE-GATED ION CHANNELS	EFFECTS OF ACUTE ETHANOL
$GABA_A$ receptor-operated channels	Enhancement
Glycine receptor-operated channels	Enhancement
NMDA receptor-operated channels	Inhibition
Nicotinic ACh receptor-operated channels	Enhancement
$5HT_3$ receptor-operated channels	Enhancement
G protein–coupled inwardly rectifying K^+ channels	Enhancement
Voltage-gated Ca^{2+} channels	Inhibition
Large conductance, Ca^{2+}/voltage-activated K^+ channels (BK, slo1-containing subunits)	Enhancement

These ligand- and voltage-activated ion channels can be modulated by 50 mM ethanol or less. The enhancement or inhibition of channel function recorded here represents an overall consensus of the acute ethanol effects observed in multiple studies. Results depend on ethanol concentration, time of exposure, channel subunit composition, brain region, cell type, posttranslational modifications, and other factors.

Consequences of Ethanol Consumption on CNS Function

The transient CNS effects of heavy ethanol consumption that produce a "hangover"—the next-morning syndrome of headache, thirst, nausea, and cognitive impairment—may reflect mechanisms associated with ethanol withdrawal, dehydration, or mild acidosis. Insomnia is a common and persistent problem in AUD, even after weeks of abstinence (Brower, 2015). Insomnia should be treated because it may be a factor contributing to relapse. Ethanol affects respiration and muscle relaxation, and heavy drinking can produce sleep apnea, especially in older alcohol-dependent subjects.

Alcohol use disorder causes shrinkage of the brain due to loss of both white and gray matter, and chronic heavy drinking increases the risk of developing *alcoholic dementia*. The cognitive deficits and brain atrophy observed soon after a heavy drinking period partially reverse over the subsequent weeks to months following abstinence. Furthermore, alcohol abuse reduces overall brain metabolism, which reverses during detoxification. The magnitude of the hypometabolic state is determined by the number of years of use and the patient's age.

Wernicke-Korsakoff syndrome consists of two neuropsychiatric disorders: Wernicke encephalopathy, which is largely reversible, and Korsakoff psychosis, which is generally not reversible. These syndromes are now considered a unitary disorder called *Wernicke-Korsakoff syndrome* that occurs subsequent to inadequate intake of thiamine, likely due to the poor dietary habits of patients with AUD. Thiamine deficiency, alone, can lead to Wernicke-Korsakoff syndrome (Scalzo et al., 2015).

Wernicke encephalopathy is characterized by a confusional state, ataxia, abnormal eye movements, blurred vision, double vision, nystagmus, and tremor. It is associated with a prolonged history of heavy drinking and an inadequate nutritional state. The neurological syndrome (ataxia, opthalmoplegia, and nystagmus) can be reversed in its early stages by high doses of thiamine, but the learning and memory impairments respond more slowly and incompletely. Untreated Wernicke encephalopathy leads to death in up to 20% of cases, and 85% of those who survive the encephalopathy go on to develop Korsakoff psychosis, characterized by severe anterograde and retrograde amnesia (Thomson et al., 2012) that is largely irreversible. Wernicke-Korsakoff syndrome is a medical emergency, and early treatment with intravenous thiamine (followed by oral maintenance treatment) is essential to reverse the Wernicke symptoms and prevent progression or reduce the severity of the Korsakoff state.

Neuroendocrine System

Both acute and chronic ethanol exposure alter endocrine regulation via the hypothalamo-pituitary-adrenal, hypothalamo-pituitary-gonadal, and hypothalamo-pituitary-thyroid axes (Molina et al., 2014). Some of the resulting endocrine-related disorders include hypothyroidism, growth retardation, diabetes, as well as hypogonadism and abnormal sexual function, discussed in the next section. Overall, alcohol abuse contributes to an impaired ability to respond to psychological and physical stressors and to maintain homeostasis.

Sexual Function

Many drugs of abuse, including ethanol, have disinhibiting effects that may initially increase libido. Despite the notion that ethanol enhances sexual function, the opposite effect generally prevails, as Shakespeare's Porter noted. Both acute and chronic ethanol use can lead to impotence in men. Increased BECs lead to decreased sexual arousal, increased ejaculatory latency, and decreased orgasmic pleasure. The incidence of sexual dysfunction may be as high as 70% in those with AUD. In addition, testicular atrophy and decreased fertility may occur. Many females with AUD complain of decreased libido, decreased vaginal lubrication, and menstrual cycle abnormalities. Their ovaries often are small and without follicular development; some data suggest that fertility rates are lower in women with AUD. Gynecomastia is associated with alcoholic liver disease and is related to an increased estrogen-to-testosterone ratio. Altered levels of reproductive hormones also affect bone metabolism.

Bone

Ethanol interferes with Ca^{2+} and bone metabolism by several processes. Acute ethanol exposure transiently decreases parathyroid hormone, resulting in increased loss of calcium. Chronic ethanol intake can disturb vitamin D metabolism and decrease Ca^{2+} absorption. Ethanol is also directly toxic to bone-forming cells and inhibits their activity. AUD is associated with decreased bone mineral density and mass and increased prevalence of osteoporosis, leading to increased risk of fractures. Anabolic hormones, particularly testosterone, are important in regulating bone remodeling and bone mass. The impaired hypothalamo-pituitary-gonadal axis and decreased testosterone levels observed in AUD further contribute to compromised bone health (Molina et al., 2014).

Body Temperature

Ingestion of ethanol causes a feeling of warmth due to enhanced cutaneous vasodilatation. Heat is transferred from the body core to the periphery and the core temperature falls due to an effect of ethanol on the central temperature-regulating mechanism in the hypothalamus. Intake of high ethanol doses may lead to pronounced decreases in body temperature, especially in cold ambient temperatures. Alcohol is a major risk factor contributing to deaths from hypothermia.

Diuresis

Ethanol inhibits the release of vasopressin (antidiuretic hormone) from the posterior pituitary gland, resulting in enhanced diuresis. Alcohol-dependent individuals in withdrawal exhibit increased vasopressin release and a consequential retention of water, as well as dilutional hyponatremia.

Cardiovascular System

There is a complex J-shaped relationship between ethanol consumption and heart disease, a leading cause of death and disability. In general, light-to-moderate ethanol intake decreases risks for coronary artery disease, congestive heart failure, and stroke, whereas high intake increases cardiovascular risk (O'Keefe et al., 2014). Epidemiological studies suggested that gender, ethanol consumption, and drinking patterns affect the association risk for IHD. AUD elevates the risk for IHD, but there is a beneficial association with IHD risk in people who consume less than 30 g per day without episodes of heavy drinking (Roerecke and Rehm, 2014). However, ethanol consumption recommendations from clinicians should remain guarded when judging the overall risk-benefit relationship given the wide range of effects and potential for other ethanol-related problems, presence of other disease states, and the lack of randomized controlled trials on ethanol's long-term effects. The risk-to-benefit ratio of drinking is also higher in younger individuals.

Serum Lipoproteins and Cardiovascular Effects

Epidemiological studies suggest that wine consumption (20–30 g ethanol per day) may confer a cardioprotective effect, resulting in decreased risk of CHD compared with abstainers. In contrast, daily consumption of greater amounts of ethanol leads to an increased incidence of arrhythmias, cardiomyopathy, and hemorrhagic stroke (Movva and Figueredo, 2013).

One possible mechanism by which ethanol could reduce the risk of CHD is through its effects on blood lipids. Changes in plasma lipoprotein levels, particularly increases in HDL (see Chapter 33), are linked with the protective effects of ethanol. HDL binds cholesterol and returns it to the liver for elimination or reprocessing, decreasing tissue cholesterol accumulation. Ethanol-induced increases in HDL cholesterol could thus decrease cholesterol accumulation in arterial walls, lessening the risk of infarction. HDL is found as two subfractions, HDL2 and HDL3. Increased levels of HDL2 (and possibly HDL3) are associated with reduced risk of myocardial infarction. Levels of both subfractions increase following ethanol consumption and decrease when consumption ceases. In addition to the antiatherogenic effects of low doses of ethanol, the flavonoids found in red wine (and purple grape juice) may play an additional role by protecting LDL from oxidative damage.

Hypertension

Heavy alcohol use can raise diastolic and systolic blood pressure. Consumption of 30 g of ethanol per day is associated with elevations in diastolic-systolic blood pressure, 1.5–2.3 mm Hg in men and 2.1–3.2 mm Hg in women.

Cardiac Arrhythmias and Cardiomyopathy

Ethanol-induced arrhythmias may be related to electrolyte abnormalities, prolongation of the QT interval, and hyperadrenergic states. Atrial arrhythmias associated with chronic alcohol use include supraventricular tachycardia, atrial fibrillation, and atrial flutter. Alcoholic cardiomyopathy is a specific disease that is classified among the acquired forms of dilated cardiomyopathy, causing left ventricular dysfunction and dilatation that may or may not be associated with right ventricular dysfunction. In general, studies suggest that consuming more than 80 g of alcohol per day over at least 5 years, in the absence of other causes of cardiomyopathy, constitutes a diagnosis of alcoholic cardiomyopathy (Guzzo-Merello et al., 2014). Women are more sensitive to alcohol than men and develop alcoholic cardiomyopathy at a lower total dose of ethanol. Lowering blood pressure with angiotensin-converting enzyme inhibitors, in particular, may be beneficial in alcoholic cardiomyopathy (Guzzo-Merello et al., 2014).

Stroke

A meta-analysis showed that low alcohol intake reduces risk of total stroke, ischemic stroke, and stroke mortality, while heavy intake increases risk of total stroke (Zhang et al., 2014). Clinical studies indicated an increased incidence of hemorrhagic and ischemic stroke in persons who drink more than 40–60 g alcohol per day. Proposed etiological factors include the following:

- Alcohol-induced cardiac arrhythmias and associated thrombus formation
- High blood pressure from chronic alcohol consumption and subsequent cerebral artery degeneration
- Acute increases in systolic blood pressure and alterations in cerebral artery tone
- Head trauma

Lungs

As in the heart and other organs, chronic alcohol abuse causes oxidative injury in the lungs. AUD increases risk of acute respiratory distress syndrome and pneumonia (Molina et al., 2014). Alcohol impairs the pulmonary response to injury, infection, and inflammation, resulting in an overall imbalance in the immune response.

Skeletal Muscle

Chronic ethanol abuse is associated with decreased muscle mass and strength, even when adjusted for other factors such as age, nicotine use, and chronic illness. Heavy doses of ethanol may irreversibly damage muscle, reflected by a marked increase in the activity of creatine kinase in plasma. Muscle biopsies from heavy drinkers also reveal decreased glycogen stores and reduced pyruvate kinase activity. Approximately 50% of chronic drinkers have skeletal muscle myopathy, which is much greater than the incidence of alcohol cirrhosis (Molina et al., 2014).

GI Tract and Digestive System

The GI system mediates ethanol absorption and metabolism and is a target for alcohol-induced pathophysiology, such as impaired esophageal and gastric motility, altered acid secretion, impaired nutrient absorption, and disrupted intestinal barrier function.

Esophagus

Alcohol is one of multiple factors associated with esophageal reflux, Barrett esophagus, traumatic rupture of the esophagus, Mallory-Weiss tears, and esophageal cancer. Either tobacco or alcohol use is associated with a 20%–30% increased likelihood of the development of esophageal squamous cell carcinoma; however, the concomitant use of both drugs increases the risk 3-fold. There is little change in esophageal function at low BECs, but at higher BECs peristalsis and lower esophageal sphincter pressure decrease. Patients with chronic reflux esophagitis may respond to proton pump inhibitors, as well as abstinence from alcohol.

Stomach

Heavy ethanol use can disrupt the gastric mucosal barrier and cause acute and chronic gastritis. Ethanol concentrations up to 5% stimulate gastric acid secretion, whereas concentrations above 5% have no effect. Alcohol concentrations above 15% inhibit gastric motility and retard emptying of stomach contents. Clinical symptoms of high concentrations of ethanol intake include acute epigastric pain that is relieved with antacids or histamine H_2 receptor antagonists.

Intestines

Many individuals with AUD have chronic diarrhea caused by malabsorption in the small intestine. The rectal fissures and pruritus ani that are associated with heavy drinking are likely related to chronic diarrhea. Diarrhea is caused by structural and functional changes in the small intestine; for example, the intestinal mucosa has flattened villi, and digestive enzyme levels often are decreased. These changes are usually reversible after a period of abstinence.

Pancreas

Heavy alcohol use is the most common cause of both acute and chronic pancreatitis in the U.S. Acute alcoholic pancreatitis, involving acinar cells, is characterized by the abrupt onset of abdominal pain, nausea, vomiting, and increased levels of serum or urine pancreatic enzymes. Treatment usually involves intravenous fluid replacement (often with nasogastric suction) and opioid pain medication. Similar to alcoholic cirrhosis, chronic pancreatitis results from progressive cellular destruction and fibrosis. Chronic pancreatitis is treated by replacing the resulting endocrine and exocrine deficiencies. Hyperglycemia can develop as a sequela of pancreatitis and often requires insulin to control blood sugar levels (see Chapter 47). Pancreatic enzyme capsules containing lipase, amylase, and proteases may be necessary to treat malabsorption (see Chapter 50). The alcohol-induced risk for chronic pancreatitis is increased in smokers, which further exacerbates the risk of pancreatic cancer (Molina et al., 2014).

Liver

As the main organ involved in ethanol metabolism, the liver is a primary target for the pathological effects of ethanol. Alcohol misuse is responsible for approximately 50% of liver disease in the U.S. Ethanol produces dose-dependent hepatic injuries that progress from fat accumulation (steatosis) and inflammation to collagen deposition (fibrosis) to loss of liver cells (cirrhosis). The clinical stages of alcoholic liver disease are hepatosteatosis, alcoholic hepatitis, and cirrhosis. Accumulation of fat in the liver is an early event and can occur in normal individuals after the ingestion of relatively small amounts of ethanol. The generation of excess NADH, via metabolism of ethanol and acetaldehyde by ADH and ALDH, inhibits the tricarboxylic acid cycle and the oxidation of fat, leading to steatosis (see Figure 23–1). Steatosis is usually reversible with abstinence.

Hepatic stellate cells play an important role in the development of alcohol-mediated liver fibrosis. Fibrosis, resulting from tissue necrosis and chronic inflammation, is the underlying cause of alcoholic cirrhosis. The histological hallmark of cirrhosis is the formation of intracytoplasmic bodies called Mallory bodies, which may be related to an altered intermediate filament cytoskeleton.

Patients with AUD and alcoholic liver disease show changes in the composition of their intestinal microbiomes, increased intestinal permeability, and increased levels of gut-derived microbial products (Hartmann et al., 2015). Chronic ethanol exposure in animals and humans increases the circulating concentration of LPS, and the severity of hepatic injury correlates with serum levels of LPS. LPS activates TLRs and induces a complex signaling cascade, causing release of reactive oxygen species, chemokines, and pro-inflammatory cytokines.

Treatment of alcoholic hepatitis involves abstinence from alcohol and administration of corticosteroids, but corticosteroids only reduce mortality in the short term (Louvet and Mathurin, 2015). Improved treatment options may come from compounds that target the gut microbiome (see previous discussion), liver inflammation/regeneration, and oxidative stress. Probiotics, antibiotics, anti-inflammatory agents, immunosuppressants, growth factors, and antioxidants are examples of some of the different compounds undergoing clinical trials.

Cancers

Ethanol consumption is strongly linked to cancers of the oral cavity, pharynx, larynx, esophagus, colorectum (especially in men), and breast (women); there is also some evidence for an increased risk of liver cancer (Roswall and Weiderpass, 2015). Alcohol dependence plays a role in approximately 3.6% of all cancer cases and a similar percentage of cancer-related deaths (Boffetta et al., 2006). Two- to three-fold increases in cancer susceptibility are seen in individuals who chronically consume 50 g of alcohol per day, and concomitant smoking has a synergistic effect. As mentioned, individuals deficient in ALDH2 activity are particularly vulnerable to esophageal cancer. A notable complication in the treatment of cancer patients with AUD is that ethanol can interfere in the metabolism of some chemotherapeutic agents. The effects of acetaldehyde, a demonstrated carcinogen in animal models, and oxidative stress are widely cited mechanisms for the increased rate of carcinogenesis among individuals with AUD. Evidence also points to a role for aberrant DNA methylation patterns and other epigenetic modifications that control genome activity as mechanisms in alcohol-induced cancer development and progression. Epigenetics refers to processes that affect gene expression without changes in DNA sequence.

Hematological and Immunological Effects

Chronic excessive ethanol use is associated with different anemias, including microcytic, macrocytic, normochromic, and sideroblastic anemias, the last of which may respond to vitamin B_6 supplementation. Ethanol use also is associated with reversible thrombocytopenia. Ethanol affects granulocytes and lymphocytes, causing leukopenia, alteration of lymphocyte subsets, decreased T-cell mitogenesis, and changes in immunoglobulin production. In some patients with AUD, depressed leukocyte migration into inflamed areas may contribute to poor resistance to some infections (e.g., *Klebsiella* pneumonia, listeriosis, and tuberculosis). Some effects of ethanol-induced innate immune mechanisms that spread from the periphery to brain are described in the inflammatory sequence of events depicted in the following section.

Neuroimmune Mechanisms

The interplay between brain, behavior, and immunity in the etiology and progression of drug abuse is a rapidly developing area of research. Chronic ethanol consumption increases the levels of innate immune signaling molecules that reach the brain, producing alterations in brain physiology and behavior (Mayfield et al., 2013). Binge drinking increases levels of LPS, disrupting tight junctions and contributing to a leaky gut that permits bacteria and endotoxins to enter the circulation and exacerbate liver inflammation (Crews and Vetreno, 2015). This in turn releases pro-inflammatory cytokines that are transported across the blood-brain barrier, eliciting long-lasting neuroimmune responses. Within brain microglia, the actions of innate immune cytokines, activated TLRs, etc., are amplified via complex signaling loops, one of which leads to activation of the transcription factor NF-κB. NF-κB then regulates transcription of pro-inflammatory immune-related genes. Ethanol-induced microglia activation and induction of neuroimmune genes can thus be initiated systemically, through blood-borne molecules, as well as locally in the brain through neuronal-glial signaling. Neuroimmune mechanisms appear to be involved in later stages of heavy drinking and may contribute to neuronal apoptosis. Ethanol-induced neuroimmune activation also occurs in the developing brain, which may be relevant in FASDs (Drew and Kane, 2014).

Teratogenic Effects: Fetal Alcohol Spectrum Disorders

Ethanol is the most common teratogen in humans. Children born to mothers who are heavy drinkers display mental deficits and a common pattern of distinct dysmorphology known as FAS. The diagnosis of FAS is typically based on the observance of a triad of abnormalities associated with a history of prenatal ethanol exposure (Dorrie et al., 2014):

- A cluster of craniofacial abnormalities
- CNS dysfunction (structural or functional)
- Pre- or postnatal growth deficiencies (weight or height)

Fetal alcohol spectrum disorder is not a diagnostic term used by clinicians but rather an umbrella term that encompasses all of the disabilities caused by prenatal alcohol exposure. For example, children who do not meet all of the criteria for a diagnosis of FAS may show physical or mental deficits consistent with partial phenotypes, including *partial FAS, ARND,* and *ARBD* (Dorrie et al., 2014). The incidence of FAS is about 0.5–2 per 1000 live births in the general U.S. population, while the incidence of FAS, ARND, and ARBD combined is at least 1%. Higher rates of FAS occur in African and Native American women. Children of binge-drinking mothers show severe mental and behavioral deficits, likely due to the high peak BECs (Dorrie et al., 2014).

The FAS craniofacial abnormalities associated with maternal drinking in the first trimester consist of microcephaly, shortened palpebral fissures, thin upper lip, smooth philtrum, and epicanthal folds. Magnetic resonance imaging studies demonstrate decreased volumes in the basal ganglia, corpus callosum, cerebrum, and cerebellum that correlate with the facial abnormalities. CNS dysfunction attributed to in utero ethanol exposure consists of hyperactivity; attention and mental deficits; learning disabilities; language, memory, and motor disorders; and psychiatric conditions. FAS is the number one preventable cause of cognitive and attention deficits in the Western world, with afflicted children consistently scoring lower than their peers on a variety of IQ tests. Although the evidence is not conclusive, it has been suggested that even moderate alcohol consumption (28 g per day) in the second trimester of pregnancy is correlated with impaired academic performance of children at age 6. Maternal age also may be a factor: Pregnant women over age 30 who drink alcohol create greater risks to their children than do younger women who consume similar amounts of alcohol. In addition, the intake of high amounts of alcohol, particularly during the first trimester, greatly increases the chances of spontaneous abortion. Current recommendations are to drink no alcohol during pregnancy.

Clinical Uses of Ethanol

As mentioned, systemically administered ethanol is confined to the treatment of poisoning by methanol or ethylene glycol. In addition, dehydrated alcohol is injected in close proximity to nerves or sympathetic ganglia to relieve the long-lasting pain related to trigeminal neuralgia, inoperable carcinoma, and other conditions. Epidural, subarachnoid, and lumbar paravertebral injections of ethanol are also administered for inoperable pain. For example, lumbar paravertebral ethanol injections destroy sympathetic ganglia and thereby cause vasodilation and pain relief and promote healing of lesions in patients with vascular disease of the lower extremities.

Drug Interactions

Due to synergistic effects, great care must be taken when using sedatives to treat patients who have ingested heavy doses of ethanol or other CNS depressants. Acute ethanol intoxication decreases general anesthetic requirements, and elective surgery should be postponed in intoxicated patients. In contrast, chronic ethanol exposure increases anesthetic requirements largely due to pharmacodynamic cross-tolerance. An additional complication is the use of neuromuscular blockers and sedative/anesthetic agents in patients with AUD presenting with compromised liver function. This is particularly true for patients administered succinylcholine and benzodiazepines.

Pharmacokinetic interactions between ethanol and other drugs also occur. *Acute administration* of ethanol inhibits the function of enzymes responsible for metabolizing a variety of different drugs, including codeine, morphine, phenytoin, some benzodiazepines, tolbutamide, and warfarin, among others. Because ethanol inhibits CYP2E1, any drug also metabolized by this CYP isozyme will be metabolized at a slower rate in the presence of ethanol. In contrast, the *chronic administration* of ethanol acts as an enzyme inducer, particularly of CYP2E1, increasing the rate of metabolism of phenytoin, warfarin, propranolol, and benzodiazepines.

Comorbidity of Alcohol Use Disorder With Other Diseases

Many systemic diseases are related to chronic alcohol abuse, such as cardiovascular and liver diseases, as well as several types of cancers. AUD appears to increase the risk for diabetes mellitus, hypertension, stroke, osteoporosis, pancreatitis, and many other diseases. In this section, we focus on comorbid mental health conditions that are often present in patients with AUD or other substance use disorders.

Psychiatric Diseases

Patients diagnosed with a mood or anxiety disorder are about twice as likely to suffer from a drug abuse disorder and vice versa. In addition, AUD or other drug abuse disorders often occur in people with schizophrenia, leading to increased social and medical problems and complicating the course and treatment of schizophrenia. Patients with AUD and comorbid psychiatric disorders require treatment strategies that address both conditions. Although SSRIs have not been shown to be effective treatments for AUD in patients without a comorbid mental disorder, SSRIs and other antidepressants may decrease intake when AUD and depression co-occur; if alcohol use occurs as a consequence of depression, treating the underlying problem can decrease drinking.

Post-Traumatic Stress Disorder

Post-traumatic stress disorder is characterized by extreme hyperarousal and hyperstress responsiveness that contributes in a major way to the classic symptom cluster of reexperiencing, avoidance, and arousal. The prevalence of AUD in individuals with PTSD may be as high as 30% (Ouimette et al., 2005). The study of PTSD neurocircuitry has evolved from animal work on fear circuits and shows significant overlap with the symptoms of hyperresponsiveness to stress observed during alcohol withdrawal. One attractive hypothesis of the functional neurocircuitry changes that occur in PTSD is that of a brain-state shift from mild stress, in which the prefrontal cortex inhibits the amygdala, to extreme stress, in which the amygdala dominates (Pitman et al., 2012). Relative cortical dominance conveys resilience, while relative amygdala dominance conveys vulnerability; similar arguments can be made for the resilience and vulnerability to alcoholism, as elaborated by studies of the neurobiology of the withdrawal–negative affect stage of the alcohol addiction cycle.

Alcohol Use Disorder, Genetics, and Pharmacogenetics

Similar to other complex trait disorders, the development and progression of AUD is influenced by the interaction of multiple genetic and environmental factors. Environmental and cultural factors include stress, drinking patterns within one's culture and peer group, availability of alcohol, and attitudes toward drunkenness. These influences contribute to the initial decision to drink and the transition from casual drinking to alcohol-related problems. The heritability of AUD is estimated to be 50%–60%, as judged by family and twin studies. Long-term alcohol abuse and dependence are linked to persistent changes in gene expression (Mayfield et al., 2008).

As discussed previously, SNPs of *ADH* and *ALDH* may explain why some populations have a lower risk for AUD. Genetic variants of *ADH* that exhibit high activity and variants of *ALDH* that exhibit low activity protect against heavy drinking, likely because ethanol consumption by individuals expressing these variants results in accumulation of acetaldehyde, producing a variety of unpleasant effects.

Many additional genes modulate responses to ethanol, including variants of the following: μ-opioid receptor (*OPRM1*), dopamine transporter (*SLC6A3*), serotonin transporter (*SLC6A4*), dopamine receptor D2 (*DRD2*), α_2 subunit of the $GABA_A$ receptor (*GABRA2*), and α_3 subunit of the glycine receptor (*GLRA3*) (Jones et al., 2015). Other candidate genes include corticotropin-releasing hormone receptor 1 (*CRHR1*) and corticotropin-releasing hormone binding protein (*CRHBP*), which are important in brain stress pathways. Ethanol also induces the expression of neuroimmune-related genes, producing increased levels of immune markers detectable in postmortem brains from individuals with AUD (e.g., high-mobility group box 1, interleukin 1β, and TLRs), which may mediate long-term changes in brain function and neurodegeneration. Polymorphisms of genes encoding interleukin 1β and other immune molecules are associated with susceptibility to alcohol dependence (Crews and Vetreno, 2015).

Some of the pharmacotherapies for AUD, discussed in the next section, may be more effective in individuals carrying particular genetic variants. Clinical advances through pharmacogenetic studies of AUD may make the goal of precision medicine a possibility, but this will require rigorous methodological and statistical analyses. Each individual has unique neurobiological, genetic, and environmental profiles that affect treatment outcome, making individualized strategies not only feasible, but also necessary to move treatment of AUD into mainstream medicine (Litten et al., 2015).

Because AUD involves multifactorial processes with genetic and environmental determinants, as well as neuroadaptations related to disease progression, moving beyond studying the significance of individual candidate genes must include a systems approach to identify the relevant gene and protein networks operating at different stages of the disease. (Gorini et al., 2014).

Pharmacotherapy of Alcohol Use Disorder

Currently, three drugs are FDA approved for the treatment of AUD: disulfiram, naltrexone, and acamprosate (Table 23–2). They have reasonable efficacy, with effect sizes similar to those of antidepressant drugs for depression; unfortunately, they are not routinely prescribed (Jonas et al., 2014). Their efficacies may be influenced by an individual's genetic makeup, and genotyping is likely to become important in future treatment strategies. Benzodiazepines are the treatment of choice for management of acute alcohol withdrawal and to prevent the progression from minor withdrawal symptoms to major ones, such as seizures and delirium tremens (see Chapter 24).

TABLE 23–2 ■ ORAL MEDICATIONS FOR TREATING ALCOHOL ABUSE

MEDICATION	USUAL DOSE	MECHANISM/EFFECT
Disulfiram	250 mg/d (range of 125–500 mg/d)	• Inhibits ALDH with resulting ↑ acetaldehyde after drinking. Abstinence is reinforced to avoid the resulting adverse reaction.
Naltrexone	50 mg/d	• μ-opioid receptor antagonist; may ↓ drinking through ↓ feelings of reward with alcohol or ↓ craving.
Acamprosate	666 mg three times daily	• Unknown mechanism, may block hyperglutamatergic state and may ↓ mild protracted abstinence syndromes with ↓ feelings of a "need" for alcohol.

Disulfiram

Disulfiram (tetraethylthiuram disulfide), the first drug approved to treat alcohol abuse, is relatively nontoxic when taken in the absence of ethanol. It inhibits ALDH activity and increases the blood acetaldehyde concentration by 5–10 times compared to the level measured when ethanol is administered alone. Disulfiram irreversibly inactivates cytosolic and mitochondrial forms of ALDH to varying degrees. It is unlikely that disulfiram itself is responsible for ALDH inactivation in vivo because several active metabolites of the drug, especially diethylthiomethylcarbamate, behave as suicide-substrate inhibitors of ALDH in vitro. These metabolites reach significant concentrations in plasma following the administration of disulfiram.

Alcohol consumption by individuals previously treated with disulfiram gives rise to marked signs and symptoms of acetaldehyde poisoning. At BECs of 5–10 mg%, mild effects are noted, increasing markedly in severity as the BEC reaches 50 mg%. If the patient attains a BEC of 125–150 mg%, loss of consciousness may occur. Within 5–10 min, the face feels hot and soon afterward becomes flushed and scarlet in appearance. As the vasodilation spreads over the whole body, intense throbbing is felt in the head and neck, and a pulsating headache may develop. Respiratory difficulties, nausea, copious vomiting, sweating, thirst, chest pain, considerable hypotension, orthostatic syncope, marked uneasiness, weakness, vertigo, blurred vision, and confusion are observed. The facial flush is then replaced by pallor, and blood pressure may fall to levels seen in shock. Thus, the use of disulfiram requires careful medical supervision and should only be attempted in motivated patients committed to maintaining abstinence. Patients must learn to avoid disguised forms of alcohol that may be present in sauces, fermented vinegar, cough syrups, and even aftershave lotions. Disulfiram treatment results in poor compliance, possibly because of the adverse effects that result if taken with ethanol.

Disulfiram should not be administered until the patient has abstained from alcohol for at least 12 h. In the initial phase of treatment, a maximal daily dose of 500 mg is given for 1–2 weeks. Maintenance dosage then ranges from 125 to 500 mg daily depending on tolerance to side effects. Unless sedation is prominent, the daily dose should be taken in the morning, the time when the resolve not to drink may be strongest. Sensitization to alcohol may last as long as 14 days after the last ingestion of disulfiram because of the slow rate of restoration of ALDH.

Disulfiram or its metabolites can inhibit many enzymes with sulfhydryl groups, producing a wide spectrum of biological effects. Hepatic CYPs are inhibited, thereby interfering with the metabolism of phenytoin, chlordiazepoxide, barbiturates, warfarin, and other drugs.

Naltrexone

Naltrexone, a μ-opioid receptor antagonist, is chemically related to naloxone but has higher oral bioavailability and a longer duration of action when administered orally. It is also approved for treatment of opioid overdose and dependence (see Chapters 18 and 24). There is evidence that naltrexone blocks activation of brain receptors by opioid peptides that are thought to be critical for the rewarding effects of drugs of abuse.

Naltrexone reduces craving and decreases relapse to heavy drinking. Meta-analyses indicated that naltrexone is better than placebo, especially in reducing risk of heavy drinking. It is typically administered after detoxification at a dose of 50 mg/d for several months. Adherence to this regimen is important to ensure the therapeutic value of naltrexone but is a problem for some patients. A long-acting depot formulation of naltrexone is available for monthly injection. Naltrexone implants lasting several months are available outside the U.S.

The most common side effect of naltrexone is nausea, which subsides if the patient abstains from alcohol. There is some evidence of dysphoria associated with administration of naltrexone, and it is contraindicated in patients with depressive disorders. Doses of naltrexone exceeding 300 mg can cause liver damage; the drug is contraindicated in patients with liver failure or acute hepatitis and should be used only after careful consideration in patients with active liver disease. Naltrexone cannot be given to patients taking opioids, but it is used following opioid detoxification for prevention of relapse to opioid dependence.

Acamprosate

Acamprosate (*N*-acetylhomotaurine) may work by blocking a hyperglutamatergic state in the alcoholic brain, but the exact molecular target has remained elusive. It is FDA-approved for the treatment of AUD and is generally well tolerated by patients, with mild diarrhea being the main side effect. Double-blind, placebo-controlled studies demonstrated that acamprosate decreases drinking frequency and reduces relapse drinking in abstinent individuals but may not be effective in those who are currently drinking or misusing other drugs. Meta-analyses of randomized clinical trials showed that acamprosate is associated with reduced relapse in drinking (Jonas et al., 2014). For dosing, see Table 23–2.

Other Agents

Baclofen (used in France) has shown positive results for the treatment of AUD in some studies but is not FDA-approved for this use. Three other drugs described next, although not FDA-approved for AUD, are either approved in Europe or may prove useful based on emerging evidence.

Nalmefene, an opioid receptor antagonist structurally similar to naltrexone, is used to treat opioid overdose and may also be used to manage addictive behaviors. It is approved in Europe for as-needed use (18 mg) to reduce heavy drinking. It has several advantages over naltrexone, including longer duration of action, lack of dose-dependent liver toxicity, and higher affinity of binding to μ– and κ–opioid receptors. Nalmefene reduces the total amount of alcohol consumed and the number of heavy drinking days in alcohol-dependent patients (van den Brink et al., 2014). Nalmefene was used for opioid overdose in the U.S. but has been discontinued.

Gabapentin, which interacts with the α2δ subunit of neuronal voltage-gated Ca^{2+} channels, is primarily used to treat epileptic seizures and neuropathic pain. A clinical trial showed that gabapentin (particularly the daily 1800-mg dose) improved rates of abstinence and no heavy drinking days in alcohol-dependent adults, decreased the number of heavy drinking days and number of drinks consumed per week, and decreased the severity of craving, insomnia, and dysphoria (Mason et al., 2014). Additional studies are needed to determine if gabapentin or other agents can be repurposed to treat AUD. For additional information on gabapentin, see Chapter 17.

Varenicline, which is approved for smoking cessation, also reduces alcohol consumption in preclinical and clinical models (Rahman et al., 2014). Varenicline acts as a partial agonist at α3β4, α4β2, and α6β2 subtypes of nAChRs and as a high-efficacy agonist at α7 nAChRs. Given the role of nAChRs in mediating the rewarding properties of ethanol and drugs of abuse, their blockade may offer pharmacological targets for treating patients with AUD who are heavy smokers. For more information on varenicline, consult Chapter 11.

Acknowledgment: *Marc A. Schuckit contributed to this chapter in a previous edition of this book, and some of his text has been retained in the current edition.*

Drug Facts for Your Personal Formulary: *Drugs Used to Treat Alcohol Use Disorder*

Drugs	Therapeutic Uses	Clinical Pharmacology and Tips
Disulfiram	• AUD	ALDH inhibitor. Causes adverse effects from increased acetaldehyde when taken with alcohol. Poor patient compliance.
Naltrexone	• AUD • Opioid dependence after opioid detoxification	μ-opioid receptor antagonist. Nausea, liver damage at high doses. Available in oral and long-acting injectable formulations. Contraindicated in patients with liver disease or taking opioids concurrently.
Acamprosate	• AUD	Unknown mechanism, may block hyperglutamatergic state. May work best in abstinent alcoholics.
Benzodiazepines	• Management of alcohol withdrawal • Anxiety/panic/seizure disorders • Insomnia • Anesthetic premedication	↑ GABA binding at $GABA_A$ receptors. Chlordiazepoxide, lorazepam, diazepam, oxazepam, midazolam, and clorazepate are used in the U.S. to manage alcohol withdrawal symptoms.
Fomepizole	• Methanol poisoning	ADH inhibitor.
Drugs Not FDA Approved for Treatment of AUD But Approved Elsewhere or Found Clinically Useful		
Gabapentin	• AUD • Epileptic seizures and neuropathic pain	Blocks neuronal voltage-gated Ca^{2+} channels. Reduced alcohol cravings in a clinical trial.
Varenicline	• ↓ alcohol consumption in clinical trials • Smoking cessation	Partial or full agonist at some central nAChR subtypes.
Nalmefene	• AUD • Opioid overdose/dependence	μ- and κ-opioid receptor antagonist. Approved in Europe for as-needed use to decrease drinking. Advantages over naltrexone: no liver toxicity, longer duration of action, higher affinity. Approved for opioid overdose but was discontinued in the U.S.
Baclofen	• AUD • Spasticity	$GABA_B$ receptor agonist, skeletal muscle relaxant, and antispasmodic agent.

Bibliography

American Psychiatric Association. *Diagnostic and Statistical Manual of Mental Disorders*. 5th ed. American Psychiatric Association Publishing, Arlington, VA, **2013**.

Boffetta P, et al. The burden of cancer attributable to alcohol drinking. *Int J Cancer*, **2006**, *119*:884–887.

Brower KJ. Assessment and treatment of insomnia in adult patients with alcohol use disorders. *Alcohol*, **2015**, *49*:417–427.

CDC. Alcohol and public health, **2017**. Available at: http://www.cdc.gov/alcohol. Accessed May 13, 2017.

CDC. Vital Signs: Binge Drinking Prevalence, Frequency, and Intensity Among Adults—United States, 2010. *Morbidity and Mortality Weekly Report*, **2012**, *61*;14–19.

Chen CH, et al. Targeting aldehyde dehydrogenase 2: new therapeutic opportunities. *Physiol Rev*, **2014**, *94*:1–34.

Crews FT, Vetreno RP. Mechanisms of neuroimmune gene induction in alcoholism. *Psychopharmacology* (Berl), **2016**, *233*:1543–1557.

Dorrie N, et al. Fetal alcohol spectrum disorders. *Eur Child Adolesc Psychiatry*, **2014**, *23*:863–875.

Drew PD, Kane CJ. Fetal alcohol spectrum disorders and neuroimmune changes. *Int Rev Neurobiol*, **2014**, *118*:41–80.

Edenberg HJ, et al. Association of alcohol dehydrogenase genes with alcohol dependence: a comprehensive analysis. *Hum Mol Genet*, **2006**, *15*:1539–1549.

Gorini G, et al. Proteomic approaches and identification of novel therapeutic targets for alcoholism. *Neuropsychopharmacology*, **2014**, *39*:104–130.

Grant BF, et al. Epidemiology of DSM-5 Alcohol Use Disorder: Results From the National Epidemiologic Survey on Alcohol and Related Conditions III. *JAMA Psychiatry*, **2015**, *72*:757–766.

Guzzo-Merello G, et al. Alcoholic cardiomyopathy. *World J Cardiol*, **2014**, *6*:771–781.

Hartmann P, et al. Alcoholic liver disease: the gut microbiome and liver cross talk. *Alcohol Clin Exp Res*, **2015**, *39*:763–775.

Heinz A, et al. Reward craving and withdrawal relief craving: assessment of different motivational pathways to alcohol intake. *Alcohol Alcohol*, **2003**, *38*:35–39.

Howard RJ, et al. Seeking structural specificity: direct modulation of pentameric ligand-gated ion channels by alcohols and general anesthetics. *Pharmacol Rev*, **2014**, *66*:396–412.

Jonas DE, et al. Pharmacotherapy for adults with alcohol use disorders in outpatient settings: a systematic review and meta-analysis. *JAMA*, **2014**, *311*:1889–1900.

Jones JD, et al. The pharmacogenetics of alcohol use disorder. *Alcohol Clin Exp Res*, **2015**, *39*:391–402.

Koob GF. Neurocircuitry of alcohol addiction: synthesis from animal models. *Hand Clin Neurol*, **2014**, *125*:33–54.

Koob GF. Alcohol use disorders: tracts, twins, and trajectories. *Am J Psychiatry*, **2015**, *172*:499–501.

Litten RZ, et al. Heterogeneity of alcohol use disorder: understanding mechanisms to advance personalized treatment. *Alcohol Clin Exp Res*, **2015**, *39*:579–584.

Louvet A, Mathurin P. Alcoholic liver disease: mechanisms of injury and targeted treatment. *Nature Rev Gastroenterol Hepatol*, **2015**, *12*:231–242.

Mason BJ, et al. Gabapentin treatment for alcohol dependence: a randomized clinical trial. *JAMA Int Med*, **2014**, *174*:70–77.

Mayfield J, et al. Neuroimmune signaling: a key component of alcohol abuse. *Curr Opin Neurobiol*, **2013**, *23*:513–520.

Mayfield RD, et al. Genetic factors influencing alcohol dependence. *Br J Pharmacol*, **2008**, *154*:275–287.

Molina PE, et al. Alcohol abuse: critical pathophysiological processes and contribution to disease burden. *Physiology*, **2014**, *29*:203–215.

Movva R, Figueredo VM. Alcohol and the heart: to abstain or not to abstain? *Int J Cardiol*, **2013**, *164*:267–276.

NIAAA. Apparent Per Capita Alcohol Consumption: National, State, And Regional Trends, 1977–2013. *Surveillance Report* #102, **2015**. Available at: https://pubs.niaaa.nih.gov/publications/surveillance102/cons13.htm. Accessed May 13, 2017.

O'Keefe JH, et al. Alcohol and cardiovascular health: the dose makes the poison … or the remedy. *Mayo Clin Proc*, **2014**, *89*:382–393.

Ouimette P, et al. Consistency of retrospective reports of *DSM-IV* criterion A traumatic stressors among substance use disorder patients. *J Trauma Stress*, **2005**, *18*:43–51.

Pava MJ, Woodward JJ. A review of the interactions between alcohol and the endocannabinoid system: implications for alcohol dependence and future directions for research. *Alcohol*, **2012**, *46*:185–204.

Pitman RK, et al. Biological studies of post-traumatic stress disorder. *Nat Rev Neurosci*, **2012**, *13*:769–787.

Rahman S, et al. Nicotinic receptor modulation to treat alcohol and drug dependence. *Front Neurosci*, **2014**, *8*:426.

Roerecke M, Rehm J. Alcohol consumption, drinking patterns, and ischemic heart disease: a narrative review of meta-analyses and a systematic review and meta-analysis of the impact of heavy drinking occasions on risk for moderate drinkers. *BMC Med*, **2014**, *12*:182.

Roswall N, Weiderpass E. Alcohol as a risk factor for cancer: existing evidence in a global perspective. *J Prev Med Public Health*, **2015**, *48*:1–9.

Scalzo SJ, et al. Wernicke-Korsakoff syndrome not related to alcohol use: a systematic review. *J Neurol Neurosurg Pyschiatry*, **2015**, *86*:1362–1368.

Schuckit MA. Comorbidity between substance use disorders and psychiatric conditions. *Addiction*, **2006**, *101*:76–88.

Schuckit MA. Alcohol-use disorders. *Lancet*, **2009**, *373*:492–501.

Thomson AD, et al. The evolution and treatment of Korsakoff's syndrome: out of sight, out of mind? *Neuropsychol Rev*, **2012**, *22*:81–92.

Trudell JR, et al. Alcohol dependence: molecular and behavioral evidence. *Trends Pharmacol Sci*, **2014**, *35*:317–323.

van den Brink W, et al. Long-term efficacy, tolerability and safety of nalmefene as-needed in patients with alcohol dependence: a 1-year, randomised controlled study. *J Psychopharmacol*, **2014**, *28*:733–744.

Volkow ND, et al. Profound decreases in dopamine release in striatum in detoxified alcoholics: possible orbitofrontal involvement. *J Neurosci*, **2007**, *27*:12700–12706.

White AM, et al. Converging patterns of alcohol use and related outcomes among females and males in the United States, 2002 to 2012. *Alcohol Clin Exp Res*, **2015**, *39*:1712–1726.

Zhang C, et al. Alcohol intake and risk of stroke: a dose-response meta-analysis of prospective studies. *Int J Cardiol*, **2014**, *174*:669–677.

Drug Use Disorders and Addiction

Charles P. O'Brien

第二十四章 药物滥用障碍和成瘾

THE CONFUSING TERMINOLOGY OF DRUG USE DISORDERS

ORIGINS OF SUBSTANCE USE DISORDERS
- Agent (Drug) Variables
- Host (User) Variables
- Environmental Variables

PHARMACOLOGICAL PHENOMENA
- Tolerance
- Physical Dependence
- Withdrawal Syndrome

CLINICAL ISSUES: CNS DEPRESSANTS
- Ethanol
- Benzodiazepines
- Barbiturates
- Nicotine
- Opioids

CLINICAL ISSUES: COCAINE AND OTHER PSYCHOSTIMULANTS
- Cocaine
- Amphetamine and Related Agents
- Caffeine
- Cannabinoids (Marijuana)
- Psychedelic Agents

中文导读

本章主要介绍：药物滥用障碍术语的困惑；物质滥用障碍的起源，包括制剂（药物）因素、主体（用药者）因素和环境因素；药理学现象，包括耐受性、躯体依赖性和戒断综合征；临床问题，包括中枢神经系统抑制药，如乙醇、苯二氮䓬类、巴比妥类、尼古丁和阿片类药物；可卡因和其他精神兴奋药的临床问题，包括可卡因、苯丙胺及其相关药物、咖啡因、大麻素（大麻）和致幻剂。

Abbreviations

AIDS: acquired immune deficiency syndrome
CDC: U.S. Centers for Disease Control and Prevention
CNS: central nervous system
DA: dopamine
DAT: dopamine transporter
DEA: Drug Enforcement Agency
DMT: *N, N*-dimethyltryptamine
DOM: dimethoxymethylamphetamine
EEG: electroencephalogram
FDA: U.S. Food and Drug Administration
GABA: γ-aminobutyric acid
GI: gastrointestinal
GPCR: G protein–coupled receptor
5HT: serotonin
LSD: lysergic acid diethylamide
MDA: methylenedioxyamphetamine
MDMA: methylenedioxymethamphetamine
MOR: μ opioid receptor
NE: norepinephrine
NMDA: *N*-methyl-D-aspartate
PCP: phenycyclidine
Δ-9-THC: Δ-9-tetrahydrocannabinol

The Confusing Terminology of Drug Use Disorders

The terminology of drug dependence, abuse, and addiction has long elicited confusion that stems from the fact that repeated use of certain prescribed medications can produce neuroplastic changes resulting in two distinctly abnormal states. The first state is *dependence*, or "physical" dependence, produced when there is progressive pharmacological adaptation to the drug resulting in tolerance. Tolerance is a normal reaction that is often mistaken for a sign of "addiction." In the tolerant state, repeating the same dose of a drug produces a smaller effect. If the drug is abruptly stopped, a withdrawal syndrome ensues in which the adaptive responses are now unopposed by the drug. The appearance of withdrawal symptoms is the cardinal sign of "physical" dependence. *Addiction*, the second abnormal state produced by repeated drug use, occurs in only a minority of those who initiate drug use; addiction leads progressively to compulsive, out-of-control drug use.

Addiction can be considered as a form of maladaptive memory. Addiction begins with the administration of substances (e.g., cocaine) or behaviors (e.g., the thrill of gambling) that directly and intensely activate brain reward circuits. Activation of these circuits motivates normal behavior, and most humans simply enjoy the experience without being compelled to repeat it. For some (~16% of those who try cocaine), the experience produces strong conditioned associations to environmental cues that signal the availability of the drug or the behavior. The individual becomes drawn into compulsive repetition of the experience, focusing on the immediate pleasure despite negative long-term consequences and neglect of important social responsibilities. The distinction between dependence and addiction is important because patients with pain sometimes are deprived of adequate opioid medication by their physician simply because they have shown evidence of tolerance or they exhibit withdrawal symptoms if the analgesic medication is stopped or reduced abruptly. The most recent revision of the classification system (*Diagnostic and Statistical Manual of Mental Disorders, Fifth Edition*; see American Psychiatric Association, 2013) makes a clear distinction between normal tolerance and a drug use disorder involving compulsive drug seeking.

Origins of Substance Use Disorders

Most of those who initiate use of a drug with addiction potential do not develop a drug use disorder. Many variables operate simultaneously to influence the likelihood that a beginning drug user will lose control and develop an addiction. These variables can be organized into three categories: agent (drug), host (user), and environment (Table 24–1).

Agent (Drug) Variables

Reinforcement refers to the capacity of drugs to produce effects that make the user wish to take them again. The more strongly reinforcing a drug is, the greater is the likelihood that the drug will be abused. Reinforcing properties of drugs are associated with their capacity to increase neuronal activity in brain reward areas (see Chapters 13 and 14). Cocaine, amphetamine, ethanol, opiates, cannabinoids, and nicotine reliably increase extracellular fluid DA levels in the ventral striatum, specifically the nucleus accumbens region. In contrast, drugs that block DA receptors generally produce bad feelings (i.e., *dysphoric effects*). Despite strong correlative findings, a precise causal relationship between DA and euphoria/dysphoria has not been established, and other findings emphasize additional roles of 5HT, glutamate, NE, endogenous opioids, and GABA in mediating the reinforcing effects of drugs.

The abuse liability of a drug is enhanced by rapidity of onset. When coca leaves are chewed, cocaine is absorbed slowly; this produces low cocaine levels in the blood and few, if any, behavioral problems. Crack cocaine, sold illegally and at a low price ($1–$3 per dose in 2016), is alkaloidal cocaine (free base) that can be readily vaporized by heating. Simply inhaling the vapors produces blood levels comparable to those resulting from intravenous cocaine owing to the large surface area for absorption

TABLE 24–1 ■ MULTIPLE SIMULTANEOUS VARIABLES AFFECTING ONSET AND CONTINUATION OF DRUG ABUSE AND ADDICTION

Agent (drug)
Availability
Cost
Purity/potency
Mode of administration
Chewing (absorption *via* oral mucous membranes)
Gastrointestinal
Intranasal
Subcutaneous and intramuscular
Intravenous
Inhalation
Speed of onset and termination of effects (pharmacokinetics: combination of agent and host)
Host (user)
Heredity
Innate tolerance
Speed of developing acquired tolerance
Likelihood of experiencing intoxication as pleasure
Metabolism of the drug (nicotine and alcohol data already available)
Psychiatric symptoms
Prior experiences/expectations
Propensity for risk-taking behavior
Environment
Social setting
Community attitudes
Peer influence, role models
Availability of other reinforcers (sources of pleasure or recreation)
Employment or educational opportunities
Conditioned stimuli: environmental cues become associated with drugs after repeated use in the same environment

into the pulmonary circulation following inhalation. Thus, inhalation of crack cocaine is much more addictive than chewing, drinking, or sniffing cocaine. The risk for developing addiction among those who try nicotine is about twice that for those who try cocaine (Table 24–2). This does not imply that the pharmacological addiction liability of nicotine is twice that of cocaine. Rather, there are other variables listed in Table 24-1 in the categories of Agent (e.g., mode of administration), Host, and Environment that influence the development of addiction.

Host (User) Variables

Effects of drugs vary among individuals. Polymorphism of genes that encode enzymes involved in absorption, metabolism, and excretion of a drug and its receptor-mediated responses may contribute to the effects of the drug across the addiction cycle (e.g., euphoria, reinforcement, etc.) (see Chapters 2 through 7). Innate tolerance to alcohol may represent a biological trait that contributes to the development of alcoholism. While innate tolerance increases vulnerability to alcoholism, impaired metabolism may *protect* against it (see Chapter 23). Similarly, individuals who inherit a gene associated with slow nicotine metabolism may experience unpleasant effects when beginning to smoke and reportedly have a lower probability of becoming nicotine dependent.

Psychiatric disorders constitute another category of host variables. People with anxiety, depression, insomnia, or even shyness may find that certain drugs give them relief. However, the apparent beneficial effects are transient, and repeated use of the drug may lead to tolerance and eventually compulsive, uncontrolled drug use. While psychiatric symptoms are seen commonly in drug abusers presenting for treatment, most of these symptoms begin *after* the person starts abusing drugs. Thus, drugs of abuse appear to produce more psychiatric symptoms than they relieve.

TABLE 24–2 ■ USE, ADDICTION, AND RISK AMONGST USERS OF TOBACCO, ETHANOL, AND ILLICIT DRUGS IN THE U.S., 1992–1994

AGENT	EVER USED[a] (%)	ADDICTION (%)	RISK OF ADDICTION (%)
Tobacco	75.6	24.1	31.9
Alcohol	91.5	14.1	15.4
Illicit drugs	51.0	7.5	14.7
Cannabis	46.3	4.2	9.1
Cocaine	16.2	2.7	16.7
Stimulants	15.3	1.7	11.2
Anxiolytics	12.7	1.2	9.2
Analgesics	9.7	0.7	7.5
Psychedelics	10.6	0.5	4.9
Heroin	1.5	0.4	23.1
Inhalants	6.8	0.3	3.7

[a]The ever-used and addiction percentages are those of the general population. The risk of addiction is specific to the drug indicated and refers to the percentage who met criteria for addiction among those who reported having used the agent at least once (i.e., each value in the rightmost column was obtained by expressing the number in the Addiction column as a percentage of the number in the Ever Used column, subject to errors of rounding).

Data source: Anthony JC, et al. Comparative epidemiology of dependence on tobacco, alcohol, controlled substances and the inhalants: basic findings from the National Comorbidity Survey. *Exp Clin Psychopharmacol*, **1994**, *2*:244–268. This study was repeated in 2001–2003: Degenhardt L, et al. Epidemiological patterns of drug use in the United States: evidence from the National Comorbidity Survey Replication, 2001–2003. doi:10.1016/j.drugalcdep.2007.03.007. Accessed July 10, 2016. The National Institute on Drug Abuse conducted a related study in 2014: available at: https://www.drugabuse.gov/national-survey-drug-use-health. Accessed July 10, 2016.

Environmental Variables

Initiating and continuing illegal drug use is influenced significantly by societal norms and peer pressure.

Pharmacological Phenomena

Tolerance

Tolerance, the most common response to repetitive use of the same drug, can be defined as the reduction in response to the drug after repeated administrations. Consider an idealized drug dose-response curve (Figure 24–1). As the dose of the drug increases, the observed effect of the drug increases. With repeated use of the drug, however, the curve shifts to the right (tolerance). There are many forms of tolerance, likely arising through multiple mechanisms.

Tolerance to some drug effects develops much more rapidly than to other effects of the same drug. For example, tolerance develops rapidly to the euphoria produced by opioids such as heroin, and addicts tend to increase their dose to reexperience that elusive "high." In contrast, tolerance to the GI effects of opioids develops more slowly. The discrepancy between tolerance to euphorigenic effects (rapid) and tolerance to effects on vital functions such as respiration and blood pressure (slow) can lead to potentially fatal overdoses.

We can define multiple aspects of tolerance and give examples of some general mechanisms and dosing schedules that contribute:

- *Innate tolerance* refers to genetically determined lack of sensitivity to a drug the first time that it is experienced.
- *Acquired tolerance* can be divided into three major types—*pharmacokinetic, pharmacodynamic,* and *learned tolerance*—and includes acute, reverse, and cross-tolerance.
  1. *Pharmacokinetic* or *dispositional tolerance* refers to changes in the distribution or metabolism of a drug after repeated administrations, such that a given dose produces a lower blood concentration than the same dose did on initial exposure. The most common mechanism is an increase in the rate of metabolism of the drug. For example, chronic administration of barbiturates induces hepatic CYPs 1A2, 2C9, 2C19, and 3A4, thereby enhancing the metabolism of drugs that are substrates for these enzymes.
  2. *Pharmacodynamic tolerance* refers to adaptive changes that have taken place within systems affected by the drug so that response to a given concentration of the drug is altered (usually reduced). Examples include drug-induced changes in receptor density or efficiency of receptor coupling to signal transduction pathways (see Chapter 3).

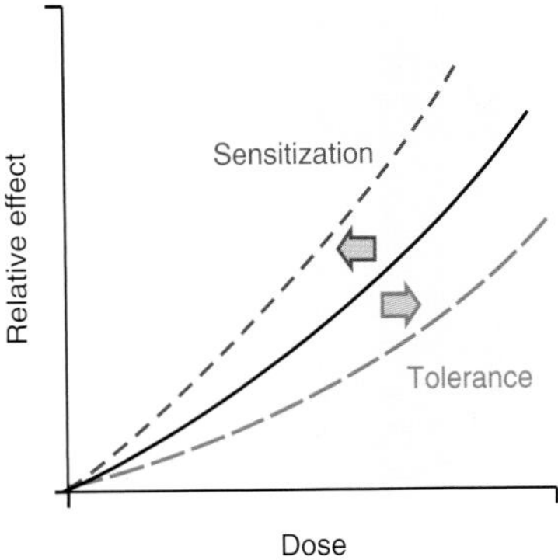

Figure 24–1 *Shifts in a dose-response curve with tolerance and sensitization.* The solid black curve describes the dose-response relationship to initial doses (the "control" curve). With tolerance, there is a shift of the curve to the right such that higher doses are required to achieve equivalent effects. With sensitization, the dose response shifts leftward, and a given dose produces a greater effect than in the control case.

3. *Learned tolerance* refers to a reduction in the effects of a drug due to compensatory mechanisms that are acquired by past experiences. One type of learned tolerance is called *behavioral tolerance.* A common example is learning to walk a straight line despite the motor impairment produced by alcohol intoxication. At higher levels of intoxication, behavioral tolerance is overcome, and the behavioral deficits are obvious.

- *Conditioned tolerance* (situation-specific tolerance) develops when environmental cues or situations consistently are paired with the administration of a drug. When a drug affects homeostatic balance by producing sedation and changes in blood pressure, pulse rate, gut activity, and so on, there is usually a reflexive counteraction or adaptation in the direction of maintaining the status quo. If a drug always is taken in the presence of specific environmental cues (e.g., smell of drug preparation and sight of syringe), these cues begin to predict the effects of the drug, and the adaptations begin to occur, which will prevent the full manifestation of the drug's effects (i.e., cause tolerance). This mechanism follows classical (Pavlovian) principles of learning and results in drug tolerance under circumstances where the drug is "expected."
- *Acute tolerance* refers to rapid tolerance developing with repeated use on a single occasion, such as in a "binge." For example, repeated doses of cocaine over several hours produce a decrease in response to subsequent doses of cocaine during the binge. This is the opposite of *sensitization*, observed with an intermittent-dosing schedule.
- *Sensitization* or *reverse tolerance* refers to an increase in response with repetition of the same dose of the drug. Sensitization results in a shift to the left of the dose-response curve (see Figure 24–1). Sensitization, in contrast to acute tolerance during a binge, requires a longer interval between doses, usually about 1 day. Sensitization can occur with stimulants such as cocaine or amphetamine.
- *Cross-tolerance* occurs when repeated use of a drug in a given category confers tolerance not only to that drug but also to other drugs in the same pharmacological category. Understanding cross-tolerance is important in the medical management of persons dependent on a drug.
- *Detoxification* is a form of treatment of drug dependence that involves giving gradually decreasing doses of the drug to prevent withdrawal symptoms, thereby weaning the patient from the drug of dependence. Detoxification can be accomplished with any medication in the same category as the initial drug of dependence. For example, users of heroin show cross-tolerance to other opioids. Thus, the detoxification of heroin-dependent patients can be accomplished with any medication that activates MORs.

These issues of tolerance, while straightforward, seem to produce a dangerous misunderstanding among self-medicating opioid users. Degrees of tolerance depend on the type of opioid, its half-life, and the route of administration. The typical addicted user is craving the "high" and seems willing to risk overdose by going beyond the safe level. This is especially dangerous when they have progressed to intravenous injection. Accidental overdose has become so common in the U.S. that death in this manner now exceeds the toll for traffic accidents in young people (Rudd et al., 2016).

Physical Dependence

Physical dependence is a state that develops as a result of the adaptation (tolerance) produced by a resetting of homeostatic mechanisms in response to repeated drug use. A person in this adapted or physically dependent state requires continued administration of the drug to maintain normal function. If administration of the drug is stopped abruptly, there is another imbalance, and the affected systems must readjust to a new equilibrium without the drug.

Withdrawal Syndrome

Withdrawal signs and symptoms occur when drug administration in a physically dependent person is terminated abruptly. The appearance of a withdrawal syndrome when administration of the drug is terminated is the only actual evidence of physical dependence. The type of withdrawal symptoms depends on the pharmacological category of the drug of dependence. Thus, withdrawal of a stimulant causes sedation during withdrawal. Withdrawal of an opioid produces craving for the opioid and physical symptoms, such as nausea, vomiting, and diarrhea, that are the opposite of the opioid's effects.

Pharmacokinetic variables are of considerable importance in the amplitude and duration of the withdrawal syndrome. Tolerance, physical dependence, and withdrawal are all biological phenomena. They are the natural consequences of drug use and can be produced in experimental animals and in any human being who takes certain medications repeatedly. These symptoms in themselves do not imply that the individual is involved in drug misuse or addiction. *Patients who take medicine for appropriate medical indications and in correct dosages still may show tolerance, physical dependence, and withdrawal symptoms* if the drug is stopped abruptly rather than gradually. A physician prescribing a medication that normally produces tolerance must understand the difference between dependence and addiction and be mindful of withdrawal symptoms if the dose is reduced.

Clinical Issues: CNS Depressants

Abuse of multiple drugs in combination is common. Alcohol is so widely available that it is combined with practically all other categories of drugs. Some combinations reportedly are taken because of their interactive effects. When confronted with a patient exhibiting signs of overdose or withdrawal, the physician must be aware of these possible combinations because each drug may require a different and specific treatment.

Ethanol

More than 90% of American adults report experience with ethanol (commonly called "alcohol"). Ethanol is classified as a depressant because it produces sedation and sleep. However, the initial effects of alcohol, particularly at lower doses, often are perceived as stimulation owing to a suppression of inhibitory systems (see Chapter 23). Heavy use of ethanol causes development of tolerance and physical dependence sufficient to produce an alcohol withdrawal syndrome when intake is stopped (Table 24–3).

Tolerance, Physical Dependence, and Withdrawal

The symptoms of mild intoxication by alcohol vary among individuals. Some experience motor incoordination and sleepiness. Others initially become stimulated. As the blood level increases, the sedating effects increase, with eventual coma and death occurring at high blood alcohol levels. The innate tolerance to alcohol varies greatly among individuals and is related to family history of alcoholism (Wilhelmsen et al., 2003). Experience with alcohol can produce greater tolerance (acquired tolerance) such that extremely high blood levels (300–400 mg/dL) can be found in alcoholics who do not appear grossly sedated. In these cases, the

TABLE 24–3 ■ ALCOHOL WITHDRAWAL SYNDROME
Alcohol craving
Tremor, irritability
Nausea
Sleep disturbance
Tachycardia
Hypertension
Sweating
Perceptual distortion
Seizures (6–48 h after last drink)
Visual (and occasionally auditory or tactile) hallucinations (12–48 h after last drink)
Delirium tremens (48–96 h after last drink; rare in uncomplicated withdrawal)
Severe agitation, confusion
Fever, profuse sweating
Tachycardia, dilated pupils
Nausea, diarrhea

lethal dose does not increase proportionately to the sedating dose; thus, the margin of safety is decreased.

Heavy consumers of alcohol acquire tolerance and also develop a state of physical dependence. This often leads to drinking in the morning to restore blood alcohol levels diminished during the night. The alcohol withdrawal syndrome generally depends on the size of the average daily dose and usually is "treated" by resumption of alcohol ingestion. Withdrawal symptoms are experienced frequently but usually are not severe or life threatening until they occur in conjunction with other problems, such as infection, trauma, malnutrition, or electrolyte imbalance. In the setting of such complications, the syndrome of *delirium tremens* becomes likely.

Alcohol addiction produces cross-tolerance to other sedatives, such as benzodiazepines. This tolerance is operative in abstinent alcoholics, but while the alcoholic is drinking, the sedating effects of alcohol add to those of other sedatives. This is particularly true for benzodiazepines, which are relatively safe in overdose when given alone but potentially are lethal in combination with alcohol. The chronic use of alcohol and other sedatives is associated with the development of depression and the risk of suicide. Cognitive deficits have been reported in alcoholics tested while sober. These deficits usually improve with abstinence. More severe recent memory impairment is associated with specific brain damage caused by nutritional deficiencies common in alcoholics (e.g., thiamine deficiency). Medical complications of alcohol abuse and dependence include liver disease, cardiovascular disease, endocrine and GI effects, and malnutrition, in addition to the CNS dysfunctions outlined previously. Ethanol readily crosses the placental barrier, producing the fetal alcohol syndrome, a major cause of mental retardation (see Chapter 23).

Pharmacological Interventions

Detoxification. Although most mild cases of alcohol withdrawal never come to medical attention, severe cases require general evaluation; attention to hydration and electrolytes; vitamins, especially high-dose thiamine; and a sedating medication that has cross-tolerance with alcohol. To block or diminish the symptoms described in Table 24–3, a short-acting benzodiazepine such as oxazepam can be used at a dose of 15–30 mg every 6–8 h according to the stage and severity of withdrawal; some authorities recommend a long-acting benzodiazepine unless there is demonstrated liver impairment. Anticonvulsants such as carbamazepine have been shown to be effective in alcohol withdrawal, but not as well as benzodiazepines.

Pharmacotherapy. Detoxification is the first step of treatment. Complete abstinence is the objective of long-term treatment, and this is best accomplished by a combination of relapse prevention, anticraving medication, and cognitive behavioral therapy. Disulfiram has been useful in some programs that focus behavioral efforts to promote ingestion of the medication. Disulfiram blocks aldehyde dehydrogenase, resulting in the accumulation of acetaldehyde (Figure 23–1), which produces an unpleasant flushing reaction and nausea when alcohol is ingested. Knowledge that this unpleasant reaction will ensue may help the patient to resist the urge to resume drinking alcohol. However, disulfiram has not proven to be effective in controlled clinical trials because so many patients choose to stop the medication rather than the alcohol.

Naltrexone is an opioid receptor antagonist that blocks the endorphin activation properties of alcohol. Chronic administration of naltrexone decreased the rate of relapse to heavy drinking in randomized clinical trials. The effect varied from strong to weak, but overall, reduction in heavy drinking was a consistent finding (Pettinati et al., 2006).

Naltrexone works best in combination with behavioral treatment programs that encourage adherence to medication and abstinence from alcohol. A depot preparation with a duration of 30 days is now available; it greatly improves medication adherence. Depot naltrexone can also be used in the prevention of relapse in opioid addiction (Lee et al., 2016).

Recent studies of alcohol detoxification have reported that gabapentin can aid in the transition to the abstinent state, possibly by improvement in sleep. Acamprosate, a competitive inhibitor of the NMDA-type glutamate receptor (see Table 23–2), appears to normalize the dysregulated neurotransmission associated with chronic ethanol intake and thereby to attenuate one of the mechanisms that lead to relapse.

Benzodiazepines

Benzodiazepines are used mainly for the treatment of anxiety disorders and insomnia (see Chapters 15 and 17). These agents are widely used, and abuse of prescription benzodiazepines is not uncommon. They may also be combined with alcohol or methadone in the treatment of opioid addiction. The proportion of patients who become tolerant and physically dependent on benzodiazepines increases after several months of use, and abrupt reduction of the dose or stopping the medication produces withdrawal symptoms (Table 24–4).

It can be difficult to distinguish benzodiazepine withdrawal symptoms from the reappearance of the anxiety symptoms for which the benzodiazepine was originally prescribed. Some patients may increase their dose over time as tolerance develops to the sedative effects. Antianxiety benefits, however, seem to continue to occur long after tolerance to the sedating effects. Moreover, some patients continue to take the medication for years in appropriate doses according to medical directions and are able to function effectively as long as they take the medication. Patients with a history of alcohol or other drug abuse problems have an increased risk for the development of benzodiazepine abuse and should rarely, if ever, be treated with benzodiazepines on a chronic basis.

Pharmacological Interventions

If patients receiving long-term benzodiazepine treatment by prescription wish to stop their medication, the process may take months of gradual dose reduction. Withdrawal symptoms may occur during this outpatient detoxification, but in most cases the symptoms are mild. Patients who have been on low doses of benzodiazepines for years usually have no adverse effects. If anxiety symptoms return, a nonbenzodiazepine such as buspirone may be prescribed. Some authorities recommend transferring the patient to a benzodiazepine with a long $t_{1/2}$ during detoxification; others recommend the anticonvulsants carbamazepine and phenobarbital. The specific benzodiazepine receptor antagonist flumazenil is useful in the treatment of overdose and in reversing the effects of long-acting benzodiazepines used in anesthesia.

Abusers of high doses of benzodiazepines usually require inpatient detoxification. Frequently, benzodiazepine abuse is part of a combined dependence involving alcohol, opioids, and cocaine. Detoxification can be a complex clinical pharmacological challenge requiring knowledge of the pharmacokinetics of each drug. One approach to complex detoxification is to focus on the CNS depressant drug and temporarily hold the opioid component constant with a low dose of methadone or buprenorphine. A long-acting benzodiazepine such as diazepam or clorazepate or a long-acting barbiturate such as phenobarbital can be used to block the sedative withdrawal symptoms. After detoxification, the prevention of relapse requires a long-term outpatient rehabilitation program similar to the treatment of alcoholism. No specific medications have been found to be useful in the rehabilitation of sedative abusers, but specific psychiatric disorders such as depression or schizophrenia, if present, require appropriate medications.

TABLE 24–4 ■ BENZODIAZEPINE WITHDRAWAL SYMPTOMS

Following moderate-dose usage
Anxiety, agitation
Increased sensitivity to light and sound
Paresthesias, strange sensations
Muscle cramps
Myoclonic jerks
Sleep disturbance
Dizziness
Following high-dose usage
Seizures
Delirium

Barbiturates

Abuse problems with barbiturates resemble those seen with benzodiazepines in many ways, and treatment of abuse and addiction to barbiturates should be handled similarly to interventions for the abuse of alcohol and benzodiazepines. Because drugs in this category frequently are prescribed as hypnotics for patients complaining of insomnia, physicians should be aware of the problems that can develop when the hypnotic agent is withdrawn and of possible causes for insomnia that are treatable by other means. Insomnia often is a symptom of an underlying chronic problem, such as depression or respiratory dysfunction. Long-term prescription of sedative medications can change the physiology of sleep and should be avoided. When the sedative is stopped, there is a rebound effect with worsened insomnia. Whether from prescribed hypnotic or self-administered alcohol, medication-induced rebound insomnia requires detoxification by gradual dose reduction. Physicians should not recommend a bedtime drink of alcohol to relieve insomnia; the result is usually disordered sleep.

Nicotine

Nicotine and agents for smoking cessation are discussed in Chapter 11. Because nicotine provides the reinforcement for cigarette smoking, the most common cause of preventable death and disease in the U.S., it is arguably the most dangerous dependence-producing drug. Although more than 80% of smokers express a desire to quit, only 35% try to stop each year, and fewer than 5% are successful in unaided attempts to quit.

Tobacco (nicotine) addiction is influenced by multiple variables. Nicotine itself produces reinforcement; users compare nicotine to stimulants such as cocaine or amphetamine, although its effects are of lower magnitude. While there are many casual users of alcohol and cocaine, few individuals who smoke cigarettes smoke a small enough quantity (≤5 cigarettes per day) to avoid dependence. Nicotine is absorbed readily through the skin, mucous membranes, and lungs. The pulmonary route produces discernible CNS effects in as little as 7 sec. Thus, each puff produces some discrete reinforcement. With 10 puffs per cigarette, the 1-pack-per-day smoker reinforces the habit 200 times daily.

In dependent smokers, the urge to smoke correlates with a low blood nicotine level, as though smoking were a means to achieve a certain nicotine level and thus avoid nicotine withdrawal symptoms (Table 24–5). Depressed mood (dysthymic disorder, affective disorder) is associated with nicotine dependence, but it is not known whether depression can predispose one to begin smoking or whether depression develops secondarily during the course of nicotine dependence.

Pharmacological Interventions

The nicotine withdrawal syndrome can be alleviated by nicotine replacement therapy (e.g., nicotine inhaler and nasal spray, nicotine gum or lozenge, or nicotine transdermal patch). Different methods of nicotine delivery provide different blood nicotine levels over varying time courses (Figure 24–2). These methods suppress the symptoms of nicotine withdrawal. Although these treatments result in more smokers achieving abstinence, most resume smoking over the ensuing weeks or months. A sustained-release preparation of the antidepressant bupropion (see Chapter 15) improves abstinence rates among smokers and remains a useful option. The cannabinoid CB_1 receptor inverse agonist rimonabant improves abstinence rates and reduces the weight gain seen frequently in ex-smokers; unfortunately, rimonabant was found in clinical trials to be linked to depressive and neurologic symptoms and is not approved in the U.S.

Varenicline, a partial agonist at the α4β2 subtype of the nicotinic acetylcholine receptor, reduces cigarette craving and improves long-term abstinence rates. It has high receptor affinity, thus blocking access to nicotine, so if the treated smoker relapses, there is little reward, and abstinence is more likely to be maintained. In one clinical trial, the abstinence rate for varenicline at 1 year was 36.7% versus 7.9% for placebo (Williams et al., 2007). There were initial reports of suicidal ideation in patients treated with this medication, but more recent studies in larger populations have failed to replicate these reports. See Chapter 11 for the pharmacology of varenicline.

TABLE 24–5 ■ NICOTINE WITHDRAWAL SYMPTOMS
Irritability, impatience, hostility
Anxiety
Dysphoric or depressed mood
Difficulty in concentrating
Restlessness
Decreased heart rate
Increased appetite or weight gain

Opioids

Opioid drugs are used primarily for the treatment of pain (see Chapter 20). Some of the CNS mechanisms that reduce the perception of pain also produce a state of well-being or euphoria. Thus, opioid drugs also are taken outside medical settings for the purpose of obtaining mood elevation or euphoria. Such use entails a high risk of overdose.

Death by Overdose

Heroin is the most frequently abused illicit opioid. Although there is no legal supply of heroin in the U.S., the drug is widely available on the illicit market. The purity of street heroin in the U.S. has increased over the past decade from about 4 mg heroin per 100-mg bag (range 0–8 mg/100 mg; the rest was nonopioid filler such as quinine) to a purity of 45%–75%, with some samples testing as high as 90%. This increase in purity has led to increased levels of physical dependence among heroin addicts. Users who interrupt regular dosing now develop more severe withdrawal symptoms. The more potent supplies can be smoked or administered nasally (snorted), making heroin use accessible to people who would not insert a needle into their veins. The increased potency of heroin has also contributed to more deaths by overdose.

Legal opioids are also abused. During early 21st century, there was increased interest among members of the medical profession in asking patients about pain, giving it a numerical rating, and treating it aggressively

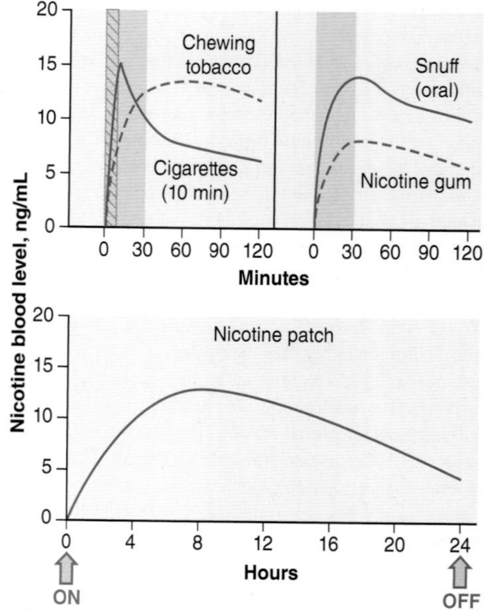

Figure 24–2 *Blood levels of nicotine resulting from different delivery systems.* In the upper panels, the shaded areas indicate the periods of nicotine delivery (30 min except for cigarettes, 10 min). In the lower panel, the arrows indicate the times of application and removal of a nicotine patch. These idealized curves are based on the findings of experiments by Benowitz et al., 1988, and Srivastava et al., 1991.

with prescription opioids as the agents of choice. In some cases, there was clear overprescribing, especially of extended-release forms of oxycodone, which have been linked to abuse, addiction, and overdose, and FDA approval of another long-acting formulation of oxycodone has provoked controversy (Manchikanti et al., 2014). Opioid overdose has become a common cause of death in many communities, and the latest reports are worrisome, indicating that death from opioid overdose is now about 25,000 annually (DEA, 2015; Rudd et al., 2016). In response, the CDC announced more stringent guidelines for physicians to limit the prescription of opioids for chronic pain (Dowell et al., 2016; see Chapter 20).

Tolerance, Dependence, and Withdrawal

Injection of a heroin solution produces a variety of sensations, described as warmth, taste, or high and intense pleasure ("rush") often compared with sexual orgasm. There are some differences among the opioids in their acute effects; for instance, morphine produces a prominent histamine-releasing effect (causing itching), and meperidine is notable for producing excitation or confusion. Even experienced opioid addicts, however, cannot distinguish between heroin and the common opioid hydromorphone, often used for pain in hospitalized patients. The popularity of heroin may be due to its widespread availability on the illicit market and its rapid onset of effect.

After intravenous injection, the effects begin in less than a minute. Heroin has high lipid solubility, crosses the blood-brain barrier quickly, and is deacetylated to the active metabolites 6-monoacetyl morphine and morphine. After the intense euphoria, which lasts from 45 sec to several minutes, there is a period of sedation and tranquility ("on the nod") lasting up to an hour. The effects of heroin wear off in 3–5 h, depending on the dose. Experienced users may inject two to four times daily. Thus, the heroin addict is constantly oscillating between being "high" and feeling the sickness of early withdrawal (as depicted in Figure 24–3). This produces many problems in the homeostatic systems regulated at least in part by endogenous opioids.

Based on patient reports, tolerance develops early to the euphoria-producing effects of heroin and other opioids. There also is tolerance to the respiratory depressant, analgesic, sedative, and emetic properties. Heroin users tend to increase their daily dose, depending on their financial resources and the availability of the drug. Overdose is likely to occur when potency of the street sample is unexpectedly high or when the heroin is mixed with a far more potent opioid, such as fentanyl.

Addiction to heroin or other short-acting opioids produces behavioral disruptions and usually becomes incompatible with a productive life. Apart from the behavioral changes and the risk of overdose, chronic use of opioids is relatively nontoxic in and of itself. Nonetheless, the mortality rate for street heroin users is high. Heroin users commonly acquire bacterial infections producing skin abscesses, endocarditis; pulmonary infections, especially tuberculosis; and viral infections producing hepatitis C and AIDS.

Another factor is the use of opioids frequently in combination with other drugs, such as heroin and cocaine ("speedball"). Users report improved euphoria because of the combination, and there is evidence of an interaction: Cocaine reduces the signs of opiate withdrawal, and heroin may reduce the irritability seen in chronic users of cocaine.

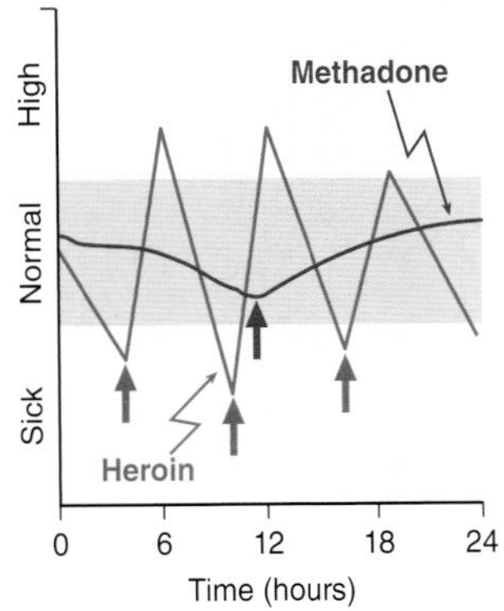

Figure 24–3 *Comparative time courses of response to heroin and methadone.* A person who injects heroin (↑) several times per day oscillates between being sick and being high (red line). In contrast, a methadone patient (purple line) remains in the "normal" range (blue band) with little fluctuation after dosing once per day. Ordinate values represent the subject's mental and physical state, not plasma levels of the drug.

Pharmacological Interventions

Withdrawal and Detoxification. The first stage of treatment addresses physical dependence and consists of detoxification. The opioid withdrawal syndrome (Table 24–6) is unpleasant but not life threatening. It begins within 6–12 h after the last dose of a short-acting opioid and as long as 72–84 h after a long-acting opioid medication. The duration and intensity of the syndrome are related to the clearance of the individual drug. Heroin withdrawal is brief (5–10 days) and intense. Methadone withdrawal is slower in onset and lasts longer.

Opioid withdrawal signs and symptoms can be treated by three different approaches. *The first and most commonly used approach* consists of transfer to a prescription opioid medication and then gradual dose reduction. It is convenient to change the patient from a short-acting opioid such as heroin to a long-acting one such as methadone. The initial dose of methadone is typically 20–30 mg. The first day's total dose can be determined by the response and then reduced by 20% per day during the course of detoxification.

A second approach to detoxification involves the use of oral clonidine, an α_2 adrenergic agonist that decreases adrenergic neurotransmission from the locus ceruleus. This medication is approved for the treatment of hypertension but is commonly used off label to reduce symptoms of opioid withdrawal. Many of the autonomic symptoms of opioid withdrawal result from the loss of opioid suppression of the locus ceruleus system during the abstinence syndrome. Clonidine can alleviate many of these symptoms but not the generalized aches and opioid craving. Lofexidine, a similar medication, is FDA-approved for use as an opioid withdrawal suppressant. With clonidine and lofexidine, the dose must be titrated according to the stage and severity of withdrawal; postural hypotension is commonly a side effect.

A third method of treating opioid withdrawal involves activation of the endogenous opioid system without medication. The techniques proposed include acupuncture and several methods of CNS activation using transcutaneous electrical stimulation. While attractive theoretically, this method is not yet deemed practical.

Long-Term Management. If patients are simply discharged from the hospital after withdrawal from opioids, there is a high probability of a quick return to compulsive opioid use. Numerous factors influence relapse. The withdrawal syndrome does not end in 5–7 days; a *protracted withdrawal syndrome* (see Table 24–6) persists for up to 6 months.

TABLE 24–6 ■ CHARACTERISTICS OF OPIOID WITHDRAWAL

SYMPTOMS	SIGNS
Regular withdrawal	
Craving for opioids	Pupillary dilation
Restlessness, irritability	Sweating
Increased sensitivity to pain	Piloerection ("gooseflesh")
Nausea, cramps	Tachycardia
Muscle aches	Vomiting, diarrhea
Dysphoric mood	Increased blood pressure
Insomnia, anxiety	Yawning
	Fever
Protracted withdrawal	
Anxiety	Cyclic changes in weight, pupil size, respiratory center sensitivity
Insomnia	
Drug craving	

Physiological measures tend to oscillate as though a new set point were being established; during this phase, outpatient drug-free treatment has a low probability of success, even when the patient has received intensive prior treatment while protected from relapse in a residential program.

The most successful treatment of heroin addiction consists of stabilization on methadone in accordance with state and federal regulations. Patients who relapse repeatedly during drug-free treatment can be transferred directly to methadone without requiring detoxification. The dose of methadone must be sufficient to prevent withdrawal symptoms for at least 24 h.

The introduction of buprenorphine, a partial agonist at the MOR, represents a major change in the treatment of opiate addiction. This drug produces minimal withdrawal symptoms when discontinued and has a low potential for overdose, a long duration of action, and the ability to block heroin effects. Treatment can take place in a qualified physician's private office rather than in a special center, as required for methadone. When taken sublingually, buprenorphine is active; unfortunately, it also can be dissolved and injected (abused). As a solution to this problem, a buprenorphine-naloxone combination is available. When taken orally (sublingually), the naloxone moiety is not effective, but if the patient abuses the medication by injecting a solution of it, the naloxone will block or diminish the subjective high that could be produced by buprenorphine alone.

Antagonist Treatment. Naltrexone is an antagonist with a high affinity for MOR; it will competitively block the effects of heroin or MOR agonists. Naltrexone will not satisfy craving or relieve protracted withdrawal symptoms, but it can be used after detoxification for patients with high motivation to remain opioid free. Recently, an extended-release depot version of naltrexone has become available (Lee et al., 2016) .

Clinical Issues: Cocaine and Other Psychostimulants

Cocaine

In the U.S. in 2014–2015, the number of people aged 12 years or older who are regular users of cocaine (at least monthly) in 2009 was about 1.5 million (FDA, 2016). About 60% of these met the criteria for dependence or abuse defined by the *Diagnostic and Statistical Manual of Mental Disorders* (American Psychiatric Association, 2013). Cocaine abuse occurs about twice as frequently in men as in women. Not all users become addicts. A key factor in addiction is the widespread availability of relatively inexpensive cocaine in the alkaloidal form (free base, "crack"), suitable for smoking, and in the hydrochloride powder form, suitable for nasal or intravenous use.

The reinforcing effects of cocaine and cocaine analogues correlate best with their effectiveness in inhibiting DAT, the transporter that recovers DA from the synapse. This leads to increased DA concentrations at critical brain sites. However, cocaine also blocks both NE and 5HT reuptake, and chronic use of cocaine leads to changes in these neurotransmitter systems as well. Cocaine produces a dose-dependent increase in heart rate and blood pressure accompanied by increased arousal, improved performance on tasks of vigilance and alertness, and a sense of self-confidence and well-being. Higher doses produce euphoria, which has a brief duration and often is followed by a desire for more drug. Repeated doses of cocaine may lead to involuntary motor activity, stereotyped behavior, and paranoia. Irritability and increased risk of violence are found among heavy chronic users. The $t_{1/2}$ of cocaine in plasma is about 50 min, but inhalant (crack) users typically desire more cocaine after 10–30 min.

COCAINE

The major route for cocaine metabolism involves hydrolysis of its two ester groups. Tissue esterases and spontaneous hydrolysis remove the methyl ester to produce benzoylecgonine (30–40%); removal of the benzoyl moiety by butyrylcholinesterase yields ecgonine methyl ester (~50%). As a pharmacokinetic approach to treating cocaine toxicity and abuse, catalytic antibodies and mutations of human butyrylcholinesterase and a bacterial cocaine esterase have been developed that speed cocaine metabolism in animal models (Schindler and Goldberg, 2012).

Benzoylecgonine, produced on loss of the methyl group, represents the major urinary metabolite and can be found in the urine for 2–5 days after a binge. As a result, the benzoylecgonine test is a valid method for detecting cocaine use; the metabolite remains detectable in the urine of heavy users for up to 10 days. Ethanol is frequently abused with cocaine, as it reduces the irritability induced by cocaine. Dual addiction to alcohol and cocaine is common. When cocaine and alcohol are taken concurrently, cocaine may be transesterified to cocaethylene, which is equipotent to cocaine in blocking DA reuptake.

Addiction is the most common complication of cocaine abuse. In general, stimulants tend to be abused much more irregularly than opioids, nicotine, and alcohol. Binge use is common, and a binge may last hours to days, terminating only when supplies of the drug are exhausted.

Toxicity

Other risks of cocaine, beyond the potential for addiction, include cardiac arrhythmias, myocardial ischemia, myocarditis, aortic dissection, cerebral vasoconstriction, and seizures. Death from trauma also is associated with cocaine use. Cocaine may induce premature labor and abruptio placentae. Cocaine has been reported to produce a prolonged and intense orgasm if taken prior to intercourse, and users often indulge in compulsive and promiscuous sexual activity. However, chronic cocaine use reduces sexual drive. Chronic use is also associated with psychiatric disorders, including anxiety, depression, and psychosis.

Tolerance, Dependence, and Withdrawal

In intermittent users of cocaine, the euphoric effect typically is not subject to sensitization. On the contrary, most experienced users become desensitized and, over time, require more cocaine to obtain euphoria (i.e., tolerance develops). Because cocaine typically is used intermittently, even heavy users go through frequent periods of withdrawal or "crash." The symptoms of withdrawal seen in users admitted to hospitals are listed in Table 24–7. Careful studies of cocaine users during withdrawal showed gradual diminution of these symptoms over 1–3 weeks. Residual depression, often seen after cocaine withdrawal, should be treated with antidepressant agents if it persists (see Chapter 15).

Pharmacological Interventions

Because cocaine withdrawal is generally mild, treatment of withdrawal symptoms usually is not required. The major problem in treatment is not detoxification but helping the patient to resist the urge to resume compulsive cocaine use. Rehabilitation programs involving individual and group psychotherapy based on the principles of Alcoholics Anonymous and behavioral treatments based on reinforcing cocaine-free urine tests result in significant improvement in the majority of cocaine users.

Animal models suggest that enhancing GABAergic inhibition can reduce reinstatement of cocaine self-administration, and a controlled clinical trial of topiramate showed a significant reduction in cocaine use. Topiramate also reduced the relapse rate in alcoholics, prompting current studies in patients dually dependent on cocaine and alcohol. Baclofen, a $GABA_B$ agonist, was found in a single-site trial to reduce relapse in cocaine addicts but was not effective in a multisite trial. Modafinil is currently

TABLE 24–7 ■ COCAINE WITHDRAWAL SYMPTOMS AND SIGNS
Dysphoria, depression
Sleepiness, fatigue
Cocaine craving
Bradycardia

being tested in clinical trials of cocaine, methamphetamine, alcohol, and other substance abuse disorders. A mild stimulant approved for treating narcolepsy, modafinil has had several positive clinical trials for use in cocaine withdrawal (Morgan et al., 2016). The medication reduces the euphoria produced by cocaine and relieves cocaine withdrawal symptoms. It remains under investigation for this purpose.

A novel approach to cocaine addiction employs a vaccine that produces cocaine-binding antibodies. Cocaine itself is not antigenic in humans; however, a conjugate of the cocaine metabolite, nor-cocaine, with the B subunit of cholera toxin has been constituted as a vaccine, and it causes a vigorous immune response with the production of antibodies (immunoglobulin G) that neutralize cocaine in the bloodstream. Initial reports were promising, but in a recent trial the vaccine did not demonstrate the expected efficiency (Kosten et al., 2014). For now, behavioral therapy remains the treatment of choice, with medication indicated for specific coexisting disorders such as depression.

Amphetamine and Related Agents

Subjective effects similar to those of cocaine are produced by *amphetamine, dextroamphetamine, methamphetamine, phenmetrazine, methylphenidate*, and *diethylpropion*. Amphetamines increase synaptic DA, NE, and 5HT primarily by stimulating presynaptic release of stored neurotransmitter (see Chapter 8). Intravenous or smoked methamphetamine produces an abuse/dependence syndrome similar to that of cocaine, although clinical deterioration may progress more rapidly. Methamphetamine addiction has become a major public health problem in the U.S. Behavioral and medical treatments for methamphetamine addiction are similar to those used for cocaine.

Caffeine

Caffeine, a mild stimulant, is the most widely used psychoactive drug in the world. It is present in soft drinks, coffee, tea, cocoa, chocolate, and numerous prescription and over-the-counter drugs.

Caffeine can inhibit cyclic nucleotide phosphodiesterases, mildly increases NE and DA release, and enhances neural activity in numerous brain areas. Caffeine is absorbed from the digestive tract, is distributed rapidly throughout all tissues, and easily crosses the placental barrier. Caffeine is metabolized largely by CYP1A2, yielding a mean biological half-life of ~5 h, a number that can vary widely. For instance, tobacco smoking reduces it by ~40%; oral contraceptives double it; fluvoxamine increases caffeine's half-life tenfold. Many of caffeine's effects are believed to occur by means of competitive antagonism at adenosine receptors. Adenosine is a neuromodulator (see Chapter 14) that resembles caffeine structurally. The mild sedating effects that occur when adenosine activates particular adenosine receptor subtypes can be antagonized by caffeine. Tolerance occurs rapidly to the stimulating effects of caffeine. Thus, a mild withdrawal syndrome has been produced in controlled studies by abruptly discontinuing the intake of as little as one to two cups of coffee per day. Caffeine withdrawal consists of feelings of fatigue and sedation. With higher doses, headaches and nausea have been reported during withdrawal; vomiting is rare.

Cannabinoids (Marijuana)

The cannabis plant has been cultivated for centuries for its presumed medicinal and psychoactive properties. The smoke from burning cannabis contains many chemicals, including 61 different cannabinoids that have been identified. One of these, Δ9-THC, produces most of the characteristic pharmacological effects of smoked marijuana. In the U.S., marijuana use remains prohibited by federal law, but it is approved in thirteen states as medicine and in eight states for recreational purposes. This is leading to increased marijuana use and a greater number of marijuana-associated auto accidents. The issues of whether and how to control the use of marijuana have not been resolved. In addition, the potencies of available botanical forms have generally not been standardized, and the dangers inherent in inhaling a smoke replete with organic molecules have not been defined for marijuana smoke.

The human cannabinoid endogenous ligand/receptor/signaling systems are described in Chapter 14 (see Figure 14–17). This system is stimulated by exogenous Δ9-THC. The pharmacological effects of Δ9-THC vary with the dose, route of administration, experience of the user, vulnerability to psychoactive effects, and setting of use. Intoxication with marijuana produces changes in mood, perception, and motivation, but the effects most frequently sought are a "high" and a "mellowing out." Effects vary with dose, but typically last about 2 h. During the high, cognitive functions, perception, reaction time, learning, and memory are impaired. Coordination and tracking behavior may be impaired for several hours beyond the perception of the high. Marijuana also produces complex behavioral changes such as giddiness and increased hunger. Unpleasant reactions such as panic or hallucinations and even acute psychosis may occur. These reactions are seen commonly with higher doses and with oral ingestion rather than smoked marijuana. Numerous clinical reports suggest that marijuana use may precipitate a recurrence of psychosis in people with a history of schizophrenia. One of the most controversial putative effects of marijuana is the production of an "amotivational syndrome." This syndrome is not an official diagnosis but has been used to describe young people who drop out of social activities and show little interest in school, work, or other goal-directed activity. At the cellular level, there is no evidence that marijuana damages brain cells or produces any permanent functional changes. There is evidence that the CB_1 receptor, a highly abundant GPCR in the mammalian brain, can deliver neuroprotective signals in animal models of striatal damage (Blázquez et al., 2015).

Marijuana has medicinal effects, including antiemetic properties that relieve side effects of anticancer chemotherapy. It also has muscle-relaxing effects, anticonvulsant properties, and the capacity to reduce the elevated intraocular pressure of glaucoma. These medical benefits come at the cost of the psychoactive effects that often impair normal activities. Dronabinol is an approved formulation of Δ9-THC (see Chapters 14 and 50).

Tolerance, Dependence, and Withdrawal

Tolerance to most of the effects of marijuana can develop rapidly after only a few doses, but also disappears rapidly. Withdrawal symptoms are not seen in clinical populations. Human subjects develop a withdrawal syndrome when they receive regular oral doses of the agent (Table 24–8). This syndrome, however, is only seen clinically in persons who use marijuana on a daily basis and then suddenly stop. Marijuana abuse and addiction have no specific treatments. Heavy users may suffer from accompanying depression and thus may respond to antidepressant medication.

Psychedelic Agents

There are two main categories of psychedelic compounds, indoleamines and phenethylamines. The indoleamine hallucinogens include LSD, DMT, and psilocybin. The phenethylamines include mescaline, DOM, MDA, and MDMA. Both groups have a relatively high affinity for $5HT_2$ receptors (see Chapter 13), but they differ in their affinity for other subtypes of 5HT receptors. There is a good correlation between the relative affinity of these compounds for $5HT_2$ receptors and their potency as hallucinogens in humans. LSD interacts with most brain 5HT receptors as an agonist/partial agonist and elicits sensory distortions (especially visual) and hallucinations at doses as low as 1 μg/kg. Current hypotheses of the mechanism of action of LSD and other hallucinogens focus on $5HT_{2A}$ receptor–mediated disruption of thalamic gating with sensory overload of the cortex (Nichols, 2016).

TABLE 24–8 ■ MARIJUANA WITHDRAWAL SYNDROME
Restlessness
Irritability
Mild agitation
Insomnia
Sleep EEG disturbance
Nausea, cramping

LSD

LSD is the most potent hallucinogenic drug, more than 3000 times more potent than mescaline. LSD is sold on the illicit market in a variety of forms. A popular contemporary system involves postage stamp–size papers impregnated with varying doses of LSD (50–300 μg or more).

The effects of hallucinogenic drugs are variable, even in the same individual on different occasions. LSD is absorbed rapidly after oral administration, with effects beginning at 40–60 min, peaking at 2–4 h, and gradually returning to baseline over 6–8 h. At a dose of 100 μg, LSD produces perceptual distortions and sometimes hallucinations; mood changes, including elation, paranoia, or depression; intense arousal; and sometimes a feeling of panic. Signs of LSD ingestion include pupillary dilation, increased blood pressure and pulse, flushing, salivation, lacrimation, and hyperreflexia. Visual effects are prominent. Colors seem more intense, and shapes may appear altered. The subject may focus attention on unusual items, such as the pattern of hairs on the back of the hand.

A "bad trip" usually consists of severe anxiety, although at times it can be marked by intense depression and suicidal thoughts. Visual disturbances usually are prominent. There are no documented toxic fatalities from LSD use, but fatal accidents and suicides have occurred during or shortly after intoxication. Prolonged psychotic reactions lasting 2 days or more may occur after the ingestion of a hallucinogen. Schizophrenic episodes may be precipitated in susceptible individuals, and there is some evidence that chronic use of these drugs is associated with the development of persistent psychotic disorders. Claims about the potential of psychedelic drugs for enhancing psychotherapy and for treating addictions and other mental disorders are not supported by controlled studies; there is no generally accepted indication for these drugs as medications.

Tolerance, Physical Dependence, and Withdrawal. Frequent, repeated use of psychedelic drugs is unusual; thus, tolerance is not commonly seen. Tolerance does develop to the behavioral effects of LSD after three or four daily doses, but no withdrawal syndrome has been observed.

Pharmacological Intervention. Because of the unpredictability of psychedelic drug effects, any use carries some risk. Users may require medical attention because of bad trips. Severe agitation may respond to diazepam (20 mg orally). "Talking down" by reassurance also is effective and is the management of first choice. Antipsychotic medications (see Chapter 16) may intensify the experience and thus are contraindicated. A particularly troubling aftereffect of LSD and similar drugs is the occasional occurrence of episodic visual disturbances. These originally were called "flashbacks" and resembled the experiences of prior LSD trips. Flashbacks belong to an official diagnostic category called the *hallucinogen persisting perception disorder*. The symptoms include false fleeting perceptions in the peripheral fields, flashes of color, geometric pseudohallucinations, and positive afterimages. The visual disorder appears stable in half the cases and represents an apparently permanent alteration of the visual system. Precipitants include stress, fatigue, emergence into a dark environment, marijuana, antipsychotic agents, and anxiety states.

MDMA ("Ecstasy") and MDA

MDMA and MDA are phenylethylamines that have stimulant as well as psychedelic effects.

Acute effects are dose dependent and include feelings of energy, altered sense of time, and pleasant sensory experiences with enhanced perception. Negative effects include tachycardia, dry mouth, jaw clenching, and muscle aches. At higher doses, visual hallucinations, agitation, hyperthermia, and panic attacks have been reported. A typical oral dose is one or two 100-mg tablets, producing effects lasting 3–6 h, although dosage and potency of street samples are variable (~100 mg of active drug per tablet).

Phencyclidine

PCP was developed originally as an anesthetic in the 1950s and later was abandoned because of a high frequency of postoperative delirium with hallucinations. It was classified as a dissociative anesthetic because, in the anesthetized state, the patient remains conscious with staring gaze, flat facies, and rigid muscles. PCP became a drug of abuse in the 1970s, first in an oral form and then in a smoked version enabling a better regulation of the dose.

As little as 50 μg/kg produces emotional withdrawal, concrete thinking, and bizarre responses to projective testing. Catatonic posturing also is produced and resembles that of schizophrenia. Abusers taking higher doses may appear to be reacting to hallucinations and may exhibit hostile or assaultive behavior. Anesthetic effects increase with dosage; stupor or coma may occur with muscular rigidity, rhabdomyolysis, and hyperthermia. Intoxicated patients in the emergency room may progress from aggressive behavior to coma, with elevated blood pressure and enlarged, nonreactive pupils. PCP binds with high affinity to sites located in the cortex and limbic structures, blocking NMDA-type glutamate receptors (see Table 14–2 and Figures 14–12 and 14–13). There is evidence that NMDA receptors are involved in ischemic neuronal death caused by high levels of excitatory amino acids; as a result, there is interest in PCP analogues that block NMDA receptors but with fewer psychoactive effects. Both PCP and ketamine ("special K"), another "club drug," produce similar effects by altering the distribution of the neurotransmitter glutamate.

Medical Intervention. Overdose must be treated by life support; there is no antagonist of PCP effects and no proven way to enhance excretion, although acidification of the urine has been proposed. PCP coma may last 7–10 days. The agitated or psychotic state produced by PCP can be treated with diazepam. Prolonged psychotic behavior requires antipsychotic medication. Because of the anticholinergic activity of PCP, antipsychotic agents with significant anticholinergic effects such as chlorpromazine should be avoided.

Bibliography

American Psychiatric Association. *Diagnostic and Statistical Manual of Mental Disorders*. 5th ed. American Psychiatric Publishing, Arlington, VA, **2013**.

Benowitz NL, et al. Nicotine absorption and cardiovascular effects with smokeless tobacco use: comparison with cigarettes and nicotine gum. *Clin Pharmacol Ther*, **1988**, *44*:23–28.

Blázquez C, et al. The CB_1 cannabinoid receptor signals striatal neuroprotection via a PI3K/Akt/mTORC1/BDNF pathway. *Cell Death Differ*, **2015**, *22*:1618–1629.

DEA. 2015 National Drug Threat Assessment Summary. **2015**. Available at: https://www.dea.gov/docs/2015%20NDTA%20Report.pdf. Accessed July 13, 2016.

Dowell D, et al. CDC guideline for prescribing opioids for chronic pain—United-States, 2016. *MMWR Recomm Rep*, **2016**, *65*(No. RR-1):1–49. doi:http://dx.doi.org/10.15585/mmwr.rr6501e1. Accessed July 13, 2016.

FDA. What is the scope of cocaine use in the United States? **2016**. Available at: https://www.drugabuse.gov/publications/research-reports/cocaine/what-scope-cocaine-use-in-united-states. Accessed July 12, 2016.

Kosten TR, et al. Vaccine for cocaine dependence: a randomized double-blind placebo-controlled efficacy trial. *Drug Alcohol Depend*, **2014**, *140*:42–47.

Lee JD, et al. Extended-release naltrexone to prevent opioid relapse in criminal justice offenders. *N Engl J Med*, **2016**, *374*:1232–1242.

Manchikanti L, et al. Zohydro™ approval by Food and Drug Administration: controversial or frightening? A health policy review. *Pain Physician*, **2014**, *17*:E437–E450.

McLellan AT, et al. Drug dependence, a chronic medical illness: Implications for treatment, insurance, and outcomes evaluation. *JAMA*, **2000**, *13*:1689–1695.

Morgan PT, et al. Modafinil and sleep architecture in an inpatatient-outpatient treatment study of cocaine dependence. *Drug Alcohol Depend*, **2016**, *160*:49–56.

Nichols DE. Psychedelics. *Pharmacol Rev*, **2016**, *68*:264–355.

Pettinati HM, et al. The status of naltrexone in the treatment of alcohol dependence. *J Clin Psychopharmacol*, **2006**, *26*:610–625.

Rudd RA, et al. Increases in drug and opioid overdose deaths—United States, 2000–2014. *Am J Transplant*, **2016**, *16*:1323–1327.

Schindler CW, Goldberg SR. Accelerating cocaine metabolism as an approach to the treatment of cocaine abuse and toxicity. *Future Med Chem*, **2012**;*4*:163–175.

Srivastava ED, et al. Sensitivity and tolerance to nicotine in smokers and nonsmokers. *Psychopharmacology*, **1991**, *105*:63–68.

Wilhelmsen KC, et al. The search for genes related to a low-level response to alcohol determined by alcohol challenges. *Alcohol Clin Exp Res*, **2003**, *27*:1041–1047.

Williams KE, et al. A double-blind study evaluating the long-term safety of varenicline for smoking cessation. *Curr Med Res Opin*, **2007**, *23*:793–801.

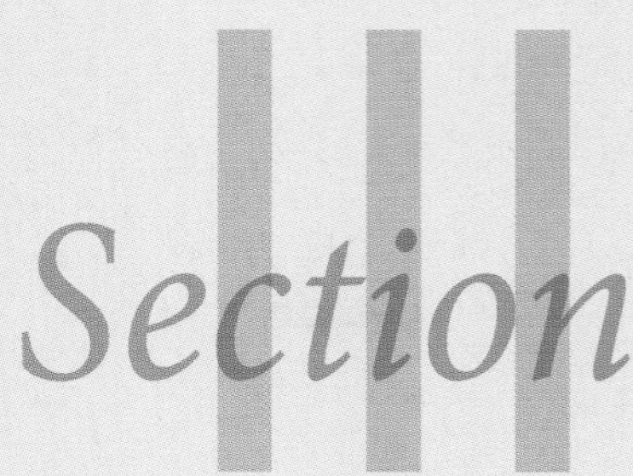

Modulation of Pulmonary, Renal, and Cardiovascular Function

第三篇 肺、肾和心血管功能的调节

Drugs Affecting Renal Excretory Function

Edwin K. Jackson

第二十五章　影响肾脏排泄功能的药物

PART I: RENAL PHYSIOLOGY AND DIURETIC DRUG ACTION

- Renal Anatomy and Physiology
- Principles of Diuretic Action
- Inhibitors of Carbonic Anhydrase
- Osmotic Diuretics
- Inhibitors of Na^+-K^+-$2Cl^-$ Symport: Loop Diuretics, High-Ceiling Diuretics
- Inhibitors of Na^+-Cl^- Symport: Thiazide-Type and Thiazide-Like Diuretics
- Inhibitors of Renal Epithelial Na^+ Channels: K^+-Sparing Diuretics
- Antagonists of Mineralocorticoid Receptors: Aldosterone Antagonists, K^+-Sparing Diuretics
- Inhibitors of the Nonspecific Cation Channel: Natriuretic Peptides
- Adenosine Receptor Antagonists
- Clinical Use of Diuretics

PART II: WATER HOMEOSTASIS AND THE VASOPRESSIN SYSTEM

- Vasopressin Physiology
- Vasopressin Receptor Agonists
- Diseases Affecting the Vasopressin System
- Clinical Use of Vasopressin Agonists
- Clinical Use of Vasopressin Antagonists

中文导读

本章主要介绍：肾脏生理和利尿药作用，包括肾脏解剖学和生理学、利尿药作用原理、碳酸酐酶抑制药、渗透性利尿药、Na^+-K^+-$2Cl^-$同向转运抑制药（髓袢利尿药和高效利尿药）、Na^+-Cl^-同向转运抑制药（噻嗪类利尿药及其类似物）、肾上皮细胞Na^+通道阻滞药（保钾利尿药）、盐皮质激素受体拮抗药（醛固酮拮抗药和保钾利尿药）、非特异性阳离子通道阻滞药（利钠肽）、腺苷受体拮抗药、利尿药的临床应用；水稳态和血管升压素系统，包括升压素的生理学、升压素受体激动药、影响升压素系统的疾病、升压素激动药和拮抗药的临床应用。

Abbreviations

AA: arachidonic acid
ACTH: corticotropin (previously adrenocorticotropic hormone)
ADH: antidiuretic hormone
AIP: aldosterone-induced protein
Aldo: aldosterone
Ang: angiotensin
ANP: atrial natriuretic peptide
ATL: ascending thin limb
AVP: arginine vasopressin
BL: basolateral membrane
BNP: brain natriuretic peptide
CA: carbonic anhydrase
cGMP: cyclic guanosine monophosphate
CHF: congestive heart failure
CNGC: cyclic nucleotide-gated cation channel
CNP: C-type natriuretic peptide
CNT: connecting tubule
COX: cyclooxygenase
DAG: diacyglycerol
DCT: distal convoluted tubule
DDAVP: 1-deamino-8-D-AVP (desmopressin)
DI: diabetes insipidus
DTL: descending thin limb
ECFV: extracellular fluid volume
ENaC: epithelial Na^+ channel
ENCC1 or TSC: the absorptive Na^+-Cl^- symporter
ENCC2, NKCC2, or BSC1: the absorptive Na^+-K^+-$2Cl^-$
ENCC3, NKCC1, or BSC2: the secretory symporter
FDA: Food and Drug Administration
FF: filtration fraction
GFR: glomerular filtration rate
GPCR: G protein–coupled receptor
GTP: guanosine triphosphate
HCTZ: hydrochlorothiazide
HDL: high-density lipoprotein
HSD: 11-β-hydroxysteroid dehydrogenase
IMCD: inner medullary collecting duct
IP_3: inositol trisphosphate
LDL: low-density lipoprotein
LM: luminal membrane
LOX: lipoxygenase
LT: leukotriene
MR: mineralocorticoid receptor
MRA: mineralocorticoid receptor antagonist
mRNA: messenger RNA
NP: natriuretic peptide
NPA: asparagine-proline-alanine
NPR_: natriuretic peptide receptor _ (e.g., NPRA, B, or C)
NSAID: nonsteroidal anti-inflammatory drug
OAT: organic anion transporter
PA: phosphatidic acid
PG: prostaglandin
PK_ : protein kinase _ (e.g. PKA, PKB, PKG)
PL_ : phospholipase _ (e.g., PLC, PLD)
PTH: parathyroid hormone
PVN: paraventricular nucleus
RAAS: renin-angiotensin-aldosterone system
RAS: renin-angiotensin system
RBF: renal blood flow
SGK-1: serum and glucocorticoid-stimulated kinase 1
SIADH: syndrome of inappropriate secretion of ADH
SNS: sympathetic nervous system
SON: supraoptic nucleus
TAL: thick ascending limb
TGF: tubuloglomerular feedback
TX: thromboxane
VP: vasopressin
VRUT: vasopressin-regulated urea transporter
vWD: von Willebrand disease
WCV: water channel-containing vesicle

The kidney filters the extracellular fluid volume across the renal glomeruli an average of 12 times a day, and the renal nephrons precisely regulate the fluid volume of the body and its electrolyte content via processes of secretion and reabsorption. Disease states such as hypertension, heart failure, renal failure, nephrotic syndrome, and cirrhosis may disrupt this balance. Diuretics increase the rate of urine flow and Na^+ excretion and are used to adjust the volume or composition of body fluids in these disorders. Precise regulation of body fluid osmolality is also essential. It is controlled by a finely tuned homeostatic mechanism that operates by adjusting both the rate of water intake and the rate of solute-free water excretion by the kidneys—that is, water balance. Abnormalities in this homeostatic system can result from genetic diseases, acquired diseases, or drugs and may cause serious and potentially life-threatening deviations in plasma osmolality.

Part I of this chapter first describes renal physiology, then introduces diuretics with regard to mechanism and site of action, effects on urinary composition, and effects on renal hemodynamics, and then integrates diuretic pharmacology with a discussion of mechanisms of edema formation and the role of diuretics in clinical medicine. Specific therapeutic applications of diuretics are presented in Chapters 28 (hypertension) and 29 (heart failure). *Part II* of this chapter describes the vasopressin system that regulates water homeostasis and plasma osmolality and factors that perturb those mechanisms and examines pharmacological approaches for treating disorders of water balance.

Part I: Renal Physiology and Diuretic Drug Action

Renal Anatomy and Physiology

The basic urine-forming unit of the kidney is the nephron. The initial part of the nephron, the renal (Malpighian) corpuscle, consists of a capsule (Bowman's capsule) and a tuft of capillaries (the glomerulus) residing within the capsule. The glomerulus receives blood from an afferent arteriole, and blood exits the glomerulus via an efferent arteriole. Ultrafiltrate produced by the glomerulus collects in the space between the glomerulus and capsule (Bowman's space) and enters a long tubular portion of the nephron, where the ultrafiltrate is reabsorbed and conditioned. Each human kidney is composed of about 1 million nephrons. Figure 25–1 illustrates subdivisions of the nephron.

Glomerular Filtration

In the glomerular capillaries, a portion of plasma water is forced through a filter that has three basic components: the fenestrated capillary endothelial cells, a basement membrane lying just beneath the endothelial cells, and the filtration slit diaphragms formed by epithelial cells that cover the basement membrane on its urinary space side. Solutes of small size flow with filtered water (solvent drag) into Bowman's space, whereas formed elements and macromolecules are retained by the filtration barrier.

Overview of Nephron Function

The kidney filters large quantities of plasma, reabsorbs substances that the body must conserve, and leaves behind or secretes substances that must be eliminated. The changing architecture and cellular differentiation along the length of a nephron are crucial to these functions (see Figure 25–1). The two kidneys in humans together produce about 120 mL

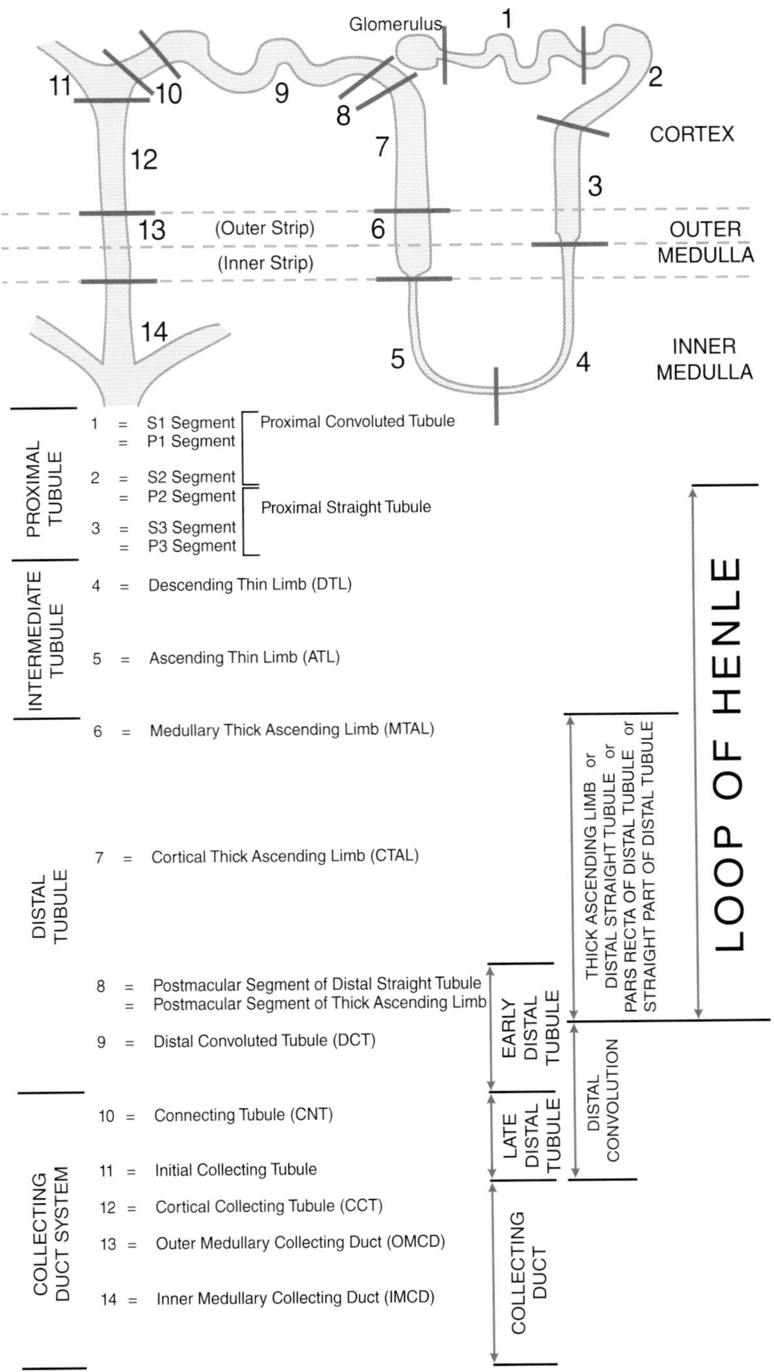

Figure 25–1 *Anatomy and nomenclature of the nephron.*

of ultrafiltrate/min, yet only 1 mL of urine/min of urine; more than 99% of the glomerular ultrafiltrate is reabsorbed at a staggering energy cost. The kidneys consume 7% of total-body O_2 intake despite comprising only 0.5% of body weight.

The proximal tubule is contiguous with Bowman's capsule and takes a tortuous path until finally forming a straight portion that dives into the renal medulla. Normally, about 65% of filtered Na^+ is reabsorbed in the proximal tubule, and because this part of the tubule is highly permeable to water, reabsorption is essentially isotonic. Between the outer and inner strips of the outer medulla, the tubule abruptly changes morphology to become the DTL, which penetrates the inner medulla, makes a hairpin turn, and then forms the ATL. At the juncture between the inner and outer medulla, the tubule once again changes morphology and becomes the TAL. Together, the proximal straight tubule, DTL, ATL, and TAL segments are known as the *loop of Henle*.

The DTL is highly permeable to water, yet its permeabilities to NaCl and urea are low. In contrast, the ATL is permeable to NaCl and urea but is impermeable to water. The TAL actively reabsorbs NaCl but is impermeable to water and urea. Approximately 25% of filtered Na^+ is reabsorbed in the loop of Henle, mostly in the TAL, which has a large reabsorptive capacity. The TAL passes between the afferent and efferent arterioles and makes contact with the afferent arteriole by means of a cluster of specialized columnar epithelial cells known as the *macula densa*. The macula densa is strategically located to sense concentrations of NaCl leaving the loop of Henle. If the concentration of NaCl is too high, the macula densa sends a chemical signal (perhaps adenosine or ATP) to the afferent arteriole of the same nephron, causing it to constrict, thereby reducing the GFR. This homeostatic mechanism, known as *TGF*, protects the organism from salt and volume wasting. The macula densa also regulates renin release from the adjacent juxtaglomerular cells in the wall of the afferent arteriole.

Approximately 0.2 mm past the macula densa, the tubule changes morphology once again to become the DCT. Like the TAL, the DCT actively transports NaCl and is impermeable to water. Because these characteristics impart the capacity to produce dilute urine, the TAL and the DCT are collectively called the *diluting segment of the nephron*, and the tubular fluid in the DCT is hypotonic regardless of hydration status. However, unlike the TAL, the DCT does not contribute to the countercurrent-induced hypertonicity of the medullary interstitium (described in material that follows).

The collecting duct system (segments 10–14 in Figure 25–1) is an area of fine control of ultrafiltrate composition and volume. It is here that final adjustments in electrolyte composition are made, a process modulated by the adrenal steroid *aldosterone*. Vasopressin (also called ADH) modulates water permeability of this part of the nephron as well. The more distal portions of the collecting duct pass through the renal medulla, where the interstitial fluid is markedly hypertonic. In the absence of ADH, the collecting duct system is impermeable to water, and dilute urine is excreted. In the presence of ADH, the collecting duct system is permeable to water, and water is reabsorbed. The movement of water out of the tubule is driven by the steep concentration gradient that exists between tubular fluid and medullary interstitium.

The hypertonicity of the medullary interstitium plays a vital role in the capacity of mammals and birds to concentrate urine, which is accomplished by a combination of the unique topography of the loop of Henle and the specialized permeabilities of the loop's subsegments. The "passive countercurrent multiplier hypothesis" proposes that active transport in the TAL concentrates NaCl in the interstitium of the outer medulla. Because this segment of the nephron is impermeable to water, active transport in the ascending limb dilutes the tubular fluid. As the dilute fluid passes into the collecting duct system, water is extracted if, and only if, ADH is present. Because the cortical and outer medullary collecting ducts have low permeability to urea, urea is concentrated in the tubular fluid. The IMCD, however, is permeable to urea, so urea diffuses into the inner medulla, where it is trapped by countercurrent exchange in the vasa recta (medullary capillaries that run parallel to the loop of Henle). Because the DTL is impermeable to salt and urea, the high urea concentration in the inner medulla extracts water from the DTL and concentrates NaCl in the tubular fluid of the DTL. As the tubular fluid enters the ATL, NaCl diffuses out of the salt-permeable ATL, thus contributing to the hypertonicity of the medullary interstitium.

General Mechanism of Renal Epithelial Transport

There are multiple mechanisms by which solutes may cross cell membranes (see Figure 5–4). The kinds of transport achieved in a nephron segment depend mainly on which transporters are present and whether they are embedded in the luminal or basolateral membrane. Figure 25–2 presents a general model of renal tubular transport that be summarized as follows:

1. Na^+, K^+-ATPase (sodium pump) in the basolateral membrane transports Na^+ into the intercellular and interstitial spaces and K^+ into the cell, establishing an electrochemical gradient for Na^+ across the cell membrane directed inward.
2. Na^+ can diffuse down this Na^+ gradient across the luminal membrane via Na^+ channels and via membrane symporters that use the energy stored in the Na^+ gradient to transport solutes out of the tubular lumen and into the cell (e.g., Na^+-glucose, Na^+-$H_2PO_4^-$, and Na^+-amino acid) and antiporters (e.g., Na^+-H^+) that move solutes into the lumen as Na^+ moves down its gradient and into the cell.
3. Na^+ exits the basolateral membrane into intercellular and interstitial spaces via the Na^+ pump.
4. The action of Na^+-linked symporters in the luminal membrane causes the concentration of substrates for these symporters to rise in the epithelial cell. These substrate/solute gradients then permit simple diffusion or mediated transport (e.g., symporters, antiporters, uniporters, and channels) of solutes into the intercellular and interstitial spaces.
5. Accumulation of Na^+ and other solutes in the intercellular space creates a small osmotic pressure differential across the epithelial cell. In water-permeable epithelium, water moves into the intercellular spaces driven by the osmotic pressure differential. Water moves through aqueous pores in both the luminal and the basolateral cell membranes, as well as through tight junctions (paracellular pathway). Bulk water flow carries some solutes into the intercellular space by solvent drag.
6. Movement of water into the intercellular space concentrates other solutes in the tubular fluid, resulting in an electrochemical gradient for these substances across the epithelium. Membrane-permeable solutes then move down their electrochemical gradients into the intercellular space by both the transcellular (e.g., simple diffusion, symporters, antiporters, uniporters, and channels) and paracellular pathways. Membrane-impermeable solutes remain in the tubular lumen and are excreted in the urine with an obligatory amount of water.
7. As water and solutes accumulate in the intercellular space, hydrostatic pressure increases, thus providing a driving force for bulk water flow. Bulk water flow carries solute out of the intercellular space into the interstitial space and, finally, into the peritubular capillaries.

Organic Acid and Organic Base Secretion

The kidney is a major organ involved in the elimination of organic chemicals from the body. Organic molecules may enter the renal tubules by glomerular filtration or may be actively secreted directly into tubules. The proximal tubule has a highly efficient transport system for organic acids and an equally efficient but separate transport system for organic bases. Current models for these secretory systems are illustrated in Figure 25–3. Both systems are powered by the sodium pump in the basolateral membrane, involve secondary and tertiary active transport, and use a facilitated diffusion step. There are many organic acid and organic base transporters (see Chapter 5). A family of OATs links countertransport of organic anions with dicarboxylates (Figure 25–3A).

Renal Handling of Specific Anions and Cations

Reabsorption of Cl^- generally follows reabsorption of Na^+. In segments of the tubule with low-resistance tight junctions (i.e., "leaky" epithelium), such as the proximal tubule and TAL, Cl^- movement can occur paracellularly. Cl^- crosses the luminal membrane by antiport with formate and oxalate (proximal tubule), symport with Na^+/K^+ (TAL), symport with Na^+ (DCT), and antiport with HCO_3^- (collecting duct system). Cl^- crosses the basolateral membrane via symport with K^+ (proximal tubule and TAL), antiport with Na^+/HCO_3^- (proximal tubule), and Cl^- channels (TAL, DCT, collecting duct system).

Of filtered K^+, 80%–90% is reabsorbed in the proximal tubule (diffusion and solvent drag) and TAL (diffusion), largely through the paracellular pathway. The DCT and collecting duct system secrete variable amounts of K^+ by a channel-mediated pathway. Modulation of the rate of K^+ secretion in the collecting duct system, particularly by aldosterone, allows urinary K^+ excretion to be matched with dietary intake. The transepithelial potential difference V_T, lumen positive in the TAL and lumen negative in the collecting duct system, drives K^+ reabsorption and secretion, respectively.

Most of the filtered Ca^{2+} (~70%) is reabsorbed by the proximal tubule by passive diffusion through a paracellular route. Another 25% of filtered Ca^{2+} is reabsorbed by the TAL in part by a paracellular route driven by the lumen-positive V_T and in part by active transcellular Ca^{2+} reabsorption modulated by PTH (see Chapter 43). Most of the remaining Ca^{2+} is reabsorbed in DCT by a transcellular pathway. The transcellular pathway in the

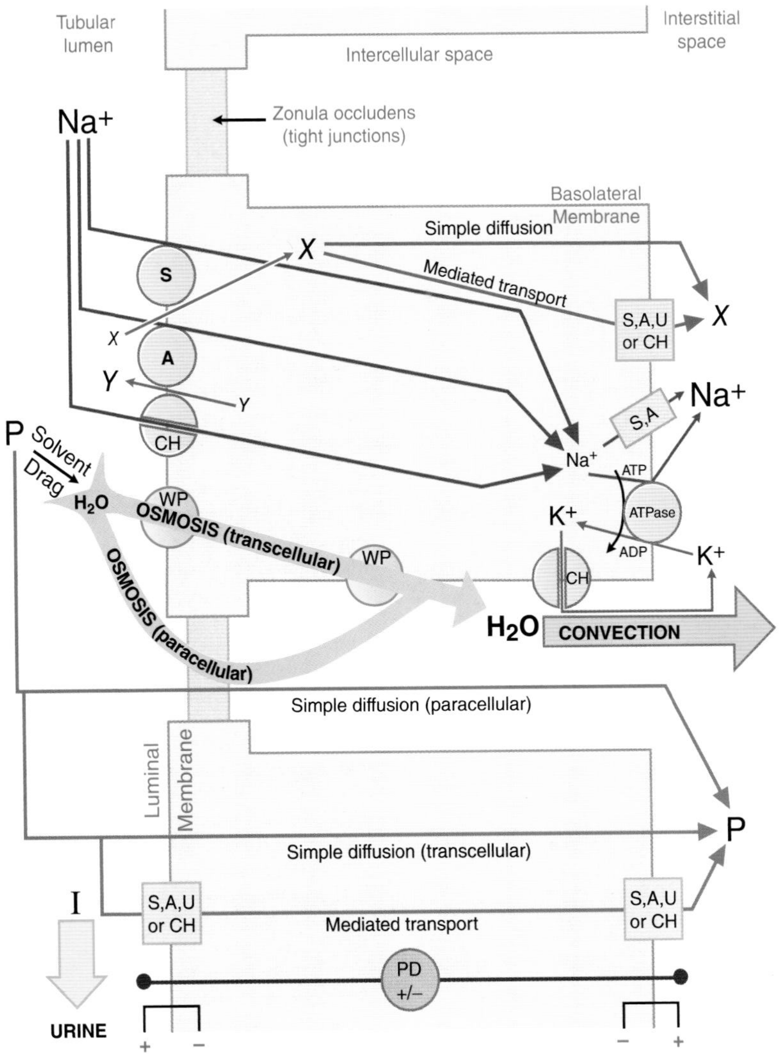

Figure 25–2 *Generic mechanism of renal epithelial cell transport* (see text for details). A, antiporter; ATPase, Na^+, K^+-ATPase (sodium pump); CH, ion channel; *I*, membrane-impermeable solutes; *P*, membrane-permeable solutes; PD, potential difference across indicated membrane or cell; S, symporter; U, uniporter; WP, water pore; *X* and *Y*, transported solutes.

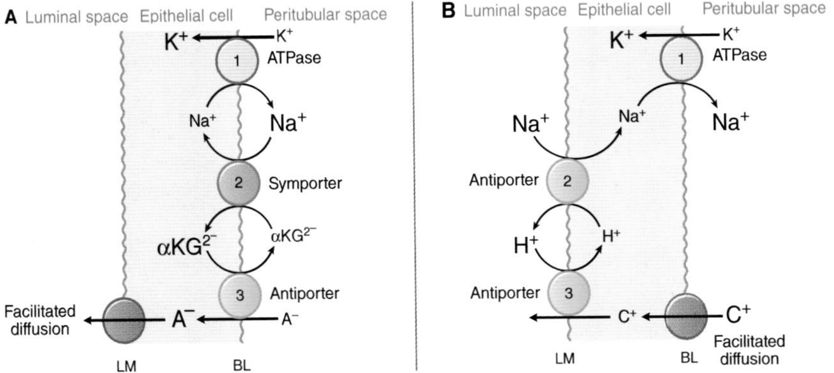

Figure 25–3 *Mechanisms of organic acid* (**A**) *and organic base* (**B**) *secretion in the proximal tubule.* The numbers 1, 2, and 3 refer to primary, secondary, and tertiary active transport, respectively. A^-, organic acid (anion); C^+, organic base (cation); αKG^{2-}, α-ketoglutarate but also other dicarboxylates. BL and LM indicate basolateral and luminal membranes, respectively.

TAL and DCT involves passive Ca^{2+} influx across the luminal membrane through Ca^{2+} channels (TRPV5, **transient receptor potential cation channel V5**), followed by Ca^{2+} extrusion across the basolateral membrane by a Ca^{2+}-ATPase. Also, in DCT and CNT, Ca^{2+} crosses the basolateral membrane by Na^+-Ca^{2+} exchanger (antiport). P_i is largely reabsorbed (80% of filtered load) by the proximal tubule. The Na^+-P_i symporter uses the free energy of the Na^+ electrochemical gradient to transport P_i into the cell. The Na^+-P_i symporter is inhibited by PTH.

The renal tubules reabsorb HCO_3^- and secrete protons (tubular acidification), thereby participating in acid-base balance. These processes are described in the section on carbonic anhydrase inhibitors.

Principles of Diuretic Action

Diuretics are drugs that increase the rate of urine flow; clinically useful diuretics also increase the rate of Na^+ excretion (natriuresis) and of an accompanying anion, usually Cl^-. Most clinical applications of diuretics are directed toward reducing extracellular fluid volume by decreasing total-body NaCl content.

Although continued diuretic administration causes a sustained net deficit in total-body Na^+, the time course of natriuresis is finite because renal compensatory mechanisms bring Na^+ excretion in line with Na^+ intake, a phenomenon known as *diuretic braking*. These compensatory mechanisms include activation of the sympathetic nervous system, activation of the renin-angiotensin-aldosterone axis, decreased arterial blood pressure (which reduces pressure natriuresis), renal epithelial cell hypertrophy, increased renal epithelial transporter expression, and perhaps alterations in natriuretic hormones such as ANP. The net effects on extracellular volume and body weight are shown in Figure 25–4.

Diuretics may modify renal handling of other cations (e.g., K^+, H^+, Ca^{2+}, and Mg^{2+}), anions (e.g., Cl^-, HCO_3^-, and $H_2PO_4^-$), and uric acid. In addition, diuretics may alter renal hemodynamics indirectly. Table 25–1 compares the general effects of the major diuretic classes.

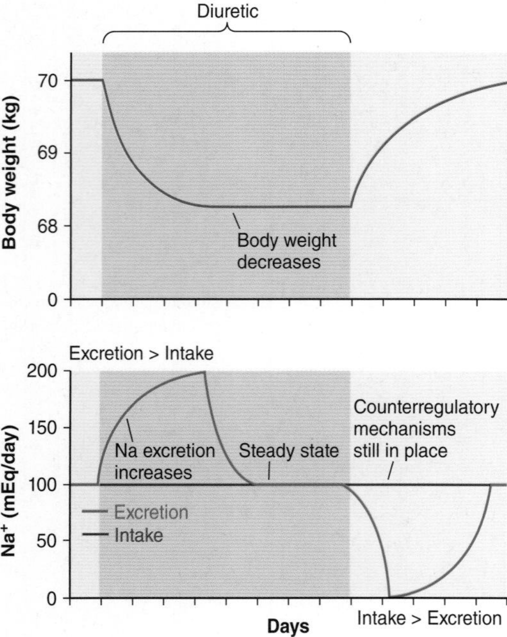

Figure 25–4 *Changes in extracellular fluid volume and weight with diuretic therapy.* The period of diuretic administration is shown in the shaded box along with its effects on body weight in the upper part of the figure and Na^{2+} excretion in the lower half of the figure. Initially, when Na^{2+} excretion exceeds intake, body weight and ECFV decrease. Subsequently, a new steady state is achieved where Na^+ intake and excretion are equal but at a lower ECFV and body weight. This results from activation of the RAAS and SNS, "the braking phenomenon." When the diuretic is discontinued, body weight and ECFV rise during a period when Na^{2+} intake exceeds excretion. A new steady state is then reached as stimulation of the RAAS and SNS wane.

Inhibitors of Carbonic Anhydrase

There are three orally administered carbonic anhydrase inhibitors—*acetazolamide, dichlorphenamide,* and *methazolamide* (Table 25–2).

Mechanism and Site of Action

Proximal tubular epithelial cells are richly endowed with the zinc metalloenzyme carbonic anhydrase, which is found in the luminal and basolateral membranes (type IV carbonic anhydrase), as well as in the cytoplasm (type II carbonic anhydrase) (Figure 25–5). Carbonic anhydrase plays a role in $NaHCO_3$ reabsorption and acid secretion.

In the proximal tubule, the free energy in the Na^+ gradient established by the basolateral Na^+ pump is used by a Na^+-H^+ antiporter (Na^+-H^+ exchanger type 3) in the luminal membrane to transport H^+ into the tubular lumen in exchange for Na^+. In the lumen, H^+ reacts with filtered HCO_3^- to form H_2CO_3, which decomposes rapidly to CO_2 and water in the presence of carbonic anhydrase in the brush border. Carbonic anhydrase reversibly accelerates this reaction several thousand fold. CO_2 is lipophilic and rapidly diffuses across the luminal membrane into the epithelial cell, where it reacts with water to form H_2CO_3, a reaction catalyzed by cytoplasmic carbonic anhydrase. Continued operation of the Na^+-H^+ antiporter maintains a low proton concentration in the cell, so H_2CO_3 ionizes spontaneously to form H^+ and HCO_3^-, creating an electrochemical gradient for HCO_3^- across the basolateral membrane. The electrochemical gradient for HCO_3^- is used by a Na^+-HCO_3^- symporter (also known as the Na^+-HCO_3^- cotransporter) in the basolateral membrane to transport $NaHCO_3$ into the interstitial space. The net effect of this process is transport of $NaHCO_3$ from the tubular lumen to the interstitial space, followed by movement of water (isotonic reabsorption). Removal of water concentrates Cl^- in the tubular lumen, and consequently, Cl^- diffuses down its concentration gradient into the interstitium by the paracellular pathway.

Carbonic anhydrase inhibitors potently inhibit both the membrane-bound and cytoplasmic forms of carbonic anhydrase, and can cause nearly complete abolition of $NaHCO_3$ reabsorption in the proximal tubule. However, due to the large excess of carbonic anhydrase activity in proximal tubules, a large fraction of the enzyme activity must be inhibited before an effect on electrolyte excretion is observed. Although the proximal tubule is the major site of action of carbonic anhydrase inhibitors, carbonic anhydrase also is involved in secretion of titratable acid in the collecting duct system, which is a secondary site of action for this class of drugs.

Effects on Urinary Excretion

Inhibition of carbonic anhydrase is associated with a rapid rise in urinary HCO_3^- excretion to about 35% of filtered load. This, along with inhibition of titratable acid and NH_4^+ secretion in the collecting duct system, results in an increase in urinary pH to about 8 and development of metabolic acidosis. However, even with a high degree of inhibition of carbonic anhydrase, 65% of HCO_3^- is rescued from excretion. The loop of Henle has large reabsorptive capacity and captures most of the Cl^- and a portion of the Na^+. Thus, only a small increase in Cl^- excretion occurs, HCO_3^- being the major anion excreted along with the cations Na^+ and K^+. The fractional excretion of Na^+ may be as much as 5%, and the fractional excretion of K^+ can be as much as 70%. The increased excretion of K^+ is in part secondary to increased delivery of Na^+ to the distal nephron, as described in the section on inhibitors of Na^+ channels. The effects of carbonic anhydrase inhibitors on renal excretion are self-limiting, probably because the resulting metabolic acidosis decreases the filtered load of HCO_3^- to the point that the uncatalyzed reaction between CO_2 and water is sufficient to achieve HCO_3^- reabsorption.

Effects on Renal Hemodynamics

By inhibiting proximal reabsorption, carbonic anhydrase inhibitors increase delivery of solutes to the macula densa. This triggers TGF, which increases afferent arteriolar resistance and reduces RBF and GFR.

TABLE 25–1 ■ EXCRETORY AND RENAL HEMODYNAMIC EFFECTS OF DIURETICS[a]

DIURETIC MECHANISM (Primary site of action)	CATIONS					ANIONS			URIC ACID		RENAL HEMODYNAMICS			
	Na^{+}	K^{+}	H^{+}[b]	Ca^{2+}	Mg^{2+}	Cl^{-}	HCO_3^{-}	$H_2PO_4^{-}$	*ACUTE*	*CHRONIC*	RBF	GFR	FF	TGF
Inhibitors of CA (proximal tubule)	+	++	–	NC	V	(+)	++	++	I	–	–	–	NC	+
Osmotic diuretics (loop of Henle)	++	+	I	+	++	+	+	+	+	I	+	NC	–	I
Inhibitors of Na^{+}-K^{+}-$2Cl^{-}$ symport (thick ascending limb)	++	++	+	++	++	++	+[c]	+[c]	+	–	V(+)	NC	V(–)	–
Inhibitors of Na^{+}-Cl^{-} symport (distal convoluted tubule)	+	++	+	V(–)	V(+)	+	+[c]	+[c]	+	–	NC	V(–)	V(–)	NC
Inhibitors of renal epithelial Na^{+} channels (late distal tubule, collecting duct)	+	–	–	–	–	+	(+)	NC	I	–	NC	NC	NC	NC
Antagonists of mineralocorticoid receptors (late distal tubule, collecting duct)	+	–	–	I	–	+	(+)	I	I	–	NC	NC	NC	NC

[a]Except for uric acid, changes are for acute effects of diuretics in the absence of significant volume depletion, which would trigger complex physiological adjustments.
[b]H^{+} includes titratable acid and NH_4^{+}.
[c]In general, these effects are restricted to those individual agents that inhibit carbonic anhydrase. However, there are notable exceptions in which symport inhibitors increase bicarbonate and phosphate (e.g., metolazone, bumetanide). ++, +, (+),–, NC, V, V(+), V(–) and I indicate marked increase, mild-to-moderate increase, slight increase, decrease, no change, variable effect, variable increase, variable decrease, and insufficient data, respectively. For cations and anions, the indicated effects refer to absolute changes in fractional excretion.

TABLE 25–2 ■ INHIBITORS OF CARBONIC ANHYDRASE

DRUG	RELATIVE POTENCY	ORAL AVAILABILITY	$t_{1/2}$ (hours)	ROUTE OF ELIMINATION
Acetazolamide	1	~100%	6–9	R
Dichlorphenamide	30	ID	ID	ID
Methazolamide	>1; <10	~100%	~14	~25% R, ~75% M

ID, insufficient data; M, metabolism; R, renal excretion of intact drug.

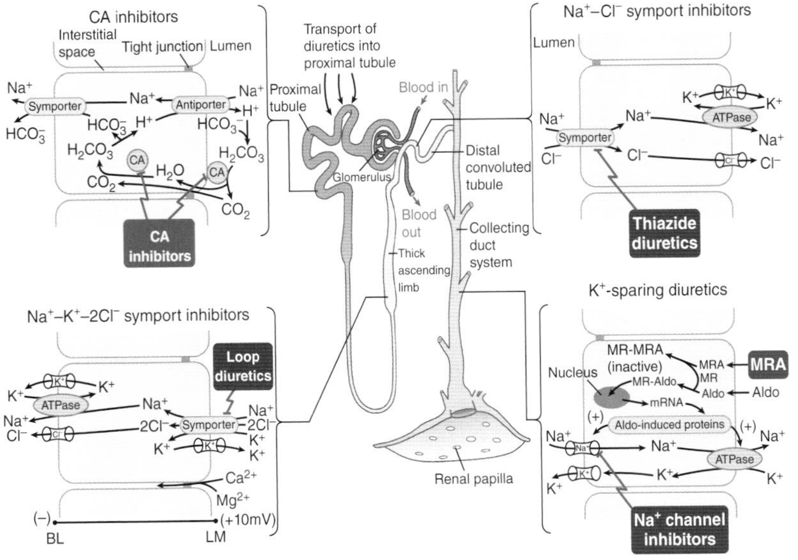

Figure 25–5 *Sites and mechanisms of action of diuretics.* Three important features are noteworthy: 1. Transport of solute across epithelial cells in all nephron segments involves highly specialized proteins, which for the most part are apical and basolateral membrane integral proteins. 2. Diuretics target and block the action of epithelial proteins involved in solute transport. 3. The site and mechanism of action of a given class of diuretics are determined by the specific protein inhibited by the diuretic.

Other Actions

These agents have extrarenal sites of action. Carbonic anhydrase in the ciliary processes of the eye mediates formation of HCO_3^- in aqueous humor. Inhibition of carbonic anhydrase decreases the rate of formation of aqueous humor and consequently reduces intraocular pressure. Acetazolamide frequently causes paresthesias and somnolence, suggesting an action of carbonic anhydrase inhibitors in the CNS. The efficacy of acetazolamide in epilepsy is due in part to the production of metabolic acidosis; however, direct actions of acetazolamide in the CNS also contribute to its anticonvulsant action. Owing to interference with carbonic anhydrase activity in erythrocytes, carbonic anhydrase inhibitors increase CO_2 levels in peripheral tissues and decrease CO_2 levels in expired gas. Acetazolamide causes vasodilation by opening vascular Ca^{2+}-activated K^+ channels; however, the clinical significance of this effect is unclear.

ADME

See Table 25–2 for pharmacokinetic data.

Therapeutic Uses

The efficacy of carbonic anhydrase inhibitors as single agents is low. The combination of acetazolamide with diuretics that block Na^+ reabsorption at more distal sites in the nephron causes a marked natriuretic response in patients with low basal fractional excretion of Na^+ (<0.2%) who are resistant to diuretic monotherapy. Even so, the long-term usefulness of carbonic anhydrase inhibitors often is compromised by the development of metabolic acidosis. The major indication for carbonic anhydrase inhibitors is open-angle glaucoma (Scozzafava and Supuran, 2014). Two products developed specifically for this use are dorzolamide and brinzolamide, which are available only as ophthalmic drops. Carbonic anhydrase inhibitors also may be employed for secondary glaucoma and preoperatively in acute-angle closure glaucoma to lower intraocular pressure before surgery (see Chapter 69). Orally administered acetazolamide also is used for the treatment of glaucoma (see Chapter 69) and absence seizures (see Chapter 21). Acetazolamide can provide symptomatic relief in patients with *high-altitude illness* or *mountain sickness* (Ritchie et al., 2012). Carbonic anhydrase inhibitors are also useful in patients with familial periodic paralysis. Dichlorphenamide is now approved for treating this syndrome. The mechanism for the beneficial effects of carbonic anhydrase inhibitors in altitude sickness and familial periodic paralysis may relate to the induction of a metabolic acidosis. Finally, carbonic anhydrase inhibitors can be useful for correcting metabolic alkalosis, especially one caused by diuretic-induced increases in H^+ excretion.

Toxicity, Adverse Effects, Contraindications, Drug Interactions

Serious toxic reactions to carbonic anhydrase inhibitors are infrequent; however, these drugs are sulfonamide derivatives and, like other sulfonamides, may cause bone marrow depression, skin toxicity, sulfonamide-like renal lesions, and allergic reactions. With large doses, many patients exhibit drowsiness and paresthesias. Most adverse effects, contraindications, and drug interactions are secondary to urinary alkalinization or metabolic acidosis, including (1) diversion of ammonia of renal origin from urine into the systemic circulation, a process that may induce or worsen hepatic encephalopathy (the drugs are contraindicated in patients with hepatic cirrhosis); (2) calculus formation and ureteral colic owing to precipitation of calcium phosphate salts in alkaline urine; (3) worsening of metabolic or respiratory acidosis (the drugs are contraindicated in patients with hyperchloremic acidosis or severe chronic obstructive pulmonary disease); and (4) reduction of the urinary excretion rate of weak organic bases.

Osmotic Diuretics

Osmotic diuretics (Table 25–3) are freely filtered at the glomerulus, undergo limited reabsorption by the renal tubule, and are relatively inert pharmacologically. Osmotic diuretics are administered in doses large enough to increase significantly the osmolality of plasma and tubular fluid. Of the osmotic diuretics listed, only glycerin and mannitol are currently available in the U.S.

TABLE 25–3 ■ OSMOTIC DIURETICS

DRUG	ORAL AVAILABILITY	$t_{1/2}$ (hours)	ROUTE OF ELIMINATION
Glycerin	Orally active	0.5–0.75	~80% M, ~20% U
Isosorbide[a]	Orally active	5–9.5	R
Mannitol	Negligible	0.25–1.7[b]	~80% R, ~20% M + B
Urea[a]	Negligible	1.2	R

B, excretion of intact drug into bile; M, metabolism; R, renal excretion of intact drug; U, unknown pathway of elimination.
[a]Not available in the U.S.
[b]In renal failure, 6–36 h.

Mechanism and Site of Action

Osmotic diuretics act in both the proximal tubule and the loop of Henle, with the latter the primary site of action. In the proximal tubule, osmotic diuretics act as nonreabsorbable solutes that limit the osmosis of water into the interstitial space and thereby reduce the luminal Na^+ concentration to the point that net Na^+ reabsorption ceases. By extracting water from intracellular compartments, osmotic diuretics expand extracellular fluid volume, decrease blood viscosity, and inhibit renin release. These effects increase RBF, and the increase in renal medullary blood flow removes NaCl and urea from the renal medulla, thus reducing medullary tonicity. A reduction in medullary tonicity causes a decrease in the extraction of water from the DTL, which in turn limits the concentration of NaCl in the tubular fluid entering the ATL. This latter effect diminishes the passive reabsorption of NaCl in the ATL. In addition, osmotic diuretics inhibit Mg^{2+} reabsorption in the TAL.

Effects on Urinary Excretion

Osmotic diuretics increase urinary excretion of nearly all electrolytes, including Na^+, K^+, Ca^{2+}, Mg^{2+}, Cl^-, HCO_3^-, and phosphate.

Effects on Renal Hemodynamics

Osmotic diuretics increase RBF by a variety of mechanisms, but total GFR is little changed.

ADME

Pharmacokinetic data on the osmotic diuretics are gathered in Table 25–3. Where available, glycerin and isosorbide can be given orally, whereas mannitol and urea must be administered intravenously (with the exception that mannitol powder is used by inhalation for diagnosis of bronchial hyperreactivity).

Therapeutic Uses

One use for mannitol is in the treatment of dialysis disequilibrium syndrome. Overly removing solutes from the extracellular fluid by hemodialysis results in a reduction in the osmolality of extracellular fluid. Consequently, water moves from the extracellular compartment into the intracellular compartment, causing hypotension and CNS symptoms (headache, nausea, muscle cramps, restlessness, CNS depression, and convulsions). Osmotic diuretics increase the osmolality of the extracellular fluid compartment and thereby shift water back into the extracellular compartment. By increasing the osmotic pressure of plasma, osmotic diuretics extract water from the eye and brain. Osmotic diuretics are used to control intraocular pressure during acute attacks of glaucoma and for short-term reductions in intraocular pressure both preoperatively and postoperatively in patients who require ocular surgery. Also, mannitol is used to reduce cerebral edema and brain mass before and after neurosurgery and to control intracranial pressure in patients with traumatic brain injury (Wakai et al., 2013). Mannitol is often used to treat or prevent acute kidney injury; however, it is questionable regarding whether mannitol improves renal outcomes (Nigwekar and Waikar, 2011). Other FDA-approved uses of mannitol include enhancement of urinary excretion of salicylates, barbiturates, bromides, and lithium following overdose;

for the diagnosis of bronchial hyperreactivity (by oral inhalation); and for antihemolytic urologic irrigation during transurethral procedures.

Toxicity, Adverse Effects, Contraindications, and Drug Interactions

Osmotic diuretics are distributed in the extracellular fluid and contribute to the extracellular osmolality. Thus, water is extracted from intracellular compartments, and the extracellular fluid volume becomes expanded. In patients with heart failure or pulmonary congestion, this may cause frank pulmonary edema. Extraction of water also causes hyponatremia, which may explain the common adverse effects, including headache, nausea, and vomiting. Conversely, loss of water in excess of electrolytes can cause hypernatremia and dehydration. Osmotic diuretics are contraindicated in patients who are anuric owing to severe renal disease. Urea may cause thrombosis or pain if extravasation occurs, and it should not be administered to patients with impaired liver function because of the risk of elevation of blood ammonia levels. Both mannitol and urea are contraindicated in patients with active cranial bleeding. Glycerin is metabolized and can cause hyperglycemia.

Inhibitors of Na^+-K^+-$2Cl^-$ Symport: Loop Diuretics, High-Ceiling Diuretics

The loop and high-ceiling diuretics inhibit activity of the Na^+-K^+-$2Cl^-$ symporter in the TAL of the loop of Henle, hence the moniker *loop diuretics*. Although the proximal tubule reabsorbs about 65% of filtered Na^+, diuretics acting only in the proximal tubule have limited efficacy because the TAL has the capacity to reabsorb most of the rejectate from the proximal tubule. In contrast, inhibitors of Na^+-K^+-$2Cl^-$ symport in the TAL, sometimes called *high-ceiling diuretics*, are highly efficacious because (1) about 25% of the filtered Na^+ load normally is reabsorbed by the TAL, and (2) nephron segments past the TAL do not possess the resorptive capacity to rescue the flood of rejectate exiting the TAL.

Of the inhibitors of Na^+-K^+-$2Cl^-$ symport (Table 25–4), only furosemide, bumetanide, ethacrynic acid, and torsemide are available in the U.S. Furosemide and bumetanide contain a sulfonamide moiety. Ethacrynic acid is a phenoxyacetic acid derivative; torsemide is a sulfonylurea. Furosemide and bumetanide are available as oral and injectable formulations. Torsemide is available as an oral formulation; ethacrynate sodium is available as an injectable solution and ethacrynic acid as an oral tablet.

Mechanism and Site of Action

These agents act primarily in the TAL, where the flux of Na^+, K^+, and Cl^- from the lumen into epithelial cells is mediated by a Na^+-K^+-$2Cl^-$ symporter (Figure 25–5). Inhibitors of this symporter block its function (Bernstein and Ellison, 2011; Wile, 2012), bringing salt transport in this segment of the nephron to a virtual standstill. There is evidence that these drugs attach to the Cl^- binding site located in the symporter's transmembrane domain; however, more recent studies challenge this view. Inhibitors of Na^+-K^+-$2Cl^-$ symport also inhibit Ca^{2+} and Mg^{2+} reabsorption in the TAL by abolishing the transepithelial potential difference that is the dominant driving force for reabsorption of these cations.

Na^+-K^+-$2Cl^-$ symporters are found in many secretory and absorbing epithelia. There are two varieties of Na^+-K^+-$2Cl^-$ symporters. The "absorptive" symporter (called *ENCC2, NKCC2*, or *BSC1*) is expressed only in the kidney, is localized to the apical membrane and subapical intracellular vesicles of the TAL, and is regulated by the cyclic AMP/PKA pathway. The "secretory" symporter (called *ENCC3, NKCC1*, or *BSC2*) is a "housekeeping" protein that is expressed widely and, in epithelial cells, is localized to the basolateral membrane. The affinity of loop diuretics for the secretory symporter is somewhat less than for the absorptive symporter (e.g., 4-fold difference for bumetanide). Mutations in the Na^+-K^+-$2Cl^-$ symporter cause a form of inherited hypokalemic alkalosis called Bartter syndrome.

Effects on Urinary Excretion

Loop diuretics increase urinary Na^+ and Cl^- excretion profoundly (i.e., up to 25% of the filtered Na^+ load) and markedly increase Ca^{2+} and Mg^{2+} excretion. Furosemide has weak carbonic anhydrase–inhibiting activity and thus increases urinary excretion of HCO_3^- and phosphate. All inhibitors of Na^+-K^+-$2Cl^-$ symport increase urinary K^+ and titratable acid excretion. This effect is due in part to increased Na^+ delivery to the distal tubule (the mechanism by which increased distal Na^+ delivery enhances K^+ and H^+ excretion is discussed in the section on Na^+ channel inhibitors). Other mechanisms contributing to enhanced K^+ and H^+ excretion include flow-dependent enhancement of ion secretion by the collecting duct, non-osmotic vasopressin release, and activation of the RAS axis.

Acutely, loop diuretics increase uric acid excretion; their chronic administration results in reduced uric acid excretion. Chronic effects of loop diuretics on uric acid excretion may be due to enhanced proximal tubule transport or secondary to volume depletion or to competition between diuretic and uric acid for the organic acid secretory mechanism in the proximal tubule. Asymptomatic hyperuricemia is a common consequence of loop diuretics, but painful episodes of gout are rarely reported (Bruderer et al., 2014). By blocking active NaCl reabsorption in the TAL, inhibitors of Na^+-K^+-$2Cl^-$ symport interfere with a critical step in the mechanism that produces a hypertonic medullary interstitium. Therefore, loop diuretics block the kidney's ability to concentrate urine. Also, because the TAL is part of the diluting segment, inhibitors of Na^+-K^+-$2Cl^-$ symport markedly impair the kidney's ability to excrete a dilute urine during water diuresis.

Effects on Renal Hemodynamics

If volume depletion is prevented by replacing fluid losses, inhibitors of Na^+-K^+-$2Cl^-$ symport generally increase total RBF and redistribute RBF to the midcortex. The mechanism of the increase in RBF is not known but may involve PGs: NSAIDs attenuate the diuretic response to loop diuretics in part by preventing PG-mediated increases in RBF. Loop diuretics block TGF by inhibiting salt transport into the macula densa so that the macula densa no longer detects NaCl concentrations in the tubular fluid.

TABLE 25–4 ■ INHIBITORS OF Na^+-K^+-$2Cl^-$ SYMPORT (LOOP DIURETICS, HIGH-CEILING DIURETICS)

DRUG	RELATIVE POTENCY	ORAL AVAILABILITY	$t_{1/2}$ (hours)	ROUTE OF ELIMINATION
Furosemide	1	~60%	~1.5	~65% R, ~35% M[a]
Bumetanide	40	~80%	~0.8	~62% R, ~38% M
Ethacrynic acid	0.7	~100%	~1	~67% R, ~33% M
Torsemide	3	~80%	~3.5	~20% R, ~80% M
Azosemide[b]	1	~12%	~2.5	~27% R, ~63% M
Piretanide[b]	3	~80%	0.6–1.5	~50% R, ~50% M

M, metabolism; R, renal excretion of intact drug.
[a]Metabolism of furosemide occurs predominantly in the kidney.
[b]Not available in the U.S.

Therefore, unlike carbonic anhydrase inhibitors, loop diuretics do not decrease the GFR by activating TGF. Loop diuretics are powerful stimulators of renin release. This effect is due to interference with NaCl transport by the macula densa and, if volume depletion occurs, to reflex activation of the sympathetic nervous system and stimulation of the intrarenal baroreceptor mechanism.

Other Actions

Loop diuretics, particularly furosemide, acutely increase systemic venous capacitance and thereby decrease left ventricular filling pressure. This effect, which may be mediated by PGs and requires intact kidneys, benefits patients with pulmonary edema even before diuresis ensues. High doses of inhibitors of Na^+-K^+-$2Cl^-$ symport can inhibit electrolyte transport in many tissues. This effect is clinically important in the inner ear and can result in ototoxicity, particularly in patients with preexisting hearing impairment.

ADME

Table 25–4 presents some pharmacokinetic properties of the agents. Because these drugs are bound extensively to plasma proteins, delivery of these drugs to tubules by filtration is limited. However, they are secreted efficiently by the organic acid transport system in the proximal tubule and thereby gain access to the Na^+-K^+-$2Cl^-$ symporter in the luminal membrane of the TAL. Approximately 65% of furosemide is excreted unchanged in urine, and the remainder is conjugated to glucuronic acid in the kidney. Thus, in patients with renal disease, the elimination $t_{1/2}$ of furosemide is prolonged. Bumetanide and torsemide have significant hepatic metabolism, so liver disease can prolong the elimination $t_{1/2}$ of these loop diuretics. Oral bioavailability of furosemide varies (10%–100%). In contrast, oral availabilities of bumetanide and torsemide are reliably high.

As a class, loop diuretics have short elimination half-lives; prolonged-release preparations are not available. Consequently, often the dosing interval is too short to maintain adequate levels of loop diuretics in the tubular lumen. Note that torsemide has a longer $t_{1/2}$ than other agents available in the U.S. As the concentration of loop diuretic in the tubular lumen declines, nephrons begin to avidly reabsorb Na^+, which often nullifies the overall effect of the loop diuretic on total-body Na^+. This phenomenon of "postdiuretic Na^+ retention" can be overcome by restricting dietary Na^+ intake or by more frequent administration of the loop diuretic.

Therapeutic Uses

A major use of loop diuretics is in the treatment of acute pulmonary edema. A rapid increase in venous capacitance in conjunction with brisk natriuresis reduces left ventricular filling pressures and thereby rapidly relieves pulmonary edema. Loop diuretics also are used widely for treatment of chronic CHF when diminution of extracellular fluid volume is desirable to minimize venous and pulmonary congestion (see Chapter 29). Diuretics cause a significant reduction in mortality and the risk of worsening heart failure, as well as an improvement in exercise capacity. Although furosemide is the most commonly used loop diuretic for the treatment of heart failure, patients with heart failure have fewer hospitalizations and better quality of life with torsemide than with furosemide, perhaps because of its more reliable absorption and due to other ancillary pharmacological effects (Buggey et al., 2015).

Although diuretics are used widely for treatment of hypertension (see Chapter 28), in patients with normal renal function, Na^+-K^+-$2Cl^-$ symport inhibitors are not considered first-line diuretics for the treatment of hypertension. This is due to the lower antihypertensive efficacy of loop diuretics in such patients and the lack of data demonstrating a reduction in cardiovascular events. However, in patients with a low GFR (<30 mL/min) or with resistant hypertension, loop diuretics are the diuretics of choice.

The edema of nephrotic syndrome often is refractory to less-potent diuretics, and loop diuretics often are the only drugs capable of reducing the massive edema associated with this renal disease. Loop diuretics also are employed in the treatment of edema and ascites of liver cirrhosis; however, care must be taken not to induce volume contraction. In patients with a drug overdose, loop diuretics can be used to induce forced diuresis to facilitate more rapid renal elimination of the offending drug. Loop diuretics, combined with isotonic saline administration to prevent volume depletion, are used to treat hypercalcemia. Loop diuretics interfere with the kidney's capacity to produce concentrated urine. Consequently, loop diuretics combined with hypertonic saline are useful for the treatment of life-threatening hyponatremia. Loop diuretics also are used to treat edema associated with chronic kidney disease, in which the dose-response curve may be right shifted, requiring higher doses of the loop diuretic.

Toxicity, Adverse Effects, Contraindications, Drug Interactions

Most adverse effects are due to abnormalities of fluid and electrolyte balance. Overzealous use of loop diuretics can cause serious depletion of total-body Na^+. This may manifest as hyponatremia or extracellular fluid volume depletion associated with hypotension, reduced GFR, circulatory collapse, thromboembolic episodes, and, in patients with liver disease, hepatic encephalopathy. Increased Na^+ delivery to the distal tubule, particularly when combined with activation of the renin-angiotensin system, leads to increased urinary K^+ and H^+ excretion, causing a hypochloremic alkalosis. If dietary K^+ intake is not sufficient, hypokalemia may develop, and this may induce cardiac arrhythmias, particularly in patients taking cardiac glycosides. Increased Mg^{2+} and Ca^{2+} excretion may result in hypomagnesemia (a risk factor for cardiac arrhythmias) and hypocalcemia (rarely leading to tetany). Loop diuretics should be avoided in postmenopausal osteopenic women, in whom increased Ca^{2+} excretion may have deleterious effects on bone metabolism.

Loop diuretics can cause ototoxicity that manifests as tinnitus, hearing impairment, deafness, vertigo, and a sense of fullness in the ears. Hearing impairment and deafness are usually, but not always, reversible. Ototoxicity occurs most frequently with rapid intravenous administration and least frequently with oral administration. To avoid ototoxicity, the rate of furosemide infusions should not exceed 4 mg/min. Ethacrynic acid appears to induce ototoxicity more often than do other loop diuretics and should be reserved for use only in patients who cannot tolerate other loop diuretics. Loop diuretics also can cause hyperuricemia (occasionally leading to gout) and hyperglycemia (infrequently precipitating diabetes mellitus) and can increase plasma levels of LDL cholesterol and triglycerides while decreasing plasma levels of HDL cholesterol. Other adverse effects include skin rashes, photosensitivity, paresthesias, bone marrow depression, and GI disturbances. Contraindications to the use of loop diuretics include severe Na^+ and volume depletion, hypersensitivity to sulfonamides (for sulfonamide-based loop diuretics), and anuria unresponsive to a trial dose of loop diuretic.

Drug interactions may occur when loop diuretics are coadministered with the following:

- Aminoglycosides, carboplatin, paclitaxel, and others (synergism of ototoxicity)
- Anticoagulants (increased anticoagulant activity)
- Digitalis glycosides (increased digitalis-induced arrhythmias)
- Lithium (increased plasma levels of Li^+)
- Propranolol (increased plasma levels of propranolol)
- Sulfonylureas (hyperglycemia)
- Cisplatin (increased risk of diuretic-induced ototoxicity)
- NSAIDs (blunted diuretic response and salicylate toxicity with high doses of salicylates)
- Probenecid (blunted diuretic response)
- Thiazide diuretics (synergism of diuretic activity of both drugs, leading to profound diuresis)
- Amphotericin B (increased potential for nephrotoxicity and intensification of electrolyte imbalance)

Inhibitors of Na^+-Cl^- Symport: Thiazide-Type and Thiazide-Like Diuretics

The term *thiazide diuretics* generally refers to all inhibitors of Na^+-Cl^- symport, so named because the original inhibitors of Na^+-Cl^- symport were benzothiadiazine derivatives. The class now includes diuretics that are benzothiadiazine derivatives (*thiazide* or *thiazide-type diuretics*) and drugs that are pharmacologically similar to thiazide diuretics but differ structurally (*thiazide-like diuretics*). Table 25–5 lists diuretics in this drug class that are currently available in the United States.

Mechanism and Site of Action

Thiazide diuretics inhibit NaCl transport in the DCT; the proximal tubule may represent a secondary site of action. Figure 25–5 illustrates the current model of electrolyte transport in the DCT. Transport is powered by a Na^+ pump in the basolateral membrane. Free energy in the electrochemical gradient for Na^+ is harnessed by a Na^+-Cl^- symporter in the luminal membrane that moves Cl^- into the epithelial cell against its electrochemical gradient. Cl^- then exits the basolateral membrane passively by a Cl^- channel. Thiazide diuretics inhibit the Na^+-Cl^- symporter (called *ENCC1* or *TSC*) that is expressed predominantly in kidney and localized to the apical membrane of DCT epithelial cells. Expression of the symporter is regulated by aldosterone. Mutations in the Na^+-Cl^- symporter cause a form of inherited hypokalemic alkalosis called Gitelman syndrome.

Effects on Urinary Excretion

Inhibitors of Na^+-Cl^- symport increase Na^+ and Cl^- excretion. However, thiazides are only moderately efficacious (i.e., maximum excretion of filtered Na^+ load is only 5%) because about 90% of the filtered Na^+ load is reabsorbed before reaching the DCT. Some thiazide diuretics also are weak inhibitors of carbonic anhydrase, an effect that increases HCO_3^- and phosphate excretion and probably accounts for their weak proximal tubular effects. Inhibitors of Na^+-Cl^- symport increase K^+ and titratable acid excretion by the same mechanisms discussed for loop diuresis. Acute thiazide administration increases uric acid excretion. However, uric acid excretion is reduced following chronic administration by similar mechanisms discussed for loop diuretics. In addition, thiazides may be transported from the basolateral compartment to the luminal compartment via the OAT4 antiporter in the apical membrane (Palmer, 2011; see Chapter 5). Acute effects of inhibitors of Na^+-Cl^- symport on Ca^{2+} excretion are variable; when administered chronically, thiazide diuretics decrease Ca^{2+} excretion. The mechanism involves increased proximal reabsorption owing to volume depletion, as well as direct effects of thiazides to increase Ca^{2+} reabsorption in the DCT. Thiazide diuretics may cause mild magnesuria; long-term use of thiazide diuretics may cause magnesium deficiency, particularly in the elderly. Because inhibitors of Na^+-Cl^- symport inhibit transport in the cortical diluting segment, thiazide diuretics attenuate the kidney's ability to excrete dilute urine during water diuresis. However, because the DCT is not involved in the mechanism that generates a hypertonic medullary interstitium, thiazide diuretics do not alter the kidney's ability to concentrate urine during hydropenia. In general, inhibitors of Na^+-Cl^- symport do not affect RBF and only variably reduce GFR owing to increases in intratubular pressure. Thiazides have little or no influence on TGF.

ADME

Table 25–5 lists pharmacokinetic parameters of Na^+-Cl^- symport inhibitors. Note the wide range of half-lives for these drugs. Sulfonamides, as organic acids, are secreted into the proximal tubule by the organic acid secretory pathway. Because thiazides must gain access to the tubular lumen to inhibit the Na^+-Cl^- symporter, drugs such as probenecid can attenuate the diuretic response to thiazides by competing for transport into the proximal tubule. However, plasma protein binding varies considerably among thiazide diuretics, and this parameter determines the contribution that filtration makes to tubular delivery of a specific thiazide.

Therapeutic Uses

Thiazide diuretics are used for the treatment of edema associated with diseases of the heart (CHF), liver (hepatic cirrhosis), and kidney (nephrotic syndrome, chronic renal failure, and acute glomerulonephritis). With the possible exceptions of metolazone and indapamide, most thiazide diuretics are ineffective when the GFR is less than 30–40 mL/min. Thiazide diuretics decrease blood pressure in hypertensive patients and are used widely for the treatment of hypertension in combination with other antihypertensive drugs (Tamargo et al., 2014) (see Chapter 28). Thiazide diuretics are inexpensive, as efficacious as other classes of antihypertensive agents, and well tolerated. Thiazides can be administered once daily, do not require dose titration, and have few contraindications. Moreover, thiazides have additive or synergistic effects when combined with other classes of antihypertensive agents. Although hydrochlorothiazide is the 10th most prescribed drug in the United States and is prescribed 20 times more often than chlorthalidone (Roush et al., 2014), there is strong evidence that chlorthalidone and other thiazide-like diuretics, such as indapamide, reduce blood pressure and cardiovascular events in hypertensive patients more so than does hydrochlorothiazide (Olde Engberink et al., 2015; Roush et al., 2014, 2015). This is likely due to the longer half-life of *thiazide-like* diuretics compared to hydrochlorothiazide, resulting in better 24-h control of arterial blood pressure by chlorthalidone.

Thiazide diuretics, which reduce urinary Ca^{2+} excretion, sometimes are employed to treat Ca^{2+} nephrolithiasis and may be useful for treatment of osteoporosis (see Chapter 44). Thiazide diuretics also are the mainstay for treatment of nephrogenic DI, reducing urine volume by up to 50%. Although it may seem counterintuitive to treat a disorder of increased urine volume with a diuretic, thiazides reduce the kidney's ability to excrete free water: They increase proximal tubular water reabsorption (secondary to volume contraction) and block the ability of the

TABLE 25–5 ■ INHIBITORS OF Na^+-Cl^- SYMPORT (THIAZIDE DIURETICS)

DRUG	RELATIVE POTENCY	ORAL AVAILABILITY	$t_{1/2}$ (hours)	ROUTE OF ELIMINATION
Thiazide diuretics				
Bendroflumethiazide	10	~100%	3–3.9	~30% R, ~70% M
Chlorothiazide	0.1	9%–56% (dose-dependent)	~1.5	R
Hydrochlorothiazide	1	~70%	~2.5	R
Methyclothiazide	10	ID	ID	M
Thiazide-like diuretics				
Chlorthalidone	1	~65%	~47	~65% R, ~10% B, ~25% U
Indapamide	20	~93%	~14	M
Metolazone	10	~65%	8–14	~80% R, ~10% B, ~10% M

B, excretion of intact drug into bile; ID, insufficient data; M, metabolism; R, renal excretion of intact drug; U, unknown pathway of elimination.

DCT to form dilute urine. This last effect results in an increase in urine osmolality. Because other halides are excreted by renal processes similar to those for Cl^-, thiazide diuretics may be useful for the management of Br^- intoxication.

Toxicity, Adverse Effects, Contraindications, Drug Interactions

Thiazide diuretics rarely cause CNS (e.g., vertigo, headache), GI, hematological, and dermatological (e.g., photosensitivity and skin rashes) disorders. The incidence of erectile dysfunction is greater with Na^+-Cl^- symport inhibitors than with several other antihypertensive agents (Grimm et al., 1997), but usually is tolerable. As with loop diuretics, most serious adverse effects of thiazides are related to abnormalities of fluid and electrolyte balance. These adverse effects include extracellular volume depletion, hypotension, hypokalemia, hyponatremia, hypochloremia, metabolic alkalosis, hypomagnesemia, hypercalcemia, and hyperuricemia (Palmer, 2011). Thiazide diuretics have caused fatal or near-fatal hyponatremia (Rodenburg et al., 2013), and some patients are at recurrent risk of hyponatremia when rechallenged with thiazides.

Thiazide diuretics also decrease glucose tolerance and unmask latent diabetes mellitus (Palmer, 2011). The mechanism of impaired glucose tolerance appears to involve reduced insulin secretion and alterations in glucose metabolism. Hyperglycemia is reduced when K^+ is given along with the diuretic. Importantly, thiazide-induced diabetes mellitus is not associated with the same cardiovascular disease risk as incident diabetes (Barzilay et al., 2012). Thiazide-induced hypokalemia also impairs the antihypertensive effect and cardiovascular protection afforded by thiazides in patients with hypertension. Thiazide diuretics also may increase plasma levels of LDL cholesterol, total cholesterol, and total triglycerides. Thiazide diuretics are contraindicated in individuals who are hypersensitive to sulfonamides. Thiazide diuretics may diminish the effects of anticoagulants, uricosuric agents used to treat gout, sulfonylureas, and insulin and may increase the effects of anesthetics, diazoxide, digitalis glycosides, lithium, loop diuretics, and vitamin D. The effectiveness of thiazide diuretics may be reduced by NSAIDs, nonselective or selective COX-2 inhibitors, and bile acid sequestrants (reduced absorption of thiazides). Amphotericin B and corticosteroids increase the risk of hypokalemia induced by thiazide diuretics.

In a potentially lethal interaction, thiazide diuretic–induced K^+ depletion may contribute to fatal ventricular arrhythmias associated with drugs that prolong the QT interval (i.e., quinidine, dofetilide, arsenic trioxide, see also Chapter 30).

Inhibitors of Renal Epithelial Na^+ Channels: K^+-Sparing Diuretics

Triamterene and amiloride are the only two drugs of this class in clinical use. Both drugs cause small increases in NaCl excretion and usually are employed for their antikaliuretic actions to offset the effects of other diuretics that increase K^+ excretion. Consequently, triamterene and amiloride, along with spironolactone and eplerenone (described in the next section), often are classified as *potassium* (K^+)*–sparing diuretics*.

Both drugs are organic bases, are transported by the organic base secretory mechanism in the proximal tubule, and have similar mechanisms of action (Figure 25–5). Principal cells in the late distal tubules and collecting ducts (particularly cortical collecting tubules) have, in their luminal membranes, ENaCs that provide a conductive pathway for Na^+ entry into the cell down the electrochemical gradient created by the basolateral Na^+ pump. The higher permeability of the luminal membrane for Na^+ depolarizes the luminal membrane but not the basolateral membrane, creating a lumen-negative transepithelial potential difference. This transepithelial voltage provides an important driving force for the secretion of K^+ into the lumen via K^+ channels (ROMK [Kir1.1] and BK channels) (Garcia and Kaczorowski, 2014) in the luminal membrane; however, the overall regulation of K^+ secretion in the late distal tubule and collecting duct involves multiple signaling mechanisms (Welling, 2013). Carbonic anhydrase inhibitors, loop diuretics, and thiazide diuretics increase Na^+ delivery to the late distal tubule and collecting duct, a situation that often is associated with increased K^+ and H^+ excretion.

Amiloride and triamterene block ENaCs in the luminal membrane of principal cells in late distal tubules and collecting ducts by binding to a site in the channel pore. ENaCs consist of three subunits (α, β, and γ) (Kellenberger and Schild, 2015). Although the α subunit is sufficient for channel activity, maximal Na^+ permeability is induced when all three subunits are coexpressed in the same cell, probably forming a tetrameric structure consisting of two α subunits, one β subunit, and one γ subunit. Incompletely understood, complex mechanisms, including proteolytic cleavage, regulate ENaC activation (Kellenberger and Schild, 2015).

Effects on Urinary Excretion

The late distal tubule and collecting duct have a limited capacity to reabsorb solutes; thus, Na^+ channel blockade in this part of the nephron increases Na^+ and Cl^- excretion rates only mildly (~2% of filtered load). Blockade of Na^+ channels hyperpolarizes the luminal membrane, reducing the lumen-negative transepithelial voltage. Because the lumen-negative potential difference normally opposes cation reabsorption and facilitates cation secretion, attenuation of the lumen-negative voltage decreases K^+, H^+, Ca^{2+}, and Mg^{2+} excretion rates. Volume contraction may increase reabsorption of uric acid in the proximal tubule; hence, chronic administration of amiloride and triamterene may decrease uric acid excretion. Amiloride and triamterene have little or no effect on renal hemodynamics and do not alter TGF.

ADME

Table 25–6 lists pharmacokinetic data for amiloride and triamterene. Amiloride is eliminated predominantly by urinary excretion of intact drug. Triamterene is metabolized in the liver to an active metabolite, 4-hydroxytriamterene sulfate, and this metabolite is excreted in urine. Therefore, triamterene toxicity may be enhanced in both hepatic disease and renal failure.

Therapeutic Uses

Because of the mild natriuresis induced by Na^+ channel inhibitors, these drugs seldom are used as sole agents in treatment of edema or hypertension; their major utility is in combination with other diuretics. Coadministration of a Na^+ channel inhibitor augments the diuretic and antihypertensive response to thiazide and loop diuretics. More important, the ability of Na^+ channel inhibitors to reduce K^+ excretion tends to offset the kaliuretic effects of thiazide and loop diuretics and to result in normal plasma K^+ values.

TABLE 25–6 ■ INHIBITORS OF RENAL EPITHELIAL Na^+ CHANNELS (K^+-SPARING DIURETICS)

DRUG	RELATIVE POTENCY	ORAL BIOAVAILABILITY	$t_{1/2}$ (hours)	ROUTE OF ELIMINATION
Amiloride	1	15%–25%	~21	R
Triamterene	0.1	~50%	~4	M

M, metabolism; R, renal excretion of intact drug; however, triamterene is transformed into an active metabolite that is excreted in the urine.

Liddle syndrome (described later in this chapter) can be treated effectively with Na^+ channel inhibitors. Aerosolized amiloride has been shown to improve mucociliary clearance in patients with cystic fibrosis. By inhibiting Na^+ absorption from the surfaces of airway epithelial cells, amiloride augments hydration of respiratory secretions and thereby improves mucociliary clearance. Amiloride also is useful for lithium-induced nephrogenic DI because it blocks Li^+ transport into collecting tubule cells (Kortenoeven et al., 2009).

Toxicity, Adverse Effects, Contraindications, Drug Interactions

The most dangerous adverse effect of renal Na^+ channel inhibitors is hyperkalemia, which can be life threatening. Consequently, amiloride and triamterene are contraindicated in patients with hyperkalemia, as well as in patients at increased risk of developing hyperkalemia (e.g., patients with renal failure, patients receiving other K^+-sparing diuretics, patients taking angiotensin-converting enzyme inhibitors, or patients taking K^+ supplements). Even NSAIDs can increase the likelihood of hyperkalemia in patients receiving Na^+ channel inhibitors. Routine monitoring of the serum K^+ level is essential in patients receiving K^+-sparing diuretics. Cirrhotic patients are prone to megaloblastosis because of folic acid deficiency, and triamterene, a weak folic acid antagonist, may increase the likelihood of this adverse event. Triamterene also can reduce glucose tolerance and induce photosensitization and has been associated with interstitial nephritis and renal stones. Both drugs can cause CNS, GI, musculoskeletal, dermatological, and hematological adverse effects. The most common adverse effects of amiloride are nausea, vomiting, diarrhea, and headache; those of triamterene are nausea, vomiting, leg cramps, and dizziness.

Antagonists of Mineralocorticoid Receptors: Aldosterone Antagonists, K^+-Sparing Diuretics

Mineralocorticoids cause salt and water retention and increase K^+ and H^+ excretion by binding to specific MRs. Two MR antagonists are available in the U.S., spironolactone and eplerenone (Table 25–7).

Mechanism and Site of Action

Epithelial cells in late distal tubule and collecting duct (particularly cortical collecting tubule) contain cytosolic MRs with high aldosterone affinity. When aldosterone binds to MRs, the MR-aldosterone complex translocates to the nucleus, where it regulates the expression of multiple gene products called aldosterone-induced proteins (AIPs) (Figure 25–6). AIPs affect the production, destruction, localization, and activation of multiple components of the system that mediates Na^+ reabsorption in late distal tubules and collecting ducts (Figure 25–6A). Consequently, transepithelial NaCl transport is enhanced, and the lumen-negative transepithelial voltage is increased. The latter effect increases the driving force for K^+ and H^+ secretion into the tubular lumen.

Drugs such as spironolactone and eplerenone competitively inhibit the binding of aldosterone to the MR. Unlike the MR-aldosterone complex, the MR-spironolactone or MR-eplerenone complex is not able to induce the synthesis of AIPs. Because spironolactone and eplerenone block the biological effects of aldosterone, these agents also are referred to as *aldosterone antagonists*. MR antagonists are the only diuretics that do not require access to the tubular lumen to induce diuresis.

TABLE 25–7 ■ MINERALOCORTICOID RECEPTOR ANTAGONISTS (ALDOSTERONE ANTAGONISTS, K^+-SPARING DIURETICS)

DRUG	ORAL AVAILABILITY	$t_{1/2}$ (hours)	ROUTE OF ELIMINATION
Spironolactone	~65%	~1.6	M
Canrenone[a]	80%	3.7–22	M
Potassium canrenoate[a]	100%	3.7–22	M
Eplerenone	69%	~5	M

M, metabolism.
[a]Not available in U.S.

Both the β and β subunits of ENaC have a specific region in their C terminus called the PY motif. The PY motif interacts with the ubiquitin ligase Nedd4-2 (Figure 25–6B), a protein that ubiquitinates ENaC and targets it for destruction by the proteasome. Aldosterone increases the expression of SGK-1; SGK-1 phosphorylates and inactivates Nedd4-2. Thus, aldosterone results in attenuated internalization and proteasome-mediated degradation of ENaC, leading to increased expression of ENaC in the luminal membrane. Liddle syndrome, an autosomal-dominant, monogenic disease characterized by sodium retention and severe hypertension, is caused by mutations in the PY motif of either the β or γ subunit of ENaC, leading to MR-independent overexpression of ENaC. Thus, Liddle syndrome is responsive to ENaC inhibitors but not to MR antagonists.

Effects on Urinary Excretion

The effects of MR antagonists on urinary excretion are similar to those induced by renal ENaC inhibitors. However, unlike Na^+ channel inhibitors, the clinical efficacy of MR antagonists is a function of endogenous aldosterone levels. The higher the endogenous aldosterone level, the greater the effects of MR antagonists on urinary excretion. MR antagonists have little or no effect on renal hemodynamics and do not alter TGF.

Other Actions

Spironolactone has some affinity toward progesterone and androgen receptors and thereby induces side effects such as gynecomastia, impotence, and menstrual irregularities. Owing to its 9,11-epoxide group, eplerenone has very low affinity for progesterone and androgen receptors (<1% and <0.1%, respectively) compared with spironolactone. High spironolactone concentrations can interfere with steroid biosynthesis by inhibiting steroid hydroxylases, but these effects have limited clinical relevance.

ADME

Spironolactone is absorbed partially (~65%), is metabolized extensively (even during its first passage through the liver), undergoes enterohepatic recirculation, and is highly protein bound. Although spironolactone per se has a short $t_{1/2}$ (~1.6 h), it is metabolized to a number of active compounds (including canrenone; see discussion that follows) that have long half-lives. The $t_{1/2}$ of spironolactone is prolonged to 9 h in patients with cirrhosis. Eplerenone has good oral availability and is eliminated primarily by metabolism by CYP3A4 to inactive metabolites, with a $t_{1/2}$ of about 5 h. Canrenone and K^+-canrenoate also are in clinical use (not available in the U.S.). Canrenoate is not active but is converted to canrenone.

Therapeutic Uses

The MR antagonists often are coadministered with thiazide or loop diuretics in the treatment of edema and hypertension. Such combinations result in increased mobilization of edema fluid while causing lesser perturbations of K^+ homeostasis. MR antagonists are particularly useful in the treatment of resistant hypertension due to primary hyperaldosteronism (adrenal adenomas or bilateral adrenal hyperplasia) and of refractory edema associated with secondary aldosteronism (cardiac failure, hepatic cirrhosis, nephrotic syndrome, and severe ascites). MR antagonists are considered diuretics of choice in patients with hepatic cirrhosis. MR antagonists, added to standard therapy, substantially reduce morbidity and mortality in patients with heart failure with reduced ejection fraction (see Chapter 29) (D'Elia and Krum, 2014).

The MR antagonists may reduce mortality in patients with systolic dysfunction following a myocardial infarction if treated within 3 to 6 days (Roush et al., 2014). In patients with diastolic dysfunction with preserved ejection fraction, the use of MR antagonists is controversial. In such patients, MR antagonists improve left ventricular end-diastolic filling, left ventricular remodeling, and neurohumoral activation but do not improve maximal exercise capacity, quality of life, mortality, or hospitalization for heart failure (Edelmann et al., 2013; Pitt et al., 2014). MR antagonists also may reduce ventricular arrhythmias and sudden cardiac death.

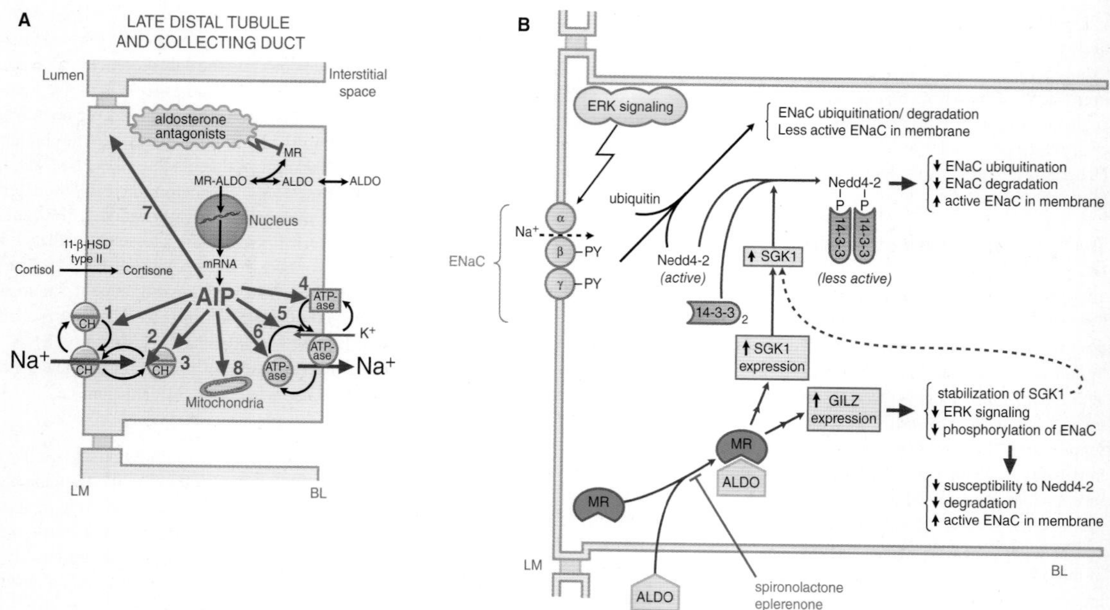

Figure 25–6 *Effects of aldosterone on late distal tubule and collecting duct and diuretic mechanism of aldosterone antagonists.*

A. Overview of aldosterone's influences on Na⁺ retention. Via interaction with the mineralocorticoid receptor (MR), aldosterone affects myriad renal pathways that handle Na^+. Key to numbered items influenced by ALDO:

1. Activation of membrane-bound Na^+ channels
2. Na^+ channel (ENaC) removal from the membrane inhibited
3. *De novo* synthesis of Na^+ channels
4. Activation of membrane-bound Na^+,K^+-ATPase
5. Redistribution of Na^+,K^+-ATPase from cytosol to membrane
6. *De novo* synthesis of Na^+,K^+-ATPase
7. Changes in permeability of tight junctions
8. Increased mitochondrial production of ATP

Cortisol also has affinity for the mineralocorticoid receptor but is inactivated in the cell by 11-β-hydroxysteroid dehydrogenase (HSD) type II.

B. Details of aldosterone's influences on membrane ENaC. ERK signaling phosphorylates components of ENaC, making them susceptible to interaction with Nedd4-2, a ubiquitin-protein ligase that ubiquitinates ENaC, leading to its degradation. The Nedd4-2 interaction with ENaC occurs via several proline-tyrosine-proline (PY) motifs of ENaC. ALDO enhances expression of the serum and glucocorticoid-regulated kinase-1 (SGK1) and the glucocorticoid-induced leucine zipper protein (GILZ; TSC22D3). SGK-1 phosphorylates and inactivates Nedd4-2; 14-3-3 dimers bind to the phosphorylated sites in Nedd4-2 and stabilize them. Phosphorylated Nedd4-2 no longer interacts well with the PY motifs of ENaC. As a result, ENaC is not ubiquitinated and remains in the membrane, leading to increased Na^+ entry into the cell. GILZ stabilizes SGK1, enhancing its effects, and decreases ERK signaling and ENaC phosphorylation, events that prime ENaC for degradation; these effects all lead to less ubiquitination and more active ENaC in the cell membranes of the distal tubule and collecting duct. For details see Ronzaud and Staub (2014) and Ronchetti et al. (2015).

Abbreviations: AIP, aldosterone-induced proteins; ALDO, aldosterone; CH, ion channel; BL, basolateral membrane; LM, luminal membrane; MR, mineralocorticoid receptor.

The MR antagonists reduce proteinuria in patients with chronic kidney disease, and the use of these drugs in kidney diseases is under intense investigation (Bauersachs et al., 2015). Spironolactone, but not eplerenone, is widely considered to be an antiandrogenic compound and has been used to treat hirsutism and acne; however, evidence for efficacy is weak (Brown et al., 2009), and these uses are not FDA-approved. Biochemical studies suggested that spironolactone is a partial agonist of androgen receptors (Nirdé et al., 2001) and can exert antiandrogenic or androgenic effects depending on context (e.g., the prevailing levels of endogenous androgenic steroids). Indeed, a recent case report described spironolactone-induced worsening of prostate cancer attributed to androgen receptor stimulation (Sundar and Dickinson, 2012).

Toxicity, Adverse Effects, Contraindications, Drug Interactions

Hyperkalemia is the principal risk of MR antagonists. Therefore, these drugs are contraindicated in patients with hyperkalemia and in those at increased risk of developing hyperkalemia. MR antagonists also can induce metabolic acidosis in cirrhotic patients. Salicylates may reduce the tubular secretion of canrenone and decrease diuretic efficacy of spironolactone. Spironolactone may alter the clearance of cardiac glycosides. Owing to its affinity for other steroid receptors, spironolactone may cause gynecomastia, impotence, decreased libido, and menstrual irregularities. Spironolactone also may induce diarrhea, gastritis, gastric bleeding, and peptic ulcers (the drug is contraindicated in patients with peptic ulcers). CNS adverse effects include drowsiness, lethargy, ataxia, confusion, and headache. Spironolactone may cause skin rashes and, rarely, blood dyscrasias. Strong inhibitors of CYP3A4 may increase plasma levels of eplerenone, and such drugs should not be administered to patients taking eplerenone and vice versa. Other than hyperkalemia and GI disorders, the rate of adverse events for eplerenone is similar to that of placebo.

Inhibitors of the Nonspecific Cation Channel: Natriuretic Peptides

Four NPs are relevant with respect to human physiology: ANP, BNP, CNP, and urodilatin. The IMCD is a major site of action of NPs.

Three NPs—ANP, BNP, and CNP—share a common homologous 17-member amino acid ring formed by a disulfide bridge between cysteine residues, although they are products of different genes. Urodilatin, also structurally similar, arises from altered processing of the same precursor molecule as ANP and has four additional amino acids at the N terminus. ANP and BNP are produced by the heart in response to wall stretch, CNP is of endothelial and renal cell origin; urodilatin is found in the kidney and urine. NPRs, classified as types A, B, and C, are membrane monospans. NPRA (binds ANP and BNP) and NPRB (binds CNP) have intracellular domains with guanylate cyclase activity and a protein kinase element. NPRC (binds all NPs) has a truncated intracellular domain and may help with NP clearance. The various NPs have somewhat overlapping effects, causing natriuresis, inhibition of production of renin and aldosterone, and vasodilation (the result of cGMP elevation in vascular smooth muscle). A human recombinant BNP, nesiritide, with the same 32–amino acid structure as the endogenous peptide produced by the ventricular myocardium, is available for clinical use.

Mechanism and Site of Action

The IMCD is the final site along the nephron where Na^+ is reabsorbed. Up to 5% of the filtered Na^+ load can be reabsorbed here. The effects of nesiritide and other NPs are mediated via effects of cGMP on Na^+ transporters (Figure 25–7). Two types of Na^+ channels are expressed in IMCD. *The first* is a high conductance, 28-pS, nonselective, CNGC. This channel is inhibited by intracellular cGMP and by NPs via their capacity to stimulate membrane-bound guanylyl cyclase activity and elevate cellular cGMP. The *second* type of Na^+ channel expressed in the IMCD is the low-conductance, 4-pS, highly selective Na^+ channel ENaC. The majority of Na^+ reabsorption in the IMCD is mediated via CNGC.

Effects on Urinary Excretion and Renal Hemodynamics

Nesiritide inhibits Na^+ transport in both the proximal and distal nephron but its primary effect is in the IMCD. Urinary Na^+ excretion increases with nesiritide, but the effect may be attenuated by upregulation of Na^+ reabsorption in upstream segments of the nephron. GFR increases in response to nesiritide in normal subjects, but in treated patients with CHF, GFR may increase, decrease, or remain unchanged.

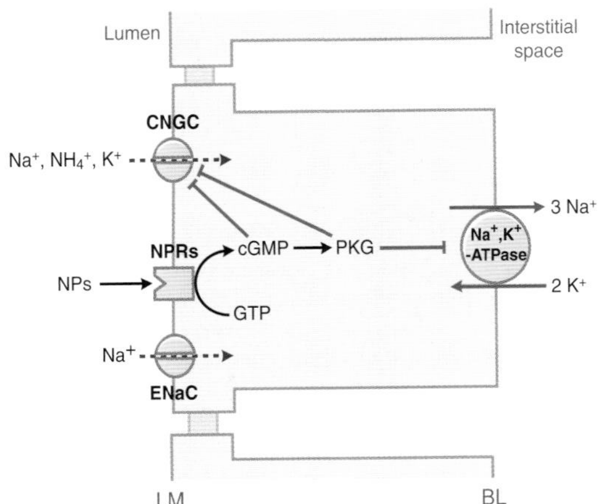

Figure 25–7 *The IMCD Na⁺ transport and its regulation.* Na^+ enters the IMCD cell in one of two ways: via ENaC and through a CNGC that transports Na^+, K^+, and NH_4^+ and is gated by cGMP. Na^+ then exits the cell via the Na^+,K^+-ATPase. The CNGC is the primary pathway for Na^+ entry and is inhibited by NPs. NPs bind to cell surface NPRs A, B, and C. The A and B receptors are isoforms of particulate guanylyl cyclase that synthesize cGMP. The CNGC is inhibited by cGMP directly and indirectly through PKG. PKG activation also inhibits Na^+ exit via the Na^+,K^+-ATPase. ENaC is a low-conductance, 4-pS, highly selective Na^+ channel that plays a minor role in IMCD Na^+ transport (see Figure 25–6).

Other Actions

Administration of nesiritide decreases systemic and pulmonary resistances and left ventricular filling pressure and induces a secondary increase in cardiac output.

ADME

Natriuretic peptides are administered intravenously. Nesiritide has a distribution $t_{1/2}$ of 2 min and a mean terminal $t_{1/2}$ of 18 min. Clearance occurs via at least two mechanisms: internalization and subsequent degradation mediated by NPCR, and metabolism by extracellular proteases (Potter, 2011). There is no need to adjust the dose for renal insufficiency.

Therapeutic Uses

Human recombinant ANP (carperitide, available only in Japan) and BNP (nesiritide) are the available therapeutic agents of this class. Urodilatin (ularitide) is in development. Nesiritide is indicated for the management of acutely decompensated CHF. In patients who have dyspnea with minimal activity or at rest, nesiritide reduces pulmonary capillary wedge pressure and improves short-term symptoms of dyspnea. However, the ASCEND-HF trial found that nesiritide does not change mortality and rehospitalization and has only a small effect on dyspnea (O'Connor et al., 2011). Thus, nesiritide is not recommended for routine use in the broad population of patients with acute heart failure (O'Connor et al., 2011).

Toxicity, Adverse Effects, Contraindications, Drug Interactions

Nesiritide can cause hypotension, and there are concerns about adverse renal effects. However, the ASCEND-HF trial did not demonstrate worsening of renal function in nesiritide-treated patients with heart failure (O'Connor et al., 2011).

Adenosine Receptor Antagonists

There are four adenosine receptor subtypes (A_1, A_{2A}, A_{2B}, and A_3). A_1, A_{2A}, and A_{2B} receptors regulate aspects of renal physiology. The A_1 receptor is expressed in the proximal tubule and stimulates reabsorption of Na^+. Consequently, antagonists of A_1 receptors cause diuresis/natriuresis, yet are K^+ sparing. Several naturally occurring methylxanthines (e.g., caffeine, theophylline, and theobromine) are A_1 receptor antagonists (albeit nonselective) and consequently cause diuresis. Pamabrom is a mild diuretic consisting of a one-to-one mixture of 8-bromotheophylline and 2-amino-2-methyl-1-propanol; 8-bromotheophylline, a methylxanthine, is the active component of pamabrom. Pamabrom is the diuretic ingredient in several over-the-counter products marketed for relief of premenstrual syndrome. Little is known regarding the pharmacology, diuretic mechanism of action, and efficacy of pamabrom. However, because 8-bromotheophylline is a methylxanthine, it is possible that the mild diuresis induced by pamabrom is related to blockade of renal A_1 receptors.

Clinical Use of Diuretics

Site and Mechanism of Diuretic Action

An understanding of the sites and mechanisms of action of diuretics enhances comprehension of the clinical aspects of diuretic pharmacology. Figure 25–5 provides a summary view of the sites and mechanisms of actions of diuretics.

The Role of Diuretics in Clinical Medicine

Figure 25–8 illustrates interrelationships among renal function, Na^+ intake, water homeostasis, distribution of extracellular fluid volume, and mean arterial blood pressure and suggests three fundamental strategies for mobilizing edema fluid:

- Correction of the underlying disease
- Restriction of Na^+ intake
- Administration of diuretics

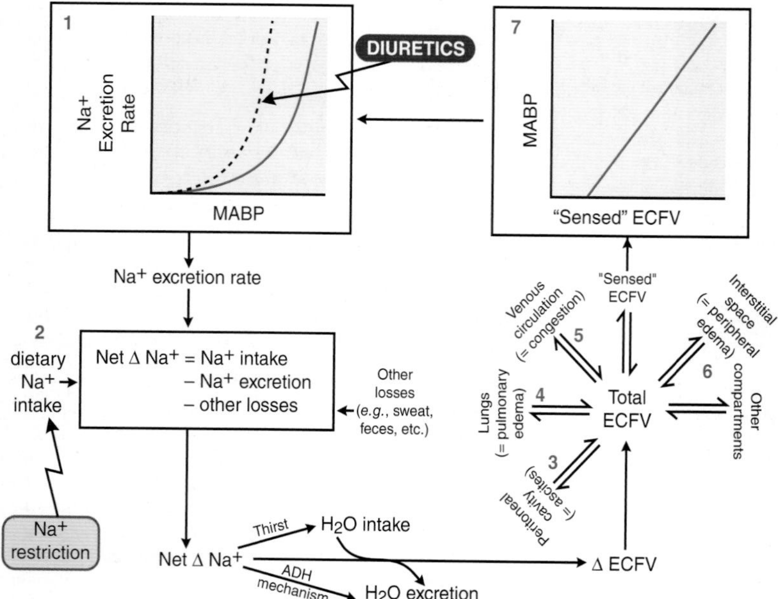

Figure 25–8 *Interrelationships amongst renal function, Na+ intake, water homeostasis, distribution of extracellular fluid volume, and mean arterial blood pressure.* Starting at upper left panel (#1), read this figure counterclockwise. Complex interrelationships exist amongst the cardiovascular system, kidneys, CNS, and capillary beds such that perturbations at one of these sites can affect all other sites. A primary law of the kidney is that Na^+ excretion is a steep function of mean arterial blood pressure (MABP) such that small increases in MABP cause marked increases in Na^+ excretion; this is known as the "pressure-natriuresis" relationship (upper left). Over any given time interval, the net change in total-body Na^+ is the dietary Na^+ intake minus the urinary excretion rate and other losses (lower left). If the pressure-natriuresis curve is right-shifted, a net positive Na^+ balance occurs, and the extracellular Na^+ concentration increases, thus stimulating water intake (thirst) and reducing urinary water output (via ADH release). These changes expand the extracellular fluid volume (ECFV), and the enlarged ECFV is distributed amongst many body compartments (lower right). ECFV on the arterial side of the circulation pressurizes the arterial tree ("sensed" ECFV), and increases MABP (upper right), thus increasing Na^+ excretion (and completing the loop). This loop cycles until net Na^+ accumulation is zero; i.e., in the long run, Na^+ intake must equal Na^+ loss.

These considerations explain the fundamental mechanisms of edema formation:

1. Rightward shift of renal pressure natriuresis curve.
2. Excessive dietary Na^+ intake.
3. Increased distribution of ECFV to peritoneal cavity (e.g., liver cirrhosis with increased hepatic sinusoidal hydrostatic pressure) leading to ascites formation.
4. Increased distribution of ECFV to lungs (e.g., left-sided heart failure with increased pulmonary capillary hydrostatic pressure) leading to pulmonary edema.
5. Increased distribution of ECFV to venous circulation (e.g., right-sided heart failure) leading to venous congestion.
6. Peripheral edema caused by altered Starling forces causing increased distribution of ECFV to interstitial space (e.g., diminished plasma proteins in nephrotic syndrome, severe burns, and liver disease).
7. Increased MABP resulting from "Sensed" ECFV on the arterial side of the heart.

These perturbations leading to edema can be addressed by: **A.** Correcting the underlying disease; **B.** Administering diuretics to left-shift the renal pressure-natriuresis relationship; **C.** Restricting dietary Na^+ intake.

ECFV, extracellular fluid volume; MABP, mean arterial blood pressure.

Figure 25–9 presents a useful synthesis, Brater's algorithm, a logically compelling algorithm for diuretic therapy (specific recommendations for drug, dose, route, and drug combinations) in patients with edema caused by renal, hepatic, or cardiac disorders (Brater, 1998).

The clinical situation dictates whether a patient should receive diuretics and what therapeutic regimen should be used (type of diuretic, dose, route of administration, and speed of mobilization of edema fluid). Massive pulmonary edema in patients with acute left-sided heart failure is a medical emergency requiring rapid, aggressive therapy, including intravenous administration of a loop diuretic. In this setting, use of oral diuretics is inappropriate. Conversely, mild pulmonary and venous congestion associated with chronic heart failure is best treated with an oral loop or thiazide diuretic, the dosage of which should be titrated carefully to maximize the benefit-to-risk ratio. Loop and thiazide diuretics decrease morbidity and mortality in patients with heart failure (Faris et al., 2002): MR antagonists also demonstrate reduced morbidity and mortality in patients with heart failure receiving optimal therapy with other drugs (Roush et al., 2014).

Periodic administration of diuretics to cirrhotic patients with ascites may eliminate the necessity for or reduce the interval between paracenteses, adding to patient comfort and sparing protein reserves that are lost during paracenteses. Although diuretics can reduce edema associated with chronic renal failure, increased doses of more powerful loop diuretics usually are required. In nephrotic syndrome, diuretic response often is disappointing. In chronic renal failure and cirrhosis, edema will not pose an immediate health risk but can greatly reduce quality of life. In such cases, only partial removal of edema fluid should be attempted, and fluid should be mobilized slowly using a diuretic regimen that accomplishes the task with minimal perturbation of normal physiology.

Diuretic resistance refers to edema that is or has become refractory to a given diuretic. If diuretic resistance develops against a less-efficacious diuretic, a more efficacious diuretic should be substituted, such as a loop diuretic for a thiazide. However, resistance to loop diuretics can be due to several causes. NSAID coadministration is a common preventable cause of diuretic resistance. PG production, especially PGE_2, is an important counterregulatory mechanism in states of reduced renal perfusion such as volume contraction, CHF, and cirrhosis characterized by activation of

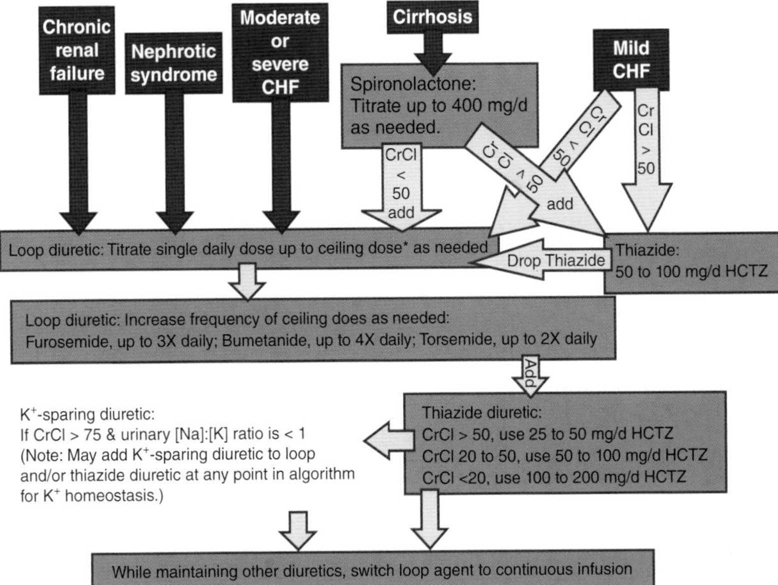

Figure 25–9 *"Brater's algorithm" for diuretic therapy of chronic renal failure, nephrotic syndrome, CHF, and cirrhosis.* Follow algorithm until adequate response is achieved. If adequate response is not obtained, advance to the next step. For illustrative purposes, the thiazide diuretic used is HCTZ. An alternative thiazide-type diuretic may be substituted with dosage adjusted to be pharmacologically equivalent to the recommended dose of HCTZ. *Do not combine two K^+-sparing diuretics due to the risk of hyperkalemia.* CrCl indicates creatinine clearance in milliliters per minute, and ceiling dose refers to the smallest dose of diuretic that produces a near-maximal effect. *Ceiling doses of loop diuretics and dosing regimens for continuous intravenous infusions of loop diuretics are disease-state specific. Doses are for adults only.

the RAAS and sympathetic nervous system. NSAID administration can block PG-mediated effects that counterbalance the RAAS and sympathetic nervous system, resulting in salt and water retention. Diuretic resistance also occurs with COX-2–selective inhibitors.

In chronic renal failure, a reduction in RBF decreases delivery of diuretics to the kidney, and accumulation of endogenous organic acids competes with loop diuretics for transport at the proximal tubule. Consequently, diuretic concentration at the active site in the tubular lumen is diminished. In nephrotic syndrome, binding of diuretics to luminal albumin was postulated to limit response; however, the validity of this concept has been challenged. In hepatic cirrhosis, nephrotic syndrome, and heart failure, nephrons may have diminished diuretic responsiveness because of increased proximal tubular Na^+ reabsorption, leading to diminished Na^+ delivery to distal nephrons.

Faced with resistance to loop diuretics, the clinician has several options:

- Bed rest may restore drug responsiveness by improving the renal circulation.
- An increase in dose of loop diuretic may restore responsiveness; however, nothing is gained by increasing the dose above that which causes a near-maximal effect (the ceiling dose) of the diuretic.
- Administration of smaller doses more frequently or a continuous intravenous infusion of a loop diuretic will increase the length of time that an effective diuretic concentration is at the active site.
- Use of combination therapy to sequentially block more than one site in the nephron may result in a synergistic interaction between two diuretics. For example, a combination of a loop diuretic with a K^+-sparing or a thiazide diuretic may improve therapeutic response; however, nothing is gained by the administration of two drugs of the same type. Thiazide diuretics with significant proximal tubular effects (e.g., metolazone) are particularly well suited for sequential blockade when coadministered with a loop diuretic.
- Reducing salt intake will diminish postdiuretic Na^+ retention, which can nullify previous increases in Na^+ excretion.
- Scheduling of diuretic administration shortly before food intake will provide effective diuretic concentration in the tubular lumen when salt load is highest.

Part II: Water Homeostasis and the Vasopressin System

Vasopressin Physiology

Arginine vasopressin (ADH in humans) is the main hormone that regulates body fluid osmolality. The hormone is released by the posterior pituitary whenever water deprivation causes an increased plasma osmolality or whenever the cardiovascular system is challenged by hypovolemia or hypotension. Vasopressin acts primarily in the renal collecting duct to increase the permeability of the cell membrane to water, thus permitting water to move passively down an osmotic gradient across the collecting duct into the extracellular compartment.

Vasopressin is a potent vasopressor/vasoconstrictor. It is also a neurotransmitter; among its actions in the CNS are apparent roles in the secretion of ACTH and in regulation of the cardiovascular system, temperature, and other visceral functions. Vasopressin also promotes release of coagulation factors by vascular endothelium and increases platelet aggregability.

Anatomy of the Vasopressin System

The antidiuretic mechanism in mammals involves two anatomical components: a CNS component for synthesis, transport, storage, and release of vasopressin and a renal collecting duct system composed of epithelial cells that respond to vasopressin by increasing their water permeability. The CNS component of the antidiuretic mechanism is called the *hypothalamoneurohypophyseal system* and consists of neurosecretory neurons with perikarya located predominantly in two specific hypothalamic nuclei, the SON and PVN. Long axons of magnocellular neurons in SON and PVN terminate in the neural lobe of the posterior pituitary (neurohypophysis), where they release vasopressin and oxytocin (see Figure 42–1).

Synthesis of Vasopressin

Vasopressin and oxytocin are synthesized mainly in the perikarya of magnocellular neurons in the SON and PVN. However, parvicellular neurons in the PVN also synthesize vasopressin, as do some non-CNS cells (see discussion that follows). Vasopressin synthesis appears to be regulated solely at the transcriptional level. In humans, a 168–amino acid preprohormone (Figure 25–10) is synthesized and then packaged into membrane-associated granules. The prohormone contains three domains: vasopressin (residues 1–9), vasopressin-neurophysin (residues 13–105), and vasopressin-glycopeptide (residues 107–145). The vasopressin domain is linked to the vasopressin-neurophysin domain through a GLY-LYS-ARG-processing signal, and the vasopressin-neurophysin is linked to the vasopressin-glycopeptide domain by an ARG-processing signal. In secretory granules, an endopeptidase, exopeptidase, monooxygenase, and lyase act sequentially on the prohormone to produce vasopressin, vasopressin-neurophysin (sometimes referred to as neurophysin II), and vasopressin-glycopeptide. The synthesis and transport of vasopressin depend on the preprohormone conformation. In particular, vasopressin-neurophysin binds vasopressin and is critical for correct processing, transport, and storage of vasopressin. Genetic mutations in either the signal peptide or vasopressin-neurophysin give rise to central DI.

Vasopressin also is synthesized by the heart and adrenal gland. In the heart, elevated wall stress increases vasopressin synthesis several-fold and may contribute to impaired ventricular relaxation and coronary vasoconstriction. Vasopressin synthesis in the adrenal medulla stimulates catecholamine secretion from chromaffin cells and may promote adrenal cortical growth and stimulate aldosterone synthesis.

Regulation of Vasopressin Secretion

Hyperosmolality. An increase in plasma osmolality is the principal physiological stimulus for vasopressin secretion by the posterior pituitary. The osmolality threshold for secretion is about 280 mOsm/kg. Below the threshold, vasopressin is barely detectable in plasma, and above the threshold, vasopressin levels are a steep and relatively linear function of plasma osmolality. Indeed, a 2% elevation in plasma osmolality causes a 2- to 3-fold increase in plasma vasopressin levels, which in turn causes increased solute-free water reabsorption, with an increase in urine osmolality. Increases in plasma osmolality above 290 mOsm/kg lead to an intense desire for water (thirst). Thus, the vasopressin system affords the organism longer thirst-free periods and, in the event that water is unavailable, allows the organism to survive longer periods of water deprivation. Above a plasma osmolality of approximately 290 mOsm/kg, plasma vasopressin levels exceed 5 pM. Since urinary concentration is maximal (~1200 mOsm/kg) when vasopressin levels exceed 5 pM, further defense against hypertonicity depends entirely on water intake rather than on decreases in water loss.

Hepatic Portal Osmoreceptors. An oral salt load activates hepatic portal osmoreceptors, leading to increased vasopressin release. This mechanism augments plasma vasopressin levels even before the oral salt load increases plasma osmolality.

Hypovolemia and Hypotension. Vasopressin secretion is regulated hemodynamically by changes in effective blood volume or arterial blood pressure. Regardless of the cause (e.g., hemorrhage, Na^+ depletion, diuretics, heart failure, hepatic cirrhosis with ascites, adrenal insufficiency, or hypotensive drugs), reductions in effective blood volume or arterial blood pressure are associated with high circulating vasopressin concentrations. However, unlike osmoregulation, hemodynamic regulation of vasopressin secretion is exponential; that is, small decreases (5%) in blood volume or pressure have little effect on vasopressin secretion, whereas larger decreases (20%–30%) can increase vasopressin levels to 20–30 times normal (exceeding the vasopressin concentration required to induce maximal antidiuresis). Vasopressin is one of the most potent vasoconstrictors known, and the vasopressin response to hypovolemia or hypotension serves as a mechanism to stave off cardiovascular collapse during periods of severe blood loss or hypotension. Hemodynamic regulation of vasopressin secretion does not disrupt osmotic regulation; rather, hypovolemia/hypotension alters the set point and slope of the plasma osmolality-plasma vasopressin relationship.

Neuronal pathways that mediate hemodynamic regulation of vasopressin release are different from those involved in osmoregulation. Baroreceptors in the left atrium, left ventricle, and pulmonary veins sense blood volume (filling pressures), and baroreceptors in the carotid sinus and aorta

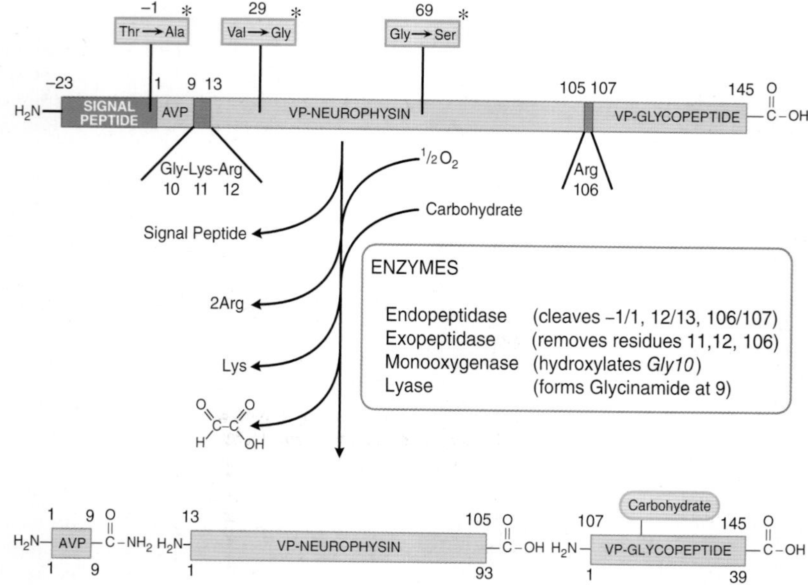

Figure 25–10 *Processing of human AVP preprohormone.* More than 40 mutations in the single gene on chromosome 20 that encodes AVP preprohormone give rise to central DI. *Boxes indicate mutations leading to central DI.

monitor arterial blood pressure. Nerve impulses reach brainstem nuclei predominantly through the vagal trunk and glossopharyngeal nerve; these signals are ultimately relayed to the SON and PVN.

Hormones and Neurotransmitters. Vasopressin-synthesizing magnocellular neurons have a large array of receptors on both perikarya and nerve terminals; therefore, vasopressin release can be accentuated or attenuated by chemical agents acting at both ends of the magnocellular neuron (Iovino et al., 2014). Also, hormones and neurotransmitters can modulate vasopressin secretion by stimulating or inhibiting neurons in nuclei that project, either directly or indirectly, to the SON and PVN (Iovino et al., 2014). Because of these complexities, modulation of vasopressin secretion by most hormones or neurotransmitters is unclear. Several agents stimulate vasopressin secretion, including acetylcholine (by nicotinic receptors), histamine (by H_1 receptors), dopamine (by both D_1 and D_2 receptors), glutamine, aspartate, cholecystokinin, neuropeptide Y, substance P, vasoactive intestinal polypeptide, PGs, and AngII. Inhibitors of vasopressin secretion include ANP, γ-aminobutyric acid, and opioids (particularly dynorphin via κ receptors). The effects of AngII have received the most attention. AngII synthesized in the brain and circulating AngII may stimulate vasopressin release. Inhibition of the conversion of AngII to AngIII blocks AngII-induced vasopressin release, suggesting that AngIII is the main effector peptide of the brain renin-angiotensin system controlling vasopressin release.

Pharmacological Agents. A number of drugs alter urine osmolality by stimulating or inhibiting vasopressin secretion. In most cases, the mechanism is not known. Stimulators of vasopressin secretion include vincristine, cyclophosphamide, tricyclic antidepressants, nicotine, epinephrine, and high doses of morphine. Lithium, which inhibits the renal effects of vasopressin, also enhances vasopressin secretion. Inhibitors of vasopressin secretion include ethanol, phenytoin, low doses of morphine, glucocorticoids, fluphenazine, haloperidol, promethazine, oxilorphan, and butorphanol. Carbamazepine has a renal action to produce antidiuresis in patients with central DI but actually inhibits vasopressin secretion by a central action. Ethanol inhibits vasopressin secretion (see Chapter 23).

Vasopressin Receptors

Cellular vasopressin effects are mediated mainly by interactions of the hormone with the three types of receptors: V_{1a}, V_{1b}, and V_2. All are GPCRs. The V_{1a} receptor is the most widespread subtype of vasopressin receptor; it is found in vascular smooth muscle, adrenal gland, myometrium, bladder, adipocytes, hepatocytes, platelets, renal medullary interstitial cells, vasa recta in the renal microcirculation, epithelial cells in the renal cortical collecting duct, spleen, testis, and many CNS structures. V_{1b} receptors have a more limited distribution and are found in the anterior pituitary, several brain regions, pancreas, and adrenal medulla. V_2 receptors are located predominantly in principal cells of the renal collecting duct system but also are present on epithelial cells in TAL and on vascular endothelial cells.

Figure 25–11 summarizes the current model of V_1 receptor-effector coupling. Vasopressin binding to V_1 receptors activates the G_q-PLC-IP_3 pathway, thereby mobilizing intracellular Ca^{2+} and activating PKC, ultimately causing biological effects that include immediate responses (e.g., vasoconstriction, glycogenolysis, platelet aggregation, and ACTH release) and growth responses in smooth muscle cells.

Principal cells in renal collecting duct have V_2 receptors on their basolateral membranes that couple to G_S to stimulate adenylyl cyclase activity (Figure 25–12). The resulting activation of the cyclic AMP/PKA pathway triggers an increased rate of insertion of water channel-containing vesicles (WCVs) into the apical membrane and a decreased rate of endocytosis of WCVs from the apical membrane. Because WCVs contain preformed functional water channels (aquaporin 2), their net shift into apical membranes in response to V_2 receptor stimulation greatly increases water permeability of the apical membrane (Nejsum, 2005) (see Figures 25–12 and 25–13).

V_2 receptor activation also increases urea permeability by 400% in the terminal portions of the IMCD. V_2 receptors increase urea permeability by

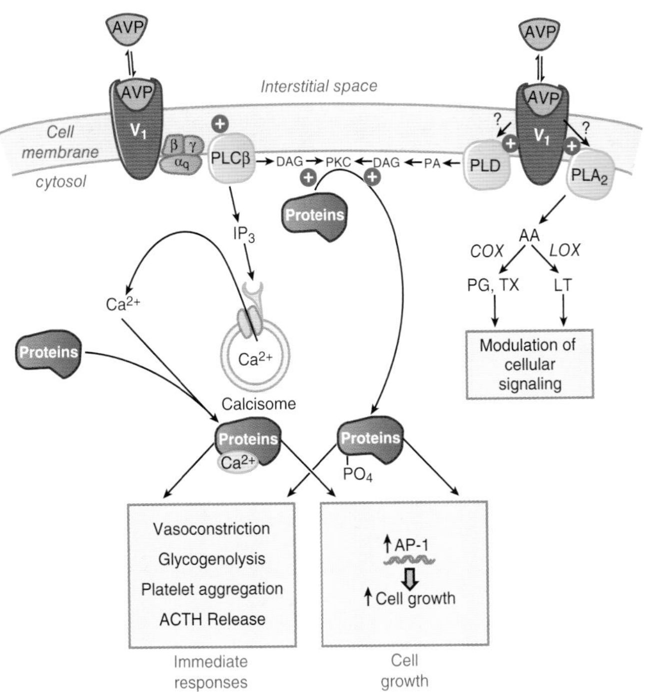

Figure 25–11 *Mechanism of V_1 receptor-effector coupling.* Binding of AVP to V_1 vasopressin receptors (V_1) stimulates membrane-bound phospholipases. Stimulation of G_q activates the PLCβ-IP_3/DAG-Ca^{2+}-PKC pathway. Activation of V_1 receptors also causes influx of extracellular Ca^{2+} by an unknown mechanism. PKC and Ca^{2+}/calmodulin-activated protein kinases phosphorylate cell-type–specific proteins, leading to cellular responses. A further component of the AVP response derives from the production of eicosanoids secondary to the activation of PLA_2; the resulting mobilization of AA provides substrate for eicosanoid synthesis by the COX and LOX pathways, leading to local production of PGs, TXs, and LT, which may activate myriad signaling pathways, including those linked to G_S and G_q.

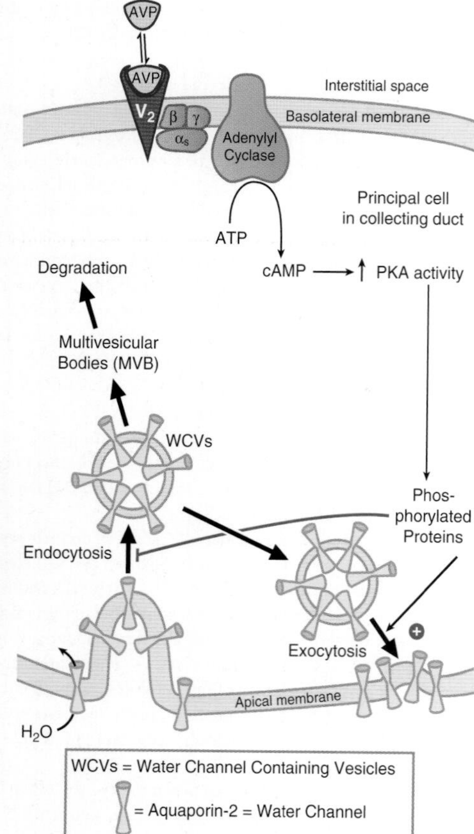

Figure 25–12 *Mechanism of V_2 receptor-effector coupling.* Binding of AVP to the V_2 receptor activates the G_s-adenylyl cyclase-cAMP-PKA pathway and shifts the balance of aquaporin 2 trafficking toward the apical membrane of the principal cell of the collecting duct, thus enhancing water permeability. Although phosphorylation of *Ser256* of aquaporin 2 is involved in V_2 receptor signaling, other proteins located in both the water channel–containing vesicles and the apical membrane of the cytoplasm also may be involved.

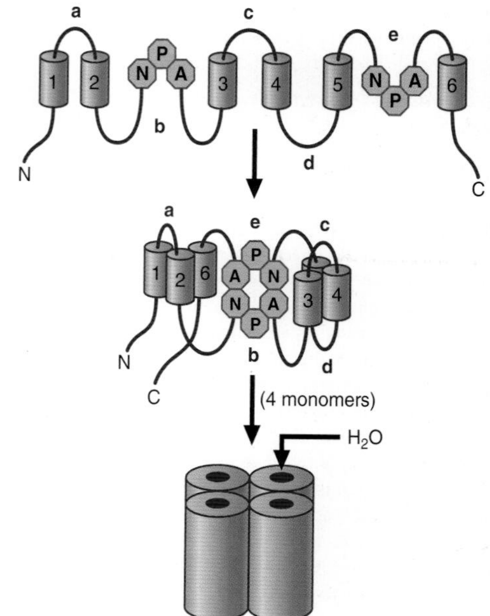

Figure 25–13 *Structure of aquaporins.* Aquaporins have six transmembrane domains, and the NH_2 and COOH termini are intracellular. Loops b and e each contain an NPA sequence. Aquaporins fold with transmembrane domains 1, 2, and 6 in close proximity and transmembrane domains 3, 4 and 5 in juxtaposition. The long b and e loops dip into the membrane, and the NPA sequences align to create a pore through which water can diffuse. Most likely, aquaporins form a tetrameric oligomer. At least seven aquaporins are expressed at distinct sites in the kidney. Aquaporin 1, abundant in the proximal tubule and DTL, is essential for concentration of urine. Aquaporin 2, exclusively expressed in the principal cells of the connecting tubule and collecting duct, is the major vasopressin-regulated water channel. Aquaporin 3 and aquaporin 4 are expressed in the basolateral membranes of collecting duct principal cells and provide exit pathways for water reabsorbed apically by aquaporin 2. Aquaporin 7 is in the apical brush border of the straight proximal tubule. Aquaporins 6–8 are also expressed in kidney; their functions remain to be clarified. Vasopressin regulates water permeability of the collecting duct by influencing the trafficking of aquaporin 2 from intracellular vesicles to the apical plasma membrane (Figure 25–12). AVP-induced activation of the cAMP-PKA pathway also enhances expression of aquaporin 2 mRNA and protein; chronic dehydration thus causes upregulation of aquaporin 2 and water transport in the collecting duct.

activating a vasopressin-regulated urea transporter (termed *VRUT, UT1,* or *UTA1*), most likely by PKA-induced phosphorylation. Kinetics of vasopressin-induced water and urea permeability differ, and vasopressin-induced regulation of VRUT does not entail vesicular trafficking to the plasma membrane.

V_2 receptor activation also increases Na^+ transport in TAL and collecting duct. Increased Na^+ transport in TAL is mediated by three mechanisms that affect the Na^+-K^+-$2Cl^-$ symporter: rapid phosphorylation of the symporter, translocation of the symporter into the luminal membrane, and increased expression of symporter protein. The multiple mechanisms by which vasopressin increases water reabsorption are summarized in Figure 25–14.

Renal Actions of Vasopressin

Several sites of vasopressin action in kidney involve both V_1 and V_2 receptors. V_1 receptors mediate contraction of mesangial cells in the glomerulus and contraction of vascular smooth muscle cells in vasa recta and efferent arterioles. V_1 receptor–mediated reduction of inner medullary blood flow contributes to the maximum concentrating capacity of the kidney. V_1 receptors also stimulate PG synthesis by medullary interstitial cells. Because PGE_2 inhibits adenylyl cyclase in collecting ducts, stimulation of PG synthesis by V_1 receptors may counterbalance V_2 receptor–mediated antidiuresis. V_1 receptors on principal cells in cortical collecting ducts may inhibit V_2 receptor–mediated water flux by activation of PKC. V_2 receptors mediate the most prominent response to vasopressin, which is increased water permeability of the collecting duct at concentrations as low as 50 fM. Thus, V_2 receptor–mediated effects of vasopressin occur at concentrations far lower than are required to engage V_1 receptor–mediated actions. Other renal actions mediated by V_2 receptors include increased urea transport in the IMCD and increased Na^+ transport in the TAL; both effects contribute to the urine-concentrating ability of the kidney. V_2 receptors also increase Na^+ transport in cortical collecting ducts, and this may synergize with aldosterone to enhance Na^+ reabsorption during hypovolemia.

Pharmacological Modification of the Antidiuretic Response to Vasopressin

The NSAIDs, particularly indomethacin, enhance the antidiuretic response to vasopressin. Because PGs attenuate antidiuretic responses to vasopressin and NSAIDs inhibit PG synthesis, reduced PG production probably accounts for potentiation of vasopressin's antidiuretic response.

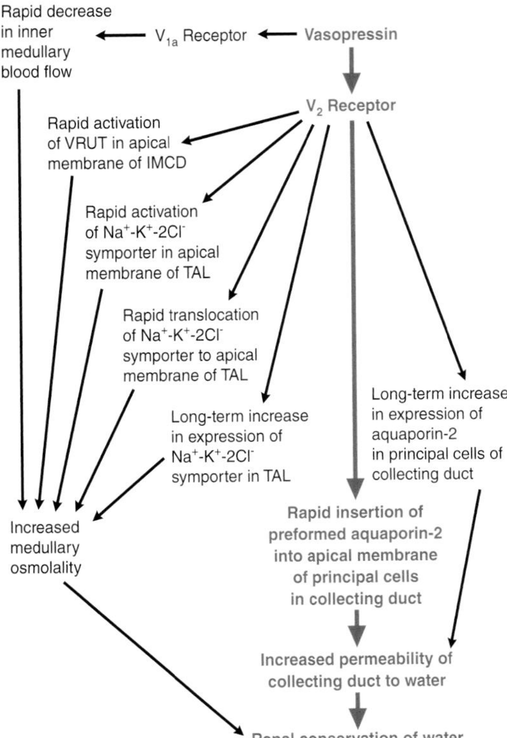

Figure 25–14 *Mechanisms by which vasopressin increases the renal conservation of water.* Red and black arrows denote major and minor pathways, respectively.

Carbamazepine and chlorpropamide also enhance antidiuretic effects of vasopressin by unknown mechanisms. In rare instances, chlorpropamide can induce water intoxication. A number of drugs inhibit the antidiuretic actions of vasopressin. Lithium is of particular importance because of its use in the treatment of manic-depressive disorders (Kishore and Ecelbarger, 2013). Acutely, Li^+ appears to reduce V_2 receptor–mediated stimulation of adenylyl cyclase. Also, Li^+ increases plasma levels of PTH, a partial antagonist to vasopressin. In most patients, the antibiotic demeclocycline attenuates the antidiuretic effects of vasopressin, probably owing to decreased accumulation and action of cyclic AMP (Kortenoeven et al., 2013).

Nonrenal Actions of Vasopressin

Cardiovascular System. The cardiovascular effects of vasopressin are complex. Vasopressin is a potent vasoconstrictor (V_1 receptor mediated), and resistance vessels throughout the circulation may be affected. Vascular smooth muscle in the skin, skeletal muscle, fat, pancreas, and thyroid gland appears most sensitive, with significant vasoconstriction also occurring in the GI tract, coronary vessels, and brain. Despite the potency of vasopressin as a direct vasoconstrictor, vasopressin-induced pressor responses in vivo are minimal and occur only with vasopressin concentrations significantly higher than those required for maximal antidiuresis. To a large extent, this is due to circulating vasopressin actions on V_1 receptors to inhibit sympathetic efferents and potentiate baroreflexes. In addition, V_2 receptors cause vasodilation in some blood vessels.

Vasopressin helps to maintain arterial blood pressure during episodes of severe hypovolemia/hypotension. The effects of vasopressin on the heart (reduced cardiac output and heart rate) are largely indirect and result from coronary vasoconstriction, decreased coronary blood flow, and alterations in vagal and sympathetic tone. Some patients with coronary insufficiency experience angina even in response to the relatively small amounts of vasopressin required to control DI, and vasopressin-induced myocardial ischemia has led to severe reactions and even death.

CNS. Vasopressin likely plays a role as a neurotransmitter or neuromodulator. Although vasopressin can modulate CNS autonomic systems controlling heart rate, arterial blood pressure, respiration rate, and sleep patterns, the physiological significance of these actions is unclear. While vasopressin is not the principal corticotropin-releasing factor, vasopressin may provide for sustained activation of the hypothalamic-pituitary-adrenal axis during chronic stress. Studies in both laboratory animals and humans indicated that vasopressin and oxytocin are key regulators of social and emotional behaviors (Benarroch, 2013). CNS effects of vasopressin appear to be mediated predominantly by V_1 receptors.

Blood Coagulation. Activation of V_2 receptors by desmopressin or vasopressin increases circulating levels of procoagulant factor VIII and of von Willebrand factor. These effects are mediated by extrarenal V_2 receptors. Presumably, vasopressin stimulates secretion of von Willebrand factor and of factor VIII from storage sites in vascular endothelium. However, because release of von Willebrand factor does not occur when desmopressin is applied directly to cultured endothelial cells or to isolated blood vessels, intermediate factors are likely to be involved.

Other Nonrenal Effects. At high concentrations, vasopressin stimulates smooth muscle contraction in the uterus (by oxytocin receptors) and GI tract (by V_1 receptors). Vasopressin is stored in platelets, and activation of V_1 receptors stimulates platelet aggregation. Also, activation of V_1 receptors on hepatocytes stimulates glycogenolysis.

Vasopressin Receptor Agonists

A number of vasopressin-like peptides occur naturally across the animal kingdom (Table 25–8); all are nonapeptides. In all mammals except swine, the neurohypophyseal peptide is 8-arginine vasopressin, and the terms vasopressin, AVP, and ADH are used interchangeably. There are also a number of synthetic peptides with receptor-subtype specificity, and one nonpeptide agonist.

Many vasopressin analogues were synthesized with the goal of increasing duration of action and selectivity for vasopressin receptor subtypes (V_1 vs. V_2 receptors, which mediate pressor responses and antidiuretic responses, respectively). Thus, the antidiuretic-to-vasopressor ratio for the V_2–selective agonist, DDAVP, also called desmopressin, is about 3000 times greater than that for vasopressin; thus, desmopressin is the preferred drug for the treatment of central DI. Substitution of valine for glutamine in position 4 further increases the antidiuretic selectivity, and the antidiuretic-to-vasopressor ratio for deamino [Val^4, D-Arg^8]AVP is about 11,000 times greater than that for vasopressin.

Increasing V_1 selectivity has proved more difficult than increasing V_2 selectivity. Vasopressin receptors in the adenohypophysis that mediate vasopressin-induced ACTH release are neither classical V_1 nor V_2 receptors. Because vasopressin receptors in the adenohypophysis appear to share a common signal-transduction mechanism with classical V_1 receptors, and because many vasopressin analogues with vasoconstrictor activity release ACTH, V_1 receptors have been subclassified into V_{1a} (vascular/hepatic) and V_{1b} (pituitary) receptors (also called V_3 receptors). There are selective agonists for V_{1a} and V_{1b} receptors.

The chemical structure of oxytocin is closely related to that of vasopressin: Oxytocin is [Ile^3, Leu^8]AVP. With such structural similarities, it is not surprising that vasopressin and oxytocin agonists and antagonists can bind to each other's receptors. Therefore, most of the available peptide vasopressin agonists and antagonists have some affinity for oxytocin receptors; at high doses, they may block or mimic the effects of oxytocin.

Diseases Affecting the Vasopressin System

Diabetes Insipidus

Diabetes insipidus is a disease of impaired renal water conservation owing either to inadequate vasopressin secretion from the neurohypophysis (central DI) or to insufficient renal vasopressin response (nephrogenic DI). Very rarely, DI can be caused by an abnormally high degradation rate

TABLE 25–8 ■ VASOPRESSIN RECEPTOR AGONISTS

$$\mathrm{H_2C^{1}(S\!-\!)\!-\!HC(A)\!-\!C(\!=\!O)\!-\!W^{2}\!-\!X^{3}\!-\!Y^{4}\!-\!Asn^{5}\!-\!Cys^{6}(\!-\!S\!-\!)\!-\!Pro^{7}\!-\!Z^{8}\!-\!Gly^{9}\!-\!(NH_2)}$$

Naturally occurring vasopressin-like peptides	A	W	X	Y	Z
A. *Vertebrates*					
1. Mammals					
AVP[a] (humans and other mammals)	NH_2	Tyr	Phe	Gln	Arg
Lypressin[a] (pigs, marsupials)	NH_2	Tyr	Phe	Gln	Lys
Phenypressin (macropodids)	NH_2	Phe	Phe	Gln	Arg
2. Nonmammalian vertebrates					
Vasotocin	NH_2	Tyr	Ile	Gln	Arg
B. *Invertebrates*					
1. Arginine conopressin (*Conus striatus*)	NH_2	Ile	Ile	Arg	Arg
2. Lysine conopressin (*Conus geographicus*)	NH_2	Phe	Ile	Arg	Lys
3. Locust subesophageal ganglia peptide	NH_2	Leu	Ile	Thr	Arg
Synthetic vasopressin peptides					
A. *V_1-selective agonists*					
1. V_{1a}-selective: [Phe², Ile³, Orn⁸] AVP	NH_2	Phe	Ile	Gln	Orn
2. V_{1b}-selective: Deamino [D-3-(3′-pyridyl)-Ala²] AVP	H	D-3-(3′-pyridyl)-Ala²	Phe	Gln	Arg
B. *V_2-selective agonists*					
1. Desmopressin*a* (DDAVP)	H	Tyr	Phe	Gln	D-Arg
2. Deamino [Val⁴, D-Arg⁸] AVP	H	Tyr	Phe	Val	D-Arg
Nonpeptide agonist					
A. *OPC-51803*					

[a]Available for clinical use.

of vasopressin by circulating vasopressinases. Pregnancy may accentuate or reveal central or nephrogenic DI by increasing plasma levels of vasopressinase and by reducing renal sensitivity to vasopressin. Patients with DI excrete large volumes (>30 mL/kg per day) of dilute (<200 mOsm/kg) urine and, if their thirst mechanism is functioning normally, are polydipsic. Central DI can be distinguished from nephrogenic DI by administration of desmopressin, which will increase urine osmolality in patients with central DI but have little or no effect in patients with nephrogenic DI. DI can be differentiated from primary polydipsia by measuring plasma osmolality, which will be low to low-normal in patients with primary polydipsia and high to high-normal in patients with DI.

Central DI. Head injury, either surgical or traumatic, in the region of the pituitary or hypothalamus may cause central DI. Postoperative central DI may be transient, permanent, or triphasic (recovery followed by permanent relapse). Other causes include hypothalamic or pituitary tumors, cerebral aneurysms, CNS ischemia, and brain infiltrations and infections. Central DI may also be idiopathic or familial. Familial central DI usually is autosomal dominant (chromosome 20), and vasopressin deficiency occurs several months or years after birth and worsens gradually. Autosomal dominant central DI is linked to mutations in the vasopressin preprohormone gene that cause the prohormone to misfold and oligomerize improperly. Accumulation of mutant vasopressin precursor causes neuronal death, hence the dominant mode of inheritance. Rarely, familial central DI is autosomal recessive owing to a mutation in the vasopressin peptide itself that gives rise to an inactive vasopressin mutant.

Antidiuretic peptides are the primary treatment of central DI, with desmopressin the peptide of choice. For patients with central DI who cannot tolerate antidiuretic peptides because of side effects or allergic reactions, other treatment options are available. Chlorpropamide, an oral sulfonylurea, potentiates the action of small or residual amounts of circulating vasopressin and will reduce urine volume in more than half of all patients with central DI. Doses of 125–500 mg daily appear effective in patients with partial central DI. If polyuria is not controlled satisfactorily with chlorpropamide alone, addition of a thiazide diuretic to the regimen usually results in an adequate reduction in urine volume. Carbamazepine (800–1000 mg daily in divided doses) also reduces urine volume in patients with central DI. Long-term use may induce serious adverse effects; therefore, carbamazepine is used rarely to treat central DI. These agents are not effective in nephrogenic DI, which indicates that functional V_2 receptors are required for the antidiuretic effect. Because carbamazepine inhibits and chlorpropamide has little effect on vasopressin secretion, it is likely that carbamazepine and chlorpropamide act directly on the kidney to enhance V_2 receptor–mediated antidiuresis.

Nephrogenic DI. Nephrogenic DI may be congenital or acquired. Hypercalcemia, hypokalemia, postobstructive renal failure, Li^+, foscarnet, clozapine, demeclocycline, and other drugs can induce nephrogenic DI. As many as one in three patients treated with Li^+ may develop nephrogenic DI. X-linked nephrogenic DI is caused by mutations in the gene encoding the V_2 receptor, which maps to Xq28. Mutations in the V_2 receptor gene may cause impaired routing of the V_2 receptor to the cell surface, defective coupling of the receptor to G proteins, or decreased receptor affinity for vasopressin. Autosomal recessive and dominant nephrogenic DI result from inactivating mutations in aquaporin 2. These findings indicate that aquaporin 2 is essential for the antidiuretic effect of vasopressin in humans.

Although the mainstay of treatment of nephrogenic DI is assurance of an adequate water intake, drugs also can be used to reduce polyuria. Amiloride blocks Li^+ uptake by the Na^+ channel in the collecting duct system and may be effective in patients with mild-to-moderate concentrating defects. Thiazide *diuretics* reduce the polyuria of patients with DI and often are used to treat nephrogenic DI. In infants with nephrogenic DI, use of thiazides may be crucial because uncontrolled polyuria may exceed the child's capacity to imbibe and absorb fluids. It is possible that the natriuretic action of thiazides and resulting extracellular fluid volume depletion play an important role in thiazide-induced antidiuresis. The antidiuretic effects appear to parallel the thiazide's ability to cause natriuresis, and the drugs are given in doses similar to those used to mobilize edema fluid. In patients with DI, a 50% reduction of urine volume is a good response to thiazides. Moderate restriction of Na^+ intake can enhance the antidiuretic effectiveness of thiazides.

A number of case reports described the effectiveness of indomethacin in the treatment of nephrogenic DI; however, other PG synthase inhibitors (e.g., ibuprofen) appear to be less effective. The mechanism of the effect may involve a decrease in GFR, an increase in medullary solute concentration, or enhanced proximal fluid reabsorption. Also, because PGs attenuate vasopressin-induced antidiuresis in patients with at least a partially intact V_2 receptor system, some of the antidiuretic response to indomethacin may be due to diminution of the PG effect and enhancement of vasopressin effects on the principal cells of collecting duct.

Syndrome of Inappropriate Secretion of Antidiuretic Hormone

A disease of impaired water excretion with accompanying hyponatremia and hypoosmolality, SIADH caused by the *inappropriate* secretion of vasopressin. Clinical manifestations of plasma hypotonicity resulting from SIADH may include lethargy, anorexia, nausea and vomiting, muscle cramps, coma, convulsions, and death. A multitude of disorders can induce SIADH, including malignancies, pulmonary diseases, CNS injuries/diseases (e.g., head trauma, infections, and tumors), and general surgery.

Three drug classes are commonly implicated in drug-induced SIADH: psychotropic medications (e.g., selective serotonin reuptake inhibitors, haloperidol, and tricyclic antidepressants), sulfonylureas (e.g., chlorpropamide), and vinca alkaloids (e.g., vincristine and vinblastine). Other drugs strongly associated with SIADH include clonidine, cyclophosphamide, enalapril, felbamate, ifosfamide, methyldopa, pentamidine, and vinorelbine. Many other drugs have been implicated. In a normal individual, an elevation in plasma vasopressin per se does not induce plasma hypotonicity because the person simply stops drinking owing to an osmotically induced aversion to fluids. Therefore, plasma hypotonicity only occurs when excessive fluid intake (oral or intravenous) accompanies inappropriate secretion of vasopressin.

Treatment of hypotonicity in the setting of SIADH includes water restriction, intravenous administration of hypertonic saline, loop diuretics (which interfere with kidney's concentrating ability), and drugs that inhibit the effect of vasopressin to increase water permeability in collecting ducts. To inhibit vasopressin's action in collecting ducts, demeclocycline, a tetracycline, has been the preferred drug, but tolvaptan and conivaptan, V_2 receptor antagonists, are now available (see next section and Table 25–9).

Although Li^+ can inhibit the renal actions of vasopressin, it is effective in only a minority of patients, may induce irreversible renal damage when used chronically, and has a low therapeutic index. Therefore, Li^+ should be considered for use only in patients with symptomatic SIADH who cannot be controlled by other means or in whom tetracyclines are contraindicated (e.g., patients with liver disease). It is important to stress that the majority of patients with SIADH do not require therapy because plasma Na^+ stabilizes in the range of 125–132 mM; such patients usually are asymptomatic. Only when symptomatic hypotonicity ensues, generally when plasma Na^+ levels drop below 120 mM, should therapy with demeclocycline be initiated. Because hypotonicity, which causes an influx of water into cells with resulting cerebral swelling, is the cause of symptoms, the goal of therapy is simply to increase plasma osmolality toward normal.

Other Water-Retaining States

In patients with CHF, cirrhosis, or nephrotic syndrome, *effective* blood volume often is reduced, and hypovolemia frequently is exacerbated by the liberal use of diuretics. Because hypovolemia stimulates vasopressin release, patients may become hyponatremic owing to vasopressin-mediated retention of water. The development of potent orally active V_2 receptor antagonists and specific inhibitors of water channels in the collecting duct has provided a new therapeutic strategy not only in patients with SIADH but also in the more common setting of hyponatremia in patients with heart failure, liver cirrhosis, and nephrotic syndrome.

Clinical Use of Vasopressin Agonists

Two antidiuretic peptides are available for clinical use in the U.S.:

TABLE 25–9 ■ VASOPRESSIN RECEPTOR ANTAGONISTS

Peptide antagonists

$H_2C(CH_2-CH_2)_2C(S)-CH_2-C(=O)$ [1] –X[2]–Phe[3]–Y[4]–Asn[5]–Cys[6]–Pro[7]–Arg[8]–Z[9], with S of residue 1 bonded to S of Cys[6]

Antagonist	X	Y	Z
A. *V_1-selective antagonists*			
V_{1a}-selective antagonist $d(CH_2)_5[Tyr(Me)^2]$ AVP	Tyr—OMe	Gln	Gly (NH_2)
V_{1b}-selective antagonist dP $[Tyr(Me)^2]$ AVP[a,b]	Tyr—OMe	Gln	Gly (NH_2)
B. *V_2-selective antagonists*[a]			
1. des Gly-NH_2^9-$d(CH_2)_5[D\text{-}Ile^2, Ile^4]$ AVP	D-Ile	Ile	—
2. $d(CH_2)_5[D\text{-}Ile^2, Ile^4, Ala\text{-}NH_2^9]$ AVP	D-Ile	Ile	Ala(NH_2)

Nonpeptide antagonists

A. *V_{1a}-selective antagonists* OPC-21268 SR 49059 (relcovaptan)	B. *V_{1b}-selective antagonists* SSR 149415 (nelivaptan)
C. *V_2-selective antagonists* SR 121463 (satavaptan) VPA-985 (lixivaptan) OPC-31260 (mozavaptan) OPC-41061 (tolvaptan)[c]	D. *V_{1a}-/V_2-selective antagonists* YM-471 YM 087 (conivaptan)[c] JTV-605 CL-385004

[a]Also blocks V_{1a} receptor.
[b]V_2 antagonistic activity in rats; however, antagonistic activity may be less or nonexistent in other species. Also, with prolonged infusion may exhibit significant agonist activity.
[c]Available for clinical use in United States.

- *Vasopressin* (synthetic 8-L-arginine vasopressin) is available as a sterile aqueous solution; it may be administered intravenously, subcutaneously, intramuscularly, intranasally, intraosseously (off label), intra-arterially, or endotracheally (off label; unreliable).
- *Desmopressin acetate* (synthetic DDAVP) is available as a sterile aqueous solution packaged for intravenous or subcutaneous injection, in a solution for intranasal administration with either a nasal spray pump or rhinal tube delivery system, and in tablets for oral administration.

Therapeutic Uses

The therapeutic uses of vasopressin and its congeners can be divided into two main categories according to the vasopressin receptor involved: V_1 receptor mediated and V_2 receptor mediated.

V_1 receptor–mediated therapeutic applications are based on the rationale that V_1 receptors cause GI and vascular smooth muscle contraction. *Vasopressin is the main agent used.* V_1 receptor–mediated GI smooth muscle contraction has been used to treat postoperative ileus and abdominal distension and to dispel intestinal gas before abdominal roentgenography to avoid interfering gas shadows. V_1 receptor–mediated vasoconstriction of the splanchnic arterial vessels reduces blood flow to the portal system and thereby attenuates pressure and bleeding in esophageal varices. Although endoscopic variceal banding ligation is the treatment of choice for bleeding esophageal varices, V_1 receptor agonists have been used in an emergency setting until endoscopy can be performed. Simultaneous administration of nitroglycerin with V_1 receptor agonists may attenuate the cardiotoxic effects of V_1 agonists while enhancing their beneficial splanchnic effects. Also, V_1 receptor agonists have been used during abdominal surgery in patients with portal hypertension to diminish the risk of hemorrhage during the procedure. V_1 receptor–mediated vasoconstriction has been used to reduce bleeding during acute hemorrhagic gastritis, burn wound excision, cyclophosphamide-induced hemorrhagic cystitis, liver transplant, cesarean section, and uterine myoma resection. Vasopressin levels in patients with vasodilatory shock are inappropriately low, and such patients are extraordinarily sensitive to the pressor actions of V_1 receptor agonists. Therefore, V_1 receptor agonists are indicated for the treatment of hypotension in patients with vasodilatory shock that responds insufficiently to therapy with fluids and catecholamines (Serpa Neto et al., 2012). Vasopressin combined with epinephrine and steroids showed improved outcomes after in-hospital cardiac arrest (Layek et al., 2014).

V_2 receptor–mediated therapeutic applications are based on the rationale that V_2 receptors cause water conservation and release of blood coagulation factors. *Desmopressin is the standard drug of choice.* Central, but not nephrogenic, DI can be treated with V_2 receptor agonists, and polyuria and polydipsia usually are well controlled by these agents. Some patients experience transient DI (e.g., in head injury or surgery in the area of the pituitary); however, therapy for most patients with DI is lifelong. Desmopressin is the drug of choice for the vast majority of patients. The duration of effect from a single intranasal dose is from 6 to 20 h; twice-daily administration is effective in most patients. The usual intranasal dosage in adults is 10–40 μg daily either as a single dose or divided into two or three doses. In view of the high cost of the drug and the importance of avoiding water intoxication, the schedule of administration should be adjusted to the minimal amount required. In some patients, chronic allergic rhinitis or other nasal pathology may preclude reliable peptide absorption following nasal administration. Oral administration of desmopressin in doses of 0.1–1.2 mg/d provides adequate desmopressin blood levels to control polyuria. Subcutaneous or intravenous administration of 2–4 μg daily of desmopressin also is effective in central DI.

Vasopressin has little, if any, place in the long-term therapy of DI because of its short duration of action and V_1 receptor–mediated side effects. Vasopressin can be used as an alternative to desmopressin in the initial diagnostic evaluation of patients with suspected DI and to control polyuria in patients with DI who recently have undergone surgery or experienced head trauma. Under these circumstances, polyuria may be transient, and long-acting agents may produce water intoxication.

Desmopressin is used in bleeding disorders. In most patients with type I vWD and in some with type IIn vWD, desmopressin will elevate von Willebrand factor and shorten bleeding time. However, desmopressin generally is ineffective in patients with types IIa, IIb, and III vWD. Desmopressin may cause a marked transient thrombocytopenia in individuals with type IIb vWD and is contraindicated in such patients. Desmopressin also increases factor VIII levels in patients with mild-to-moderate hemophilia A. Desmopressin is not indicated in patients with severe hemophilia A, those with hemophilia B, or those with factor VIII antibodies. In patients with renal insufficiency, desmopressin shortens bleeding time and increases circulating levels of factor VIII coagulant activity, factor VIII–related antigen, and ristocetin cofactor. It also induces the appearance of larger von Willebrand factor multimers. Desmopressin is effective in some patients with liver cirrhosis- or drug-induced (e.g., heparin, hirudin, and antiplatelet agents) bleeding disorders. Desmopressin, given intravenously at a dose of 0.3 μg/kg, increases factor VIII and von Willebrand factor for more than 6 h. Desmopressin can be given at intervals of 12–24 h depending on the clinical response and severity of bleeding. Tachyphylaxis to desmopressin usually occurs after several days (owing to depletion of factor VIII and von Willebrand factor storage sites) and limits its usefulness to preoperative preparation, postoperative bleeding, excessive menstrual bleeding, and emergency situations.

Another V_2 receptor–mediated therapeutic application is the use of desmopressin for primary nocturnal enuresis. Bedtime administration of desmopressin tablets provides a high response rate that is sustained with long-term use and that accelerates the cure rate. Intranasal desmopressin is no longer recommended for the treatment of primary nocturnal enuresis because of increased risk of hyponatremia. Desmopressin also relieves post–lumbar puncture headache, probably by causing water retention and thereby facilitating rapid fluid equilibration in the CNS.

ADME

When vasopressin and desmopressin are given orally, they are inactivated quickly by trypsin. Inactivation by peptidases in various tissues (particularly liver and kidney) results in a plasma $t_{1/2}$ of vasopressin of 17–35 min. Following intramuscular or subcutaneous injection, antidiuretic effects of vasopressin last 2–8 h. The $t_{1/2}$ of desmopressin is 75 min to 3.5 h.

Toxicity, Adverse Effects, Contraindications, Drug Interactions

Most adverse effects are mediated through V_1 receptor activation on vascular and GI smooth muscle; such adverse effects are much less common and less severe with desmopressin than with vasopressin. After injection of large doses of vasopressin, marked facial pallor owing to cutaneous vasoconstriction is observed commonly. Increased intestinal activity is likely to cause nausea, belching, cramps, and an urge to defecate. Vasopressin should be administered with extreme caution in individuals suffering from vascular disease, especially coronary artery disease. Other cardiac complications include arrhythmia and decreased cardiac output. Peripheral vasoconstriction and gangrene were encountered in patients receiving large doses of vasopressin.

The major V_2 receptor–mediated adverse effect is water intoxication. Many drugs, including carbamazepine, chlorpropamide, morphine, tricyclic antidepressants, and NSAIDs, can potentiate the antidiuretic effects of these peptides. Several drugs, such as Li^+, demeclocycline, and ethanol, can attenuate the antidiuretic response to desmopressin. Desmopressin and vasopressin should be used cautiously in disease states in which a rapid increase in extracellular water may impose risks (e.g., in angina, hypertension, and heart failure) and should not be used in patients with acute renal failure. Patients receiving desmopressin to maintain hemostasis should be advised to reduce fluid intake. Also, it is imperative that these peptides not be administered to patients with primary or psychogenic polydipsia because severe hypotonic hyponatremia will ensue. Mild facial flushing and headache are the most common adverse effects. Allergic reactions ranging from urticaria to anaphylaxis may occur with desmopressin or vasopressin. Intranasal administration may cause local adverse effects in the nasal passages, such as edema, rhinorrhea, congestion, irritation, pruritus, and ulceration.

Clinical Use of Vasopressin Antagonists

Table 25–9 summarizes the selectivity of vasopressin receptor antagonists. Only tolvaptan and conivaptan are currently available in the United States.

Therapeutic Uses

When the kidney perceives the arterial blood volume to be low (as in the disease states of CHF, cirrhosis, and nephrosis), AVP perpetuates a state of total body salt and water excess. V_2 receptor antagonists or "aquaretics" may have a therapeutic role in these conditions, especially in patients with concomitant hyponatremia. They are also effective in hyponatremia associated with SIADH. Aquaretics increase renal free water excretion with little or no change in electrolyte excretion. Because they do not affect Na^+ reabsorption, they do not stimulate the TGF mechanism with its associated consequence of reducing GFR.

Tolvaptan is a selective oral V_2 receptor antagonist FDA-approved for clinically significant hypervolemic and euvolemic hyponatremia. Conivaptan is a nonselective V_{1a} receptor/V_2 receptor antagonist that is FDA-approved for the treatment of hospitalized patients with euvolemic and hypervolemic hyponatremia. Conivaptan is available only for intravenous infusion. Expert panels have yet to reach a consensus regarding the appropriate use of V_2 receptor antagonists (Berl, 2015).

ADME

Tolvaptan has a $t_{1/2}$ of 2.8–12 h and less than 1% is excreted in the urine. Tolvaptan is a substrate and inhibitor of P-glycoprotein and is eliminated entirely by CYP3A4 metabolism. Conivaptan is highly protein bound, has a terminal elimination $t_{1/2}$ of 5–12 h, is metabolized via CYP3A, and is partially excreted by the kidney.

Toxicity, Adverse Effects, Contraindications, Drug Interactions

The most dangerous adverse effect of V_2 receptor antagonists is due to their pharmacological action to increase free water excretion. This may correct hyponatremia too rapidly, resulting in serious and even fatal consequences (osmotic demyelination syndrome). Indeed, tolvaptan is labeled with a black-box warning against too rapid correction of hyponatremia and with the recommendation to initiate therapy in a hospital setting capable of close monitoring of serum Na^+. V_2 receptor antagonists should not be used with hypertonic saline. Antagonism of V_2 receptors can also cause polyuria, which likely explains the increased incidence of dehydration, hypotension, dizziness, pyrexia, increased thirst, and xerostomia with this class of drugs. Both tolvaptan and conivaptan can cause adverse GI adverse effects. Tolvaptan can cause liver damage; therefore, administration of tolvaptan generally should be limited to 30 days, and tolvaptan should not be used in patients with liver disease. Both tolvaptan and conivaptan can induce headaches, hypokalemia, and hyperglycemia, and both are contraindicated in anuria (no benefit) and in patients receiving drugs that inhibit CYP3A4 (e.g., clarithromycin, ketoconazole).

Acknowledgment: *Robert F. Reilly contributed to this chapter in the prior edition of this book. We have retained some of his text in the current edition.*

Drug Facts for Your Personal Formulary: *Diuretics and Agents Regulating Renal Excretion*

Drug	Major Therapeutic Uses	Clinical Pharmacology and Tips
Carbonic Anhydrase Inhibitors		
Acetazolamide Dichlorphenamide	• Glaucoma • Epilepsy • Altitude sickness • Diuretic resistance • Metabolic alkalosis • Familial periodic paralysis	• Ineffective as diuretic monotherapy because effects on renal excretion are self-limiting • Dichlorphenamide drug of choice for familial periodic paralysis
Osmotic Diuretics		
Mannitol	• Elevated intraocular pressure • Elevated intracranial pressure • Dialysis disequilibrium syndrome • Diagnosis of bronchial hyperreactivity • Urologic irrigation • Management of some overdoses	• Frequently used to treat or prevent acute kidney injuries, efficacy unclear • Expansion of extracellular fluid volume may cause pulmonary edema
Inhibitors of Na^+-K^+-$2Cl^-$ Symport (Loop Diuretics; High-Ceiling Diuretics)		
Bumetanide Ethacrynic acid Furosemide Torsemide	• Acute pulmonary edema • Edema associated with congestive heart failure, liver cirrhosis, chronic kidney disease, and nephrotic syndrome • Hyponatremia • Hypercalcemia • Hypertension	• Higher doses needed with impaired renal function • Torsemide may be superior to furosemide in heart failure • Increased risk of ototoxicity with ethacrynic acid compared to other loop diuretics • Risk for hypokalemia and arrhythmia when combined with QT-prolonging drugs
Inhibitors of Na^+-Cl^- Symport (Thiazide Diuretics)		
Thiazide type Chlorothiazide Hydrochlorothiazide Methyclothiazide ***Thiazide-like*** Chlorthalidone Indapamide Metolazone	• Hypertension • Edema associated with congestive heart failure, liver cirrhosis, chronic kidney disease, and nephrotic syndrome • Nephrogenic diabetes insipidus • Kidney stones caused by Ca^{2+} crystals	• Among first choice for treating hypertension • Thiazide-like have longer half-lives than thiazide-type and thus may be superior for hypertension • Higher doses needed for treating edema in patients with impaired renal function • Frequently combined with a loop diuretic to effect "sequential blockade" of tubular transport • Risk for hypokalemia and arrhythmia when combined with QT-prolonging drugs • Cause metabolic disturbances (e.g., elevate plasma glucose and LDL) • May cause severe hyponatremia in some patients

Drug Facts for Your Personal Formulary: *Diuretics and Agents Regulating Renal Excretion (continued)*

Drug	Major Therapeutic Uses	Clinical Pharmacology and Tips
Inhibitors of Renal Epithelial Na^+ Channels (K^+-Sparing Diuretics)		
Amiloride Triamterene	• Hypertension • Edema associated with congestive heart failure, liver cirrhosis, and chronic kidney disease • Liddle syndrome • Lithium-induced nephrogenic diabetes insipidus	• Low efficacy as monotherapy for edema • Frequently combined with loop or thiazide diuretics to prevent hypokalemia and increase diuresis • Risk of hyperkalemia in renal insufficiency or when combined with angiotensin-converting enzyme inhibitors or angiotensin-receptor antagonists
Mineralocorticoid Receptor Antagonists (Aldosterone Antagonists; K^+-Sparing Diuretics)		
Eplerenone Spironolactone	• Hypertension • Edema associated with congestive heart failure, liver cirrhosis, chronic kidney disease • Primary hyperaldosteronism • Acute myocardial infarction (eplerenone) • Heart failure (in combination with standard therapy) • Polycystic ovary disease	• Endogenous aldosterone levels determine therapeutic efficacy • Sometimes combined with loop or thiazide diuretics to prevent hypokalemia and increase diuresis • Diuretics of choice for treating resistant hypertension due to primary hyperaldosteronism and for refractory edema due to secondary aldosteronism (e.g., heart failure, hepatic cirrhosis). • High risk for hyperkalemia in chronic renal insufficiency • Eplerenone contraindicated with potent inhibitors of CYP3A4 (e.g., ketoconazole, itraconazole) • Spironolactone active metabolite has long half-life requiring slow dose adjustments (over days)
Inhibitors of the Nonspecific Cation Channel (Naturietic Peptide Analogues)		
Nesiritide	• Hospitalized patients with acutely decompensated congestive heart failure (New York Heart Association class IV)	• Intravenous only • Clinical benefit remains questionable • High risk of serious hypotension
Vasopressin Receptor Agonist		
V_1 receptor-agonist Vasopressin	• Postoperative abdominal distention • Abdominal roentgenography • Bleeding • Cardiac arrest • Hypovolemic shock	• Contraindicated in nephrogenic diabetes insipidus • Not for long-term therapy of central diabetes insipidus • Use with extreme caution in patients with vascular disease
V_2 receptor-agonist Desmopressin (DDAVP)	• Central diabetes insipidus • Primary nocturnal enuresis • Prevention of blood loss in patients with specific bleeding disorders	• Contraindicated in nephrogenic diabetes insipidus • Drug of choice for central diabetes insipidus • Can be administered orally at high doses • Major adverse effect is water intoxication
Vasopressin Receptor Antagonists		
Conivaptan Tolvaptan	• Treatment of hypervolemic and euvolemic hyponatremia	• Risk of too rapid correction with serious consequences (osmotic demyelination syndrome) • Close monitoring of serum Na^+ required

ACEI, angiotensin converting enzyme inhibitor; ARB, angiotensin receptor antagonist; DDAVP, Desmopressin; LDL, low density lipoprotein.

Bibliography

Barzilay JI, et al. Long-term effects of incident diabetes mellitus on cardiovascular outcomes in people treated for hypertension: the ALLHAT Diabetes Extension Study. *Circ Cardiovasc Qual Outcomes*, **2012**, *5*:153–162.

Bauersachs J, et al. Mineralocorticoid receptor activation and mineralocorticoid receptor antagonist treatment in cardiac and renal diseases. *Hypertension*, **2015**, *65*:257–263.

Benarroch EE. Oxytocin and vasopressin: social neuropeptides with complex neuromodulatory functions. *Neurology*, **2013**, *80*:1521–1528.

Berl T. Vasopressin antagonists. *N Engl J Med*, **2015**, *372*:2207–2216.

Bernstein PL, Ellison DH. Diuretics and salt transport along the nephron. *Semin Nephrol*, **2011**, *31*:475–482.

Brater DC. Diuretic therapy. *N Engl J Med*, **1998**, *339*:387–395.

Brown J, et al. Spironolactone versus placebo or in combination with steroids for hirsutism and/or acne. *Cochrane Database Syst Rev*, **2009**, (2):CD000194.

Bruderer S, et al. Use of diuretics and risk of incident gout: a population-based case-control study. *Arthritis Rheumatol*, **2014**, *66*:185–196.

Buggey J, et al. A reappraisal of loop diuretic choice in heart failure patients. *Am Heart J*, **2015**, *169*:323–333.

D'Elia E, Krum H. Mineralcorticoid antagonists in heart failure. *Heart Fail Clin*, **2014**, *10*:559–564.

Edelmann F, et al. Effect of spironolactone on diastolic function and exercise capacity in patients with heart failure with preserved ejection fraction: the Aldo-DHF randomized controlled trial. *JAMA*, **2013**, *309*:781–791.

Faris R, et al. Current evidence supporting the role of diuretics in heart failure: a meta analysis of randomised controlled trials. *Int J Cardiol*, **2002**, *82*:149–158.

Garcia ML, Kaczorowski GJ. Targeting the inward-rectifier potassium channel ROMK in cardiovascular disease. *Curr Opin Pharmacol*, **2014**, *15*:1–6.

Grimm RH Jr, et al. Long-term effects on sexual function of five antihypertensive drugs and nutritional hygienic treatment in hypertensive men and women. Treatment of Mild Hypertension Study (TOMHS). *Hypertension*, **1997**, *29*:8–14.

Iovino M, et al. Molecular mechanisms involved in the control of neurohypophyseal hormones secretion. *Curr Pharm Des*, **2014**,

20:6702–6713.

Kellenberger S, Schild L. International Union of Basic and Clinical Pharmacology. XCI. Structure, function, and pharmacology of acid-sensing ion channels and the epithelial Na+ channel. *Pharmacol Rev*, **2015**, *67*:1–35.

Kishore BK, Ecelbarger CM. Lithium: a versatile tool for understanding renal physiology. *Am J Physiol Renal Physiol*, **2013**, *304*:F1139–F1149.

Kortenoeven MLA, et al. Amiloride blocks lithium entry through the sodium channel thereby attenuating the resultant nephrogenic diabetes insipidus. *Kidney Int*, **2009**, *76*:44–53.

Kortenoeven MLA, et al. Demeclocycline attenuates hyponatremia by reducing aquaporin-2 expression in the renal inner medulla. *Am J Physiol Renal Physiol*, **2013**, *305*:F1705–F1718.

Layek A, et al. Efficacy of vasopressin during cardio-pulmonary resuscitation in adult patients: a meta-analysis. *Resuscitation*, **2014**, *85*:855–863.

Nejsum LN. The renal plumbing system: aquaporin water channels. *Cell Mol Life Sci*, **2005**, *62*:1692–1706.

Nigwekar SU, Waikar SS. Diuretics in acute kidney injury. *Semin Nephrol*, **2011**, *31*:523–534.

Nirdé P, et al. Antimineralocorticoid 11β-substituted spirolactones exhibit androgen receptor agonistic activity: a structure function study. *Mol Pharmacol*, **2001**, *59*:1307–1313.

O'Connor CM, et al. Effect of nesiritide in patients with acute decompensated heart failure. *N Engl J Med*, **2011**, *365*:32–43.

Olde Engberink RHG, et al. Effects of thiazide-type and thiazide-like diuretics on cardiovascular events and mortality: systematic review and meta-analysis. *Hypertension*, **2015**, *65*:1033–1040.

Palmer BF. Metabolic complications associated with use of diuretics. *Semin Nephrol*, **2011**, *31*:542–552.

Pitt B, et al. Spironolactone for heart failure with preserved ejection fraction. *N Engl J Med*, **2014**, *370*:1383–1392.

Potter LR. Natriuretic peptide metabolism, clearance and degradation. *FEBS J*, **2011**, *278*:1808–1817.

Ritchie ND, et al. Acetazolamide for the prevention of acute mountain sickness—a systematic review and meta-analysis. *J Travel Med*, **2012**, *19*:298–307.

Rodenburg EM, et al. Thiazide-associated hyponatremia: a population-based study. *Am J Kidney Dis*, **2013**, *62*:67–72.

Ronchetti S, et al. GILZ as a mediator of the anti-inflammatory effects of glucocorticoids. Front Endocrinol (Lausanne) 2015, 6: article 170. doi: 10.3389/fendo.2015.00170, Accessed April 10, 2017.

Ronzaud C, Staub O. Ubiquitylation and control of renal Na+ balance and blood pressure. *Physiology*, **2014**, *29*:16–26.

Roush GC, et al. Diuretics: a review and update. *J Cardiovasc Pharmacol Ther*, **2014**, *19*:5–13.

Roush GC, et al. Head-to-head comparisons of hydrochlorothiazide with indapamide and chlorthalidone: antihypertensive and metabolic effects. *Hypertension*, **2015**, *65*:1041–1046.

Scozzafava A, Supuran CT. Glaucoma and the applications of carbonic anhydrase inhibitors. *Subcell Biochem*, **2014**, *75*:349–359.

Serpa Neto A, et al. Vasopressin and terlipressin in adult vasodilatory shock: a systematic review and meta-analysis of nine randomized controlled trials. *Crit Care*, **2012**, *16*:R154.

Sundar S, Dickinson PD. Spironolactone, a possible selective androgen receptor modulator, should be used with caution in patients with metastatic carcinoma of the prostate. *BMJ Case Rep*, **2012,** *25*:2012.

Tamargo J, et al. Diuretics in the treatment of hypertension. Part 1: thiazide and thiazide-like diuretics. *Expert Opin Pharmacother*, **2014**, *15*:527–547.

Wakai A, et al. Mannitol for acute traumatic brain injury. *Cochrane Database Syst Rev*, **2013**, (8):CD001049.

Welling PA. Regulation of renal potassium secretion: molecular mechanisms. *Semin Nephrol*, **2013**, *33*:215–228.

Wile D. Diuretics: a review. *Ann Clin Biochem*, **2012**, *49*:419–431.

Renin and Angiotensin

Randa Hilal-Dandan

第二十六章 肾素和血管紧张素

中文导读

本章主要介绍：肾素-血管紧张素系统（RAS），包括历史、经典RAS、RAS中的新范例；肾素-血管紧张素系统的组成，包括肾素、肾素分泌的调控、血管紧张素原、血管紧张素转换酶、血管紧张素转换酶2、血管紧张素Ⅱ生物合成的替代途径、血管紧张素肽及其受体、局部（组织）肾素-血管紧张素系统、肾素（原）受体；血管紧张素Ⅱ的功能和作用，包括血管紧张素Ⅱ增加外周阻力的机制、调节肾功能的机制、改变心血管结构的机制，以及RAS在饮食Na^+摄入极值情况下对长时程维持动脉血压的作用；肾素-血管紧张素系统抑制药，包括血管紧张素转换酶抑制药、血管紧张素Ⅱ受体阻滞药、直接肾素抑制药、药物降压对RAS功能的影响。

Abbreviations

ACE: angiotensin-converting enzyme
ACEI: angiotensin-converting enzyme inhibitor
Ac-SDKP: *N*-acetyl-seryl-aspartyl-lysyl-proline
ACTH: corticotropin (formerly adrenocorticotropic hormone)
Ang: angiotensin
ARB: angiotensin receptor blocker
ATR: angiotensin receptor
BP: blood pressure
cAMP: cyclic AMP
CNS: central nervous system
COX: cyclooxygenase
DRI: direct renin inhibitor
FDA: Food and Drug Administration
GFR: glomerular filtration rate
GI: gastrointestinal
GPCR: G protein–coupled receptor
HCTZ: hydrochlorothiazide
JG: juxtaglomerular
LDL: low-density lipoprotein
MrgD: Mas-related G protein–coupled receptor D
NE: norepinephrine
NO: nitric oxide
NOS: nitric oxide synthase
NSAID: nonsteroidal anti-inflammatory drug
PAI-1: plasminogen activator inhibitor type 1
PCP: prolylcarboxylpeptidase
PG: prostaglandin
PI_3K: phosphoinositide 3-kinase
PL: phospholipase
PRA: plasma renin activity
PRC: plasma renin concentration
(pro)renin: renin and prorenin
PRR: (pro)renin receptor
RAS: renin-angiotensin system
RBF: renal blood flow
ROS: reactive O_2 species
TGF: transforming growth factor
TPR: total peripheral resistance

The Renin-Angiotensin System

The RAS participates in the pathophysiology of hypertension, congestive heart failure, myocardial infarction, and diabetic nephropathy. This realization has led to a thorough exploration of the RAS and the development of new approaches for inhibiting its actions. This chapter discusses the physiology, biochemistry, and cellular and molecular biology of the classical RAS and novel RAS components and pathways. The chapter also discusses the basic pharmacology of drugs that interrupt the RAS, and the clinical utility of inhibitors of the RAS. Therapeutic applications of drugs covered in this chapter are also discussed in Chapters 27–29.

History

In 1898, Tiegerstedt and Bergman found that crude saline extracts of the kidney contained a pressor substance that they named *renin.* In 1934, Goldblatt and his colleagues demonstrated that constriction of the renal arteries produced persistent hypertension in dogs. In 1940, Braun-Menéndez and his colleagues in Argentina and Page and Helmer in the U.S. reported that renin was an enzyme that acted on a plasma protein substrate to catalyze the formation of the actual pressor material, a peptide, that was named *hypertensin* by the former group and *angiotonin* by the latter. Ultimately, the pressor substance was renamed *angiotensin,* and the plasma substrate was called *angiotensinogen.*

In the mid-1950s, two forms of angiotensin were recognized, a decapeptide (AngI) and an octapeptide (AngII) formed by proteolytic cleavage of AngI by an enzyme termed *ACE.* The octapeptide was the more active form, and its synthesis in 1957 by Schwyzer and by Bumpus made the material available for intensive study. Later research showed that the kidneys are an important site of aldosterone action, and that angiotensin potently stimulates the production of aldosterone in humans. Moreover, renin secretion increased with depletion of Na^+. Thus, the RAS became recognized as a mechanism to stimulate aldosterone synthesis and secretion and an important homeostatic mechanism in the regulation of blood pressure and electrolyte composition.

In the early 1970s, polypeptides were discovered that either inhibited the formation of AngII or blocked AngII receptors. These inhibitors revealed important physiological and pathophysiological roles for the RAS and inspired the development of a new and broadly efficacious class of antihypertensive drugs: the orally active ACE inhibitors. Studies with ACE inhibitors uncovered roles for the RAS in the pathophysiology of hypertension, heart failure, vascular disease, and renal failure. Selective and competitive antagonists of AngII receptors were subsequently developed that yielded losartan, the first orally active, highly selective, and potent nonpeptide AngII receptor antagonist (Dell'Italia, 2011). Subsequently, many other AngII receptor antagonists have been developed; more recently, aliskiren, a direct renin inhibitor, was approved for antihypertensive therapy.

Classical RAS

Through the actions of AngII, the RAS participates in blood pressure regulation, aldosterone release, Na^+-reabsorption from renal tubules, electrolyte and fluid homeostasis, and cardiovascular remodeling. AngII is derived from angiotensinogen in two proteolytic steps. First, the enzyme renin, released into the circulation from the JG cells in the kidneys, cleaves the decapeptide AngI from the amino terminus of angiotensinogen (renin substrate). Then, an ACE, located on the endothelial cell lining of the vasculature, removes the carboxy-terminal dipeptide of AngI to produce the octapeptide AngII. These enzymatic steps are summarized in Figure 26–1. AngII acts by binding to two distinct heptaspanning GPCRs, AT_1 and AT_2.

New Paradigms in the RAS

The RAS has expanded from being solely an endocrine system to include a paracrine, autocrine/intracrine hormonal system with several new components and active pathways. The current understanding of the RAS involves local (tissue) RAS; alternative pathways for AngII synthesis (*ACE independent* and *renin independent*); an ACE2/Ang(1–7)/Mas receptor axis that opposes the vasoconstrictor effects of ACE/AngII/AT_1 receptor axis; an AngIV/AT_4 receptor axis that is important in brain functions and cognition; multiple biologically active angiotensin peptides such Ang(1–9), AngIII, Ang(3–7), angiotensin A, and alamandine; multiple receptors for angiotensin (AT_1, AT_2, AT_4; Mas; and MrgD); and the PRR. Differential activation of these multiple arms of the RAS may underlie the pathophysiological outcome in cardiovascular and renal disease (Campbell, 2014; Santos, 2014).

Components of the Renin-Angiotensin System

Renin

Renin is the major determinant of the rate of AngII production; its secretion is regulated by several mechanisms (Figures 26–1 through 26–3). Renin is synthesized, stored, and secreted by exocytosis into the renal arterial circulation by the granular JG cells located in the walls of the afferent arterioles that enter the glomeruli. Renin is an aspartyl protease that cleaves the bond between residues 10 and 11 at the amino terminus of angiotensinogen to generate AngI. The active form of renin is a

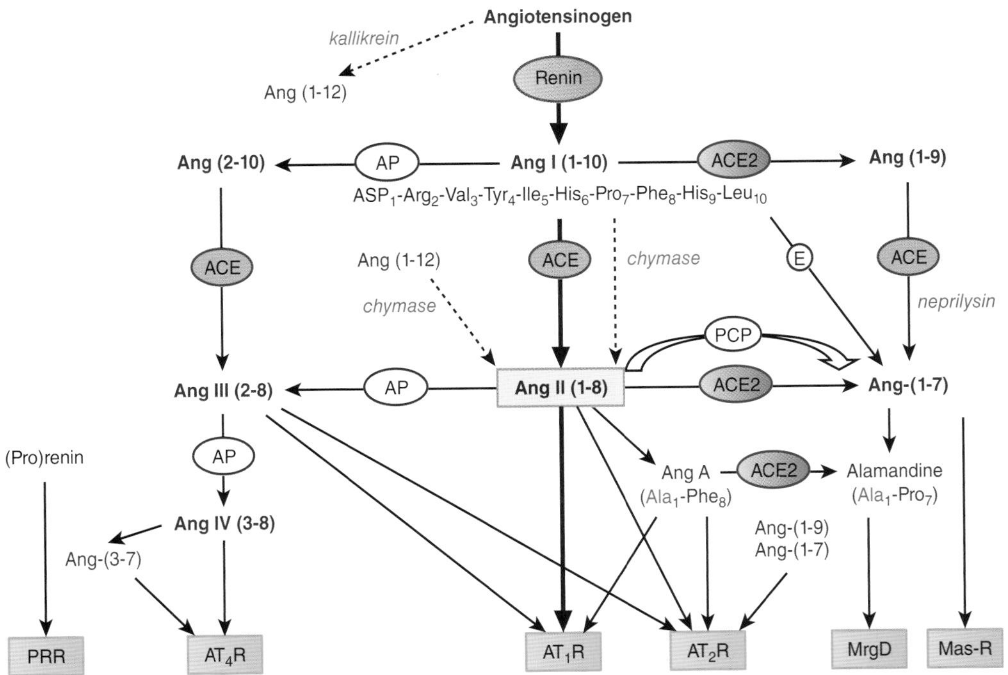

Figure 26–1 *Components of the RAS.* The heavy arrows show the classical pathway, and the light arrows indicate alternative pathways. Receptors involved: AT_1, AT_2, AT_4, Mas, MrgD, and PRR. AP, aminopeptidase; E, endopeptidases; PCP, prolylcarboxylpeptidase.

glycoprotein that contains 340 amino acids. It is synthesized as a pre-proenzyme that is processed to prorenin.

Prorenin may be activated in two ways (Figure 26–2): *proteolytically*, by proconvertase 1 or cathepsin B enzymes that remove 43 amino acids (propeptide) from its amino terminus to uncover the active site of renin; and *nonproteolytically*, when prorenin binds to the PRR, resulting in conformational changes that unfold the propeptide and expose the active catalytic site of the enzyme (Nguyen and Danser, 2008). Both renin and prorenin are stored in the JG cells and, when released, circulate in the blood. The concentration of prorenin in the circulation is about 10-fold greater than that of the active enzyme. The $t_{1/2}$ of circulating renin is about 15 min.

Control of Renin Secretion

Renin is secreted by the granular cells within the JG apparatus and is regulated by the following pathways (Figure 26–3):

1. The macula densa pathway
2. The intrarenal baroreceptor pathway
3. The β_1 adrenergic receptor pathway

The Macula Densa Pathway

The macula densa pathway provides an important function for salt and water regulation by the RAS. The macula densa lies adjacent to the JG cells and is composed of specialized columnar epithelial cells in the wall of that portion of the cortical thick ascending limb that passes between the afferent and efferent arterioles of the glomerulus. A change in NaCl reabsorption by the macula densa results in the transmission to nearby JG cells of chemical signals that modify renin release. Increases in NaCl flux across the macula densa inhibit renin release, whereas decreases in NaCl flux stimulate renin release.

Adenosine, ATP, and PGs modulate the macula densa pathway (Figure 26–4). ATP and adenosine *inhibit renin release* when NaCl

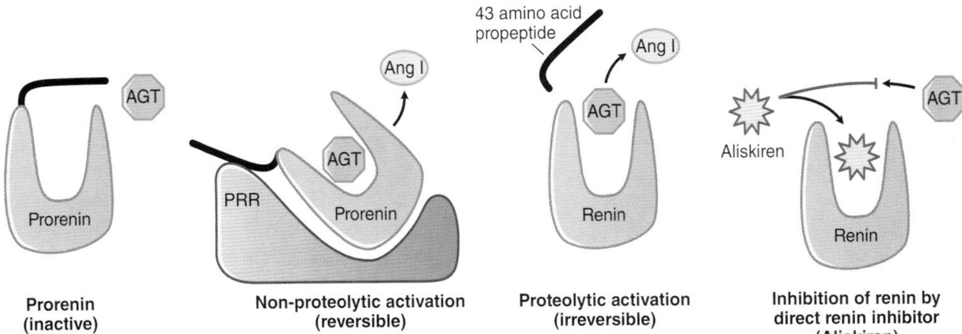

Figure 26–2 *Biological activation of prorenin and pharmacological inhibition of renin.* Prorenin is inactive; accessibility of AGT (angiotensinogen) to the catalytic site is blocked by the propeptide (black segment). The blocked catalytic site can be activated nonproteolytically by the binding of prorenin to the PRR or by proteolytic removal of the propeptide. The competitive renin inhibitor aliskiren has a higher affinity (~0.1 μm) for the active site of renin than does AGT (~1 μm).

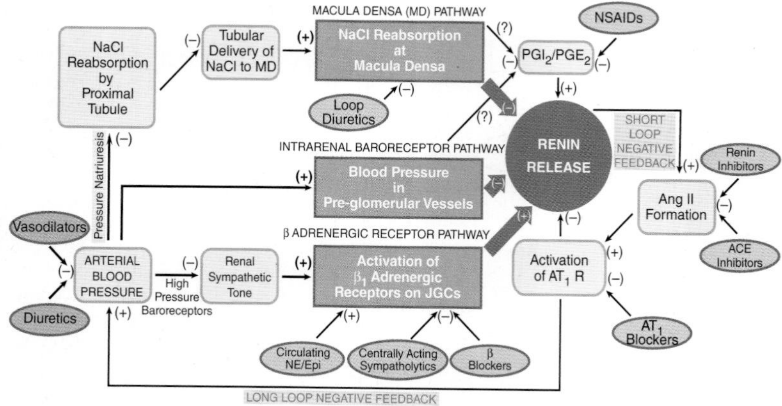

Figure 26–3 *Physiological pathways, feedback loops, and pharmacological regulation of the RAS.* Schematic portrayal of the three major physiological pathways regulating renin release. See text for details.

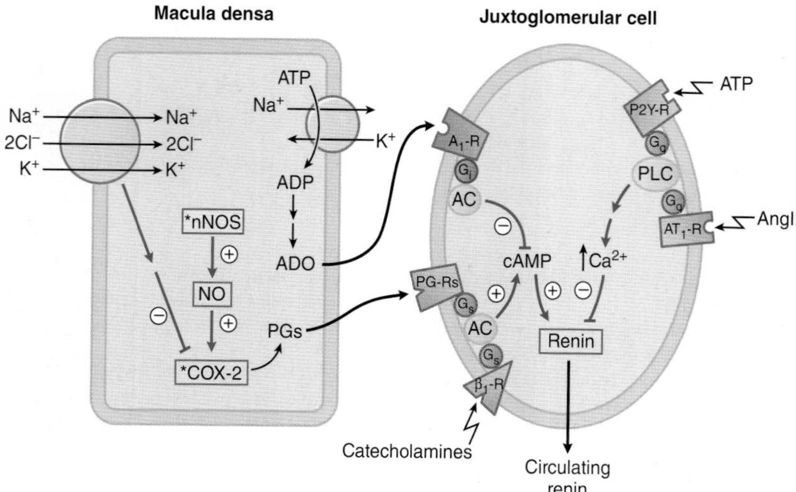

Figure 26–4 *Regulation of JG cell renin release by the macula densa.* Mechanisms by which the MD regulates renin release. Changes in tubular delivery of NaCl to the MD cause appropriate signals to be conveyed to the JG cells. Sodium depletion upregulates nNOS and COX-2 in the MD to enhance production of PGs. PGs and catecholamines stimulate adenylyl cyclase (AC) and cAMP production and thence renin release from the JG cells. Increased NaCl transport depletes ATP and increases adenosine (ADO) levels. Adenosine diffuses to the JG cells and inhibits cAMP production and renin release via G_i-coupled A_1 receptors. Increased NaCl transport in the MD augments the efflux of ATP, which may inhibit renin release directly by binding to P2Y receptors and activating the G_q-PLC-IP_3-Ca^{2+} pathway in JG cells. Circulating AngII also inhibits renin release on JG cells via G_q-coupled AT_1 receptors.
*Expression upregulated by chronic Na^+ depletion.

transport *increases.* ATP acts via P2Y receptors to enhance Ca^{2+} release, and adenosine acts via the A_1 adenosine receptor to inhibit adenylyl cyclase activity and cyclic AMP production. PGE_2 and PGI_2 *stimulate renin release* when NaCl transport *decreases* through enhancing cyclic AMP formation. PG production is enhanced by inducible cyclooxygenase 2 (COX-2) and nNOS. The expression of COX-2 and nNOS is upregulated by chronic dietary Na^+ restriction; selective inhibition of either COX-2 or nNOS inhibits renin release (Peti-Peterdi et al., 2010).

Regulation of the macula densa pathway is more dependent on the luminal concentration of Cl^- than Na^+. NaCl transport into the macula densa is mediated by the Na^+-K^+-$2Cl^-$ symporter (Figure 26–4), and the half-maximal concentrations of Na^+ and Cl^- required for transport via this symporter are 2–3 and 40 mEq/L, respectively. Because the luminal concentration of Na^+ at the macula densa usually is much greater than the level required for half-maximal transport, physiological variations in luminal Na^+ concentrations at the macula densa have little effect on renin release (i.e., the symporter remains saturated with respect to Na^+). Conversely, physiological changes in Cl^- concentrations (20–60 mEq/L) at the macula densa profoundly affect macula densa–mediated renin release.

The Intrarenal Baroreceptor Pathway

Increases and decreases in blood pressure or renal perfusion pressure in the preglomerular vessels inhibit and stimulate renin release, respectively. The immediate stimulus to secretion is believed to be reduced tension within the wall of the afferent arteriole. The release of renal PGs and biomechanical coupling via stretch-activated ion channels may mediate in part the intrarenal baroreceptor pathway.

The β_1 Adrenergic Receptor Pathway

The β_1 adrenergic receptor pathway is regulated by the release of NE from postganglionic sympathetic nerves; activation of β_1 receptors on JG cells increases cyclic AMP and enhances renin secretion. Treatment with β blockers reduces renin secretion and PRA.

Feedback Regulation

Renin release is subject to feedback regulation (Figure 26–3). Increased renin secretion enhances the formation of AngII, which stimulates AT_1 receptors on JG cells to inhibit renin release, an effect termed *short-loop negative feedback.* Inhibition of renin release due to AngII-dependent increase in blood pressure is termed *long-loop negative feedback.* AngII increases arterial blood pressure via AT_1 receptors; this effect inhibits renin release by the following:

1. Activating high-pressure baroreceptors, thereby reducing renal sympathetic tone
2. Increasing pressure in the preglomerular vessels
3. Reducing NaCl reabsorption in the proximal tubule (pressure natriuresis), which increases tubular delivery of NaCl to the macula densa

Drugs That Affect Renin Secretion

Renin release is influenced by arterial blood pressure, dietary salt intake, and pharmacological agents (Figures 26–3 and 26–4). Loop diuretics stimulate renin release and increase PRC by decreasing arterial blood pressure and by blocking the reabsorption of NaCl at the macula densa. *NSAIDs* inhibit PG synthesis and thereby decrease renin release. ACE inhibitors, ARBs, and renin inhibitors interrupt both the short- and long-loop negative-feedback mechanisms and therefore increase renin release and PRC. Centrally acting sympatholytic drugs, as well as β_1 adrenergic receptor antagonists, decrease renin secretion by reducing activation of β_1 adrenergic receptors on JG cells.

Angiotensinogen

The substrate for renin is angiotensinogen, an abundant globular glycoprotein. AngI is cleaved by renin from the amino terminus of angiotensinogen. Human angiotensinogen contains 452 amino acids and is synthesized as preangiotensinogen, which has a 24– or 33–amino acid signal peptide. Angiotensinogen is synthesized and secreted primarily by the liver, although angiotensinogen transcripts occur in many tissues, including the heart, kidneys, pancreas, adipocytes, and certain regions of the CNS. Biosynthesis of angiotensinogen is stimulated by inflammation, insulin, estrogens, glucocorticoids, thyroid hormone, and AngII. During pregnancy, plasma levels of angiotensinogen increase several-fold owing to increased estrogen.

Circulating levels of angiotensinogen are approximately equal to the K_m of renin for its substrate (~1 μM). Consequently, the rate of AngII synthesis, and therefore blood pressure, can be influenced by changes in angiotensinogen levels. Oral contraceptives containing estrogen increase circulating levels of angiotensinogen and can induce hypertension. A missense mutation in the angiotensinogen gene (M235T in angiotensinogen) that increases plasma levels of angiotensinogen is associated with essential and pregnancy-induced hypertension (Sethi et al., 2003). Urinary angiotensinogen levels are considered an index for local intrarenal RAS activation and are elevated in patients with hypertension and progressive renal disease (Kobori and Urushihara, 2013).

Angiotensin-Converting Enzyme

Angiotensin-converting enzyme (ACE, kininase II, dipeptidyl carboxypeptidase) is an ectoenzyme and glycoprotein with an apparent molecular weight of 170 kDa. Human ACE contains 1277 amino acid residues and has two homologous domains, each with a catalytic site and a Zn^{2+}-binding region. ACE has a large amino-terminal extracellular domain, a short carboxyl-terminal intracellular domain, and a 22–amino acid transmembrane hydrophobic region that anchors the ectoenzyme. ACE is rather nonspecific and cleaves dipeptide units from substrates with diverse amino acid sequences. Preferred substrates have only one free carboxyl group in the carboxyl-terminal amino acid, and proline must not be the penultimate amino acid; thus, the enzyme does not degrade AngII. ACE is identical to kininase II, the enzyme that inactivates bradykinin and other potent vasodilator peptides. Although slow conversion of AngI to AngII occurs in plasma, the very rapid metabolism that occurs in vivo is due largely to the activity of membrane-bound ACE present on the luminal surface of endothelial cells throughout the vascular system (Guang et al., 2012).

The *ACE* gene contains an insertion/deletion polymorphism in intron 16 that explains the large phenotypic variance in serum ACE levels. The deletion allele, associated with higher levels of serum ACE and increased metabolism of bradykinin, may confer an increased risk of hypertension, cardiac hypertrophy, atherosclerosis, and diabetic nephropathy (Sayed-Tabatabaei et al., 2006; Hadjadj et al., 2001).

Angiotensin-Converting Enzyme 2

A carboxypeptidase, ACE2, cleaves one amino acid from the carboxyl terminal to convert AngII to Ang(1–7). ACE2 may also convert AngI to Ang(1–9), which is then converted to Ang(1–7) by ACE, neprilysin, and endopeptidases (Santos, 2014). ACE2 contains a single catalytic domain that is 42% identical to the two catalytic domains of ACE. AngII is the preferred substrate for ACE2, with 400-fold higher affinity than AngI (Guang et al., 2012).

The counterregulation of the actions of AngII by ACE2 occur in at least two ways:

1. It decreases AngII levels and limits its effects by metabolizing it to Ang(1–7).
2. It increases levels of Ang(1–7), which acts on Mas receptors to oppose AngII actions (Figure 26–5).

Angiotensin-converting enzyme 2 is not inhibited by the standard ACE inhibitors and has no effect on bradykinin. Reduced expression or deletion of ACE2 is associated with hypertension, defects in cardiac contractility, and elevated levels of AngII. Inhibition of AT_1 receptors by ARBs increases the expression of ACE2. Overexpression of the ACE2 gene decreases blood pressure and prevents AngII-induced cardiac hypertrophy in hypertensive rats. ACE2 is protective against diabetic nephropathy through the Ang(1–7)/Mas receptor pathway (Varagic et al., 2014). Ang(1–9), which is generated from AngI by ACE2, may also have vasodilating and protective

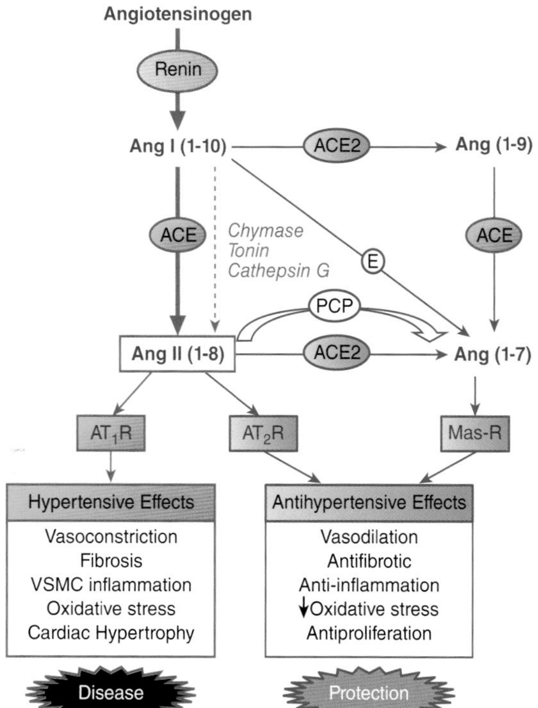

Figure 26–5 *Schematic diagram of opposing arms in the RAS.* Therapeutic interventions aim to inhibit the ACE/AngII/AT_1 receptor axis (red) and enhance ACE2/Ang(1–7)/Mas receptor axis (green). VSMC: vascular smooth muscle cells.

effects by activating AT_2 receptors (Etelvino et al., 2014). In addition, ACE2 metabolizes Apelin peptides, serves as a receptor for the severe acute respiratory syndrome coronavirus (SARS), and has been reported to interact with and regulate amino acid transporters (Kuba et al., 2013).

Alternative Pathways for Angiotensin II Biosynthesis

Angiotensin II may be generated through ACE-independent pathways or "ACE escape." Angiotensinogen is converted to AngI, or directly to AngII by cathepsin G and tonin. Enzymes that convert AngI to AngII include cathepsin G, chymostatin-sensitive AngII-generating enzyme, and chymase. Chymase contributes to tissue conversion of AngI and Ang(1–12) to AngII, particularly in the heart and kidneys. The major source of chymase is mast cells (Ferrario et al., 2014; Paul et al., 2006).

Angiotensinases

Angiotensinases include aminopeptidases, endopeptidases, carboxypeptidases, and other peptidases that metabolize angiotensin peptides; none is specific.

Angiotensin Peptides and Their Receptors

Table 26–1 shows the RAS peptides, their receptors, and overall effects of the receptor-peptide interactions.

AngII-AT_1 Receptor Axis

Angiotensin II binds to specific GPCRs, designated AT_1 and AT_2. The hypertensive, renal, and hypertrophic effects of AngII are mediated by activation of the AT_1 receptor (Dell'Italia, 2011). The AT_1 receptor gene contains a polymorphism (A1166C) associated with hypertension, hypertrophic cardiomyopathy, and coronary artery vasoconstriction. Moreover, the C allele synergizes with the ACE deletion allele with regard to increased risk of coronary artery disease (Álvarez et al., 1998). Preeclampsia is associated with the development of agonistic autoantibodies against the AT_1 receptor in some cases (Xia et al., 2013).

AngII-AT_1 Receptor-Effector Coupling. The AT_1 receptors link to a large array of signal transduction systems to produce effects that vary with cell type and that are a combination of primary and secondary responses. AT_1 receptors couple to several heterotrimeric G proteins, including G_q, $G_{12/13}$, and G_i, and the GPCR characteristics of being substrates for phosphorylation and desensitization by G protein-coupled receptor kinases (GRKs), interacting with β-arrestin, and being subsequently internalized.

TABLE 26–1 ■ RAS PEPTIDES AND THEIR IDENTIFIED RECEPTORS

RECEPTOR	RAS PEPTIDE	EFFECT
AT_1	AngII, AngIII, AngA, Ang(1–12)	Vasoconstriction hypertrophy Fibrosis, nephropathy
AT_2	AngII, AngIII, Ang(1–7), Ang(1–9), AngA	Vasodilation, antihypertrophy, antifibrosis Natriuresis
Mas	Ang(1–7)	Vasodilation, antihypertrophy, antifibrosis Natriuresis
MrgD	Alamandine	Vasodilation, antihypertrophy, antifibrosis
AT_4	AngIV, Ang(3–7)	Neuroprotection Cognition Renal vasodilation Natriuresis
PRR	Prorenin, renin	Hypertrophy, fibrosis Apoptosis

In most cell types, AT_1 receptors couple to G_q to activate the PLCβ-IP_3-Ca^{2+} pathway. Secondary to G_q activation, activation of PKC, PLA_2, and PLD and eicosanoid production, Ca^{2+}-dependent and MAP kinases, Ca^{2+}-calmodulin–dependent activation of NOS may occur. Activation of G_i may occur and will reduce the activity of adenylyl cyclase, lowering cellular cyclic AMP content; however, there also is evidence for $G_q \rightarrow G_s$ cross talk such that activation of the AT_1-G_q-PLC pathway enhances cyclic AMP production. The βγ subunits of G_i and activation of $G_{12/13}$ lead to activation of tyrosine kinases and small G proteins such as Rho. Ultimately, the Jak/STAT pathway may be activated and a variety of transcriptional regulatory factors induced. By these mechanisms, angiotensin influences the expression of a host of gene products relating to cell growth and the production of components of the extracellular matrix. Through AT_1 receptors, AngII also stimulates the activity of a membrane-bound NADH/NADPH oxidase that generates ROS. ROS may contribute to some of the biochemical effects (activation of MAP kinase, tyrosine kinase, and phosphatases; inactivation of NO; and expression of monocyte chemoattractant protein-1) and physiological effects (acute effects on renal function, chronic effects on blood pressure, and vascular hypertrophy and inflammation) of AngII (Mehta and Griendling, 2007). The relative importance of these myriad signal transduction pathways in mediating biological responses to AngII is tissue specific. The AT_1 receptor is structurally flexible and may be activated, independently of AngII binding, by conformational changes such as mechanical stress (Kim et al., 2012). Functions of the AT_1 receptor may be modified by dimerization with AT_2 receptor, the bradykinin B_2 receptor, the $β_2$ adrenergic receptor, and the apelin receptor (Goupil et al., 2013).

AngII-AT_2 Receptor Axis

Activation of the AT_2 receptors counteracts many of the effects of the AT_1 receptors by having antiproliferative, anti-inflammatory, vasodilatory, natriuretic, and antihypertensive effects (Figure 26–5). The AT_2 receptors are distributed widely in fetal tissues, but their distribution is more restricted in adults. Expression of AT_2 receptors is upregulated in cardiovascular diseases, including heart failure, cardiac fibrosis, and ischemic heart disease (Jones et al., 2008). Signaling through the AT_2 receptor is mediated by G protein–dependent ($G_{iα2}$ and $G_{iα3}$) and G protein–independent pathways. Consequences of AT_2 receptor activation include activation of phosphotyrosine phosphatases that inhibit MAP kinases and ERK 1/2; inhibition of Ca^{2+} channel functions; and enhancing NO, cyclic GMP, and bradykinin production. The AT_2 receptors can bind the AT_1 receptors to antagonize and reduce their expression; and the AT_2 receptors can form heterodimers with the bradykinin B_2 receptor to enhance NO production (Jones et al., 2008; Padia and Carey, 2013).

Angiotensin (1–7)/Mas Receptor Axis

The ACE2/Ang(1–7)/Mas receptor axis is a negative regulator of the pressor, profibrotic, and antinatriuretic effects of the ACE/AngII/AT_1 receptor axis of the RAS (Figure 26–5). Ang(1–7) is generated in several ways (Figure 26–1):

- from AngII by ACE2;
- from AngII by carboxypeptidases;
- from AngI by endopeptidases; and
- from AngI by a two-step conversion, by ACE2 to Ang(1–9) and then to Ang(1–7) by ACE or neprilysin.

The antihypertensive effects of Ang(1–7) are mediated through binding to the Mas receptors, although Ang(1–7) can bind and activate AT_2 receptors (Gironacci et al., 2014). Activation of the Mas receptor by Ang(1–7) induces vasodilation, stimulates PI_3K/Akt pathway that promotes NO production, potentiates the vasodilatory effects of bradykinin, and inhibits AngII-induced activation of ERK1/2 and NFκB; it has antiangiogenic, antiproliferative, and antithrombotic effects; and it is renoprotective and cardioprotective in cardiac ischemia and heart failure (Fraga-Silva et al., 2013; Varagic et al., 2014).

The *Mas* proto-oncogene encodes an orphan GPCR. Knockout of the *Mas* gene in mice causes increased vascular resistance and cardiac dysfunction (Santos, 2014; Varagic et al., 2014). The Mas receptor is present in the brain, and its activation is associated with improved memory and cognition (Gironacci et al., 2014).

The capacity of Ang(1–7) to counterbalance the actions of AngII may depend on the ratio of ACE-AngII-AT_1 receptor activity to ACE2-Ang(1–7)-Mas receptor activity (see Figure 26–5; Santos, 2014; Romero et al., 2015). Pharmacologically enhancing the ACE2-Ang(1–7)-Mas receptor pathway using ACE2 activators and specific Mas receptor agonists could provide new avenues for modulating RAS in cardiovascular and renal disease.

Angiotensin III

Angiotensin III, also called Ang(2–8), can be formed by the action of aminopeptidase A on AngII or by the action of ACE on Ang(2–10). AngIII binds to both AT_1 and AT_2 receptors, causing effects qualitatively similar to those of AngII. AngII and AngIII stimulate aldosterone secretion with equal potency; however, AngIII is less efficacious in elevating blood pressure (25%) and stimulating the adrenal medulla (10%). Data from model systems make clear that AngIII and the shorter angiotensin-derived peptides have significant activity, especially at the AT_2 receptor, and that there may be instances where AngIII is the active endogenous ligand (Bosnyak et al., 2011).

Angiotensin IV/AT_4 Receptor Axis

Angiotensin IV, also called Ang(3–8), is formed from AngIII through the catalytic action of aminopeptidase N. Central and peripheral actions of AngIV are mediated through a specific AT_4 receptor that was identified as IRAP (insulin-regulated aminopeptidase) (see Figure 26–1). This receptor is a single transmembrane protein (1025 amino acids) that colocalizes with the glucose transporter type 4. AT_4 receptors are detectable in a number of tissues, such as heart, vasculature, adrenal cortex, and brain regions processing sensory and motor functions. AngIV-dependent AT_4 receptor activation regulates cerebral blood flow, is neuroprotective, and facilitates long-term potentiation, memory consolidation, and cognition (Wright et al., 2013). AngIV binding to the AT_4 receptor inhibits the catalytic activity of IRAP and enables accumulation of various neuropeptides linked to memory potentiation. Other actions include renal vasodilation, natriuresis, neuronal differentiation, hypertrophy, inflammation, and extracellular matrix remodeling. Analogues of AngIV are being developed for their therapeutic potential in Alzheimer disease and head injury (Albiston et al., 2007; Wright et al., 2013).

New Physiologically Active Angiotensin Peptides

New biologically active angiotensin peptides and their receptors have been identified (Table 26–1). These peptides include Ang(1–9), AngA and alamandine, Ang(3–7), and proangiotensin/Ang(1–12) (Ferrario et al., 2014). Ang(1–9) is generated from AngI by the action of ACE2, carboxypeptidase A, and cathepsin. Ang(1–9) has cardioprotective and antipressor effects reportedly mediated through binding to AT_2 receptors and the release of NO (Etelvino et al., 2014). Alamandine is produced from Ang(1–7) by the decarboxylation of the Asp_1 residue into Ala_1 residue on the N-terminal. Alamandine acts through the *MrgD* to mediate vasodilatory and antifibrotic effects similar to Ang(1–7). Alamandine is an ACE substrate and may act as an ACE inhibitor. Alamandine is elevated in patients with chronic renal disease (Etelvino et al., 2014).

Angiotensin A is an octapeptide produced by decarboxylation of the Asp_1 residue of AngII into Ala_1. AngA binds to both AT_1 and AT_2 receptors and has effects similar to, but less potent than, AngII. AngA is reported to be elevated in patients with end-stage renal disease (Ferrario et al., 2014). Ang(3–7) is generated from AngIV and binds AT_4 receptors (Wright et al., 2013). Proangiotensin or Ang(1–12) is generated from angiotensinogen through a nonrenin pathway and can be converted to AngII through action of chymase. Ang(1–12) can bind to the AT_1 receptors and may be a precursor for autocrine/intracrine production of AngII (Ferrario et al., 2014).

Local (Tissue) Renin-Angiotensin System

Local (tissue) RAS is a tissue-based AngII-producing system that plays a role in hypertrophy, nephropathy, inflammation, remodeling, and apoptosis. ACE is present on the luminal face of vascular endothelial cells throughout the circulation; circulating (pro)renin can bind the PRR in the arterial wall and other tissues to mediate local generation of AngII (Campbell, 2014; Paul et al., 2016). Tissue RAS is also an autocrine and intracrine mechanism that can generate AngII and other bioactive angiotensin peptides independently of the renal/hepatic-based system. Many tissues—including the brain, pituitary, blood vessels, heart, kidney, and adrenal gland—produce renin, angiotensinogen, ACE and ACE2, chymase, PRR, and angiotensins I, II, III, IV, Ang(1–7) and the AT_1, AT_2, and Mas receptors (Campbell, 2014; Ferrario et al., 2014). Selective activation of the local RAS components is tissue specific and likely affects the pathophysiological outcomes in disease.

The (Pro) Renin Receptor

(Pro)renin/PRR binding enhances tissue-RAS activity and induces profibrotic intracellular signaling events that are independent of AngII production (Figure 26–6). The PRR is abundant in the heart, brain, eye, adrenals, placenta, adipose tissue, liver, and kidneys. The PRR gene is located in the locus p11.4 of the X chromosome and is named ATP6ap2 (ATPase-6 accessory protein 2). Knockout of the PRR gene is lethal, indicating an important role for PRR in development. In humans, mutations in the PRR gene are associated with mental retardation and epilepsy (Nguyen and Danser, 2008). Human PRR is a single transmembrane protein of 350 amino acids (~37 kDa). PRR is composed of N-terminal extracellular domain that binds (pro)renin, a transmembrane domain and a cytosolic

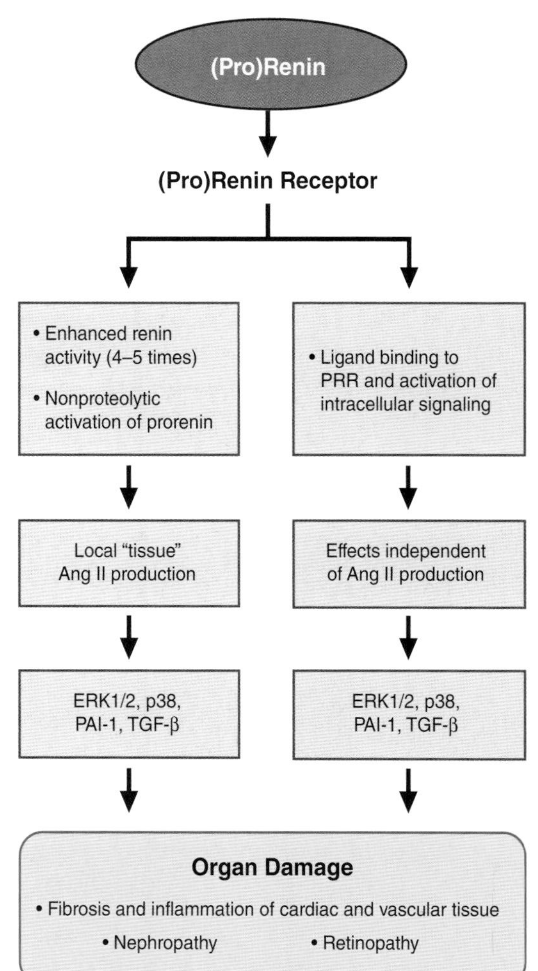

Figure 26–6 *(Pro)renin/PRR interaction activates AngII-dependent and AngII-independent signaling pathways.* See text for details.

domain that are associated with Vacuolar-H+-ATPase (V-ATPase) activity (Nguyen, 2011). Cleavage of the extracellular domain of PRR by furin or ADAM19 produces the N-terminal segment, soluble PRR, found in plasma and urine. Increased levels of urinary soluble PRR correlate with elevated urinary angiotensinogen levels, a biomarker of intrarenal RAS activity (Oshima et al., 2014).

(Pro)renin receptor binds (pro)renin with nanomolar affinity and high specificity to enhance the tissue-RAS. Binding of (pro)renin to PRR augments the catalytic activity of renin and induces nonproteolytic activation of prorenin by unfolding the 43 amino acid–prorenin prosegment and exposing the enzymatic cleft (Figure 26–2). Bound, activated (pro)renin catalyzes the conversion of angiotensinogen to AngI, with the consequent formation of AngII. The binding of (pro)renin to PRR also induces profibrotic signaling events that are *AngII independent* (Figure 26–6), including activation of ERK1/2, p38, tyrosine kinases, COX-2, TGF-β gene expression, and PAI-1 (Nguyen and Danser, 2008). These signaling pathways are not blocked by ACE inhibitors or AT_1 receptor antagonists and are reported to contribute to fibrosis, nephrosis, and end-organ damage (Kaneshiro et al., 2007). Overexpression of the human PRR in transgenic animals increases plasma aldosterone levels in the absence of changes in plasma renin levels and induces hypertension and nephropathy. Rats overexpressing PRR exhibit increased expression of COX-2 in the macula densa and develop proteinuria and glomerulosclerosis that increase with aging (Kaneshiro et al., 2007).

Circulating plasma concentrations of (pro)renin are elevated 100-fold in diabetic patients and are associated with increased risk of nephropathy, renal fibrosis, and retinopathy (Nguyen and Danser, 2008). The blockade of PRR by administration of a peptide antagonist, known as "handle region peptide" (HRP), was reported to be protective in animal models against diabetic nephropathy and retinopathy (Oshima et al, 2014); however, the efficacy and specificity of HRP was not strongly confirmed by other groups (reviewed by Binger and Muller, 2013; Nguyen, 2011). The pathophysiological significance of (pro)renin/PRR interaction outside the local tissue RAS is still unclear (Lu et al., 2016).

The PRR participates in many functions that are independent of (pro)renin binding. PRR functions as an accessory protein essential for V-ATPase activity, which is required for intracellular acidity, receptor-mediated endocytosis, and activation of lysosomal and autophagosomal enzymes (Oshima et al., 2014). Cardiomyocyte-specific PRR knockout mice and podocyte-specific PRR knockout mice develop lethal organ-specific failure due loss of V-ATPase and the dysregulation of intracellular acidification and autophagic functions (Binger and Muller, 2013). PRR also participates in the activation of Wnt/β-catenin and Wnt/planar cell polarity signaling pathways that are important in cell polarization in the plane of tissue (Nguyen, 2011). PRR reportedly can regulate LDL uptake and metabolism. In hepatocytes, silencing PRR expression decreased cellular LDL uptake by decreasing expression of LDL receptor and sortelin 1 protein, a regulator of LDL uptake and metabolism and a PRR-interacting protein (Lu et al., 2016). (Pro)renin also binds to mannose-6-phosphate receptor, an insulin-like growth factor II receptor that functions as a clearance receptor (Nguyen and Danser, 2008).

Functions and Effects of Angiotensin II

Angiotensin II increases total peripheral resistance (TPR) and alters renal function and cardiovascular structure (Figure 26–7). Modest increases in plasma concentrations of AngII acutely raise blood pressure; on a molar basis, AngII is about 40 times more potent than NE; the EC_{50} of AngII for acutely raising arterial blood pressure is about 0.3 nM. When a single moderate dose of AngII is injected intravenously, systemic blood pressure begins to rise within seconds, peaks rapidly, and returns to normal within minutes (Figure 26–8). This *rapid pressor response* to AngII is due to a swift increase in TPR—a response that helps to maintain arterial blood pressure in the face of an acute hypotensive challenge (e.g., blood loss or vasodilation). Although AngII increases cardiac contractility directly (via opening voltage-gated Ca^{2+} channels in cardiac myocytes) and increases heart rate indirectly (via facilitation of sympathetic tone, enhancing adrenergic neurotransmission, and provoking adrenal catecholamine release), the rapid increase in arterial blood pressure activates a baroreceptor reflex

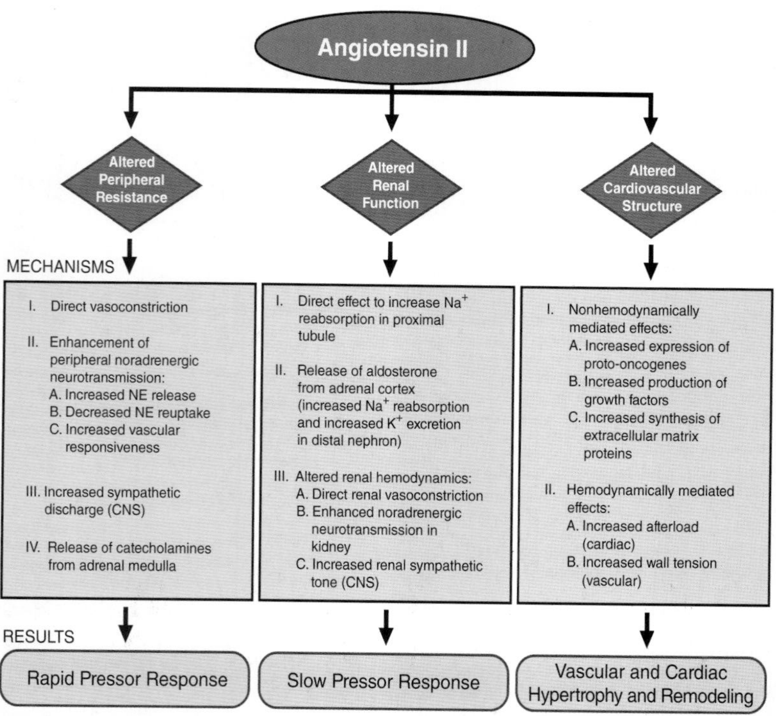

Figure 26–7 *Major physiological effects of AngII.*

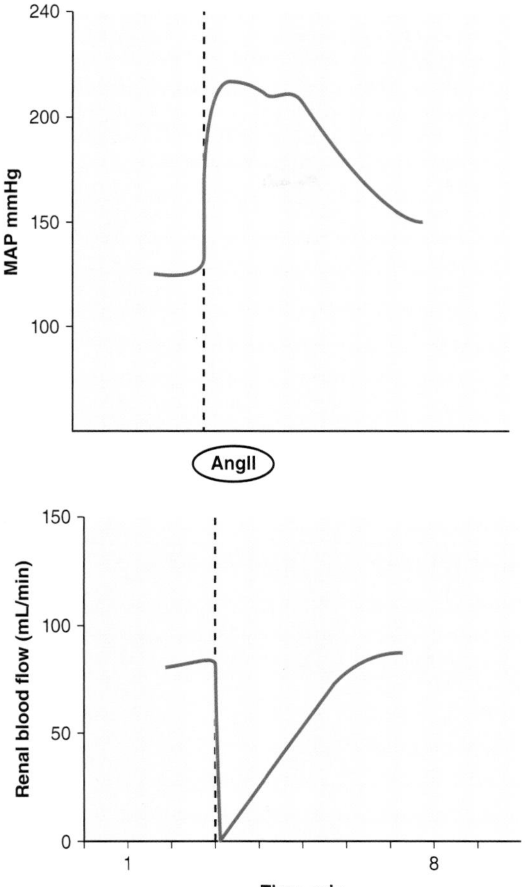

Figure 26–8 *Effect of an intravenous bolus of AngII on arterial BP and RBF.* Angiotensin was added at the time indicated by the dashed vertical line.

that decreases sympathetic tone and increases vagal tone. Thus, depending on the physiological state, AngII may increase, decrease, or not change cardiac contractility, heart rate, and cardiac output. Changes in cardiac output therefore contribute little, if at all, to the rapid pressor response induced by AngII.

AngII also causes a *slow pressor response* that helps to stabilize arterial blood pressure over the long term. A continuous infusion of initially subpressor doses of AngII gradually increases arterial blood pressure, with the maximum effect requiring days to achieve. This slow pressor response probably is mediated by a decrement in renal excretory function that shifts the renal pressure–natriuresis curve to the right (see the next section). AngII stimulates the synthesis of endothelin 1 and superoxide anion, which may contribute to the slow pressor response.

In addition to its effects on arterial blood pressure, AngII stimulates remodeling of the cardiovascular system, causing hypertrophy of vascular and cardiac cells and increased synthesis and deposition of collagen by cardiac fibroblasts.

Mechanisms by Which Angiotensin II Increases Total Peripheral Resistance

Angiotensin II increases peripheral resistance via direct and indirect effects on blood vessels (Figure 26–7).

Direct Vasoconstriction

Angiotensin II constricts precapillary arterioles and, to a lesser extent, postcapillary venules by activating AT_1 receptors located on vascular smooth muscle cells and stimulating the G_q-PLC-IP_3-Ca^{2+} pathway. AngII has differential effects on vascular beds. Direct vasoconstriction is strongest in the kidneys (Figure 26–8) and somewhat less in the splanchnic bed. AngII-induced vasoconstriction is much less in vessels of the brain and still weaker in those of the lung and skeletal muscle. Nevertheless, high circulating concentrations of AngII may decrease cerebral and coronary blood flow.

Enhancement of Peripheral Noradrenergic Neurotransmission

Angiotensin II, binding to AT_1 receptors, augments NE release from sympathetic nerve terminals by inhibiting the reuptake of NE into nerve terminals and by enhancing the vascular response to NE in model systems (see Chapter 12). High concentrations of the peptide stimulate ganglion cells directly.

Effects on the CNS

Angiotensin II increases sympathetic tone. Small amounts of AngII infused into the vertebral arteries cause an increase in arterial blood pressure. This response reflects effects of the hormone on circumventricular nuclei that are not protected by a blood-brain barrier (e.g., area postrema, subfornical organ, organum vasculosum of the lamina terminalis). Circulating AngII also attenuates baroreceptor-mediated reductions in sympathetic discharge, thereby increasing arterial pressure. The CNS is affected both by blood-borne AngII and by AngII formed within the brain. The brain contains all components of the RAS. AngII also causes a centrally mediated dipsogenic (thirst) effect and enhances the release of vasopressin from the neurohypophysis.

Release of Catecholamines From the Adrenal Medulla

Angiotensin II stimulates the release of catecholamines from the adrenal medulla by promoting Ca^{2+} entry secondary to depolarization of chromaffin cells.

Mechanisms by Which Angiotensin II Regulates Renal Function

Angiotensin II has pronounced effects on renal function, reducing the urinary excretion of Na^+ and water while increasing the excretion of K^+. The overall effect of AngII on the kidneys is to shift the renal pressure–natriuresis curve to the right (Figure 26–9).

Direct Effects of AngII on Na^+ Reabsorption in the Renal Tubules

Very low concentrations of AngII stimulate Na^+/H^+ exchange in the proximal tubule—an effect that increases Na^+, Cl^-, and bicarbonate reabsorption. Approximately 20%–30% of the bicarbonate handled by the nephron may be affected by this mechanism. AngII also increases the expression

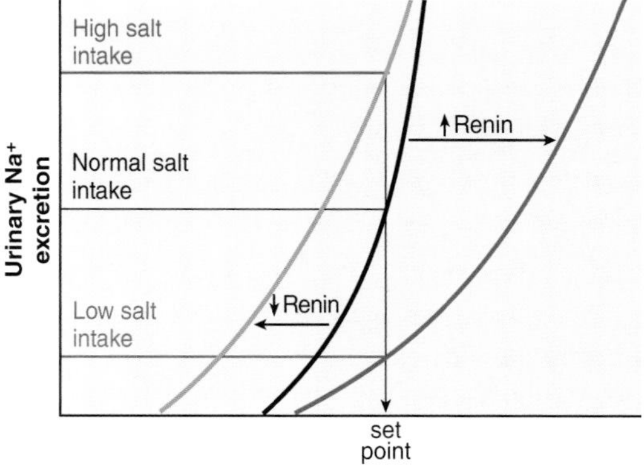

Figure 26–9 *Pressure-natriuresis curve: effects of Na^+ intake on renin release (AngII formation) and arterial blood pressure.* Inhibition of the RAS will cause a large drop in blood pressure in Na^+-depleted individuals. (Modified with permission from Jackson EK, Branch RA, Margolius HS, Oates JA. Physiological functions of the renal prostaglandin, renin, and kallikrein systems. In: Seldin DW, Giebisch GH, eds. *The Kidney: Physiology and Pathophysiology*. Vol 1. Lippincott Williams & Wilkins, Philadelphia, **1985**, 624.)

of the Na^+–glucose symporter in the proximal tubule. Paradoxically, at high concentrations, AngII may inhibit Na^+ transport in the proximal tubule. AngII also directly stimulates the Na^+-K^+-$2Cl^-$ symporter in the thick ascending limb. The proximal tubule secretes angiotensinogen, and the connecting tubule releases renin, so a paracrine tubular RAS may contribute to Na^+ reabsorption.

Release of Aldosterone From the Adrenal Cortex

Angiotensin II stimulates the zona glomerulosa of the adrenal cortex to increase the synthesis and secretion of aldosterone and augments responses to other stimuli (e.g., ACTH, K^+). Increased output of aldosterone is elicited by concentrations of AngII that have little or no acute effect on blood pressure. Aldosterone acts on the distal and collecting tubules to cause retention of Na^+ and excretion of K^+ and H^+. The stimulant effect of AngII on aldosterone synthesis and release is enhanced under conditions of hyponatremia or hyperkalemia and is reduced when concentrations of Na^+ and K^+ in plasma are altered in the opposite directions.

Altered Renal Hemodynamics

Angiotensin II reduces renal blood flow and renal excretory function by directly constricting the renal vascular smooth muscle, by enhancing renal sympathetic tone (a CNS effect), and by facilitating renal adrenergic transmission (an intrarenal effect). AngII-induced vasoconstriction of preglomerular microvessels is enhanced by endogenous adenosine owing to signal transduction systems activated by AT_1 and the adenosine A_1 receptor.

Angiotensin II influences the GFR by several mechanisms:

- Constriction of the afferent arterioles, which reduces intraglomerular pressure and tends to reduce GFR
- Contraction of mesangial cells, which decreases the capillary surface area within the glomerulus available for filtration and also tends to decrease GFR
- Constriction of efferent arterioles, which increases intraglomerular pressure and tends to increase GFR

Normally, AngII slightly reduces GFR; however, with renal artery hypotension, the effects of AngII on the efferent arteriole predominate so that AngII increases GFR. Thus, blockade of the RAS may cause acute renal failure in patients with bilateral renal artery stenosis or in patients with unilateral stenosis who have only a single kidney.

Mechanisms by Which Angiotensin II Alters Cardiovascular Structure

Pathological alterations involving cardiovascular hypertrophy and remodeling increase morbidity and mortality. The cells involved include vascular smooth muscle cells, cardiac myocytes, and fibroblasts. AngII induces hypertrophy of cardiac myocytes; stimulates the migration, proliferation, and hypertrophy of vascular smooth muscle cells; increases extracellular matrix production by vascular smooth muscle cells; and increases extracellular matrix production by cardiac fibroblasts. In addition, AngII alters extracellular matrix formation and degradation indirectly by increasing aldosterone production and mineralocorticoid receptor activation. The adverse cardiovascular remodeling induced by AngII can be reduced but not entirely prevented by mineralocorticoid receptor antagonists.

Hemodynamically Mediated Effects of Angiotensin II on Cardiovascular Structure

In addition to the direct cellular effects of AngII on cardiovascular structure, changes in cardiac preload (volume expansion owing to Na^+ retention) and afterload (increased arterial blood pressure) probably contribute to cardiac hypertrophy and remodeling. Arterial hypertension also contributes to hypertrophy and remodeling of blood vessels.

Role of the RAS in Long-Term Maintenance of Arterial Blood Pressure Despite Extremes in Dietary Na^+ Intake

Arterial blood pressure is a major determinant of Na^+ excretion. This is illustrated graphically by plotting urinary Na^+ excretion versus mean arterial blood pressure (Figure 26–9), a plot known as the *renal pressure–natriuresis curve*. Over the long term, Na^+ excretion must equal Na^+ intake; therefore, the set point for long-term levels of arterial blood pressure can be obtained as the intersection of a horizontal line representing Na^+ intake with the renal pressure–natriuresis curve. The RAS plays a major role in maintaining a constant set point for long-term levels of arterial blood pressure despite extreme changes in dietary Na^+ intake. When dietary Na^+ intake is low, renin release is stimulated, and AngII acts on the kidneys to shift the renal pressure–natriuresis curve to the right. Conversely, when dietary Na^+ is high, renin release is inhibited, and the withdrawal of AngII shifts the renal pressure–natriuresis curve to the left. When modulation of the RAS is blocked by drugs, changes in salt intake markedly affect long-term levels of arterial blood pressure.

Other Effects of the RAS

Expression of the RAS is required for the development of normal kidney morphology, particularly the maturational growth of the renal papilla. AngII causes a marked anorexigenic effect and weight loss, and high circulating levels of AngII may contribute to the anorexia, wasting, and cachexia of heart failure (Paul et al., 2006; Yoshida et al., 2013).

Inhibitors of the Renin-Angiotensin System

Drugs that interfere with the RAS play a prominent role in the treatment of cardiovascular disease. Besides β_1 blockers that inhibit renin release, the following three classes of inhibitors of the RAS are utilized therapeutically (Figure 26–10):

1. ACE inhibitors
2. Angiotensin receptor blockers
3. Direct renin inhibitors

All of these classes of agents will reduce the actions of AngII and lower blood pressure, but each has different effects on the individual components of the RAS (Table 26–2). Representative structures of agents inhibiting the RAS and reducing the effects of AngII are shown in Figure 26–11, near the end of the chapter.

Angiotensin-Converting Enzyme Inhibitors

History

In the 1960s, Ferreira and colleagues found that venom extract from the Brazilian pit viper (*Bothrops jararaca*) contains factors that intensify

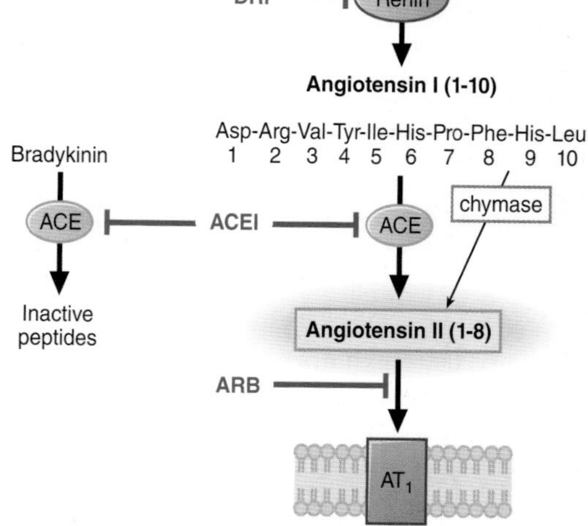

Figure 26–10 *Inhibitors of the RAS.*

TABLE 26–2 ■ EFFECTS OF ANTIHYPERTENSIVE AGENTS ON COMPONENTS OF THE RAS

	DRIs	ACEIs	ARBs	DIURETICS	β_1-BLOCKERS
PRC	↑	↑	↑	↑	↓
PRA	↓	↑	↑	↑	↓
AngI	↓	↑	↑	↑	↓
AngII	↓	↓	↑	↑	↓
ACE activity	↔	Inhibition	↔		
Aldosterone	↓	↓	↓	↑	↓/↔
Bradykinin	↔	↑	↔		
AT_1R	↔	↔	Inhibition		
AT_2R	↔	↔	Stimulation		

vasodilator responses to bradykinin. These bradykinin-potentiating factors are peptides that inhibit kininase II, an enzyme that inactivates bradykinin. Erdös and coworkers established that ACE and kininase II are the same enzyme, which catalyzes both the synthesis of AngII and the destruction of bradykinin. Based on these findings, the nonapeptide teprotide (snake venom peptide that inhibits kininase II and ACE) was later synthesized and tested in human subjects. It lowered blood pressure in many patients with essential hypertension and exerted beneficial effects in patients with heart failure. The orally effective ACE inhibitor *captopril* was developed by analysis of the inhibitory action of teprotide, inference about the action of ACE on its substrates, and analogy with carboxypeptidase A, which was known to be inhibited by D-benzylsuccinic acid. Ondetti, Cushman, and colleagues argued that inhibition of ACE might be produced by succinyl amino acids that corresponded in length to the dipeptide cleaved by ACE. This led to the synthesis of a series of carboxy alkanoyl and mercapto alkanoyl derivatives that are potent competitive inhibitors of ACE.

Pharmacological Effects

The ACE inhibitors inhibit the conversion of AngI to AngII. Inhibition of AngII production lowers blood pressure and enhances natriuresis. ACE is an enzyme with many substrates; thus, there are other consequences of its inhibition, including inhibition of the degradation of bradykinin, which has beneficial antihypertensive and protective effects. ACE inhibitors increase by 5-fold the circulating levels of the natural stem cell regulator Ac-SDKP, which may also contribute to the cardioprotective effects of ACE inhibitors (Rhaleb et al., 2001). ACE inhibitors will increase renin release and the rate of formation of AngI by interfering with both short- and long-loop negative feedbacks on renin release (Figure 26–3). Accumulating AngI is directed down alternative metabolic routes, resulting in the increased production of vasodilator peptides such as Ang(1–9) and Ang(1–7) (Figures 26–1 and 26–5).

Clinical Pharmacology

The ACE inhibitors can be classified into three broad groups based on chemical structure:

1. Sulfhydryl-containing ACE inhibitors structurally related to captopril
2. Dicarboxyl-containing ACE inhibitors structurally related to enalapril (e.g., lisinopril, benazepril, quinapril, moexipril, ramipril, trandolapril, perindopril, Figure 26–11)
3. Phosphorus-containing ACE inhibitors structurally related to fosinopril

Many ACE inhibitors are ester-containing prodrugs that are 100–1000 times less potent but have better oral bioavailability than the active molecules. Currently, 11 ACE inhibitors are available for clinical use in the U.S. They differ with regard to potency, whether ACE inhibition is primarily a direct effect of the drug itself or the effect of an active metabolite, and pharmacokinetics.

All ACE inhibitors block the conversion of AngI to AngII and have similar therapeutic indications, adverse-effect profiles, and contraindications. Because hypertension usually requires lifelong treatment, quality-of-life issues are an important consideration in comparing antihypertensive drugs. With the exceptions of fosinopril, trandolapril, and quinapril (which display balanced elimination by the liver and kidneys), ACE inhibitors are cleared predominantly by the kidneys. Impaired renal function significantly diminishes the plasma clearance of most ACE inhibitors, and dosages of these drugs should be reduced in patients with renal impairment. *Elevated PRA renders patients hyperresponsive to ACE inhibitor–induced hypotension, and initial dosages of all ACE inhibitors should be reduced in patients with high plasma levels of renin (e.g., patients with heart failure and during salt depletion including diuretic use).* ACE inhibitors differ markedly in tissue distribution, and it is possible that this difference could be exploited to inhibit some local (tissue) RAS while leaving others relatively intact.

Captopril. Captopril is a potent ACE inhibitor with a K_i of 1.7 nM. Given orally, captopril is absorbed rapidly and has a bioavailability of about 75%. Bioavailability is reduced by 25%–30% with food. Peak concentrations in plasma occur within an hour, and the drug is cleared rapidly, with a $t_{1/2}$ of about 2 h. Most of the drug is eliminated in urine, 40%–50% as captopril and the rest as captopril disulfide dimers and captopril–cysteine disulfide. The oral dose of captopril ranges from 6.25 to 150 mg 2–3 times daily, with 6.25 mg thrice daily or 25 mg twice daily appropriate for the initiation of therapy for heart failure or hypertension, respectively.

Enalapril. Enalapril maleate is a prodrug that is hydrolyzed by esterases in the liver to produce enalaprilat, the active dicarboxylic acid. Enalaprilat is a potent inhibitor of ACE with a K_i of 0.2 nM. Enalapril is absorbed rapidly when given orally and has an oral bioavailability of about 60% (not reduced by food). Although peak concentrations of enalapril in plasma occur within an hour, enalaprilat concentrations peak only after 3–4 h. Enalapril has a $t_{1/2}$ of about 1.3 h, but enalaprilat, because of tight binding to ACE, has a plasma $t_{1/2}$ of about 11 h. Elimination is by the kidneys as either intact enalapril or enalaprilat. The oral dosage of enalapril ranges from 2.5 to 40 mg daily, with 2.5 and 5 mg daily appropriate for the initiation of therapy for heart failure and hypertension, respectively.

Enalaprilat. Enalaprilat is not absorbed orally but is available for intravenous administration when oral therapy is not appropriate. For hypertensive patients, the dosage is 0.625–1.25 mg given intravenously over 5 min. This dosage may be repeated every 6 h.

Lisinopril. Lisinopril is the lysine analogue of enalaprilat; unlike enalapril, lisinopril itself is active. In vitro, lisinopril is a slightly more potent ACE inhibitor than is enalaprilat. Lisinopril is absorbed slowly, variably, and incompletely (~30%) after oral administration (not reduced by food); peak concentrations in plasma are achieved in about 7 h. It is excreted unchanged by the kidney with a plasma $t_{1/2}$ of about 12 h. Lisinopril does not

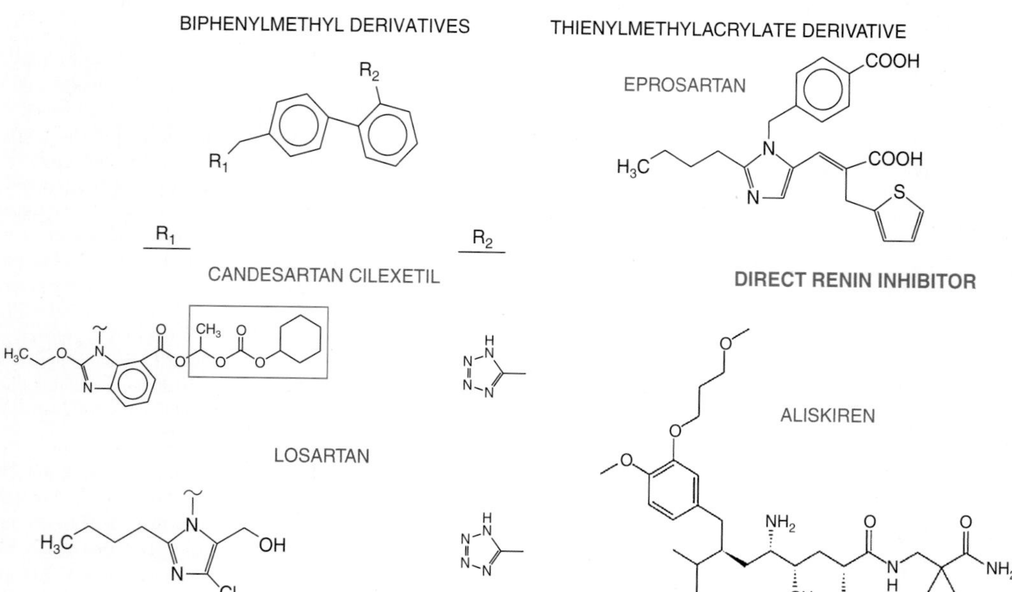

Figure 26–11 *Structures of representative RAS inhibitors.* Enalapril and candesartan cilexetil are pro-drugs, relatively inactive until in vivo esterases remove the region within the red box, replacing it with a hydrogen atom to form the active drug.

accumulate in tissues. The oral dosage of lisinopril ranges from 5 to 40 mg daily (single or divided dose), with 5 and 10 mg daily appropriate for the initiation of therapy for heart failure and hypertension, respectively. A daily dose of 2.5 mg with close medical supervision is recommended for patients with heart failure who are hyponatremic or have renal impairment.

Benazepril. Cleavage of the ester moiety by hepatic esterases transforms benazepril, a prodrug, into benazeprilat. Benazepril is absorbed rapidly but incompletely (37%) after oral administration (only slightly reduced by food). Benazepril is nearly completely metabolized to benazeprilat and to the glucuronide conjugates of benazepril and benazeprilat, which are excreted into the urine and bile; peak concentrations of benazepril and benazeprilat in plasma are achieved in 0.5–1 and 1–2 h, respectively. Benazeprilat has an effective plasma $t_{1/2}$ of 10–11 h. With the exception of the lungs, benazeprilat does not accumulate in tissues. The oral dosage of benazepril ranges from 5 to 80 mg daily (single or divided dose).

Fosinopril. Cleavage of the ester moiety by hepatic esterases transforms fosinopril into fosinoprilat. Fosinopril is absorbed slowly and incompletely (36%) after oral administration (rate but not extent reduced by food). Fosinopril is largely metabolized to fosinoprilat (75%) and to the glucuronide conjugate of fosinoprilat. These are excreted in both the urine and the bile; peak concentrations of fosinoprilat in plasma are achieved in about 3 h. Fosinoprilat has an effective plasma $t_{1/2}$ of about 11.5 h, a figure not significantly altered by renal impairment. The oral dosage of fosinopril ranges from 10 to 80 mg daily (single or divided dose). The initial dose is reduced to 5 mg daily in patients with Na^+ or water depletion or renal failure.

Trandolapril. An oral dose of trandolapril is absorbed without reduction by food and produces plasma levels of trandolapril (10% bioavailability) and trandolaprilat (70% bioavailability). Trandolaprilat is about 8 times more potent than trandolapril as an ACE inhibitor. Glucuronides of trandolapril and deesterification products are recovered in the urine (33%, mostly trandolaprilat) and feces (66%). Peak concentrations of trandolaprilat in plasma are achieved in 4–10 h.

Trandolaprilat displays biphasic elimination kinetics, with an initial $t_{1/2}$ of about 10 h (the major component of elimination), followed by a more prolonged $t_{1/2}$ (owing to slow dissociation of trandolaprilat from tissue ACE). Plasma clearance of trandolaprilat is reduced by both renal and hepatic insufficiency. The oral dosage ranges from 1 to 8 mg daily (single or divided dose). The initial dose is 0.5 mg in patients who are taking a diuretic or who have renal impairment.

Quinapril. Cleavage of the ester moiety by hepatic esterases transforms quinapril, a prodrug, into quinaprilat. Quinapril is absorbed rapidly (peak concentrations are achieved in 1 h), and the rate, but not extent, of oral absorption (60%) may be reduced by food (delayed peak). Quinaprilat and other minor metabolites of quinapril are excreted in the urine (61%) and feces (37%). Peak concentrations of quinaprilat in plasma are achieved in about 2 h. Conversion of quinapril to quinaprilat is reduced in patients with diminished liver function. The initial $t_{1/2}$ of quinaprilat is about 2 h; a prolonged terminal $t_{1/2}$ of about 25 h may be due to high-affinity binding of the drug to tissue ACE. The oral dosage of quinapril ranges from 5 to 80 mg daily.

Ramipril. Orally administered ramipril is absorbed rapidly (peak concentrations in 1 h; the rate but not extent of its oral absorption (50%–60%) is reduced by food. Ramipril is metabolized to ramiprilat by hepatic esterases and to inactive metabolites that are excreted predominantly by the kidneys. Peak concentrations of ramiprilat in plasma are achieved in about 3 h. Ramiprilat displays triphasic elimination kinetics ($t_{1/2}$ values: 2–4, 9–18, and more than 50 h) This triphasic elimination is due to extensive distribution to all tissues (initial $t_{1/2}$), clearance of free ramiprilat from plasma (intermediate $t_{1/2}$), and dissociation of ramiprilat from tissue ACE (long terminal $t_{1/2}$). The oral dosage of ramipril ranges from 1.25 to 20 mg daily (single or divided dose).

Moexipril. Moexipril's antihypertensive activity is due to its deesterified metabolite, moexiprilat. Moexipril is absorbed incompletely, with bioavailability as moexiprilat of about 13%. Bioavailability is markedly decreased by food. The time to peak plasma concentration of moexiprilat is almost 1.5 h; the elimination $t_{1/2}$ varies between 2 and 12 h. The recommended dosage range is 7.5–30 mg daily (single or divided doses). The dosage range is halved in patients who are taking diuretics or who have renal impairment.

Perindopril. Perindopril erbumine is a prodrug, and 30%–50% of systemically available perindopril is transformed to perindoprilat by hepatic esterases. Although the oral bioavailability of perindopril (75%) is not affected by food, the bioavailability of perindoprilat is reduced by about 35%. Perindopril is metabolized to perindoprilat and to inactive metabolites that are excreted predominantly by the kidneys. Peak concentrations of perindoprilat in plasma are achieved in 3–7 h. Perindoprilat displays biphasic elimination kinetics with half-lives of 3–10 h (the major component of elimination) and 30–120 h (owing to slow dissociation of perindoprilat from tissue ACE). The oral dosage ranges from 2 to 16 mg daily (single or divided dose).

Therapeutic Uses of ACE Inhibitors

The ACE inhibitors are effective in the treatment of cardiovascular disease, heart failure, and diabetic nephropathy.

ACE Inhibitors in Hypertension. Inhibition of ACE lowers systemic vascular resistance and mean, diastolic, and systolic blood pressures in various hypertensive states except when high blood pressure is due to primary aldosteronism (see Chapter 28). The initial change in blood pressure tends to be positively correlated with PRA and AngII plasma levels prior to treatment. However, some patients may show a sizable reduction in blood pressure that correlates poorly with pretreatment values of PRA. It is possible that increased local (tissue) production of AngII or increased responsiveness of tissues to normal levels of AngII makes some hypertensive patients sensitive to ACE inhibitors despite normal PRA.

The long-term fall in systemic blood pressure observed in hypertensive individuals treated with ACE inhibitors is accompanied by a leftward shift in the renal pressure–natriuresis curve (Figure 26–9) and a reduction in TPR in which there is variable participation by different vascular beds. The kidney is a notable exception: Because the renal vessels are extremely sensitive to the vasoconstrictor actions of AngII, ACE inhibitors increase renal blood flow via vasodilation of the afferent and efferent arterioles. Increased renal blood flow occurs without an increase in GFR; thus, the filtration fraction is reduced.

The ACE inhibitors cause systemic arteriolar dilation and increase the compliance of large arteries, which contributes to a reduction of systolic pressure. Cardiac function in patients with uncomplicated hypertension generally is little changed, although stroke volume and cardiac output may increase slightly with sustained treatment. Baroreceptor function and cardiovascular reflexes are not compromised, and responses to postural changes and exercise are little impaired. Even when substantial lowering of blood pressure is achieved, heart rate and concentrations of catecholamines in plasma generally increase only slightly, if at all. This perhaps reflects an alteration of baroreceptor function with increased arterial compliance and the loss of the normal tonic influence of AngII on the sympathetic nervous system.

Aldosterone secretion is reduced, but not seriously impaired, by ACE inhibitors. Aldosterone secretion is maintained at adequate levels by other steroidogenic stimuli, such as ACTH and K^+. The activity of these secretagogues on the zona glomerulosa of the adrenal cortex requires very small trophic or permissive amounts of AngII, which always are present because ACE inhibition never is complete. Excessive retention of K^+ is encountered in patients taking supplemental K^+, in patients with renal impairment, or in patients taking other medications that reduce K^+ excretion.

The ACE inhibitors alone normalize blood pressure in about 50% of patients with mild-to-moderate hypertension. Ninety percent of patients with mild-to-moderate hypertension will be controlled by the combination of an ACE inhibitor and a Ca^{2+} channel blocker, a β_1 adrenergic receptor blocker, or a diuretic. Diuretics augment the antihypertensive response to ACE inhibitors by rendering the patient's blood pressure renin dependent. Several ACE inhibitors are marketed in fixed-dose combinations with a thiazide diuretic or Ca^{2+} channel blocker for the management of hypertension.

ACE Inhibitors in Left Ventricular Systolic Dysfunction. Unless contraindicated, ACE inhibitors should be given to all patients with impaired left ventricular systolic function whether or not they have symptoms of overt heart failure (see Chapter 29). Several large clinical studies demonstrated that inhibition of ACE in patients with systolic dysfunction prevents or delays the progression of heart failure, decreases the incidence of sudden death and myocardial infarction, decreases hospitalization, and improves quality of life. Inhibition of ACE commonly reduces afterload and systolic wall stress, and both cardiac output and cardiac index increase, as do indices of stroke work and stroke volume. In systolic dysfunction, AngII decreases arterial compliance, and this is reversed by ACE inhibition. Heart rate generally is reduced. Systemic blood pressure falls, sometimes steeply at the outset, but tends to return toward initial levels. Renovascular resistance falls sharply, and renal blood flow increases. Natriuresis occurs as a result of the improved renal hemodynamics, the reduced stimulus to the secretion of aldosterone by AngII, and the diminished direct effects of AngII on the kidney. The excess volume of body fluids contracts, which reduces venous return to the right side of the heart. A further reduction results from venodilation and an increased capacity of the venous bed.

Although AngII has little acute venoconstrictor activity, long-term infusion of AngII increases venous tone, perhaps by central or peripheral interactions with the sympathetic nervous system. The response to ACE inhibitors also involves reductions of pulmonary arterial pressure, pulmonary capillary wedge pressure, and left atrial and left ventricular filling volumes and pressures. Consequently, preload and diastolic wall stress are diminished. The better hemodynamic performance results in increased exercise tolerance and suppression of the sympathetic nervous system. Cerebral and coronary blood flows usually are well maintained, even when systemic blood pressure is reduced. In heart failure, ACE inhibitors reduce ventricular dilation and tend to restore the heart to its normal elliptical shape. ACE inhibitors may reverse ventricular remodeling via changes in preload/afterload by preventing the growth effects of AngII on myocytes and by attenuating cardiac fibrosis induced by AngII and aldosterone.

ACE Inhibitors in Acute Myocardial Infarction. The beneficial effects of ACE inhibitors in acute myocardial infarction are particularly large in hypertensive and diabetic patients. Unless contraindicated (e.g., cardiogenic shock or severe hypotension), ACE inhibitors should be started immediately during the acute phase of myocardial infarction and can be administered along with thrombolytics, aspirin, and β adrenergic receptor antagonists (ACE Inhibitor Myocardial Infarction Collaborative Group, 1998). In high-risk patients (e.g., large infarct, systolic ventricular dysfunction), ACE inhibition should be continued long term (see Chapters 27 and 28).

ACE Inhibitors in Patients Who Are at High Risk of Cardiovascular Events. Patients at high risk of cardiovascular events benefit considerably from treatment with ACE inhibitors (Heart Outcomes Prevention Study Investigators, 2000). ACE inhibition significantly decreases the rate of myocardial infarction, stroke, and death in patients who do not have left ventricular dysfunction but have evidence of vascular disease or diabetes and one other risk factor for cardiovascular disease. In patients with coronary artery disease but without heart failure, ACE inhibition reduces cardiovascular disease death and myocardial infarction (European Trial, 2003).

ACE Inhibitors in Diabetes Mellitus and Renal Failure. Diabetes mellitus is the leading cause of renal disease. In patients with type 1 diabetes mellitus and diabetic nephropathy, ACE inhibitors prevent or delay the progression of renal disease, affording renoprotection, as defined by changes in albumin excretion. The renoprotective effects of ACE inhibitors in type 1 diabetes are in part independent of blood pressure reduction. In addition, ACE inhibitors may decrease retinopathy progression in type 1 diabetics and attenuate the progression of renal insufficiency in patients with a variety of nondiabetic nephropathies (Ruggenenti et al., 2010).

Several mechanisms participate in the renal protective effects of ACE inhibitors. Increased glomerular capillary pressure induces glomerular injury, and ACE inhibitors reduce this parameter by decreasing arterial blood pressure and by dilating renal efferent arterioles. ACE inhibitors increase the permeability selectivity of the filtering membrane, thereby diminishing exposure of the mesangium to proteinaceous factors that may stimulate mesangial cell proliferation and matrix production, two processes that contribute to expansion of the mesangium in diabetic nephropathy. Because AngII is a growth factor, reductions in the intrarenal levels of AngII may further attenuate mesangial cell growth and matrix production. ACE inhibitors increase Ang(1–7) levels by preventing its metabolism by ACE. Ang(1–7) binds to Mas receptors and has protective and antifibrotic effects (Santos, 2014). In the setting of diabetes, at the level of renal epithelial podocytes, activation of AT_1 receptors leads to activation of protein kinase signaling cascades, cytoskeletal rearrangements, retraction of podocyte processes, and a reduction in proteins of the slit diaphragm, all resulting in increased permeability of the renal epithelium to proteins (proteinuria). ACE inhibitors reduce these effects of AngII (Márquez et al., 2015).

ACE Inhibitors in Scleroderma Renal Crisis. The use of ACE inhibitors considerably improves survival of patients with scleroderma renal crisis.

Adverse Effects of ACE Inhibitors

In general, ACE inhibitors are well tolerated. The drugs do not alter plasma concentrations of uric acid or Ca^{2+} and may improve insulin sensitivity and glucose tolerance in patients with insulin resistance and decrease cholesterol and lipoprotein (a) levels in proteinuric renal disease.

Hypotension. A steep fall in blood pressure may occur following the first dose of an ACE inhibitor in patients with elevated PRA. Care should be exercised in patients who are salt depleted, are on multiple antihypertensive drugs, or have congestive heart failure.

Cough. In 5%–20% of patients, ACE inhibitors induce a bothersome, dry cough mediated by the accumulation in the lungs of bradykinin, substance P, or PGs. Thromboxane antagonism, aspirin, and iron supplementation reduce cough induced by ACE inhibitors. ACE dose reduction or switching to an ARB is sometimes effective. Once ACE inhibitors are stopped, the cough disappears, usually within 4 days.

Hyperkalemia. Significant K^+ retention is rarely encountered in patients with normal renal function. However, ACE inhibitors may cause hyperkalemia in patients with renal insufficiency or diabetes or in patients taking K^+-sparing diuretics, K^+ supplements, β receptor blockers, or NSAIDs.

Acute Renal Failure. Inhibition of ACE can induce acute renal insufficiency in patients with bilateral renal artery stenosis, stenosis of the artery to a single remaining kidney, heart failure, or volume depletion owing to diarrhea or diuretics.

Angioedema. In 0.1%–0.5% of patients, ACE inhibitors induce rapid swelling in the nose, throat, mouth, glottis, larynx, lips, or tongue. Once ACE inhibitors are stopped, angioedema disappears within hours; meanwhile, the patient's airway should be protected, and if necessary, epinephrine, an antihistamine, or a glucocorticoid should be administered. African Americans have a 4.5 times greater risk of ACE inhibitor–induced angioedema than Caucasians. Although rare, angioedema of the intestine (visceral angioedema) characterized by emesis, watery diarrhea, and abdominal pain also has been reported. ACE inhibitor–associated angioedema is a class effect, and patients who develop this adverse event should not be prescribed any other drugs within the ACE inhibitor class.

Fetopathic Potential. If a pregnancy is diagnosed, it is imperative that ACE inhibitors be discontinued as soon as possible. ACE inhibitors and ARBs have been associated with renal developmental defects when administered in the third trimester of pregnancy, and potentially earlier. The fetopathic effects may be due in part to fetal hypotension. This possible adverse effect should be discussed with any woman of childbearing potential, as should the necessity of appropriate birth control measures.

Skin Rash. The ACE inhibitors occasionally cause a maculopapular rash that may itch, but that may resolve spontaneously or with antihistamines.

Other Side Effects. Extremely rare but reversible side effects include *dysgeusia* (an alteration in or loss of taste), *neutropenia* (symptoms include sore throat and fever), *glycosuria* (spillage of glucose into the urine in the absence of hyperglycemia), *anemia,* and *hepatotoxicity.*

Drug Interactions. Antacids may reduce the bioavailability of ACE inhibitors; capsaicin may worsen ACE inhibitor–induced cough; NSAIDs, including aspirin, may reduce the antihypertensive response to ACE inhibitors; and K^+-sparing diuretics and K^+ supplements may exacerbate ACE inhibitor–induced hyperkalemia. ACE inhibitors may increase plasma levels of digoxin and lithium and hypersensitivity reactions to allopurinol.

Angiotensin II Receptor Blockers

HISTORY

Attempts to develop therapeutically useful AngII receptor antagonists date to the early 1970s. Initial endeavors concentrated on angiotensin peptide analogues. Saralasin, 1-sarcosine, 8-isoleucine AngII, and other 8-substituted angiotensins are potent AngII receptor antagonists but were of no clinical value because of lack of oral bioavailability and unacceptable partial agonist activity. A breakthrough came in the early 1980s with the synthesis and testing of a series of imidazole-5-acetic acid derivatives that attenuated pressor responses to AngII in rats. Two compounds, S-8307 and S-8308, proved to be highly specific, albeit very weak, nonpeptide AngII receptor antagonists that were devoid of partial agonist activity (Dell'Italia, 2011). Through a series of stepwise modifications, the orally active, potent, and selective nonpeptide AT_1 receptor antagonist losartan was developed and approved for clinical use in the U.S. in 1995. Since then, seven additional AT_1 receptor antagonists (see Drug Facts for Your Personal Formulary table) have been approved. Although these AT_1 receptor antagonists are devoid of partial agonist activity, structural modifications as minor as a methyl group can transform a potent antagonist into an agonist (Perlman et al., 1997).

Pharmacological Effects

The AngII receptor blockers bind to the AT_1 receptor with high affinity and are more than 10,000-fold selective for the AT_1 receptor over the AT_2 receptor. Although binding of ARBs to the AT_1 receptor is competitive, the inhibition by ARBs of biological responses to AngII often is functionally insurmountable. Insurmountable antagonism has the theoretical advantage of sustained receptor blockade even with increased levels of endogenous ligand and with missed doses of drug. ARBs inhibit most of the biological effects of AngII, which include AngII-induced (1) contraction of vascular smooth muscle; (2) rapid pressor responses; (3) slow pressor responses; (4) thirst; (5) vasopressin release; (6) aldosterone secretion; (7) release of adrenal catecholamines; (8) enhancement of noradrenergic neurotransmission; (9) increases in sympathetic tone; (10) changes in renal function; and (11) cellular hypertrophy and hyperplasia. ARBs reduce arterial blood pressure in animals with renovascular and genetic hypertension, as well as in transgenic animals overexpressing the renin gene. ARBs, however, have little effect on arterial blood pressure in animals with low-renin hypertension (e.g., rats with hypertension induced by NaCl and deoxycorticosterone) (Csajka et al., 1997).

Do ARBs Have Therapeutic Efficacy Equivalent to That of ACE Inhibitors?

Although both ARBs and ACE inhibitors of drugs block the RAS, they differ in several important aspects:

- *ARBs reduce activation of AT_1 receptors more effectively than do ACE inhibitors.* ACE inhibitors reduce the biosynthesis of AngII by the action of ACE, but do not inhibit AngII generation via chymase and other ACE-independent AngII-producing pathways. ARBs block the actions of AngII via the AT_1 receptor regardless of the biochemical pathway leading to AngII formation.
- In contrast to ACE inhibitors, *ARBs permit activation of AT_2 receptors.* ACE inhibitors increase renin release, but block the conversion of AngI to AngII. ARBs also stimulate renin release; however, with ARBs, this translates into a several-fold increase in circulating levels of AngII. Because ARBs block AT_1 receptors, this increased level of AngII is available to activate AT_2 receptors.
- *ACE inhibitors and ARBs increase Ang(1-7) levels by different mechanisms.* ACE is involved in the clearance of Ang(1-7), so inhibition of ACE increases Ang(1-7) levels. With ARBs, AngII, the preferred substrate of ACE2, is converted to Ang(1-7).
- *ACE inhibitors increase the levels of a number of ACE substrates, including bradykinin and Ac-SDKP.*

Whether the pharmacological differences between ARBs and ACE inhibitors result in significant differences in therapeutic outcomes is an open question.

Clinical Pharmacology

Oral bioavailability of ARBs generally is low (<50%) except for azilsartan (~60%) and irbesartan (~70%), and protein binding is high (>90%).

Candesartan Cilexetil. Candesartan cilexetil is an inactive ester prodrug that is completely hydrolyzed to the active form, candesartan, during absorption from the GI tract (Figure 26–11). Peak plasma levels are obtained 3–4 h after oral administration; the plasma $t_{1/2}$ is about 9 h. Plasma clearance of candesartan is due to renal elimination (33%) and biliary excretion (67%). The plasma clearance of candesartan is affected by renal insufficiency but not by mild-to-moderate hepatic insufficiency. Candesartan cilexetil should be administered orally once or twice daily for a total daily dose of 4–32 mg.

Eprosartan. Peak plasma levels are obtained 1–2 h after oral administration; the plasma $t_{1/2}$ is 5–9 h. Eprosartan is metabolized in part to the glucuronide conjugate. Clearance is by renal elimination and biliary excretion. The plasma clearance of eprosartan is affected by both renal insufficiency and hepatic insufficiency. The recommended dosage of eprosartan is 400–800 mg/d in one or two doses.

Irbesartan. Peak plasma levels are obtained about 1.5–2 h after oral administration; the plasma $t_{1/2}$ is 11–15 h. Irbesartan is metabolized in part to the glucuronide conjugate, and the parent compound and its glucuronide conjugate are cleared by renal elimination (20%) and biliary excretion (80%). The plasma clearance of irbesartan is unaffected by either renal or mild-to-moderate hepatic insufficiency. The oral dosage of irbesartan is 150–300 mg once daily.

Losartan. Approximately 14% of an oral dose of losartan is converted by CYP2C9 and CYP3A4 to the 5-carboxylic acid metabolite, EXP 3174, which is more potent than losartan as an AT_1 receptor antagonist. Peak plasma levels of losartan and EXP 3174 occur about 1–3 h after oral administration, and the plasma half-lives are 2.5 and 6–9 h, respectively. The plasma clearances of losartan and EXP 3174 are via the kidney and liver (metabolism and biliary excretion) and are affected by hepatic but not renal insufficiency. Losartan should be administered orally once or twice daily for a total daily dose of 25–100 mg. Losartan is a competitive antagonist of the thromboxane A_2 receptor and attenuates platelet aggregation. EXP 3179, another metabolite of losartan without angiotensin receptor effects, reduces COX-2 messenger RNA upregulation and COX-dependent PG generation (Krämer et al., 2002) (Figure 26–11).

Olmesartan Medoxomil. Olmesartan medoxomil is an inactive ester prodrug that is completely hydrolyzed to the active form, olmesartan, during absorption from the GI tract. Peak plasma levels are obtained 1.4–2.8 h after oral administration; the plasma $t_{1/2}$ is 10–15 h. Plasma clearance of olmesartan is due to both renal elimination and biliary excretion. Although renal impairment and hepatic disease decrease the plasma clearance of olmesartan, no dose adjustment is required in patients with mild-to-moderate renal or hepatic impairment. The oral dosage of olmesartan medoxomil is 20–40 mg once daily.

Telmisartan. Peak plasma levels are obtained 0.5–1 h after oral administration; the plasma $t_{1/2}$ is about 24 h. Telmisartan is cleared from the circulation mainly by biliary secretion of intact drug. The plasma clearance of telmisartan is affected by hepatic but not renal insufficiency. The recommended oral dosage of telmisartan is 40–80 mg once daily.

Valsartan. Peak plasma levels occur 2–4 h after oral administration; food markedly decreases absorption; the plasma $t_{1/2}$ is about 9 h. Valsartan is cleared from the circulation by the liver (~70% of total clearance), and hepatic insufficiency will reduce clearance. The oral dosage of valsartan is 80–320 mg once daily.

Azilsartan Medoxomil. The prodrug is hydrolyzed in the GI tract into the active form, azilsartan. The drug is available in 40- and 80-mg once-daily doses. At the recommended dose of 80 mg once a day, azilsartan medoxomil is superior to the maximal doses of valsartan and olmesartan in lowering blood pressure. Bioavailability of azilsartan is about 60% and is not affected by food. Peak plasma concentrations C_{max} are achieved within 1.5–3 h. The elimination $t_{1/2}$ is about 11 h. Azilsartan is metabolized mostly by CYP2C9 into inactive metabolites. Elimination of the drug is 55% in feces and 42% in urine. About 15% of the dose is eliminated as unchanged azilsartan in urine. Plasma clearance is not affected by renal or hepatic insufficiency.

Angiotensin Receptor–Neprilysin Inhibitor. A combination of sacubitril and valsartan, marketed as Entresto, is a first-in-class drug that combines the AT_1 receptor antagonistic moiety of valsartan with the neprilysin inhibitor moiety of sacubitril. The complex (sacubitril, valsartan, Na^+, and water [1:1:3:2.5]) dissociates into sacubitril and valsartan after oral administration. Sacubitril bioavailability is about 60%, and it is highly protein bound (94%–97%). Sacubitril is further metabolized by esterases into the active metabolite LBQ657, which has a $t_{1/2}$ of 11 h. The neprilysin inhibitor blocks the breakdown of natriuretic peptides ANP, BNP, and CNP, as well as AngI and bradykinin. The drug combination lowers vascular resistance and increases blood flow. In clinical trial, this combination agent was reported to be superior to enalapril in decreasing the risk of deaths from cardiovascular causes and heart failure by 20% (McMurray et al., 2014).

Entresto is approved for treatment of heart failure with reduced ejection fraction, with a recommended dose of 100–400 mg daily, divided into two doses. Because the ACE/neprilysin inhibitor omapatrilat demonstrated an increased risk of angioedema, use of Entresto is contraindicated in conjunction with an ACE inhibitor or in patients with a history of angioedema during ACE inhibitor or ARB use. The drug should not be used in conjunction with an ARB or ACE inhibitor, and in patients with diabetes should not be used in conjunction with aliskiren. Potential adverse effects discussed for valsartan also apply to this sacubutril-valsartan combination.

A New Class of ARBs in Development. *A β-arrestin-biased AT_1 receptor blocker,* TRV027 is a ligand that binds AT_1 receptor and blocks G protein–coupled signaling while engaging β-arrestin. β-Arrestin functions as an adaptor protein that participates in receptor desensitization and internalization. In animal models, β-arrestin–biased AT_1 receptor ligand increases myocyte contractility and protects against apoptosis (Kim et al., 2012). In phase II clinical studies, TRV027 decreased mean arterial pressure and was well tolerated. The safety and efficacy of TRV027 is being tested in the BLAST-HF study in patients with acute heart failure (Felker et al., 2015).

Therapeutic Uses of ARBs

All ARBs are approved for the treatment of hypertension. ARBs are renoprotective in type 2 diabetes mellitus, and many experts now consider them the drugs of choice for renoprotection in diabetic patients.

Irbesartan and losartan are approved for diabetic nephropathy, losartan is approved for stroke prophylaxis, and valsartan and candesartan are approved for heart failure and to reduce cardiovascular mortality in clinically stable patients with left ventricular failure or left ventricular dysfunction following myocardial infarction. The efficacy of ARBs in lowering blood pressure is comparable with that of ACE inhibitors and other established antihypertensive drugs, with a favorable adverse-effect profile. ARBs also are available as fixed-dose combinations with HCTZ or amlodipine (see Chapters 27–29).

The Losartan Intervention for Endpoint (LIFE) Reduction in Hypertension Study demonstrated the superiority of an ARB compared with a $β_1$ adrenergic receptor antagonist with regard to reducing stroke in hypertensive patients with left ventricular hypertrophy (Dahlöf et al., 2002). Also, irbesartan appears to maintain sinus rhythm in patients with persistent, long-standing atrial fibrillation (Madrid et al., 2002). Losartan is reported to be safe and highly effective in the treatment of portal hypertension in patients with cirrhosis and portal hypertension without compromising renal function (Schneider et al., 1999).

The ELITE (Evaluation of Losartan in the Elderly) study and a follow-up study (ELITE II) concluded that in elderly patients with heart failure, losartan is as effective as captopril in improving symptoms (Pitt et al., 2000). The VALIANT (Valsartan in Acute Myocardial Infarction) trial demonstrated that valsartan is as effective as captopril in patients with myocardial infarction complicated by left ventricular systolic dysfunction with regard to all-cause mortality (Pfeffer et al., 2003). Both valsartan and candesartan reduce mortality and morbidity in patients with heart failure (reviewed by Makani et al., 2013). Current recommendations are to use ACE inhibitors as first-line agents for the treatment of heart failure and to reserve ARBs for treatment of heart failure in patients who cannot tolerate or have an unsatisfactory response to ACE inhibitors.

The ARBs are renoprotective in type 2 diabetes mellitus, and many experts now consider them the drugs of choice for renoprotection in diabetic patients.

Dual Inhibition of the RAS. At present, there is contradictory evidence regarding the advisability of combining an ARB and an ACE inhibitor in patients with heart failure, with one study indicating that a combination of ARB and ACE inhibitors decreases morbidity and mortality in patients with heart failure, and another showing that combination therapy is associated with increased adverse effects and no added benefits (Dell'Italia, 2011; Makani et al., 2013; ONTARGET Investigators, 2008).

Adverse Effects

The ARBs are generally well tolerated. The incidence of angioedema and cough with ARBs is less than that with ACE inhibitors. As with ACE inhibitors, ARBs have teratogenic potential and should be discontinued in pregnancy. In patients whose arterial blood pressure or renal function is highly dependent on the RAS (e.g., renal artery stenosis), ARBs can cause hypotension, oliguria, progressive azotemia, or acute renal failure. ARBs may cause hyperkalemia in patients with renal disease or in patients taking K^+ supplements or K^+-sparing diuretics. ARBs enhance the blood pressure–lowering effect of other antihypertensive drugs, a desirable effect but one that may necessitate dosage adjustment. There are rare postmarketing reports of anaphylaxis, abnormal hepatic function, hepatitis, neutropenia, leukopenia, agranulocytosis, pruritus, urticaria, hyponatremia, alopecia, and vasculitis, including Henoch-Schönlein purpura.

Direct Renin Inhibitors

Angiotensinogen is the only specific substrate for renin. DRIs inhibit the cleavage of AngI from angiotensinogen by renin, an enzymatic reaction that is the rate-limiting step for the subsequent generation of AngII. Aliskiren is the only DRI approved for clinical use.

HISTORY

Earlier renin inhibitors were orally inactive peptide analogues of the prorenin propeptide or analogues of renin-substrate cleavage site. Orally active, first-generation renin inhibitors (*enalkiren, zankiren, CGP38560A,* and *remikiren*) were effective in reducing AngII levels, but none of them made it past clinical trials due to their low potency, poor bioavailability, and short $t_{1/2}$. Low-molecular-weight renin inhibitors were designed based on molecular modeling and crystallographic structural information of renin-substrate interaction (Wood et al., 2003). This led to the development of aliskiren, a second-generation renin inhibitor that is FDA approved for the treatment of hypertension. Aliskiren has blood pressure–lowering effects similar to those of ACE inhibitors and ARBs.

Pharmacological Effects

Aliskiren is a low-molecular-weight nonpeptide and a potent competitive inhibitor of renin. It binds the active site of renin to block conversion of angiotensinogen to AngI, thus reducing the consequent production of AngII. Aliskiren has a 10,000-fold higher affinity to renin (IC_{50} ~ 0.6 nM) than to any other aspartic peptidases. In healthy volunteers, aliskiren (40–640 mg/d) induces a dose-dependent decrease in blood pressure, reduces PRA and AngI and AngII levels, but increases PRC by 16- to 34-fold due to the loss of the short-loop negative feedback by AngII (Figure 26–3; Table 26–2). Aliskiren also decreases plasma and urinary aldosterone levels and enhances natriuresis (Nussberger et al., 2002).

Clinical Pharmacology

Aliskiren is recommended as a single oral dose of 150 or 300 mg/d. Bioavailability of aliskiren is low (~2.5%), but its high affinity and potency compensate for the low bioavailability. Peak plasma concentrations are reached within 3–6 h. The $t_{1/2}$ is 20–45 h. Steady state in plasma is achieved in 5–8 days. Plasma protein binding is 50% and is independent of concentration. Aliskiren is a substrate for P-glycoprotein, which contributes low bioavailability. Fatty meals significantly decrease the absorption of aliskiren. Hepatic metabolism by CYP3A4 is minimal. Elimination is mostly as unchanged drug in feces. About 25% of the absorbed dose appears in the urine as the parent drug.

Therapeutic Uses of Aliskiren

Therapeutic uses of aliskiren are discussed in Chapter 28.

Adverse Effects and Contraindications

Aliskiren is well tolerated, and adverse events are mild or comparable to placebo with no gender difference. Adverse effects include mild GI symptoms such as diarrhea at high doses (600 mg daily), abdominal pain, dyspepsia, and gastroesophageal reflux; headache; nasopharyngitis; dizziness; fatigue; upper respiratory tract infection; back pain; angiodema; and cough (much less common than with ACE inhibitors). Other adverse

Drug Facts for Your Personal Formulary: *Inhibitors of the RAS*

Drugs	Therapeutic Uses	Clinical Pharmacology and Tips
Angiotensin-Converting Enzyme Inhibitors • Inhibit the conversion of AngI to AngII		
Captopril Lisinopril Enalapril Benazepril Quinapril Ramipril Moexipril	• Inhibit AngII production, thus lowering arteriolar resistance • Hypertension • Acute myocardial infarction • Congestive heart failure • Diabetic nephropathy • Scleroderma renal crisis	• Antihypertensive effects potentiated by inhibition of ACE-catalyzed breakdown of bradykinin • Antihypertensive effects potentiated by increase in Ang(1–7) levels and activation of Ang(1–7)/Mas receptor pathway • Increase PRC and PRA • Adverse effects include cough in 5%–20% of patients, angioedema, hypotension, hyperkalemia, skin rash, neutropenia, anemia, fetopathic syndrome • Contraindicated in patients with renal artery stenosis and should be used with caution in patients with impaired renal function or hypovolemia • Should be stopped during pregnancy
Enalaprilat (IV)		• Intravenous administration
Fosinopril Trandolapril Perindopril		• Undergo both hepatic and renal elimination and should be used with caution in patients with renal or hepatic impairment
Angiotensin Receptor Blockers • Block AT_1 receptors		
Losartan Valsartan Eprosartan Irbesartan Candesartan Olmesartan Telmisartan Azilsartan	• Block the vasoconstrictor and profibrotic effects of AngII by inhibiting AT_1 receptors while permitting vasodilation through activation of AT_2 receptors • Hypertension • Congestive heart failure • Diabetic nephropathy	• Antihypertensive effects potentiated by activation of the AT_2 receptors • Antihypertensive effects potentiated by ACE2-dependent conversion of AngII to Ang(1–7) and activation of vasodilation via Ang(1–7)/Mas receptor pathway • Increase PRC and PRA • Adverse effects include hyperkalemia and hypotension • Contraindicated in patients with renal insufficiency • Should be stopped during pregnancy
Direct Renin Inhibitors • Inhibit renin and thus the conversion of angiotensinogen to AngI		
Aliskiren	• Decrease AngI and AngII levels • Hypertension	• Therapeutic value unclear; no evidence for superiority over ACEIs or ARBs • Increase PRC but decrease PRA • Contraindicated in diabetic nephropathy, pregnancy or renal insufficiency

effects include rash, hypotension, hyperkalemia in diabetics on combination therapy, elevated uric acid, renal stones, and gout. Like other RAS inhibitors, aliskiren is not recommended in pregnancy.

Drug Interactions. Aliskiren does not interact with drugs that interact with CYPs. Aliskiren reduces absorption of furosemide by 50%. Irbesartan reduces the C_{max} of aliskiren by 50%. Aliskiren plasma levels are increased by drugs, such as ketoconazole, atorvastatin, and cyclosporine, that inhibit P-glycoprotein.

Effect of Pharmacological Blood Pressure Reduction on Function of the RAS

The RAS responds to alterations in blood pressure with compensatory changes (Figure 26–3). Thus, pharmacological agents that lower blood pressure will alter the feedback loops that regulate the RAS and cause changes in the levels and activities of the system's components. These changes, summarized in Table 26–2, should be taken into account when interpreting laboratory evaluation of patients. Furthermore, during aliskiren treatment, the assay for PRA will be inhibited by persistence of aliskiren in this ex vivo reaction, whereas the renin concentration radioimmunoassay will not be inhibited.

Bibliography

ACE Inhibitor Myocardial Infarction Collaborative Group. Indications for ACE inhibitors in the early treatment of acute myocardial infarction: systematic overview of individual data from 100,000 patients in randomized trials. *Circulation*, **1998**, *97*:2202–2212.

Albiston AL, et al. Therapeutic targeting of insulin-regulated aminopeptidase: heads and tails? *Pharmacol Ther*, **2007**, *116*:417–427.

Álvarez R, et al. Angiotensin-converting enzyme and angiotensin II receptor 1 polymorphisms: association with early coronary disease. *Cardiovasc Res*, **1998**, *40*:375–379.

Binger KJ, Muller DN. Autopahgy and the (pro)renin receptor. *Front Endocrinol*, **2013**, *4*:155.

Bosnyak S, et al. Relative affinity of angiotensin peptides and novel ligands at AT_1 and AT_2 receptors. *Clin Sci* (Lond), **2011**, *121*:297–303.

Campbell DJ. Clinical relevance of local renin angiotensin systems. *Front Endocrinol*, **2014**, *5*:113.

Csajka C, et al. Pharmacokinetic-pharmacodynamic profile of angiotensin II receptor antagonists. *Clin Pharmacokinet*, **1997**, *32*:1–29.

Dahlöf B, et al., for the LIFE Study Group. Cardiovascular morbidity and mortality in the Losartan Intervention for Endpoint reduction in hypertension study (LIFE): a randomized trial against atenolol. *Lancet*, **2002**, *359*:995–1003.

Dell'Italia LJ. Translational success stories: angiotensin receptor 1 antagonists in heart failure. *Circ Res*, **2011**, *109*:437–452.

Etelvino GM, et al. New components of the renin-angiotensin system: alamandine and the MAS-related G protein coupled receptor D. *Curr Hypertens Rep*, **2014**, *16*:433.

EURopean trial On reduction of cardiac events with Perindopril in stable coronary Artery disease (EUROPA) Investigators. Efficacy of perindopril in reduction of cardiovascular events among patients with stable coronary artery disease: randomised, double-blind, placebo-controlled, multicentre trial (the EUROPA study). *Lancet*, **2003**, *362*:782–788.

Felker GM, et al. Heart failure therapeutics on the basis of a biased ligand of the angiotensin-2 type 1 receptor: rationale and design of the BLAST-AHF Study (Biased Ligand of the Angiotensin Receptor Study in Acute Heart Failure). *JACC Heart Fail*, **2015**, *3*:193–201.

Ferrario CM, et al. An evolving story of angiotensin-II-forming pathways in rodents and humans. *Clin Sci*, **2014**, *126*:461–469.

Fraga-Silva RA, et al. Opportunities for targeting the angiotensin-converting enzyme 2/angiotensin-(1–7)/Mas receptor pathway in hypertension. *Curr Hypertens Rep*, **2013**, *15*:31–38.

Gironacci MM, et al. Protective axis of the renin-angiotensin system in the brain. *Clin Sci*, **2014**, *127*:295–306.

Goupil E, et al. GPCR heterodimers: asymmetries in ligand binding and signaling output offer new targets for drug discovery. *Br J Pharmacol*, **2013**, *168*:1101–1103.

Guang C, et al. Three key proteases—angiotensin-I-converting enzyme (ACE), ACE2 and renin—within and beyond the renin-angiotensin system. *Arch Cardiovasc Dis*, **2012**, *105*:373–385.

Hadjadj S, et al. Prognostic value of angiotensin-I converting enzyme *I/D* polymorphism for nephropathy in type 1 diabetes mellitus: a prospective study. *J Am Soc Nephrol*, **2001**, *12*:541–549.

Heart Outcomes Prevention Study Investigators. Effects of an angiotensin-converting-enzyme inhibitor ramipril on cardiovascular events in high-risk patients. The Heart Outcomes Prevention Evaluation Study Investigators. *N Engl J Med*, **2000**, *342*:145–153 (published erratum appears in *N Engl J Med*, **2000**, *342*:478).

Jones E, Vinh A, et al. AT2 receptors: functional relevance in cardiovascular disease. *Pharmacol Ther*, **2008**, *120*:292–316.

Kaneshiro Y, et al. Slowly progressive, angiotensin II-independent glomerulosclerosis in human (pro)renin receptor-transgenic rats. *J Am Soc Nephrol*, **2007**, *18*:1789–1795.

Kim KS, et al. β-Arrestin-biased AT1R stimulation promotes cell survival during acute cardiac injury. *Am J Physiol Heart Circ Physiol*, **2012**, *303*:H1001–H1010.

Kobori H, Urushihara M. Augmented intrarenal and urinary angiotensinogen in hypertension and kidney disease. *Pflugers Arch*, **2013**, *465*:3–12.

Krämer C, et al. Angiotensin II receptor-independent antiinflammatory and angiaggregatory properties of losartan: role of the active metabolite EXP3179. *Circ Res*, **2002**, *90*:770–776.

Krum H, et al. Losing ALTITUDE? How should ASTRONAUT launch into ATMOSPHERE. *Eur J Heart Fail*, **2013**, *15*:1205–1207.

Kuba K, et al. Multiple functions of angiotensin-converting enzyme 2 and its relevance in cardiovascular diseases. *Circ J*, **2013**, *77*:301–308.

Lu X, et al. Identification of the (pro)renin receptor as a novel regulator of low-density lipoprotein metabolism. *Circ Res*, **2016**, *118*: 222–229.

Madrid AH, et al. Use of irbesartan to maintain sinus rhythm in patients with long-lasting persistent atrial fibrillation: a prospective and randomized study. *Circulation*, **2002**, *106*:331–336.

Makani H, et al. Efficacy and safety of dual blockade of the renin-angiotensin system: meta-analysis of randomized trials. *BMJ*, **2013**, *346*:1360.

Márquez E, et al. Renin-angiotensin system within the diabetic podocyte. *Am J Physiol Renal Physiol*, **2015**, *308*:1–10.

McMurray JJ, et al. Angiotensin-neprilysin inhibition versus enalapril in heart failure. *N Engl J Med*, **2014**, *371*:993–1004.

McMurray JJ, et al. Aliskiren, ALTITUDE, and the implications for ATMOSPHERE. *Eur J Heart Fail*, **2012**, *14*:341–343.

McMurray JJ, et al. Effects of the oral direct renin inhibitor aliskiren in patients with symptomatic heart failure. *Circ Heart Fail*, **2008**, *1*:17–24.

Mehta PK, Griendling KK. Angiotensin II cell signaling: physiological and pathological effects in the cardiovascular system. *Am J Physiol Cell Physiol*, **2007**, *292*:C82–C97.

Nguyen G. Renin and prorenin receptor in hypertension: what's new? *Curr Hypertens Rep*, **2011**, *13*:79–85.

Nguyen G, Danser AH. Prorenin and (pro)renin receptor: a review of available data from in vitro studies and experimental models in rodents. *Exp Physiol*, **2008**, *93*:557–563.

Nussberger J, et al. Angiotensin II suppression in humans by the orally active renin inhibitor aliskiren (SPP100): comparison with enalapril. *Hypertension*, **2002**, *39*:E1–E8.

Oh BH, et al. Aliskiren, an oral renin inhibitor, provides dose-dependent efficacy and sustained 24-hour blood pressure control in patients with hypertension. *J Am Coll Cardiol*, **2007**, *49*:1157–1163.

ONTARGET Investigators. Telmisartan, ramipril, or both in patients at high risk for vascular events. *N Engl J Med*, **2008**, *358*:1547–1559.

Oparil S, et al. Efficacy and safety of combined use of aliskiren and valsartan in patients with hypertension: a randomised, double-blind trial. *Lancet*, **2007**, *370*:221–229.

Oshima Y, et al. Roles of the (pro)renin receptor in the kidney. *World J Nephrol*, **2014**, *3*:302–307.

Padia SH, Carey RM. AT2 receptors: beneficial counter-regulatory role in cardiovascular and renal function. *Pflugers Arch*, **2013**, *465*:99–110.

Parving HH, et al., ALTITUDE Investigators. Cardiorenal end points in a trial of aliskiren for type 2 diabetes. *N Engl J Med*, **2012**, *367*:2204–2213.

Parving HH, et al. Aliskiren combined with losartan in type 2 diabetes and nephropathy. *N Engl J Med*, **2008**, *358*:2433–2246.

Paul M, et al. Physiology of local renin angiotensin systems. *Physiol Rev*, **2006**, *86*:747–803.

Perlman S, et al. Dual agonistic and antagonistic property of nonpeptide angiotensin AT_1 ligands: susceptibility to receptor mutations. *Mol Pharmacol*, **1997**, *51*:301–311.

Peti-Peterdi J, Harris RC. Macula densa sensing and signaling mechanisms of renin release. *J Am Soc Nephrol*, **2010**, *21*:1093–1096.

Pfeffer MA, et al., for the Valsartan in Acute Myocardial Infarction Trial Investigators. Valsartan, captopril, or both in myocardial infarction complicated by heart failure, left ventricular dysfunction, or both. *N Engl J Med*, **2003**, *349*:1893–1906.

Pitt B, et al., on behalf of the ELITE II investigators. Effect of losartan compared with captopril on mortality in patients with symptomatic heart failure: randomized trial—the Losartan Heart Failure Survival Study ELITE II. *Lancet*, **2000**, *355*:1582–1587.

Rhaleb N-E, et al. Long-term effect of *N*-acetyl-seryl-aspartyl-lysly-proline on left ventricular collagen deposition in rats with two-kidney, one-clip hypertension. *Circulation*, **2001**, *103*:3136–3141.

Ruggenenti P, et al. The RAAS in the pathogenesis and treatment of diabetic nephropathy. *Nat Rev Nephrol*, **2010**, *6*:319–330.

Sanoski CA. Aliskiren: an oral direct renin inhibitor for the treatment of hypertension. *Pharmacotherapy*, **2009**, *29*:193–212.

Santos RA. Angiotensin-(1–7). *Hypertension*, **2014**, *63*:1138–1134.

Sayed-Tabatabaei FA, et al. ACE polymorphisms. *Circ Res*, **2006**, *98*:1123–1133.

Schneider AW, et al. Effect of losartan, an angiotensin II receptor antagonist, on portal pressure in cirrhosis. *Hepatology*, **1999**, *29*:334–339.

Sethi AA, et al. Angiotensinogen single nucleotide polymorphisms, elevated blood pressure, and risk of cardiovascular disease. *Hypertension*, **2003**, *41*:1202–1211.

Solomon SD, et al. Effect of the direct renin inhibitor aliskiren, the angiotensin receptor blocker losartan, or both on left ventricular mass in patients with hypertension and left ventricular hypertrophy. *Circulation*, **2009**, *119*:530–537.

Solomon SD, et al. Effect of the direct renin inhibitor aliskiren on left ventricular remodelling following myocardial infarction with systolic dysfunction. *Eur Heart J*, **2011**, *32*:1227–1234.

Varagic J, et al. ACE2 AngiotenisnII/Angiotensin-(1–7) balance in cardiorenal injury. *Curr Hypertens Rep*, **2014**,*16*:420.

Wood JM, et al. Structure-based design of aliskiren, a novel orally effective renin inhibitor. *Biochem Biophys Res Commun*, **2003**, *308*:698–705.

Wright JW, et al. A role for the brain RAS in Alzheimer's and Parkinson's diseases. *Front Endocrinol*, **2013**,*4*:158.

Xia Y, Kellems RE. Angiotensin receptor agonistic autoantibodies and hypertension: preeclampsia and beyond. *Circ Res*, **2013**, *113*:78–87.

Yoshida et al. Molecular mechanisms and signaling pathways of angiotensin II-induced muscle wasting: potential therapeutic targets for cardiac cachexia. *Int J Biochem Cell Biol*, **2013**, *45*:2322–2232.

Treatment of Ischemic Heart Disease

Thomas Eschenhagen

第二十七章　缺血性心脏病的治疗

中文导读

本章主要介绍：缺血性心脏病的病理生理学；心绞痛的病理生理学特点；缺血性心脏病的药物治疗，包括有机硝酸盐、钙离子通道阻滞药、β肾上腺素受体拮抗药（β阻滞药）、抗血小板药、抗整合素药、抗血栓药和其他抗心绞痛药；治疗策略，包括稳定型冠状动脉疾病、急性冠状动脉综合征、跛行与周围血管疾病的治疗；机械药理学治疗（药物洗脱血管内支架）。

Abbreviations

ACE: angiotensin-converting enzyme
ACEI: angiotensin-converting enzyme inhibitor
ACS: acute coronary syndrome
ALDH2: mitochondrial aldehyde dehydrogenase
ARB: angiotensin receptor blocker
AV: atrioventricular
CABG: coronary artery bypass grafting
CAD: coronary artery disease
COX-1: cyclooxygenase isoform 1
CYP: cytochrome P450
EC_{50}: half-maximal effective concentration
EMA: European Medicines Agency
eNOS: endothelial NOS
FDA: U.S. Food and Drug Administration
FFA: free fatty acid
GI: gastrointestinal
GTN: glyceryl trinitrate (nitroglycerin)
HCM: hypertrophic cardiomyopathy
HCN: hyperpolarization-activated cyclic nucleotide–gated
HMG-CoA: 3-hydroxy-3-methylglutaryl coenzyme A
iNOS: inducible NOS
IP_3: inositol 1,4,5-trisphosphate
ISDN: isosorbide dinitrate
ISMN: isosorbide-5-mononitrate
MI: myocardial infarction
nNOS: neuronal NOS
NO: nitric oxide
NOS: nitric oxide synthase
NSTEMI: non–ST-elevation myocardial infarction
PDE: cyclic nucleotide phosphodiesterase
Pgp: P-glycoprotein
PLC: phospholipase C
rTPA: recombinant tissue plasminogen activator
SA: sinoatrial
SNS: sympathetic nervous system
STEMI: ST-segment elevation myocardial infarction
Tn: troponin
TxA_2: thromboxane A_2

Pathophysiology of Ischemic Heart Disease

The pathophysiological understanding of ischemic heart disease has seen major changes over the past two decades—from a concept of localized calcification causing progressive constrictions of coronary arteries, ischemia, and exercise-induced angina pectoris to a systemic inflammatory disease of the arteries, including the coronaries (therefore the CAD name). A key finding in this change of paradigm was that most infarct-causing occlusions occur at small-to-medium plaques ("active plaques") by thrombosis rather than at hemodynamically relevant stenoses by progressive narrowing. Thus, in addition to the mere size of an obstructing plaque, the inflammatory activity of the atherosclerotic process, the stability of the plaque, and platelet reactivity appear to determine the prognosis (Libby et al., 2002).

Atherosclerosis encompasses increased lipid deposition in the subendothelial space (early plaque), endothelial dysfunction with decreased production of NO, less vasodilation and increased risk of platelet adhesion, influx of lipid scavenger cells (mainly macrophages), necrosis, sterile inflammation, proliferation of smooth muscle cells, and calcification and narrowing of the blood vessel by increasing plaque formation. If the endothelium covering of the plaque or the cell layer enclosing the necrotic core of the plaque disrupt, thrombogenic materials such as collagen are presented to the bloodstream, causing platelet adhesion, fibrin deposition, thrombus formation, and closure of the blood vessel.

Triggering factors can be not only acute inflammation (e.g., influenza), but also blood pressure peaks during physical exercise or emotional stress (e.g., demonstrated during a life-threatening emergency and in avid fans during football games). Importantly, the process is dynamic, and the net thrombus formation is the result of the balance between thrombosis and thrombolysis by the fibrinolytic system (plasminogen). The degree and the duration of coronary obstruction and thereby of the ischemia of downstream myocardium (and its size) determine the degree of necrosis of muscle tissue, that is, infarct size.

Taken together, important factors that determine the progress of CAD are the concentration of lipids in the blood, endothelial function, blood pressure (as a mechanical factor predisposing to plaque rupture), the activity of the inflammatory system, and the reactivity of pro- and antithrombotic systems. Patients with CAD should be advised not only to exercise regularly, stop smoking, and have blood pressure and body weight well controlled, but also to be treated with statins, aspirin, and β adrenergic receptor antagonists (β blockers) and have annual vaccinations against influenza. The widespread implementation of this combination drug regimen and the considerably improved treatment of ACSs likely account for the continuous reduction in MIs and age-corrected cardiovascular lethality in Western countries (−42% between 2000 and 2011; Mozaffarian et al., 2015). Interestingly, the incidence of the classical large STEMI is declining as that of smaller non-STEMI increases. This raises the hypothesis that the dominant pathogenesis of acute coronary thrombosis may have changed from the rupture of lipid-rich, inflammatory plaques (in the prestatin era) to the erosion of stable plaques (Libby and Pasterkamp, 2015).

Antiplatelet agents, fibrinolytic drugs, anticoagulants, and statins (HMG-CoA reductase inhibitors) are systematically discussed in Chapters 32 and 33. This chapter concentrates on pharmacotherapy for angina pectoris and myocardial ischemia.

Pathophysiology of Angina Pectoris

Angina pectoris, the primary symptom of ischemic heart disease, is caused by transient episodes of myocardial ischemia that are due to an imbalance in the myocardial oxygen supply-demand relationship. This imbalance may be caused by an increase in myocardial oxygen demand (which is determined by heart rate, ventricular contractility, and ventricular wall tension) or by a decrease in myocardial oxygen supply (primarily determined by coronary blood flow, but occasionally modified by the oxygen-carrying capacity of the blood), or sometimes by both (Figure 27–1). Because blood flow is inversely proportional to the fourth power of the artery's luminal radius, the progressive decrease in vessel radius that characterizes coronary atherosclerosis can impair coronary blood flow and lead to symptoms of angina when myocardial O_2 demand increases, as with exertion (the so-called typical and most prevalent form of angina pectoris). In some patients, anginal symptoms may occur without any increase in myocardial O_2 demand, but rather as a consequence of an abrupt reduction in blood flow, as might result from coronary thrombosis (unstable angina or ACS) or localized vasospasm (variant or Prinzmetal angina). Regardless of the precipitating factors, the sensation of angina is similar in most patients. Typical angina is experienced as a heavy, pressing substernal discomfort (rarely described as a "pain"), often radiating to the left shoulder, flexor aspect of the left arm, jaw, or epigastrium. However, a significant minority of patients note discomfort in a different location or of a different character. Women, the elderly, and diabetics are more likely to experience myocardial ischemia with atypical symptoms. In most patients with typical angina, whose symptoms are provoked by exertion, the symptoms are relieved by rest or by administration of sublingual nitroglycerin.

Angina pectoris is a common symptom, affecting 8 million Americans (Mozaffarian et al., 2015). Angina pectoris may occur in a stable pattern over many years or may become unstable, increasing in frequency or

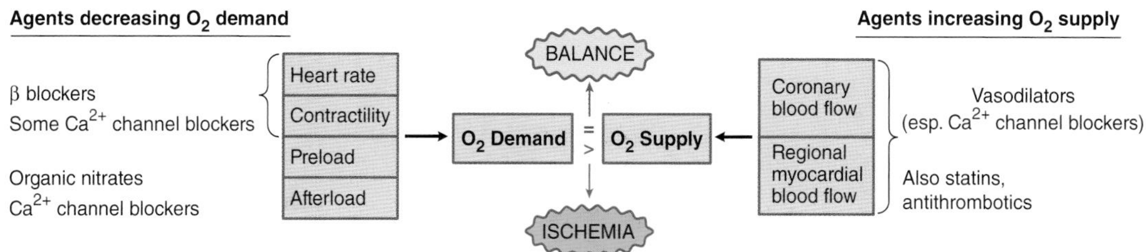

Figure 27–1 *Pharmacological modification of the major determinants of myocardial O_2 supply.* When myocardial O_2 requirements exceed O_2 supply, an ischemic episode results. This figure shows the primary hemodynamic sites of action of pharmacological agents that can reduce O_2 demand (left side) or enhance O_2 supply (right side). Some classes of agents have multiple effects. Stents, angioplasty, and coronary bypass surgery are mechanical interventions that increase O_2 supply. Both pharmacotherapy and mechanotherapy attempt to restore a dynamic balance between O_2 demand and O_2 supply.

severity and even occurring at rest. In typical stable angina, the pathological substrate is usually fixed atherosclerotic narrowing of an epicardial coronary artery, on which exertion or emotional stress superimposes an increase in myocardial O_2 demand. In variant angina, focal or diffuse coronary vasospasm episodically reduces coronary flow. Patients also may display a mixed pattern of angina with the addition of altered vessel tone on a background of atherosclerotic narrowing. In most patients with unstable angina, rupture of an atherosclerotic plaque, with consequent platelet adhesion and aggregation, decreases coronary blood flow. Superimposed thrombosis may lead to the complete abrogation of blood flow. Atherosclerotic plaques with thinner fibrous caps appear to be more "vulnerable" to rupture.

Myocardial ischemia also may be *silent*, with electrocardiographic, echocardiographic, or radionuclide evidence of ischemia appearing in the absence of symptoms. While some patients have only silent ischemia, most patients who have silent ischemia have symptomatic episodes as well. The precipitants of silent ischemia appear to be the same as those of symptomatic ischemia. We now know that the *ischemic burden* (i.e., the total time a patient is ischemic each day) is greater in many patients than was recognized previously. In most trials, the agents that are efficacious in typical angina also are efficacious in reducing silent ischemia. β Blockers appear to be more effective than the Ca^{2+} channel blockers in the prevention of episodes. Therapy directed at abolishing all silent ischemia has not been shown to be of additional benefit over conventional therapy.

Pharmacotherapy of Ischemic Heart Disease

The principal pharmacological agents used in the treatment of angina are nitrovasodilators, β blockers (see Chapter 12), and Ca^{2+} channel blockers. In patients with typical exercise-induced angina on the basis of CAD, these antianginal agents improve the balance of myocardial O_2 supply and O_2 demand principally by reducing myocardial O_2 demand by decreasing heart rate, myocardial contractility, or ventricular wall stress. Increased O_2 supply by dilating the coronary vasculature may play an additional role and is the major effect of nitrovasodilators and Ca^{2+} channel blockers in variant angina.

By contrast, the principal therapeutic goal in ACSs with unstable angina is to prevent or reduce coronary thrombus formation and increase myocardial blood flow; strategies include the use of antiplatelet agents and *heparin*, often accompanied by efforts to restore flow by mechanical means, including percutaneous coronary interventions using coronary stents, or (less commonly) emergency coronary bypass surgery. The principal therapeutic aim in variant or Prinzmetal angina is to prevent coronary vasospasm.

Antianginal agents may provide prophylactic or symptomatic treatment, but β blockers also reduce mortality, apparently by decreasing the incidence of sudden cardiac death associated with myocardial ischemia and infarction. The chronic use of organic nitrate vasodilators, which are highly efficacious in treatment of angina, is not associated with improvements in cardiac mortality, and some investigators have suggested that chronic use of nitroglycerin may have adverse cardiovascular effects (Parker, 2004).

Besides symptomatic relief from angina pain conferred by antianginal drugs, patients with CAD should be treated with drugs that can reduce the progression of atherosclerosis and reduce the risk of coronary thrombosis and MI. *Aspirin* is used routinely in patients with myocardial ischemia, and daily aspirin at low doses reduces the incidence of clinical events (Fihn et al., 2012). The optimal dose appears to be between 75 and 150 mg/d (Montalescot et al., 2013), although most large studies have been done with a 325-mg dose. The oral ADP receptor antagonist clopidogrel was slightly superior to aspirin in patients with chronic atherosclerotic vascular disease and had a favorable safety profile (CAPRIE Steering Committee, 1996). When used in combination with aspirin in patients with ACS, clopidogrel reduced the cardiovascular death rate by 20%, but increased the incidence of major bleeding events by 38% (Yusuf et al., 2001). In patients with stable cardiovascular disease, clopidogrel conferred no benefit over aspirin and was associated with signs of harm in patients with multiple risk factors (Bhatt et al., 2006). Guidelines therefore recommend clopidogrel only as an alternative in patients with aspirin intolerance and advise against the routine use of dual platelet inhibition in patients with stable disease (Fihn et al., 2012; Montalescot et al., 2013). In contrast, dual platelet inhibition is routinely given in patients who underwent coronary artery stenting. The recommended time (1–12 months) varies depending on the intervention (e.g., bare metal vs. drug-eluting stent) and the risk profile of patients. The newer ADP receptor antagonists prasugrel and ticagrelor have a more useful pharmacokinetic profile and seem to have a better benefit/risk ratio than clopidogrel in the postintervention treatment phase (Cannon et al., 2010; Wiviott et al., 2007) but are not generally recommended as alternatives to clopidogrel in patients with stable CAD. Statins reduce mortality in patients with CAD. Although high-risk patients (including those with high plasma LDL cholesterol levels) have the greatest absolute benefit, the relative risk reduction of approximately 25% appears largely independent of baseline cholesterol blood levels. Statins should therefore be given to all patients with CAD. It is unclear whether ACEIs or angiotensin receptor blockers (see Chapter 26) reduce mortality or other end points in patients with CAD when given routinely in addition to aspirin, statins, and β blockers, but they are recommended for subgroups of patients with CAD with reduced left ventricular systolic function, hypertension, diabetes, or chronic kidney disease (Montalescot et al., 2013).

Coronary artery bypass surgery and percutaneous coronary interventions such as angioplasty and coronary artery stent deployment commonly complement pharmacological treatment. In some subsets of patients, percutaneous or surgical revascularization may have a survival advantage over medical treatment alone (Kappetein et al., 2011). Intracoronary drug delivery using drug-eluting coronary stents represents an intersection of mechanical and pharmacological approaches in the treatment of CAD.

Organic Nitrates

The organic nitrate agents are prodrugs that are sources of NO. NO activates the soluble isoform of guanylyl cyclase, thereby increasing intracellular levels of cGMP. In turn, cGMP promotes the dephosphorylation of the myosin light chain and the reduction of cytosolic Ca^{2+} and leads to the relaxation of smooth muscle cells in a broad range of tissues (see Figures 3-13, 3-17, and 44-7). The NO-dependent relaxation of vascular smooth muscle leads to vasodilation; NO-mediated guanylyl cyclase activation also inhibits platelet aggregation and relaxes smooth muscle in the bronchi and GI tract.

The broad biological response to nitrovasodilators reflects the existence of endogenous NO-modulated regulatory pathways. The endogenous synthesis of NO in humans is catalyzed by a family of NOSs that oxidize the amino acid L-arginine to form NO, plus L-citrulline as a coproduct. There are three distinct mammalian NOS isoforms: *nNOS*, *eNOS*, and *iNOS* (see Chapter 3), and they are involved in processes as diverse as neurotransmission, vasomotion, and immunomodulation. In several vascular disease states, pathways of endogenous NO-dependent regulation appear to be deranged (reviewed in [Dudzinski et al., 2006]).

HISTORICAL PERSPECTIVE

Nitroglycerin was first synthesized in 1846 by Sobrero, who observed that a small quantity placed on the tongue elicited a severe headache. The explosive properties of nitroglycerin also were soon noted, and control of this unstable compound for military and industrial use was not realized until Alfred Nobel devised a process to stabilize the nitroglycerin and patented a specialized detonator in 1863. The vast fortune that Nobel accrued from the nitroglycerin detonator patent provided the funds later used to establish the Nobel prizes. In 1857, T. Lauder Brunton of Edinburgh (no relation to the editor of this volume) administered *amyl nitrite*, a known vasodepressor, by inhalation and noted that anginal pain was relieved within 30–60 sec. The action of amyl nitrite was transitory, however, and the dosage was difficult to adjust. Subsequently, William Murrell surmised that the action of nitroglycerin mimicked that of amyl nitrite and established the use of sublingual nitroglycerin for relief of the acute anginal attack and as a prophylactic agent to be taken prior to exertion. The empirical observation that organic nitrates could dramatically and safely alleviate the symptoms of angina pectoris led to their widespread acceptance by the medical profession. Indeed, Alfred Nobel himself was prescribed nitroglycerin by his physicians when he developed angina in 1890. Basic investigations defined the role of NO in both the vasodilation produced by nitrates and endogenous vasodilation. The importance of NO as a signaling molecule in the cardiovascular system and elsewhere was recognized by the awarding of the 1998 Nobel Prize in Medicine/Physiology to the pharmacologists Robert Furchgott, Louis Ignarro, and Ferid Murad.

Chemistry

Organic nitrates are polyol esters of nitric acid, whereas organic nitrites are esters of nitrous acid (Table 27–1). Nitrate esters (—C—O—NO_2) and nitrite esters (—C—O—NO) are characterized by a sequence of carbon-oxygen-nitrogen, whereas nitro compounds possess carbon-nitrogen bonds (C—NO_2). Thus, GTN is not a nitro compound, and it is erroneously called nitroglycerin; however, this nomenclature is both widespread and official. Amyl nitrite is a highly volatile liquid that must be administered by inhalation and is of limited therapeutic utility. Organic nitrates of low molecular mass (such as GTN) are moderately volatile, oily liquids, whereas the high-molecular-mass nitrate esters (e.g., erythrityl tetranitrate, ISDN, and isosorbide mononitrate) are solids. In the pure form (without an inert carrier such as lactose), nitroglycerin is explosive. The organic nitrates and nitrites, collectively termed *nitrovasodilators*, must be metabolized (reduced) to produce gaseous NO, which appears to be the active principle of this class of compounds. NO gas also can be directly administered by inhalation.

Pharmacological Properties

Mechanism of Action. Nitrites, organic nitrates, nitroso compounds, and a variety of other nitrogen oxide–containing substances (including *nitroprusside;* see further in the chapter) lead to the formation of the reactive gaseous free radical NO and related NO-containing compounds. NO gas also may be administered by inhalation. Surprisingly, more than 140 years after its introduction in the therapy of angina pectoris, the mode of action of organic nitrates is still incompletely understood (Mayer and Beretta, 2008). Established mechanisms of GTN bioactivation and action include a nonenzymatic reaction with L-cysteine, formation of nitrite and NO by ALDH2 (Chen et al., 2002), activation of soluble guanylyl cyclase, and generation of cGMP. The bioactivation of other nitrovasodilators such as ISDN and ISMN is ALDH2 independent, suggesting the involvement of other enzymes, such as CYPs, xanthine oxidoreductase, and cytosolic ALDH isoforms (Munzel et al., 2014). The action of NO on soluble guanylyl cyclase seems to be elicited in substantial part by S-nitrosothiol. The different ALDH2 dependence of GTN and ISDN is clinically relevant because individuals of Asian origin carry an inactive ALDH2 variant and do not respond adequately to GTN but do respond to ISDN (Stamler, 2008).

The NO-stimulated elevation of cGMP activates PKG and modulates the activities of cyclic nucleotide PDEs (PDEs 2, 3, and 5) in a variety of cell types. In smooth muscle, the net result is reduced phosphorylation of myosin light chain, reduced Ca^{2+} concentration in the cytosol, and relaxation (Figure 44–7). Reduced phosphorylation of myosin light chain is the result of decreased myosin light-chain kinase activity and increased myosin light-chain phosphatase activity and promotes vasorelaxation and smooth muscle relaxation in many tissues. cGMP is a substrate for PDE 5, whose inhibition by sildenafil and related compounds potentiates the action of nitrovasodilators (see *Toxicity and Untoward Responses*).

Hemodynamic Effects. The nitrovasodilators promote relaxation of vascular smooth muscle. For reasons not understood, GTN dilates large blood vessels (>200-μm diameter) more potently than small vessels, explaining why low doses of GTN preferentially dilate veins and conductance arteries and leave the tone of the small-to-medium arterioles (that regulate resistance) unaffected. This profile has important consequences for the antianginal efficacy of nitrovasodilators. At low-to-medium doses, preferential venodilation decreases venous return, leading to a fall in left and right ventricular chamber size and end-diastolic pressures, reduced wall stress, and thereby reduced cardiac O_2 demand (see discussion that follows). Systemic vascular resistance and arterial pressure are not or only mildly decreased, leaving coronary perfusion pressure unaffected. Heart rate remains unchanged or may increase slightly in response to a decrease in blood pressure. Pulmonary vascular resistance and cardiac output are slightly reduced. Doses of GTN that do not alter systemic arterial pressure may still produce arteriolar dilation in the face and neck, resulting in a facial flush, or dilation of meningeal arterial vessels, causing headache.

Higher doses of organic nitrates cause further venous pooling and may decrease arteriolar resistance as well, thereby decreasing systolic and diastolic blood pressure and causing pallor, weakness, dizziness, and activation of compensatory sympathetic reflexes. This can happen to such an extent that coronary flow is compromised, and the sympathetic increase in myocardial O_2 demand overrides the beneficial action of the nitrovasodilators, leading to ischemia. In addition, sublingual nitroglycerin administration may produce bradycardia and hypotension, probably owing to activation of the Bezold-Jarisch reflex.

In patients with autonomic dysfunction and an inability to increase sympathetic outflow (multiple-system atrophy and pure autonomic failure are the most common forms, much less commonly seen in the autonomic dysfunction associated with diabetes), the fall in blood pressure consequent to the venodilation produced by nitrates cannot be compensated. In these clinical contexts, nitrates may reduce arterial pressure and coronary perfusion pressure significantly, producing potentially life-threatening hypotension and even aggravating angina.

TABLE 27–1 ■ ORGANIC NITRATES AVAILABLE FOR CLINICAL USE

AGENT	PREPARATIONS, DOSES, ADMINISTRATION[a]	
Nitroglycerin (glyceryl trinitrate)	T: 0.3–0.6 mg as needed	O: 2.5–5 cm, topically every 4–8 h
	S: 0.4 mg per spray as needed	D: 1 disk (2.5–15 mg) for 12–16 h/d
	C: 2.5–9 mg 2–4 times daily	IV: 10–20 μg/min; ↑ 10 μg/min to max of 400 μg/min
	B: 1 mg every 3–5 h	
Isosorbide dinitrate	T: 2.5–10 mg every 2–3 h	T(O): 5–40 mg every 8 h
	T(C): 5–10 mg every 2–3 h	C: 40–80 mg every 12 h
Isosorbide-5-mononitrate	T: 10–40 mg twice daily	C: 60–120 mg daily

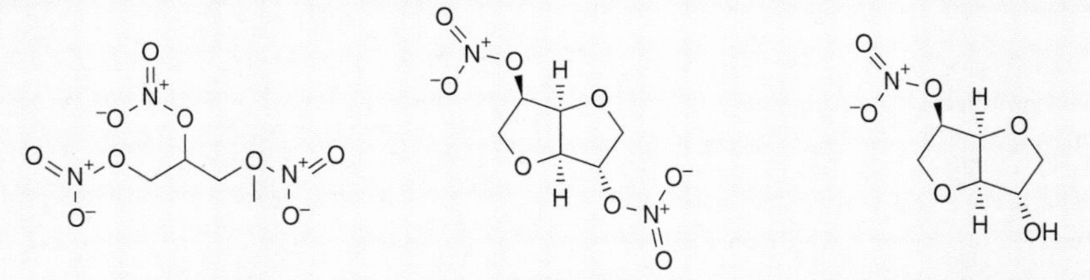

Nitroglycerin (glyceryl trinitrate, GTN)

Isosorbide dinitrate (ISDN)

Isosorbide-5-mononitrate (ISMN)

[a]B, buccal (transmucosal) tablet; C, sustained-release capsule or tablet; D, transdermal disk or patch; IV, intravenous injection; O, ointment; S, lingual spray; T, tablet for sublingual use; T(C), chewable tablet; T(O), oral tablet or capsule.

ADME. As outlined previously, nitrovasodilators differ in their dependence on ALDH2 for bioactivation (note ALDH2 deficiency in many Asians). In addition, their pharmacokinetic profiles exhibit therapeutically relevant differences in sublingual resorption, onset of action, and half-life (Table 27–1).

Nitroglycerin. Peak concentrations of GTN are found in plasma within 4 min of sublingual administration; the drug has a $t_{1/2}$ of 1–3 min. The onset of action of GTN may be even more rapid if delivered as a sublingual spray rather than as a sublingual tablet. Glyceryl dinitrate metabolites, which have about one-tenth the vasodilator potency, appear to have half-lives of about 40 min.

Isosorbide Dinitrate. Sublingual administration of ISDN produces maximal plasma concentrations of the drug by 6 min, and the fall in concentration is rapid ($t_{1/2}$ of about 45 min). The primary initial metabolites, isosorbide-2-mononitrate and ISMN, have longer half-lives (3–6 h) and are presumed to contribute to the therapeutic efficacy of the drug. ISDN is therefore suitable both for standby and sustained therapy.

Isosorbide-5-Mononitrate. This agent is available in tablet form. ISMN does not undergo significant first-pass metabolism, so it has high bioavailability after oral administration, but its onset of action is too slow for acute treatment of angina.

Inhaled NO. Nitric oxide gas administered by inhalation appears to exert most of its therapeutic effects on the pulmonary vasculature because of the rapid inactivation of NO by hemoglobin in the blood. It is approved for the treatment of pulmonary hypertension in hypoxemic neonates, where it reduced morbidity and mortality (Bloch et al., 2007), and is currently tested in patients with pulmonary arterial hypertension.

Mechanisms of Antianginal Efficacy of Organic Nitrates

When GTN is injected directly into the coronary circulation of patients with CAD, anginal attacks (induced by electrical pacing) are not aborted even when coronary blood flow is increased. In contrast, sublingual administration of GTN does relieve anginal pain in the same patients, indicating that the major antianginal effect of nitrovasodilators is mediated by preload reduction rather than coronary artery dilation.

This interpretation is supported by studies in exercising patients showing that angina occurs at the same value of the *triple product* (Aortic pressure × Heart rate × Ejection time, which is roughly proportional to myocardial consumption of O_2) with or without nitroglycerin. Thus, the beneficial effect of nitroglycerin has to result from reduced cardiac O_2 demand rather than an increase in the delivery of O_2 to ischemic regions of myocardium. However, these results do not preclude the possibility that a favorable redistribution of blood flow to ischemic subendocardial myocardium may contribute to relief of pain in a typical anginal attack, and they do not preclude the possibility that direct coronary vasodilation may be the major effect of nitroglycerin in situations where vasospasm compromises myocardial blood flow.

Effects on Myocardial O_2 Requirements. The major determinants of myocardial O_2 consumption are left ventricular wall tension, heart rate, and myocardial contractility (Figure 27–1). Ventricular wall tension is affected by preload and afterload. *Preload* is determined by the diastolic pressure that distends the ventricle (ventricular end-diastolic pressure). Increasing end-diastolic volume augments the ventricular wall tension (by the law of Laplace, tension is proportional to pressure times radius). Increasing venous capacitance with nitrates decreases venous return to the heart, decreases ventricular end-diastolic volume, and thereby decreases O_2 consumption. An additional benefit of reducing preload is that it increases the pressure gradient for perfusion across the ventricular wall, which favors subendocardial perfusion. *Afterload* is the impedance against which the ventricle must eject. In the absence of aortic valvular disease, afterload is related to peripheral resistance. Decreasing peripheral arteriolar resistance reduces afterload and thus myocardial work and O_2 consumption. The distensibility of the large conductance arteries such as the aorta may play an additional role.

Nitrovasodilators preferentially decrease preload by dilating venous capacitance vessels. The decrease in afterload is generally small and mainly observed at higher doses. The effect on aortic stiffness appears complex (Soma et al., 2000). NO and nitrovasodilators can directly modulate the inotropic or chronotropic state of the heart via cGMP and its stimulatory effect on PDE2 (thereby reducing cAMP) or an inhibitory effect on the cAMP-specific PDE3 (thereby increasing cAMP). An inotropic response depends on the extent to which the PDE isoforms are expressed in the appropriate cells and in the proper subcellular compartment (Steinberg and Brunton, 2001). Small NO concentrations favor a positive inotropic effect (Kojda et al., 1997); however, the effect size is small and its significance unclear. Because nitrates affect several of the primary determinants of myocardial O_2 demand, their net effect usually is to decrease myocardial O_2 consumption. In addition, an improvement in the lusitropic state of the heart may be seen with more rapid early diastolic filling. This may be secondary to the relief of ischemia rather than primary, or it may be due to a reflex increase in sympathetic activity. Nitrovasodilators also increase cGMP in platelets, with consequent inhibition of platelet function. While this may contribute to their antianginal efficacy, the effect appears to be modest and in some settings may be confounded by the potential of nitrates to alter the pharmacokinetics of heparin, reducing its antithrombotic effect.

Effects on Total and Regional Coronary Blood Flow. When considering the effect of vasodilators in the ischemic heart, it is important to realize that myocardial ischemia itself is a powerful stimulus to coronary vasodilation and part of an autoregulatory mechanism. In the presence of atherosclerotic coronary artery narrowing, ischemia distal to the lesion stimulates vasodilation of downstream resistance arterioles and thereby helps maintain adequate perfusion of the ischemic area under rest. If the stenosis is severe, much of the capacity to dilate is used to maintain resting blood flow. Further dilation may not be possible, neither under exercise nor with therapeutically applied vasodilators. In contrast, nonselective vasodilators such as adenosine or dipyridamole (which inhibits adenosine transmembrane transport and thereby increases extracellular concentrations) can worsen the perfusion of ischemic areas by dilating the relatively constricted arterioles of the healthy myocardium, leading to redistribution of blood flow away from the ischemic myocardium ("steal phenomenon"). Accordingly, dipyridamole is not used therapeutically but can be used as a stress test to provoke angina pectoris (Bodi et al., 2007).

Nitrovasodilators, in contrast, do not have a major effect on the smaller resistance arteries (and therefore do not cause steal phenomena) but can dilate the large, epicardial sections of the coronary arteries upstream of a stenosis and also in a stenosis (concept of the "dynamic stenosis"; Brown et al., 1981) and thereby increase blood flow distal to the narrowing. Collateral flow to ischemic regions also is increased. As outlined previously, GTN also reduces wall stress that opposes blood flow to the subendocardium, which is particularly sensitive to ischemia.

In patients with angina owing to coronary artery spasm, the capacity of nitrovasodilators to dilate epicardial coronary arteries, particularly regions affected by spasm, is the primary mechanism of their beneficial effect.

Other Effects. The nitrovasodilators also relax smooth muscles of the bronchial tract, the gallbladder, biliary ducts, and sphincter of Oddi and the GI tract. Spontaneous motility decreased by nitrates both in vivo *and* in vitro. The effect may be transient and incomplete in vivo, but abnormal "spasm" frequently is reduced. Indeed, many incidences of atypical chest pain and "angina" are due to biliary or esophageal spasm, and these also can be relieved by nitrates. Nitrates can also relax ureteral and uterine smooth muscle, but these responses are of uncertain clinical significance.

Tolerance

Frequently repeated or continuous exposure to high doses of nitrovasodilators lead to tolerance, that is, marked attenuation in the magnitude of most of their pharmacological effects. The magnitude of tolerance is a function of dosage and frequency of use. Tolerance may result from a reduced capacity of the vascular smooth muscle to convert nitroglycerin to NO, *true vascular tolerance*, or to the activation of mechanisms extraneous to the vessel wall, *pseudotolerance* (Munzel et al., 1995). Multiple mechanisms have been proposed to account for nitrate tolerance, including volume expansion, neurohumoral activation, cellular depletion of sulfhydryl groups, and the generation of free radicals (Parker and Parker, 1998). A reactive intermediate formed during the generation of NO from organic nitrates may itself damage and inactivate the enzymes of the activation pathway (Munzel et al., 1995; Parker, 2004). Inactivation of ALDH2 (Sydow et al., 2004) and S-nitrosylation of soluble guanylyl cyclase (Sayed et al., 2008) are seen in models of nitrate tolerance and could explain cross-tolerance to different (nitro)vasodilators. Other changes observed in the setting of nitroglycerin tolerance include an enhanced response to vasoconstrictors such as angiotensin II, serotonin, and phenylephrine. Prolonged administration of GTN is associated with plasma volume expansion, which may be reflected by a decrease in hematocrit. Unfortunately, attempts to prevent nitrate tolerance based on these mechanisms (e.g., antioxidants, coapplication of vasodilators or diuretics) failed in clinical trials.

A clinically important lesson of research on nitrate tolerance is that prolonged treatment with nitrates may not only induce a loss of response to nitrates, but also actually decrease angina threshold in the interval (Parker et al., 1995). A special form of GTN tolerance is observed in individuals exposed to GTN in the manufacture of explosives. If protection is inadequate, workers may experience severe headaches, dizziness, and postural weakness during the first several days of employment ("Monday disease"). Tolerance then develops and can lead to organic nitrate dependence. Workers without demonstrable organic vascular disease have been reported to have an increase in the incidence of ACSs during the 24- to 72-h periods away from the work environment. It seems prudent not to withdraw nitrates abruptly from a patient who has received such therapy chronically.

Therapy should be designed to prevent tolerance. High doses should be avoided and therapy interrupted for 8–12 h daily, which allows the return of efficacy. In patients with exertional angina, it is usually most convenient to omit dosing at night either by adjusting dosing intervals of oral or buccal preparations or by removing cutaneous GTN. Patients whose anginal pattern suggests its precipitation by increased left ventricular filling pressures (e.g., in association with orthopnea or paroxysmal nocturnal dyspnea) may benefit from continuing nitrates at night and omitting them during a quiet period of the day. Some patients develop an increased frequency of nocturnal angina when a nitrate-free interval is employed using GTN patches; such patients may require another class of antianginal agent during this period. Continuous intravenous administration of GTN regularly induces tolerance and should therefore be avoided. Tolerance also has been seen with ISMN and ISDN; an eccentric twice-daily dosing schedule appears to maintain efficacy (Parker and Parker, 1998). Molsidomine, a direct NO donor, is approved in many European countries and is claimed to induce less tolerance than the organic nitrates, but the supporting evidence is weak. A recent study failed to demonstrate beneficial effects of molsidomine on endothelial dysfunction (Barbato et al., 2015).

Toxicity and Untoward Responses

Untoward responses to the therapeutic use of organic nitrates are almost all secondary to actions on the cardiovascular system. Headache is common and can be severe, usually decreasing over a few days if treatment is continued and often controlled by decreasing the dose. Transient episodes of dizziness, weakness, and other manifestations associated with postural hypotension may develop, particularly if the patient is standing immobile, and may progress occasionally to loss of consciousness, a reaction that appears to be accentuated by alcohol. It also may be seen with very low doses of nitrates in patients with autonomic dysfunction. Even in severe nitrate syncope, positioning and other measures that facilitate venous return are the only therapeutic measures required. All the organic nitrates occasionally can produce drug rash.

Interaction of Nitrates With PDE5 Inhibitors. Erectile dysfunction is a frequently encountered problem whose risk factors parallel those of CAD. Thus, many men desiring therapy for erectile dysfunction already may be receiving (or may require, especially if they increase physical activity) antianginal therapy. The combination of sildenafil and other PDE5 inhibitors with organic nitrate vasodilators can cause extreme hypotension.

Cells in the corpus cavernosum produce NO during sexual arousal in response to nonadrenergic, noncholinergic neurotransmission (Burnett et al., 1992). NO stimulates the formation of cGMP, which leads to relaxation of smooth muscle of penile arteries that fill the corpus cavernosum, leading to engorgement of the corpus cavernosum and erection. The accumulation of cGMP is enhanced by inhibition of the cGMP-specific PDE5 family. Sildenafil and congeners inhibit PDE5 and have been demonstrated to improve erectile function in patients with erectile dysfunction.

Not surprisingly, PDE5 inhibitors have assumed the status of widely used recreational drugs. Sildenafil is also FDA and EMA approved in patients with pulmonary arterial hypertension in whom the drug decreased pulmonary vascular resistance and enhanced exercise capacity. PDE5 inhibitors also are being studied in patients with congestive heart failure, but a recent trial in patients with preserved ejection fraction failed (Redfield et al., 2013; Chapter 28). Tadalafil and vardenafil share similar therapeutic efficacy and side-effect profiles with sildenafil; tadalafil has a longer time to onset of action and a longer therapeutic $t_{1/2}$ than the other PDE5 inhibitors (Table 45–1). Sildenafil has been the most thoroughly characterized of these compounds, but all three PDE5 inhibitors are contraindicated for patients taking organic nitrate vasodilators, and the PDE5 inhibitors should be used with caution in patients taking α- or β blockers (see Chapter 12).

The side effects of sildenafil and other PDE5 inhibitors are largely predictable on the basis of their effects on PDE5. Headache, flushing, and rhinitis may be observed, as well as dyspepsia owing to relaxation of the lower esophageal sphincter. Sildenafil and vardenafil also weakly inhibit PDE6, the enzyme involved in photoreceptor signal transduction (Figure 69–9), and can produce visual disturbances, most notably changes in the perception of color hue or brightness. In addition to visual disturbances, sudden one-sided hearing loss has also been reported. Tadalafil inhibits PDE11, a widely distributed PDE isoform, but the clinical importance of this effect is not clear. The most important toxicity of all these PDE5 inhibitors is hemodynamic. When given alone to men with severe CAD, these drugs induce only a modest (<10%) decrease of blood pressure (Herrmann et al., 2000). However, PDE5 inhibitors and nitrates act synergistically to cause profound increases in cGMP and dramatic reductions in blood pressure (>25 mm Hg). *PDE5 inhibitors should therefore not be prescribed to patients receiving any form of nitrate* (Cheitlin et al., 1999); in prescribing nitrates, the physician should warn the patient that PDE5 inhibitors and nitrates must not be used concurrently, and that no PDE5 inhibitor should be used in the 24 h prior to initiating nitrate therapy. A period of longer than 24 h may be needed following administration of a PDE5 inhibitor for safe use of nitrates, especially with tadalafil, due to its prolonged $t_{1/2}$. In the event that patients develop significant hypotension following combined administration of sildenafil and a nitrate, fluids and α adrenergic receptor agonists, if needed, may be used for support.

Sildenafil, tadalafil, and vardenafil are metabolized via CYP3A4, and their toxicity may be enhanced in patients who receive inhibitors of this enzyme, including macrolide and imidazole antibiotics, and antiretroviral agents (see individual chapters and Chapter 6). PDE5 inhibitors also may prolong cardiac repolarization by blocking the I_{Kr}. Although these interactions and effects are important clinically, the overall incidence and profile of adverse events observed with PDE5 inhibitors, when used without nitrates, are consistent with the expected background frequency of the same events in the treated population. In patients with CAD whose exercise capacity indicates that sexual activity is unlikely to precipitate angina and who are not currently taking nitrates, the use of PDE5 inhibitors can be considered.

Therapeutic Uses

Stable Angina Pectoris. Diseases that predispose to CAD and angina should be treated as part of a comprehensive therapeutic program with the primary goal being to prolong life. Conditions such as hypertension, anemia, thyrotoxicosis, obesity, heart failure, cardiac arrhythmias, and acute emotional stress can precipitate anginal symptoms in many patients. Patients should be counseled to stop smoking, lose weight, and maintain a low-fat, high-fiber diet; hypertension and hyperlipidemia should be corrected; and daily aspirin (or clopidogrel if aspirin is not tolerated) and statins (see Chapter 33) should be prescribed. Exposure to sympathomimetic agents (e.g., those in nasal decongestants and other sources) and serotonin receptor agonists used in the treatment of migraine (sumatriptan and similar) should be avoided. The use of drugs that modify the perception of pain is a poor approach to the treatment of angina because the underlying myocardial ischemia is not relieved.

Table 27–1 lists the preparations and dosages of the nitrites and organic nitrates. The rapidity of onset, the duration of action, and the likelihood of developing tolerance are related to the method of administration.

Short-Acting Nitrates for Standby Therapy. GTN is the most commonly used drug for the rapid release of angina and can be applied as tablets, capsules, sublingual powder, spray, and aerosol. The onset of action is within 1–2 min (fastest with the spray), and the effects are undetectable by 1 h after administration. An initial dose of 0.3 mg GTN often relieves pain within 3 min. ISDN, but not ISMN, is an alternative to GTN. It has a slower onset of action (3–4 min), but a longer duration (>1 h). Anginal pain may be prevented when the drugs are used prophylactically immediately prior to exercise or stress. The smallest effective dose should be prescribed. Patients should be instructed to seek medical attention immediately if three tablets of GTN taken over a 15-min period do not relieve a sustained attack because this situation may be indicative of MI, unstable angina, or another cause of the pain.

Longer-Acting Nitrates for the Prophylaxis of Angina. Nitrates can also be used to provide prophylaxis against anginal episodes in patients who have more than occasional angina. However, such patients should be offered revascularizing therapy. Moreover, chronic treatment with nitrates is not associated with a prognostic benefit and may induce tolerance and endothelial dysfunction as discussed previously. Nitrates must therefore be considered a second choice compared to β blockers. Sustained-release oral preparations of ISDN, ISMN, and GTN are available. Sustained-release ISDN and ISMN are typically given in two doses administered 6–7 h apart, followed by a nitrate-free interval of at least 8 h.

Variant (Prinzmetal) Angina. The large coronary arteries normally contribute little to coronary resistance. However, in variant angina, coronary constriction results in reduced blood flow and ischemic pain. Multiple mechanisms have been proposed to initiate vasospasm, including endothelial cell injury. Whereas long-acting nitrates alone are occasionally efficacious in abolishing episodes of variant angina, additional therapy with Ca^{2+} channel blockers usually is required. Ca^{2+} channel blockers, but not nitrates, have been shown to influence mortality and the incidence of MI favorably in variant angina; they should generally be included in therapy.

Congestive Heart Failure. The utility of nitrovasodilators to relieve pulmonary congestion and to increase cardiac output in congestive heart failure is addressed in Chapter 28.

Unstable Angina Pectoris (Acute Coronary Syndromes, see discussion that follows). Resistance to nitrates classifies angina symptoms as "unstable" and is a characteristic feature of ACSs, typically caused by transient or permanent thrombotic occlusion of coronary vessels. Nitrates do not modify this process specifically and are second-line drugs.

Ca^{2+} Channel Blockers

Voltage-gated Ca^{2+} channels (L-type or slow channels) mediate the entry of extracellular Ca^{2+} into smooth muscle and cardiac myocytes and SA and AV nodal cells in response to electrical depolarization. In both smooth muscle and cardiac myocytes, Ca^{2+} is a trigger for contraction, albeit by different mechanisms. Ca^{2+} channel antagonists, also called *Ca^{2+} entry blockers* or *Ca^{2+} channel blockers*, inhibit Ca^{2+} influx. In vascular smooth muscle, this leads to relaxation, especially in arterial beds, in cardiac myocytes to negative inotropic effects. All Ca^{2+} channel blockers exert these two principal actions, but the ratio differs according to the class as does the presence of chronotropic and dromotropic effects.

HISTORICAL PERSPECTIVE

The work in the 1960s of Fleckenstein and colleagues led to the concept that drugs can alter cardiac and smooth muscle contraction by blocking the entry of Ca^{2+} into myocytes (Fleckenstein et al., 1969). Godfraind and associates showed that the effect of the diphenylpiperazine analogues in preventing agonist-induced vascular smooth muscle contraction could be overcome by raising the concentration of Ca^{2+} in the extracellular medium (Godfraind et al., 1986). Hass and Hartfelder reported in 1962 that verapamil, a coronary vasodilator, possessed negative inotropic and chronotropic effects that were not seen with other vasodilatory agents, such as GTN. In 1967, Fleckenstein suggested that the negative inotropic effect resulted from inhibition of excitation-contraction coupling and that the mechanism involved reduced movement of Ca^{2+} into cardiac myocytes. Verapamil was the first clinically available Ca^{2+} channel blocker; it is a congener of papaverine. Many other Ca^{2+} entry blockers with a wide range of structures are now available.

Chemistry

The multiple Ca^{2+} channel blockers that are approved for clinical use in the U.S. have diverse chemical structures. Clinically used Ca^{2+} channel blockers include the phenylalkylamine verapamil, the benzothiazepine diltiazem, and numerous dihydropyridines, including amlodipine, clevidipine, felodipine, isradipine, lercanidine, nicardipine, nifedipine, nimodipine, and nisoldipine. The structures and relative specificities of representative drugs are shown in Table 27–2. Although these drugs are commonly grouped together as "calcium channel blockers," there are fundamental differences among verapamil, diltiazem, and the dihydropyridines with respect to pharmacodynamics, drug interactions, and toxicities.

Mechanisms of Action

An increased concentration of cytosolic Ca^{2+} causes increased contraction in both cardiac and vascular smooth muscle cells. In cardiac myocytes, the entry of extracellular Ca^{2+} causes a larger Ca^{2+} release from intracellular stores (Ca^{2+}-induced Ca^{2+} release) and thereby initiates the contraction twitch. In smooth muscle cells, entry of Ca^{2+} plays a dominant role, but the release of Ca^{2+} from intracellular storage sites also contributes to contraction of vascular smooth muscle, particularly in some vascular beds. In contrast to cardiac muscle, smooth muscles typically contract tonically. Cytosolic Ca^{2+} concentrations can be increased by diverse contractile stimuli in vascular smooth muscle cells. Many hormones and autocoids increase Ca^{2+} influx through so-called receptor-operated channels, whereas increases in external concentrations of K^+ and depolarizing electrical stimuli increase Ca^{2+} influx through voltage-gated, or "potential operated," channels. The Ca^{2+} channel blockers produce their effects by binding to the α_1 subunit of the L-type voltage-gated Ca^{2+} channels and reducing Ca^{2+} flux through the channel. The vascular and cardiac effects of some of the Ca^{2+} channel blockers are summarized in the next section and in Table 27–2.

Voltage-gated channels contain domains of homologous sequence that are arranged in tandem within a single large subunit. In addition to the major channel-forming subunit (termed α_1), Ca^{2+} channels contain several other associated subunits (termed α_2, β, γ, and δ) (Schwartz, 1992). Voltage-gated Ca^{2+} channels have been divided into at least three subtypes based on their conductances and sensitivities to voltage (Schwartz, 1992; Tsien et al., 1988). The channels best characterized to date are the L, N, and T subtypes. Only the L-type channel is sensitive to the dihydropyridine Ca^{2+} channel blockers. All approved Ca^{2+} channel blockers bind to the α_1 subunit of the L-type Ca^{2+} channel, which is the main pore-forming unit of the channel. This approximately 250,000-Da subunit is associated with a disulfide-linked $\alpha_2\delta$ subunit of about 140,000 Da and a smaller intracellular β subunit. The α_1 subunits share a common topology of four homologous domains, each of which is composed of six putative transmembrane segments (S1–S6). The α_2, δ, and β subunits modulate the α_1 subunit (see Figure 14–2). The phenylalkylamine Ca^{2+} channel blocker verapamil binds to transmembrane segment 6 of domain IV (IVS6), the benzothiazepine Ca^{2+} channel blocker diltiazem binds to the cytoplasmic bridge between domain III (IIIS) and domain IV (IVS), and the dihydropyridine Ca^{2+} channel blockers (nifedipine and several others) bind to transmembrane segments of both domains III and IV. These three separate receptor sites are linked allosterically.

Pharmacological Actions

Vascular Tissue. Depolarization of vascular smooth muscle cells depends primarily on the influx of Ca^{2+}. At least three distinct mechanisms may be responsible for contraction of vascular smooth muscle cells. First, voltage-gated Ca^{2+} channels open in response to depolarization of

TABLE 27–2 ■ COMPARATIVE CV EFFECTS OF Ca^{2+} CHANNEL BLOCKERS[a]

DRUG CLASS: EXAMPLE	VASODILATION	↓ CARDIAC CONTRACTILITY	↓ AUTOMATICITY (SA NODE)	↓ CONDUCTION (AV NODE)
***Phenylalkylamine*:** Verapamil	4	4	5	5
***Benzothiazepine*:** Diltiazem	3	2	5	4
***Dihydropyridine*[b]:** Amlodipine	5	1	1	0

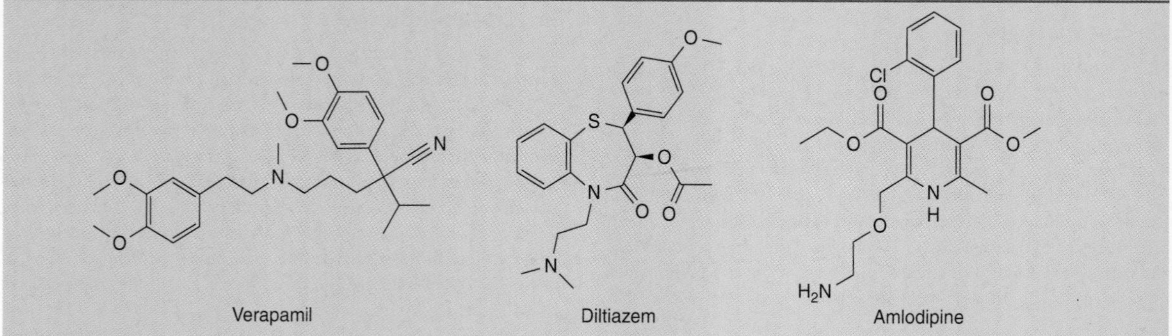

Verapamil

Diltiazem

Amlodipine

[a]Relative effects are ranked from *no effect* (0) to *prominent* (5).

[b]See text for individual characteristics of the numerous dihydropyridines.

the membrane, and extracellular Ca^{2+} moves down its electrochemical gradient into the cell. After closure of Ca^{2+} channels, a finite period of time is required before the channels can open again in response to a stimulus. Second, agonist-induced contractions that occur without depolarization of the membrane result from stimulation of the G_q-PLC-IP_3 pathway, resulting in the release of intracellular Ca^{2+} from the sarcoplasmic reticulum (Chapter 3). Emptying of intracellular Ca^{2+} stores may trigger further influx of extracellular Ca^{2+} (store-operated Ca^{2+} entry), but its relevance in smooth muscle is unresolved. Third, receptor-operated Ca^{2+} channels allow the entry of extracellular Ca^{2+} in response to receptor occupancy. An increase in cytosolic Ca^{2+} results in enhanced binding of Ca^{2+} to calmodulin. The Ca^{2+}-calmodulin complex in turn activates myosin light-chain kinase, with resulting phosphorylation of the myosin light chain. Such phosphorylation promotes interaction between actin and myosin and leads to sustained contraction of smooth muscle. Ca^{2+} channel blockers inhibit the voltage-dependent Ca^{2+} channels in vascular smooth muscle and decrease Ca^{2+} entry. All Ca^{2+} channel antagonists relax arterial smooth muscle and thereby decrease arterial resistance, blood pressure, and cardiac afterload. Although experimentally large conductance veins of pig appear similarly or even more sensitive to Ca^{2+} channel blockers than arteries (Magnon et al., 1995), Ca^{2+} channel blockers do not affect cardiac preload significantly when given at normal doses in patients. This suggests that capacitance veins that determine venous return to the heart are resistant to the relaxing effect of Ca^{2+} channel antagonists.

Cardiac Cells. The mechanisms of excitation-contraction coupling in cardiac myocytes of the working myocardium differ from those in vascular smooth muscle in that increases in intracellular Ca^{2+} are fast and transient (Chapter 28). They are initiated by a fast and short (<5 ms) Na^+ influx through voltage-gated Na^+ channels that causes depolarization of the membrane and opening of L-type Ca^{2+} channels. Repolarizing K^+ currents terminate the cardiac action potential and Ca^{2+} influx. Within the cardiac myocyte, Ca^{2+} binds to troponin C, relieving the inhibitory effect of the troponin complex on the contractile apparatus and permitting productive interaction of actin and myosin, leading to contraction. By inhibiting Ca^{2+} influx, Ca^{2+} channel blockers reduce the peak size of the systolic Ca^{2+} transient and thereby produce a negative inotropic effect. Although this is true of all classes of Ca^{2+} channel blockers, the greater degree of peripheral vasodilation seen with the dihydropyridines is accompanied by a baroreceptor reflex–mediated increase in sympathetic tone sufficient to overcome the negative inotropic effect.

In the SA and AV nodes, depolarization largely depends on the movement of Ca^{2+} through the slow channel. The effect of a Ca^{2+} channel blocker on AV conduction and on the rate of the sinus node pacemaker depends on whether the agent delays the recovery of the slow channel (Schwartz, 1992). Although nifedipine reduces the slow inward current in a dose-dependent manner, it does not affect the rate of recovery of the slow Ca^{2+} channel. Although nifedipine has clear negative chronotropic effects in isolated preparations (at ~ 5-fold higher concentrations than needed for negative inotropy), at doses used clinically, nifedipine does not directly affect pacemaking or conduction through the AV node. Rather, it stimulates the heart indirectly by eliciting reflex sympathetic activation in response to a lowering of blood pressure (Figure 27–2).

In contrast, verapamil not only reduces the magnitude of the Ca^{2+} current through the slow channel, but also decreases the rate of recovery of the channel. In addition, channel blockade caused by verapamil (and to a lesser extent by diltiazem) is enhanced as the frequency of stimulation increases, a phenomenon known as *frequency dependence* or *use dependence*. Verapamil and diltiazem depress the rate of the sinus node pacemaker and slow AV conduction at clinically used doses; the latter effect is the basis for their use in the treatment of supraventricular tachyarrhythmias (see Chapter 30). Verapamil also inhibits fast Na^+ and repolarizing K^+ currents (I_{Kr}). The contribution of these actions to the clinical profile is unclear, but note that verapamil, despite the effect on I_{Kr}, has not been associated with torsades des pointes arrhythmias as have other I_{Kr} blockers.

Integrated Cardiovascular Effects of Different Ca^{2+} Channel Antagonists. The hemodynamic profiles of the Ca^{2+} channel blockers approved for clinical use differ and depend mainly on the ratio of vasodilating and negative inotropic and chronotropic effects on the heart (Figure 27–2). The dihydropyridines dilate blood vessels at several-fold lower concentrations than those required for decreasing myocardial force; the ratio is close to one for diltiazem and verapamil. The published selectivity values differ widely, depending on the type of blood vessel and the mode of precontraction used for the comparison (Table 27–2 and Figure 27–3). The differences between the relatively vasoselective

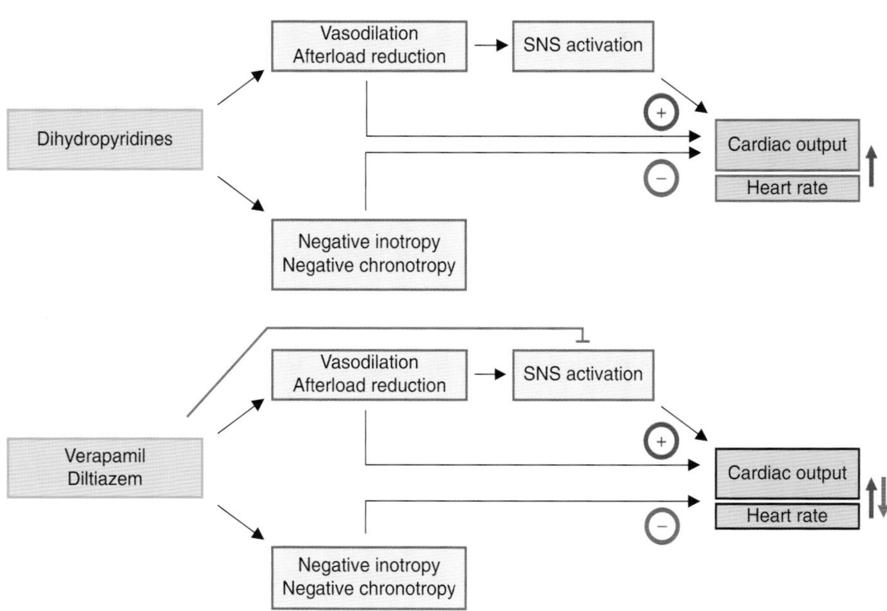

Figure 27–2 *Comparison of the integrated actions of Ca^{2+} channel blockers.* Due to different potencies and efficacies at various sites of action within the cardiovascular system, dihydropyridines produce integrated effects that are not identical to those of verapamil and diltiazem. Verapamil can have direct inhibitory effects on the SNS. The thickness of the arrow indicates the relative strength of the effect.

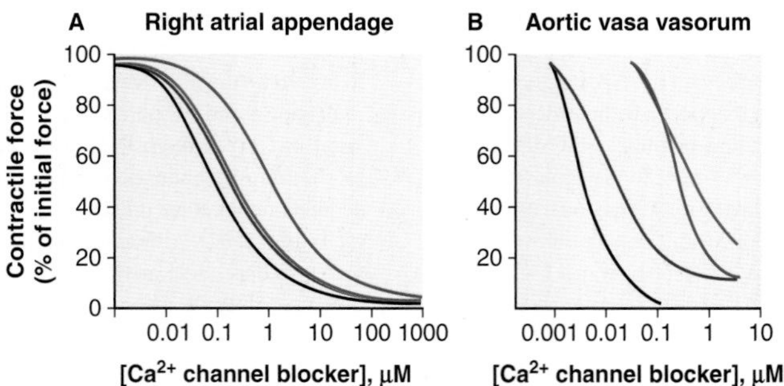

Figure 27–3 *Potency of Ca^{2+} channel blockers at different sites.* Effects were assessed on the contractile force of human right atrial appendages (**A**) and human arteries from aortic vasa vasorum precontracted with high-K^+ concentrations (**B**). Felodipine (black), nifedipine (blue), amlodipine (green) are more potent on vascular muscle, inhibiting contraction of atrial muscle at concentrations about 10 times higher than those needed to reduce contraction in vascular tissue. Verapamil (red) inhibits atrial muscle force development at 20% of the concentration required to reduce contraction in vascular tissue. The vascular selectivities of the various Ca^{2+} channel blockers (EC_{50} on atrial appendage/EC_{50} on vasa vasorum) are as follows: felodipine, 12; nifedipine, 7, amlodipine, 5; verapamil, 0.2. (Figure is based on data of Angus et al., 2000.)

dihydropyridines and the much less-selective diltiazem and verapamil have important consequences because the decrease in arterial blood pressure elicits reflex sympathetic activation, resulting in the stimulation of heart rate, AV conduction velocity, and myocardial force, just the opposite of the direct effect of Ca^{2+} channel blockers. While direct and indirect effects normally balance each other in case of verapamil and diltiazem, sympathetic stimulation often prevails in dihydropyridines, causing an increase in heart rate and contractility. Cardiac depressant effects of dihydropyridines may be unmasked, though, in the presence of β blockers and in patients with heart failure.

The dihydropyridines in clinical use—amlodipine, clevidipine, felodipine, isradipine, lercanidipine, nicardipine, nifedipine, nimodipine, and nisoldipine—share most pharmacodynamic properties. Differences with regard to vascular selectivity or subvascular selectivity have been intensely addressed in the past, but claims of large vasoselectivity factors were based on indirect comparisons (Godfraind et al., 1992). Overall, the clinical relevance of vasoselectivity ratios appears questionable; actual differences are probably not great (Figure 27–3). In any event, the drugs exert their antianginal effect mainly by peripheral arterial vasodilation and afterload reduction and not by coronary artery dilation (exception in variant angina).

Verapamil, like the dihydropyridines, causes little effect on venous return and preload, but has more direct negative inotropic and chronotropic effects than the dihydropyridines at doses that produce arteriolar dilation and afterload reduction (Figure 27–2). Thus, the consequences of a reflex increase in adrenergic tone are generally offset by the direct cardiodepressant effects of the drug. In patients without heart failure, oral administration of verapamil reduces peripheral vascular resistance and blood pressure with minimal changes in heart rate. Ventricular performance is not impaired and actually may improve, especially if ischemia limits performance. In contrast, in patients with heart failure, intravenous verapamil can cause a marked decrease in contractility and left ventricular function. The antianginal effect of verapamil, like that of all Ca^{2+} channel blockers, is due primarily to a reduction in myocardial O_2 demand. The negative dromotropic effect has no relevance for the improvement of exercise but can cause second-degree AV block, particularly when given in combination with β blockers (contraindicated). Diltiazem's effects lie in between those of dihydropyridines and verapamil.

The effects of Ca^{2+} channel blockers on diastolic ventricular relaxation (the lusitropic state of the ventricle) are complex. Nifedipine, diltiazem, and verapamil impaired parameters of ventricular relaxation in dogs, especially when given into the coronary arteries (Walsh and O'Rourke, 1985). However, reflex stimulation of sympathetic tone accelerates relaxation, which may outweigh a direct negative lusitropic effect. Likewise, a reduction in afterload will improve the lusitropic state. In addition, if ischemia is improved, the negative lusitropic effect will be reduced. The sum total of these effects in any given patient cannot be determined a priori.

ADME and Drug Interactions. Ca^{2+} channel blockers exhibit clinically relevant differences in pharmacokinetics (Figure 27–4). Immediate-release nifedipine is quickly absorbed after oral intake and produces only a briefly elevated blood level of the drug ($t_{1/2}$ ~ 1.8 h) that is associated with an abrupt decrease in blood pressure, reflex activation of the sympathetic nervous system, and tachycardia. This can cause a typical flush and can increase the risk of angina pectoris by abruptly decreasing coronary perfusion pressure concomitantly with tachycardia. Sustained-release preparations of nifedipine somewhat reduce fluctuations of plasma concentration. By contrast, amlodipine has slow absorption and a prolonged effect. With a plasma $t_{1/2}$ of 35–50 h, plasma levels and effect increase over 7–10 days of daily administration of a constant dose, resulting in a C_p with modest peaks and troughs. Such a profile allows the body to adapt and is associated with less reflex tachycardia. Felodipine, nitrendipine, lercanidipine, and isradipine have similar profiles for chronic treatment (Table 27–2). Clevidipine is available for intravenous administration and has a very rapid ($t_{1/2}$ ~ 2 min) onset and offset of action. It is metabolized

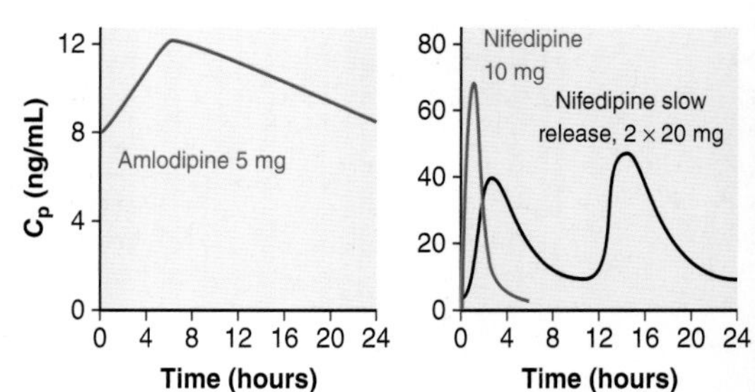

Figure 27–4 *Minimizing daily fluctuations in C_p values of Ca^{2+} channel blockers.* Graphs show plasma levels (C_p values) of amlodipine (left) and of nifedipine (right) in immediate-release (red) and slow-release (black) preparations; doses were administered at zero time. Plasma levels of amlodipine and nifedipine slow-release formulations were assessed after repeated application; thus, C_p values do not start at zero. Note the much smaller differences between trough and peak plasma concentrations in case of amlodipine compared to the rapid and brief pulse in plasma concentration of immediate-release nifedipine and the relatively large fluctuations even with the slow-release form of nifedipine. The plasma $t_{1/2}$ of amlodipine is about 39 h; that of nifedipine is about 1.8 h. A large fluctuation in C_p may result in adverse effects at the maximum and lack of efficacy at the minimum (see Figure 2–9A). (For original data, see Bainbridge et al., 1993; Debbas et al., 1986; and van Harten et al., 1987.)

by esterases in blood. It may be useful in controlling blood pressure in severe or perioperative hypertension as an alternative to GTN, sodium nitroprusside, or nicardipine.

The bioavailability of all Ca^{2+} channel blockers is reduced, in some cases markedly, by first-pass metabolism by CYP3A4 enzymes in the intestinal epithelium and the liver. This has two consequences:

- The bioavailability of these drugs may be increased by strong inhibitors of CYP3A4, such as macrolide and imidazole antibiotics, antiretroviral agents, and grapefruit juice (see Chapter 6). Bioavailability is reduced by inducers of CYP3A4, such as rifampin, carbamazepine, and hypericum (St. John's wort).
- Some Ca^{2+} channel blockers (particularly verapamil) are strong CYP3A4 inhibitors and cause clinically relevant drug interactions with other CYP3A4 substrates, such as simvastatin and atorvastatin.

Moreover, verapamil is a relatively efficient inhibitor of the intestinal and renal ABC transport protein Pgp (also called MDR1 and ABCB1; see Chapter 5) and can thereby increase plasma levels of digoxin, cyclosporine, and loperamide and other agents that are exported by Pgp. This high potential of verapamil for drug-drug interactions is a clear disadvantage and one of the reasons for its declining use. In patients with hepatic cirrhosis, the bioavailabilities and half-lives of the Ca^{2+} channel blockers may be increased, and dosage should be decreased accordingly. The half-lives of these agents also may be longer in older patients.

Toxicity and Untoward Responses. The profile of adverse reactions to the Ca^{2+} channel blockers varies among the drugs in this class. Immediate-release capsules of nifedipine often cause headache, flushing, and dizziness and can actually worsen myocardial ischemia. Dizziness and flushing are much less of a problem with the sustained-release formulations and with the dihydropyridines having a long $t_{1/2}$ and providing more constant plasma drug concentrations. Peripheral edema may occur in some patients with Ca^{2+} channel blockers but is not the result of generalized fluid retention; rather, it most likely results from increased hydrostatic pressure in the lower extremities owing to precapillary dilation and reflex postcapillary constriction (Epstein and Roberts, 2009). Other adverse effects of these drugs are due to actions in nonvascular smooth muscle. For example, Ca^{2+} channel blockers can cause or aggravate gastroesophageal reflux. Constipation is a common side effect of verapamil but occurs less frequently with other Ca^{2+} channel blockers. Urinary retention is a rare adverse effect. Uncommon adverse effects include rash and elevations of liver enzymes.

Although bradycardia, transient asystole, and exacerbation of heart failure have been reported with verapamil, these responses usually have occurred after intravenous administration of verapamil in patients with disease of the SA node, AV nodal conduction disturbances, or in the presence of β-blockade. The use of intravenous verapamil with an intravenous β blocker is contraindicated because of the increased propensity for AV block or severe depression of ventricular function. Patients with ventricular dysfunction, SA or AV nodal conduction disturbances, and systolic blood pressures below 90 mmHg should not be treated with verapamil or diltiazem, particularly intravenously. Verapamil may also exacerbate AV nodal conduction disturbances observed with digoxin, both for pharmacodynamic and pharmacokinetic reasons (Pgp inhibition; see previous discussion). When used with quinidine, verapamil may cause excessive hypotension, again due to pharmacodynamic and pharmacokinetic reasons (quinidine is CYP3A4 substrate and Pgp inhibitor).

Therapeutic Uses

Variant Angina. Variant angina results from reduced blood flow (a consequence of transient localized vasoconstriction) rather than increased O_2 demand. Drug-induced causes (e.g., cocaine, amphetamines, sumatriptan, and related antimigraine drugs) should be excluded. Ca^{2+} channel blockers are effective in about 90% of patients (Montalescot et al., 2013). These agents are considered first-line treatment and may be combined with nitrovasodilators (Amsterdam et al., 2014).

Exertional Angina. Ca^{2+} channel blockers also are effective in the treatment of exertional, or exercise-induced, angina. Numerous double-blind, placebo-controlled studies have shown that these drugs decrease the number of anginal attacks and attenuate exercise-induced ST-segment depression, but evidence for life-prolonging efficacy is lacking. They are therefore considered the drugs of choice if β blockers do not achieve sufficient symptomatic benefit or are not tolerated (Montalescot et al., 2013).

The Ca^{2+} channel blockers reduce the *double product*, Heart rate × Systolic blood pressure, an approximate index of myocardial O_2 demand. Because these agents reduce the level of the double product at a given external workload, and because the value of the double product at peak exercise is not altered, the beneficial effect of Ca^{2+} channel blockers likely derives from a decrease in O_2 demand rather than an increase in coronary flow.

Concurrent therapy of a dihydropyridine with a β blocker has proven more effective than either agent given alone in exertional angina, presumably because the β blocker suppresses reflex tachycardia. This concurrent drug therapy is particularly attractive because the dihydropyridines do not delay AV conduction and will not enhance the negative dromotropic effects associated with β receptor blockade. In contrast, the concurrent administration of verapamil or diltiazem with a β blocker is contraindicated for the potential for AV block, severe bradycardia, and decreased left ventricular function.

Unstable Angina (Acute Coronary Syndrome). In the past, Ca^{2+} channel blockers were routinely administered in patients presenting with unstable angina and ACS without persistent ST elevation. Reports about trends for harm with immediate-release nifedipine or nifedipine infusion in the absence of β blockers have led to the recommendation not to use dihydropyridines without concurrent therapy with β blockers. Verapamil and diltiazem are recommended only for patients who continue to show signs of ischemia, do not tolerate β blockers, have no clinically significant left ventricular dysfunction, and show no signs of disturbed AV conduction (Amsterdam et al., 2014).

Other Uses. The use of verapamil and diltiazem (but not dihydropyridines) as antiarrhythmic agents in supraventricular tachyarrhythmias is discussed in Chapter 30; their use for the treatment of hypertension is discussed in Chapter 28. Ca^{2+} channel blockers are contraindicated in patients with heart failure with reduced ejection fraction, but amlodipine and felodipine did not worsen the prognosis and can therefore be administered if indicated for other reasons (Chapter 29). Verapamil improves left ventricular outflow obstruction and symptoms in patients with HCM. Diltiazem has shown early promising results in a clinical study in asymptomatic HCM mutation carriers (Ho et al., 2015). Verapamil also has been used in the prophylaxis of migraine headaches but is considered a second-choice drug. Nimodipine has been approved for use in patients with neurological deficits secondary to cerebral vasospasm after the rupture of a congenital intracranial aneurysm, but clinical evidence for greater effectiveness than verapamil or magnesium is sparse. Nifedipine, diltiazem, amlodipine, and felodipine appear to provide symptomatic relief in Raynaud disease. The Ca^{2+} channel blockers cause relaxation of the myometrium in vitro and may be effective in reducing preterm uterine contractions in preterm labor (see Chapter 44).

β Blockers

β blockers are the only drug class that is effective in reducing the severity and frequency of attacks of exertional angina and in improving survival in patients who have had an MI. They are therefore recommended as first-line treatment of patients with stable CAD (Montalescot et al., 2013) and unstable angina/ACS (Hamm et al., 2011). Recent meta-analyses raised doubts about the mortality-reducing effects of β blockers in the MI reperfusion era (Bangalore et al., 2014); however, some of the results, such as the slightly increased heart failure frequency in patients receiving β blockers, contradicted numerous well-controlled prospective trials (see Chapter 29) and raised doubts about the validity of the analysis. Thus, the issue has not been definitively resolved. β Blockers are not useful for vasospastic angina and, if used in isolation, may worsen that condition. β Blockers appear equally effective in the treatment of exertional angina (Fihn et al., 2012;

Montalescot et al., 2013), but very short-acting agents or drug formulations giving rise to large fluctuations of plasma concentrations (e.g., unformulated metoprolol) should be avoided for treatment of chronic CAD.

The effectiveness of β blockers in the treatment of exertional angina is attributable primarily to a fall in myocardial O_2 consumption at rest and during exertion. The decrease in myocardial O_2 consumption is due to a negative chronotropic effect (particularly during exercise), a negative inotropic effect, and a reduction in arterial blood pressure (particularly systolic pressure) during exercise. A decrease in heart rate prolongs the time of myocardial perfusion during diastole. Moreover, there is evidence that β blockers can increase blood flow toward ischemic regions by increasing coronary collateral resistance and preventing blood from being shunted away from the ischemic myocardium during maximal coronary vasodilation (Billinger et al., 2001), a "reverse steal or Robin Hood phenomenon" (see previous discussion).

Not all actions of β blockers are beneficial in all patients. The decreases in heart rate and contractility cause increases in the systolic ejection period and left ventricular end-diastolic volume; these alterations tend to increase O_2 consumption. However, the net effect of β blockade usually is to decrease myocardial O_2 consumption, particularly during exercise. Nevertheless, in patients with limited cardiac reserve who are critically dependent on adrenergic stimulation, β blockade can result in profound decreases in left ventricular function. Despite this, several β blockers demonstrably reduce mortality in patients with congestive heart failure, and β blockers have become standard therapy for many such patients (see Chapters 12 and 29).

Numerous β blockers are approved for clinical use. Standard compounds for the treatment of angina are β_1-selective and without intrinsic sympathomimetic activity (e.g., atenolol, bisoprolol, or metoprolol). Chapter 12 presents their pharmacology in detail.

Antiplatelet, Anti-integrin, and Antithrombotic Agents

Antiplatelet agents represent the cornerstone of therapy for ACS (Amsterdam et al., 2014; Roffi et al., 2015) and are systematically discussed in Chapter 32. They interfere either with two signaling pathways (TxA_2 and ADP) that cooperatively promote platelet aggregation in an auto- and paracrine manner or with a major common pathway of platelet aggregation, the GpIIb/IIIa fibrinogen receptor. Aspirin inhibits platelet aggregation by irreversibly inactivating the thromboxane-synthesizing COX-1 in platelets, thereby reducing production of TxA_2. Aspirin, given at doses of 160–325 mg at the onset of treatment of ACS, improves survival (Yeghiazarians et al., 2000). The thienopyridines are ADP receptor ($P2Y_{12}$ receptor) antagonists that block the proaggregatory effect of ADP, which is stored in vesicles within platelets and released when platelets adhere to prothrombotic structures. The proaggregatory synergism of TxA_2 and ADP on platelet aggregation and thrombus formation accounts for the potentiating effect of adding a thienopyridine to aspirin.

The addition of the thienopyridine clopidogrel to aspirin therapy reduces mortality in patients with ACS. Newer thienopyridines (prasugrel, ticagrelor, cangrelor) with favorable pharmacokinetic properties have been approved for the treatment of ACS. All three appear superior to clopidogrel in treating patients with ACS; contributing factors likely include faster onset of action and less-variable pharmacokinetics. Ticagrelor is a direct, reversible $P2Y_{12}$ receptor antagonist, while clopidogrel and prasugrel are both prodrugs. The hepatic activation of prasugrel is more stable and faster than that of clopidogrel. Cangrelor is the first $P2Y_{12}$ receptor antagonist for intravenous application, producing very rapid inhibition of platelet aggregation. Recent guidelines recommend ticagrelor and prasugrel as the primary choice in patients with ACS and clopidogrel as an alternative in patients who cannot receive the former or are on oral anticoagulation therapy (e.g., for stroke prevention in atrial fibrillation). The place of cangrelor is not yet fully defined (Roffi et al., 2015).

The optimal timing of the initiation of dual platelet treatment is controversial and depends on the likely clinical course. If conservative treatment is likely and the patient is not at an increased risk of bleeding, aspirin and a parenteral anticoagulant (see discussion that follows) should be given as soon as possible, with the addition of a $P2Y_{12}$ receptor antagonist as soon as the diagnosis of NSTEMI has been made. Dual platelet inhibition for 1 year is currently recommended for all patients after NSTEMI or STEMI and revascularization, independently of the type of revascularization and type of stent used (Roffi et al., 2015). Due to the irreversible (aspirin, clopidogrel, and prasugrel) or prolonged (ticagrelor) modes of action, the risk of bleeding remains increased for extended periods after withdrawal of these drugs. Nonemergency major noncardiac surgeries should therefore be postponed for 5 (ticagrelor, clopidogrel) or 7 days (prasugrel, aspirin) after intake of the last dose.

Anti-integrin agents directed against the platelet integrin GPIIb/IIIa (including abciximab, tirofiban, and eptifibatide) are highly effective by blocking the final effector pathway of platelet aggregation; however, these agents have a small therapeutic index and must be administered parenterally. Meta-analyses of studies in patients with ACS showed that the use of GpIIb/IIIa inhibitors in addition to heparin was associated with about a 10% reduction in mortality, but with an increase in bleeding. Because most of these trials were conducted before the widespread use of the newer and more effective thienopyridines prasugrel and ticagrelor, the current value of the GpIIb/IIIa antagonists is not clear. Guidelines recommend them in patients on prasugrel or ticagrelor only in bailout situations (Roffi et al., 2015).

Heparin, in its unfractionated form and as low-molecular-weight heparin (e.g., enoxaparin), also reduces symptoms and prevents infarction in unstable angina (Yeghiazarians et al., 2000). Fondaparinux, a heparinoid pentasaccharide, antithrombin III-dependent Factor Xa inhibitor has the best efficacy-safety profile of all anticoagulants and is therefore currently first choice. Thrombin inhibitors, such as hirudin or bivalirudin, directly inhibit even clot-bound thrombin, are not affected by circulating inhibitors, and function independently of antithrombin III. Bivalirudin provides no benefit over heparin in ACS (Valgimigli et al., 2015). Thrombolytic agents such as rTPA are of no benefit in unstable angina. The new oral anticoagulants (factor IIa inhibitor dabigatran and factor Xa inhibitors rivaroxaban, apixaban, and edoxaban) have no established place in the treatment of CAD.

Other Antianginal Agents

Ranolazine

Ranolazine is FDA and EMA approved as a second-line agent for the treatment of chronic angina. The drug may be used with a variety of other agents, including β blockers, Ca^{2+} channel blockers, ACEIs, ARBs, and therapeutic agents for lowering lipids and reducing platelet aggregation.

Mechanism of Action. The mechanism of ranolazine's therapeutic efficacy in angina is uncertain. Its anti-ischemic and antianginal effects occur independently of reductions in heart rate and arterial blood pressure or changes in coronary blood flow. Ranolazine inhibits several cardiac ion fluxes, including I_{Kr} and I_{Na}. Preferential inhibition of late I_{Na} may explain its cardiac effects (Hasenfuss and Maier, 2008). The late I_{Na} contributes to arrhythmias in patients with the rare long QT 3 syndrome (Chapter 30), and is increased in heart failure and ischemia. Reduction of the late I_{Na} could explain in part the elevated cytosolic Na^+ concentrations in cardiac myocytes in these conditions, leading to higher diastolic Ca^{2+} concentrations, Ca^{2+} overload, arrhythmias, and problems with diastolic relaxation. Inhibition of late I_{Na} by ranolazine could reduce $[Na^+]_i$-dependent Ca^{2+} overload and its detrimental effects on myocardial ATP hydrolysis and cardiac function.

Other mechanisms of action have been proposed. Ranolazine reduces cardiac fatty acid oxidation and stimulates glucose metabolism without inhibiting carnitine palmityl transferase 1, and on this basis ranolazine was initially categorized as a metabolic modulator (McCormack et al., 1998). However, the effect is small, occurs at ranolazine concentrations more than 5-fold higher than do therapeutic effects, and can be assessed in the absence of fatty acid oxidation (Belardinelli et al., 2006). Ranolazine has weak β receptor blocking activity (Letienne et al., 2001) that may contribute to its anti-anginal activity.

In a large prospective trial of patients with incomplete revascularization after percutaneous coronary intervention, anti-ischemic therapy with ranolazine did not improve the prognosis of these high-risk patients (Weisz et al., 2016). Clinical trials are currently testing ranolazine in HCM and heart failure with preserved ejection fraction.

ADME and Adverse Effects. Ranolazine, supplied as extended-release tablets, is administered without regard to meals at 500 to 1000 mg twice daily; higher doses are poorly tolerated. The drug's oral bioavailability is about 75%; inhibitors of Pgp (e.g., digoxin, cyclosporine; see Chapter 5) can increase absorption of ranolazine and increase exposure to both ranolazine and the competing drug. Ranolazine's terminal $t_{1/2}$ is about 7 h; with repeated dosing, a steady-state C_p is reached in 3 days. Ranolazine is metabolized mainly by CYP3A4 and to a lesser extent by CYP2D6; unchanged drug (5%) and metabolites are excreted in the urine. Ranolazine should not be used together with strong CYP3A4 inhibitors (e.g., macrolide and imidazole antibiotics, HIV protease inhibitors), and doses need to be limited when moderate CYP3A4 inhibitors such as verapamil, diltiazem, and erythromycin are used in combination. Inducers of CYP3A4 (e.g., rifampin, carbamazepine, and hypericum) can decrease ranolazine plasma levels, requiring dose adjustment. Ranolazine can affect plasma levels of other CYP3A4 substrates, including doubling levels of simvastatin and its active metabolite and requiring dose adjustment; dose reduction may be needed for other CYP3A4 substrates (e.g., lovastatin), especially for those with a narrow therapeutic range (e.g., cyclosporine, tacrolimus, sirolimus). Coadministration of ranolazine may increase exposure to other substrates of CYP2D6, such as tricyclic antidepressant drugs and antipsychotic agents.

The most frequent adverse effects are dizziness, headache, nausea, and constipation. Some CNS effects (e.g., dizziness, blurry vision, and confusional state) are reminiscent of class I antiarrhythmics. QT prolongations have to be considered, but no torsades des pointes arrhythmias or related events have been reported.

Ivabradine

Ivabradine is EMA approved for treating stable angina and heart failure in patients in whom β blockers are not tolerated or are insufficiently effective in reducing heart rate and FDA-approved only for the treatment of heart failure (Chapter 29). Ivabradine is a selective blocker of hyperpolarization-activated HCN ion channels involved in the generation of automaticity in the SA node. By reducing the pacemaker current I_f through HCN channels, the compound dose dependently reduces heart rate and, differently from β blockers, does not affect cardiac contractile force. The antianginal effect is explained solely by reduction of heart rate and thereby O_2 demand (Figure 27–1).

A typical, often transient, side effect are phosphenes, transient enhanced lightness in restricted areas of the visual field, that are explained by effects on retinal HCN channels (3%–5% of cases). In a recent study in patients with chronic angina and normal left ventricular function, the addition of ivabradine to β blockers did not confer benefit but was associated with a trend for more cardiovascular end points and an increase in symptomatic bradycardia, atrial fibrillation, and QT prolongation (Fox et al., 2014). The data raise doubts about the hypothesis that heart rate reduction per se is associated with better cardiovascular outcome and has led to restrictions on use of ivabradine (e.g., contraindication for concurrent therapy with verapamil or diltiazem).

Nicorandil

Nicorandil is a nitrate ester of nicotinamide developed as an antianginal agent and currently is approved in many Asian and European countries (but not in the U.S. and Germany) for the treatment of stable angina pectoris. Nicorandil is not available in the U.S.

Mechanism of Action and Pharmacological Effects. Nicorandil has nitrate-like (cGMP-dependent) properties and acts as an agonist at ATP-sensitive potassium (K_{ATP}) channels. Its vasodilating action is potentiated by PDE5 inhibitors and only partially blocked by inhibitors of K_{ATP} channels, such as glibenclamide, suggesting that both properties participate in nicorandil's effect. Nicorandil dilates both arterial and venous vascular beds, leading to decreases in afterload and preload of the heart. In the absence of direct effects on contractile force of the ventricles, the decrease in afterload causes cardiac output to increase. The last effect is stronger than that seen after administration of nitrovasodilators and partially explained by (reflex) tachycardia. Thus, the hemodynamic profile of nicorandil lies in between that of nitrovasodilators and dihydropyridine Ca^{2+} channel blockers. Its antianginal effect is described to be stable, but early studies reported a clear decrease or loss of antianginal effect after 2 weeks of oral treatment (Meany et al., 1989; Rajaratnam et al., 1999).

Experimental and clinical studies indicated that nicorandil has cardioprotective effects (Matsubara et al., 2000), mimicking that of ischemic preconditioning, a phenomenon that short periods of ischemia preceding prolonged stopping of perfusion (as in MI) reduce myocardial injury. While the exact mechanisms are not fully understood, a central role of mitochondrial K_{ATP} channels is assumed (Ardehali and O'Rourke, 2005; Sato et al., 2000). Retrospective studies indicated a survival-prolonging effect of chronic treatment with nicorandil in patients with stable CAD, but sufficiently powered prospective studies are lacking.

ADME and Adverse Effects. Nicorandil is rapidly absorbed after sublingual or oral administration and has a short $t_{1/2}$ (1 h), which does not provide relevant trough levels at the usual regimen of twice-daily dosing at 20 mg/dose. Besides nitrate-like headache and hypotension (note contraindication of concurrent PDE5 inhibitors), nicorandil has been associated with the appearance of ulcerations. They were first described in 1997 (Boulinguez et al., 1997) as large, painful buccal apthosis and seem to extend to a 40%–60% increased risk of GI ulcerations and perforations (Lee et al., 2015).

Trimetazidine

Trimetazidine was developed as an antianginal agent. Its effect is thought to be due to inhibition of long-chain 3-ketoacyl coenzyme A thiolase, the final enzyme in the FFA β-oxidation pathway. This leads to a partial shift from FFA to glucose oxidation in the heart, which provides less ATP but requires less O_2 and may therefore be beneficial in ischemia (Ussher et al., 2014). Numerous small studies provided evidence for the efficacy of the compound to reduce angina and increase exercise tolerance, particularly in patients with diabetes and heart failure (e.g., Tuunanen et al., 2008); as with nicorandil, large randomized studies to define the true therapeutic value of this compound are lacking.

Trimetazidine can cause GI upset, nausea, and vomiting, and, rarely, it has been associated with thrombocytopenia, agranulocytosis, and liver dysfunction. More important, trimetazidine may increase the risk of movement disorders such as Parkinson disease, particularly in older patients with decreased kidney function. This serious effect has led to use restrictions by the EMA and the recommendation to use trimetazidine only as second-line treatment of stable angina in patients inadequately controlled by or intolerant to first-line antianginal therapies. Trimetazidine is not available in the U.S.

Therapeutic Strategies

Stable Coronary Artery Disease

Guidelines

Task forces from the American College of Cardiology and the American Heart Association (Fihn et al., 2012) and the European Society of Cardiology (Montalescot et al., 2013) have published guidelines that are useful in the selection of appropriate initial therapy for patients with chronic stable angina pectoris. All patients with CAD should receive at least one drug for angina relief in addition to fast- and short-acting nitrovasodilators (GTN, ISDN) and, for event prevention, aspirin and a statin. ACEIs should be considered in patients with CAD who have left ventricular dysfunction or diabetes (Table 27–3).

TABLE 27-3 ■ MANAGEMENT OF PATIENTS WITH STABLE CORONARY ARTERY DISEASE

TREATMENT LEVEL	ANGINA RELIEF	EVENT PREVENTION
All patients	Short-acting nitrates as standby medication	Education: Lifestyle management, control of risk factors
First-line treatment	β Blockers or diltiazem/verapamil	Aspirin + statins; consider ACEIs or ARBs
	Long-acting dihydropyridine if heart rate low or there are issues of intolerance/contraindications	
	β Blockers + dihydropyridines if angina persists	
	For vasospastic angina, consider dihydropyridines or long-acting nitrates; avoid β blockers	
Second-line treatment (first line in some cases, according to comorbidities and tolerance)	Add or switch to ivabradine, long-acting nitrates, nicorandil, ranolazine[a], or trimetazidine[a]	Consider clopidogrel in cases of aspirin intolerance
Invasive therapy	Consider angiography and stenting or CABG	

[a]In patients with diabetes mellitus.
Source: Adapted from the European Society for Cardiology Guidelines; for details, see Montalescot et al., **2013**.

The evidence for clinically relevant differences between the three main classes of antianginal drugs is not compelling. A meta-analysis of publications that compared two or more antianginal therapies concluded that β blockers are associated with fewer episodes of angina per week and a lower rate of withdrawal due to adverse events than is nifedipine. However, differences did not extend to Ca^{2+} channel blockers other than nifedipine. Of note, no significant differences were observed in outcome between *long-acting* nitrates, Ca^{2+} channel blockers, and β blockers. Nevertheless, guidelines recommend that β blockers be considered first-line treatment of chronic angina relief; Ca^{2+} channel blockers with heart rate–lowering effects (diltiazem, verapamil) are alternatives. Dihydropyridines should be considered in patients who do not tolerate β blockers. In case of persistent angina, a combination of a dihydropyridine and a β blocker should be considered.

Second-Line Treatment

Longer-acting organic nitrates/nitrate formulation (e.g., cutaneous GTN) or ranolazine, and, in non-U.S. countries, ivabradine, trimetazidine, and nicorandil may be considered as adjunct therapy in patients whose angina is not adequately controlled by first-line drugs. β Blockers can block the baroreceptor-mediated reflex tachycardia and positive inotropic effects that may occur with nitrates, whereas nitrates, by increasing venous capacitance, can attenuate the increase in left ventricular end-diastolic volume associated with β-blockade. Concurrent administration of nitrates also can alleviate the increase in coronary vascular resistance associated with blockade of β adrenergic receptors. Ranolazine and trimetazidine have a direct effect on the myocardium and likely act independently of hemodynamic effects. They can therefore be well combined with all other antianginal drugs where permitted. Ivabradine is a possible alternative to β blockers but is associated with toxicity when added to β blockers, verapamil, or diltiazem (Fox et al., 2014).

Ca^{2+} Channel Blockers and Nitrates. In severe exertional or vasospastic angina, the combination of a nitrate and a Ca^{2+} channel blocker may provide additional relief over that obtained with either type of agent alone. Because nitrates primarily reduce preload, whereas Ca^{2+} channel blockers reduce afterload, the net effect on reduction of O_2 demand should be additive; however, excessive vasodilation and hypotension can occur.

Acute Coronary Syndromes

The term *ACS* refers to chest pain with or without MI (i.e., myocardial necrosis). The latter diagnosis is essentially based on the presence or absence of increases in plasma levels of cardiac troponin (I or T). With tests becoming more and more sensitive, the number of MI diagnoses has increased, while that of unstable angina (i.e., chest pain without necrosis) has decreased. The term *unstable angina pectoris* is used for angina symptoms that present for the first time, change their usual pattern, occur at rest, or are resistant to nitrates.

Common to most clinical presentations of ACS is a disruption of a coronary plaque, leading to local platelet aggregation and thrombosis at the arterial wall, with subsequent partial or total occlusion of the vessel. Less commonly, vasospasm in minimally atherosclerotic coronary vessels may account for unstable angina. The pathophysiological principles that underlie therapy for exertional angina—which are directed at decreasing myocardial O_2 *demand*—have limited efficacy in the treatment of ACSs characterized by an insufficiency of myocardial O_2 (blood) *supply*. The most important interventions are as follows:

- Antiplatelet agents, including aspirin and thienopyridines (e.g., clopidogrel, prasugrel, or ticagrelor)
- Antithrombin agents such as heparin or fondaparinux
- Anti-integrin therapies that directly inhibit platelet aggregation mediated by glycoprotein GPIIb/IIIa
- Primary angioplasty with percutaneously deployed intracoronary stents or, if not possible for logistical reasons, fibrinolysis with rTPA
- Coronary bypass surgery for selected patients

The β blockers reduce O_2 consumption and arrhythmias and have been associated with a moderate reduction in mortality in ACS but should be avoided in patients with compromised ventricular function or decreased blood pressure (Roffi et al., 2015). Nitrates are useful in reducing vasospasm and in reducing myocardial O_2 consumption by decreasing ventricular wall stress. Intravenous administration of nitroglycerin allows high concentrations of drug to be attained rapidly. Because nitroglycerin is degraded rapidly, the dose can be titrated quickly and safely using intravenous administration. If coronary vasospasm is present, intravenous nitroglycerin is likely to be effective, although the addition of a Ca^{2+} channel blocker may be required to achieve complete control in some patients. If a patient has consumed a PDE5 inhibitor within the preceding 24 h, there is a risk of profound hypotension, and nitrates should be withheld in favor of an alternate antianginal therapy.

While these principles apply to the entire group of patients with ACS, specific treatment algorithms and the value of different drug classes in ACS depend on the exact diagnosis and should be chosen according to recent guidelines (Amsterdam et al., 2014; Roffi et al., 2015).

ST-elevation myocardial infarction is generally due to a complete obstruction of a large coronary artery. The mainstay in these patients is immediate reperfusion by primary angioplasty and stenting or, in the absence of invasive options, fibrinolytic therapy.

Non-ST-elevation myocardial infarction can present with variable symptoms and electrocardiographic signs and is likely due to transient obstruction of larger coronary arteries or occlusion of small branches, leading to disseminated myocardial necrosis. Primary angioplasty is also indicated in these patients.

Unstable angina is differentiated from NSTEMI by the absence of increased plasma troponin concentrations. These patients have a better long-term prognosis and benefit less from early invasive procedures and intensified antiplatelet therapy. Mainstays are β blockers and nitrovasodilators (in the absence of contraindications such as hypotension). Short-acting Ca^{2+} channel blockers (e.g., nifedipine; see Figure 27–4) should normally be avoided in ACS because of a strong reflex activation of the sympathetic nervous system, but they are the first choice if vasospasm is the underlying cause.

Claudication and Peripheral Vascular Disease

Most patients with peripheral vascular disease also have CAD, and the therapeutic approaches for peripheral and coronary arterial diseases overlap (Rooke et al., 2011). Mortality in patients with peripheral vascular disease is most commonly due to cardiovascular disease (Regensteiner and Hiatt, 2002), and treatment of CAD remains the central focus of therapy. Many patients with advanced peripheral arterial disease are more limited by the consequences of peripheral ischemia than by myocardial ischemia. In the cerebral circulation, arterial disease may be manifest as stroke or transient ischemic attacks. The painful symptoms of peripheral arterial disease in the lower extremities (claudication) typically are provoked by exertion, with increases in skeletal muscle O_2 demand exceeding blood flow that is impaired by proximal stenoses. When flow to the extremities becomes critically limiting, peripheral ulcers and rest pain from tissue ischemia can become debilitating.

Most of the therapies shown to be efficacious for treatment of CAD also have a salutary effect on progression of peripheral artery disease (Hirsch et al., 2006). Antiplatelet therapy using aspirin (75–325 mg) and clopidogrel (75 mg) are recommended, although the evidence for beneficial effects on cardiovascular or total mortality are mixed (Rooke et al., 2011). Oral anticoagulation is ineffective and increases bleeding risks. ACEIs and statins have been recommended for patients with peripheral artery disease (Hirsch et al., 2006), but the evidence for prognostic benefits is much weaker than in CAD. Interestingly, neither intensive treatment of diabetes mellitus nor antihypertensive therapy appears to alter the progression of symptoms of claudication. Other risk factor and lifestyle modifications remain cornerstones of therapy for patients with claudication; physical exercise, rehabilitation, and smoking cessation (possibly supported by drug treatment with varenicline or bupropion) have proven efficacy.

Drugs used specifically in the treatment of lower extremity claudication include pentoxifylline and cilostazol. Pentoxifylline is a methylxanthine derivative that is called a *rheologic modifier* for its effects on increasing the deformability of red blood cells. However, the effects of pentoxifylline on lower extremity claudication appear to be modest and not sufficiently supported by prospective evidence (Salhiyyah et al., 2015).

Cilostazol is an inhibitor of PDE3 and promotes accumulation of intracellular cAMP in many cells, including blood platelets. Cilostazol-mediated increases in cAMP inhibit platelet aggregation and promote vasodilation. The drug is metabolized by CYP3A4 and has important drug interactions with other drugs metabolized via this pathway (see Chapter 6). Cilostazol has been mainly studied in Asian populations and seems to improve symptoms of claudication, but the effect on cardiovascular mortality remains unclear (Bedenis et al., 2014). As a PDE3 inhibitor, cilostazol is in the same drug class as milrinone, which had been used orally as an inotropic agent for patients with heart failure. Milrinone therapy was associated with an increase in sudden cardiac death, and the oral form of the drug was withdrawn from the market. Concerns about several other inhibitors of PDE3 (inamrinone, flosequinan) followed. Cilostazol therefore is labeled as being contraindicated in patients with heart failure, although it is not clear that cilostazol itself leads to increased mortality in such patients. Cilostazol has been reported to increase nonsustained ventricular tachycardia; headache is the most common side effect.

Other treatments for claudication, including naftidrofuryl, propionyl levocarnitine, and prostaglandins, have been explored in clinical trials, and there is some evidence that some of these therapies may be efficacious.

Mechanopharmacological Therapy: Drug-Eluting Endovascular Stents

Intracoronary stents can ameliorate angina and reduce adverse events in patients with ACSs. However, the long-term efficacy of intracoronary stents is limited by subacute luminal restenosis within the stent, which, in bare metal stents, occurs in 20%–30% of patients during the first 6–9 months of follow-up (Montalescot et al., 2013). The pathways that lead to "in-stent restenosis" are complex, but smooth muscle proliferation within the lumen of the stented artery is a common pathological finding. Local antiproliferative therapies at the time of stenting have been explored over many years; several drug-eluting stents and, more recently, biodegradable stents have been introduced in the market. The drugs currently used in intravascular stents are paclitaxel, sirolimus (rapamycin), and the two sirolimus derivatives everolimus and zatarolimus. Paclitaxel is a tricyclic diterpene that inhibits cellular proliferation by binding to and stabilizing polymerized microtubules. Sirolimus is a hydrophobic macrolide that binds to the cytosolic immunophilin FKBP12; the FKBP12-sirolimus complex inhibits the protein kinase mTOR, the mammalian target of rapamycin (see Figure 35–2), thereby inhibiting cell cycle progression (Figure 65–2). Paclitaxel and sirolimus differ markedly in their mechanisms of action but share common chemical properties as hydrophobic small molecules. Stent-induced damage to the vascular endothelial cell layer can lead to thrombosis. The inhibition of cellular proliferation by paclitaxel and sirolimus or derivatives not only affects vascular smooth muscle cell proliferation but also attenuates the formation of an intact endothelial layer within the stented artery and thereby markedly reduces the rate of restenosis compared with bare metal stents. Dual antiplatelet therapy (aspirin, typically with clopidogrel) is recommended for one year after intracoronary stenting with drug-eluting stents, similar to bare metal stents. Evidence for the benefit of even longer periods is limited.

Acknowledgment: *Thomas Michel and Brian B. Hoffman contributed to this chapter in recent editions of this book. We have retained some of their text in the current edition.*

Bibliography

Amsterdam EA, et al. 2014 AHA/ACC guideline for the management of patients with non-ST-elevation acute coronary syndromes: a report of the American College of Cardiology/American Heart Association Task Force on Practice Guidelines. *J Am Coll Cardiol*, **2014**, *64*:e139–e228.

Angus JA, et al. Quantitative analysis of vascular to cardiac selectivity of L- and T-type voltage-operated calcium channel antagonists in human tissues. *Clin Exp Pharmacol Physiol*, **2000**, *27*:1019–1021.

Ardehali H, O'Rourke B. Mitochondrial K(ATP) channels in cell survival and death. *J Mol Cell Cardiol*, **2005**, *39*:7–16.

Bainbridge AD, et al. A comparative assessment of amlodipine and felodipine ER: pharmacokinetic and pharmacodynamic indices. *Eur J Clin Pharmacol*, **1993**, *45*:425–430.

Bangalore S, et al. Clinical outcomes with beta-blockers for myocardial infarction: a meta-analysis of randomized trials. *Am J Med*, **2014**, *127*:939–953.

Barbato E, et al. Long-term effect of molsidomine, a direct nitric oxide donor, as an add-on treatment, on endothelial dysfunction in patients with stable angina pectoris undergoing percutaneous coronary intervention: results of the MEDCOR trial. *Atherosclerosis*, **2015**, *240*:351–354.

Drug Facts for Your Personal Formulary: *Coronary Artery Disease*

Drug	Therapeutic Uses	Major Toxicity and Clinical Pearls
Organic Nitrates		
Glyceryl trinitrate (GTN, nitroglycerin) Isosorbide dinitrate (ISDN) Isosorbide mononitrate (ISMN)	• Angina (sublingual) • Acute pulmonary edema (IV) • Acute hypertension (IV)	• NO-mediated vasodilation of large (venous, arterial) > small (resistance) vessels ⇒ preferential preload reduction without steal effect • Short-acting formulations of GTN or ISDN are standby drugs for all patients with CAD • First choice for vasospastic angina, along with Ca^{2+} channel blockers • Second choice for the prevention of exertional angina (longer-acting formulations) • Adverse effects: headache, dizziness, postural hypotension, syncope • Tolerance after > 16 h (leave nitrate-free interval of > 8 h) • Do not use concurrently with PDE5 inhibitor
Molsidomine	• Angina	• Direct NO donor • Second choice for the prevention of angina • Adverse effects same as above • No documented advantage over GTN/ISDN/ISMN
Inhaled NO	• Pulmonary hypertension in neonates	• Relatively selective effect on pulmonary vascular bed
Ca^{2+} Channel Blockers		
Dihydropyridines Amlodipine Felodipine Lercanidipine Nifedipine Nitrendipine ***Others*** Diltiazem Verapamil	• Angina • Hypertension • Rate control in atrial fibrillation (verapamil, diltiazem)	• Preferential arterial vasodilation ⇒ afterload reduction • First choice for vasospastic angina (dihydropyridines) • Second choice for preventing exertional angina • Immediate-release nifedipine and short-acting dihydropyridines can cause tachycardia and hypotension and trigger angina • Diltiazem and verapamil can ↓ heart rate and AV conduction; should not be used with β blockers • CYP3A4-mediated drug interactions with verapamil and diltiazem • Other unwanted effects: peripheral edema (dihydropyridines), obstipation (verapamil)
β Blockers		
Atenolol Bisoprolol Carvedilol Metoprolol Nadolol Nebivolol Many others	• Angina • Heart failure • Hypertension • Widely used for other indications (prevention of arrhythmias, rate control in atrial fibrillation, migraine, etc.)	• First choice for prevention of exertional angina • Only antianginal drug class with proven prognostic benefits in CAD • Adverse effects: bradycardia, AV block, bronchospasm, peripheral vasoconstriction, worsening of acute heart failure, depression, worsening of psoriasis • Polymorphic CYP2D6 metabolism (metoprolol) • Additional vasodilation (carvedilol, nebivolol)
Ranolazine		
	• Angina	• Inhibits late Na^+ and other cardiac ion currents • Has weak β blocking and metabolic effects • Second choice in the prevention of exertional angina • CYP3A4-dependent metabolism
Ivabradine		
	• Angina • Heart failure	• Selectively ↓ heart rate by inhibiting HCN currents in SA node • Second choice in the prevention of exertional angina; approved in patients not tolerating β blockers or having heart rate > 75 under β blockers • Unwanted effects: bradycardia, QT prolongation, atrial fibrillation, phosphenes • Contraindication: combination with diltiazem or verapamil
Nicorandil		
	• Angina	• Dual nitrate-like and I_{KATP}-stimulatory action • Hemodynamic profile between nitrates and dihydropyridines; ↓ afterload more than nitrates • Second choice in the prevention of exertional angina • Adverse effects: hypotension, headache, buccal and GI ulcers • Do not combine with PDE5 inhibitor
Trimetazidine		
	• Angina	• Metabolic shift from fatty acid to glycolytic metabolism in the heart • Second choice in the prevention of exertional angina • May increase the incidence of Parkinson disease

Drug Facts for Your Personal Formulary: *Coronary Artery Disease (continued)*

Drug	Therapeutic Uses	Major Toxicity and Clinical Pearls
Antiplatelet, Anti-integrin, and Antithrombotic Drugs		
Aspirin $P2Y_{12}$ receptor antagonists (clopidogrel, prasugrel, ticagrelor cangrelor [IV])	• Prevention of thrombotic events (MI, stroke) • Acute coronary syndromes • Prevention of stent thrombosis	• ↓ Platelet aggregation by inhibiting COX-1–mediated TxA_2 production (aspirin) or ADP receptors ($P2Y_{12}$ receptor antagonists) • Oral use only: clopidogrel, prasugrel, ticagrelor • Irreversible action: aspirin, clopidogrel, prasugrel • Prodrugs: clopidogrel, prasugrel • Variable, CYP2C9-dependent metabolism (clopidogrel) • Withdraw 5–7 days before surgery • First choice in NSTEMI and STEMI • Dual platelet inhibition after stenting
Abciximab Eptifibatide Tirofiban	• Percutaneous coronary interventions	• Antibody (abciximab) or small molecule antagonists at platelet GpIIb/IIIa receptor • Parenteral use only • Highly efficient platelet inhibition • Therapeutic value in the era of highly effective dual platelet inhibition unclear
Heparin Low-molecular-weight heparins (e.g., enoxaparine)	• Acute coronary syndromes • Percutaneous coronary interventions	• Endogenous polysaccharide, inhibits thrombin (factor IIa) and factor Xa in an antithrombin III–dependent manner • Parenteral use only • Heparin: short $t_{1/2}$, complex pharmacokinetics, low bioavailability after subcutaneous. injection • Low-molecular-weight heparin: longer half-life, renal excretion; accumulation in renal insufficiency • Heparin-induced thrombocytopenia
Fondaparinux	• Acute coronary syndromes • Percutaneous coronary interventions	• Synthetic pentasaccharide, antithrombin III-dependent, factor Xa inhibitor • Most favorable efficacy-safety ratio
Bivalirudin Lepirudin	• Percutaneous coronary interventions (bivalirudin) • Heparin-induced thrombocytopenia (HIT II) recombinant lepirudin	• Direct thrombin (factor IIa) inhibitors • Parenteral use only • Advantage of bivalirudin over heparin unclear

Bedenis R, et al. Cilostazol for intermittent claudication. *Cochrane Database Syst Rev*, **2014**, (10):CD003748.

Belardinelli L, et al. Inhibition of the late sodium current as a potential cardioprotective principle: effects of the late sodium current inhibitor ranolazine. *Heart*, **2006**, *92*:iv6-iv14.

Bhatt DL, et al. Clopidogrel and aspirin versus aspirin alone for the prevention of atherothrombotic events. *N Engl J Med*, **2006**, *354*:1706–1717.

Billinger M, et al. Collateral and collateral-adjacent hyperemic vascular resistance changes and the ipsilateral coronary flow reserve. Documentation of a mechanism causing coronary steal in patients with coronary artery disease. *Cardiovasc Res*, **2001**, *49*:600–608.

Bloch KD, et al. Inhaled NO as a therapeutic agent. *Cardiovasc Res*, **2007**, *75*:339–348.

Bodi V, et al. Prognostic value of dipyridamole stress cardiovascular magnetic resonance imaging in patients with known or suspected coronary artery disease. *J Am Coll Cardiol*, **2007**, *50*:1174–1179.

Boulinguez S, et al. Giant buccal aphthosis caused by nicorandil [in French]. *Presse Med*, **1997**, *26*:558.

Brown BG, et al. The mechanisms of nitroglycerin action: stenosis vasodilatation as a major component of the drug response. *Circulation*, **1981**, *64*:1089–1097.

Burnett AL, et al. Nitric oxide: a physiologic mediator of penile erection. *Science*, **1992**, *257*:401–403.

Cannon CP, et al. Comparison of ticagrelor with clopidogrel in patients with a planned invasive strategy for acute coronary syndromes (PLATO): a randomised double-blind study. *Lancet*, **2010**, *375*:283–293.

CAPRIE Steering Committee. A randomised, blinded, trial of clopidogrel versus aspirin in patients at risk of ischaemic events (CAPRIE). CAPRIE Steering Committee. *Lancet*, **1996**, *348*:1329–1339.

Cheitlin MD, et al. ACC/AHA expert consensus document. Use of sildenafil (Viagra) in patients with cardiovascular disease. American College of Cardiology/American Heart Association. *J Am Coll Cardiol*, **1999**, *33*:273–282.

Chen Z, et al. Identification of the enzymatic mechanism of nitroglycerin bioactivation. *Proc Natl Acad Sci U S A*, **2002**, *99*:8306–8311.

Debbas NM, et al. The bioavailability and pharmacokinetics of slow release nifedipine during chronic dosing in volunteers. *Br J Clin Pharmacol*, **1986**, *21*:385–388.

Dudzinski DM, et al. The regulation and pharmacology of endothelial nitric oxide synthase. *Annu Rev Pharmacol Toxicol*, **2006**, *46*:235–276.

Epstein BJ, Roberts ME. Managing peripheral edema in patients with arterial hypertension. *Am J Ther*, **2009**, *16*:543–553.

Fihn SD, et al. 2012 ACCF/AHA/ACP/AATS/PCNA/SCAI/STS guideline for the diagnosis and management of patients with stable ischemic heart disease. *Circulation*, **2012**, *126*:e354–e471.

Fleckenstein A, et al. Selective inhibition of myocardial contractility by competitive divalent Ca^{++} antagonists (iproveratril, D 600, prenylamine) [in German]. *Naunyn Schmiedebergs Arch Pharmakol*, **1969**, *264*:227–228.

Fox K, et al. Ivabradine in stable coronary artery disease. *N Engl J Med*, **2014**, *371*:2435.

Godfraind T, et al. Calcium antagonism and calcium entry blockade. *Pharmacol Rev*, **1986**, *38*:321–416.

Godfraind T, et al. Selectivity scale of calcium antagonists in the human cardiovascular system based on in vitro studies. *J Cardiovasc Pharmacol*, **1992**, *20*(suppl 5):S34–S41.

Hamm CW, et al. ESC guidelines for the management of acute coronary syndromes in patients presenting without persistent ST-segment elevation: the Task Force for the Management of Acute Coronary Syndromes (ACS) in Patients Presenting Without Persistent ST-Segment Elevation of the European Society of Cardiology (ESC). *Eur Heart J*, **2011**, *32*:2999–3054.

Hasenfuss G, Maier LS. Mechanism of action of the new anti-ischemia drug ranolazine. *Clin Res Cardiol*, **2008**, *97*:222–226.

Herrmann HC, et al. Hemodynamic effects of sildenafil in men with severe coronary artery disease. *N Engl J Med*, **2000**, *342*:1622–1626.

Hirsch AT, et al. ACC/AHA 2005 Practice guidelines for the management of patients with peripheral arterial disease (lower extremity, renal, mesenteric, and abdominal aortic): a collaborative report. *Circulation*, **2006**, *113*:e463–e654.

Ho CY, et al. Diltiazem treatment for pre-clinical hypertrophic cardiomyopathy sarcomere mutation carriers: a pilot randomized trial to modify disease expression. *JACC Heart Fail*, **2015**, *3*:180–188.

Kappetein AP, et al. Comparison of coronary bypass surgery with drug-eluting stenting for the treatment of left main and/or three-vessel disease: 3-year follow-up of the SYNTAX trial. *Eur Heart J*, **2011**, *32*:2125–2134.

Kojda G, et al. Positive inotropic effect of exogenous and endogenous NO in hypertrophic rat hearts. *Br J Pharmacol*, **1997**, *122*: 813–820.

Lee CC, et al. Use of nicorandil is associated with increased risk for gastrointestinal ulceration and perforation—a nationally representative population-based study. *Sci Rep*, **2015**, *5*:11495.

Letienne R, et al. Evidence that ranolazine behaves as a weak beta1- and beta2-adrenoceptor antagonist in the rat [correction of cat] cardiovascular system. *Naunyn Schmiedeberg's Arch Pharmacol*, **2001**, *363*:464–471.

Libby P, Pasterkamp G. Requiem for the "vulnerable plaque." *Eur Heart J*, **2015**, *36*:2984–2987.

Libby P, et al. Inflammation and atherosclerosis. *Circulation*, **2002**, *105*:1135–1143.

Magnon M, et al. Intervessel (arteries and veins) and heart/vessel selectivities of therapeutically used calcium entry blockers: variable, vessel-dependent indexes. *J Pharmacol Exp Ther*, **1995**, *275*:1157–1166.

Matsubara T, et al. Three minute, but not one minute, ischemia and nicorandil have a preconditioning effect in patients with coronary artery disease. *J Am Coll Cardiol*, **2000**, *35*:345–351.

Mayer B, Beretta M. The enigma of nitroglycerin bioactivation and nitrate tolerance: news, views and troubles. *Br J Pharmacol*, **2008**, *155*:170–184.

McCormack JG, et al. Ranolazine: a novel metabolic modulator for the treatment of angina. *Gen Pharmacol*, **1998**, *30*:639–645.

Meany TB, et al. Exercise capacity after single and twice-daily doses of nicorandil in chronic stable angina pectoris. *Am J Cardiol*, **1989**, *63*:66J–70J.

Montalescot G, et al. 2013 ESC guidelines on the management of stable coronary artery disease: the Task Force on the Management of Stable Coronary Artery Disease of the European Society of Cardiology. *Eur Heart J*, **2013**, *34*:2949–3003.

Mozaffarian D, et al. Heart disease and stroke statistics—2015 update: a report from the American Heart Association. *Circulation*, **2015**, *131*:e29–e322.

Munzel T, et al. Evidence for enhanced vascular superoxide anion production in nitrate tolerance. A novel mechanism underlying tolerance and cross-tolerance. *J Clin Invest*, **1995**, *95*:187–194.

Munzel T, et al. Organic nitrates: update on mechanisms underlying vasodilation, tolerance and endothelial dysfunction. *Vascul Pharmacol*, **2014**, *63*:105–113.

Parker JD. Nitrate tolerance, oxidative stress, and mitochondrial function: another worrisome chapter on the effects of organic nitrates. *J Clin Invest*, **2004**, *113*:352–354.

Parker JD, et al. Intermittent transdermal nitroglycerin therapy. Decreased anginal threshold during the nitrate-free interval. *Circulation*, **1995**, *91*:973–978.

Parker JD, Parker JO. Nitrate therapy for stable angina pectoris. *N Engl J Med*, **1998**, *338*:520–531.

Rajaratnam R, et al. Attenuation of anti-ischemic efficacy during chronic therapy with nicorandil in patients with stable angina pectoris. *Am J Cardiol*, **1999**, *83*:1120–1124, A1129.

Redfield MM, et al. Effect of phosphodiesterase-5 inhibition on exercise capacity and clinical status in heart failure with preserved ejection fraction: a randomized clinical trial. *JAMA*, **2013**, *309*:1268–1277.

Regensteiner JG, Hiatt WR. Current medical therapies for patients with peripheral arterial disease: a critical review. *Am J Med*, **2002**, *112*:49–57.

Roffi M, et al. 2015 ESC Guidelines for the management of acute coronary syndromes in patients presenting without persistent ST-segment elevation: Task Force for the Management of Acute Coronary Syndromes in Patients Presenting Without Persistent ST-Segment Elevation of the European Society of Cardiology (ESC). *Eur Heart J*, **2016**, *37*:267–315.

Rooke TW, et al. 2011 ACCF/AHA focused update of the guideline for the management of patients with peripheral artery disease (updating the 2005 guideline): a report of the American College of Cardiology Foundation/American Heart Association Task Force on Practice Guidelines. *J Am Coll Cardiol*, **2011**, *58*:2020–2045.

Salhiyyah K, et al. Pentoxifylline for intermittent claudication. *Cochrane Database Syst Rev*, **2015**, (9):CD005262.

Sato T, et al. Nicorandil, a potent cardioprotective agent, acts by opening mitochondrial ATP-dependent potassium channels. *J Am Coll Cardiol*, **2000**, *35*:514–518.

Sayed N, et al. Nitroglycerin-induced S-nitrosylation and desensitization of soluble guanylyl cyclase contribute to nitrate tolerance. *Circ Res*, **2008**, *103*:606–614.

Schwartz A. Molecular and cellular aspects of calcium channel antagonism. *Am J Cardiol*, **1992**, *70*:6F–8F.

Soma J, et al. Sublingual nitroglycerin delays arterial wave reflections despite increased aortic "stiffness" in patients with hypertension: a Doppler echocardiography study. *J Am Soc Echocardiogr*, **2000**, *13*:1100–1108.

Stamler JS. Nitroglycerin-mediated S-nitrosylation of proteins: a field comes full cycle. *Circ Res*, **2008**, *103*:557–559.

Steinberg SF, Brunton LL. Compartmentation of G protein-coupled signaling pathways in cardiac myocytes. *Annu Rev Pharmacol Toxicol*, **2001**, *41*:751–773.

Sydow K, et al. Central role of mitochondrial aldehyde dehydrogenase and reactive oxygen species in nitroglycerin tolerance and cross-tolerance. *J Clin Invest*, **2004**, *113*:482–489.

Tsien RW, et al. Multiple types of neuronal calcium channels and their selective modulation. *Trends Neurosci*, **1988**, *11*:431–438.

Tuunanen H, et al. Trimetazidine, a metabolic modulator, has cardiac and extracardiac benefits in idiopathic dilated cardiomyopathy. *Circulation*, **2008**, *118*:1250–1258.

Ussher JR, et al. Treatment with the 3-ketoacyl-CoA thiolase inhibitor trimetazidine does not exacerbate whole-body insulin resistance in obese mice. *J Pharmacol Exp Ther*, **2014**, *349*:487–496.

Valgimigli M, et al. Bivalirudin or unfractionated heparin in acute coronary syndromes. *N Engl J Med*, **2015**, *373*:997–1009.

van Harten J, et al. Negligible sublingual absorption of nifedipine. *Lancet*, **1987**, *2*:1363–1365.

Walsh RA, O'Rourke RA. Direct and indirect effects of calcium entry blocking agents on isovolumic left ventricular relaxation in conscious dogs. *J Clin Invest*, **1985**, *75*:1426–1434.

Weisz G, et al. Ranolazine in Patients With Incomplete Revascularisation After Percutaneous Coronary Intervention (RIVER-PCI): a multicentre, randomised, double-blind, placebo-controlled trial. *Lancet*, **2016**, *387*:136–145.

Wiviott SD, et al. Prasugrel versus clopidogrel in patients with acute coronary syndromes. *N Engl J Med*, **2007**, *357*:2001–2015.

Yeghiazarians Y, et al. Unstable angina pectoris. *N Engl J Med*, **2000**, *342*:101–114.

Yusuf S, et al. Effects of clopidogrel in addition to aspirin in patients with acute coronary syndromes without ST-segment elevation. *N Engl J Med*, **2001**, *345*:494–502.

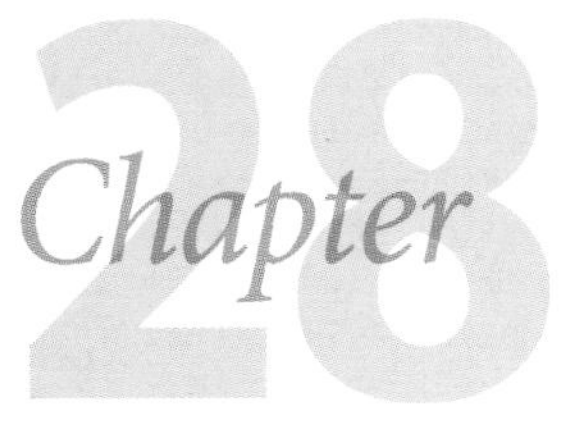

Treatment of Hypertension

Thomas Eschenhagen

第二十八章 高血压的治疗

中文导读

本章主要介绍：流行病学及治疗办法，包括降压治疗的原则；利尿药，包括苯并噻二嗪及相关化合物、其他利尿类降压药、保钾利尿药、利尿药相关药物相互作用；抗交感神经药，包括β肾上腺素受体拮抗药（β阻滞药）、α_1-肾上腺素受体拮抗药（α_1阻滞药）、α_1和β肾上腺受体拮抗药、中枢抗交感神经药；Ca^{2+}通道阻滞药；肾素-血管紧张素系统抑制药，包括血管紧张素转换酶抑制药、AT_1受体阻滞药、直接肾素抑制药；血管舒张药，包括肼屈嗪、ATP敏感型钾离子通道开启药（米诺地尔）、硝普钠和二氮嗪；高血压的非药物治疗；个体化治疗中抗高血压药的选择；急性降压治疗；难治性高血压。

Abbreviations

ACE: angiotensin-converting enzyme
ACEI: angiotensin-converting enzyme inhibitor
Aldo: aldosterone
AngII: angiotensin II
ANP: atrial natriuretic peptide
ARB: angiotensin receptor blocker
AT_1: type 1 receptor for angiotensin II
ATPase: adenosine triphosphatase
AV: atrioventricular
BB: β blocker
β blocker: β adrenergic receptor antagonist
BNP: brain natriuretic peptide
BP: blood pressure
CAD: coronary artery disease
CCB: Ca^{2+} channel blocker
CNS: central nervous system
COX-2: cyclooxygenase 2
DOPA: 3,4-dihydroxyphenylalanine
DRI: direct renin inhibitor
ENaC: epithelial Na^+ channel
ESC: European Society of Cardiology
GI: gastrointestinal
GFR: glomerular filtration rate
HDL: high-density lipoprotein
HF: heart failure
HTN: hypertension
ISA: intrinsic sympathomimetic activity
ISDN: isosorbide dinitrate
JNC8: Eighth Joint National Committee
MI: myocardial infarction
MRA: mineralocorticoid receptor antagonist
NCC: NaCl cotransporter
NE: norepinephrine
NO: nitric oxide
NSAID: nonsteroidal anti-inflammatory drug
RAAS: renin-angiotensin-aldosterone system
RAS: renin-angiotensin system
SA: sinoatrial
SNS: sympathetic nervous system
VMAT2: vesicular catecholamine transporter 2

Epidemiology and Treatment Algorithms

Hypertension is the most common cardiovascular disease. Elevated arterial pressure causes hypertrophy of the left ventricle and pathological changes in the vasculature. As a consequence, hypertension is the principal cause of stroke; a major risk factor for CAD and its attendant complications, MI and sudden cardiac death; and a major contributor to heart failure, renal insufficiency, and dissecting aneurysm of the aorta. The prevalence of hypertension increases with age; for example, about 50% of people between the ages of 60 and 69 years old have hypertension, and the prevalence further increases beyond age 70. According to a recent survey in the U.S., 81.5% of those with hypertension are aware they have it, 74.9% are being treated, yet only 52.5% are considered controlled (Go et al., 2014). The success of hypertension treatment programs, such as one organized in a large integrated healthcare delivery system in the U.S. (Jaffe et al., 2013), show that these figures can be substantially improved by electronic hypertension registries tracking hypertension control rates, regular feedback to providers, development and frequent updating of an evidence-based treatment guideline, promotion of single-pill combination therapies, and follow-up blood pressure checks. Between 2001 and 2009, this program increased the number of patients with a diagnosis of hypertension by 78%, as well as the proportion of subjects meeting target blood pressure goals from 44% to more than 84% (Jaffe et al., 2013).

Hypertension is defined as a sustained increase in blood pressure of 140/90 mmHg or higher, a criterion that characterizes a group of patients whose risk of hypertension-related cardiovascular disease is high enough to merit medical attention. Actually, the risk of both fatal and nonfatal cardiovascular disease in adults is lowest with systolic blood pressures of less than 120 mmHg and diastolic blood pressures less than 80 mmHg; these risks increase incrementally as systolic and diastolic blood pressures rise. Recognition of this continuously increasing risk prevents a simple definition of hypertension (Go et al., 2014) (Table 28–1). Although many of the clinical trials classified the severity of hypertension by diastolic pressure, progressive elevations of systolic pressure are similarly predictive of adverse cardiovascular events; at every level of diastolic pressure, risks are greater with higher levels of systolic blood pressure. Indeed, in patients more than 50 years old, systolic blood pressures predict adverse outcomes better than do diastolic pressures. Pulse pressure, defined as the difference between systolic and diastolic pressure, may add additional predictive value (Pastor-Barriuso et al., 2003). This may be at least in part due to higher-than-normal pulse pressure indicating adverse remodeling of blood vessels, representing an accelerated decrease in blood vessel compliance normally associated with aging and atherosclerosis. Isolated systolic hypertension (sometimes defined as systolic blood pressure greater than 140–160 mmHg with diastolic blood pressure less than 90 mmHg) is largely confined to people older than 60 years.

The presence of pathological changes in certain target organs heralds a worse prognosis than the same level of blood pressure in a patient lacking these findings. For instance, retinal hemorrhages, exudates, and papilledema in the eyes indicate a far worse short-term prognosis for a given level of blood pressure. Left ventricular hypertrophy defined by electrocardiogram, or more sensitively by echocardiography or cardiac magnetic resonance imaging, is associated with a substantially worse long-term outcome that includes a higher risk of sudden cardiac death. The risk of cardiovascular disease, disability, and death in hypertensive patients also is increased markedly by concomitant cigarette smoking, diabetes, or elevated LDL; the coexistence of hypertension with these risk factors increases cardiovascular morbidity and mortality to a degree that is compounded by each additional risk factor.

The purpose of treating hypertension is to decrease cardiovascular risk; thus, other dietary and pharmacological interventions may be required to treat these additional risk factors. Effective pharmacological treatment of patients with hypertension decreases morbidity and mortality from cardiovascular disease, reducing the risk of strokes, heart failure, and CAD (Rosendorff et al., 2015). The reduction in risk of MI may be less significant.

Principles of Antihypertensive Therapy

Nonpharmacological therapy, or lifestyle-related changes, is an important component of treatment of all patients with hypertension (James et al., 2014; Mancia et al., 2013). In some grade 1 hypertensives (Figure 28–1), blood pressure may be adequately controlled by a combination of weight loss (in overweight individuals), restricting sodium intake (to 5–6 g/d), increasing aerobic exercise (>30 min/d), moderating consumption of alcohol (ethanol/day ≤ 20–30 g in men [two drinks], ≤ 10–20 g in women [one drink]), smoking cessation, increased consumption of fruits, vegetables, and low-fat dairy products.

The majority of patients require drug therapy for adequate blood pressure control (Figure 28–1). Optimal blood pressure goals for drug therapy are still debated, and current guidelines from cardiovascular societies differ slightly (James et al., 2014). Recently, a large comparative study in nondiabetics with increased cardiovascular risk was prematurely stopped because the group of patients treated with antihypertensives to a systolic blood pressure target of 120 mmHg, with an average of 2.8 drugs, experienced a 25% lower rate of cardiovascular end points and total mortality

TABLE 28–1 ■ AMERICAN HEART ASSOCIATION CRITERIA FOR HYPERTENSION IN ADULTS

CLASSIFICATION	BLOOD PRESSURE (mmHg)	
	SYSTOLIC	DIASTOLIC
Normal	<120	and < 80
Prehypertension	120–139	or 80–89
Hypertension, stage 1	140–159	or 90–99
Hypertension, stage 2	≥160	or ≥ 100
Hypertensive crisis	>180	or > 110

than the group targeted to the current standard goal target of 140 mmHg (SPRINT Research Group, 2015). The rate of adverse effects such as hypotension and worsening of renal function were higher in the intensified treatment group, yet this did not translate to a signal for real harm. The data will likely lead to a reexamination of current guideline-recommended blood pressure targets.

Arterial pressure is the product of cardiac output and peripheral vascular resistance (Figure 28–2). Drugs lower blood pressure by actions on peripheral resistance, cardiac output, or both. Drugs may decrease the cardiac output by inhibiting myocardial contractility or by decreasing ventricular filling pressure. Reduction in ventricular filling pressure may be achieved by actions on the venous tone or on blood volume via renal effects. Drugs can decrease peripheral resistance by acting on smooth muscle to cause relaxation of resistance vessels or by interfering with the activity of systems that produce constriction of resistance vessels (e.g., the sympathetic nervous system, the RAS). In patients with isolated systolic hypertension, complex hemodynamics in a rigid arterial system contribute to increased blood pressure; drug effects may be mediated not only by changes in peripheral resistance but also via effects on large artery stiffness (Franklin, 2000).

Antihypertensive drugs can be classified according to their sites or mechanisms of action (Table 28–2, Figure 28–2). The hemodynamic consequences of long-term treatment with antihypertensive agents (Table 28–3) provide a rationale for potential complementary effects of concurrent therapy with two or more drugs. Concurrent use of drugs from different classes is a strategy for achieving effective control of blood pressure while minimizing dose-related adverse effects.

It generally is not possible to predict the responses of individuals with hypertension to any specific drug. For example, for some antihypertensive drugs, about two-thirds of patients will have a meaningful clinical response, whereas about one-third of patients will not respond to the same drug. Racial origin and age may have modest influence on the likelihood of a favorable response to a particular class of drugs. Polymorphisms in genes involved in the metabolism of antihypertensive drugs have been

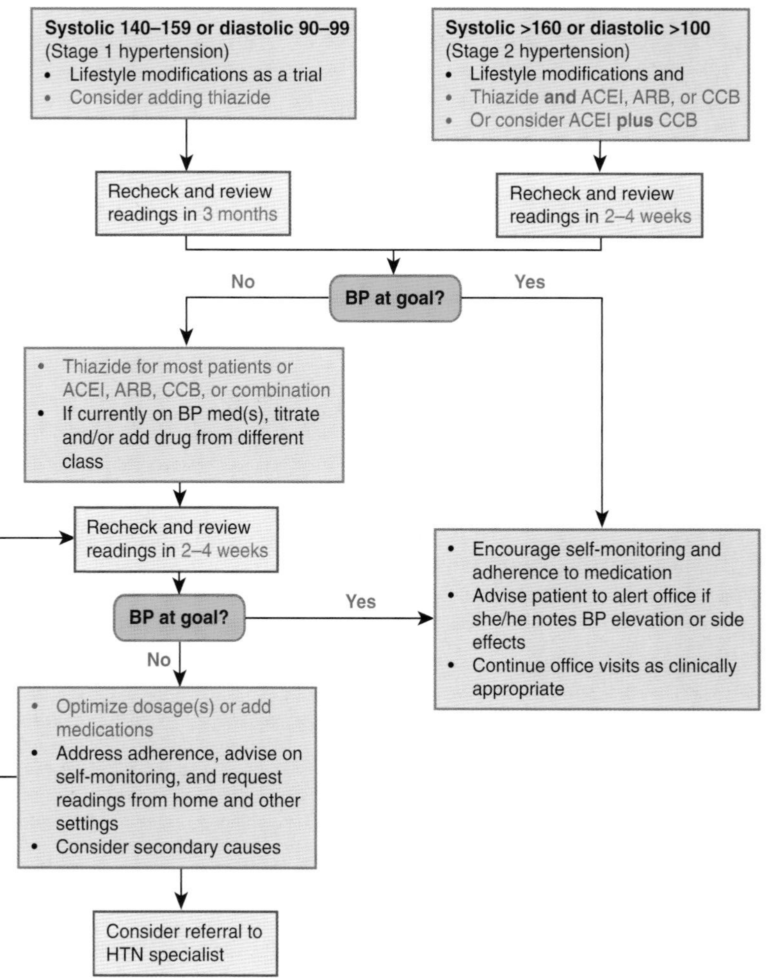

Figure 28–1 *Treatment algorithm for adults with hypertension.* Algorithm is based on recommendations of the American Heart Association and the American College of Cardiology (Go et al., 2013).

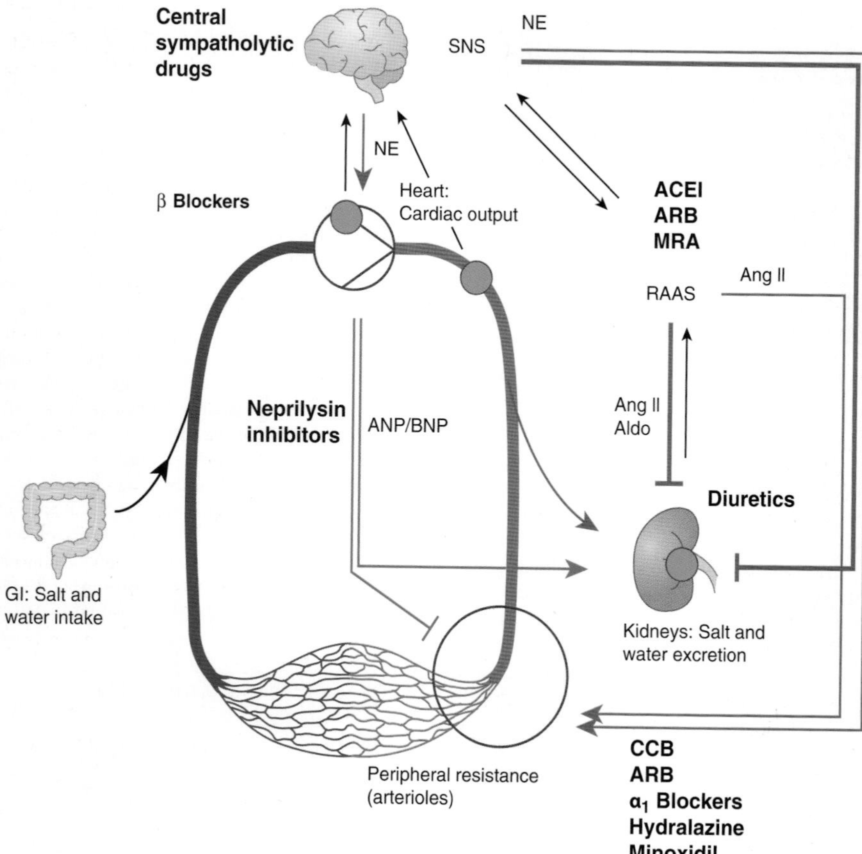

Figure 28–2 *Principles of blood pressure regulation and its modification by drugs.* Cardiac output and peripheral arteriolar resistance, the major determinants of arterial blood pressure, are regulated by myriad mechanisms, including the SNS (main peripheral neurotransmitter NE), the balance between salt intake by the intestine (GI) and salt excretion by the kidneys, the RAAS (main agonists AngII and Aldo), and natriuretic peptides produced in the heart (ANP and BNP). Sensors (green circles) provide afferent input on pressure in the heart and great vessels and on salt concentrations in the kidney. Note positive feedback between the SNS and RAAS via β_1-stimulated renin release and AngII-stimulated NE release. Drug classes are indicated in boldface type at their main site of action. Arrows indicate blood pressure-increasing (red) and -decreasing (green) effects. Neprilysin inhibitors (e.g., sacubitril) are in clinical testing for hypertension and have been approved for the treatment of heart failure (in combination with an ARB).

identified in the CYPs (phase I metabolism) and in phase II metabolism, such as catechol-*O*-methyltransferase (see Chapters 6 and 7). While these polymorphisms can change the pharmacokinetics of specific drugs quite markedly (e.g., five times higher plasma concentrations of metoprolol in CYP2D6 poor metabolizers), differences in efficacy are smaller (Rau et al., 2009) and of unknown clinical relevance. Polymorphisms that influence pharmacodynamic responses to antihypertensive drugs, including ACE inhibitors and diuretics, have also been identified, but evidence for clinically meaningful differences in drug response is sparse. Genome-wide scanning has identified several genetic variants associated with hypertension, but the effect sizes are much smaller than that of clinically established risk factors such as overweight.

Diuretics

An early strategy for the management of hypertension was to alter Na^+ balance by restriction of salt in the diet. Pharmacological alteration of Na^+ balance became practical with the development of the orally active thiazide diuretics (see Chapter 25). These and related diuretic agents have antihypertensive effects when used alone, and they enhance the efficacy of virtually all other antihypertensive drugs. Thus, this class of drugs remains important in the treatment of hypertension.

The exact mechanism for reduction of arterial blood pressure by diuretics is not certain. The initial action of thiazide diuretics decreases extracellular volume by interacting with a thiazide-sensitive NCC (*SLC12A3*) expressed in the distal convoluted tubule in the kidney, enhancing Na^+ excretion in the urine, and leading to a decrease in cardiac output. However, the hypotensive effect is maintained during long-term therapy due to decreased vascular resistance; cardiac output returns to pretreatment values, and extracellular volume returns to almost normal due to compensatory responses such as activation of the RAS. The explanation for the long-term vasodilation induced by thiazide diuretics is unknown. *Hydrochlorothiazide* may open Ca^{2+}-activated K^+ channels, leading to hyperpolarization of vascular smooth muscle cells, which leads in turn to closing of L-type Ca^{2+} channels and lower probability of opening, resulting in decreased Ca^{2+} entry and reduced vasoconstriction. Hydrochlorothiazide also inhibits vascular carbonic anhydrase, which, hypothetically, could alter smooth muscle cell systolic pH and thereby cause opening of Ca^{2+}-activated K^+ channels with the consequences noted previously.

The relevance of these findings—largely assessed in vitro—to the observed antihypertensive effects of thiazides is speculative. The major action of these drugs on SLC12A3—expressed predominantly in the distal convoluted tubules and not in vascular smooth muscle or the heart—suggests that these drugs decrease peripheral resistance as an indirect effect of negative Na^+ balance. That thiazides lose efficacy in treating

TABLE 28–2 ■ CLASSES OF ANTIHYPERTENSIVE DRUGS

Diuretics (Chapter 25) • *Thiazides and related agents*: chlorothiazide, chlorthalidone, hydrochlorothiazide, indapamide • *Loop diuretics*: bumetanide, furosemide, torsemide • *K^+-sparing diuretics*: amiloride, triamterene, MRA spironolactone
Sympatholytic drugs (Chapter 12) • *β Blockers*: atenolol, bisoprolol, esmolol, metoprolol, nadolol, nebivolol, propranolol, timolol • *α Blockers*: prazosin, terazosin, doxazosin, phenoxybenzamine • *Mixed α/β blockers*: labetalol, carvedilol • *Centrally acting sympatholytic agents*: clonidine, guanabenz, guanfacine, methyldopa, moxonidine, reserpine
Ca^{2+} channel blockers (Chapter 27): amlodipine, clevidipine, diltiazem, felodipine, isradipine, lercanidipine, nicardipine, nifedipine,[a] nisoldipine, verapamil
Renin-angiotensin antagonists **(Chapter 26)** • *Angiotensin-converting enzyme inhibitors*: benazepril, captopril, enalapril, fosinopril, lisinopril, moexipril, perindopril, quinapril, ramipril, trandolapril • *AngII receptor blockers*: candesartan, eprosartan, irbesartan, losartan, olmesartan, telmisartan, valsartan • *Direct renin inhibitor*: aliskiren
Vasodilators **(Chapters 27 and 28)** • *Arterial*: diazoxide, fenoldopam, hydralazine, minoxidil • *Arterial and venous*: nitroprusside

[a]Only extended-release nifedipine is approved for hypertension.

hypertension in patients with coexisting renal insufficiency is compatible with this hypothesis. Moreover, carriers of rare functional mutations in SLC12A3 that decrease renal Na^+ reabsorption have lower blood pressure than appropriate controls (Ji et al., 2008); in a sense, this is an experiment of nature that may mimic the therapeutic effect of thiazides.

Benzothiadiazines and Related Compounds

Benzothiadiazines ("thiazides") and related diuretics are the most frequently used class of antihypertensive agents in the U.S. Following the discovery of *chlorothiazide*, a number of oral diuretics were developed that have an arylsulfonamide structure and block the NCC. Some of these are not benzothiadiazines but have structural features and molecular functions that are similar to the original benzothiadiazine compounds; consequently, they are designated as members of the thiazide class of diuretics. For example, chlorthalidone (also written as chlortalidone), one of the nonbenzothiadiazines, is widely used in the treatment of hypertension, as is indapamide.

Regimen for Administration of the Thiazide-Class Diuretics in Hypertension

Because members of the thiazide class have similar pharmacological effects, they generally have been viewed as interchangeable with appropriate adjustment of dosage (see Chapter 25). However, the pharmacokinetics and pharmacodynamics of these drugs differ, so they may not necessarily have the same clinical efficacy in treating hypertension. In a direct comparison, the antihypertensive efficacy of chlorthalidone was greater than that of hydrochlorothiazide, particularly during the night (Ernst et al., 2006), suggesting the much longer $t_{1/2}$ of chlorthalidone (>24 h) compared to hydrochlorothiazide (several hours) gave more stable blood pressure reductions. In light of the considerable clinical trial data supporting the capacity of chlorthalidone to diminish adverse cardiovascular events—in comparison to that available for currently used low doses of hydrochlorothiazide—there is a growing concern that chlorthalidone may be an underutilized drug in hypertensive patients requiring a diuretic.

Antihypertensive effects can be achieved in many patients with as little as 12.5 mg daily of chlorthalidone or hydrochlorothiazide. Furthermore, when used as monotherapy, the maximal daily dose of thiazide-class diuretics usually should not exceed 25 mg of hydrochlorothiazide or chlorthalidone (or equivalent). Even though more diuresis can be achieved with higher doses, some evidence suggests that doses higher than this are not generally more efficacious in lowering blood pressure in patients with normal renal function. Low doses of either thiazide reduce the risk of adverse effects such as K^+ wasting and inhibition of uric acid excretion, indicating an improved risk-to-benefit ratio at low doses of a thiazide. However, other studies suggested that low doses of hydrochlorothiazide have inadequate effects on blood pressure when monitored in a detailed manner (Lacourciere et al., 1995).

Clinical trials of antihypertensive therapy in the elderly demonstrated the best outcomes for cardiovascular morbidity and mortality when 25 mg of hydrochlorothiazide or chlorthalidone was the maximum dose given; if this dose did not achieve the target blood pressure reduction, a

TABLE 28–3 ■ HEMODYNAMIC EFFECTS OF LONG-TERM ADMINISTRATION OF ANTIHYPERTENSIVE AGENTS

	HEART RATE	CARDIAC OUTPUT	TOTAL PERIPHERAL RESISTANCE	PLASMA VOLUME	PLASMA RENIN ACTIVITY
Diuretics	↔	↔	↓	–↓	↑
Sympatholytic agents					
Centrally acting	–↓	–↓	↓	–↑	–↓
α_1 Blockers	–↑	–↑	↓	–↑	↔
β Blockers					
No ISA	↓	↓	–↓	–↑	↓
ISA[a]	↓↑	↔	↓	–↑	–↓
Arteriolar vasodilators	↑	↑	↓	↑	↑
Ca^{2+} channel blockers	↓ or ↑	↓ or ↑	↓	–↑	–↑
ACEIs	↔	↔	↓	↔	↑
AT_1 receptor blockers	↔	↔	↓	↔	↑
Renin inhibitor	↔	↔	↓	↔	↓ (but renin ↑)

↑, increased; ↓, decreased; –↑, increased or no change; –↓, decreased or no change; ↔, unchanged.

[a]Heart rate can be increased at rest and decreased under exercise as a result of ISA. During rest, ISA may increase resting heart rate; during exercise, β adrenergic antagonism predominates, attenuating heart rate acceleration by NE.

second drug was initiated (1991; Dahlof et al., 1991). A case-control study found a dose-dependent increase in the occurrence of sudden death at doses of hydrochlorothiazide greater than 25 mg daily (Siscovick et al., 1994), supporting the hypothesis that higher diuretic doses are associated with increased cardiovascular mortality as long as hypokalemia is not corrected. Thus, if adequate blood pressure reduction is not achieved with the 25-mg daily dose of hydrochlorothiazide or chlorthalidone, the addition of a second drug is indicated rather than an increase in the dose of diuretic.

Urinary K^+ loss can be a problem with thiazides. ACE inhibitors and ARBs will attenuate diuretic-induced loss of K^+ to some degree, and this is a consideration if a second drug is required to achieve further blood pressure reduction beyond that attained with the diuretic alone. Because the diuretic and hypotensive effects of these drugs are greatly enhanced when they are given in combination, care should be taken to initiate combination therapy with low doses of each of these drugs (Vlasses et al., 1983). Administration of ACE inhibitors or ARBs together with other K^+-sparing agents or with K^+ supplements requires great caution; combining K^+-sparing agents with each other or with K^+ supplementation can cause potentially dangerous hyperkalemia in some patients.

In contrast to the limitation on the dose of thiazide-class diuretics used as monotherapy, the treatment of severe hypertension that is unresponsive to three or more drugs may require larger doses of the thiazide-class diuretics. Indeed, hypertensive patients may become refractory to drugs that block the sympathetic nervous system or to vasodilator drugs, because these drugs engender a state in which the blood pressure is very volume dependent. Therefore, it is appropriate to consider the use of thiazide-class diuretics in doses of 50 mg of daily hydrochlorothiazide equivalent when treatment with appropriate combinations and doses of three or more drugs fails to yield adequate control of the blood pressure. Alternatively, there may be a need to use higher-capacity diuretics such as furosemide, especially if renal function is not normal.

The effectiveness of thiazides as diuretics or antihypertensive agents is progressively diminished when the glomerular filtration rate falls below 30 mL/min. One exception is metolazone, which retains efficacy in patients with this degree of renal insufficiency.

Most patients will respond to thiazide diuretics with a reduction in blood pressure within about 4–6 weeks. Therefore, doses should not be increased more often than every 4–6 weeks. There is no way to predict the antihypertensive response from the duration or severity of the hypertension in a given patient, although diuretics are unlikely to be effective as sole therapy in patients with stage 2 hypertension (Table 28–1). Because the effect of thiazide diuretics is additive with that of other antihypertensive drugs, combination regimens that include these diuretics are common and rational. A wide range of fixed-dose combination products containing a thiazide are marketed for this purpose. Diuretics also have the advantage of minimizing the retention of salt and water that is commonly caused by vasodilators and some sympatholytic drugs. Omitting or underutilizing a diuretic is a frequent cause of "resistant hypertension."

Adverse Effects and Precautions

The adverse effects of diuretics are discussed in Chapter 25. Some of these determine whether a patient can tolerate and adhere to diuretic treatment.

The K^+ depletion produced by thiazide-class diuretics is dose dependent and variable among individuals, such that a subset of patients may become substantially K^+ depleted on diuretic drugs. Given chronically, even small doses lead to some K^+ depletion, which is a well-known risk factor for ventricular arrhythmias by reducing cardiac repolarization reserve. The last has recently been used to explain that insults in a particular repolarization current do not necessarily result in QT interval prolongation, the principle clinical measure of repolarization (see Chapter 30). Hypokalemia directly reduces repolarization reserve by decreasing several K^+ conductances (inward rectifier I_{K1}, delayed rectifier I_{Kr}, and the transient outward current I_{to}) and increases the binding activity of I_{Kr}-inhibiting drugs such as dofetilide (Yang and Roden, 1996). Hypokalemia also reduces the activity of the Na^+,K^+-ATPase (the Na^+ pump), causing intracellular accumulation of Na^+ and Ca^{2+}, further increasing the risk of afterdepolarizations (Pezhouman et al., 2015). Consequently, hypokalemia increases the risk of drug-induced polymorphic ventricular tachycardia (torsade de pointes; see Chapter 30) and the risk for ischemic ventricular fibrillation, the leading cause of sudden cardiac death and a major contributor to cardiovascular mortality in treated hypertensive patients. There is a positive correlation between diuretic dose and sudden cardiac death and an inverse correlation between the use of adjunctive K^+-sparing agents and sudden cardiac death (Siscovick et al., 1994). Thus, hypokalemia needs to be avoided by, for example, combining a thiazide with inhibitors of the RAS or with a K^+-sparing diuretic.

Thiazides have residual carbonic anhydrase–inhibiting activity, thereby reducing Na^+ reabsorption in the proximal tubule. The increased presentation of Na^+ at the macula densa leads to a reduced glomerular filtration rate via tubuloglomerular feedback. While this effect is clinically not meaningful in patients with normal renal function, it reduces diuretic effectiveness and may gain importance in patients with reduced kidney function. RAS inhibitors and Ca^{2+} channel blockers interfere with tubuloglomerular feedback, providing one explanation for the synergistic effect on blood pressure. Erectile dysfunction is a troublesome adverse effect of the thiazide-class diuretics, and physicians should inquire specifically regarding its occurrence in conjunction with treatment with these drugs. Gout may be a consequence of the hyperuricemia induced by these diuretics. The occurrence of either of these adverse effects is a reason for considering alternative approaches to therapy. However, precipitation of acute gout is relatively uncommon with low doses of diuretics. Hydrochlorothiazide may cause rapidly developing, severe hyponatremia in some patients. Thiazides inhibit renal Ca^{2+} excretion, occasionally leading to hypercalcemia; although generally mild, this can be more severe in patients subject to hypercalcemia, such as those with primary hyperparathyroidism. The thiazide-induced decreased Ca^{2+} excretion may be used therapeutically in patients with osteoporosis or hypercalciuria.

Thiazide diuretics have also been associated with changes in plasma lipids and glucose tolerance that have led to some concern. The clinical significance of the changes has been disputed because the clinical studies demonstrated comparable efficacy of the thiazide diuretic chlortalidone in reducing cardiovascular risk (ALLHAT Officers, 2002).

All thiazide-like drugs cross the placenta. While they have no direct adverse effects on the fetus, administration of a thiazide during pregnancy increases a risk of transient volume depletion that may result in placental hypoperfusion. Because the thiazides appear in breast milk, they should be avoided by nursing mothers.

Other Diuretic Antihypertensive Agents

The thiazide diuretics are more effective antihypertensive agents than are the loop diuretics, such as furosemide and bumetanide, in patients who have normal renal function. This differential effect is most likely related to the short duration of action of loop diuretics. In fact, a single daily dose of loop diuretics does not cause a significant net loss of Na^+ for an entire 24-h period because the strong initial diuretic effect is followed by a rebound mediated by activation of the RAS. Unfortunately, loop diuretics are frequently and inappropriately prescribed as a once-a-day medication in the treatment not only of hypertension, but also of congestive heart failure and ascites. The high efficacy of loop diuretics to produce a rapid and profound natriuresis can be detrimental for the treatment of hypertension. When a loop diuretic is given twice daily, the acute diuresis can be excessive and lead to more side effects than occur with a slower-acting, milder thiazide diuretic. Loop diuretics may be particularly useful in patients with azotemia or with severe edema associated with a vasodilator such as minoxidil.

K^+-Sparing Diuretics

Amiloride and triamterene are K^+-sparing diuretics that have little value as antihypertensive monotherapy but are important in combination with thiazides to antagonize urinary K^+ loss and the concomitant risk of ventricular arrhythmias. They act by reversibly inhibiting the ENaC in the distal tubule membrane, the transporter responsible for the reabsorption of Na^+ in exchange for K^+. The importance of ENaC for hypertension is illustrated by the fact that an inherited form of hypertension, Liddle syndrome, is due to hyperactivity of ENaC. Gene expression of ENaC is mineralocorticoid sensitive, explaining the antihypertensive and K^+-sparing effect of another class of K^+-sparing diuretics, the MRAs spironolactone and eplerenone. In contrast to the immediate and short-term inhibition of ENaC by amiloride and triamterene, the action of MRAs is delayed for about 3 days and is long lasting because MRAs regulate the density of the channel protein in the tubule membrane.

The MRAs have a particular role in hypertension and heart failure (see Chapter 27) because small doses of spironolactone are often highly effective in patients with "resistant hypertension." First described decades ago (Ramsay et al., 1980), the concept was recently validated in a prospective, placebo-controlled trial comparing spironolactone (25–50 mg) with bisoprolol or doxazosin as add-ons in patients with uncontrolled hypertension despite triple standard antihypertensive therapy (Williams et al., 2015). Spironolactone had about a 2-fold larger blood pressure–lowering effect (8.7 vs. 4.8 and 4 mmHg, respectively). The efficacy of the MRA spironolactone in resistant hypertension supports a primary role of Na^+ retention in this condition. Some of the effect may be related to the so-called aldosterone-escape phenomenon, or a return to pre-RAS-inhibitor plasma aldosterone levels with extended time of treatment, observed under treatment with RAS inhibitors. Primary hyperaldosteronism occurs in a significant fraction of patients with resistant hypertension (Calhoun et al., 2002).

Spironolactone has some significant adverse effects, especially in men (e.g., erectile dysfunction, gynecomastia, benign prostatic hyperplasia). Eplerenone is a more specific, though less-potent, MRA with reduced side effects.

All K^+-sparing diuretics should be used cautiously, with frequent measurements of plasma K^+ concentrations in patients predisposed to hyperkalemia. Patients should be cautioned regarding the possibility that concurrent use of K^+-containing salt substitutes could produce hyperkalemia. Renal insufficiency is a relative contraindication to the use of K^+-sparing diuretics. Concomitant use of an ACE inhibitor or an ARB magnifies the risk of hyperkalemia with these agents.

Diuretic-Associated Drug Interactions

Because the antihypertensive effects of diuretics are additive with those of other antihypertensive agents, a diuretic commonly is used in combination with other drugs. The K^+- and Mg^{2+}-depleting effects of the thiazides and loop diuretics can potentiate arrhythmias that arise from digitalis toxicity. Corticosteroids can amplify the hypokalemia produced by the diuretics. NSAIDs (see Chapter 38) that inhibit the synthesis of prostaglandins reduce the antihypertensive effects of diuretics and all other antihypertensives. The renal effects of selective COX-2 inhibitors are similar to those of the traditional NSAIDs. NSAIDs and RAS inhibitors reduce plasma concentrations of aldosterone and can potentiate the hyperkalemic effects of a K^+-sparing diuretic. All diuretics can decrease the clearance of Li^+, resulting in increased plasma concentrations of Li^+ and potential toxicity.

Sympatholytic Agents

With the demonstration in 1940 that bilateral excision of the thoracic sympathetic chain could lower blood pressure, there was a search for effective chemical sympatholytic agents. Many of the early sympatholytic drugs were poorly tolerated and had limiting adverse side effects, particularly on mood. A number of sympatholytic agents are currently in use (Table 28–2). Antagonists of α and β adrenergic receptors have been mainstays of antihypertensive therapy.

β Blockers

β Adrenergic receptor antagonists (β blockers) were not expected to have antihypertensive effects when they were first investigated in patients with angina, their primary indication. However, *pronethalol*, a drug that was never marketed, was found to reduce arterial blood pressure in hypertensive patients with angina pectoris. This antihypertensive effect was subsequently demonstrated for *propranolol* and all other β blockers. The basic pharmacology of these drugs is discussed in Chapter 12; characteristics relevant to their use in hypertension are described here.

Locus and Mechanism of Action

Antagonism of β adrenergic receptors affects the regulation of the circulation through a number of mechanisms, including a reduction in myocardial contractility and heart rate (i.e., cardiac output; see Figure 27–1). Antagonism of $β_1$ receptors of the juxtaglomerular complex reduces renin secretion and RAS activity. This action likely contributes to the antihypertensive action. Some members of this large, heterogeneous class of drugs have additional effects unrelated to their capacity to bind to β adrenergic receptors. For example, labetalol and carvedilol are also $α_1$ blockers, and nebivolol promotes endothelial cell–dependent vasodilation via activation of NO production (Pedersen and Cockcroft, 2006) (see Figure 12–4).

Pharmacodynamic Differences

The β blockers vary in their selectivity for the $β_1$ receptor subtype, presence of partial agonist or intrinsic sympathomimetic activity, and vasodilating capacity. While all of the β blockers are effective as antihypertensive agents, these differences influence the clinical pharmacology and spectrum of adverse effects of the various drugs. The antihypertensive effect resides in antagonism of the $β_1$ receptor, while major unwanted effects result from antagonism of $β_2$ receptors (e.g., peripheral vasoconstriction, bronchoconstriction, hypoglycemia). Standard therapies are $β_1$ blockers without intrinsic sympathomimetic activity (e.g., atenolol, bisoprolol, metoprolol). They produce an initial reduction in cardiac output (mainly $β_1$) and a reflex-induced rise in peripheral resistance, with little or no acute change in arterial pressure. In patients who respond with a reduction in blood pressure, peripheral resistance gradually returns to pretreatment values or less. Generally, persistently reduced cardiac output and possibly decreased peripheral resistance account for the reduction in arterial pressure. Nonselective β blockers (e.g., propranolol) have stronger adverse effects on peripheral vascular resistance by also blocking $β_2$ receptors that normally mediate vasodilation. Vasodilating β blockers (e.g., carvedilol, nebivolol) may be preferred in patients with peripheral artery disease. Drugs with intrinsic sympathomimetic activity (e.g., pindolol, xamoterol) are not recommended for the treatment of hypertension or any other cardiovascular disease because they actually increase nighttime mean heart rate due to their direct partial agonistic activity.

Pharmacokinetic Differences

Lipophilic β blockers (metoprolol, bisoprolol, carvedilol, propranolol) appear to have more antiarrhythmic efficacy than the hydrophilic compounds (atenolol, nadolol, labetalol), possibly related to a central mode of action. Many β blockers have relatively short plasma half-lives and require more than once-daily dosing (metoprolol, propranolol, carvedilol), a significant disadvantage in the treatment of hypertension. They should generally be prescribed in sustained-release forms. Bisoprolol and nebivolol have $t_{1/2}$ values of 10–12 h and thus achieve sufficient trough levels at once-daily dosing. Hepatic metabolism of metoprolol, carvedilol, and nebivolol is CYP2D6 dependent. The relevance is probably greatest in case of metoprolol, for which CYP2D6 poor metabolizers (~7% of the Caucasian population) show 5-fold higher drug exposure and 2-fold higher heart rate decreases than the majority of extensive metabolizers (Rau et al., 2009).

Effectiveness in Hypertension

Meta-analyses have suggested that β blockers reduce the incidence of MI similar to other antihypertensives but are only be about half as effective in preventing stroke (Lindholm et al., 2005). This has led to downgrading of this class of drugs in certain national guidelines (e.g., U.K. standards); however, many of the studies supporting this conclusion were conducted with atenolol, which may not be the ideal β blocker. Atenolol may not lower central (aortic) blood pressure as effectively as it appears when conventionally measured in the brachial artery using a standard arm cuff (Williams et al., 2006). Indeed, atenolol, in contrast to bisoprolol, carvedilol, metoprolol, or nebivolol, has not been positively tested in heart failure trials. Prospective studies of hypertensive agents have not compared different β blockers head to head; therefore, the clinical relevance of pharmacological differences in this heterogeneous drug class remains unclear. Results of a detailed meta-analysis of 147 randomized trials of blood pressure reduction showed that, regardless of blood pressure before treatment, lowering systolic blood pressure by 10 mmHg or diastolic blood pressure by 5 mmHg using any of the main classes of antihypertensive drugs significantly reduced coronary events and stroke without an increase in nonvascular mortality (Law et al., 2009).

Adverse Effects and Precautions

The adverse effects of β blockers are discussed in Chapter 12. These drugs should be avoided in patients with reactive airway disease (e.g., asthma) or with SA or AV nodal dysfunction or in combination with other drugs that inhibit AV conduction, such as verapamil. The risk of hypoglycemic reactions may be increased in diabetics taking insulin, but type 2 diabetes is not a contraindication. β Blockers increase concentrations of triglycerides in plasma and lower those of HDL cholesterol without changing total cholesterol concentrations. The long-term consequences of these effects are unknown.

Sudden discontinuation of β blockers can produce a withdrawal syndrome that is likely due to upregulation of β receptors during blockade, causing enhanced tissue sensitivity to endogenous catecholamines—potentially exacerbating the symptoms of CAD. The result, especially in active patients, can be rebound hypertension. Thus, β blockers should not be discontinued abruptly, except under close observation; dosage should be tapered gradually over 10–14 days prior to discontinuation.

Epinephrine can produce severe hypertension and bradycardia when a nonselective β blocker is present. The hypertension is due to the unopposed stimulation of α adrenergic receptors when vascular β_2 receptors are blocked. The bradycardia is the result of reflex vagal stimulation. Such paradoxical hypertensive responses to β blockers have been observed in patients with hypoglycemia or pheochromocytoma, during withdrawal from *clonidine*, following administration of epinephrine as a therapeutic agent, or in association with the illicit use of cocaine.

Therapeutic Uses

The β blockers provide effective therapy for all grades of hypertension. Marked differences in their pharmacokinetic properties should be considered; once-daily dosing is preferred for better compliance. Populations that tend to have a lesser antihypertensive response to β blockers include the elderly and African Americans. However, intraindividual differences in antihypertensive efficacy are generally much larger than statistical evidence of differences between racial or age-related groups. Consequently, these observations should not discourage the use of these drugs in individual patients in groups reported to be less responsive.

The β blockers usually do not cause retention of salt and water, and administration of a diuretic is not necessary to avoid edema or the development of tolerance. However, diuretics do have additive antihypertensive effects when combined with β blockers. The combination of a β blocker, a diuretic, and a vasodilator is effective for patients who require a third antihypertensive drug. β Blockers (i.e., bisoprolol, carvedilol, metoprolol, or nebivolol) are highly preferred drugs for hypertensive patients with conditions such as MI, ischemic heart disease, or congestive heart failure and may be preferred for younger patients with signs of increased sympathetic drive. However, for other hypertensive patients, particularly older patients with a high risk for stroke, enthusiasm for their early use in treatment has diminished.

α_1 Blockers

The availability of drugs that selectively block α_1 adrenergic receptors without affecting α_2 adrenergic receptors adds another group of antihypertensive agents. The pharmacology of these drugs is discussed in detail in Chapter 12. Prazosin, terazosin, and doxazosin are the agents available for the treatment of hypertension. Phenoxybenzamine, an irreversible α blocker ($\alpha_1 > \alpha_2$), is used in the treatment of catecholamine-producing tumors (pheochromocytoma).

Pharmacological Effects

Initially, α_1 blockers reduce arteriolar resistance and increase venous capacitance; this causes a sympathetically mediated reflex increase in heart rate and plasma renin activity. During long-term therapy, vasodilation persists, but cardiac output, heart rate, and plasma renin activity return to normal. Renal blood flow is unchanged during therapy with an α_1 blocker. The α_1 blockers cause a variable amount of postural hypotension, depending on the plasma volume. Retention of salt and water occurs in many patients during continued administration, and this attenuates the postural hypotension. The α_1 blockers reduce plasma concentrations of triglycerides and total LDL cholesterol and increase HDL cholesterol. These potentially favorable effects on lipids persist when a thiazide-type diuretic is given concurrently. The long-term consequences of these small, drug-induced changes in lipids are unknown.

Therapeutic Uses

α_1 Blockers are not recommended as monotherapy for hypertensive patients, primarily as a consequence of the ALLHAT study (see further discussion). Consequently, they are used primarily in conjunction with diuretics, β blockers, and other antihypertensive agents. β Blockers enhance the efficacy of α_1 blockers. α_1 Blockers are not the drugs of choice in patients with pheochromocytoma because a vasoconstrictor response to epinephrine can still result from activation of unblocked vascular α_2 adrenergic receptors. α_1 Blockers are attractive drugs for hypertensive patients with benign prostatic hyperplasia because they also improve urinary symptoms.

Adverse Effects

The use of doxazosin as monotherapy for hypertension increases the risk for developing congestive heart failure (ALLHAT Officers, 2002). This may be a class effect that represents an adverse effect of all of the α_1 blockers and has led to recommendations not to use this class of drugs in patients with heart failure. Interpretation of the outcome of the ALLHAT study is controversial, but the commonly held belief that the higher rate of apparent heart failure development in the groups of patients treated with a nondiuretic was caused by withdrawal of prestudy diuretics has not been substantiated (Davis et al., 2006).

A major precaution regarding the use of the α_1 blockers for hypertension is the so-called first-dose phenomenon, in which symptomatic orthostatic hypotension occurs within 30–90 min (or longer) of the initial dose of the drug or after a dosage increase. This effect may occur in up to 50% of patients, especially in patients who are already receiving a diuretic. After the first few doses, patients develop a tolerance to this marked hypotensive response.

Combined α_1 and β Blockers

Carvedilol (see Chapter 12) is a nonselective β blocker with α_1-antagonist activity. Carvedilol is approved for the treatment of hypertension and symptomatic heart failure. The ratio of α_1- to β-antagonist potency for carvedilol is approximately 1:10. The drug dissociates slowly from its receptor, explaining why the duration of action is longer than the short $t_{1/2}$ (2.2 h) and why its effect can hardly be overcome by catecholamines. Carvedilol undergoes oxidative metabolism and glucuronidation in the liver; the oxidative metabolism occurs via CYP2D6. As with labetalol, the long-term efficacy and side effects of carvedilol in hypertension are predictable based on its properties as a β and α_1 blocker. Carvedilol reduces mortality in patients with congestive heart failure (Chapter 29). Due to the vasodilating effect, it is a β blocker of choice in patients with peripheral artery disease.

Labetalol (see Chapter 12) is an equimolar mixture of four stereoisomers. One isomer is an α_1 blocker, another is a nonselective β blocker with partial agonist activity, and the other two isomers are inactive. Labetalol has efficacy and adverse effects that would be expected with any combination of an α_1 and a β blocker. It has the disadvantages that are inherent in fixed-dose combination products: The extent of α_1- to β-blockade is somewhat unpredictable and varies from patient to patient. Labetalol is FDA-approved for eclampsia, preeclampsia, hypertension, and hypertensive emergencies. The main indication for labetalol is hypertension in pregnancy, for which it is one of the few compounds known to be safe (Magee et al., 2016).

Centrally Acting Sympatholytic Drugs

Methyldopa

Methyldopa, a centrally acting antihypertensive agent, is a prodrug that exerts its antihypertensive action via an active metabolite. Although used frequently as an antihypertensive agent in the past, methyldopa's adverse effect profile limits its current use largely to treatment of hypertension in pregnancy, where it has a record for safety.

Methyldopa (α-methyl-3,4-dihydroxy-L-phenylalanine), an analogue of DOPA, is metabolized by the L-aromatic amino acid decarboxylase in adrenergic neurons to α-methyldopamine, which then is converted to α-methylnorepinephrine, the pharmacologically active metabolite. α-Methylnorepinephrine is stored in the secretory vesicles of adrenergic neurons, substituting for NE, such that the stimulated adrenergic neuron now discharges α-methylnorepinephrine instead of NE. α-Methylnorepinephrine acts in the CNS to inhibit adrenergic neuronal outflow from the brainstem, probably via acting as an agonist at presynaptic α_2 adrenergic receptors in the brainstem, attenuating NE release and thereby reducing the output of vasoconstrictor adrenergic signals to the peripheral sympathetic nervous system.

ADME. Because methyldopa is a prodrug that is metabolized in the brain to the active form, its C_p has less relevance for its effects than that for many other drugs. C_{pmax} occurs 2–3 h following an oral dose. The drug is eliminated with a $t_{1/2}$ of about 2 h. Methyldopa is excreted in the urine primarily as the sulfate conjugate (50%–70%) and as the parent drug (25%). Other minor metabolites include methyldopamine, methylnorepinephrine, and their *O*-methylated products. The $t_{1/2}$ of methyldopa is prolonged to 4–6 h in patients with renal failure.

Despite its rapid absorption and short $t_{1/2}$, the peak effect of methyldopa is delayed for 6–8 h, even after intravenous administration, and the duration of action of a single dose is usually about 24 h; this permits once- or twice-daily dosing. The discrepancy between the effects of methyldopa and the measured concentrations of the drug in plasma is most likely related to the time required for transport into the CNS, conversion to the active metabolite storage of α-methyl NE, and its subsequent release in the vicinity of relevant α_2 receptors in the CNS. Methyldopa is a good example of a complex relationship between a drug's pharmacokinetics and its pharmacodynamics. Patients with renal failure are more sensitive to the antihypertensive effect of methyldopa, but it is not known if this is due to alteration in excretion of the drug or to an increase in transport into the CNS.

Therapeutic Uses. Methyldopa is a preferred drug for treatment of hypertension during pregnancy based on its effectiveness and safety for both mother and fetus (Magee et al., 2016). The usual initial dose of methyldopa is 250 mg twice daily; there is little additional effect with doses greater than 2 g/d. Administration of a single daily dose of methyldopa at bedtime minimizes sedative effects, but administration twice daily is required for some patients.

Adverse Effects and Precautions. Methyldopa produces sedation that is largely transient. A diminution in psychic energy may persist in some patients, and depression occurs occasionally. Methyldopa may produce dryness of the mouth. Other adverse effects include diminished libido, parkinsonian signs, and hyperprolactinemia that may become sufficiently pronounced to cause gynecomastia and galactorrhea. Methyldopa may precipitate severe bradycardia and sinus arrest.

Methyldopa also produces some adverse effects that are not related to its therapeutic action in the CNS. Hepatotoxicity, sometimes associated with fever, is an uncommon but potentially serious toxic effect of methyldopa. At least 20% of patients who receive methyldopa for a year develop a positive Coombs test (antiglobulin test) that is due to autoantibodies directed against the Rh antigen on erythrocytes. The development of a positive Coombs test is not necessarily an indication to stop treatment with methyldopa; however, 1%–5% of these patients will develop a hemolytic anemia that requires prompt discontinuation of the drug. The Coombs test may remain positive for as long as a year after discontinuation of methyldopa, but the hemolytic anemia usually resolves within a matter of weeks. Severe hemolysis may be attenuated by treatment with glucocorticoids. Adverse effects that are even rarer include leukopenia, thrombocytopenia, red cell aplasia, lupus erythematosus–like syndrome, lichenoid and granulomatous skin eruptions, myocarditis, retroperitoneal fibrosis, pancreatitis, diarrhea, and malabsorption.

Clonidine and Moxonidine

The detailed pharmacology of the α_2 adrenergic agonists clonidine and moxonidine is discussed in Chapter 12. These drugs stimulate α_{2A} adrenergic receptors in the brainstem, resulting in a reduction in sympathetic outflow from the CNS (MacMillan et al., 1996). The hypotensive effect correlates directly with the decrease in plasma concentrations of NE. Patients who have had a spinal cord transection above the level of the sympathetic outflow tracts do not display a hypotensive response to clonidine. At doses higher than those required to stimulate central α_{2A} receptors, these drugs can activate α_{2B} receptors on vascular smooth muscle cells (MacMillan et al., 1996). This effect accounts for the initial vasoconstriction that is seen when overdoses of these drugs are taken and may be responsible for the loss of therapeutic effect that is observed with high doses. A major limitation in the use of these drugs is the paucity of information about their efficacy in reducing the risk of cardiovascular consequences of hypertension.

Pharmacological Effects. The α_2 adrenergic agonists lower arterial pressure by effects on both cardiac output and peripheral resistance. In the supine position, when the sympathetic tone to the vasculature is low, the major effect is a reduction in heart rate and stroke volume; however, in the upright position, when sympathetic outflow to the vasculature is normally increased, these drugs reduce vascular resistance. This action may lead to postural hypotension. The decrease in cardiac sympathetic tone leads to a reduction in myocardial contractility and heart rate that could promote congestive heart failure in susceptible patients.

Therapeutic Uses. The CNS effects are such that this class of drugs is not a leading option for monotherapy of hypertension. Indeed, there is no fixed place for these drugs in the treatment of hypertension. They effectively lower blood pressure in some patients who have not responded adequately to combinations of other agents. The greater clinical experience exists with clonidine. A recent study with moxonidine in patients with hypertension and paroxysmal atrial fibrillation indicated that the drug reduced the incidence of atrial fibrillation (Giannopoulos et al., 2014). Clonidine may be effective in reducing early morning hypertension in patients treated with standard antihypertensives. Overall, enthusiasm for α_2 receptor antagonists is diminished by the relative absence of evidence demonstrating reduction in risk of adverse cardiovascular events.

Clonidine has been used in hypertensive patients for the diagnosis of pheochromocytoma. The failure of clonidine to suppress the plasma concentration of NE to less than 500 pg/mL 3 h after an oral dose of 0.3 mg of clonidine suggests the presence of such a tumor. A modification of this test, wherein overnight urinary excretion of NE and epinephrine is measured after administration of a 0.3-mg dose of clonidine at bedtime, may be useful when results based on plasma NE concentrations are equivocal.

Adverse Effects and Precautions. Many patients experience persistent and sometimes intolerable adverse effects with these drugs. Sedation and xerostomia are prominent adverse effects. The xerostomia may be accompanied by dry nasal mucosa, dry eyes, and swelling and pain of the parotid gland. Postural hypotension and erectile dysfunction may be prominent in some patients. Clonidine may produce a lower incidence of dry mouth and sedation when given transdermally, perhaps because high peak concentrations are avoided. Moxonidine has additional activity at central imidazoline receptors and may produce less sedation than clonidine, but direct comparisons are lacking. Less-common CNS side effects include sleep disturbances with vivid dreams or nightmares, restlessness, and depression. Cardiac effects related to the sympatholytic action of these drugs include symptomatic bradycardia and sinus arrest in patients with dysfunction of the SA node and AV block in patients with AV nodal disease or in patients taking other drugs that depress AV conduction. Some 15%–20% of patients who receive transdermal clonidine may develop contact dermatitis.

Sudden discontinuation of clonidine and related α_2 adrenergic agonists may cause a withdrawal syndrome consisting of headache, apprehension, tremors, abdominal pain, sweating, and tachycardia. Arterial blood pressure may rise to levels above those present prior to treatment, but the withdrawal syndrome may occur in the absence of an overshoot in pressure. Symptoms typically occur 18–36 h after the drug is stopped and are associated with increased sympathetic discharge, as evidenced by elevated plasma and urine concentrations of catecholamines and metabolites. The frequency of occurrence of the withdrawal syndrome is not known, but withdrawal symptoms are likely dose related and more dangerous in patients with poorly controlled hypertension. Rebound hypertension also has been seen after discontinuation of transdermal administration of clonidine (Metz et al., 1987).

Treatment of the withdrawal syndrome depends on the urgency of reducing the arterial blood pressure. In the absence of life-threatening target organ damage, patients can be treated by restoring the use of clonidine. If a more rapid effect is required, *sodium nitroprusside* or a combination of an α and β blocker is appropriate. β Blockers should not be used alone in this setting because they may accentuate the hypertension by allowing unopposed α adrenergic vasoconstriction caused by activation of the sympathetic nervous system and elevated circulating catecholamines.

Because perioperative hypertension has been described in patients in whom clonidine was withdrawn the night before surgery, surgical patients who are being treated with an α_2 adrenergic agonist either should be switched to another drug prior to elective surgery or should receive their morning dose or transdermal clonidine prior to the procedure. All patients who receive one of these drugs should be warned of the potential danger of discontinuing the drug abruptly, and patients suspected of being noncompliant with medications should not be given α_2 adrenergic agonists for hypertension.

Adverse drug interactions with α_2 adrenergic agonists are rare. Diuretics predictably potentiate the hypotensive effect of these drugs. Tricyclic antidepressants may inhibit the antihypertensive effect of clonidine, but the mechanism of this interaction is not known.

Reserpine

Reserpine is an alkaloid extracted from the root of *Rauwolfia serpentina*, a climbing shrub indigenous to India. Ancient Hindu Ayurvedic writings describe medicinal uses of the plant; Sen and Bose described its use in the Indian biomedical literature. However, rauwolfia alkaloids were not used in Western medicine until the mid-1950s. Reserpine was the first drug found to interfere with the function of the sympathetic nervous system in humans, and its use began the modern era of effective pharmacotherapy of hypertension.

Mechanism of Action. Reserpine binds tightly to adrenergic storage vesicles in central and peripheral adrenergic neurons and remains bound for prolonged periods of time. The interaction inhibits the vesicular catecholamine transporter VMAT2, so that nerve endings lose their capacity to concentrate and store NE and dopamine. Catecholamines leak into the cytoplasm, where they are metabolized. Consequently, little or no active transmitter is released from nerve endings, resulting in a pharmacological sympathectomy. Recovery of sympathetic function requires synthesis of new storage vesicles, which takes days to weeks after discontinuation of the drug. Because reserpine depletes amines in the CNS as well as in the peripheral adrenergic neuron, it is probable that its antihypertensive effects are related to both central and peripheral actions.

Pharmacological Effects. Both cardiac output and peripheral vascular resistance are reduced during long-term therapy with reserpine.

ADME. Few data are available on the pharmacokinetic properties of reserpine because of the lack of an assay capable of detecting low concentrations of the drug or its metabolites. Reserpine that is bound to isolated storage vesicles cannot be removed by dialysis, indicating that the binding is not in equilibrium with the surrounding medium. Because of the irreversible nature of reserpine binding, the amount of drug in plasma is unlikely to bear any consistent relationship to drug concentration at the site of action. Free reserpine is entirely metabolized; therefore, none of the parent drug is excreted unchanged.

Toxicity and Precautions. Most adverse effects of reserpine are due to its effect on the CNS. Sedation and inability to concentrate or perform complex tasks are the most common adverse effects. More serious is the occasional psychotic depression that can lead to suicide. Depression usually appears insidiously over many weeks or months and may not be attributed to the drug because of the delayed and gradual onset of symptoms. Reserpine must be discontinued at the first sign of depression. Reserpine-induced depression may last several months after the drug is discontinued. The risk of depression is likely dose related. Depression is uncommon, but not unknown, with doses of 0.25 mg/d or less. The drug should never be given to patients with a history of depression. Other adverse effects include nasal stuffiness and exacerbation of peptic ulcer disease, which is uncommon with small oral doses.

Therapeutic Uses. Reserpine at low doses, in combination with diuretics, is effective in the treatment of hypertension, especially in the elderly. Several weeks are necessary to achieve maximum effect. In elderly patients with isolated systolic hypertension, reserpine (at 0.05 mg/d) was used as an alternative to atenolol together with a diuretic (Perry et al., 2000; SHEP Cooperative Research Group, 1991). However, with the availability of newer drugs that have proven life-prolonging effects and are well tolerated, the use of reserpine has largely diminished, and it is no longer recommended for the treatment of hypertension (Mancia et al., 2013).

Ca^{2+} Channel Blockers

The Ca^{2+} channel–blocking agents are an important group of drugs for the treatment of hypertension. The general pharmacology of these drugs is presented in Chapter 27. The basis for their use in hypertension comes from the understanding that hypertension generally is the result of increased peripheral vascular resistance. Because contraction of vascular smooth muscle is dependent on the free intracellular concentration of Ca^{2+}, inhibition of transmembrane movement of Ca^{2+} through voltage-sensitive Ca^{2+} channels can decrease the total amount of Ca^{2+} that reaches intracellular sites. Indeed, all of the Ca^{2+} channel blockers lower blood pressure by relaxing arteriolar smooth muscle and decreasing peripheral vascular resistance. As a consequence of a decrease in peripheral vascular resistance, the Ca^{2+} channel blockers evoke a baroreceptor reflex–mediated sympathetic discharge. In the case of the dihydropyridines, tachycardia may occur from the adrenergic stimulation of the SA node; this response is generally quite modest except when the drug is administered rapidly. Tachycardia is typically minimal or absent with verapamil and diltiazem because of the direct negative chronotropic effect of these two drugs. Indeed, the concurrent use of a β blocker may magnify negative chronotropic effects of these drugs or cause heart block in susceptible patients. Consequently, the concurrent use of β blockers with either verapamil or diltiazem should be avoided.

The Ca^{2+} channel blockers are among the preferred drugs for the treatment of hypertension, both as monotherapy and in combination with other antihypertensives, because they have a well-documented effect on cardiovascular end points and total mortality. The combination of amlodipine and the ACE inhibitors perindopril proved superior to the combination of the β blocker atenolol and hydrochlorothiazide (Dahlof et al., 2005), and amlodipine was superior to hydrochlorothiazide as the combination partner for the ACEI benazepril (Jamerson et al., 2008).

The Ca^{2+} channel blockers most studied and used for the treatment of hypertension are long-acting dihydropyridines with sufficient 24-h efficacy at once-daily dosing (e.g., amlodipine, felodipine, lercanidipine, and sustained-release formulations of others). Peripheral edema (ankle edema) are the main unwanted effects. Fewer patients appear to experience this harmless, but possibly distracting, side effect with newer compounds such as lercanidipine (Makarounas-Kirchmann et al., 2009), but the commonly used combination with RAS inhibitors has the same effect (Messerli et al., 2000). Immediate-release nifedipine and other short-acting dihydropyridines have no place in the treatment of hypertension. Verapamil and diltiazem also have short half-lives, more cardiac side effects, and a high drug interaction potential (verapamil > diltiazem) and are therefore not first-line antihypertensives.

Compared with other classes of antihypertensive agents, there may be a greater frequency of achieving blood pressure control with Ca^{2+} channel blockers as monotherapy in elderly subjects and in African Americans, population groups in which the low renin status is more prevalent. However, intrasubject variability is more important than relatively small differences between population groups. Ca^{2+} channel blockers are effective in lowering blood pressure and decreasing cardiovascular events in the elderly with isolated systolic hypertension (Staessen et al., 1997) and may be a preferred treatment in these patients.

Inhibitors of the Renin-Angiotensin System

Angiotensin II is an important regulator of cardiovascular function (see Chapter 26). The capacity to reduce the effects of AngII with pharmacological agents has been an important advance in the treatment of hypertension and its sequelae. Chapter 26 presents the basic physiology of the RAS and the pharmacology of inhibitors of the RAS. Table 26–2 summarizes the effects of a variety of antihypertensive agents on components of the RAS and warrants careful study.

Angiotensin-Converting Enzyme Inhibitors

The ability to reduce levels of AngII with orally effective ACE inhibitors represents an important advance in the treatment of hypertension. Captopril was the first such agent to be developed for the treatment of hypertension. Since then, enalapril, lisinopril, quinapril, ramipril, benazepril, moexipril, fosinopril, trandolapril, and perindopril have become available. These drugs are useful for the treatment of hypertension because of their efficacy and a favorable adverse effect profile that enhances patient adherence. Chapter 26 presents the pharmacology of ACE inhibitors in detail.

The ACE inhibitors appear to confer a special advantage in the treatment of patients with diabetes, slowing the development and progression of diabetic glomerulopathy. They also are effective in slowing the progression of other forms of chronic renal disease, such as glomerulosclerosis, which coexists with hypertension in many patients. An ACE inhibitor is the preferred initial agent in these patients. Patients with hypertension and ischemic heart disease are candidates for treatment with ACE inhibitors. Administration of ACE inhibitors in the immediate post-MI period has been shown to improve ventricular function and reduce morbidity and mortality (see Chapter 27).

The endocrine consequences of inhibiting the biosynthesis of AngII are of importance in a number of facets of hypertension treatment. Because ACE inhibitors blunt the rise in aldosterone concentrations in response to Na^+ loss, the normal role of aldosterone to oppose diuretic-induced natriuresis is diminished. Consequently, ACE inhibitors tend to enhance the efficacy of diuretic drugs. This means that even very small doses of diuretics may substantially improve the antihypertensive efficacy of ACE inhibitors; conversely, the use of high doses of diuretics together with ACE inhibitors may lead to excessive reduction in blood pressure and to Na^+ loss in some patients.

Attenuation of aldosterone production by ACE inhibitors also influences K^+ homeostasis; there is a small and clinically unimportant rise in serum K^+ when these agents are used alone in patients with normal renal function. However, substantial retention of K^+ can occur in some patients with renal insufficiency. Furthermore, the potential for developing hyperkalemia should be considered when ACE inhibitors are used with other drugs that can cause K^+ retention, including the K^+-sparing diuretics (amiloride, triamterene, and the MRAs spironolactone and eplerenone), NSAIDs, K^+ supplements, and β blockers. Some patients with diabetic nephropathy may be at greater risk of hyperkalemia.

There are several cautions in the use of ACE inhibitors in patients with hypertension. Cough is a common (~5%) adverse effect and a reason to switch to AT_1 receptor blockers. Angioedema is a rare but serious and potentially fatal adverse effect of the ACE inhibitors. Patients starting treatment with these drugs should be explicitly warned to discontinue their use with the advent of any signs of angioedema. Due to the risk of severe fetal adverse effects, ACE inhibitors are contraindicated during pregnancy, a fact that should be communicated to women of childbearing age.

In most patients, there is little or no appreciable change in glomerular filtration rate following the administration of ACE inhibitors. However, in renovascular hypertension, the glomerular filtration rate is generally maintained as the result of increased resistance in the postglomerular arteriole caused by AngII. Accordingly, in patients with bilateral renal artery stenosis or stenosis in a sole kidney, the administration of an ACE inhibitor will reduce the filtration fraction and cause a substantial reduction in glomerular filtration rate. In some patients with preexisting renal disease, the glomerular filtration may decrease with an ACE inhibitor. Thus, it should be kept in mind that ACE inhibitors, while inhibiting the progression of chronic kidney disease, carry a risk of reversible drug-induced impairment of glomerular filtration. Serum creatinine levels and K^+ should therefore be monitored in the first weeks after establishing therapy. Increases of serum creatinine of greater than 20% predict the presence of renal artery stenosis (van de Ven et al., 1998) and are a reason to discontinue the treatment with ACE inhibitors.

The ACE inhibitors lower the blood pressure to some extent in most patients with hypertension. Following the initial dose of an ACE inhibitor, there may be a considerable fall in blood pressure in some patients; this response to the initial dose is a function of plasma renin activity prior to treatment. The potential for a large initial drop in blood pressure is the reason for using a low dose to initiate therapy, especially in patients who may have a very active RAS supporting blood pressure, such as patients with diuretic-induced volume contraction or congestive heart failure. It should also be realized that, generally, no reason exists for normalizing blood pressure in a few days in patients with a lifelong disease. Attempts to do so increase the frequency of side effects and decrease compliance. With continuing treatment, there usually is a progressive fall in blood pressure that in most patients does not reach a maximum for several weeks. The blood pressure seen during chronic treatment is not strongly correlated with the pretreatment plasma renin activity. Young and middle-aged Caucasian patients have a higher probability of responding to ACE inhibitors; elderly African American patients as a group are more resistant to the hypotensive effect of these drugs. While most ACE inhibitors are approved for once-daily dosing for hypertension, a significant fraction of patients has a response that lasts less than 24 h and may require twice-daily dosing for adequate control of blood pressure (e.g., enalapril, ramipril). Captopril, with its very short duration of action, is not a good choice in the treatment of hypertension.

AT_1 Receptor Blockers

The importance of AngII in regulating cardiovascular function has led to the development of nonpeptide antagonists of the AT_1 subtype of AngII receptor. Losartan, candesartan, irbesartan, valsartan, telmisartan, olmesartan, and eprosartan have been approved for the treatment of hypertension. The pharmacology of AT_1 receptor blockers is presented in detail in Chapter 26. By antagonizing the effects of AngII, these agents relax smooth muscle and thereby promote vasodilation, increase renal salt and water excretion, reduce plasma volume, and decrease cellular hypertrophy. Given the central role of AT_1 receptors for the action of AngII, it is not surprising that AT_1 receptor blockers have the same pharmacological profile as ACE inhibitors with one notable exception. AT_1 receptor blockers do not inhibit the ACE-mediated degradation of bradykinin and substance P and thereby cause no cough.

Initial hopes for superiority of AT_1 receptor blockers over ACE inhibitors have not been fulfilled. They were based on the idea that the AT_2

subtype elicits beneficial effects of AngII (e.g., antigrowth and antiproliferative responses). Because the AT_1 receptor mediates feedback inhibition of renin release, renin and AngII concentrations are increased during AT_1 receptor antagonism, leading to increased stimulation of uninhibited AT_2 receptors. Despite considerable interest, not much evidence supports any extra benefit from AT_1 blockade versus ACE inhibition, and attempts to show greater reductions in cardiovascular events by AT_1 receptor blockers or by the combination of an AT_1 receptor blocker plus an ACE inhibitor over ACE inhibitor alone failed. ON-TARGET, one of the largest studies to date in patients with high vascular risk (70% hypertension) showed that telmisartan caused less cough and angioedema than ramipril (1.1% vs. 4.2%, and 0.1% vs. 0.3%) but had identical efficacy. The combination, although not more efficacious, was associated with greater worsening of renal function (13.5% vs. 10.2%), hypotension, and syncope (Yusuf et al., 2008).

Therapeutic Uses

The AT_1 receptor blockers have a sufficient 24-h effect at once-daily dosing (except losartan). The full effect of AT_1 receptor blockers on blood pressure typically is not observed until about 4 weeks after the initiation of therapy. If blood pressure is not controlled by an AT_1 receptor blocker alone, a second drug acting by a different mechanism (e.g., a diuretic or Ca^{2+} channel blocker) may be added. The combination of an ACE inhibitor and an AT_1 receptor blocker is not recommended for the treatment of hypertension.

Adverse Effects and Precautions

Adverse effects of ACE inhibitors that result from inhibiting AngII-related functions (see previous discussion and Chapter 26) also occur with AT_1 receptor blockers. These include hypotension, hyperkalemia, and reduced renal function, including that associated with bilateral renal artery stenosis and stenosis in the artery of a solitary kidney. Hypotension is most likely to occur in patients in whom the blood pressure is highly dependent on AngII, including those with volume depletion (e.g., with diuretics), renovascular hypertension, cardiac failure, and cirrhosis; in such patients, initiation of treatment with low doses and attention to blood volume are essential. Hyperkalemia may occur in conjunction with other factors that alter K^+ homeostasis, such as renal insufficiency, ingestion of excess K^+, and the use of drugs that promote K^+ retention. Cough and angioedema occur rarely. ACE inhibitors and AT_1 receptor blockers should not be administered during pregnancy and should be discontinued as soon as pregnancy is detected.

Direct Renin Inhibitors

Aliskiren, the first orally effective direct renin inhibitor is FDA-approved for the treatment of hypertension. The detailed pharmacology of aliskiren is covered in Chapter 26. Aliskiren is an effective antihypertensive drug but has not been studied sufficiently in monotherapy of hypertension. A large study comparing a placebo or aliskiren added to a background of an ARB or an ACE inhibitor was stopped prematurely for a trend toward increased cardiovascular events in the aliskiren treatment group (McMurray et al., 2012). The combination also induced more renal worsening, hypotension, and hyperkalemia. This mirrors previous studies with ARB/ACE inhibitor combinations and indicates that complete blockade of the RAS system achieves more harm than benefit.

Pharmacology

The initial renin inhibitors were peptide analogues of sequences either in renin itself or included the renin cleavage site in angiotensinogen. While effective in inhibiting renin and lowering blood pressure, these peptide analogues were effective only parenterally. However, aliskiren is effective following oral administration; it directly and competitively inhibits the catalytic activity of renin, leading to diminished production of AngI, AngII, and aldosterone—with a resulting fall in blood pressure. Aliskiren along with ACE inhibitors and AT_1 receptor blockers lead to an adaptive increase in the plasma concentrations of renin; however, because aliskiren inhibits renin activity, plasma renin activity does not increase as occurs with these other classes of drugs (Table 26–2). Nevertheless, the aldosterone escape known from ACE inhibitors and AT_1 receptor blockers has also been observed under continuous treatment with aliskiren (Bomback et al., 2012).

ADME

Aliskiren is poorly absorbed, with an oral bioavailability of less than 3%. Taking the drug with a high-fat meal may substantially decrease plasma concentrations. Aliskiren has an elimination $t_{1/2}$ of at least 24 h. Elimination of the drug may be primarily through hepatobiliary excretion with limited metabolism via CYP3A4.

Therapeutic Uses

Given the unclear effectiveness and safety of aliskiren monotherapy, the place of this drug in the treatment of hypertension remains clouded. The combination of aliskiren with other RAS inhibitors is contraindicated, and the European Society of Cardiology guideline does not recommend its use (Mancia et al., 2013).

Toxicity and Precautions

Aliskiren is generally well tolerated. Diarrhea may occur, especially at higher-than-recommended doses. The incidence of cough may be higher than for placebo but substantially less than found with ACE inhibitors. Aliskiren has been associated with several cases of angioedema in clinical trials (Frampton and Curran, 2007). Drugs acting on the RAS may damage the fetus and should not be used in pregnant women.

Vasodilators

Hydralazine

Hydralazine (1-hydrazinophthalazine) was one of the first orally active antihypertensive drugs to be marketed in the U.S.; however, the drug initially was used infrequently because of tachycardia and tachyphylaxis. With a better understanding of the compensatory cardiovascular responses that accompany use of arteriolar vasodilators, hydralazine was combined with sympatholytic agents and diuretics with greater therapeutic success. Nonetheless, its role in the treatment of hypertension has markedly diminished with the introduction of new classes of antihypertensive agents.

Mechanism of Action

Hydralazine directly relaxes arteriolar smooth muscle with little effect on venous smooth muscle. The molecular mechanisms mediating this action are not clear but may ultimately involve a reduction in intracellular Ca^{2+} concentrations. While a variety of changes in cellular signaling pathways are influenced by hydralazine, precise molecular targets that explain its capacity to dilate arteries remain uncertain. Potential mechanisms include inhibition of inositol trisphosphate–induced release of Ca^{2+} from intracellular storage sites, opening of high-conductance Ca^{2+}-activated K^+ channels in smooth muscle cells, and activation of an arachidonic acid, COX, and prostacyclin pathway that would explain sensitivity to NSAIDs (Maille et al., 2016).

Hydralazine-induced vasodilation is associated with powerful stimulation of the sympathetic nervous system, likely due to baroreceptor-mediated reflexes, resulting in increased heart rate and contractility, increased plasma renin activity, and fluid retention. These effects tend to counteract the antihypertensive effect of hydralazine.

Pharmacological Effects

Most of the effects of hydralazine are confined to the cardiovascular system. The decrease in blood pressure after administration of hydralazine is associated with a selective decrease in vascular resistance in the coronary, cerebral, and renal circulations, with a smaller effect in skin and muscle. Because of preferential dilation of arterioles over veins, postural hypotension is not a common problem; hydralazine lowers blood pressure similarly in the supine and upright positions.

ADME

Following oral administration, hydralazine is well absorbed via the GI tract. Hydralazine is *N*-acetylated in the bowel and the liver, contributing to the drug's low bioavailability (16% in fast acetylators and 35% in slow acetylators). The rate of acetylation is genetically determined; about half of the U.S. population acetylates rapidly, and half does so slowly. The acetylated compound is inactive; thus, the dose necessary to produce a systemic effect is larger in fast acetylators. Because the systemic clearance exceeds hepatic blood flow, extrahepatic metabolism must occur. Indeed, hydralazine rapidly combines with circulating α-keto acids to form hydrazones, and the major metabolite recovered from the plasma is hydralazine pyruvic acid hydrazone. This metabolite has a longer $t_{1/2}$ than hydralazine but appears to be relatively inactive. Although the rate of acetylation is an important determinant of the bioavailability of hydralazine, it does not play a role in the systemic elimination of the drug, probably because hepatic clearance is so high that systemic elimination is principally a function of hepatic blood flow. The peak concentration of hydralazine in plasma and the peak hypotensive effect of the drug occur within 30–120 min of ingestion. Although its $t_{1/2}$ in plasma is about 1 h, the hypotensive effect of hydralazine can last as long as 12 h. There is no clear explanation for this discrepancy.

Therapeutic Uses

Hydralazine is no longer a first-line drug in the treatment of hypertension on account of its relatively unfavorable adverse-effect profile. The drug has a role as a combination pill containing isosorbide dinitrate (BiDil) in the treatment of heart failure (see Chapter 29). Hydralazine may have utility in the treatment of some patients with severe hypertension, can be part of evidence-based therapy in patients with congestive heart failure (in combination with nitrates for patients who cannot tolerate ACE inhibitors or AT_1 receptor blockers), and may be useful in the treatment of hypertensive emergencies, especially preeclampsia, in pregnant women. Hydralazine should be used with great caution in elderly patients and in hypertensive patients with CAD because of the possibility of precipitating myocardial ischemia due to reflex tachycardia. The usual oral dosage of hydralazine is 25–100 mg twice daily. Off-label twice-daily administration is as effective as administration four times a day for control of blood pressure, regardless of acetylator phenotype. The maximum recommended dose of hydralazine is 200 mg/d to minimize the risk of drug-induced lupus syndrome.

Toxicity and Precautions

Two types of adverse effects occur after the use of hydralazine. The first, which are extensions of the pharmacological effects of the drug, include headache, nausea, flushing, hypotension, palpitations, tachycardia, dizziness, and angina pectoris. Myocardial ischemia can occur on account of increased O_2 demand induced by the baroreceptor reflex–induced stimulation of the sympathetic nervous system. Following parenteral administration to patients with CAD, the myocardial ischemia may be sufficiently severe and protracted to cause frank MI. For this reason, parenteral administration of hydralazine is not advisable in hypertensive patients with CAD, hypertensive patients with multiple cardiovascular risk factors, or older patients. In addition, if the drug is used alone, there may be salt retention with development of high-output congestive heart failure. When combined with a β blocker and a diuretic, hydralazine is better tolerated, although adverse effects such as headache are still commonly described and may necessitate discontinuation of the drug.

The second type of adverse effect is caused by immunological reactions, of which the drug-induced lupus syndrome is the most common. Administration of hydralazine also can result in an illness that resembles serum sickness, hemolytic anemia, vasculitis, and rapidly progressive glomerulonephritis. The mechanism of these autoimmune reactions is unknown, although it may involve the drug's capacity to inhibit DNA methylation (Arce et al., 2006). The drug-induced lupus syndrome usually occurs after at least 6 months of continuous treatment with hydralazine, and its incidence is related to dose, gender, acetylator phenotype, and race. In one study, after 3 years of treatment with hydralazine, drug-induced lupus occurred in 10% of patients who received 200 mg daily, 5% who received 100 mg daily, and none who received 50 mg daily (Cameron and Ramsay, 1984). The incidence is four times higher in women than in men, and the syndrome is seen more commonly in Caucasians than in African Americans. The rate of conversion to a positive antinuclear antibody test is faster in slow acetylators than in rapid acetylators, suggesting that the native drug or a nonacetylated metabolite is responsible. However, the majority of patients with positive antinuclear antibody tests do not develop the drug-induced lupus syndrome, and hydralazine need not be discontinued unless clinical features (arthralgia, arthritis, and fever) of the syndrome appear. Discontinuation of the drug is all that is necessary for most patients with the hydralazine-induced lupus syndrome, but symptoms may persist in a few patients, and administration of corticosteroids may be necessary.

Hydralazine also can produce a pyridoxine-responsive polyneuropathy. The mechanism appears to be related to the ability of hydralazine to combine with pyridoxine to form a hydrazone. This side effect is unusual with doses of 200 mg/d or less.

K_{ATP} Channel Openers: Minoxidil

The discovery in 1965 of the hypotensive action of minoxidil was a significant advance in the treatment of hypertension; the drug has proven to be efficacious in patients with the most severe and drug-resistant forms of hypertension.

Locus and Mechanism of Action

Minoxidil is not active in vitro but must be metabolized by hepatic sulfotransferase to the active molecule, minoxidil *N-O* sulfate; the formation of this active metabolite is a minor pathway in the metabolic disposition of minoxidil. Minoxidil sulfate relaxes vascular smooth muscle in isolated systems where the parent drug is inactive. Minoxidil sulfate activates the ATP-modulated K^+ channel permitting K^+ efflux, and causes hyperpolarization and relaxation of smooth muscle.

Pharmacological Effects

Minoxidil produces arteriolar vasodilation with essentially no effect on the capacitance vessels; the drug resembles hydralazine and diazoxide in this regard. Minoxidil increases blood flow to skin, skeletal muscle, the GI tract, and the heart more than to the CNS. The disproportionate increase in blood flow to the heart may have a metabolic basis in that administration of minoxidil is associated with a reflex increase in myocardial contractility and in cardiac output. The cardiac output can increase markedly, as much as 3- to 4-fold. The principal determinant of the elevation in cardiac output is the action of minoxidil on peripheral vascular resistance to enhance venous return to the heart; by inference from studies with other drugs, the increased venous return probably results from enhancement of flow in the regional vascular beds, with a fast time constant for venous return to the heart (Ogilvie, 1985). The adrenergically mediated increase in myocardial contractility contributes to the increased cardiac output but is not the predominant causal factor.

The effects of minoxidil on the kidney are complex. Minoxidil is a renal artery vasodilator, but systemic hypotension produced by the drug occasionally can decrease renal blood flow. Renal function usually improves in patients who take minoxidil for the treatment of hypertension, especially if renal dysfunction is secondary to hypertension. Minoxidil is a potent stimulator of renin secretion. This effect is mediated by a combination of renal sympathetic stimulation and activation of the intrinsic renal mechanisms for regulation of renin release.

Discovery of K^+_{ATP} channels in a variety of cell types and in mitochondria is prompting consideration of K^+_{ATP} channel modulators as therapeutic agents in many cardiovascular diseases (Pollesello and Mebazaa, 2004). Minoxidil, similar to other K^+_{ATP} channel openers such as diazoxide, pinacidil, and nicorandil, may have protective effects on the heart during ischemia/reperfusion (Sato et al., 2004). It also promotes the synthesis of vascular elastin in rats (Slove et al., 2013), a potentially interesting therapeutic effect.

ADME

Minoxidil is well absorbed from the GI tract. Although peak concentrations of minoxidil in blood occur 1 h after oral administration, the maximal hypotensive effect of the drug occurs later, possibly because formation of the active metabolite is delayed.

The bulk of the absorbed drug is eliminated as a glucuronide; about 20% is excreted unchanged in the urine. The extent of biotransformation of minoxidil to its active metabolite, minoxidil *N-O* sulfate, has not been evaluated in humans. Minoxidil has a plasma $t_{1/2}$ of 3–4 h, but its duration of action is 24 h and occasionally even longer. It has been proposed that persistence of minoxidil in vascular smooth muscle is responsible for this discrepancy, but without knowledge of the pharmacokinetic properties of the active metabolite, an explanation for the prolonged duration of action cannot be given.

Therapeutic Uses

Systemic minoxidil is best reserved for the treatment of severe hypertension that responds poorly to other antihypertensive medications, especially in male patients with renal insufficiency. Minoxidil has been used successfully in the treatment of hypertension in both adults and children. Minoxidil should never be used alone; it must be given concurrently with a diuretic to avoid fluid retention, with a sympatholytic drug (e.g., β blocker) to control reflex cardiovascular effects and an inhibitor of the RAS to prevent remodeling effects on the heart. The drug usually is administered either once or twice a day, but some patients may require more frequent dosing for adequate control of blood pressure. The initial daily dose of minoxidil may be as little as 1.25 mg, which can be increased gradually to 40 mg in one or two daily doses.

Adverse Effects and Precautions

The adverse effects of minoxidil, which can be severe, fall into three major categories: fluid and salt retention, cardiovascular effects, and hypertrichosis. Retention of salt and water results from increased proximal renal tubular reabsorption, which is secondary to reduced renal perfusion pressure and to reflex stimulation of renal tubular α adrenergic receptors. Similar antinatriuretic effects can be observed with the other arteriolar dilators (e.g., diazoxide and hydralazine). Although administration of minoxidil causes increased secretion of renin and aldosterone, this is not an important mechanism for retention of salt and water in this case. Fluid retention usually can be controlled by the administration of a diuretic. However, thiazides may not be sufficiently efficacious, and it may be necessary to use a loop diuretic, especially if the patient has any degree of renal dysfunction.

The cardiac consequences of the baroreceptor-mediated activation of the sympathetic nervous system during minoxidil therapy are similar to those seen with hydralazine; there is an increase in heart rate, myocardial contractility, and myocardial O_2 consumption. Thus, myocardial ischemia can be induced by minoxidil in patients with CAD. The cardiac sympathetic responses are attenuated by concurrent administration of a β blocker. The adrenergically induced increase in renin secretion also can be ameliorated by a β blocker or an ACE inhibitor, with enhancement of blood pressure control.

The increased cardiac output evoked by minoxidil has particularly adverse consequences in those hypertensive patients who have left ventricular hypertrophy and diastolic dysfunction. Such poorly compliant ventricles respond suboptimally to increased volume loads, with a resulting increase in left ventricular filling pressure. This probably is a major contributor to the increased pulmonary artery pressure seen with minoxidil (and hydralazine) therapy in hypertensive patients and is compounded by the retention of salt and water caused by minoxidil. Cardiac failure can result from minoxidil therapy in such patients; the potential for this complication can be reduced but not prevented by effective diuretic therapy. Pericardial effusion is an uncommon but serious complication of minoxidil. Mild and asymptomatic pericardial effusion is not an indication for discontinuing minoxidil, but the situation should be monitored closely to avoid progression to tamponade. Effusions usually clear when the drug is discontinued but can recur if treatment with minoxidil is resumed.

Flattened and inverted T waves frequently are observed in the electrocardiogram following the initiation of minoxidil treatment. These are not ischemic in origin and are seen with other drugs that activate K^+ channels. In model systems, *pinacidil* is associated with a lowered ventricular fibrillation threshold and increased spontaneous ventricular fibrillation in the ischemic canine heart, and minoxidil causes cardiac antiarrhythmias in the rabbit; whether such findings translate to events in humans is unknown.

Excess hair growth occurs in patients who receive minoxidil for an extended period and is probably a consequence of K^+ channel activation. Growth of hair occurs on the face, back, arms, and legs and is particularly offensive to women. Frequent shaving or depilatory agents can be used to manage this problem. Topical minoxidil is marketed over the counter for the treatment of male pattern baldness and hair thinning and loss on the top of the head in women. The topical use of minoxidil also can cause measurable cardiovascular effects in some individuals.

Other side effects of the drug are rare and include rashes, Stevens-Johnson syndrome, glucose intolerance, serosanguineous bullae, formation of antinuclear antibodies, and thrombocytopenia.

Sodium Nitroprusside

Although sodium nitroprusside has been known since 1850 and its hypotensive effect in humans was described in 1929, its safety and usefulness for the short-term control of severe hypertension were not demonstrated until the mid-1950s. Several investigators subsequently demonstrated that sodium nitroprusside also was effective in improving cardiac function in patients with left ventricular failure (see Chapter 29).

Sodium nitroprusside

Mechanism of Action

Nitroprusside is a nitrovasodilator that acts by releasing NO. NO activates the guanylyl cyclase–cyclic guanosine monophosphate–protein kinase G pathway, leading to vasodilation, mimicking the production of NO by vascular endothelial cells, which is impaired in many hypertensive patients. The mechanism of release of NO from nitroprusside is not clear and likely involves both enzymatic and nonenzymatic pathways. Tolerance develops to *nitroglycerin* but not to nitroprusside. The pharmacology of the organic nitrates, including nitroglycerin, is presented in Chapter 27.

Pharmacological Effects

Nitroprusside dilates both arterioles and venules, and the hemodynamic response to its administration results from a combination of venous pooling and reduced arterial impedance. In subjects with normal left ventricular function, venous pooling affects cardiac output more than does the reduction of afterload; cardiac output tends to fall. In contrast, in patients with severely impaired left ventricular function and diastolic ventricular distention, the reduction of arterial impedance is the predominant effect, leading to a rise in cardiac output (see Chapter 29).

Sodium nitroprusside is a nonselective vasodilator, and regional distribution of blood flow is little affected by the drug. In general, renal blood flow and glomerular filtration are maintained, and plasma renin activity increases. Unlike minoxidil, hydralazine, diazoxide, and other arteriolar vasodilators, sodium nitroprusside usually causes only a modest increase in heart rate and an overall reduction in myocardial O_2 demand.

ADME

Sodium nitroprusside is an unstable molecule that decomposes under strongly alkaline conditions or when exposed to light. The drug must be protected from light and given by continuous intravenous infusion to be effective. Its onset of action is within 30 sec; the peak hypotensive effect occurs within 2 min, and when the infusion of the drug is stopped, the effect disappears within 3 min.

Sodium nitroprusside is available in vials that contain 50 mg. The contents of the vial should be dissolved in 2–3 mL of 5% dextrose in water. Because the compound decomposes in light, only fresh solutions should be used, and the bottle should be covered with an opaque wrapping. The drug must be administered as a controlled continuous infusion, and the patient must be closely observed. The majority of hypertensive patients respond to an infusion of 0.25–1.5 μg/kg/min. Higher infusion rates are necessary to produce controlled hypotension in normotensive patients under surgical anesthesia. Patients who are receiving other antihypertensive medications usually require less nitroprusside to lower blood pressure. If infusion rates of 10 μg/kg/min do not produce adequate reduction of blood pressure within 10 min, the rate of administration of nitroprusside should be reduced to minimize potential toxicity.

The metabolism of nitroprusside by smooth muscle is initiated by its reduction, which is followed by the release of cyanide and then NO. Cyanide is further metabolized by hepatic rhodanase to form thiocyanate, which is eliminated almost entirely in the urine. The mean elimination $t_{1/2}$ for thiocyanate is 3 days in patients with normal renal function and much longer in patients with renal insufficiency.

Therapeutic Uses

Sodium nitroprusside is used primarily to treat hypertensive emergencies but also can be used in situations when short-term reduction of cardiac preload or afterload is desired. Nitroprusside has been used to lower blood pressure during acute aortic dissection; to improve cardiac output in congestive heart failure, especially in hypertensive patients with pulmonary edema that does not respond to other treatment (see Chapter 29); and to decrease myocardial O_2 demand after acute MI. In addition, nitroprusside is used to induce controlled hypotension during anesthesia to reduce bleeding in surgical procedures. In the treatment of acute aortic dissection, it is important to administer a β blocker with nitroprusside because reduction of blood pressure with nitroprusside alone can increase the rate of rise in pressure in the aorta as a result of increased myocardial contractility, thereby enhancing propagation of the dissection.

Toxicity and Precautions

The short-term adverse effects of nitroprusside are due to excessive vasodilation, with hypotension and its consequences. Close monitoring of blood pressure and the use of a continuous variable-rate infusion pump will prevent an excessive hemodynamic response to the drug in the majority of cases.

Less commonly, toxicity may result from conversion of nitroprusside to cyanide and thiocyanate. Toxic accumulation of cyanide leading to severe lactic acidosis usually occurs when sodium nitroprusside is infused at a rate greater than 5 μg/kg/min but also can occur in some patients receiving doses on the order of 2 μg/kg/min for a prolonged period. The limiting factor in the metabolism of cyanide appears to be the availability of sulfur-containing substrates in the body (i.e., mainly thiosulfate). The concomitant administration of sodium thiosulfate can prevent accumulation of cyanide in patients who are receiving higher-than-usual doses of sodium nitroprusside; the efficacy of the drug is unchanged. The risk of thiocyanate toxicity increases when sodium nitroprusside is infused for more than 24–48 h, especially if renal function is impaired. Signs and symptoms of thiocyanate toxicity include anorexia, nausea, fatigue, disorientation, and toxic psychosis. The plasma concentration of thiocyanate should be monitored during prolonged infusions of nitroprusside and should not be allowed to exceed 0.1 mg/mL. Rarely, excessive concentrations of thiocyanate may cause hypothyroidism by inhibiting iodine uptake by the thyroid gland. In patients with renal failure, thiocyanate can be removed readily by hemodialysis.

Nitroprusside can worsen arterial hypoxemia in patients with chronic obstructive pulmonary disease because the drug interferes with hypoxic pulmonary vasoconstriction and therefore promotes mismatching of ventilation with perfusion.

Diazoxide

Diazoxide was used in the treatment of hypertensive emergencies but fell out of favor at least in part due to the risk of marked falls in blood pressure when large bolus doses of the drug were used. Other drugs are now preferred for parenteral administration in the control of hypertension. Diazoxide also is administered orally to treat patients with various forms of hypoglycemia (see Chapter 47).

Nonpharmacological Therapy of Hypertension

Nonpharmacological approaches to the treatment of hypertension may suffice in patients with modestly elevated blood pressure. Such approaches also can augment the effects of antihypertensive drugs in patients with more marked initial elevations in blood pressure. The indications and efficacy of various lifestyle modifications in hypertension were reviewed in recent guidelines (James et al., 2014; Mancia et al., 2013).

- Reduction in body weight for people who are modestly overweight or frankly obese may be useful (Goodpaster et al., 2010).
- Restricting sodium consumption lowers blood pressure in some patients.
- Restriction of ethanol intake to modest levels (daily consumption < 20 g in women, < 40 g in men) may lower blood pressure.
- Increased physical activity improves control of hypertension.
- Renal denervation may be effective in patients with well-defined resistant hypertension (Azizi et al., 2015).
- Bariatric surgery in grossly overweight individuals may normalize blood pressure and increase life expectancy (Sjostrom et al., 2007).

Selection of Antihypertensive Drugs in Individual Patients

Choice of antihypertensive drugs for individual patients may be complex; there are many sources of influence that modify therapeutic decisions. While results derived from randomized, controlled clinical trials are the optimal foundation for rational therapeutics, sorting through the multiplicity of those results and addressing how to apply them to an individual patient can be vexing. While therapeutic guidelines can be useful in reaching appropriate therapeutic decisions, it often is difficult for clinicians to apply guidelines at the point of care, and guidelines often do not provide enough information about recommended drugs. In addition, intense marketing of specific drugs to both clinicians and patients may confound optimal decision-making. Moreover, persuading patients to continue taking drugs that may be expensive for an asymptomatic disease is a challenge. Clinicians may be reluctant to prescribe and patients reluctant to consume the number of drugs that may be necessary to adequately control blood pressure. For these and other reasons, perhaps one-half of patients being treated for hypertension have not achieved therapeutic goals in blood pressure lowering.

Choice of an antihypertensive drug should be driven by the likely benefit in an individual patient, taking into account concomitant diseases such as diabetes mellitus, problematic adverse effects of specific drugs, and cost. The last factor is losing relevance as the most important antihypertensive drug classes (diuretics, Ca^{2+} channel blockers, ACE inhibitors/AT_1 receptor blockers, and β blockers) are out of patent protection and available as low-cost generics.

After a long debate about blood pressure–independent effects of certain antihypertensive drug classes, there is a consensus that blood pressure lowering per se is the most important goal of antihypertensive treatment. This conclusion is based on a number of large comparative prospective trials that, overall, did not show major differences in outcome depending on drug class (reviewed by Mancia et al., 2013). The JNC8 guidelines formulated a preference for an initial therapy with thiazide diuretics, Ca^{2+} channel blockers, and ACE inhibitor/ARB in the general non-black population (including diabetics) and a preference for thiazides and Ca^{2+} channel blockers in black patients (James et al., 2014). The ESC guidelines state that "although meta-analyses occasionally appear, claiming superiority of one class of agents over another for some outcomes, this largely depends on the selection bias of trials, and the largest meta-analyses available do not show clinically relevant differences between drug classes."

TABLE 28–4 ■ ANTIHYPERTENSIVE AGENTS PREFERRED IN SPECIFIC PATIENT POPULATIONS

MEDICAL CONDITION	PREFERRED ANTIHYPERTENSIVE AGENTS
Left ventricular hypertrophy	ACEI, ARB, CCB
Asymptomatic atherosclerosis	CCB
Microalbuminuria	ACEI, ARB
Renal dysfunction	ACEI, ARB
Previous stroke	ACEI, ARB, diuretics
Previous myocardial infarction	ACEI, ARB, BB
Coronary artery disease	ACEI, ARB, BB
Angina pectoris	BB, CCB
Heart failure	ACEI, ARB, BB, diuretics, MRA
Aortic aneurysm	BB
Atrial fibrillation, prevention	ACEI, ARB, BB
Atrial fibrillation, rate control	BB, CCB (nondihydropyridines)
End-stage renal disease, proteinuria	ACEI
Peripheral artery disease	ACEI, CCB
Isolated systolic hypertension	ACEI, ARB, CCB, diuretics
Metabolic syndrome	ACEI, ARB, CCB
Diabetes mellitus	ACEI, ARB, CCB, diuretics
Diabetes mellitus with proteinuria	ACEI, ARB
Hyperaldosteronism	MRA
Pregnancy	BB, CCB, α-methyldopa
Black ethnicity	CCB, diuretics

The drug choices depicted represent a combined view from nine guidelines that differ; thus, the table is, necessarily, a didactic simplification (for details, consult Kjeldsen et al., 2014).

They conclude "that diuretics (including thiazides, chlorthalidone and indapamide), β blockers, calcium channel blockers, ACE inhibitors and AT_1-receptor blockers are all suitable for the initiation and maintenance of antihypertensive treatment, either as monotherapy or in some combinations" (Mancia et al., 2013). Major guideline recommendations around the world have been recently compared (Kjeldsen et al., 2014) and are the basis of recommendations for a compilation of drug choices in Table 28–4.

A number of pharmacological principles should be considered for optimizing the antihypertensive drug regimen.

1. **Pharmacokinetics:** Hypertension is a chronic, often lifelong disease without major symptoms but with serious complications, making compliance to antihypertensive drugs a factor of utmost prognostic importance. Antihypertensives should be chosen that exhibit relatively even plasma concentrations at once-daily dosing, achieving sufficient 24-h control of blood pressure and trough-peak effect ratios greater than 50%. The longer the half-life, the less the variation of plasma concentrations (e.g., chlorthalidone vs. hydrochlorothiazide). Drugs with stable pharmacokinetics, that is, low drug interaction potential and no pharmacogenetic influence, are preferred (e.g., bisoprolol vs. metoprolol).
2. **Drug combinations:** Two-thirds of patients with hypertension require two or more antihypertensives for sufficient blood pressure control (<140/90 mmHg). It is therefore reasonable to start combining drugs at low-to-medium doses instead of increasing the dose of a single drug. Prescribing fixed drug combinations (e.g., a Ca^{2+} channel blocker + ACE inhibitor or an ACE inhibitor + diuretic) improves compliance.
3. **Strength of scientific evidence:** Data from large prospective trials provide a high level of confidence for a beneficial risk-benefit ratio and are a reason to use one drug over another.
4. **Pharmacodynamic considerations:** Although not formally tested in prospective trials, certain drug combinations make more sense than others. Thiazide diuretics increase the antihypertensive actions of all other classes, but their combination with RAS inhibitors makes particular sense as their K^+-sparing effect and thus their main risk are reduced by members of this class.
5. **Adverse drug effects and contraindications:** The major classes of antihypertensives are generally well tolerated and, in placebo-controlled trials, showed rates of adverse effects in the range of placebo with some notable exceptions that need to be taken into consideration when choosing a specific drug for a specific patient (Table 28–5). The rate of adverse effects such as hypotension or bradycardia can be largely reduced by starting antihypertensives at low doses and employing a slow dose-escalation strategy.
6. **Compelling indications:** A number of compelling indications exist for specific antihypertensive agents on account of other serious, underlying cardiovascular disease (Table 28–4). These include heart failure, CAD, post-MI, chronic kidney disease, or diabetes. For example, a hypertensive patient with congestive heart failure ideally should be treated with a diuretic, β blocker, ACE inhibitor/AT_1 receptor blocker, and, in selected patients, spironolactone because of the benefit of these drugs in congestive heart failure, even in the absence of hypertension (see Chapter 29). Similarly, ACE inhibitors/AT_1 receptor blockers should be first-line drugs in the treatment of diabetics with hypertension in view of these drugs' well-established benefits in diabetic nephropathy.
7. **Comorbidities:** Some patients have other diseases that could influence the choice of antihypertensive drugs. For example, a hypertensive patient with symptomatic benign prostatic hyperplasia might benefit from having an α_1 blocker as part of his therapeutic program because α_1 blockers are efficacious in both diseases. Similarly, a patient with recurrent migraine attacks might particularly benefit from use of a β blocker because a number of drugs in this class are efficacious in preventing migraine attacks. Women with a high risk of osteoporosis may benefit from the Ca^{2+}-increasing effect of thiazide diuretics. On the other hand, in pregnant hypertensives, some drugs that are otherwise little used (e.g., methyldopa) may be preferred and popular drugs (e.g., ACE inhibitors) need to be avoided on account of concerns about safety.
8. **Second- and third-line hypertensives:** In the vast majority of cases, hypertension can well be controlled by antihypertensives of the five major classes with or without spironolactone at low doses. However, patients with chronic kidney disease often require the additional use of drugs such as hydralazine or minoxidil. The place of clonidine/moxonidine or α_1 blockers in the treatment of hypertension is not well defined.

Acute Antihypertensive Treatment

The considerations mentioned apply to patients with hypertension who need treatment to reduce long-term risk, not patients in immediately life-threatening settings due to hypertension. While there are limited clinical trial data, clinical judgment favors rapidly lowering blood pressure in patients with life-threatening complications of hypertension, such as encephalopathy or pulmonary edema due to severe hypertension. However, rapid reduction in blood pressure has considerable risks for the patients; if blood pressure is decreased too quickly or extensively, cerebral blood flow may diminish due to adaptations in the cerebral circulation that protect the brain from the sequelae of very high blood pressures. The temptation to treat patients merely on the basis of increased blood pressure should be resisted. Appropriate therapeutic decisions need to encompass how well a patient's major organs are reacting to the very high blood pressures. While many drugs have been used parenterally to rapidly decrease blood pressure in emergencies (including nitroprusside, enalaprilat, esmolol, fenoldopam, labetalol, clevidipine and nicardipine, hydralazine, and phentolamine), the clinical

TABLE 28–5 ■ COMPELLING AND POSSIBLE CONTRAINDICATIONS[a] TO ANTIHYPERTENSIVE DRUGS

DRUG CLASS	COMPELLING	POSSIBLE CONTRAINDICATION/PRECAUTION
Diuretics (thiazides)	Gout	Metabolic syndrome Glucose intolerance Pregnancy Hypercalcemia Hypokalemia Erectile dysfunction
Mineralocorticoid receptor antagonists (MRA)	Hyperkalemia Serum creatinine >2.5 mg/dL in men, >2.0 mg/dL in women)	Situations associated with higher risk of hyperkalemia (ACEI, ARB, diabetes)
ACE inhibitors	Pregnancy Angioneurotic edema Hyperkalemia Bilateral renal artery stenosis	Women with child-bearing potential
Angiotensin receptor blockers	Pregnancy Hyperkalemia Bilateral renal artery stenosis	Women with child-bearing potential
Ca^{2+} channel blockers (dihydropyridines)		Tachycardia/arrhythmia Heart failure
Ca^{2+} channel blockers (verapamil, diltiazem)	AV block (grade 2-3) Severe LV dysfunction Heart failure	Co-medication with CYP3A4- or Pgp–dependent drugs (e.g. statins, digoxin)
β Blockers	Asthma AV block (grade 2-3)	Metabolic syndrome Glucose intolerance Athletes and physically active patients Chronic obstructive lung disease Psoriasis Depression
α Blockers	Heart failure	
Central sympatholytic drugs	Depression AV block (grade 2-3)	Erectile dysfunction Xerostomia

[a]*Possible contraindications and precautions* noted in column 3 are not formal contraindications, but rather patient characteristics that should be considered on an individual basis and that may mitigate against use of a class of drugs (e.g., metabolic syndrome and glucose intolerance for diuretics and β blockers). Similarly, some patients with chronic obstructive lung disease can be treated with β_1 blockers without deterioration of lung function, whereas other patients may experience significant bronchoconstriction with β blockers.

significance of differing actions of many of these drugs in this setting is largely unknown (Perez et al., 2009).

Resistant Hypertension

Some patients with hypertension fail to respond to recommended antihypertensive treatments. There are many potential explanations. To achieve stringent control of hypertension, many patients require two, three, or four appropriately selected drugs used at optimal doses. Exhibiting *an abundance of caution* and *therapeutic inertia*, clinicians may be reluctant to prescribe sufficient numbers of medications that exploit the drugs' full dose-response curves; conversely, patients may not adhere to the recommended pharmacological regimen. Sometimes, multiple drugs in the same therapeutic class that act by the same mechanism are combined; that is generally not a rational approach. Excess salt intake and the tendency of some antihypertensive drugs, especially vasodilators, to promote salt retention may mitigate falls in blood pressure; consequently, inadequate diuretic treatment commonly is found in patients with resistant hypertension. A relevant fraction of patients with resistant hypertension has primary hyperaldosteronism and benefits from the addition of daily spironolactone at 25–50 mg (Williams et al., 2015). Patients may take prescription drugs, over-the-counter drugs, or herbal preparations that oppose the actions of antihypertensive drugs (e.g., NSAIDs, sympathomimetic decongestants, cyclosporine, erythropoietin, ephedra [also called ma huang], or licorice). Illicit drugs such as cocaine and amphetamines may raise blood pressure. The physician must inquire about a patient's other medications and supplements and individualize the antihypertensive regimen.

Acknowledgment: *Thomas Michel and Brian B. Hoffman contributed to this chapter in recent editions of this book. We have retained some of their text in the current edition.*

Bibliography

ALLHAT Officers. Major outcomes in high-risk hypertensive patients randomized to angiotensin-converting enzyme inhibitor or calcium channel blocker vs. diuretic: the Antihypertensive and Lipid-Lowering Treatment to Prevent Heart Attack Trial (ALLHAT). *JAMA*, **2002**, *288*:2981–2997.

Arce C, et al. Hydralazine target: from blood vessels to the epigenome. *J Transl Med*, **2006**, *4*:10.

Azizi M, et al. Optimum and stepped care standardised antihypertensive treatment with or without renal denervation for resistant hypertension (DENERHTN): a multicentre, open-label, randomised controlled trial. *Lancet*, **2015**, *385*:1957–1965.

Bomback AS, et al. Aldosterone breakthrough during aliskiren, valsartan, and combination (aliskiren + valsartan) therapy. *J Am Soc Hypertens*, **2012**, *6*:338–345.

Calhoun DA, et al. Hyperaldosteronism among black and white subjects

Drug Facts for Your Personal Formulary: *Antihypertensives*

Antihypertensive Drug	Therapeutic Uses	Major Toxicity and Clinical Pearls
Diuretics		
Thiazide type Chlorothiazide Hydrochlorothiazide ***Thiazide-like*** Chlorthalidone Indapamide Metolazone	• Hypertension • Edema associated with HF, liver cirrhosis, chronic kidney disease, nephrotic syndrome • Nephrogenic diabetes insipidus • Kidney stones caused by Ca^{2+} crystals	• First choice for treating HTN • Chlorthalidone may be superior to hydrochlorothiazide in HTN • Lose efficacy at GFR < 30–40 mL/min (exceptions: indapamide, metolazone) • Potentiate effect of loop diuretics in HF (sequential tubular blockade) • Risk of hypokalemia and arrhythmia when combined with QT-prolonging drugs • Combine with ACEI/ARB or K+-sparing diuretic/MRA to prevent hypokalemia
Loop diuretics Bumetanide Furosemide Torsemide	• Acute pulmonary edema • Edema associated with HF, liver cirrhosis, chronic kidney disease, nephrotic syndrome • Hyponatremia • Hypercalcemia • Hypertension	• Not first choice for treating HTN with normal renal function: action too short and followed by rebound • Indicated acutely in malignant HTN and GFR < 30–40 mL/min • Torsemide may be superior to furosemide in HF • Risk of hypokalemia and arrhythmia when combined with QT-prolonging drugs
Sympatholytic Drugs		
β_1 Blockers Atenolol Bisoprolol Metoprolol Nebivolol Many others	• Hypertension • Heart failure (bisoprolol, metoprolol, nebivolol) • Widely used for other indications (angina, prevention of arrhythmias, rate control in atrial fibrillation, migraine, etc.)	• Role as first choice in the treatment of HTN debated; clear indication for angina, HF, atrial fibrillation, etc. • Bradycardia and AV block • Bronchospasm, peripheral vasoconstriction • Worsening of *acute* heart failure • Depression • Worsening of psoriasis • Polymorphic CYP2D6 metabolism (metoprolol) • Nebivolol NO-mediated vasodilation
Nonselective β blocker Propranolol	• Hypertension • Migraine	• Not first choice for treating HTN • Unwanted effects via blockade of β_2 receptors
α_1 Blockers Alfuzosin Doxazosin Prazosin Tamsulosin Silodosin	• Benign prostate hyperplasia • Hypertension	• Not first choice for treating HTN • Higher rate of HF development (?) • Tachyphylaxis • Phenoxybenzamine (irreversible α_1/α_2 blockade) used in pheochromocytoma
α_1 and β blockers Carvedilol Labetalol	• Hypertension • Heart failure (carvedilol)	• β blocker of choice in patients with peripheral artery disease • Among first choices for treating HF • Labetalol first choice for HTN in pregnancy
Central sympatholytic drugs Methyldopa Clonidine/moxonidine Reserpine Guanfacine	• Hypertension	• Not first choice in treating HTN • Fatigue, depression • Nasal congestion
Ca^{2+} Channel Blockers		
Dihydropyridines Amlodipine, felodipine Nifedipine Clevidipine, isradipine Lercanidipine, nitrendipine ***Others*** Diltiazem, verapamil	• Hypertension • Angina • Rate control in atrial fibrillation (verapamil, diltiazem)	• Extended-release, long-acting dihydropyridines among first choice in HTN • Diltiazem and verapamil: only if effects on heart rate and AV conduction are wanted, not in combination with β blockers; beware CYP3A4-mediated drug interactions
Inhibitors of the Renin-Angiotensin System		
ACE inhibitors Benazepril Captopril Enalapril Lisinopril Quinapril Ramipril Moexipril Fosinopril Trandolapril Perindopril	• Hypertension • Heart failure • Diabetic nephropathy	• Among first choice for treating HTN • Short-acting captopril only for initiation of therapy; enalapril and ramipril twice daily • Cough in 5%–10% of patients, angioedema • Hypotension, hyperkalemia, skin rash, neutropenia, anemia, fetopathic syndrome • Contraindications: pregnancy, renal artery stenosis; caution in patients with impaired renal function or hypovolemia • Fosinopril: hepatic and renal elimination, thus eliminated in patients with HF and low renal perfusion

Drug Facts for Your Personal Formulary: *Antihypertensives (continued)*

Antihypertensive Drug	Therapeutic Uses	Major Toxicity and Clinical Pearls
Inhibitors of the Renin-Angiotensin System		
Angiotensin receptor blockers Candesartan Eprosartan Irbesartan Losartan Olmesartan Telmisartan Valsartan Azilsartan	• Hypertension • Heart failure • Diabetic nephropathy	• Same as ACEI, less cough or angioedema • No evidence for superiority over ACEI • In combination with ACEI, more harm than benefit • Contraindicated in pregnancy
Direct renin inhibitors Aliskiren	• Hypertension	• Therapeutic value unclear; no evidence for superiority over ACEIs or ARBs • Combination with RAS inhibitors contraindicated
Vasodilators		
Hydralazine	• Hypertension • Heart failure in African Americans (fixed combination with ISDN)	• Not first choice in treating HTN • Adverse effects: headache, nausea, flushing, hypotension, palpitations, tachycardia, dizziness, and angina pectoris; generally combined with β blocker to reduce baroreceptor reflex effects • Use cautiously in patients with CAD • Lupus syndrome at high doses
Minoxidil	• Hypertension • Alopecia	• Reserve antihypertensive in patients with renal insufficiency • Water retention, tachycardia, angina, pericardial effusion • Use in combination with diuretic, β blocker, and RAS inhibitor • Hypertrichosis
Sodium nitroprusside	• Hypertensive emergencies	• Only short-term intravenously • Adverse effect: hypotension • Cyanide intoxication

with resistant hypertension. *Hypertension*, **2002**, *40*:892–896.

Cameron HA, Ramsay LE. The lupus syndrome induced by hydralazine: a common complication with low dose treatment. *Br Med J (Clin Res Ed)*, **1984**, *289*:410–412.

Dahlof B, et al. Morbidity and mortality in the Swedish Trial in Old Patients with Hypertension (STOP-Hypertension). *Lancet*, **1991**, *338*:1281–1285.

Dahlof B, et al. Prevention of cardiovascular events with an antihypertensive regimen of amlodipine adding perindopril as required versus atenolol adding bendroflumethiazide as required, in the Anglo-Scandinavian Cardiac Outcomes Trial-Blood Pressure Lowering Arm (ASCOT-BPLA): a multicentre randomised controlled trial. *Lancet*, **2005**, *366*:895–906.

Davis BR, et al. Role of diuretics in the prevention of heart failure: the Antihypertensive and Lipid-Lowering Treatment to Prevent Heart Attack Trial. *Circulation*, **2006**, *113*:2201–2210.

Ernst ME, et al. Comparative antihypertensive effects of hydrochlorothiazide and chlorthalidone on ambulatory and office blood pressure. *Hypertension*, **2006**, *47*:352–358.

Frampton JE, Curran MP. Aliskiren: a review of its use in the management of hypertension. *Drugs*, **2007**, *67*:1767–1792.

Franklin SS. Is there a preferred antihypertensive therapy for isolated systolic hypertension and reduced arterial compliance? *Curr Hypertens Rep*, **2000**, *2*:253–259.

Giannopoulos G, et al. Central sympathetic inhibition to reduce postablation atrial fibrillation recurrences in hypertensive patients: a randomized, controlled study. *Circulation*, **2014**, *130*:1346–1352.

Go AS, et al. An effective approach to high blood pressure control: a science advisory from the American Heart Association, the American College of Cardiology, and the Centers for Disease Control and Prevention. *Hypertension*, **2014**, *63*:878–885.

Goodpaster BH, et al. Effects of diet and physical activity interventions on weight loss and cardiometabolic risk factors in severely obese adults: a randomized trial. *JAMA*, **2010**, *304*:1795–1802.

Jaffe MG, et al. Improved blood pressure control associated with a large-scale hypertension program. *JAMA*, **2013**, *310*:699–705.

Jamerson K, et al. Benazepril plus amlodipine or hydrochlorothiazide for hypertension in high-risk patients. *N Engl J Med*, **2008**, *359*:2417–2428.

James PA, et al. 2014 evidence-based guideline for the management of high blood pressure in adults: report from the panel members appointed to the Eighth Joint National Committee (JNC 8). *JAMA*, **2014**, *311*:507–520.

Ji W, et al. Rare independent mutations in renal salt handling genes contribute to blood pressure variation. *Nat Genet*, **2008**, *40*:592–599.

Kjeldsen S, et al. Updated national and international hypertension guidelines: a review of current recommendations. *Drugs*, **2014**, *74*:2033–2051.

Lacourciere Y, et al. Antihypertensive effects of amlodipine and hydrochlorothiazide in elderly patients with ambulatory hypertension. *Am J Hypertens*, **1995**, *8*:1154–1159.

Law MR, et al. Use of blood pressure lowering drugs in the prevention of cardiovascular disease: meta-analysis of 147 randomised trials in the context of expectations from prospective epidemiological studies. *Brit Med J*, *338*:b1665.

Lindholm LH, et al. Should beta blockers remain first choice in the treatment of primary hypertension? A meta-analysis. *Lancet*, **2005**, *366*:1545–1553.

MacMillan LB, et al. Central hypotensive effects of the alpha2a-adrenergic receptor subtype. *Science*, **1996**, *273*:801–803.

Magee LA, et al. Do labetalol and methyldopa have different effects on pregnancy outcome? Analysis of data from the Control of Hypertension In Pregnancy Study (CHIPS) trial. *BJOG*, **2016**, *123*:1143–1151.

Maille N, et al. Mechanism of hydralazine-induced relaxation in resistance arteries during pregnancy: hydralazine induces vasodilation via a prostacyclin pathway. *Vascul Pharmacol*, **2016**, *78*:36–42.

Makarounas-Kirchmann K, et al. Results of a meta-analysis comparing the tolerability of lercanidipine and other dihydropyridine calcium channel blockers. *Clin Ther*, **2009**, *31*:1652–1663.

Mancia G, et al. 2013 ESH/ESC guidelines for the management of arterial hypertension: the Task Force for the Management of Arterial Hypertension of the European Society of Hypertension (ESH) and of the European Society of Cardiology (ESC). *Eur Heart J*, **2013**, *34*:2159–2219.

McMurray JJ, et al. Aliskiren, ALTITUDE, and the implications for ATMOSPHERE. *Eur J Heart Fail*, **2012**, *14*:341–343.

Messerli FH, et al. Comparison of efficacy and side effects of combination therapy of angiotensin-converting enzyme inhibitor (benazepril) with calcium antagonist (either nifedipine or amlodipine) versus high-dose calcium antagonist monotherapy for systemic hypertension. *Am J Cardiol*, **2000**, *86*:1182–1187.

Metz S, et al. Rebound hypertension after discontinuation of transdermal clonidine therapy. *Am J Med*, **1987**, *82*:17–19.

Ogilvie RI. Comparative effects of vasodilator drugs on flow distribution and venous return. *Can J Physiol Pharmacol*, **1985**, *63*:1345–1355.

Pastor-Barriuso R, et al. Systolic blood pressure, diastolic blood pressure, and pulse pressure: an evaluation of their joint effect on mortality. *Ann Intern Med*, **2003**, *139*:731–739.

Pedersen ME, Cockcroft JR. The latest generation of beta-blockers: new pharmacologic properties. *Curr Hypertens Rep*, **2006**, *8*:279–286.

Perez MI, et al. Effect of early treatment with anti-hypertensive drugs on short and long-term mortality in patients with an acute cardiovascular event. *Cochrane Database Syst Rev*, **2009**, (4):CD006743.

Perry HM Jr, et al. Effect of treating isolated systolic hypertension on the risk of developing various types and subtypes of stroke: the Systolic Hypertension in the Elderly Program (SHEP). *JAMA*, **2000**, *284*:465–471.

Pezhouman A, et al. Molecular basis of hypokalemia-induced ventricular fibrillation. *Circulation*, **2015**, *132*:1528–1537.

Pollesello P, Mebazza A. ATP-depenedent potassium channels as key targets for the treatment of myocardial and vascular dysfunction. *Curr Opin Crit Care*, **2004**, *10*:436–441.

Ramsay LE, et al. Diuretic treatment of resistant hypertension. *Br Med J*, **1980**, *281*:1101–1103.

Rau T, et al. Impact of the CYP2D6 genotype on the clinical effects of metoprolol: a prospective longitudinal study. *Clin Pharmacol Ther*, **2009**, *85*:269–272.

Rosendorff C, et al. Treatment of hypertension with coronary artery disease: a scientific statement from the American Heart Association, American College of Cardiology, and American Society of Hypertension. *Circulation*, *131*:e435–e470.

Sato T, et al. Minoxidil opens mitochondrial K(ATP) channels and confers cardioprotection. *Br J Pharmacol*, **2004**, *141*:360–366.

SHEP Cooperative Research Group. Prevention of stroke by antihypertensive drug treatment in older persons with isolated systolic hypertension. Final results of the Systolic Hypertension in the Elderly Program (SHEP). *JAMA*, **1991**, *265*:3255–3264.

Siscovick DS, et al. Diuretic therapy for hypertension and the risk of primary cardiac arrest. *N Engl J Med*, **1994**, *330*:1852–1857.

Sjostrom L, et al. Effects of bariatric surgery on mortality in Swedish obese subjects. *N Engl J Med*, **2007**, *357*:741–752.

Slove S, et al. Potassium channel openers increase aortic elastic fiber formation and reverse the genetically determined elastin deficit in the BN rat. *Hypertension*, **2013**, *62*:794–801.

SPRINT Research group. A randomized trial of intensive versus standard blood-pressure control. *N Engl J Med*, **2015**, *373*:2103–2116.

Staessen JA, et al. Randomised double-blind comparison of placebo and active treatment for older patients with isolated systolic hypertension. The Systolic Hypertension in Europe (Syst-Eur) Trial Investigators. *Lancet*, **1997**, *350*:757–764.

van de Ven PJ, et al. Angiotensin converting enzyme inhibitor-induced renal dysfunction in atherosclerotic renovascular disease. *Kidney Int*, **1998**, *53*:986–993.

Vlasses PH, et al. Comparative antihypertensive effects of enalapril maleate and hydrochlorothiazide, alone and in combination. *J Clin Pharmacol*, **1983**, *23*:227–233.

Williams B, et al. Differential impact of blood pressure-lowering drugs on central aortic pressure and clinical outcomes: principal results of the Conduit Artery Function Evaluation (CAFE) study. *Circulation*, **2006**, *113*:1213–1225.

Williams B, et al. Spironolactone versus placebo, bisoprolol, and doxazosin to determine the optimal treatment for drug-resistant hypertension (PATHWAY-2): a randomised, double-blind, crossover trial. *Lancet*, **2015**, *386*:2059–2068.

Yang T, Roden DM. Extracellular potassium modulation of drug block of IKr. Implications for torsade de pointes and reverse use-dependence. *Circulation*, **1996**, *93*:407–411.

Yusuf S, et al. Telmisartan, ramipril, or both in patients at high risk for vascular events. *N Engl J Med*, **2008**, *358*:1547–1559.

Therapy of Heart Failure

Thomas Eschenhagen

第二十九章　心力衰竭的治疗

中文导读

本章主要介绍：心力衰竭的病理生理学，包括心力衰竭的定义、多种心脏疾病的共同终末途径、病理生理机制、保留射血分数的心力衰竭、心力衰竭分期、心力衰竭的预防和治疗；药物治疗慢性收缩性心力衰竭（B期和C期），包括治疗原则Ⅰ（神经体液调节）、治疗原则Ⅱ（预负荷减少）、治疗原则Ⅲ（后负荷减少）、治疗原则Ⅳ（增加心肌收缩力）和治疗原则Ⅴ（心率降低）；急性失代偿性心力衰竭的药物治疗，包括利尿药、血管舒张药、正性肌力药、肌丝钙敏化药（左西孟旦和匹莫苯丹）、用于心力衰竭的其他药物、标准联合治疗；心力衰竭药物研发的经验教训，包括失败药物的教训、治疗急性心力衰竭的教训、最新进展和新方法。

Abbreviations

ACC: American College of Cardiology
ACE: angiotensin-converting enzyme
ACEI: angiotensin-converting enzyme inhibitor
ACh: acetylcholine
ADH: antidiuretic hormone (vasopressin)
ADR: adverse drug reaction
AF: atrial fibrillation
AHA: American Heart Association
AngII: angiotensin II
ANP: atrial natriuretic peptide
ARB: AT_1 angiotensin receptor antagonist (blocker)
ARNI: angiotensin receptor/neprilysin inhibitor
AV: atrioventricular
AVP: arginine vasopressin
BB: β blocker
BNP: brain-type natriuretic peptide
CAD: coronary artery disease
CCB: calcium channel blocker
CG: cardiac glycoside
CHF: congestive heart failure
CM: cardiomyopathy
CNP: C-type natriuretic peptide
COX: cyclooxygenase
CPT1: Carnitine palmitoyltransferase 1
CRT: cardiac resynchronization therapy
CYP: cytochrome P450
DCM: dilated cardiomyopathy
DM: diabetes mellitus
ECG: electrocardiogram
EF: ejection fraction
EMA: European Medicines Agency
eNOS: endothelial nitric oxide synthase
EPI: epinephrine
ESC: European Society of Cardiology
ET: endothelin
FDA: Food and Drug Administration
GC: guanylyl cyclase
GDMT: guideline-directed medical therapy
GFR: glomerular filtration rate
GI: gastrointestinal
GPCR: G protein–coupled receptor
GTN: glycerol trinitrate
HCM: hypertrophic cardiomyopathy
HCN: hyperpolarization-activated, cyclic nucleotide–gated cation channel
HF: heart failure
HFpEF: heart failure with preserved ejection fraction (diastolic heart failure)
HFrEF: heart failure with reduced ejection fraction (systolic heart failure)
HMG CoA: 3-hydroxy-3-methylglutaryl coenzyme A
HRQOL: health-related quality of life
HTN: hypertension
ICD: implantable cardioverter-defibrillator
ISDN: isosorbide 2,5′-dinitrate
ISMN: isosorbide 5′-mononitrate
LV: left ventricular
LVH: left ventricular hypertrophy
MCS: mechanical circulatory support
MI: myocardial infarction
MRA: mineralocorticoid receptor antagonist
NCX: Na^+/Ca^{2+} exchanger
NE: norepinephrine
NO: nitric oxide
NSAID: nonsteroidal anti-inflammatory drug
NYHA: New York Heart Association
PD: pharmacodynamic
PDE: cyclic nucleotide phosphodiesterase
PKA: protein kinase A
PLB: phospholamban
PLM: phospholemman
RAAS: renin-angiotensin-aldosterone system
ROS: reactive oxygen species
RyR: ryanodine receptor
SERCA: sarco/endoplasmic reticulum Ca^{2+} ATPase
sGC: soluble guanylyl cyclase
SL: sarcolemma
SNS: sympathetic nervous system
SR: sarcoplasmic reticulum
TnC: troponin C
TNF: tumor necrosis factor
TnI: inhibitory subunit of troponin

Heart failure is responsible for more than half a million deaths annually in the U.S. Its prevalence is increasing worldwide, likely due to improved survival of those who have had an acute myocardial infarction and an aging population. Median survival rates after the first hospitalization associated with heart failure are worse than those of most cancers, but have improved over the past 30 years (1.3 to 2.3 years in men and 1.3 to 1.7 years in women) (Jhund et al., 2009). This positive trend was associated with a 2- to 3-fold higher prescription rate of ACEIs and ARBs, β receptor antagonists (β blockers), and MRAs, suggesting that improved drug therapy has contributed to enhanced survival of heart failure.

Pathophysiology of Heart Failure

Definitions

Heart failure is a state in which the heart is unable to pump blood at a rate commensurate with the requirements of the body's tissues or can do so only at elevated filling pressure. This leads to symptoms that define the heart failure syndrome clinically. Low output (forward failure) causes fatigue, dizziness, muscle weakness, and shortness of breath, which is aggravated by physical exercise. Increased filling pressure leads to congestion of the organs upstream of the heart (backward failure), clinically apparent as peripheral or pulmonary edema, maldigestion, and ascites.

Most patients with heart failure are diagnosed exclusively on the basis of symptoms; that is, their heart function has never been directly measured (e.g., by echocardiography). Under these circumstances, it is not possible to differentiate between HFrEF (or systolic heart failure) and HFpEF (or diastolic heart failure, see discussion that follows). Other diseases associated with similar symptoms can therefore be wrongly categorized as heart failure (e.g., chronic obstructive pulmonary disease).

Common Final Pathway of Multiple Cardiac Diseases

Heart failure is not a single disease entity but a clinical syndrome that represents the final pathway of multiple cardiac diseases. The most common reason for systolic heart failure today is ischemic heart disease causing either acute (myocardial infarction) or chronic loss of viable heart muscle mass. Other reasons include chronic arterial hypertension and valvular diseases (both are decreasing in incidence due to improved therapy), genetically determined primary heart muscle defects (cardiomyopathies), viral infections (cytomegalovirus and possibly parvovirus), and toxins. The last encompass excessive alcohol, cocaine, amphetamines, and cancer drugs such as doxorubicin or trastuzumab, the monoclonal antibody directed against the growth factor receptor Her-2/Erb-B2 (see Chapter 67).

Pathophysiological Mechanisms

The pathophysiology of systolic heart failure is relatively well understood. The mechanisms of HFpEF are much less clear, but surely differ and are discussed further in this chapter. The pathophysiology of heart failure is complex and involves four major interrelated systems (Figure 29–1):

- the heart itself
- the vasculature
- the kidney
- neurohumoral regulatory circuits

The Heart Itself: Cardiomyopathy of the Overload

Any overload of the myocardium—loss of relevant muscle mass, which overloads the remaining healthy myocardium; chronic hypertension; or valvular defects—will eventually lead to the organ's failure to produce sufficient cardiac output. This concept can be extended to the genetically determined cardiomyopathies in which essentially any defect in an organelle of cardiac myocytes can lead to primary myocyte contractile dysfunction and then, secondarily, to the picture commonly seen in the cardiomyopathy of the overload. Not surprisingly, the most common cardiomyopathies (HCM, DCM) are due to mutations in genes encoding proteins of the contractile machinery, the sarcomere, proteins anchoring the sarcomere to the plasma membrane, or proteins mediating and maintaining cell-cell contact.

The overload (or the primary contractile defect) leads to alterations of the heart that can partially compensate but that come at a price. Because cardiac myocytes essentially stop replicating in the early postnatal period, the usual response to overload is not myocyte division but rather hypertrophy, growing in size and assembling more sarcomeres that can contribute to contractile force development. Whereas hypertrophy is principally a normal response to physiological needs such as body growth, pregnancy, and physical exercise ("physiological hypertrophy"), hypertrophy in response to chronic overload comes with features that make it a major risk factor for the development of heart failure ("pathological hypertrophy"). A direct consequence of cardiac myocyte hypertrophy is a reduced capillary/myocyte ratio (i.e., less O_2 and nutrient supply per myocyte), causing an energy deficit and metabolic reprogramming. Altered gene expression of ion channels, Ca^{2+}-regulating proteins, and contractile proteins can be interpreted as partially beneficial, energy-saving adaptations; on the other hand, the adaptations also aggravate contractile failure and favor arrhythmias. Concurrently, fibroblasts proliferate and deposit increased amounts of extracellular matrix (e.g., collagen). This fibrosis in heart failure also favors arrhythmias, increases the stiffness of the heart, and interrupts myocyte-to-myocyte communication (coordinated conduction and force transmission). Finally, overload leads to cardiac myocyte death by apoptosis or necrosis. Collectively, these adverse adaptations are called *pathological remodeling*.

Some of these alterations are direct, heart-intrinsic consequences of overload (e.g., hypertrophy, altered gene expression); others are secondary to neurohumoral activation and thereby susceptible to neurohumoral blocking agents (see discussion that follows and Figure 29–1).

The Vasculature

A critical parameter of cardiac function is the stiffness of the vasculature. It determines the resistance against which the heart has to expel the blood and increases with aging. Heart failure may be the consequence of premature aging of the vasculature (Strait and Lakatta, 2012). Aging-induced loss of elasticity of the great blood vessels reduces their compliance, that is, the elasticity that permits vessels to extend in systole and contract in diastole. Good compliance reduces peak systolic pressure and increases diastolic pressure, which favors perfusion in diastole. It is negatively correlated with pulse pressure, that is, the difference between systolic and

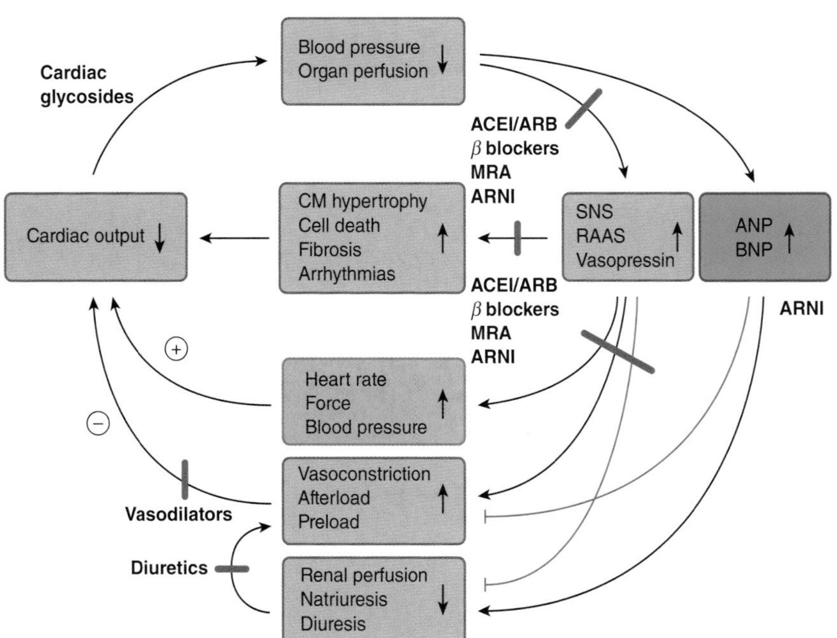

Figure 29–1 *Pathophysiologic mechanisms of systolic heart failure (HFrEF) and therapeutic interventions.* Any major decrease in cardiac contractile function leads to activation of neurohumoral systems, including the SNS, the RAAS, and vasopressin (ADH) secretion, which acutely stabilize blood pressure and organ perfusion by stimulating cardiac output, constricting resistance vessels, decreasing kidney perfusion, and increasing Na^+ and H_2O retention. Unfortunately, these responses are maladaptive, causing chronic overloading and overstimulation of the failing heart. Direct hypertrophic, pro-apoptotic, fibrotic, and arrhythmogenic effects of NE and AngII further accelerate the deleterious process. Note that the concomitant activation of the ANP/BNP system is the consequence of stretch and increased wall stress in the heart and has opposite and beneficial effects. See Abbreviations list at beginning of chapter.

diastolic blood pressure, which is low in children and high in the elderly. Arterial hypertension and diabetes mellitus are the major reasons for premature stiffening of blood vessels, which imposes increased afterload to the heart and contributes to heart failure. Theoretically, stiffening and loss of compliance could be directly tackled by drugs (see section Recent Developments; Novel Approaches).

Another critical aspect of vascular function is the ability to adapt the vessel diameter to hemodynamic and neurohumoral stimuli, a function that is governed by cross talk between luminal endothelial and underlying smooth muscle cells (Chapter 28). The main signaling pathway involves receptors that increase intracellular Ca^{2+} levels in endothelial cells, which activates eNOS to produce NO. This gaseous transmitter diffuses into smooth muscle cells and activates sGC to produce cGMP, which causes relaxation of vascular smooth muscle. Heart failure is always accompanied by endothelial dysfunction, which is a disturbed balance between vasodilating NO and proconstrictor ROS. ROS, by inactivating the two critical enzymes eNOS and sGC and converting NO in peroxynitrite, a strong ROS, favor vasoconstriction. Several common cardiovascular drugs (ACEIs/ARBs, MRAs, statins) improve endothelial function by reducing ROS production. PDE5 inhibitors have similar consequences by inhibiting cGMP degradation in smooth muscle cells and thereby promoting relaxation.

The Kidney

The kidney regulates Na^+ and H_2O excretion and thereby intravascular volume. Under normal conditions, autoregulatory and neurohumoral mechanisms ensure an adequate GFR and diuresis over a wide range of renal perfusion pressures. Prominent mechanisms with relevance for heart failure are (1) the AngII-mediated regulation of filtration rate by regulating the diameter of efferent glomerular arteriole; (2) the regulation of kidney perfusion by a balance between constrictor-promoting effects of AngII (via AT_1 receptors) and vasopressin (AVP, via V_1 receptors) and the vasodilating influence of prostaglandins (hence the deleterious effects of NSAIDs); (3) the aldosterone-mediated regulation of Na^+ reabsorption in the distal tubule; and (4) AVP-regulated water transport in the collecting ducts (via V_2 receptors). In heart failure, all mechanisms are dysregulated and constitute therapeutic targets of ACEIs/ARBs, MRAs, and diuretics. Newer agents, such as adenosine A_1 receptor antagonists and AVP receptor antagonists, have failed to exert therapeutic benefit in clinical studies.

Neurohumoral Regulation and HFrEF

The decrease in cardiac output in heart failure leads to the activation of the SNS and the RAAS and increases in plasma levels of AVP and ET (Figure 29–1). This concerted response ensures the perfusion of centrally important organs such as the brain and the heart (at the expense of kidney, liver, and skeletal muscle perfusion) in situations of acute blood loss. These responses are components of the "fight-or-flight response" and provide useful short-term physiological responses to alarm and danger. Chronically, however, neurohumoral activation exerts deleterious effects that constitute a vicious cycle in heart failure. Vasoconstriction initially not only stabilizes blood pressure but also increases afterload, which is the resistance against which the heart works to expel blood (see Figures 29–4 and 27–1). Because of the decreased contractile reserve, the failing heart is particularly sensitive to increases in afterload (see Figure 29–4); such increases further decrease cardiac output. Decreased kidney perfusion and increased aldosterone production reduce diuresis and promote volume overload, which increases cardiac preload, dilation, and ventricular wall stress, a major determinant of cardiac O_2 consumption. Tachycardic and positive inotropic actions of catecholamines not only acutely increase cardiac output but also promote arrhythmias and increase O_2 consumption in a failing, energy-depleted heart. AngII, NE, and ET accelerate pathological cardiac remodeling (hypertrophy, fibrosis, and cell death). Aldosterone has prominent profibrotic actions. This spectrum of adverse consequences of chronic neurohumoral activation explains why inhibitors of these systems (ACEIs/ARBs, β blockers, and MRAs) exert long-term, life-prolonging effects in heart failure and are the cornerstones of current

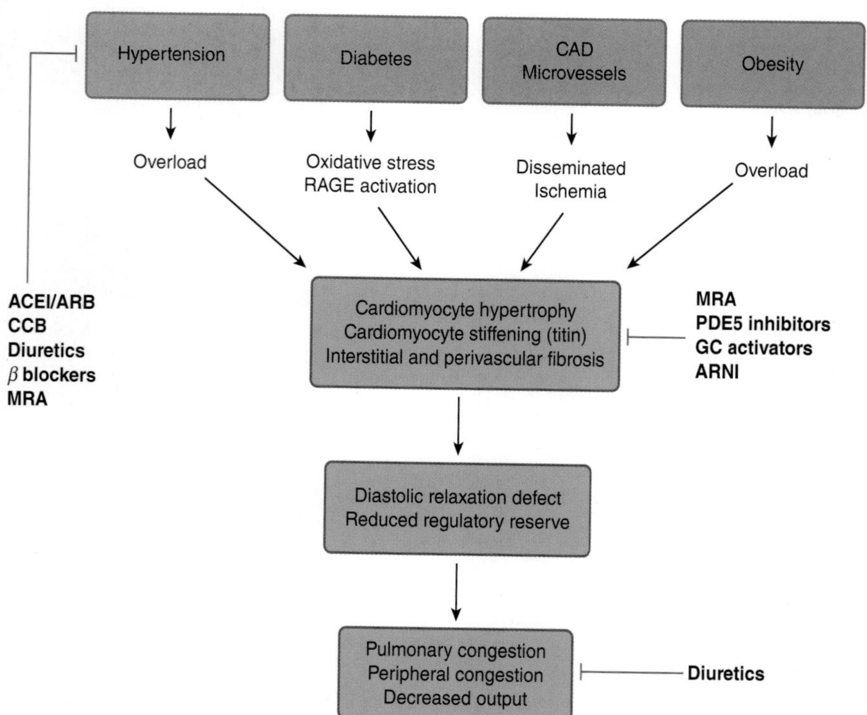

Figure 29–2 *Pathophysiological mechanisms of diastolic heart failure HFpEF and possible therapeutic interventions.* Unlike the case with HFrEF, the pharmacological agents shown have not been proven to have clinical efficacy toward HFpEF, although these agents can help to control underlying diseases, such as hypertension, diabetes, and obesity. Only exercise training has proven effective in increasing maximal exercise capacity. RAGE; receptor for advanced glycosylation end-products.

therapy.

Unexpectedly, ET and AVP receptor antagonists provide no beneficial effect in patients with heart failure, despite promising results in preclinical studies. Clinical trials suggested that neurohumoral activation in response to altered cardiac function may be sufficiently inhibited by the standard combination therapy, leaving no room for improvement from the addition of ET and AVP antagonists; however, recent data indicate that additional benefit may accrue via another therapeutic route: a drug combination called ARNIs. The FDA has approved a fixed-dose combination of the ARB valsartan with the neprilysin inhibitor sacubitril. Valsartan blocks AT_1 receptors, reducing the deleterious effects of AngII. Sacubitril inhibits the degradation of the natriuretic peptides ANP and BNP. The valsartan-sacubitril combination appears superior to the ACEI enalapril, reducing the rates of hospitalization and death from all cardiovascular causes in patients with HFrEF (Hubers and Brown, 2016).

This finding reflects the fact that neurohumoral activation in heart failure includes one system that exerts beneficial effects: the natriuretic peptides. Normally, ANP and BNP are expressed in the atria and released on increased preload (stretch). During heart failure, ANP and BNP are also produced by the ventricles, such that plasma levels are elevated. Indeed, BNP is used as a biomarker of heart failure. ANP and BNP stimulate the plasma membrane guanylyl cyclase. In the kidney, elevated cGMP has diuretic effects. Elevated cellular cGMP mediates vasodilation in the vasculature and, in the heart, antihypertrophic, antifibrotic, and compliance-increasing effects related to phosphorylation of titin. Enhancing these effects by inhibiting the degradation of ANP/BNP likely explains the clinical benefits of sacubitril-valsartan.

Heart Failure With Preserved Ejection Fraction

Systematic echocardiographic determination of left ventricular EF in thousands of patients with heart failure revealed that about 50% had no reduction; that is, they exhibited EF values greater than 50%. Still, patients had typical heart failure symptoms, including acute decompensation with pulmonary edema and a survival prognosis not much better or even identical to patients with reduced EF (systolic heart failure or HFrEF). These data point to a different pathophysiology in which abnormalities of the diastolic and not the systolic component of cardiac function prevail. Due to difficulties in defining diastolic function by standard techniques, the term *HFpEF* has been introduced and applies to patients with typical heart failure symptoms and "normal" (>50%) or only mildly reduced EF.

Even more than HFrEF, HFpEF is a multifactorial disease (Figure 29–2). HFpEF is typically associated with arterial hypertension, ischemic heart disease, diabetes mellitus, and obesity (metabolic syndrome); it is more frequent in women than men and shows a strong increase in prevalence with age. Hearts of patients with HFpEF are generally not dilated, wall thickness is enlarged (hypertrophy), and left atrial size often is enlarged as a sign of chronically elevated end-diastolic pressures. Central to the pathophysiology of HFpEF is, presumably, compromised diastolic relaxation of the left ventricle, which causes congestion of the lung, shortness of breath, or pulmonary edema. Clinical decompensation is often associated with strongly elevated blood pressure.

Molecular alterations include increased myocardial fibrosis (causing a permanent relaxation deficit) as well as more dynamic changes, such as reduced phosphorylation of titin, the sarcomeric protein that spans the large region from the Z to the M band. Titin contains several molecular spring domains whose elastic modulus determines the passive tension of cardiomyocytes, particularly at low-to-medium levels of stretch. At higher levels of stretch, the extracellular matrix becomes involved. Titin stiffness is determined by its isoforms and by cGMP-dependent phosphorylation, suggesting that agents that increase cellular cGMP might be beneficial in HFpEF. However, the PDE5 inhibitor sildenafil, which preserves and elevates cellular cGMP in some cells (see Chapters 3, 31, and 45), failed to show benefit (Redfield et al., 2013). This lack of efficacy is, unfortunately, also true for all other pharmacological interventions in HFpEF, including ACEIs, ARBs, and spironolactone. Exercise training is presently the only intervention that significantly increases maximal physical activity in HFpEF patients. In the absence of evidence-based clinical trial data, current therapy recommendations concentrate on optimal treatment of the underlying diseases, such as hypertension, diabetes, and obesity.

Heart Failure Staging

Heart failure was one of the first diseases for which guidelines described specific therapies for each stage of the disease. An early classification of the stages of heart failure was that of the NYHA, a classification still in use: class I (left ventricular dysfunction, no symptoms); class II (symptoms at medium-to-high levels of physical exercise); class III (symptoms at low levels of physical exercise); and class IV (symptoms at rest or daily life physical activities such as brushing teeth). The more recent guidelines of the AHA and ACC extended this classification by taking into account that

- heart failure is part of the cardiovascular continuum with preventable risk factors (stage A)
- an asymptomatic stage exists that requires treatment to delay transition to symptomatic heart failure (stage B)
- patients oscillate between different degrees of symptoms and therefore between class II and III (class C, which generally includes NYHA class II/III patients)
- a final stage of the disease requires different treatment and special considerations, such as heart transplantation and left ventricular assist device implantation (stage D).

This chapter uses the AHA/ACC classification (Yancey et al., 2013) but also considers the recent guidelines of the European Society of Cardiology (Ponikowski et al., 2016), which provide more specific treatment algorithms, and the 2016 AHA/ACC update (Yancy et al., 2016). Treatment guidelines are summarized in Figure 29–3.

Prevention and Treatment

Ischemic heart disease, hypertension, and valvular diseases are the most prevalent causes of heart failure. People at high risk (stage A) should therefore be consequently treated with drugs with an established effect on the natural course of these diseases, in conjunction with appropriate lifestyle changes. Studies in thousands of patients have reproducibly shown that blood pressure lowering in hypertensive patients and lipid-lowering with statins in dyslipidemic patients reduce not only the incidence of myocardial infarction and death but also the incidence of heart failure. The data are weaker for antidiabetic drugs, but consensus exists that blood glucose should be controlled with a hemoglobin A_{1C} goal of 7%–7.5%.

Treatment of heart failure has seen a dramatic change over the past decades. Until the late 1980s, drugs and drug dosing were symptom oriented and based on pathophysiological considerations of *acute* systolic heart failure. Treatment was mainly directed toward symptom relief and short-term improvement of hemodynamic function. With the era of randomized clinical trials, which mainly tested effects of drugs on long-term morbidity (hospitalizations) and mortality, much of the former beliefs have proven to be wrong. For example, positive inotropic drugs (sympathomimetics and PDE inhibitors) that exert acute symptomatic benefit reduce life expectancy when given chronically. In contrast, β blockers decrease cardiac output acutely and may make people feel weak at the start of therapy but prolong life expectancy when given in increasing doses for extended periods. Vasodilators once seemed a logical choice for heart failure, but pure vasodilators such as the α_1 receptor antagonist prazosin or the nitrate ISDN, in combination with the vasodilator hydralazine, do not positively affect the prognosis in Caucasians (see further discussion). Thus, clinical trials have established important principles for assessing efficacy of therapies for heart failure:

1. Drugs for the treatment of chronic heart failure should reduce the patient morbidity and mortality.
2. Short-term drug effects poorly predict the outcome of randomized clinical trials and optimal therapies for heart failure.
3. Considerations of stage of disease are critical.
4. New drugs for heart failure should be compared to the most effective current combination therapy, a principle often ignored in preclinical

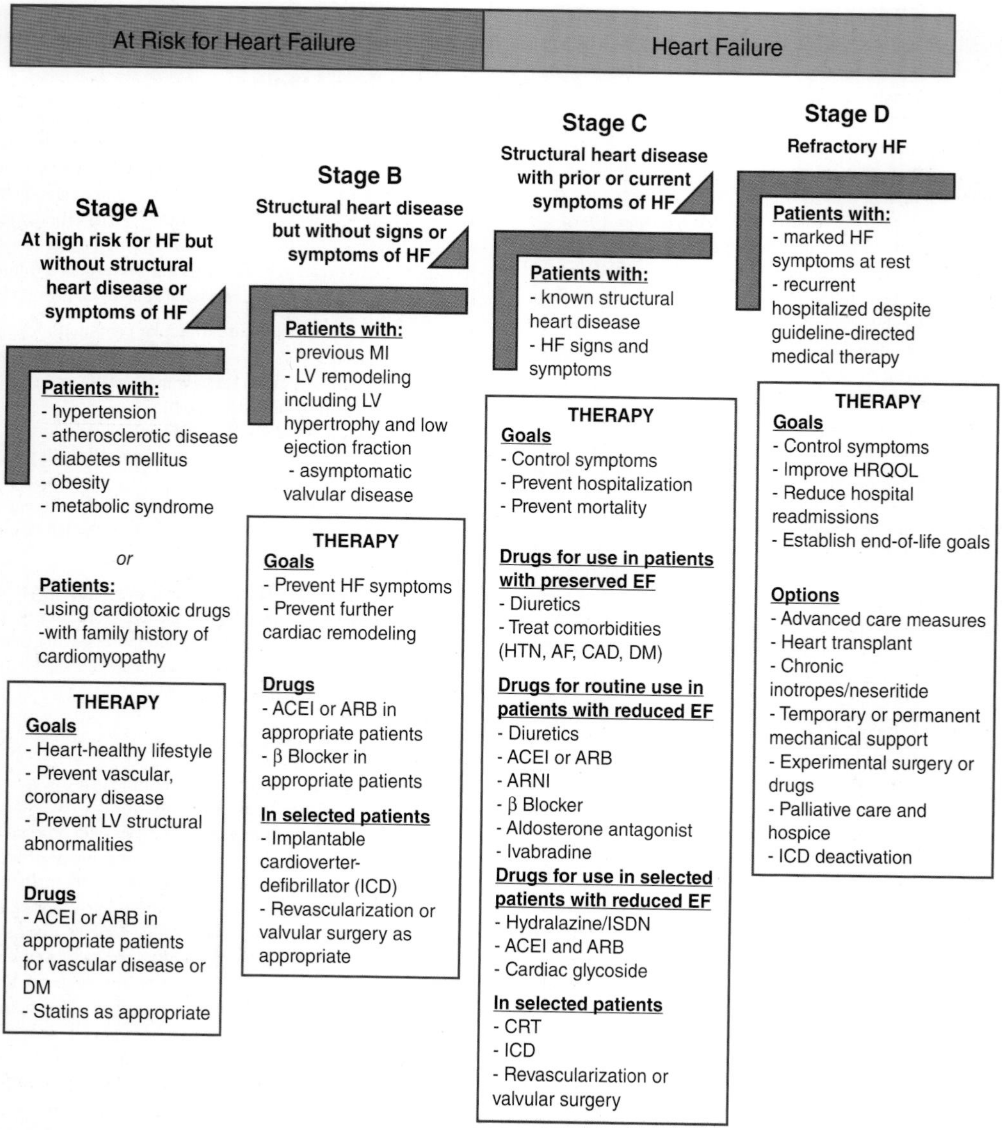

At Risk for Heart Failure		Heart Failure	
Stage A At high risk for HF but without structural heart disease or symptoms of HF	**Stage B** Structural heart disease but without signs or symptoms of HF	**Stage C** Structural heart disease with prior or current symptoms of HF	**Stage D** Refractory HF
Patients with: - hypertension - atherosclerotic disease - diabetes mellitus - obesity - metabolic syndrome *or* **Patients:** -using cardiotoxic drugs -with family history of cardiomyopathy	**Patients with:** - previous MI - LV remodeling including LV hypertrophy and low ejection fraction - asymptomatic valvular disease	**Patients with:** - known structural heart disease - HF signs and symptoms	**Patients with:** - marked HF symptoms at rest - recurrent hospitalized despite guideline-directed medical therapy
THERAPY **Goals** - Heart-healthy lifestyle - Prevent vascular, coronary disease - Prevent LV structural abnormalities **Drugs** - ACEI or ARB in appropriate patients for vascular disease or DM - Statins as appropriate	**THERAPY** **Goals** - Prevent HF symptoms - Prevent further cardiac remodeling **Drugs** - ACEI or ARB in appropriate patients - β Blocker in appropriate patients **In selected patients** - Implantable cardioverter-defibrillator (ICD) - Revascularization or valvular surgery as appropriate	**THERAPY** **Goals** - Control symptoms - Prevent hospitalization - Prevent mortality **Drugs for use in patients with preserved EF** - Diuretics - Treat comorbidities (HTN, AF, CAD, DM) **Drugs for routine use in patients with reduced EF** - Diuretics - ACEI or ARB - ARNI - β Blocker - Aldosterone antagonist - Ivabradine **Drugs for use in selected patients with reduced EF** - Hydralazine/ISDN - ACEI and ARB - Cardiac glycoside **In selected patients** - CRT - ICD - Revascularization or valvular surgery	**THERAPY** **Goals** - Control symptoms - Improve HRQOL - Reduce hospital readmissions - Establish end-of-life goals **Options** - Advanced care measures - Heart transplant - Chronic inotropes/neseritide - Temporary or permanent mechanical support - Experimental surgery or drugs - Palliative care and hospice - ICD deactivation

Figure 29–3 *AHA/ACC 2013 Heart Failure Treatment Guidelines: stages in the development of HF and recommended therapy by stage.* (See Yancy et al., 2013 and 2016, for details.)

animal work.

5. Nonpharmacological treatment options such as cardiac resynchronization devices and intracardiac defibrillator/cardioverters are important for their documented lifesaving effect in selected patient populations.

Attention to these principles for assessing long-term efficacy of heart failure therapies has provided evidence-based principles of treatment.

HISTORICAL PERSPECTIVE

A series of landmark studies over three decades has established the current thinking on the treatment of patients with chronic HFrEF. These studies are not reviewed here, but interested readers may wish to consult the evidence that supports current therapies. These studies, often indicated by an acronym, are summarized in Table 29–1.

Drug Treatment of Chronic Systolic Heart Failure (Stages B and C)

Treatment Principle I: Neurohumoral Modulation

Dampening neurohumoral activation and its deleterious consequences on the heart, blood vessels, and kidney is the cornerstone of heart failure therapy. Therapy consists of ACEIs/ARBs, β blockers, and MRAs. Further activation of the natriuretic peptide system adds benefit (Figure 29–1). A systematic discussion of the drugs is found in Chapters 12, 25, 26, 27, and 28.

Angiotensin-Converting Enzyme Inhibitors

Angiotensin II, the most active angiotensin peptide, is largely derived from angiotensinogen in two proteolytic steps. First, *renin*, an enzyme released from the kidneys, cleaves the decapeptide AngI from the amino terminus of angiotensinogen (renin substrate). Then, ACE removes a

TABLE 29–1 ■ LANDMARK STUDIES IN THE TREATMENT OF PATIENTS WITH CHRONIC HEART FAILURE WITH REDUCED EJECTION FRACTION

STUDY (as cited in Bibliography)	STUDY POPULATION	NO. OF SUBJECTS	BASELINE DRUGS (% of patients on each)	DRUG EFFECT (on all-cause mortality)
Cohn et al., 1986	Men, impaired cardiac function and exercise capacity	642	CG, D	ISDN/hydralazine ↓ 34% Prazosin +/- vs. placebo
CONSENSUS Trial Study Group, 1987	Severe HF, NYHA class IV	253	D 100, CG 93, BB 2, spironolactone 52, vasodilators ~ 50	Enalapril ↓ 40% vs. placebo
SOLVD Investigators, 1991	NYHA II–III, left EF < 35%	2569	D 86, CG 67, BB 7.5, vasodilators 51	Enalapril ↓ 16% vs. placebo
SOLVD Investigators, 1992	NYHA I, left EF < 35%	4228	Vasodilators 46, D 17, CG 13	Enalapril ↓ 8% (n.s.) vs. placebo (heart failure development ↓ 20%)
Digitalis Investigation Group, 1997	NYHA II–III	6800	D 81, ACE 95, nitrates 43	Digoxin +/- (HF hospitalizations ↓ 27%)
RALES (Pitt et al., 1999)	Severe HF, left EF < 35%	1663	D 100, ACEI 94, CG 72, BB 10	Spironolactone ↓ 30% vs. placebo
MERIT-HF Investigators, 1999	NYHA II–IV	3991	ACEI/ARB 95, D 90, CG 63	Metoprolol CR/XL ↓ 34% vs. placebo
PARADIGM-HF (McMurray et al., 2014)	NYHA II–IV	8442	BB 93, MRA 56, CG 30, ICD 15, CRT 7, D 80	Sacubitril/valsartan ↓ 16% vs. enalapril

D, diuretics; n.s., nonsignificant; NYHA indicates classification of HF according to the NYHA.

carboxy-terminal dipeptide (His[9]-Leu[10]) from AngI, yielding the active octapeptide, AngII (Figure 26–1). Thus, ACEIs reduce circulating levels of AngII. All patients with heart failure (stages B and C; NYHA I–IV) should receive an ACEI.

Mechanism of Action. AngII interacts with two heptahelical GPCRs, AT_1 and AT_2, and has four major cardiovascular actions that are all mediated by the AT_1 receptor:

- vasoconstriction
- stimulation of aldosterone release from the adrenal glands
- direct hypertrophic and proliferative effects on cardiomyocytes and fibroblasts, respectively
- stimulation of NE release from sympathetic nerve endings and the adrenal medulla

Physiological Effects. The ACEIs lower the circulating level of AngII and thereby reduce its deleterious effects. Thus, ACEIs not only act as vasodilators but also reduce aldosterone levels and thereby act as an indirect diuretic, have direct antiremodeling effects on the heart, and produce sympatholytic effects (thus moderating the reflex tachycardia that accompanies vasodilation and the lowering of blood pressure).

The ACEIs have important renal effects. When renal perfusion pressure is reduced, AngII constricts renal efferent arterioles, and this serves to maintain glomerular filtration pressure and GFR. Thus, under circumstances in which renal perfusion pressure is compromised, inhibition of the RAAS may induce a sudden and marked decrease in GFR. For this reason, ACEIs are contraindicated in bilateral renal artery stenosis. Likewise, because patients with heart failure often have low renal perfusion pressures, aggressive treatment with ACEIs may induce acute renal failure. To avoid this, for patients with heart failure patients, ACEIs should be initiated at very low doses; blood pressure, blood creatinine, and K^+ levels should be monitored; and the ACEI dose slowly increased over weeks toward target levels (for agents that have been carefully evaluated in clinical trials; Table 29–2). The potentially dangerous acute effects become beneficial with long-term use of ACEIs because the (small) chronic lowering of glomerular pressures protects the glomerulus from fibrotic degeneration.

The ACEI-induced lowering of aldosterone levels causes reduced expression of the aldosterone-dependent epithelial Na^+ channel (ENaC) in the distal tubule (see Figure 25-6). This target of K^+-sparing diuretics (see discussion that follows) normally mediates Na^+ reabsorption and K^+ excretion. Lower levels of ENaC lead to less absorption of Na^+ and less excretion of K^+. Thus, ACEIs favor hyperkalemia, which can be detrimental in patients with renal insufficiency but is normally beneficial for patients with heart failure who more often present with hypokalemia, a condition that promotes cardiac arrhythmias. ACEIs shift the balance of vascular smooth muscle tone toward vasodilation and thereby increase renal blood flow, another reason for their chronic protective effects on the kidney. This effect also explains why NSAIDs, which reduce the production of vasodilating prostaglandins, antagonize effects of ACEIs and should be avoided in patients with heart failure.

Other Actions, Good and Adverse. Angiotensin-converting enzyme has other actions, including the inactivation of bradykinin and substance P. ACEIs increase bradykinin and substance P levels, with two prominent consequences: cough, the most frequent ADR (~5%); and angioedema, a rare (~0.7%), but life-threatening condition presenting with swelling of the skin and mucous membranes of the throat and asphyxia (three times more common amongst African Americans). Experimental evidence suggests that increases in bradykinin contribute to the therapeutic efficacy of ACEIs and may explain why ARBs, which do not increase bradykinin (and therefore cause no cough), have not been consistently associated with improved survival in patients with HFrEF (Ponikowski et al., 2016).

The ACEIs are generally well tolerated in the majority of patients. Important ADRs are the following:

- dry cough, necessitating a change to ARBs;
- creatinine plasma concentration increase (<20%, normal; 20%–50%: careful observation and reduction of ACEI dosage; > 50%, stop ACEI and consult specialist for diagnosis of renal artery);
- hyperkalemia (small increase normal, but requires careful observation in patients with diabetes, renal insufficiency, or comedication with MRAs, K^+-sparing diuretics, or NSAIDs);
- angioedema (stop drug immediately, treat with antihistamines, corticosteroids, or, in severe case, EPI); and
- allergic skin reactions.

TABLE 29–2 ■ PROPERTIES AND THERAPEUTIC DAILY DOSES OF ACEIs AND ARBs APPROVED AND CLINICALLY EVALUATED FOR THE THERAPY OF HFrEF[a]

CLASS/ Drug	HALF-LIFE (h)	STARTING DOSE (mg)	TARGET DOSE (mg)	IMPORTANT ADVERSE EFFECTS, INTERACTIONS, AND CONTRAINDICATIONS
ACE inhibitors				
Captopril	1.7	3 × 6.25	3 × 50	**Adverse effects**: Cough (~5%), ↑ serum creatinine (<25% is normal; if > 50%, possibility of renal artery stenosis), hyperkalemia, hypotension, angioedema **Interactions**: Increased rate of hyperkalemia in combination with K^+-sparing diuretics, K^+ supplements, cyclosporine, NSAIDs (PD), reduced efficacy in combination with NSAIDs (PD), ↑ [Li^+] in serum (PK), ↑ hypoglycemic risk in combination with insulin or oral antidiabetics; increased effect in renal insufficiency (PK) **Contraindications**: Bilateral renal artery stenosis
Enalapril	11	2 × 2.5	2 × 20	
Lisinopril	13	1 × 2.5–5	1 × 20–35	
Ramipril	13–17	1 × 2.5	1 × 10	
Trandolapril	15–23	1 × 0.5	1 × 4	
Angiotensin receptor blockers				
Candesartan	9	1 × 4–8	1 × 32	**Adverse effects:** Similar to ACE, but no cough **Interactions and contraindications:** As ACEI
Losartan	6–9	1 × 50	1 × 150	
Valsartan	6	2 × 40	2 × 160	

[a]Plasma half-lives partially apply to active metabolites (e.g., losartan). PD, pharmacodynamic; PK, pharmacokinetic.

Angiotensin Receptor Antagonists

The ARBs are systematically discussed in Chapter 26. They are highly selective, competitive receptor antagonists at the AT_1 receptor, which mediates the major effects of AngII. They are therapeutic alternatives to ACEIs and second choice in all stages of heart failure in patients who do not tolerate ACEIs. Given the central role of the AT_1 receptor for the actions of AngII, it is not surprising that ARBs show the same pharmacological profile as ACEIs with the exception of not inducing cough. The unopposed activity of AT_2 receptor pathways in the presence of AT_1 blockade by an ARB seems to confer no therapeutic advantage to ARBs over ACEIs. Moreover, the addition of an ARB to therapy with an ACEI does not affect the prognosis of patients with heart failure but does increase hypotension, hyperkalemia, and renal dysfunction. A negative interaction between ACEIs and ARBs appears to extend to patients with higher renal risk. There is, therefore, no routine indication for this combination.

β Adrenergic Receptor Antagonists

Major Effects of β Adrenergic Antagonists. The sympathetic neurotransmitters NE (released at adrenergic nerve varicosities) and EPI (secreted by the adrenal medulla) are strong stimuli of heart function. They increase heart rate (positive chronotropic effect) and force of contraction (positive inotropic effect) and thereby augment cardiac output. They quicken the rate of force development (increased +dP/dt, positive clinotropy) and accelerate cardiac muscle relaxation (greater −dP/dt, positive lusitropic effect, which aids ventricular filling during diastole. Acceleration of the atrial-ventricular conduction rate (positive dromotropic effect) shortens the heart cycle and allows higher beating rates. Catecholamines enhance cardiac myocyte automaticity and lower the threshold for arrhythmias (positive bathmotropic effect). All these acute effects are mediated by β_1 receptors and, to a smaller extent, β_2 receptors. Extracardiac effects include bronchodilation (β_2), vasodilation (β_2) as well as vasoconstriction (α_1 receptors, which dominate at higher concentrations of catecholamines), stimulation of hepatic glycogen metabolism and gluconeogenesis (β_2), and, importantly, stimulation of renin release from the macula densa (β_1). Thus, activation of the SNS coactivates the RAAS, and, as outlined previously, activation of the RAAS activates the SNS by stimulation of NE release (see Chapters 12 and 26).

The β blockers competitively reduce β receptor–mediated actions of catecholamines and thus, depending on the activation level of the SNS, reduce heart rate and force, slow relaxation, slow AV conduction, suppress arrhythmias, lower renin levels, and, depending on their selectivity for the β_1 receptor, permit more or less bronchoconstriction, vasoconstriction, and lowering of hepatic glucose production.

Why Use β Blockers in Heart Failure? In light of the above actions, the efficacy of β blockers in heart failure came as a surprise and had to overcome resistance in the medical community. How can a drug with cardiodepressant actions on heart function be beneficial in a clinical situation in which the heart is already dysfunctional and depending on catecholamines to maintain cardiac output? The first therapeutic application of β blockers at low doses was to a Swedish cohort of patients with heart failure with cardiac decompensation and heart rate greater than 120 beats/min; the goal was to reduce heart rate and cardiac energy consumption (Waagstein et al., 1975). The success of the experiment led to large clinical trials that showed an impressive 35% prolongation of life expectancy in patients treated with β blockers (Table 29–1), on top of effects of ACEIs, diuretics, and digoxin.

Key to the understanding of the success of β blockers in heart failure were two lessons. *First*, therapy must be initiated in a clinically stable condition and at very low doses (1/8 of target), and dose escalation requires time (e.g., doubling every 4 weeks in ambulatory settings; "start low, go slow"). Under these conditions, the heart has time to adapt to decreasing stimulation by catecholamines and to find a new equilibrium at a lower adrenergic drive. Importantly, β blockers do not fully block the receptors; rather, they are competitive antagonists that shift the concentration-response curve of catecholamines to the right (see Figure 3–4).

Second, although the acute effects of catecholamines can be lifesaving, that level of β adrenergic stimulation applied chronically, as the SNS does in response to heart failure, is deleterious. Positive chronotropic, inotropic, and lusitropic effects all come at the price of overproportional increase in energy consumption. This is irrelevant in situations of acute blood loss or other stresses, but critical if persistent. The heart reacts to chronic sympathetic stimulation by a heart failure–specific gene program (e.g., downregulation of β adrenergic receptor density; upregulation of inhibitory G proteins; and decreases of SR Ca^{2+}-ATPase, the fast isoform of myosin heavy chain, and repolarizing K^+ currents), changes that come at the price of decreased dynamic range and increased propensity for arrhythmias. Reversal of the heart failure gene program by β blockers (Lowes et al., 2002) likely contributes to the paradoxical increase in left ventricular EF after 3–6 months of therapy and to the reduced rate of arrhythmogenic sudden cardiac death noted in the large studies. In a simple view, β blockers protect the heart from the adverse long-term consequences of adrenergic overstimulation, for example, increased energy consumption, fibrosis, arrhythmias, and cell death. Lower heart rates not only save energy but also improve contractile function because the failing heart, in contrast to the healthy human heart, has a negative force-frequency relation (Pieske et al., 1995). In addition, β blockers improve perfusion of the myocardium by prolonging diastole, thereby reducing ischemia.

Available Agents. Four β blockers have been successfully tested in randomized clinical trials (Table 29–1): the β_1-selective agents metoprolol (MERIT-HF Investigators, 1999) and bisoprolol (CIBIS-II Investigators, 1999) and the third-generation agents with additional actions, carvedilol and nebivolol. Carvedilol is a nonselective β blocker and an α_1 receptor antagonist. Nebivolol (Flather et al., 2005) is β_1 selective and has additional vasodilatory actions that may be NO mediated (Figure 12–4; Table 12–4). Early evidence of superiority of carvedilol over metoprolol (Poole-Wilson et al., 2003) has not been confirmed.

Pharmacokinetic Considerations. There are important pharmacokinetic differences amongst these β blockers (Table 29–3), distinctions that are relevant because successful therapy of heart failure (and most other chronic cardiovascular diseases) requires stable plasma concentrations over the entire day (trough levels before next dose application > 50% of maximum).

Metoprolol has a too short $t_{1/2}$ (3–5 h) and should be prescribed only as the zero-order prolonged-release formulation used by all successful clinical studies. Standard extended-release formulations likely do not suffice. A further disadvantage of metoprolol is its dependency on the polymorphic CYP2D6 for its metabolism. CYP2D6 "poor metabolizers," about 8% of the Caucasian population, exhibit C_{Pmax} levels of metoprolol 5-fold higher than those of standard metabolizers; in a prospective longitudinal study, that difference correlated with 2-fold differences in heart rate responses (Rau et al., 2009). Bisoprolol has a sufficiently long plasma $t_{1/2}$ (10–12 h) for once-daily dosing and is not metabolized by CYP2D6. Carvedilol has a shorter $t_{1/2}$ (6–10 h) and requires twice-daily dosing. An advantageous peculiarity of carvedilol is that it dissociates only slowly from β receptors and therefore acts longer than its plasma $t_{1/2}$ suggests. Carvedilol metabolism depends on CYP2D6, but less so than metoprolol. Nebivolol plasma concentrations are 10- to 15-fold higher in CYP2D6 poor metabolizers, but this is without clinical consequence, likely because the first metabolite is similarly active as the parent compound. Nebivolol is not approved in the U.S. for the treatment of heart failure, but it is approved in 71 countries worldwide, including Europe (patients > 70 years of age).

Clinical Use. All patients with symptomatic heart failure (stage C, NYHA II–IV) and all patients with left ventricular dysfunction (stage B, NYHA I) after myocardial infarction should be treated with a β blocker. The therapy with β blockers should be initiated only in clinically stable patients at very low doses, generally 1/8 of the final target dose, and titrated upward every 4 weeks. Even when initiated properly, a tendency to retain fluid exists that may require diuretic dose adjustment. The improvement of left ventricular function generally takes 3–6 months, and in this period, patients should be carefully monitored.

The β blockers should not be administered in new-onset or acutely decompensated heart failure. If patients are hospitalized with acute decompensation under current therapy with β blockers, doses often have to be reduced or the drug discontinued until clinical stabilization, after which therapy should again be initiated.

Precautions. Formally, β blockers have long lists of adverse drug responses and contraindications. Practically, however, they are generally well tolerated if properly initiated. If doses are increased too rapidly, fall of blood pressure, fluid retention, and dizziness are common and require dose reduction.

The major cardiovascular responses associated with use of β blockers are the following:

- *Heart rate lowering,* a desirable effect that indicates proper dosing (no decrease indicates insufficient dosing). A reasonable target resting heart rate is 60–70/min.
- *AV block* (beware preexisting conduction disturbance; consider pacemaker implantation).
- *Bronchoconstriction.* Allergic asthma is a contraindication for all β blocker use; however, chronic obstructive lung disease is not, because the β_2 receptor–dependent dynamic range is low in these patients, and studies have documented safety. Nonetheless, only β_1-selective compounds should be used in patients with chronic obstructive pulmonary disease.
- *Peripheral vasoconstriction (cold extremities).* Initial vasoconstriction turns into vasodilation under chronic therapy with β blockers. Cold extremities are generally not a problem in patients with heart failure. Yet, patients with peripheral artery disease or symptoms of claudication or Raynaud disease should be carefully monitored and treated with carvedilol if a β blocker is employed.

Mineralocorticoid Receptor Antagonists

The third group of drugs with a documented life-prolonging effect in patients with heart failure is MRAs. They should be given in low doses to all patients in stage C (NYHA class II–IV), that is, with symptomatic HFrEF, despite the fact that the combination of ACEIs/ARBs, and MRA is formally contraindicated due to the risk of hyperkalemia. The safety of a low-dose MRA (25 mg vs. a standard of 100 mg spironolactone) was demonstrated in a large randomized trial in a patient cohort with severe heart failure (NYHA III–IV), with the MRA added to ACEIs, diuretics, and digoxin (Pitt, 2004). Later studies with eplerenone in less-severe heart failure essentially confirmed the efficacy of this class of drugs.

Mechanism of Action. The MRAs act as antagonists of nuclear receptors of aldosterone (Figure 25-6). They are K^+-sparing diuretics (see discussion that follows) but gained more importance in the treatment of heart failure for their additional efficacy in suppressing the consequences of neurohumoral activation. Aldosterone, as the second major actor of the RAAS, promotes Na^+ and fluid retention, loss of K^+ and Mg^{2+}, sympathetic activation, parasympathetic inhibition, myocardial and vascular fibrosis, baroreceptor dysfunction, and vascular damage, all adverse effects in the setting of heart failure. Aldosterone plasma levels decrease under therapy with ACEIs or ARBs, but quickly increase again, a phenomenon called *aldosterone escape*. It is likely explained by incomplete blockade of the RAAS (e.g., AngI can be converted to AngII by chymase, in addition to ACE; see Figure 26–1) and by the fact that aldosterone secretion is regulated not only by AngII but also by sodium and potassium plasma Na^+ and

TABLE 29–3 ■ PROPERTIES AND THERAPEUTIC DOSES OF β BLOCKERS APPROVED AS THERAPY OF HFrEF

β BLOCKER	β_1 SELECTIVE	VASODILATION	HALF-LIFE (h)	START DOSE (mg)	TARGET DOSE (mg)	METABOLISM BY CYPs[a]
Bisoprolol	Yes	No	10–12	1 × 1.25	1 × 10	None
Carvedilol	No	Yes	6–10	2 × 3.125	2 × 25	CYP2D6
Metoprolol succinate[a]	Yes	No	>12[b]	1 × 12.5[a]	1 × 200	CYP2D6
Nebivolol	Yes	Yes	10	1 × 1.25	1 × 10	CYP2D6

[a]CYP2D6 indicates dependence on polymorphic CYP2D6 metabolism, likely less relevant for nebivolol because the first metabolite is active.
[b]Clinical studies in heart failure have mainly used metoprolol succinate in a slow-release formulation (zero order of kinetics); metoprolol, itself, has a $t_{1/2}$ of 3–5 h.

K^+. MRAs inhibit all the effects of aldosterone, of which the reduction in fibrosis is most pronounced in animal models.

Clinical Use; Adverse Responses. Currently, two MRAs are available, spironolactone and eplerenone. Only eplerenone is FDA-approved for the therapy of heart failure because no economic interest exists for the approval of spironolactone, which is free of patent protection. Nevertheless, guidelines recommend both. Spironolactone is a nonspecific steroid hormone receptor antagonist with similar affinity for progesterone and androgen receptors; it causes gynecomastia (painful breast swelling, 10% of patients) in men and dysmenorrhea in women. Eplerenone is selective for the mineralocorticoid receptor and therefore does not cause gynecomastia.

The most important ADR of both MRAs is hyperkalemia. Under the well-controlled conditions of clinical trials, serious hyperkalemia (>5.5 mmol/L) occurred in 12% in the eplerenone group and in 7% in the placebo group (Zannad et al., 2011). Rates may be higher in clinical practice when risk conditions, comedication, and dose restrictions are not well controlled (Juurlink et al., 2004). Guidelines for the use of MRAs in patients with heart failure are:

- Administer no more than 50 mg/d.
- Do not use if the GFR is less than 30 mL/min (creatinine ~ 2 mg/dL).
- Be careful with elderly patients, in whom improvement in prognosis may be less relevant than prevention of serious side effects.
- Be careful with diabetics, who carry a higher risk of hyperkalemia.
- Do not combine with NSAIDs, which are contraindicated in heart failure but are frequently prescribed for chronic degenerative diseases of the musculoskeletal system.
- Do not combine with other K^+-sparing diuretics.

Angiotensin Receptor and Neprilysin Inhibitors

The latest addition to standard combination therapy of heart failure is sacubitril/valsartan. It is made by cocrystallizing the well-known ARB valsartan with sacubritril, a prodrug that, after deesterization, inhibits neprilysin, a peptidase mediating the enzymatic degradation and inactivation of natriuretic peptides (ANP, BNP, CNP), bradykinin, and substance P. Thus, the drug combines inhibition of the RAAS with activation of a beneficial axis of neurohumoral activation, the natriuretic peptides. Consequently, the ARNI is expected to promote the beneficial effects natriuresis, diuresis, and vasodilation of arterial and venous blood vessels and to inhibit thrombosis, fibrosis, cardiac myocyte hypertrophy, and renin release. Augmentation of ANP/BNP levels by inhibiting degradation is probably a better pharmacological principle than giving the agonist BNP (neseritide; see under acute heart failure) directly because it enhances *endogenous* regulation of plasma and tissue levels. Sacubitril/valsartan causes smaller increases in bradykinin and substance P than omapatrilat, an earlier drug combining a neprilysin inhibitor and an ACEI. This difference may explain why sacubitril/valsartan is not associated with an increased rate of angioedema, the adverse effect that stopped the development of omapatrilat. A large head-to-head comparison study in patients with stable heart failure showed superiority of sacubitril/valsartan over enalapril (McMurray et al., 2014).

Treatment Principle II: Preload Reduction

Fluid overload with increased filling pressures (increased preload) and dilation of the ventricles in heart failure is the consequence of decreased kidney perfusion and activation of the RAAS. Normally, increased preload and stretch of the myofilaments increase contractile force in an autoregulatory manner, the positive force-length relationship or Frank-Starling mechanism. However, the failing heart in congestion operates at the flat portion of this relationship (Figure 29–4) and cannot generate sufficient force with increasing preload, leading to edema in the lungs and the periphery.

Diuretics increase Na^+ and water excretion by inhibiting transporters in the kidney and thereby improve symptoms of CHF by moving patients to lower cardiac filling pressures along the same ventricular function curve. Diuretics are an integral part of the combination therapy of symptomatic forms of heart failure. Prognostic efficacy of diuretics in heart failure will remain an academic question, simply because randomization for a trial of diuretics would be ethically impermissible. Diuretics should *not* be given to patients without congestion because they activate the RAAS and may accelerate a vicious downward spiral. On the other hand, in severe heart failure, diuretic resistance may occur for various reasons and cause clinical deterioration (Table 29–4).

Loop Diuretics

Loop diuretics (furosemide, torasemide, bumetanide; Table 29–5) inhibit the Na^+-K^+-2Cl symporter in the ascending limb of the loop of Henle, where up to 15% of the primary filtrate (~150 L/d) is reabsorbed, explaining their strong diuretic action. The increase in Na^+ and fluid delivery to distal nephron segments has two consequences:

- It is sensed in the macula densa and normally activates tubuloglomerular feedback to decrease GFR. This autoregulation explains the quick loss of efficacy of older diuretics of the carbonic anhydrase inhibitor class (e.g., acetazolamide), acting in the proximal tubule. Thiazides (see discussion that follows) are derived from this class and cause a small decrease in the GFR. Loop diuretics inhibit the feedback mechanism because it is mediated by the Na^+-K^+-2Cl symporter; they exhibit stable action and do not affect the GFR.
- It leads to increased ENaC-mediated reabsorption of Na^+ and, in exchange, to more K^+ excretion in the distal tubule, explaining the main side effect, hypokalemia.

The bioavailability of orally administered furosemide ranges from 40% to 70%. High drug doses are often required to initiate diuresis in patients with worsening symptoms or in those with impaired GI absorption, as may occur in severely hypervolemic patients with CHF-induced GI edema. Oral bioavailabilities of bumetanide and torasemide are greater than 80%, and as a result, these agents are more consistently absorbed than furosemide. Furosemide and bumetanide are short-acting drugs. The $t_{1/2}$ of furosemide in normal kidney function is about 1 h (increases in terminal kidney failure to > 24 h), and rebound Na^+ retention normally requires dosing twice a day or more. Bumetanide reaches maximal plasma concentrations in 0.5–2 h and has a $t_{1/2}$ of 1–1.5 h. Torasemide has a slower onset of action (maximal effect 1–2 h after ingestion) and a plasma $t_{1/2}$ of

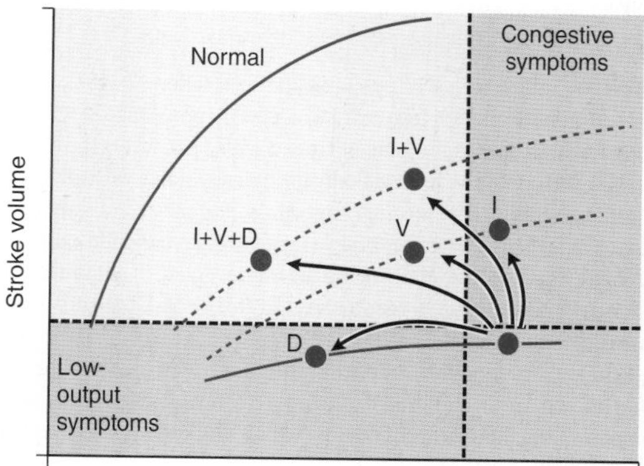

Figure 29–4 *Hemodynamic responses to pharmacologic interventions in heart failure.* The relationships between diastolic filling pressure (preload) and stroke volume (ventricular performance) are illustrated for a normal heart (green line; the Frank-Starling relationship) and for a patient with heart failure with systolic dysfunction (red line). Note that positive inotropic agents (I), such as CGs or dobutamine, move patients to a higher ventricular function curve (lower dashed line), resulting in greater cardiac work for a given level of ventricular filling pressure. Vasodilators (V), such as ACEIs or nitroprusside, also move patients to improved ventricular function curves while reducing cardiac filling pressures. Diuretics (D) improve symptoms of CHF by moving patients to lower cardiac filling pressures along the same ventricular function curve.

TABLE 29–4 ■ CAUSES OF DIURETIC RESISTANCE IN HEART FAILURE

Noncompliance with medical regimen; excess dietary Na^+ intake
Decreased renal perfusion and glomerular filtration rate due to *Excessive vascular volume depletion and hypotension due to aggressive diuretic or vasodilator therapy* *Decline in cardiac output due to worsening heart failure, arrhythmias, or other primary cardiac causes* *Selective reduction in glomerular perfusion pressure following initiation (or dose increase) of ACEI therapy*
Nonsteroidal anti-inflammatory drugs
Primary renal pathology (e.g., cholesterol emboli, renal artery stenosis, drug-induced interstitial nephritis, obstructive uropathy)
Reduced or impaired diuretic absorption due to gut wall edema and reduced splanchnic blood flow

3–4 h. Kidney failure does not critically affect the elimination of bumetanide or torasemide.

Thiazide Diuretics

Thiazide diuretics (hydrochlorothiazide, chlorthalidone; Table 29–5) have a limited role in heart failure for their low maximal diuretic effect and loss of efficacy at a GFR below 30 mL/min. However, combination therapy with loop diuretics is often effective in those refractory to loop diuretics alone, as refractoriness is often caused by upregulation of the Na^+-Cl cotransporter in the distal convoluted tubule, the main target of thiazide diuretics (see Chapter 25). Thiazides are associated with a greater degree of K^+ wasting per fluid volume reduction than loop diuretics, and combination therapy requires careful monitoring of K^+ loss.

K^+-Sparing Diuretics

K^+-Sparing diuretics (see Chapter 25) inhibit apical Na^+ channels in distal segments of the tubulus directly (ENaC; e.g., amiloride, triamterene) or reduce its gene expression (MRAs spironolactone and eplerenone). These agents are weak diuretics, but they are often used in the treatment of hypertension in combination with thiazides or loop diuretics to reduce K^+ and Mg^{2+} wasting. The prognostic efficacy of MRAs, which is at least partially independent of its K^+-sparing activity, make amiloride and triamteren largely dispensable in the therapy of heart failure. They should not be combined with ACEIs and MRAs.

Treatment Principle III: Afterload Reduction

The failing heart is exquisitely sensitive to increased arterial resistance (i.e., afterload) (Figure 29–5). Vasodilators, therefore, should have beneficial effects on patients with heart failure by reducing afterload and allowing the heart to expel blood against lower resistance. However, clinical trials with pure vasodilators were mainly disappointing, whereas inhibitors of the RAAS, vasodilators with a broader mode of action, were successful. Likely reasons include reflex tachycardia and tachyphylaxis (prazosin, ISDN) and negative inotropic effects (dihydropyridine calcium channel antagonists).

Hydralazine–Isosorbide Dinitrate

A remarkable exception is the therapeutic effect of a fixed combination of hydralazine and ISDN. In a pioneering trial, Cohn and colleagues showed moderate efficacy of this combination in patients with heart failure (Cohn et al., 1986). The benefit was restricted to improvement in the cohort of

TABLE 29–5 ■ PROPERTIES AND THERAPEUTIC DOSES OF DIURETICS FOR THE THERAPY OF HFrEJ[a]

DIURETIC	START DOSE (mg)	COMMON DAILY DOSE (mg)	TIME TO START OF EFFECT (h)	HALF-LIFE (h)	ADVERSE EFFECTS AND INTERACTIONS
Loop diuretics					
Bumetanide	0.5–1	1–5	0.5	1–1.5	**Adverse effects**: Hypokalemia, hyponatremia, hypomagnesemia, hyperuricemia, hypocalcemia (loop diuretics, hypercalcemia (thiazides), glucose intolerance **Interactions**: ↑[Li+] in serum (PK) and cardiac glycoside toxicity (PD, hypokalemia), anion exchanger resins (PK), non-steroidal anti-inflammatory drugs (NSAID), and glucocorticoids (PD) can ↓ effect of diuretics.
Furosemide	20–40	40–240	0.5	1	
Torasemide	5–10	10–20	1	3–4	
Thiazides					
Chlorthalidone	50	50–100	2	50	
Hydrochlorothiazide	25	12.5–100	1–2	6–8	
Potassium-sparing diuretics					
Eplerenone, spironolactone	50[b]	100–200[b]	2–6	24–36	**Adverse effects**: Hyperkalemia (all), gynecomasty, erectile dysfunction, and menstrual bleeding disorders (spironolactone) **Interactions**: ↑ Risk of hyperkalemia when given with ACE or ARB (use 50% lower dose), also with cyclosporine and NSAIDs **Contraindication**: Renal insufficiency with creatinine clearance < 30 mL/min
Amiloride	5[b]	10–20[b]	2	10–24	
Triamterene	50[b]	200[b]	2	8–16	

[a]Dosing recommendations were adapted from ESC guidelines (Ponikowski et al., 2016). [b]50% dose reduction when co-administered with RAS blocker.

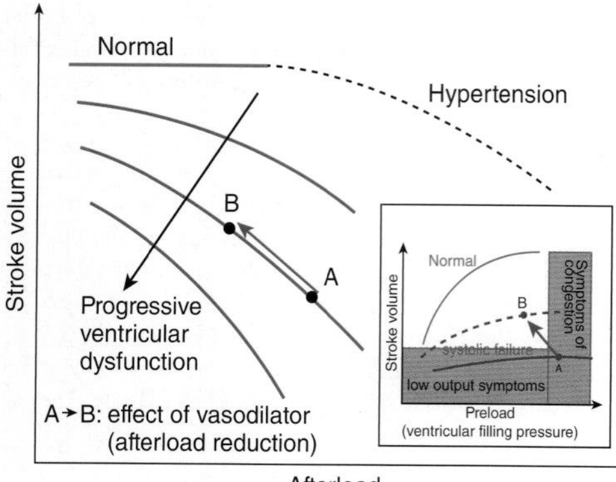

Figure 29–5 *Stroke volume versus afterload (outflow resistance): effects of heart failure. Increasing the resistance to ventricular outflow, a basic determinant of afterload, has little effect on stroke volume in normal hearts until high levels of outflow resistance (top curve).* However, in patients with systolic ventricular dysfunction (lower curves), an increase in outflow resistance elicits a noticeable decrease in cardiac performance (= stroke volume) that is progressive with increasing failure. Such an increase in outflow resistance can occur as a compensatory response by the SNS and RAAS to decreased cardiac function and depressed arterial pressure as a result of heart failure. A higher resistance to ventricular outflow increases peak pressure development in the left ventricle in opening the aortic valve, thereby increasing ventricular wall stress and end-systolic volume. This can cause end-diastolic volume to increase. In the normal heart, increasing ventricular stretch enhances cardiac contractile performance (stroke volume); this is the Frank-Starling effect (inset). However, in the failing heart, the positive contractile response embodied in the Frank-Starling effect is poor and provides only a small increase in stroke volume. Reducing outflow resistance with agents that reduce systemic vascular resistance, such as arterial vasodilators, can shift cardiac performance to a larger stroke volume in patients with myocardial dysfunction (from A to B). Such an increase in stroke volume may provide sufficient output and compensate for the decrease in systemic vascular resistance and moderate the fall in systemic arterial pressure due to the vasodilator. For details, see Figure 29–4 and the work of Klabunde (2015).

African Americans. In a second trial in African Americans only, the combination conferred a 43% survival benefit (Taylor et al., 2004). It was FDA-approved in 2006, the first ethnically restricted approval.

As an orally available organic nitrate, ISDN, similar to GTN and ISMN, preferentially dilates large blood vessels, for instance, venous capacitance and arterial conductance vessels (Chapter 27). The main effect is "venous pooling" and reduction of diastolic filling pressure (preload) with little effect on systemic vascular resistance (which is regulated by small-to-medium arterioles). Sustained monotherapy is compromised by nitrate tolerance (i.e., loss of effect and induction of a pro-constrictory state with high levels of ROS). Hydralazine is a direct vasodilator whose mechanism of action remains unresolved (Chapter 28). It was suggested that hydralazine prevents nitrate tolerance by reducing ROS-mediated inactivation of NO (Munzel et al., 2005), an action that could explain the efficacy of this drug combination in heart failure amongst African Americans. A test of this hypothesis in patients with NYHA class II–III heart failure (Chirkov et al., 2010) failed to confirm the hypothesis. The relevant differences in responsiveness between African American and Caucasian patients with heart failure have not been explained.

The fixed-combination formulation in use contains 37.5 mg hydralazine and 20 mg ISDN and is uptitrated to a target dose of 2 tablets, thrice daily. Patients will also generally be taking a β blocker. Hypotension may be dose limiting. Frequent adverse effects include dizziness and headache. Adherence to the thrice-daily dosing regimen may impose practical problems (Cohn et al., 1986), and hydralazine doses greater than 200 mg have been associated with lupus erythematosus.

Treatment Principle IV: Increasing Cardiac Contractility

The failing heart is unable to generate force sufficient to meet the needs of the body for perfusion of oxygenated blood (Figure 29-1). Historically, physicians attempted to stimulate force generation with positive inotropic drugs. Unfortunately, when used chronically, these agents do not improve life expectancy or cardiac performance. Rather, chronic use of positive inotropes is associated with excess mortality. Of the available inotropic agents, only CGs are used in the treatment of chronic heart failure; this is for two reasons: history and one large trial in patients with NYHA class II–III heart failure showing that digoxin reduced the rate of heart failure–associated hospitalizations without increasing mortality (Table 29–1).

Inotropic Agents and the Regulation of Cardiac Contractility

Cardiac myocytes contract and develop force in response to membrane depolarization and subsequent increases in intracellular Ca^{2+} concentrations (Figure 29–6). The mechanisms of this *excitation-contraction coupling* are the basis for understanding the mode of action of positive inotropic drugs and cardiac myocyte function in general. Most currently employed positive inotropes and novel compounds in development act by increasing the concentration of free intracellular Ca^{2+} ($[Ca^{2+}]_i$). Ca^{2+} "sensitizers" (e.g., levosimendan) sensitize myofilaments to Ca^{2+}; that is, they shift the sigmoidal relationship between free Ca^{2+} concentration and force to the left.

Na^+/K^+ ATPase Inhibitors. Cardiac glycosides inhibit the plasma membrane Na^+/K^+ ATPase, a key enzyme that actively pumps Na^+ out and K^+ into the cell and thereby maintains the steep concentration gradients of Na^+ and K^+ across the plasma membrane. Inhibition of this enzyme slightly reduces the Na^+ gradient across the myocyte membrane, reducing the driving force for Ca^{2+} extrusion by the NCX, thereby providing more Ca^{2+} for storage in the SR and subsequent release to activate contraction. The details are explained by Figure 29–6 and its legend.

cAMP-Dependent Inotropes. The strongest stimulation of the heart is achieved by receptor-mediated stimulation of adenylyl cyclase. This explains the use of dobutamine, EPI, and NE in cardiogenic shock (see discussion that follows). Inhibition of cAMP degradation by PDE inhibitors such as milrinone or enoximone elevates cellular cAMP concentrations and activates the cAMP-PKA pathway and other cAMP-responsive systems (see Chapter 3). This concerted action results in higher peak Ca^{2+} concentrations in systole and thereby peak force (Figure 29–6). All cAMP-dependent inotropes hasten contraction (positive clinotropic effect) and relaxation (positive lusitropic effect), allowing sufficient perfusion of the ventricles in diastole under catecholamine stimulation and with the concomitant tachycardia. On the downside, acceleration of contraction during catecholamine stimulation, by promoting net Ca^{2+} entry per unit of time, increases the utilization of ATP for Ca^{2+} reuptake into the SR via the SERCA and to restore the membrane potential by the activity of the Na^+/K^+ ATPase.

Myofilament Ca^{2+} Sensitizers. Calcium sensitizers increase the affinity of the myofilaments for Ca^{2+}, for example, by inducing a conformational change in TnC. They enhance force for a given $[Ca^{2+}]_i$ and do not elevate $[Ca^{2+}]_i$ with its potentially deleterious pro-arrhythmic and energy-increasing consequences. But, increased myofilament Ca^{2+} sensitivity also causes reduced dissociation of Ca^{2+} from the myofilaments in diastole and prolongation of relaxation ("negative lusitropic effect"). This effect can aggravate the already-compromised diastolic function in heart failure. It could also lead to delayed Ca^{2+} release from myofilaments in diastole and arrhythmias (Schober et al., 2012). Calcium sensitizers failed to improve prognosis in clinical trials of patients with chronic heart failure. However, levosimendan is approved in some countries for the treatment of acute heart failure. It has additional selective and potent inhibitory effects on PDE III, whose positive lusitropic consequence appears to antagonize the negative lusitropic effect of Ca^{2+} sensitization. Agonists of G_q-coupled receptors (α_1, AT_1, ET_A) also increase myofilament Ca^{2+} sensitivity, likely due to increased myosin light chain phosphorylation. The positive inotropic effect is smaller than that of β receptor stimulation, develops more slowly, and is independent of cAMP.

Cardiac Glycosides

Actions and Therapeutic Use of Digoxin. ***Positive Inotropic Effect.*** CGs at therapeutic concentrations mildly inhibit the cardiac Na^+/K^+ ATPase, causing an increase in intracellular $[Na^+]$. Increased $[Na^+]_i$ inhibits Ca^{2+} extrusion via the NCX resulting in higher intracellular $[Ca^{2+}]$ and enhanced contractility (Figure 29–6). The increased contractility and hence cardiac output provides symptomatic relief in patients with heart failure (Figure 29–1). With the main trigger for neurohumoral activation removed, sympathetic nerve tone and, consequently, heart rate and peripheral vascular resistance drop. These decreases in preload and afterload reduce chamber dilation and thereby wall stress, a strong determinant of myocardial O_2 consumption. Increased renal perfusion lowers renin production and increases diuresis, further decreasing preload.

Electrophysiological Actions. CGs at therapeutic concentrations shorten action potentials by accelerating the inactivation of L-type Ca^{2+} channels due to higher $[Ca^{2+}]_i$. Shorter action potentials (= refractory period) favor reentry arrhythmias, a reason that CGs promote atrial fibrillation. With the loss of intracellular K^+ and increase in intracellular Na^+, the resting membrane potential (determined largely by the K^+ current, now diminished) moves to less-negative values with two consequences. Diastolic depolarization and automaticity are enhanced, and, due to partial inactivation of Na^+ channels, impulse propagation is strongly reduced. Both phenomena promote reentry arrhythmias. At even higher CG concentrations, SR Ca^{2+} overload reaches a point at which Ca^{2+} is spontaneously released at amounts large enough to initiate Ca^{2+} waves and, via the NCX, depolarization of the cell (Figure 29–6). The typical ECG signs at this stage of CG intoxication are extrasystoles and bigeminies with a high risk of ventricular fibrillation.

Extracardiac Effects. CGs also inhibit Na^+/K^+ ATPase in other excitable tissues. (1) At low plasma concentrations, CGs stimulate vagal efferents and sensitize baroreceptor reflex mechanisms, causing increased parasympathetic and decreased sympathetic tone. The beneficial effect of digoxin at low plasma concentrations (Rathore et al., 2003), at which positive inotropic effects are minor, suggests that the neurohumoral actions of CGs may be therapeutically more relevant than the direct positive inotropic effects. (2) CGs at higher plasma concentrations increase Ca^{2+} concentrations in vascular smooth muscle cells and cause vasoconstriction. In patients with heart failure, vasodilation normally prevails due to the decrease in sympathetic nervous tone, but the direct vascular effect explains mesenteric artery ischemia or occlusion, a rare but severe adverse effect of CGs.

Indirect Actions. The vagotonic and sympatholytic effects of CGs cause bradycardia and AV prolongation (negative dromotropic effect) and can promote atrial flutter and fibrillation. Fibrillation is explained by the ACh-induced shortening of atrial action potentials, which is further enhanced by the direct CG effect described previously. On the other hand, CGs are therapeutically used for frequency control of permanent atrial fibrillation because of their negative dromotropic effects.

Interactions With K^+, Ca^{2+}, and Mg^{2+}. Hyperkalemia reduces and hypokalemia increases the binding affinity of CG to the Na^+/K^+ ATPase. In addition, hypokalemia reduces repolarizing K^+ currents, with the consequence of increased spontaneous diastolic depolarization and automaticity. Hypokalemia is therefore a major risk factor for arrhythmogenic effects of CGs. Hypercalcemia as well as hypomagnesemia favor SR Ca^{2+} overload and spontaneous Ca^{2+} release events. Control of serum electrolytes is therefore mandatory.

Adverse Effects. The therapeutic index of CG is extremely narrow, about 2, as documented in the DIG trial: plasma concentrations between 0.5 and 0.8 ng/mL are associated with beneficial effects, and concentrations of 1.2 ng/mL and greater are associated with a tendency toward increased mortality (Rathore et al., 2003). The most frequent and most serious adverse effects are arrhythmias. In CG overdosing, patients exhibit arrhythmias (90%), GI symptoms (~55%), and neurotoxic symptoms (~12%). The most frequent causes of toxicity are renal insufficiency and overdosing.

Cardiac toxicity in healthy persons presents as extreme bradycardia, atrial fibrillation, and AV block, whereas ventricular arrhythmias are rare. In patients with structural heart disease, frequent signs of CG toxicity are ventricular extrasystoles, bigeminy, ventricular tachycardia, and fibrillation. In principle, however, every type of arrhythmia can be CG induced. GI adverse effects are anorexia, nausea, and vomiting, mainly as a result of CG effects on chemosensors in the area postrema. Spastic contraction of the mesenteric artery can rarely lead to severe diarrhea and life-threatening necrosis of the intestine. Headache, fatigue, and sleeplessness can be early symptoms of CG toxicity.

Typical, albeit not too common (10%), are visual effects: altered color perception and coronas (halos). Some have speculated that the visual effects of digitalis intoxication contributed to the qualities of late paintings by Vincent van Gogh, who may have been treated for neurological complaints with foxglove by Dr. Paul Gachet, whose portraits by van Gogh (painted in June 1890) show the doctor seated next to a sprig of the plant, a natural source of CGs and used widely in the 19th century (Lee, 1981).

Therapy of CG Toxicity. Cessation of CG medication normally suffices as therapy of CG toxicity. However, severe arrhythmias, such as extreme bradycardia or complex ventricular arrhythmias, require active therapy.

- Extreme sinus bradycardia, sinoatrial block, or AV block grade II or III: Atropine (0.5–1 mg) IV. If not successful, a temporary pacemaker may be necessary.
- Tachycardic ventricular arrhythmias and hypokalemia: K^+ infusion (40–60 mmol/d). Consider that high K+ can aggravate AV conduction defects.
- An effective antidote for digoxin toxicity is antidigoxin immunotherapy. Purified Fab fragments from ovine antidigoxin antisera (Digibind) are usually dosed by the estimated total dose of digoxin ingested to achieve a fully neutralizing effect.

HISTORICAL PERSPECTIVE

The British botanist William Withering (1741–1799) systematically described the actions of *Digitalis purpurea* in patients with heart failure ("dropsy") and gave exact dosing recommendations (Skou 1986). Oswald Schmiedeberg (1833–1921), working in Strasbourg, France, isolated the first chemical entities from foxglove leaves; one of these entities was digitoxin. Until diuretics became available, CGs were the only heart failure drugs. CGs encompass many chemical entities, but only digoxin, its derivatives β-acetyl digoxin, methyldigoxin, and digitoxin are in clinical use in most countries. Until the 1980s, CGs were dosed according to therapeutic effects (e.g., improved diuresis [Withering considered CGs as diuretics], reduction of heart size [verifiable by X-ray], or alterations of the surface ECG) and to symptoms of overdosing, such as nausea and altered color perception (yellow-green). Now, serum digoxin concentrations can be measured by radioimmunoassay. Digoxin has therapeutic efficacy (including a small survival benefit) only at serum concentrations between 0.5 and 0.8 ng/mL (Rathore et al., 2003). Concentrations greater than 1.2 ng/mL are associated with increased mortality. Serum digoxin concentrations greater than 0.8 ng/mL should be avoided.

Treatment Principle V: Heart Rate Reduction

Heart rate is a strong determinant of cardiac energy consumption, and higher heart rates in patients with heart failure are associated with poor prognosis (Bohm et al., 2010). Partial agonists at β receptors such as xamoterol increase nocturnal heart rate (i.e., they prevent the physiological dip) and are associated with excess mortality in patients with heart failure (Xamoterol Study Group, 1990). Conversely, β blockers lower heart rate and improve survival prognosis.

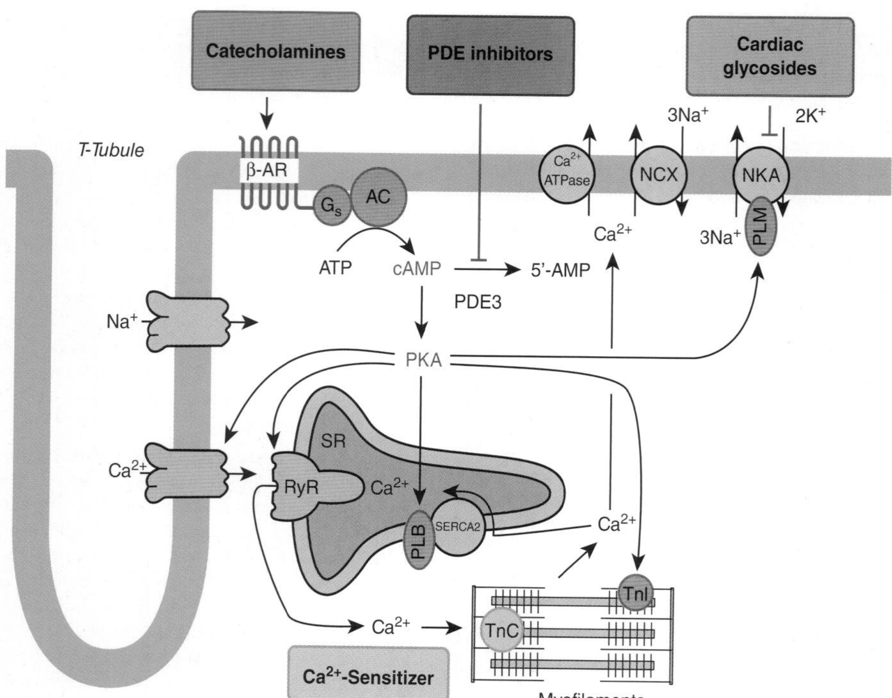

Figure 29–6 *Cardiac excitation-contraction coupling and its regulation by positive inotropic drugs.* The cardiac cycle is initiated by membrane depolarization, which causes the opening of voltage-dependent Na^+ and L-type Ca^{2+} channels, permitting Na^+ and Ca^{2+} flow down their electrochemical gradients into the myocyte. Thus, Na^+ and Ca^{2+} enter the cardiac myocyte during each cycle of membrane depolarization, triggering the release, through the RyR, of larger amounts of Ca^{2+} from internal stores in the SR. The resulting increase in intracellular Ca^{2+} interacts with troponin C and activates interactions between actin and myosin that result in sarcomere shortening. The electrochemical gradient for Na^+ across the sarcolemma is maintained by active transport of Na^+ out of the cell by the sarcolemmal Na^+/K^+ ATPase (NKA). The bulk of cytosolic Ca^{2+} (70%) is pumped back into the SR by a Ca^{2+}-ATPase, SERCA2. The remainder is removed from the cell by either a sarcolemmal Ca^{2+}-ATPase or a high-capacity NCX. The NCX exchanges three Na^+ for a Ca^{2+}, using the electrochemical potential of Na^+ to drive Ca^{2+} extrusion. The β adrenergic agonists (acting at βAR, the β adrenergic receptor) and PDE inhibitors, by increasing intracellular cAMP levels, activate PKA, which phosphorylates PLB in the SR, the α subunit of the L-type Ca^{2+} channel, and regulatory components of the RyR, as well as TnI. As a result, the probabilities of opening of the L-type Ca^{2+} channel and the RyR2 Ca^{2+} channel are increased; SERCA2 inhibition by PLB is released, with the result that SERCA2 accumulates Ca^{2+} into the SR faster, more avidly, and to a higher concentration; and relaxation occurs at slightly higher $[Ca^{2+}]_i$ due to slightly reduced sensitivity of the troponin complex to Ca^{2+}. The net effect of these phosphorylations is a positive inotropic effect: a faster rate of tension development to a higher level of tension, followed by a faster rate of relaxation. CGs, by inhibiting the Na^+/K^+ ATPase, reduce Na^+ extrusion from the cell, thereby permitting $[Na^+]_{in}$ to rise, reducing the inward gradient for Na^+ that drives Ca^{2+} extrusion by NCX. As a consequence, Ca^{2+} accumulates in the SR, and a positive inotropic effect follows, as noted previously for the effect of increased cellular cAMP. See the text for details of additional effects of CGs. Note that, under steady-state conditions, the amount of Ca^{2+} leaving the cell exactly matches the amount entering it. As NCX exchanges three Na^+ for every Ca^{2+}, it creates a depolarizing current. This makes not only the direction of transport dependent on the chemical gradients of Na^+ and Ca^{2+} across the membrane but also the membrane potential. Thus, the direction of Na^+-Ca^{2+} exchange may briefly reverse during depolarization, when the electrical gradient across the sarcolemma is transiently reversed. PLM is an tonic inhibitor of the Na^+/K^+ ATPase, which supplies the driving force (an appropriately low $[Na^+]_{in}$) for maintaining low diastolic Ca^{2+}. Phosphorylation of PLM by PKA removes this inhibitory influence, thereby stimulating the activity of the Na^+/K^+ ATPase and limiting $[Na^+]_{in}$ and $[Ca^{2+}]_{in}$. This may reduce the tendency toward arrhythmias during adrenergic stimulation (see Pavlovic et al., 2013).

Ivabradine

The circumstantial evidence for beneficial effects of heart rate lowering led to the development of ivabradine, a selective inhibitor of cardiac pacemaker channels (HCNs). The compound is approved in Europe for the treatment of heart failure and stable angina pectoris in patients not tolerating β blockers or in whom β blockers did not sufficiently lower heart rate (<75/min). Approval was based on a study showing a decrease in hospitalization and heart failure mortality, but not total or cardiovascular mortality (Swedberg et al., 2010). Of note, the effect of ivabradine was not superior to that of digoxin in an earlier study (Digitalis Investigation Group, 1997). In a recent large study in patients with stable angina (85% on β blockers), ivabradine conferred no benefit but led to phosphenes (typical transient enhanced brightness in a restricted area of the visual field) and increased the rate of bradycardia, atrial fibrillation, and QT prolongation (Fox et al., 2014), casting doubts about the role of the compound in ischemic heart disease. Ivabradine is not approved in the U.S.

Drug Treatment of Acutely Decompensated Heart Failure

Acutely decompensated heart failure is a leading cause of hospitalization in patients older than 65 and represents a sentinel prognostic event in the natural course of the disease, with a high recurrence rate and a 1-year mortality rate of about 30%. Even in decompensated heart failure, about 50% of patients exhibit preserved left ventricular function (HFpEF). The HFpEF cohort is older, more likely to be female and hypertensive, and with less coronary artery disease than the HFrEF cohort. Therapeutically, it is important to quickly identify and treat specific reasons for decompensation. These include, besides acute myocardial ischemia, uncorrected high blood pressure, atrial fibrillation and other arrhythmias, pulmonary embolism, and kidney failure, as well as several pharmacological reasons: nonadherence to heart failure medication and Na^+/fluid restriction, negative inotropic drugs (e.g., verapamil, diltiazem, nifedipine, β blockers), and NSAIDs and COX-2 inhibitors.

The therapy of acutely decompensated heart failure aims at fast symptom relief, short-term survival, fast recompensation, and reduction of readmission rates. It is less evidence-based than the therapy of chronic heart failure, and no single drug given to patients experiencing acute decompensation has yet been shown to improve the long-term prognosis. The main principles (besides nonpharmacological treatment modalities such as O_2 and noninvasive or [rarely] invasive ventilatory support) are diuretics and vasodilators, with positive inotropes in selected cases and mechanical support systems as an ultimate step.

Diuretics

Patients with dyspnea and signs of fluid overload/congestion should be promptly treated with an intravenous loop diuretic such as furosemide that exerts an acute vasodilator and slightly delayed but still fast diuretic effect. Optimal doses and regimens need to be adapted to the clinical picture. An intravenous bolus of 40–80 mg furosemide is a common starting dose, often continued by an infusion of furosemide at a daily dose equal to the (oral) daily dose prescribed before hospitalization. Doses may need to be escalated according to symptoms and diuresis. Additional use of a thiazide diuretic in small doses can break a relative resistance to loop diuretics but requires careful monitoring of K^+ losses. Excessive doses of furosemide must be avoided because they can cause hypotension, a reduction in GFR, electrolyte disturbance, and further neurohumoral activation.

Vasodilators

Vasodilators such as *nitroglycerin* and *nitroprusside* reduce preload and afterload. The reduction in preload (= diastolic filling pressure) moves the patient to the left on the stroke volume-preload relationship, similar to the effect of diuretic-induced volume reduction (Figure 29–3). The accompanying reduction in chamber dimension reduces wall stress and thus O_2 consumption. The additional reduction in afterload allows the heart to expel blood against a lower output resistance (Figure 29–4). These mechanisms explain why vasodilators (which have no inotropic efficacy and lower blood pressure) increase stroke volume. Yet, robust evidence for symptomatic benefit or improved clinical outcome is lacking. They are probably best suited for patients with hypertension and should be avoided in patients with systolic blood pressure less than 110 mm Hg (Ponikowski et al., 2016). The main risk is hypotension, which is negatively associated with favorable outcomes in patients with acutely decompensated heart failure (Patel et al., 2014).

Neseritide, recombinant human BNP, dilates arterial and venous blood vessels by stimulating the membrane-bound guanylyl cyclase to produce more cGMP. By this mechanism, it decreases preload and afterload and reduces pulmonary capillary wedge pressure. It is approved for the treatment of acutely decompensated heart failure in the U.S., but not in several European countries. Early clinical studies and a meta-analysis raised concerns that the use of neseritide was associated with an increased risk for renal failure and death when compared to a noninotrope control therapy (Sackner-Bernstein et al., 2005). This risk was not confirmed in a more recent study (O'Connor et al., 2011), but beneficial effects (dyspnea relief) were also modest.

Positive Inotropic Agents

Stimulating the heart's force of contraction in a situation of critically diminished cardiac output may appear to be the most intuitive intervention. Yet, inotropes in acutely decompensated heart failure are associated with worse outcome and should therefore be restricted to patients with critically low cardiac output and perfusion of vital organs. Hypotension less than 85 mm Hg has been suggested as a practical limit (Ponikowski et al., 2016). Reasons for the adverse consequences of positive inotropes are probably complex. All inotropic agents increase cardiac energy expenditure (greater and faster force development ⇒ more ATP consumption ⇒ greater O_2 demand), which carries the risk of diffuse cardiac myocyte death. In acutely decompensated heart failure, the risk is exaggerated by the low perfusion pressure, any preexisting coronary artery disease, and the likely presence of cardiac myocyte hypertrophy and myocyte-endothelial cell mismatch. Tachycardia, aggravated by many inotropes, adds to the problem by strongly increasing energy expenditure and reducing the time for coronary perfusion in diastole. All positive inotropes increase the risk of arrhythmias.

Dobutamine

Dobutamine is the β adrenergic agonist of choice for the management of patients with acute CHF with systolic dysfunction. Dobutamine has relatively well-balanced cardiac and vascular actions: stimulation of cardiac output with less tachycardia than EPI and with a concomitant decrease in pulmonary artery wedge pressure. Dobutamine is a racemic mixture of (−) and (+) enantiomers. The (−) enantiomer is a potent agonist at α_1 adrenergic receptors and a weak agonist at β_1 and β_2 receptors. The (+) enantiomer is a potent β_1 and β_2 agonist without much activity at α_1 adrenergic receptors. Dobutamine has no activity at dopamine receptors. At infusion rates that result in a positive inotropic effect in humans, the β_1 adrenergic effect in the myocardium predominates. In the vasculature, the α_1 adrenergic agonist effect of the (−) enantiomer appears to be offset by the vasodilating effects of the (+) enantiomer at β_2 receptors. Thus, the principal hemodynamic effect of dobutamine is an increase in stroke volume from positive inotropy, augmented by a small decrease in systemic vascular resistance and, therefore, afterload. Lowering of pulmonary artery capillary pressure is considered an advantage compared to other catecholamines, as is the smaller chronotropic effect (reasons for which are not clear).

Continuous dobutamine infusions are typically initiated at 2–3 μg/kg/min and uptitrated until the desired hemodynamic response is achieved. Pharmacologic tolerance may limit infusion efficacy beyond 4 days; therefore, addition or substitution a PDE3 inhibitor may be necessary to maintain adequate circulatory support. The major side effects of dobutamine are tachycardia and supraventricular/ventricular arrhythmias, which may require a reduction in dosage. The concurrent use of β blockers is a common cause of blunted clinical responsiveness to dobutamine. It can be overcome by higher doses in case of bisoprolol and metoprolol, but not as easily for carvedilol, which has a very slow dissociation rate.

Epinephrine

The natural sympathetic agonist is mainly produced by the adrenal gland and systemically released. It is a balanced β_1, β_2, and α_1 adrenergic agonist and has a similar net hemodynamic effect as dobutamine, but with a stronger tachycardic effect, which makes it a second-choice inotrope in acutely decompensated heart failure.

Norepinephrine

The main sympathetic neurotransmitter released from sympathetic nerve endings is a potent β_1 and α_1 agonist and weak β_2 receptor agonist. This profile causes the positive inotropism accompanied by prominent vasoconstriction and increased afterload. Vasoconstriction of coronary blood vessels promotes ischemia; increased afterload may impede cardiac output (Figure 29–4). However, the stronger blood pressure–increasing effect of NE may be needed in persistent hypotension despite adequate cardiac filling pressures. Moreover, the increase in mean blood pressure leads to a reflex increase in parasympathetic nervous tone that can antagonize the direct tachycardic effect of NE and actually cause bradycardia.

Dopamine

The pharmacologic and hemodynamic effects of DA vary with concentration. Low doses (≤2 μg/kg lean body mass/min) induce cAMP-dependent vascular smooth muscle vasodilation by direct stimulation of D2 receptors. Activation of D2 receptors on sympathetic nerves in the peripheral circulation also inhibits NE release and reduces α adrenergic stimulation of vascular smooth muscle, particularly in splanchnic and renal arterial beds. This is the pharmacological basis for the "low-dose DA infusion" historically used to increase renal blood flow and maintain an adequate GFR and diuresis in hospitalized patients with CHF with impaired renal function refractory to diuretics. However, mainly negative clinical studies argue against the validity of this concept (Chen et al., 2013; Vargo et al., 1996). At intermediate infusion rates (2–5 μg/kg/min), dopamine directly stimulates cardiac β receptors to enhance myocardial contractility. At higher infusion rates (5–15 μg/kg/min), α adrenergic receptor stimulation–mediated peripheral arterial and venous constriction occurs. The complex profile and negative clinical data on low-dose infusion make DA a second or third choice in the treatment of heart failure.

Phosphodiesterase Inhibitors

The cAMP-PDE inhibitors decrease cellular cAMP degradation, resulting in elevated levels of cAMP. This results in positive inotropic and chronotropic effects in the heart and dilation of resistance and capacitance vessels, effectively decreasing preload and afterload (thus the term *inodilator*). PDE inhibitors may be more advantageous than catecholamines in patients on β blockers and in patients with high systemic or pulmonary artery resistance. Hypotension is often dose limiting; tachycardic and arrhythmogenic effects are similar to those of catecholamines.

Milrinone and Enoximone. Parenteral formulations of milrinone and enoximone are used for short-term circulation support in advanced CHF. Enoximone (not available in the U.S.) is a relative selective inhibitor of PDE3, the cGMP-inhibited cAMP PDE and main isoform involved in inotropic control in human heart. Milrinone inhibits human heart PDE3 and PDE4 with similar potency (Bethke et al., 1992). By increasing intracellular cAMP concentrations, they have similar actions as the β receptor agonists dobutamine and EPI, but tend to lower systemic and pulmonary vascular resistance more than do the catecholamines. It should be kept in mind that PDE inhibitors potentiate the actions of β receptor agonists, both beneficial and detrimental. The loading dose of milrinone is ordinarily 25–75 μg/kg, and the continuous infusion rate ranges from 0.375 to 0.75 μg/kg/min. Bolus doses of enoximone at 0.5–1.0 mg/kg over 5–10 min are followed by an infusion of 5–20 μg/kg/min. The elimination half-lives of milrinone and enoximone in normal individuals are 0.5–1 h and 2–3 h, respectively, but can be increased in patients with severe CHF.

Myofilament Calcium Sensitizers (Levosimendan, Pimobendan)

In some countries but not in the U.S., calcium sensitizers are approved for the short-term treatment of acutely decompensated heart failure (e.g., levosimendan in Sweden, pimobendan in Japan). Calcium sensitizers increase the sensitivity of contractile myofilaments to Ca^{2+} by binding to and inducing a conformational change in the thin-filament regulatory protein troponin C. This causes an increased force for a given cytosolic Ca^{2+} concentration, theoretically without raising the $[Ca^{2+}]_{cytosol}$. However, a variety of other effects has been ascribed to pimobendan and levosimendan, including inhibition of PDEs, inhibition of the production of pro-inflammatory cytokines, and opening of ATP-dependent potassium channels. Clinical data provide evidence for symptomatic benefit and reductions in the length of stay in the hospital but do not support a better safety profile of levosimendan compared to catecholamines or classical PDE inhibitors (Mebazaa et al., 2007). Increased rates of arrhythmia and death are likely related to the PDE3 inhibitor activity of these compounds.

Other Drugs Used in Heart Failure

The vasopressin receptor antagonist tolvaptan is FDA-approved for the treatment of therapy-resistant hyponatremia, a common and difficult-to-treat complication in decompensated heart failure. Studies in a more general cohort of patients with heart failure failed to show convincing beneficial effects of this compound. Severe thirst and dehydration are common side effects. Heparin or other anticoagulants are routinely used in hospitalized patients with heart failure to prevent thromboembolism.

Role of Standard Combination Therapy

The majority of patients hospitalized with acutely decompensated heart failure have preexisting heart failure and respective maintenance therapy. Guidelines suggest reviewing a patient's existing therapy on admission to determine whether recent changes in the medication could be causally related to an exacerbation of cardiac disease. If not, the standard heart failure medication (ACEI, β blocker, MRA, diuretic) should be continued in the absence of hemodynamic instability or contraindications (Yancey et al., 2013).

Lessons From Heart Failure Drug Development

Heart failure is an attractive but difficult indication for drug development. The number of drug development failures over the past two decades largely exceeded that of successes, indicating our incomplete understanding of the pathophysiology of heart failure, but sometimes also signaling problematic trial design. Even negative trials have helped to better understand the disease. Examples of drugs that have been tested in large prospective trials and failed are listed in Table 29–6.

TABLE 29–6 ■ FAILURES IN DRUG DEVELOPMENT FOR HEART FAILURE

DRUG (type)	YEAR OF PUBLICATION	REASON FOR FAILURE
Milrinone (PDE inhibitor)	1991	Increased mortality
Pimobendan (PDE inhibitor)	1996	Trend toward increased mortality
Flosequinan (unclear)	1993	Increased mortality
Vesnarinone (unclear)	1998	Increased mortality, arrhythmias
Moxonidine (central antisympathetic)	1998	Increased mortality
Infliximab (TNFα blocker)	2003	Increased mortality
Etanercept (TNFα blocker)	2004	Trend toward increased mortality
Bosentan (ET receptor blocker)	2005	Liver toxicity, trend toward benefit over time (?)
Etomoxir (CPT1 blocker)	2007	Liver toxicity
Omapatrilat (dual ACEI and neprilysin inhibitor)	2002	Angioedema, no clear benefit
ARB + ACEI	2003 and 2008	No benefit, more angioedema and renal side effects
Rosuvastatin (HMG CoA reductase inhibitor)	2007	No benefit
Tolvaptan (vasopressin V2 receptor blocker)	2009	No benefit
Rolophylline (adenosine A_1 receptor blocker)	2009	No benefit, seizures

Lessons From Failed Drugs

The failure of *positive inotropic agents* (PDE inhibitors, catecholamines, calcium sensitizers, mixed-acting compounds such as flosequinan or vesnarinone; Cohn et al., 1998) to improve long-term outcome of patients with heart failure has induced a paradigm shift toward drugs that unload the heart and reduce neurohumoral activation, the current standard. It demonstrated that further stimulating the failing heart may transiently improve symptoms but increase mortality. But, simply reducing the load without protecting the heart from the adverse consequences of the activated SNS and RAAS also seems inefficient, as exemplified by the neutral effect of the α_1 receptor antagonist *prazosin* in the VeHeFT-I trial (Cohn et al., 1986). *Moxonidine*, a centrally acting α_2/imidazole agonist with similar sympatholytic actions as clonidine, should have had efficacy similar to that of β blockers, but moxonidine increased mortality in a larger prospective trial (Cohn et al., 2003). It is unclear whether doses and dose titration were too aggressive or whether the principle of central sympatholysis is unsafe in heart failure. Multiple lines of laboratory and clinical evidence suggested that heart failure has an important inflammatory component; yet, two blockers of TNF, *infliximab* and *etanercept*, induced harm rather than benefit in patients with chronic heart failure (Chung et al., 2003; Mann et al., 2004).

Endothelin 1, a potent vasoconstrictor, is upregulated in heart failure and could play an adverse role in heart failure, similar to that of AngII. Nonselective ET receptor antagonists such as *bosentan* had striking efficacy in postinfarct rodent models and are successfully used in pulmonary hypertension (Chapter 31). However, bosentan showed no efficacy in patients with chronic heart failure (Packer et al., 2005). *Omapatrilat*, a dual inhibitor of ACE and neprilysin, can decrease AngII and increase ANP/BNP, conditions promoting vasodilation, diuresis, and antihypertrophic effects; however, expectations that omapatrilat would be more efficacious than an ACEI in heart failure were not confirmed in a prospective study (Packer et al., 2002).

Numerous clinical trials have tested the idea that adding an ARB or the renin inhibitor *aliskiren* to standard therapy that includes an ACEI would be beneficial by more completely inhibiting the RAAS. With the exception of one trial (McMurray et al., 2003), studies of these combinations consistently showed a lack of benefit and an increase in adverse effects, particularly decreased renal function and hyperkalemia. The premise was that if some inhibition of the RAAS is good, more would be better; perhaps the premise was wrong.

Statins were proposed to have anti-inflammatory, antihypertrophic, and pro-angiogenic effects independent of their cholesterol-lowering effect (Liao and Laufs, 2005). Trials testing this hypothesis by adding statins to standard treatment of chronic heart failure demonstrated that the combination was safe but had no added beneficial effect on mortality (Kjekshus et al., 2007). An antagonist of the V_2 vasopressin receptor tolvaptan was ineffective in patients with chronic stable heart failure (Udelson et al., 2007). The discrepancy to several positive preclinical and early clinical studies suggests that the vasopressin axis of the neurohumoral activation program in heart failure may be sufficiently addressed by standard combination therapy, leaving no room for further improvement.

Lessons From Treating Acute Heart Failure

The drugs currently recommended (furosemide, nitroglycerin, dobutamine) for the treatment of acutely decompensated heart failure have never been tested in adequately powered prospective clinical trials. All novel drugs tested either in comparison to standard inotropes or noninotropes or as an add-on have failed to show convincing superiority or benefit in terms of symptoms, duration of hospitalization, and 30-day mortality. The A_1 adenosine receptor antagonist *rolophylline* should produce several beneficial effects on the kidney, including inhibition of tubular reabsorption of Na^+ and water, dilation of the afferent arteriole, and inhibition of tubular-glomerular feedback, but its addition to standard therapy in patients with acute heart failure with impaired kidney function produced no salutary renal or cardiac effects and caused unacceptable adverse effects such as seizures, a typical side effect of central A_1 adenosine antagonism known also from theophylline (Massie et al., 2010).

Recent Developments; Novel Approaches

Numerous pharmacological and nonpharmacological treatment options are being tested in preclinical and clinical studies (https://www.clinicaltrials.gov). They range from cell and gene therapies to food supplements (vitamins, polyunsaturated fatty acid) and intravenous iron to classical small molecules. In the CUPID2 trial, gene therapy, in the form of an intracoronary infusion of adeno-associated virus 1/SERCA2, did not provide any benefit in HFrEF (Greenberg et al., 2016). *Serelaxin*, recombinant human *relaxin 2*, is a naturally occurring peptide with 53 amino acids discovered in 1926 as an ovarian hormone inducing relaxation of the uterus during pregnancy. Its actions on the cardiovascular system include increased arterial compliance, cardiac output, and renal blood flow, characteristics of a promising drug for the treatment of acutely decompensated heart failure. However, the promising results of an earlier study (Teerlink et al., 2013) were not confirmed in a larger phase III trial (announced online March 2017).

Guanylyl cyclases are established targets for natriuretic peptides (the membrane form, mGC) and NO and organic nitrates (the soluble form, sGC). *Riociugat* is a direct, heme-dependent stimulator of sGC; *cinaciguat* is a heme-independent activator of sGC. Oxidative inactivation of sGC is believed to be a common pathology in cardiovascular disease and a reason for endothelial dysfunction. sGC activators have maintained (or even enhanced) effects at sGC enzymes inactivated by oxidation. Riociguat is approved for the treatment of pulmonary artery hypertension and chronic thromboembolic pulmonary hypertension (see Chapter 31). A prospective study with cinaciguat was prematurely stopped because the drug not only lowered pulmonary wedge pressure and increased cardiac output, but also markedly increased the rate of symptomatic hypotension (Erdmann et al., 2013), a classical problem of vasodilator therapy in acute heart failure.

Heart failure is often associated with anemia, a predictor of a poor prognosis. Yet, correction of anemia by an erythropoietin derivative, *darbapoetin* alpha, did not affect any clinical end point but increased the rate of thromboembolic events and ischemic strokes in patients with heart failure and mild-to-moderate anemia (Swedberg et al., 2013). However, intravenous iron, added to standard therapy in patients with NYHA class II–III heart failure, iron deficiency, and hemoglobin levels of 9.5–13.5 g/dL, improved quality of life, NYHA class, and physical exercise capacity (Anker et al., 2009). The beneficial effects seemed to be independent of the presence of anemia and may be related to other roles of iron in the body. Larger prospective studies are needed to confirm the effects.

Acknowledgment: *Henry Ooi, Wilson Colucci, Bradley A. Maron, James C. Fang, and Thomas P. Rocco have contributed to this chapter in recent editions of this book. We have retained some of their text in the current edition.*

Bibliography

Anker SD, et al. Ferric carboxymaltose in patients with heart failure and iron deficiency. *N Engl J Med*, **2009**, *361*:2436–2448.

Bethke T, et al. Phosphodiesterase inhibition by enoximone in preparations from nonfailing and failing human hearts. *Arzneimittelforschung*, **1992**, *42*:437–445.

Bohm M, et al. Heart rate as a risk factor in chronic heart failure (SHIFT): the association between heart rate and outcomes in a randomised placebo-controlled trial. *Lancet*, **2010**, *376*:886–894.

Chen HH, et al. Low-dose dopamine or low-dose nesiritide in acute heart failure with renal dysfunction: the ROSE acute heart failure randomized trial. *JAMA*, **2013**, *310*:2533–2543.

Chirkov YY, et al. Hydralazine does not ameliorate nitric oxide resistance in chronic heart failure. *Cardiovasc Drugs Ther*, **2010**, *24*:131–137.

Chung ES, et al. Randomized, double-blind, placebo-controlled, pilot trial of infliximab, a chimeric monoclonal antibody to tumor necrosis factor-alpha, in patients with moderate-to-severe heart failure: results of the anti-TNF Therapy Against Congestive Heart Failure (ATTACH) trial. *Circulation*, **2003**, *107*:3133–3140.

Drug Facts for Your Personal Formulary: *Heart Failure Drugs*

Drug	Therapeutic Uses	Major Toxicity and Clinical Pearls
Inhibitors of the Renin-Angiotensin System		
ACE Inhibitors Benazepril Captopril Enalapril Lisinopril Quinapril Ramipril	• Heart failure • Hypertension • Diabetic nephropathy	• First choice in treating heart failure • Short-acting captopril only for initiation of therapy; enalapril requires twice-daily dosing • Cough in 5%–10% of patients, angioedema • Hypotension, hyperkalemia, skin rash, neutropenia, anemia, fetopathic syndrome • Contraindicated in patients with renal artery stenosis; caution in patients with impaired renal function or hypovolemia
Fosinopril Trandolapril Perindopril		• Both hepatic and renal elimination, caution in patients with renal or hepatic impairment
Angiotensin Receptor Blockers Candesartan Eprosartan Irbesartan Losartan Olmesartan Telmisartan Valsartan	• Hypertension • Heart failure • Diabetic nephropathy	• Only in cases of intolerance to ACEI • Unwanted effects as ACEI, but no cough or angioedema • No evidence for superiority over ACEI • In combination with ACEI more harm than benefit
β Blockers		
Bisoprolol Carvedilol Metoprolol Nebivolol	• Heart failure • Hypertension • Widely used for angina, prevention of arrhythmias, rate control in atrial fibrillation, migraine	• First choice in the treatment of heart failure • Start low (1/10 target dose), go slow (2- to 4-weekly doubling) • Adverse effects: bradycardia, AV block, bronchospasm, peripheral vasoconstriction, worsening of acute heart failure, depression, worsening of psorias • Polymorphic CYP2D6 metabolism (metoprolol)
Mineralocorticoid Receptor Antagonists		
Eplerenone Spironolactone	• Heart failure • Hypertension • Hyperaldosteronism, hypokalemia, ascites	• First choice in treating symptomatic heart failure • Low doses (25–50 mg) • Most serious side effect is hyperkalemia • Spironolactone causes painful breast swelling and impotence in men, dysmenorrhea in women due to nonselective binding to sex hormone receptors
Neprilysin Inhibitor/Angiotensin Receptor Blocker		
Sacubitril/valsartan	• Heart failure	• Superior to the ACEI enalapril • May become first choice in treating heart failure • ↓ Degradation of natriuretic peptides, ↑ their beneficial actions • Hypotension
Diuretics		
Thiazide Type Chlorothiazide Hydrochlorothiazide ***Thiazide-like*** Chlorthalidone Indapamide Metolazone	• Edema associated with congestive heart failure, liver cirrhosis, chronic kidney disease, and nephrotic syndrome • Hypertension • Nephrogenic diabetes insipidus • Kidney stones caused by Ca^{2+} crystals	• Symptomatic treatment of milder forms of heart failure • Loose efficacy at GFR < 30–40 mL/min (exception indapamide and metolazone) • Potentiate effect of loop diuretics in severe heart failure (sequential tubulus blockade) • Risk for hypokalemia and arrhythmia when combined with QT-prolonging drugs
Loop Diuretics Bumetanide Furosemide Torasemide	• Acute pulmonary edema (intravenous) • Edema associated with congestive heart failure, liver cirrhosis, chronic kidney disease, and nephrotic syndrome • Hyponatremia • Hypercalcemia • Hypertension with renal insufficiency	• Symptomatic treatment of severe heart failure and acute decompensation • Often required in treating severe chronic heart failure, twice-daily dosing or more • Torasemide may be superior to furosemide in heart failure • Risk for hypokalemia and arrhythmia when combined with QT-prolonging drugs
Vasodilators		
ISDN/hydralazine	• Heart failure in African Americans	• Approved only for African Americans • Adverse effects: headache, nausea, flushing, hypotension, palpitations, tachycardia, dizziness, angina pectoris; ⇒ use in combination with β blocker • Compliance problems • Lupus syndrome

Drug Facts for Your Personal Formulary: *Heart Failure Drugs (continued)*

Drug	Therapeutic Uses	Major Toxicity and Clinical Pearls
Positive Inotropes		
Digoxin Digitoxin	• Heart failure	• Not first choice in treating heart failure • May exert benefits in heart failure and atrial fibrillation • Low therapeutic index: proarrhythmic, nausea, diarrhea, visual disturbances • Digoxin kidney dependent, digitoxin not • Half-life 1.5 (digoxin) or 7 days (digitoxin) • Plasma concentration: 0.5–0.8 ng/mL (digoxin) or 10–25 ng/mL (digitoxin)
Heart Rate Reduction		
Ivabradine	• Heart failure	• Not first choice in treating heart failure • May exert benefits in patients not tolerating β blockers or having heart rate > 75 under β blockers • Unwanted effects: bradycardia, QT prolongation, atrial fibrillation, phosphenes
Intravenous Vasodilators: Acute decompensated heart failure		
Nitroglycerin Sodium nitroprusside	• Acute decompensated heart failure	• May ↑ cardiac output in acute congestion (↑ filling pressure and dilation) via ↓ preload and afterload • NO releaser, stimulates soluble guanylyl cyclase • Avoid if systolic blood pressure < 110 mmHg • Prognostic benefit unclear
Neseritide	• Acute decompensated heart failure	• Recombinant human BNP • Stimulates membrane-bound guanylyl cyclase • May ↑ cardiac output via ↓ preload and afterload • Therapeutic benefit unclear
Intravenous Positive Inotropes: Acutely decompensated heart failure		
Dobutamine Dopamine Epinephrine Norepinephrine	• Acute decompensated heart failure	• β_1 receptor-mediated stimulation of cardiac output and, depending on drug, complex vascular actions • Last option in patients with systolic blood pressure <85 mmHg • ↑ Cardiac energy consumption and risk of arrhythmia • Use of catecholamines correlates with poor prognosis; use lowest possible doses for shortest possible time • Dobutamine causes less tachycardia than EPI and less afterload increase than NE • Role of low-dose dopamine unclear
Enoximone Milrinone	• Acute decompensated heart failure	• PDE3/4 inhibitors, ↑ cellular cAMP • ↑ Cardiac output and dilate blood vessels ("inodilator") • May be used in patients on β blockers and with high peripheral and pulmonary arterial resistance • Blood pressure decrease is dose limiting • Risks and prognostic effects: same as catecholamines (above)
Levosimendan	• Acute decompensated heart failure	• Combined Ca^{2+} sensitizer (troponin C binding) and PDE3 inhibitor • ↑ Cardiac output and ↓ vascular resistance ("inodilator") • Advantages over catecholamines or simple PDE inhibitors unclear

CIBIS-II Investigators. The Cardiac Insufficiency Bisoprolol Study II (CIBIS-II): a randomised trial. *Lancet,* **1999**, *353*:9–13.

Cohn JN, et al. Effect of vasodilator therapy on mortality in chronic congestive heart failure. Results of a Veterans Administration Cooperative Study. *N Engl J Med,* **1986**, *314*:1547–1552.

Cohn JN, et al. A dose-dependent increase in mortality with vesnarinone among patients with severe heart failure. Vesnarinone Trial Investigators. *N Engl J Med,* **1998**, *339*:1810–1816.

Cohn JN, et al. Adverse mortality effect of central sympathetic inhibition with sustained-release moxonidine in patients with heart failure (MOXCON). *Eur J Heart Fail,* **2003**, *5*:659–667.

CONSENSUS Trial Study Group. Effects of enalapril on mortality in severe congestive heart failure. Results of the Cooperative North Scandinavian Enalapril Survival Study (CONSENSUS). *N Engl J Med,* **1987**, *316*:1429–1435.

Digitalis Investigation Group. The effect of digoxin on mortality and morbidity in patients with heart failure. *N Engl J Med,* **1997**, *336*:525–533.

Erdmann E, et al. Cinaciguat, a soluble guanylate cyclase activator, unloads the heart but also causes hypotension in acute decompensated heart failure. *Eur Heart J,* **2013**, *34*:57–67.

Flather MD, et al. Randomized trial to determine the effect of nebivolol on mortality and cardiovascular hospital admission in elderly patients with heart failure (SENIORS). *Eur Heart J,* **2005**, *26*:215–225.

Fox K, et al. Ivabradine in stable coronary artery disease. *N Engl J Med,* **2014**, *371*:2435.

Greenberg B, et al. Calcium Upregulation by Percutaneous Administration of Gene Therapy in Patients With Cardiac Disease (CUPID 2): a randomised, multinational, double-blind, placebo-controlled, phase 2b trial. *Lancet,* **2016**, *387*:1178–1186.

Hubers SA, Brown NJ. Combined angiotensin receptor antagonism and neprilysin inhibition. *Circulation,* **2016**, *133*:1115–1124.

Jhund PS, et al. Long-term trends in first hospitalization for heart failure and subsequent survival between 1986 and 2003: a population study of 5.1 million people. *Circulation,* **2009**, *119*:515–523.

Juurlink D, et al. Rates of hyperkalemia after publication of the Randomized Aldactone Evaluation Study. *N Engl J Med,* **2004**, *351*:543–551.

Kjekshus J, et al. Rosuvastatin in older patients with systolic heart failure. *N Engl J Med*, **2007**, *357*:2248–2261.

Klabunde RE. Cardiovascular physiology concepts: ventricular systolic dysfunctions. **2015**. Available at: http://www.cvphysiology.com/Heart%20Failure/HF005. Accessed February 26, 2017.

Lee TC. Van Gogh's vision: digitalis intoxication? *JAMA*, **1981**, *245*: 727–729.

Liao JK, Laufs U. Pleiotropic effects of statins. *Annu Rev Pharmacol Toxicol*, **2005**, *45*:89–118.

Lowes BD, et al. Myocardial gene expression in dilated cardiomyopathy treated with beta-blocking agents. *N Engl J Med*, **2002**, *346*:1357–1365.

Mann DL, et al. Targeted anticytokine therapy in patients with chronic heart failure: results of the Randomized Etanercept Worldwide Evaluation (RENEWAL). *Circulation*, **2004**, *109*:1594–1602.

Massie BM, et al. Rolofylline, an adenosine A_1-receptor antagonist, in acute heart failure. *N Engl J Med*, **2010**, *363*:1419–1428.

McMurray JJ, et al. Effects of candesartan in patients with chronic heart failure and reduced left-ventricular systolic function taking angiotensin-converting-enzyme inhibitors: the CHARM-Added trial. Lancet, **2003**, *362*:767–771.

McMurray JJ, et al. Angiotensin-neprilysin inhibition versus enalapril in heart failure. *N Engl J Med*, **2014**, *371*:993–1004.

Mebazaa A, et al. Levosimendan vs dobutamine for patients with acute decompensated heart failure: the SURVIVE Randomized Trial. *JAMA*, **2007**, *297*:1883–1891.

MERIT-HF Investigators. Effect of metoprolol CR/XL in chronic heart failure: Metoprolol CR/XL Randomised Intervention Trial in Congestive Heart Failure (MERIT-HF). *Lancet*, **1999**, *353*:2001–2007.

Munzel T, et al. Explaining the phenomenon of nitrate tolerance. *Circ Res*, **2005**, *97*:618–628.

O'Connor CM, et al. Effect of nesiritide in patients with acute decompensated heart failure. *N Engl J Med*, **2011**, *365*:32–43.

Packer M, et al. Comparison of omapatrilat and enalapril in patients with chronic heart failure: the Omapatrilat Versus Enalapril Randomized Trial of Utility in Reducing Events (OVERTURE). *Circulation*, **2002**, *106*:920–926.

Packer M, et al. Clinical effects of endothelin receptor antagonism with bosentan in patients with severe chronic heart failure: results of a pilot study. *J Card Fail*, **2005**, *11*:12–20.

Patel PA, et al. Hypotension during hospitalization for acute heart failure is independently associated with 30-day mortality: findings from ASCEND-HF. *Circ Heart Fail*, **2014**, *7*:918–925.

Pavlovic D, et al. Novel regulation of cardiac Na pump via phospholemman. *J Mol Cell Cardiol*, **2013**, *61*:83–93.

Pieske B, et al. Alterations in intracellular calcium handling associated with the inverse force-frequency relation in human dilated cardiomyopathy. *Circulation*, **1995**, *92*:1169–1178.

Pitt B. Effect of aldosterone blockade in patients with systolic left ventricular dysfunction: implications of the RALES and EPHESUS studies. *Mol Cell Endocrinol*, **2004**, *217*:53–58.

Pitt B, et al. The effect of spironolactone on morbidity and mortality in patients with severe heart failure. *N Engl J Med*, **1999**, *341*: 709–717.

Ponikowski P, et al. 2016 European Society of Cardiology Guidelines for the diagnosis and treatment of acute and chronic heart failure. *Eur Heart J*, **2016**, *37*:2129–2200.

Poole-Wilson PA, et al. Comparison of carvedilol and metoprolol on clinical outcomes in patients with chronic heart failure in the Carvedilol Or Metoprolol European Trial (COMET): randomised controlled trial. *Lancet*, **2003**, *362*:7–13.

Rathore SS, et al. Association of serum digoxin concentration and outcomes in patients with heart failure. *JAMA*, **2003**, *289*:871–878.

Rau T, et al. Impact of the CYP2D6 genotype on the clinical effects of metoprolol: a prospective longitudinal study. *Clin Pharmacol Ther*, **2009**, *85*:269–272.

Redfield MM, et al. Effect of phosphodiesterase-5 inhibition on exercise capacity and clinical status in heart failure with preserved ejection fraction: a randomized clinical trial. *JAMA*, **2013**, *309*:1268–1277.

Sackner-Bernstein JD, et al. Short-term risk of death after treatment with nesiritide for decompensated heart failure: a pooled analysis of randomized controlled trials. *JAMA*, **2005**, *293*:1900–1905.

Schober T, et al. Myofilament Ca sensitization increases cytosolic Ca binding affinity, alters intracellular Ca homeostasis, and causes pause-dependent Ca-triggered arrhythmia. *Circ Res*, **2012**, *111*:170–179.

Skou JC. William Withering—the man and his work. In: Erdmann E, Greeff K, Skou JC, eds. *Cardiac Glycosides 1785–1985*. Springer-Verlag, Berlin, **1986**, 1–10.

SOLVD Investigators. Effect of enalapril on survival in patients with reduced left ventricular ejection fractions and congestive heart failure. *N Engl J Med*, **1991**, *325*:293–302.

SOLVD Investigators. Effect of enalapril on mortality and the development of heart failure in asymptomatic patients with reduced left ventricular ejection fractions. *N Engl J Med*, **1992**, *327*:685–691.

Strait JB, Lakatta EG. Aging-associated cardiovascular changes and their relationship to heart failure. *Heart Fail Clin*, **2012**, *8*:143–164.

Swedberg K, et al. Ivabradine and outcomes in chronic heart failure (SHIFT): a randomised placebo-controlled study. *Lancet*, **2010**, *376*: 875–885.

Swedberg K, , et al. Treatment of anemia with darbepoetin alfa in systolic heart failure. *N Engl J Med*, **2013**, *368*:1210–1219.

Taylor AL, et al. Combination of isosorbide dinitrate and hydralazine in blacks with heart failure. *N Engl J Med*, **2004**, *351*:2049–2057.

Teerlink JR, et al. Serelaxin, recombinant human relaxin-2, for treatment of acute heart failure (RELAX-AHF): a randomised, placebo-controlled trial. *Lancet*, **2013**, *381*:29–39.

Udelson JE, et al. Multicenter, randomized, double-blind, placebo-controlled study on the effect of oral tolvaptan on left ventricular dilation and function in patients with heart failure and systolic dysfunction. *J Am Coll Cardiol*, **2007**, *49*:2151–2159.

Vargo DL, et al. Dopamine does not enhance furosemide-induced natriuresis in patients with congestive heart failure. *J Am Soc Nephrol*, **1996**, *7*:1032–1037.

Waagstein F, et al. Effect of chronic beta-adrenergic receptor blockade in congestive cardiomyopathy. *Br Heart J*, **1975**, *37*:1022–1036.

Xamoterol Study Group. Xamoterol in severe heart failure. *Lancet*, **1990**, *336*:1–6.

Yancy CW, et al. 2013 ACCF/AHA guideline for the management of heart failure: a report of the American College of Cardiology Foundation/American Heart Association Task Force on practice guidelines. *Circulation*, **2013**, *128*:e240–e327. doi:10.1161/CIR.0b013e31829e8776. Accessed March 7, 2017.

Yancy CW, et al. 2016 ACCF/AHA/HFSA focused update on new pharmcological therapy for heart failure: an update of the 2013 guideline for the management of heart failure. *Circulation*, **2016**, *135*:e282–e293. doi:10.1161/CIR.0000000000000435. http://circ.ahajournals.org/content/early/2016/05/18/CIR.0000000000000435. Accessed March 7, 2017.

Zannad F, et al. Eplerenone in patients with systolic heart failure and mild symptoms. *N Engl J Med*, **2011**, *364*:11–21.

Antiarrhythmic Drugs

Bjorn C. Knollmann and Dan M. Roden

第三十章　抗心律失常药

中文导读

本章主要介绍：心脏电生理学原理，包括静息状态心肌细胞（K^+通透膜）、心脏的动作电位、细胞内离子稳态的保持、遗传性心律失常性疾病、心脏动作电位异质性、冲动传播和心电图、不应性和传导衰竭；心律失常发生机制，包括自律性升高、后去极化和触发自律性、折返、常见的心律失常及其机制；抗心律失常药的作用机制，包括状态依赖性的离子通道阻滞药、抗心律失常药分类；抗心律失常药临床应用原则，包括识别和消除诱发因素、明确治疗目标、减少风险，以及将心脏电生理学作为“移动靶”的考虑；抗心律失常药，包括腺苷、胺碘酮、溴苄胺、地高辛、丙吡胺、多非利特、决奈达隆、艾司洛尔、氟卡尼、伊布利特、利多卡因、镁、美西律、普鲁卡因胺、普罗帕酮、奎尼丁、索他洛尔和维那卡兰。

Abbreviations

AF: atrial fibrillation/flutter
4-AP: 4-aminopyridine
AV: atrioventricular
β blocker: β adrenergic receptor antagonist
CPVT: catecholaminergic polymorphic ventricular tachycardia
DAD: delayed afterdepolarization
DC: direct current
EAD: early afterdepolarization
ECG: electrocardiogram
ERP: effective refractory period
GX: glycine xylidide
HERG: *human ether-a-go-go related gene*
ICD: implantable cardioverter-defibrillator
IV: intravenous
LQTS: long QT syndrome
LV: left ventricle
NCX: Na^+-Ca^{2+} exchanger
PSVT: paroxysmal supraventricular tachycardia
RV: right ventricle
RyR2: ryanodine receptor type 2
SA: sinoatrial
SERCA2: SR-Ca^{2+} ATPase
SR: sarcoplasmic reticulum
VF: ventricular fibrillation
VT: ventricular tachycardia
WPW: Wolff-Parkinson-White

Cardiac cells undergo depolarization and repolarization about 60 times per minute to form and propagate cardiac action potentials. The shape and duration of each action potential are determined by the activity of ion channel protein complexes in the membranes of individual cells, and the genes encoding most of these proteins and their regulators now have been identified. Action potentials in turn provide the primary signals to release Ca^{2+} from intracellular stores and to thereby initiate contraction. Thus, each normal heartbeat results from the highly integrated electrophysiological behavior of multiple proteins on the surface and within multiple cardiac cells. Disordered cardiac rhythm can arise from influences such as inherited variation in ion channel or other genes, ischemia, sympathetic stimulation, or myocardial scarring. Available antiarrhythmic drugs suppress arrhythmias by blocking flow through specific ion channels or by altering autonomic function. An increasingly sophisticated understanding of the molecular basis of normal and abnormal cardiac rhythm may lead to identification of new targets for antiarrhythmic drugs and perhaps improved therapies (Dobrev et al., 2012; Van Wagoner et al., 2015).

Arrhythmias can range from incidental, asymptomatic clinical findings to life-threatening abnormalities. Mechanisms underlying cardiac arrhythmias have been identified in cellular and animal experiments. For some human arrhythmias, precise mechanisms are known, and treatment can be targeted specifically to those mechanisms. In other cases, mechanisms can be only inferred, and the choice of drugs is based largely on results of prior experience. Antiarrhythmic drug therapy has two goals: termination of an ongoing arrhythmia or prevention of an arrhythmia. Unfortunately, antiarrhythmic drugs may not only help control arrhythmias but also can cause them, even during long-term therapy. Thus, prescribing antiarrhythmic drugs requires that precipitating factors be excluded or minimized, that a precise diagnosis of the type of arrhythmia (and its possible mechanisms) be made, that the prescriber has reason to believe that drug therapy will be beneficial, and that the risks of drug therapy can be minimized.

Principles of Cardiac Electrophysiology

The flow of ions across cell membranes generates the currents that make up cardiac action potentials. Factors that determine the magnitude of individual currents and their modulation by drugs include transmembrane potential, time since depolarization, or the presence of specific ligands (Nerbonne and Kass, 2005; Priori et al., 1999). Further, because the function of many channels is time and voltage dependent, even a drug that targets a single ion channel may, by altering the trajectory of the action potential, alter the function of other channels. Most antiarrhythmic drugs affect more than one ion current, and many exert ancillary effects, such as modification of cardiac contractility or autonomic nervous system function. Thus, antiarrhythmic drugs usually exert multiple actions and can be beneficial or harmful in individual patients (Priori et al., 1999; Roden, 1994).

The Cardiac Cell at Rest: a K^+-Permeable Membrane

Ions move across cell membranes in response to electrical and concentration gradients, not through the lipid bilayer but through specific ion channels or transporters. The normal cardiac cell at rest maintains a transmembrane potential approximately 80 to 90 mV negative to the exterior; this gradient is established by pumps, especially the Na^+, K^+–ATPase, and fixed anionic charges within cells. There are both an electrical and a concentration gradient that would move Na^+ ions into resting cells (Figure 30–1). However, Na^+ channels, which allow Na^+ to move along this gradient, are closed in the cardiac cell at rest, so Na^+ does not enter normal resting cardiac cells. In contrast, a specific type of K^+ channel protein (the inward rectifier channel) remains open at negative resting potentials. Hence, K^+ can move through these channels across the cell membrane at negative potentials in response to either electrical or concentration gradients (Figure 30–1). For each individual ion, there is an equilibrium potential E_x at which there is no net driving force for the ion to move across the membrane. E_x can be calculated using the Nernst equation:

$$E_x = -(RT/FZx) \ln([x]_i/[x]_o) \quad (30\text{–}1)$$

where Zx is the valence of the ion, T is the absolute temperature, R is the gas constant, F is Faraday's constant, $[x]_o$ is the extracellular concentration

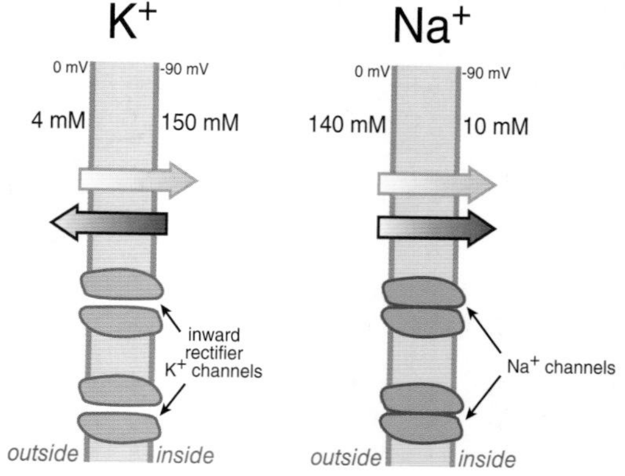

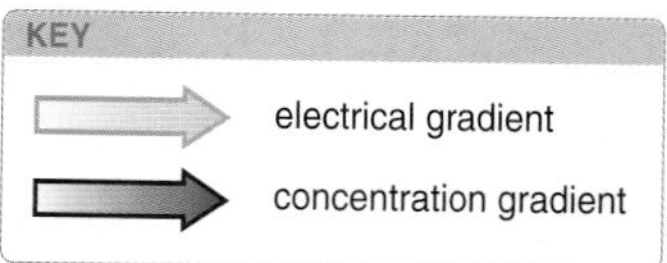

Figure 30–1 *Electrical and chemical gradients for K^+ and for Na^+ in a resting cardiac cell.* Inward rectifier K^+ channels are open (left), allowing K^+ ions to move across the membrane and the transmembrane potential to approach E_K. In contrast, Na^+ does not enter the cell despite a large net driving force because Na^+ channel proteins are in the closed conformation (right) in resting cells.

of the ion, and $[x]_i$ is the intracellular concentration. For typical values for K^+, $[K]_o$ = 4 mM and $[K]_i$ = 150 mM, the calculated K^+ equilibrium potential E_K is −96 mV. There is thus no net force driving K^+ ions into or out of a cell when the transmembrane potential is −96 mV, which is close to the resting potential. If $[K]_o$ is elevated to 10 mM, as might occur in diseases such as renal failure or myocardial ischemia, the calculated E_K rises to −70 mV. In this situation, there is excellent agreement between changes in theoretical E_K owing to changes in $[K]_o$ and the actual measured transmembrane potential, indicating that the normal cardiac cell at rest is permeable to K^+ (because inward rectifier channels are open) and that $[K]_o$ is the major determinant of resting potential.

The Cardiac Action Potential

Transmembrane current through voltage-gated ion channels is the primary determinant of cardiac action potential morphology and duration. Channels are macromolecular complexes consisting of a pore-forming transmembrane structure (which may be a single protein, often termed an α subunit, or a multimer), as well as function-modifying β subunits and other accessory proteins. Common features of the pore-forming structure include a voltage-sensing domain, a selectivity filter, a conducting pore, and an inactivating particle (Figure 30–2; see also Figure 22–2). In response to changes in local transmembrane potential, ion channels undergo conformational changes, allowing for, or preventing, the flow of ions through the conducting pore along their electrochemical gradient, generally in time-, voltage-, or ligand-dependent fashion.

To initiate an action potential, a cardiac myocyte at rest is depolarized above a threshold potential, usually via gap junctions by a neighboring myocyte. On membrane depolarization, Na^+ channel proteins change conformation from the "closed" (resting) state to the "open" (conducting) state (Figure 30–2), allowing up to 10^7 Na^+ ions/s to enter each cell and moving the transmembrane potential toward E_{Na} (+65 mV). This surge of Na^+ ions lasts only about a millisecond, after which the Na^+ channel protein rapidly changes conformation from the open state to an "inactivated," nonconducting state (Figure 30–2). The maximum upstroke slope of phase 0 (dV/dt_{max}, or V_{max}) of the action potential (Figure 30–3) is largely governed by Na^+ current and is a major determinant of conduction velocity of a propagating action potential. Under normal conditions, Na^+ channels, once inactivated, cannot reopen until they reassume the closed conformation. However, a small population of Na^+ channels may continue to open during the action potential plateau in some cells (Figure 30–3), providing further inward current, often termed a "late" Na^+ current. As the cell membrane repolarizes, the negative membrane potential moves Na^+ channel proteins from inactivated to closed conformations, from which they are again available to open and depolarize the cell. The relationship between Na^+ channel availability and transmembrane potential is an important determinant of conduction and refractoriness in many cells, as discussed in the material that follows.

The changes in transmembrane potential generated by the inward Na^+ current produce, in turn, a series of openings (and in some cases subsequent inactivation) of other channels (Figure 30–3). For example, when a cell is depolarized by the Na^+ current, "transient outward" K^+ channels quickly change conformation to enter an open, or conducting, state; because the transmembrane potential at the end of phase 0 is positive to E_K, the opening of transient outward channels results in an outward, or repolarizing, K^+ current (termed I_{TO}), which contributes to the phase 1 "notch" seen in some action potentials (e.g., more prominent in epicardium than in endocardium). Transient outward K^+ channels, like Na^+ channels, inactivate rapidly. During the phase 2 plateau of a normal cardiac action potential, inward, depolarizing currents, primarily through L-type Ca^{2+} channels, are balanced by outward, repolarizing currents primarily through K^+ ("delayed rectifier") channels. Delayed rectifier currents (collectively termed I_K) increase with time, whereas Ca^{2+} currents inactivate (and so decrease with time); as a result, cardiac cells repolarize (phase 3) several hundred milliseconds after the initial Na^+ channel opening.

A common mechanism whereby drugs prolong cardiac action potentials and provoke arrhythmias is inhibition of a specific delayed rectifier current, I_{Kr}, generated by expression of *KCNH2* (formerly termed the *HERG*). The ion channel protein generated by *KCNH2* expression differs from other ion channels in important structural features that make it much more susceptible to drug block; understanding these structural constraints is an important first step to designing drugs lacking I_{Kr}-blocking properties (Mitcheson et al., 2000). Avoiding I_{Kr}/*KCNH2* channel block has become a major issue in drug development (Roden, 2004).

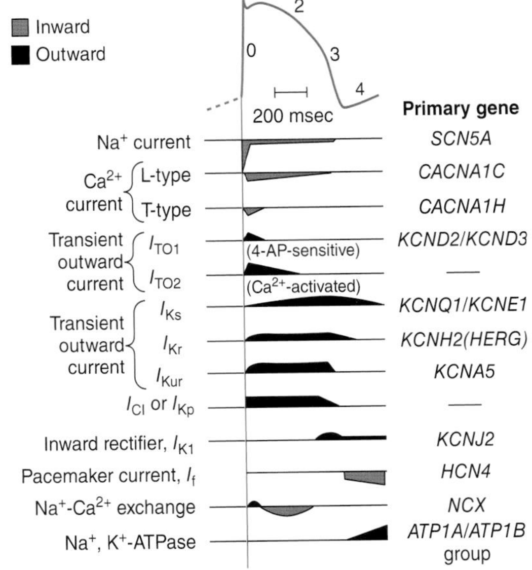

Figure 30–3 *The relationship between an action potential from the conducting system and the time course of the currents that generate it.* The current magnitudes are not to scale; the Na^+ current is ordinarily 50 times larger than any other current, although the portion that persists into the plateau (phase 2) is small. Multiple types of Ca^{2+} current, transient outward current I_{TO}, and delayed rectifier I_K have been identified. Each represents a different channel protein, usually associated with ancillary (function-modifying) subunits. 4-AP is a widely used in vitro blocker of K^+ channels. I_{TO2} may be a Cl^- current in some species. Components of I_K have been separated on the basis of how rapidly they activate: slowly (I_{Ks}), rapidly (I_{Kr}), or ultrarapidly (I_{Kur}). The voltage-activated, time-independent current may be carried by Cl^- (I_{Cl}) or K^+ (I_{Kp}, *p* for plateau). The genes encoding the major pore-forming proteins have been cloned for most of the channels shown here and are listed in the right-hand column.

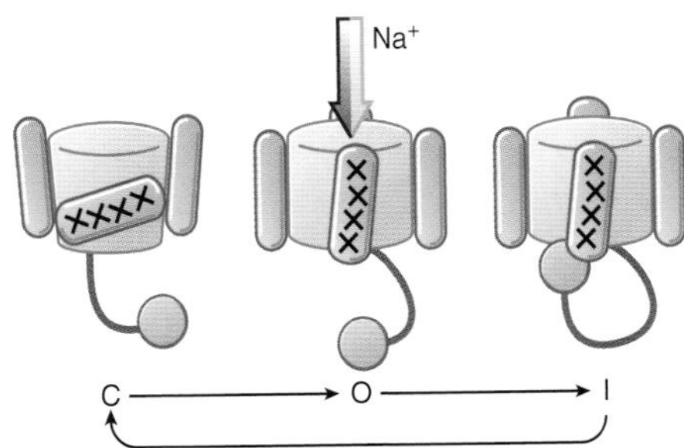

Figure 30–2 *Voltage-dependent conformational changes determine current flow through Na^+ channels.* At hyperpolarized potentials, the channel is in a closed conformation, and no current can flow (left). As depolarization begins, the voltage sensor (indicated here as ++++) moves, thus altering channel conformation and opening the pore, allowing conduction (middle). As depolarization is maintained, an intracellular particle blocks current flow, making the channel nonconducting in this inactivated state (right).

Maintenance of Intracellular Ion Homeostasis

With each action potential, the cell interior gains Na^+ ions and loses K^+ ions. An ATP-requiring Na^+-K^+ exchange mechanism, or pump, is activated in most cells to maintain intracellular homeostasis. This Na^+, K^+–ATPase extrudes three Na^+ ions for every two K^+ ions shuttled from the exterior of the cell to the interior; as a result, the act of pumping itself is electrogenic, generating a net outward (repolarizing) current.

Normally, intracellular Ca^{2+} is maintained at very low levels (<100 nM). In cardiac myocytes, the entry of Ca^{2+} during each action potential through L-type Ca^{2+} channels is a signal to the SR to release its Ca^{2+} stores, and thus initiate Ca^{2+}-dependent contraction, a process termed excitation-contraction coupling. The efflux of Ca^{2+} from the SR occurs through ryanodine receptor release channels (RyR2) and subsequent removal of intracellular Ca^{2+} occurs by both SERCA2, which moves Ca^{2+} ions back into the SR, and an electrogenic NCX on the cell surface, which exchanges three Na^+ ions from the exterior for each Ca^{2+} ion extruded.

Genetic Arrhythmia Diseases

Rare congenital arrhythmia diseases such as the LQTS and CPVT can cause sudden death due to fatal arrhythmias, often in young subjects. The identification of disease genes not only has resulted in improved care of affected patients and their families but also has contributed importantly to our understanding of the normal action potential, arrhythmia mechanisms, and potential antiarrhythmic drug targets (Keating and Sanguinetti, 2001). For example, mutations in the cardiac Na^+ channel gene *SCN5A* can cause one form of LQTS by destabilizing fast inactivation, increasing late Na^+ current, thereby prolonging action potentials, and thus the QT interval (as discussed in material that follows). Drugs inhibiting this abnormal current may be antiarrhythmic in this form of LQTS (Remme and Wilde, 2013), and drugs increasing late Na^+ current may cause arrhythmias (Yang et al., 2014). Inhibitors may include not only antiarrhythmics such as mexiletine or flecainide discussed in this chapter, but also the antianginal agent ranolazine (see Chapter 28), which appears to be a late Na^+ current blocker.

Similarly, mutations in the *RyR2* gene encoding an intracellular Ca^{2+} release channel (or less commonly in other genes regulating RyR2 function) cause CPVT by generating "leaky" RyR2 channels, perturbing intracellular Ca^{2+} homeostasis and causing DAD-dependent arrhythmias described further in this chapter. Drugs such as flecainide and propafenone that inhibit these abnormal RyR2 channels appear to prevent CPVT in mouse models and in humans (Watanabe et al., 2009). Intriguingly, some arrhythmias in acquired heart disease have been attributed to increased late Na^+ current or leaky RyR2 channels. Thus, studies in the rare congenital arrhythmia syndromes may point to new avenues for drug development in more common arrhythmias in acquired heart disease (Knollmann and Roden, 2008 Priori et al., 1999).

Action Potential Heterogeneity in the Heart

The general description of the action potential and the currents that underlie it must be modified for certain cell types (Figure 30–4), primarily due to variability in the expression of ion channels and electrogenic ion transport pumps. The resultant diversity of action potentials in different regions of the heart plays a role in understanding the pharmacological profiles of antiarrhythmic drugs. In the ventricle, action potential duration varies across the wall of each chamber, as well as apicobasally, largely as a consequence of varying densities of repolarizing currents. In the neighboring His-Purkinje conduction system, action potentials are longer, probably due to decreased K^+ currents, increased "late" Na^+ currents, and differences in intercellular Ca^{2+} handling (Dun and Boyden, 2008).

Atrial cells have shorter action potentials than ventricular cells because of larger early repolarization currents such as I_{TO}. Atrial cells also express an additional repolarizing K^+ channel that is activated by the neurotransmitter acetylcholine and accounts for action potential shortening with vagal stimulation. Cells of the sinus and AV nodes lack substantial Na^+ currents, and depolarization is achieved by inward current generated by opening of Ca^{2+} channels. In addition, these cells, as well as cells from the conducting system, normally display the phenomenon of spontaneous diastolic, or phase 4, depolarization and thus spontaneously reach

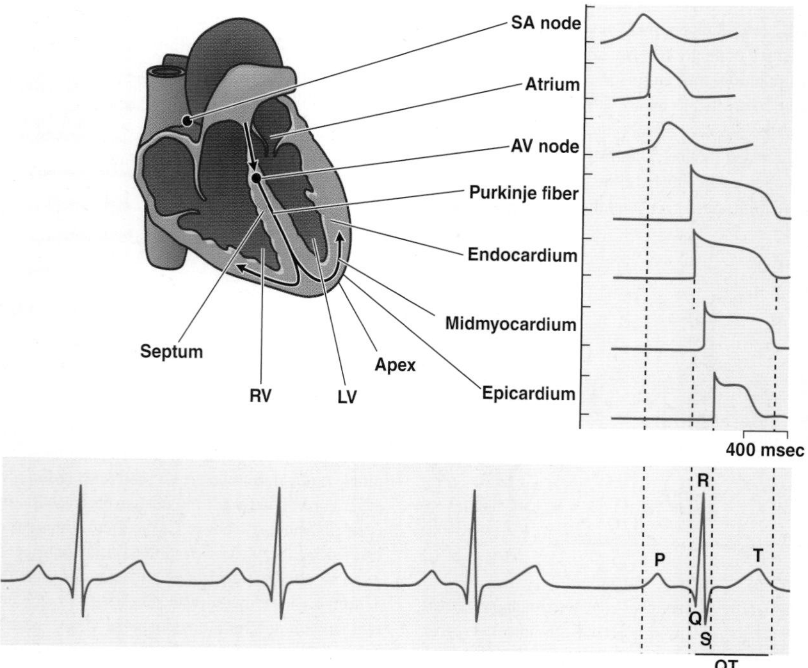

Figure 30–4 *Normal impulse propagation.* A schematic of the human heart with example action potentials from different regions of the heart (top) for a normal beat and their corresponding contributions to the macroscopic ECG (bottom). (Reproduced with permission from Nerbonne JM, Kass RS. Molecular physiology of cardiac repolarization. *Physiol Rev*, **2005**, 85:1205–1253. Used with permission of the American Physiological Society.)

threshold for regeneration of action potentials. The rate of spontaneous firing usually is fastest in sinus node cells, which therefore serve as the natural pacemaker of the heart. The slow diastolic depolarization that underlies pacemaker activity is generated by a nonselective channel that conducts both Na^+ and K^+ and is activated at hyperpolarized membrane potentials (Cohen and Robinson, 2006). In diseased cells, pacemaker-like activity can arise from spontaneous Ca^{2+} release from the SR, followed by membrane depolarization due to activation of NCX.

Certain ion channels are expressed only in some tissues or become active only under specific pathophysiologic conditions. For example, the T-type Ca^{2+} channel may be important in diseases such as hypertension and play a role in pacemaker activity (Ono and Iijima, 2010). A T-type-selective Ca^{2+} channel antagonist, *mibefradil* was commercially available briefly in the late 1990s but was withdrawn because of concerns over potentially life-threatening pharmacokinetic interactions with many other drugs. A second example is a channel that transports Cl^- ions and results in repolarizing currents (I_{Cl}) (Duan, 2013); some of these are observed only in association with pathophysiological conditions. A third example is the K^+ channel that are quiescent when intracellular ATP stores are normal and become active when these stores are depleted. Such ATP-inhibited K^+ channel may become particularly important in repolarizing cells during states of metabolic stress such as myocardial ischemia (Tamargo et al., 2004).

Impulse Propagation and the Electrocardiogram

Normal cardiac impulses originate in the sinus node. Impulse propagation in the heart depends on the magnitude of the depolarizing current (usually Na^+ current) and the geometry and density of cell-cell electrical connections (Kleber and Saffitz, 2014). Cardiac cells are relatively long and thin and well coupled through specialized gap junction proteins at their ends, whereas lateral ("transverse") gap junctions are sparser. As a result, impulses spread along cells two to three times faster than across cells. This "anisotropic" (direction-dependent) conduction may be a factor in the genesis of certain arrhythmias described in the material that follows (Priori et al., 1999).

Once impulses leave the sinus node, they propagate rapidly throughout the atria, resulting in atrial systole and the P wave of the surface ECG (Figure 30–4). Propagation slows markedly through the AV node, where the inward current (through Ca^{2+} channels) is much smaller than the Na^+ current in atria, ventricles, or the subendocardial conducting system. This conduction delay, represented as the PR interval on the ECG, allows the atrial contraction to propel blood into the ventricle, thereby optimizing cardiac output.

Once impulses exit the AV node, they enter the conducting system, where Na^+ currents are larger than in any other tissue, and propagation is correspondingly faster, up to 0.75 m/s longitudinally. Activation spreads from the His-Purkinje system on the endocardium of the ventricles throughout the rest of the ventricles, stimulating coordinated ventricular contraction. This electrical activation manifests itself as the QRS complex on the ECG. Ventricular repolarization is presented on the surface ECG as the T wave. The time from initial depolarization in the ventricle until the end of repolarization is termed the QT interval. Lengthening of ventricular action potentials prolongs the QT interval and may be associated with arrhythmias in LQTS and other settings.

Refractoriness and Conduction Failure

In atrial, ventricular, and His-Purkinje cells, if a restimulation occurs very early during the plateau of an action potential, no Na^+ channels are available to open, so no inward current results, and no new action potential is generated: At this point, the cell is termed *refractory* (Figure 30–5). On the other hand, if a stimulus occurs after the cell has repolarized completely, Na^+ channels have recovered from inactivation, and a normal Na^+ channel–dependent upstroke results with the same amplitude as the previous upstroke (Figure 30–5A). When a stimulus occurs during phase 3 of the action potential, the upstroke of the premature action potential is slower and of smaller magnitude. The magnitude depends on the number of Na^+ channels that have recovered from inactivation (Figure 30–5A), which in turn is dependent on the membrane potential. Thus, refractoriness is determined by the voltage-dependent recovery of Na^+ channels from inactivation.

Refractoriness frequently is measured by assessing whether premature stimuli applied to tissue preparations (or the whole heart) result in propagated impulses. While the magnitude of the Na^+ current is one major determinant of propagation of premature beats, cellular geometry also is important in multicellular preparations. Propagation from cell to cell requires current flow from the first site of activation and consequently can fail if inward current is insufficient to drive activation in many neighboring cells. The *ERP* is the longest interval at which a premature stimulus fails to generate a propagated response and often is used to describe drug effects in intact tissue.

The situation is different in tissue whose depolarization is largely controlled by Ca^{2+} channel current, such as the AV node. Because Ca^{2+} channels have a slower recovery from inactivation, these tissues are often referred to as *slow response* (Figure 30–5C), in contrast to *fast response* in the remaining cardiac tissues. Even after a Ca^{2+} channel–dependent action potential has repolarized to its initial resting potential, not all Ca^{2+} channels are available for reexcitation. Therefore, an extra stimulus applied shortly after repolarization is complete generates a reduced Ca^{2+} current, which may propagate slowly to adjacent cells prior to extinction. An extra stimulus applied later will result in a larger Ca^{2+} current and faster propagation. Thus, in Ca^{2+} channel–dependent tissues, which include not only the AV node but also tissues whose underlying characteristics have been altered by factors such as myocardial ischemia, refractoriness is prolonged, and propagation occurs slowly. Conduction that exhibits such dependence on the timing of premature stimuli is termed *decremental*. Slow conduction in the heart, a critical factor in the genesis of reentrant arrhythmias (see further discussion), also can occur when Na^+ currents are depressed

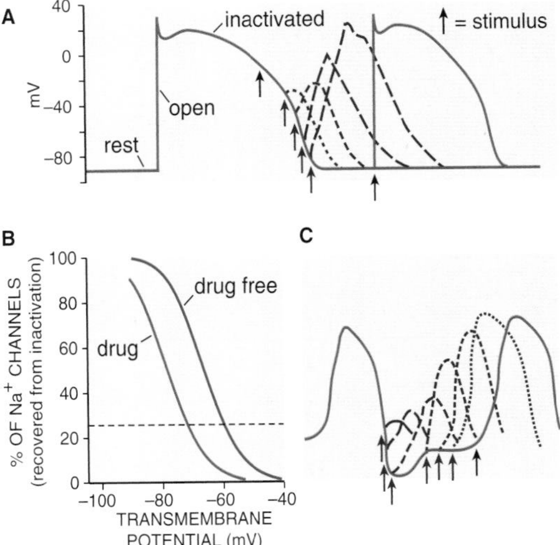

Figure 30–5 *Qualitative differences in responses of nodal and conducting tissues to premature stimuli.* **A.** With a very early premature stimulus (black arrow) in ventricular myocardium, all Na^+ channels still are in the inactivated state, and no upstroke results. As the action potential repolarizes, Na^+ channels recover from the inactivated to the resting state, from which opening can occur. The phase 0 upstroke slopes of the premature action potentials (purple) are greater with later stimuli because recovery from inactivation is voltage-dependent. **B.** The relationship between transmembrane potential and degree of recovery of Na^+ channels from inactivation. The dotted line indicates 25% recovery. Most Na^+ channel–blocking drugs shift this relationship to the left. **C.** In Ca^{2+}-dependent slow-response tissues such as the AV node, premature stimuli delivered even after full repolarization of the action potential are depressed; recovery from inactivation is time-dependent.

by disease or membrane depolarization (e.g., elevated $[K]_o$), resulting in decreased steady-state Na^+ channel availability (Figure 30–5B).

Mechanisms of Cardiac Arrhythmias

An arrhythmia is by definition a perturbation of the normal sequence of impulse initiation and propagation. Failure of impulse initiation, in the sinus node, may result in slow heart rates (bradyarrhythmias), whereas failure in the normal propagation of action potentials from atrium to ventricle results in dropped beats (commonly referred to as heart block) and usually reflects an abnormality in either the AV node or the His-Purkinje system. These abnormalities may be caused by drugs (Table 30–1) or by structural heart disease; in the latter case, permanent cardiac pacing may be required.

Abnormally rapid heart rhythms (tachyarrhythmias) are common clinical problems that may be treated with antiarrhythmic drugs. Three major underlying mechanisms have been identified: enhanced automaticity, triggered automaticity, and reentry. These are often interrelated mechanisms as abnormal beats arising from one mechanism can elicit a second; for example, a triggered automatic beat can initiate reentry.

Enhanced Automaticity

Enhanced automaticity may occur in cells that normally display spontaneous diastolic depolarization—the sinus and AV nodes and the His-Purkinje system. β Adrenergic stimulation, hypokalemia, and mechanical stretch of cardiac muscle cells increase phase 4 slope and so accelerate pacemaker rate, whereas *acetylcholine* reduces pacemaker rate both by decreasing phase 4 slope and by hyperpolarization (making the maximum diastolic potential more negative). In addition, automatic behavior may occur in sites that ordinarily lack spontaneous pacemaker activity; for example, depolarization of ventricular cells (e.g., by ischemia) may produce "abnormal" automaticity. When impulses propagate from a region of enhanced normal or abnormal automaticity to excite the rest of the heart, more complex arrhythmias may result from the induction of reentry.

TABLE 30–1 ■ DRUG-INDUCED CARDIAC ARRHYTHMIAS

ARRHYTHMIA	DRUG	LIKELY MECHANISM	TREATMENT*	CLINICAL FEATURES
Sinus bradycardia, AV block	Digoxin	↑Vagal tone	Antidigoxin antibodies, temporary pacing	Atrial tachycardia may also be present
Sinus bradycardia, AV block	Verapamil, diltiazem	Ca^{2+} channel block	Ca^{2+}, temporary pacing	
Sinus bradycardia	β Blockers	Sympatholytic	Isoproterenol	
AV block	Clonidine Methyldopa		Temporary pacing	
Sinus tachycardia Any other tachycardia	β Blocker withdrawal	Upregulation of β receptors with chronic therapy; β blocker withdrawal →↑β effects	β Blockade	Hypertension, angina also possible
↑Ventricular rate in atrial flutter	Quinidine Flecainide Propafenone	Conduction slowing in atrium, with enhanced (quinidine) or unaltered AV conduction	AV nodal blockers	QRS complexes often widened at fast rates
↑Ventricular rate in atrial fibrillation in patients with WPW syndrome	Digoxin Verapamil	↓ Accessory pathway refractoriness	IV procainamide DC cardioversion	Ventricular rate can exceed 300 beats/min
Multifocal atrial tachycardia	Theophylline	↑Intracellular Ca^{2+} and DADs	Withdraw theophylline ?Verapamil	Often in advanced lung disease
Polymorphic VT with ↑QT interval (torsades de pointes)	Quinidine Sotalol Procainamide Disopyramide Dofetilide Ibutilide "Noncardioactive" drugs (see text) Amiodarone (rare)	EAD-related triggered activity	Cardiac pacing Isoproterenol Magnesium	Hypokalemia, bradycardia frequent Related to ↑ plasma concentrations, except for quinidine
Frequent or difficult to terminate VT ("incessant" VT)	Flecainide Propafenone Quinidine (rarer)	Conduction slowing in reentrant circuits	Na^+ bolus reported effective in some cases	Most often in patients with advanced myocardial scarring
Atrial tachycardia with AV block; ventricular bigeminy, others	Digoxin	DAD-related triggered activity (± ↑ vagal tone)	Antidigoxin antibodies	Coexistence of abnormal impulses with abnormal sinus or AV nodal function
Ventricular fibrillation	Inappropriate use of IV verapamil	Severe hypotension and/or myocardial ischemia	Cardiac resuscitation (DC cardioversion)	Misdiagnosis of VT as PSVT and inappropriate use of verapamil

*In each of these cases, recognition and withdrawal of the offending drug(s) are mandatory ↑, increase; ↓, decrease; ?, unclear.

Afterdepolarizations and Triggered Automaticity

Under some pathophysiological conditions, a normal cardiac action potential may be interrupted or followed by an abnormal depolarization (Figure 30–6). If this abnormal depolarization reaches threshold, it may, in turn, give rise to secondary upstrokes that can propagate and create abnormal rhythms. These abnormal secondary upstrokes occur only after an initial normal, or "triggering," upstroke and thus are termed *triggered rhythms*.

Two major forms of triggered rhythms are recognized. In the first case, under conditions of intracellular or SR Ca^{2+} overload (e.g., myocardial ischemia, adrenergic stress, digitalis intoxication, or CPVT), a normal action potential may be followed by a *DAD* (Figure 30–6A); as discussed previously, enhanced NCX current is thought to be a common mechanism underlying DADs. If this afterdepolarization reaches threshold, a secondary triggered beat or beats may occur. DAD amplitude is increased in vitro by rapid pacing, and clinical arrhythmias thought to correspond to DAD-mediated triggered beats are more frequent when the underlying cardiac rate is rapid (Priori et al., 1999).

In the second type of triggered activity, the key abnormality is marked prolongation of the cardiac action potential. When this occurs, phase 3 repolarization may be interrupted by an EAD (Figure 30–6B). EAD-mediated triggering in vitro and clinical arrhythmias are most common when the underlying heart rate is slow, extracellular K^+ is low, and certain drugs that prolong action potential duration (antiarrhythmics and others) are present. EAD-related triggered upstrokes probably reflect inward current through Na^+ or Ca^{2+} channels. Due to their intrinsically longer action potential, EADs are induced more readily in Purkinje cells and in endocardial than in epicardial cells.

When cardiac repolarization is markedly prolonged, polymorphic ventricular tachycardia with a long QT interval, termed *torsades de pointes*, may occur. This arrhythmia is thought to be caused by EADs, which trigger functional reentry (discussed next) owing to heterogeneity of action potential durations across the ventricular wall (Priori et al., 1999). Congenital LQTS, a disease in which *torsades de pointes* causes syncope or death, is most often caused by mutations in the genes encoding the Na^+ channels (10%) or the channels underlying the repolarizing currents I_{Kr} and I_{Ks} (80-90%) (Nerbonne and Kass, 2005).

Reentry

Reentry occurs when a cardiac impulse travels in a path such as to return to its original site and reactivate the original site, thus perpetuating rapid reactivation independent of normal sinus node function. Key features enabling reentrant excitation are a pathway; heterogeneity of electrophysiologic properties, notably refractoriness, along the pathway; and slow conduction.

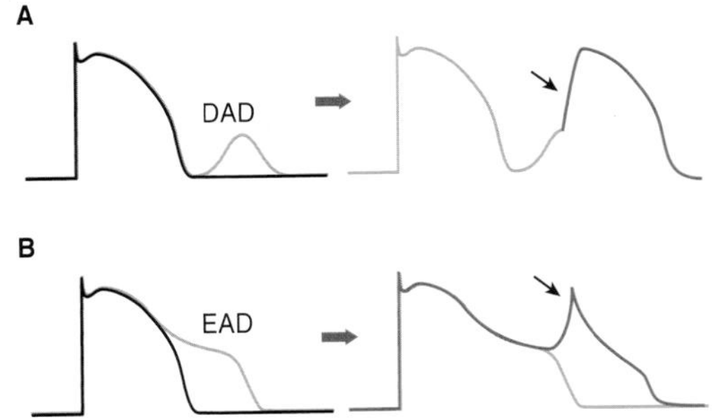

Figure 30–6 *Afterdepolarizations and triggered activity.* **A.** Delayed afterdepolarization arising after full repolarization. DADs are typically caused by spontaneous Ca^{2+} release from the SR under conditions of Ca^{2+} overload. The extracytosolic Ca^{2+} is removed from the cytosol by the electrogenic Na-Ca exchanger, which produces Na^+ influx and causes a cell membrane depolarization in the form of a DAD. A DAD that reaches threshold results in a triggered upstroke (black arrow, right). **B.** Early afterdepolarization interrupting phase 3 repolarization. Multiple ion channels and transporters can contribute to EADs (e.g., Na^+ channel, L-type Ca^{2+} channel, Na-Ca exchanger). Under some conditions, triggered beat(s) can arise from an EAD (black arrow, right).

Anatomically Defined Reentry

The prototypical example of reentry is the WPW syndrome in which patients have an accessory connection between the atrium and ventricle (Figure 30–7). With each sinus node depolarization, impulses can excite the ventricle via the normal structures (AV node) or the accessory pathway, and this often results in an unusual and characteristic QRS complex in normal sinus rhythm. Importantly, the electrophysiological properties of the AV node and accessory pathways are different: Accessory pathways usually consist of nonnodal tissue with longer refractory periods and without decremental conduction. Thus, with a premature atrial beat (e.g., from abnormal automaticity), conduction may fail in the accessory pathway but continue, albeit slowly, in the AV node and then through the His-Purkinje system; there the propagating impulse may encounter the ventricular end of the accessory pathway when it is no longer refractory. The likelihood that the accessory pathway is no longer refractory increases as AV nodal conduction slows, demonstrating how slow conduction enables reentry. When the impulse reenters the atrium, it then can reenter the ventricle via the AV node, reenter the atrium via the accessory pathway, and so on (Figure 30–7).

Reentry of this type, referred to as *AV reentrant tachycardia*, is determined by the following:

1. The presence of an anatomically defined circuit
2. Heterogeneity in refractoriness among regions in the circuit
3. Slow conduction in one part of the circuit

Similar "anatomically defined" reentry commonly occurs in the region of the AV node (*AV nodal reentrant tachycardia*), in the atrium (*atrial flutter*), and in scarred ventricle (*ventricular tachycardia*). The term *PSVT* includes both AV reentry and AV nodal reentry, which share many clinical features.

While antiarrhythmic drugs or electrical cardioversion are used to terminate reentry acutely (discussed further in the chapter and Table 30–2), the primary therapy for anatomically defined reentry is radio-frequency ablation because its consistent pathway often makes it possible to identify and ablate critical segments of this pathway effectively, curing the patient and obviating the need for long-term drug therapy. Radio-frequency

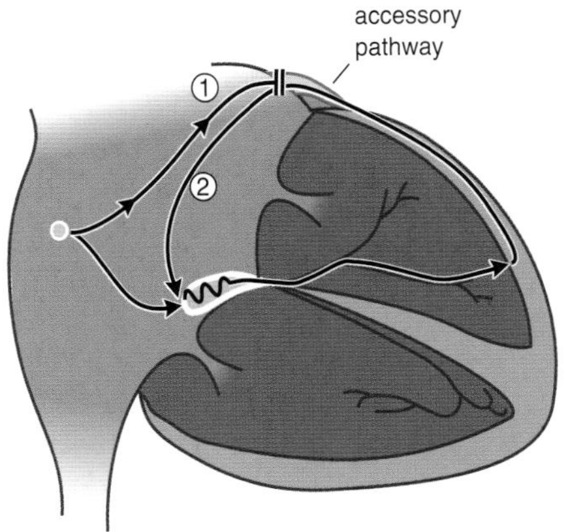

Figure 30–7 *Atrioventricular reentrant tachycardia in the WPW syndrome.* In these patients, an accessory AV connection is present (light blue). A premature atrial impulse blocks in the accessory pathway (1) and propagates slowly through the AV node and conducting system. On reaching the accessory pathway (by now no longer refractory), the impulse reenters the atrium (2), where it then can reenter the ventricle via the AV node and become self-sustaining (see Figure 30–9C). AV nodal blocking drugs readily terminate this tachycardia. Recurrences can be prevented by drugs that prevent atrial premature beats, by drugs that alter the electrophysiological characteristics of tissue in the circuit (e.g., they prolong AV nodal refractoriness), and by nonpharmacological ablation techniques that selectively destroy the accessory pathway.

ablation is carried out through a catheter advanced to the interior of the heart and requires minimal convalescence.

Functionally Defined Reentry

Reentry also may occur in the absence of a distinct, anatomically defined pathway (Figure 30–8). For example, a premature beat from within the ventricular wall may encounter refractory tissue in only one direction, allowing for conduction throughout the rest of the wall until the originally refractory area recovers, reexcites, and then propagates back through the original location of the premature beat. Another example is localized ischemia or other electrophysiological perturbations that result in an area of sufficiently slow conduction in the ventricle that impulses exiting from that area find the rest of the myocardium reexcitable, in which case reentry may ensue. Atrial fibrillation and VF are extreme examples of "functionally defined" reentry: Cells are reexcited as soon as they are repolarized sufficiently to allow enough Na^+ channels to recover from inactivation. The abnormal activation pathway subsequently provides abnormal spatial heterogeneity of repolarization that can cause other reentrant circuits to form. In atrial fibrillation, these can persist for years, and rotor-like activity can sometimes be recorded, presumably reflecting reentrant circuits that can be transiently stable or meander around the atrium.

Common Arrhythmias and Their Mechanisms

The primary tool for diagnosis of arrhythmias is the ECG. More sophisticated approaches sometimes are used, such as recording from specific regions of the heart during artificial induction of arrhythmias by specialized pacing techniques. Table 30–2 lists common arrhythmias, their likely mechanisms, and approaches that should be considered for their acute termination and for long-term therapy to prevent recurrence. Examples of some arrhythmias discussed here are shown in Figure 30–9. Some arrhythmias, notably VF, are treated not pharmacologically but with DC cardioversion—the application of a large electric current across the chest.

TABLE 30–2 ■ A MECHANISTIC APPROACH TO ANTIARRHYTHMIC THERAPY

ARRHYTHMIA	COMMON MECHANISM	ACUTE THERAPY[a]	CHRONIC THERAPY[a]
Premature atrial, nodal, or ventricular depolarizations	Unknown	None indicated	None indicated
Atrial fibrillation	Disorganized "functional" reentry Continual AV node stimulation and irregular, often rapid, ventricular rate	1. Control ventricular response: AV node block[b] 2. Restore sinus rhythm: DC cardioversion	1. Control ventricular response: AV nodal block[b] 2. Maintain normal rhythm: K^+ channel block, Na^+ channel block, Na^+ channel block with $\tau_{recovery}$ >1 sec
Atrial flutter	Stable reentrant circuit in the right atrium Ventricular rate often rapid and irregular	Same as atrial fibrillation Same as atrial fibrillation	Same as atrial fibrillation AV nodal blocking drugs especially desirable to avoid ↑ ventricular rate Ablation in selected cases[c]
Atrial tachycardia	Enhanced automaticity, DAD-related automaticity, or reentry in atrium	Adenosine sometimes effective Same as atrial fibrillation	Same as atrial fibrillation Ablation of tachycardia "focus"[c]
AV nodal reentrant tachycardia (PSVT)	Reentrant circuit within or near AV node	AV nodal block[b] Less commonly: ↑ vagal tone (digitalis, edrophonium, phenylephrine)	*AV nodal block Flecainide Propafenone *Ablation[c]
Arrhythmias associated with WPW syndrome: 1. AV reentry (PSVT)	Reentry (Figure 30–7)	Same as AV nodal reentry *DC cardioversion	K^+ channel block Na^+ channel block with $\tau_{recovery}$ >1 sec *Ablation[c]
2. Atrial fibrillation with atrioventricular conduction via accessory pathway	Very rapid rate due to nondecremental properties of accessory pathway	*Procainamide Lidocaine	K^+ channel block Na^+ channel block with $\tau_{recovery}$ >1 sec (AV nodal blockers can be harmful)
VT in patients with remote myocardial infarction	Reentry near the rim of the healed myocardial infarction	Amiodarone Procainamide DC cardioversion Adenosine[e]	*ICD[d] Amiodarone K^+ channel block Na^+ channel block
VT in patients without structural heart disease	DADs triggered by ↑ sympathetic tone	Verapamil[e] β Blockers[e] *DC cardioversion	Verapamil[e] β Blockers[e]
VF	Disorganized reentry	Lidocaine Amiodarone Procainamide Pacing	*ICD[d] Amiodarone K^+ channel block Na^+ channel block
Torsades de pointes, congenital or acquired; (often drug related)	EAD-related triggered activity	Magnesium Isoproterenol	β Blockade Pacing

*Indicates treatment of choice. [a]Acute drug therapy is administered intravenously; chronic therapy implies long-term oral use. [b]AV nodal block can be achieved clinically by adenosine, Ca^{2+} channel block, β adrenergic receptor blockade, or increased vagal tone (a major antiarrhythmic effect of digitalis glycosides). [c]Ablation is a procedure in which tissue responsible for the maintenance of a tachycardia is identified by specialized recording techniques and then selectively destroyed, usually by high-frequency radio waves delivered through a catheter placed in the heart. [d]ICD, implanted cardioverter–defibrillator: a device that can sense VT or VF and deliver pacing and/or cardioverting shocks to restore normal rhythm. [e]These may be harmful in reentrant VT and so should be used for acute therapy only if the diagnosis is secure.

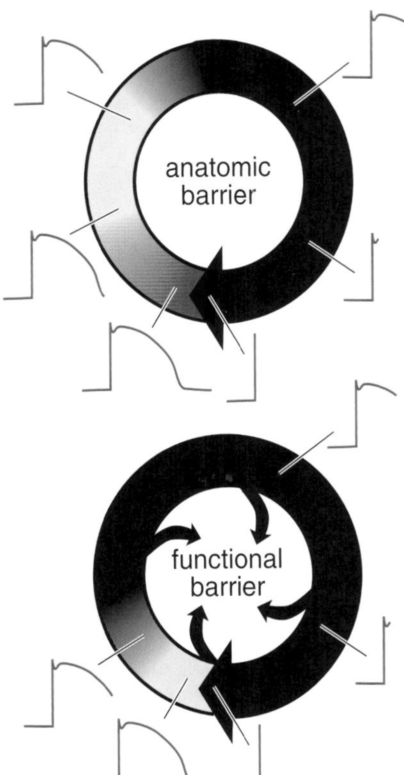

Figure 30–8 *Two types of reentry.* The border of a propagating wavefront is denoted by a heavy black arrowhead. In anatomically defined reentry (top), a fixed pathway is present (e.g., Figure 30–7). The black area denotes tissue in the reentrant circuit that is completely refractory because of the recent passage of the propagating wavefront; the gray area denotes tissue in which depressed upstrokes can be elicited (see Figure 30–5A), and the dark red area represents tissue in which restimulation would result in action potentials with normal upstrokes. The dark red area is termed an *excitable gap*. In functionally defined, or "leading circle," reentry (bottom), there is no anatomic pathway and no excitable gap. Rather, the circulating wavefront creates an area of inexcitable tissue at its core. In this type of reentry, the circuit does not necessarily remain in the same anatomic position during consecutive beats. During mapping of excitation sequences in the heart, this type of activity may be manifest as one or more "rotors."

This technique also can be used to immediately restore normal rhythm in less-serious cases; if the patient is conscious, a brief period of general anesthesia is required. ICDs, devices that are capable of detecting VF and automatically delivering a defibrillating shock, are used increasingly in patients judged to be at high risk for VF. Often, drugs are used with these devices if defibrillating shocks, which are painful, occur frequently.

Mechanisms of Antiarrhythmic Drug Action

Antiarrhythmic drugs almost invariably have multiple effects in patients, and their effects on arrhythmias can be complex. A drug can modulate other targets in addition to its primary site of action. At the same time, a single arrhythmia may result from multiple underlying mechanisms (e.g., torsades de pointes [Figure 30–9H] can result either from increased Na^+ channel late currents or decreased inward rectifier currents). Thus, antiarrhythmic therapy should be tailored to target the most relevant underlying arrhythmia mechanism, where it is known. Drugs may be antiarrhythmic by suppressing the initiating mechanism or by altering reentrant circuits. In some cases, drugs may suppress an initiator but nonetheless promote reentry (see discussion that follows).

Drugs may slow automatic rhythms by altering any of the four determinants of spontaneous pacemaker discharge (Figure 30–10): (1) increase maximum diastolic potential, (2) decrease phase 4 slope, (3) increase threshold potential, or (4) increase action potential duration. *Adenosine* and acetylcholine may increase maximum diastolic potential, and β blockers (see Chapter 12) may decrease phase 4 slope. Blockade of Na^+ or Ca^{2+} channels usually results in altered threshold, and blockade of cardiac K^+ channels prolongs the action potential.

Antiarrhythmic drugs may suppress arrhythmias owing to DADs or EADs by two major mechanisms:

1. inhibition of the development of afterdepolarizations; and
2. interference with the inward current (usually through Na^+ or Ca^{2+} channels), which is responsible for the upstroke

Thus, arrhythmias owing to DADs (i.e., due to *digitalis* toxicity or CPVT) may be inhibited by *verapamil* (which blocks the development of DAD by reducing Ca^{2+} influx into the cell, thereby decreasing SR Ca^{2+} load and the likelihood of spontaneous Ca^{2+} release from the SR) or by Na^+ channel–blocking drugs, which elevate the threshold required to produce the abnormal upstroke. In CPVT, more effective than *verapamil* is combined RyR2 and Na^+ channel block by agents such as *flecainide* or *propafenone*. Similarly, two approaches are used in arrhythmias related to EAD-triggered beats (Tables 30–1 and 30–2). EADs can be inhibited by shortening action potential duration; in practice, heart rate is accelerated by *isoproterenol* infusion or by pacing. Triggered beats arising from EADs can be inhibited by Mg^{2+} without normalizing repolarization in vitro or QT interval through mechanisms that are not well understood. In most forms of congenital LQTS, torsades de pointes occurs with adrenergic stress; therapy includes β adrenergic blockade (which does not shorten the QT interval but may prevent EADs) as well as pacing to shorten action potentials.

In anatomically determined reentry, drugs may terminate the arrhythmia by blocking propagation of the action potential. Conduction usually fails in a "weak link" in the circuit. In the example of the WPW-related arrhythmia described previously, the weak link is the AV node, and drugs that prolong AV nodal refractoriness and slow AV nodal conduction, such as Ca^{2+} channel blockers, β blockers, or adenosine, are likely to be effective. On the other hand, slowing conduction in functionally determined reentrant circuits may change the pathway without extinguishing the circuit. In fact, slow conduction generally promotes the development of reentrant arrhythmias, whereas the most likely approach for terminating functionally determined reentry is prolongation of refractoriness (Knollmann and Roden, 2008; Priori et al., 1999; Task Force, 1991). In atrial and ventricular myocytes, refractoriness can be prolonged by delaying the recovery of Na^+ channels from inactivation. Drugs that act by blocking Na^+ channels generally shift the voltage dependence of recovery from block (Figure 30–5B) and so prolong refractoriness (Figure 30–11).

Drugs that increase action potential duration without direct action on Na^+ channels (e.g., by blocking delayed rectifier currents) also will prolong refractoriness (Figure 30–11). Particularly in SA or AV nodal tissues, Ca^{2+} channel blockade prolongs refractoriness. Drugs that interfere with cell-cell coupling also theoretically should increase refractoriness in multicellular preparations; *amiodarone*, a drug with a multiplicity of electrophysiologic actions that may be antiarrhythmic, may exert this effect in diseased tissue. Acceleration of conduction in an area of slow conduction also could inhibit reentry; *lidocaine* may exert such an effect, and peptides that suppress experimental arrhythmias by increasing gap junction conductance have been described. Arrhythmia-prone hearts often display abnormal anatomy and histology, notably enhanced fibrosis, and some evidence suggests anti-inflammatory or antifibrotic interventions could thus be antiarrhythmic by preventing these changes (Van Wagoner et al., 2015).

State-Dependent Ion Channel Block

Knowing the structural and molecular determinants of ion channel permeation and drug block has provided key information for analyzing the

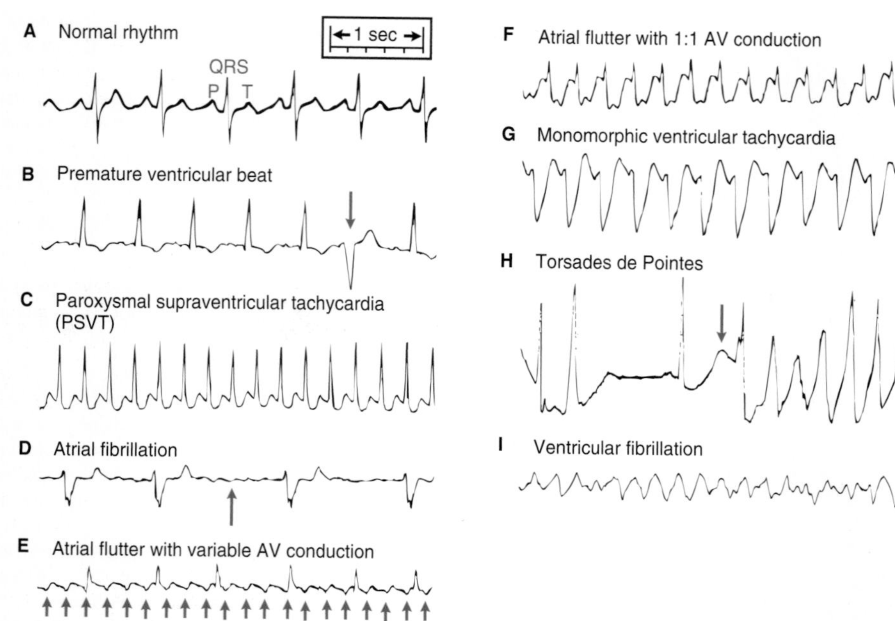

Figure 30–9 *Electrocardiograms showing normal and abnormal cardiac rhythms.* The P, QRS, and T waves in normal sinus rhythm are shown in panel **A**. Panel **B** shows a premature beat arising in the ventricle (arrow). PSVT is shown in panel **C**; this is most likely reentry using an accessory pathway (see Figure 30–7) or reentry within or near the AV node. In atrial fibrillation (panel **D**), there are no P waves, and the QRS complexes occur irregularly (and at a slow rate in this example); electrical activity between QRS complexes shows small undulations (arrow) corresponding to fibrillatory activity in the atria. In atrial flutter (panel **E**), the atria beat rapidly, approximately 250 beats/min (arrows) in this example, and the ventricular rate is variable. If a drug that slows the rate of atrial flutter is administered, 1:1 AV conduction (panel **F**) can occur. In monomorphic VT (panel **G**), identical wide QRS complexes occur at a regular rate, 180 beats per min. The electrocardiographic features of the torsades de pointes syndrome (panel **H**) include a very long QT interval (>600 ms in this example, arrow) and VT in which each successive beat has a different morphology (polymorphic VT). Panel **I** shows the disorganized electrical activity characteristic of VF.

actions of available and new antiarrhythmic compounds (MacKinnon, 2003). A key concept is that ion channel–blocking drugs bind to specific sites on the ion channel proteins to modify function (e.g., decrease current). The affinity of the ion channel protein for the drug on its target site generally varies as the ion channel protein shuttles among functional conformations (or ion channel "states"; see Figure 30–2). Physicochemical characteristics, such as molecular weight and lipid solubility, are important determinants of this state-dependent binding. State-dependent binding has been studied most extensively in the case of Na^+ channel–blocking drugs. Most useful agents of this type block open or inactivated Na^+ channels and have little affinity for channels in the resting state. Most Na^+ channel blockers bind to a local anesthetic binding site in the pore of Nav1.5 (Fozzard et al., 2005). Thus, during each action potential, drugs bind to Na^+ channels and block them, and with each diastolic interval, drugs dissociate, and the block is released. Allosteric mechanisms have also been described whereby drug binding to a site distant from the pore nevertheless alters channel conformation and thus permeation though the pore.

As illustrated in Figure 30–12, the dissociation rate is a key determinant of steady-state block of Na^+ channels. When heart rate increases, the time available for dissociation decreases, and steady-state Na^+ channel block increases. The rate of recovery from block also slows as cells are depolarized, as in ischemia. This explains the finding that Na^+ channel blockers depress Na^+ current, and hence conduction, to a greater extent in ischemic tissues than in normal tissues. Open- versus inactivated-state block also may be important in determining the effects of some drugs. Increased action potential duration, which results in a relative increase in time spent in the inactivated state, may increase block by drugs that bind to inactivated channels, such as lidocaine or amiodarone.

The rate of recovery from block often is expressed as a time constant ($\tau_{recovery}$, the time required to complete approximately 63% of an exponentially determined process to be complete). In the case of drugs such as lidocaine, $\tau_{recovery}$ is so short (<<1 sec) that recovery from block is very rapid, and substantial Na^+ channel block occurs only in rapidly driven tissues, particularly in ischemia. Conversely, drugs such as *flecainide* have such long $\tau_{recovery}$ values (>10 sec) that roughly the same numbers of Na^+ channels are blocked during systole and diastole. As a result, slowing of conduction occurs even in normal tissues at normal rates.

Classifying Antiarrhythmic Drugs

Classifying drugs by common electrophysiological properties emphasizes the connection between basic electrophysiological actions and antiarrhythmic effects (Vaughan Williams, 1992). To the extent that the clinical actions of drugs can be predicted from their basic electrophysiological properties, such classification schemes have merit. However, as each compound is better characterized in a range of in vitro and in vivo test systems, it becomes apparent that differences in pharmacological effects occur even among drugs that share the same classification, some of which may be responsible for the observed clinical differences in responses to drugs of the same broad "class" (Table 30–3).

An alternative way of approaching antiarrhythmic therapy is to attempt to classify arrhythmia mechanisms and then to target drug therapy to the electrophysiological mechanism most likely to terminate or prevent the arrhythmia (Priori et al., 1999; Task Force, 1991) (Table 30–2). This approach has been further enhanced by an increasing understanding of arrhythmia mechanisms in genetic diseases such as LQTS and CPVT, so a genetic framework represents a complementary approach for improving antiarrhythmic drug development and therapy (Knollmann and Roden, 2008).

Na^+ Channel Block

The extent of Na^+ channel block depends critically on heart rate and membrane potential, as well as on drug-specific physicochemical characteristics

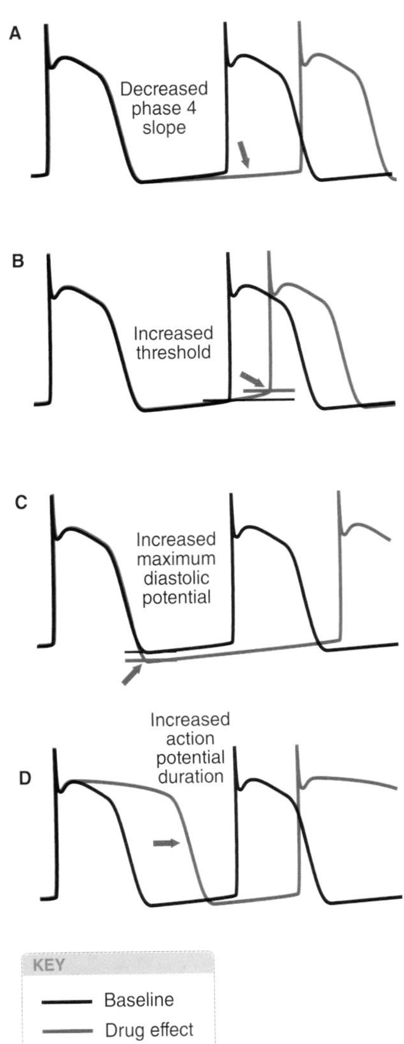

Figure 30–10 *Four ways to reduce the rate of spontaneous discharge.* The horizontal lines in panels **B** and **C** mark the threshold potentials for triggering an action potential before and after drug application.

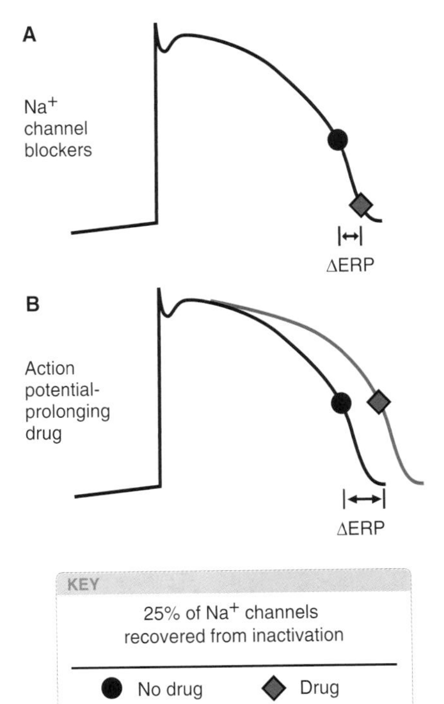

Figure 30–11 *Two ways to increase refractoriness.* In this figure, the black dot indicates the point at which a sufficient number of Na^+ channels (an arbitrary 25%; see Figure 30–5B) have recovered from inactivation to allow a premature stimulus to produce a propagated response in the absence of a drug. Block of Na^+ channels (**A**) shifts voltage dependence of recovery (see Figure 30–5B) and so delays the point at which 25% of channels have recovered (red diamond), prolonging the ERP. Note that if the drug also dissociates slowly from the channel (see Figure 30–12), refractoriness in fast-response tissues actually can extend beyond full repolarization ("postrepolarization refractoriness"). Drugs that prolong the action potential (**B**) also will extend the point at which an arbitrary percentage of Na^+ channels have recovered from inactivation, even without directly interacting with Na^+ channels.

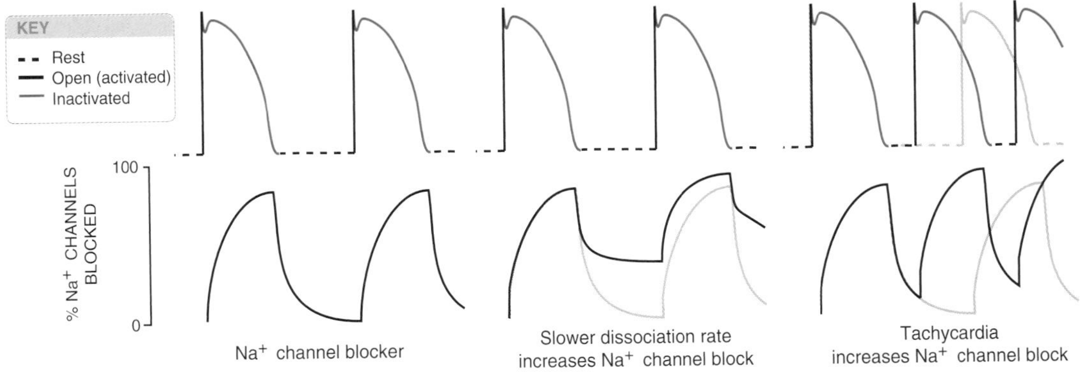

Figure 30–12 *Recovery from block of Na^+ channels during diastole.* This recovery is the critical factor determining extent of steady-state Na^+ channel block. Na^+ channel blockers bind to (and block) Na^+ channels in the open or inactivated states, resulting in phasic changes in the extent of block during the action potential. As shown in the middle panel, a decrease in the rate of recovery from block increases the extent of block. Different drugs have different rates of recovery, and depolarization reduces the rate of recovery. The right panel shows that increasing heart rate, which results in relatively less time spent in the rest state and also increases the extent of block. (Reproduced with permission from Roden DM, et al. Clinical pharmacology of antiarrhythmic agents. In: Josephson ME, ed. *Sudden Cardiac Death*. Blackwell Scientific, London, **1993**, 182–185.)

TABLE 30–3 ■ MAJOR ELECTROPHYSIOLOGIC ACTIONS OF ANTIARRHYTHMIC DRUGS

DRUG	Na^+ CHANNEL BLOCK		↑APD	Ca^{2+} CHANNEL BLOCK	AUTONOMIC EFFECTS	OTHER EFFECTS
	$\tau_{RECOVERY}$[1], *SECONDS*	STATE DEPENDENCE[1]				
Lidocaine	0.1	I > O				
Phenytoin	0.2	I				
Mexiletine[a]	0.3					
Procainamide	1.8	O	√		Ganglionic blockade (especially intravenous)	√: Metabolite prolongs APD
Quinidine	3	O	√	(x)	α Blockade, vagolytic Anticholinergic	
Disopyramide[b]	9	O	√		Anticholinergic	
Propafenone[b]	11	O ≈ I	√		β Blockade (variable clinical effect)	√ RyR2 channel block
Flecainide[a]	11	O	(x)	(x)		
β Blockers: Propanolol[b]					β Blockade	Na^+ channel block in vitro
Sotalol[b]			√		β Blockade	
Amiodarone, dronedarone	1.6	I	√	(x)	Noncompetitive β blockade	Antithyroid action
Dofetilide			√			
Ibutilide			√			
Verapamil[a]				√		
Diltiazem[a]				√		
Digoxin					√: Vagal stimulation	√: Inhibition of Na^+, K^+-ATPase
Adenosine					√: Adenosine receptor activation	√: Activation of outward K^+ current
Magnesium				?√		Mechanism not well understood

√Indicates an effect that is important in mediating the clinical action of a drug. (x)Indicates a demonstrable effect whose relationship to drug action in patients is less well established. [a]Indicates drugs prescribed as racemates, and the enantiomers are thought to exert similar electrophysiologic effects. [b]Indicates racemates for which clinically relevant differences in the electrophysiologic properties of individual enantiomers have been reported (see text). One approach to classifying drugs is:

Class	*Major action*
I	Na^+ channel block
II	β blockade
III	action potential prolongation (usually by K^+ channel block)
IV	Ca^{2+} channel block

Drugs are listed here according to this scheme. It is important to bear in mind, however, that many drugs exert multiple effects that contribute to their clinical actions. It is occasionally clinically useful to subclassify Na^+ channel blockers by their rates of recovery from drug-induced block ($\tau_{recovery}$) under physiologic conditions. Because this is a continuous variable and can be modulated by factors such as depolarization of the resting potential, these distinctions can become blurred: class Ib, $\tau_{recovery}$ <1 s; class Ia, $\tau_{recovery}$ 1–10 s; class Ic, $\tau_{recovery}$ >10 s. These class and subclass effects are associated with distinctive ECG changes, characteristic "class" toxicities, and efficacy in specific arrhythmia syndromes (see text). [1]These data are dependent on experimental conditions, including species and temperature. The $\tau_{recovery}$ values cited here are from Courtney (1987). O, open-state blocker; I, inactivated-state blocker.

that determine $\tau_{recovery}$ (Figure 30–12). The description that follows applies when Na^+ channels are blocked, that is, at rapid heart rates in diseased tissue with a rapid-recovery drug such as *lidocaine* or even at normal rates in normal tissues with a slow-recovery drug such as *flecainide*. When Na^+ channels are blocked, threshold for excitability is decreased; that is, greater membrane depolarization is required to open enough Na^+ channels to overcome K^+ currents at the resting membrane potential and elicit an action potential. This change in threshold probably contributes to the clinical finding that Na^+ channel blockers tend to increase both pacing threshold and the energy required to defibrillate the fibrillating heart. These deleterious effects may be important if antiarrhythmic drugs are used in patients with pacemakers or implanted defibrillators. Na^+ channel block decreases conduction velocity in nonnodal tissue and increases QRS duration. Usual doses of flecainide prolong QRS intervals by 25% or more during normal rhythm, whereas lidocaine increases QRS intervals only at very fast heart rates. Drugs with $\tau_{recovery}$ values greater than 10 sec (e.g., *flecainide*) also tend to prolong the PR interval; it is not known whether this represents additional Ca^{2+} channel block (see discussion that follows) or block of fast-response tissue in the region of the AV node. Drug effects on the PR interval also are highly modified by autonomic effects. For example, *quinidine* actually tends to shorten the PR interval largely as a result of its vagolytic properties. Action potential duration is either unaffected or is shortened by Na^+ channel block; some Na^+ channel–blocking drugs do prolong cardiac action potentials but by other mechanisms, usually K^+ channel block (Table 30–3).

By increasing threshold, Na^+ channel block decreases automaticity (Figure 30–10B) and can inhibit triggered activity arising from DADs or EADs. Many Na^+ channel blockers also decrease phase 4 slope (Figure 30–10A). In anatomically defined reentry, Na^+ channel blockers may decrease conduction sufficiently to extinguish the propagating reentrant wavefront. However, as described previously, conduction slowing owing to Na^+ channel block may exacerbate reentry. Block of Na^+ channels also shifts the voltage dependence of recovery from inactivation (Figure 30–5B) to more negative potentials, thereby tending to increase refractoriness. Thus, whether a given drug exacerbates or suppresses reentrant arrhythmias depends on the balance between its effects on refractoriness and on conduction in a particular reentrant circuit. *Lidocaine* and *mexiletine* have short $\tau_{recovery}$ values and are not useful in atrial fibrillation or flutter, whereas *quinidine*, *flecainide*, *propafenone*, and similar agents are effective in some patients. Many of these agents owe part of their antiarrhythmic activity to blockade of K^+ channels.

Na^+ Channel Blocker Toxicity

Conduction slowing in potential reentrant circuits can account for toxicity of drugs that block the Na^+ channel (Table 30–1). For example, Na^+ channel block decreases conduction velocity and hence slows atrial flutter rate. Normal AV nodal function permits a greater number of impulses to penetrate the ventricle, and heart rate actually may increase (Figure 30–9). Thus, with Na^+ channel blocker therapy, atrial flutter rate may drop from 300 per min, with 2:1 or 4:1 AV conduction (i.e., a heart rate of 150 or 75 beats per min), to 220 per min, but with 1:1 transmission to the ventricle (i.e., a heart rate of 220 beats per min), with potentially disastrous consequences. This form of drug-induced arrhythmia is especially common during treatment with quinidine because the drug also increases AV nodal conduction through its vagolytic properties; flecainide, propafenone, and occasionally amiodarone also have been implicated. Therapy with Na^+ channel blockers in patients with reentrant ventricular tachycardia after a myocardial infarction can increase the frequency and severity of arrhythmic episodes. Although the mechanism is unclear, slowed conduction allows the reentrant wavefront to persist within the tachycardia circuit. Such drug-exacerbated arrhythmia can be difficult to manage, and deaths owing to intractable drug-induced ventricular tachycardia have been reported. In this setting, Na^+ infusion may be beneficial. Drug-exacerbated ventricular tachycardia or VF also likely accounts for increased mortality with Na^+ channel blockers compared to placebo in patients convalescing from acute myocardial infarction in the CAST (Echt et al., 1991). Several Na^+ channel blockers (e.g., *procainamide* and quinidine) have been reported to exacerbate neuromuscular paralysis by D-tubocurarine (see Chapter 11).

Action Potential Prolongation

Most drugs that prolong the action potential do so by blocking I_{Kr} (Roden et al., 1993), although increased late Na^+ current also produces this effect (Lu et al., 2012; Yang et al., 2014). Both drug effects increase action potential duration and reduce normal automaticity (Figure 30–10D). Increased action potential duration, seen as an increase in QT interval, increases refractoriness (Figure 30–11) and therefore should be an effective way of treating reentry (Task Force, 1991). Experimentally, K^+ channel block produces a series of desirable effects: reduced defibrillation energy requirement, inhibition of VF owing to acute ischemia, and increased contractility (Roden, 1993; Singh, 1993). As shown in Table 30–3, many K^+ channel–blocking drugs also interact with β adrenergic receptors (sotalol) or other channels (e.g., amiodarone and quinidine). Amiodarone and sotalol appear to be at least as effective as drugs with predominant Na^+ channel–blocking properties in both atrial and ventricular arrhythmias. "Pure" action potential–prolonging drugs (e.g., dofetilide and ibutilide) also are available (Murray, 1998; Torp-Pedersen et al., 1999).

Toxicity of Drugs That Prolong the Action Potential

Most of these agents disproportionately prolong cardiac action potentials and the QT interval when underlying heart rate is slow and can cause torsades de pointes (Table 30–1, Figure 30–9). While this effect usually is seen with QT-prolonging antiarrhythmic drugs, it can occur more rarely with drugs that are used for noncardiac indications. For such agents, the risk of torsades de pointes may become apparent only after widespread use postmarketing, and recognition of this risk has been a common cause for drug withdrawal (Roden, 2004). Sex hormones modify cardiac ion channels and help account for the clinically observed increased incidence of drug-induced torsades de pointes in women (Tadros et al., 2014).

Ca^{2+} Channel Block

The major electrophysiological effects resulting from block of cardiac Ca^{2+} channels are in nodal tissues. Dihydropyridines, such as nifedipine, which are used commonly in angina and hypertension (see Chapters 27 and 28), preferentially block Ca^{2+} channels in vascular smooth muscle; their cardiac electrophysiological effects, such as heart rate acceleration, result principally from reflex sympathetic activation secondary to peripheral vasodilation. Only verapamil, diltiazem, and bepridil (no longer available in the U.S.) block Ca^{2+} channels in cardiac cells at clinically used doses. These drugs generally slow heart rate (Figure 30–10A), although hypotension, if marked, can cause reflex sympathetic activation and tachycardia. The velocity of AV nodal conduction decreases, so the PR interval increases. AV nodal block occurs as a result of decremental conduction, as well as increased AV nodal refractoriness. These effects form the basis of the antiarrhythmic actions of Ca^{2+} channel blockers in reentrant arrhythmias whose circuit involves the AV node, such as AV reentrant tachycardia (Figure 30–7).

Another important indication for antiarrhythmic therapy is to reduce the ventricular rate in atrial flutter or fibrillation. Parenteral verapamil and diltiazem are approved for temporary control of rapid ventricular rate in atrial flutter or fibrillation and for rapid conversion of PSVT to sinus rhythm (where their use has largely been supplanted by adenosine). Oral verapamil or diltiazem may be used to control the ventricular rate in chronic atrial flutter or fibrillation and for prophylaxis of repetitive PSVT. Unlike β blockers, Ca^{2+} channel blockers have not been shown to reduce mortality after myocardial infarction (Singh, 1990). In contrast to other Ca^{2+} channel blockers, bepridil increases action potential duration in many tissues and can exert an antiarrhythmic effect in atria and ventricles. However, because bepridil can cause torsades de pointes, it is not prescribed widely and has been discontinued in the U.S.

Verapamil and Diltiazem

The major adverse effect of intravenous verapamil or diltiazem is hypotension, particularly with bolus administration. This was a particular problem when the drugs were used mistakenly in patients with ventricular tachycardia (in which Ca^{2+} channel blockers usually are not effective) misdiagnosed as PSVT; the drugs are now rarely used for this indication. Hypotension also is frequent in patients receiving other vasodilators and in patients with underlying left ventricular dysfunction, which the drugs can exacerbate. Severe sinus bradycardia or AV block also occurs, especially in susceptible patients, such as those also receiving β blockers. With oral therapy, these adverse effects tend to be less severe. Constipation can occur with oral verapamil.

Verapamil is prescribed as a racemate. L-Verapamil is the more potent Ca^{2+} channel blocker. However, with oral therapy, the L-enantiomer undergoes more extensive first-pass hepatic metabolism. For this reason, a given concentration of verapamil prolongs the PR interval to a greater extent when administered intravenously (where concentrations of the L- and D-enantiomers are equivalent) than when administered orally. Diltiazem also undergoes extensive first-pass hepatic metabolism, and both drugs have metabolites that exert Ca^{2+} channel–blocking actions. In clinical practice, adverse effects during therapy with verapamil or diltiazem are determined largely by underlying heart disease and concomitant therapy; plasma concentrations of these agents are not measured routinely. Both drugs can increase serum digoxin concentration, although the magnitude of this effect is variable; excess slowing of ventricular response may occur in patients with atrial fibrillation.

Blockade of β Adrenergic Receptors

β Adrenergic stimulation increases the magnitude of the Ca^{2+} current and slows its inactivation; increases the magnitude of the repolarizing current I_{Ks}; increases pacemaker current (thereby increasing sinus rate; DiFrancesco, 1993); increases the Ca^{2+} stored in the SR (thereby increasing likelihood of spontaneous Ca^{2+} release and DADs); and under pathophysiological conditions, can increase both DAD- and EAD-mediated arrhythmias. The increases in plasma epinephrine associated with severe stress (e.g., acute myocardial infarction or resuscitation after cardiac arrest) lower serum K^+, especially in patients receiving chronic diuretic therapy. β blockers inhibit these effects and can be antiarrhythmic by reducing heart rate, decreasing intracellular Ca^{2+} overload, and inhibiting afterdepolarization-mediated automaticity. Epinephrine-induced hypokalemia appears to be mediated by β_2 adrenergic receptors and is blocked by "noncardioselective" antagonists such as propranolol (see Chapter 12). In acutely ischemic tissue, β blockers increase the energy required to fibrillate the heart, an antiarrhythmic action. These effects may contribute to the reduced short-term and long-term mortality observed in trials of chronic therapy with β blockers—after myocardial infarction (Singh, 1990).

As with Ca^{2+} channel blockers and digitalis, β blockers increase AV nodal conduction time (increased PR interval) and prolong AV nodal refractoriness; hence, they are useful in terminating reentrant arrhythmias that involve the AV node and in controlling ventricular response in atrial fibrillation or flutter. In many (but not all) patients with the congenital LQTS, in all patients with the CPVT syndrome, as well as in many other patients, arrhythmias are triggered by physical or emotional stress; β blockers may be useful in these cases (Roden and Spooner, 1999; Schwartz et al., 2000). β blockers also reportedly are effective in controlling arrhythmias owing to Na^+ channel blockers; this effect may be due in part to slowing of the heart rate, which then decreases the extent of rate-dependent conduction slowing by Na^+ channel block.

Adverse effects of β blockade include fatigue, bronchospasm, hypotension, impotence, depression, aggravation of heart failure, worsening of symptoms owing to peripheral vascular disease, and masking of the symptoms of hypoglycemia in diabetic patients (see Chapter 12). In patients with arrhythmias owing to excess sympathetic stimulation (e.g., pheochromocytoma or *clonidine* withdrawal), β blockers can result in unopposed α adrenergic stimulation, with resulting severe hypertension or α adrenergic–mediated arrhythmias. In such patients, arrhythmias should be treated with both α and β blockers or with a drug such as labetalol that combines α- and β-blocking properties. Abrupt discontinuation of chronic β-blocker therapy can lead to "rebound" symptoms, including hypertension, increased angina, and arrhythmias; thus, β blockers are tapered over 2 weeks prior to discontinuation of chronic therapy (see Chapters 12 and 27–29).

Selected β Blockers

It is likely that most β blockers share antiarrhythmic properties. Some, such as propranolol, also exert Na^+ channel–blocking effects at high concentrations. Similarly, drugs with intrinsic sympathomimetic activity may be less useful as antiarrhythmics (Singh, 1990). Acebutolol is as effective as quinidine in suppressing ventricular ectopic beats, an arrhythmia that many clinicians no longer treat. Sotalol (see its discussion in a separate section) is more effective for many arrhythmias than other β blockers, probably because of its K^+ channel–blocking actions. Esmolol (see separate discussion that follows) is a β_1-selective agent that has a very short elimination half-life. Intravenous esmolol is useful in clinical situations in which immediate β adrenergic blockade is desired. Some β blockers (e.g., propranolol) are CYP2D6 substrates; thus, efficacy may vary across individuals (Chapter 7). Many clinicians now favor nadolol when β blockade is needed in congenital arrhythmias (CPVT, LQTS).

Principles in the Clinical Use of Antiarrhythmic Drugs

Drugs that modify cardiac electrophysiology often have a very narrow margin between the doses required to produce a desired effect and those associated with adverse effects. Moreover, antiarrhythmic drugs can induce new arrhythmias with possibly fatal consequences. Nonpharmacological treatments, such as cardiac pacing, electrical defibrillation, or ablation of targeted regions, are indicated for some arrhythmias; in other cases, no therapy is required, even though an arrhythmia is detected. Therefore, the fundamental principles of therapeutics described here must be applied to optimize antiarrhythmic therapy.

1. Identify and Remove Precipitating Factors

Factors that commonly precipitate cardiac arrhythmias include hypoxia, electrolyte disturbances (especially hypokalemia), myocardial ischemia, and certain drugs. Antiarrhythmics, including cardiac glycosides, are not the only drugs that can precipitate arrhythmias (Table 30–1). For example, *theophylline* can cause multifocal atrial tachycardia, which sometimes can be managed simply by reducing the dose of theophylline. Torsades de pointes can arise during therapy not only with action potential–prolonging antiarrhythmics but also with other "noncardiovascular" drugs not ordinarily classified as having effects on ion channels (Roden, 2004). The incidence can vary from 1% to 3% in patients receiving sotalol or dofetilide to very rare (<1/50,000) with some noncardiovascular drugs. Drugs with a very wide range of clinical indications have been implicated: These include some antibiotics (including antibacterials, antiprotozoals, antivirals, and antifungals), antipsychotics, antihistamines, antidepressants, and methadone. The website https://crediblemeds.org maintains a list of drugs (and levels of evidence) that have been implicated in this adverse effect.

2. Establish the Goals of Treatment

Some Arrhythmias Should Not Be Treated: The CAST Example

Abnormalities of cardiac rhythm are readily detectable by a variety of recording methods. However, the mere detection of an abnormality does not equate with the need for therapy. This was illustrated in CAST. The presence of asymptomatic ventricular ectopic beats is a known marker for increased risk of sudden death owing to VF in patients convalescing from myocardial infarction. In CAST, patients whose ventricular ectopic beats were suppressed by the potent Na^+ channel blocker encainide (no longer marketed) or flecainide were randomly assigned to receive those drugs or placebo. Unexpectedly, the mortality rate was 2- to 3-fold higher among patients treated with the drugs than those treated with placebo (Echt et al., 1991). While the explanation for this effect is not known, several lines of evidence suggest that, in the presence of these drugs, transient episodes of myocardial ischemia or sinus tachycardia can cause marked conduction slowing (because these drugs have a very long $\tau_{recovery}$), resulting in fatal reentrant ventricular tachyarrhythmias.

One consequence of this pivotal clinical trial was to reemphasize the concept that therapy should be initiated only when a clear benefit to the patient can be identified. When symptoms are obviously attributable to an ongoing arrhythmia, there usually is little doubt that termination of the arrhythmia will be beneficial; when chronic therapy is used to prevent recurrence of an arrhythmia, the risks may be greater (Roden, 1994). *Among the antiarrhythmic drugs discussed here, only β adrenergic blockers and, to a lesser extent, amiodarone* (Connolly, 1999) *demonstrably reduce mortality during long-term therapy.*

Symptoms Due to Arrhythmias

Some patients with an arrhythmia may be asymptomatic; in this case, establishing any benefit for treatment will be difficult. Some patients may present with presyncope, syncope, or even cardiac arrest, which may be due to brady- or tachyarrhythmias. Other patients may present with a sensation of irregular heartbeats (i.e., palpitations) that can be minimally symptomatic in some individuals and incapacitating in others. The irregular heartbeats may be due to intermittent premature contractions or to sustained arrhythmias such as atrial fibrillation (which results in an irregular ventricular rate) (Figure 30–9). Finally, patients may present with symptoms owing to decreased cardiac output attributable to arrhythmias. The most common symptom is breathlessness either at rest or on exertion. Occasionally, sustained or frequent tachycardias may produce no "arrhythmia" symptoms (such as palpitations) but will depress contractile function; these patients may present with heart failure due to "tachycardia-induced cardiomyopathy", a condition that can be controlled by treating the arrhythmia.

Choosing Among Therapeutic Approaches

In choosing among available therapeutic options, it is important to establish clear therapeutic goals. For example, three options are available in patients with atrial fibrillation: (1) reduce the ventricular response using AV nodal-blocking agents such as digitalis, verapamil, diltiazem, or β blockers (Table 30–1); (2) restore and maintain normal rhythm using drugs such as flecainide or amiodarone; or (3) decide not to implement antiarrhythmic therapy, especially if the patient truly is asymptomatic. Most patients with atrial fibrillation also benefit from anticoagulation to reduce stroke incidence regardless of symptoms (Dzeshka and Lip, 2015) (see Chapter 32).

Factors that contribute to choice of therapy include not only symptoms but also the type and extent of structural heart disease, the QT interval prior to drug therapy, the coexistence of conduction system disease, and the presence of noncardiac diseases (Table 30–4). In the rare patient with the WPW syndrome and atrial fibrillation, the ventricular response can be extremely rapid and can be accelerated paradoxically with digitalis or Ca^{2+} channel blockers; deaths owing to drug therapy have been reported under these circumstances.

The frequency and reproducibility of arrhythmia should be established prior to initiating therapy because inherent variability in the occurrence of arrhythmias can be confused with a beneficial or adverse drug effect. Techniques for this assessment include recording cardiac rhythm for prolonged periods or evaluating the response of the heart to artificially induced premature beats. It is important to recognize that drug therapy may be only partially effective. A marked decrease in the duration of paroxysms of atrial fibrillation may be sufficient to render a patient asymptomatic even if an occasional episode still can be detected.

TABLE 30–4 ■ PATIENT-SPECIFIC ANTIARRHYTHMIC DRUG CONTRAINDICATIONS

CONDITION	EXCLUDE/USE WITH CAUTION
Cardiac	
Heart failure	Disopyramide, flecainide
Sinus or AV node dysfunction	Digoxin, verapamil, diltiazem, β blockers, amiodarone
Wolff–Parkinson–White syndrome (risk of extremely rapid rate if atrial fibrillation develops)	Digoxin, verapamil, diltiazem
Infranodal conduction disease	Na^+ channel blockers, amiodarone
Aortic/subaortic stenosis	Bretylium
History of myocardial infarction	Flecainide
Prolonged QT interval	Quinidine, procainamide, disopyramide, sotalol, dofetilide, ibutilide, amiodarone
Cardiac transplant	Adenosine
Noncardiac	
Diarrhea	Quinidine
Prostatism, glaucoma	Disopyramide
Arthritis	Chronic procainamide
Lung disease	Amiodarone
Tremor	Mexiletine
Constipation	Verapamil
Asthma, peripheral vascular disease, hypoglycemia	β blockers, propafenone

3. Minimize Risks

Antiarrhythmic Drugs Can Cause Arrhythmias

One well-recognized risk of antiarrhythmic therapy is the possibility of provoking new arrhythmias, with potentially life-threatening consequences. Antiarrhythmic drugs can provoke arrhythmias by different mechanisms (Table 30–1). These drug-provoked arrhythmias must be recognized because further treatment with antiarrhythmic drugs often exacerbates the problem, whereas withdrawal of the causative agent is curative. Thus, establishing a precise diagnosis is critical, and targeting therapies at underlying mechanisms of the arrhythmias may be required. For example, treating a ventricular tachycardia with verapamil not only may be ineffective but also can cause catastrophic cardiovascular collapse.

Monitoring of Plasma Concentration

Some adverse effects of antiarrhythmic drugs result from excessive plasma drug concentrations. Measuring plasma concentration and adjusting the dose to maintain the concentration within a prescribed therapeutic range may minimize some adverse effects. In many patients, serious adverse reactions relate to interactions involving antiarrhythmic drugs (often at usual plasma concentrations), transient factors such as electrolyte disturbances or myocardial ischemia, and the type and extent of the underlying heart disease (Roden, 1994). Factors such as generation of unmeasured active metabolites, variability in elimination of enantiomers (which may exert differing pharmacological effects), and disease- or enantiomer-specific abnormalities in drug binding to plasma proteins can complicate the interpretation of plasma drug concentrations.

Patient-Specific Contraindications

Another way to minimize the adverse effects of antiarrhythmic drugs is to avoid certain drugs in certain patient subsets altogether. For example, patients with a history of congestive heart failure are particularly prone to develop heart failure during *disopyramide* therapy. In other cases, adverse effects of drugs may be difficult to distinguish from exacerbations of underlying disease. Amiodarone may cause interstitial lung disease; its use therefore is undesirable in a patient with advanced pulmonary disease in whom the development of this potentially fatal adverse effect would be difficult to detect. Specific diseases that constitute relative or absolute contraindications to specific drugs are listed in Table 30–4.

4. Consider the Electrophysiology of the Heart as a "Moving Target"

Cardiac electrophysiology varies dynamically in response to external influences such as changing autonomic tone, myocardial ischemia, and myocardial stretch (Priori et al., 1999). For example, myocardial ischemia results in changes in extracellular K^+ that make the resting potential less negative, inactivate Na^+ channels, decrease Na^+ current, and slow conduction. In addition, myocardial ischemia can result in the formation and release of metabolites such as lysophosphatidylcholine, which can alter ion channel function; ischemia also may activate channels that otherwise are quiescent, such as the ATP-inhibited K^+ channels. Thus, in response to myocardial ischemia, a normal heart may display changes in resting potential, conduction velocity, intracellular Ca^{2+} concentrations, and repolarization, any one of which then may create arrhythmias or alter response to antiarrhythmic therapy.

Antiarrhythmic Drugs

Summaries of important electrophysiological and pharmacokinetic features of the drugs considered here are presented in Tables 30–3 and 30–5. Ca^{2+} channel blockers and β blockers are discussed in Chapters 12 and 27 to 29. The drugs are presented in alphabetical order. Prescribing patterns have changed over the past several decades in part because fewer suppliers market older drugs, such as quinidine or procainamide, which are therefore increasingly difficult to obtain, a problem for a small number of patients who may still benefit from treatment (Inama et al., 2010; Viskin et al., 2013).

TABLE 30–5 ■ PHARMACOKINETIC CHARACTERISTICS AND DOSES OF ANTIARRHYTHMIC DRUGS

DRUG	BIOAVAILABILITY	PROTEIN BINDING >80%	ELIMINATION			ELIMINATION[a] $t_{1/2}$	ACTIVE METABOLITE(S)	THERAPEUTIC[b] PLASMA CONCENTRATION	USUAL DOSES[c]	
	REDUCED FIRST-PASS METABOLISM		RENAL	HEPATIC	OTHER				LOADING DOSES	MAINTENANCE DOSES
Adenosine[d]					√	<10 s	√		6–12 mg (IV only) 800–1600 mg/d × 1–3 wk (IV: 1000 mg over 24 h)	
Amiodarone		√		√		wk	√	0.5-2 μg/mL		100-200 mg/day IV: 0.5 mg/min
Digoxin	–80%		√			36 h		0.5-2.0 ng/mL	0.6–1 mg over 12–24 h	0.0625–0.5 mg/24 h
Diltiazem	√			√		4 h	(x)		0.25 mg/kg over 10 min (IV)	5-15 mg/h (IV); 180-360 mg/d in 3-4 divided doses (immediate release); 120-180 mg/24 h (extended release)[e]
Disopyramide	>80%		√	√		4-10 h	(x)	2-5 μg/mL		150 mg/6 h (immediate release); 300 mg (controlled release[f]
Dofetilide	>80%		√	(x)		7-10 h				0.5 mg/12 h
Dronedarone	√	>98%	√			13-19 h	√			400 mg/12 h
Esmolol					√	5-10 min			0.5 mg/kg over 1 min (IV)	0.05-0.3 mg/kg/min for 4 min (IV)
Flecainide	>80%			√		10-18 h		0.2-1 μg/mL		50-100 mg/12 h
Ibutilide	√								1 mg (IV) over 10 min; may repeat once 10 min later	
Lidocaine	√	√		√		120 min	(x)	1.5-5 μg/mL	50-100 mg administered at a rate of 25-50 mg/min (IV)	1-4 mg/min (IV)
Mexiletine	>80%			√		9-15 h		0.5-2 μg/mL	400 mg	200 mg/8 h
Procainamide	>80%		√	√		3-4 h	√	4-8 μg/mL	500-600 mg (IV), given at 20 mg/min	2-6 mg/min (IV); 250 mg q3h; 500-1000 mg q6h
(*N*-Acetyl procainamide)	(>80%)		(√)			(6-10 h)		(10-20 μg/mL)		

Propafenone	√			√		2-32 h	√	<1 μg/mL		150 mg/8h (immediate release); 225 mg/12h (extended release)
Propranolol	√	√	√			4 h			1-3 mg administered no faster than 1 mg/min, may repeat[e] after 2 min (IV)	10-30 mg q6-8h (immediate release)
Quinidine	>80%	–80%	(x)	√		4-10 h	√	2-5 μg/mL		648 mg (gluconate) every 8h
Sotalol	>80%		√			8 h		<5 μg/mL (?)		80-160 mg/12h
Verapamil	√	√		√		3-7 h	√		5-10 mg given over 2 min or more (IV)	40-120 mg/6-8h (immediate release)

√ Indicates an effect that affects the clinical action of the drug. (x): metabolite or route of elimination probably of minor clinical importance. [a]The elimination $t_{1/2}$ is one, but not the only, determinant of how frequently a drug must be administered to maintain a therapeutic effect and avoid toxicity (Chapter 2). For some drugs with short elimination half-lives, infrequent dosing is nevertheless possible, e.g., verapamil. Formulations that allow slow release into the GI tract of a rapidly eliminated compound (available for many drugs, including procainamide, disopyramide, verapamil, diltiazem, and propranolol) also allow infrequent dosing. [b]The therapeutic range is bounded by a plasma concentration below which no therapeutic effect is likely, and an upper concentration above which the risk of adverse effects increases. Many serious adverse reactions to antiarrhythmic drugs can occur at "therapeutic" concentrations in susceptible individuals. When only an upper limit is cited, a lower limit has not been well defined. Variable generation of active metabolites may further complicate the interpretation of plasma concentration data (Chapter 2). [c]Oral doses are presented unless otherwise indicated. Doses are presented as suggested ranges in adults of average build; lower doses are less likely to produce toxicity. Lower maintenance dosages may be required in patients with renal or hepatic disease. Loading doses are only indicated when a therapeutic effect is desired before maintenance therapy would bring drug concentrations into a therapeutic range—that is, for acute therapy (e.g., lidocaine, verapamil, adenosine) or when the elimination $t_{1/2}$ is extremely long (amiodarone). [d] Bioavailability reduced by incomplete absorption. [e]Indicates suggested dosage using slow-release formulation. IV, intravenous.

Adenosine

Adenosine is a naturally occurring nucleoside that is administered as a rapid intravenous bolus for the acute termination of reentrant supraventricular arrhythmias (Link, 2012). Rare cases of ventricular tachycardia in patients with otherwise-normal hearts are thought to be DAD mediated and can be terminated by adenosine. Adenosine also has been used to produce controlled hypotension during some surgical procedures and in the diagnosis of coronary artery disease. Intravenous ATP appears to produce effects similar to those of adenosine.

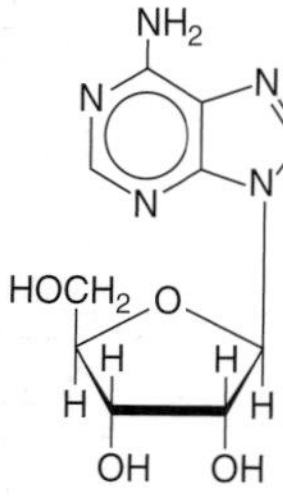

ADENOSINE

Pharmacological Effects

The effects of adenosine are mediated by its interaction with specific G protein–coupled adenosine receptors. Adenosine activates acetylcholine-sensitive K^+ current in the atrium and sinus and AV nodes, resulting in shortening of action potential duration, hyperpolarization, and slowing of normal automaticity (Figure 30–10C). Adenosine also inhibits the electrophysiological effects of increased intracellular cyclic AMP that occur with sympathetic stimulation. Because adenosine thereby reduces Ca^{2+} currents, it can be antiarrhythmic by increasing AV nodal refractoriness and by inhibiting DADs elicited by sympathetic stimulation.

Administration of an intravenous bolus of adenosine to humans transiently slows sinus rate and AV nodal conduction velocity and increases AV nodal refractoriness. A bolus of adenosine can produce transient sympathetic activation by interacting with carotid baroreceptors; a continuous infusion can cause hypotension.

Adverse Effects

A major advantage of adenosine therapy is that adverse effects are short-lived because the drug is transported into cells and deaminated so rapidly. Transient asystole (lack of any cardiac rhythm whatsoever) is common but usually lasts less than 5 sec and is in fact the therapeutic goal. Most patients feel a sense of chest fullness and dyspnea when therapeutic doses (6 to 12 mg) of adenosine are administered. Rarely, an adenosine bolus can precipitate atrial fibrillation, presumably by heterogeneously shortening atrial action potentials, or bronchospasm.

Clinical Pharmacokinetics

Adenosine is eliminated with a half-life of seconds by carrier-mediated uptake, which occurs in most cell types, including the endothelium, followed by metabolism by adenosine deaminase. Adenosine probably is the only drug whose efficacy requires a rapid bolus dose, preferably through a large central intravenous line; slow administration results in elimination of the drug prior to its arrival at the heart.

The effects of adenosine are potentiated in patients receiving *dipyridamole*, an adenosine-uptake inhibitor, and in patients with cardiac transplants owing to denervation hypersensitivity. Methylxanthines (see Tables 14-7, 40-2, and 40-3, and Figure 40-5) such as theophylline and caffeine block adenosine receptors; therefore, larger-than-usual doses are required to produce an antiarrhythmic effect in patients who have consumed these agents in beverages or as therapy.

Amiodarone

Amiodarone exerts a multiplicity of pharmacological effects, none of which is clearly linked to its arrhythmia-suppressing properties. Amiodarone is a structural analogue of thyroid hormone, and some of its antiarrhythmic actions and its toxicity may be attributable to interaction with nuclear thyroid hormone receptors. Amiodarone is highly lipophilic, is concentrated in many tissues, and is eliminated extremely slowly; consequently, adverse effects may resolve very slowly. In the U.S., the drug is indicated for oral therapy in patients with recurrent ventricular tachycardia or VF resistant to other drugs. In addition, the intravenous form is a first-line drug for management of ventricular tachycardia or VF causing cardiac arrest (Dorian et al., 2002). Trials of oral amiodarone have shown a modest beneficial effect on mortality after acute myocardial infarction (Amiodarone Trials Meta-Analysis Investigators, 1997). Despite uncertainties about its mechanisms of action and the potential for serious toxicity, amiodarone is used widely in the treatment of common arrhythmias such as atrial fibrillation (Roy et al., 2000).

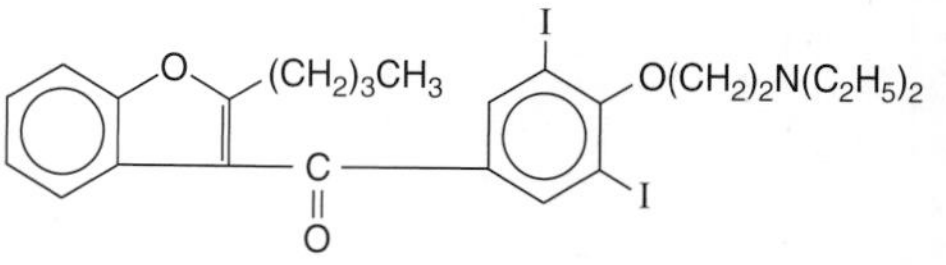

AMIODARONE

Pharmacological Effects

Studies of the acute effects of amiodarone in in vitro systems are complicated by its insolubility in water, necessitating the use of solvents such as dimethyl sulfoxide, which can have electrophysiological effects on its own. Amiodarone's effects may be mediated by perturbation of the lipid environment of the ion channels. Amiodarone blocks inactivated Na^+ channels and has a relatively rapid rate of recovery (time constant ≈ 1.6 sec) from block. It also decreases Ca^{2+} current and transient outward delayed rectifier and inward rectifier K^+ currents and exerts a noncompetitive adrenergic-blocking effect. Amiodarone potently inhibits abnormal automaticity and, in most tissues, prolongs action potential duration. Amiodarone decreases conduction velocity by Na^+ channel block and by a poorly understood effect on cell-cell coupling that may be especially important in diseased tissue. Prolongations of the PR, QRS, and QT intervals and sinus bradycardia are frequent during chronic therapy. Amiodarone prolongs refractoriness in all cardiac tissues; Na^+ channel block, delayed repolarization owing to K^+ channel block, and inhibition of cell-cell coupling all may contribute to this effect.

Adverse Effects

Hypotension owing to vasodilation and depressed myocardial performance are frequent with the intravenous form of amiodarone and may be due in part to the solvent. While depressed contractility can occur during long-term oral therapy, it is unusual. Despite administration of high doses that would cause serious toxicity if continued long term, adverse effects are unusual during oral drug-loading regimens, which typically require several weeks. Occasional patients develop nausea during the loading phase, which responds to a decrease in daily dose.

Adverse effects during long-term therapy reflect both the size of daily maintenance doses and the cumulative dose, suggesting that tissue accumulation may be responsible. The most serious adverse effect during chronic amiodarone therapy is pulmonary fibrosis, which can be rapidly progressive and fatal. Underlying lung disease, doses of 400 mg/d or more, and recent pulmonary insults such as pneumonia appear to be risk factors. Serial chest X-rays or pulmonary function studies may detect early amiodarone toxicity, but monitoring plasma concentrations has not been useful. With low doses, such as 200 mg/d or less as used in atrial fibrillation, pulmonary toxicity is less common (Zimetbaum, 2007). Other adverse effects during long-term therapy include corneal microdeposits (which often are asymptomatic), hepatic dysfunction, neuromuscular symptoms (most commonly peripheral neuropathy or proximal muscle weakness), photosensitivity, and hypo- or hyperthyroidism. The multiple effects of amiodarone on thyroid function are discussed further in Chapter 43. Treatment consists of withdrawal of the drug and supportive measures, including corticosteroids, for life-threatening pulmonary toxicity; reduction of dosage may be sufficient if the drug is deemed necessary and the adverse effect is not life threatening. Despite the marked QT prolongation and bradycardia typical of chronic amiodarone therapy, torsades de pointes and other drug-induced tachyarrhythmias are unusual.

Clinical Pharmacokinetics

Amiodarone's oral bioavailability is about 30%, presumably due to poor absorption. This incomplete bioavailability is important in calculating equivalent dosing regimens when converting from intravenous to oral therapy. The drug distributes into lipid; heart tissue-to-plasma concentration ratios of greater than 20:1 and lipid-to-plasma ratios of greater than 300:1 have been reported. After the initiation of amiodarone therapy, increases in refractoriness, a marker of pharmacological effect, require several weeks to develop. Amiodarone undergoes hepatic metabolism by CYP3A4 to desethyl-amiodarone, a metabolite with pharmacological effects similar to those of the parent drug. When amiodarone therapy is withdrawn from a patient who has been receiving therapy for several years, plasma concentrations decline with a half-life of weeks to months. The mechanisms of amiodarone and desethyl-amiodarone elimination are not well established.

A therapeutic plasma amiodarone concentration range of 0.5 to 2 μg/mL has been proposed. However, efficacy apparently depends as much on duration of therapy as on plasma concentration, and elevated plasma concentrations do not predict toxicity. Because of amiodarone's slow accumulation in tissue, a high-dose oral loading regimen (e.g., 800 to 1600 mg/d) usually is administered for several weeks before maintenance therapy is started. The maintenance dose is adjusted based on adverse effects and the arrhythmias being treated. If the presenting arrhythmia is life threatening, dosages of more than 300 mg/d normally are used unless unequivocal toxicity occurs. On the other hand, maintenance doses of 200 mg/d or less are used if recurrence of an arrhythmia would be tolerated, as in patients with atrial fibrillation, because amiodarone slows the ventricular rate during atrial fibrillation.

Dosage adjustments are not required in hepatic, renal, or cardiac dysfunction. Amiodarone potently inhibits the hepatic metabolism or renal elimination of many compounds. Mechanisms identified to date include inhibition of CYP3A4, CYP2C9, and P-glycoprotein (see Chapters 5 and 6). Dosages of warfarin, other antiarrhythmics (e.g., flecainide, procainamide, and quinidine), or digoxin usually require reduction during amiodarone therapy.

Bretylium

Bretylium is a quaternary ammonium compound that prolongs cardiac action potentials and interferes with reuptake of norepinephrine by sympathetic neurons. In the past, bretylium was used to treat VF and prevent its recurrence; the drug is currently not available in the U.S.

Digoxin

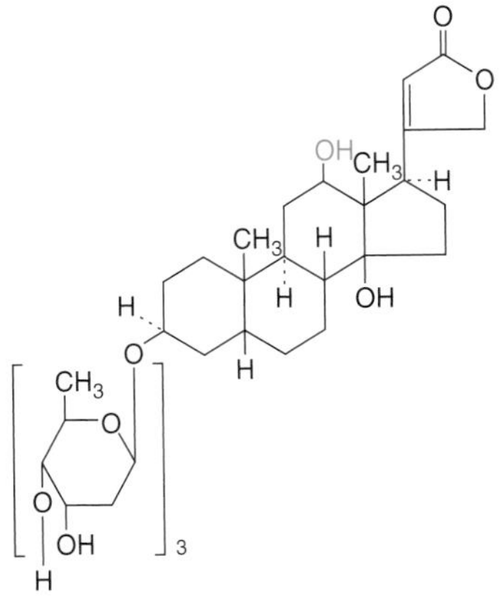

DIGOXIN

Pharmacological Effects

Digitalis glycosides exert positive inotropic effects and have been used in heart failure; now, they are rarely prescribed (see Chapter 29). Their inotropic action results from increased intracellular Ca^{2+}, which also forms the basis for arrhythmias related to cardiac glycoside intoxication. Cardiac glycosides increase phase 4 slope (i.e., increase the rate of automaticity), especially if $[K]_o$ is low. These drugs (e.g., digoxin) also exert prominent vagotonic actions, resulting in inhibition of Ca^{2+} currents in the AV node and activation of acetylcholine-mediated K^+ currents in the atrium. Thus, the major "indirect" electrophysiological effects of cardiac glycosides are hyperpolarization, shortening of atrial action potentials, and increases in AV nodal refractoriness. The last action accounts for the utility of digoxin in terminating reentrant arrhythmias involving the AV node and in controlling ventricular response in patients with atrial fibrillation. Cardiac glycosides may be especially useful in the last situation because many such patients have heart failure, which can be exacerbated by other AV nodal–blocking drugs such as Ca^{2+} channel blockers or β blockers. However, sympathetic drive is increased markedly in many patients with advanced heart failure, so digitalis is not very effective in decreasing the rate; on the other hand, even a modest decrease in rate can ameliorate heart failure.

Similarly, in other conditions in which high sympathetic tone drives rapid AV conduction (e.g., chronic lung disease and thyrotoxicosis), digitalis therapy may be only marginally effective in slowing the rate. In heart transplant patients, in whom innervation has been ablated, cardiac glycosides are ineffective for rate control. Increased sympathetic activity and hypoxia can potentiate digitalis-induced changes in automaticity and DADs, thus increasing the risk of digitalis toxicity. A further complicating feature in thyrotoxicosis is increased digoxin clearance.

The major ECG effects of cardiac glycosides are PR prolongation and a nonspecific alteration in ventricular repolarization (manifested by depression of the ST segment), whose underlying mechanism is not well understood.

Adverse Effects

Because of the low therapeutic index of cardiac glycosides, their toxicity is a common clinical problem (see Chapter 29). Arrhythmias, nausea, disturbances of cognitive function, and blurred or yellow vision are the usual manifestations. Elevated serum concentrations of digitalis, hypoxia (e.g., owing to chronic lung disease), and electrolyte abnormalities (e.g., hypokalemia, hypomagnesemia, and hypercalcemia) predispose patients to digitalis-induced arrhythmias. While digitalis intoxication can cause virtually any arrhythmia, certain types of arrhythmias are characteristic. Arrhythmias that should raise a strong suspicion of digitalis intoxication are those in which DAD-related tachycardias occur along with impairment of sinus node or AV nodal function. Atrial tachycardia with AV block is classic, but ventricular bigeminy (sinus beats alternating with beats of ventricular origin), "bidirectional" ventricular tachycardia (a rare entity), AV junctional tachycardias, and various degrees of AV block also can occur. With severe intoxication (e.g., with suicidal ingestion), severe hyperkalemia owing to poisoning of Na^+, K^+–ATPase and profound bradyarrhythmias, which may be unresponsive to pacing therapy, are seen. In patients with elevated serum digitalis levels, the risk of precipitating VF by DC cardioversion probably is increased; in those with therapeutic blood levels, DC cardioversion can be used safely.

Minor forms of cardiac glycoside intoxication may require no specific therapy beyond monitoring cardiac rhythm until symptoms and signs of toxicity resolve. Sinus bradycardia and AV block often respond to intravenous atropine, but the effect is transient. Mg^{2+} has been used successfully in some cases of digitalis-induced tachycardia. Any serious arrhythmia should be treated with antidigoxin Fab fragments (Digibind, Digifab), which are highly effective in binding digoxin and digitoxin and greatly enhance their renal excretion (see Chapter 29). Serum glycoside concentrations rise markedly with antidigitalis antibodies, but these represent bound (pharmacologically inactive) drug. Temporary cardiac pacing may be required for advanced sinus node or AV node dysfunction. Digitalis exerts direct arterial vasoconstrictor effects, which can be especially deleterious in patients with advanced atherosclerosis who receive intravenous drug; mesenteric and coronary ischemia have been reported.

Clinical Pharmacokinetics

The only digitalis glycoside used in the U.S. is digoxin. Digitoxin (various generic preparations) also is used for chronic oral therapy outside the U.S. Digoxin tablets are incompletely (75%) bioavailable. In some patients, intestinal microflora may metabolize digoxin, markedly reducing bioavailability. In these patients, higher-than-usual doses are required for clinical efficacy; toxicity is a serious risk if antibiotics are administered that destroy intestinal microflora. Inhibition of P-glycoprotein (see further discussion) also may play a role in cases of toxicity. Digoxin is 20% to 30% protein bound.

The antiarrhythmic effects of digoxin can be achieved with intravenous or oral therapy. However, digoxin undergoes relatively slow distribution to effector site(s); therefore, even with intravenous therapy, there is a lag of several hours between drug administration and the development of measurable antiarrhythmic effects such as PR interval prolongation or slowing of the ventricular rate in atrial fibrillation. To avoid intoxication, a loading dose of approximately 0.6 to 1 mg digoxin is administered over 24 h. Measurement of postdistribution serum digoxin concentration and adjustment of the daily dose (0.0625 to 0.5 mg) to maintain concentrations of 0.5 to 2 ng/mL are useful during chronic digoxin therapy (Table 30–5). Some patients may require and tolerate higher concentrations, but with an increased risk of adverse effects.

The elimination half-life of digoxin ordinarily is about 36 h, so maintenance doses are administered once daily. Renal elimination of unchanged drug accounts for about 80% of digoxin elimination. Digoxin doses should be reduced (or dosing interval increased) and serum concentrations monitored closely in patients with impaired excretion owing to renal failure or in patients who are hypothyroid. Digitoxin undergoes primarily hepatic metabolism and may be useful in patients with fluctuating or advanced renal dysfunction. Digitoxin metabolism is accelerated by drugs such as phenytoin and rifampin that induce hepatic metabolism. Digitoxin's elimination half-life is even longer than that of digoxin (about 7 days); it is highly protein bound, and its therapeutic range is 10 to 30 ng/mL.

Amiodarone, quinidine, verapamil, diltiazem, cyclosporine, itraconazole, propafenone, and flecainide decrease digoxin clearance, likely by inhibiting P-glycoprotein, the major route of digoxin elimination (Fromm et al., 1999). New steady-state digoxin concentrations are approached after four to five half-lives (i.e., in about a week). Digitalis toxicity results so often with quinidine or amiodarone that it is routine to decrease the dose of digoxin if these drugs are started. In all cases, digoxin concentrations should be measured regularly and the dose adjusted if necessary. Hypokalemia, which can be caused by many drugs (e.g., diuretics, amphotericin B, and corticosteroids), will potentiate digitalis-induced arrhythmias.

Disopyramide

Disopyramide exerts electrophysiological effects very similar to those of quinidine, but the drugs have different adverse effect profiles. Disopyramide can be used to maintain sinus rhythm in patients with atrial flutter or atrial fibrillation and to prevent recurrence of ventricular tachycardia or VF. Because of its negative inotropic effects, it is sometimes used in hypertrophic cardiomyopathy. Disopyramide is prescribed as a racemate.

Pharmacological Actions and Adverse Effects

The in vitro electrophysiological actions of *S*-(+)-disopyramide are similar to those of quinidine. The *R*-(−)-enantiomer produces similar Na^+ channel block but does not prolong cardiac action potentials. Unlike quinidine, racemic disopyramide does not antagonize α adrenergic receptors, but does exert prominent anticholinergic actions that account for many of its adverse effects. These include precipitation of glaucoma, constipation, dry mouth, and urinary retention; the last is most common in males with prostatism but also can occur in females. Disopyramide can cause torsades de pointes and also commonly depresses contractility, which can precipitate heart failure. In patients with hypertrophic cardiomyopathy, this depression contractility may be exploited to therapeutic advantage to decrease dynamic outflow tract obstruction (Sherrid and Arabadjian, 2012).

Clinical Pharmacokinetics

Disopyramide is well absorbed. Binding to plasma proteins is concentration dependent, so a small increase in total concentration may represent a disproportionately larger increase in free drug concentration. Disopyramide is eliminated by both hepatic metabolism (to a weakly active metabolite) and renal excretion of unchanged drug. The dose should be reduced in patients with renal dysfunction. Higher-than-usual dosages may be required in patients receiving drugs that induce hepatic metabolism, such as phenytoin.

Dofetilide

Dofetilide prolongs action potentials and the QT interval by potently blocking the I_{Kr} channel. Increased late Na^+ current, likely due to inhibition of phosphoinositide 3–kinase (Yang et al., 2014), may also contribute. The drug has virtually no extracardiac pharmacological effects. Dofetilide is effective in maintaining sinus rhythm in patients with atrial fibrillation. In the DIAMOND studies (Torp-Pedersen et al., 1999), dofetilide did not affect mortality in patients with advanced heart failure or in those convalescing from acute myocardial infarction. Dofetilide currently is available through a restricted distribution system that includes only physicians, hospitals, and other institutions that have received special educational programs covering proper dosing and in-hospital treatment initiation.

Adverse Effects

Torsades de pointes occurred in 1%–3% of patients in clinical trials where strict exclusion criteria (e.g., hypokalemia) were applied and continuous ECG monitoring was used to detect marked QT prolongation in the hospital. Other adverse effects were no more common than with placebo during premarketing clinical trials.

Clinical Pharmacokinetics

Most of a dose of dofetilide is excreted unchanged by the kidneys. In patients with mild-to-moderate renal failure, decreases in dosage based on creatinine clearance are required to minimize the risk of torsades de pointes. The drug should not be used in patients with advanced renal failure or with inhibitors of renal cation transport. Dofetilide also undergoes minor hepatic metabolism.

Dronedarone

Dronedarone is a noniodinated benzofuran derivative of amiodarone that is FDA-approved for the treatment of atrial fibrillation and atrial flutter. In randomized placebo-controlled trials, it was effective in maintaining sinus rhythm and reducing the ventricular response rate during episodes of atrial fibrillation (Patel et al., 2009). Compared to amiodarone, dronedarone treatment is associated with significantly fewer adverse events, but it is also significantly less effective in maintaining sinus rhythm. Dronedarone decreased hospital admissions compared to placebo in patients with a history of atrial fibrillation (Hohnloser et al., 2009). In other studies, however, the drug increased mortality in patients with permanent atrial fibrillation (Connolly et al., 2011) and in those with severe heart failure (Kober et al., 2008).

Pharmacological Effects

Like amiodarone, dronedarone is a blocker of multiple ion currents, including the rapidly activating delayed-rectifier K^+ current (I_{Kr}), the slowly activating delayed-rectifier K^+ current (I_{Ks}), the inward rectifier K^+ current (I_{K1}), the acetylcholine-activated K^+ current, the peak Na^+ current, and the L-type Ca^{2+} current. It has stronger antiadrenergic effects than amiodarone.

Adverse Effects and Drug Interactions

The most common adverse reactions are diarrhea, nausea, abdominal pain, vomiting, and asthenia. Dronedarone causes dose-dependent prolongation of the QTc interval, but torsades de pointes is rare. Dronedarone is metabolized by CYP3A and is a moderate inhibitor of CYP3A, CYP2D6, and P-glycoprotein. Potent CYP3A4 inhibitors such as ketoconazole may increase dronedarone exposure by as much as 25-fold. Consequently, dronedarone should not be coadministered with potent CYP3A4 inhibitors (e.g., antifungals, macrolide antibiotics). Coadministration with other drugs metabolized by CYP2D6 (e.g., metoprolol) or P-glycoprotein (e.g., digoxin) may result in increased drug concentrations. Dronedarone may cause severe liver injury; the FDA recommends monitoring of hepatic enzymes.

Esmolol

Esmolol is a β_1-selective agent that is metabolized by erythrocyte esterases and so has a very short elimination half-life (9 min). Intravenous esmolol is useful in clinical situations in which immediate β adrenergic blockade is desired (e.g., for rate control of rapidly conducted atrial fibrillation). Because of esmolol's very rapid elimination, adverse effects due to β adrenergic blockade—should they occur—dissipate rapidly when the drug is stopped. Although methanol is a metabolite of esmolol, methanol intoxication has not been a clinical problem. The pharmacology of esmolol is described in further detail in Chapter 12.

Flecainide

The effects of flecainide therapy are thought to be attributable to the drug's very long $\tau_{recovery}$ from Na^+ channel block. Suppression of DADs triggered by RyR2 Ca^{2+} release may also contribute to flecainide's antiarrhythmic effect. In CAST, flecainide increased mortality in patients convalescing from myocardial infarction (Echt et al., 1991). However, it continues to be approved for certain arrhythmias in patients in whom structural heart disease is absent (Henthorn et al., 1991); this includes the maintenance of sinus rhythm in patients with supraventricular arrhythmias, including atrial fibrillation, as well as life-threatening ventricular arrhythmias, such as sustained ventricular tachycardia. Clinical case series suggested long-term flecainide efficacy in two congenital ventricular arrhythmia syndromes: type 3 LQTS due to mutations that cause late Na^+ currents and CPVT due to mutations that cause "leaky" RyR2 SR Ca^{2+} release channels. Supported by data from a recent randomized clinical trial (Kannankeril et al. 2017), flecainide has become the drug of choice for preventing arrhythmias in CPVT patients uncontrolled by β blockers.

Pharmacological Effects

Flecainide blocks Na^+ current and delayed rectifier K^+ current (I_{Kr}) in vitro at similar concentrations, 1 to 2 μM. It also blocks Ca^{2+} currents in vitro. Action potential duration is shortened in Purkinje cells, probably owing to block of late-opening Na^+ channels, but is prolonged in ventricular cells, probably owing to block of delayed rectifier current. Flecainide does not cause EADs in vitro but has been associated with rare cases of torsades de pointes. In atrial tissue, flecainide disproportionately prolongs action potentials at fast rates, an especially desirable antiarrhythmic drug effect; this effect contrasts with that of quinidine, which prolongs atrial action potentials to a greater extent at slower rates. Flecainide prolongs the duration of PR, QRS, and QT intervals even at normal heart rates. Flecainide is also an open channel blocker of RyR2 Ca^{2+} release channels and prevents arrhythmogenic Ca^{2+} release from the SR and hence DADs in isolated myocytes (Hilliard et al., 2010). The RyR2 channel block by flecainide targets directly the underlying molecular defect in patients with mutations in the RyR2 gene and the cardiac calsequestrin gene, which may explain why flecainide suppresses ventricular arrhythmias in patients with CPVT refractory to β blocker therapy (Watanabe et al., 2009; Kannankeril et al, 2017).

Adverse Effects

Flecainide produces few subjective complaints in most patients; dose-related blurred vision is the most common noncardiac adverse effect. It can exacerbate congestive heart failure in patients with depressed left ventricular performance. The most serious adverse effects are provocation or exacerbation of potentially lethal arrhythmias. These include acceleration of ventricular rate in patients with atrial flutter, increased frequency of episodes of reentrant ventricular tachycardia, and increased mortality in patients convalescing from myocardial infarction. As discussed previously, it is likely that all these effects can be attributed to Na^+ channel block. Flecainide also can cause heart block in patients with conduction system disease.

Clinical Pharmacokinetics

Flecainide is well absorbed. The elimination $t_{1/2}$ is shorter with urinary acidification (10 h) than with urinary alkalinization (17 h), but it is nevertheless sufficiently long to allow dosing twice daily (Table 30–5). Elimination occurs by both renal excretion of unchanged drug and hepatic metabolism to inactive metabolites. The latter is mediated by the polymorphically distributed enzyme CYP2D6. However, even in patients in whom this pathway is absent because of genetic polymorphism or inhibition by other drugs (e.g., quinidine or fluoxetine), renal excretion ordinarily is sufficient to prevent drug accumulation. In the rare patient with renal dysfunction and lack of active CYP2D6, flecainide may accumulate to toxic plasma concentrations. Flecainide is a racemate, but there are no differences in the electrophysiological effects or disposition kinetics of its enantiomers. Some reports have suggested that plasma flecainide concentrations greater than 1 μg/mL should be avoided to minimize the risk of flecainide toxicity; however, in susceptible patients, the adverse electrophysiological effects of flecainide therapy can occur at therapeutic plasma concentrations.

Ibutilide

Ibutilide is an I_{Kr} blocker that in some systems also activates an inward Na^+ current (Murray, 1998). The action potential–prolonging effect of the drug may arise from either mechanism. Ibutilide is administered as a rapid infusion (1 mg over 10 min) for the immediate conversion of atrial fibrillation or flutter to sinus rhythm. The drug's efficacy rate is higher in patients with atrial flutter (50%–70%) than in those with atrial fibrillation (30%–50%). In atrial fibrillation, the conversion rate is lower in those in whom the arrhythmia has been present for weeks or months compared with those in whom it has been present for days. The major toxicity with ibutilide is torsades de pointes, which occurs in up to 6% of patients and requires immediate cardioversion in up to one-third of these. The drug undergoes extensive first-pass metabolism, so it is not used orally. It is eliminated by hepatic metabolism and has a $t_{1/2}$ of 2–12 h (average 6 h).

Lidocaine

Lidocaine is a local anesthetic that also is useful in the acute intravenous therapy of ventricular arrhythmias. When lidocaine was administered to all patients with suspected myocardial infarction, the incidence of VF was reduced. However, survival to hospital discharge tended to be decreased, perhaps because of lidocaine-exacerbated heart block or congestive heart failure. Therefore, lidocaine no longer is administered routinely to all patients in coronary care units.

Pharmacological Effects

Lidocaine blocks both open and inactivated cardiac Na^+ channels. In vitro studies suggested that lidocaine-induced block reflects an increased likelihood that the Na^+ channel protein assumes a nonconducting conformation in the presence of drug (Balser et al., 1996). Recovery from block is rapid, so lidocaine exerts greater effects in depolarized (e.g., ischemic) or rapidly driven tissues. Lidocaine is not useful in atrial arrhythmias, possibly because atrial action potentials are so short that the Na^+ channel is in the inactivated state only briefly compared with diastolic (recovery) times, which are relatively long. In some studies, lidocaine increased current through inward rectifier channels, but the clinical significance of this effect is not known. Lidocaine can hyperpolarize Purkinje fibers depolarized by low $[K]_o$ or stretch; the resulting increased conduction velocity may be antiarrhythmic in reentry.

Lidocaine decreases automaticity by reducing the slope of phase 4 and altering the threshold for excitability. Action potential duration usually is unaffected or is shortened; such shortening may be due to block of the few Na^+ channels that inactivate late during the cardiac action potential. Lidocaine usually exerts no significant effect on PR or QRS duration; QT is unaltered or slightly shortened. The drug exerts little effect on hemodynamic function, although rare cases of lidocaine-associated exacerbations of heart failure have been reported, especially in patients with very poor left ventricular function. For additional information on lidocaine, see Chapter 22 on local anesthetics.

Adverse Effects

When a large intravenous dose of lidocaine is administered rapidly, seizures can occur. When plasma concentrations of the drug rise slowly above the therapeutic range, as may occur during maintenance therapy, tremor, dysarthria, and altered levels of consciousness are more common. Nystagmus is an early sign of lidocaine toxicity.

Clinical Pharmacokinetics

Lidocaine is well absorbed but undergoes extensive though variable first-pass hepatic metabolism; thus, oral use of the drug is inappropriate. In theory, therapeutic plasma concentrations of lidocaine may be maintained by intermittent intramuscular administration, but the intravenous route is preferred (Table 30–5). Lidocaine's metabolites, GX and monoethyl GX, are less potent as Na^+ channel blockers than the parent drug. GX and lidocaine appear to compete for access to the Na^+ channel, suggesting that with infusions during which GX accumulates, lidocaine's efficacy may be diminished. With infusions lasting longer than 24 h, the clearance of lidocaine falls—an effect that may result from competition between parent drug and metabolites for access to hepatic drug-metabolizing enzymes.

Plasma concentrations of lidocaine decline biexponentially after a single intravenous dose, indicating that a multicompartment model is necessary to analyze lidocaine disposition. The initial drop in plasma lidocaine following intravenous administration occurs rapidly, with a $t_{1/2}$ of about 8 min, and represents distribution from the central compartment to peripheral tissues. The terminal elimination $t_{1/2}$ of about 2 h represents drug elimination by hepatic metabolism. Lidocaine's efficacy depends on maintenance of therapeutic plasma concentrations in the central compartment. Therefore, the administration of a single bolus dose of lidocaine can result in transient arrhythmia suppression that dissipates rapidly as the drug is distributed and concentrations in the central compartment fall. To avoid this distribution-related loss of efficacy, a loading regimen of 3 to 4 mg/kg over 20–30 min is used (e.g., an initial 100 mg followed by 50 mg every 8 min for three doses). Subsequently, stable concentrations can be maintained in plasma with an infusion of 1 to 4 mg/min, which replaces drug removed by hepatic metabolism. The time to steady-state lidocaine concentrations is approximately 8–10 h. If the maintenance infusion rate is too low, arrhythmias may recur hours after the institution of apparently successful therapy. On the other hand, if the rate is too high, toxicity may result. In either case, routine measurement of plasma lidocaine concentration at the time of expected steady state is useful in adjusting maintenance infusion rate.

In heart failure, the central volume of distribution is decreased, so the total loading dose should be decreased. Because lidocaine clearance also is decreased, the rate of the maintenance infusion should be decreased. Lidocaine clearance also is reduced in hepatic disease, during treatment with *cimetidine* or β blockers, and during prolonged infusions. Frequent measurement of plasma lidocaine concentration and dose adjustment to ensure that plasma concentrations remain within the therapeutic range (1.5 to 5 μg/mL) are necessary to minimize toxicity in these settings. Lidocaine is bound to the acute-phase reactant α_1-acid glycoprotein. Diseases such as acute myocardial infarction are associated with increases in α_1-acid glycoprotein and protein binding and hence a decreased proportion of free drug. These findings may explain why some patients require and tolerate higher-than-usual total plasma lidocaine concentrations to maintain antiarrhythmic efficacy.

Magnesium

The intravenous administration of 1 to 2 g $MgSO_4$ reportedly is effective in preventing recurrent episodes of torsades de pointes, even if the serum Mg^{2+} concentration is normal (Brugada, 2000). However, controlled studies of this effect have not been performed. The mechanism of action is unknown because the QT interval is not shortened; an effect on the inward current, possibly a Ca^{2+} current, responsible for the triggered upstroke arising from EADs (black arrow, Figure 30–6B) is possible. Intravenous Mg^{2+} also has been used successfully in arrhythmias related to digitalis intoxication.

Large placebo-controlled trials of intravenous Mg^{2+} to improve outcome in acute myocardial infarction have yielded conflicting results (ISIS-4 Collaborative Group, 1995; Woods and Fletcher, 1994). While oral Mg^{2+} supplements may be useful in preventing hypomagnesemia, there is no evidence that chronic Mg^{2+} ingestion exerts a direct antiarrhythmic action.

Mexiletine

Mexiletine is an analogue of lidocaine that has been modified to reduce first-pass hepatic metabolism and permit chronic oral therapy. The electrophysiological actions are similar to those of lidocaine. Tremor and nausea, the major dose-related adverse effects, can be minimized by taking the drugs with food.

Mexiletine undergoes hepatic metabolism, which is inducible by drugs such as phenytoin. Mexiletine is approved for treating ventricular arrhythmias; combinations of mexiletine with quinidine or sotalol may increase efficacy while reducing adverse effects. In vitro studies and clinical case series have suggested a role for mexiletine (or flecainide; see previous discussion) in correcting the aberrant late inward Na^+ current in type 3 congenital LQTS (Napolitano et al., 2006).

Procainamide

Procainamide is an analogue of the local anesthetic procaine (see Figure 22–1). It exerts electrophysiological effects similar to those of quinidine but lacks quinidine's vagolytic and α adrenergic blocking activity. Procainamide is better tolerated than quinidine when given intravenously. Loading and maintenance intravenous infusions are used in the acute therapy of many supraventricular and ventricular arrhythmias. However, long-term oral treatment is poorly tolerated and often is stopped owing to adverse effects.

Pharmacological Effects

Procainamide is a blocker of open Na^+ channels with an intermediate $\tau_{recovery}$ from block. It also prolongs cardiac action potentials in most tissues, probably by blocking outward K^+ current(s). Procainamide decreases automaticity, increases refractory periods, and slows conduction. The major metabolite, *N*-acetyl procainamide, lacks the Na^+ channel–blocking activity of the parent drug but is equipotent in prolonging action potentials. Because the plasma concentrations of *N*-acetyl procainamide often exceed those of procainamide, increased refractoriness and QT prolongation during chronic procainamide therapy may be partly attributable to the metabolite. However, it is the parent drug that slows conduction and produces QRS interval prolongation. Although hypotension may occur at high plasma concentrations, this effect usually is attributable to ganglionic blockade rather than to any negative inotropic effect, which is minimal.

Adverse Effects

Hypotension and marked slowing of conduction are major adverse effects of high concentrations (>10 μg/mL) of procainamide, especially during intravenous use. Dose-related nausea is frequent during oral therapy and may be attributable in part to high plasma concentrations of *N*-acetyl procainamide. Torsades de pointes can occur, particularly when plasma concentrations of *N*-acetyl procainamide rise to greater than 30 μg/mL. Procainamide produces potentially fatal bone marrow aplasia in 0.2% of patients; the mechanism is not known, but high plasma drug concentrations are not suspected.

During long-term therapy, most patients will develop biochemical evidence of the drug-induced lupus syndrome, such as circulating antinuclear antibodies. Therapy need not be interrupted merely because of the presence of antinuclear antibodies. However, 25%–50% of patients eventually develop symptoms of the lupus syndrome; common early symptoms are rash and small-joint arthralgias. Other symptoms of lupus, including pericarditis with tamponade, can occur, although renal involvement is unusual. The lupus-like symptoms resolve on cessation of therapy or during treatment with *N*-acetyl procainamide (see discussion that follows).

Clinical Pharmacokinetics

Procainamide is eliminated rapidly ($t_{1/2}$ ~ 3–4 h) by both renal excretion of unchanged drug and hepatic metabolism. The major pathway for hepatic metabolism is conjugation by *N*-acetyl transferase, whose activity is determined genetically, to form *N*-acetyl procainamide. *N*-Acetyl procainamide is eliminated by renal excretion ($t_{1/2}$ ~ 6–10 h) and is not significantly converted back to procainamide. Because of the relatively rapid elimination rates of both the parent drug and its major metabolite, oral procainamide usually is administered as a slow-release formulation. In patients with renal failure, procainamide or *N*-acetyl procainamide can accumulate to potentially toxic plasma concentrations. Reduction of procainamide dose and dosing frequency and monitoring of plasma concentrations of both compounds are required in this situation. Because the parent drug and metabolite exert different pharmacological effects, the past practice of using the sum of their concentrations to guide therapy is inappropriate.

In individuals who are "slow acetylators," the procainamide-induced lupus syndrome develops more often and earlier during treatment than among rapid acetylators. In addition, the symptoms of procainamide-induced lupus resolve during treatment with *N*-acetyl procainamide. Both these findings support results of in vitro studies suggesting that it is chronic exposure to the parent drug (or an oxidative metabolite) that results in the lupus syndrome; these findings also provided one rationale for the further development of *N*-acetyl procainamide and its analogues as antiarrhythmic agents (Roden, 1993).

Propafenone

Propafenone is a Na^+ channel blocker with a relatively slow time constant for recovery from block (Funck-Brentano et al., 1990). Some data suggest that, like flecainide, propafenone also blocks K^+ channels. Its major electrophysiological effect is to slow conduction in fast-response tissues. The drug is prescribed as a racemate; while the enantiomers do not differ in their Na^+ channel–blocking properties, *S*-(+)-propafenone is a β adrenergic receptor antagonist in vitro and in some patients. Propafenone prolongs PR and QRS durations. Chronic therapy with oral propafenone is used to maintain sinus rhythm in patients with supraventricular tachycardias, including atrial fibrillation; like other Na^+ channel blockers, it also can be used in ventricular arrhythmias, but with only modest efficacy. *R*-(−) propafenone blocks RyR2 channels and may be an alternative to flecainide in CPVT (Hwang et al, 2011).

Adverse Effects

Adverse effects during propafenone therapy include acceleration of ventricular response in patients with atrial flutter, increased frequency or severity of episodes of reentrant ventricular tachycardia, exacerbation of heart failure, and the adverse effects of β adrenergic blockade, such as sinus bradycardia and bronchospasm (see previous discussion and Chapter 12).

Clinical Pharmacokinetics

Propafenone is well absorbed and is eliminated primarily by CYP2D6-mediated hepatic metabolism (see Chapter 6). In most subjects ("extensive metabolizers"), propafenone undergoes extensive first-pass hepatic metabolism to 5-hydroxy propafenone, a metabolite equipotent to propafenone as a Na^+ channel blocker but much less potent as a β adrenergic receptor antagonist. A second metabolite, *N*-desalkyl propafenone, is formed by non-CYP2D6–mediated metabolism and is a less-potent blocker of Na^+ channels and β adrenergic receptors. CYP2D6-mediated metabolism of propafenone is saturable, so small increases in dose can increase plasma propafenone concentration disproportionately. In "poor metabolizer" subjects, in whom CYP2D6 activity is low or absent, first-pass hepatic metabolism is much less than in extensive metabolizers, and plasma propafenone concentrations will be much higher after an equal dose. The incidence of adverse effects during propafenone therapy is significantly higher in poor metabolizers.

CYP2D6 activity can be inhibited markedly by a number of drugs, including quinidine and fluoxetine. In extensive metabolizer subjects receiving such drugs or in poor metabolizer subjects, plasma propafenone concentrations of more than 1 μg/mL are associated with clinical effects of β adrenergic receptor blockade, such as reduction of exercise heart rate. It is recommended that dosage in patients with moderate-to-severe liver disease should be reduced to approximately 20%–30% of the usual dose, with careful monitoring. It is not known if propafenone doses must be decreased in patients with renal disease. A slow-release formulation allows twice-daily dosing.

Quinidine

As early as the 18th century, the bark of the cinchona plant was used to treat "rebellious palpitations" (Levy and Azoulay, 1994). Studies in the early 20th century identified quinidine, a diastereomer of the antimalarial quinine, as the most potent of the antiarrhythmic substances extracted from the cinchona plant, and by the 1920s, quinidine was used as an antiarrhythmic agent. Quinidine is used to maintain sinus rhythm in patients with atrial flutter or atrial fibrillation and to prevent recurrence of ventricular tachycardia or VF (Grace and Camm, 1998). Quinidine may be especially useful in preventing recurrent VF in unusual congenital arrhythmias syndromes such as Brugada syndrome or short QT syndrome (Inama et al., 2010; Viskin et al., 2013).

$CH_2=CH$ HO N H H CH_3O N

QUINIDINE

Pharmacological Effects

Quinidine blocks Na^+ current and multiple cardiac K^+ currents. It is an open-state blocker of Na^+ channels, with a $\tau_{recovery}$ in the intermediate (~3-sec) range; as a consequence, QRS duration increases modestly, usually by 10%–20%, at therapeutic dosages. At therapeutic concentrations, quinidine commonly prolongs the QT interval up to 25%, but the effect is highly variable. At concentrations as low as 1 μM, quinidine blocks Na^+ current and the rapid component of delayed rectifier (I_{Kr}); higher concentrations block the slow component of delayed rectifier, inward rectifier, transient outward current, and L-type Ca^{2+} current.

Quinidine's Na^+ channel–blocking properties result in an increased threshold for excitability and decreased automaticity. As a consequence of its K^+ channel–blocking actions, quinidine prolongs action potentials in most cardiac cells, most prominently at slow heart rates. In some cells, such as midmyocardial cells and Purkinje cells, quinidine consistently elicits EADs at slow heart rates, particularly when $[K]_o$ is low (Priori et al., 1999). Quinidine prolongs refractoriness in most tissues, probably as a result of both prolongation of action potential duration and Na^+ channel blockade.

In intact animals and humans, quinidine also produces α adrenergic receptor blockade and vagal inhibition. Thus, the intravenous use of quinidine is associated with marked hypotension and sinus tachycardia. Quinidine's vagolytic effects tend to inhibit its direct depressant effect on AV nodal conduction, so the effect of drug on the PR interval is variable. Moreover, quinidine's vagolytic effect can result in increased AV nodal transmission of atrial tachycardias such as atrial flutter (Table 30–1).

Adverse Effects

Noncardiac. Diarrhea is the most common adverse effect during quinidine therapy, occurring in 30%–50% of patients; the mechanism is not known. Diarrhea usually occurs within the first several days of quinidine therapy but can occur later. Diarrhea-induced hypokalemia may potentiate torsades de pointes due to quinidine.

A number of immunological reactions can occur during quinidine therapy. The most common is thrombocytopenia, which can be severe but which resolves rapidly with discontinuation of the drug. Hepatitis, bone marrow depression, and lupus syndrome occur rarely. None of these effects is related to elevated plasma quinidine concentrations.

Quinidine also can produce cinchonism, a syndrome that includes headache and tinnitus. In contrast to other adverse responses to quinidine therapy, cinchonism usually is related to elevated plasma quinidine concentrations and can be managed by dose reduction.

Cardiac. Of patients receiving quinidine therapy, 2%–8% will develop marked QT interval prolongation and torsades de pointes. In contrast to effects of sotalol, *N*-acetyl procainamide, and many other drugs, quinidine-associated torsades de pointes generally occurs at therapeutic or even subtherapeutic plasma concentrations. The reasons for individual susceptibility to this adverse effect are not known.

At high plasma concentrations of quinidine, marked Na^+ channel block can occur, with resulting ventricular tachycardia. This adverse effect occurs when very high doses of quinidine are used to try to convert atrial fibrillation to normal rhythm; this aggressive approach to quinidine dosing has been abandoned, and quinidine-induced ventricular tachycardia is unusual.

Quinidine can exacerbate heart failure or conduction system disease. However, in most patients with congestive heart failure, quinidine is well tolerated, perhaps because of its vasodilating actions.

Clinical Pharmacokinetics

Quinidine is well absorbed and is 80% bound to plasma proteins, including albumin and, like lidocaine, the acute-phase reactant α_1-acid glycoprotein. As with lidocaine, greater-than-usual doses (and total plasma quinidine concentrations) may be required to maintain therapeutic concentrations of free quinidine in high-stress states such as acute myocardial infarction. Quinidine undergoes extensive hepatic oxidative metabolism, and approximately 20% is excreted unchanged by the kidneys. One metabolite, 3-hydroxyquinidine, is nearly as potent as quinidine in blocking cardiac Na^+ channels and prolonging cardiac action potentials. Concentrations of unbound 3-hydroxyquinidine equal to or exceeding those of quinidine are tolerated by some patients. Other metabolites are less potent than quinidine, and their plasma concentrations are lower; thus, they are unlikely to contribute significantly to the clinical effects of quinidine.

There is substantial individual variability in the range of dosages required to achieve therapeutic plasma concentrations of 2 to 5 μg/mL. Some of this variability may be assay dependent because not all assays exclude quinidine metabolites. In patients with advanced renal disease or congestive heart failure, quinidine clearance is decreased only modestly. Thus, dosage requirements in these patients are similar to those in other patients.

Drug Interactions

Quinidine is a potent inhibitor of CYP2D6. As a result, the administration of quinidine to patients receiving drugs that undergo extensive CYP2D6-mediated metabolism may result in altered drug effects owing to accumulation of parent drug and failure of metabolite formation. For example, inhibition of CYP2D6-mediated metabolism of *codeine* to its active metabolite *morphine* results in decreased analgesia. On the other hand, inhibition of CYP2D6-mediated metabolism of propafenone results in elevated plasma propafenone concentrations and increased β adrenergic receptor blockade. Quinidine reduces the clearance of digoxin; inhibition of P-glycoprotein–mediated digoxin transport has been implicated (Fromm et al., 1999). Dextromethorphan, a CYP2D6 substrate that undergoes extensive first-pass bioinactivation, has shown promise in treatment of various neurological disorders, notably pseudobulbar affect. A combination of dextromethorphan and very low-dose quinidine (30 mg) inhibits the first-pass metabolism, achieves higher systemic concentrations than monotherapy, and is now approved for use in pseudobulbar affect (Olney and Rosen, 2010).

Quinidine metabolism is induced by drugs such as *phenobarbital* and phenytoin. In patients receiving these agents, very high doses of quinidine may be required to achieve therapeutic concentrations. If therapy with the inducing agent is then stopped, quinidine concentrations may rise to very high levels, and its dosage must be adjusted downward. Cimetidine and verapamil also elevate plasma quinidine concentrations, but these effects usually are modest.

Sotalol

Sotalol is a nonselective β adrenergic receptor antagonist that also prolongs cardiac action potentials by inhibiting delayed rectifier and possibly other K^+ currents (Hohnloser and Woosley, 1994). Sotalol is prescribed as a racemate; the L-enantiomer is a much more potent β adrenergic receptor antagonist than the D-enantiomer, but the two are equipotent as K^+ channel blockers. In the U.S., sotalol is approved for use in patients with both ventricular tachyarrhythmias and atrial fibrillation or flutter. Clinical trials suggest that it is at least as effective as most Na^+ channel blockers in ventricular arrhythmias.

Sotalol prolongs action potential duration throughout the heart and QT interval on the ECG. It decreases automaticity, slows AV nodal conduction, and prolongs AV refractoriness by blocking both K^+ channels and β adrenergic receptors, but it exerts no effect on conduction velocity in fast-response tissue. Sotalol causes EADs and triggered activity in vitro and can cause torsades de pointes, especially when the serum K^+ concentration is low. Unlike the situation with quinidine, the incidence of torsades de pointes (1.5%–2% incidence) seems to depend on the dose of sotalol; indeed, torsades de pointes is the major toxicity with sotalol overdose. Occasional cases occur at low dosages, often in patients with renal dysfunction, because sotalol is eliminated by renal excretion of unchanged drug. The other adverse effects of sotalol therapy are those associated with β adrenergic receptor blockade (see previous discussion and Chapter 12).

Vernakalant

Vernakalant is an inhibitor of multiple ion channels and prolongs atrial refractory periods without significantly affecting ventricular refractoriness. Intravenous vernakalant has modest efficacy in terminating atrial fibrillation (Roy et al., 2008) and is available for this indication in several European countries, but not the U.S. Consult the 12th edition of this text for more information on this drug.

Acknowledgment: *Kevin J Simpson and Robert S. Kass contributed to this chapter in the previous edition of this book. We have retained some of their text in the current edition.*

Drug Facts for Your Personal Formulary: *Antiarrhythmic Agents*

Antiarrhythmic Drug	Therapeutic Uses	Major Toxicity and Clinical Pearls
Class IA: Na^+ Channel Blockers • Slow to intermediate off rate • Concomitant class III action (prolong QT)		
Procainamide	• Acute treatment of AF, VT, and VF • Chronic treatment to prevent AF, VT, and VF	• 40% of patients discontinue within 6 months of therapy due to side effects: hypotension (especially from intravenous use), nausea • QT prolongation and torsades de pointes due to accumulation of active *N*-acetyl metabolite • Lupus-like syndrome (25%–50% with chronic use), especially in genetic slow acetylators • Oral drug no longer widely available
Quinidine	• Chronic treatment to prevent AF, VT, and VF	• Diarrhea (30%–50% of patients); diarrhea-induced hypokalemia may potentiate torsades de pointes • Marked QT prolongation and high risk (~1%–5%) of torsades de pointes at therapeutic or subtherapeutic concentrations • Immune thrombocytopenia (~1%) • Cinchonism: tinnitus, flushing, blurred vision, dizziness, diarrhea • Potent inhibitor of *CYP2D6* and *ABCB1*: altered effects of digitalis, many antidepressants, and others
Disopyramide	• Chronic treatment to prevent AF, VT, and VF	• Anticholinergic effects (dry eyes, urinary retention, constipation) • Long QT (torsades de pointes) • Depression of contractility can precipitate or worsen heart failure; paradoxically, this can be useful in hypertrophic cardiomyopathy to reduce outflow tract obstruction
Class IB: Na^+ Channel Blockers • Fast off rate • Little effect on ECG		
Lidocaine	• Acute treatment of VT and VF	• CNS: seizures and tinnitus • CNS: tremor, hallucinations, drowsiness, coma
Mexiletine	• Chronic treatment to prevent VT and VF	• Tremor and nausea
Class IC: Na^+ Channel Blockers • Slow off rate • Prolong PR and broaden QRS intervals		
Flecainide	• Chronic treatment to prevent PSVT, AF, VT, and VF in the absence of structural heart disease • Available in some countries for intravenous use in PSVT, AF • Useful in CPVT uncontrolled by β-blockers	• Much better tolerated than class IA or IB agents • Risk of severe proarrhythmia in patients with structural heart disease; increased mortality in patients with myocardial infarction (CAST) • Blurred vision • Can worsen heart failure
Propafenone	• Chronic treatment to prevent PSVT, AF, VT, and VF in the absence of structural heart disease • Available in some countries for intravenous use in PSVT, AF • Alternative to flecainide for CPVT	• Also has β adrenergic blocking effects (worsening of heart failure and bronchospasm), especially prominent in *CYP2D6* poor metabolizers • Risk of severe proarrhythmia in patients with structural heart disease
Class II: β Blockers		
Nadolol Propranolol Metoprolol Many others	• Chronic treatment to prevent arrhythmias in congenital LQTS and CPVT • Rate control in AF • Widely used for other indications (angina, hypertension, migraine, etc.)	• β Adrenergic blocking effects (worsening of heart failure, bradycardia, bronchospasm) • Nadolol preferred by many for LQTS and CPVT
Esmolol	• Acute treatment to control rate in AF	• Ultrashort $t_{1/2}$, intravenous use only
Class III: K^+ Channel Blocker • Increase refractory period (prolong QT)		
Amiodarone	• Drug of choice for acute treatment of VT and VF and to slow ventricular rate and convert AF • Chronic treatment to prevent AF, VT, and VF	• Hypotension, depressed ventricular function and torsades de pointes (*rare*) with intravenous administration • Pulmonary fibrosis with chronic therapy, which can be fatal (requires periodic monitoring of lung function) • Many other adverse effects: corneal microdeposits, hepatotoxicity, neuropathies, photosensitivity, thyroid dysfunction • Note: tissue half-life of several months • Inhibitor of many drug-metabolizing and transport systems, with high potential for drug interactions

Drug Facts for Your Personal Formulary: *Antiarrhythmic Agents(continued)*

Antiarrhythmic Drug	Therapeutic Uses	Major Toxicity and Clinical Pearls
Class III: K^+ Channel Blocker • Increase refractory period (prolong QT)		
Dronedarone	• Chronic treatment to prevent AF	• Amiodarone analogue with lower efficacy than amiodarone • GI disturbances, risk for fatal hepatotoxicity • Increases mortality in patients with severe heart failure
Sotalol	• Chronic treatment to prevent AF, VT, and VF	• Also has β adrenergic blocking effects • High risk (~1%–5%) of torsades de pointes
Dofetilide	• Chronic treatment to prevent AF	• Few adverse effects except high risk (~1%–5%) of torsades de pointes
Ibutilide	• Acute treatment to convert AF	• High risk (~1%–5%) of torsades de pointes
Class IV: Ca^{2+} Channel Blockers • Nondihydropyridine • Inhibit SA and AV nodes • Prolong PR		
Diltiazem, Verapamil	• Acute intravenous use to convert PSVT and for rate control in AF • Chronic treatment to prevent PSVT and control rate in AF	• Hypotension (intravenous) • Sinus bradycardia or AV block especially in combination with β-blockers • Constipation • Worsening of heart failure
Antiarrhythmic Drugs With Miscellaneous Mechanisms		
Adenosine (activates A receptors)	Drug of choice for acute treatment PSVT	• Short $t_{1/2}$ (<5 sec) • Transient asystole • Transient dyspnea • Transient atrial fibrillation (rare)
$MgSO_4$	• Acute treatment of torsades de pointes	
Digoxin (Na^+-K^+–ATPase inhibitor)	• Ventricular rate control in atrial fibrillation • Modest positive inotropic effect	• Adverse effects common and include GI symptoms, visual/cognitive dysfunction, and arrhythmias, typically supraventricular arrhythmias with heart block or atrial or ventricular extrasystoles • Severe toxicities (e.g., with overdose) can be treated with antibody • Probably mortality neutral

Bibliography

Amiodarone Trials Meta-Analysis Investigators. Effect of prophylactic amiodarone on mortality after acute myocardial infarction and in congestive heart failure—meta-analysis of individual data from 6500 patients in randomised trials. *Lancet*, **1997**, *350*:1417–1424.

Balser JR, et al. Local anesthetics as effectors of allosteric gating: lidocaine effects on inactivation-deficient rat skeletal muscle Na channels. *J Clin Invest*, **1996**, *98*:2874–2886.

Brugada P. Magnesium: an antiarrhythmic drug, but only against very specific arrhythmias. *Eur Heart J*, **2000**, *21*:1116.

Cohen IS, Robinson RB. Pacemaker currents and automatic rhythms: toward a molecular understanding. *Handb Exp Pharmacol*, **2006**, *171*:41–71.

Connolly SJ. Evidence-based analysis of amiodarone efficacy and safety. *Circulation*, **1999**, *100*:2025–2034.

Connolly SJ, et al. Dronedarone in high-risk permanent atrial fibrillation. *N Engl J Med*, **2011**, *365*:2268–2276.

Courtney, KR. Progress and prospects for optimum antiarrhythmic drug design. *Cardiovasc Drug Ther*, **1987**, *1*:117–123.

DiFrancesco D. Pacemaker mechanisms in cardiac tissue. *Annu Rev Physiol*, **1993**, *55*:455–472.

Dobrev D, et al. Novel molecular targets for atrial fibrillation therapy. *Nat Rev Drug Discov*, **2012**, *11*(4):275–291.

Dorian P, et al. Amiodarone as compared with lidocaine for shock-resistant ventricular fibrillation. *N Engl J Med*, **2002**, *346*:884–890.

Duan DD. Phenomics of cardiac chloride channels. *Compr Physiol*, **2013**, *3*:667–692.

Dun W, Boyden PA. The purkinje cell; 2008 style. *J Mol Cell Cardiol*, **2008**, *45*(5):617–624.

Dzeshka MS, Lip GY. Non-vitamin K oral anticoagulants in atrial fibrillation: where are we now? *Trends Cardiovasc Med*, **2015**, *25*: 315–336.

Echt DS, et al. Mortality and morbidity in patients receiving encainide, flecainide, or placebo. *N Engl J Med*, **1991**, *324*:781–788.

Fozzard HA, et al. Mechanism of local anesthetic drug action on voltage-gated sodium channels. *Curr Pharm Des*, **2005**, *11*(21):2671–2686.

Fromm MF, et al. Inhibition of P-glycoprotein-mediated drug transport: a unifying mechanism to explain the interaction between digoxin and quinidine. *Circulation*, **1999**, *99*: 552–557.

Funck-Brentano C, et al. Propafenone. *N Engl J Med*, **1990**, *322*:518–525.

Grace AA, Camm J. Quinidine. *N Engl J Med*, **1998**, *338*:35–45.

Henthorn RW, et al. Flecainide acetate prevents recurrence of symptomatic paroxysmal supraventricular tachycardia. The Flecainide Supraventricular Tachycardia Study Group. *Circulation*, **1991**, *83*: 119–125.

Hilliard FA, et al. Flecainide inhibits arrhythmogenic Ca(2+) waves by open state block of ryanodine receptor Ca(2+) release channels and reduction of Ca(2+) spark mass. *J Mol Cell Cardiol*, **2010**, *48*:293–301.

Hohnloser SH, et al. Effect of dronedarone on cardiovascular events in atrial fibrillation. *N Engl J Med*, **2009**, *360*:668–678.

Hohnloser SH, Woosley RL. Sotalol. *N Engl J Med*, **1994**, *331*:31–38.

Hwang HS, et al. Inhibition of cardiac Ca^{2+} release channels (RyR2) determines efficacy of class I antiarrhythmic drugs in catecholaminergic polymorphic ventricular tachycardia. *Circ Arrhythm Electrophysiol*, **2011**, *4*:128–135.

Inama G, et al. "Orphan drugs" in cardiology: nadolol and quinidine. *J Cardiovasc Med*, **2010**, *11*:143–144.

ISIS-4 Collaborative Group. ISIS-4: a randomised factorial trial assessing early oral captopril, oral mononitrate, and intravenous magnesium sulphate in 58,050 patients with suspected acute myocardial infarction. ISIS-4 (Fourth International Study of Infarct Survival) Collaborative Group. *Lancet*, **1995**, *345*:669–685.

Kannankeril PJ, et al. Efficacy of flecainide in the treatment of catecholaminergic polymorphic ventricular tachycardia: a randomized clinical trial. *JAMA Cardiol*. Published online May 10, 2017. doi:10.1001/jamacardio.2017.1320

Keating MT, Sanguinetti MC. Molecular and cellular mechanisms of cardiac arrhythmias. *Cell*, **2001**, *104*:569–580.

Kleber AG, Saffitz JE. Role of the intercalated disc in cardiac propagation and arrhythmogenesis. *Front Physiol*, **2014**, *5*:404.

Knollmann BC, Roden DM. A genetic framework for improving arrhythmia therapy. *Nature*, **2008**, *451*:929–936.

Kober L, et al. Increased mortality after dronedarone therapy for severe heart failure. *N Engl J Med*, **2008**, *358*:2678–2687.

Levy S, Azoulay S. Stories about the origin of quinquina and quinidine. *J Cardiovasc Electrophysiol*, **1994**, *5*:635–636.

Link MS. Clinical practice. Evaluation and initial treatment of supraventricular tachycardia. *N Engl J Med*, **2012**, *367*:1438–1448.

Lu Z, et al. Suppression of phosphoinositide 3-kinase signaling and alteration of multiple ion currents in drug-induced long QT syndrome. *Sci Transl Med*, **2012**, *4*:131.

MacKinnon R. Potassium channels. *FEBS Lett*, **2003**, *555*:62–65.

Mitcheson JS, et al. A structural basis for drug-induced long QT syndrome. *Proc Natl Acad Sci U S A*, **2000**, *97*:12329–12333.

Murray KT. Ibutilide. *Circulation*, **1998**, *97*:493–497.

Napolitano C, et al. Gene-specific therapy for inherited arrhythmogenic diseases. *Pharmacol Ther*, **2006**, *100*:1–13.

Nerbonne JM, Kass RS. Molecular physiology of cardiac repolarization. *Physiol Rev*, **2005**, *85*:1205–1253.

Olney N, Rosen H. AVP-923, a combination of dextromethorphan hydrobromide and quinidine sulfate for the treatment of pseudobulbar affect and neuropathic pain. *IDrugs*, **2010**, *13*:254–265.

Ono K, Iijima T. Cardiac T-type Ca(2+) channels in the heart. *J Mol Cell Cardiol*, **2010**, *48*:65–70.

Patel C, et al. Dronedarone. *Circulation*, **2009**, *120*:636–644.

Priori SG, et al. Genetic and molecular basis of cardiac arrhythmias: impact on clinical management. Study group on molecular basis of arrhythmias of the Working Group on Arrhythmias of the European Society of Cardiology. *Eur Heart J*, **1999**, *20*:174–195.

Remme CA, Wilde AA. Late sodium current inhibition in acquired and inherited ventricular (dys)function and arrhythmias. *Cardiovasc Drugs Ther*, **2013**, *27*:91–101.

Roden DM. Current status of class III antiarrhythmic drug therapy. *Am J Cardiol*, **1993**, *72*:44B–49B.

Roden DM. Drug-induced prolongation of the QT interval. *N Engl J Med*, **2004**, *350*:1013–1022.

Roden DM. Risks and benefits of antiarrhythmic therapy. *N Engl J Med*, **1994**, *331*:785–791.

Roden DM, et al. Clinical pharmacology of antiarrhythmic agents. In: Josephson ME, ed. *Sudden Cardiac Death*. Blackwell Scientific, London, **1993**, 182–185.

Roden DM, Spooner PM. Inherited long QT syndromes: a paradigm for understanding arrhythmogenesis. *J Cardiovasc Electrophysiol*, **1999**, *10*:1664–1683.

Roy D, et al. Vernakalant hydrochloride for rapid conversion of atrial fibrillation: a phase 3, randomized, placebo-controlled trial. *Circulation*, **2008**, *117*:1518–1525.

Roy D, et al. Amiodarone to prevent recurrence of atrial fibrillation. Canadian Trial of Atrial Fibrillation Investigators. *N Engl J Med*, **2000**, *342*:913–920.

Schwartz PJ, et al. Long QT syndrome. In: Zipes DP, Jalife J, eds. *Cardiac Electrophysiology: From Cell to Bedside*. 3rd ed. Saunders, Philadelphia, **2000**, 615–640.

Sherrid MV, Arabadjian M. A primer of disopyramide treatment of obstructive hypertrophic cardiomyopathy. *Prog Cardiovas Dis*, **2012**, *54*:483–492.

Singh BN. Advantages of beta blockers versus antiarrhythmic agents and calcium antagonists in secondary prevention after myocardial infarction. *Am J Cardiol*, **1990**, *66*:9C–20C.

Singh BN. Arrhythmia control by prolonging repolarization: the concept and its potential therapeutic impact. *Eur Heart J*, **1993**, *14*(suppl H):14–23.

Tadros R, et al. Sex differences in cardiac electrophysiology and clinical arrhythmias: epidemiology, therapeutics, and mechanisms. *Can J Cardiol*, **2014**, *30*:783–792. Erratum in: *Can J Cardiol*, **2014**, *30*:1244.

Tamargo J, et al. Pharmacology of cardiac potassium channels. *Cardiovasc Res*, **2004**, *62*:9–33.

Task Force of the Working Group on Arrhythmias of the European Society of Cardiology. The Sicilian gambit: a new approach to the classification of antiarrhythmic drugs based on their actions on arrhythmogenic mechanisms. *Circulation*, **1991**, *84*:1831–1851.

Torp-Pedersen C, et al. Dofetilide in patients with congestive heart failure and left ventricular dysfunction. Danish Investigations of Arrhythmia and Mortality on Dofetilide Study Group. *N Engl J Med*, **1999**, *341*:857–865.

Van Wagoner DR, et al. Progress toward the prevention and treatment of atrial fibrillation: a summary of the Heart Rhythm Society Research Forum on the Treatment and Prevention of Atrial Fibrillation, Washington, DC, December 9–10, 2013. *Heart Rhythm*, **2015**, *12*:e5–e29.

Vaughan Williams EM. Classifying antiarrhythmic actions: by facts or speculation. *J Clin Pharmacol*, **1992**, *32*:964–977.

Viskin S, et al. Quinidine, a life-saving medication for Brugada syndrome, is inaccessible in many countries. *J Am Coll Cardiol*, **2013**, *61*:2383–2387.

Watanabe H, et al. Flecainide prevents catecholaminergic polymorphic ventricular tachycardia in mice and humans. *Nat Med*, **2009**, *15*:380–383.

Woods KL, Fletcher S. Long-term outcome after intravenous magnesium sulphate in suspected acute myocardial infarction: the second Leicester Intravenous Magnesium Intervention Trial (LIMIT-2). *Lancet*, **1994**, *343*:816–819.

Yang T, et al. Screening for acute IKr block is insufficient to detect torsades de pointes liability: role of late sodium current. *Circulation*, **2014**, *130*:224–234.

Zimetbaum P. Amiodarone for atrial fibrillation. *N Engl J Med*, **2007**, *356*:935–941.

Treatment of Pulmonary Arterial Hypertension

Dustin R. Fraidenburg, Ankit A. Desai, and Jason X.-J. Yuan

第三十一章　肺动脉高压的治疗

INTRODUCTION TO PULMONARY HYPERTENSION
- Pulmonary Hypertension Classification
- Pulmonary Arterial Hypertension
- Pulmonary Hypertension Associated With Other Disease States
- Routes of Drug Delivery to the Pulmonary Circulation

MECHANISMS OF PULMONARY ARTERIAL HYPERTENSION

CLINICAL USE OF DRUGS FOR PULMONARY HYPERTENSION

PHARMACOTHERAPY FOR PULMONARY HYPERTENSION
- Stimulators of cGMP and PKG Signaling
- Prostacyclin Receptor Agonists
- Endothelin and Endothelin Receptor Antagonists
- Receptor Tyrosine Kinase Inhibitors
- Calcium Channels and Their Blockers
- A Pharmacologist's View of Signal Integration in PAH

中文导读

本章主要介绍：肺动脉高压导论，包括肺动脉高压分类、肺动脉高压、肺动脉高压与其他疾病状态的关系、给药到肺循环的途径；肺动脉高压的发病机制；肺动脉高压治疗药物的临床应用；肺动脉高压的药物治疗，包括刺激cGMP和PKG信号、前列环素受体激动药、内皮素和内皮素受体拮抗药、受体酪氨酸激酶抑制药、钙通道及其阻滞药、PAH信号整合的药理学观点。

Introduction to Pulmonary Hypertension

The pulmonary circulation plays a unique and essential role in gas exchange and, in particular, oxygenation of venous blood. It is a low-resistance and low-pressure circulatory system; the mean PAP in a healthy man is about 12 mm Hg. PAP is a function of CO and PVR. PH is defined as the mean PAP of 25 mm Hg or greater at rest. In patients with PH, pressure overload (i.e., increased afterload) places additional stress on the RV, leading to RV dysfunction and hypertrophy, and in some cases right heart failure. Patients present with a range of symptoms, including dyspnea, fatigue, chest pain, and syncope. PH is a complication of many chronic diseases and is estimated to affect as much as 10%–20% of the general population (McLaughlin et al., 2009).

Pulmonary Hypertension Classification

Pulmonary hypertension is a primary disorder of the pulmonary vasculature and a complication of other cardiopulmonary, vascular, and inflammatory diseases. Based on shared pathophysiological and pathological characteristics as well as response to therapies, PH can be classified into five groups (Simonneau et al., 2013):

1. PAH
2. PH owing to left heart disease
3. PH owing to lung diseases or hypoxia
4. Chronic thromboembolic PH
5. PH with unclear multifactorial mechanisms

Abbreviations

ATPase: adenosine triphosphatase
BMPR2: bone morphogenetic protein receptor type 2
$[Ca^{2+}]_{cyt}$: cytosolic free Ca^{2+} concentration
CCB: calcium channel blocker
COPD: chronic obstructive pulmonary disease
CTEPH: chronic thromboembolic pulmonary hypertension
CYP: cytochrome P450
DAG: diacylglycerol
EC: endothelial cell
ECE: endothelin-converting enzyme
EGF: epidermal growth factor
ERA: endothelin receptor antagonist
ET: endothelin-1
FDA: Food and Drug Administration
HCN: hyperpolarization-activated cyclic nucleotide–gated
HIV: human immunodeficiency virus
HPAP: heritable pulmonary arterial hypertension
HPV: hypoxic pulmonary vasoconstriction
5HT: serotonin
IP_3: inositol triphosphate
IPAH: idiopathic pulmonary arterial hypertension
IPR: prostacyclin receptor
LV: left ventricle
mGC: membrane guanylate cyclase
6MWT: six-minute walk testing
NO: nitric oxide
NO_2: nitric dioxide
NYHA: New York Heart Association
PA: pulmonary artery
PAEC: pulmonary arterial endothelial cell
PAH: pulmonary arterial hypertension
Pao_2: partial pressure of arterial O_2
PAOP: pulmonary artery occlusion pressure
PAP: pulmonary arterial pressure
PASMC: pulmonary artery smooth muscle cell
PDE: phosphodiesterase
PDGF: platelet-derived growth factor
PGI_2: prostacyclin, prostaglandin I_2
PH: pulmonary hypertension
PIP_2: phosphatidylinositol 4,5-biphosphate
PKA: protein kinase A
PKG: protein kinase G
PLC: phospholipase C
PVR: pulmonary vascular resistance
RAP: right atrial pressure
ROC: receptor-operated Ca^{2+} channel
RV: right ventricle
RVF: right ventricular failure
RVH: right ventricular hypertrophy
RVSP: right ventricular systolic pressure
sGC: soluble guanylate cyclase
SR: sarcoplasmic reticulum
SVR: systemic vascular resistance
TKR: tyrosine kinase receptor
TxA_2: thromboxane A_2
VDCC: voltage-dependent Ca^{2+} channel
VEGF: vascular endothelial growth factors
VIP: vasoactive intestinal peptide
VSM: vascular smooth muscle

Pulmonary Arterial Hypertension

Pulmonary arterial hypertension is a rare, progressive, and fatal disease in which vascular changes in the small arteries and arterioles lead to progressive increases in PVR, resulting in increased PAP (McLaughlin et al., 2009). In patients with PAH, elevated afterload increases stress on the RV, leading to right heart dysfunction and failure, the major cause of morbidity and mortality in this population. The disease is defined clinically by hemodynamic parameters measured during a right heart catheterization: mean PAP 25 mm Hg or greater, accompanied by normal pulmonary venous pressure measured as pulmonary artery occlusion pressure or left ventricular end-diastolic pressure of 15 mm Hg or less. The median survival in untreated disease is 2.8 years, yet with modern therapies, the median survival has been estimated to be about 9 years (Benza et al., 2012). This group of patients is the most well-studied subset and the primary target of available therapeutics (Frumkin, 2012).

Pulmonary Hypertension Associated With Other Disease States

Other PH groups represent the majority of recognized cases of PH. The presence of PH in these more common diseases portends a much poorer prognosis, often identifying people with multiple comorbidities, late-stage presentations, or more severe disease. While recognition of PH in heart and lung disease carries important prognostic implications, to date there are no approved targeted therapies for PH in these other disease states, with the exception of CTEPH. While surgical pulmonary thromboendarterectomy is the treatment of choice in CTEPH, nonsurgical patients or those with persistent PH following surgery respond to pulmonary vasodilator therapy (Fedullo et al., 2011; Ghofrani, et al., 2013).

Routes of Drug Delivery to the Pulmonary Circulation

The pulmonary circulation permits delivery of drugs through multiple routes. The pulmonary circulation runs in series with the systemic circulation, receiving the entire CO in each cardiac cycle. Thus, exposure of pulmonary tissue to drugs is excellent and reliable. Continuous intravenous infusion is used to deliver high concentrations of drugs that exhibit short half-lives to the pulmonary circulation while avoiding first-pass metabolism. Alternatively, drug administration by subcutaneous pump may be used to lower risk of adverse effects. Oral delivery remains a safe, effective, and reliable route for many classes of drugs used to treat PAH. The small pulmonary arteries and precapillary arterioles are also unique in their close proximity to the alveoli and lower airways. Hence, inhalational delivery of therapeutic compounds can directly target the lung vasculature and pulmonary circulation, limit systemic side effects, and preferentially affect well-ventilated parts of the lung to improve ventilation-perfusion matching (see Chapter 40).

Mechanisms of Pulmonary Arterial Hypertension

Pulmonary arterial hypertension is thought to arise from pathophysiological changes in the small pulmonary arteries and arterioles. Regardless of the initial etiological trigger, the putative mechanisms contributing to elevated PVR and PAP include the following:

- pulmonary vascular remodeling
- sustained pulmonary vasoconstriction
- in situ thrombosis
- pulmonary vascular wall stiffening

Each of these mechanisms (Figure 31–1) can contribute to the development and progression of PAH and forms the basis for drug therapy for this disease. Accordingly, an effective therapy for PAH would (1) cause pulmonary vasodilation; (2) exert antiproliferative or proapoptotic effects on highly proliferative cells in the pulmonary vascular wall (e.g., fibroblasts, myofibroblasts, and smooth muscle cells); (3) prevent or resolve in situ thrombosis in small arteries and precapillary arterioles; (4) exert antifibrotic effects to attenuate extracellular matrix stiffness; and (5) reduce pulmonary vascular

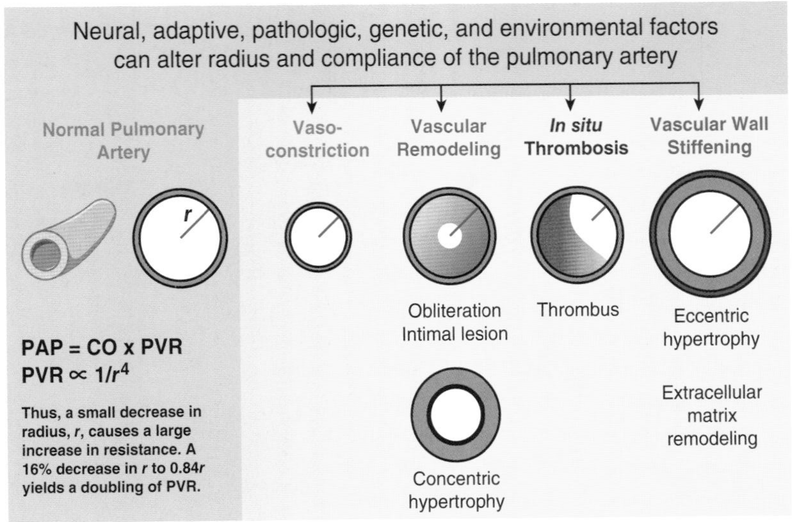

Figure 31–1 *Major pathogenic components in the development of PAH.* Vascular remodeling occurs as changes in the intraluminal radius with or without changes in the vascular wall thickness. Changes in intraluminal radius of small pulmonary arteries and arterioles have dramatic effects on the PVR. Pathogenic factors contributing to the development and progression of PAH include sustained vasoconstriction, pulmonary vascular remodeling, in situ thrombosis, and vascular wall stiffening.

wall stiffness due to myogenic tone and cholesterol-associated membrane stiffness (Mandegar et al., 2004; Morrell et al., 2009).

Although the cellular and molecular mechanisms leading to these changes in the pulmonary vasculature are complex, an imbalance of vasoactive mediators, mitogenic and angiogenic factors, and pro- and antiapoptotic proteins plays an important role in PAH development. Relative deficiencies of vasodilators (e.g., NO and prostacyclin) deleteriously accompany an excess of vasoconstrictors (e.g., ET-1 and TxA_2). NO released by the vascular ECs normally promotes the production of cyclic GMP in the PASMCs, resulting in PASMC relaxation and pulmonary vasodilation. PGI_2, also released from the vascular endothelium, promotes the synthesis of cAMP, causing PASMC relaxation and pulmonary vasodilation. In addition, NO and PGI_2 both have antiproliferative and anticoagulant effects that inhibit concentric pulmonary vascular wall thickening and in situ thrombosis. ET-1 is a potent vasoconstrictor secreted by ECs; it exerts vasoconstrictive and proliferative effects on PASMCs. Other vasoactive mediators such as TxA_2, 5HT, and VIP appear to play a role in the development of PAH, but the therapeutic potential of targeting these substances has not been well established. Table 31–1 summarizes the changes in these vasoactive mediators and the likely contributions of those changes to the development of PAH.

Sustained vasoconstriction and pulmonary vascular remodeling also result from functional and transcriptional changes in membrane receptors and ion channels on the surface of PASMCs. Several GPCRs and TKRs are implicated in the development and progression of PAH. Increased cytosolic $[Ca^{2+}]$ is an important common pathway by which receptor activation and downstream cellular signaling cascades exert their effects in the pulmonary vasculature. A rise in $[Ca^{2+}]_{cyt}$ in PASMCs is a major trigger for PASMC contraction and an important mediator for PASMC proliferation, migration, and vascular remodeling. In addition, ion channels, particularly Ca^{2+}-permeable cation channels and K^+-permeable channels (e.g., KCNA5 and KCNK3) in the plasma membrane of PASMCs, can directly influence $[Ca^{2+}]_{cyt}$ (Mandegar et al., 2004). Ion channels and transporters, such as VDCCs, ROCs, store-operated Ca^{2+} channels, and the Na^+-Ca^{2+} exchanger, are implicated in the development of PAH; all are potential therapeutic targets. Downregulation of K^+-permeable channels in PASMCs leads to membrane depolarization and opening of VDCCs, enhancing Ca^{2+} influx, with a consequent increase in $[Ca^{2+}]_{cyt}$ and further sustained vasoconstriction and vascular remodeling (Kuhr et al., 2012).

TABLE 31–1 ■ ROLES OF VASOACTIVE MEDIATORS IN PAH

EFFECTOR	Δ IN PAH	CONSEQUENCE OF ALTERED [EFFECTOR] ON		
		VASCULAR CONTRACTION	THROMBUS FORMATION	CELL PROLIFERATION
NO	↓	↑	↑	–/↑
PGI_2	↓	↑	↑	↑
TxA_2	↑	↑	↑	↑
VIP	↓	↑	↑	↑
5HT	↑	↑	↑	↑
ET	↑	↑	–[a]	↑

↑, increased, ↓, decreased; -, no change.
[a]↓ in plexiform lesions.

Clinical Use of Drugs for Pulmonary Hypertension

Treatment of PAH must include a proper assessment of symptoms, functional classification, and RV performance for optimal selection of appropriate agents. The most widely used criterion for initiating treatment is the presence of symptoms and impairments in functional capacity, as measured by functional classification. This classification measures the physical limitations imposed on a particular patient from the disease, progressing from class I through class IV (from no impairment through mounting functional limitation to inability to perform physical activity). Clinical trials suggested that class II patients may benefit from therapy, with greater benefit seen in class III. While overall number of patients is low, patients with the most severe functional impairments, class IV, fare far worse. RV dysfunction results from increased PVR, in part, and is the major contributor to morbidity and mortality in this population; therefore, assessment of the RV often is used in conjunction with functional assessment to guide therapy (Figure 31–2).

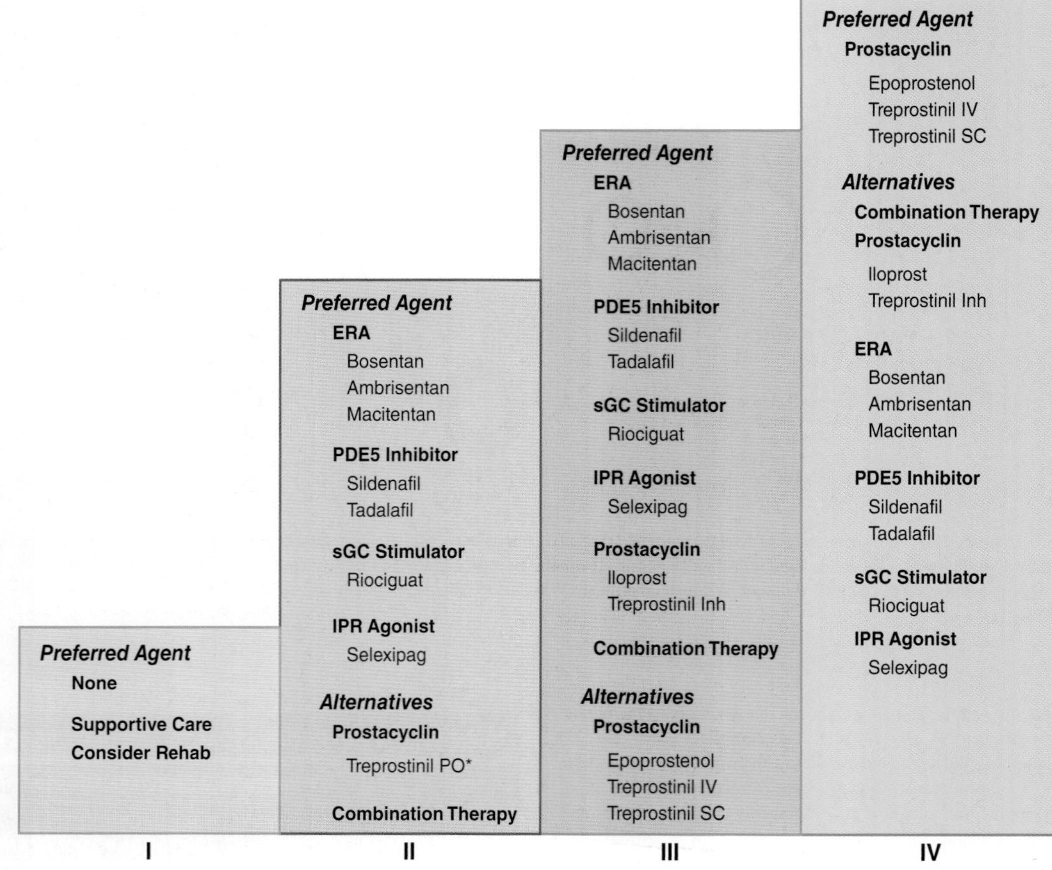

Figure 31–2 *Clinical use of PAH drugs based on functional class.* Treatment of PAH is generally based on the patient's functional classification at the time of presentation. Four functional classes have been defined for PAH: (I) no symptoms or functional limitation; (II) slight limitation of physical activity; (III) marked limitation of physical activity; and (IV) symptoms with any activity or at rest. In patients with no functional limitation, there is no specific therapy that has shown benefit in clinical trials. Expert guidelines recommend only supportive care and physical rehabilitation in this group. Patients with symptoms consistent with functional classes II and III have the best evidence for therapeutic benefits. First-line therapeutics include oral agents such as ERAs, PDE5 inhibitors, sGC stimulators, and the IPR antagonist selexipag. Inhaled PGI_2 analogues can also be considered. The oral formulation of treprostinil has been approved for use in minimally symptomatic individuals but should be reserved for use only as monotherapy. The most severely limited patients, those in functional class IV, or those with evidence of right heart dysfunction should be started on the most potent vasodilators, which include the intravenous and subcutaneous formulations of PGI_2 analogues. Alternatively, combination therapy using multiple agents has been shown to be effective in small clinical trials and one phase 3 clinical trial combining ambrisentan and tadalafil. *approved for monotherapy only.

Goals of treatment include improvement in symptoms, such as dyspnea, fatigue, chest pain, or syncope; improved functional capacity, including 6-min walk distance; and improvement in pulmonary and RV hemodynamics. Oral formulations, either ERAs, PDE5 inhibitors, or sGC stimulators, are usually employed as first-line agents due to ease of use. Treatment of the most severe PAH patients generally involves parenteral therapy with epoprostenol or treprostinil, the most potent pulmonary vasodilators, yet controversy exists on the initial treatment of patients with moderate-to-severe functional limitations. Sequential combination therapy with the addition of separate classes of medications is often utilized for severe or progressive disease (Ghofrani and Humbert, 2014). Modest effects with single agents may be enhanced with the use of up-front combinations and could lead to more dramatic improvements in both symptoms and hemodynamics (Sitbon et al., 2014; Galie et al., 2015).

Pulmonary hypertension is a complex disease process often complicating common diseases of the heart and lungs and heralding poor outcomes. Despite this, PAH, and more recently CTEPH, are the only two subtypes of PH with safe and effective pharmacotherapy. Supportive care therapies described in other chapters include volume management with diuretics (e.g., furosemide), anticoagulants (e.g., warfarin) for patients at high risk for thrombotic disease, supplemental oxygen therapy for hypoxic patients, and inotropic therapy (e.g., digoxin) to improve cardiac contractility in patients with RV dysfunction.

Pharmacotherapy for Pulmonary Hypertension

Pharmacotherapy for PH targets the major pathogenic mechanisms of the disease—pulmonary vascular remodeling (e.g., concentric pulmonary vascular thickening and intraluminal obliteration), sustained pulmonary vasoconstriction, in situ thrombosis, and pulmonary vascular wall stiffening—with the goals of attenuating the development and progression of PAH and reversing these pathologic changes in patients with established PAH. Currently available PAH therapeutics are classified based on their cellular and molecular mechanisms (see Humbert and Ghofrani, 2016):

- NO and stimulators of cGMP and PKG signaling
- membrane receptor agonists
- membrane receptor antagonists
- ion channel blockers and openers

Stimulators of cGMP and PKG Signaling

Nitric oxide is synthesized mainly in vascular ECs and diffuses into vascular smooth muscle cells (PASMCs) to activate sGC. Activated sGC generates cGMP, which in turn is inactivated by cyclic nucleotide PDE5 to 5′-GMP (Figure 31–3). cGMP is an important intracellular second messenger that signals through (1) cGMP-dependent PKG, the principal downstream mediator of cGMP, and (2) cyclic nucleotide–gated and hyperpolarization-activated cyclic nucleotide–gated (HCN) channels (Craven and Zagotta, 2006). Increased cellular cGMP exerts relaxant and antiproliferative effects on PASMCs and myofibroblasts through activation of cGMP-gated K^+ channels, inhibition of Ca^{2+}-permeable channels (e.g., L-type VDCCs, transient receptor potential cation channels), and attenuation of several specific intracellular signaling cascades that are related to cell proliferation, growth, and migration (cAMP [via activated PKA] has similar effects). The drugs currently available for the treatment of PAH in this category include inhaled NO, stimulators and activators of sGC, and inhibitors of PDE5.

The enzymic catalysts of cGMP formation in tissues are sGC and particulate (plasma membrane) mGC. NO stimulates sGC, while the natriuretic peptides stimulate mGC (see Chapter 3 for information on the structure and mechanisms of activation of these enzymes). The sGC is the source of cGMP synthesis on which therapeutics agents for PAH rely. In the lung, activation of the cGMP-PKG pathway causes relaxation of smooth muscle, inhibits proliferation of bronchial smooth muscle and vascular smooth muscle cells, and has an antiproliferative effect (and can induce apoptosis) in pulmonary vascular smooth muscle cells and ECs (Figure 31–3).

Nitric Oxide

Nitric oxide is biosynthesized from the terminal nitrogen of L-arginine by the enzyme nitric oxide synthase (see Chapter 3) Endogenous NO levels are reduced in patients with PAH, PH associated with connective tissue disease, COPD, and interstitial lung disease (Girgis et al., 2005; Kawaguchi et al., 2006).

ADME. NO is a soluble gas. *Inhaled NO* is a gaseous blend of NO and N_2 (0.01% and 99.99%, respectively, for 100 ppm NO). NO must be compressed and stored with an inert gas such as N_2 to minimize the exposure to O_2, decreasing the risk of the accumulation of NO_2. Inhaled NO increases the PaO_2 by preferentially vasodilating better-ventilated lung regions from poorly inflated lung areas (i.e., with low ventilation/perfusion [V/Q] ratios). Inhaled NO is generally administered continuously or with a pulsing device that is rapidly triggered with the onset of inspiration; careful monitoring of response is warranted (Griffiths and Evans, 2005). Inhaled NO is a selective pulmonary vasodilator. Its acute and relatively specific effects on PAP and PVR are due to its route of administration and short half-life (2–6 sec), which is primarily a result of the rapid inactivation of NO by hemoglobin binding and oxidation to nitrite; the nitrite interacts with oxyhemoglobin, leading to the formation of nitrate and met-hemoglobin (Bueno et al., 2013). Nitrate has been identified as the predominant NO metabolite excreted in the urine, accounting for more than 70% of the NO dose inhaled (Ichinose et al., 2004).

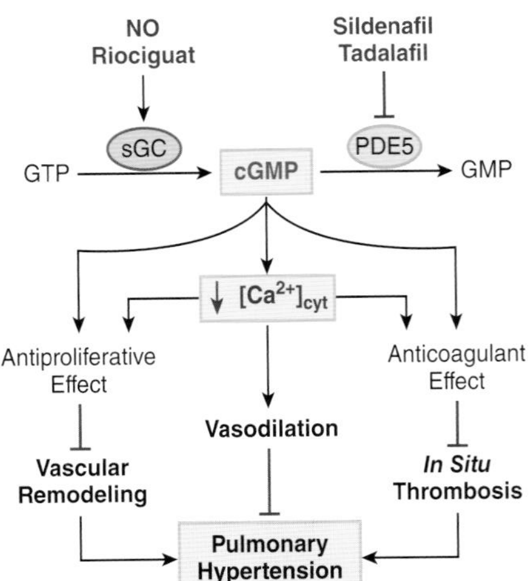

Figure 31–3 *Stimulators of NO/cGMP signaling.* NO stimulates sGC to produce cGMP, which has vasodilating effects through decreased $[Ca^{2+}]_{cyt}$ as well as anticoagulant and antiproliferative effects that are both dependent and independent of $[Ca^{2+}]_{cyt}$. cGMP is degraded primarily by PDE5 in PASMCs, which is targeted by the PDE5 inhibitors sildenafil and tadalafil.

Clinical Use. NO can acutely lower PAP and PVR without altering systemic arterial pressure. Inhaled NO is used for the treatment of term and near-term neonates with persistent pulmonary hypertension of the newborn and acute hypoxemic respiratory failure (Abman, 2013). Acute vasodilator testing is another well-established but off-label use of inhaled NO in adult patients with PAH. Vasodilator testing is performed in the course of deciding whether a patient might derive clinical benefit from Ca^{2+} channel blockade therapy (e.g., *nifedipine*) (Abman, 2013). In the treatment of PH, a 30% decrease in PVR during the inhalation of NO (10 ppm for 10 min) has been used to identify an association with vascular responsiveness and a favorable response to CCBs in a small cohort of patients with primary PH (McLaughlin et al., 2009).

Adverse Effects and Precautions. High doses of inhaled NO (500–1000 ppm) are lethal. However, NO doses of less than 40 ppm are well tolerated chronically for up to 6 months and do not cause methemoglobinemia in adults who have normal methemoglobin reductase activity (Griffiths and Evans, 2005). In neonates, methemoglobin accumulation has been investigated during the first 12 h of exposure to 0, 5, 20, and 80 ppm of inhaled NO (Abman, 2013). Methemoglobin concentrations increased during the first 8 h of NO exposure. The mean methemoglobin level remained below 1% in the placebo group and in the 5- and 20-ppm groups, but reached approximately 5% in the 80-ppm inhaled NO group.

Drug interactions between properly dosed NO and other medications are not expected, but side effects may include noisy breathing, hematuria, or possibly atelectasis. Overdosage with inhaled NO manifests as elevations in methemoglobin and pulmonary toxicities associated with inspired NO_2, including acute respiratory distress syndrome. Elevations in methemoglobin reduce the O_2 delivery capacity of the circulation. Based on clinical studies, NO_2 levels greater than 3 ppm or methemoglobin levels greater than 7% are treated by reducing the dose of, or discontinuing, inhaled NO therapy (Abman, 2013). Methemoglobinemia that does not resolve after reduction or discontinuation of inhaled NO therapy can be treated with intravenous vitamin C, intravenous methylene blue, or blood transfusion, based on the clinical situation.

Inhaled NO gas has limitations: Dosing must be individualized and frequently adjusted; delivery is cumbersome and expensive; off-target effects from reactive nitrogen species are possible; and rebound PH may appear when the NO administration is interrupted. The oxidative product of NO metabolism, the inorganic anion nitrite NO_2^- is relatively stable compared to NO ($t_{1/2}$ = 51 min); NO_2^- can be reduced back to NO under physiological and pathological hypoxia by enzymatic and nonenzymatic processes and thus can serve as an intravascular endocrine reservoir of potential NO bioactivity (Bueno et al., 2013). Other NO donor drugs such as sodium nitroprusside and nitroglycerin offer protective benefits in PVR or remodeling, but when administered intravenously, however, these drugs have limited use given their significant systemic vasodilating effects.

Riociguat

In patients with NO deficiency due to dysfunctional endothelial nitric oxide synthase or arginine insufficiency, activation of sGC increases signaling through the cGMP-PKG pathway and exerts a therapeutic effect (Stasch and Evgenov, 2013). Riociguat, a direct activator of sGC, has recently been approved.

Mechanism of Action. Riociguat is the first-in-class stimulator of sGC. The agent exhibits a dual mode of action; it sensitizes sGC to endogenous NO, and it also directly stimulates sGC independently of NO.

ADME. The drug has excellent oral absorption, and the plasma concentration peaks approximately 1.5 h after oral intake (Stasch and Evgenov, 2013). Food does not affect the bioavailability of riociguat; its volume of distribution is about 30 L. Riociguat is metabolized by CYPs 1A1, 3A, 2C8, and 2J2. The action of CYP1A1 forms the major and active metabolite, M1, which is converted to an inactive *N*-glucuronide. The terminal elimination half-life is about 12 h in patients with PAH (7 h in healthy subjects) (Stasch and Evgenov, 2013).

Clinical Use. Riociguat at doses up to 2.5 mg given three times daily for 12 weeks increased walking distance and significantly delayed time to clinical worsening for patients with PAH (Ghofrani, 2013). Riociguat was also effective in patients with CTEPH, for whom improvements in walking distance were apparent from week 2 onward (Ghofrani, et al., 2013).

Adverse Reactions and Precautions. Concurrent use of riociguat with nitroglycerin or PDE5 inhibitors can cause severe hypotension and syncope (Stasch and Evgenov, 2013). Serious adverse effects include embryo-fetal toxicity, hypotension, and bleeding. Other common adverse reactions include headache, dyspepsia, dizziness, nausea, diarrhea, vomiting, anemia, reflux, constipation, palpitations, nasal congestion, epistaxis, dysphagia, abdominal distension, and peripheral edema (Ghofrani, et al., 2013; Ghofrani, et al., 2013; Stasch and Evgenov, 2013).

PDE5 Inhibitors

Cyclic nucleotide PDEs comprise a superfamily of enzymes that hydrolyze 3′-5′ cyclic nucleotides to their cognate 5′ monophosphates (Omori and Kotera, 2007). PDE5, an isoform that is relatively specific for cGMP, is abundant in PASMCs (Kass et al., 2007). The physiological importance of PDE5 in the regulation of smooth muscle tone has been most effectively demonstrated by the successful clinical use of its specific inhibitors in the treatment of erectile dysfunction and PAH (Galiè et al., 2005; Ravipati et al., 2007).

Sildenafil. Mechanism of Action. Sildenafil, which structurally mimics the purine ring of cGMP, is a competitive and selective inhibitor of PDE5. Sildenafil has a relatively high selectivity (>1000-fold) for human PDE5 over other PDEs. By inhibiting cGMP hydrolysis, sildenafil elevates cellular levels of cGMP and augments signaling through the cGMP-PKG pathway, *provided guanylyl cyclase is active.*

ADME. The drug is rapidly absorbed and reaches a peak plasma concentration 1 h after oral administration. Sildenafil is cleared by the hepatic CYP3A (major route) and CYP2C9 (minor). Sildenafil and its major active metabolite, *N*-desmethyl sildenafil, have terminal half-lives of about 4 h. Both the parent compound and the major metabolite are highly bound to plasma proteins (96%) (Cockrill and Waxman, 2013). Metabolites are predominantly excreted into the feces (73%–88%) and to a lesser extent into the urine; unmetabolized drug is not detected in urine or feces (Muirhead et al., 2002). Clearance is reduced in the elderly (>65 years), leading to an increase in area-under-the-curve values for the parent drug and the *N*-desmethyl metabolite.

Clinical Use and Adverse Effects and Precautions. Sildenafil, 5 to 20 mg three times per day improves exercise capacity, functional class, and hemodynamics. In addition to improved exercise capacity and hemodynamic parameters, sildenafil (initiated at 20 mg three times daily, titrated to 40–80 mg three times daily) plus long-term epoprostenol therapy also resulted in delayed time to clinical worsening of PAH in clinical studies.

Dose adjustments for reduced renal and hepatic function are usually not necessary except for severe hepatic and renal impairment (Cockrill and Waxman, 2013). Concomitant administration of potent CYP3A inducers (e.g., bosentan) will generally cause substantial decreases in plasma levels of sildenafil. The mean reduction in the bioavailability of sildenafil (80 mg three times a day) when coadministered with epoprostenol was 28% (Cockrill and Waxman, 2013). CYP3A inhibitors (e.g., protease inhibitors used in HIV therapy, erythromycin, and cimetidine) inhibit sildenafil metabolism, thereby prolonging the $t_{1/2}$ and elevating blood levels of sildenafil. Consistent with its mechanism of action, potentiation of cGMP signaling, sildenafil and other PDE5 inhibitors potentiate the hypotensive effects of nitrate vasodilators, producing dangerously low blood pressure. Thus, the administration of PDE5 inhibitors to patients receiving organic nitrates is contraindicated. In any event, the patient's underlying cardiovascular status and concurrent use of hypotensive agents (e.g., nitrate vasodilators, α adrenergic antagonists) must be considered prior to use of this class of drugs.

Headache (16%) and flushing (10%) are the most frequently reported side effects. Patients taking sildenafil or vardenafil may notice a transient blue-green tinting of vision due to inhibition of retinal PDE6, which is involved in phototransduction (see Figure 69-9).

Other PDE5 Inhibitors. *Vardenafil* is structurally similar to sildenafil and a potent inhibitor of PDE5. Although not FDA-approved for PAH in the U.S., its clinical efficacy in PAH appears similar to that of sildenafil (Cockrill and Waxman, 2013). *Tadalafil*, another PDE5 inhibitor used for the treatment of PAH, differs structurally from sildenafil and has a longer half-life (Cockrill and Waxman, 2013). See Table 45–2 for comparative pharmacokinetic data of PDE5 inhibitors.

Prostacyclin Receptor Agonists

Prostacyclin is mainly synthesized in and released from vascular ECs and exerts relaxant and antiproliferative effects on vascular smooth muscle cells. Similar to NO, endogenous PGI_2 is considered an endothelium-derived relaxing factor. Decreased PGI_2 synthesis occurs in patients with idiopathic PAH, a finding that provided the rationale for using PGI_2 and its analogues for treatment of PAH (Christman et al., 1992).

Mechanism of Action. Prostacyclin binds to the IPR in the plasma membrane of PASMCs and activates the G_s-AC-cAMP-PKA pathway (Figure 31–4). PKA continues the signaling cascade by (1) decreasing $[Ca^{2+}]_{cyt}$ via activating K^+ channels (which causes membrane hyperpolarization and repolarization, leading to closure of VDCCs) and (2) inhibiting myosin light chain kinase, thereby causing smooth muscle relaxation and vasodilation (Olschewski et al., 2004). Activated PKA can also exert an antiproliferative effect on PASMCs by inhibiting the signaling cascades of hedgehog, ERK/p21, and Akt/mTOR. Inhibition of cyclic nucleotide PDEs, mainly PDE3 and PDE4, enhances the cAMP-PKA–mediated relaxant and antiproliferative effects on vascular smooth muscle cells.

Epoprostenol (Prostacyclin)

Clinical Use, Adverse Effects and Precautions. The first synthetic PGI_2, epoprostenol, has dose-dependent inhibitory effects on both SVR and PVR, paired with increases in cardiac output, for patients with PAH (Rubin et al., 1982). Epoprostenol's short half-life (3–5 min) requires the use of a drug delivery pump system for continuous intravenous infusion to achieve long-term efficacy in the treatment of PAH. In a clinical trial, epoprostenol treatment caused significant improvements in pulmonary hemodynamics, patient symptoms, and survival over a 12-week period (Barst et al., 1996).

Epoprostenol is light and temperature sensitive, although a more recent thermostable formulation is now available that permits its use at room temperature (20°C–25°C). This agent remains a mainstay of PAH treatment, particularly in advanced stages of the disease. Adverse effects of epoprostenol are similar for the entire class of PGI_2 analogues and include myalgias and pain in the extremities, jaw pain, nausea, headaches, abdominal discomfort, diarrhea, flushing, dizziness, and systemic hypotension. Side effects are generally dose dependent, and slow titration is required for the drug to be sufficiently tolerated.

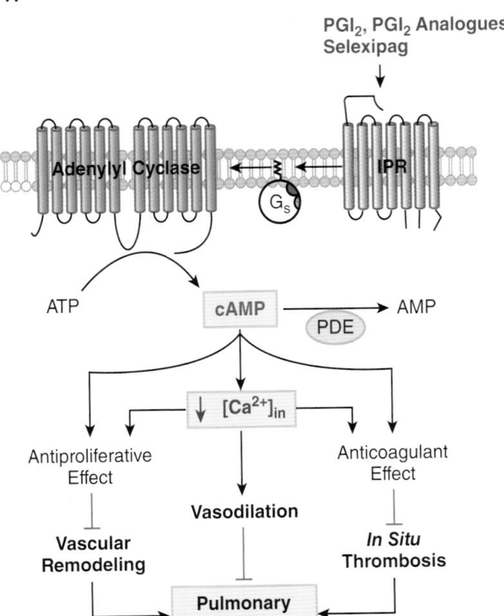

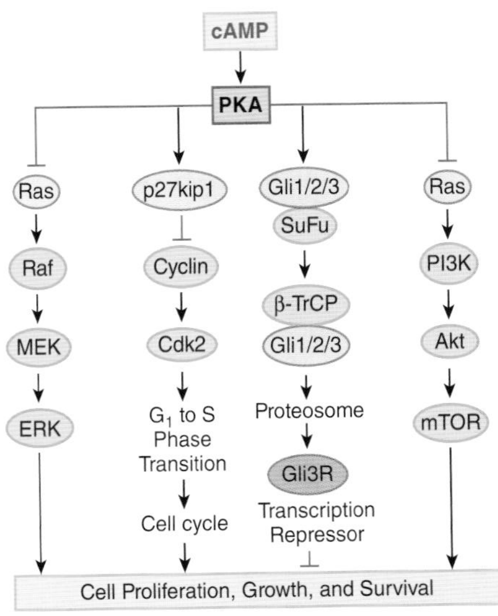

Figure 31–4 *Membrane receptor agonists that increase cAMP.* Therapies targeting the IPR, including PGI_2, PGI_2 analogues, and selexipag, increase cAMP through stimulation of its production by AC. The vasodilating properties of cAMP are produced through decreased $[Ca^{2+}]_{cyt}$ as well as anticoagulant and antiproliferative effects that are both dependent and independent of $[Ca^{2+}]_{cyt}$. The antiproliferative effects of cAMP (panel **B**) are shown through numerous distinct pathways, many of which are currently under investigation as novel therapies.

Treprostinil

Clinical Use. Treprostinil, a PGI_2 analogue with longer half-life than that of epoprostenol, is available for continuous intravenous infusion, subcutaneous infusion, inhalation, and oral delivery. The risk of bacteremia or other catheter-related complications can be reduced by subcutaneous delivery. Subcutaneous treprostinil has similar efficacy to intravenous formulations of epoprostenol and treprostinil (Simonneau et al., 2002). Adverse effects related to delivery into the subcutaneous tissue of the lower abdomen are common, including pain and erythema in a majority of patients; these effects subside over time.

Compared to intravenous treprostinil, the inhaled formulation has more potent pulmonary vasodilating effects, but patients find the dosing scheme complex: Multiple breaths are taken through a nebulizer or inhaler four times a day and slowly titrated up to a maximum of nine breaths four times a day. Inhaled treprostinil has comparable hemodynamic effects to inhaled iloprost with a longer duration of effect in patients with PAH. The most common adverse effect related to inhalation is transient coughing.

Monotherapy with extended-release oral formulations of treprostinil are effective in patients with PAH with moderate functional impairments (Jing et al., 2013). The dose is given twice a day, starting at 0.25 mg and titrating up every 3 days to a maximum of 21 mg twice a day. Serum concentrations at a steady dose of 3.5 mg twice daily are thought to approximate therapeutic levels of intravenous treprostinil. Oral treprostinil fails to show any significant improvement in 6-min walk distance for patients on baseline treatment with either an ERA or PDE5 inhibitor and is therefore not recommended in patients already treated (Tapson et al., 2012).

Iloprost

Clinical Use, Adverse Effects and Precautions. The first PGI_2 analogue available in an inhaled formulation, iloprost was designed to target the pulmonary vasculature with minimal systemic side effects. Inhalation has potent vasodilative effects on the pulmonary circulation, with less systemic vasodilation than intravenous PGI_2 (Olschewski et al., 1996). The effects of a single inhalation decline to baseline over 60–120 min, and current dosing strategies suggest 6–9 inhalations daily. The dose is generally titrated from 2.5 mg/inhalation to 5 mg after the first 2–4 weeks. Minor side effects common to the PGI_2 class include headache and jaw pain. Side effects specific to the inhaled formulation are cough, although this appears to resolve over time.

Beraprost

The first orally available PGI_2 analogue, beraprost, showed promise in early trials, but long-term trials showed no benefit over 12 months of therapy (Barst et al., 2003). As a result, beraprost is not approved for use in the U.S. or E.U.

Selexipag

Selexipag is an orally active, selective IPR agonist that is chemically distinct and has different kinetic properties compared to other PGI_2 analogues.

ADME. Selexipag is rapidly absorbed and hydrolyzed in the liver ($t_{1/2}$ = 1–2 h) to an active metabolite, ACT-333679 (Kaufmann et al., 2015). The active metabolite has a longer half-life, 10–14 h, allowing twice-daily dosing.

Clinical Use, Adverse Effects, and Precautions. The drug is taken at a starting dose of 200 μg and titrated upward weekly to a maximum dose of 1600 μg twice daily. In phase 3 clinical trials, selexipag reduced the risk of morbidity and mortality in patients with PAH (Simonneau et al., 2012; Sitbon et al., 2015). Selexipag was added to existing pulmonary vasodilator therapy in a majority of patients in the clinical trials for this agent. Adverse effects of selexipag are similar to those of PGI_2 analogues and include headache, jaw pain, nausea, dizziness, flushing, nasopharyngitis, and vomiting. Adverse effects appear to be more common when the drug is taken while fasting and wane over time.

Endothelin and Endothelin Receptor Antagonists

Endothelin 1

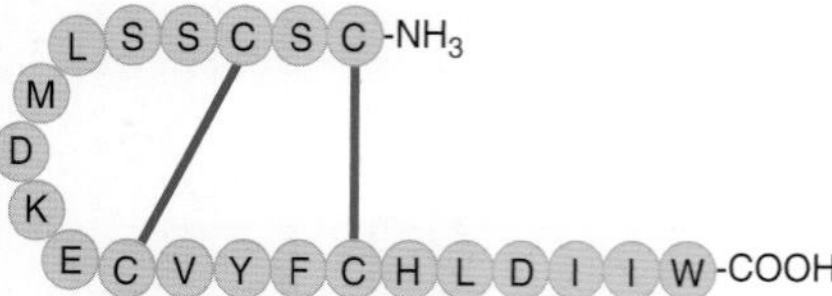

Amino Acid Sequence of Human Endothelin 1

Biosynthesis. Endothelins are a trio of 21 amino acid peptides, each the product of a different gene, produced through a pre-pro and pro-peptide sequence by ECE activities (ECE-1, ECE-2). ECE-1 is the rate-limiting step in ET-1 synthesis. Each mature ET peptide contains two disulfide bridges. ET-1, the predominant form, is encoded by the *EDN1* gene and produced in vascular ECs, although other cell types can also produce endothelin. A variety of cytokines, angiotensin II, and mechanical stress enhance ET-1 production. NO and PGI_2 reduce *EDN1* gene expression. ETs interact with two GPCRs, the ET_A and ET_B receptors, as described in the material that follows. ET-1 is cleared by interaction with the ET_B receptor and via proteolytic degradation by neutral endopeptidase NEP24.11. Davenport and colleagues (2016) have reviewed key concepts of the biosynthesis, signaling, and pharmacology of ETs.

Endothelin Signaling. Endothelin 1 was discovered as a potent, endothelium-derived, constricting factor (Yanagisawa et al., 1988). The constrictor response is mediated by the ET_A receptor, which is localized on PASMCs. The ET_B receptor is present on both PASMCs and PAEC. Binding of ET-1 to ET_A receptor on PASMCs activates the G_q-PLC-IP_3-Ca^{2+} and DAG-Ca^{2+}-PKC pathways (Figure 31–5 and Chapter 3). IP_3 activates the Ca^{2+} release channel on intracellular Ca^{2+} storage organelles, thereby mobilizing Ca^{2+} and increasing $[Ca^{-+}]_{cyt}$. DAG can reportedly activate ROCs on the plasma membrane, enhance Ca^{2+} influx, and contribute to the increased $[Ca^{2+}]_{cyt}$. The elevated cytosolic Ca^{2+} produces vasoconstriction (Figure 3–14). ET-1 is also a mitogenic factor that exerts proliferative effects on many types of cells, including vascular smooth muscle cells and myofibroblasts via intracellular signaling cascades (e.g., PI3K/Akt/mTOR and Ras/ERK/p21 pathways) (Davenport et al., 2016). The activation of ET_B receptors on ECs mediates vasodilation by increasing production of NO and PGI_2 and can inhibit ET-1 production.

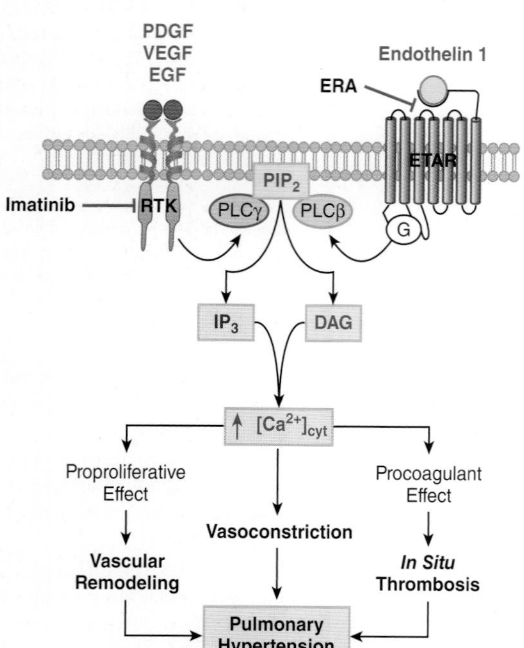

Figure 31–5 *Agents that inhibit receptor-mediated activation of phospholipase C.* The potent vasoconstricting agent ET-1 exerts effect on PASMCs primarily through the endothelin receptor ET_A, a GPCR. Stimulation of the receptor leads to activation of PLC and production of IP_3 and DAG, both of which lead to increased $[Ca^{2+}]_{cyt}$. Similarly, distinct receptor tyrosine kinases, such as PDGF, VEGF, and EGF, can lead to increased IP_3 and DAG and subsequent increases in $[Ca^{2+}]_{cyt}$ through a similar, yet distinct, pathway.

Rationale for Antagonizing ET's Effects in PAH. Endothelin 1 is implicated as a contributory factor in idiopathic PAH (Giaid et al., 1993): Plasma ET-1 levels are increased up to 10-fold in patients with PAH and correlate well with severity of disease and the elevation of right atrial pressure. There are no clinically available specific inhibitors of ECE-1, the rate-limiting step in ET-1 synthesis, but a number of orally effective small molecule antagonists of ET receptors have been developed. Despite the opposing effects of ET_A and ET_B receptor activation, pharmacological targeting of specific ET_A receptors has not led to significantly altered clinical responses compared to dual antagonism (e.g., antagonism of ET-1 binding to both ET_A and ET_B receptors) in treating PAH.

Endothelin Receptor Antagonists

Available ET receptor antagonists (ERAs) are bosentan, macitentan, and ambrisentan.

Commonalities. Endothelin antagonists generally share adverse effects. Common side effects of the class include headache, pulmonary edema, and nasal congestion/pharyngitis, with a risk of testicular atrophy and infertility. Bosentan and ambrisentan may increase liver transaminases, which should be monitored closely, and the drugs are contraindicated in patients with moderate-to-severe liver disease; the elevation of liver enzymes generally resolves after discontinuation of treatment.

The three available ET antagonists are metabolized by CYP3A4 and to some extent by CYPs 2C9 and 2C19. Repeated bosentan dosing elicits induction of CYPs 3A4 and 2C9, reducing exposure to drugs that are also metabolized by these CYPs (contraceptives, warfarin, some statins; coadministration with cyclosporine and glyburide is contraindicated); likewise, coadministration of bosentan or macitentan with a CYP inducer such as rifampin should be avoided. Inhibitors of these CYPs (e.g., ketoconazole and ritonoavir) can increase bosentan and macitentan exposure (O'Callaghan et al., 2011).

The ERAs are potent teratogens and should be used with caution in women of childbearing age. These agents must not be used in pregnant patients. Documentation of a negative pregnancy test prior to initiation of therapy and a clear contraceptive plan are recommended, and fertile women must use two acceptable methods of birth control while taking ET antagonists.

Bosentan. Bosentan is a nonpeptide, orally effective, competitive antagonist of ET_A and ET_B receptors. In patients with PAH with mild-to-severe functional impairment (functional classes II–IV), bosentan improves symptoms, functional capacity, and pulmonary hemodynamic parameters (Rubin et al., 2002). Bosentan is usually started at 62.5 mg twice daily, increasing to 125 mg twice daily after 4 weeks. Bosentan is metabolized by hepatic CYPs 2C9 and 3A4 with a $t_{1/2}$ of about 5 h, with excretion of metabolites in the bile.

Macitentan. Macitentan is an orally active, competitive ET_A and ET_B receptor antagonist. At a dose of 10 mg daily, macitentan improves the time to disease progression or death in PAH and improves symptoms, functional capacity, and pulmonary hemodynamic measurements (Pulido et al., 2013). The drug is relatively well tolerated and has thus far not been associated with elevation of liver-associated enzymes, but caution is recommended. Macitentan is metabolized by CYPs to an active metabolite; the $t_{1/2}$ of the parent compound is about 16 h, that of the active metabolite about 48 h, such that the metabolite contributes about 40% of the total pharmacologic activity over time.

Ambrisentan. Unlike bosentan and macitentan, ambrisentan is a relatively selective ET_A antagonist (approximately 4000 times greater affinity for ET_A than ET_B). Ambrisentan is initiated at a dose of 5 mg daily and increased to a maximum of 10 mg daily. The $t_{1/2}$ is 9 h at steady state. Liver-associated enzyme abnormalities are much less common than with bosentan, yet monitoring of liver function tests is still recommended. Elimination is largely via nonrenal pathways that have not been extensively characterized. There is some metabolism by CYPs 3A4 and 2C19, followed by glucuronidation; thus, drug interactions might be expected, although clinically relevant interactions have not been reported.

Receptor Tyrosine Kinase Inhibitors

Many growth factors and mitogenic factors are reportedly upregulated in tissues of patients with PAH. Elevations of ET-1, ATP, VIP, PDGF, VEGFs, EGF, fibroblast growth factor, and insulin-like growth factor in lung tissue, vascular smooth muscle cells, and peripheral blood have been assessed in PAH (Budhiraja et al., 2004; Du et al., 2003; Schermuly et al., 2005). These myriad mitogenic factors can activate TKRs, such as PDGF and EGF receptors. Activation of these receptors induces cell proliferation, growth, migration, and contraction in PASMCs, PAECs, and pulmonary vascular fibroblasts. With these actions as a rationale, antagonists of TKRs have been tried as therapeutics for PAH (Moreno-Vinasco et al, 2008; Gomberg-Maitland et al, 2010).

Imatinib

Imatinib was initially developed as targeted treatment of chronic myelogenous leukemia by targeting the ABL TKR; the compound is now known to have many other targets, one of which is the PDGF receptor that has been linked to vascular smooth muscle hypertrophy in the development of PAH (Humbert et al., 1998). Imatinib as add-on therapy for refractory PAH has shown efficacy in both case reports and a clinical trial, although serious adverse reactions, particularly subdural hematoma, are of concern (Hoeper et al., 2013). Larger clinical trials are needed before imatinib can be used in PAH treatment regimens.

Calcium Channels and Their Blockers

An increase in $[Ca^{2+}]_{cyt}$ in PASMCs causes pulmonary vasoconstriction and is an important stimulant of proliferation, migration, and vascular remodeling. $[Ca^{2+}]_{cyt}$ in PASMCs can be increased by Ca^{2+} influx through membrane Ca^{2+} channels and Ca^{2+} mobilization through the Ca^{2+} release channels/IP_3 receptors in the SR membrane. $[Ca^{2+}]_{cyt}$ can be decreased in three ways: by Ca^{2+} extrusion via the Ca^{2+}/Mg^{2+} ATPase (the Ca^{2+} pump in the plasma membrane), export of Ca^{2+} by the Na^+/Ca^{2+} exchanger, and by sequestration of cytosolic Ca^{2+} into the SR by SR Ca^{2+}-ATPase. There are three classes of Ca^{2+}-permeable channels functionally expressed in the plasma membrane of PASMCs: (1) VDCCs, (2) ROCs, and (3) store-operated Ca^{2+} channels. These are targets in the current therapy of PAH and putative targets for therapeutics of the future.

Voltage-Gated Ca^{2+} Channel Blockers

A rare subset of patients (typically less than 5%–15% of all group I PAH confirmed by right heart catheterization) is considered vasoreactive, which is defined as a significant decrease in mean PAP (>10 mm Hg drop to absolute mean PAP < 40 mm Hg) while preserving cardiac output during the administration of inhaled NO or intravenous injection of PGI_2 or adenosine (Rich and Brundage, 1987). Vasoreactive patients can achieve prolonged survival, sustained functional improvement, and hemodynamic improvement with CCB therapy (Hemnes et al., 2015; Rich and Brundage, 1987). The utility of CCB therapy in patients with vasoreactive PAH was supported by a series of well-designed observational studies (Hemnes et al., 2015; Rich and Brundage, 1987; Sitbon et al., 2005).

Clinical Use. Therapy with CCB can be initiated with a low dose of long-acting nifedipine, amlodipine, diltiazem, or verapamil. The dose is then increased to the maximal tolerated dose. Systemic blood pressure, heart rate, and oxygen saturation should be carefully monitored during titration. Sustained-release preparations of nifedipine, verapamil, and diltiazem are available that minimize the adverse effects of therapy, especially systemic hypotension. Patients who respond (defined as asymptomatic or minimal symptoms) to CCB therapy with a dihydropyridine or diltiazem are typically reassessed for sustaining the response (Figure 31–6).

Adverse Effects and Precautions. Adverse effects are common with CCB therapy. Systemic vasodilation may cause hypotension, while pulmonary vasodilation may reduce HPV. Loss or inhibition of HPV can worsen V/Q mismatch and cause hypoxemia. CCBs may also be associated with deterioration of RV function because of their inhibitory effect on VDCC in cardiomyocytes. The pharmacology of CCBs is discussed in detail in Chapter 27.

PAH Drugs in Development

In addition to the PAH drugs in clinical use, there are many repurposed drugs and newly developed drugs that have therapeutic benefits in experimental models of PH. These agents have potential as future therapies for PAH:

- antagonists of $5HT_{2B}$ receptors and transporters (e.g., LY393558);
- allosteric antagonists of Ca^{2+}-sensing receptors (e.g., NPS2143 and calhex 231);
- openers or activators of Ca^{2+}-activated and voltage-gated K^+ channels and ATP-sensitive K^+ channels (e.g., cromakalim);
- inhibitors of the PI3K/Akt1/mTOR signaling cascades (e.g., perifosine, ipatasertib, and rapamycin derivatives sirolimus, temsirolimus, everolimus, deforolimus);
- inhibitors of the Notch signaling pathway (e.g., DAPT and MK-0752);
- VIP;
- blockers of transient receptor potential cation channels (e.g., 2-APB, ML204, aniline-thiazoles);
- extracellular elastase inhibitors (e.g., elafin and sivelestat);
- Rho kinase inhibitors (e.g., fasudil); and
- angiopoietin 1 inhibitors (e.g., trebananib).

Some of these drugs are already in phase 3 clinical trials; others are still in preclinical development.

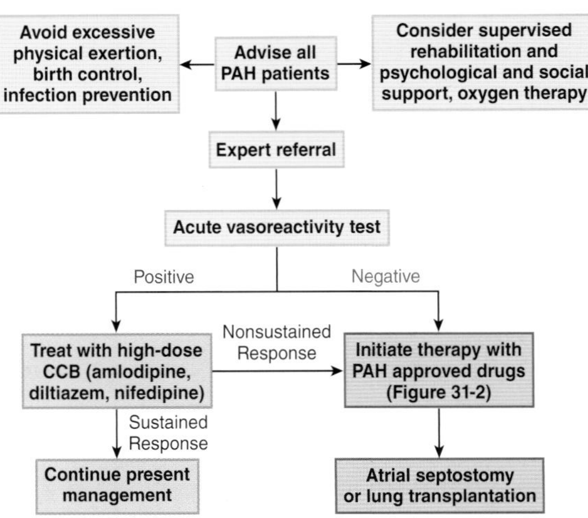

Figure 31–6 *Treatment algorithm for use of CCBs in PAH.* Vasoreactivity testing is used to identify the minority of patients who may have a substantial benefit from high-dose CCB therapy. These individuals must be monitored closely to ensure a sustained response. Patients without a positive vasodilator response should potentially be started on therapies approved for PAH based on symptoms at presentation. The patients with the most severe disease who fail to respond to therapy may need referral for surgical intervention to treat their disease.

A Pharmacologist's View of Signal Integration in PAH

As noted, an imbalance of vasoactive mediators, mitogenic and angiogenic factors, and pro- and antiapoptotic proteins plays an important role in PAH development. The pharmacological agents employed in PAH are focused on restoring the balance between contraction and proliferation on the one hand and relaxation and antiproliferation on the other, as summarized in Figure 31–7.

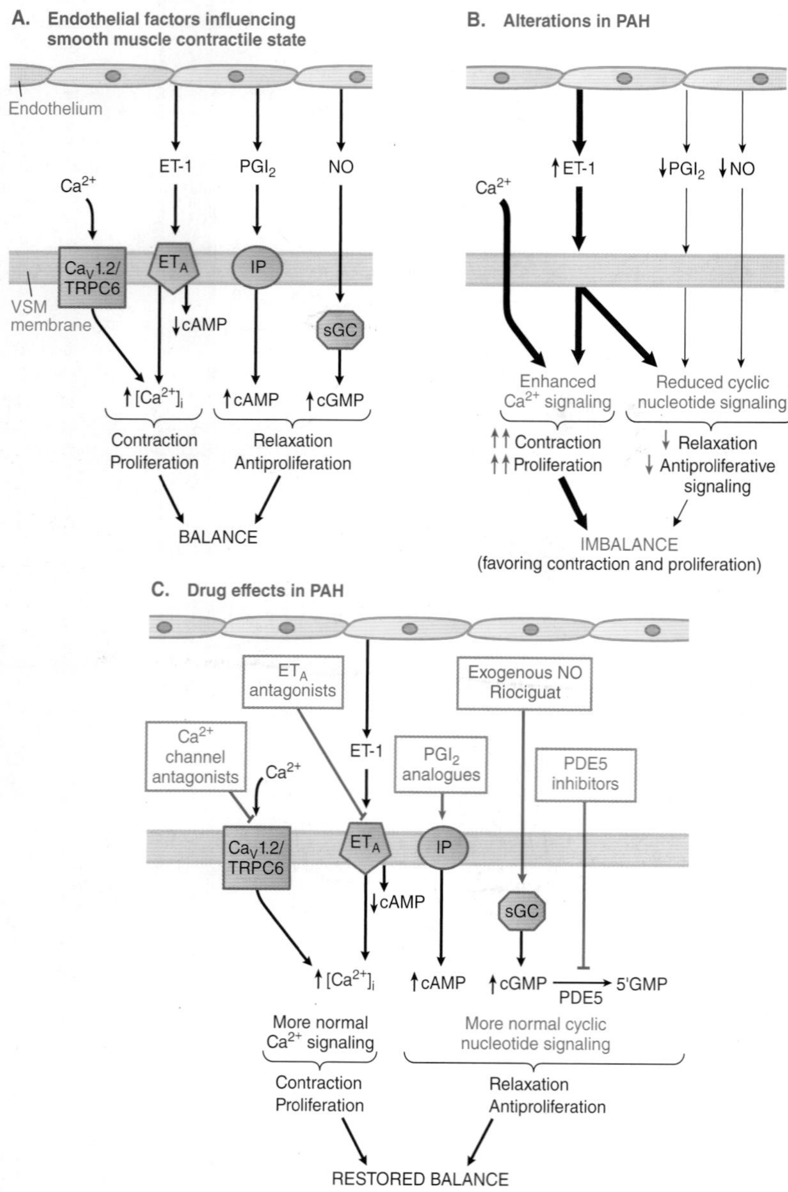

Figure 31–7 *Interactions between endothelium and vascular smooth muscle in PAH.* **A. Balance.** In normal pulmonary artery, there is a balance between constrictor and relaxant influences that may be viewed as competition between Ca^{2+} signaling pathways and cyclic nucleotide signaling pathways in VSM. ET-1 binds to the ET_A receptor on VSM cells and activates the G_q-PLC-IP_3 pathway to increase cytosolic Ca^{2+}; ET-1 may also couple to G_i to inhibit cAMP production. As VSM cells depolarize, Ca^{2+} may enter via the L-type Ca^{2+} channel ($Ca_v1.2$) or transient receptor potential cation channel (TRPC6). ECs also produce relaxant factors, PGI_2, and NO. NO stimulates the sGC, causing accumulation of cGMP in VSM cells; PGI_2 binds to the IPR and stimulates cAMP production; elevation of these cyclic nucleotides promotes VSM relaxation (see Figures 31-3, 40-4 and 45-6). **B. Imbalance.** In PAH, ET-1 production is enhanced, production of PGI_2 and NO is reduced, and the balance is shifted toward constriction and proliferation of VSM. **C. Restored balance.** In treating PAH, ET_A receptor antagonists can reduce the constrictor effects of ET-1, and Ca^{2+} channel antagonists can further reduce Ca^{2+}-dependent contraction. Exogenous PGI_2 and NO can be supplied to promote vasodilation (relaxation of VSM); the sGC can be activated pharmacologically (riociguat); inhibition of PDE5 can enhance the relaxant effect of elevated cGMP by inhibiting the degradation of cGMP. Thus, these drugs can reduce Ca^{2+} signaling and enhance cyclic nucleotide signaling, restoring the balance between the forces of contraction/proliferation and relaxation/antiproliferation. Remodeling and deposition of extracellular matrix by adjacent fibroblasts is influenced positively and negatively by the same contractile and relaxant signaling pathways, respectively. Effects of pharmacological agonists are noted by green arrows, effects of antagonists by red T-bars.

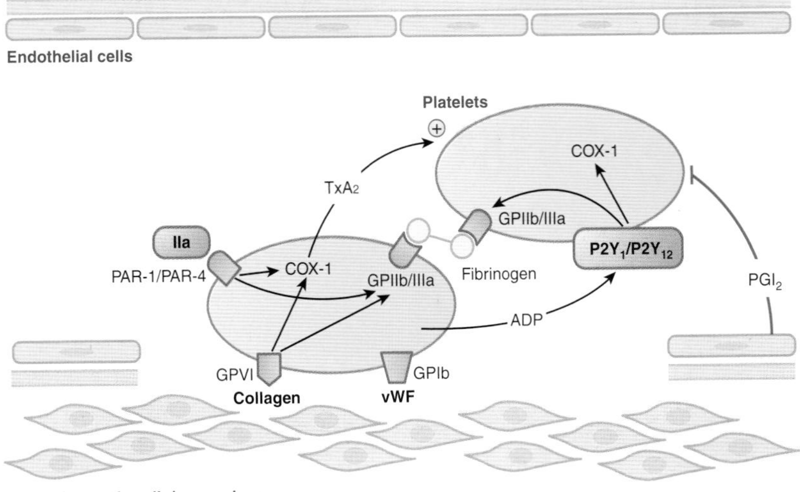

Figure 32–1 *Platelet adhesion and aggregation.* GPVI and GPIb are platelet receptors that bind to collagen and vWF, causing platelets to adhere to the subendothelium of a damaged blood vessel. PAR-1 and PAR-4 are PARs that respond to thrombin (IIa); $P2Y_1$ and $P2Y_{12}$ are receptors for ADP; when stimulated by agonists, these receptors activate the fibrinogen-binding protein GPIIb/IIIa and COX-1 to promote platelet aggregation and secretion. TxA_2 is the major product of COX-1 involved in platelet activation. Prostacyclin (PGI_2), synthesized by endothelial cells, inhibits platelet activation.

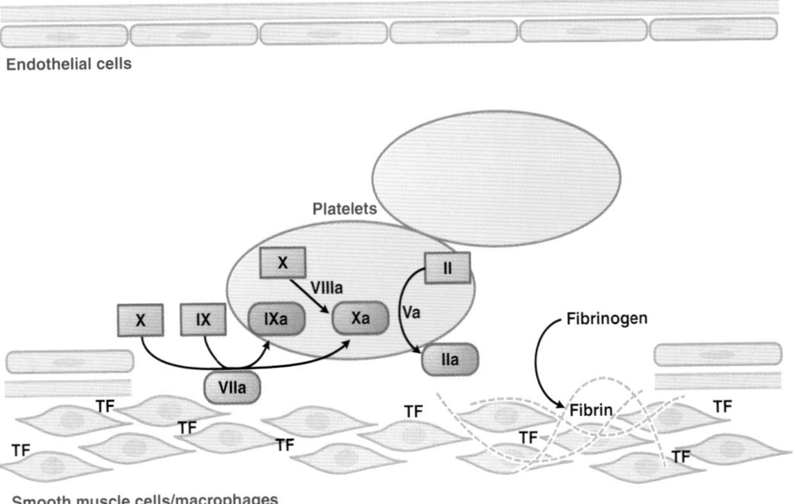

Figure 32–2 *Major reactions of blood coagulation.* Shown are interactions among proteins of the "extrinsic" (TF and factor VII), "intrinsic" (factors IX and VIII), and "common" (factors X, V, and II) coagulation pathways that are important in vivo. Boxes enclose the coagulation factor zymogens (indicated by Roman numerals); the rounded boxes represent the active proteases. Activated coagulation factors are followed by the letter *a*: II, prothrombin; IIa, thrombin.

Factor VIII and Factor V Are Procofactors

Factor VIII circulates in plasma bound to *von Willebrand factor*, which serves to stabilize it. Factor V circulates in plasma, is stored in platelets in a partially activated form, and is released when platelets are activated. Thrombin releases von Willebrand factor from factor VIII and activates factors V and VIII to yield factor Va and VIIIa, respectively. Once activated, the cofactors bind to the surface of activated platelets and serve as receptors; factor VIIIa serves as the receptor for factor IXa, while factor Va serves as the receptor for factor Xa. In addition to binding factors IXa and Xa, factors VIIIa and Va bind their substrates, factors X and prothrombin (factor II), respectively.

Activation of Prothrombin

By cleaving two peptide bonds on prothrombin, factor Xa converts it to thrombin. In the presence of factor Va, a negatively charged phospholipid surface, and Ca^{2+} (the so-called prothrombinase complex), factor Xa activates prothrombin with 10^9-fold greater efficiency. This maximal rate of activation only occurs when prothrombin and factor Xa contain Gla residues at their amino terminals, which endows them with the capacity to bind calcium and interact with the anionic phospholipid surface.

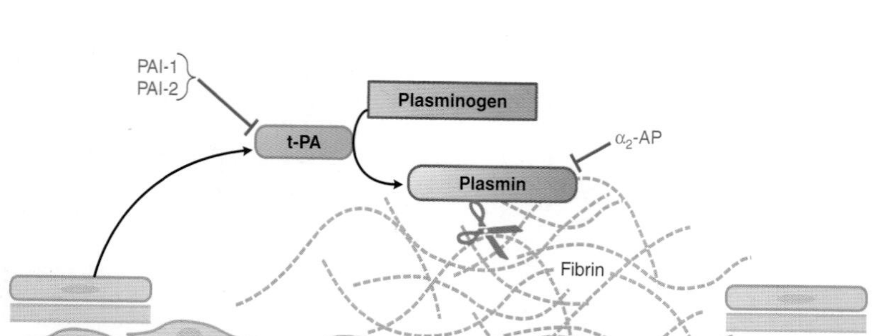

Figure 32–3 *Fibrinolysis.* Endothelial cells secrete t-PA at sites of injury. t-PA binds to fibrin and converts plasminogen to plasmin, which digests fibrin. PAI-1 and PAI-2 inactivate t-PA; α_2-AP inactivates plasmin.

Initiation of Coagulation

TF exposed at sites of vessel wall injury initiates coagulation via the *extrinsic pathway*. The small amount of factor VIIa circulating in plasma binds subendothelial TF and the TF–factor VIIa complex, then activates factors X and IX (see Figure 32–2). When bound to TF in the presence of anionic phospholipids and Ca^{2+} (extrinsic tenase), factor VIIa activity is increased 30,000-fold over that of factor VIIa alone.

The *intrinsic pathway* is initiated in vitro when factor XII, prekallikrein, and high-molecular-weight kininogen interact with kaolin, glass, or another negatively charged surface to generate small amounts of factor XIIa. Factor XII can be activated in vivo by contact of the blood with medical devices, such as mechanical heart valves or extracorporeal circuits, or by cell-free DNA, neutrophil extracellular traps, which are web-like structures composed of DNA and histones extruded from activated neutrophils, or inorganic polyphosphates released from activated platelets. Factor XIIa activates factor XI and the resultant factor XIa, then activates factor IX. Factor IXa activates factor X in a reaction accelerated by factor VIIIa, anionic phospholipids, and Ca^{2+}. Optimal thrombin generation depends on the formation of this factor IXa complex (intrinsic tenase) because it activates factor X more efficiently than the TF–factor VIIa complex.

Activation of factor XII is not essential for hemostasis, as evidenced by the fact that patients deficient in factor XII, prekallikrein, or high-molecular-weight kininogen do not have excessive bleeding. Factor XI deficiency is associated with a variable and usually mild bleeding disorder. In contrast, congenital deficiency of factor VIII or IX results in hemophilia A or B, respectively, and is associated with spontaneous bleeding, which can be fatal.

Fibrinolysis

The fibrinolysis pathway is summarized in Figure 32–3. The fibrinolytic system dissolves intravascular *fibrin* through the action of *plasmin*. To initiate fibrinolysis, plasminogen activators convert single-chain plasminogen, an inactive precursor, into two-chain *plasmin* by cleavage of a specific peptide bond. There are two distinct plasminogen activators: *t-PA* and *u-PA*, which is also known as urokinase. Although both activators are synthesized by endothelial cells, t-PA predominates under most conditions and drives intravascular fibrinolysis, while synthesis of u-PA mainly occurs in response to inflammatory stimuli and promotes extravascular fibrinolysis.

The fibrinolytic system is regulated such that unwanted fibrin thrombi are removed, while fibrin in wounds is preserved to maintain hemostasis. t-PA is released from endothelial cells in response to various stimuli. Released t-PA is rapidly cleared from blood or inhibited by *PAI-1* and, to a lesser extent, by *PAI-2*. Therefore, t-PA exerts little effect on circulating plasminogen in the absence of fibrin, and circulating α_2*-antiplasmin* rapidly inhibits any plasmin that is generated. The catalytic efficiency of t-PA activation of plasminogen increases more than 300-fold in the presence of fibrin, which promotes plasmin generation on its surface.

Plasminogen and plasmin bind to lysine residues on fibrin via five loop-like regions near their amino termini, which are known as *kringle domains*. To inactivate plasmin, α_2-antiplasmin binds to the first of these kringle domains and then blocks the active site of plasmin. Because the kringle domains are occupied when plasmin binds to fibrin, plasmin on the fibrin surface is protected from inhibition by α_2-antiplasmin and can digest the fibrin. Once the fibrin clot undergoes degradation, α_2-antiplasmin rapidly inhibits any plasmin that escapes from this local milieu. To prevent premature clot lysis, factor XIIIa mediates covalent cross-linking of small amounts of α_2-antiplasmin onto fibrin.

When thrombi occlude major arteries or veins, therapeutic doses of plasminogen activators are sometimes administered to rapidly degrade the fibrin and restore blood flow. In high doses, these plasminogen activators promote the generation of so much plasmin that the inhibitory controls are overwhelmed. Plasmin is a relatively nonspecific protease; in addition to degrading fibrin, it degrades several coagulation factors. Reduction in the levels of these coagulation proteins impairs the capacity for thrombin generation, which can contribute to bleeding. In addition, unopposed plasmin tends to dissolve fibrin in hemostatic plugs as well as that in pathological thrombi, a phenomenon that also increases the risk of bleeding. Therefore, fibrinolytic drugs can produce hemorrhage as their major side effect.

Coagulation In Vitro

Whole blood normally clots in 4–8 min when placed in a glass tube. Under these conditions, contact of the blood with glass activates factor XII, thereby initiating coagulation via the *intrinsic pathway*. Clotting is prevented if a chelating agent such as EDTA or citrate is added to bind Ca^{2+}. Recalcified plasma normally clots in 2–4 min. The clotting time after recalcification is shortened to 26–33 sec by the addition of negatively charged phospholipids and particulate substances, such as kaolin (aluminum silicate) or celite (diatomaceous earth), which activate factor XII; the measurement of this is termed the *aPTT*. Alternatively, recalcified plasma clots in 12–14 sec after addition of "thromboplastin" (a mixture of TF and phospholipid) and calcium; the measurement of this is termed the *PT*.

Natural Anticoagulant Mechanisms

Platelet activation and coagulation do not normally occur within an intact blood vessel. Thrombosis is prevented by several regulatory mechanisms that require healthy vascular endothelium. Nitric oxide and prostacyclin synthesized by endothelial cells inhibit platelet activation (see Chapter 37).

Antithrombin is a plasma protein that inhibits coagulation enzymes of the extrinsic, intrinsic, and common pathways. Heparan sulfate proteoglycans synthesized by endothelial cells enhance the activity of antithrombin by about 1000-fold. Another regulatory system involves protein C, a plasma zymogen that is homologous to factors II, VII, IX, and X; its activity depends on the binding of Ca^{2+} to Gla residues within its amino terminal domain. Protein C binds to EPCR, which presents it to the thrombin-thrombomodulin complex for activation. Activated protein C then dissociates from EPCR, and, in combination with protein S, its nonenzymatic Gla-containing cofactor, activated protein C degrades factors Va and VIIIa. Without these activated cofactors, the rates of activation of prothrombin and factor X are greatly diminished, and thrombin generation is attenuated. Congenital or acquired deficiency of protein C or protein S is associated with an increased risk of venous thrombosis.

Tissue factor pathway inhibitor is a natural anticoagulant found in the lipoprotein fraction of plasma or bound to endothelial cell surface. TFPI first binds and inhibits factor Xa, and this binary complex then inhibits factor VIIa bound to TF. By this mechanism, factor Xa regulates its own generation.

Parenteral Anticoagulants: Heparin, LMWHs, Fondaparinux

Heparin and Its Standardization

Heparin, a glycosaminoglycan found in the secretory granules of mast cells, is synthesized from UDP-sugar precursors as a polymer of alternating D-glucuronic acid and *N*-acetyl-D-glucosamine residues. Heparin is commonly extracted from porcine intestinal mucosa, which is rich in mast cells, and preparations may contain small amounts of other glycosaminoglycans. Various commercial heparin preparations have similar biological activity (~150 USP units/mg). A USP unit reflects the quantity of heparin that prevents 1 mL of citrated sheep plasma from clotting for 1 h after calcium addition. European manufacturers measure potency with an anti–factor Xa assay. To determine heparin potency, residual factor Xa activity in the sample is compared with that detected in controls containing known concentrations of an international heparin standard. When assessed this way, heparin potency is expressed in international units per milligram. Effective October 1, 2009, the new USP unit dose was harmonized with the international unit dose. As a result, the new USP unit dose is about 10% less potent than the old one, which results in a requirement for somewhat higher heparin doses to achieve the same level of anticoagulation.

Heparin Derivatives

Derivatives of heparin in current use include LMWH and fondaparinux (see their comparison in Table 32–1).

Mechanism of Action. Heparin, LMWHs, and fondaparinux have no intrinsic anticoagulant activity; rather, these agents bind to antithrombin and accelerate the rate at which it inhibits various coagulation proteases. Synthesized in the liver, antithrombin circulates in plasma at an approximate concentration of 2.5 μM. Antithrombin inhibits activated coagulation factors, particularly thrombin and factor Xa, by serving as a "suicide substrate." Thus, inhibition occurs when the protease attacks a specific Arg–Ser peptide bond in the reactive center loop of antithrombin and becomes trapped as a stable 1:1 complex. Heparin binds to antithrombin via a specific pentasaccharide sequence that contains a 3-*O*-sulfated glucosamine residue (Figure 32–4).

Pentasaccharide binding to antithrombin induces a conformational change in antithrombin that renders its reactive site more accessible to the target protease (Figure 32–5). This conformational change accelerates the rate of factor Xa inhibition by at least two orders of magnitude but has no effect on the rate of thrombin inhibition. To enhance the rate of thrombin inhibition by antithrombin, heparin serves as a catalytic template to which both the inhibitor and the protease bind. Only heparin molecules composed of 18 or more saccharide units (molecular weight > 5400) are of sufficient length to bridge antithrombin and thrombin together. Consequently, by definition, heparin catalyzes the rates of factor Xa and thrombin inhibition to a similar extent, as expressed by an anti–factor Xa to anti–factor IIa (thrombin) ratio of 1:1 (Figure 32–5A). In contrast, at least half of LMWH molecules (mean molecular weight of 5000, which corresponds with about 17 saccharide units) are too short to provide this bridging function and have no effect on the rate of thrombin inhibition by antithrombin (Figure 32–5B). Because these shorter molecules still induce the conformational change in antithrombin that accelerates inhibition of factor Xa, LMWH has greater anti–factor Xa activity than anti–factor IIa activity, and the ratio ranges from 3:1 to 2:1 depending on the preparation. Fondaparinux, a synthetic analogue of the pentasaccharide sequence in heparin or LMWH that mediates their interaction with antithrombin, has only anti–factor Xa activity because it is too short to bridge antithrombin to thrombin (Figure 32–5C).

Heparin, LMWH, and fondaparinux act in a catalytic fashion. After binding to antithrombin and promoting the formation of covalent complexes between antithrombin and target proteases, the heparin, LMWH,

TABLE 32–1 ■ COMPARISON OF THE FEATURES OF SUBCUTANEOUS HEPARIN, LOW-MOLECULAR-WEIGHT HEPARIN, AND FONDAPARINUX

FEATURES	HEPARIN	LMWH	FONDAPARINUX
Source	Biological	Biological	Synthetic
Mean molecular weight (Da)	15,000	5000	1500
Target	Xa and IIa	Xa and IIa	Xa
Subcutaneous			
Bioavailability (%)	30 (at low doses)	90	100
$t_{1/2}$ (h)	1–8[a]	4	17
Renal excretion	No	Yes	Yes
Antidote effect	Complete	Partial	None
Thrombocytopenia	<5%	<1%	<0.1%

[a]Half-life $t_{1/2}$ is dose dependent; half-life is 1 h with 5000 units given subcutaneously and can extend to 8 h with higher doses.

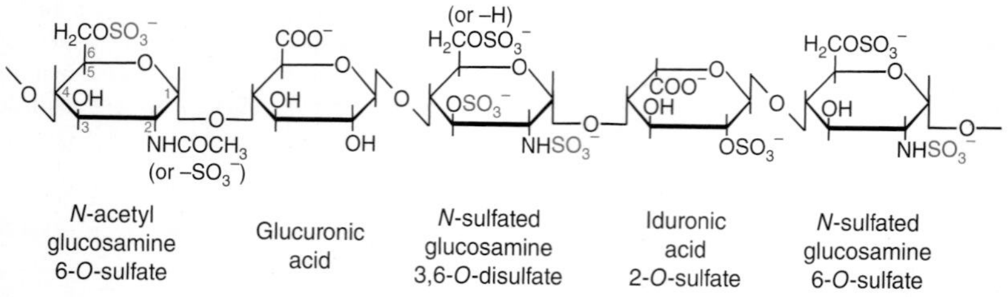

$H_2COSO_3^-$ … $NHCOCH_3$ (or $-SO_3^-$)
N-acetyl glucosamine 6-*O*-sulfate

COO^- … OH
Glucuronic acid

(or –H) $H_2COSO_3^-$ … OSO_3^- … $NHSO_3^-$
N-sulfated glucosamine 3,6-*O*-disulfate

COO^- … OH … OSO_3^-
Iduronic acid 2-*O*-sulfate

$H_2COSO_3^-$ … OH … $NHSO_3^-$
N-sulfated glucosamine 6-*O*-sulfate

Figure 32–4 *The antithrombin-binding pentasaccharide structure of heparin.* Sulfate groups required for binding to antithrombin are indicated in red.

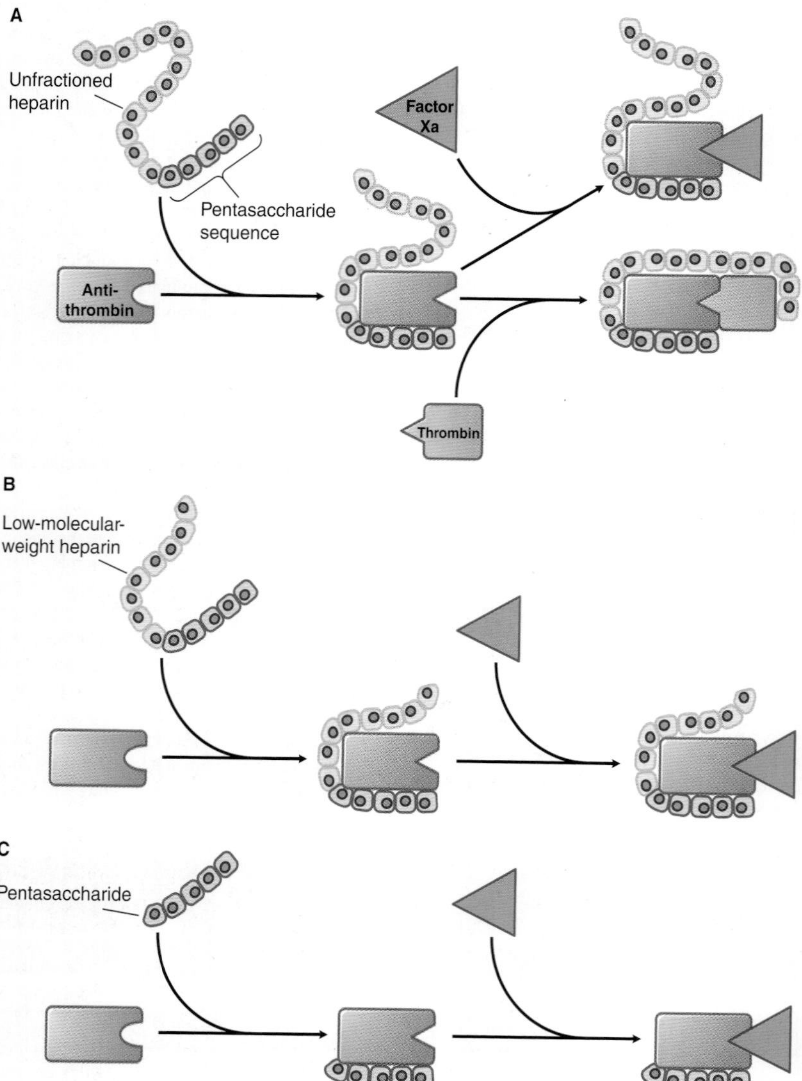

Figure 32–5 *Mechanism of action of heparin, LMWH, and fondaparinux, a synthetic pentasaccharide.* **A.** Heparin binds to antithrombin via its pentasaccharide sequence. This induces a conformational change in the reactive center loop of antithrombin that accelerates its interaction with factor Xa. To potentiate thrombin inhibition, heparin must simultaneously bind to antithrombin and thrombin. Only heparin chains composed of at least 18 saccharide units (MW ~ 5400 Da) are of sufficient length to perform this bridging function. With a mean MW of approximately 15,000 Da, virtually all of the heparin chains are long enough to do this. **B.** LMWH has greater capacity to potentiate factor Xa inhibition by antithrombin than thrombin because at least half of the LMWH chains (mean MW ~ 4500–5000 Da) are too short to bridge antithrombin to thrombin. **C.** The pentasaccharide accelerates only factor Xa inhibition by antithrombin; the pentasaccharide is too short to bridge antithrombin to thrombin.

or fondaparinux dissociates from the complex and can then catalyze other antithrombin molecules.

Platelet factor 4, a cationic protein released from α-granules during platelet activation, binds heparin and prevents it from interacting with antithrombin. This phenomenon may limit the activity of heparin in the vicinity of platelet-rich thrombi. Because LMWH and fondaparinux have a lower affinity for platelet factor 4, these agents may retain their activity in the vicinity of such thrombi to a greater extent than heparin.

Miscellaneous Pharmacological Effects. High doses of heparin can interfere with platelet aggregation and prolong the bleeding time. In contrast, LMWH and fondaparinux have little effect on platelets. Heparin "clears" lipemic plasma in vivo by causing the release of lipoprotein lipase into the circulation. Lipoprotein lipase hydrolyzes triglycerides to glycerol and free fatty acids. The clearing of lipemic plasma may occur at concentrations of heparin below those necessary to produce an anticoagulant effect.

Clinical Use. Heparin, LMWH, or fondaparinux can be used to initiate treatment of deep vein thrombosis and pulmonary embolism. They also can be used for the initial management of patients with unstable angina or acute myocardial infarction (Gara et al., 2013; Roffi et al., 2015). For most of these indications, LMWH or fondaparinux has replaced continuous heparin infusions because of their pharmacokinetic advantages, which permit subcutaneous administration once or twice daily in fixed or weight-adjusted doses without coagulation monitoring. Thus, LMWH or fondaparinux can be used for out-of-hospital management of patients with deep vein thrombosis or pulmonary embolism.

Heparin or LMWH is used during coronary balloon angioplasty with or without stent placement to prevent thrombosis. Fondaparinux is not used in this setting because of the risk of catheter thrombosis, a complication caused by catheter-induced activation of factor XII; longer heparin molecules are better than shorter ones for blocking this process. Cardiopulmonary bypass circuits also activate factor XII, which can cause clotting of the oxygenator. Heparin remains the agent of choice for surgery requiring cardiopulmonary bypass. Heparin or LMWH also is used to treat selected patients with disseminated intravascular coagulation. Subcutaneous administration of low-dose heparin or LMWH is often used for thromboprophylaxis in immobilized medically ill patients (Kahn et al., 2012) or in those who have undergone major surgery (Falck-Ytter et al., 2012; Gould et al., 2012).

Unlike the oral anticoagulants, heparin, LMWH, and fondaparinux do not cross the placenta and have not been associated with fetal malformations, making them the drugs of choice for anticoagulation during pregnancy. Heparin, LMWH, and fondaparinux do not appear to increase fetal mortality or prematurity. If possible, the drugs should be discontinued 24 h before delivery to minimize the risk of postpartum bleeding.

ADME. Heparin, LMWH, and fondaparinux are not absorbed through the GI mucosa and must be given parenterally. Heparin is given by continuous intravenous infusion, intermittent infusion every 4–6 h, or subcutaneous injection every 8–12 h. Heparin has an immediate onset of action when given intravenously. In contrast, there is considerable variation in the bioavailability of heparin given subcutaneously, and the onset of action is delayed by 1–2 h. LMWH and fondaparinux are absorbed more uniformly after subcutaneous injection. The $t_{1/2}$ of heparin in plasma depends on the dose administered. When doses of 100, 400, or 800 units/kg of heparin are injected intravenously, the half-lives are about 1, 2.5, and 5 h, respectively. Heparin appears to be cleared and degraded primarily by the reticuloendothelial system; a small amount of intact heparin appears in the urine.

Both LMWH and fondaparinux have longer biological half-lives than heparin, 4–6 and 17 h, respectively. Because these smaller heparin fragments are cleared almost exclusively by the kidneys, the drugs can accumulate in patients with renal impairment and lead to bleeding. Both LMWH and fondaparinux are contraindicated in patients with a creatinine clearance below 30 mL/min. In addition, thromboprophylaxis with fondaparinux is contraindicated in patients undergoing hip fracture, hip replacement, knee replacement, or abdominal surgery who have a body weight less than 50 kg.

Administration and Monitoring. Full-dose heparin usually is administered by continuous intravenous infusion. Treatment of venous thromboembolism is initiated with a fixed-dose bolus injection of 5000 units or with a weight-adjusted bolus, followed by 800–1600 units/h delivered by an infusion pump. Therapy is monitored by measuring the aPTT. The therapeutic range for heparin is considered to be that which is equivalent to a plasma heparin level of 0.3–0.7 units/mL, as determined with an anti–factor Xa assay. An aPTT that is two or three times the normal mean aPTT value generally is assumed to be therapeutic. The aPTT should be measured initially and the infusion rate adjusted every 6 h. Once a steady dosage schedule has been established, daily aPTT monitoring usually is sufficient. Very high doses of heparin are required to prevent clotting in patients undergoing percutaneous coronary intervention or cardiac surgery with cardiopulmonary bypass. The aPTT is infinitely prolonged with these high doses of heparin, so a less-sensitive coagulation test, the ACT, is employed to monitor therapy in this situation.

For therapeutic purposes, heparin also can be administered subcutaneously on a twice-daily basis. A total daily dose of about 35,000 units administered as divided doses every 8–12 h usually is sufficient to achieve an aPTT of twice the control value (measured midway between doses). For low-dose heparin therapy (to prevent venous thromboembolism in hospitalized medical or surgical patients), a subcutaneous dose of 5000 units is given two or three times daily.

Heparin Resistance. Patients who fail to achieve a therapeutic aPTT with daily doses of heparin of 35,000 units or more are considered to have heparin resistance, which may reflect pseudo- or true resistance. Concomitant measurement of the aPTT and the anti–factor Xa level distinguishes between these two possibilities. With heparin pseudoresistance, the anti–factor Xa level is therapeutic despite the subtherapeutic aPTT, whereas with true heparin resistance both the anti–factor Xa level and the aPTT are subtherapeutic. Pseudoresistance to heparin occurs if the aPTT is shorter than the control value prior to initiating heparin treatment because of high concentrations of factor VIII and fibrinogen. True heparin resistance occurs because of high plasma levels of proteins that compete with antithrombin for heparin binding or because of antithrombin deficiency. Heparin does not require dose adjustment in patients with pseudoresistance because the anti–factor Xa level is therapeutic. In contrast, with true resistance, heparin doses need to be increased until a therapeutic aPTT or anti-factor Xa level is achieved. Patients with severe antithrombin deficiency may require antithrombin concentrate to achieve therapeutic anticoagulation with heparin.

LMWH Preparations

Enoxaparin and dalteparin are the LMWH preparations marketed in the U.S.; tinzaparin is available in other countries. The composition of these agents differs, as do their dosing regimens. Because LMWH produces a relatively predictable anticoagulant response, monitoring is not done routinely. Patients with renal impairment may require monitoring with an anti–factor Xa assay because this condition can prolong the $t_{1/2}$ and slow the elimination of LMWH. Obese patients, pregnant women, and children given LMWH also may require monitoring.

Fondaparinux

Fondaparinux, a synthetic pentasaccharide, is administered by subcutaneous injection, reaches peak plasma levels in 2 h, has a $t_{1/2}$ of 17 h, and is excreted in the urine. Because of the risk of accumulation and subsequent bleeding, fondaparinux should not be used in patients with a creatinine clearance less than 30 mL/min. Fondaparinux can be given subcutaneously once a day at a fixed or weight-adjusted dose without coagulation monitoring. Fondaparinux is much less likely than heparin or LMWH to trigger heparin-induced thrombocytopenia, and the drug has been used successfully to treat patients with this condition. Fondaparinux is approved for thromboprophylaxis in patients undergoing hip or knee surgery or surgery for hip fracture and for initial therapy of patients with deep vein thrombosis or pulmonary embolism. In some countries, but not the U.S., fondaparinux also is licensed as an alternative to heparin or LMWH in patients with acute coronary syndrome. For this indication and for thromboprophylaxis, fondaparinux is administered subcutaneously once daily at a dose of 2.5 mg.

Bleeding. The major untoward effect of heparin, LMWH, and fondaparinux is bleeding. Major bleeding occurs in 1%–5% of patients treated with intravenous heparin for venous thromboembolism. The incidence of bleeding is somewhat less in patients treated with LMWH for this indication. Often, an underlying cause for bleeding is present, such as recent surgery, trauma, peptic ulcer disease, or platelet dysfunction due to concomitant administration of aspirin or other antiplatelet drugs.

The anticoagulant effect of heparin disappears within hours of discontinuation of the drug. Mild bleeding due to heparin usually can be controlled without administration of an antagonist. If life-threatening hemorrhage occurs, heparin can rapidly be reversed by the intravenous infusion of *protamine sulfate* (a mixture of basic polypeptides isolated from salmon sperm), which binds tightly to heparin and neutralizes its anticoagulant effect. Protamine also interacts with platelets, fibrinogen, and other plasma proteins and may cause an anticoagulant effect of its own. Therefore, one should give the minimal amount of protamine required to neutralize the heparin present in the plasma. This amount is 1 mg of protamine for every 100 units of heparin remaining in the patient; protamine is given intravenously at a slow rate (up to a maximum of 50 mg over 10 min). Protamine binds only long heparin molecules. Therefore, protamine only partially reverses the anticoagulant activity of LMWH and has no effect on that of fondaparinux.

Heparin-Induced Thrombocytopenia. Heparin-induced thrombocytopenia (platelet count < 150,000/mL or a 50% decrease from the pretreatment value) occurs in about 0.5% of medical patients 5–10 days after initiation of therapy with heparin. Although the incidence is lower, thrombocytopenia also occurs with LMWH and rarely with fondaparinux. Life-threatening thrombotic complications that can lead to limb amputation, which occurs in up to one-half of the affected heparin-treated patients and may precede the onset of thrombocytopenia. Women are twice as likely as men to develop this condition, and heparin-induced thrombocytopenia is more common in surgical patients than medical patients.

Venous thromboembolism occurs most commonly, but arterial thrombosis causing limb ischemia, myocardial infarction, or stroke also occurs. Bilateral adrenal hemorrhage, skin lesions at the site of subcutaneous heparin injection, and a variety of systemic reactions may accompany heparin-induced thrombocytopenia. The development of immunoglobulin G antibodies against complexes of heparin with platelet factor 4 (or, rarely, other chemokines) causes most of these reactions.

Heparin or LMWH should be discontinued immediately if unexplained thrombocytopenia or any of the clinical manifestations mentioned occur 5 or more days after beginning therapy, regardless of the dose or route of administration. The diagnosis of heparin-induced thrombocytopenia can be confirmed with a heparin-dependent platelet activation assay or an immunoassay for antibodies that react with heparin–platelet factor 4 complexes. Because thrombotic complications may occur after cessation of therapy, an alternative anticoagulant such as bivalirudin or argatroban (see the next section) or fondaparinux should be administered to patients with heparin-induced thrombocytopenia. LMWH should be avoided because it cross-reacts with heparin antibodies. *Warfarin may precipitate venous limb gangrene or skin necrosis in patients with heparin-induced thrombocytopenia and should not be used until the platelet count returns to normal.*

Other Toxicities. Abnormalities of hepatic function tests occur frequently in patients who are receiving heparin or LMWH. Osteoporosis occurs occasionally in patients who have received therapeutic doses of heparin (>20,000 units/d) for extended periods (e.g., 3–6 months). The risk of osteoporosis is lower with LMWH or fondaparinux than it is with heparin. Heparin can inhibit the synthesis of aldosterone by the adrenal glands and occasionally causes hyperkalemia.

Other Parenteral Anticoagulants

Desirudin and Lepirudin

Desirudin and lepirudin (not available in the U.S.) are recombinant forms of hirudin. Desirudin is indicated for thromboprophylaxis in patients undergoing elective hip replacement surgery. Both desirudin and lepirudin are also used for treating thrombosis in the setting of heparin-induced thrombocytopenia (Kelton et al., 2013). Desirudin and lepirudin are eliminated by the kidneys; the $t_{1/2}$ is about 2 h after subcutaneous administration and about 10 min after intravenous infusion. Both drugs should be used cautiously in patients with decreased renal function, and serum creatinine and aPTT should be monitored daily.

Bivalirudin

Bivalirudin is a synthetic 20–amino acid polypeptide that directly inhibits thrombin. Bivalirudin is administered intravenously and is used as an alternative to heparin in patients undergoing coronary angioplasty or cardiopulmonary bypass surgery (Barria Perez et al. 2016). Patients with heparin-induced thrombocytopenia or a history of this disorder also can be given bivalirudin instead of heparin during coronary angioplasty. The $t_{1/2}$ of bivalirudin is 25 min; dosage reductions are recommended for patients with renal impairment.

Argatroban

Argatroban, a synthetic compound based on the structure of L-arginine, binds reversibly to the active site of thrombin. Argatroban is administered intravenously and has a $t_{1/2}$ of 40–50 min. It is metabolized in the liver and excreted in the bile. Therefore, argatroban can be used in patients with renal impairment, but dose reduction is required for patients with hepatic insufficiency. Argatroban is licensed for the prophylaxis or treatment of patients with, or at risk of developing, heparin-induced thrombocytopenia (Grouzi, 2014). In addition to prolonging the aPTT, argatroban prolongs the PT, which can complicate the transitioning of patients from argatroban to warfarin. A factor X assay can be used instead of the PT to monitor warfarin in these patients.

Vitamin K Antagonist

Warfarin

Warfarin or other vitamin K antagonists are commonly used oral anticoagulants.

Mechanism of Action

Coagulation factors II, VII, IX, and X and proteins C and S are synthesized in the liver and are biologically inactive unless 9–13 of the amino-terminal Glu residues are γ-carboxylated to form the Ca^{2+}-binding Gla domain. This carboxylation reaction requires CO_2, O_2, and reduced vitamin K and is catalyzed by γ-glutamyl carboxylase (Figure 32–6). Carboxylation is coupled to the oxidation of vitamin K to its corresponding epoxide form. Reduced vitamin K must be regenerated from the epoxide form for sustained carboxylation and synthesis of functional proteins. The enzyme that catalyzes this reaction, VKOR is inhibited by therapeutic doses of warfarin.

At therapeutic doses, warfarin decreases the functional amount of each vitamin K–dependent coagulation factor made by the liver by 30%–70%. Warfarin has no effect on the activity of fully γ-carboxylated factors already in the circulation, and these must be cleared before it can produce an anticoagulant effect. The approximate $t_{1/2}$ values of factors VII, IX, X, and II are 6, 24, 36, and 50 h, respectively, while the $t_{1/2}$ values of protein C and protein S are 8 and 24 h, respectively. Because of the long $t_{1/2}$ of some of the coagulation factors, in particular factor II, the full antithrombotic effect of warfarin is not achieved for 4 to 5 days. For this reason, warfarin must be overlapped with a rapidly acting parenteral anticoagulant, such as heparin, LMWH, or fondaparinux, in patients with thrombosis or at high risk for thrombosis.

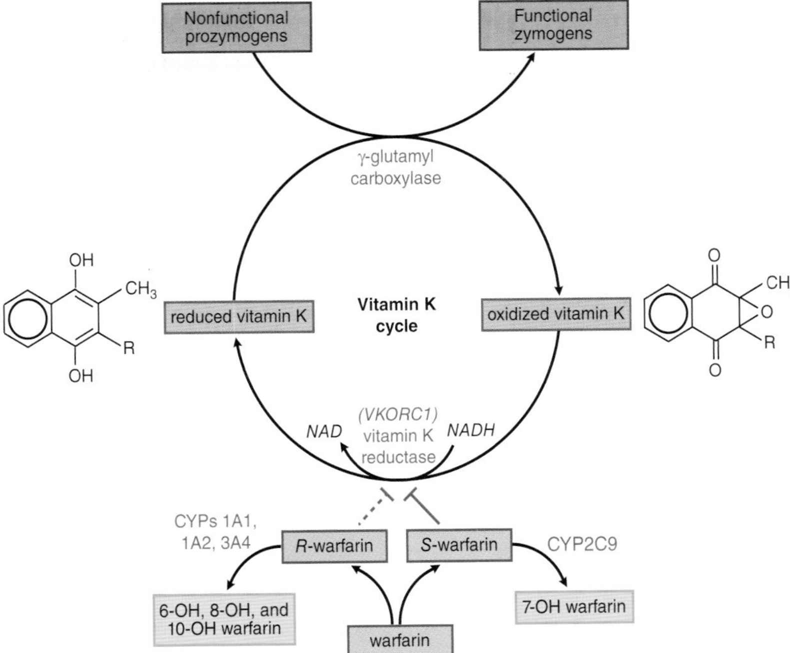

Figure 32–6 *The vitamin K cycle and mechanism of action of warfarin.* In the racemic mixture of *S*- and *R*-enantiomers, *S*-warfarin is more active. By blocking VKOR encoded by the *VKORC1* gene, warfarin inhibits the conversion of oxidized vitamin K epoxide into its reduced form, vitamin K hydroquinone. This inhibits vitamin K–dependent γ-carboxylation of factors II, VII, IX, and X because reduced vitamin K serves as a cofactor for a γ-glutamyl carboxylase that catalyzes the γ-carboxylation process whereby prozymogens are converted to zymogens capable of binding Ca^{2+} and interacting with anionic phospholipids. *S*-Warfarin is metabolized by *CYP2C9*; common genetic polymorphisms in this enzyme increase warfarin metabolism. Polymorphisms in the VKORC1 increase the susceptibility of the enzyme to warfarin-induced inhibition. Thus, patients expressing polymorphisms in these two enzymes require reduction of warfarin dosage (see Table 32–2).

ADME

The bioavailability of warfarin is nearly complete when the drug is administered orally, intravenously, or rectally. Generic warfarin tablets may vary in their rate of dissolution, and this may cause some variation in the rate and extent of absorption. Food in the GI tract also can decrease the rate of absorption. Plasma warfarin concentrations peak in 2–8 h. Warfarin is administered as a racemic mixture of *S*- and *R*-warfarin. *S*-Warfarin is 3- to 5-fold more potent than *R*-warfarin and is mainly metabolized by CYP2C9. Inactive metabolites of warfarin are excreted in urine and stool. The $t_{1/2}$ varies (25–60 h), but the duration of action of warfarin is 2–5 days.

Table 32–2 summarizes the effects of known genetic factors on warfarin dose requirements. Polymorphisms in two genes, *CYP2C9* and *VKORC1* account for most of the genetic contribution to variability in warfarin response (International Warfarin Pharmacogenetics Consortium, 2009; McClain et al., 2008). *CYP2C9* variants affect warfarin pharmacokinetics, whereas *VKORC1* variants affect warfarin pharmacodynamics. Common variations in the *CYP2C9* gene (designated *CYP2C9*2* and **3*), encode an enzyme with decreased activity and thus are associated with higher drug concentrations and reduced warfarin dose requirements. *VKORC1* variants are more prevalent than those of *CYP2C9*, particularly in Asians, followed by European Americans and African Americans (Limdi et al., 2015). The warfarin dose requirement is decreased in patients with these variants (Shi et al., 2015). Point-of-care methods for *CYP2C9* and *VKORC1* genotyping and algorithms that incorporate genotype information have been developed to facilitate precision dosing of warfarin. It remains uncertain, however, whether precision dosing improves clinical outcome compared with usual warfarin management.

Clinical Use

Vitamin K antagonists are used to prevent the progression or recurrence of acute deep vein thrombosis or pulmonary embolism following an initial course of heparin, LMWH, or fondaparinux (Kearon et al., 2016). They also are effective in preventing stroke or systemic embolization in patients with atrial fibrillation, mechanical heart valves, or ventricular assist devices.

Prior to initiation of therapy, laboratory tests are used in conjunction with the history and physical examination to uncover hemostatic defects that might make the use of warfarin more dangerous (e.g., congenital coagulation factor deficiency, thrombocytopenia, hepatic or renal insufficiency, vascular abnormalities). Thereafter, the INR calculated from the patient's PT is used to monitor the extent of anticoagulation and compliance. Therapeutic INR ranges for various clinical indications have been established and reflect the extent of anticoagulation that reduces the morbidity from thromboembolic disease while minimally increasing the risk of serious hemorrhage. For most indications, an INR range of 2–3 is used. A higher INR range (2.5–3.5) is recommended for patients with mechanical heart valves in the mitral position or for patients with mechanical valves in another position who have concomitant atrial fibrillation or a prior history of stroke.

For treatment of acute venous thromboembolism, heparin, LMWH, or fondaparinux usually is continued for at least 5 days after warfarin therapy is begun. The parenteral agent is stopped when the INR is in the therapeutic range on 2 consecutive days. This overlap allows for adequate depletion of vitamin K–dependent coagulation factors with long half-lives, especially factor II. Frequent INR measurements are indicated at the onset of therapy to ensure that a therapeutic effect is obtained. Once a stable dose of warfarin has

TABLE 32–2 ■ EFFECT OF *CYP2C9* GENOTYPES AND *VKORC1* HAPLOTYPES ON WARFARIN DOSING

GENOTYPE/HAPLOTYPE	FREQUENCY (%) CAUCASIANS	AFRICAN AMERICANS	ASIANS	DOSE REDUCTION COMPARED WITH WILD TYPE (%)
CYP2C9				
*1/*1	70	90	95	—
*1/*2	17	2	0	22
*1/*3	9	3	4	34
*2/*2	2	0	0	43
*2/*3	1	0	0	53
*3/*3	0	0	1	76
VKORC1				
Non-A/non-A	37	82	7	—
Non-A/A	45	12	30	26
A/A	18	6	63	50

Polymorphisms in two genes, *CYP2C9* and *VKORC1*, largely account for the genetic contribution to the variability in warfarin response. *CYP2C9* variants affect warfarin pharmacokinetics. *CYP2C9* metabolizes warfarin, and the non-*1/*1 variants are less active than *CYP2C9**1/*1, necessitating a reduction in dose. *VKORC1* variants affect warfarin pharmacodynamics. *VKORC1* is the target of coumarin anticoagulants such as warfarin. The non-A/A and A/A forms have decreased requirements for warfarin.

Source: Ghimire LV, Stein CM. Warfarin pharmacogenetics. Goodman and Gilman Online.

been identified, the INR can be monitored every 3 to 4 weeks.

Dosage

The usual adult dosage of warfarin is 2–5 mg/d for 2–4 days, followed by 1–10 mg/d as indicated by measurements of the INR (see the functional definition of INR in the section on clinical use). A lower initial dose should be given to patients with an increased risk of bleeding, including the elderly.

Interactions

Warfarin interactions can be caused by drugs, foods, or genetic factors that alter (1) uptake or metabolism of warfarin or vitamin K; (2) synthesis, function, or clearance of clotting factors; or (3), the integrity of any epithelial surface. Reduced warfarin efficacy can occur because of reduced absorption (e.g., binding to cholestyramine in the GI tract) or increased hepatic clearance from induction of hepatic enzymes (e.g., *CYP2C9* induction by barbiturates, carbamazepine, or rifampin). Warfarin has a decreased volume of distribution and a short $t_{1/2}$ with hypoproteinemia, such as occurs with nephrotic syndrome. Relative warfarin resistance can also be caused by ingestion of large amounts of vitamin K–rich foods or supplements or by increased levels of coagulation factors during pregnancy.

Drug interactions that enhance the risk of hemorrhage in patients taking warfarin include decreased metabolism due to *CYP2C9* inhibition by amiodarone, azole antifungals, cimetidine, clopidogrel, cotrimoxazole, disulfiram, fluoxetine, isoniazid, metronidazole, sulfinpyrazone, tolcapone, or zafirlukast. Relative deficiency of vitamin K may result from inadequate diet (e.g., postoperative patients on parenteral fluids), especially when coupled with the elimination of intestinal flora by antimicrobial agents. Gut bacteria synthesize vitamin K and are an important source of this vitamin. Consequently, antibiotics can cause an increase in the INR in patients on warfarin. Low concentrations of coagulation factors may result from impaired hepatic function, congestive heart failure, or hypermetabolic states, such as hyperthyroidism; generally, these conditions enhance the effect of warfarin on the INR. Serious interactions that do not alter the INR include inhibition of platelet function by agents such as *aspirin* and gastritis or frank ulceration induced by anti-inflammatory drugs. Agents may have more than one effect (e.g., clofibrate increases the rate of turnover of coagulation factors and inhibits platelet function).

Hypersensitivity to Warfarin

About 10% of patients require less than 1.5 mg/d of warfarin to achieve an INR of 2–3. These patients often possess variants of *CYP2C9* or *VKORC1*; these affect the pharmacokinetics or pharmacodynamics of warfarin, respectively. Supplementation with low daily doses of vitamin K renders these patients less sensitive to warfarin and may result in more stable dosing.

Adverse Effects

Bleeding. The most common side effect of warfarin is bleeding. The risk of bleeding increases with the intensity and duration of anticoagulant therapy, the use of other medications that interfere with hemostasis, and the presence of an anatomical source of bleeding. The incidence of major bleeding episodes is generally less than 3% per year in patients treated to a target INR of 2–3. The risk of intracranial hemorrhage increases dramatically with an INR greater than 4, although up to two-thirds of intracranial bleeds on warfarin occur when the INR is therapeutic.

If the INR is above the therapeutic range and the patient is not bleeding or in need of a surgical procedure, warfarin can be held temporarily and restarted at a lower dose once the INR is within the therapeutic range. If the INR is 10 or greater, vitamin K_1 can be given orally at a dose of 2.5 to 5 mg. These doses of oral vitamin K_1 generally cause the INR to decrease substantially within 24–48 h without rendering the patient resistant to further warfarin therapy. Higher doses or parenteral administration may be required if more rapid correction of the INR is necessary. The effect of vitamin K_1 is delayed for at least several hours because reversal of anticoagulation requires synthesis of fully carboxylated coagulation factors. If immediate hemostatic competence is necessary because of serious bleeding or profound warfarin overdosage, adequate concentrations of vitamin K–dependent coagulation factors can be restored by transfusion of four-factor prothrombin complex concentrate, supplemented with 10 mg of vitamin K_1, given by slow intravenous infusion. Vitamin K_1 administered intravenously carries the risk of anaphylactoid reactions. Patients who receive high doses of vitamin K_1 may become unresponsive to warfarin for several days, but heparin or LMWH can be given if continued anticoagulation is required.

Birth Defects. Administration of warfarin during pregnancy causes birth defects and abortion. CNS abnormalities have been reported following exposure during the second and third trimesters. Fetal or neonatal hemorrhage and intrauterine death may occur, even when maternal INR values are within the therapeutic range. Vitamin K antagonists should not be used during pregnancy, but heparin or LMWH can be used safely.

Skin Necrosis. Warfarin-induced skin necrosis is a rare complication characterized by the appearance of skin lesions 3–10 days after treatment is initiated. The lesions typically are on the extremities, but adipose tissue, the penis, and the female breast also may be involved. Skin necrosis occurs in patients with protein C or S deficiency or in those with heparin-induced thrombocytopenia.

Other Toxicities. A reversible, sometimes painful, blue-tinged discoloration of the plantar surfaces and sides of the toes that blanches with pressure and fades with elevation of the legs (purple toe syndrome) may develop 3–8 weeks after initiation of therapy with warfarin; cholesterol emboli released from atheromatous plaques have been implicated as the cause. Other infrequent reactions include alopecia, urticaria, dermatitis, fever, nausea, diarrhea, abdominal cramps, and anorexia.

Direct Oral Anticoagulants

Direct Oral Thrombin Inhibitor

Dabigatran

Dabigatran etexilate is a synthetic prodrug with a molecular weight of 628 Da.

Mechanism of Action. Dabigatran etexilate is rapidly converted to dabigatran by plasma esterases. Dabigatran competitively and reversibly blocks the active site of free and clot-bound thrombin. In turn, this blocks thrombin-mediated conversion of fibrinogen to fibrin, feedback activation of coagulation, and platelet activation.

ADME. Dabigatran has oral bioavailability of about 6%, a peak onset of action in 2 h, and a plasma $t_{1/2}$ of 12–14 h. Dabigatran is given twice a day in capsule form. The bioavailability of the drug is altered if capsules are chewed or broken prior to ingestion. Therefore, the capsules should be swallowed whole. Circulating dabigatran is 35% bound to plasma proteins. Around 80% of absorbed dabigatran is excreted unchanged by the kidneys. A dosage reduction is required when dabigatran is administered to patients with severe renal impairment (creatinine clearance 15 to 30 mL/min). Dosage recommendations are not available for patients with a creatinine clearance below 15 mL/min.

When given in fixed doses, dabigatran etexilate produces such a predictable anticoagulant response that routine coagulation monitoring is unnecessary. Although dabigatran prolongs the aPTT, the values plateau with higher drug levels. Dabigatran has an unreliable effect on the INR. The thrombin time is too sensitive to use to monitor dabigatran therapy because the test is markedly prolonged with even low levels of drug. To circumvent this problem, a diluted thrombin time assay has been developed. By comparing the results with those obtained with dabigatran calibrators, this test can be used to quantify plasma dabigatran concentrations.

Therapeutic Uses. Dabigatran is licensed for treatment of acute venous thromboembolism after at least 5 days of parenteral anticoagulation with heparin, LMWH, or fondaparinux (Schulman et al., 2009) and for secondary prevention of venous thromboembolism (Beyer-Westendorf and Ageno, 2015; Gomez-Outes et al., 2015). Dabigatran also is licensed for stroke prevention in patients with nonvalvular atrial fibrillation (Connolly et al., 2009). It is contraindicated in patients with mechanical heart valves (Eikelboom et al., 2013). In some countries, lower-dose regimens of once-daily dabigatran are licensed for thromboprophylaxis after knee or hip arthroplasty. Dabigatran is contraindicated for stroke prevention in patients with mechanical heart valves.

Adverse Effects. Bleeding is the major side effect of dabigatran. In elderly patients with atrial fibrillation, the annual risk of major bleeding with dabigatran 150 mg twice daily is similar to that with warfarin, about 3.0%. However, the risk of intracranial bleeding is reduced by 70% with dabigatran compared with warfarin. In contrast, the risk of GI bleeding is higher with dabigatran, particularly in those over 75 years of age. Additional risks for bleeding with dabigatran include renal impairment and concurrent use of antiplatelet agents or nonsteroidal anti-inflammatory drugs.

Drug Interactions. Dabigatran is a substrate for P-glycoprotein, so drugs that inhibit or induce P-glycoprotein have the potential to increase or decrease plasma dabigatran concentrations, respectively. Verapamil, dronedarone, quinidine, ketoconazole, and clarithromycin can increase dabigatran concentrations, while rifampicin may decrease the concentration.

Direct Oral Factor Xa Inhibitors

Rivaroxaban, Apixaban, and Edoxban

Mechanism of Action. Rivaroxaban, apixaban, and edoxaban inhibit free and clot-associated factor Xa, which results in reduced thrombin generation. In turn, platelet aggregation and fibrin formation are suppressed.

ADME. Rivaroxaban has 80% oral bioavailability, a peak onset of action in 3 h, and a plasma $t_{1/2}$ of 7–11 h. Maximum absorption of rivaroxaban occurs in the stomach, and when given in therapeutic doses, the drug should be administered with a meal to enhance absorption. Rivaroxaban is provided in tablet form; the tablet can be crushed and delivered via nasogastric tube. Rivaroxaban is 95% plasma protein bound. About one-third of the drug is excreted unchanged in the urine; the remainder is metabolized by the hepatic CYP3A4 system, and inactive metabolites are excreted equally in the urine and feces. Rivaroxaban exposure is increased in patients with renal impairment or severe hepatic dysfunction. The therapeutic dose of rivaroxaban is reduced from 20 mg once daily to 15 mg once daily if the creatinine clearance is 15–50 mL/min. The drug should not be used in those with a lower creatinine clearance.

The bioavailability of apixaban is around 50%, and peak concentrations are achieved 1 to 3 h after ingestion. Food does not affect absorption, and the drug can be administered as a whole tablet or the tablet can be crushed in water and delivered via a nasogastric tube. Apixaban is 87% plasma protein bound, and about 27% of the drug is cleared unchanged via the kidneys. Apixaban is metabolized by the hepatic CYP3A4 system, and metabolites are excreted in the bile, intestines, and urine. The usual dose of apixaban is 5 mg twice daily. The dose is reduced to 2.5 mg twice daily in patients who have two of the following three characteristics: age over 80 years, body weight of 60 kg or less, or serum creatinine concentration of 1.5 mg/dL or higher. In patients with acute venous thromboembolism, patients start apixaban at a dose of 10 mg twice daily for 7 days, and the dose is then decreased to 5 mg twice daily thereafter. For those requiring treatment beyond 6 to 12 months, the apixaban dose can be decreased to 2.5 mg twice daily.

The bioavailability of edoxaban is 62%, and peak drug concentrations are achieved 1 to 2 h after ingestion. Food does not affect absorption. Edoxaban is 55% protein bound. Of the absorbed edoxaban, about 50% is eliminated as unchanged drug in the urine. There is minimal hepatic metabolism, and liver disease does not affect drug pharmacodynamics. Drug exposure is increased by renal impairment, low body weight, and concomitant intake of potent P-glycoprotein inhibitors. Therefore, the dose of edoxaban should be reduced from 60 to 30 mg once daily in patients with a creatinine clearance between 15 and 50 mL/min, in those with a body weight of 60 kg or less, or in those taking quinidine, dronedarone, rifampin, erythromycin, ketoconazole, or cyclosporine. Edoxaban is contraindicated in those with a creatinine clearance below 15 mL/min. Edoxaban is also not recommended in patients with a high creatinine clearance over 95 mL/min because of increased risk of ischemic stroke compared with warfarin.

Rivaroxaban, apixaban, and edoxaban are given in fixed doses and do not require routine coagulation monitoring. The drugs affect the PT more than the aPTT, but they prolong the PT to a variable extent, and this test does not provide a reliable measure of their anticoagulant activity. Anti–factor Xa assays using specific drug calibrators can be used to measure drug levels. Renal function should be assessed at least yearly in patients taking oral factor Xa inhibitors or more frequently in patients with renal dysfunction.

Therapeutic Uses. Rivaroxaban, apixaban, and edoxaban are licensed for stroke prevention in patients with atrial fibrillation (Giugliano et al., 2013; Granger et al., 2011; Patel et al., 2011) and for treatment of acute deep vein thrombosis or pulmonary embolism (Beyer-Westendorf and Ageno, 2015; Gomez-Outes et al., 2015). For the last indication, edoxaban is only started after a minimum 5-day course of treatment with heparin, LMWH, or fondaparinux (Hokusai VTE Investigators, 2013). In contrast, rivaroxaban and apixaban can be started immediately without the need for heparin bridging (EINSTEIN investigators, 2010, 2012; Granziera et al., 2016). Rivaroxaban and apixaban are also licensed for postoperative thromboprophylaxis in patients undergoing hip or knee arthroplasty (Falck-Ytter et al., 2012); for this indication, the drugs are given at doses of 10 mg once daily and 2.5 mg twice daily, respectively. All three drugs are contraindicated for stroke prevention in patients with mechanical heart valves.

Adverse Effects. As with all anticoagulants, the major adverse effect is bleeding. Rates of intracranial bleeding with rivaroxaban, apixaban, and edoxaban are at least 50% lower than that with warfarin. Rates of bleeding in other sites are similar or lower than those with warfarin. The sole exception is the GI tract; rates of GI bleeding with rivaroxaban and edoxaban, but not apixaban, are higher than that with warfarin. The explanation for this difference is uncertain, but it may reflect the capacity of unabsorbed anticoagulant in the gut to promote bleeding from preexisting lesions. Despite the increased risk of GI bleeding, rates of life-threatening and fatal bleeding are lower with all of the oral factor Xa inhibitors than with warfarin. Like with other anticoagulants, the risk of bleeding with rivaroxaban, apixaban, or edoxaban is increased in patients taking concomitant antiplatelet agents or nonsteroidal anti-inflammatory agents.

Drug Interactions. All of the oral factor Xa inhibitors are substrates for P-glycoprotein. Consequently, potent inhibitors or inducers of P-glycoprotein will increase or decrease drug concentrations, respectively. Rivaroxaban and apixaban are metabolized by CYP3A4, whereas edoxaban undergoes only minimal CYP3A4-mediated metabolism. Plasma levels of rivaroxaban and apixaban are reduced by potent inducers of both P-glycoprotein and CYP3A4, such as carbamazepine, phenytoin, rifampin, and St. John's wort and increased by potent inhibitors, such as dronedarone, ketoconazole, itraconazole, ritonavir, clarithromycin, erythromycin, and cyclosporine.

Reversal Agents for Direct Oral Anticoagulants

Life-threatening bleeding can occur with the direct oral anticoagulants, and patients taking these drugs may require urgent surgery or interventions. Therefore, the availability of specific reversal agents streamlines the management of such patients. Idarucizumab, the reversal agent for dabigatran, is licensed. Andexanet alfa, a reversal agent for rivaroxaban, apixaban, and edoxaban, is in advanced phase 3 evaluation, while ciraparantag, a potential reversal agent for all of the direct anticoagulants, is at an earlier stage of development.

If specific reversal agents are not available, prothrombin complex concentrate, activated prothrombin complex concentrate, or recombinant factor VIIa have been recommended to manage patients taking dabigatran, rivaroxaban, apixaban, or edoxaban who present with life-threatening bleeding, such as intracranial or pericardial bleeding. In patients taking dabigatran who present with serious bleeding in the setting of acute renal failure, hemodialysis can be used to remove dabigatran from the circulation. Dialysis is of no value for removal of rivaroxaban, apixaban or edoxaban because of their higher protein binding.

Idarucizumab

A specific reversal agent for dabigatran, idarucizumab is a humanized mouse monoclonal antibody fragment directed against dabigatran. The antibody binds dabigatran with an affinity 350-fold higher than that of dabigatran for thrombin, and the essentially irreversible idarucizumab-dabigatran complex is cleared by the kidneys. Idarucizumab is infused as two intravenous boluses, each of 2.5 g. It rapidly reverses the anticoagulant effects of dabigatran, and patients have then safely undergone major surgery (Pollack et al., 2015).

Andexanet Alfa

Designed as a decoy for the oral factor Xa inhibitors, andexanet alfa is a recombinant analogue of factor Xa that has the active site serine residue replaced with an alanine residue to eliminate catalytic activity and the Gla domain removed to preclude its incorporation in the prothrombinase complex. Andexanet is administered as an intravenous bolus followed by a 2-h infusion. By sequestering circulating factor Xa inhibitors, andexanet rapidly reverses the anti–factor Xa activity produced by these agents and restores thrombin generation (Siegal et al., 2015). Higher doses of andexanet are needed to reverse rivaroxaban or edoxaban than apixaban. An ongoing phase 3 study is evaluating the effect of andexanet in patients taking these agents who present with serious bleeding.

Ciraparantag

Ciraparantag is a synthetic, small cationic molecule that is reported to bind dabigatran, rivaroxaban, apixaban, and edoxaban, as well as heparin and LMWH. In healthy volunteers given edoxaban, an intravenous bolus of ciraparantag restored the whole-blood clotting time to normal. Ciraparantag has yet to be evaluated in patients.

Fibrinolytic Drugs

Fibrinolytic drugs initiate the fibrinolytic pathway, which is summarized in Figure 32–3. These agents include recombinant t-PA and its variants, urokinase and streptokinase, although the latter are rarely used.

Tissue Plasminogen Activator

Tissue plasminogen activator is a serine protease and a poor plasminogen activator in the absence of fibrin. When bound to fibrin, t-PA activates fibrin-bound plasminogen several 100-fold more rapidly than it activates plasminogen in the circulation. Because it has little activity except in the presence of fibrin, physiological t-PA concentrations of 5–10 ng/mL do not induce systemic plasmin generation. With therapeutic infusion of recombinant t-PA, the concentrations rise to 300–3000 ng/mL, which can induce systemic fibrinogen degradation. Clearance of t-PA primarily occurs via hepatic metabolism, and its $t_{1/2}$ is about 5 min. t-PA is effective for treatment of acute myocardial infarction (Gara et al., 2013), acute ischemic stroke, and life-threatening pulmonary embolism (Meyer et al., 2014).

For coronary thrombolysis, t-PA is given as a 15-mg intravenous bolus, followed by 0.75 mg/kg over 30 min (not to exceed 50 mg) and 0.5 mg/kg (up to 35 mg accumulated dose) over the following hour. Recombinant variants of t-PA include *reteplase* and *tenecteplase*. They differ from native t-PA by having longer plasma half-lives that allow convenient bolus dosing. In addition, in contrast to t-PA, tenecteplase is relatively resistant to inhibition by PAI-1. Despite these apparent advantages, these agents are similar to t-PA in efficacy and toxicity.

Hemorrhagic Toxicity of Thrombolytic Therapy

The major toxicity of all thrombolytic agents is hemorrhage. It is due to (1) degradation of fibrin in hemostatic plugs at sites of vascular injury or (2) the systemic lytic state that results from the systemic generation of plasmin, which degrades fibrinogen and other coagulation factors, especially factors V and VIII. Contraindications to fibrinolytic therapy are listed in Table 32–3.

If heparin is used concurrently with t-PA, serious hemorrhage will occur in 2%–4% of patients. Intracranial hemorrhage is the most serious problem and can occur in up to 1% of patients. For this reason, mechanical reperfusion is preferred over systemic thrombolysis in patients with acute myocardial infarction with ST-segment elevation. In patients with acute ischemic stroke, the current standard of care is mechanical thrombus extraction, which can be done with or without adjunctive t-PA or tenecteplase.

TABLE 32–3 ■ ABSOLUTE AND RELATIVE CONTRAINDICATIONS TO FIBRINOLYTIC THERAPY

Absolute Contraindications

- Prior intracranial hemorrhage
- Known structural cerebral vascular lesion
- Known malignant intracranial neoplasm
- Ischemic stroke within 3 months
- Suspected aortic dissection
- Active bleeding or bleeding diathesis (excluding menses)
- Significant closed-head trauma or facial trauma within 3 months

Relative Contraindications

- Uncontrolled hypertension (systolic blood pressure > 180 mm Hg or diastolic blood pressure > 110 mm Hg)
- Traumatic or prolonged CPR or major surgery within 3 weeks
- Recent (within 2–4 weeks) internal bleeding
- Noncompressible vascular punctures
- For streptokinase: prior exposure (more than 5 days ago) or prior allergic reaction to streptokinase
- Pregnancy
- Active peptic ulcer
- Current use of warfarin and INR > 1.7

Inhibitors of Fibrinolysis

ε-Aminocaproic Acid and Tranexamic Acid

ε-Aminocaproic acid and tranexamic acid are lysine analogues that compete for lysine binding sites on plasminogen and plasmin, thereby blocking their interaction with fibrin. Therefore, these agents inhibit fibrinolysis and can reverse states that are associated with excessive fibrinolysis.

The main problem with their use is that thrombi that form during treatment are not degraded. For example, in patients with hematuria, ureteral obstruction by clots may lead to renal failure after treatment with ε-aminocaproic acid or tranexamic acid. ε-Aminocaproic acid has been used intravenously to reduce bleeding after prostatic surgery and orally to reduce bleeding after tooth extractions in hemophiliacs. ε-Aminocaproic acid is absorbed rapidly after oral administration, and 50% is excreted unchanged in the urine within 12 h. For intravenous use, a loading dose of 4–5 g is given over 1 h, followed by an infusion of 1–1.25 g/h until bleeding is controlled. No more than 30 g should be given in a 24-h period. Rarely, the drug causes myopathy and muscle necrosis.

Tranexamic acid is given intravenously in trauma resuscitation and in patients with massive hemorrhage (CRASH2 trial investigators, 2010). It is also used to reduce operative bleeding in patients undergoing hip or knee arthroplasty or cardiac surgery. There appears to be little or no increased risk of thrombosis. Tranexamic acid is excreted in the urine; therefore, dose reduction is necessary in patients with renal impairment. Oral tranexamic acid is approved for treatment of heavy menstrual bleeding, usually given at a dose of 1 g four times daily for 4 days.

Antiplatelet Drugs

Platelet aggregates form the initial hemostatic plug at sites of vascular injury. Platelets also contribute to the pathological thrombi that lead to myocardial infarction, stroke, and peripheral arterial thrombosis. Potent inhibitors of platelet function have been developed in recent years. These drugs act by discrete mechanisms (Figure 32–7); thus, in combination, their effects are additive or even synergistic.

Aspirin

In platelets, the major COX-1 product is TxA_2, a labile inducer of platelet aggregation and a potent vasoconstrictor. Aspirin blocks production of TxA_2 by acetylating a serine residue near the active site of platelet COX-1.

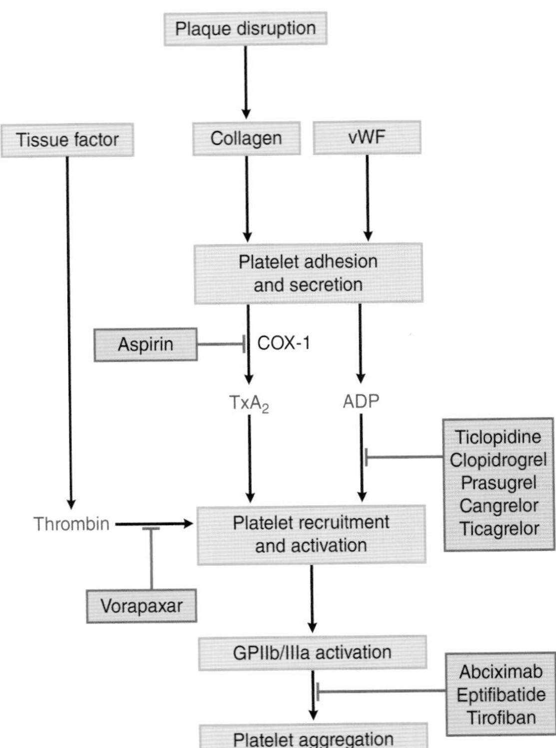

Figure 32–7 *Sites of action of antiplatelet drugs.* Aspirin inhibits TxA_2 synthesis by irreversibly acetylating COX-1. Reduced TxA_2 release attenuates platelet activation and recruitment to the site of vascular injury. Ticlopidine, clopidogrel, and prasugrel irreversibly block $P2Y_{12}$, a key ADP receptor on the platelet surface; cangrelor and ticagrelor are reversible inhibitors of $P2Y_{12}$. Abciximab, eptifibatide, and tirofiban inhibit the final common pathway of platelet aggregation by blocking fibrinogen and vWF from binding to activated GPIIb/IIIa. Vorapaxar inhibits thrombin-mediated platelet activation by targeting PAR-1, the major thrombin receptor on platelets.

Because platelets do not synthesize new proteins, the action of aspirin on platelet COX-1 is permanent, lasting for the lifetime of the platelet (7–10 days). Thus, repeated doses of aspirin produce a cumulative effect on platelet function.

Complete inactivation of platelet COX-1 is achieved with a daily aspirin dose of 75 mg. Therefore, aspirin is maximally effective as an antithrombotic agent at doses much lower than those required for other actions of the drug. Numerous trials indicated that aspirin, when used as an antithrombotic drug, is maximally effective at doses of 50–325 mg/d. Higher doses do not improve efficacy and potentially are less efficacious because of inhibition of prostacyclin production, which can be largely spared by using lower doses of aspirin. Higher doses also increase toxicity, especially bleeding. Therefore, daily aspirin doses of 100 mg or less are used for most indications (Cohen et al., 2015; Ittaman et al., 2014). Nonsteroidal anti-inflammatory drugs that are reversible inhibitors of COX-1 have not been shown to have antithrombotic efficacy and in fact may even interfere with low-dose aspirin regimens (see Chapters 37 and 38).

Dipyridamole

Dipyridamole interferes with platelet function by increasing the intracellular concentration of cyclic AMP. This effect is mediated by inhibition of phosphodiesterase or by blockade of uptake of adenosine, thereby increasing the dwell time of adenosine at cell surface adenosine A_2 receptors that link to the stimulation of platelet adenylyl cyclase. Dipyridamole is a vasodilator that, in combination with warfarin, inhibits embolization from prosthetic heart valves. Dipyridamole is approved for secondary prevention of stroke when it is combined with low-dose aspirin.

$P2Y_{12}$ Receptor Antagonists

Clopidogrel

Clopidogrel is a thienopyridine prodrug that inhibits the $P2Y_{12}$ receptor. Platelets contain two purinergic receptors, $P2Y_1$ and $P2Y_{12}$; both are G protein–coupled receptors for ADP. The ADP-activated platelet $P2Y_1$ receptor couples to the G_q-PLC-IP_3–Ca^{2+} pathway and induces a shape change and aggregation. The $P2Y_{12}$ receptor couples to G_i and, when activated by ADP, inhibits adenylyl cyclase, resulting in lower levels of intracellular cyclic AMP and thereby less cyclic AMP–dependent inhibition of platelet activation. Both receptors must be stimulated to result in maximal platelet activation.

Clopidogrel is an irreversible inhibitor of $P2Y_{12}$. It has largely replaced ticlopidine because clopidogrel is more potent and less toxic, with thrombocytopenia and leukopenia occurring only rarely. Clopidogrel is a prodrug that requires metabolic activation in the liver. Therefore, it has a slow onset of action. It also has a slow offset of action because of its irreversible effect on $P2Y_{12}$. Metabolic activation of clopidogrel can be affected by polymorphisms in *CYP2C19* that result in reduced or absent CYP2C19 activity. These polymorphisms contribute to the variable effect of clopidogrel on ADP-induced platelet aggregation. Inhibition of platelet activation is seen 2 h postingestion of a loading dose of clopidogrel, and platelets are affected for the remainder of their life span.

Therapeutic Uses. Clopidogrel is somewhat better than aspirin for secondary prevention of stroke, and the combination of clopidogrel plus aspirin is superior to aspirin alone for prevention of recurrent ischemia in patients with unstable angina. The FDA-approved indications for clopidogrel are to reduce the rate of stroke, myocardial infarction, and death in patients with recent myocardial infarction or stroke, established peripheral artery disease, or acute coronary syndrome (Amsterdam et al., 2014; Gara et al., 2013; Park et al., 2016; Roffi et al., 2015; Zhang et al., 2015). Clopidogrel is often used in combination with aspirin after coronary stent implantation.

Adverse Effects. Clopidogrel increases the risk of bleeding, particularly when combined with aspirin or an anticoagulant. Thrombotic thrombocytopenic purpura can occur but is rare.

Drug Interactions. CYP219 inhibition by proton pump inhibitors (e.g., omeprazole, lansoprazole, deslansprazole, and pantoprazole) may reduce conversion to the active metabolite of clopidogrel, which may contribute to the lower efficacy of clopidogrel when coadministered with proton pump inhibitors.

Prasugrel

The newest member of the thienopyridine class, prasugrel is a prodrug that requires metabolic activation in the liver. However, because the activation of prasugrel is more efficient than that of clopidogrel, prasugrel has a more rapid onset of action, and it produces greater and more predictable inhibition of ADP-induced platelet aggregation.

Prasugrel is rapidly and completely absorbed from the gut. It is hydrolyzed in the intestine to a thiolactone, which is then converted to the active metabolite in the liver. Virtually all of the absorbed prasugrel undergoes activation; by comparison, only 15% of absorbed clopidogrel undergoes metabolic activation. Because the active metabolites of prasugrel bind irreversibly to the $P2Y_{12}$ receptor, its effect lasts the lifetime of the platelets. This slow offset of action can be problematic if patients require urgent surgery. Prasugrel is inactivated by methylation or conjugation with cysteine. Moderate renal or hepatic impairment does not appear to change the drug pharmacodynamics.

Therapeutic Uses. Prasugrel is indicated to reduce the rate of thrombotic cardiovascular events (including stent thrombosis) in patients with acute coronary syndrome who are managed with percutaneous coronary intervention (Gara et al., 2013; Guimaraúes and Tricoci, 2015; Lhermusier and Waksman, 2015). The incidence of cardiovascular death, myocardial infarction, and stroke is significantly lower with prasugrel than with clopidogrel, mainly reflecting a reduction in the incidence of nonfatal myocardial infarction. The incidence of stent thrombosis is also lower with prasugrel than with clopidogrel.

Adverse Effects. Prasugrel is associated with higher rates of fatal and life-threatening bleeding than clopidogrel. Because patients with a history of a prior stroke or transient ischemic attack are at particularly high risk of intracranial bleeding, the drug is contraindicated in such patients. Patients over 75 years of age should not be prescribed prasugrel because of the increased bleeding risk. After a loading dose of 60 mg, prasugrel is given once daily at a dose of 10 mg. The daily dose should be reduced to 5 mg in patients weighing less than 60 kg. No dose adjustment is required in patients with hepatic or renal impairment. If patients present with serious bleeding, platelet transfusion may be beneficial. Prasugrel has been reported to cause thrombotic thrombocytopenic purpura.

Drug Interactions. Concomitant administration of prasugrel with an anticoagulant or nonsteroidal anti-inflammatory drugs increases the risk of bleeding.

Ticagrelor

Ticagrelor is an orally active, reversible inhibitor of $P2Y_{12}$. The drug is given twice daily and not only has a more rapid onset and offset of action than clopidogrel, but also produces greater and more predictable inhibition of ADP-induced platelet aggregation. The bioavailability of ticagrelor is about 36%. It can be given as a whole tablet or crushed in water and administered via a nasogastric tube. Ticagrelor is metabolized by hepatic CYP3A4.

Therapeutic Uses. Ticagrelor is FDA-approved for reduction in the risk of cardiovascular death, myocardial infarction, and stroke in patients with acute coronary syndrome (Gara et al., 2013) or a history of myocardial infarction (Dobesh and Oestreich, 2014). In contrast to prasugrel in patients with acute coronary syndrome, which is only indicated in those undergoing percutaneous intervention, ticagrelor is indicated in those undergoing intervention and in those managed medically.

Adverse Effects. Dyspnea is reported in 17% of patients. This is often transient and not associated with pulmonary disease. Ticagrelor is associated with a higher risk of intracranial bleeding than clopidogrel and is contraindicated in patients with a history of prior intracranial bleeding. Platelet transfusion is ineffective in patients taking ticagrelor who present with serious bleeding, and a neutralizing antibody is under investigation for urgent reversal.

Drug Interactions. Concomitant aspirin at a dose greater than 100 mg daily may reduce the effectiveness of ticagrelor. Potent inhibitors of CYP3A (such as ketoconazole, itraconazole, voriconazole, clarithromycin, nefazodone, ritonavir, saquinavir, nelfinavir, indinavir, atazanavir, and telithromycin) and strong inducers of CYP3A (such as rifampin, phenytoin, carbamazepine, and phenobarbital) should be avoided. Ticagrelor increases serum concentrations of simvastatin and lovastatin and may affect digoxin metabolism.

Cangrelor

Cangrelor is a parenteral reversible inhibitor of $P2Y_{12}$. When administered intravenously as a bolus followed by an infusion, cangrelor inhibits ADP-induced platelet aggregation within minutes, and its effect on platelet aggregation disappears within 1 h of discontinuation of the drug. Cangrelor has a short half-life because it is rapidly dephosphorylated in the circulation to an inactive metabolite.

Therapeutic Use. Cangrelor is indicated for reduction in the risk of periprocedural myocardial infarction, repeat coronary revascularization, and stent thrombosis in patients undergoing percutaneous coronary intervention who have not been treated with an oral $P2Y_{12}$ inhibitor and are not given a glycoprotein IIb/IIIa antagonist (Keating et al., 2015).

Adverse Effects. The risk of bleeding with cangrelor is greater than that with clopidogrel during the coronary intervention.

Drug Interactions. Coadministered clopidogrel or prasugrel will have no antiplatelet effect. Administration of ticagrelor, prasugrel, or clopidogrel should be delayed until the cangrelor infusion is stopped.

Thrombin Receptor Inhibitor

There are two major thrombin receptors on the platelet surface, PAR-1 and PAR-4, respectively. Thrombin binds to these G protein–coupled receptors and cleaves them at their amino terminals. The newly created amino terminals then serve as tethered ligands to activate the receptors. PAR-1 is activated by lower concentrations of thrombin than are required to activate PAR-4.

Vorapaxar

Vorapaxar is a competitive antagonist of PAR-1 and inhibits thrombin-induced platelet aggregation. The drug is 90% bioavailable and has a rapid onset of action and a circulating half-life of 3 or 4 days. However, because vorapaxar remains tightly bound to PAR-1 on platelets, its effect on thrombin-induced platelet aggregation can persist for up to 4 weeks after the drug is stopped. Vorapaxar is metabolized in the liver by CYP3A4.

Therapeutic Uses. Vorapaxar is given orally in combination with either aspirin or clopidogrel. It is indicated for the reduction of thrombotic cardiovascular events in patients with a history of myocardial infarction or peripheral artery disease (Arif et al., 2015; Moschonas et al., 2015).

Adverse Effects. Vorapaxar increases the risk of bleeding and is contraindicated in patients with a history of intracranial bleeding, stroke, or transient ischemic attack.

Drug Interactions. Potent CYP3A4 inducers, such as rifampin, reduce drug exposure, while strong CYP3A4 inhibitors, such as ketoconazole, increase drug exposure. Antacids and pantoprazole reduce drug exposure.

Glycoprotein IIb/IIIa Inhibitors

Glycoprotein IIb/IIIa is a platelet-surface integrin, designated $\alpha_{IIb}\beta_3$ by the integrin nomenclature. This dimeric glycoprotein undergoes a conformational transformation when platelets are activated to serve as a receptor for fibrinogen and von Willebrand factor, which anchor platelets to each other, thereby mediating aggregation (Figure 32-1). Thus, inhibitors of this receptor are potent antiplatelet agents that act by a mechanism distinct from that of aspirin or $P2Y_{12}$ or PAR-1 inhibitors. Three agents are approved for use at present; their features are highlighted in Table 32-4. The use of these agents has decreased with the availability of potent $P2Y_{12}$ inhibitors such as prasugrel and ticagrelor.

Abciximab

Abciximab is the Fab fragment of a humanized monoclonal antibody directed against the $\alpha_{IIb}\beta_3$ receptor. It also binds to the vitronectin receptor on platelets, vascular endothelial cells, and smooth muscle cells.

The antibody is administered to patients undergoing percutaneous coronary intervention and, when used in conjunction with aspirin and heparin, has been shown to prevent recurrent myocardial infarction and death (Gara et al., 2013; Roffi et al., 2015). The $t_{1/2}$ of the circulating antibody is about 30 min, but antibody remains bound to the $\alpha_{IIb}\beta_3$ receptor and inhibits platelet aggregation as measured in vitro for 18–24 h after infusion. It is given as a 0.25-mg/kg bolus followed by an infusion of 0.125 μg/kg/min (maximum 10 μg/kg/min) for 12 to 24 h.

Adverse Effects. The major side effect of abciximab is bleeding, and the contraindications to its use are similar to those for the fibrinolytic agents listed in Table 32-4. The frequency of major hemorrhage in clinical trials varies from 1% to 10%, depending on the intensity of concomitant anticoagulation with heparin. Thrombocytopenia with a platelet count below 50,000 occurs in about 2% of patients and may be due the formation of antibodies directed against neoepitopes induced by bound antibody. Because the duration of action is long, if major bleeding occurs, platelet transfusion may reverse the aggregation defect because free antibody concentrations fall rapidly after cessation of infusion.

Eptifibatide

Eptifibatide is a cyclic peptide inhibitor of the fibrinogen binding site on $\alpha_{IIb}\beta_3$. It is administered intravenously and blocks platelet aggregation. In patients undergoing percutaneous coronary intervention, eptifibatide is typically given as a double intravenous bolus of 180 μg/kg (spaced 10 min apart), followed by an infusion of 2 μg/kg/min for 18 to 24 h. The drug is cleared by the kidneys and has a short plasma half-life of 10 to 15 min. Like abciximab, eptifibatide is mainly used in patients undergoing primary percutaneous coronary intervention for acute ST-segment elevation myocardial infarction, although it also can be used in patients with unstable angina.

Adverse Effects. The major side effect is bleeding. Thrombocytopenia occurs in 0.5%–1% of patients and is less frequent than with abciximab.

Tirofiban

Tirofiban is an intravenously administered nonpeptide, small-molecule inhibitor of $\alpha_{IIb}\beta_3$. It has a short duration of action and is used for management of patients with non–ST-segment elevation acute coronary syndrome. Tirofiban is administered as an intravenously bolus of 25 μg/kg followed by an infusion of 0.15 μg/kg/min for up to 18 h. The infusion dose is reduced by half in patients with a creatinine clearance below 60 mL/min. Like the other agents in this class, the major side effect of tirofiban is bleeding, and it may induce thrombocytopenia.

The Role of Vitamin K

Green plants are a nutritional source of vitamin K for humans, in whom vitamin K is an essential cofactor in the γ-carboxylation of multiple glutamate residues of several clotting factors and anticoagulant proteins. The vitamin K–dependent formation of Gla residues permits the appropriate interactions of clotting factors, Ca^{2+}, and membrane phospholipids and modulator proteins (see Figures 32–1, 32–2, and 32–3). Vitamin K antagonists (coumarin derivatives) block Gla formation and thereby inhibit clotting; excess vitamin K_1 can reverse the effects.

Vitamin K activity is associated with at least two distinct natural substances, designated as vitamin K_1 and vitamin K_2. Vitamin K_1, or *phytonadione* (also referred to as *phylloquinone*), is 2-methyl-3-phytyl-1,4-naphthoquinone; it is found in plants and is the only natural vitamin K available for therapeutic use. Vitamin K_2 actually is a series of compounds (the *menaquinones*) in which the phytyl side chain of phytonadione has been replaced by a side chain built up of 2–13 prenyl units.

TABLE 32–4 ■ FEATURES OF GPIIb/IIIa ANTAGONISTS

FEATURE	ABCIXIMAB	EPTIFIBATIDE	TIROFIBAN
Description	Fab fragment of humanized mouse monoclonal antibody	Cyclical KGD-containing heptapeptide	Nonpeptidic RGD-mimetic
Specific for GPIIb/IIIa	No	Yes	Yes
Plasma $t_{1/2}$	Short (minutes)	Long (2.5 h)	Long (2.0 h)
Platelet-bound $t_{1/2}$	Long (days)	Short (seconds)	Short (seconds)
Renal clearance	No	Yes	Yes

Considerable synthesis of menaquinones occurs in gram-positive bacteria; indeed, intestinal flora synthesizes the large amounts of vitamin K contained in human and animal feces. Menadione is at least as active on a molar basis as phytonadione.

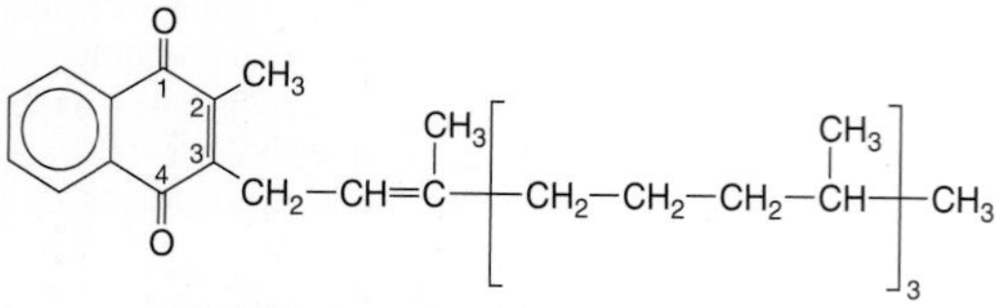

PHYTONADIONE (vitamin K_1, phylloquinone)

Physiological Functions and Pharmacological Actions

Phytonadione and menaquinones promote the biosynthesis of the clotting factors II (prothrombin), VII, IX, and X as well as the anticoagulant proteins C and S and protein Z (a cofactor to the inhibitor of Xa).

Figure 32–6 summarizes the coupling of the vitamin K cycle with glutamate carboxylation. The γ-glutamyl carboxylase and epoxide reductase are integral membrane proteins of the endoplasmic reticulum and function as a multicomponent complex. With respect to proteins affecting blood coagulation, these reactions occur in the liver, but γ-carboxylation of glutamate also occurs in lung, bone, and other cell types. Mutations in γ-glutamyl carboxylase lead to bleeding disorders.

Human Requirements

In patients rendered vitamin K deficient by a starvation diet and antibiotic therapy for 3–4 weeks, the minimum daily requirement is estimated to be 0.03 μg/kg of body weight and possibly as high as 1 μg/kg, which is approximately the recommended intake for adults (70 μg/d).

Symptoms of Deficiency

The major clinical manifestation of vitamin K deficiency is bleeding. Ecchymoses, epistaxis, hematuria, GI bleeding, and postoperative hemorrhage are common; intracranial hemorrhage may occur. Hemoptysis is uncommon. The presence of vitamin K–dependent proteins in bone such as osteocalcin and matrix Gla protein may explain why fetal bone abnormalities can occur with maternal warfarin administration in the first trimester of pregnancy. Vitamin K plays a role in adult skeletal maintenance and the prevention of osteoporosis. Low concentrations of the vitamin are associated with decreased bone mineral density and subsequent fractures; vitamin K supplementation increases the carboxylation state of osteocalcin and improves bone mineral density, but the relationship between these effects is unclear. Bone mineral density in adults does not appear to be changed with long-term warfarin therapy, but new bone formation may be affected.

Toxicity

Phytonadione and the menaquinones are nontoxic. Menadione and its derivatives (synthetic forms of vitamin K) may produce hemolytic anemia and kernicterus in neonates and should not be used as therapeutic forms of vitamin K.

ADME

The mechanism of intestinal absorption of compounds with vitamin K activity varies depending on their solubility. In the presence of bile salts, phytonadione and the menaquinones are adequately absorbed from the intestine, phytonadione by an energy-dependent, saturable process in proximal portions of the small intestine and menaquinones by diffusion in the distal small intestine and the colon. After absorption, phytonadione is incorporated into chylomicrons in close association with triglycerides and lipoproteins. The low phytonadione levels in newborns may partly reflect the low plasma lipoprotein concentrations at birth and may lead to an underestimation of vitamin K tissue stores. After absorption, phytonadione and menaquinones are concentrated in the liver, but the concentration of phytonadione declines rapidly. Menaquinones, produced in the distal bowel, are less biologically active because of their long side chain. Very little vitamin K accumulates in other tissues. There is only modest storage of vitamin K in the body. Consequently, when lack of bile interferes with absorption of vitamin K, there is progressive reduction in the levels of the vitamin K–dependent clotting factors over the course of several weeks.

Therapeutic Uses

Vitamin K is used therapeutically to correct the bleeding tendency or hemorrhage associated with its deficiency. Vitamin K deficiency can result from inadequate intake, absorption, or utilization of the vitamin or as a consequence of the action of warfarin.

Phytonadione is available in tablet form and in a dispersion with buffered polysorbate and propylene glycol or polyoxyethylated fatty acid derivatives and dextrose. Phytonadione may be given by any route; however, the subcutaneous route should be avoided in patients with a coagulopathy because of the risk of bleeding. The oral route is preferred, but if more rapid reversal is required, phytonadione can be given by slow intravenous infusion; it should not be given rapidly because severe reactions resembling anaphylaxis can occur.

Inadequate Intake

After infancy, hypoprothrombinemia due to dietary deficiency of vitamin K is extremely rare. The vitamin is present in many foods and is synthesized by intestinal bacteria. Occasionally, the use of a broad-spectrum antibiotic may itself produce hypoprothrombinemia that responds readily to small doses of vitamin K and reestablishment of normal bowel flora. Hypoprothrombinemia can occur in patients receiving prolonged intravenous alimentation; to prevent this, it is recommended that such patients receive 1 mg of phytonadione per week (the equivalent of about 150 μg/day).

Hypoprothrombinemia of the Newborn

Healthy newborn infants have decreased plasma concentrations of vitamin K–dependent clotting factors for a few days after birth, the time required for adequate dietary intake of the vitamin and for establishment of normal intestinal flora. Measurements of non-γ-carboxylated prothrombin suggest that vitamin K deficiency occurs in about 3% of live births.

Hemorrhagic disease of the newborn has been associated with breastfeeding; human milk has low concentrations of vitamin K. In addition, the microbiome of breast-fed infants may lack microorganisms that synthesize the vitamin. Commercial infant formulas are supplemented with vitamin K. In the neonate with hemorrhagic disease of the newborn, administration of vitamin K raises the concentration of these clotting factors to levels normal for newborns and controls the bleeding tendency within about 6 h. Routine administration of 1 mg phytonadione intramuscularly at birth is required by law in the U.S. The dose may have to be increased or repeated if the mother has received warfarin or anticonvulsant drug therapy or if the infant develops a bleeding diathesis. Alternatively, some clinicians treat mothers who are receiving anticonvulsants with oral vitamin K prior to delivery (20 mg/d for 2 weeks).

Inadequate Absorption

Vitamin K is poorly absorbed in the absence of bile. Thus, hypoprothrombinemia may be associated with intrahepatic or extrahepatic biliary obstruction or with defective intestinal absorption of fat from other causes.

Biliary Obstruction or Fistula

Bleeding that accompanies obstructive jaundice or a biliary fistula responds promptly to the administration of vitamin K. Oral phytonadione administered with bile salts is both safe and effective and should be used in the care of the jaundiced patient, both preoperatively and postoperatively. In the absence of significant hepatocellular disease, the prothrombin level rapidly returns to normal. If oral administration is not feasible, a parenteral preparation should be used. The usual daily dose of vitamin K is 10 mg.

Malabsorption Syndromes

Among the disorders that result in inadequate absorption of vitamin K from the intestinal tract are cystic fibrosis, celiac disease, Crohn disease, ulcerative colitis, dysentery, and extensive resection of bowel. Because drugs that reduce the bacterial population of the bowel are used frequently in many of these disorders, the availability of the vitamin may be further reduced. For immediate correction of the deficiency, parenteral vitamin K should be given.

Inadequate Utilization

Hepatocellular disease or long-standing biliary obstruction may be accompanied or followed by hypoprothrombinemia. If inadequate secretion of bile salts is contributing to the syndrome, some benefit may be obtained from the parenteral administration of 10 mg of phytonadione daily. Paradoxically, administration of large doses of vitamin K or its analogues in an attempt to correct the hypoprothrombinemia can be associated with severe hepatitis or cirrhosis, which may contribute to a further reduction in the level of prothrombin.

Drug- and Venom-Induced Hypoprothrombinemia

Warfarin and its congeners act as competitive antagonists of vitamin K and interfere with the hepatic biosynthesis of Gla-containing clotting factors. The treatment of bleeding caused by oral anticoagulants was described previously. Vitamin K may be of help in combating the bleeding and hypoprothrombinemia that follow the bite of the tropical American pit viper or other species whose venom degrades or inactivates prothrombin.

Drug Facts for Your Personal Formulary: *Agents That Modify Blood Coagulation*

Drugs	Therapeutic Uses	Clinical Pharmacology and Tips
Unfractionated Heparin		
Heparin	• Prophylaxis/treatment of venous thromboembolism • Acute coronary syndrome • Percutaneous coronary intervention • Cardiopulmonary bypass surgery • Disseminated intravascular coagulation	• Administered SC 2–3 times daily for thromboprophylaxis • Administered IV for immediate onset of action with aPTT monitoring • Can be used in renal impairment • Can be used in pregnancy
Low-Molecular-Weight Heparin		
Enoxaparin Dalteparin Tinzaparin (not in the U.S.)	• Prophylaxis against venous thrombosis • Initial treatment of venous thromboembolism • Maintenance treatment in patients with cancer-associated venous thromboembolism • Acute coronary syndrome	• Administered SC once or twice daily • Routine anti-factor Xa monitoring not required • Dosage adjustment required when CrCL < 30 mL/min • Can be used in pregnancy
Fondaparinux		
Fondaparinux	• Prophylaxis against venous thromboembolism • Initial treatment of venous thromboembolism • Heparin-induced thrombocytopenia • Acute coronary syndrome in some countries	• Once-daily SC injection • Lower dose used for thromboprophylaxis and in acute coronary syndrome • Contraindicated if CrCL < 30 mL/min • Use in pregnancy less established than for low-molecular-weight heparin • Routine anti-factor Xa monitoring not required
Other Anticoagulants		
Desirudin	• Thromboprophylaxis after hip arthroplasty	• Twice-daily SC injection • Dosage adjustment required with renal impairment
Bivalirudin	• Percutaneous coronary intervention • Heparin-induced thrombocytopenia	• Administered IV • ACT or aPTT monitoring • Requires dose reduction with renal impairment
Argatroban	• Heparin-induced thrombocytopenia	• Hepatic metabolism • Can be used in renal impairment • Increases INR, which can complicate transition to warfarin
Vitamin K Antagonist		
Warfarin	• Treatment of venous thromboembolism in tandem with parenteral anticoagulation • Secondary prevention of venous thromboembolism • Prevention of stroke in atrial fibrillation • Prevention of stroke in patient with mechanical heart valves or ventricular assist devices	• Oral vitamin K antagonist • Narrow therapeutic index • Requires regular INR monitoring • Multiple drug interactions • Dietary vitamin K interactions • Can be used in renal failure • Contraindicated in pregnancy
Direct Oral Thrombin Inhibitor		
Dabigatran etexilate	• Treatment of acute venous thromboembolism after at least 5 days of parenteral anticoagulation • Secondary prevention of venous thromboembolism • Prevention of stroke in atrial fibrillation • Thromboprophylaxis after hip or knee arthroplasty	• Fixed twice-daily oral dosing (once daily if used for thromboprophylaxis) • Reduce the dose with CrCL 15–30 mL/min • Contraindicated if CrCL < 15 mL/min • Use with caution in patients with recent bleeding, especially GI bleeding • Can be reversed with idarucizumab

Drug Facts for Your Personal Formulary: *Agents That Modify Blood Coagulation (continued)*

Drugs	Therapeutic Uses	Clinical Pharmacology and Tips
Direct Oral Factor Xa Inhibitors		
Rivaroxaban	• Treatment of acute venous thromboembolism • Secondary prevention of venous thromboembolism • Prevention of stroke in atrial fibrillation • Thromboprophylaxis after hip or knee arthroplasty • Prevention of recurrent ischemia in stabilized acute coronary syndrome patients (not in North America)	• Fixed oral dosing (once daily with the exception of initial treatment of venous thromboembolism, which starts with twice-daily dosing for 21 days and once daily thereafter, or secondary prevention after acute coronary syndrome where the drug is given twice daily) • Avoid in patients with renal/hepatic dysfunction • Use with caution in patients with recent bleeding, especially GI bleeding
Apixaban	• Treatment of acute venous thromboembolism • Secondary prevention of venous thromboembolism • Prevention of stroke in atrial fibrillation • Thromboprophylaxis after hip or knee arthroplasty	• Fixed oral dosing (twice daily, higher dose for the first 7 days for acute venous thromboembolism) • Reduce dose for stroke prophylaxis if any two of age > 80 years, body weight < 60 kg, or serum creatinine ≥ 1.5 mg/dL • Use with caution in patients with recent bleeding, especially GI bleeding
Edoxaban	• Treatment of acute venous thromboembolism after at least 5 days of parenteral anticoagulation • Secondary prevention of venous thromboembolism • Prevention of stroke in atrial fibrillation	• Fixed once-daily dosing • Reduce the dose if any of CrCL 15–50 mL/min, body weight < 60 kg, or concomitant potent P-glycoprotein inhibitor • Not recommended for patients with CrCL < 15 mL/min • Contraindicated if CrCL > 95 mL/min • Use with caution in patients with recent bleeding, especially GI bleeding
Reversal Agents for Direct Oral Anticoagulants		
Idarucizumab	• Reversal of dabigatran	• Humanized Fab fragment against dabigatran • Bolus IV administration • Rapid and complete reversal
Andexanet alfa	• Reversal of rivaroxaban, apixaban, or edoxaban	• Recombinant analogue of factor Xa • Acts as a decoy for oral factor Xa inhibitors • Given as IV bolus followed by 2-h IV infusion • In phase 3 evaluation
Ciraparantag	• Reversal of dabigatran, rivaroxaban, apixaban, or edoxaban	• Synthetic small molecule • Binds target drugs • In phase 2 evaluation
Fibrinolytic Drugs		
Alteplase	• Thrombolysis in acute ischemic stroke, massive pulmonary embolism, or myocardial infarction	• IV bolus followed by an infusion • Risk of major bleeding, including intracranial bleeding
Reteplase	• Thrombolysis in myocardial infarction	• Two IV boluses • Risk of major bleeding, including intracranial bleeding
Tenecteplase	• Thrombolysis in pulmonary embolism and myocardial infarction	• Single IV bolus • Risk of major bleeding, including intracranial bleeding
Inhibitors of Fibrinolysis		
ε-Aminocaproic acid	• Reduce intraoperative bleeding	• Inhibits plasmin-mediated degradation of fibrin • IV infusion
Tranexamic acid	• Major head injury • Major trauma resuscitation • Reduce intraoperative bleeding • Topical application for dental bleeding and epistaxis • Menorrhagia	• Inhibits plasmin-mediated degradation of fibrin • Available in oral or IV form • Given orally in patients undergoing dental procedures or in women with menorrhagia and IV in patients with major trauma or undergoing major orthopedic surgery
Antiplatelet Drugs		
Aspirin	• Acute myocardial infarction or acute ischemic stroke • Secondary prevention in patients with stroke, coronary artery disease, or peripheral artery disease	• COX-1 inhibitor (selectivity > 100x over COX-2) • Antithrombotic effect achieved with low doses (<100 mg daily) • Reduced toxicity with lower doses
Dipyridamole	• Secondary prevention of stroke when combined with aspirin	• Available as a fixed-dose combined tablet with aspirin
Clopidogrel	• Acute coronary syndrome • Secondary prevention in patients with myocardial infarction, stroke, or peripheral artery disease	• Irreversible inhibitor of $P2Y_{12}$ • Given once daily • Variable response because common genetic polymorphisms attenuate metabolic activation • Proton pump inhibitors reduce conversion to active metabolite

Drug Facts for Your Personal Formulary: *Agents That Modify Blood Coagulation (continued)*

Drugs	Therapeutic Uses	Clinical Pharmacology and Tips
Antiplatelet Drugs		
Prasugrel	• After coronary intervention for acute coronary syndrome	• Irreversible inhibitor of $P2Y_{12}$ • Given once daily • More predictable inhibition of ADP-induced platelet activation than clopidogrel because of more efficient metabolic activation • Contraindicated in patients with cerebrovascular disease, prior intracranial bleed, or > 75 years of age • Reduce dose in patients weighing < 60 kg • Higher bleeding risk than clopidogrel
Ticagrelor	• Acute coronary syndrome with or without coronary intervention	• Reversible inhibitor of $P2Y_{12}$ • Given twice daily • Does not require metabolic activation • Higher bleeding risk than clopidogrel • Contraindicated in patients with a history of intracranial bleeding
Cangrelor	• Percutaneous coronary intervention	• $P2Y_{12}$ inhibitor • Rapid onset and offset IV agent • Higher bleeding risk than clopidogrel • Coadministration of clopidogrel or prasugrel with cangrelor will have no antiplatelet effect
Vorapaxar	• Secondary prevention in patients with a history of myocardial infarction or peripheral artery disease	• PAR-1 antagonist • Contraindicated in patients with cerebrovascular disease or prior intracranial bleed
Abciximab	• Coronary intervention for acute coronary syndrome	• Glycoprotein IIb/IIIa antagonist • Up to 10% bleeding risk • Can cause thrombocytopenia
Eptifibatide	• Coronary intervention for acute coronary syndrome	• Glycoprotein IIb/IIIa antagonist • Up to 10% bleeding risk • Can cause thrombocytopenia • Contraindicated in renal failure
Tirofiban	• Coronary intervention for acute coronary syndrome	• Glycoprotein IIb/IIIa antagonist • Up to 10% bleeding risk • Reduce dose if CrCL ≤ 60 mL/min
Vitamin Supplementation		
Vitamin K	• Reversal of warfarin • Hypoproteinemia of the newborn • Biliary obstruction • Malnutrition	• Oral or SC administration preferred • Can be given by slow IV infusion but high risk of adverse events

Bibliography

Amsterdam EA, et al. 2014 AHA/ACC guideline for the management of patients with non-ST-elevation acute coronary syndromes. A report of the American College of Cardiology/American Heart Association Task Force on Practice Guidelines. *J Am Coll Cardiol*, **2014**, *64*:e139–e228.

Arif SA, et al. Vorapaxar for reduction of thrombotic cardiovascular events in myocardial infarction and peripheral artery disease. *Am J Health Syst Pharm*, **2015**, *72*:1615–1622.

Barria Perez AE, et al. Meta-analysis of effects of bivalirudin versus heparin on myocardial ischemic and bleeding outcomes after percutaneous coronary intervention. *Am J Cardiol*, **2016**, *117*:1256–1266.

Beyer-Westendorf J, Ageno W. Benefit-risk profile of non-vitamin K antagonist oral anticoagulants in the management of venous thromboembolism. *Thromb Haemost*, **2015**, *113*:231–246.

Cohen AT, et al. The use of aspirin for primary and secondary prevention in venous thromboembolism and other cardiovascular disorders. *Thromb Res*, **2015**, *135*:217–225.

Connolly SJ, et al. Dabigatran versus warfarin in patients with atrial fibrillation. *N Engl J Med*, **2009**, *361*:1139–1151.

CRASH2 trial investigators. Effects of tranexamic acid on death, vascular occlusive events, and blood transfusion in trauma patients with significant haemorrhage (CRASH-2): a randomised, placebo-controlled trial. *Lancet*, **2010**, *376*:23–32.

Dobesh PP, Oestreich JH. Ticagrelor: pharmacokinetics, pharmacodynamics, clinical efficacy, and safety. *Pharmacotherapy*, **2014**, *34*:1077–1090.

Eikelboom JW, et al. Dabigatran versus warfarin in patients with mechanical heart valves. *N Engl J Med*, **2013**, *369*:1206–1214.

EINSTEIN investigators. Oral rivaroxaban for symptomatic venous thromboembolism. *N Engl J Med*, **2010**, *363*:2499–2510.

EINSTEIN investigators. Oral rivaroxaban for the treatment of symptomatic pulmonary embolism. *N Engl J Med*, **2012**, *366*:1287–1297.

Falck-Ytter Y, et al. Prevention of venous thromboembolism in orthopedic surgery patients: antithrombotic therapy and prevention of thrombosis, 9th ed: American College of Chest Physicians evidence-based clinical practice guidelines. *Chest*, **2012**, *141*:e278S–e325S.

Gara PT, et al. 2013 ACCF/AHA guideline for the management of ST-elevation myocardial infarction: a report of the American College of Cardiology Foundation/American Heart Association Task Force on

Practice Guidelines. *Circulation*, **2013**, *127*:e362–e425.

Giugliano RP, et al. Edoxaban versus warfarin in patients with atrial fibrillation. *N Engl J Med*, **2013**, *369*:2093–2104.

Gomez-Outes A, et al. Direct-acting oral anticoagulants: pharmacology, indications, management, and future perspectives. *Eur J Haematol*, **2015**, *95*:389–404.

Gould MK, et al. Prevention of venous thromboembolism in nonorthopedic surgical patients: antithrombotic therapy and prevention of thrombosis, 9th ed: American College of Chest Physicians evidence-based clinical practice guidelines. *Chest*, **2012**, *141*:e227S–e277S.

Granger CB, et al. Apixaban versus warfarin in patients with atrial fibrillation. *N Engl J Med*, **2011**, *365*:981–992.

Granziera S, et al. Direct oral anticoagulants and their use in treatment and secondary prevention of acute symptomatic venous thromboembolism. *Clin Appl Thromb Hemost*, **2016**, *22*:209–221.

Grouzi E. Update on argatroban for the prophylaxis and treatment of heparin-induced thrombocytopenia type II. *J Blood Med*, **2014**, *5*:131–141.

Guimaraúes PO, Tricoci P. Ticagrelor, prasugrel, or clopidogrel in ST-segment elevation myocardial infarction: which one to choose? *Expert Opin Pharmacother*, **2015**, *16*:1983–1995.

Hokusai VTE investigators. Edoxaban versus warfarin for the treatment of symptomatic venous thromboembolism. *N Engl J Med*, **2013**, *369*:1406–1415.

International Warfarin Pharmacogenetics Consortium. Estimation of the warfarin dose with clinical and pharmacogenetic data. *N Engl J Med*, **2009**, *360*:753–764.

Ittaman SV, et al. The role of aspirin in the prevention of cardiovascular disease. *Clin Med Res*, **2014**, *12*:147–154.

Kahn SR, et al. Prevention of VTE in nonsurgical patients: Antithrombotic therapy and prevention of thrombosis, 9th ed: American College of Chest Physicians evidence-based clinical practice guidelines. *Chest*, **2012**, *141*:e195S–e226S.

Kearon C, et al. Antithrombotic therapy for VTE disease: chest guideline and expert panel report. *Chest*, **2016**, *149*:315–352.

Keating G. Cangrelor: a review in percutaneous coronary intervention. *Drug*, **2015**, *75*:1425–1434.

Kelton JG, et al. Nonheparin anticoagulants for heparin-induced thrombocytopenia. *N Engl J Med*, **2013**, *368*:737–744.

Lhermusier T, Waksman R. Prasugrel hydrochloride for the treatment of acute coronary syndromes. *Expert Opin Pharmacother*, **2015**, *16*:585–596.

Limdi NA, et al. Race influences warfarin dose changes associated with genetic factors. *Blood*, **2015**, *126*:539–545.

McClain MR, et al. A rapid-ACCE review of CYP2C9 and VKORC1 alleles testing to inform warfarin dosing in adults at elevated risk for thrombotic events to avoid serious bleeding. *Genet Med*, **2008**, *10*:89–98.

Meyer G, et al. Fibrinolysis for patients with intermediate-risk pulmonary embolism. *N Engl J Med*, **2014**, *370*:1402–1411.

Moschonas IC, et al. Protease-activated receptor-1 antagonists in long-term antiplatelet therapy. Current state of evidence and future perspectives. *Int J Cardiol*, **2015**, *185*:9–18.

Park Y, et al. Update on oral antithrombotic therapy for secondary prevention following non-ST segment elevation myocardial infarction. *Trends Cardiovasc Med*, **2016**, *26*:321–334.

Patel MR, et al. Rivaroxaban versus warfarin in nonvalvular atrial fibrillation. *N Engl J Med*, **2011**, *365*:883–891.

Pollack CV, et al. Idarucizumab for dabigatran reversal. *N Engl J Med*, **2015**, *373*:511–520.

Roffi M, et al. 2015 ESC guidelines for the management of acute coronary syndromes in patients presenting without persistent ST-segment elevation. *Eur Heart J*, **2015**, doi:10.1093/eurheartj/ehv320.

Schulman S, et al. Dabigatran versus warfarin in the treatment of acute venous thromboembolism. *N Engl J Med*, **2009**, *361*:2342–2352.

Shi C, et al. Pharmacogenetics-based versus conventional dosing of warfarin: a meta-analysis of randomized controlled trials. *PLoS One*, **2015**, *10*:e0144511.

Siegal DM, et al. Andexanet alfa for the reversal of factor Xa inhibitor activity. *N Engl J Med*, **2015**, *373*:2413–2424.

Zhang Q, et al. Aspirin plus clopidogrel as secondary prevention after stroke or transient ischemic attack: a systematic review and meta-analysis. *Cerebrovasc Dis*, **2015**, *39*:13–22.

Drug Therapy for Dyslipidemias

Holly E. Gurgle and Donald K. Blumenthal

第三十三章　血脂异常的药物治疗

PLASMA LIPOPROTEIN METABOLISM
- Chylomicrons
- Chylomicron Remnants
- Very Low-Density Lipoproteins
- Low-Density Lipoproteins
- High-Density Lipoproteins
- Lipoprotein (a)

ATHEROSCLEROTIC CARDIOVASCULAR DISEASE RISK ASSESSMENT

STATIN DRUG THERAPY

NONSTATIN DRUG THERAPIES
- Bile Acid Sequestrants
- Niacin (Nicotinic Acid)
- Fibric Acid Derivatives
- Inhibitor of Cholesterol Absorption
- Omega-3 Fatty Acid Ethyl Esters
- PCSK9 Inhibitors
- Inhibitor of Microsomal Triglyceride Transfer
- Inhibitor of Apolipoprotein B-100 Synthesis

中文导读

本章主要介绍：血浆脂蛋白代谢，包括乳糜微粒、乳糜微粒残余颗粒、极低密度脂蛋白、低密度脂蛋白、高密度脂蛋白和脂蛋白α；动脉粥样硬化性心血管疾病；疾病风险评估；他汀类药物治疗；非他汀类药物治疗，包括胆汁酸螯合剂、烟酸（尼克酸）、苯氧酸衍生物、胆固醇吸收抑制药、Omega-3脂肪酸乙酯、PCSK9抑制药、微粒体甘油三酯转移抑制药、载脂蛋白B-100合成抑制药。

Dyslipidemia is a major cause of ASCVDs, such as CHD, ischemic cerebrovascular disease, and peripheral vascular disease. Cardiovascular disease represents the number one cause of death among adults in many developed nations (Mozaffarian et al., 2015). Both genetic disorders and lifestyle contribute to the dyslipidemias, including hypercholesterolemia and low levels of HDL-C.

Classes of drugs that modify cholesterol levels include the following:

- Inhibitors of HMG-CoA reductase (*statins*)
- Bile acid–binding resins
- Nicotinic acid (*niacin*)
- Fibric acid derivatives (*fibrates*)
- Inhibitor of cholesterol absorption (*ezetimibe*)
- Omega-3 fatty acid ethyl esters (fish oil)
- PCSK9 inhibitors
- MTP inhibitor (*lomitapide*)
- Inhibitor of apolipoprotein B-100 synthesis (*mipomersen*)

The 2014 ACC/AHA Guideline on the Treatment of Blood Cholesterol to Reduce Atherosclerotic Cardiovascular Risk in Adults (Stone et al., 2014) recommends a substantial shift in approach to cholesterol management compared to the ATPIII (Grundy et al., 2004; NCEP, 2002). Whereas ATPIII advocated treating to specific lipoprotein targets, the 2014 ACC/AHA guideline focuses on offering fixed doses of statins to patients in four statin benefit groups to reduce morbidity and mortality. Since the 2014 release of the ACC/AHA guideline, several additional

Abbreviations

ACAT-2: type 2 isozyme of acyl coenzyme A:cholesterol acyltransferase
ACC: American College of Cardiology
AHA: American Heart Association
ALT: alanine aminotransferase
apo(a): apolipoprotein (a)
ASCVD: atherosclerotic cardiovascular disease
AST: aspartate aminotransferase
ATPIII: 2002 Third Report of the Expert Panel on Detection, Evaluation, and Treatment of High Blood Cholesterol in Adults
CETP: cholesteryl ester transfer protein
CHD: coronary heart disease
DHA: docosahexaenoic acid
DM: diabetes mellitus
EPA: eicosapentaenoic acid
ER: extended release
FH: familial hypercholesterolemia
FRS: Hard CHD Framingham Risk Score
HDL: high-density lipoprotein
HDL-C: high-density lipoprotein cholesterol
heFH: heterozygous familial hypercholesterolemia
HL: hepatic lipase
HMG-CoA: 3-hydroxy-3-methylglutaryl coenzyme A
hoFH: homozygous familial hypercholesterolemia
HSL: hormone-sensitive lipase
IDL: intermediate-density lipoprotein
LCAT: lecithin:cholesterol acyltransferase
LDL: low-density lipoprotein
LDL-C: low-density lipoprotein cholesterol
LDLR: LDL receptor
LP(a): lipoprotein (a)
LPL: lipoprotein lipase
LRP: LDL receptor–related protein
MTP: microsomal triglyceride transfer protein
NCEP: National Cholesterol Education Program
NHLBI: National Heart, Lung, and Blood Institute
NLA: National Lipid Association
NPC1L1: Niemann-Pick C1-like 1 protein
OTC: over the counter
PCE: pooled cohort equation
PCSK9: proprotein convertase subtilisin/kexin type 9
PPAR: peroxisome proliferator–activated receptor
SR: scavenger receptor
SREBP: sterol regulatory element–binding protein
USPSTF: U.S. Preventive Services Task Force
VLDL: very low-density lipoprotein

expert consensus recommendations have been published, providing alternative opinions on cholesterol management (Jacobson et al., 2015) and recommendations regarding the role of nonstatin cholesterol treatments (Lloyd-Jones et al., 2016) in reduction of ASCVD risk (see Table 33–1).

Plasma Lipoprotein Metabolism

Lipoproteins are macromolecular assemblies that contain lipids and proteins. The lipid constituents include free and esterified cholesterol, triglycerides, and phospholipids. The protein components, known as *apolipoproteins* or *apoproteins*, provide structural stability to the lipoproteins and also may function as ligands in lipoprotein-receptor interactions or as cofactors in enzymatic processes that regulate lipoprotein metabolism. The major classes of lipoproteins and their properties are summarized in Table 33–2. Apoproteins have well-defined roles in plasma lipoprotein metabolism (Table 33–3). Mutations in lipoproteins or their receptors can lead to familial dyslipidemias and premature death due to accelerated atherosclerosis.

In all spherical lipoproteins, the most water-insoluble lipids (cholesteryl esters and triglycerides) are core components, and the more polar, water-soluble components (apoproteins, phospholipids, and unesterified cholesterol) are located on the surface. Except for apo(a), the lipid-binding regions of all apoproteins contain amphipathic helices that interact with the polar, hydrophilic lipids (such as surface phospholipids) and with the aqueous plasma environment in which the lipoproteins circulate. Differences in the non–lipid-binding regions determine the functional specificities of the apolipoproteins.

Figure 33–1 summarizes the pathways involved in the uptake and transport of dietary fat and cholesterol, pathways that involve the lipoprotein structures described next.

Chylomicrons

Chylomicrons are synthesized from the fatty acids of dietary triglycerides and cholesterol absorbed by epithelial cells in the small intestine. Chylomicrons are the largest and lowest-density plasma lipoproteins. In normolipidemic individuals, chylomicrons are present in plasma for 3–6 h after a fat-containing meal has been ingested. Intestinal cholesterol absorption is mediated by *NPC1L1*, which appears to be the target of *ezetimibe*, a cholesterol absorption inhibitor.

After their synthesis in the endoplasmic reticulum, triglycerides are transferred by *MTP* to the site where newly synthesized apo B-48 is available to form chylomicrons. Apo B-48, synthesized only by intestinal epithelial cells, is unique to chylomicrons and functions primarily as a structural component of chylomicrons. Dietary cholesterol is esterified by the ACAT-2. ACAT-2 is found in the intestine and in the liver, where cellular free cholesterol is esterified before triglyceride-rich lipoproteins (chylomicrons and *VLDLs*) are assembled.

After entering the circulation via the thoracic duct, chylomicrons are metabolized initially at the capillary luminal surface of tissues that synthesize LPL (see Figure 33–1), including adipose tissue, skeletal and cardiac

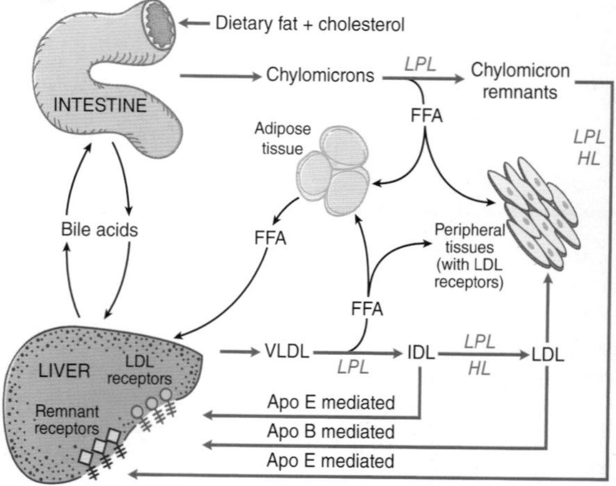

Figure 33–1 *The major pathways involved in the metabolism of chylomicrons synthesized by the intestine and VLDL synthesized by the liver.* Chylomicrons are converted to chylomicron remnants by the hydrolysis of their triglycerides by LPL. Chylomicron remnants are rapidly cleared from the plasma by the liver. "Remnant receptors" include the LRP, LDL receptors, and perhaps other receptors. FFA released by LPL is used by muscle tissue as an energy source or taken up and stored by adipose tissue.

TABLE 33–1 ■ COMPARISON OF KEY CLINICAL GUIDELINES FOR THE MANAGEMENT OF CHOLESTEROL IN ADULTS

	ATPIII 2004	ACC/AHA 2014	NLA 2015	USPSTF 2016
Risk assessment strategy	10-year FRS; CHD risk factors	10-year PCE	ASCVD risk factors used; FRS, PCE, or other	10-year PCE
Candidates for treatment	Patients above LDL goal	Patients in four statin benefit groups	Patients above LDL goal	Primary prevention in patients with risk
Recommended statin intensity	Titrated to achieve LDL goal	Moderate-to-high intensity	Titrated to achieve LDL goal	Low-to-moderate intensity
Recommendations	*Risk groups and LDL goals:* • High risk (LDL goal < 100, < 70 optional) if CHD, risk equivalent, or FRS ≥ 20% • Moderate-high risk (LDL goal < 130, < 100 optional) if ≥ 2 risk factors or FRS 10% to < 20% • Moderate risk (LDL goal <130, therapy started if LDL >160) if ≥2 risk factors or FRS <10% • Lower risk (LDL goal <160, therapy started if LDL >190) if 0 or 1 risk factor	*Four statin benefit groups:* • If ≥ 21 years old, clinical ASCVD, high-intensity statin (or moderate if > 75 years old) • If ≥ 21 years old and LDL ≥ 190, high-intensity statin • 40–75 years old with DM and LDL 70–189, moderate intensity (or high intensity if ASCVD ≥ 7.5%) • 40–75 years old with LDL 70–189, moderate-to-high intensity if ASCVD ≥ 7.5%	*Risk groups and LDL goals:* • Very high risk (LDL goal < 70) if ASCVD or DM + multiple risk factors or end-organ damage • High risk (LDL goal < 100) if 3 or more risk factors, DM + 0–1 risk factors, chronic kidney disease, LDL > 190, or high risk per calculator • Moderate risk (LDL goal < 100) if ≥ 2 risk factors or high risk per calculator • Low risk (LDL goal < 100) if 0–1 risk factors	• Statins recommended if 10-year risk ≥ 10% and 40 to 75 years old • Patient-specific approach if 10-year risk 7.5% to < 10% and with 1 or more cardiovascular risk factors • Statins not recommended if ≥ 75 years old

Refer to Table 33–4 for discussion of ASCVD risk factors.

Source: Data from ATPIII (Grundy et al., 2004; NCEP, 2002), ACC/AHA (Stone et al., 2014), NLA (Jacobson et al., 2015), USPSTF (2016).

TABLE 33–2 ■ CHARACTERISTICS OF PLASMA LIPOPROTEINS

LIPOPROTEIN CLASS	DENSITY (g/mL)	MAJOR LIPID CONSTITUENT	TG:CHOL	SIGNIFICANT APOPROTEINS	SITE OF SYNTHESIS	CATABOLIC PATHWAY
Chylomicrons and remnants	<1.006	Dietary triglycerides and cholesterol	10:1	B-48, E, A-I, A-IV, C-I, C-II, C-III	Intestine	Triglyceride hydrolysis by LPL; apo E–mediated remnant uptake by liver
VLDL	<1.006	"Endogenous" or hepatic triglycerides	5:1	B-100, E, C-I, C-II, C-III	Liver	Triglyceride hydrolysis by LPL
IDL	1.006–1.019	Cholesteryl esters and "endogenous" triglycerides	1:1	B-100, E, C-II, C-III	Product of VLDL catabolism	50% converted to LDL mediated by HL; 50% apo E–mediated uptake by liver
LDL	1.019–1.063	Cholesteryl esters	NS	B-100	Product of VLDL catabolism	Apo B-100-mediated uptake by LDL receptor (~75% in liver)
HDL	1.063–1.21	Phospholipids, cholesteryl esters	NS	A-I, A-II, E, C-I, C-II, C-III	Intestine, liver, plasma	Complex: transfer of cholesteryl ester to VLDL and LDL; uptake of HDL cholesterol by hepatocytes
Lp(a)	1.05–1.09	Cholesteryl esters	NS	B-100, apo(a)	Liver	Unknown

CHOL, cholesterol; NS, not significant (triglyceride is < 5% of LDL and HDL); TG, triglyceride.

muscle, and breast tissue of lactating women. The resulting free fatty acids are taken up and used by the adjacent tissues. The interaction of chylomicrons and LPL requires apo C-II as a cofactor.

Chylomicron Remnants

After LPL-mediated removal of much of the dietary triglycerides, the *chylomicron remnants*, with all of the dietary cholesterol, detach from the capillary surface and within minutes are removed from the circulation by the liver (see Figure 33–1). First, the remnants are sequestered by the interaction of apo E with heparan sulfate proteoglycans on the surface of hepatocytes and are processed by *HL*, further reducing the remnant triglyceride content. Next, apo E mediates remnant uptake by interacting with the hepatic *LDL* receptor or the *LRP*.

During the initial hydrolysis of chylomicron triglycerides by LPL, apo A-I and phospholipids are shed from the surface of chylomicrons and remain in the plasma. This is one mechanism by which nascent (precursor) HDL are generated. Chylomicron remnants are not precursors of LDL, but the dietary cholesterol delivered to the liver by remnants

TABLE 33–3 ■ APOLIPOPROTEINS

APOLIPOPROTEIN (MW in kDa)	AVERAGE CONCENTRATION (mg/dL)	SITES OF SYNTHESIS	FUNCTIONS
apo A-I (~29)	130	Liver, intestine	Structural in HDL; LCAT cofactor; ligand of ABCA1 receptor; reverse cholesterol transport
apo A-II (~17)	40	Liver	Forms -*S*-*S*- complex with apo E-2 and E-3, which inhibits E-2 and E-3 binding to lipoprotein receptors
apo A-V (~40)	<1	Liver	Modulates triglyceride incorporation into hepatic VLDL; activates LPL
apo B-100 (~513)	85	Liver	Structural protein of VLDL, IDL, LDL; LDL receptor ligand
apo B-48 (~241)	Fluctuates according to dietary fat intake	Intestine	Structural protein of chylomicrons
apo C-I (~6.6)	6	Liver	LCAT activator; modulates receptor binding of remnants
apo C-II (8.9)	3	Liver	Lipoprotein lipase cofactor
apo C-III (8.8)	12	Liver	Modulates receptor binding of remnants
apo E (34)	5	Liver, brain, skin, gonads, spleen	Ligand for LDL receptor and receptors binding remnants; reverse cholesterol transport (HDL with apo E)
apo (a) (Variable)	Variable (under genetic control)	Liver	Modulator of fibrinolysis

increases plasma LDL levels by reducing LDL receptor–mediated catabolism of LDL by the liver.

Very Low-Density Lipoproteins

The VLDLs are produced in the liver when triglyceride production is stimulated by an increased flux of free fatty acids or by increased *de novo* synthesis of fatty acids by the liver. Apo B-100, apo E, and apo C-I, C-II, and C-III are synthesized constitutively by the liver and incorporated into VLDLs (see Table 33–3). Triglycerides are synthesized in the endoplasmic reticulum, and along with other lipid constituents, are transferred by MTP to the site in the endoplasmic reticulum where newly synthesized apo B-100 is available to form nascent (precursor) VLDL. Small amounts of apo E and the C apoproteins are incorporated into nascent particles within the liver before secretion, but most of these apoproteins are acquired from plasma HDL after the VLDLs are secreted by the liver. Mutations of MTP that result in the inability of triglycerides to be transferred to either apo B-100 in the liver or apo B-48 in the intestine prevent VLDL and chylomicron production and cause the genetic disorder *abetalipoproteinemia*.

Plasma VLDL is catabolized by LPL in the capillary beds in a process similar to the lipolytic processing of chylomicrons (see Figure 33–1). When triglyceride hydrolysis is nearly complete, the VLDL remnants, usually termed *IDLs*, are released from the capillary endothelium and reenter the circulation. Apo B-100–containing small VLDLs and IDLs, which have a $t_{1/2}$ of less than 30 min, have two potential fates. About 40%–60% are cleared from the plasma by the liver via apo B-100– and apo E–mediated interaction with LDL receptors and LRP. LPL and HL convert the remainder of the IDLs to LDLs by removal of additional triglycerides. The C apoproteins, apo E, and apo A-V redistribute to HDL.

Apolipoprotein E plays a major role in the metabolism of triglyceride-rich lipoproteins (chylomicrons, chylomicron remnants, VLDLs, and IDLs). About half of the apo E in the plasma of fasting subjects is associated with triglyceride-rich lipoproteins, and the other half is a constituent of HDL.

Low-Density Lipoproteins

Virtually all of the LDL particles in the circulation are derived from VLDL. The LDL particles have a $t_{1/2}$ of 1.5–2 days. In subjects without hypertriglyceridemia, two-thirds of plasma cholesterol is found in the LDL. Plasma clearance of LDL is mediated primarily by LDL receptors (apo B-100 binds LDL to its receptor); a small component is mediated by nonreceptor clearance mechanisms.

The most common cause of autosomal dominant hypercholesterolemia involves mutations of the LDL receptor gene. Defective or absent LDL receptors cause high levels of plasma LDL and *FH*. Treatment of hoFH, which is associated with accelerated ASCVD and premature death at the age of 30 or before, is treated by inhibiting apo B-100 synthesis with *mipomersen*, as well as by inhibiting cholesterol synthesis with statins. LDL becomes atherogenic when modified by oxidation, a required step for LDL uptake by the SRs of macrophages. This process leads to foam cell formation in arterial lesions. At least two SRs are involved (SR-AI/II and CD36). SR-AI/II appears to be expressed more in early atherogenesis, and CD36 expression is greater as foam cells form during lesion progression. The liver expresses a large complement of LDL receptors and removes about 75% of all LDL from the plasma. Consequently, manipulation of hepatic LDL receptor gene expression is a most effective way to modulate plasma LDL-C levels. *The most effective dietary alteration (decreased consumption of saturated fat and cholesterol) and pharmacological treatment (statins) for hypercholesterolemia act by enhancing hepatic LDL receptor expression.*

High-Density Lipoproteins

The HDLs are protective lipoproteins that decrease the risk of CHD; thus, high levels of HDL are desirable. This protective effect may result from the participation of HDL in reverse cholesterol transport, the process by which excess cholesterol is acquired from cells and transferred to the liver for excretion. HDL effects also include putative anti-inflammatory, antioxidative, platelet antiaggregatory, anticoagulant, and profibrinolytic activities. Apo A-I is the major HDL apoprotein and its plasma concentration is a more powerful inverse predictor of CHD risk than is the HDL-C level. Apo A-I synthesis is required for normal production of HDL.

Mutations in the apo A-I gene that cause HDL deficiency often are associated with accelerated atherogenesis. In addition, two major subclasses of mature HDL particles in the plasma can be differentiated by their content of the major HDL apoproteins, apo A-I and apo A-II. Epidemiologic evidence in humans suggests that apo A-II may be atheroprotective.

The membrane transporter ABCA1 facilitates the transfer of free cholesterol from cells to HDL. After free cholesterol is acquired by the pre-β1 HDL, it is esterified by LCAT. The newly esterified and nonpolar cholesterol moves into the core of the particle, which becomes progressively more spherical, larger, and less dense with continued cholesterol acquisition and esterification. As the cholesteryl ester content of the particle (now called HDL_2) increases, the cholesteryl esters of these particles begin to be exchanged for triglycerides derived from any of the triglyceride-containing lipoproteins (chylomicrons, VLDLs, remnant lipoproteins, and LDLs). This exchange, mediated by the CETP, accounts for the removal of about two-thirds of the cholesterol associated with HDL in humans. The transferred cholesterol subsequently is metabolized as part of the lipoprotein into which it was transferred. Treatments that target CETP and the ABC transporters have yielded equivocal results in humans. While CETP inhibitors effectively reduce LDL, they also paradoxically increase the frequency of adverse cardiovascular events (angina, revascularization, myocardial infarction, heart failure, and death).

The triglyceride that is transferred into HDL_2 is hydrolyzed in the liver by HL, a process that regenerates smaller, spherical HDL_3 particles that recirculate and acquire additional free cholesterol from tissues containing excess free cholesterol. HL activity is regulated and modulates HDL-C levels. Androgens increase HL gene expression/activity, which accounts for the lower HDL-C values observed in men than in women. Estrogens reduce HL activity, but their impact on HDL-C levels in women is substantially less than that of androgens on HDL-C levels in men. HL appears to have a pivotal role in regulating HDL-C levels, as HL activity is increased in many patients with low HDL-C levels.

Lipoprotein (a)

Lipoprotein (a) [Lp(a)] is composed of an LDL particle that has a second apoprotein, apo(a), in addition to apo B-100. Apo(a) of Lp(a) is structurally related to plasminogen and appears to be atherogenic.

TABLE 33–4 ■ RISK FACTORS FOR ATHEROSCLEROTIC CARDIOVASCULAR DISEASE

Age
Male > 45 years of age or female > 55 years of age
Family history of premature CHD[a]
A first-degree relative (male < 55 years of age or female < 65 years of age when the first CHD clinical event occurs)
Current cigarette smoking
Defined as smoking within the preceding 30 days
Hypertension
Systolic blood pressure ≥ 140, diastolic pressure ≥ 90 or use of antihypertensive medication, irrespective of blood pressure
Low HDL-C
< 40 mg/dL (consider < 50 mg/dL as "low" for women)
Obesity
Body mass index > 25 kg/m^2 and waist circumference > 40 inches (men) or > 35 inches (women)
Type 2 diabetes mellitus[b]

[a]CHD defined as myocardial infarction, coronary death, or a coronary revascularization procedure.
[b]Diabetes mellitus is considered a high or very high risk condition for ASCVD.
Source: Data from 2015 NLA recommendations, part 1 (Jacobson et al, 2015).

Atherosclerotic Cardiovascular Disease Risk Assessment

Therapy for dyslipidemias is based on reducing the risk of fatal and nonfatal atherosclerotic cardiovascular events, including myocardial infarction and stroke. A flowchart that illustrates the assessment and management of ASCVD risk is shown in Figure 33–2.

The major conventional risk factors for ASCVD are elevated LDL-C, reduced HDL-C, cigarette smoking, hypertension, type 2 diabetes mellitus, advancing age, and a family history of premature CHD events (men < 55 years; women < 65 years) in a first-degree relative (Table 33–4).

Primary prevention involves management of risk factors to prevent a first-ever ASCVD event. Secondary prevention is aimed at patients who have had a prior ASCVD event (myocardial infarction, stroke, or revascularization) and whose risk factors must be treated aggressively. In addition to cholesterol management, a comprehensive approach to ASCVD risk reduction includes smoking cessation, weight management, physical activity, healthy eating habits, antiplatelet use, and glucose and blood pressure management. All treatment plans to reduce ASCVD risk must include patient counseling to effect lifestyle changes. Secondary causes of dyslipidemias (Table 33–5), including medications that affect cholesterol, should also be considered prior to initiating treatment. Patients should also be evaluated for metabolic syndrome, which affects more than one in three adults and includes insulin resistance, obesity, hypertension, low HDL-C levels, a procoagulant state, vascular inflammation, and substantially increased risk of cardiovascular disease.

The PCE, published as part of the 2014 ACC/AHA guideline on the assessment of cardiovascular risk, was developed based on data from nine

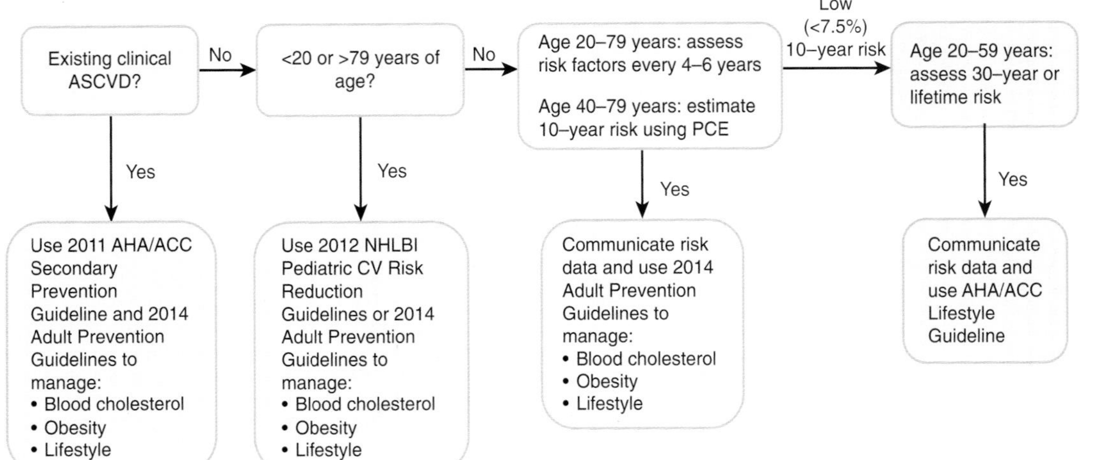

Figure 33–2 *Flowchart for assessing and managing ASCVD risk.* This chart is based on the 2014 ACC/AHA guideline on the assessment of cardiovascular risk. Refer to Table 33–1 and the ACC/AHA guidelines (Stone et al., 2014) for additional details.

TABLE 33–5 ■ SECONDARY CAUSES OF DYSLIPIDEMIA

SECONDARY CAUSE	ELEVATED LDL-C	ELEVATED TRIGLYCERIDES
Disorders and Conditions		
Diabetes mellitus		+
Nephrotic syndrome	+	+
Excess alcohol use		+
Pregnancy	+	+
Menopause transition (declining estrogen levels)	+	+
Chronic kidney disease	+	+
Hypothyroidism	+	+
Obstructive liver disease	+	
Metabolic syndrome		+
HIV infection	+	+
Autoimmune disorders	+	+
Polycystic ovary syndrome	+	+
Drug Therapies		
Oral estrogens		+
Some progestins	+	
Glucocorticoids	+	+
Immunosuppressive drugs	+	+
Thiazide diuretics	+	+
Anabolic steroids	+	
Thiazolidinediones	+	
Rosiglitazone		+
β blockers (especially non-β_1 selective)		+
Fibric acids (in severe hypertriglyceridemia)	+	
Bile acid sequestrants		+
Amiodarone	+	
Danazol	+	
Isotretinoin	+	
Long chain ω-3 fatty acids (in severe hypertriglyceridemia) with docosahexanoate)	+	
Tamoxifen		+
Raloxifene		+
Interferon		+
Atypical antipsychotic drugs (clozapine, olanzapine)		+
Protease inhibitors		+
L-Asparaginase		+
Cyclophosphamide		+

Source: Data from 2015 NLA recommendations, part 1 (Jacobson et al, 2015).

NHLBI-funded cohort studies and included data from geographically and racially diverse patient populations. The PCE estimates an individual patient's 10-year risk of ASCVD (defined as nonfatal myocardial infarction, CHD death, or fatal or nonfatal stroke) based on age, gender, total cholesterol, HDL-C, race, systolic blood pressure, smoking status, and history

TABLE 33–6 ■ CLASSIFICATION OF PLASMA LIPID LEVELS (mg/dL)

Non–HDL-C	
<130	Desirable
130–159	Above desirable
160–189	Borderline high
190–219	High
≥220	Very high
HDL-C	
<40	Low (consider < 50 mg/dL as low for women)
>60	High (desirable because of negative risk)
LDL-C	
<70	Optimal for very high risk[a]
<100	Desirable
100–129	Above desirable
130–159	Borderline high
160–189	High
≥190	Very high
Triglycerides	
<150	Normal
150–199	Borderline high
200–499	High
≥500	Very high

[a]Some consider LDL < 70 the optimal goal for patients with CHD or risk equivalents.

Source: Reproduced with permission from Jacobson TA, et al. National lipid association recommendations for patient-centered management of dyslipidemia: part 1—full report. *J Clin Lipidol*, **2015**, *9*:129–169.

of diabetes, and hypertension. The ASCVD risk assessment calculator using the PCE is available online (https://tools.acc.org/ASCVD-Risk-Estimator/) and as a mobile app. Cardiovascular risk assessment calculators have also been developed for lifetime risk of cardiovascular disease.

Statin Drug Therapy

Although an understanding of optimal lipoprotein levels is helpful (see ranges in Table 33–6), the 2014 ACC/AHA guideline recommends the use of fixed statin doses for at-risk patients, instead of titration to specific lipoprotein goals. The ACC/AHA guidelines identify four statin benefit groups or patient populations most likely to benefit from statin therapy. Patients with known history of clinical ASCVD and those with elevated LDL-C greater than or equal to 190 mg/dL should be offered statins.

For primary prevention in patients 40 through 79 years of age with LDL 70 to 189 mg/dL, use of the PCE is recommended to identify patients more likely to benefit from treatment. Table 33–1 summarizes ACC/AHA recommendations for use of statins in adults. In November 2016, the USPSTF released recommendations for the use of statins in primary prevention populations (USPSTF, 2016). These recommendations build on those in the ACC/AHA guideline in helping to further identify higher-risk primary prevention patients. USPSTF also questions the use of higher-intensity statins in the 2014 ACC/AHA guideline and instead recommends low- to moderate-intensity statins for primary prevention patients.

Because the overwhelming body of evidence for ASCVD risk reduction with lipid-lowering therapies is from statin trials, evidence-based statin therapy of appropriate intensity is the hallmark of drug therapy of dyslipidemias. These drugs are competitive inhibitors of HMG-CoA reductase, which catalyzes an early, rate-limiting step in cholesterol biosynthesis.

Higher doses of the more potent statins (e.g., atorvastatin, simvastatin, and rosuvastatin) also can reduce triglyceride levels caused by elevated VLDL levels. Figure 33–3 shows a representative statin structure and the reaction catalyzed by HMG-CoA reductase.

Mechanism of Action

Statins exert their major effect—reduction of LDL levels—through a mevalonic acid–like moiety that competitively inhibits HMG-CoA reductase. By reducing the conversion of HMG-CoA to mevalonate, statins inhibit an early and rate-limiting step in cholesterol biosynthesis. Statins affect blood cholesterol levels by inhibiting hepatic cholesterol synthesis, which results in increased expression of the LDL receptor gene. Some studies suggested that statins also can reduce LDL levels by enhancing the removal of LDL precursors (VLDL and IDL) and by decreasing hepatic VLDL production. The reduction in hepatic VLDL production induced by statins is thought to be mediated by reduced synthesis of cholesterol, a required component of VLDLs.

ADME

After oral administration, intestinal absorption of the statins is variable (30%–85%). All the statins, except simvastatin and lovastatin, are administered in the β-hydroxy acid form, which is the form that inhibits HMG-CoA reductase. Simvastatin and lovastatin are administered as inactive lactones that must be transformed in the liver to their respective β-hydroxy acids, simvastatin acid, and lovastatin acid. There is extensive first-pass hepatic uptake of all statins, mediated primarily by the organic anion transporter OATP1B1 (see Chapter 5). *Hepatic cholesterol synthesis is maximal between midnight and 2:00* AM. *Thus, statins with* $t_{1/2}$ *of 4 h or less (all but atorvastatin and rosuvastatin) should be taken in the evening.* Atorvastatin and rosuvastatin both have longer half-lives and may be taken at other times of day to optimize adherence.

Due to extensive first-pass hepatic uptake, systemic bioavailability of the statins and their hepatic metabolites varies between 5% and 30% of administered doses. The metabolites of all statins, except fluvastatin and pravastatin, have some HMG-CoA reductase inhibitory activity. Under steady-state conditions, small amounts of the parent drug and its metabolites produced in the liver can be found in the systemic circulation. In the plasma, more than 95% of statins and their metabolites are protein bound, with the exception of pravastatin and its metabolites, which are only 50% bound. Peak plasma concentrations of statins are achieved in 1–4 h. The $t_{1/2}$ of the parent compounds are 1–4 h, except in the case of atorvastatin and rosuvastatin, which have half-lives of about 20 h, and simvastatin with a $t_{1/2}$ of about 12 h. The longer $t_{1/2}$ of atorvastatin and rosuvastatin may contribute to their greater cholesterol-lowering efficacy. The liver biotransforms all statins, and more than 70% of statin metabolites are excreted by the liver, with subsequent elimination in the feces.

Therapeutic Effects

Triglyceride Reduction by Statins

Triglyceride levels greater than 250 mg/dL are reduced substantially by statins, and the percentage reduction achieved is similar to the percentage reduction in LDL-C.

Effect of Statins on HDL-C Levels

Most studies of patients treated with statins have systematically excluded patients with low HDL-C levels. In studies of patients with elevated LDL-C levels and gender-appropriate HDL-C levels (40–50 mg/dL for men; 50–60 mg/dL for women), an increase in HDL-C of 5%–10% was observed, irrespective of the dose or statin employed. However, in patients with reduced HDL-C levels (<35 mg/dL), statins may differ in their effects on HDL-C levels. More studies are needed to ascertain whether the effects of statins on HDL-C in patients with low HDL-C levels are clinically significant.

Effects of Statins on LDL-C Levels

Dose-response relationships for all statins demonstrate that the efficacy of LDL-C lowering is log linear; LDL-C is reduced by about 6% (from baseline) with each doubling of the dose. Maximal effects on plasma cholesterol levels are achieved within 7–10 days. The statins are effective in almost all patients with high LDL-C levels. The exception is patients with *hoFH*, who have very attenuated responses to the usual doses of statins because both alleles of the LDL receptor gene code for dysfunctional LDL receptors.

Adverse Effects and Drug Interactions

Hepatotoxicity

Serious hepatotoxicity is rare and unpredictable, with a rate of about 1 case per million person-years of use. ACC/AHA guidelines recommend measuring ALT at baseline prior to initiation of statins. However since 2012, the FDA has no longer recommended routine monitoring of ALT or other liver enzymes following the initiation of statin therapy because routine periodic monitoring does not appear to be effective in detecting or preventing serious liver injury. Liver enzymes should be evaluated in patients with clinical symptoms suggestive of liver injury following initiation or changes in statin treatment (FDA, 2012).

Myopathy

The major adverse effect associated with statin use is myopathy. Myopathy refers to a broad spectrum of muscle complaints, ranging from mild muscle soreness or weakness (myalgia) to life-threatening rhabdomyolysis.

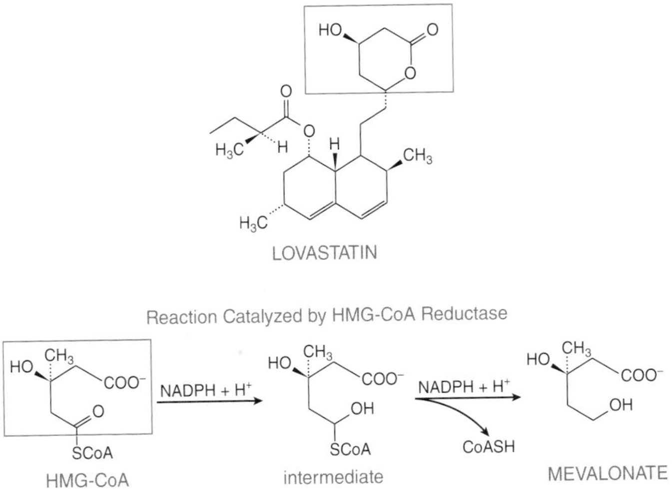

Figure 33–3 *Lovastatin and the HMG-CoA reductase reaction.*

The risk of muscle adverse effects increases in proportion to statin dose and plasma concentrations. Consequently, factors inhibiting statin catabolism are associated with increased myopathy risk, including advanced age (especially > 80 years of age), hepatic or renal dysfunction, perioperative periods, small body size, and untreated hypothyroidism. Measurements of creatinine kinase are not routinely necessary unless the patient also is taking a drug that enhances the risk of myopathy. Concomitant use of drugs that diminish statin catabolism or interfere with hepatic uptake is associated with increased risk of myopathy and rhabdomyolysis. The most common statin interactions occur with fibrates, especially *gemfibrozil* (38%), and with *cyclosporine* (4%), *digoxin* (5%), *warfarin* (4%), macrolide antibiotics (3%), and azole antifungals (1%). Other drugs that increase the risk of statin-induced myopathy include niacin (rare), HIV protease inhibitors, *amiodarone*, and *nefazodone*.

Gemfibrozil, the drug most commonly associated with statin-induced myopathy, both inhibits uptake of the active hydroxy acid forms of statins into hepatocytes by OATP1B1 and interferes with the transformation of most statins by glucuronidases. Coadministration of gemfibrozil nearly doubles the plasma concentration of the statin hydroxy acids. When statins are administered with niacin, the myopathy probably is caused by an enhanced inhibition of skeletal muscle cholesterol synthesis (a pharmacodynamic interaction). In 2016, the FDA withdrew approval for statin drug combinations containing fibrates or niacin (FDA, 2016).

Drugs that interfere with statin oxidation are those metabolized primarily by CYP3A4 and include certain macrolide antibiotics (e.g., *erythromycin*); azole antifungals (e.g., *itraconazole*); cyclosporine; *nefazodone*, a phenylpiperazine antidepressant; HIV protease inhibitors; and amiodarone. These pharmacokinetic interactions are associated with increased plasma concentrations of statins and their active metabolites. Atorvastatin, lovastatin, and simvastatin are primarily metabolized by CYPs 3A4 and 3A5. Fluvastatin is mostly (50%–80%) metabolized by CYP2C9 to inactive metabolites, but CYP3A4 and CYP2C8 also contribute to its metabolism. Pravastatin, however, is not metabolized to any appreciable extent by the CYP system and is excreted unchanged in the urine. Because pravastatin, fluvastatin, and rosuvastatin are not extensively metabolized by CYP3A4, these statins may be less likely to cause myopathy when used with one of the predisposing drugs. However, the benefits of combined therapy with any statin should be carefully weighed against the risk of myopathy.

Other Considerations

The choice of statins should be patient specific and based on factors such as cost, drug interactions, possible adverse effects, and desired intensity. Statin doses are characterized as low, moderate, or high intensity (Table 33–7), based on the degree of LDL-C lowering expected (range 30%–60%).

Rosuvastatin and pravastatin may be better tolerated than other statins and should be considered in patients with a history of myalgias with other statins. Lovastatin absorption is increased when taken with food, and patients should be encouraged to take with their evening meal. According to a 2012 FDA warning, simvastatin should not be used in combination with cyclosporine, HIV protease inhibitors, erythromycin, or gemfibrozil. In patients taking amlodipine or amiodarone, the daily dose of simvastatin should not exceed 20 mg. No more than 10 mg of simvastatin should be used in combination with diltiazem or verapamil. Concerns have been raised about possible cognitive impairment with statins, although review of the published data do not suggest that statins harm cognition. In contrast, other studies suggested statins may have a role in the prevention of dementias. Statins, especially at higher doses, likely confer a small increased risk of developing diabetes. However, the beneficial effects of statins on ASCVD events and mortality outweigh any increased risk conferred by promoting the development of diabetes. Atorvastatin is often the statin of choice for patients with severe renal dysfunction as it does not require dose adjustment.

Some statins have been approved for use in children with heFH. Atorvastatin, lovastatin, and simvastatin are indicated for children 11 years and older. Pravastatin is approved for children 8 years and older. *Statins are contraindicated during pregnancy and should be discontinued prior to conception if possible.* Data regarding statin use while breastfeeding are limited, and use should be discouraged.

TABLE 33–7 ■ INTENSITY OF STATINS BY APPROXIMATE REDUCTIONS IN LDL-C WITH DAILY DOSING

HIGH-INTENSITY STATINS	MODERATE-INTENSITY STATINS	LOW-INTENSITY STATINS
LOWER LDL-C BY APPROXIMATELY 50% OR MORE	LOWER LDL-C BY APPROXIMATELY 30% TO LESS THAN 50%	LOWER LDL-C, ON AVERAGE, BY LESS THAN 30%
Atorvastatin 40–80 mg **Rosuvastatin 20–40 mg**	**Atorvastatin 10–20 mg** **Fluvastatin 40 mg twice daily** Fluvastatin XL 80 mg **Lovastatin 40 mg** Pitavastatin 2–4 mg **Pravastatin 40–80 mg** **Rosuvastatin 5–10 mg** **Simvastatin 20–40 mg**	Fluvastatin 20–40 mg **Lovastatin 20 mg** Pitavastatin 1 mg **Pravastatin 10–20 mg** Simvastatin 10 mg

Bold type signifies statins and doses used in randomized controlled trials demonstrating a reduction in major cardiovascular events or death.

Source: Data from Table 5 in 2014 ACC/AHA guidelines (Stone et al., 2014) and Table 2 in "2016 ACC Expert Consensus Decision Pathway on the Role of Non-Statin Therapies" (Lloyd-Jones et al., 2016).

Nonstatin Drug Therapies

The 2014 ACC/AHA guideline focuses on the use of statins to reduce ASCVD risk. However, several important clinical trials have evaluated whether fibrates, niacin, ezetimibe, and fish oil result in further reductions in ASCVD risk when used in addition to statins (ACCORD, 2010; AIM-HIGH, 2011; Cannon et al., 2015; HPS2-THRIVE, 2014; ORIGIN, 2012). The National Lipid Association released recommendations in 2015 that continued to emphasize specific LDL goals and encouraged the use of nonstatin therapies in addition to statins in high-risk individuals (Jacobson et al., 2015). In April 2016, the FDA withdrew approval for niacin ER or fenofibrate when used in addition to statins, citing studies that demonstrated no additional reduction in ASCVD events versus monotherapy with a statin (FDA, 2016). In July 2016, the ACC also released an expert consensus decision pathway to aid clinicians in the use of nonstatins (bile acid sequestrants, PCSK9 inhibitors, or ezetimibe) in addition to statins for the management of ASCVD risk (Lloyd-Jones et al., 2016). The use of nonstatins in high-risk patient populations requires careful shared decision-making.

Elevated triglycerides are an important risk factor for pancreatitis. Treatment with agents most effective at reducing levels of triglycerides (fibrate or fish oil) are recommended in patients with very elevated triglycerides (>1000 mg/dL) to reduce the risk of pancreatitis. These therapies may be used in addition to statin treatment if the patient otherwise has risk factors for ASCVD that make the patient an appropriate candidate for statin therapy.

Bile Acid Sequestrants

Cholestyramine, Colestipol, Colesevelam

The bile acid sequestrants cholestyramine and colestipol are among the oldest of the hypolipidemic drugs and are probably the safest because they are not absorbed from the intestine. These resins also are recommended for patients 11–20 years of age. Although statins are remarkably effective as monotherapy, the resins could be utilized as a second agent if statin therapy does not lower LDL-C levels sufficiently or in cases of statin intolerance.

Mechanism of Action. The bile acid sequestrants are highly positively charged and bind negatively charged bile acids. Because of their large size, the resins are not absorbed, and the bound bile acids are excreted in the stool. Because more than 95% of bile acids are normally reabsorbed, interruption of this process depletes the pool of bile acids, and hepatic bile acid synthesis increases. As a result, hepatic cholesterol content declines, stimulating the production of LDL receptors, an effect similar to that of statins. The increase in hepatic LDL receptors increases LDL clearance and lowers LDL-C levels, but this effect is partially offset by the enhanced cholesterol synthesis caused by upregulation of HMG-CoA reductase. Inhibition of reductase activity by a statin substantially increases the effectiveness of the resins. The resin-induced increase in bile acid production is accompanied by an increase in hepatic triglyceride synthesis, which is of consequence in patients with significant hypertriglyceridemia (baseline triglyceride level > 250 mg/dL). Use of colesevelam to lower LDL-C levels in hypertriglyceridemic patients should be accompanied by frequent (every 1–2 weeks) monitoring of fasting triglyceride levels.

Effects on Lipoprotein Levels. The reduction in LDL-C by resins is dose dependent. Doses of 8–12 g of cholestyramine or 10–15 g of colestipol are associated with 12%–18% reductions in LDL-C. Colesevelam lowers LDL-C by 18% at its maximum dose. Maximal doses (24 g of cholestyramine, 30 g of colestipol) may reduce LDL-C by as much as 25% but will cause GI side effects, which are often unacceptable. One to 2 weeks is sufficient to attain maximal LDL-C reduction by a given resin dose. In patients with normal triglyceride levels, triglycerides may increase transiently and then return to baseline. When used with a statin, resins are usually prescribed at submaximal doses due to poor tolerability.

Preparations and Use. The powdered forms of cholestyramine (4 g/dose) and colestipol (5 g/dose) are either mixed with a fluid (water or juice) and drunk as a slurry or mixed with crushed ice in a blender. Ideally, patients should take the resins before breakfast and before supper, starting with 1 scoop or packet twice daily and increasing the dosage after several weeks or longer as needed and as tolerated. Patients generally will not take more than 2 doses (scoops or packets) twice daily. Colesevelam hydrochloride is available as a solid tablet containing 0.625 g of colesevelam and as a powder in packets of 3.75 g or 1.875 g. The starting dose is either 3 tablets taken twice daily with meals or all 6 tablets taken with a meal. The tablets should be taken with a liquid. The maximum daily dose is 7 tablets (4.375 g).

Adverse Effects and Drug Interactions. The resins are generally safe, as they are not systemically absorbed. Because they are administered as chloride salts, rare instances of hyperchloremic acidosis have been reported. Severe hypertriglyceridemia is a contraindication to the use of cholestyramine and colestipol because these resins increase triglyceride levels. At present, there are insufficient data on the effect of colesevelam on triglyceride levels.

Drinking a slurry of powdered cholestyramine or colestipol produces a gritty sensation that is unpleasant but generally tolerated. Colestipol is available in a tablet form. Colesevelam is available as a hard capsule that absorbs water and creates a soft, gelatinous material that allegedly minimizes the potential for GI irritation. Patients taking cholestyramine and colestipol complain of bloating and dyspepsia. These symptoms can be substantially reduced if the drug is completely suspended in liquid several hours before ingestion. Constipation may occur but sometimes can be prevented by adequate daily water intake and psyllium. Colesevelam may be less likely than colestipol to cause the dyspepsia, bloating, and constipation.

The effect of cholestyramine and colestipol on the absorption of most drugs has not been studied. Cholestyramine and colestipol bind and interfere with the absorption of many drugs, including some thiazides, *furosemide, propranolol, L-thyroxine*, digoxin, warfarin, and some of the statins. Colesevelam does not appear to interfere with the absorption of fat-soluble vitamins or of drugs such as digoxin, lovastatin, warfarin, *metoprolol, quinidine*, and *valproic acid*. Colesevelam reduces the maximum concentration and the area under the curve of sustained-release *verapamil* by 31% and 11%, respectively. In the absence of information to the contrary, prudence suggests that patients take other medications 1 h before or 3–4 h after a dose of colesevelam or colestipol. The safety and efficacy of colesevelam have not been studied in pediatric patients or pregnant women.

Niacin (Nicotinic Acid)

Niacin is a water-soluble B-complex vitamin that functions as a vitamin only after conversion to NAD or NADP, in which it occurs as an amide. Both niacin and its amide may be given orally as a source of niacin for its functions as a vitamin, but only niacin affects lipid levels. The hypolipidemic effects of niacin require larger doses than are required for its vitamin effects.

NICOTINIC ACID   NICOTINAMIDE

Mechanism of Action

In adipose tissue, niacin inhibits the lipolysis of triglycerides by HSL, thereby reducing transport of free fatty acids to the liver and decreasing hepatic triglyceride synthesis. Niacin may exert its effects on lipolysis by stimulating a G protein–coupled receptor (GPR109A) that couples to G_i and inhibits cyclic AMP production in adipocytes. In the liver, niacin reduces triglyceride synthesis by inhibiting both the synthesis and the esterification of fatty acids, effects that increase apo B degradation. Reduction of triglyceride synthesis reduces hepatic VLDL production, which accounts for the reduced LDL levels. Niacin also enhances LPL activity, an action that promotes the clearance of chylomicrons and VLDL triglycerides. Niacin raises HDL-C levels by decreasing the fractional clearance of apo A-I in HDL rather than by enhancing HDL synthesis.

ADME

The doses of regular (crystalline) niacin used to treat dyslipidemia are almost completely absorbed, and peak plasma concentrations (up to 0.24 mmol) are achieved within 30–60 min. The $t_{1/2}$ is about 60 min, which necessitates dosing two to three times daily. At lower doses, most niacin is taken up by the liver; only the major metabolite, nicotinuric acid, is found in the urine. At higher doses, a greater proportion of the drug is excreted in the urine as unchanged nicotinic acid.

Effects on Plasma Lipoprotein Levels

Regular or crystalline niacin in doses of 2–6 g/d reduces triglycerides by 35%–50% (as effectively as fibrates and statins); the maximal effect occurs within 4–7 days. Reductions of 25% in LDL-C levels are possible with doses of 4.5–6 g/d; 3–6 weeks are required for maximal effect. Niacin is the most effective agent available for increasing HDL-C (30%–40%), but the effect is less in patients with HDL-C levels less than 35 mg/dL. Niacin also is the only lipid-lowering drug that reduces Lp(a) levels significantly. Despite salutary effect on lipids, niacin's side effects limit its use (see Adverse Effects).

Therapeutic Use

Niacin is indicated for hypertriglyceridemia and elevated LDL-C. There are two commonly available forms of niacin. Crystalline niacin (immediate release or regular) refers to niacin tablets that dissolve quickly after ingestion. Sustained-release niacin refers to preparations that continuously release niacin for 6–8 h after ingestion. Niacin ER is the only preparation of niacin that is FDA-approved for treating dyslipidemia and that requires a prescription.

Crystalline niacin tablets are available OTC in a variety of strengths, from 50- to 500-mg tablets. The dose may be increased stepwise every 7 days to a total daily dose of 1.5–2 g. After 2–4 weeks at this dose, transaminases, serum albumin, fasting glucose, and uric acid levels should be measured. After a stable dose is attained, blood should be drawn every 3–6 months to monitor for the various toxicities. OTC, sustained-release niacin preparations, and niacin ER are effective up to a total daily dose of 2 g. All doses of sustained-release niacin, but particularly doses above 2 g/d, have been reported to cause hepatotoxicity, which may occur soon after beginning therapy or after several years of use. The potential for severe liver damage should preclude use of OTC preparations in most patients. Niacin ER may be less likely to cause hepatotoxicity.

Concurrent use of niacin and a statin can cause myopathy. Two randomized trials evaluating niacin as add-on therapy to a statin versus statin monotherapy demonstrated no further reduction in ASCVD risk, despite improved lipoprotein parameters. Given this evidence, the FDA removed the indication for niacin use in addition to statin therapy and withdrew approval for statin combination formulations containing niacin (FDA, 2016). Niacin could still be considered as monotherapy in a statin-intolerant patient.

Adverse Effects

Two of niacin's side effects, flushing and dyspepsia, limit patient compliance. The cutaneous effects include flushing and pruritus of the face and upper trunk, skin rashes, and acanthosis nigricans. Flushing and associated pruritus are prostaglandin-mediated, thus taking an aspirin each day can alleviate the flushing in many patients. Flushing is worse when therapy is initiated or the dosage is increased but ceases in most patients after 1–2 weeks of a stable dose. Flushing is more likely to occur when niacin is consumed with hot beverages or with alcohol. Flushing is minimized if therapy is initiated with low doses (100–250 mg twice daily) and if the drug is taken after a meal. Dry skin, a frequent complaint, can be dealt with by using skin moisturizers, and acanthosis nigricans can be dealt with by using lotions containing *salicylic acid*. Dyspepsia and rarer episodes of nausea, vomiting, and diarrhea are less likely to occur if the drug is taken after a meal. Patients with any history of peptic ulcer disease should not take niacin.

The most common, medically serious side effects are hepatotoxicity, manifested as elevated serum transaminases, and hyperglycemia. Both regular (crystalline) niacin and sustained-release niacin, which was developed to reduce flushing and itching, have been reported to cause severe liver toxicity. Niacin ER appears to be less likely to cause severe hepatotoxicity, perhaps simply because it is administered once daily. The incidence of flushing and pruritus with this preparation is not substantially different from that with regular niacin. Severe hepatotoxicity is more likely to occur when patients take more than 2 g of sustained-release OTC preparations. Affected patients experience flu-like fatigue and weakness; usually, aspartate transaminase and ALT are elevated, serum albumin levels decline, and total cholesterol and LDL-C levels decline substantially.

In patients with diabetes mellitus, niacin should be used cautiously because niacin-induced insulin resistance can cause severe hyperglycemia. If niacin is prescribed for patients with known or suspected diabetes, blood glucose levels should be monitored at least weekly until proven to be stable. Niacin also elevates uric acid levels and may reactivate gout. A history of gout is a relative contraindication for niacin use. Rarer reversible side effects include toxic amblyopia and toxic maculopathy. Atrial tachyarrhythmias and atrial fibrillation have been reported, more commonly in elderly patients. *Niacin, at doses used in humans, has been associated with birth defects in experimental animals and should not be taken by pregnant women.*

Fibric Acid Derivatives

Clofibrate is a halogenated fibric acid derivative. Gemfibrozil is a nonhalogenated acid that is distinct from the halogenated fibrates. A number of fibric acid analogues (e.g., fenofibrate, *bezafibrate, ciprofibrate*) have been developed and are used in Europe and elsewhere.

Mechanism of Action

The mechanisms by which fibrates lower lipoprotein levels, or raise HDL levels, remain unclear. Many of the effects of these compounds on blood lipids are mediated by their interaction with PPARs, which regulate gene transcription. Fibrates bind to PPARα and reduce triglycerides through PPARα-mediated stimulation of fatty acid oxidation, increased LPL synthesis, and reduced expression of apo C-III. Increased LPL synthesis would enhance the clearance of triglyceride-rich lipoproteins. Reduced hepatic production of apo C-III, which serves as an inhibitor of lipolysis and receptor-mediated clearance, would enhance the clearance of VLDLs. Fibrate-mediated increases in HDL-C are due to PPARα stimulation of apo A-I and apo A-II expression, which increases HDL levels. Fenofibrate is more effective than gemfibrozil at increasing HDL levels. Most fibrates have potential antithrombotic effects, including inhibition of coagulation and enhancement of fibrinolysis.

ADME

Fibrates are absorbed rapidly and efficiently (>90%) when given with a meal but less efficiently when taken on an empty stomach. Peak plasma concentrations are attained within 1–4 h. More than 95% of these drugs in plasma are bound to protein, nearly exclusively to albumin. The $t_{1/2}$ of fibrates range from 1.1 (gemfibrozil) to 20 h (fenofibrate). The drugs are widely distributed throughout the body, and concentrations in liver, kidney, and intestine exceed the plasma level. Gemfibrozil is transferred across the placenta. The fibrate drugs are excreted predominantly as glucuronide conjugates (60%–90%) in the urine, with smaller amounts appearing in the feces. Excretion of these drugs is impaired in renal failure.

Effects on Lipoprotein Levels

Effects of fibric acid agents on lipoprotein levels differ widely, depending on the starting lipoprotein profile, the presence or absence of a genetic hyperlipoproteinemia, the associated environmental influences, and the specific fibrate used. Patients with type III hyperlipoproteinemia (*dysbetalipoproteinemia*) are among the most sensitive responders to fibrates. Elevated triglyceride and cholesterol levels are dramatically lowered, and tuberoeruptive and palmar xanthomas may regress completely. Angina and intermittent claudication also improve.

In patients with mild hypertriglyceridemia (e.g., triglycerides < 400 mg/dL), fibrate treatment decreases triglyceride levels by up to 50% and increases HDL-C concentrations by about 15%; LDL-C levels may be unchanged or increase. Normotriglyceridemic patients with heFH usually experience little change in LDL levels with gemfibrozil; with the other fibric acid agents, reductions as great as 20% may occur in some patients. Fibrates usually are the drugs of choice for treating severe hypertriglyceridemia and the chylomicronemia syndrome. While the primary therapy is to remove alcohol and lower dietary fat intake as much as possible, fibrates assist by increasing triglyceride clearance and decreasing hepatic triglyceride synthesis. In patients with chylomicronemia syndrome, fibrate maintenance therapy and a low-fat diet keep triglyceride levels well below 1000 mg/dL and thus prevent episodes of pancreatitis.

Therapeutic Use

Gemfibrozil usually is administered as a 600-mg dose taken twice daily, 30 min before the morning and evening meals. Fenofibrate is available in tablets of 48 and 145 mg or capsules containing 67, 134, and 200 mg. The choline salt of fenofibric acid is available in capsules of 135 and 45 mg. Equivalent doses of fenofibrate formulations are 135 mg of choline salt, 145-mg tablets, and 200-mg capsules. Fibrates are the drugs of choice for treating hyperlipidemic subjects with type III hyperlipoproteinemia, as well as subjects with severe hypertriglyceridemia (triglycerides > 1000 mg/dL) who are at risk for pancreatitis. A randomized clinical trial of fenofibrate added on to background statin therapy resulted in no further reduction of ASCVD risk (ACCORD, 2010). In 2016, the FDA withdrew approval for use of fenofibrate in addition to statin therapy for ASCVD risk reduction.

Adverse Effects and Drug Interactions

Fibric acid compounds usually are well tolerated. GI side effects occur in up to 5% of patients. Infrequent side effects include rash, urticaria, hair loss, myalgias, fatigue, headache, impotence, and anemia. Minor increases in liver transaminases and alkaline phosphatase have been reported. Clofibrate, bezafibrate, and fenofibrate reportedly potentiate the action of warfarin. Careful monitoring of the prothrombin time and reduction in dosage of warfarin may be appropriate.

A myopathy syndrome occasionally occurs in subjects taking clofibrate, gemfibrozil, or fenofibrate and may occur in up to 5% of patients treated with a combination of gemfibrozil and higher doses of statins. Gemfibrozil inhibits hepatic uptake of statins by OATP1B1 and competes for the same glucuronosyl transferases that metabolize most statins. Thus, levels of both drugs may be elevated when they are coadministered. Patients taking this combination should be followed at 3-month intervals with careful history and determination of creatine kinase values until a stable pattern is established. Patients taking fibrates with rosuvastatin should be followed especially closely even if low doses (5–10 mg) of rosuvastatin are employed. Fenofibrate is glucuronidated by enzymes that are not involved in statin glucuronidation; thus, fenofibrate-statin combinations are less likely to cause myopathy than combination therapy with gemfibrozil and statins.

All of the fibrates increase the lithogenicity of bile. Clofibrate use has been associated with increased risk of gallstone formation. Renal failure is a relative contraindication to the use of fibric acid agents, as is hepatic dysfunction. *Fibrates should not be used by children or pregnant women.*

Inhibitor of Cholesterol Absorption

Ezetimibe is the first compound approved for lowering total and LDL-C levels that inhibits cholesterol absorption by enterocytes in the small intestine. It lowers LDL-C levels by about 20% and may be used as adjunctive therapy with statins.

Mechanism of Action

Ezetimibe inhibits luminal cholesterol uptake by jejunal enterocytes, by inhibiting the transport protein NPC1L1. In human subjects, ezetimibe reduces cholesterol absorption by 54%, precipitating a compensatory increase in cholesterol synthesis that can be inhibited with a cholesterol synthesis inhibitor (e.g., a statin). The consequence of inhibiting intestinal cholesterol absorption is a reduction in the incorporation of cholesterol into chylomicrons; this diminishes the delivery of cholesterol to the liver by chylomicron remnants. The diminished remnant cholesterol content may decrease atherogenesis directly, as chylomicron remnants are very atherogenic lipoproteins. Reduced delivery of intestinal cholesterol to the liver by chylomicron remnants stimulates expression of the hepatic genes regulating LDL receptor expression and cholesterol biosynthesis. The greater expression of hepatic LDL receptors enhances LDL-C clearance from the plasma. Ezetimibe reduces LDL-C levels by 15%–20%.

ADME

Ezetimibe is highly water insoluble, precluding studies of its bioavailability. After ingestion, it is glucuronidated in the intestinal epithelium and absorbed and then enters an enterohepatic recirculation. Pharmacokinetic studies indicated that about 70% is excreted in the feces and about 10% in the urine (as a glucuronide conjugate). Bile acid sequestrants inhibit absorption of ezetimibe, and the two agents should not be administered together.

Therapeutic Use

Ezetimibe is available as a 10-mg tablet that may be taken at any time during the day, with or without food. Ezetimibe may be taken in combination with other dyslipidemia medications except bile acid sequestrants, which inhibit its absorption.

The role of ezetimibe as monotherapy of patients with elevated LDL-C levels is generally limited to the small group of statin-intolerant patients. The actions of ezetimibe are complementary to those of statins. Dual therapy with these two classes of drugs prevents both the enhanced cholesterol synthesis induced by ezetimibe and the increase in cholesterol absorption induced by statins, providing additive reductions in LDL-C levels. A combination tablet containing ezetimibe, 10 mg, and various doses of simvastatin (10, 20, 40, and 80 mg) has been approved. LDL reduction at the highest simvastatin dose plus ezetimibe is similar to that of high-intensity statins.

Adverse Effects and Drug Interactions

Other than rare allergic reactions, specific adverse effects have not been observed in patients taking ezetimibe. *Because all statins are contraindicated in pregnant and nursing women, combination products containing ezetimibe and a statin should not be used by women in childbearing years in the absence of contraception.*

Omega-3 Fatty Acid Ethyl Esters

Mechanism of Action

Omega-3 fatty acids, commonly EPA and DHA ethyl esters, reduce VLDL triglycerides and are used as an adjunct to diet for treatment of adult patients with severe hypertriglyceridemia. The recommended daily oral dose for patients with severe hypertriglyceridemia is 3–4 g/d administered with food.

ADME

The small intestine absorbs EPA and DHA, which are mainly oxidized in the liver, similar to fatty acids derived from dietary sources. The $t_{1/2}$ of elimination is approximately 50 to 80 h.

Therapeutic Use

Fish oil or other products containing omega-3 fatty acids are among the most common OTC herbal, vitamin, or nutritional supplements purchased by consumers each year. Doses and formulations of OTC items vary considerably. The AHA recommends that consumers eat a variety of fish at least twice a week and that fish oil supplements should only be considered for individuals with heart disease or high triglyceride levels in consultation with a medical professional. In addition to OTC fish oil products, several prescription-only products are available, generally at higher doses than those used OTC (1–1.2 g) and containing a combination of EPA and DHA. Icosapent ethyl, an ethyl ester derivative of EPA, does not contain DHA. Mixtures containing both EPA and DHA have increased LDL-C in patients with severe hypertriglyceridemia, whereas studies of EPA-only products suggest they may not significantly increase LDL-C while still reducing triglycerides. Controversy exists about when to treat hypertriglyceridemia. Modifiable secondary causes of high triglycerides such as uncontrolled diabetes and excessive alcohol intake should always be addressed prior to initiating therapy. While prescription omega-3 products generally have FDA indications for triglycerides 500 mg/dL or greater, many professional organizations advocate that such products be limited to patients with levels of 1000 mg/dL or greater who are at greatest risk for pancreatitis. The ORIGIN trial found no additional reduction in ASCVD risk associated with the use of omega-3 fatty acids versus background therapy with statins alone, calling into question the common use of fish oil supplements for "heart protection" by consumers.

Adverse Effects and Drug Interactions

Adverse effects may include arthralgia, nausea, fishy burps, dyspepsia, and increased LDL. Because omega-3 fatty acids may prolong bleeding time, patients taking anticoagulants should be monitored.

PCSK9 Inhibitors

Mechanism of Action

Proprotein convertase subtilisin/kexin type 9 is a protease that binds to the LDL receptor on the surface of hepatocytes and enhances lysosomal degradation of the LDL receptor, resulting in higher plasma LDL concentrations. Loss-of-function mutations of PCSK9 are associated with reduced LDL and lowered risk of ASCVD. Conversely, mutations leading to increased PCSK9 expression result in increased LDL levels and higher risk of ASCVD events. Two PCSK9 inhibitors, *alirocumab* and *evolocumab*, antibodies to PCSK9, are FDA-approved as adjunctive therapy to diet and maximally tolerated statin therapy in adult patients with hoFH and heFH or established ASCVD requiring additional LDL lowering. Evolocumab and alirocumab are fully humanized monoclonal antibodies that bind free PCSK9, thereby interfering with its binding to the LDL receptor, leading to increased liver clearance of LDL from the circulation and lower serum LDL levels (see Figure 33–4).

Although studies are ongoing, ORION-1 describes a novel RNA interference therapeutic, inclisiran, that targets PCSK9 mRNA and thus blocks PCSK9 protein synthesis (Ray et al., 2017). Early clinical trials showed promise for an RNA interference therapeutic (ALN-PCS) that targets

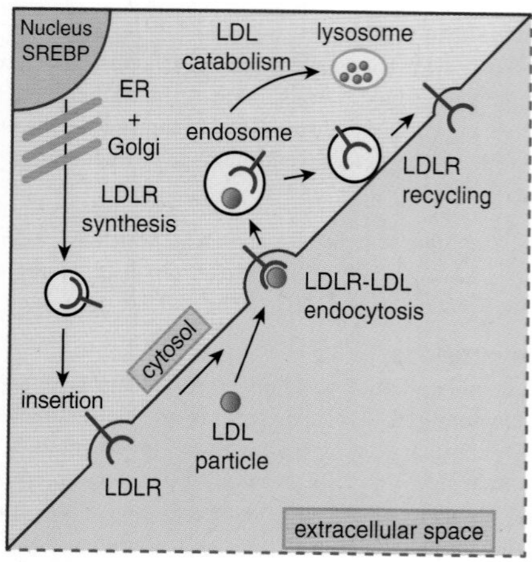

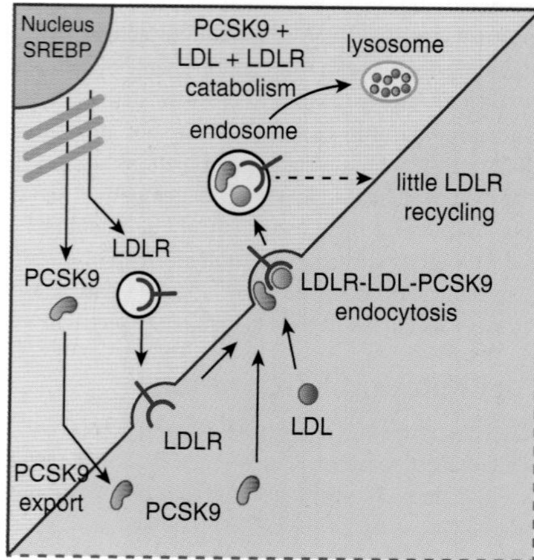

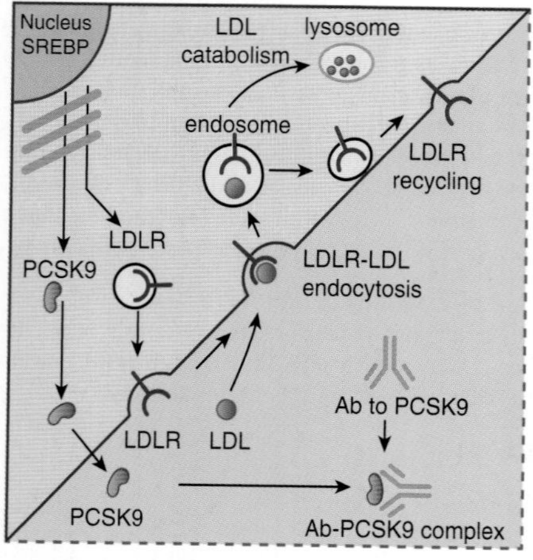

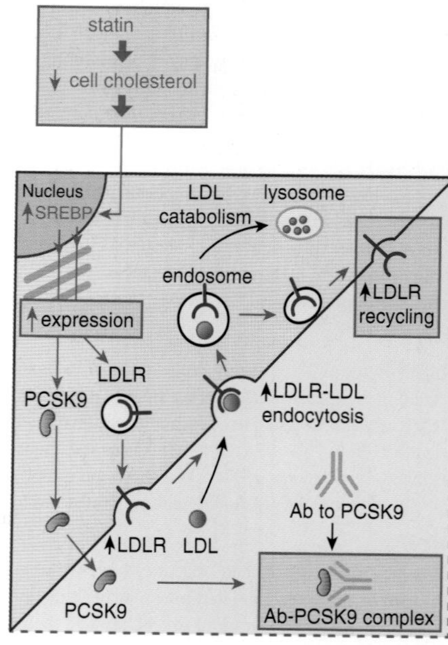

Figure 33–4 *LDL catabolism: effects of PCSK9, antibody to PCSK9, and statins.* Hepatic LDL uptake varies with the density of LDLRs in the hepatocyte membrane. The extent of LDLR synthesis and recycling affect the availability of LDLRs, variables that PCSK9, antibody to PCSK9, and statins can influence. **A.** *In the absence of PCSK9,* the LDLR is synthesized and inserted into the plasma membrane, where it binds LDL. The LDLR-LDL complex enters the hepatocyte by endocytosis. The complex dissociates within the endosome, the LDL entering the lysosomal pathway (degradation), and the LDLR being recycled to the membrane. **B.** *In the presence of PCSK9 biosynthesis,* however, PCSK9 is exported into the circulation. At the surface of the hepatocyte, PCSK9 interacts with the LDLR-LDL complex, entering the endosome and preventing the dissociation of LDLRs from LDL. As a consequence, the entire LDLR-LDL-PCSK9 complex enters the lysosomal pathway for degradation. Little or no LDLR is recycled, and future LDL uptake is reduced. There are gain-of-function mutations that enhance PCSK9 activity (see text). **C.** *In the presence of PCSK9 and antibody to PCSK9,* antibody to PCSK9 (Ab^{PCSK9}) prevents the binding of PCSK9 to the LDLR-LDL complex, returning the fate of the LDLR-LDL complex to that described in **A**, lysosomal degradation of LDL and recycling of LDLR to the membrane. **D.** *In the presence of PCSK9, antibody to PCSK9, and a statin,* levels of LDLR are increased by two different mechanisms. Statins, by inhibiting HMG-CoA reductase, reduce cell cholesterol, thereby activating SREBP and upregulating transcription of genes under its control; those include genes for LDLR and PCSK9. Expression of LDLR and PCSK9 increases. The newly synthesized LDLR molecules are inserted into the plasma membrane; the newly synthesized PCSK9 is exported. *In the absence of Ab^{PCSK9}*, the increased extracellular PCSK9 will bind to LDLR-LDL complexes, cause their lysosomal destruction, and thereby counteract some the statin's effect on circulating LDL and its uptake by hepatic LDLRs. *In the presence of antibody to PCSK9*, however, PCSK9 is complexed by Ab^{PCSK9} and rendered inactive, permitting an increase in LDLR presence on the hepatocyte membrane and an increase in recycling of used LDLR to the membrane. Thus, by protecting LDLRs from degradation and enhancing synthesis of new LDLRs, the combination of a statin and Ab^{PCSK9} can have a greater LDL-lowering effect than would the statin alone.

PCSK9 mRNA and thus blocks PCSK9 protein synthesis. Low-volume subcutaneous injections of inclisiran resulted in persistent reductions in LDL-C and other atherogenic lipids for 180 days, suggesting that a biannual subcutaneous dosing regimen might be possible.

ADME

The PCSK9 inhibitors are administered as subcutaneous injections either every 2 weeks or once monthly, depending on the dose and indication. Evolocumab is administered as a 140-mg injection every 2 weeks or 420 mg once monthly. For hoFH, evolocumab 420 mg is administered once monthly or every 2 weeks, and alirocumab (75 mg or 150 mg) is administered once every 2 weeks. Administration requirements and storage of these medications are barriers when compared with the ease of oral dosage forms of other medications.

The LDL-C plasma levels may be measured 4 to 8 weeks after initiating therapy or changing doses. These medications inhibit PCSK9 availability for 2 to 3 weeks after administration (half-life of elimination is 11 to 20 days), after which LDL levels begin to rise. Limited data are available in individuals with renal or hepatic impairment, although dose adjustments are not expected to be necessary. *PCKS9 inhibitors should not be used in pregnancy because transmission across the placenta is expected. It is not known to what degree the medications will be present in breast milk, so use during lactation is not recommended.*

Therapeutic Use

The effects of PCSK9 inhibitors are complementary to those of statins. While statins interfere with cholesterol production and stimulate the production of LDL receptors, PCSK9 inhibitors enable more LDL receptors to be available on the surface of liver cells. PCSK9 inhibitors reduce LDL-C in a dose-dependent manner by as much as 70% when used as monotherapy or by as much as 60% in patients already on statin therapy. Indications and approvals of these agents vary between countries. Currently, PCSK9 inhibitors are not FDA-approved for treatment of dyslipidemias in statin-intolerant patients without known ASCVD, although they are being used in this population elsewhere. Among patients with known ASCVD and LDL >70 despite treatment with moderate-high intensity statins, the addition of evolucumab further reduced the risk of ASCVD events, but not death, in the FOURIER trial (Sabatine et al., 2017). Given the high cost of treatment with PCSK9 inhibitors versus relatively inexpensive statin treatment, cost-effectiveness studies will also need to be conducted in a variety of patient populations to provide further recommendations on the patients most likely to benefit from these therapies. Currently, and because of cost-effectiveness, treatment with maximally tolerated doses of statins and ezetimibe is recommended prior to initiation of PCKS9 inhibitors.

Adverse Effects and Drug Interactions

Several clinical trials have identified a small (<1%) risk of neurocognitive effects in patients treated with PCSK9 inhibitors compared to placebo. Additional studies are under way to better understand the long-term neurocognitive effects of these medications, if any. Unlike other medications used to treat dyslipidemias, PCSK9 inhibitors do not appear to substantially increase the risk of myopathies when used as monotherapy or in combination with statins. Similar to other monoclonal antibodies, risk of infections, including nasopharyngitis, urinary tract infections, or upper respiratory infections, is slightly increased. Injection site reactions are the most frequent adverse effect, although these occur in less than 10% of patients. There are no expected drug interactions with PCSK9 inhibitors.

Inhibitor of Microsomal Triglyceride Transfer

Lomitapide

Mechanism of Action. Lomitapide mesylate is the first drug that acts by inhibiting MTP, which is essential for the formation of VLDLs.

ADME. Lomitapide is administered with water and without food (or at least 2 h after the evening meal) because administration with food may increase risk of GI adverse effects. The drug is metabolized by CYP3A4 and is contraindicated with inhibitors of CYP3A4.

Therapeutic Use. Lomitapide is FDA-approved as an adjunct to diet for lowering LDL-C, total cholesterol, apo B, and non–HDL-C lipoproteins in patients with hoFH. Lomitapide reduces LDL by up to 50% and should be used in combination with maximally tolerated statin therapy. The recommended starting oral dose (5 mg/d) is titrated upward at 4-week intervals to a maximum dose of 60 mg daily. The long-term cardiovascular effects of lomitapide are currently unknown.

Adverse Effects and Drug Interactions. Reported adverse effects commonly include significant diarrhea, vomiting, and abdominal pain in most patients. A strict low-fat diet may improve tolerability. Serious concerns also exist regarding hepatotoxicity and liver steatosis. In clinical trials, a third of patients experienced elevations in ALT or AST greater than three times the upper limit of normal. Lomitapide also increases hepatic fat, with or without concomitant increases in transaminases. The agent is used under an FDA risk evaluation and mitigation strategy due to its concerning side-effect profile. Lomitapide may be embryotoxic, and women of childbearing potential should have a negative pregnancy test before starting treatment and use effective contraception during treatment.

Inhibitor of Apolipoprotein B-100 Synthesis

Mipomersen

Mechanism of Action. Mipomersen is the first antisense oligonucleotide inhibitor of apo B-100 synthesis. Mipomersen binds to the mRNA of apo B-100 in a sequence-specific manner, which results in degradation or disruption of the apo B-100 mRNA, thereby reducing expression of apo B-100 protein.

ADME. The recommended dose is 1 mL of a 200-mg/mL solution, injected subcutaneously, once a week. It is metabolized in tissues by endonucleases to form shorter oligonucleotides available for further metabolism by exonucleases. The $t_{1/2}$ is 1 to 2 months. Maximal LDL reduction occurs after 6 months of treatment. Use is contraindicated in individuals with liver disease.

Therapeutic Use. In 2013, mipomersen was approved by the FDA as an addition to lipid-lowering medications and diet for patients with hoFH. However, given the side-effect profile of the medication, it was not approved elsewhere, including in Europe. LDL levels are reduced 30% to 50% with this treatment, although the discontinuation rates were high in clinical trials with this drug.

Adverse Effects and Drug Interactions. Injection site reactions are common (80%) and include erythema, pain, itching, and hematoma. Other common adverse effects include flu-like symptoms (30%), fatigue, and headache (15%). The agent is used under an FDA risk evaluation and mitigation strategy due to concerns about hepatotoxicity. Elevations in liver enzymes greater than three times the upper limit of normal occurred in approximately 10%–15% of patients in clinical trials.

Acknowledgement: *Thomas P. Bersot and Robert W. Mahley contributed to this chapter in recent editions of this book. We have retained some of their text in the current edition.*

Drug Facts for Your Personal Formulary: *Therapy for Dyslipidemias*

Drugs	Therapeutic Uses	Clinical Pharmacology and Tips
HMG-CoA Reductase Inhibitors (Statins)		
Atorvastatin Simvastatin Rosuvastatin Lovastatin Pravastatin Fluvastatin Pitavastatin	• The most effective and best-tolerated agents to treat dyslipidemias, especially elevated LDL-C	• *Safety of statins during pregnancy has not been established.* Women wishing to conceive and nursing mothers should not take statins. During their childbearing years, women taking statins should use highly effective contraception. • Hepatotoxicity (one case per million person-years of use); measure liver enzymes (ALT) at baseline and thereafter only when clinically indicated. • Myopathy and rhabdomyolysis (one death per million prescriptions (30-day supply); risk ↑ with dose and concomitant administration of drugs that interfere with statin catabolism or hepatic uptake.
Bile Acid–Binding Resins (Bile Acid Sequestrants)		
Cholestyramine Colestipol Colesevelam	• Probably safest lipid-lowering drugs (not absorbed systemically) • Recommended for patients 11–20 years of age	• Common GI side effects: bloating, dyspepsia, constipation. • Cholestyramine and colestipol bind and interfere with absorption of many drugs; administer all other drugs either 1 h before or 3–4 h after dose of a bile acid resin. • Severe hypertriglyceridemia is a contraindication to the use of cholestyramine and colestipol; they ↑ triglyceride levels.
Nicotinic Acid		
Niacin	• Favorably affects all lipid parameters; most effective agent for increasing HDL-C; also lowers triglycerides and reduces LDL-C	• *Should not be taken by pregnant women.* • Flushing, pruritus, and dyspepsia limit patient compliance. • Rarer episodes of nausea, vomiting, and diarrhea. • Hepatotoxicity, manifested as ↑ serum transaminases. • Hyperglycemia and niacin-induced insulin resistance; in patients with known or suspected diabetes, blood glucose levels should be monitored at least weekly until stable. • Concurrent use of niacin and a statin can cause myopathy and is contraindicated. • Contraindicated if any history of peptic ulcer disease. • Gout is a relative contraindication.
Fibric Acid (Fibrates)		
Gemfibrozil Fenofibrate *Not in the U.S.:* Ciprofibrate Bezafibrate	• Usual drugs of choice for treating chylomicronemia, hyperlipidemia with type III hyperlipoproteinemia, severe hypertriglyceridemia (triglycerides > 1000 mg/dL)	• GI side effects occur in up to 5% of patients. • *Fibrates should not be used by children or pregnant women.* • A myopathy syndrome may occur in subjects taking clofibrate, gemfibrozil, or fenofibrate. • The FDA has withdrawn approval for coadministration of fibrates with statins. • Renal failure and hepatic dysfunction are relative contraindications to the use of fibrates.
Cholesterol Absorption Inhibitor		
Ezetimibe	• Monotherapy in patients with ↑ LDL-C who are statin intolerant • Combination with statin ⇒ additive reductions in LDL-C	• Bile-acid sequestrants inhibit absorption of ezetimibe; avoid concurrent use. • *Combination products containing ezetimibe and a statin should not be used by women in childbearing years in the absence of contraception.* • Generally well tolerated agent.
PCSK9 Inhibitors (Monoclonal Antibodies)		
Alirocumab Evolocumab	• Adjunct to diet and maximally tolerated statin therapy for adults with hoFH, heFH or clinical ASCVD who require additional lowering of LDL-C	• Hypersensitivity or injection site reactions are possible. • Most effective agents at reducing LDL-C. • Like other monoclonal antibodies, influenza-like symptoms, nasopharyngitis, upper respiratory infections may occur. • Used in addition to maximally tolerated statin doses (complementary mechanism; see Figure 33–4).
Omega-3 Fatty Acid Ethyl Esters		
Omega-3 fatty acids (EPA and DHA)	• Adjunct for treating severe hypertriglyceridemia (triglycerides > 1000 mg/dL)	• Adverse effects may include arthralgia, nausea, fishy burps, dyspepsia, and increased LDL. • Since omega-3-fatty acids may prolong bleeding time, patients taking anticoagulants should be monitored.
Inhibitor of Apo B-100 Synthesis (Antisense Oligonucleotide)		
Mipomersen	• Used as an adjunct to lipid-lowering agents and diet in patients with hoFH	• Common adverse effects include injection site reactions, flu-like symptoms, headache, and elevation of liver enzymes. • The agent is used under an FDA risk evaluation and mitigation strategy.
Inhibitor of Liver Microsomal Triglyceride Transfer Protein		
Lomitapide	• Used as an adjunct to diet for lowering LDL-C, total cholesterol, apo B, and non–HDL-C in patients with hoFH	• In patients with hoFH, treatment can reduce LDL-C by 40%–50%. • Adverse effects include GI symptoms, elevation of serum liver enzymes, and increased liver fat in most patients. • The agent is used under an FDA risk evaluation and mitigation strategy.

Bibliography

ACCORD Study Group. Effects of combination lipid therapy in type 2 diabetes mellitus. *N Engl J Med,* **2010**, *362*:1563–1574.

AIM-HIGH Investigators. Niacin in patients with low HDL cholesterol levels receiving intensive statin therapy. *N Engl J Med,* **2011**, *365*: 2255–2267.

Cannon CP, et al. IMPROVE-IT Investigators. Ezetimibe added to statin therapy after acute coronary syndromes. *N Engl J Med,* **2015**, *372*:2387–2397.

FDA. FDA drug safety communication: important safety label changes to cholesterol-lowering statin drugs. **January 2012**. Available at: https://www.fda.gov/drugs/drugsafety/ucm293101.htm. Accessed February 27, 2017.

FDA. Withdrawal of approval of indications related to the coadministration with statins in applications for niacin extended-release tablets and fenofibric acid delayed-release capsules. **April 2016**. Available at: https://www.federalregister.gov/documents/2016/04/18/2016-08887/abbvie-inc-et-al-withdrawal-of-approval-of-indications-related-to-the-coadministration-with-statins. Accessed February 27, 2017.

Grundy SM, et al. Implications of recent clinical trials for the National Cholesterol Education Program Adult Treatment Panel III Guidelines. *J Am Coll Cardiol,* **2004**, *44*:720–732.

HPS2-THRIVE Collaborative Group. Effects of extended-release niacin with laropiprant in high-risk patients. *N Engl J Med,* **2014**, *371*:203–212.

Jacobson TA, et al. National lipid association recommendations for patient-centered management of dyslipidemia—full report. *J Clin Lipidol,* **2015**, *9*:129–169.

Lloyd-Jones DM, et al. 2016 ACC expert consensus decision pathway on the role of non-statin therapies for LDL-cholesterol lowering in the management of atherosclerotic cardiovascular disease risk. *J Am Coll Cardiol,* **2016**, *68*:92–125.

Mozaffarian D, et al. Heart disease and stroke statistics—2015 update: a report from the American Heart Association. *Circulation,* **2015**, *131*:e29–e322.

National Cholesterol Education Program (NCEP). Third report of the National Cholesterol Education Program (NCEP) Expert Panel on Detection, Evaluation, and Treatment of High Blood Cholesterol in Adults (Adult Treatment Panel III) final report. *Circulation,* **2002**, *106*:3143–3421.

ORIGIN Trial Investigators. n–3 Fatty acids and cardiovascular outcomes in patients with dysglycemia. *N Engl J Med,* **2012**, *367*:309–318.

Ray KK, et al. Inclisiran in patients at high cardiovascular risk with elevated LDL cholesterol. *N Engl J Med,* **2017**, *376*:1430-1440.

Sabatine MS, et al. Evolocumab and clinical outcomes in patients with cardiovascular disease. *N Engl J Med,* **2017**, *376*:1713-1722.

Stone NJ, et al. 2013 ACC/AHA guideline on the treatment of blood cholesterol to reduce atherosclerotic cardiovascular risk in adults: a report of the American College of Cardiology/American Heart Association Task Force on Practice Guidelines. *Circulation,* **2014**, *129*(25)(suppl 2):S1–S45.

USPSTF. Statin use for the primary prevention of cardiovascular disease in adults US Preventive Services Task Force recommendation statement. *JAMA,* **2016**, *316*:1997–2007.

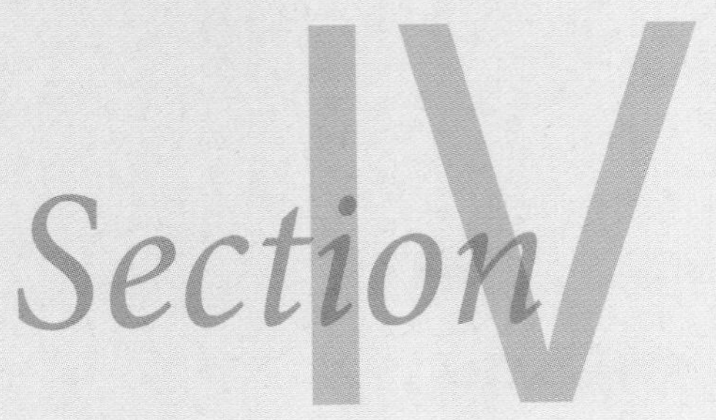

Inflammation, Immunomodulation, and Hematopoiesis

第四篇　炎症、免疫调节和造血

Introduction to Immunity and Inflammation

Nancy Fares-Frederickson and Michael David

第三十四章　免疫和炎症导论

CELLS AND ORGANS OF THE IMMUNE SYSTEM
- Hematopoiesis
- Cells of the Innate Immune System
- Cells of the Adaptive Immune System
- Organs of the Immune System

INNATE IMMUNITY
- Anatomical Barriers
- Pathogen Recognition
- Pathogen Clearance

ADAPTIVE IMMUNITY
- Initiation of the Adaptive Immune Response
- Pathogen Recognition
- Pathogen Receptors: BCRs and TCRs
- Antigen Processing and Presentation
- Lymphocyte Development and Tolerance
- Primary Responses
- Leukocyte Extravasation: Diapedesis
- Immunological Memory
- Summary: Innate and Adaptive Immunity in Infectious Diseases

INFLAMMATION
- What Is Inflammation, and What Purpose Does It Serve?
- Acute Inflammatory Response
- Chronic Inflammation

IMMUNE SYSTEM–RELATED CONDITIONS
- Hypersensitivity Reactions
- Autoimmunity, Immune Deficiency, and Transplant Rejection
- Cancer Immunotherapy

中文导读

本章主要介绍：免疫系统中的细胞和器官，包括造血功能、先天免疫系统细胞、适应性免疫系统细胞和免疫系统器官；先天免疫，包括解剖学屏障、病原体识别和病原体清除；适应性免疫，包括适应性免疫反应的启动、病原体识别、病原体受体（BCRs和TCRs）、抗原处理和呈递、淋巴细胞的发育和耐受性、初级反应、白细胞外渗（渗出）、免疫记忆、有关传染病的先天免疫和适应性免疫的总结；炎症，包括什么是炎症及其作用、急性炎症反应及慢性炎症；免疫系统相关状况，包括过敏反应，自身免疫、免疫缺陷和移植排斥反应，癌症免疫治疗。

Abbreviations

Ag: antigen
APC: antigen presenting cell
BCR: B-cell receptor
C#: complement component # (e.g. C3, C5)
CD: cluster of differentiation
CLL: chronic lymphocytic leukemia
CR#: complement receptor #
CTL: cytotoxic T lymphocyte
CTLA-4: cytotoxic T-lymphocyte–associated protein 4
DC: dendritic cell
HLA: human leukocyte antigen
HSC: hematopoietic stem cell
IFN: interferon
Ig: immunoglobulin
IL: interleukin
iNOS: inducible nitric oxide synthase: NOS2
IRF#: interferon regulatory factor #
ISG: interferon-stimulated gene
ISRE: interferon-stimulated response element
LTB_4: Leukotriene B_4
MADCAM-1: mucosal vascular addressin cell adhesion molecule 1
MALT: mucosa-associated lymphoid tissue
MHC: major histocompatibility complex
NK cell: natural killer cell
NO: nitric oxide
NSAID: nonsteroidal anti-inflammatory drug
PAMP: pathogen-associated molecular pattern
PD1: programmed cell death protein 1
PRR: pattern recognition receptor
Rh: rhesus
ROS: reactive oxygen species
ST: short term
TAP: transporter associated with antigen processing
T_C: cytotoxic T cell
TCR: T-cell receptor
T_{FH}: follicular helper T cells
T_H: helper T cell
TLR: toll-like receptor
TNF-α: tumor necrosis factor alpha
T_{Reg}: T-regulatory cells

The introduction of pathogens and foreign proteins into the human body can stimulate immune recognition, leading to inflammatory and allergic responses. Aspects of these responses are subject to pharmacological modulation. Before describing the actions of pharmacological agents affecting allergy and immunity, this chapter describes the cellular and molecular basis of immune and allergic responses and the points of pharmacological intervention. Subsequent chapters in this section cover in detail the classes of agents that can alter allergic and immune responses, as well as the biology and pharmacology of inflammation.

Cells and Organs of the Immune System

Hematopoiesis

All blood cells, including immune cells, originate from pluripotent hematapoietic stem cells (HSCs) of the bone marrow. HSCs are a population of undifferentiated progenitor cells that are capable of self-renewal. On exposure to cytokines and contact with the surrounding stromal cells, HSCs can differentiate into megakaryocytes (the source of platelets), erythrocytes (red blood cells), and leukocytes (white blood cells). This process is known as hematopoiesis (Figure 34–1).

The HSC pool can be divided in two populations: long-term (LT) and short-term (ST) HSCs. LT-HSCs are capable of lifelong self-renewal, allowing for continuous hematopoiesis throughout life. ST-HSCs have limited self-renewing capability, and differentiate into multipotent progenitors—the common myeloid progenitor (CMP) and the common lymphoid progenitor (CLP). The CMP gives rise to the myeloid lineage of cells that includes megakaryocytes; erythrocytes; granulocytes (neutrophils, eosinophils, basophils, mast cells); monocytes; macrophages; and dendritic cells (DCs).. In contrast, the CLP gives rise to the lymphoid lineage of cells that includes natural killer (NK) cells, B lymphocytes (B cells), and T lymphocytes (T cells) (Doulatov et al., 2012; Eaves, 2015).

Cells of the Innate Immune System

Innate immunity refers to the host defense mechanisms that are immediately available on exposure to pathogens.

Granulocytes

Granulocytes have characteristic cytoplasmic granules containing substances that, in addition to killing invading pathogens, enhance inflammation at the site of infection or injury. Neutrophils are the most abundant of the granulocytes and are generally the first cells to arrive at the site of injury. They are specialized at engulfing and killing pathogens—a process known as phagocytosis. Like neutrophils, eosinophils are also motile phagocytic cells. These cells defend against parasitic organisms such as helminths by releasing the contents of their granules, which are thought to damage the parasite membrane. Basophils and mast cells have granules that contain histamine and other pharmacologically active substances. In addition to their protective function, these cells can become dysregulated during the generation of allergic responses, in which they play an important role (see Hypersensitivity Reactions).

Mononuclear Phagocytes

Mononuclear phagocytes consist of monocytes and macrophages. Monocytes circulate in the blood and then migrate into tissues where they differentiate into macrophages, increase 5- to 10-fold in size, and acquire enhanced phagocytic and microbicidal activity. Macrophages engulf and eliminate pathogens, dead cells, and cellular debris. Macrophages can remain motile and travel throughout the tissues by amoeboid movements, and they can also take up residence in specific tissues, becoming tissue-resident macrophages. In addition to their role as phagocytes, macrophages release pro-inflammatory molecules, such as cytokines and eicosanoids, that recruit other immune cells to the site of infection (see Inflammation).

Natural Killer Cells

Natural killer cells are cytotoxic, granular lymphocytes that target tumor and virus-infected cells. NK cell receptors selectively target damaged or infected host cells by recognizing abnormal expression of surface molecules seen on damaged, but not healthy, cells.

Dendritic Cells

Dendritic cells are specialized cells that reside in tissues and stimulate adaptive immune responses. Immature DCs patrol peripheral tissues and sample their environment for infection by capturing pathogens through phagocytosis, receptor-mediated endocytosis, and pinocytosis. After maturation, DCs shift from a phenotype that promotes antigen capture, to one that supports antigen presentation. Mature DCs migrate from the peripheral tissues to lymphoid organs and present antigens to activate helper and cytotoxic T cells (see Antigen Processing and Presentation).

Cells of the Adaptive Immune System

Adaptive immunity (also known as the acquired immune system) represents a branch of the immune system that is characterized by antigen specificity and immunological memory. It is mediated by B and T lymphocytes following exposure to specific antigens and is more complex than innate immunity in that it requires prior antigen processing and recognition to launch lymphocyte responses. Furthermore, in contrast to innate immune responses, which occur within hours after infection, B- and T-lymphocyte responses take days to develop.

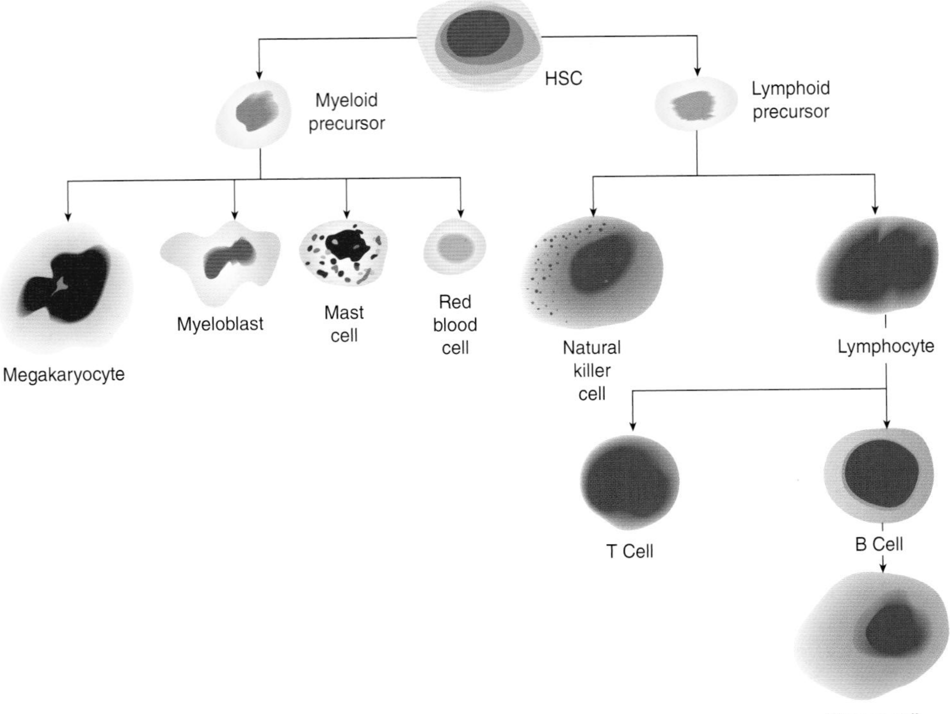

Figure 34–1 *Development of myeloid and lymphoid lineage cells from HSCs in the bone marrow.* HSCs give rise to lineage-specific precursors, which differentiate into all myeloid and lymphoid cells.

B Cells

The B lymphocytes, also known as B cells, express cell surface pathogen receptors called immunoglobulins. When a naïve B cell (one that has not previously encountered antigen) detects a pathogen through binding of its immunoglobulin, it begins to proliferate. Its progeny can differentiate into plasma cells or memory B cells. Plasma cells are short-lived effector cells that specialize in secreting antibodies—the soluble form of immunoglobulins. Memory B cells are long-lived and persist for years following an infection. Because memory B cells express the same immunoglobulin as their parent B cell, they mount an enhanced secondary response to a pathogen on reinfection and are the basis for B cell–mediated immunity.

T Cells

The T lymphocytes, also known as T cells, express cell surface pathogen receptors called TCRs. Unlike immunoglobulins, which independently recognize antigens, TCRs only recognize antigens presented on MHC molecules on the surface of DCs or other APCs. T cells are divided into two subpopulations—T_C cells and T_H cells. T_C cells or killer T cells destroy host cells that are infected with intracellular pathogens, whereas T_H cells secrete cytokines that help enhance the function of other immune cells to mediate pathogen clearance. Activated T cells can differentiate into effector cells—cells that carry out immediate functions to help clear the infection—or memory cells. Memory T cells, like memory B cells, persist for years following an infection and mount an enhanced response on reexposure to the same pathogen (see Immunological Memory).

Organs of the Immune System

The organs of the immune system are divided into two categories based on their function: *primary lymphoid organs* and *secondary lymphoid organs.* Lymphocyte maturation and development take place in the primary lymphoid organs, whereas secondary lymphoid organs provide sites for mature lymphocytes to interact with APCs. These lymphoid organs are interconnected by blood and lymphatic vessels.

Primary Lymphoid Organs

The bone marrow and thymus make up the primary lymphoid organs. Both B-cell and T-cell precursors originate in the bone marrow from HSCs. B cells complete their maturation in the bone marrow, whereas T-cell precursors migrate to the thymus to complete their development.

The bone marrow tissue is composed of a meshwork of stromal cells (e.g., endothelial cells, adipocytes, fibroblasts, osteoclasts, osteoblasts, and macrophages). Immature B cells proliferate and differentiate within the bone marrow with direct (cell-cell contact) and indirect (cytokine release) help from stromal cells. IL-1, IL-6, and IL-7 are the most important cytokines guiding the B-cell differentiation process (Hoggatt et al., 2016).

The thymus is a bilobe organ that sits above the heart. Each lobe is divided into smaller lobules that consist of an outer compartment (cortex) and an inner compartment (medulla). Both the cortex and the medulla contain a stromal cell network comprising epithelial cells, DCs, and macrophages that present self-antigens to maturing T cells. This stromal cell network is responsible for the maturation process, and the cytokines IL-1, IL-2, IL-6, and IL-7 also play an important role in this process. The thymus begins to atrophy after puberty (as the thymic stroma is eventually replaced with adipose tissue), causing a decline in T-cell output. By age 35, T-cell production drops to 20% compared to that of newborn levels, and by age 65 this number further decreases to 2% (Palmer, 2013). Importantly, once the periphery is seeded with mature T cells, the host is equipped with a diversity of naïve T cells that will respond to any pathogen encounter, irrespective of diminished thymic output.

Secondary Lymphoid Organs

The secondary lymphoid organs, including the spleen, lymph nodes, and mucosa-associated lymphoid tissue MALT, are the sites where adaptive immune responses are initiated. The spleen is the largest lymphoid organ, consisting of red pulp and white pulp. The red pulp is a sponge-like tissue where old or damaged erythrocytes are recycled, whereas the white pulp region consists of lymphocytes. The spleen is the only lymphoid organ that is not connected to the lymphatic vessels. Instead, immune cells enter and exit the spleen through blood vessels.

Lymph nodes are round, specialized structures that are positioned along the lymphatic vessels like beads on a chain. They collect the lymph (containing immune cells and antigens) that drains from the skin and internal organs and provide the physical location where antigen presentation and lymphocyte activation occur. The MALTs are loosely organized lymphoid tissues located in the submucosal surfaces of the gastrointestinal (GI) tract, respiratory system, and urinary tract (Neely and Flajnik, 2016).

The Lymphatic System

The "lymphatic system" or "lymphatics" represent a network of lymphatic vessels (similar to the circulatory system's veins and capillaries) that are connected to lymph nodes. Similar to their circulatory counterparts, small lymph capillaries are made up of single endothelial cell layers, whereas in larger lymph vessels the endothelial cells are surrounded by layers of smooth muscle cells. Additional parts of the lymphatic system are the tonsils, adenoids, spleen, and thymus. The lymphatics collect plasma continuously leaking out from blood vessels into the interstitial spaces and return this fluid, now called lymph, to the blood (after filtration in the lymph nodes) into the subclavian veins located on either side of the neck near the clavicles. Unlike blood movement, which is driven by a pump and flows throughout the body in a continuous loop, lymph flows in only one direction—upward toward the neck—and movement originates from rhythmic contractions of the smooth muscle cells, with directionality achieved via semilunar valves inside the vessels. The lymphatics therefore have an important function in regulating both immune and fluid homeostasis.

The B and T cells, unlike other blood cells, traffic through the body via both blood and lymph (hence the term *lymphocyte*). After completing their development in the primary lymphoid organs, B and T cells enter the bloodstream. When lymphocytes reach blood capillaries that empty into secondary lymphoid tissues, they enter these tissues. If a naïve lymphocyte encounters antigen, it will remain in the secondary lymphoid tissue and become activated. Otherwise, if no antigen is detected, the lymphocyte then exits through the efferent lymph and reenters the bloodstream. This pattern of movement between the blood and lymph is referred to as lymphocyte recirculation, and it allows the lymphocyte population to continuously monitor the secondary lymphoid organs for signs of infection (Masopust and Schenkel, 2013; Thomas et al., 2016).

Innate Immunity

Innate immunity refers to the defense mechanisms that are immediately available on exposure to pathogens. These mechanisms consist of anatomical barriers, soluble mediators, and cellular responses. To establish an infection, a pathogen must first penetrate a host's anatomical barriers, including the skin and mucous membranes. If a pathogen manages to breach these anatomical barriers, the cellular innate immune response initiates rapidly, within a matter of minutes, to activate further mechanisms of the immune response.

Anatomical Barriers

The skin and mucosal surfaces form the first line of defense against pathogens. The skin is made up of a thin outer layer (epidermis) of tightly packed epithelial cells and an inner layer (dermis) of connective tissue containing blood vessels, sebaceous glands, and sweat glands. The respiratory, GI, and urogenital tracts are lined by mucous membranes. Like skin, mucous membranes consist of an outer layer of epithelial cells and an underlying layer of connective tissue. These anatomical surfaces act as more than just passive barriers against pathogens. All epithelial surfaces secrete antimicrobial peptides called host defense peptides (HDPs). HDPs kill bacteria, fungi, and viruses by disrupting their membranes (Hancock et al., 2016). The sebum secreted by the sebaceous glands contains fatty acids and lactic acids that inhibit bacterial growth on the skin. Mucosal surfaces are continuously covered in mucus (a viscous fluid secreted by epithelial cells of mucous membranes) containing antimicrobial substances that trap foreign microorganisms and help limit the spread of infection. In the respiratory tract, this mucous is continually removed by the action of cilia on epithelial cells. In addition, all these anatomical surfaces harbor commensal microorganisms. These commensals help protect against disease by preventing colonization by harmful microorganisms. These physical, mechanical, chemical, and microbiological barriers prevent a majority of pathogens from gaining access to the cells and tissues of the body (Belkaid and Tamoutounour, 2016).

However, some pathogens manage to breach these barriers. Microbes can enter the skin through scratches, wounds, or insect bites, such as those from mosquitoes (e.g., *Plasmodium falciparum,* the protozoan species predominantly responsible for malaria); ticks (e.g., *Borrelia burgdorferi,* the bacterium responsible for Lyme disease); and fleas (e.g., *Yersinia pestis,* the bacterium responsible for bubonic plague). Many pathogens enter the body by penetrating mucous membranes. One example is the influenza virus, which expresses a surface molecule that allows it to attach to and invade cells in the mucous membranes of the respiratory tract.

Once a pathogen breaches these anatomical barriers, the innate immune system first responds by detecting the pathogen. This initiates an inflammatory response—mediated by soluble effectors such as complement, eicosanoids, and cytokines—that results in the recruitment of immune cells to the site of infection, direct lysis or phagocytosis of pathogens, and eventual activation of the adaptive immune response.

Pathogen Recognition

The first phase of an innate immune response involves pathogen detection, which is mediated by secreted and cell surface pathogen receptors. Innate immune cells recognize broad structural patterns that are conserved within microbial species but are absent from host tissues. These broad structural patterns are referred to as *PAMPs* and the receptors that recognize them are called *PRRs*. PRRs can be broadly divided into three classes: secreted, endocytic, and signaling PRRs.

Secreted PRRs and the Complement System

Secreted PRRs are opsonins (molecules that enhance phagocytosis) that bind to microbial cell walls and tag them for destruction by the complement system or by phagocytes. C-reactive protein and mannose-binding lectin are two examples of secreted PRRs; both are components of the acute-phase response (see Inflammation).

The plasma proteins known as the complement system are some of the first to act following pathogen entry into host tissues. Over 30 proteins make up the complement system. These proteins circulate in blood and interstitial fluid in inactive forms that become activated in sequential cascades in response to interaction with molecular components of pathogens, leading to the activation of C3, which plays the most important role in pathogen detection and clearance. Complement activation leads to the cleavage of C3 into C3b and C3a fragments. The large C3b fragment (an opsonin) attaches to pathogen surfaces in a process called complement fixation and can activate C5 and a lytic pathway that can damage the plasma membrane of adjacent cells and microorganisms. The C5a fragment attracts macrophages and neutrophils and can activate mast cells. The small C3a fragment (anaphylatoxin) also promotes inflammation. Thus, complement fixation has two functions: the formation of protein complexes that damage the pathogen's membrane and marking the pathogen for destruction by phagocytes (Morgan and Harris, 2015).

PAMPs, PRRs, and the Induction of Interferons

Cells of the innate immune system—predominantly dendritic cells and macrophages—recognize broad structural patterns that are conserved within microbial species but are absent from host tissues. These patterns are called *pathogen-associated molecular patterns* (PAMPs); *Pattern recognition receptors* (PRRs) recognize PAMPS. There are three broad classes of PRRs: secreted, endocytic, and signaling PRRs.

Activation of signaling PRRs results in the production of cytokines that orchestrate the early immune response. The most well-studied group of signaling PRRs are the 11 Toll-like receptors (TLRs), each of which displays specificity for a distinct PAMP (e.g., TLR4 recognizes lipopolysaccharide (LPS); TLR3 binds double-stranded RNA [dsRNA]; TLR9 interacts with foreign DNA, etc.). Another receptor group, C-type lectin-like receptors, recognizes unique carbohydrate structures on invading microorganisms. Other signaling PRRs are cytosolic, such as retinoic acid–inducible gene (RIG)-I-like receptors (RLRs) that are activated by cytoplasmic double-stranded and 5′-triphosphorylated RNA species, and the nucleotide-binding oligomerization domain (NOD)-like receptor (NLRs) that detect cytosolic endotoxins. Signaling through most PRRs leads to broad cytokine responses, mediated by nuclear factor kappa B (NF-κB) and resulting in the production of pro-inflammatory cytokines such as interleukin (IL) 1, IL-6, IL-12, and tumor necrosis factor alpha (TNF-α).

In response to attack by viruses, bacteria, parasites, and tumor cells, membrane-bound and cytosolic (endosomal) signaling PRRs, including TLRs, work via several convergent pathways to stimulate the production of yet another class of cytokines, the interferons (IFNs). There are three types of IFNs: type I IFN (mainly IFN-α and IFN-β, plus other minor forms such as IFN-ε or IFN-ω); type II IFN (IFN-γ); and type III IFN (IFN-λ). IFNs are about 145 amino acid glycoproteins, with molecular masses of approximately 19–24 kDa, depending on the extent of glycosylation. Viral infections are the major inducers of the transcription of genes encoding type I IFNs. Pathways leading to IFN production are complex. The contemporary model now encompasses the concept that PRRs trigger intracellular signaling cascades that involve receptor-associated adapters (e.g., TRIM, TIRAP, MyD88, etc.) and the assembly of a signalosome containing various kinases (e.g., TBK1, IKKε, TAK, ASK1, etc.). Activation of these kinases in response to pathogen recognition leads to the phosphorylation and activation of the latent cytoplasmic transcription factors termed interferon regulatory factors (IRFs). Activation of IRF3 and IRF7, sometimes in combination with other transcription factors, activates transcription of the genes encoding type I IFNs.

Actions of IFNs

The IFNs are unique among the cytokine superfamily in that they produce an array of pleiotropic effects when they bind to their specific receptor. IFNs convey antiviral, antiproliferative, and immunomodulatory functions onto their target cells.

The IFNs are the most crucial cytokines in the defense against invading microorganisms, particularly viruses. IFN-α, IFN-β, and the more recently discovered IFN-λ, are vital elements in these defense mechanisms. Type I IFNs promote the production of interferon-stimulated genes (ISGs) in infected and neighboring cells, the products of which induce an intracellular antimicrobial program that limits the spread of infectious pathogens. Type I IFNs also augment antigen presentation, costimulation, and cytokine production by innate immune cells, leading to enhanced adaptive immune responses.

Produced by activated helper T (T_H) and natural killer (NK) cells, IFN-γ enhances the microbicidal activity of macrophages by inducing mammalian inducible nitric oxide synthase (iNOS, also called NOS2), thereby increasing their production of nitric oxide (NO) and their capacity to kill intracellular pathogens. Furthermore, $CD8^+$ T cells utilize IFN-γ to directly kill infected cells and tumors. Indeed, IFN-γ contributes significantly to the adaptive immune system, where it also influences developmental processes such as immunoglobulin (Ig) isotype switching in B cells and T_H1 cell differentiation.

Cellular Signaling in Responses to IFNs

Interferon signaling is a complex mechanism that elicits the appropriate antimicrobial program in target cells. IFNs bind to distinct heteromeric membrane receptors. Binding of the type I IFNs to their specific cell surface receptors leads to cross tyrosine phosphorylation, recruitment and activation of the STAT (Janus kinase/signal transducer and activator of transcription) pathway. Several members of the STAT family of transcription factors and IRF9 cooperatively form the DNA binding protein complex ISGF3, which is required for expression of ISGs through activation of the interferon-stimulated response element (ISRE) in their promoters. Transcriptional induction of these immediate early response genes facilitates the establishment of an antiviral state, achieves antiproliferation in normal and tumor cells, and influences adaptive immune responses (e.g., via modulation of IL-2 production and expression of the α chain [CD25] of the IL-2R complex; see Figure 35–2).

Numerous genes contain an ISRE. Their gene products are components of the antiviral defense: 2′-5′ poly-A-synthase, dsRNA activated protein kinase (PKR), cell surface proteins such as ICAM and the major histocompatibility complex (MHC) I and II classes, chemokines (e.g., ISG15 and the IP10), and myriad genes of unknown function. More recently, numerous micro-RNAs have been added to the repertoire of IFN-induced response genes that contribute to control of pathogens.

Endocytic PRRs

Endocytic PRRs are expressed on the surface of phagocytic cells. These receptors mediate the uptake and transport of microbes into lysosomes, where they are degraded. The degraded microbial peptides are processed and presented to T cells by members of the MHC family of cell surface proteins. (In humans, the MHC is also called *human leukocyte antigen* or *HLA*). The mannose, glucan, and scavenger receptors are part of this class of receptors.

Signaling PRRs

On PAMP detection, signaling PRRs trigger intracellular signaling cascades that eventually result in the production of cytokines that orchestrate the early immune response. The most-studied group of signaling PRRs are the TLRs. TLRs are a family of PRRs that recognize a variety of microbial products. These transmembrane proteins are composed of an extracellular domain that detects pathogens and a cytoplasmic signaling domain that relays information to the nucleus. TLRs are expressed on the plasma membranes and endosomes of immune cells.

Signaling through TLRs leads to activation of two distinct signal transduction pathways (see PAMPs, PRRs, and the Induction of Interferons on next page). Most TLRs signal through a pathway that promotes the activation of the transcription factor NF-κB and the production of pro-inflammatory cytokines such as IL-1, IL-6, IL-12, and TNF-α. The exception is TLR3, which signals through a pathway that leads to the activation of the transcription factor IRF3, and the production of interferon (IFN) types I and III TLR4 is unique in that it signals through both pathways (Cao, 2016).

Type I (IFN-α and IFN-β) and type III (IFN-λ) IFNs promote the production of ISGs in infected and neighboring cells, the products of which induce an intracellular antimicrobial program that limits the spread of infectious pathogens, particularly viruses. Type I IFNs also augment antigen presentation and cytokine production by innate immune cells, leading to enhanced adaptive immune responses (Gonzalez-Navajas et al., 2012).

Pathogen Clearance

Pathogens vary in the manner by which they live and replicate within their hosts. Extracellular pathogens replicate on epithelial surfaces, or within the interstitial spaces, blood, and lymph of their host. Intracellular pathogens establish infections within host cells, either in the cytoplasm or in cellular vesicles. Depending on the nature of the infection, different immune cells and effector mechanisms are involved in the control and elimination of the pathogen.

Extracellular Pathogens

Unlike pathogens that replicate within host cells, extracellular pathogens are accessible to soluble effector proteins. Pathogens that replicate within interstitial spaces, blood, and lymph are detected by secreted PRRs and complement proteins. Complement fixation triggers direct lysis of the pathogen and enhances pathogen uptake by phagocytic cells. The phagocytic cells involved in the clearance of extracellular pathogens are macrophages and neutrophils. Tissue-resident macrophages are long-lived cells that are present from the start of an infection. They engulf pathogens and release inflammatory mediators to alert host cells of an attack. Neutrophils, in contrast, are short-lived, circulating phagocytes. Inflammatory cues, such as those released by macrophages, recruit neutrophils to the site of infection, where they soon become the dominant phagocyte.

On entry into host tissues, the first immune cells a pathogen encounters are the tissue-resident macrophages. Macrophages phagocytize microorganisms in a nonspecific fashion through their phagocytic receptors. Proteins of the complement system enhance this process by binding to receptors expressed by macrophages. One such receptor is complement receptor 1 (CR1). CR1 molecules interact with C3b fragments that have been deposited on the pathogen's surface, facilitating the engulfment and destruction of the pathogen.

In addition to engulfing invading pathogens, macrophages alert host cells of an infection. TLR4 engagement on macrophages leads to the production of pro-inflammatory cytokines such as IL-1, IL-6, IL-12, TNF-α, and CXCL8 (see Inflammation). These cytokines recruit immune cells, the most prominent of which are neutrophils, to the infected tissue (Lavin et al., 2015).

Circulating neutrophils have an average life span of less than 2 days. Mature neutrophils are kept in the bone marrow for up to 5 days before being released into circulation, ensuring a large reserve that can be summoned during an infection. When neutrophils sense inflammatory signals such as cytokines, chemokines, eicosanoids, ROS, or NO, they migrate to the site of infection, where they engulf and kill the invading pathogen. In addition, neutrophils can release extracellular DNA nets that trap bacterial pathogens (von Kockritz-Blickwede and Nizet, 2009). Neutrophils die within 2 h of entry into infected tissues, forming the characteristic pus that develops at sites of infection (Kruger et al., 2015).

Intracellular Pathogens

The NK cells provide an early defense against intracellular pathogens. Like neutrophils, these circulating leukocytes migrate from the blood to the site of infection in response to inflammatory cues. Once at the site of infection, NK cells target and kill infected host cells.

The NK cells express receptors that deliver either activating or inhibitory signals. The ligands for the activating NK cell receptors are typically cell surface proteins whose expression is altered during infection or trauma. Healthy cells are protected from attack by NK cells because the signals generated from the inhibitory NK cell receptors dominate those generated from the activating receptors. In contrast, interaction between NK cells and infected or damaged cells shifts the balance of inhibitory and activating signals to favor an attack. This system allows NK cells to discriminate between healthy cells that should be protected and infected cells that should be destroyed.

The NK cells are stimulated by cytokines, including type I IFNs, IL-12, and TNF-α. IFN-α and IFN-β enhance NK cell cytotoxicity and induce NK cell proliferation, whereas IL-12 enhances cytokine production. The key cytokine produced by NK cells is IFN-γ, also called type II IFN. One function of IFN-γ is to activate macrophages. Activated macrophages exhibit enhanced microbicidal activity. One mechanism of their microbicidal activity is the induction of iNOS and the production of prodigious amounts of NO (Bjorkstrom et al., 2016).

Adaptive Immunity

Adaptive immunity refers to the arm of the immune response that changes (adapts) with each new infection. The cells responsible for adaptive immunity are B cells and T cells. The effector mechanisms used by B and T cells are similar to those used by innate immune cells; however, the important distinction between innate and adaptive immunity lies in their mode of pathogen recognition. Whereas the PRRs of the innate immune response recognize broad microbial patterns, B cells and T cells express receptors that recognize highly specific molecular structures. Following pathogen exposure, B and T cells with receptors that recognize the invading pathogen proliferate robustly and differentiate into effector lymphocytes. Soon after pathogen clearance, a large number of effector B and T cells die, but a small population of memory cells survives. Those cells have the ability to mount a rapid and specific response on reexposure to the same pathogen. This memory response, unique to adaptive immunity, is the basis for vaccination (see Chapter 36).

Initiation of the Adaptive Immune Response

The skin and mucosal surfaces prevent the majority of pathogens from entering host tissues and causing infections. Innate immune responses generally eliminate microorganisms that breach these barriers, typically within a few days. However, some pathogens establish an infection that cannot be controlled entirely by the innate immune response. In these cases, pathogen clearance requires the adaptive immune response.

Dendritic cells provide an essential link between innate and adaptive immunity. DCs engulf pathogens at the site of infection and travel to the lymphoid organs. Once there, they activate T cells by presenting them with fragments of the engulfed pathogen loaded on MHC molecules (see section on Antigen Processing and Presentation).

Pathogen Recognition

The innate immune system detects pathogens by a fixed repertoire of soluble and cell-surface receptors that recognize broad structures shared by different pathogens. The genes encoding these pathogen receptors are inherited from one generation to the next in a stable form.

The adaptive immune system uses a more focused strategy of pathogen recognition. B and T cells recognize pathogens by using cell surface receptors of one molecular type: BCRs and TCRs. In contrast to the stably inherited genes encoding innate immune pathogen receptors, the genes encoding BCRs and TCRs rearrange during the course of lymphocyte development. This gene rearrangement enables the development of millions of pathogen receptors with unique binding sites, each expressed by a small subset of lymphocytes. On pathogen exposure, only those lymphocytes with receptors that recognize specific components of the invading pathogen (referred to as the receptor's *cognate antigen*) are selected to proliferate and differentiate into effector cells.

Pathogen Receptors: BCRs and TCRs

The BCRs and TCRs are structurally related molecules. The BCR, also called immunoglobulin, is composed of two identical heavy chains and two identical light chains. Each polypeptide chain expresses an amino-terminal variable region, which contains the antigen-binding site, and a carboxy-terminal constant region. Immunoglobulins are anchored in the B-cell membrane by two transmembrane regions at the end of each heavy chain. Immunoglobulins are initially surface bound but become soluble when a B cell differentiates into a plasma cell. The soluble forms of immunoglobulins are called antibodies.

The TCR is composed of an α chain (TCRα) and a β chain (TCRβ), both anchored in the T-cell membrane by a transmembrane region. The α and β chains consist of a variable region that contains the antigen-binding site and a constant region. In contrast to immunoglobulins, TCRs remain membrane bound and are not secreted.

Both BCRs and TCRs develop through gene rearrangement. This genetic recombination process (which B cells complete in the bone marrow and T cells in the thymus) is a defining feature of the adaptive immune system. The human BCR and its soluble derivative, the antibody, are composed from genes of three loci, the *IG heavy chain*, the *IG κ light chain*, and the *IG λ light chain*, yielding a repertoire of more than 10^{11} possible combinations. In close resemblance, the TCR comprises either an α and a β chain (most common) or a γ and a δ chain. Two of the key enzymes involved are RAG1 and RAG2 (RAG, recombination-activating gene; deficiencies in these enzymes result in a complete absence of mature lymphocytes) and the terminal deoxynucleotidyl transferase, albeit the full complexity of the DNA repair machinery is required to accomplish a productive rearrangement. Failure to do so will lead to the elimination of the unsuccessful B or T cells by programmed cell death (Nemazee, 2006). These recombination and subsequent somatic hypermutation events are vital for an optimally performing adaptive immune system. They remain unutilized as pharmacological targets.

Antigen Processing and Presentation

Immunoglobulins are capable of recognizing antigens in their native form. TCRs, in contrast, only recognize processed antigen fragments presented by specialized molecules encoded by the MHC (Figure 34–2). The MHC was first identified as a genetic complex that determines an organism's ability to accept or reject transplanted tissue. Further studies highlighted the importance of MHC molecules in generating T_H- and T_C-cell responses.

There are two types of MHC molecules involved in antigen presentation: MHC class I and MHC class II. These structurally related molecules are expressed on different cell types but perform parallel functions in priming T-cell responses.

MHC Class I

MHC class I molecules consist of a transmembrane glycoprotein α chain noncovalently associated with a $β_2$m molecule. MHC class I molecules are expressed on the surface of nearly all nucleated cells and present peptides from endogenous antigens to CD8 T_C cells.

MHC Class II

MHC class II molecules consist of two noncovalently associated transmembrane glycoproteins, an α chain and a β chain. MHC class II molecules are primarily expressed on the surface of professional APCs (DCs, macrophages, B cells) and present peptides from exogenous antigens to CD4 T_H cells.

Antigen Processing for Presentation by MHC

Unlike immunoglobulins, which recognize a wide range of molecular structures in their native form, TCRs can only recognize antigens in the form of a peptide bound to an MHC molecule. For a pathogen to be recognized by a T cell, pathogen-derived proteins need to be degraded into peptides—an event referred to as antigen processing (Figure 34-2). Endogenous antigens, those derived from intracellular pathogens, are processed by the cytosolic pathway for presentation by MHC class I molecules. Proteins in the cytosol are degraded into peptides by the proteosome. The resultant peptides are then transported out of the cytosol and into the ER by a protein called the *TAP*, which is embedded in the ER membrane. Once newly synthesized MHC class I α chains and $β_2$m molecules are translocated into the ER membrane, the α chains and $β_2$m molecules associate and bind peptide, forming a peptide-MHC complex. These peptide-MHC complexes make their way to the plasma membrane in membrane-enclosed vesicles of the Golgi apparatus.

Exogenous antigens, those derived from extracellular pathogens, are processed by the endocytic pathway for presentation by MHC class II molecules. In this pathway, extracellular pathogens are internalized by host cells through endocytosis or phagocytosis and are degraded by

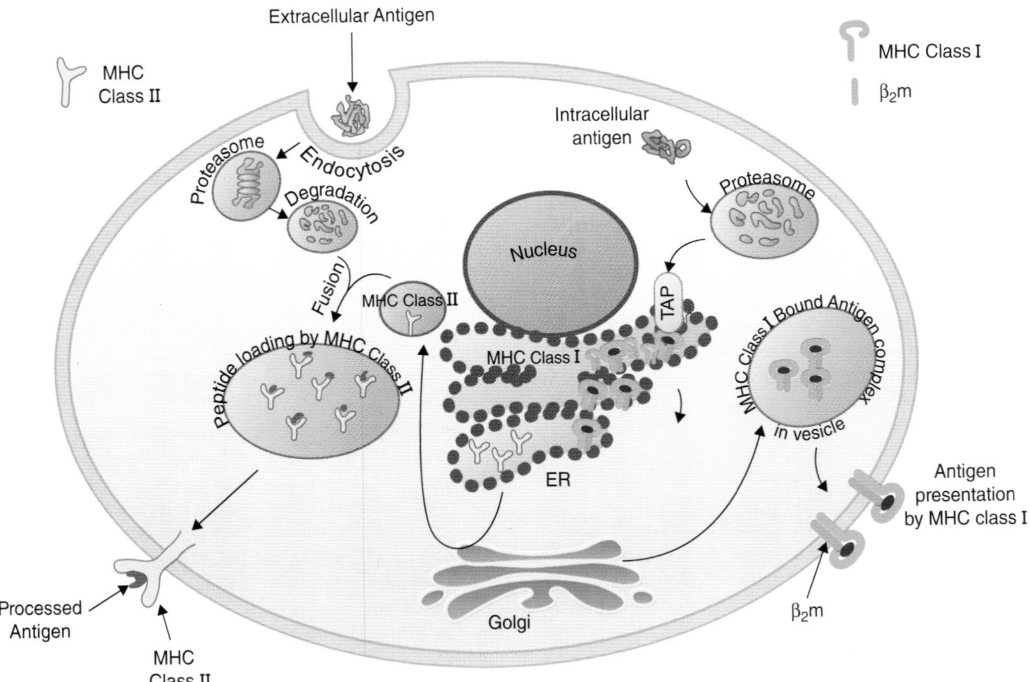

Figure 34–2 *Antigen processing and presentation via the MHC class I and II pathways.* Endogenous peptides from a variety of sources are processed by proteasomes; the resulting peptides are transported via the TAP complex into the ER, where they encounter MHC class I-$β_2$M ($β_2$-microglobulin) heterodimers. After the peptide loading of the MHC class I complex, the final peptide–MHC class I complexes migrate through the Golgi and are delivered to the cell surface to engage CD8⁺ T cells. Exogenous antigens are endocytosed and processed by a lysosome/proteasome. The MHC class II complex is assembled in the ER, migrates through the Golgi, and subsequently fuses with the vesicle containing processed antigen fragments. These peptide cleavage products are loaded into the peptide-binding groove of the MHC class II, and the peptide–MHC class II complexes are transported to the cell surface and presented to CD4⁺ T cells.

proteolytic enzymes within endocytic vesicles. Newly synthesized MHC class II α and β chains are translocated into the ER membrane, where they associate with a third chain, called the invariant chain. The invariant chain prevents MHC class II molecules from binding peptides in the ER and delivers MHC class II molecules to endocytic vesicles. Once in the endocytic vesicles, MHC class II molecules bind peptide and are carried to the cell surface by outgoing vesicles.

All T cells require peptide-MHC presentation by professional APCs for activation (see Primary Responses). If an intracellular pathogen does not infect a professional APC, CD8 T_C-cell responses can be generated through a third pathway of antigen presentation called *cross-presentation*. Cross-presentation involves the uptake of extracellular material by professional APCs and its delivery to the MHC class I presentation pathway instead of the MHC class II presentation pathway via a mechanism that remains incompletely understood (Blum et al., 2013).

Note that protein degradation occurs continuously, even in the absence of infection. In uninfected cells, MHC molecules carry self-peptides—derived from normal cellular protein turnover—to the cell surface. While these peptide-MHC complexes do not normally provoke an immune response, recognition of these self-peptides by autoreactive T cells can result in the development of *autoimmunity* (see *Autoimmunity: A Breach of Tolerance*).

Lymphocyte Development and Tolerance

Innate immune PRRs are fixed receptors that recognize broad microbial structures or structures associated with damaged host cells. These receptors rarely, if ever, recognize self-antigens expressed by healthy cells. In contrast, because BCRs and TCRs develop from gene rearrangement, receptors that recognize self-antigens expressed by healthy host cells can arise. The goal of lymphocyte development is to produce cells with functional pathogen receptors but eliminate cells whose receptors recognize self-antigens. Next, we describe the processes of B-cell and T-cell development and highlight the mechanisms that maintain self-tolerance.

B-Cell Development

B-cell development takes place in the bone marrow and is driven by interaction with bone marrow stromal cells and the local cytokine environment. B-cell development can be broadly divided into pro-B-, pre-B-, immature B-, and mature B-cell stages. BCR gene rearrangement starts at the early pro-B stage and continues throughout the pre-B stage. By the immature B-cell stage, B cells express fully rearranged IgM immunoglobulins on their cell surface. At this stage, immature B cells leave the bone marrow and complete their maturation in the periphery. Mature B cells express both IgM and IgD immunoglobulins on their cell surfaces (LeBien and Tedder, 2008).

Because B-cell activation depends on help from CD4 T_H cells, negative selection of T cells whose receptors recognize self-antigens also ensures that B cells whose receptors bind to the same self-antigen will not be activated. Consequently, B cells do not undergo as rigorous of a selection process as T cells. However, B cells whose receptors recognize components of the bone marrow are negatively selected and die by apoptosis.

T-Cell Development

Unlike B cells, which develop in the bone marrow, T-cell precursors complete their development in the thymus. T-cell precursors enter the thymus as $CD4^-$ $CD8^-$ DN (double negative) cells, not yet committed to the T-cell lineage.

The DN T cells can be divided into four subsets—DN1 to DN4—based on the expression of certain cell surface molecules. Gene rearrangement of the TCRB chain begins during the DN2 stage and continues through the DN3 stage. After β-chain rearrangement is complete, the newly synthesized β-chain combines with a protein known as the pre-Tα chain, forming the pre-TCR. DN3 cells then progress to the DN4 stage and express both the CD4 and CD8 coreceptors. These cells are now referred to as $CD4^+CD8^+$ DP (double positive) cells. DP T cells proliferate rapidly, generating clones of cells expressing the same β chain. After this period of rapid proliferation, T cells begin to rearrange their α-chain genes. Because cells within each clone can rearrange a different α chain, they generate a more diverse population than if the original cell had rearranged both the β chain and α chain before proliferating. Once a DP T cell expresses a fully rearranged TCR, it undergoes the processes of positive and negative selection.

The T cells migrate into the thymic cortex to undergo positive selection. The purpose of positive selection is to select for T cells whose TCRs can interact with an individual's own MHC molecules. In the cortex, T cells interact with cortical thymic epithelial cells, which express both MHC class I and MHC class II molecules. T cells with TCRs that do not recognize self-MHC molecules die by apoptosis. T cells with TCRs that can successfully bind to self-MHC molecules are signaled to survive and proceed to the thymic medulla. As a result of positive selection, DP thymocytes mature into single-positive T cells that express just one coreceptor (CD4 or CD8). T cells that successfully interact with MHC class I molecules develop into CD8 T cells, whereas T cells that interact with MHC class II molecules become CD4 cells.

After positive selection, T cells migrate to the thymic medulla to undergo negative selection. The purpose of negative selection is to eliminate T cells whose TCRs recognize self-antigens. This is accomplished by medullary thymic epithelial cells, which promiscuously express self-peptides on their MHC molecules. If T cells interact with self-peptides with high affinity, they are deleted by apoptosis (Shah and Zuniga-Pflucker, 2014).

The positive and negative selection processes responsible for generating self-MHC restricted and self-tolerant T cells are rigorous. It is estimated that over 98% of thymocytes die by apoptosis within the thymus, with the majority failing at the positive selection stage. The T cells that manage to successfully complete both positive and negative selection leave the thymus and take up residence in the secondary lymphoid structures.

Primary Responses

The processes of lymphocyte development and gene rearrangement generate millions of unique lymphocytes that each express pathogen receptors of a single specificity. During an infection, only a small portion of these B and T cells express receptors that can recognize the invading pathogen. To increase their numbers, each lymphocyte that recognizes the invading pathogen becomes activated and proliferates, giving rise to clones expressing identical immunoglobulins or TCRs. These processes, referred to as *clonal selection* and *clonal expansion*, are essential features of lymphocyte activation and differentiation, and facilitate the effector mechanisms that B and T cells use to combat infection.

B-Cell Activation and Antibody Production

In the majority of primary immune responses, B-cell activation and subsequent antibody production are dependent on help from CD4 T_H cells. When circulating B cells home to secondary lymphoid tissues, they first enter at the T-cell zone. If a B cell encounters its specific antigen, cross-linking of the BCR and coreceptor induces a signal transduction cascade that mediates changes in cell surface expression of adhesion molecules and chemokine receptors, preventing the B cells from leaving the T-cell zone.

After immunoglobulins bind their cognate antigen, they internalize the antigen by receptor-mediated endocytosis and process the antigen for display by MHC class II molecules. If a CD4 T_H cell recognizes its antigen, the B and T cell form a conjugate pair. This cognate interaction facilitates the delivery of T cell–derived cytokines to B cells. The most important of these cytokines is IL-4, which is essential for B-cell proliferation and differentiation into antibody-secreting plasma cells.

The initial antibodies produced by plasma cells are of generally low affinity. They help to keep the infection under control until a stronger antibody response is generated. Antibody quality improves over the course of the infection due to two processes: somatic hypermutation and isotype switching. Somatic hypermutation introduces random single-nucleotide substitutions throughout the immunoglobulin variable regions. These changes can result in immunoglobulin molecules with increased affinity for the pathogen. B cells producing these improved immunoglobulin molecules outcompete for binding to the invading pathogen and are preferentially selected to become plasma cells. As an infection proceeds, antibodies of higher affinity are produced—a process referred to as *affinity maturation* (Di Noia and Neuberger, 2007).

Isotype Switching. Immunoglobulins can be divided into five classes (isotypes) called IgA, IgD, IgE, IgG, and IgM. These isotypes differ in their heavy-chain constant regions and have specialized effector functions. IgM is the first antibody secreted following B-cell activation and marks pathogens for destruction by the complement system. As an infection proceeds, antibodies with additional effector functions are generated by isotype switching. Isotype switching is a process by which proliferating B cells rearrange their DNA to change their immunoglobulin constant regions. This process is strongly influenced by cytokines secreted by the B cell's cognate T cell (Xu et al., 2012).

Role of Antibodies in Pathogen Clearance. Antibodies can aid in pathogen clearance in a number of ways. They can bind to a pathogen (or toxin) and prevent it from interacting with host cells. These antibodies are called neutralizing antibodies. Antibodies can also function as opsonins—coating of pathogens with antibodies can facilitate their engulfment by phagocytic cells, which often express receptors for the constant regions of antibodies. In addition, antibody deposition can activate the complement system, leading to the direct lysis of pathogens.

T-Cell Activation

Naïve T cells first encounter antigen presented by DCs in the secondary lymphoid tissues. For T cells to become fully activated, they need to receive two signals (Figure 34–3):

- a primary signal generated through ligation of the TCR
- a costimulatory signal generated through ligation of a T-cell surface protein called CD28

Both of these signals must be delivered by ligands on the same APC.

The primary signal is generated when the TCR engages a peptide-MHC complex. The TCR associates with an accessory molecule called CD3, forming the TCR-CD3 complex. CD3 does not influence the interaction of the TCR with its antigen but participates in the signal transduction that occurs after antigen engagement. The T-cell coreceptors CD4 and CD8 bind to the conserved regions of MHC molecules, strengthening and stabilizing the interaction between the TCR and the peptide-MHC complex. CD4 and CD8 also participate in signal transduction.

The costimulatory signal is generated when CD28 binds to its ligands, called B7-1 (CD80) and B7-2 (CD86). These costimulatory B7 molecules are only expressed on activated professional APCs, highlighting their importance in T-cell activation.

Engagement of the TCR complex activates signal transduction cascades that induce the expression of multiple genes, including NFAT, AP-1, and NF-κB. One of the most important downstream targets of these genes is IL-2, a cytokine that is essential for T-cell proliferation and survival. The IL-2 receptor, CD25, is expressed on activated T cells. When T cells become activated, they begin to express a cell surface protein called CTLA-4. This protein resembles CD28 and binds to the costimulatory B7 molecules with higher affinity than does CD28. Whereas CD28 ligation promotes T-cell activation, CTLA-4 ligation dampens T-cell activation. This inhibitory molecule serves to keep T-cell responses in check (Brownlie and Zamoyska, 2013). In addition to CTLA-4, T cells upregulate expression of other inhibitory coreceptors such as PD1 and PSGL-1 that help to fine-tune the ensuing T-cell response (Attanasio et al., 2016; Tinoco et al., 2016).

T-Cell Anergy. For a naïve T cell to become fully activated, it must receive a signal through the TCR and CD28. If a T cell engages a peptide-MHC complex in the absence of a sufficient costimulatory signal, it enters a state of nonresponsiveness referred to as clonal anergy. Anergy is defined by the

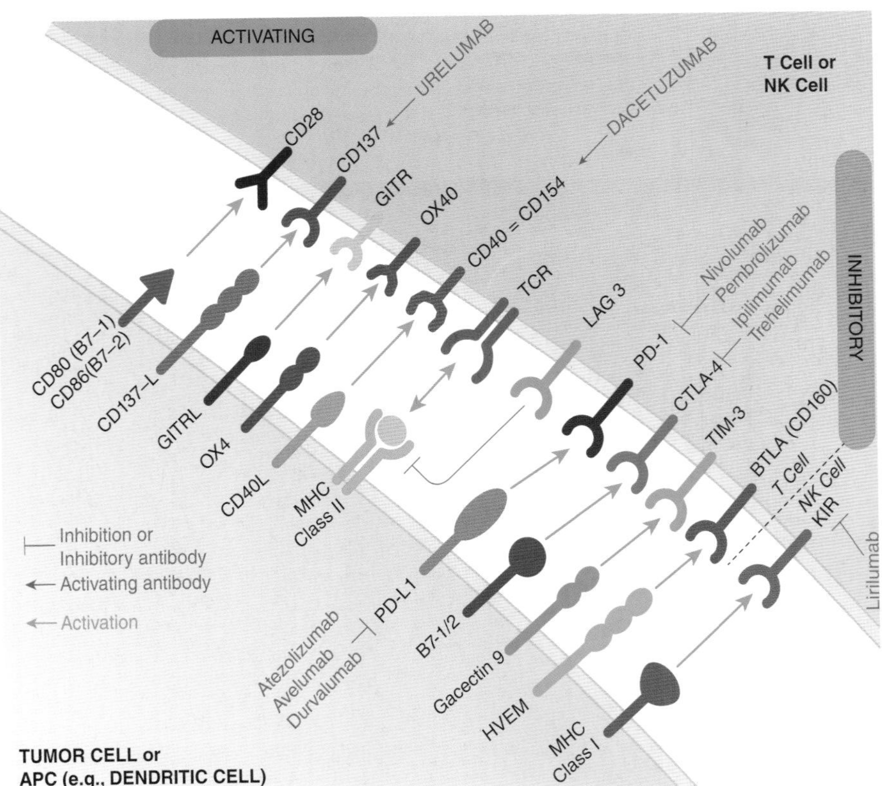

Figure 34–3 *T-cell receptor signaling.* TCR signaling on CD4+ cells after engagement with an MHC class II–peptide complex is enhanced by activating coreceptors (green-shaded area) or attenuated by inhibitory coreceptors (red-shaded area) after these bind their respective ligands on APCs or tumor cells. Numerous activating (→) or blocking (—|) monoclonal antibodies interfere with this fine-tuning of TCR signaling, thus allowing for the pharmacological modulation of the resulting immune response.

inability of T cells to proliferate after engaging a peptide-MHC complex due to a lack of IL-2 production and signaling (see Figure 35–2).

CD4 T_H-Cell Differentiation and Effector Functions. Following activation, naïve CD4 T_H cells can differentiate into specialized T_H-cell subsets. These T_H-cell subsets display unique patterns of cytokine production and perform distinct effector functions. The initial studies on T_H-cell differentiation generated a biphasic model in which activated T_H cells differentiate into either T_H1 cells, which defend mainly against intracellular pathogens, or T_H2 cells, which aid in the clearance of extracellular pathogens. More recent models of T_H-cell differentiation have been expanded to include T_H9, T_H17, T_H22, T_{FH}, and T_{Reg} cells (DuPage and Bluestone, 2016).

As their name implies, CD4 T_H cells help activate other immune cells. T_H1 cells secrete IFN-γ and TNF-α, which activate macrophages to kill pathogens located within their phagosomes. These cytokines also activate CD8 T_C cells to kill infected host cells. T_H2 cells, which produce IL-4 and IL-5, defend against extracellular pathogens by enhancing humoral immunity. IL-4 activates B cells to differentiate into antibody-secreting plasma cells. T_H2-derived cytokines also induce class switching to IgA and IgE. Another subset of CD4 T_H cell, the T_{Reg} cell, is responsible for maintaining peripheral tolerance. Through various mechanisms, these cells suppress the proliferation of effector T cells, keeping the T-cell response under control.

CD8 T_C-Cell Effector Functions. The main role of CD8 T_C cells is to induce cytolysis of infected host cells expressing peptide-MHC class I complexes. Activated CD8 T_C cells kill their target cells by two distinct pathways: the granule exocytosis pathway and the Fas-FasL pathway. The granule exocytosis pathway involves the release of perforin and granule enzymes (granzymes A and B). Perforin molecules form pores in the target cell membrane, allowing the granzyme molecules to enter the cell. Upregulation of FasL (CD95L) on activated T_C cells induces the aggregation of Fas (CD95) on target cells. Both of these pathways activate the caspase cascade in the target cell, resulting in programmed cell death.

In addition to their cytolytic activity, activated CD8 T_C cells release pro-inflammatory cytokines, including IFN-γ and TNF-α. These cytokines further aid in pathogen clearance by enhancing the activity of macrophages and neutrophils (Harty et al., 2000).

Leukocyte Extravasation: Diapedesis

Leukocytes fulfill most of their immunological functions outside the bloodstream in the surrounding tissues. Consequently, traversing the blood endothelial cell layer barrier is a crucial step in this process. Extravasation (diapedesis) refers to the movement of leukocytes out of the blood into the site of infection or physical tissue damage (Figure 34–4). In the case of blood monocytes, extravasation also occurs in the absence of pathophysiological events and facilitates their conversion into tissue macrophages. On a molecular level, diapedesis can be dissected into four mechanistic steps: *chemoattraction, rolling adhesion, tight adhesion,* and *transmigration* (Vestweber, 2015).

While initially believed to play its most important role in innate immunity, diapedesis has garnered more attention in recent years as a pharmacological target in the treatment of chronic (inflammatory) autoimmune diseases such as *multiple sclerosis* or *Crohn disease* (see Autoimmunity). The leukocyte cell surface adhesion molecule $\alpha_4\beta_1$ integrin (VLA-4) that facilitates extravasation of CD4⁺ T cells interacts with VCAM-1 on vascular endothelial cells. Natalizumab is a humanized monoclonal antibody directed against α_4 integrin whose interference with the $\alpha_4\beta_1$ integrin–VCAM-1 interaction leads to a blockade of autoreactive T-cell diapedesis into the brain and thus prevents attack on the myelin composing the nerve shielding. Similarly, natalizumab-mediated prevention of $\alpha_4\beta_7$ integrin

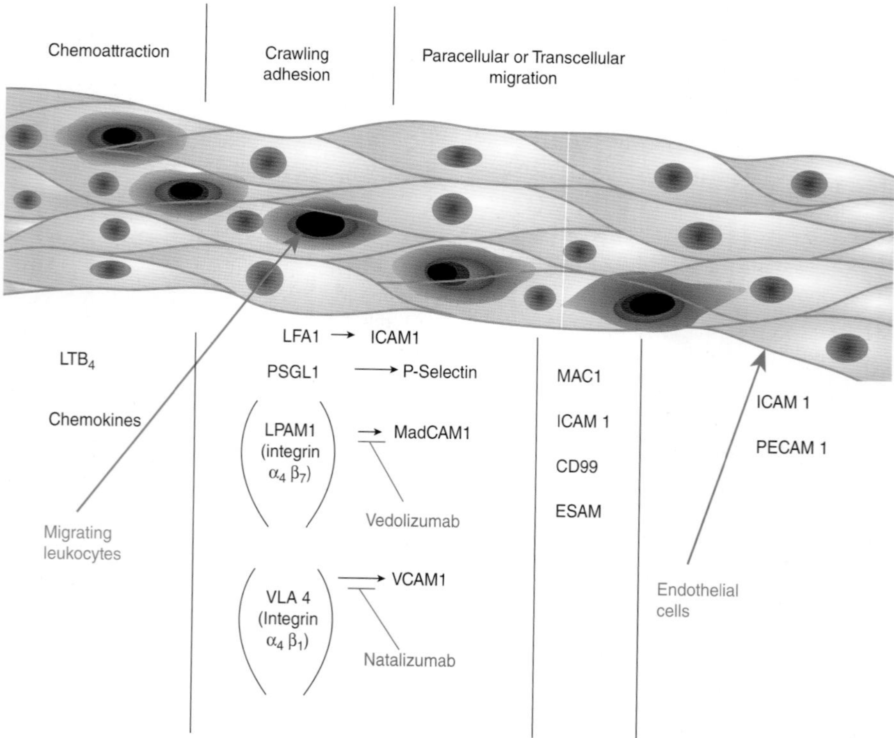

Figure 34–4 *Leukocyte diapedesis.* Leukocytes are recruited to the site of injury or infection by various chemoattractants. The expression of specific, complementary adhesion molecules on the surfaces of both the endothelial cells and the leukocytes facilitates the initial capture and subsequently the "rolling" binding of the leukocyte. After engagement of additional adhesion molecules, the leukocyte enters the subendothelial space, either by squeezing between endothelial cells (paracellular migration) or via movement through individual endothelial cells (transcellular migration). CAM, cellular adhesion molecule; ESAM, endothelial CAM; VCAM-1, vascular CAM 1; MADCAM-1, mucosal vascular addressin CAM 1; ICAM, inter-CAM; PSGL-1, P-selectin glycoprotein ligand 1; CD99, cluster of differentiation 99 antigen; MAC-1, macrophage-1 antigen.

binding to the adhesion molecule MADCAM-1 found on endothelial cells of venules is responsible for the efficacy of the drug against Crohn disease. Another monoclonal antibody recently approved for the treatment of Crohn disease and ulcerative colitis is vedolizumab, which produces fewer side effects due to its $\alpha_4\beta_7$-restricted binding specificity. Preventing entry of effector cells to inflammatory sites through the use of neutralizing antibodies has shown high therapeutic potential in multiple disease settings.

Immunological Memory

The B- and T-cell numbers decline after pathogen clearance, leaving behind a small population of memory cells. These memory cells have the ability to mount an enhanced secondary immune response on reexposure to the same pathogen.

Due to their expression of certain cell surface molecules, memory T cells are more sensitive to TCR-mediated activation by peptide-MHC complexes than naïve T cells. In addition, memory T cells have less-stringent requirements for costimulatory signals, allowing them to respond to peptide-MHC complexes displayed on cells that lack the costimulatory B7 molecules (Farber et al., 2014). Memory B cells produce better antibodies than naïve B cells because they express immunoglobulins that underwent somatic hypermutation and isotype switching during the first antigen encounter (Kurosaki et al., 2015). Combined, these properties allow for a faster and stronger secondary immune response, features that form the foundation of vaccination and subsequent "booster" or "refresher" inoculations (see Chapter 36).

Summary: Innate and Adaptive Immunity in Infectious Diseases

As described, the innate and adaptive immune systems work together to keep the host healthy. The innate immune response is the body's first line of defense and eliminates the majority of pathogens on its own. In the case that the innate immune system is insufficient to eliminate the pathogen, it keeps the infection in check until the adaptive immune system is able to mount a response. Pathogens will be cleared (acute infections), or they may evade the immune response and persist (chronic infections). Chronic infections such as HIV/AIDS and hepatitis B and C lead to immune system suppression that results in susceptibility to secondary infections or cancers associated with infection.

Inflammation

What Is Inflammation, and What Purpose Does It Serve?

The inflammatory response, or inflammation, is a physiologic response to tissue injury and infection, although it should be clear that *inflammation* is not a synonym for *infection*. The Romans described the characteristics of this response almost 2000 years ago: pain (*dolor*), heat (*calor*), redness (*rubor*), and swelling (*tumor*). Within minutes of tissue injury and infection, plasma proteins mediate an increase in vascular diameter (vasodilation) and vascular permeability. Vasodilation increases blood flow to the area of injury, resulting in the heating and reddening of the tissue. Increased vascular permeability allows leakage of fluid from the blood vessels into the damaged tissue, resulting in swelling (edema). Within a few hours of these vascular changes, leukocytes arrive at the site of injury. They adhere to activated endothelial cells in the inflamed region and pass through the capillary walls into the tissue (extravasation). These leukocytes phagocytize the invading pathogens and release soluble mediators—cytokines, prostaglandins, leukotrienes—that further contribute to the inflammatory response and the recruitment and activation of effector cells.

Inflammation can be acute, as in response to tissue injury, or it may be chronic, leading to progressive tissue destruction, as seen in chronic infections, autoimmunity, and certain cancers. Next, we discuss both forms of inflammation, including their triggers, the soluble mediators and cell types involved, and the resulting tissue pathology.

Acute Inflammatory Response

The acute inflammatory response provides protection following tissue injury and infection by restricting damage to the localized site, recruiting immune cells to eliminate the invading pathogen, and initiating the process of wound repair.

Following tissue damage, a number of plasma proteins are activated, including those of the clotting and kinin systems. The enzymatic cascade of the clotting system produces fibrin strands that accumulate to form clots, limiting the spread of infection into the blood. The enzymatic cascade of the kinin system results in the production of bradykinin—a peptide that induces vasodilation and enhanced vascular permeability (see Chapter 39). In addition, the complement products C3a and C5a bind to receptors on local mast cells, facilitating their degranulation. The resulting release of histamine, prostaglandins, and leukotrienes contributes to vascular changes by inducing vasodilation and enhancing vascular permeability. Prostaglandins and leukotrienes also serve as chemoattractants for neutrophils (see Chapter 37).

Within a few hours of these vascular changes, neutrophils bind to the endothelial cells of the inflamed region and extravasate into the tissue (see previous section, Diapedesis). They phagocytize the invading pathogens and release soluble inflammatory mediators, including macrophage inflammatory proteins (MIPs) 1α and 1β, which are chemokines that attract macrophages to the site of inflammation. Macrophages arrive at the damaged tissue 5 to 6 h after the onset of the inflammatory response. Activated macrophages secrete three major pro-inflammatory cytokines: IL-1, IL-6, and TNF-α. These cytokines induce coagulation, increase vascular permeability, and promote the acute-phase response. IL-1 and TNF-α also induce increased expression of adhesion molecules on endothelial cells, allowing for circulating leukocytes (neutrophils, macrophages, granulocytes, and lymphocytes) to interact with the endothelium and extravasate into the inflamed tissues. Acute inflammation displays a rapid onset following tissue injury and resolves relatively quickly. The resulting tissue pathology is typically mild and localized.

Chronic Inflammation

Chronic inflammation results from continuous exposure to the offending element. This can be due to pathogen persistence, autoimmune diseases in which self-antigens continuously activate T cells, and cancers. The hallmark of chronic inflammation is the accumulation and activation of macrophages and lymphocytes, as well as fibroblasts that replace the original, damaged, or necrotic tissue. Soluble factors released by macrophages and lymphocytes play an important role in the development of chronic inflammation. While during acute inflammation non-protein–based soluble factors (e.g., eicosanoids, bioamines, etc.) dominate the landscape, chronic inflammation is largely caused not only by cytokines, chemokines, growth factors, and secreted/released enzymes, but also by ROS. For instance, cytotoxic T cells and Th1 cells release IFN-γ, which activates macrophages and DCs. These, in turn, release a variety of soluble factors, such as IL-6 and TNF-α, that ultimately result in tissue injury and cell death. Replacement of tissue lost this way by fibroblasts leads to fibrosis—an excessive deposition of fibrous tissue that can interfere with normal tissue function—due to excessive amounts of growth factors (platelet-derived growth factor, transforming growth factor-β), fibrogenic cytokines (IL-1 and TNF-α), and angiogenic factors (fibroblast growth factor, vascular endothelial growth factor). Chronic inflammation can also lead to the formation of granulomas—a mass of cells consisting of activated macrophages surrounded by activated lymphocytes.

Many mediators of acute and chronic inflammation have been identified, and there are myriad anti-inflammatory drugs available. The oldest class, NSAIDs, includes aspirin, which entered the market over a century ago, and the more recently introduced agents acetaminophen (1956) and ibuprofen (1969). NSAIDs target cyclooxygenase (COX), the rate-limiting enzyme in the production of prostaglandins, but can lead to an increase in leukotriene production. In contrast, glucocorticoids prevent the liberation of arachidonic acid from plasma-membrane phospholipids and thus reduce the synthesis of both classes of eicosanoids. The newest group of anti-inflammatory agents, whose use is limited to chronic inflammatory conditions, aims to eliminate pro-inflammatory cytokines through the use of monoclonal antibodies, or soluble receptors (typically a truncated receptor encompassing only the ligand-binding, extracellular domain). Infliximab, adalimumab, certolizumab, and golilumab are monoclonal antibodies that bind and neutralize TNF-α; etanercept is a TNF-α receptor fusion protein with the same goal.

Immune System–Related Conditions

There are pathologic conditions to which the immune system contributes, such as overreactions (allergy, autoimmunity, transplant rejection) or insufficient responses (immune deficiencies, cancer).

Hypersensitivity Reactions

The immune system mobilizes a number of effector mechanisms to eliminate pathogens from the body. These effector mechanisms typically generate a localized inflammatory response that effectively eliminates the pathogen, with minimal collateral damage to the surrounding tissue. Besides pathogens, humans come into contact with numerous foreign antigens, such as plant pollen and food. Contact with these environmental antigens does not elicit an immune response in the majority of individuals. However, in certain predisposed individuals, the immune system can mount a response to these generally innocuous antigens, resulting in tissue damage that ranges from mild irritation to life-threatening anaphylactic shock. These immune responses are referred to as allergic reactions or hypersensitivity reactions. Hypersensitivity reactions can be divided into four categories, type I to type IV, distinguished by the cell types and effector molecules involved (Burmester et al., 2003).

Type I Hypersensitivity: Immediate Hypersensitivity Reactions

Type I hypersensitivity reactions require that an individual first produces IgE antibodies on initial encounter with an antigen, also referred to as an allergen. After the antigen is cleared, the remaining antigen-specific IgE molecules will be bound by mast cells, basophils, and eosinophils that express receptors for the IgE constant region (FcεR1). This process is referred to as sensitization. On subsequent exposure to antigen, cross-linking of the IgE molecules on sensitized cells induces their immediate degranulation. The release of inflammatory mediators such as histamine, leukotrienes, and prostaglandins causes vasodilation, bronchial smooth muscle contraction, and mucus production similar to that seen during inflammatory responses to tissue injury and infection. Type I hypersensitivity reactions can be local or systemic. Systemic reactions against peanut or bee venom antigens can result in anaphylaxis, a potentially life-threatening condition.

Allergic asthma is an example of type I hypersensitivity. On exposure to certain allergens (typically inhaled), individuals with allergic asthma experience inflammation of the airways, characterized by tissue swelling and excessive mucus production. This narrowing of the airways makes it difficult to breathe (see Chapter 40).

Type II Hypersensitivity: Antibody-Mediated Cytotoxic Reactions

Type II hypersensitivities are antibody-mediated cytotoxic reactions. One example is the immunization to erythrocyte antigens during pregnancy. In an Rh-negative mother with an Rh-positive fetus (Rh inherited from the father), the mother forms antibodies against the Rh antigen when fetal blood cells come into contact with the maternal immune system, typically during delivery. If a subsequent pregnancy with an Rh-positive fetus occurs, maternal IgG antibodies can cross the placenta and cause hemolysis of fetal Rh-positive erythrocytes. Close monitoring and adequate symptomatic treatments (e.g., plasma exchange, intrauterine infusion, Rh immunoglobulin) are prescribed, as fetal symptoms can range from mild to potential fetal death from heart failure.

Type III Hypersensitivity: Immune Complex–Mediated Reactions

Type III hypersensitivity reactions are mediated by antibody-antigen complexes that form during an immune response (Figures 34–3 and 34–5). When not properly cleared, these immune complexes can settle into various tissues, where they induce complement activation. These immune complexes are of particular concern in the kidney, where they can lead to glomerulonephritis and kidney failure. While in the past

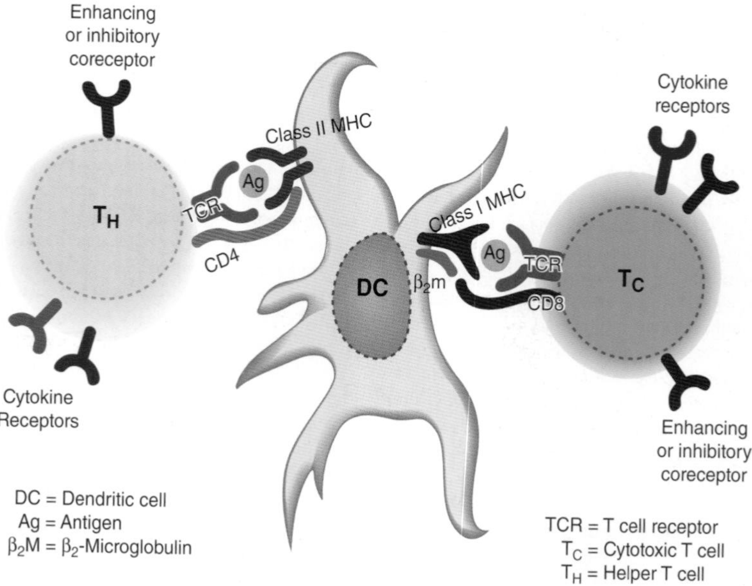

Figure 34–5 *Professional APCs.* APCs such as DCs display peptide-loaded MHC class I and class II complexes on their cell surface. CD8⁺ or CD4⁺ T cells, respectively, engage these MHC-antigen complexes, leading to signaling via the TCR. Simultaneous occupation of activating or inhibitory coreceptors, as well as various cytokine receptors, determines the ultimate T-cell response.

type III hypersensitivity reactions fell largely in the realm of autoimmune diseases (e.g., systemic lupus erythematosus), their incidence rate has significantly risen with the introduction of nonhuman or nonhumanized monoclonal antibodies as pharmacological agents (human antimouse antibodies). Murine or murine-human chimeric therapeutic monoclonal antibodies are "mistaken" by the patient's immune system as potentially dangerous, foreign antigens. The resulting immune response not only "defuses" the therapeutic antibody, but also promotes the formation of antibody(mu)-antibody(hu) or antibody(chim)-antibody(hu) complexes that trigger type III hypersensitivity reactions.

Type IV Hypersensitivity: Delayed Hypersensitivity Reactions

Unlike type I–III hypersensitivity reactions, which are antibody mediated, type IV reactions are mediated by T cells. However, all these hypersensitivity reactions are memory responses. Haptens are molecules that are too small to function as antigens on their own. These molecules penetrate the epidermis and bind to carrier proteins in the skin. Hapten-carrier complexes are detected by APCs in the skin (Langerhans cells), which then migrate to the lymph nodes and prime T-cell responses. When an individual is reexposed to the hapten, antigen-specific T cells migrate to the skin, causing local inflammation and edema. Nickel in clothing and jewelry is a common trigger of type IV hypersensitivity reactions.

Autoimmunity, Immune Deficiency, and Transplant Rejection

Just as for a regular and, appropriate immune response, autoimmunity is founded in either humoral (autoantibody) or cellular (T-cell) responses. As described in the section on lymphocyte development, the process of central tolerance limits the development of autoreactive B and T cells. This process is imperfect, and mechanisms of peripheral tolerance are in place to limit the activity of self-reactive lymphocytes that manage to escape thymic deletion. Peripheral tolerance is primarily mediated by two mechanisms: the action of T_{Reg} cells (see section on CD4 T_H-cell effector functions), and the induction of T-cell anergy. Naïve T cells require costimulatory signals to become activated. Consequently, autoreactive T cells typically will not become activated if they interact with an MHC molecule expressing self-antigen because most tissues do not express costimulatory molecules. Induction of anergy leaves T cells unresponsive, even on subsequent exposure to antigen with sufficient costimulation.

Autoimmunity: A Breach of Tolerance

Several theories exist that aim to explain the origins of individual autoimmune disorders:

CURRENT MONOCLONAL ANTIBODY NOMENCLATURE

UNIQUE PREFIX	TARGET TISSUE		SOURCE ORGANISM		CONSERVED SUFFIX
variable	*-o(s)-*	bone	*-u-*	human	-mab
	-vi(r)-	viral	*-o-*	mouse	
	-ba(c)-	bacterial	*-a-*	rat	
	-li(m)-	immune	*-e-*	hamster	
	-le(s)-	infectious lesions	*-i-*	primate	
	-ci(r)-	cardiovascular	*-xi-*	chimeric	
	-mu(l)-	musculoskeletal	*-zu-*	humanized	
	-ki(n)-	interleukin	*-axo-*	rat/murine hybrid	
	-co(l)-	colonic tumor			
	-me(l)-	melanoma			
	-ma(r)-	mammary tumor			
	-go(t)-	testicular tumor			
	-go(v)-	ovarian tumor			
	-pr(o)-	prostate tumor			
	-tu(m)-	miscellaneous tumor			
	-neu(r)-	nervous system			
	-tox(a)-	toxin as target			
Examples:					
Beva	ci		zu		mab
Ri	tu		xi		mab
Ala	ci		zu		mab
Glemba	tum		u		mab

Figure 34–6 *Current nomenclature for therapeutic monoclonal antibodies.* Current nomenclature incorporates information on the source of the antibody as well as the intended target tissue. An older nomenclature, still used by some workers, focused on the source of the antibody (Figure 34–7).

- *Molecular Mimicry.* The hypothesis of "molecular mimicry" reasons that unique pathogen-derived antigens resemble endogenous host antigens. If an infection occurs, the immune system's defensive arsenal (antibodies, CTLs, and NK cells) not only attack the pathogen-derived antigen but also assault the host's structurally similar antigen, thus causing autoimmunity in the form of "collateral damage."
- *Relationship Between Autoimmunity and the HLA System.* Individuals with specific HLA types are more likely to develop certain autoimmune diseases (e.g., type I diabetes, ankylosing spondylitis, celiac disease, systemic lupus erythematosus). A reasonable explanation for this observation might be found in the fact that particular HLA proteins are more "efficient" than others in presenting antigens and consequently might erroneously activate T cells.
- *Altered Thymic Function.* Thymic T-cell selection is crucial to central tolerance, and type I IFNs, which are highly induced during infectious events, also govern several steps in T-cell selection. Therefore, pathogen-induced disturbances to thymic events might negatively affect elimination of autoreactive T cells. Regardless of the mechanism, central tolerance has thus far not been exploited for pharmacological intervention.

Immune Deficiencies

Primary immunodeficiency encompasses genetic or developmental defects in the immune system that leave the individual susceptible to infections to various degrees. Severe forms (severe combined immunodeficiency) are typically diagnosed in early childhood and are associated with significantly reduced life expectancy. Presently, nine classes of primary immunodeficiency are recognized, totaling over 120 unique conditions. Unfortunately, current treatment options are limited to supportive therapy in the form of antiviral, antifungal, and antibacterial drugs.

Acquired immunodeficiency refers to the loss of immune function due to environmental exposure. These conditions encompass patients receiving immune-suppressive therapy for autoimmune disorders or to prevent transplant rejections. Acquired immunodeficiency is also commonly observed in patients suffering from hematopoietic malignancies, as tumor cells outcompete functional leukocytes for space in the bone marrow or blood. Probably the most common use for the term, however, is in connection with HIV infection, the underlying cause for AIDS (see Chapter 64).

Transplant Rejection

"Host-versus-graft disease" or "graft-versus-host disease" results from the immunological rejection of a transplanted tissue by the recipient's immune system, or in cases where bone marrow is transplanted, the "new" immune system might attack the host's tissues. The intensity of rejection is minimized with increased compatibility between donor and recipient; however, a lifelong regimen of immunosuppressive drugs is unavoidable (see Chapter 35).

Classical immunosuppressive therapy employs glucocorticoids (e.g., prednisone), inhibitors of T-cell activation (e.g., cyclosporine), T-cell proliferation inhibitors (e.g., mycophenolic acid) or mTOR inhibitors (e.g., sirolimus) that inhibit production of IL-2, a cytokine essential for T-cell activation and proliferation. Treatment of transplant rejection also has benefitted from advances in monoclonal antibody therapy, and antibodies directed against the IL-2 receptor (e.g., daclizumab) or CD20 (e.g., rituximab) are now available to prevent transplant rejection (Figure 35–2).

Cancer Immunotherapy

As described previously, T-cell responses are modulated by a balance between costimulatory signals, exemplified by CD28 ligation, and coinhibitory signals, such as those provided by CTLA-4 or PD1 ligation. *Immune checkpoints* refer to inhibitory (often negative-feedback) pathways that limit the amplitude and duration of an immune response. Under normal physiological conditions, immune checkpoints protect tissues from damage during an immune response and contribute to the maintenance of self-tolerance. In conditions of chronic viral infections and cancers, chronic antigen persistence results in the development of dysfunctional "exhausted" T cells. Exhausted T cells are actively suppressed by inhibitory signals that limit their effector functions and turn off their target cell–killing capacity. These inhibitory pathways resulting in T-cell exhaustion have been documented in mice, monkeys, and humans, highlighting their importance in modulating T-cell function.

Cancer cells express a variety of genetic and epigenetic alterations that distinguish them from their normal counterparts. These tumor-associated antigens can be recognized by the host immune system; antitumor T cells are generated, which then eliminate these transformed cells. However, tumors frequently develop immune resistance mechanisms that evade the host's immune attack. One of these evasion strategies involves the manipulation of immune-inhibitory pathways or immune checkpoints. Tumors avoid being destroyed by actively stimulating these inhibitory receptors to turn off antitumor T cells. Figure 34–7 provides an overview of activating and inhibitory coreceptors and the drugs (monoclonal antibodies) that target them. In general, these antibodies work by releasing the brake on antitumor T cells and reinvigorating them to kill tumors. It is important to be aware that whereas some monoclonal antibodies block their respective target (PD1), others block the respective ligand (PD-L1). The therapeutic goal is to interfere with this inhibitory interaction that is actively suppressing T cells in the tumor microenvironment.

The two immune checkpoint receptors that have been the most extensively characterized in the context of cancer immunotherapy are CTLA-4 and PD1. These inhibitory molecules are highly expressed on antitumor T cells. When bound by their respective ligands (CD80/86 and PD-L1/PD-L2) on APCs or tumor cells, these inhibitory receptors dampen the T-cell response, albeit by different intracellular pathways. As antitumor T cells express PD1, tumor cells engage it through their expression of PD-L1. The tumor effectively inactivates the T cells and the tumor continues to grow (Pardoll, 2012; Tang et al., 2016). These pathways are further discussed in the cancer therapy chapters (Chapters 65–68).

Immunotherapy to cancers holds great promise for treating patients with advanced disease, as evidenced by the success of clinical trials using this technology. Biologics to stimulate antitumor T cells have been rapidly approved by the FDA and have become the first line of treatment of cancers such as metastatic melanoma, non–small cell lung cancer, and renal cell carcinoma. In addition, anti-PD1, anti–PD-L1, and anti–CTLA-4 therapies are currently in clinical trials to assess their efficacy in head and neck cancers, breast cancer, small cell lung cancer, Hodgkin lymphoma, gastric cancer, hepatocellular carcinoma, bladder cancer, ovarian cancer, colon cancer, and Merkel cell carcinoma. It is important to note that only a small fraction of patients respond to checkpoint monotherapy, and this frequency can increase when patients are given combination therapy, such as administering both anti-PD1 and anti–CTLA-4 antibodies. Furthermore, combination strategies that include checkpoint blockade paired with radiation or chemotherapy may further increase responsiveness in cancer patients.

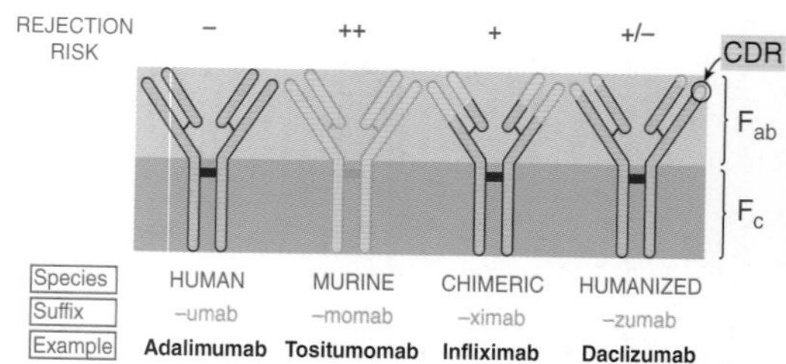

Figure 34–7 *Former nomenclature of therapeutic monoclonal antibodies.* This older nomenclature, still in use by some workers, focused primarily on the source of the antibody (murine, human, chimeric, or humanized). Current nomenclature (Figure 34–6) incorporates information on the target tissue as well. Fab, antigen-binding fragment; Fc, crystallizable fragment; CDR, complementarity-determining regions of the variable domains, also called hypervariable regions.

One consequence of checkpoint blockade is that autoreactive T cells are also unleashed after therapy. Patients can develop toxicities that include hepatic, pneumonitis, colitis, rash, vitiligo, and endocrine pathology. Greater immunotherapy efficacy will likely be achieved when drugs are developed to target other inhibitory pathways and are used in combination, but caution must be evaluated to ensure patient safety (Callahan et al., 2016).

In addition to solid tumors, liquid tumors like CLL are also being targeted by immunotherapeutic approaches. Patient T cells are engineered to express chimeric antigen receptors (CARs) comprising antibody-binding domains connected to domains that activate T cells. In the case of CLL, CAR T cells recognize CD19 on B cells, and their chimeric receptor sustains T activation. CAR T cells are engineered from patient blood, expanded in vitro; then, millions are infused into the same patient. These cells then circulate in the patient and recognize all B cells expressing CD19 and destroy them. This cellular therapy has shown promise in patients with CLL with high durable objective responses (Kalos et al., 2011).

Bibliography

Attanasio J, Wherry EJ. Costimulatory and coinhibitory receptor pathways in infectious disease. *Immunity,* **2016**, *44*:1052–1068.

Belkaid Y, Tamoutounour S. The influence of skin microorganisms on cutaneous immunity. *Nat Rev Immunol,* **2016**, *16*(6):353–66.

Bjorkstrom NK, et al. Emerging insights into natural killer cells in human peripheral tissues. *Nat Rev Immunol,* **2016**, *16*(5):310–320.

Blum JS, et al. Pathways of antigen processing. *Annu Rev Immunol,* **2013**, *31*:443–473.

Brownlie RJ, Zamoyska R. T cell receptor signalling networks: branched, diversified and bounded. *Nat Rev Immunol,* **2013**, *13*(4):257–269.

Burmester G-Rd, et al. *Color Atlas of Immunology*. Thieme flexibook. Thieme, New York, **2003**, xiv, 322.

Callahan MK, et al. Targeting T cell co-receptors for cancer therapy. *Immunity,* **2016**, *44*:1069–1078.

Cao X. Self-regulation and cross-regulation of pattern-recognition receptor signalling in health and disease. *Nat Rev Immunol,* **2016**, *16*(1):35–50.

Di Noia JM, Neuberger MS. Molecular mechanisms of antibody somatic hypermutation. *Annu Rev Biochem,* **2007**, 76:1–22.

Doulatov S, et al. Hematopoiesis: a human perspective. *Cell Stem Cell,* **2012**, *10*(2):120–136.

DuPage M, Bluestone JA. Harnessing the plasticity of CD4(+) T cells to treat immune-mediated disease. *Nat Rev Immunol,* **2016**, *16*(3):149–163.

Eaves CJ. Hematopoietic stem cells: concepts, definitions, and the new reality. *Blood,* **2015**, *125*(17):2605–2613.

Farber DL, et al. Human memory T cells: generation, compartmentalization and homeostasis. *Nat Rev Immunol,* **2014**, *14*(1):24–35.

Gonzalez-Navajas JM, et al. Immunomodulatory functions of type I interferons. *Nat Rev Immunol,* **2012**, *12*(2):125–135.

Hancock RE, et al. The immunology of host defence peptides: beyond antimicrobial activity. *Nat Rev Immunol,* **2016**, *16*(5):321–334.

Harty JT, et al. CD8+ T cell effector mechanisms in resistance to infection. *Annu Rev Immunol,* **2000**, *18*:275–308.

Hoggatt J, et al. Hematopoietic stem cell niche in health and disease. *Annu Rev Pathol,* **2016**, *11*:555–581.

Kalos M, et al. T cells with chimeric antigen receptors have potent antitumor effects and can establish memory in patients with advanced leukemia. *Sci Transl Med,* **2011**, *3*:95ra73.

Kruger P, et al. Neutrophils: between host defence, immune modulation, and tissue injury. *PLoS Pathog,* **2015**, *11*(3):e1004651.

Kurosaki T, et al. Memory B cells. *Nat Rev Immunol,* **2015**, *15*(3): 149–159.

Lavin Y, et al. Regulation of macrophage development and function in peripheral tissues. *Nat Rev Immunol,* **2015**, *15*(12):731–744.

LeBien TW, Tedder TF. B lymphocytes: how they develop and function. *Blood,* **2008**, *112*(5):1570–1580.

Masopust D, Schenkel JM. The integration of T cell migration, differentiation and function. *Nat Rev Immunol,* **2013**, *13*(5): 309–320.

Morgan BP, Harris CL. Complement, a target for therapy in inflammatory and degenerative diseases. *Nat Rev Drug Discov,* **2015**, *14*(12): 857–877.

Neely HR, Flajnik MF. Emergence and evolution of secondary lymphoid organs. *Annu Rev Cell Dev Biol,* **2016**, *32*:693–711.

Nemazee D. Receptor editing in lymphocyte development and central tolerance. *Nat Rev Immunol,* **2006**, *6*(10):728–740.

Palmer DB. The effect of age on thymic function. *Front Immunol,* **2013**. 4:316.

Pardoll DM. The blockade of immune checkpoints in cancer immunotherapy. *Nat Rev Cancer,* **2012**, *12*(4):252–264.

Shah DK, Zuniga-Pflucker JC. An overview of the intrathymic intricacies of T cell development. *J Immunol,* **2014**, *192*(9):4017–4023.

Tang H, et al. Immunotherapy and tumor microenvironment. *Cancer Lett,* **2016**, *370*(1):85–90.

Thomas SN, et al. Implications of lymphatic transport to lymph nodes in immunity and immunotherapy. *Annu Rev Biomed Eng,* **2016**, *18*:207–233.

Tinoco R, et al. PSGL-1 is an immune checkpoint regulator that promotes T cell exhaustion. *Immunity,* **2016**, *44*:1190–1203.

Vestweber D. How leukocytes cross the vascular endothelium. *Nat Rev Immunol,* **2015**, *15*(11):692–704.

von Köckritz-Blickwede M, Nizet V. Innate immunity turned inside-out: antimicrobial defense by phagocyte extracellular traps. *J Mol Med (Berl),* **2009**, *87*:775–783.

Xu Z, et al. Immunoglobulin class-switch DNA recombination: induction, targeting and beyond. *Nat Rev Immunol,* **2012**, *12*(7): 517–531.

Immunosuppressants and Tolerogens

Alan M. Krensky, Jamil R. Azzi, and David A. Hafler

第三十五章　免疫抑制药和耐受性

中文导读

本章主要介绍：免疫反应；免疫抑制，包括器官移植治疗的一般方法、糖皮质激素、钙调磷酸酶抑制药、抗增殖和抗代谢药、其他抗增殖和细胞毒性药、生物免疫抑制抗体和融合受体蛋白、单克隆抗体、自身免疫性疾病治疗的一般方法、抑制淋巴细胞功能-相关抗原、细胞因子治疗（干扰素）、靶向B细胞；耐受性，包括协同刺激的阻断、供体细胞嵌合性、抗原、可溶性人类白细胞抗原（HLA）；多发性硬化的免疫治疗，包括临床特征和病理学。

Abbreviations

ALG: antilymphocyte globulin
APC: antigen-presenting cell
ATG: antithymocyte globulin
AUC: area under the curve
CD: cluster of differentiation
CLL: chronic lymphocytic leukemia
CNS: central nervous system
CTL: cytotoxic T lymphocyte
CTLA4: cytotoxic T-lymphocyte–associated antigen 4
FKBP-12: FK506-binding protein 12
CYP: cytochrome P450
GVHD: graft-versus-host disease
HLA: human leukocyte antigen
HRPT: hypoxanthine–guanine phosphoribosyl transferase
IFN-β: interferon type I beta
Ig: immunoglobulin
IL: interleukin
IL-1RA: IL-1 receptor antagonist
IL-2R: interleukin 2 receptor
JCV: polyomavirus JC
LDL: low-density lipoprotein
LFA: lymphocyte function–associated antigen
mAb: monoclonal antibody
MHC: histocompatibility complex
MMF: mycophenolate mofetil
6-MP: 6-mercaptopurine
MPA: mycophenolic acid
MPAG: MPA glucuronide
MS: multiple sclerosis
mTOR: mammalian target of rapamycin
NFAT: nuclear factor of activated T lymphocytes
NHP: nonhuman primate
NK: natural killer
NSAID: nonsteroidal anti-inflammatory drug
PD1: programmed cell death protein 1
PD-L1: programmed death ligand 1
PML: progressive multifocal leukoencephalopathy
RA: rheumatoid arthritis
S1P-R: sphingosine-1-phosphate receptor
TCR: T-cell receptor
VZV: varicella zoster virus
WBC: white blood cell

This chapter reviews the components of the immune response and drugs that modulate immunity via immunosuppression or tolerance. Four major classes of immunosuppressive drugs are discussed: glucocorticoids (see Chapter 46), calcineurin inhibitors, antiproliferative and antimetabolic agents (see Chapter 66), and antibodies. While there are similarities, the approach to the use of immunosuppressant drugs in transplant rejection has evolved separately from the approaches used to treat autoimmune disease and thus is presented separately. Finally, the chapter ends with a brief case study of immunotherapy for the autoimmune disease MS.

The Immune Response

The immune system evolved to discriminate self from nonself. *Innate immunity* (natural immunity) is primitive, does not require priming, and is of relatively low affinity, but it is broadly reactive. *Adaptive immunity* (learned immunity) is antigen specific, depends on antigen exposure or priming, and can be of very high affinity. The two arms of immunity work closely together, with the innate immune system most active early in an immune response and adaptive immunity becoming progressively dominant over time.

The major effectors of *innate immunity* are complement, granulocytes, monocytes/macrophages, NK cells, mast cells, and basophils. The major effectors of *adaptive immunity* are B and T lymphocytes. B lymphocytes make antibodies; T lymphocytes function as helper, cytolytic, and regulatory (suppressor) cells. These cells not only are important in the normal immune response to infection and tumors but also mediate transplant rejection and autoimmunity.

Immunoglobulins (antibodies) on the B-lymphocyte surface are receptors for a large variety of specific structural conformations. In contrast, T lymphocytes recognize antigens as peptide fragments in the context of self MHC antigens (called HLAs in humans) on the surface of APCs, such as dendritic cells, macrophages, and other cell types expressing MHC class I and class II antigens. Once activated by specific antigen recognition, both B and T lymphocytes are triggered to differentiate and divide, leading to release of soluble mediators (cytokines, lymphokines) that perform as effectors and regulators of the immune response. Chapter 34 presents a more detailed view of the immune system at the levels of the molecules, cells, and organs involved in immunity.

Immunosuppression

Immunosuppressive drugs are used to dampen the immune response in organ transplantation and autoimmune disease. In transplantation, the major classes of immunosuppressive drugs used today are the following:

- Glucocorticoids
- Calcineurin inhibitors
- Antiproliferative/antimetabolic agents
- Biologicals (antibodies)

Table 35–1 summarizes the sites of action of representative immunosuppressants on T-cell activation. These drugs are successful in treating conditions such as acute immune rejection of organ transplants and autoimmune diseases. However, such therapies often require lifelong use and

TABLE 35–1 ■ SITES OF ACTION OF SELECTED IMMUNOSUPPRESSIVE AGENTS ON T-CELL ACTIVATION

DRUG	SITE (AND MECHANISM) OF ACTION
Glucocorticoids	Glucocorticoid response elements in DNA (regulate gene transcription)
Cyclosporine	Calcineurin (inhibits phosphatase activity)
Tacrolimus	Calcineurin (inhibits phosphatase activity)
Azathioprine	DNA (false nucleotide incorporation)
Mycophenolate mofetil	Inosine monophosphate dehydrogenase (inhibits activity)
Sirolimus	mTOR, protein kinase involved in cell-cycle progression (inhibits activity)
Everolimus	mTOR, protein kinase involved in cell-cycle progression (inhibits activity)
Belatacept	Costimulatory ligands (CD80 and CD86) present on antigen presenting cells (inhibits activity)
Alemtuzumab	CD52 protein, widely expressed on B cells, T cells, macrophages, NK cells (induces lysis)
Muromonab-CD3	T-cell receptor complex (blocks antigen recognition)
Daclizumab, basiliximab	IL-2R (block IL-2–mediated T-cell activation)

nonspecifically suppress the entire immune system, exposing patients in some instances to higher risks of infection and cancer. The calcineurin inhibitors and daily glucocorticoids, in particular, are nephrotoxic and diabetogenic, respectively, thus restricting their usefulness in a variety of clinical settings.

Monoclonal and polyclonal antibody preparations directed at both T cells and B cells or against cytokines such as TNF-α are important therapies providing an opportunity to more specifically target immune pathways. Finally, newer small molecules and antibodies have expanded the arsenal of immunosuppressives. In particular, mTOR inhibitors (*sirolimus, everolimus, temsirolimus*) (Budde et al., 2011; Euvrard et al., 2012), and anti-CD25 (IL-2R) antibodies (*basiliximab, daclizumab*) (Nashan, 2005) target growth factor pathways. *Belatacept* (Satyananda and Shapiro, 2014) inhibits T-cell costimulation. Thus, there are useful pharmacological tools that can substantially limit clonal expansion and potentially promote tolerance (Goldfarb-Rumyantzev et al., 2006; Krensky et al., 1990).

General Approach to Organ Transplantation Therapy

Organ transplantation therapy is organized around five general principles.

1. Carefully prepare the patient and select the best available ABO blood type–compatible HLA match for organ donation.
2. Employ multitier immunosuppressive therapy; simultaneously use several agents, each of which is directed at a different molecular target within the allograft response. Synergistic effects permit use of the various agents at relatively low doses, thereby limiting specific toxicities while maximizing the immunosuppressive effect.
3. Employ intensive induction and lower-dose maintenance drug protocols; greater immunosuppression is required to gain early engraftment or to treat established rejection than to maintain long-term immunosuppression. The early high risk of acute rejection is replaced over time by the increased risk of the medications' side effects, necessitating a slow reduction of maintenance immunosuppressive drugs.
4. Investigation of each episode of transplant dysfunction is required, including evaluation for recurrence of the disease, rejection, drug toxicity, and infection (keeping in mind that these various problems can and often do coexist).
5. Reduce dosage or withdraw a drug if its toxicity exceeds its benefit (Danovitch et al., 2007).

Biological Induction Therapy

In many transplant centers, induction therapy with biological agents is used to delay the use of the nephrotoxic calcineurin inhibitors or to intensify the initial immunosuppressive therapy in patients at high risk of rejection (i.e., repeat transplants, broadly presensitized patients, African American patients, or pediatric patients). This strategy has been an important component of immunosuppression since the 1960s, when Starzl and colleagues demonstrated the beneficial effect of antilymphocyte globulin (ALC) in the prophylaxis of rejection. Two preparations are FDA-approved for use in transplantation: lymphocyte immune globulin (Atgam) and antithymocyte globulin (ATG; Thymoglobulin) (Brennan et al., 2006; Nashan, 2005). ATG is the most frequently used depleting agent. Alemtuzumab, a humanized anti-CD52 mAb that produces prolonged lymphocyte depletion, is approved for use in CLL and MS but is increasingly used off label as induction therapy in transplantation (Jones and Coles, 2014).

Most limitations of murine-based mAbs generally were overcome by the introduction of chimeric or humanized mAbs that lack antigenicity and have a prolonged serum $t_{1/2}$. Antibodies derived from transgenic mice carrying human antibody genes are labeled "humanized" (90%–95% human) or "fully human" (100% human); antibodies derived from human cells are labeled "human." However, all three types of antibodies are of equal efficacy and safety. Chimeric antibodies generally contain about 33% mouse protein and 67% human protein and can still produce an antibody response that results in reduced efficacy and shorter $t_{1/2}$ compared to humanized antibodies.

Biological agents for induction therapy in the prophylaxis of rejection currently are used in about 70% of de novo transplant patients. Biological agents for induction can be divided into two groups: the *depleting agents* and the *immune modulators*. The depleting agents consist of lymphocyte immune globulin, ATG, and muromonab-CD3 mAb; their efficacy derives from their ability to deplete the recipient's CD3-positive cells at the time of transplantation and antigen presentation. The second group of biological agents, the anti–IL-2R mAbs, do not deplete T lymphocytes, but rather block IL-2–mediated T-cell activation by binding to the α chain of IL-2R (CD25). For patients with high levels of anti-HLA antibodies and humoral rejection, more aggressive therapies include plasmapheresis, intravenous immunoglobulin, and rituximab, a chimeric anti-CD20 mAb (Brennan et al., 2006; Chan et al., 2011; Guerra et al., 2011; Nashan, 2005; Sureshkumar et al., 2012).

Maintenance Immunotherapy

Basic immunosuppressive therapy uses multiple drugs simultaneously, typically a calcineurin inhibitor, glucocorticoids, and mycophenolate (a purine metabolism inhibitor), each directed at a discrete step in T-cell activation (Vincenti et al., 2008). Glucocorticoids, azathioprine, cyclosporine, tacrolimus, mycophenolate, sirolimus, belatacept, and various mAbs and polyclonal antibodies all are approved for use in transplantation.

Therapy for Established Rejection

Low doses of prednisone, calcineurin inhibitors, purine metabolism inhibitors, sirolimus, or belatacept are effective in preventing acute cellular rejection; they are less effective in blocking activated T lymphocytes and thus are not very effective against established, acute rejection or for the total prevention of chronic rejection. Therefore, treatment of established rejection requires the use of agents directed against activated T cells. These include glucocorticoids in high doses (pulse therapy), polyclonal antilymphocyte antibodies, or muromonab-CD3 (licensed by the FDA but not currently marketed in the U.S. due to decreased use).

Glucocorticoids

The introduction of glucocorticoids as immunosuppressive drugs in the 1960s played a key role in making organ transplantation possible. Prednisone, prednisolone, and other glucocorticoids are used alone and in combination with other immunosuppressive agents for treatment of transplant rejection and autoimmune disorders. The pharmacological properties of glucocorticoids are described in Chapter 46.

Mechanism of Action

Glucocorticoids have broad anti-inflammatory effects on multiple components of cellular immunity, but relatively little effect on humoral immunity. Glucocorticoids bind to receptors inside cells and regulate the transcription of numerous other genes (see Chapter 46). Glucocorticoids also curtail activation of NF-κB, suppress formation of pro-inflammatory cytokines such as IL-1 and IL-6, inhibit T cells from making IL-2 and proliferating, and inhibit the activation of CTLs. In addition, glucocorticoid-treated neutrophils and monocytes display poor chemotaxis and decreased lysosomal enzyme release.

Therapeutic Uses

There are numerous therapeutic indications for glucocorticoids. They commonly are combined with other immunosuppressive agents to prevent and treat transplant rejection. Glucocorticoids also are efficacious for treatment of GVHD in bone marrow transplantation. Glucocorticoids are routinely used to treat autoimmune disorders such as rheumatoid and other arthritides, systemic lupus erythematosus, systemic dermatomyositis, psoriasis and other skin conditions, asthma and other allergic disorders, inflammatory bowel disease, inflammatory ophthalmic diseases, autoimmune hematological disorders, and acute exacerbations of MS (see multiple sclerosis section). Lower-dose oral glucocorticoids, however, appear to have different biologic effects; low-dose oral prednisone made optic neuritis worse compared to high-dose intravenous solumedrol (Beck et al., 1992). In addition, glucocorticoids limit allergic reactions that occur with other immunosuppressive agents and are used in transplant recipients to block first-dose cytokine storm caused by treatment with muromonab-CD3 and to a lesser extent ATG (see Antithymocyte Globulin). Most transplant centers use an initial high dose of intravenous solumedrol with tapering to a maintenance dose of 5–10 mg/d in the long term. Currently, more than one-third of kidney transplant centers in the U.S. aim to withdraw steroids within the first 3 months after transplantation (Bergmann et al., 2012).

Toxicity

Extensive glucocorticoid use often results in disabling and life-threatening adverse effects. These effects include growth retardation in children, avascular necrosis of bone, osteopenia, increased risk of infection, poor wound healing, cataracts, hyperglycemia, and hypertension (see Chapter 46). The advent of combined glucocorticoid/calcineurin inhibitor regimens has allowed reduced doses or rapid withdrawal of steroids, resulting in lower steroid-induced morbidities (Vincenti et al., 2008).

Calcineurin Inhibitors

The most effective immunosuppressive drugs in routine use are the calcineurin inhibitors *cyclosporine* and *tacrolimus* (Figure 35–1), which target intracellular signaling pathways induced as a consequence of TCR activation (Figure 35–2). Cyclosporine and tacrolimus bind to an immunophilin (cyclophilin for cyclosporine or FKBP-12 for tacrolimus), resulting in subsequent interaction with calcineurin to block its phosphatase activity. Calcineurin-catalyzed dephosphorylation is required for movement of a component of the NFAT into the nucleus. NFAT, in turn, is required to induce a number of cytokine genes, including IL-2, a prototypic T-cell growth and differentiation factor (Verghese et al., 2014).

Tacrolimus

Tacrolimus is a macrolide antibiotic produced by *Streptomyces tsukubaensis*. Because of perceived slightly greater efficacy and ease of blood level monitoring, tacrolimus has become the preferred calcineurin inhibitor in most transplant centers (Ekberg et al., 2007).

Mechanism of Action. Like cyclosporine, tacrolimus inhibits T-cell activation by inhibiting calcineurin. Tacrolimus binds to an intracellular protein, FKBP-12, an immunophilin structurally related to cyclophilin. A complex of tacrolimus–FKBP-12, Ca^{2+}, calmodulin, and calcineurin then forms, and calcineurin phosphatase activity is inhibited (see Figure 35–2). Inhibition of phosphatase activity prevents dephosphorylation and nuclear translocation of NFAT and inhibits T-cell activation. Thus, although the

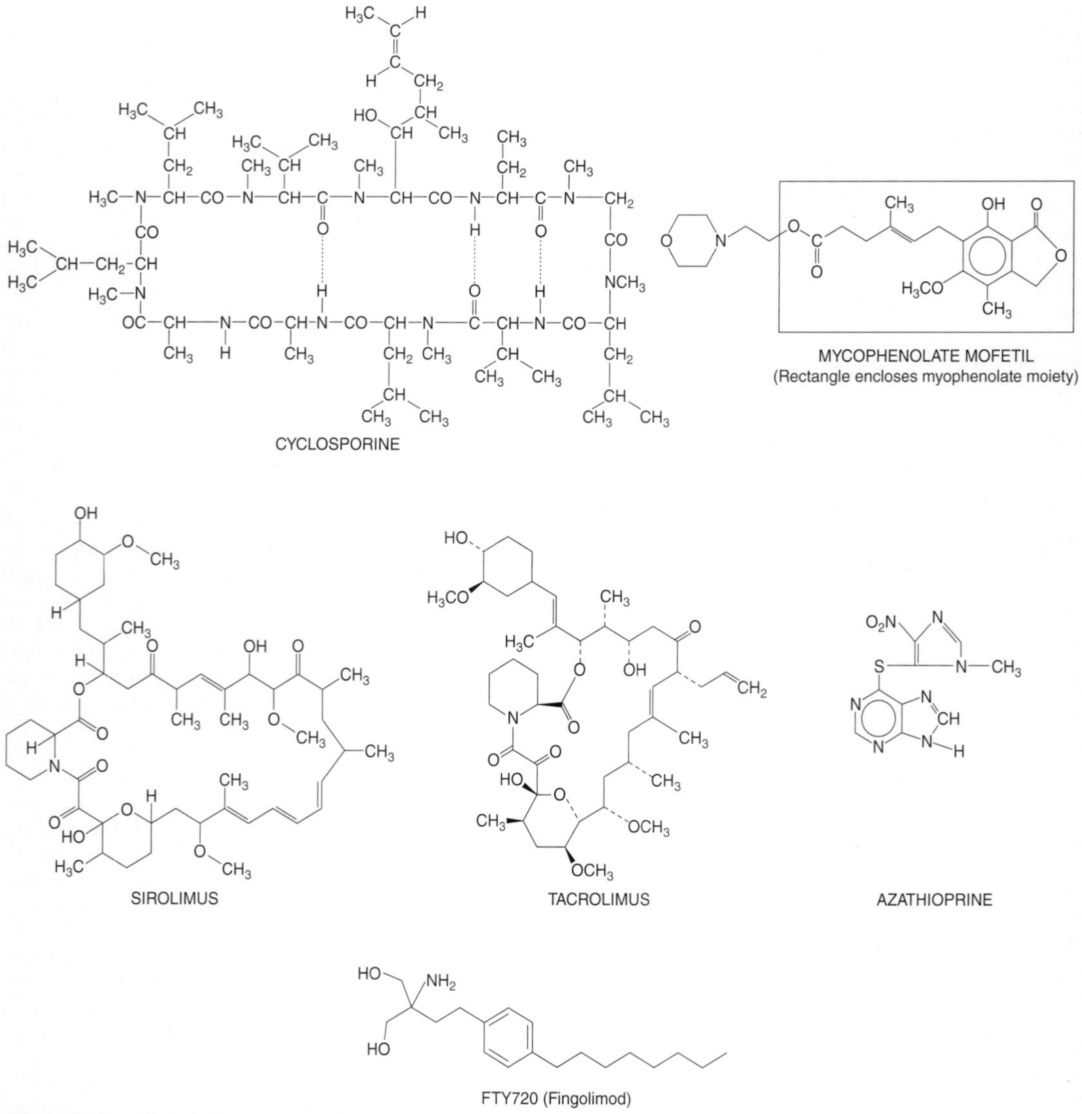

CYCLOSPORINE

MYCOPHENOLATE MOFETIL
(Rectangle encloses myophenolate moiety)

SIROLIMUS

TACROLIMUS

AZATHIOPRINE

FTY720 (Fingolimod)

Figure 35–1 *Structures of selected immunosuppressive drugs.*

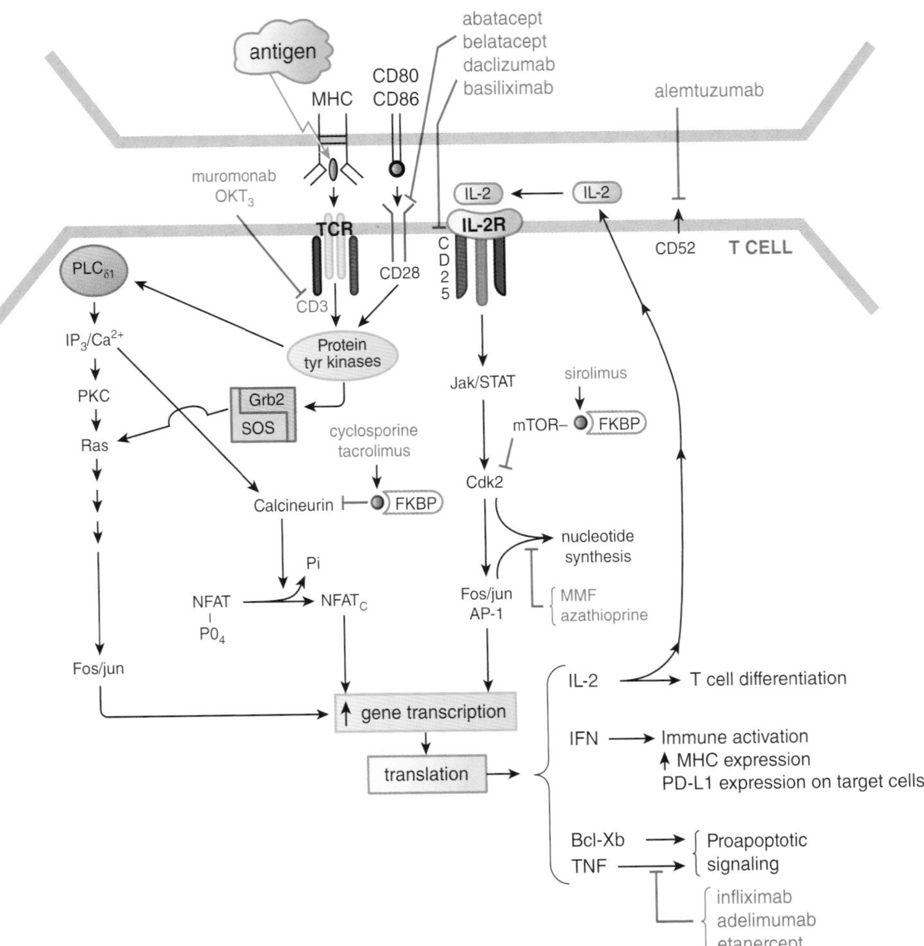

Figure 35–2 *T-cell activation and sites of action of immunosuppressive agents.* The TCR recognizes antigens bound to the MHC. A costimulatory signal is required for T-cell activation: The CD80/CD86-CD28 interaction from the APC to the T cell. Activation leads to IL-2 production (in a positive-feedback loop) and a host of other events, some of which are bracketed in the lower right-hand corner. Numerous agents are available to suppress T-cell activation. Cyclosporine and tacrolimus bind to immunophilins (cyclophilin and FKBP, respectively), forming a complex that inhibits the phosphatase calcineurin and the calcineurin-catalyzed dephosphorylation that permits translocation of NFAT into the nucleus. NFAT is required for transcription of IL-2 and other growth and differentiation–associated cytokines (lymphokines). Sirolimus (rapamycin) works downstream of the IL-2R, binding to FKBP; the FKBP-sirolimus complex binds to and inhibits the mTOR, a kinase involved in cell cycle progression (proliferation). MMF and azathioprine inhibit nucleic acid synthesis, thereby inhibiting T-cell proliferation. The antibody muromunab (OKT3) inhibits TCR function via interaction with its CD3 component. Daclizumab and basilixmab block IL-2 signaling by interacting with the alpha subunit of the IL-2R complex (CD25). Several antibodies can block the systemic effects of released TNF. Alemtuzumab, by binding to CD52, marks the cell for destruction, thereby depleting CD52^{+} cells.

intracellular receptors differ, cyclosporine and tacrolimus target the same pathway for immunosuppression.

ADME. *Tacrolimus* is available for oral administration as capsules and extended-release capsules (0.5, 1, and 5 mg); extended-release tablets (0.75, 1, and 4 mg); and a solution for injection (5 mg/mL). Sublingual tacrolimus has been used off label for the short term in patients who are unable to receive medications orally. Because of intersubject variability in pharmacokinetics, individualized dosing is required for optimal therapy. For tacrolimus, whole blood is the preferred sampling compartment; the trough drug level in whole blood seems to correlate better with clinical events for tacrolimus than for cyclosporine. Target concentrations are 10–15 ng/mL in the early preoperative period and 6–8 ng/mL at 3 months posttransplantation. Gastrointestinal absorption is incomplete and variable. Target concentrations are dependent on sampling technique and on product-release characteristics, immediate- versus extended-release forms. Food decreases the rate and extent of absorption. Plasma protein binding of tacrolimus is 75%–99%, involving primarily albumin and α_1-acid glycoprotein. The $t_{1/2}$ of tacrolimus is about 12 h. Tacrolimus is extensively metabolized in the liver by CYP3A; some of the metabolites are active. The bulk of excretion of the parent drug and metabolites is in the feces.

Therapeutic Uses. Tacrolimus is indicated for the prophylaxis of solid-organ allograft rejection in a manner similar to cyclosporine (see Cyclosporine) and is used off label as rescue therapy in patients with rejection episodes despite "therapeutic" levels of cyclosporine. Recommended initial oral doses are 0.2 mg/kg/d for adult kidney transplant patients, 0.1–0.15 mg/kg/d for adult liver transplant patients, 0.075 mg/kg/d for adult heart transplant patients, and 0.15–0.2 mg/kg/d for pediatric liver transplant patients in two divided doses 12 h apart. These dosages are intended to achieve typical blood trough levels in the 5- to 20-ng/mL range (Goring et al., 2014). Note that the oral dose of tacrolimus depends on product release characteristics (immediate- vs. extended-release formulation) and the specific cocktail of medications selected for prophylaxis.

Toxicity. Nephrotoxicity; neurotoxicity (e.g., tremor, headache, motor disturbances, seizures); GI complaints; hypertension; hyperkalemia; hyperglycemia; and diabetes all are associated with tacrolimus use. Tacrolimus has a negative effect on pancreatic islet β cells, and glucose intolerance and diabetes mellitus are well-recognized complications of tacrolimus-based immunosuppression. While combined use of calcineurin inhibitors and glucocorticoids is particularly diabetogenic, new-onset diabetes after transplantation (NODAT) incidence was significantly higher with tacrolimus compared to cyclosporine, the other calcineurin inhibitor. Obese patients, African American or Hispanic transplant recipients, or those with a family history of type 2 diabetes or obesity are especially at risk. As with other immunosuppressive agents, there is an increased risk of secondary tumors and opportunistic infections. Notably, tacrolimus does not adversely affect uric acid or LDL cholesterol. Diarrhea and alopecia are common in patients on concomitant mycophenolate therapy.

Drug Interactions. Because of its potential for nephrotoxicity, tacrolimus blood levels and renal function should be monitored closely. Coadministration with cyclosporine results in additive or synergistic nephrotoxicity; therefore, a delay of at least 24 h is required when switching a patient from cyclosporine to tacrolimus. Because tacrolimus is metabolized mainly by CYP3A, the potential interactions described in the following section for cyclosporine also apply for tacrolimus. Per the label, concomitant use of tacrolimus with cyclosporine or sirolimus is not recommended for prophylaxis against renal transplant rejection.

Cyclosporine

Cyclosporine (cyclosporin A) is a cyclic polypeptide of 11 amino acids, produced by the fungus *Beauveria nivea,* that inhibits calcineurin activity (Azzi et al., 2013).

Mechanism of Action. Cyclosporine forms a complex with cyclophilin, a cytoplasmic-receptor protein present in target cells (Figure 35–2). This complex binds to calcineurin, inhibiting Ca^{2+}-stimulated dephosphorylation of the cytosolic component of NFAT. When cytoplasmic NFAT is dephosphorylated, it translocates to the nucleus and complexes with nuclear components required for complete T-cell activation, including transactivation of IL-2 and other lymphokine genes. Calcineurin phosphatase activity is inhibited after physical interaction with the cyclosporine/cyclophilin complex.

At the level of immune system function, cyclosporine suppresses some humoral immunity but is more effective against T-cell–dependent immune mechanisms such as those underlying transplant rejection and some forms of autoimmunity. It preferentially inhibits antigen-triggered signal transduction in T lymphocytes, blunting expression of many lymphokines, including IL-2, and the expression of antiapoptotic proteins. Cyclosporine also increases expression of TGF-β, a potent inhibitor of IL-2–stimulated T-cell proliferation and generation of CTLs (Colombo and Ammirati, 2011; Molnar et al., 2015).

ADME. Because cyclosporine is lipophilic and highly hydrophobic, it is formulated for clinical administration using castor oil or other strategies to ensure solubilization. Cyclosporine can be administered intravenously or orally. The intravenous preparation is provided as a solution in an ethanol–polyoxyethylated castor oil vehicle that must be further diluted in 0.9% sodium chloride solution or 5% dextrose solution before injection. The oral dosage forms include soft gelatin capsules and oral solutions. Cyclosporine supplied in the original soft gelatin capsule is absorbed slowly, with 20%–50% bioavailability. A modified microemulsion formulation, NEORAL, has become the most widely used preparation. It has more uniform and slightly increased bioavailability compared to the original formulation. It is provided as 25- and 100-mg soft gelatin capsules and a 100-mg/mL oral solution. The original and microemulsion formulations are *not bioequivalent* and cannot be used interchangeably without heightened monitoring of drug concentrations and assessment of graft function. A second modified formulation, GENGRAF, is also marketed, and like NEORAL, is *not interchangeable* with nonmodified cyclosporine formulations. Transplant units need to educate patients that the cyclosporine preparation know as SANDIMMUNE and its generics are not the same as NEORAL and its generics, such that one preparation cannot be substituted for another without risk of inadequate immunosuppression or increased toxicity. The danger of unauthorized, inadvertent, unmonitored, or inappropriate substitution of nonequivalent formulations can result in graft loss and other adverse patient outcomes.

Blood levels taken 2 h after a dose administration (so-called C_2 levels) may correlate better with the AUC than other single points, but no single time point can simulate the exposure better than more frequent drug sampling. In practice, if a patient has clinical signs or symptoms of toxicity or if there is unexplained rejection or renal dysfunction, a pharmacokinetic profile can be used to estimate that person's systemic exposure to the drug.

Cyclosporine absorption is incomplete following oral administration and varies with the individual patient and the formulation used. Cyclosporine is distributed extensively outside the vascular compartment. After intravenous dosing, the steady-state volume of distribution reportedly is as high as 3–5 L/kg in solid-organ transplant recipients. The elimination of cyclosporine from the blood generally is biphasic, with a terminal $t_{1/2}$ of 5–18 h. After intravenous infusion, clearance is about 5–7 mL/min/kg in adult recipients of renal transplants, but results differ by age and between different patient populations. For example, clearance is slower in cardiac transplant patients and more rapid in children. Thus, the intersubject variability is so large that individual monitoring is required.

After oral administration of cyclosporine (as NEORAL), the time to peak blood concentrations is 1.5–2 h. Administration with food delays and decreases absorption. High- and low-fat meals consumed within 30 min of administration decrease the AUC by about 13% and the maximum concentration by 33%. This makes it imperative to individualize dosage regimens for outpatients. Cyclosporine is extensively metabolized in the liver by hepatic CYP3A and to a lesser degree in the GI tract and kidneys. At least 25 metabolites have been identified in human bile, feces, blood, and urine. All of the metabolites have reduced biological activity and toxicity compared to the parent drug. Cyclosporine and its metabolites are excreted principally through the bile into the feces, with about 6% excreted in the urine. Cyclosporine also is excreted in human milk. In the presence of hepatic dysfunction, dosage adjustments are required. No adjustments generally are necessary for patients on dialysis or with renal failure.

Therapeutic Uses. Clinical indications for cyclosporine are kidney, liver, heart, and other organ transplantation; rheumatoid arthritis; psoriasis; and xerophthalmia. Its use in dermatology is discussed in Chapter 70. Cyclosporine usually is combined with other agents, especially glucocorticoids and either azathioprine or mycophenolate, and, most recently, sirolimus. The dose of cyclosporine varies, depending on the organ transplanted and the other drugs used in the specific treatment protocol(s). The initial dose generally is not given before the transplant because of the concern about nephrotoxicity. For renal transplant patients, therapeutic algorithms have been developed to delay cyclosporine or tacrolimus introduction until a threshold renal function has been attained. Dosing is guided by signs of rejection (too low a dose), renal or other toxicity (too high a dose), and close monitoring of blood levels. Great care must be taken to differentiate renal toxicity from rejection in kidney transplant patients. Ultrasound-guided allograft biopsy is the best way to assess the basis for renal dysfunction. Because adverse reactions have been ascribed more frequently to the intravenous formulation, this route of administration is discontinued as soon as the patient can take the drug orally.

In rheumatoid arthritis, cyclosporine is used in severe cases that have not responded to methotrexate. Cyclosporine can be combined with methotrexate, but the levels of both drugs must be monitored closely. In psoriasis, cyclosporine is indicated for treatment of adult immunocompetent patients with severe and disabling disease for whom other systemic therapies are contraindicated or have failed. Because of its mechanism of action, there is a theoretical basis for the use of cyclosporine in a variety of other T-cell–mediated diseases. Cyclosporine reportedly is effective in Behçet's, acute ocular syndrome, endogenous uveitis, atopic dermatitis, inflammatory bowel disease, and nephrotic syndrome, even when standard therapies have failed.

Toxicity. The principal adverse reactions to cyclosporine therapy are renal dysfunction and hypertension; tremor, hirsutism, hyperlipidemia, and gum hyperplasia also are frequently encountered. Hypertension occurs in about 50% of renal transplant and almost all cardiac transplant patients. Hyperuricemia may lead to worsening of gout, increased P-glycoprotein activity, and hypercholesterolemia (see Chapters 5, 33, and 38). Nephrotoxicity occurs in the majority of patients and is the major reason for cessation or modification of therapy. Combined use of calcineurin inhibitors and glucocorticoids is particularly diabetogenic, although this seems more problematic in patients treated with tacrolimus (see previous Tacrolimus section). Cyclosporine, as opposed to tacrolimus, is more likely to produce elevations in LDL cholesterol.

Drug Interactions. Cyclosporine interacts with a wide variety of commonly used drugs, and close attention must be paid to drug interactions. Any drug that affects CYPs, especially CYP3A, may affect cyclosporine blood concentrations. Substances that inhibit this enzyme can decrease cyclosporine metabolism and increase blood concentrations. These include Ca^{2+} channel blockers (e.g., *verapamil, nicardipine*); antifungal agents (e.g., *fluconazole, ketoconazole*); antibiotics (e.g., *erythromycin*); glucocorticoids (e.g., *methylprednisolone*); HIV-protease inhibitors (e.g., *indinavir*); and other drugs (e.g., *allopurinol, metoclopramide*). Grapefruit juice inhibits CYP3A and the P-glycoprotein multidrug efflux pump and thereby can increase cyclosporine blood concentrations. In contrast, drugs that induce CYP3A activity can increase cyclosporine metabolism and decrease blood concentrations. Such drugs include antibiotics (e.g., *nafcillin, rifampin*); anticonvulsants (e.g., *phenobarbital, phenytoin*); and others (e.g., *octreotide, ticlopidine*).

Interactions between cyclosporine and sirolimus require that administration of the two drugs be separated by time. Sirolimus aggravates cyclosporine-induced renal dysfunction, while cyclosporine increases sirolimus-induced hyperlipidemia and myelosuppression. Additive nephrotoxicity may occur when cyclosporine is coadministered with *NSAIDs* and other drugs that cause renal dysfunction; elevation of methotrexate levels may occur when the two drugs are coadministered, as can reduced clearance of other drugs, including prednisolone, digoxin, and statins (Azzi et al., 2013; Ekberg et al., 2007).

Antiproliferative and Antimetabolic Drugs

Sirolimus

Sirolimus (rapamycin) is a macrocyclic lactone produced by *Streptomyces hygroscopicus*.

Mechanism of Action. Sirolimus inhibits T-lymphocyte activation and proliferation downstream of the IL-2 and other T-cell growth factor receptors (see Figure 35–2). Like cyclosporine and tacrolimus, therapeutic action of sirolimus requires formation of a complex with an immunophilin, in this case *FKBP-12*. The *sirolimus–FKBP-12 complex* does not affect calcineurin activity; rather, it binds to and inhibits the protein kinase *mTOR*, which is a key enzyme in cell cycle progression. Inhibition of mTOR blocks cell cycle progression at the $G_1 \rightarrow S$ phase transition.

In animal models, sirolimus not only inhibits transplant rejection, GVHD, and a variety of autoimmune diseases, but also has effects for several months after discontinuation, suggesting a tolerizing effect (see Tolerance). A newer indication for sirolimus is the avoidance of calcineurin inhibitors, even when patients are stable, to protect kidney function (Schena et al., 2009).

ADME. After oral administration, sirolimus is absorbed rapidly and reaches a peak blood concentration within about 1 h after a single dose in healthy subjects and within about 2 h after multiple oral doses in renal transplant patients. Systemic availability is about 15%, and blood concentrations are proportional to dose between 3 and 12 mg/m^2. A high-fat meal decreases peak blood concentration by 34%; sirolimus therefore should be taken consistently either with or without food, and blood levels should be monitored closely. About 40% of sirolimus in plasma is protein bound, especially to albumin. The drug partitions into formed elements of blood (blood-to-plasma ratio = 38 in renal transplant patients). Sirolimus is extensively metabolized by CYP3A4 and is transported by P-glycoprotein. The bulk of total excretion is via the feces. Although some of its metabolites are active, sirolimus itself is the major active component in whole blood and contributes more than 90% of the immunosuppressive effect. The blood $t_{1/2}$ after multiple doses in stable renal transplant patients is 62 h. A loading dose of three times the maintenance dose will provide nearly steady-state concentrations within 1 day in most patients.

Therapeutic Uses. Sirolimus is indicated for prophylaxis of organ transplant rejection, usually in combination with a reduced dose of calcineurin inhibitor and glucocorticoids. Sirolimus has been used with glucocorticoids and mycophenolate to avoid permanent renal damage. Sirolimus dosing regimens are relatively complex, with blood levels generally targeted between 5 and 15 ng/mL. It is recommended that the daily maintenance dose be reduced by approximately one-third in patients with hepatic impairment. Sirolimus also has been incorporated into stents to inhibit local cell proliferation and blood vessel occlusion (Moes et al., 2015).

Toxicity. The use of sirolimus in renal transplant patients is associated with a dose-dependent increase in serum cholesterol and triglycerides that may require treatment. Although immunotherapy with sirolimus per se is not considered nephrotoxic, patients treated with cyclosporine plus sirolimus have impaired renal function compared to patients treated with cyclosporine alone. Sirolimus can worsen proteinuria and should be used with caution in patients with GFR below 30% or proteinuria; these conditions can worsen renal failure. Renal function and proteinuria therefore must be monitored closely in such patients. Lymphocele, a known surgical complication associated with renal transplantation, is increased in a dose-dependent fashion by sirolimus, requiring close postoperative follow-up.

Other adverse effects include anemia, leukopenia, thrombocytopenia, mouth ulcer, hypokalemia, and GI effects. Delayed wound healing may occur with sirolimus use. This mTOR inhibitor has been shown to have anticancer effect, especially on skin cancer; it is considered the immunosuppressant of choice in patients with a history of malignancy. Temsirolimus is specifically approved for kidney (but not skin) cancer, while everolimus is approved for a variety of cancers (but not skin cancer). As with other immunosuppressive agents, there is an increased risk of infections.

Drug Interactions. Because sirolimus is a substrate for CYP3A4 and is transported by P-glycoprotein, close attention to interactions with other drugs that are metabolized or transported by these proteins is required (see Chapters 5 and 6). Dose adjustment may be required when sirolimus is coadministered with CYP3A4 and P-glycoprotein inhibitors (such as diltiazem) or strong inducers (such as rifampin) (Alberú et al., 2011; Euvrard et al., 2012).

Everolimus

Everolimus [40-O-(2-hydroxyethyl)-rapamycin] is FDA-approved for treatment of astrocytoma, breast cancer, kidney and liver transplant rejection prophylaxis, pancreatic neuroendocrine tumor, renal angiomyolipoma, and renal cell cancer. It is chemically closely related to sirolimus but has distinct pharmacokinetics. The main difference is a shorter $t_{1/2}$ and thus a shorter time to achieve steady-state concentrations of the drug. Dosage on a milligram per kilogram basis is similar to (but not the same as) that of sirolimus. In kidney transplant rejection prophylaxis, the initial dose of everolimus is 0.75 mg twice daily, with later adjustment based on serum concentrations. As with sirolimus, the combination of a calcineurin inhibitor and an mTOR inhibitor produces worse renal function at 1 year than does calcineurin inhibitor therapy alone, suggesting a drug interaction between the mTOR inhibitors and the calcineurin inhibitors that reduces rejection but enhances toxicity. The toxicity of everolimus and the potential for drug interactions seem to be the same as with sirolimus (Budde et al., 2011; Moes et al., 2015). Like sirolimus, individualization of drug dose through therapeutic drug monitoring is required.

Azathioprine

Azathioprine is a purine antimetabolite. It is an imidazolyl derivative of 6-mercaptopurine, metabolites of which can inhibit purine synthesis.

Mechanism of Action. Following exposure to nucleophiles such as glutathione, azathioprine is cleaved to 6-MP, which in turn is converted to additional metabolites that inhibit de novo purine synthesis (see Chapter 66). A fraudulent nucleotide, 6-thio-IMP, is converted to 6-thio-GMP and finally to 6-thio-GTP, which is incorporated into DNA. Cell proliferation thereby is inhibited, impairing a variety of lymphocyte functions. Azathioprine appears to be a more potent immunosuppressive agent than 6-MP (Hardinger et al., 2013).

ADME. Azathioprine is well absorbed orally and reaches maximum blood levels within 1–2 h after administration. The $t_{1/2}$ of azathioprine is about 10 min, and the $t_{1/2}$ of 6-MP is about 1 h. Other metabolites have a $t_{1/2}$ of up to 5 h. Blood levels have limited predictive value because of extensive metabolism, significant activity of many different metabolites, and high tissue levels attained. Azathioprine and mercaptopurine are moderately bound to plasma proteins and are partially dialyzable. Both are rapidly removed from the blood by oxidation or methylation in the liver or erythrocytes. Renal clearance has little impact on the biological effectiveness or toxicity.

Therapeutic Uses. Azathioprine is indicated as an adjunct for prevention of organ transplant rejection and in severe rheumatoid arthritis. The usual starting dose of azathioprine is 3–5 mg/kg/d. Lower initial doses (1 mg/kg/d) are used in treating rheumatoid arthritis. Complete blood count and liver function tests should be monitored.

Toxicity. The major side effect of azathioprine is bone marrow suppression, including leukopenia (common), thrombocytopenia (less common), or anemia (uncommon). Other important adverse effects include increased susceptibility to infections (especially varicella and herpes simplex viruses), hepatotoxicity, alopecia, GI toxicity, pancreatitis, and increased risk of neoplasia.

Drug Interactions. Xanthine oxidase, an enzyme of major importance in the catabolism of azathioprine metabolites, is blocked by allopurinol. Hence, the combination of azathioprine with allopurinol should be avoided. Adverse effects resulting from coadministration of azathioprine with other myelosuppressive agents or angiotensin-converting enzyme inhibitors include leukopenia, thrombocytopenia, and anemia as a result of myelosuppression.

Mycophenolate Mofetil

Mycophenolate mofetil is the 2-morpholinoethyl ester of MPA (Darji et al., 2008; Molnar et al., 2015).

Mechanism of Action. Mycophenolate mofetil is a prodrug that is rapidly hydrolyzed to the active drug MPA, a selective, noncompetitive, reversible inhibitor of inosine monophosphate dehydrogenase (IMPDH), an enzyme in the de novo pathway of guanine nucleotide synthesis. B and T lymphocytes are highly dependent on this pathway for cell proliferation; MPA thus selectively inhibits lymphocyte proliferation and functions, including antibody formation, cellular adhesion, and migration.

ADME. Mycophenolate mofetil undergoes rapid and complete metabolism to MPA after oral or intravenous administration. MPA is then metabolized to the inactive glucuronide MPAG. The parent drug is cleared from the blood within a few minutes. The $t_{1/2}$ of MPA is ~16 h. Most (87%) is excreted in the urine as MPAG. Plasma concentrations of MPA and MPAG are increased in patients with renal insufficiency.

Therapeutic Uses. Mycophenolate mofetil is indicated for prophylaxis of transplant rejection, and it typically is used in combination with glucocorticoids and a calcineurin inhibitor but not with azathioprine. Combined treatment with sirolimus is possible, although potential drug interactions necessitate careful monitoring of drug levels. The approved dose for liver transplantation rejection prophylaxis is 1 g twice daily. For renal transplants, 1 g is administered orally or intravenously (over 2 h) twice daily (2 g/d). A higher dose, 1.5 g twice daily (3 g/d), may be recommended for African American renal transplant patients and all liver and cardiac transplant patients. MMF is increasingly used off label in systemic lupus. MMF has been used to treat a number of different inflammatory disorders, including MS and sarcoidosis. A delayed-release formulation of MPA is available; it does not release MPA under acidic conditions (pH < 5), as in the stomach, but is soluble in neutral pH, as in the intestine. The enteric coating results in a delay in the time to reach maximum MPA concentrations (Darji et al., 2008).

Toxicity. The principal toxicities of MMF are GI and hematologic: leukopenia, pure red cell aplasia, diarrhea, and vomiting. The MPA formulation has been introduced to reduce the frequent GI upset and has had variable results. There also is an increased incidence of some infections, especially sepsis associated with cytomegalovirus. Tacrolimus in combination with MMF has been associated with activation of polyoma viruses such as BK virus, which can cause interstitial nephritis. The use of mycophenolate in pregnancy is associated with congenital anomalies and increased risk of pregnancy loss.

Drug Interactions. Tacrolimus delays elimination of MMF by impairing the conversion of MPA to MPAG. This may enhance GI toxicity. Coadministration with antacids containing aluminum or magnesium hydroxide leads to decreased absorption of MMF; thus, these drugs should not be administered simultaneously. MMF should not be administered with cholestyramine or other drugs that affect enterohepatic circulation. Such agents decrease plasma MPA concentrations, probably by binding free MPA in the intestines. Acyclovir and ganciclovir may compete with MPAG for tubular secretion, possibly resulting in increased concentrations of both MPAG and the antiviral agents in the blood, an effect that may be compounded in patients with renal insufficiency. Mycophenolate serum level monitoring is not performed routinely (Darji et al., 2008; Goldfarb-Rumyantzev et al., 2006).

Other Antiproliferative and Cytotoxic Agents

Many of the cytotoxic and antimetabolic agents used in cancer chemotherapy (see Chapter 66) are immunosuppressive due to their action on lymphocytes and other cells of the immune system. Other cytotoxic drugs that have been used both on and off label as immunosuppressive agents include methotrexate, cyclophosphamide, thalidomide, and chlorambucil. *Methotrexate* is used for prophylaxis against GVHD and treatment of rheumatoid arthritis, psoriasis, bullous pemphigoid, and some cancers. *Cyclophosphamide* and *chlorambucil* are used in leukemia and lymphomas and a variety of other malignancies. Cyclophosphamide also is FDA-approved for childhood nephrotic syndrome and is used widely off label for treatment of severe systemic lupus erythematosus, MS, and vasculitides such as Wegener granulomatosis. *Leflunomide* is a pyrimidine synthesis inhibitor indicated for the treatment of adults with rheumatoid arthritis. This drug has found increasing empirical use in the treatment of polyomavirus nephropathy seen in immunosuppressed renal transplant recipients. There are no controlled studies showing efficacy compared with control patients treated with only withdrawal or reduction of immunosuppression alone in BK virus nephropathy. The drug inhibits dihydroorotate dehydrogenase in the de novo pathway of pyrimidine synthesis. It is hepatotoxic and can cause fetal injury when administered to pregnant women.

Fingolimod

Fingolimod is the first agent in a new class of small molecules, S1P-R agonists. This S1P-R prodrug reduces recirculation of lymphocytes from the lymphatic system to the blood and peripheral tissues, thereby shunting lymphocytes away from inflammatory lesions and organ grafts.

Mechanism of Action. *Fingolimod* specifically and reversibly causes sequestration of host lymphocytes into the lymph nodes and Peyer patches and thus away from the circulation, thereby protecting lesions and grafts from T-cell–mediated attack. Fingolimod does not impair T- and B-cell functions. Sphingosine kinase 2 phosphorylates fingolimod;

the fingolimod-phosphate product is a potent agonist at S1P-Rs, producing the altered lymphocyte traffic.

Therapeutic Uses. Fingolimod is not useful for treatment of transplant rejection but is effective and FDA-approved as a first-line therapy in the MS (see section on MS; Pelletier and Hafler, 2012).

Toxicity. Lymphopenia, the predictable and most common side effect of fingolimod, reverses on discontinuation of the drug. Of greater concern is the negative chronotropic effect on the heart, which has been observed with the first dose in up to 30% of patients (Vincenti and Kirk, 2008). In most patients, the heart rate returns to baseline within 48 h, with the remainder returning to baseline thereafter.

Immunosuppression Antibodies and Fusion Receptor Protein

Polyclonal and mAbs against lymphocyte cell surface antigens are widely used for prevention and treatment of organ transplant rejection. Polyclonal antisera are generated by repeated injections of human thymocytes (ATG) or lymphocytes (ALG) into animals and then purifying the serum immunoglobulin fraction. These preparations vary in efficacy and toxicity from batch to batch.

The capacity to produce mAbs (Figure 35–3) has overcome the problems of variability in efficacy and toxicity seen with the polyclonal products, but mAbs are more limited in their target specificity. The first-generation murine mAbs have been replaced by newer humanized or fully human mAbs that lack antigenicity, have a prolonged $t_{1/2}$, and can be mutagenized to alter their affinity to Fc receptors.

Another class of biological agents being developed for both autoimmunity and transplantation are fusion receptor proteins. These agents consist of the ligand-binding domains of receptors bound to the Fc region of an immunoglobulin (usually IgG1) to provide a longer $t_{1/2}$ (Baldo, 2015). Examples of such agents include *abatacept* (CTLA4-Ig) and *belatacept* (a second-generation CTLA4-Ig), discussed in the Costimulatory Blockade section.

Antithymocyte Globulin

Antithymocyte globulin is a purified gamma globulin from the serum of rabbits immunized with human thymocytes (Thiyagarajan et al., 2013). It is provided as a sterile, freeze-dried product for intravenous administration after reconstitution with sterile water. ATG is one of many immune globulin preparations used therapeutically, generally for passive immunization (see Table 35–2 and Chapter 36).

Mechanism of Action. Antithymocyte globulin contains cytotoxic antibodies that bind to CD2, CD3, CD4, CD8, CD11a, CD18, CD25, CD44, CD45, and HLA class I and II molecules on the surface of human T lymphocytes. The antibodies deplete circulating lymphocytes by direct cytotoxicity (both complement and cell mediated) and block lymphocyte function by binding to cell surface molecules involved in the regulation of cell function.

Therapeutic Uses. Antithymocyte globulin is used for induction immunosuppression, although the approved indications are for the treatment and prophylaxis of acute renal transplant rejection in combination with other immunosuppressive agents and for the treatment of aplastic anemia. Antilymphocyte-depleting agents (Thymoglobulin, Atgam, and OKT3) are not registered for use as induction immunosuppression. A course of antithymocyte-globulin often is given to renal transplant patients with delayed graft function to avoid early treatment with the nephrotoxic calcineurin inhibitors, thereby aiding in recovery from ischemic reperfusion injury. The recommended dose of Thymoglobulin for acute rejection of renal grafts is 1.5 mg/kg/d (over 4–6 h) for 7–14 days. Mean T-cell counts fall by day 2 of therapy. The recommended dose of Atgam for acute rejection of renal grafts is 10–15 mg/kg/d for 14 days.

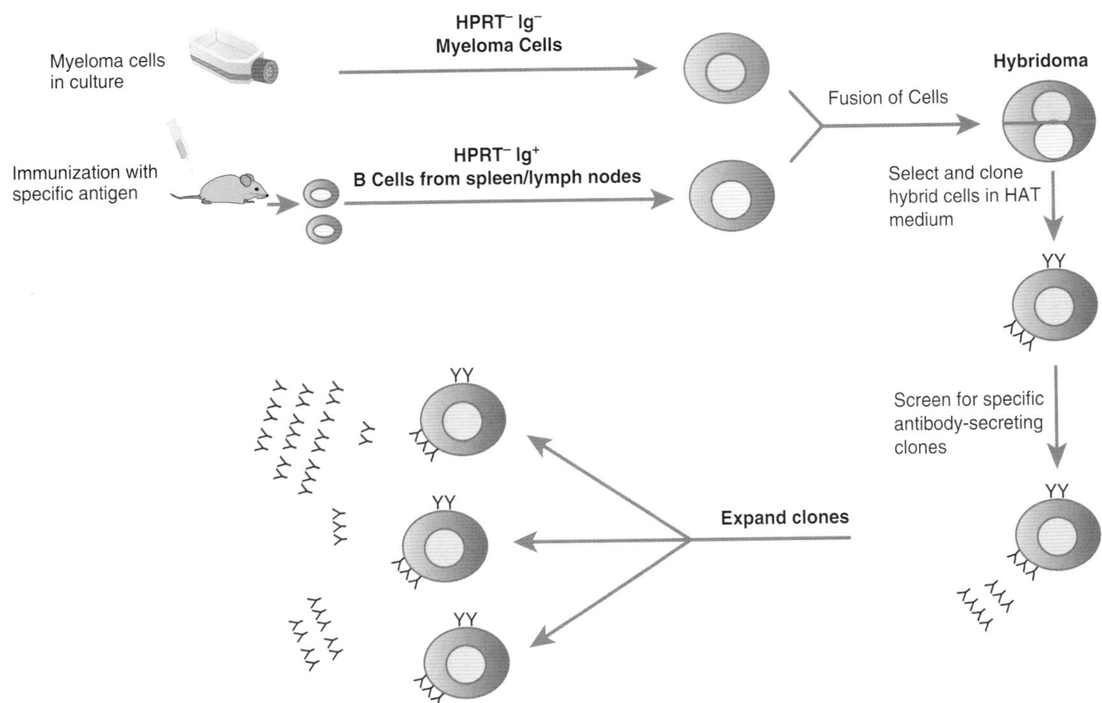

Figure 35–3 *Generation of mAbs.* Mice are immunized with the selected antigen, and the spleen or lymph node is harvested and B cells separated. These B cells are fused to a suitable B-cell myeloma selected for its ability to grow in medium supplemented with HAT (hypoxanthine, aminopterin, and thymidine). Only myeloma cells that fuse with B cells can survive in HAT-supplemented medium. The hybridomas expand in culture. Hybridomas of interest are selected based on a specific screening technique and then cloned by limiting dilution. The mAbs can be used directly as supernatants or ascites fluid for experimental use but are purified for clinical use.

TABLE 35–2 ■ SELECTED IMMUNE GLOBULIN PREPARATIONS

GENERIC NAME	COMMON SYNONYMS	ORIGIN
Antithymocyte globulin	ATG	Rabbit
Botulism immune globulin intravenous	BIG-IV	Human
Cytomegalovirus immune globulin intravenous	CMV-IGIV	Human
Hepatitis B immune globulin	HBIG	Human
Immune globulin intramuscular	Gamma globulin, IgG, IGIM	Human
Immune globulin intravenous	IVIG	Human
Immune globulin subcutaneous	IGSC	Human
Lymphocyte immune globulin	ALG, antithymocyte globulin (equine), ATG (equine)	Equine
Rabies immune globulin	RIG	Human
Rho(D) immune globulin intramuscular	Rho[D] IGIM	Human
Rho(D) immune globulin intravenous	Rho[D] IGIV	Human
Rho(D) immune globulin microdose	Rho[D] IG microdose	Human
Tetanus immune globulin	TIG	Human
Vaccinia immune globulin intravenous	VIGIV	Human

ATG also is used for acute rejection of other types of organ transplants and for prophylaxis of rejection.

Toxicity. Polyclonal antibodies are xenogeneic proteins that can elicit major side effects, including fever and chills with the potential for hypotension. Premedication with corticosteroids, acetaminophen, or an antihistamine and administration of the antiserum by slow infusion (over 4–6 h) into a large-diameter vessel minimize such reactions. Serum sickness and glomerulonephritis can occur; anaphylaxis is rare. Hematologic complications include leukopenia and thrombocytopenia. As with other immunosuppressive agents, there is an increased risk of infection and malignancy, especially when multiple immunosuppressive agents are combined. No drug interactions have been described; anti-ATG antibodies develop but do not limit repeated use.

Monoclonal Antibodies

Immunotherapy and the Nature of Costimulation and Inhibition

Multiple costimulatory and inhibitory molecules interact to regulate T-cell responses. Immune activation requires two signals that emanate from the interaction of membrane proteins on APCs and T cells (Figures 34–5A and 34–5B). A growing number of antibodies directed at these interacting proteins permits interruption of immune activation to produce a state of immune suppression. Figures 35–2 and 35–4 point out some of these antibodies, which are especially useful in preventing rejection after organ transplantation, as summarized in the material that follows.

In what might be considered an antiparallel system to activation, inhibitory regulation of T-cell activity can also result from the interaction of paired membrane ligands of APCs and T cells (Figure 35–4C). These points of negative regulation are called *immune checkpoints*. By targeting and blocking these immune checkpoints, antibodies can permit T-cell activation to proceed, unfettered by downregulation (Figure 35–4C and 35–4D). Activating immune attacks of tumor cells by blockade of immune checkpoints is producing new therapeutic options for cancer therapy (Callahan et al., 2016; Topalian et al., 2015). Chapter 67 presents the use of immunotherapy in cancer treatment.

Anti-CD3 Monoclonal Antibodies

CD3 is a component of the TCR complex on the surface of human T lymphocytes (Figure 35–2). Antibodies directed at the ε chain of CD3 have been used with considerable efficacy in human transplantation. The anti-CD3 antibody is monoclonal and targets the CD3 chain of the TCR, inducing its endocytosis and T-cell inactivation and removal through phagocytosis. The original mouse IgG2a antihuman CD3 mAb, *muromonab-CD3* (OKT3), is no longer marketed due to its side effects: It frequently causes cytokine release syndrome and severe pulmonary edema. Nevertheless, muromonab remains FDA-registered and could be reintroduced to the market at any time.

Recently, genetically altered anti-CD3 mAbs have been developed that are "humanized" to minimize the occurrence of antiantibody responses and mutated to prevent binding to Fc receptors. In initial clinical trials, a humanized anti-CD3 mAb that does not bind to Fc receptors reversed acute renal allograft rejection without causing the first-dose cytokine release syndrome. Humanized anti-CD3 mAbs are also in phase 3 trials in patients with type 1 autoimmune diabetes.

Anti-CD52 Monoclonal Antibody (Alemtuzumab)

Alemtuzumab is a depleting humanized anti-CD52 mAb.

Mechanism of Action. Alemtuzumab binds the CD52 protein that is wildly expressed on B cells and T-cells, as well as macrophages, NK cells, and some granulocytes. Alemtuzumab binding to CD52 induces an antibody-dependent lysis of cells and a profound leukopenia that may last for more than a year (Jones and Coles, 2014).

Therapeutic Uses. *Alemtuzumab* is used mainly for induction of immunosuppressive therapy and allows the avoidance of the early high dose of steroids. For transplants, the most common regimen is a single intraoperative dose of 30 mg. Alemtuzumab is also used for the treatment of refractory acute cellular- and antibody-mediated rejections with the same dose used during induction. The drug is licensed for the management of CLL and MS (CAMMS223 Investigators et al., 2008).

Toxicity. Neutropenia remains the most common adverse effect seen with *alemtuzumab*. Almost half of the patients will also experience thrombocytopenia and anemia. Another major side effect is autoimmune hemolytic anemia and other autoimmune diseases thought to be due to immune reconstitution after the profound lymphocyte depletion.

Anti-IL-2 Receptor (Anti-CD25) Antibodies

Daclizumab is a humanized murine complementarity-determining region/human IgG1 chimeric mAb. *Basiliximab* is a murine-human chimeric mAb. Both are licensed for use in conjunction with cyclosporine and corticosteroids for the prophylaxis of acute organ rejection in patients receiving renal transplants.

Mechanism of Action. The anti-CD25 mAbs bind with high affinity to the α subunit of the IL-2 receptor (Figure 35–2) and act as a receptor antagonist, inhibiting T-cell activation and proliferation without inducing cell lysis (Table 35–1). *Daclizumab* has a somewhat lower affinity but a longer $t_{1/2}$ (20 days) than *basiliximab* (Brennan et al., 2006). In addition, the induction of $CD56^+$ $CD4^+$ T cells is associated with response to therapy in patients with MS (D'Amico et al., 2015).

Therapeutic Uses. Anti-CD25 mAbs are used for induction therapy in solid-organ transplantation. They are also in phase 3 clinical trials in patients with MS. The long $t_{1/2}$ of daclizumab (20 days) results in saturation of the IL-2Rα on circulating lymphocytes for up to 120 days after transplantation. Daclizumab is administered in five doses (1 mg/kg given intravenously over 15 min in 50–100 mL of normal saline) starting immediately preoperatively and subsequently at biweekly intervals.

The $t_{1/2}$ of basiliximab is 7 days. In trials, basiliximab was administered in a fixed dose of 20 mg preoperatively and on days 0 and 4 after

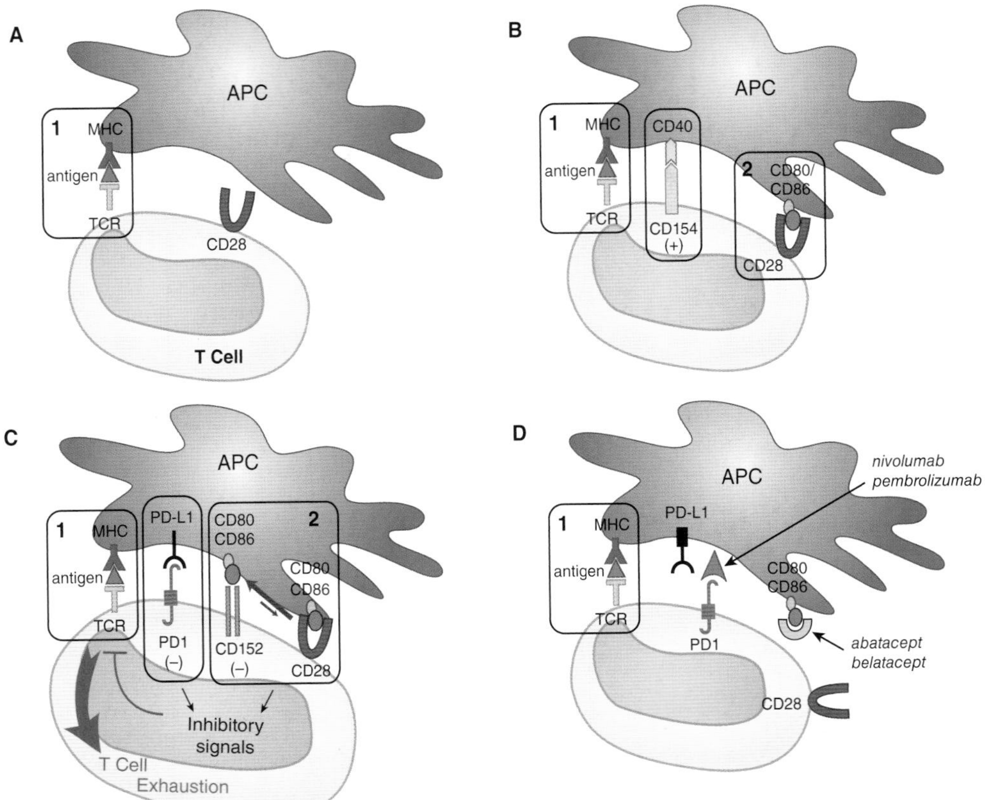

Figure 35–4 *T-cell activation: costimulation and coinhibitory checkpoints.* Numerous membrane CD proteins may be expressed on the APC and the T cell that lead to signaling interactions between ligands and receptors. These interactions can enhance or reduce the activation state of the T cell. Two signals are required for T-cell activation: presentation of an antigen ligand to the TCR and signaling by an additional "costimulatory" pair. **A.** The primary signal, *signal 1*, is the interaction of the TCR with the MHC-antigen complex on the APC. Activation requires a second, costimulatory interaction. **B.** *Signal 2*, the costimulatory interaction between CD28 on the T cell (the costimulatory receptor) and the costimulatory ligand on the APC, CD80/CD86, leads to T-cell activation. Additional costimulatory signals, such as the interaction of CD154 with CD40 on the APC, can further enhance T-cell activation (+). In the absence of costimulation, a T cell can become anergic or unresponsive. **C.** Additional APC–T-cell interactions can occur after T-cell activation, and some can be inhibitory, providing *immune checkpoints* that are important for reducing autoimmunity and for regulating the size and extent of immune responses. For example, the interaction of CD152 (CTLA4) with CD80/86 produces inhibitory signals that attenuate T-cell activation and proliferation (–). CD28 and CD152 compete for binding to CD80/CD86. As the figure suggests, the affinity of CD152 for CD80/CD86 exceeds that of CD28, and the equilibrium lies toward the formation of the inhibitory signaling complex, CD152-CD80/CD86. T cells may express varying amounts of another important modifier, PD1 (CD279). When liganded by PD-L1, PD1 produces inhibitory signals (↑ protein phosphatase activity, ↓ signaling by TCR, ↓ MAPK activity; see Figure 35–2) and reduces T-cell proliferation, leading to T-cell exhaustion, a state of hyporesponsiveness. When PD1 is highly expressed, as during conditions of chronic viral infection and cancer, suppression of T-cell activity via this pathway can be very effective; this pathway can facilitate continued viral replication and tumor progression. **D.** These immune checkpoints are useful sites for pharmacological regulation of T-cell activation. For instance, the agents abatacept and belatacept are fusion proteins that contain the CTLA4 domain of CD154 and act as decoys. These agents block costimulation of T cells by binding CD80/CD86 (see additional examples in Figure 35–2). Nivolumab and pembrolizumab are antibodies to PD1 and block interaction of PD1 with PD-L1, thereby blocking the immune suppression that would normally ensue and producing a state of immune hyperactivity. Checkpoint inhibitors that enhance immune responses are being used in cancer therapy (see Chapter 67). Antibodies can also be designed to be stimulatory ligands at checkpoints, to aid in generating a state of immune suppression that would be useful in treating autoimmune diseases.

transplantation. This regimen of basiliximab saturated IL-2R on circulating lymphocytes for 25–35 days after transplantation. Basiliximab was used with a maintenance regimen consisting of cyclosporine and prednisone and was found to be safe and effective when used in a maintenance regimen consisting of cyclosporine, MMF, and prednisone.

While daclizumab and basiliximab are comparable in effectiveness, daclizumab has a more costly dosing regimen. The higher cost has reduced demand, and daclizumab is now produced only for use in treating MS.

Toxicity. *Basiliximab* and *daclizumab* seem to be relatively safe as induction agents, with most of the clinical trials reporting adverse reactions rates comparable to placebo. No cytokine-release syndrome has been noted, but anaphylactic reactions and rare lymphoproliferative disorders and opportunistic infections may occur. No drug interactions have been described.

Belatacept, a Fusion Protein

Belatacept is a fusion protein composed of a modified Fc fragment of a human immunoglobulin linked to the extracellular domain of the CTLA4 (CD152) that is present on T cells (Figure 35–5). This second-generation CTLA4-Ig has two amino acid substitutions, increasing its affinity for CD80 (2-fold) and CD86 (4-fold), yielding a 10-fold increase in potency in vitro compared to CTLA4-Ig (Chinen et al., 2015).

Mechanism of Action. Induction of specific immune responses by T lymphocytes requires two signals: an antigen-specific signal via the

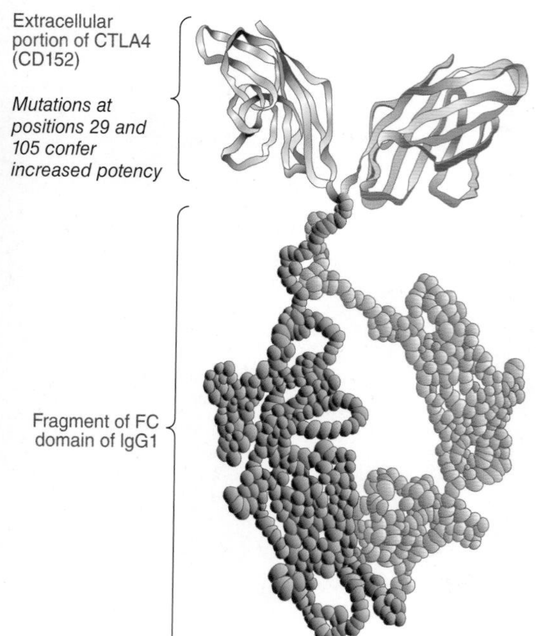

Figure 35–5 *Structure of belatacept, a CLTA4-Ig congener.* For details, see the text and Figure 35–4.

TCR and a costimulatory signal provided by the interaction of molecules such as CD28 on CD4 lymphocyte with CD80 and CD86 on APCs and CD2 engagement by LFA-3 (CD58) on CD8 cells (Figure 35–4) (Riella and Sayegh, 2013). *Belatacept* is a selective T-cell costimulation blocker that potently binds the cell surface costimulatory ligands (CD80 and CD86) present on APCs, interrupting their interaction with CD28 on T cells (signal 2). The inhibition of signal 2 inhibits T-cell activation, promoting anergy and apoptosis.

Disposition and Pharmacokinetics. *Belatacept* is the first intravenous maintenance therapy in solid-organ transplantation. Belatacept's pharmacokinetics were determined to be linear, with zero-order intravenous infusion and first-order elimination within the standard dose range of 5–10 mg/kg. The $t_{1/2}$ of *belatacept* is about 11 days.

Therapeutic Uses. Preclinical renal transplant studies showed that belatacept did not induce tolerance but did prolong graft survival. *Belatacept* is FDA approved as an alternative to calcineurin inhibitors as a strategy to prevent long-term calcineurin inhibitor toxicity (Satyananda and Shapiro, 2014; Talawila and Pengel, 2015). *Belatacept* has been approved specifically for prophylaxis of organ rejection in adult patients receiving a kidney transplant in combination with basiliximab induction, MMF, and corticosteroids.

The BENEFIT trial compared two *belatacept*-based regimens to cyclosporine and showed better kidney function and metabolic profile with belatacept-treated patients compared to cyclosporine. Patients were induced with basiliximab and maintained on MMF and a prednisone taper. While infusions of belatacept are required relatively frequently early after transplantation, it becomes once/month by the end of the first or third month, depending on the dosage regimen chosen (Masson et al., 2014).

Toxicity. An increased risk of posttransplant lymphoproliferative disorder in Epstein-Barr virus seronegative patients has been observed with *belatacept* treatment. Hence, its use is restricted to Epstein-Barr virus seropositive patients. Infusion-related reactions occur infrequently, and the drug is generally well tolerated (Masson et al., 2014).

Drug Interactions. No specific pharmacokinetic drug-drug interactions have been reported with belatacept (Pestana et al., 2012).

General Approach to Treatment of Autoimmune Diseases

Genome-wide association scans have clearly clustered genetic variants around a group of diseases that appear to be mediated by autoimmune responses (Farh et al., 2015). Therapeutically, these diseases respond well to immunosuppression and the use of mABs directed against cytokine pathways. However, these genetic investigations have revealed that a risk variant in one disease may be protective in another (Maier et al., 2009), consistent with the observation that inhibiting cytokine responses in one disease state, such as anti–TNF-α in rheumatoid arthritis, may lead to flare-ups in another disease (MS).

Anti–IL-2 Receptor (Anti-CD25) Antibodies

Anti–IL-2R mAbs discussed previously have been FDA-approved as a second line drug for patients with MS.

Anti-CD52

Mature lymphocytes express CD52 (CAMPATH-1 antigen), a negatively charged membrane dodecapeptide. *Alemtuzumab,* discussed previously, is a humanized mAb that binds to CD52 and targets the lymphocyte for destruction. In addition to the uses mentioned, alemtuzumab is approved for use in CLL and MS.

Anti-TNF Reagents

Tumor necrosis factor alpha is a pro-inflammatory cytokine that has been implicated in the pathogenesis of several immune-mediated intestinal, skin, and joint diseases. Several diseases (rheumatoid arthritis, Crohn disease) are associated with elevated levels of TNF-α. As a result, a number of anti-TNF agents have been developed as treatments.

Infliximab is a chimeric IgG1 mAb containing a human constant (Fc) region and a murine variable region. It binds with high affinity to TNF-α and prevents the cytokine from binding to its receptors. Infliximab is approved in the U.S. for treating the symptoms of rheumatoid arthritis and is typically used in combination with methotrexate in patients who do not respond to methotrexate alone. Infliximab also is approved for treatment of symptoms of moderate-to-severe Crohn disease in patients who have failed to respond to conventional therapy (see Chapter 51). Other FDA-approved indications include ankylosing spondylitis, plaque psoriasis, psoriatic arthritis, and ulcerative colitis. About 1 in 6 patients receiving infliximab experiences an infusion reaction characterized by fever, urticaria, hypotension, and dyspnea within 1–2 h after antibody administration. The development of antinuclear antibodies, and rarely a lupus-like syndrome, has been reported after treatment with infliximab (Meroni et al., 2015).

Etanercept is a fusion protein that targets TNF-α. Etanercept contains the ligand-binding portion of a human TNF-α receptor fused to the Fc portion of human IgG1 and binds to TNF-α and prevents it from interacting with its receptors. It is approved for treatment of the symptoms of rheumatoid arthritis, ankylosing spondylitis, plaque psoriasis, polyarticular juvenile idiopathic arthritis, and psoriatic arthritis. Etanercept can be used in combination with methotrexate in patients who have not responded adequately to methotrexate alone. Injection-site reactions (i.e., erythema, itching, pain, or swelling) have occurred in more than one-third of etanercept-treated patients.

Adalimumab is another anti-TNF product for intravenous use. This recombinant human IgG1 mAb is approved for use in rheumatoid arthritis, ankylosing spondylitis, Crohn disease, juvenile idiopathic arthritis, plaque psoriasis, psoriatic arthritis, and ulcerative colitis.

Golimumab is a human IgG1 (anti–TNF-α) monoclonal antibody. Golimumab alone or in combination with methotrexate is approved for treatment of moderately to severely active rheumatoid arthritis and active psoriatic arthritis. It is also approved for treatment of patients with ankylosing spondylitis and moderately to severely active ulcerative colitis. Golimumab is administered by subcutaneous injections and is available in 50- and 100-mg doses.

Certolizumab pegol is a humanized pegylated antibody specific to TNF-α. Pegylation of the Fab' fragment provides sustained activity. This agent is approved for the treatment of adults with Crohn disease and rheumatoid arthritis, active psoriatic arthritis, and active ankylosing spondylitis. It is available as 200 mg lyophilized powder or 200-mg/mL prefilled sterile injections for subcutaneous administration.

Toxicity. All anti-TNF agents (i.e., *infliximab, etanercept, adalimumab, golimumab, certolizumab*) increase the risk of serious infections, lymphomas, and other malignancies. For example, fatal hepatosplenic T-cell lymphomas have been reported in adolescent and young adult patients with Crohn disease treated with infliximab in conjunction with azathioprine or 6-MP.

IL-1 Inhibition

Plasma IL-1 levels are increased in patients with active inflammation (see Chapter 34). In addition to the naturally occurring IL-1RA, several IL-1RAs are in development, and a few have been approved for clinical use.

Anakinra is an FDA-approved recombinant, nonglycosylated form of human IL-1RA for the management of joint disease in rheumatoid arthritis. *Anakinra* is also approved for cryopyrin-associated periodic syndromes (CAPS), a group of rare inherited inflammatory diseases associated with overproduction of IL-1 that includes familial cold autoinflammatory and Muckle-Wells syndromes and for treatment of neonatal-onset multisystem inflammatory disease. It can be used alone or in combination with anti-TNF agents such as etanercept, infliximab, or adalimumab.

Canakinumab is an IL-1β mAb that is FDA approved for CAPS and active systemic juvenile idiopathic arthritis. *Canakinumab* is being evaluated for use in chronic obstructive pulmonary disease.

Rilonacept, a fusion protein that binds IL-1, is being evaluated for gout. IL-1 is an inflammatory mediator of joint pain associated with elevated uric acid crystals.

Other Interleukin Antagonists

Tocilizumab, an IL-6R, is FDA-approved for treatment of rheumatoid arthritis and systemic juvenile idiopathic arthritis; *siltuximab*, another IL-6 antagonist, is FDA approved for treatment of multicentric Castleman disease if the patient is HIV and human herpesvirus 8 negative. *Ustekinumab* is a human IL-12 and IL-23 antagonist indicated for the treatment of plaque psoriasis and psoriatic arthritis.

Secukinumab is a human anti-IL-17A antagonist indicated for treatment of plaque psoriasis.

Inhibition of Lymphocyte Function–Associated Antigen

Efalizumab is a humanized IgG1 mAb targeting the CD11a chain of LFA-1. Efalizumab binds to LFA-1 on lymphocytes and prevents LFA-1 interaction with intercellular adhesion molecule (ICAM), thereby inhibiting T-cell adhesion, trafficking, and activation. Efalizumab was approved for use in patients with psoriasis but has been withdrawn from the market because of excessive progressive multifocal leukoencephalopathy (Prater et al., 2014).

Alefacept is a human LFA-3–IgG1 fusion protein. The LFA-3 portion of alefacept binds to CD2 on T lymphocytes, blocking the interaction between LFA-3 and CD2 and interfering with T-cell activation. Alefacept is approved for use in psoriasis. Treatment with alefacept has been shown to produce a dose-dependent reduction in T-effector memory cells (CD45, RO$^+$) but not in naïve cells (CD45, RA$^+$) (Vincenti and Kirk, 2008). This effect has been related to its efficacy in psoriatic disease and is of significant interest in transplantation because T-effector memory cells are associated with costimulation blockade-resistant and depletional induction-resistant rejection. Alefacept delays rejection in NHP cardiac transplantation and has synergistic potential when used with costimulation blockade or sirolimus-based regimens in NHPs (Vincenti and Kirk, 2008). A phase II multicenter study to assess the safety and efficacy of maintenance therapy with alefacept in kidney transplant recipients showed no difference from placebo controls (Rostaing et al., 2013).

Cytokine Therapy: Interferon

For a description of IFN induction and signaling and the major actions of IFN, see Chapter 34. Interferon-β (IFN-β) was among the first cytokines used for the treatment of autoimmune diseases, particularly MS. IFNs are endogenous regulatory cytokines that increase or decrease transcriptional initiation of hundreds of genes in a cell-dependent fashion with multiple mechanisms of action, including induction of IL-10. The different IFN-β formulations have modest therapeutic efficacy, decreasing the exacerbation rate in MS by approximately 30%. They are relatively safe; fatigue is the major side effect. There are multiple preparations of IFN-β in the market that are administered either by the intramuscular or subcutaneous routes. IFN-β preparations are usually used for MS and IFN-α/γ preparations are used for infections. Three IFN-β preparations are currently on the market: AVONEX and REBIF are 1a formulations for MS; BETASERON, EXTAVIA (1β preparations) and *peginterferon* (1a) are indicated for relapsing MS. There are no significant differences between these IFN preparations, and as more efficacious drugs are now available, they should no longer be considered first-line drugs for the treatment of MS.

Targeting B Cells

Most of the advances in transplantation can be attributed to drugs designed to inhibit T-cell responses. As a result, T-cell–mediated acute rejection has been become much less of a problem, while B-cell–mediated responses such as antibody-mediated rejection and other effects of donor-specific antibodies have become more evident. Both biologicals and small molecules with B-cell–specific effects now are in development for transplantation, including humanized mAbs to CD20 and inhibitors of the two B-cell–activation factors, BLYS and APRIL, and their respective receptors. *Belimumab*, a mAb that targets BLYS, was recently approved for use in patients with systemic lupus erythromatosus.

The CD20 antibodies *rituximab* and *ocrelizumab* deplete circulating mature B lymphocytes (though they may remain to some degree in lymph nodes), and positive results from clinical trials in patients with rheumatoid arthritis and MS strongly suggest that B cells play a critical part in disease pathogenesis. Genetic fine mapping studies demonstrated a potentially pathogenic role of B cells in MS and rheumatoid arthritis that were not limited to antibody production. In particular, a definitive genetic modeling study pointed to the crucial role of B cells as APCs (Farh et al., 2015).

Tolerance

Immunosuppression has concomitant risks of opportunistic infections and secondary tumors. Therefore, the ultimate goal of research on organ transplantation and autoimmune diseases is to induce and maintain immunological tolerance, the active state of antigen-specific nonresponsiveness (Krensky and Clayberger, 1994). Tolerance, if attainable, would represent a true cure for conditions discussed previously in this section without the side effects of the various immunosuppressive therapies. The calcineurin inhibitors prevent tolerance induction in some, but not all, preclinical models. In these same model systems, *sirolimus* does not prevent tolerance and may even promote tolerance (Kawai et al., 2014; Krensky and Clayberger, 1994). In experimental animals, *sirolimus* promotes regulatory T cells, a subtype of T cells shown to suppress all immunity, and promotes tolerance. Studies in kidney transplant recipients showed that *sirolimus* spared regulatory T cells in the periphery, unlike calcineurin inhibitors, which reduced their percentage (Segundo et al., 2006).

Costimulatory Blockade

Inhibition of the costimulatory signal has been shown to induce tolerance (Figure 35–4).

Abatacept is a fusion protein (see previous discussion) that contains the binding region of CTLA4 (CD152), which is a CD28 homolog, and the Fc region of the human IgG1. CTLA4-Ig competitively inhibits CD28 binding to CD80 and CD86 and thus activation of T cells. CTLA4-Ig is effective in the treatment of rheumatoid arthritis in patients resistant to other drugs.

A second costimulatory pathway involves the interaction of CD40 on activated T cells with CD40 ligand (CD154) on B cells, endothelium, or APCs (see Figure 35–4). Among the purported activities of anti-CD154 antibody treatment is the blockade of B7 expression induced by immune activation. Two humanized anti-CD154 mAbs have been used in clinical trials in renal transplantation and autoimmune diseases. The development of these antibodies, however, is on hold because of associated thromboembolic events. An alternative approach to block the CD154-CD40 pathway is to target CD40 with mAbs. These antibodies are undergoing trials in non-Hodgkin lymphoma but are also likely to be developed for autoimmunity and transplantation.

Donor Cell Chimerism

A promising approach is induction of chimerism (coexistence of cells from two genetic lineages in a single individual) by first dampening or eliminating immune function in the recipient with ionizing radiation, drugs such as cyclophosphamide, or antibody treatment and then providing a new source of immune function by adoptive transfer (transfusion) of bone marrow or hematopoietic stem cells. On reconstitution of immune function, the recipient no longer recognizes new antigens provided during a critical period as "nonself." Such tolerance is long lived and less likely to be complicated by the use of calcineurin inhibitors.

Antigens

Specific antigens induce immunological tolerance in preclinical models of diabetes mellitus, arthritis, and MS. In vitro and preclinical in vivo studies demonstrated that one can selectively inhibit immune responses to specific antigens without the associated toxicity of immunosuppressive therapies. With these insights comes the promise of specific immune therapies to treat an array of immune disorders from autoimmunity to transplant rejection (Riedhammer and Weissert, 2015). To date, this approach has only worked in animal models of autoimmune disease.

Soluble HLA

In the precyclosporine era, blood transfusions were shown to be associated with improved outcomes in renal transplant patients. These findings gave rise to donor-specific transfusion protocols that improved outcomes. After the introduction of cyclosporine, however, these effects of blood transfusions disappeared, presumably due to the efficacy of this drug in blocking T-cell activation. Nevertheless, the existence of tolerance-promoting effects of transfusions is irrefutable. It is possible that this effect is due to HLA molecules on the surface of cells or in soluble forms. Soluble HLA and peptides corresponding to linear sequences of HLA molecules can induce immunological tolerance in animal models via a variety of mechanisms (Murphy and Krensky, 1999).

Immunotherapy for Multiple Sclerosis

Clinical Features and Pathology

Multiple sclerosis is a genetically mediated demyelinating inflammatory disease of the CNS white matter, characterized by mononuclear cell infiltration into the white matter with relative demyelination to axonal loss. Dense meningeal infiltrates are found in the subarachnoid spaces of patients, and these infiltrates are intimately associated with subpial demyelination, neuronal and neuritic damage, oligodendrocyte loss, cortical atrophy, and parenchymal microglial activation in the outer cortical layers. Inflammatory cortical demyelination occurs early in MS, preceding the appearance of classic white matter plaques with neurodegenerative changes, including oligodendrocyte loss, reactive astrocytosis, and axonal and neuronal injury within these cortical plaques on a background of inflammation. MS may be episodic or progressive and occurs with prevalence increasing from late adolescence to 35 years of age and then declining. MS is 3-fold more common in females than in males and occurs mainly in higher latitudes of the temperate climates. Epidemiologic studies suggest a role for environmental factors in the pathogenesis of MS, including low vitamin D, smoking, increases in body mass index, and high salt intake (Ransohoff et al., 2015).

Genome-wide association studies have identified genetic variants associated with MS susceptibility (International Multiple Sclerosis Genetics Consortium, et al., 2007), now with 200 variants identified. Although each of these contributes only a small increase in the complex phenotype of disease risk, the biological functions associated with individual allelic variants have been striking. Many of these variants fall within specific signaling cascades, which suggests that alterations in pathways—rather than individual genes—may be useful in predicting response to therapy. Over half of genetic variants associated with MS risk are also found in other putative autoimmune diseases, and risk alleles are primarily associated with genes that regulate immune function. Approximately 60% of probable causal variants mapped to enhancer-like elements, with preferential correspondence to stimulus-dependent CD4$^+$ T-cell enhancers. By overlapping causal single-nucleotide variants with transcription factor–binding maps generated by ENCODE, single-nucleotide variants were strongly enriched within binding sites for immune-related transcription factors (Farh et al., 2015). In patients with MS, there are activated T cells that are reactive to different myelin antigens, including myelin basic protein, and these T cells secrete pro-inflammatory cytokines, whereas in healthy controls, T cells secrete the anti-inflammatory IL-10 cytokine (Cao et al., 2015). It is difficult to vigorously find autoantibodies to myelin antigens in patients with MS, distinguishing MS from other autoimmune diseases.

Attacks are classified by type and severity and likely correspond to specific degrees of CNS damage and pathological processes. Thus, physicians refer to relapsing-remitting MS (the form in 85% of younger patients), secondary progressive MS (progressive neurological deterioration following a long period of relapsing-remitting disease), and primary progressive MS (~15% of patients, wherein deterioration with relatively little inflammation is apparent at onset).

Pharmacotherapy

There have been major advances in the treatment of MS. Table 35–3 summarizes current immunomodulatory therapies for MS. Specific therapies are aimed at resolving acute attacks, reducing recurrences and exacerbations, and slowing the progression of disability. MS exacerbations are treated with 3 to 5 days of 1000 mg of intravenous methylprednisolone, as oral prednisone alone is an ineffective treatment that increases the risk of new attacks. The so-called first-generation (but not necessarily "first-line") drugs include a variety of *IFN-β* (discussed previously in Cytokine Therapy) and random polymers that contain amino acids commonly used as MHC anchors, and TCR contact residues have been proposed as possible "universal altered peptide ligands." Glatiramer acetate (GA), a random-sequence polypeptide consisting of four amino acids (alanine [A], lysine [K], glutamate [E], and tyrosine [Y]) with an average length of 40–100 amino acids, binds efficiently to MHC class II DR molecules in vitro. In clinical trials, GA, administered subcutaneously to patients with relapsing-remitting MS, decreased the rate of exacerbations by about 30%, similar to the efficacy of IFN-β. In vivo administration of GA induces highly cross-reactive CD4$^+$ T cells that are immune deviated to secrete anti-inflammatory Th2 cytokines such as IL-4 and IL-13. Administration of GA also prevents the appearance of new lesions detectable by MRI (Duda et al., 2000). This represents one of the first successful uses of an agent that ameliorates autoimmune disease by altering signals through the TCR complex.

The long-term treatment of patients with MS is in transition, having moved from the use of first-era therapies of IFN-β and GA to more effective treatments. The anti-CD20 B cell depletion therapy with *ocrelizumab* is currently the most efficacious treatment (Hauser et al., 2017) and should in most instances be considered as a first line therapy. There is no rationale for the use of step therapy with IFN-β and GA before using the more effective drugs such as ocrelizumab and natalizumab.

TABLE 35–3 ■ EFFICACY RANKING OF APPROVED THERAPIES FOR MULTIPLE SCLEROSIS[a]

DRUG	ERA OF DEVELOPMENT	MECHANISM OF ACTION	KEY CONSIDERATIONS
Most effective			
Natalizumab	Second	Monoclonal antibody against integrin α4	Risk of PML must be assessed via presence of JCV antibodies.
Ocrelizumab	Third	mAB against CD20 (B cells)	Low risk PML, slight increase in infections
Alemtuzumab	Third	mAB against CD52	High risk of 2° thyroiditis & other autoimmune disease
Highly effective			
Fingolimod	Second	Sphingosine S1P-R modulator	Cardiac complications preclude use in individuals over the age of 50 and those with history of cardiac disease. VZV antibody testing must be conducted to mitigate risk of disseminated herpes zoster.
Dimethyl fumarate	Third	Immunomodulator	Necessary to monitor lymphocyte count as risk mitigation against PML. GI complications may limit use.
Moderately effective			
IFN-β	First	Immunomodulator	Well-characterized long-term safety and efficacy profiles. Patients should not be required to "fail" before receiving alternative treatments.
Glatiramer acetate	First	Immunomodulator	Best safety profile for pregnant women with mild disease. Patients should not be required to "fail" before receiving alternative treatments.
Teriflunomide	Third	Pyrimidine-synthesis inhibitor	Risk of teratogenicity precludes use in women who are, or intend to become, pregnant.

[a]Rankings are estimated on the basis of clinical trials, postapproval studies, and few head-to-head comparisons. The factors that determine drug efficacy in any individual patient are largely undefined, and good clinical judgment is essential for treatment selection. For details, see Ransohoff et al., 2015.

The mAb *natalizumab*, directed against the adhesion molecule α_4 integrin, antagonizes interactions with integrin heterodimers containing α_4 integrin, such as $\alpha_4\beta_1$ integrin that is expressed on the surface of activated lymphocytes and monocytes. An interaction of $\alpha_4\beta_1$ integrin with vascular cell adhesion molecule 1 is critical for T-cell trafficking from the periphery into the CNS; blocking this interaction has been highly effective in inhibiting disease exacerbations.

Similarly, the S1P agonist *fingolimod* (mechanism discussed previously) is FDA-approved as a first-line therapy in MS, decreasing the exacerbation rate by about 50%. Use of natalizumab is associated with the development of progressive multifocal leukoencephalopathy, and availability is limited to a special distribution program (Touch) administered by the manufacturer that dictates measurement of JCV antibodies. Patients negative for JCV are often recommended to begin natalizumab, while JCV-positive persons are tested for VZV to evaluate fingolimod treatment. If the result is positive, indicating VZV immunity, fingolimod can be begun. If not, fingolimod treatment should follow VZV immunization. Regarding safety, natalizumab seems to be safe in patients negative for JCV antibody. In patients with cardiac issues—particularly with bundle branch blocks—fingolimod should be avoided.

Dimethyl fumarate appears to have multiple immunomodulatory effects and is an activator of *nrf2* that mediates antioxidative response. In two pivotal phase 3 trials, dimethyl fumarate reduced relapse rates by about 50% as compared with placebo, with a significant reduction of gadolinium-enhanced lesions as well as T2 lesions on MRI. The drug seems to be safe, although gastrointestinal side effects can occasionally cause difficulties.

Monoclonal antibodies directed against CD52 (*alemtuzumab*) were recently approved for relapsing-remitting MS (discussed previously). While it appears to be highly effective and long lived in terms of response, secondary autoimmune responses that emerge in patients with MS but not in those with CLL are thyroiditis and, more rarely, idiopathic thrombocytopenic purpura. The anti-CD20 antibody *ocrelizumab* has recently completed a phase 3 trial and has the most dramatic efficacy in treating MS, leading to FDA approval. It is now considered a first line drug in the treatment of relapsing remitting MS.

With all of these agents, the earlier in the course of MS that they are used, the more effective they are in preventing disease relapses. What is not clear is whether any of these agents will prevent or diminish the later onset of secondary progressive disease, which causes more severe disability.

Drug Facts for Your Personal Formulary: *Immunosuppressants and Tolerogens*

Drugs	Therapeutic Uses	Clinical Pharmacology and Tips
Glucocorticoids		
• Prednisone The liver converts prednisone to prednisolone.	Prevent and treat transplant rejection, treat GVHD in bone marrow transplant, autoimmune disease, rheumatoid arthritis, ulcerative colitis, multiple sclerosis, systemic lupus erythematosus	• Broad effects on cellular immunity • Affects transcription of many genes; ↓ NF-κB activation, ↓ pro-inflammatory cytokines IL-1 and IL-6 • ↓ T-cell proliferation, cytotoxic T-lymphocyte activation and neutrophil and monocyte function • Can cause ↑ blood glucose, hypertension, Cushingoid habitus, ↑ weight, ↑ risk of infection, osteoporosis, glaucoma, cataracts, depression, anxiety, psychosis • Long-term treatment ⇒ adrenal suppression; withdraw slowly on alternate days

Drug Facts for Your Personal Formulary: *Immunosuppressants and Tolerogens (continued)*

Drugs	Therapeutic Uses	Clinical Pharmacology and Tips
Glucocorticoids		
• Prednisolone	Rheumatoid arthritis, uveitis, ulcerative colitis, multiple sclerosis, vasculitis, sarcoidosis, systemic lupus erythematosus	• As above
• Methylprednisolone	Systemic lupus erythematosus, multiple sclerosis	• As above
• Dexamethasone	Rheumatoid arthritis, idiopathic thrombocytopenic purpura	• As above
Calcineurin Inhibitors		
• Cyclosporine	Transplant rejection prophylaxis, transplant rejection rescue therapy, rheumatoid arthritis, psoriasis and other skin diseases, xerophthalmia	• Use algorithms to delay dosing until renal function OK in kidney transplant patients • Monitor C_p to avoid side effects • Side effects: tremor, hallucinations, drowsiness, coma, nephrotoxicity, hypertension, hirsutism, hyperlipidemia, gum hyperplasia • Metabolized by CYP3A ⇒ drug interactions • Severe interactions with antiarrhythmics
• Tacrolimus	Transplant rejection prophylaxis, transplant rejection rescue therapy	• GI absorption is incomplete and variable • Side effects include nephrotoxicity, neurotoxicity, GI complaints, and hypertension • Glucose intolerance and diabetes mellitus • Monitor blood levels to avoid nephrotoxicity
Antiproliferative and Antimetabolic Agents		
• Azathioprine	Purine metabolism inhibitor, adjunct for prevention of organ transplant rejection, rheumatoid arthritis	• Renal clearance has little effect on efficacy or toxicity • Side effects include bone marrow suppression (leukopenia > thrombocytopenia > anemia) • Susceptibility to infections, hepatotoxicity, alopecia, GI toxicity • Avoid allopurinol
• Mycophenolate mofetil	Purine metabolism inhibitor, prophylaxis of transplant rejection, used off label for systemic lupus erythematosus, multiple sclerosis, sarcoidosis	• Side effects include GI (diarrhea and vomiting) and hematologic (leukopenia, pure red cell aplasia) problems • Contraindicated in pregnancy
• Sirolimus	mTOR inhibitor, prophylaxis of organ transplant rejection, incorporated into stents to inhibit occlusion	• Monitor blood levels • Hyperlipidemia • Anemia, leukopenia, thrombocytopenia • GI effects, mouth ulcers, hyperkalemia • Anticancer effects • Metabolized by CYP3A; requires close attention to drug interactions
• Everolimus	mTOR inhibitor, astrocytoma, breast cancer, kidney and liver transplant reception prophylaxis, pancreatic neuroendocrine tumor, renal angiomyolipoma, renal cell cancer	• Pharmacokinetics distinct from sirolimus • Toxicity similar to sirolimus
• Temsirolimus	mTOR inhibitor	
T-cell costimulatory blocker		
• Belatacept	Prevention of renal transplant rejection	• Due to an increased risk of post-transplant lymphoproliferative disorder predominantly involving the CNS, progressive multifocal leukoencephalopathy, and serious CNS infections, administration of higher than the recommended doses or more frequent dosing is NOT recommended.
Antibodies		
Antilymphocyte globulin • ATGAM • Thymoglobulin	Prevention and treatment of organ transplant rejection, aplastic anemia	• Contains antibodies against numerous T-cell surface molecules • Can elicit fever, chills, and potentially hypotension; use premedication: steroid/acetaminophen/antihistamine • Serum sickness, glomerulonephritis, anaphylaxis: rare • Watch for leukopenia, thrombocytopenia
Muromonab-CD3	In trials for autoimmune diseases	• Depletes CD3-positive cells
Anti-CD25 (anti–IL-2 receptor antibodies) • Basailixmab • Daclizumab	Prophylaxis of acute organ transplant rejection, multiple sclerosis (in clinical trial)	• β Adrenergic blocking effects (worsening of heart failure and bronchospasm) • Block T-cell activation • Do not deplete • Good safety profile

Drug Facts for Your Personal Formulary: *Immunosuppressants and Tolerogens (continued)*

Drugs	Therapeutic Uses	Clinical Pharmacology and Tips
Antibodies		
• Abetacept • Belatacept	Prophylaxis of organ transplant rejection, autoimmunity trials	• CTLA4-Ig fusion protein • Risk for posttransplant lymphoproliferative disorder
Anti-CD52 • Alemtuzumab	Chronic lymphocytic leukemia, multiple sclerosis, prevention and treatment of transplant rejection	• Prolonged lymphocyte depletion (neutropenia, thrombocytopenia as side effects) • Secondary autoimmunity
Anti-CD154 (CD40 ligand)	Renal transplantation, autoimmune diseases	• Blockade of B7 protein expression • On hold due to thromboembolic events
Anti-CD20 • Rituximab • Ocrelizumab	Rheumatoid arthritis, multiple sclerosis	• Deplete circulating mature B lymphocytes
Anti-TNF • Infliximab • Etanercept • Adalimumab • Golimumab • Certolizumab	Rheumatoid arthritis, Crohn disease, ankylosing spondylitis, plaque psoriasis, psoriatic arthritis, ulcerative colitis	• Infusion reaction with fever, urticaria, hypotension, and dyspnea can occur • Risk of serious infections, lymphoma, other malignancies
Anti–IL-1 • Anakinra • Canakininumab • Rilonacept	Rheumatoid arthritis, cryopyrin-associated syndromes, evaluated in gout	
Anti–LFA-1 • Efalizumab	Psoriasis	• Withdrawn: excessive progressive multifocal leukoencephalopathy
Anti-CD2 • Alefacept	Psoriasis	
• Belimumab (anti-BLYS)	Systemic lupus erythematosus	
Anti-VLA-4 • Natalizumab	Multiple sclerosis, Crohn disease	• Targets α-4 integrin blocking T-cell traffic to organ • Progressive multifocal leukoencephalopathy
Therapy for MS (Table 35–2 Summarizes More Detailed Therapies for MS.)		
• Ocrelizumab • Natalizumab • Alemtuzumab	Multiple sclerosis	• β cell depleting. First line drug. Highly efficacious. • Anti-VLA-4, blocks T cell traffic. Very efficacious. • Anti-CD52. Highly efficacious. Second line drug due to side effects.
• IFN-β	Multiple sclerosis	• Modest efficacy but safe • No longer first-line drug
• Fingolomod	Multiple sclerosis	• S1P-R agonist • Potential cardiac complications
• Tecfidera	Multiple sclerosis	• Monitor WBCs; slight risk of progressive multifocal leukoencephalopathy
• Glatiramer acetate	Multiple sclerosis	• Potentially safe in pregnancy but less efficacious
• Teriflunomide	Multiple sclerosis	• Pyrimidine-synthesis inhibitor; pregnancy risk

WBCs, white blood cells

Bibliography

Alberú J, et al. Lower malignancy rates in renal allograft recipients converted to sirolimus-based, calcineurin inhibitor-free immunotherapy: 24-month results from the CONVERT trial. *Transplantation*, **2011**, *92*:303–310.

Azzi JR, et al. Calcineurin inhibitors: 40 years later, can't live without. *J Immunol*, **2013**, *191*:5785–5791.

Baldo BA. Chimeric fusion proteins used for therapy: indications, mechanisms, and safety. *Drug Saf*, **2015**, *38*:455–479.

Beck RW, et al. A randomized controlled trial of corticosteroids in the treatment of acute optic neuritis. The Optic Neuritis Group. *N Engl J Med*, **1992**, *326*:581–588.

Bergmann TK, et al. Clinical pharmacokinetics and pharmacodynamics of prednisolone and prednisone in solid organ transplantation. *Clin Pharmacokinet*, **2012**, *51*:711–741.

Brennan DC, et al, and The Thymoglobulin Induction Study Group. Rabbit antithymocyte globulin versus basiliximab in renal transplantation. *N Engl J Med*, **2006**, *355*:1967–1977.

Budde K, et al. Everolimus-based, calcineurin-inhibitor-free regimen in recipients of de-novo kidney transplants: an open-label, randomised, controlled trial. *Lancet*, **2011**, *377*:837–847.

Callahan MK, et al. Targeting T cell co-receptors for cancer therapy. *Immunity*, **2016**, 44:1079–1078.

CAMMS223 Investigators, et al. Alemtuzumab vs. interferon beta-1a in early multiple sclerosis. *N Engl J Med*, **2008**, *359*:1786–1801.

Cao Y, et al. Functional inflammatory profiles distinguish myelin-reactive T cells from patients with multiple sclerosis. *Sci Transl Med,* **2015**, *7*:287ra274.

Chan K, et al. Kidney transplantation with minimized maintenance: alemtuzumab induction with tacrolimus monotherapy—an open label, randomized trial. *Transplantation,* **2011**, *92*:774–780.

Chinen J, et al. Advances in basic and clinical immunology in 2014. *J Allergy Clin Immunol,* **2015**, *135*:1132–1141.

Colombo D, Ammirati E. Cyclosporine in transplantation—a history of converging timelines. *J Biol Regul Homeost Agents,* **2011**, *25*: 493–504.

D'Amico E, et al. A critical appraisal of daclizumab use as emerging therapy in multiple sclerosis. *Expert Opin Drug Saf,* **2015**, *14*:1157–1168.

Danovitch GM, et al. Immunosuppression of the elderly kidney transplant recipient. *Transplantation,* **2007**, *84*:285–291.

Darji P, et al. Conversion from mycophenolate mofetil to enteric-coated mycophenolate sodium in renal transplant recipients with gastrointestinal tract disorders. *Transplant Proc,* **2008**, *40*:2262–2267.

Duda PW, et al. Glatiramer acetate (Copaxone) induces degenerate, Th2-polarized immune responses in patients with multiple sclerosis. *J Clin Invest,* **2000**, *105*:967–976.

Ekberg H, et al. Reduced exposure to calcineurin inhibitors in renal transplantation. *N Engl J Med,* **2007**, *357*:2562–2575.

Euvrard S, et al. Sirolimus and secondary skin-cancer prevention in kidney transplantation. *N Engl J Med,* **2012**, *367*:329–339.

Farh KK, et al. Genetic and epigenetic fine mapping of causal autoimmune disease variants. *Nature,* **2015**, *518*:337–343.

Goldfarb-Rumyantzev AS, et al. Role of maintenance immunosuppressive regimen in kidney transplant outcome. *Clin J Am Soc Nephrol,* **2006**, *1*:563–574.

Goring SM, et al. A network meta-analysis of the efficacy of belatacept, cyclosporine and tacrolimus for immunosuppression therapy in adult renal transplant recipients. *Curr Med Res Opin,* **2014**, *30*:1473–1487.

Guerra G, et al. Randomized trial of immunosuppressive regimens in renal transplantation. *J Am Soc Nephrol,* **2011**, *22*:1758–1768.

Hardinger KL, et al. Selection of induction therapy in kidney transplantation. *Transpl Int,* **2013**, *26*:662–672.

Hauser SL et al, and The OPERA I and OPERA II Clinical Investigators. Ocrelizumab versus Interferon Beta-1a in Relapsing Multiple Sclerosis. *N Engl J Med,* **2017**, *376*:221–234.

International Multiple Sclerosis Genetics Consortium, et al. Risk alleles for multiple sclerosis identified by a genomewide study. *N Engl J Med,* **2007**, *357*:851–862.

Jones JL, Coles AJ. Mode of action and clinical studies with alemtuzumab. *Exp Neurol,* **2014**, *262*(pt A):37–43.

Kappos KG, et al. Wide-QRS-complex tachycardia with a negative concordance pattern in the precordial leads: are the ECG criteria always reliable? *Pacing Clin Electrophysiol,* **2006**, *29*:63–66.

Kawai T, et al. Tolerance: one transplant for life. *Transplantation,* **2014**, *98*:117–121.

Krensky AM, Clayberger C. Prospects for induction of tolerance in renal transplantation. *Pediatr Nephrol,* **1994**, *8*:772–779.

Krensky AM, et al. T-lymphocyte-antigen interactions in transplant rejection. *N Engl J Med,* **1990**, *322*:510–517.

Maier LM, et al. IL2RA genetic heterogeneity in multiple sclerosis and type 1 diabetes susceptibility and soluble interleukin-2 receptor production. *PLoS Genet,* **2009**, *5*:e1000322.

Masson P, et al. Belatacept for kidney transplant recipients. *Cochrane Database Syst Rev,* **2014**, (11):CD010699.

Meroni PL, et al. New strategies to address the pharmacodynamics and pharmacokinetics of tumor necrosis factor (TNF) inhibitors: a systematic analysis. *Autoimmunol Rev,* **2015**, *14*:812–829.

Moes DJ, et al. Sirolimus and everolimus in kidney transplantation. *Drug Discov Today,* **2015**, *20*:1243–1249.

Molnar AO, et al. Generic immunosuppression in solid organ transplantation: systematic review and meta-analysis. *BMJ,* **2015**, *350*:h3163.

Murphy B, Krensky AM. HLA-derived peptides as novel immunomodulatory therapeutics. *J Am Soc Nephrol,* **1999**, *10*:1346–1355.

Nashan B. Antibody induction therapy in renal transplant patients receiving calcineurin-inhibitor immunosuppressive regimens: a comparative review. *BioDrugs,* **2005**, *19*:39–46.

Pelletier D, Hafler DA. Fingolimod for multiple sclerosis. *N Engl J Med,* **2012**, *366*:339–347.

Pestana JO, et al. Three-year outcomes from BENEFIT-EXT: a phase III study of belatacept versus cyclosporine in recipients of extended criteria donor kidneys. *Am J Transplant,* **2012**, *12*:630–639.

Polman CH, et al. A randomized, placebo-controlled trial of natalizumab for relapsing multiple sclerosis. *N Engl J Med,* **2006**, *354*:899–910.

Prater EF, et al. A retrospective analysis of 72 patients on prior efalizumab subsequent to the time of voluntary market withdrawal in 2009. *J Drugs Dermatol,* **2014**, *13*:712–718.

Ransohoff RM, et al. Multiple sclerosis-a quiet revolution. *Nat Rev Neurol,* **2015**, *11*:134–142.

Riedhammer C, Weissert R. Antigen presentation, autoantigens, and immune regulation in multiple sclerosis and other autoimmune diseases. *Front Immunol,* **2015**, *6*:322.

Riella LV, Sayegh MH. T-cell co-stimulatory blockade in transplantation: two steps forward one step back! *Expert Opin Biol Ther,* **2013**, *13*:1557–1568.

Rostaing L, et al. Alefacept combined with tacrolimus, mycophenolate mofetil and steroids in de novo kidney transplantation: a randomized controlled trial. *Am J Transplant,* **2013**, *13*:1724–1733.

Satyananda V, Shapiro R. Belatacept in kidney transplantation. *Curr Opin Organ Transplant,* **2014**, *19*:573–577.

Schena FP, et al, and The Sirolimus CONVERT Trial Study Group. Conversion from calcineurin inhibitors to sirolimus maintenance therapy in renal allograft recipients: 24-month efficacy and safety results from the CONVERT trial. *Transplantation,* **2009**, *87*:233–242.

Segundo DS, et al. Calcineurin inhibitors, but not rapamycin, reduce percentages of $CD4^+CD25^+FOXP3^+$ regulatory T cells in renal transplant recipients. *Transplantation,* **2006**, *82*:550–557.

Sureshkumar KK, et al. Influence of induction modality on the outcome of deceased donor kidney transplant recipients discharged on steroid-free maintenance immunosuppression. *Transplantation,* **2012**, *93*:799–805.

Talawila N, Pengel LH. Does belatacept improve outcomes for kidney transplant recipients? A systematic review. *Transpl Int,* **2015**, *28*:1251–1264.

Thiyagarajan UM, et al. Thymoglobulin and its use in renal transplantation: a review. *Am J Nephrol,* **2013**, *37*:586–601.

Topalian SL, et al. Immune checkpoint blockade: a common denominator approach to cancer therapy. *Cancer Cell,* **2015**, *4*:450–461.

Verghese PS, et al. Calcineurin inhibitors in HLA-identical living related donor kidney transplantation. *Nephrol Dial Transplant,* **2014**, *29*:209–218.

Vincenti F, Kirk AD. What's next in the pipeline. *Am J Transplant,* **2008**, *8*:1972–1981.

Vincenti F, et al. A randomized, multicenter study of steroid avoidance, early steroid withdrawal or standard steroid therapy in kidney transplant recipients. *Am J Transplant,* **2008**, *8*:307–316.

Immune Globulins and Vaccines

Roberto Tinoco and James E. Crowe, Jr.

第三十六章　免疫球蛋白和疫苗

中文导读

本章主要介绍：免疫球蛋白和疫苗的发展历史；疫苗接种可诱导免疫记忆的发展；免疫策略，包括被动免疫和主动免疫；疫苗类型，包括减毒活疫苗、失活疫苗、亚单位疫苗、DNA疫苗和重组载体；免疫球蛋白，包括结构、抗体类别和功能；美国推荐的特定常规疫苗，包括细菌疫苗和病毒疫苗；母体免疫；旅行疫苗（Vaccines for Travel），包括流行性乙型脑炎病毒疫苗、黄热病疫苗、伤寒疫苗和狂犬病疫苗；特种疫苗，包括炭疽疫苗、痘苗病毒（天花疫苗）以及其他用于生物防御和特殊病原体的疫苗；国际上的疫苗，包括登革热疫苗、疟疾疫苗、卡介苗；疫苗技术的未来；疫苗安全（神话、真相和结果），包括疫苗佐剂和安全性、疫苗不会导致自闭症、防腐剂（包括硫柳汞）、疫苗不良事件、疫苗神话（myths）及其公共健康结果；疫苗许可和监管，包括免疫相关性及其机制、监管和咨询机构。

Abbreviations

ACIP: Advisory Committee on Immunization Practices
ADCC: antibody-dependent cell-mediated cytotoxicity
AID: activation-induced cytidine deaminase
aP: acellular pertussis
APC: antigen-presenting cell
ASD: autism spectrum disorder
AVA: anthrax vaccine adsorbed
BCG: bacille Calmette-Guérin
BCR: B cell receptor
CDC: Centers for Disease Control and Prevention
CoP: correlate of protection
CRM: cross-reactive material
DTaP: diphtheria and tetanus toxoids and acellular pertussis
DTP: diphtheria and tetanus toxoids and pertussis
EMA: European Medicines Agency
Fab: fragment, antigen-binding
Fc: fragment crystallizable
GBS: Guillian-Barré syndrome
H1N1: hemagglutinin type 1 and neuraminidase type 1
H2N2: hemagglutinin type 2 and neuraminidase type 2
H3N2: hemagglutinin type 3 and neuraminidase type 2
HA: hemagglutinin
HbOC: *Haemophilus influenzae* type b oligosaccharide conjugate
Hib: *Haemophilus influenzae* type b
HIV: human immunodeficiency virus
HPV: human papillomavirus
IgG: immunoglobulin, class G
IIV: inactivated influenza vaccine
IOM: Institute of Medicine
IPV: inactivated poliovirus (vaccine)
JE: Japanese encephalitis
JE-MB: Japanese encephalitis mouse brain
JE-VC: Japanese encephalitis Vero cell
mCoP: mechanistic correlates of protection
MCV4: meningococcal vaccine 4
MeV: measles virus
MMR: measles-mumps-rubella
MMRV: measles-mumps-rubella-varicella
MVA: modified vaccinia Ankara
NA: neuraminidase
nCoP: nonmechanistic correlates of protection
PCV13: pneumococcal conjugate vaccine 13 valent
PRP: polyribosylribitol phosphate
PRP-OMPC: polyribosylribitol phosphate outer membrane protein conjugate
PRP-T: polyribosylribitol phosphate tetanus
RAG: recombination-activating gene
RSV: respiratory syncytial virus
SAE: serious adverse event
SAGE: Strategic Advisory Group of Experts
SIDS: sudden infant death syndrome
TB: *Mycobacterium tuberculosis*
Td: tetanus toxoid and reduced diphtheria toxoid
Tdap: tetanus toxoid, reduced diphtheria toxoid, acellular pertussis
VDJ: variable, diversity, joining
VLP: virus-like particle
VZV: varicella zoster virus
WHO: World Health Organization

Historical Perspective

The historical impact of infectious diseases is evident in the high mortality rates in young children and adults and the disruption that these diseases have caused in emerging societies. The rise of civilization in conjunction with the domestication of plants and animals permitted people to live in denser communities with each other and with their animals. Such proximity provided ideal breeding grounds for infectious pathogens, and their spread resulted in epidemics throughout the world. As people began to question the underlying causes of disease and the apparent protection to reinfection afforded to some survivors of a disease, ideas of immunity and disease prevention were born, apparently as early as the 5th century.

The concept of immunity goes back at least to the 17th century when emperor K'ang of China documented his practice of variolation, or inoculation, of his troops and his own children with smallpox to confer protection from the disease (Hopkins, 2002). Variolation involved taking liquid from a smallpox pustule of an infected patient, cutting the skin of an uninfected person, and then introducing the inoculum. Records from the 18th century note that Africans brought to the U.S. as slaves bore scars from smallpox variolation and were under the belief that they were immune to the disease. Variolation against smallpox was also reported by Lady Mary Montagu during her time in Constantinople (1716–1718). Lady Montagu, herself a survivor of smallpox, reported that certain Turkish women would open a wound in healthy individuals and introduce the contents of a smallpox vesicle with a large needle, thereby providing a level of protection against smallpox. About 2%–3% died after variolation, whereas 20%–30% died from natural infection. Lady Montagu had herself and a son variolated and later had a daughter successfully variolated in London under the auspices of physicians of the Royal Society. Positive outcomes notwithstanding, fear of the procedure persisted.

Around the same time, in Boston, Cotton Mather and Dr. Zabdiel Boylston began a program of variolation against smallpox. The program met with general success but was opposed by many physicians, fearful that inoculation spread the disease and worried by deaths after inoculation (~2% of those inoculated). One Puritan religious leader, Edmund Massey, preached against inoculation, quoting from the book of Job (Job 2:7: "So Satan went forth from the presence of the Lord and smote Job with sore boils.") and arguing that Satan was the prime practitioner of inoculation and that such diseases as smallpox were a necessary trial of faith or punishment for sins, the fear of which "is a happy restraint upon many people" (Gross and Sepkowitz, 1998). Medical practice in Boston has come a long way since that time.

In 1796, Edward Jenner, who coined the term *vaccination*, from *vacca*, Latin for "cow," helped to advance vaccine safety. He tested the hypothesis that smallpox protection could be achieved by using cowpox, a nonfatal, self-limited disease in humans caused by a virus of the Poxviridae family that includes monkeypox and smallpox and that can spread from cows to humans. Jenner infected a boy with cowpox pus from an infected milkmaid; the boy got mildly ill from cowpox, recovered, and when challenged with smallpox collected from scabs of a smallpox patient, was unaffected, showed no symptoms, and was fully protected against the disease. Thus, it was possible to inoculate against a disease using material from a related but less-harmful disease.

By the early to mid-19th century, vaccination was accepted widely, and governments in the U.S. and Europe began to require vaccination of children. As in our own era, there was organized resistance from antivaccination groups. There was also a sense that immunity waned with time, and revaccinations were introduced, producing a sustained diminution of smallpox.

The work of Pasteur and Koch established a link between microorganisms and disease and provided the scientific understanding to develop more specific vaccines. Preservatives (glycerol was an early additive) and refrigeration increased shelf life of vaccines and permitted their wider distribution. The cells of the immune system began to be identified around 1890, followed by the discovery of antibodies and hyperimmune serum and demonstration of the efficacy of adjuvants (aluminum was the first) to increase immunogenicity (Marrack et al., 2009). In the 1950s, freeze-drying became standard, permitting worldwide distribution of purified vaccines. Through the coordinating efforts of the WHO, smallpox was declared "eliminated" in 1979.

Other scourges were attacked by vaccination in the mid-20th century. One was polio, an incurable neurological disease causing muscle wasting, paralysis, and death if the diaphragm is affected. In 1955, Jonas Salk released a vaccine against poliovirus. The Salk vaccine, an inactivated virus preparation administered by injection, was followed in 1961 by the Sabin oral vaccine, which employs an attenuated poliovirus that provides immunity to all three types of poliovirus. As a result of the polio vaccines, the annual number of cases in the U.S. fell to 161 in 1961 from 35,000 in 1955 (Hinman, 1984). Eradication of polio depends on interruption of person-to-person transmission, which requires that a high percentage of the susceptible population be inoculated. Most adults in developed countries are immune, but when a significant fraction of children is unvaccinated, there is the potential for an outbreak because wild polioviruses circulate.

These fundamental observations and experiments paved the way for the modern vaccines that have reduced mortality and morbidity rates from infectious pathogens across the globe. Modern laboratory technologies have rendered vaccines safe and highly effective against infectious pathogens and virus-transforming cancers and against neoantigens on cancerous cells. Vaccination strategies are a public health success, as shown by the complete worldwide eradication of smallpox and the elimination of polio in the Americas in 1994, Europe in 2002, and South-East Asia in 2014, with remaining endemic cases only in Pakistan, Afghanistan, and Nigeria in 2016 according to WHO. In 2016, WHO and the Pan American Health Organization declared the Americas free of endemic measles, credited to immunization campaigns. The current recommendations for childhood vaccinations are summarized in Table 36–1. The issue of nonvaccinators is presented further in the chapter.

Vaccination Induces Development of Immunological Memory

The hallmarks of an immune response to pathogens are the recognition and activation of the innate immune response that limits pathogen spread when microbes breach the host's natural protective barriers, such as the skin, the respiratory epithelium, or the GI epithelium. If the pathogen is not controlled, the innate immune system then recruits the humoral (antibody-secreting B cell) and cellular (T cell) arms of the adaptive immune response to specifically target and destroy the invading pathogen. Once the microbe is eliminated during this primary response, small numbers of pathogen-specific B and T cells survive long term, sometimes for the entire life of the host, as *memory B and T cells*. These memory cells confer host protection against reinfection with the same pathogen. During a second response, memory cells use their specific antigen receptors to recognize the invading pathogen. This results in their activation and expansion to directly kill infected cells (via T cells) or generate antibodies (via B cells) that will neutralize the pathogen.

Vaccination technology takes advantage of this paradigm. As a means of generating immunological memory, uninfected individuals are given a controlled infection or exposed to antigen that elicits an immune response. When these vaccinated individuals are subsequently infected with these pathogens in their environment, the responses of their memory T and B cells outpace the invading microbes to neutralize and prevent their spread in a much more rapid and greater magnitude secondary response.

B cell clonal expansion results in the differentiation of long-lived memory B cells and emergence of shorter-lived plasma cells that produce antibodies. During the primary response, following the vaccination, B cells will undergo this differentiation process and will initially secrete IgM antibodies. IgM antibodies are large and provide some protection. Days after the response is initiated, B cells will undergo clonal selection and will produce IgG, which is a higher-affinity antibody with enhanced pathogen neutralization capacity.

Differentiated plasma cells can also produce other antibody classes, such as IgA, IgD, and IgE, that have unique functions. IgD can be expressed on the surface of B cells; its function continues to be investigated. IgA antibodies are concentrated in mucous secretions, breast milk, and tears. IgE antibodies are important in the elimination of parasitic infections. *Because IgG antibodies have undergone a selection process that increases their affinity, these antibody types are the targets of vaccine design.* Secondary responses after vaccination therefore elicit a faster and larger B-cell response, and these B cells primarily make IgG antibodies (Clem, 2011).

Cellular immunity involving both $CD4^+$ and $CD8^+$ T cells is also a target of vaccine design. Unlike B cells, T cells target intracellular pathogens that have infected host cells. $CD4^+$ T cells or helper T cells, stimulate B cells to produce antibody. $CD8^+$ T cells kill infected cells. Like B cells, antigen-memory T cells survive long term and provide protection for future encounters with their specific antigen.

Immunization Strategies

Immunity can be achieved from either passive or active methods involving exposure to natural infection or through artificial human-made antigens. Individuals can develop antibodies from natural infection or after vaccination.

Passive

Passive immunity involves the transfer of preformed antibodies from an immune individual to a nonimmune individual to confer temporary immunity. An example of passive natural immunity is the transfer of antibodies from mother to fetus during pregnancy and through breast milk and colostrum consumed by an infant. These antibodies enter the body and provide a first line of defense to the fetus or infant, which otherwise has no immunity to any pathogen.

An example of *artificial passive immunization* is the injection of antivenom antibodies. Animals are immunized with venom antigen and their hyperimmunized serum is transfused into the patient. Antivenom can be monovalent, effective against one type of venom, or polyvalent and effective against venom from multiple species. An antivenom binds and neutralizes a toxin. Early administration after injury is

TABLE 36–1 ■ RECOMMENDED IMMUNIZATION SCHEDULE FOR CHILDREN AND ADOLESCENTS AGED 18 YEARS OR YOUNGER, U.S., 2017.

Vaccine	Birth	1 mo	2 mos	4 mos	6 mos	9 mos	12 mos	15 mos	18 mos	19-23 mos	2-3 yrs	4-6 yrs	7-10 yrs	11-12 yrs	13-15 yrs	16 yrs	17-18 yrs
Hepatitis B (HepB)	1st dose	←--- 2nd dose ---→					←--- 3rd dose ---→										
Rotavirus (RV) RV1 (2-dose series); RV5 (3-dose series)			1st dose	2nd dose	See footnote												
Diphtheria, tetanus, & acellular pertussis(DTaP: <7 yrs)			1st dose	2nd dose	3rd dose			←--- 4th dose ---→				5th dose					
Haemophilus influenzae type b (Hib)			1st dose	2nd dose	See footnote		←--- 3rd or 4th dose, See footnote ---→										
Pneumococcal conjugate (PCV13)			1st dose	2nd dose	3rd dose		←--- 4th dose ---→										
Inactivated poliovirus (IPV: <18 yrs)			1st dose	2nd dose			←--- 3rd dose ---→					4th dose					
Influenza (IIV)									Annual vaccination (IIV) 1 or 2 doses						Annual vaccination (IIV) 1 dose only		
Measles, mumps, rubella (MMR)					See footnote		←--- 1st dose ---→					2nd dose					
Varicella(VAR)							←--- 1st dose ---→					2nd dose					
Hepatitis A (HepA)								←--- 2-dose series, See footnote ---→									
Meningococcal(Hib-MenCY ≥6 weeks; MenACWY-D≥9 mos; MenACWY-CRM ≥2 mos)							See footnote							1st dose		2nd dose	
Tetanus, diphtheria, & acellular pertussis(Tdap:≥7 yrs)														Tdap			
Human papillomavirus (HPV)														See footnote			
Meningococcal B															See footnote		
Pneumococcal polysaccharide (PPSV23)														See footnote			

Range of recommended ages for all children | Range of recommended ages for catch-up immunization | Range of recommended ages for certain high-risk groups | Range of recommended ages for non-high-risk groups that may receive vaccine, subject to individual clinical decision making | No recommendation

These recommendations are reprinted from the website of the Centers for Disease Control and Prevention (CDC) and should be read with the footnotes provided on the CDC website: https://www.cdc.gov/vaccines/schedules/. **For those who fall behind or start late, provide catch-up vaccination at the earliest opportunity as indicated by the green bars. To determine minimum intervals between doses, see the catch-up schedule on the CDC website. School entry and adolescent vaccine age groups are shaded in gray.**

critical because antivenom can halt but not reverse venom damage. Even though antivenom is purified, trace proteins remain, and these can trigger anaphylaxis or serum sickness in patients. Most antivenoms are administered intravenously but can also be injected intramuscularly against stonefish and redback spider venom. Antivenoms have been developed against venomous spiders, acarids, insects, scorpions, marine animals, and snakes. Passive immunization is used for a variety of toxins and infections; a list of available immunoglobulins is shown in Table 36–2.

Active

A natural infection that stimulates the immune response in uninfected individuals may lead to development of immunological memory and protection from reinfection, as in the case of infection with the MeV. This only occurs if the individual survives the primary infection, which is not always the case for viruses like measles, influenza, or ebola. Active immunization through injection of artificial antigens elicits a controlled immune response leading to the generation of immunological memory. This type of immunization, compared to natural infection, does not cause infectious disease or compromise the life of the individual. Thus, vaccine technologies through active stimulation of the immune system ensure that the individual survives and has protection against the pathogen in the natural environment.

Vaccine Types

Advanced technologies are currently used to generate vaccines to prevent many infectious diseases and to deter infectious pathogens that cause cancer such as hepatitis viruses that can lead to hepatocellular carcinoma and HPVs, which can cause cervical, anal, vaginal, and penile cancers. Effective vaccines activate both the innate and the adaptive immune systems. There are many different types of vaccines, each with advantages and disadvantages. Vaccine design involves an understanding of the nature of the microbe, the tropism of the pathogen, and the practical need in certain regions of the world. The following section summarizes current methods used in vaccine design. For a list of vaccines approved by the U.S. Food and Drug Administration, see Table 36–3.

TABLE 36–2 ■ AVAILABLE IMMUNE GLOBULINS

Human intravenous immune globulin
Human subcutaneous immune globulin
Human hyperimmune globulins
Anthrax immune globulin, intravenous
Botulism immune globulin, intravenous
Cytomegalovirus immune globulin, intravenous
Hepatitis B immune globulin, intravenous
Rho(D) immune globulin, intravenous
Vaccinia immune globulin, intravenous
Varicella zoster immune globulin
Animal-derived immune globulin products
Equine
Lymphocyte immune globulin, antithymocyte globulin
Centruroides (scorpion) immune $F(ab')_2$ injection
Crotalidae immune $F(ab')_2$
Black widow spider antivenin
Botulism antitoxin bivalent types A and B
Botulism antitoxin heptavalent (A, B, C, D, E, F, G)
Ovine
Crotalidae polyvalent immune Fab
Digoxin immune Fab
Rabbit
Antithymocyte globulin

TABLE 36–3 ■ APPROVED VACCINES IN THE U.S.

Toxoids
Tetanus and diphtheria toxoids adsorbed for adult use
Tetanus toxoid adsorbed
Tetanus toxoid, reduced diphtheria toxoid and acellular pertussis vaccine, adsorbed
Bacterial polysaccharide
Meningococcal polysaccharide vaccine, groups A, C, Y, and W-135 combined
Pneumococcal vaccine, polyvalent
Typhoid Vi polysaccharide vaccine
Bacterial conjugate vaccines
Haemophilus b conjugate vaccine (meningococcal protein conjugate)
Haemophilus b conjugate vaccine (tetanus toxoid conjugate)
Pneumococcal 7-valent conjugate vaccine (diphtheria CRM_{197} protein)
Pneumococcal 13-valent conjugate vaccine (diphtheria CRM_{197} protein)
Meningococcal (groups A, C, Y, and W-135) oligosaccharide diphtheria CRM_{197} conjugate vaccine
Meningococcal groups C and Y and *Haemophilus* b tetanus toxoid conjugate vaccine
Meningococcal (groups A, C, Y, and W-135) polysaccharide diphtheria toxoid conjugate vaccine
Meningococcal group B vaccine
Live bacterial
BCG live
Typhoid vaccine live oral Ty21a
Cholera vaccine live oral
Inactivated bacterial
Plague vaccine
Live Viral
Measles and mumps virus vaccine, live
Measles, mumps, and rubella virus vaccine, live
Measles, mumps, rubella and varicella virus vaccine, live
Varicella virus vaccine, live
Zoster vaccine, live
Rotavirus vaccine, live, oral
Rotavirus vaccine, live, oral, pentavalent
Influenza vaccine, live, intranasal (quadrivalent, types A and types B)
Adenovirus type 4 and type 7 vaccine, live, oral
Yellow fever vaccine
Smallpox (vaccinia) vaccine, live
Inactivated or subunit viral
Poliovirus vaccine inactivated (human diploid cell)
Poliovirus vaccine inactivated (monkey kidney cell)
Hepatitis A vaccine, inactivated
Hepatitis B (recombinant) vaccine
Hepatitis A vaccine, inactivated, and Hepatitis B (recombinant) vaccine
Influenza A (H1N1) 2009 monovalent vaccine
Influenza virus vaccine, H5N1 (for national stockpile)
Influenza A (H5N1) virus monovalent vaccine, adjuvanted
Influenza virus vaccine (trivalent, types A and B)
Influenza virus vaccine (quadrivalent, types A and B)
Human papillomavirus bivalent (types 16, 18) vaccine, recombinant
Human papillomavirus quadrivalent (types 6, 11, 16, 18) vaccine, recombinant
Human papillomavirus 9-valent vaccine, recombinant
Japanese encephalitis virus vaccine, inactivated
Japanese encephalitis virus vaccine, inactivated, adsorbed
Rabies vaccine
Rabies vaccine adsorbed

Live Attenuated

Live attenuated vaccines use a weakened form of a virus that contains antigens that appropriately stimulate an immune response. Such viruses have been passaged to reduce their virulence but retain immunogenic antigens that elicit strong humoral and cellular responses and the development of memory cells after one or two doses. A virus, for example, can be isolated from humans and then used to infect monkey cells. After several passages, the virus can no longer infect human cells but retains immunogenic capacity. These attenuated viruses can elicit a robust immune response because they are similar to the natural pathogen.

Several drawbacks exist with these vaccines. Because these are live viruses, they generally must be refrigerated to retain their activity. In remote areas of the world where refrigeration is not available, obtaining and storing this type of vaccine can be limiting. Because viruses can mutate and change in the host, it may be possible that viruses can become virulent again and cause disease, although the frequency of adverse reactions using these vaccines is very low. Furthermore, attenuated vaccines cannot be utilized in immune-compromised individuals (e.g., patients with HIV or cancer). In addition, these vaccines are usually not given during pregnancy. Measles, polio, rotavirus, yellow fever, and chickenpox viruses are examples of pathogens for which live attenuated vaccines have been generated. Attenuated vaccines for bacteria are more challenging to generate than for viruses because bacteria have more complex genomes; however, recombinant DNA technology can be utilized to remove virulence but retain immunogenicity. A vaccine against *Vibrio cholera* has been generated this way (currently not approved in the U.S.). A live attenuated vaccine for tuberculosis also has been developed.

Inactivated

Polio, influenza, and rabies viruses and typhoid and plague bacteria have been utilized to generate inactivated vaccines. Killing pathogens through the use of heat, radiation, or chemicals to inactivate them generates the antigenic starting materials. The dead pathogens can no longer replicate or mutate to their disease-causing state and thus are safe. These types of vaccines are useful because they can be freeze-dried and transported without refrigeration, an important consideration in reaching developing countries. A drawback with inactivated vaccines is that they induce an immune response that is much weaker than that induced by the natural infection; thus, patients require multiple doses to sustain immunity to the pathogen. In areas where people have limited access to healthcare, ensuring that these multiple doses are delivered on time can be problematic and may result in reduced immunity to the pathogen, as in the case of poliovirus endemic disease.

Subunit Vaccines

As with inactivated vaccines, subunit vaccines do not contain live pathogens; rather, subunit vaccines use a component of the microorganism as a vaccine antigen to mimic exposure to the organism itself. Subunit vaccines typically contain *polysaccharides* or proteins (*surface proteins* or *toxoids*). Compared to live attenuated vaccines, subunit vaccines induce a less-robust immune response. The selection of antigenic subunit and the design and development of the vaccine can be lengthy and costly because the pathogen's subunit antigens and their combination must be thoroughly tested to ensure they elicit an effective immune response. Scientists can identify the more immunogenic antigens in the laboratory and manufacture these antigen molecules via recombinant DNA technology, producing *recombinant subunit vaccines*. For example, the hepatitis B vaccine is generated by the insertion into baker's yeast of hepatitis B genes coding for selected antigens. The yeast cells express these antigens, which are then purified and used in making a vaccine. A drawback to these vaccines is that even though they elicit an immune response, immunity is not guaranteed. Subunit vaccines usually are considered safe because they have no live replicating pathogen present.

Polysaccharides. Polysaccharide subunit vaccines utilize polysaccharide (sugar) antigens to induce an immune response. Bacterial cell walls are composed of peptidoglycan polysaccharides that help pathogens evade the immune system. This evasion mechanism is highly effective in infants and young children, making them more susceptible to infection. Unfortunately, these polysaccharides are not very immunogenic. Furthermore, the vaccines produced to sugar antigens cause suboptimal immune responses that result in only short-term immunity. Meningococcal infection caused by *Neisseria meningitidis* (groups A, C, W-135, and Y) and *pneumococcal* disease are polysaccharide subunit vaccines against bacterial pathogens. Conjugate subunit vaccines use a technology to bind polysaccharide from the bacterial capsule to a carrier protein, often diphtheria or tetanus toxoid. This sort of antigen combination can induce long-term protection in infants and adults. These vaccines provide protection against pathogens where plain polysaccharide vaccines fail to work in infants and also provide more long-term protection in young children and adults. The *Haemophilus influenzae* type b (Hib) and *Pneumococcal* (PCV7 valent, PCV10 valent, PCV13 valent) are conjugate subunit vaccines recommended for children (see Table 36–1). The *meningococcal A* vaccine used in Africa is also an example of a conjugate subunit vaccine.

Surface Protein Subunit Vaccines. T protein–based subunit vaccines utilize purified proteins from the pathogen to induce an immune response. Because these proteins may not be presented in native form (i.e., as in the live pathogen), antibodies generated against these antigens may not bind efficiently to the live pathogen. Acellular pertussis (aP) and hepatitis B vaccines are examples of protein-based subunit vaccines. The hepatitis B vaccine contains the hepatitis B virus envelope protein made as an antigen produced in yeast cell culture.

Toxoids. Pathogenic bacteria such as *Clostridium tetani* and *Corynebacterium diphtheria* induce disease (tetanus or diphtheria, respectively) through production of their toxins. Vaccines against these toxins, known as toxoid vaccines, are effective because they elicit an immune response that results in the production of antibodies that can bind and neutralize these toxins, preventing cell damage in the patient. Inactivated or killed toxins are used as the immunogen; however, because they are not highly immunogenic, they must be adsorbed to adjuvants (aluminum or calcium salts) to increase their capacity to stimulate the immune response. Toxoid vaccines are safe because they do not contain live pathogens. In addition, they are stable over a wide range of temperatures and humidities (Baxter, 2007).

DNA Vaccines

Sequencing the genome of a pathogen provides information that enables the production of a DNA vaccine against selected genetic material. A microbe's antigenic genes are selected and incorporated in synthetic DNA. Intramuscular or intradermal injection delivers this engineered DNA to APCs, which uptake the DNA and transcribe and translate it to produce antigenic proteins. These APCs present these antigens to both humoral and cellular immune system components to generate immunity. This type of vaccine poses no risk of infection, can easily be developed and produced, is cost-effective, is stable, and provides long-term protection (Robinson et al., 2000). Disadvantages include its limit to protein antigens and the possibility of generating tolerance to that antigen because of low immunogenicity, thereby rendering ineffective immunity.

Many of these vaccines are currently in experimental phases, but none has been licensed in the U.S. DNA vaccines for influenza virus, herpesvirus, flaviviruses like Zika virus, and others are in the early stages of development. A DNA vaccine against West Nile virus has been approved for veterinary use. Delivery platforms for enhancing efficacy of DNA vaccines (such as electroporation) are being developed. There is also an emerging research field to use RNA as a vaccine delivery platform.

Recombinant Vectors

A vector is a virus or bacterium that is used to deliver heterologous microbial genes to cells for expression in the vaccinee to elicit an immune response. Once the vector infects or transduces host cells, the selected antigens will be presented during the immune response to generate immunity. Both viruses and bacteria are being investigated as recombinant vectors for candidate vaccines. Virus vectors that have been used in candidate vaccines include many poxviruses (vaccinia virus, modified vaccinia Ankara, avian poxviruses, and others), a large number of adenoviruses (of both human and primate origin), and other families of viruses.

Immunoglobulins

Structure

Vaccination results in the expansion and differentiation of B cells into long-lived memory cells that provide long-term protection to secondary challenge, and plasma cells, which are immunoglobulin (antibody)–generating cells that produce large quantities of these proteins. Antibodies in the body are found in two forms, either membrane bound on B cells as BCRs that can deliver signals to activate and induce B-cell differentiation after antigen ligation or as soluble effector molecules that neutralize antigens throughout the body. Antibodies are heterodimeric proteins composed of two chains, the light and heavy chains. Both light and heavy chains contain variable regions in the N-terminal region of the protein that engage antigens. Naïve B cells express BCRs with low affinity to antigen. These BCRs can be selected through VDJ recombination via the activity of RAG enzymes. Antibody diversity is achieved through antigen-binding site region variation, combinatorial diversity of gene segments, and combination of light and heavy regions, an overall diversity program that can result in an antibody repertoire of potentially 10^{16} to 10^{18} different molecules, ensuring that a unique B cell in the body will exist to recognize any foreign antigen. In addition to this diversity, antibodies also can undergo class-switch recombination in which the constant region of the heavy chain can be switched, based on cytokine signals by T cells, to tailor antibody specificity and function. It is this portion of the antibody that determines the five main isotypes: IgM, IgD, IgG, IgA, and IgE. These isotypes differ in size, Fc receptor binding, ability to fix complement, and appropriate isotypes for specific pathogens (Schroeder and Cavacini, 2010).

Antibody diversity can be further enhanced on antigen recognition by B cells and help from $CD4^+$ T cells. B cells can further strengthen their antibody affinity by mutating their variable regions, and with repetitive antigen stimulation, the affinity of binding to antigen can increase further. This mechanism explains why some vaccines, like the one for hepatitis B, are most immunogenic when delivered in three doses. This repeated antigen stimulation induces somatic hypermutation of antibody variable genes to increase antibody efficacy. AID is a key enzyme in mediating class-switch recombination and somatic hypermutation. Human patients with defective AID suffer from hyper-IgM syndrome and are unable to class switch their antibodies, which makes them more susceptible to certain infections.

Manufactured antibodies can be used for passive immunization; for a list of available antibodies, see Table 36–4. Such monoclonal antibodies are biologicals that have become some of the most important drugs of our era. To date, monoclonal antibodies have been implemented most effectively for use in cancer immunotherapy and management of autoimmune diseases. Palivizumab is a humanized murine monoclonal antibody that is licensed for use in high-risk infants to prevent hospitalization due to RSV. As the cost of production of monoclonal antibodies continues to fall, more of these biologicals will likely be used for prophylaxis or treatment of infectious diseases.

Antibody Classes and Functions

Immunoglobulin M

The first antibody class expressed by B cells is IgM. IgM molecules are membrane-bound monomers found on circulating mature B cells. When mature B cells are antigen stimulated, they generate IgM pentamers that are secreted. IgM antibodies, also called natural antibodies, have low affinity as monomers, but their avidity can increase in their pentameric structure, which improves epitope binding to repeating antigens on pathogens. These antibodies are found at mucosal surfaces and constitute 10% of the antibody content of serum. These antibodies are associated with a primary immune response. IgM molecules function by coating their specific antigen to target the pathogen for destruction via phagocytosis or to induce complement fixation to kill the pathogen (Schroeder and Cavacini, 2010).

Immunoglobulin D

Like IgM molecules, IgD molecules are also expressed on naïve B cells that have not been activated by their specific antigen and thus have not undergone somatic hypermutation. They are expressed as monomers on the surface of B cells and can also be secreted; they represent less than 0.5% of the antibody in the serum (Schroeder and Cavacini, 2010). The exact function of this antibody is not fully known, but it can bind bacterial proteins through the constant region (Riesbeck and Nordstrom, 2006).

Immunoglobulin G

The IgG antibodies exist as monomers, represent about 70% of the antibody in circulation, and have been the most studied. They have the longest $t_{1/2}$ in serum and are generated with high affinity after affinity maturation. The constant region of the heavy chain can further lead to diversity in the structure of these antibodies to generate four subclasses: IgG1, IgG2, IgG3, and IgG4. These subclasses are named based on their concentrations in serum, with IgG1 the most abundant and IgG4 the least. IgG1, IgG2, and IgG3 subclasses can activate complement to opsonize pathogens, but IgG4 cannot. These antibodies can also differ in their ability and affinity to engage Fc receptors, which further enhances their effector functions. All IgG subclasses cross the placenta to provide passive immunity to the fetus.

Vaccines predominantly induce these antibody types, which become important during the secondary immune response to inactivate pathogens. Different subclasses are selected during the secondary antibody response. In designing vaccines, scientists must determine which antibody subclass will provide the optimal response. In addition to complement and opsonization, IgG antibodies can directly neutralize toxins and viruses (Schroeder and Cavacini, 2010).

Immunoglobulin A

The IgA antibody class is expressed as monomers or dimers and represents about 15% of the antibodies in serum, slightly higher than IgM antibodies. At mucosal surfaces, saliva, and breast milk, however, IgA antibodies are found at the highest concentrations (Woof and Mestecky, 2005). In late pregnancy and the early post-natal period, female mammary glands produce colostrum; more than half of the protein content of colostrum that breast-feeding neonates consume is IgA antibodies. IgA is primarily a monomer in the serum but a dimer at mucosal sites.

IgA antibodies have two subclasses, IgA1 and IgA2, that differ only slightly in their structures. IgA1 antibodies are longer than IgA2 antibodies and are therefore more sensitive to degradation. IgA2 is more stable and is found primarily in mucosal secretions, in contrast to IgA1, which predominates in serum. IgA antibodies work via direct neutralization of viruses, bacteria, and toxins to protect mucosal tissues. They prevent antigen binding to host cells that damage or infect them. IgA antibodies within cells may also prevent pathogen tropism. Even though IgA antibodies do not lead to complement fixation, neutrophils can uptake them to mediate ADCC (Schroeder and Cavacini, 2010).

Immunoglobulin E

The IgE antibody class is present at the lowest serum concentration, less than 0.01% of circulating antibodies, and has the shortest $t_{1/2}$. IgE binds to Fcγ receptors with very high affinity. Langerhans and mast cells, basophils, and eosinophils express Fcγ receptors that bind IgE antibodies. Fc receptor engagement also results in FcγR upregulation on bound cells. These antibodies recognize antigens on parasitic worms when they are cross-linked on granulocytes; the cells degranulate to release inflammatory mediators to destroy the parasite. IgE antibodies are also relevant in mediating allergic reactions by recognizing innocuous antigens, such as bee venom and peanut antigen.

TABLE 36–4 ■ THERAPEUTIC MONOCLONAL ANTIBODIES APPROVED IN THE E.U. AND THE U.S.

ANTIBODY	TARGET; *Ab Type*	THERAPEUTIC USE
Abciximab	GPIIb/IIIa; *chimeric IgG1 Fab*	Prevention of blood clots in angioplasty
Adalimumab	TNF; *human IgG1*	Rheumatoid arthritis
Ado-trastuzumab emtansine	HER2; *humanized IgG1; immunoconjugate*	Breast cancer
Alemtuzumab	CD52; *humanized IgG1*	Multiple sclerosis
Alirocumab	PCSK9; *human IgG1*	Lowering cholesterol
Atezolizumab[a]	PD-L1; *humanized IgG1*	Bladder cancer
Avelumab	PD-L1/*human IgG1*	Merkel cell carcinoma
Basiliximab	IL-2R; *chimeric IgG1*	Prevention of kidney transplant rejection
Belimumab	BLyS; *human IgG1*	Systemic lupus erythematosus
Bevacizumab	VEGF; *humanized IgG1*	Colorectal cancer
Bezlotoxumab	*Clostridium difficile* toxin B/*human IgG1*	*Clostridium difficile* infections
Blinatumomab	CD19, CD3; *murine bispecific tandem scFv*	Acute lymphoblastic leukemia
Brentuximab vedotin	CD30; *chimeric IgG1; immunoconjugate*	Hodgkin lymphoma, systemic anaplastic large cell lymphoma
Brodalumab	IL-17RA/*human IgG2*	Plaque psoriasis
Canakinumab	IL-1β; *human IgG1*	Muckle-Wells syndrome
Catumaxomab[b]	EPCAM/CD3; *rat/mouse bispecific mAb*	Malignant ascites
Certolizumab pegol	TNF; *humanized Fab, pegylated*	Crohn disease
Cetuximab	EGFR; *chimeric IgG1*	Colorectal cancer
Daclizumab	IL-2R; *humanized IgG1*	Multiple sclerosis
Daratumumab	CD38; *human IgG1*	Multiple myeloma
Denosumab	RANK-L; *human IgG2*	Bone loss
Dinutuximab	GD2; *chimeric IgG1*	Neuroblastoma
Dupilumab	IL-4Rα/*human IgG4*	Eczema
Durvalumab	PD-L1/*human IgG1*	Urothelial carcinoma
Eculizumab	C5; *humanized IgG2/4*	Paroxysmal nocturnal hemoglobinuria
Efalizumab	CD11a; *humanized IgG1*	Psoriasis
Elotuzumab	SLAMF7; *humanized IgG1*	Multiple myeloma
Evolocumab	PCSK9; *human IgG2*	Lowering cholesterol
Gemtuzumab ozogamicin[a]	CD33; *humanized IgG4*	Acute myeloid leukemia
Golimumab	TNF; *human IgG1*	Rheumatoid and psoriatic arthritis, ankylosing spondylitis
Ibritumomab tiuxetan	CD20; *murine IgG1*	Non-Hodgkin lymphoma
Idarucizumab	Dabigatran; *humanized Fab*	Dabigatran excess (reversing anticoagulation)
Infliximab	TNF; *chimeric IgG1*	Crohn disease
Ipilimumab	CTLA-4; *human IgG1*	Metastatic melanoma
Ixekizumab	IL-17a; *humanized IgG4*	Psoriasis
Mepolizumab	IL-5; *hIgG1*	Severe eosinophilic asthma
Muromonab-CD3	CD3; *murine IgG2a*	Reversal of kidney transplant rejection
Natalizumab	a4 integrin; *humanized IgG4*	Multiple sclerosis
Necitumumab	EGFR; *human IgG1*	Non–small cell lung cancer
Nivolumab	PD1; *human IgG4*	Melanoma, non–small cell lung cancer, renal cell carcinoma, non small cell carcinoma
Obiltoxaximab[a]	Protective antigen *of B. anthracis* exotoxin[c]; *chimeric IgG1*	Prevention of inhalational anthrax
Obinutuzumab	CD20; *humanized IgG1; glycoengineered*	Chronic lymphocytic leukemia
Ocrelizumab	CD20/*human IgG1*	Multiple Sclerosis
Ofatumumab	CD20; *human IgG1*	Chronic lymphocytic leukemia

(*Continued*)

TABLE 36–4 ■ THERAPEUTIC MONOCLONAL ANTIBODIES APPROVED IN THE E.U. AND THE U.S.(CONTINUED)

ANTIBODY	TARGET; *Ab Type*	THERAPEUTIC USE
Olaratumab	PDGFR/*human IgG1*	Soft tissue sarcoma
Omalizumab	IgE; *humanized IgG1*	Asthma
Palivizumab	RSV; *humanized IgG1*	Prevention of respiratory syncytial virus infection
Panitumumab	EGFR; *human IgG2*	Colorectal cancer
Pembrolizumab	PD1; *humanized IgG4*	Melanoma, non-small cell carcinoma
Pertuzumab	HER2; *humanized IgG1*	Breast cancer
Ramucirumab	VEGFR2; *human IgG1*	Gastric cancer
Ranibizumab	VEGF; *humanized IgG1 Fab*	Macular degeneration
Raxibacumab[a]	*B. anthrasis* protective antigen[c]; *human IgG1*	Prevention of inhalational anthrax
Reslizumab	IL-5; *humanized IgG4*	Asthma
Rituximab	CD20; *chimeric IgG1*	Non-Hodgkin lymphoma
Sarilumab	IL-6R/*human IgG1*	Rheumatoid arthritis
Secukinumab	IL-17a; *human IgG1*	Psoriasis
Siltuximab	IL-6; *chimeric IgG1*	Castleman disease
Tocilizumab	IL-6R; *humanized IgG1*	Rheumatoid arthritis
Tositumomab-I[131a]	CD20; *murine IgG2a*	Non-Hodgkin lymphoma
Trastuzumab	HER2; *hIgG1*	Breast cancer
Ustekinumab	IL-12/23; *human IgG1*	Psoriasis
Vedolizumab	α4β7 integrin; *humanized IgG1*	Ulcerative colitis, Crohn disease

[a]Not approved in the E.U.
[b]Not approved in the U.S.
[c]Inhibits the binding of the protective antigen to its membrane receptors, thereby preventing the intracellular entry of the anthrax lethal factor and edema factor, the enzymatic toxin components responsible for the pathogenic effects of anthrax toxin.

Patients who develop allergic reactions generate memory B cells that produce IgE antibodies to specific antigens. The granulocytes become coated with IgE antibodies and on antigen reexposure such as a bee's sting or peanuts, the antigen cross-links IgEs, leading to granulocyte degranulation, which can result in anaphylactic shock. Therapies are in development to generate and use antibodies against soluble IgE molecules to prevent their uptake by granulocytes. For a list of approved monoclonal antibodies, see Table 36–4.

Specific Conventional Vaccines Recommended in the U.S.

The CDC maintains tables listing currently recommended vaccinations for various susceptibilities throughout life. Next is a discussion of the properties and schedule of administration for the vaccinations recommended from birth to elder adulthood. The vaccines are grouped by the target type (bacterium, virus, etc.) and then by vaccine type, as discussed in the previous section. See Table 36–1 for infant and childhood vaccination schedules. For a complete list of the adult recommended immunization schedule, see Tables 36-5 and 36-6.

Vaccines for Bacteria

Bacterial Toxoid Vaccines: Diphtheria and Tetanus

Tetanus Toxoid Vaccine. Tetanus is a disease characterized by prolonged spasms and tetany caused by the toxin secreted by the bacterium *C. tetani*, which enters from environmental sources through wounds. Tetanus toxin enters the nervous system and by retrograde transport reaches the inhibitory interneurons of the spinal cord, where the active fragment cleaves synaptobrevin (see Figures 8–3 to 8–6), thereby inhibiting exocytosis of neurotransmitter from these nerve cells and resulting in uninhibited skeletal muscle contraction. The toxoid is produced by deactivating toxin isolated from the bacterium using formaldehyde. Immunization usually begins at about age 2 months, as a component of the combination vaccine DTaP that is given to infants. Tetanus toxoid is included in several combination vaccine formulations. DTaP is the vaccine used in children younger than age 7; Tdap and Td, given at later ages, are booster immunizations that offer continued protection from those diseases for adolescents and adults. In these designations, upper- and lowercase letters represent the comparative quantity of antigen present. Thus, the shared uppercase *T* indicates there is about the same amount of tetanus toxoid in DTaP, Tdap, and Td. The uppercase *D* and *P* in the childhood formulation indicate that there is more diphtheria and pertussis antigen in DTaP than in Tdap or Td.

Diphtheria Toxoid Vaccines. Diphtheria is a disease caused by a secreted toxin of the aerobic gram-positive bacterium *C. diphtheria*; toxin production is under control of the bacterial systems, but the structural gene for toxin production is contributed by a β phage that infects all pathogenic strains of *C. diphtheria*. The A subunit of the toxin is an ADP-ribosylase; following its entry into a cell, it ADP-ribosylates eukaryotic elongation factor 2 (eEF-2) and thereby inhibits protein translation in human cells (Gill et al., 1973). The throat of the victim becomes swollen and sore during infection, and the toxin causes damage to myelin sheaths in the nervous system, leading to loss of sensation or motor control. The vaccine, which has been used for nearly 80 years, is a toxoid that is produced by treating toxin with formalin. The toxoid is used to immunize infants beginning at about 2 months, typically as part of the combination DTaP vaccine. The diphtheria toxin also has been detoxified genetically by introduction of point mutations that abrogate enzymatic activity but allow retention of binding activity; for instance, the mutant diphtheria toxin protein CRM_{197} is the protein carrier for a licensed Hib vaccine.

TABLE 36–5 ■ RECOMMENDED IMMUNIZATION SCHEDULE FOR ADULTS AGED 19 YEARS OR OLDER BY AGE GROUP, U.S., 2017.

Vaccine	19–21 years	22–26 years	27–59 years	60–64 years	≥ 65 years
Influenza*	1 dose annually				
Td/Tdap*	Substitute Tdap for Td once, then Td booster every 10 yrs				
MMR*	1 or 2 doses depending on indication				
VAR*	2 doses				
HZV*				1 dose	
HPV–Female*	3 doses				
HPV–Male*	3 doses				
PCV13*	1 dose				
PPSV23*	1 or 2 doses depending on indication				1 dose
HepA*	2 or 3 doses depending on vaccine				
HepB*	3 doses				
MenACWY or MPSV*	1 or more doses depending on indication				
MenB*	2 or 3 doses depending on vaccine				
Hib*	1 or 3 doses depending on indication				

Recommended for adults who meet the age requirement, lack documentation of vaccination, or lack evidence of past infection

Recommended for adults with additional medical conditions or other indications

No recommendation

*NOTE: The above recommendations are reprinted from the website of the Centers for Disease Control and Prevention (CDC) and should be read along with the footnotes of this schedule available on the CDC website: https://www.cdc.gov/vaccines/schedules/.

TABLE 36–6 ■ RECOMMENDED IMMUNIZATION SCHEDULE FOR ADULTS AGED 19 YEARS OR OLDER BY MEDICAL CONDITION AND OTHER INDICATIONS, UNITED STATES, 2017.

Vaccine	Pregnancy*	Immuno-compromised (excluding HIV infection)*	HIV infection CD4+ count (cells/μL)*		Asplenia, persistent complement deficiencies*	Kidney failure, end-stage renal disease, on hemodialysis*	Heart or lung disease, chronic alcoholism*	Chronic liver disease*	Diabetes*	Healthcare personnel*	Men who have sex with men*
			< 200	≥ 200							
Influenza*	1 dose annually										
Td/Tdap*	1 dose Tdap each pregnancy	Substitute Tdap for Td once, then Td booster every 10 yrs									
MMR*	contraindicated			1 or 2 doses depending on indication							
VAR*	contraindicated			2 doses							
HZV*	contraindicated				1 dose						
HPV–Female*		3 doses through age 26 yrs									
HPV–Male*		3 doses through age 26 yrs			3 doses through age 21 yrs						3 doses through age 26 yrs
PCV13*		1 dose									
PPSV23*	1, 2, or 3 doses depending on indication										
HepA*	2 or 3 doses depending on vaccine										
HepB*	3 doses										
MenACWY or MPSV4*	1 or more doses depending on indication										
MenB*		2 or 3 doses depending on vaccine									
Hib*		3 doses post-HSCT recipients only	1 dose								

Recommended for adults who meet the age requirement, lack documentation of vaccination, or lack evidence of past infection

Recommended for adults with additional medical conditions or other indications

Contraindicated

No recommendation

*NOTE: The above recommendations are reprinted from the website of the Centers for Disease Control and Prevention (CDC) and should be read along with the footnotes of this schedule available on the CDC website: https://www.cdc.gov/vaccines/schedules/.

Pertussis Vaccines. Pertussis, or whooping cough, is a respiratory tract disease characterized by prolonged paroxysmal coughing and sometimes respiratory failure; it is caused by the gram-negative coccobacillus *Bordetella pertussis*. The secreted pertussis toxin has an A subunit that, once in the cell cytosol, ADP-ribisylates the α subunit of the G_i protein that couples inhibitory GPCR signaling to adenylyl cyclase to reduce cyclic AMP production. After ADP-ribosylation, G_{ia} becomes inactive, and GPCR-mediated reduction of cyclic AMP production is abolished. The physiological sequelae of this action of pertussis toxin are thought to contribute to the constellation of symptoms of whooping cough. Routine vaccination typically begins as part of the childhood combination DTaP vaccine series. It is also appropriate to immunize healthy adults, adolescents, and pregnant mothers as pertussis does occur throughout life due to waning immunity. There are two licensed pertussis vaccines, the historical inactivated organism "whole-cell" vaccine used in the past in the U.S. and still in many other countries and a second "acellular" formulation that incorporates antigen fragments derived from the organism. Both vaccines are immunogenic and protective. The whole-cell vaccine appears to induce more durable immunity, but the acellular vaccine causes about a 10-fold lower rate of side effects such as fever or injection site pain and erythema. Most developed countries now use acellular pertussis vaccine to reduce the reactivity profile, but many other countries continue to use the whole-cell vaccine successfully because the response is equally efficacious and more durable and the vaccine is economical.

Conjugated Bacterial Polysaccharide Vaccines

Haemophilus influenzae Type B Vaccine. *Haemophilus influenzae* is a major cause of life-threatening childhood bacterial diseases, including buccal, preseptal and orbital cellulitis, epiglottitis, bacteremia with sepsis, and meningitis. Universal vaccination with the Hib vaccine has nearly eliminated these diseases in the U.S. The Hib vaccine is a polysaccharide-protein conjugate that confers immunity to the disease by inducing antibodies to the capsular polysaccharide PRP. The Hib polysaccharide has been conjugated to diverse proteins, including the mutant diphtheria protein CRM_{197} (a vaccine termed HbOC); the meningococcal group B outer membrane protein C (a vaccine termed PRP-OMPC); and tetanospasmin, which is a toxoid of the *C. tetani* neurotoxin (a vaccine termed PRP-T). The vaccines all exhibit a high level of safety and immunogenicity. Interestingly, widespread immunization not only reduces disease in those vaccinated, but also reduces nasal carriage of the bacterium, resulting in reduced transmission to even those not vaccinated and providing evidence of herd immunity.

Streptococcus pneumoniae Vaccines. The gram-positive encapsulated bacterium *S. pneumoniae* causes invasive diseases in infants and young children, including meningitis, bacteremia and sepsis, and pneumonia. There are myriad *S. pneumoniae* types, based on the capsular polysaccharide; thus, polyvalent vaccines are needed. Vaccines confer immunity by inducing type-specific antipolysaccharide antibodies. Two types of vaccines are available, *polysaccharide* and *conjugate* vaccines. The 23-valent polysaccharide vaccine contains long chains of capsular polysaccharides that are collected from inactivated bacteria. Polysaccharide vaccine is used in children older than 2 years and in at-risk adults. PCVs have been developed, and increasing numbers of serotypes have been incorporated over time. The combined 13 serotypes in PCV13 protect against most invasive disease in the U.S. Infants are given a primary series of PCV13 at ages 2, 4, and 6 months, with a booster at 12 to 15 months.

Neisseria meningitidis Vaccines. *Neisseria meningitidis* is a significant cause of invasive bacterial disease in childhood, causing sepsis and meningitis. As with *S. pneumoniae*, there are diverse types of polysaccharide; thus, type-specific anticapsular polysaccharide antibodies mediate protection against invasive disease. Therefore, multivalent vaccines are required. A licensed quadrivalent polysaccharide vaccine protects against four subtypes of meningococcus—designated A, C, Y, and W-135. The polysaccharide vaccine works only in children older than 2 years. A tetra-valent meningococcal conjugate vaccine, also containing the A, C, Y, and W-135 subtypes, is used in persons 9 months to 55 years of age. In 2013, the European Commission licensed a four-component, protein-based meningococcal B vaccine (incorporating fHbp, NadA, NHBA, and PorA P1.4 proteins) to prevent septicemia and meningitis.

Vaccines for Viruses

Poliovirus Vaccines

Polio is a characterized by acute flaccid paralysis, against which the WHO and others are conducting a worldwide eradication campaign. There are two types of poliovirus vaccines in use. The first is a *live attenuated oral vaccine* in use since the early 1960s (the "Sabin vaccine"), containing attenuated poliovirus types I, II, and III, produced in monkey kidney cell tissue culture. The vaccine replicates in the intestine and induces systemic and mucosal immunity, but also is shed in the stool, sometimes transmitting to close contacts. Infection of most close contacts contributes to herd immunity in the human population. Rarely (about one case per million doses), partial revertant viruses occur that cause vaccine-associated paralytic poliomyelitis in contacts. In many parts of the world, live poliovirus vaccine is still used. The last known case of naturally acquired poliovirus disease acquired in the U.S. occurred in 1979; the U.S. discontinued use of the live vaccine in 2000. Live poliovirus vaccine is contraindicated in subjects with primary immunodeficiency. Pregnant women and children with symptomatic HIV infection should receive IPV vaccine.

The second type of vaccine is a *killed virus* preparation called *IPV* (the "Salk vaccine"). Killed vaccine induces mainly humoral immunity but still exhibits excellent efficacy against disease. IPV does not transmit virus to contacts and does not cause vaccine-associated paralysis. An enhanced-potency IPV vaccine has been available since 1998, and this IPV preparation is now a component of some combination vaccines.

Measles Virus Vaccines

The current measles vaccine is a live attenuated strain given subcutaneously. A live, "more attenuated" preparation of the Enders-Edmonston virus strain (designated the "Moraten" strain) is the MeV vaccine currently used in the U.S. Vaccination is initiated at 12 to 15 months of age in the U.S. because transplacentally acquired maternal antibodies inhibit immunogenicity of vaccine in the first year of life.

Mumps Virus Vaccine

Mumps virus causes a febrile illness most commonly associated with inflammation of the parotids and sometimes with more severe conditions, including aseptic meningitis. A live attenuated virus vaccine has been used exclusively since the 1970s. The Jeryl-Lynn vaccine (from a mixture of two strains) was isolated from the throat of the daughter of Maurice Hilleman, a noted vaccine developer. The vaccine is typically given as a component of the combination MMR or MMRV vaccine at 12 to 15 months of age.

Rubella Virus Vaccine

Rubella virus, a member of the Togaviridae family, is spread by respiratory droplets and causes a mild infection with viremia. Rubella is harmful only to fetuses, and the effects can be devastating. A rubella infection during pregnancy can cause miscarriage, preterm birth, stillbirth, or various birth defects. The risks decrease as pregnancy progresses. The main goal of rubella immunization is to prevent congenital rubella syndrome. The live attenuated rubella virus vaccine is given subcutaneously, now usually as a component of MMR or MMRV vaccine, beginning between 12 and 15 months of age. The live rubella virus vaccine strain RA 27/3 is grown in human diploid cell culture. In the U.S., universal immunization (both boys and girls) is used to reduce infection of pregnant women. As a result, rubella and congenital rubella syndrome have been eliminated in the U.S. Rubella vaccine is part of MMR or MMRV combination vaccines for universal immunization starting at 12 to 15 months, followed by a booster dose at school entry (~5 to 6 years).

Varicella Zoster Virus Vaccine

Varicella zoster virus is one of the most infectious among agents that affect humans. It is spread by the respiratory route by small aerosol particles (cough, sneeze, etc.). Infection causes a febrile syndrome with vesicular rash, sometimes complicated by pneumonia or invasive bacterial skin disease. Congenital varicella syndrome can occur if varicella infection occurs during pregnancy. The vaccine used is the Oka strain of live attenuated VZV attenuated by sequential passage in cell monolayer cultures; it was licensed for universal immunization in the U.S. in 1995. The virus in the Oka/Merck vaccine in current use in the U.S. was further passaged in MRC-5 human diploid-cell cultures. The vaccine is often given as a part of the combination MMRV vaccine.

Hepatitis A Virus Vaccines

Hepatitis A virus infection causes acute liver disease after transmission by the fecal-oral route. An inactivated vaccine is recommended for all children, starting at 1 year of age. Two hepatitis A vaccines and one hepatitis A vaccine/hepatitis B combovaccine are licensed in the U.S. The vaccine is given as a two-dose series.

Hepatitis B Virus Vaccines

Hepatitis B virus is transmitted between people by contact with blood or other bodily fluids, including by sexual contact and maternal transfer to fetus or infant. Hepatitis B virus can cause a life-threatening and sometimes chronic liver disease. All infants receive the hepatitis B vaccine. When the mother has active infection, the neonate is treated with both the vaccine and hepatitis B immune globulin. The vaccine is a recombinant protein produced in yeast that is the protective antigen, hepatitis B surface antigen (see also Chapter 63).

Rotavirus Vaccines

Throughout the world, rotavirus is the most common cause of dehydrating diarrhea in infants. Four or five types (based on the surface proteins) cause severe disease. An early live attenuated vaccine (Rotashield) was withdrawn after association with intussusception (a segmental, telescoping collapse of the intestine). Two similar vaccines are now used that are safe and immunogenic. One is an oral pentavalent human-bovine reassortant rotavirus vaccine (containing five reassortant rotaviruses developed from human and the Wistar Calf 3 bovine parent rotaviral strains) first licensed in the U.S. in 2006 (RotaTeq). This vaccine is administered in a three-dose schedule, at 2, 4, and 6 months of age. Another oral live attenuated rotavirus vaccine licensed in the U.S. is based on a single attenuated human strain (Rotarix) using a two-dose schedule, beginning at 2 months of age. Rotavirus vaccines are used for universal immunization during infancy, with care to keep the initiation of the two- or three-dose series at a young age, as the rare rotavirus-associated intussusception risk with infection appears slightly higher at older ages.

Influenza Virus Vaccines

The orthomyxovirus influenza virus is a respiratory virus spread person-to-person by large-particle aerosols and fomites. The virus circulates in humans in two major serotypes (types A and B); two distinct A subtypes, designated H1N1 and H3N2, currently cause disease ("the flu") in humans. Current seasonal influenza vaccines are trivalent, including A/H1N1, A/H3N2, and B antigens, or quadrivalent with a second type B antigen. Experimental vaccines are being tested for some avian influenza viruses (such as A/H5N1 and A/H7N9) that have infected humans and have pandemic potential. During each annual seasonal epidemic, point mutations occur in genes encoding the hemagglutinin and neuraminidase proteins, which are the principal targets for protective antibodies. This antigenic drift in circulating influenza strains has led to a process in which regulatory officials and manufacturers adjust the virus antigens in influenza vaccines every year. Occasionally, the segmented virus genome reasserts during coinfection of an animal with a human and an avian virus, a new virus arises (antigenic shift), and a pandemic occurs. Major worldwide pandemics occurred in 1918 (H1N1), 1957 (H2N2), 1968 (H3N2), and 2009 (a novel H1N1). Major adjustments of vaccines must be made in such instances.

Two principal types of influenza vaccines are licensed at present, inactivated vaccine and live attenuated virus vaccine. The inactivated vaccine is prepared by treating wild-type viruses prepared in eggs or cell culture with an inactivating agent. Inactivated vaccine often prevents more than half of serious influenza-related disease when the viruses chosen for the seasonal vaccine antigenically match the eventual epidemic virus well. The vaccine is most effective at preventing severe respiratory disease and influenza-related hospitalizations.

All persons aged 6 months and above should be vaccinated. Those at most risk of severe disease and in most need of vaccine are infants, young children, people older than 65 years, pregnant women, and those with chronic health conditions or immunodeficiency. This vaccine is contraindicated in those who have had a life-threatening allergic reaction after a dose of influenza vaccine or have a severe allergy to any component of the vaccine, some of which contain a small amount of egg protein. Some people with a history of Guillain-Barré syndrome should not receive this vaccine. The vaccine is usually given as a single dose each year, although children 6 months through 8 years of age may need two doses during a single influenza season. Some IIVs contain a small amount of the preservative thimerosal (see Preservatives, Including Thimerosal). Although any association with developmental disorders has been disproven, public concern about this topic has led to the development of thimerosal-free IIVs.

The second principal type of influenza vaccine is a trivalent or quadrivalent live attenuated virus vaccine that is administered topically by nasal spray. New vaccines are prepared each year to address antigenic drift by reasserting genes encoding the current HA and NA antigens with a virus genetic background containing internal viral genes with well-defined attenuating mutations. The vaccine is licensed in the U.S. for persons 2 to 49 years of age. In some pediatric studies, the live attenuated vaccine appeared to provide a higher level of protection than inactivated vaccine; however, CDC vaccine effectiveness data from the influenza seasons in 2013–2016 in the U.S. indicated that the quadrivalent live attenuated vaccine did not demonstrate statistically significant effectiveness in children 2–17 years of age. Therefore, the CDC provided an interim recommendation that the vaccine should not be used in any setting in the U.S. for the 2016–2017 influenza season. Practitioners should check regularly for updated guidelines from the CDC on this point.

Human Papillomavirus Vaccines

Human papillomaviruses cause nearly all cases of cervical and anal cancer and a majority of oropharyngeal cancers. Most such cancers are caused by just two of the many HPV serotypes, types 16 and 18. Remarkably, even though the virus cannot be grown efficiently in culture, effective HPV vaccines were developed using VLPs that are formed by HPV surface components. All licensed HPV vaccines protect against at least these two types and some protect against four or nine types of HPV, with effectiveness against vaginal and vulvar cancers in women, as well as most cases of anal cancer and genital warts in both females and males. HPV vaccines are recommended for all 11- and 12-year-olds to protect against HPV infection and for women 13 to 26 years old and men 13 to 21 years old not previously vaccinated. HPV vaccination is also recommended for any man who has sex with a man. The vaccines are given in a three-dose regimen on a schedule of 0, 1-2, and 6 months.

Maternal Immunization

Maternal immunization during pregnancy can enhance newborn protection after birth by providing passive immunity to the neonate. Immunizing pregnant mothers is safe and protects the child from deadly infectious pathogens early in life when the immune system is not fully developed. One of the most successful maternal immunization protocols involves injection of tetanus toxoid to stimulate the production of IgG antibodies that have high neutralizing capacity and can cross the placenta. Vaccines for group B *Streptococcus*, Hib, RSV, *Streptococcus pneumoniae*, *Bordetella pertussis*, and trivalent *IIVs* have been tested in pregnant women. For a complete list of maternal vaccines, see Table 36–7.

TABLE 36–7 ■ VACCINES THAT MAY BE USED IN MOTHERS BEFORE, DURING, OR AFTER PREGNANCY[a]

VACCINE	BEFORE PREGNANCY	DURING PREGNANCY	AFTER PREGNANCY	TYPE OF VACCINE
Influenza	Yes	Yes, during season	Yes	Inactivated
Tdap	May be recommended; better to vaccinate during pregnancy when possible	Yes, during each pregnancy	Yes, immediately postpartum, if Tdap never received in lifetime; it is better to vaccinate during pregnancy	Toxoid/inactivated
Td	May be recommended	May be recommended, but Tdap is preferred	May be recommended	Toxoid
Hepatitis A	May be recommended	May be recommended	May be recommended	Inactivated
Hepatitis B	May be recommended	May be recommended	May be recommended	Inactivated
Meningococcal	May be recommended	Base decision on risk vs. benefit; inadequate data for specific recommendation	May be recommended	Inactivated
Pneumococcal	May be recommended	Base decision on risk vs. benefit; inadequate data for specific recommendation	May be recommended	Inactivated
HPV	May be recommended (through 26 years of age)	No	May be recommended (through 26 years of age)	Inactivated
MMR	May be recommended; once received, avoid conception for 4 weeks	No	May be recommended	Live
Varicella	May be recommended; once received, avoid conception for 4 weeks	No	May be recommended	Live

[a]Adapted from CDC guidance: http://www.cdc.gov/vaccines/pregnancy/downloads/immunizations-preg-chart.pdf.

Vaccines for Travel

International travelers should ensure that their vaccination status is current for conventional vaccines, including diphtheria, tetanus, pertussis, hepatitis A and B, and poliovirus; exposures to these agents may be more common in some international settings. There are additional vaccines that may be of benefit as preventive vaccines; these are listed next.

Japanese Encephalitis Virus Vaccine

Japanese encephalitis is a serious mosquito-borne flavivirus infection (not spread person to person) that can cause mild infections with fever and headache, serious neurological sequelae, and even death. Travelers who spend a month or longer in some rural parts of Korea, Japan, China, and eastern areas of Russia should consider vaccination. Two JE vaccines are licensed in the U.S.: an inactivated mouse brain–derived JE vaccine (JE-MB) for use in travelers aged 1 year or older and an inactivated Vero cell culture–derived JE vaccine (JE-VC) for persons aged 17 years or older.

Yellow Fever Virus Vaccine

Yellow fever is a mosquito-borne flaviviral disease with a wide range of systemic symptoms. In severe cases, the disease causes hepatitis, hemorrhagic fever, and death. The CDC recommends this vaccine for children older than 9 months and adults who will be traveling to high-risk areas. There is generally a requirement for documentation of vaccination for travel to and from infected areas. The vaccine is a live attenuated virus vaccine that has been used successfully for many decades. For international travel, yellow fever virus vaccine must be approved by WHO and must be administered by an approved yellow fever vaccination center that can provide both vaccination and a validated International Certificate of Vaccination. The vaccine should be given at least 10 days before travel to an endemic area. Generally, a single dose suffices.

Typhoid Vaccine

Typhoid fever is an acute illness caused by the bacterium *S. typhi*, which is transmitted by ingestion of contaminated water or food. Typhoid vaccination is recommended for international travelers who will visit rural areas or villages that have inadequate sanitation. Symptoms include fever, headache, anorexia, and abdominal discomfort; the disease can be fatal. Treatment is challenging, and there has been an increase in the number of drug-resistant strains of *S. typhi* over the last several decades. There are two vaccines available to prevent infection: a single-dose, injectable, inactivated typhoid vaccine and an oral live typhoid vaccine that is taken in a four-dose course.

Rabies Virus Vaccine

Rabies is caused by a lyssavirus transmitted to humans from the bite of infected mammals; the untreated infection is nearly always fatal in humans. Rabies vaccination is used in two ways, first as a preventive vaccine prior to exposure and second as a postexposure intervention to prevent progression to fatal disease. Candidates for preexposure vaccination are people at high risk of exposure to natural rabies (veterinarians, animal handlers, spelunkers, et al.) or to laboratory strains or tissues (such as those involved in production of rabies biologicals). Preventive vaccination should be offered to international travelers who are likely to come in contact with animals in parts of the world where rabies is common (see CDC website). The vaccine is given in a three-dose series on days 0, 7, and 28. For those who may be repeatedly exposed to rabies virus, periodic testing for immunity is recommended, and booster doses can be administered as needed to maintain immunity. Postexposure vaccination is used in emergency settings following a bite or close exposure to an animal that may be rabid. In this setting, the vaccine is given in a four-dose series on days 0, 3, 7, and 14, concomitant with two injections of rabies immune globulin on day 0, one locally into the bite site and a second in an intramuscular injection for systemic administration of antibodies. A bite victim who has been previously vaccinated should receive two doses of rabies vaccine on days 0 and 3 but does not need rabies immune globulin.

Specialty Vaccines

There are limited-use vaccines that are offered in special circumstances to at-risk persons.

Anthrax Vaccine

Anthrax vaccine is offered to certain at-risk adults 18 to 65 years of age, including some members of the U.S. military, laboratory workers who work with anthrax, and some veterinarians or other individuals who handle animals or animal products. Anthrax is a serious disease in animals and human caused by *Bacillus anthracis*. People can contract anthrax from contact with infected animals or animal products. Usually, the cutaneous infection causes ulcers on the skin and systemic symptoms, including fever and malaise; up to 20% of untreated cases are fatal. Inhaled spores of *B. anthracis* usually cause fatal infection. AVA, given as multiple booster injections, protects against cutaneous and inhalation anthrax acquired by exposure on skin or by inhalation. The CDC recommends anthrax intramuscular booster shots 4 weeks, 6 months, 12 months, 18 months, and then annually.

Vaccinia Virus (Smallpox Vaccine)

Vaccinia vaccine is a live attenuated orthopoxvirus vaccine developed by multiple passages in cell culture to isolate viral variants that cause only limited infection in humans. The virus is produced as purified calf lymph and given percutaneously with a bifurcated needle. This vaccine was used in the first successful worldwide efforts to eradicate a human virus, variola or smallpox. Routine universal vaccinia immunization was discontinued around 1980, following the declaration by WHO that variola (smallpox) was eradicated, but the vaccine is still available. The nonemergency use of vaccinia vaccine includes vaccination of laboratory and healthcare workers exposed occupationally to vaccinia virus, to recombinant vaccinia viruses, or other orthopoxviruses that can infect humans, such as monkeypox virus and cowpox virus. Because there are still laboratory stocks of variola in research use in several countries, including the U.S., the U.S. ACIP has developed recommendations for the use of vaccinia vaccine if variola virus were used as an agent of biological terrorism or if a smallpox outbreak occurred accidentally. Large-scale use in the military and consideration of use in medical first responders in the U.S. has been implemented in recent decades. A derivative of conventional vaccinia virus vaccine has been developed that has desirable properties. MVA virus is a highly attenuated strain of vaccinia virus isolated after more than 500 passages in chicken embryo fibroblasts, during which the virus lost about 10% of the vaccinia genome and the ability to replicate productively in human and other primate cells.

Other Vaccines for Biodefense and Special Pathogens

There are a number of limited-use vaccines, such as those for workers in high-containment facilities conducting research on highly pathogenic agents that are emerging infectious diseases or potential agents for use in bioterrorism or biowarfare. Typically, these vaccines are used only under Investigational New Drug status. Examples include vaccines for Eastern equine encephalitis (EEE) virus, Venezuelan equine encephalitis (VEE) virus, Rift Valley fever virus, botulinum toxin, and others.

International Vaccines

There are additional vaccines pertinent to exposures in other countries that are licensed in some areas, but not yet in the U.S.

Dengue Virus Vaccine

Dengue fever is another mosquito-borne flaviviral disease caused by four different viral serotypes and annually affecting about 400 million people worldwide. The disease can be a mild systemic febrile illness during primary infection but can cause severe dengue disease and death during a second infection with virus of a different serotype. It is thought that cross-reactive nonneutralizing antibodies induced by one infection enhance the disease caused by subsequent infection with a heterologous serotype virus. This antibody-dependent enhancement concern has been a significant barrier to vaccine development efforts. Nevertheless, much progress has been made recently in dengue vaccine development.

There is currently no dengue vaccine approved for use in the U.S.; however, CYD-TDV developed by Sanofi Pasteur is a recombinant tetravalent (four-serotype) live attenuated virus vaccine that was first licensed in Mexico in December 2015 for use in individuals 9–45 years of age living in endemic areas. It is given as a three-dose series on a 0-, 6-, 12-month schedule. Additional dengue vaccine candidates are in clinical development.

Malaria Vaccine

The RTS,S vaccine is a recombinant protein-based malaria vaccine with AS01 adjuvant against *Plasmodium falciparum* that was developed by a large international public-private consortium and is the first malaria vaccine to complete efficacy trial testing with a positive review of the outcome. It is relevant for *P. falciparum*, which is common in sub-Saharan Africa, but does not protect against *Plasmodium vivax* malaria, which is more common in many countries outside Africa. The EMA issued a "European scientific opinion" on the vaccine, and WHO and its SAGE have advocated its use in large-scale implementation pilot tests in Africa.

BCG Vaccine

BCG vaccine is used to prevent severe disease due to *Mycobacterium tuberculosis* (TB). BCG vaccine is produced using a live attenuated bovine bacillus strain, *Mycobacterium bovis*, that has lost its ability to cause severe disease in humans. The vaccine typically is given as a single intradermal dose, often to infants near the time of birth. The efficacy of BCG vaccine against TB is uncertain in many settings, but the consensus is that the vaccine does protect against the most severe forms of disseminated TB, such as miliary disease and TB meningitis. The vaccine is a WHO essential medicine for endemic areas but is not used for universal vaccination in the U.S.

The Future of Vaccine Technology

Vaccination technology and improved methods to generate vaccines have led to the prevention of many infectious diseases. People no longer die at the high rates that prevailed before vaccines were developed. In the developing world, however, according to WHO reports, over 40% of deaths are due to infectious diseases, highlighting a continued need to improve existing vaccines, develop new vaccines, and improve delivery methods to increase efficacy. Viruses, bacteria, parasites, and antigens on cancerous cells are all future vaccine targets. New vaccines for pregnant mothers will be available to prevent diseases that can become chronic if the fetus becomes infected in utero, as is the case with malaria. Furthermore, an increasing elderly population will need access to better vaccines that can stimulate their aging immune systems, which are susceptible to infections like influenza and varicella viruses. Delivery methods are being explored to utilize nanoparticles and alternative adjuvants to improve vaccine immunogenicity so people will only need one vaccine dose rather than several. Needle-less delivery is already possible, as in the case of oral polio vaccine or via nasal sprays for influenza. Investigation continues on developing new edible vaccines using plants, microneedles, and needle-free dermal patches.

Most vaccines work through preventing disease due to acute infections; the challenge remains to develop vaccines against chronic viral infections where the host is immunosuppressed. These pathogens evade the immune system and persist in the host's own cells. To overcome these chronic pathogens, vaccines need to elicit both antibody and T cell responses, where B cells can neutralize the pathogen and T cells can actively kill and destroy infected cells. Vaccines against HPV and hepatitis B viruses protect not only from viral infection but also from developing infection-associated cancers.

New vaccines for other viral pathogens that can cause further complications are needed. For example, infection with group A streptococcus can lead to rheumatic fever, *Helicobacter pylori* may result in stomach cancer, and chlamydia infection can cause blindness and infertility. Vaccines provide effective prophylaxis; however, the frontier in vaccine technology will involve vaccines as therapies for already-established disease. Vaccines can be utilized against pathogens that become chronic, as in shingles, and also in conditions of autoimmunity and cancer, where the immune response is dysregulated. In the case of cancer, vaccines can be utilized to augment immunity to tumors to prevent their growth and metastasis. In the case of autoimmunity, the goal of this "negative vaccination" is to use vaccines to dampen immune function to prevent self-tissue destruction (Nossal, 2011).

Vaccine Safety: Myths, Truths, and Consequences

Vaccine Adjuvants and Safety

Adjuvants are substances added to vaccines to enhance the magnitude, quality, and duration of the protective immune response. Adjuvants are useful in vaccines because they stimulate the innate immune system that subsequently activates a strong adaptive immune response to ensure immune protection. Because many modern vaccines do not contain live pathogens, they must include adjuvants to ensure vaccine efficacy. Adjuvants are particularly useful in subunit protein vaccines, which often are inadequately immunogenic without enhancement.

There is extensive experience in human vaccines with two adjuvants, aluminum and monophosphoryl lipid A. Aluminum, in the form of alum, has been used for nearly 90 years in vaccines; aluminum hydroxide [$Al(OH)_3$] and aluminum phosphate ($AlPO_4$) are currently used. Aluminum is used in many childhood vaccines in the U.S. targeted to diphtheria-tetanus-pertussis, Hib and pneumococcus, hepatitis A and B, and HPV. Monophosphoryl lipid A (isolated from bacteria) has been used in the HPV vaccine Cervarix since 2009. A new influenza vaccine licensed for the 2016–2017 season included the adjuvant MF59, an oil-in-water emulsion of squalene oil. Another new influenza vaccine that is targeted to influenza H5N1 contains a new adjuvant termed AS03 (an "adjuvant system" containing α-tocopherol and squalene in an oil-in-water emulsion) and was licensed for inclusion in the U.S. pandemic influenza vaccine stockpile. Live attenuated virus vaccines do not contain adjuvants; thus, adjuvant-free vaccines include those directed against measles, mumps, rubella, chickenpox, rotavirus, polio, and live attenuated seasonal influenza virus.

Vaccines Do Not Cause Autism

Autism spectrum disorder rates have increased in the U.S. and other parts of the world in parallel with expansion in the diagnostic criteria of autism that that now include spectrum disorders with a broader array of symptoms (Hansen et al., 2015). The CDC found that 1 of 68 children in the U.S. has ASD. Patients with this disorder have development impairments that affect their communication, behavior, and social interactions. Even though some people have been concerned with a causal link between vaccines and autism, many large scientific studies have failed to detect any such link (Hviid et al., 2003; Madsen et al., 2002; Schechter and Grether, 2008; Taylor et al., 2014). The IOM (now termed the National Academy of Medicine) conducted thorough reviews and concluded that current childhood and adult vaccines are very safe. In 2014, a CDC study added to reports around the world that vaccines do not cause ASD. They concluded that the total amount of antigen received from vaccines did not differ between children with ASD and those without the disorder. Vaccination with the MMR vaccine also is not associated with development of ASD in children.

Preservatives, Including Thimerosal

Preservatives added to vaccine preparations are designed to kill or inhibit the growth of bacteria and fungi that could contaminate a vaccine vial. There are historical reports of severe adverse events or death due to bacterial contamination of multidose vials lacking preservative. The highest risk of contamination is probably due to repetitive puncture of a multidose vaccine vial that is stored over time. Therefore, The U.S. *Code of Federal Regulations* requires the addition of a preservative to multidose vials of vaccines. Preservatives eliminate or reduce contamination in this setting. Several preservatives have been incorporated into licensed vaccines, including 2-phenoxyethanol, benzethonium chloride, phenol, and thimerosal.

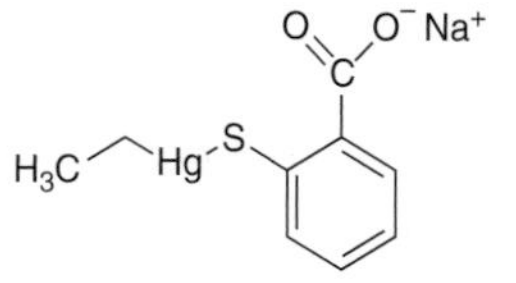

thimerosal-Na^+

Thimerosal, known to many by the trade name Merthiolate, has been one of the most commonly used preservatives; it is an organomercurial, an organic compound containing mercury. Thimerosal has been used safely since the early 20th century as a preservative in biologics, including many vaccines, and has a long history of use. Over time, concerns were raised about its safety because some organomercurials were increasingly associated with neurotoxicity, and children began receiving increasing numbers of licensed vaccines. The FDA chose to work with manufacturers toward reduction or elimination of thimerosal from childhood vaccines because of these *theoretical concerns*. As a result, thiomersal has been eliminated or reduced to trace amounts in nearly all childhood vaccines except some IIVs.

In terms of toxicity from mercury, most of the data in the field pertains to methylmercury, whereas thimerosal is a derivative of ethylmercury, which is cleared more rapidly. Thimerosal does not have significant toxic effects at the concentrations used in vaccine formulations. However, questions were raised about the potential association of thimerosal-containing vaccines in children and the occurrence of neurodevelopmental disorders, especially autism. A rather sordid history of fraud, conflict of interest, and other irregularities has been revealed pertaining to the now-debunked association studies of thimerosal and autism; decades of studies have been conducted in safety reviews around this matter.

The National Vaccine Advisory Committee, ACIP of the CDC, and the IOM's Immunization Safety Review Committee have all conducted extensive reviews of association studies, and the conclusion is that autism is not associated with the amount of thimerosal in childhood vaccines. In any event, recognizing public concern, between 2001 and 2003, thimerosal was eliminated from or reduced in childhood vaccines (except for flu) for children under 6 years old in hopes of encouraging childhood vaccination. The CDC has compiled a thorough review and list of articles relating to this issue (CDC, 2015).

Adverse Events With Vaccines

For injectable vaccines, common adverse effects include minor *local reactions* to vaccines at the injection site (pain, swelling, and redness). More widespread effects, termed *systemic reactions*, may include fever, rash, irritability, drowsiness, and other symptoms, depending on the vaccine. The profile of reactions seen in large-scale trials is carefully documented in package inserts. During vaccine candidate testing, any occurrence of serious adverse events (SAEs) are examined carefully. SAEs are events following vaccination that involve hospitalization, life-threatening events, death, disability, permanent damage, congenital anomaly/birth defect, or other conditions requiring medical intervention. Vaccines with clear association with SAEs are typically not licensed. In some cases, to increase the likelihood of detecting of rare SAEs, the FDA requires phase 4 studies (postmarketing surveillance) to follow the performance of vaccines as use expands beyond the size of the trials leading to licensure. The government also collects data after licensure through the vaccine adverse event reporting system (VAERS).

Vaccines can be withdrawn from market if concerns arise. For example, licensure for use of the live oral rotavirus vaccine Rotashield, which was recommended for routine immunization of the U.S. infants in 1998, was withdrawn in 1999 when reports in VAERS suggested an association between the vaccine and intussusception, a form of bowel obstruction.

Allergic Reactions

Allergy to components of vaccine formulations also can cause reactions. Trace amounts of antibiotics like neomycin, used to ensure sterility in some vaccines (e.g., MMR, trivalent IPV, and varicella vaccine), may cause adverse reactions. A history of anaphylactic reaction (but not local reaction) to neomycin is a contraindication to future immunization with those vaccines. Persons with a history of egg allergy should not be given an influenza vaccine prepared in eggs. Gelatin, which is used as a stabilizer in some virus vaccines like varicella and MMR vaccines, may cause allergic reaction in some.

Fainting

Fainting, or syncope, also has been reported in people after vaccination. Fainting is more common in adolescents than in children or adults and thus is more common after vaccination with HPV, MCV4, and Tdap. Immediate fainting episodes following vaccination procedures is triggered by pain or anxiety, rather than the contents of the vaccines. While fainting is not serious, falling while fainting can cause injury, with head injuries the most serious. Clinicians can give patients drinks and snacks to prevent some fainting and can prevent falls by having patients lie down or sit during the procedure. Patients who faint after vaccination will recover after a few minutes, and clinicians should observe patients for at least 15 min after vaccination (a recommendation of the CDC).

Febrile Seizure

Fevers of 102°F (38.9°C) or higher can cause children to experience febrile seizures, which are characterized by body spasms and jerky movements that may last for up to 2 min. About 5% of children will experience a febrile seizure in their lifetime, with most occurring at 14–18 months of age. Children experiencing simple febrile seizures recover quickly without long-term harm. These common seizures also are caused by febrile illnesses associated with viral infections, especially roseola, ear infections, and other common childhood illnesses. Current vaccines sometimes induce fevers, usually low grade in nature, but rarely result in febrile seizures. Although fever following vaccination with most vaccines rarely causes febrile seizure, there is a small increase in risk after MMR and MMRV vaccines. The CDC also has reported a small increase in febrile seizures after a child receives the IIV together with PCV13 vaccine or in combination with diphtheria, tetanus, or DTaP vaccines. The increase of febrile seizures when combining these vaccines is small, and the CDC does not recommend delivering them on separate days. Importantly, vaccine usage can help prevent febrile seizures by providing vaccinated children protection against measles, mumps, rubella, chickenpox, influenza, and pneumococcal infectious pathogens that may result in febrile seizures.

Guillain-Barré Syndrome

Guillian-Barré syndrome is a rare disease that affects the nervous system. Patients with GBS display muscle weakness and sometimes paralysis that results when their own immune system injures their neurons. GBS often occurs after an infection with bacteria or virus; most patients with GBS recover fully. However, some subjects can have permanent nerve damage. The incidence of GBS in the U.S. currently is about 3000–6000 cases per year; thus, it is rare in a population of about 350 million. GBS is more common in older adults, with people older than 50 years at greater risk. GBS may have several underlying causes, but scientists report that two-thirds of GBS cases occurred after patients were ill with gastroenteritis or respiratory tract infections. Infection with *Campylobacter jejuni* is the most common risk factor for the disease, but GBS also has been reported commonly after influenza virus, cytomegalovirus, or Epstein-Barr viral infection. GBS after vaccination is reported but rare.

An IOM study reported that widespread use of the 1976 swine influenza virus vaccine was associated with a small increase in risk for GBS, with an additional case of GBS per 100,000 people who were vaccinated, although later statistical review called this association into question. Current assessments are that the there is no significant risk of GBS after obtaining a seasonal influenza vaccine, or if there is an association, the risk is approximately one case per million vaccinated individuals, a low rate that is difficult to detect with certainty. Studies have shown that a person is more likely to get GBS after influenza infection than vaccination. Importantly, severe morbidity and mortality are a significant risk after influenza infection, and preventing complications and death can be achieved by getting vaccinated.

Sudden Infant Death Syndrome

Sudden infant death syndrome peaks when babies are between 2 and 4 months old, and infants are also given many vaccines during this period. The temporal overlap of peak SIDS incidence and the period of initiation of childhood vaccination series led to questions about any causal relationship between vaccines and SIDS. Numerous studies have failed to detect a causative association for vaccines and SIDS (Silvers et al., 2001). The IOM 2003 report reviewed the relationship of SIDS and vaccines and concluded that vaccines do not cause SIDS. Infant death by SIDS has decreased dramatically due to the 1992 American Academy of Pediatrics recommendations to place infants on their backs to sleep and the 1994 National Institute of Child Health and Human Development campaign efforts.

Safety of Multiple Vaccinations

Children are exposed to a large number of bacteria and viruses in their environment through food, teething of objects, and exposure to pets and to other humans. The typical viral infection results in exposure of the immune system to a dozen or more antigens; some bacteria express hundreds of antigens during infection. Each recommended childhood vaccine protects against 1 to 69 antigens. When a child is given the full recommended vaccines on the 2014 schedule, they are exposed to up to 315 antigens by age 2, which provides them critical protection against pathogens in the environment (CDC, 2016). Vaccinating patients against multiple antigens has been shown to be safe when they are delivered in combination at the same time. This strategy is advantageous for patients, especially children, because they lack immunity to most vaccine preventable diseases, so receiving this protection during the relatively vulnerable period of early development is important. The patient also has fewer doctor visits with combination or multiple vaccinations, reducing cost in terms of money and time for parents and disruption for children. Numerous studies have shown that giving various vaccine combinations does not cause chronic disease. Furthermore, each time a combination vaccine or multiple vaccination schedule is licensed, that intervention already has been tested for safety and efficacy in combination with the vaccines previously recommended for that age group. The ACIP and the Academy of Pediatrics recommend receiving multiple vaccines at the same time (CDC, 2016).

Vaccine Myths and Their Public Health Consequences

The public health success of vaccines is demonstrated by the decreased rates of mortality and morbidity due to infectious diseases contracted in childhood and adulthood. A dramatic example of success is the worldwide eradication of smallpox, a pathogen responsible for epidemics that killed 300–500 million people in the 20th century and disfigured many survivors. In the 20th century, poliovirus and MeV also incapacitated and killed infected individuals, especially young children. New generations have never seen the debilitating effects of these infectious diseases, thanks to decades of successful public health vaccination strategies. Infectious diseases, however, continue to affect the lives of many people in the developing world who have less access to healthcare or are affected by wars or famine. Recently, preventable diseases are arising again in the developed world because of vaccine myths that have reduced vaccination rates in these countries.

One of these myths concerns autism. A study that has been retracted and discredited claimed there was a link between vaccination in children and autism (Wakefield et al., 1998). Despite major shortcomings and incorrect interpretations, this study changed public perceptions regarding vaccine safety, and its influence persists. Experimental studies in different parts of the world with large cohorts, statistical power, and rigor have found no evidence that vaccines cause autism (American Academy of Pediatrics, 2017; Madsen et al., 2002). Researchers have found that autism occurs in families, may have a genetic component, and may be affected by environmental triggers such as insecticides, certain drugs, and rubella virus. The exact causes of ASDs are unknown and continue to be investigated (Landrigan, 2010).

Nonetheless, the antivaccination movement has gained momentum, with celebrities, politicians, and social media continuing to propagate erroneous vaccine information and conspiracy theories. According to the CDC, vaccination rates have fallen in many parts of the U.S. In nine U.S. states, fewer than two-thirds of children ages 19 to 35 months have been vaccinated with the recommended seven-vaccination regimen. This dismissal of scientific evidence on vaccines can have deadly consequences. Infectious epidemics due to preventable agents like poliovirus and MeV can reemerge. Unvaccinated children will be more susceptible to infection, and many of them will not survive. Furthermore, unvaccinated subjects contribute to reducing the benefits of herd immunity that protects people who cannot be vaccinated for medical reasons, such as cancer, HIV infection, and other types of immunodeficiency.

Diseases due to pertussis, polio, measles, *H. influenzae*, and rubella virus once affected hundreds of thousands of people and killed thousands. Following the introduction of universal vaccinations, the rates of these diseases decreased to near-zero levels in the U.S. Some believe that because these diseases have been nearly eliminated in the U.S., vaccination is no longer needed. This thinking is incorrect. Vaccine-preventable diseases are communicable diseases, spreading from person to person, and the causative viruses and bacteria survive in nature. People, especially the unvaccinated, can be infected, and infected individuals will spread the disease to unvaccinated individuals. A greater fraction of vaccinated individuals in a population leads to fewer opportunities for the disease to spread (herd immunity).

Parental vaccine concerns should be taken seriously, and misconceptions should be thoroughly discussed by providers to ensure that patients have scientific information and are informed about the risks associated with failure to vaccinate. By providing parental education, pediatricians and other primary care medical providers can help reduce vaccine hesitancy.

Licensure and Monitoring of Vaccines

Immune Correlates and Mechanisms

During the process of vaccine development and testing, manufacturers seek to define laboratory tests and parameters that are associated with efficacy, which have been designated immune CoPs. First, it is important theoretically to understand some features of the biological mechanism of protection to optimize development and use of vaccines. At a practical level, identification of a correlate allows monitoring of the reproducibility of vaccines during repetitive manufacture, monitoring the expected impact of new combinations of vaccine antigens on immunogenicity of existing vaccines, and other critical issues.

Plotkin and others have developed terminology for principal types of correlates (Plotkin and Gilbert, 2012). A *CoP* is a marker of immune function that statistically correlates with protection. Such markers can be simply associated with protection (termed nCoP) or alternatively may be known to measure directly the immune effectors that mediate protection (mCoP). From a practical standpoint, either an nCoP or an mCoP can enable monitoring and prediction of effective vaccination.

The ideal CoP is one that is quantitative and derives from a reproducible laboratory test that has been validated under good laboratory practice conditions. The type of protection suggested for a particular correlate may vary because vaccines may be designed to prevent differing classes of infection, such as local versus systemic infection or severe disease versus any disease. Examples of quantitative CoPs in use include a threshold of 10 mIU/mL in serum of hepatitis B antibodies detected in a standardized ELISA (enzyme-linked immunosorbent assay), serum diphtheria toxin neutralization concentration of 0.01 to 0.1 IU/mL, a serum virus neutralization dilution titer of 1/5 for yellow fever virus, or a 1/40 dilution of serum in influenza hemagglutination inhibition titer.

Regulatory and Advisory Bodies

The Center for Biologics Evaluation and Research (CBER) of the FDA regulates vaccine products in the U.S., with recommendations from its Vaccines and Related Biological Products Advisory Committee. The EMA regulates in Europe. Manufacturers conduct phase 1 (safety and immunogenicity studies) in a small number of closely monitored subjects; phase 2 studies (dose-ranging studies) typically in several hundred subjects; and then phase 3 trials (efficacy studies) typically in thousands of subjects. If successful, the sponsor submits a Biologics License Application (BLA) to the FDA, which may lead to licensure. Licensure allows use, but decisions on whether vaccines are recommended for specific populations or for universal use are made by additional advisory bodies. The CDC hosts the ACIP, a committee of public health and medical experts, which makes recommendations for use of vaccines in the U.S. Various professional medical societies also publish recommendations, for instance, the American Academy of Pediatrics publishes the *AAP Red Book*, or "Report of the Committee on Infectious Diseases of the American Academy of Pediatrics," which contains vaccine recommendations. Finally, third-party payers, such as insurance companies, affect usage through reimbursement policies; thus, issues of cost, benefit, and profitability become considerations, as examined in Chapter 1.

Bibliography

American Academy of Pediatrics. Vaccine safety: examine the evidence. January 26, **2017**. Available at: https://www.healthychildren.org/English/safety-prevention/immunizations/Pages/Vaccine-Studies-Examine-the-Evidence.aspx. Accessed March 4, 2017.

Baxter D. Active and passive immunity, vaccine types, excipients and licensing. *Occup Med (Lond)*, **2007**, *57*:552–556.

CDC. Vaccines do not cause autism. Update of November 23, **2015**. Available at: https://www.cdc.gov/vaccinesafety/concerns/autism.html. Accessed March 7, 2017.

CDC. Safety Information About Specific Vaccines. Update of January 21, **2016**. Available at: https://www.cdc.gov/vaccinesafety/vaccines/index.html. Accessed June 15, 2017.

Clem AS. Fundamentals of vaccine immunology. *J Glob Infect Dis*, **2011**, *3*:73–78.

Gill DM, et al. Diphtheria toxin, protein synthesis, and the cell. *Fed Proc*, **1973**, *32*:1508–1515.

Gross CP, Sepkowitz KA. The myth of the medical breakthrough: smallpox, vaccination, and Jenner reconsidered. *Int J Infect Dis*, **1998**, *3*:54–60.

Hansen SN, et al. Explaining the increase in the prevalence of autism spectrum disorders: the proportion attributable to changes in reporting practices. *JAMA Pediatr*, **2015**, *169*:56–62.

Hinman A. Landmark perspective: mass vaccination against polio. *JAMA*, **1984**, *251*:2994–2996.

Hopkins DR. *The Greatest Killer: Smallpox in History*. University of Chicago Press, Chicago, **2002**.

Hviid A, et al. Association between thimerosal-containing vaccine and autism. *JAMA*, **2003**, *290*:1763–1766.

Madsen KM, et al. A population-based study of measles, mumps, and rubella vaccination and autism. *N Engl J Med*, **2002**, *347*:1477–1482.

Marrack P, et al. Towards an understanding of the adjuvant action of aluminium. *Nat Rev Immunol*, **2009**, *9*:287–293.

Landrigan PJ. What causes autism? Exploring the environmental contribution. *Curr Opin Pediatr*, **2010**, *22*:219–225.

Nossal GJ. Vaccines of the future. *Vaccine*, **2011**, *29*(suppl 4):D111–D115.

Plotkin SA, Gilbert PB. Nomenclature for immune correlates of protection after vaccination. *Clin Infect Dis*, **2012**, *54*:1615–1617.

Riesbeck K, Nordstrom T. Structure and immunological action of the human pathogen *Moraxella catarrhalis* IgD-binding protein. *Crit Rev Immunol,* **2006**, *26*:353–376.

Robinson HL, et al. DNA vaccines for viral infections: basic studies and applications. *Adv Virus Res,* **2000**, *55*:1–74.

Schechter R, Grether JK. Continuing increases in autism reported to California's developmental services system: mercury in retrograde. *Arch Gen Psychiatry,* **2008**, *65*:19–24.

Schroeder HW Jr, Cavacini L. Structure and function of immunoglobulins. *J Allergy Clin Immunol,* **2010**, *125*:S41–S52.

Silvers LE, et al. The epidemiology of fatalities reported to the vaccine adverse event reporting system 1990–1997. *Pharmacoepidemiol Drug Saf,* **2001**, *10*:279–285.

Taylor LE, et al. Vaccines are not associated with autism: an evidence-based meta-analysis of case-control and cohort studies. *Vaccine,* **2014**, *32*:3623–3629.

Wakefield AJ, et al. Ileal-lymphoid-nodular hyperplasia, non-specific colitis, and pervasive developmental disorder in children. *Lancet,* **1998**, *351*: 637–641. Article retracted: *Lancet*, **2010**, *375*:445.

Woof JM, Mestecky J. Mucosal immunoglobulins. *Immunol Rev,* **2005**, *206*:64–82.

Lipid-Derived Autacoids: Eicosanoids and Platelet-Activating Factor

Emer M. Smyth, Tilo Grosser, and Garret A. FitzGerald

第三十七章　脂质衍生的自体活性物质：二十碳烯酸和血小板活化因子

中文导读

本章主要介绍：二十碳烯酸，包括二十碳烯酸的生物合成和生物合成抑制药，以及二十碳烯酸的代谢、药理性质、生理作用、药理学效应和治疗应用；血小板活化因子（PAF），包括PAF的化学及生物合成、PAF合成的位点、PAF的作用机制、PAF的生理学和病理学功能、PAF受体拮抗药。

Membrane lipids supply the substrate for the synthesis of *eicosanoids* and *platelet-activating factor* (PAF). Arachidonic acid (AA) metabolites, including *PGs*, *PGI$_2$*, *TxA$_2$*, *LTs*, and *epoxygenase products* of CYPs, collectively the eicosanoids, are not stored but are produced by most cells when a variety of physical, chemical, and hormonal stimuli activate acyl hydrolases that make arachidonate available. *Membrane glycerophosphocholine* derivatives can be modified enzymatically to produce PAF. PAF is formed by a smaller number of cell types, principally leukocytes, platelets, and endothelial cells. Eicosanoids and PAF lipids function as signaling molecules in many biological processes, including the regulation of vascular tone, renal function, hemostasis, parturition, GI mucosal integrity, and stem cell function. They are also important mediators of innate immunity and inflammation. Several classes of drugs, most notably NSAIDs (see Chapter 38), including aspirin, owe their principal therapeutic effects—relief of inflammatory pain and antipyresis—to blockade of PG formation.

Eicosanoids

Eicosanoids, from the Greek *eikosi* ("twenty") are formed from precursor essential fatty acids that contain 20 carbons and 3, 4, or 5 double bonds: 8,11,14-eicosatrienoic acid (dihomo-γ-linolenic acid), 5,8,11,14-eicosatetraenoic acid (AA; Figure 37–1), and EPA. AA is the most abundant precursor, derived from the dietary omega-6 fatty acid, linoleic acid (9,12-octadecadienoic acid), or ingested directly as a dietary constituent. EPA is a major constituent of oils from fatty fish such as salmon.

Abbreviations

AA: arachidonic acid
ACTH: corticotropin (formerly adrenocorticotrophic hormone)
BLT1/2: LTB4 receptors
cAMP: cyclic adenosine monophosphate
COX: cyclooxygenase
CYP: cytochrome P450
CysLT: cysteinyl leukotriene
CysLT1/2: CysLT receptors
DP_2: a member of the fMLP-receptor superfamily, CRTH2
DP: PGD_2 receptor
EDHF: endothelium-derived hyperpolarizing factor
EET: epoxyeicosatrienoic acid
EP: PGE_2 receptor
EPA: 5,8,11,14,17-eicosapentaenoic acid
FLAP: 5-LOX–activating protein
FP: $PGF_2\alpha$ receptor
fMLP: formyl-methionyl-leucyl-phenylalanine
GPCR: G protein–coupled receptor
HETE: hydroxyeicosatetraenoic acid
HPETE: hydroxyperoxyeicosatetraenoic acid
IL: interleukin
IP_3: inositol 1,4,5-trisphosphate
IP: PGI_2 receptor
$iPLA_2$: independent PLA_2
IsoP: isoprostane
LOX: lipoxygenase
LT: leukotriene
LX*: lipoxin*, e.g., LXA, LXB
NSAID: nonsteroidal anti-inflammatory drug
PAF: platelet-activating factor
PAF-AH: PAF acetylhydrolyase
PG: prostaglandin
PGDH: PG 15-OH dehydrogenase
PGI_2: prostacyclin
PL*: phospholipase*, e.g., PLA, PLC
PMN: polymorphonuclear leukocyte
POX: peroxidase
TNF: tumor necrosis factor
TP: TxA_2 receptor
TxA: thromboxane A

History

In 1930, American gynecologists Kurzrok and Lieb observed that strips of uterine myometrium relax or contract when exposed to semen. Subsequently, Goldblatt in England and von Euler in Sweden reported independently on smooth muscle contracting and vasodepressor activities in seminal fluid and accessory reproductive glands. In 1935, von Euler identified the active material as a lipid-soluble acid, which he named *prostaglandin*. Samuelsson, Bergström, and their colleagues elucidated the structures of PGE_1 and $PGF_1\alpha$ in 1962. In 1964, Bergström and coworkers and van Dorp and associates independently achieved biosynthesis of PGE_2 from AA. Discovery of TxA_2, PGI_2, and the LTs followed. Vane, Smith, and Willis in 1971 reported that aspirin and NSAIDs act by inhibiting PG biosynthesis. This remarkable period of discovery linked the Nobel Prize of von Euler in 1970 to that of Bergström, Samuelsson, and Vane in 1982.

Biosynthesis

Biosynthesis of eicosanoids is limited by the availability of AA and depends primarily on the release of esterified AA from membrane phospholipids or other complex lipids by acyl hydrolases, notably PLA_2. Once liberated, AA is metabolized rapidly to oxygenated products by *COXs*, *LOXs*, and CYPs (Figure 37–1).

Chemical and physical stimuli activate the Ca^{2+}-dependent translocation of group IV_A cytosolic phospholipase A_2 ($cPLA_2$) to the membrane, where it hydrolyzes the *sn*-2 ester bond of membrane phosphatidylcholine and phosphatidylethanolamine, releasing AA. Multiple additional PLA_2 isoforms (secretory [s] and Ca^{2+}-independent [i] forms) have been characterized. Under basal conditions, AA liberated by $iPLA_2$ is reincorporated into cell membranes. During stimulation, $cPLA_2$ dominates the acute release of AA, while an inducible $sPLA_2$ contributes to AA release under conditions of sustained or intense stimulation. $sPLA_2$ contributes to platelet microparticle generation of eicosanoids that then direct microparticle internalization by neutrophils driving inflammation (Duchez et al., 2015).

Products of Cyclooxygenases (Prostaglandin G/H Synthases)

Prostaglandin endoperoxide G/H synthase is called *cyclooxygenase* or *COX* colloquially. Products of this pathway are PGs, PGI_2, and TxA_2, collectively termed *prostanoids*. The pathway is described by Figure 37–1 and its legend.

Prostanoids are distinguished by substitutions on their cyclopentane rings the number of double bonds in their side chains, as indicated by numerical subscripts (dihomo-γ-linolenic acid is the precursor of *series*$_1$, AA for *series*$_2$, and EPA for *series*$_3$). Prostanoids derived from AA carry the subscript 2 and are the major series in mammals.

There are two distinct COX isoforms, COX-1 and COX-2 (Rouzer and Marnett, 2009; Smith et al., 2011). COX-1, expressed constitutively in most cells, is the dominant source of prostanoids for housekeeping functions, such as cytoprotection of the gastric epithelium (see Chapter 49). COX-2, in contrast, is upregulated by cytokines, shear stress, and growth factors and is the principal source of prostanoid formation in inflammation and cancer. However, this distinction is not absolute; both enzymes may contribute to the generation of autoregulatory and homeostatic prostanoids during physiologic and pathophysiologic processes.

With 61% amino acid identity, COX-1 and COX-2 have remarkably similar crystal structures. Both isoforms are expressed as dimers homotypically inserted into the endoplasmic reticular membrane. Through sequential COX and POX activity, both COXs convert AA to two unstable intermediates that are then converted to the prostanoids by synthases, expressed in a relatively cell-specific fashion. For example, COX-1–derived TxA_2 is the dominant product in platelets, whereas COX-2–derived PGE_2 and TxA_2 dominate in activated macrophages. Prostanoids are released from cells by diffusion, although transport may be facilitated through the multidrug resistance-associated protein (MRP) transporter (Schuster, 2002).

Lipoxygenase Products

Major products of the LOX pathways are hydroxy fatty acid derivatives known as HETEs, LTs, and LXs (Figure 37–2) (Haeggström and Funk, 2011; Powell and Rokach, 2015). LTs play a major role in the development and persistence of the inflammatory response.

The LOXs are a family of enzymes containing nonheme iron; LOXs catalyze the oxygenation of polyenic fatty acids to corresponding lipid hydroperoxides. The enzymes require a fatty acid substrate with two cis double bonds separated by a methylene group. AA, which contains several double bonds in this configuration, is metabolized to HPETEs, which vary in the site of insertion of the hydroperoxy group. HPETEs are converted to their corresponding HETEs either nonenzymatically or by a POX.

There are five active human LOXs—5(*S*)-LOX, 12(*S*)-LOX, 12(*R*)-LOX, 15(*S*)-LOX-1, and 15(*S*)-LOX-2—classified according to the site

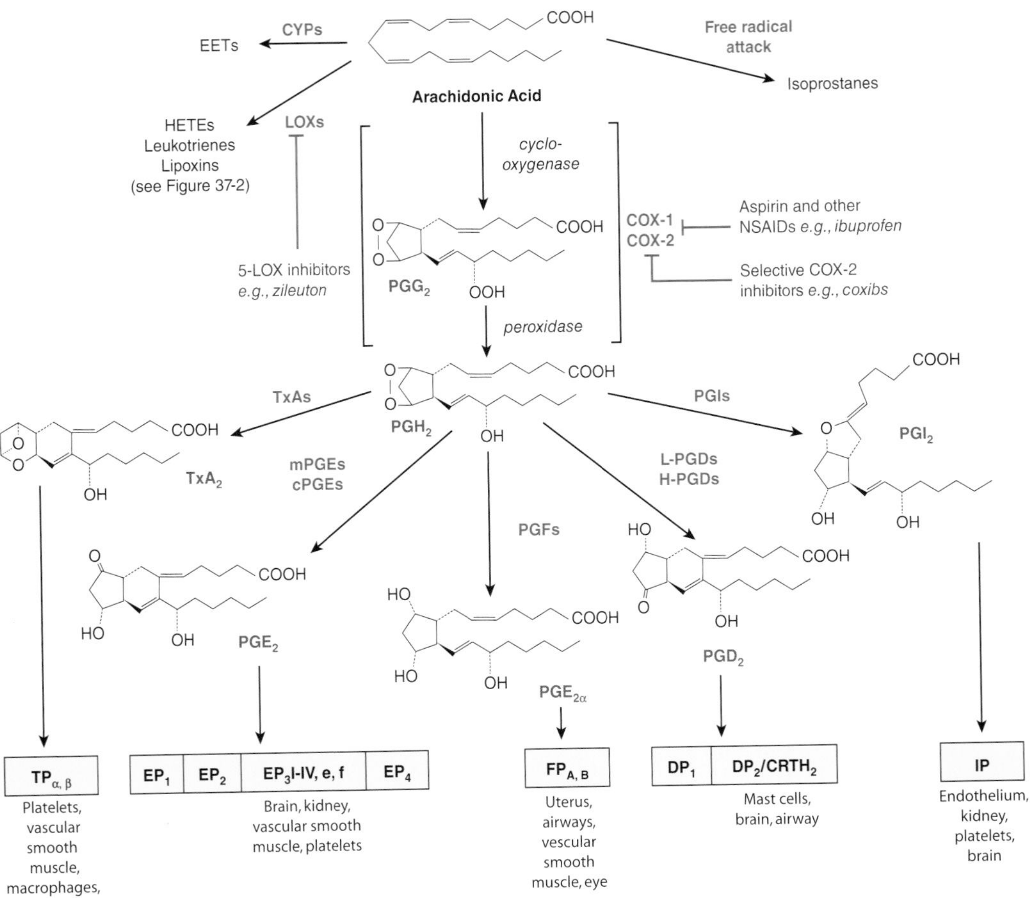

Figure 37–1 *Metabolism of AA.* Cyclic endoperoxides (PGG_2 and PGH_2) arise from the sequential COX and hydroperoxidase actions of COX-1 or COX-2 on AA released from membrane phospholipids. Subsequent products are generated by tissue-specific synthases and transduce their effects via membrane-bound receptors (blue boxes). EETs and isoprostanes are generated via CYP activity and nonenzymatic free radical attack, respectively. Aspirin and nonselective NSAIDs are nonselective inhibitors of COX-1 and COX-2 but do not affect LOX activity. See the text and the Abbreviations list for further definitions.

of hydroperoxy group insertion. Their expression is frequently cell specific; platelets have only 12(*S*)-LOX, whereas leukocytes contain both 5(*S*)- and 12(*S*)-LOX (Figure 37–2). 12(*R*)-LOX is restricted in expression mostly to the skin. The epidermal LOXs, which constitute a distinct LOX subgroup, also include 15-LOX-2 and eLOX-3, the most recently identified family member. eLOX-3 has been reported to metabolize further 12(*R*)-HETE, the product of 12(*R*)-LOX, to a specific epoxyalcohol product.

The 5-LOX pathway leads to the synthesis of the LTs. When eosinophils, mast cells, PMNs, or monocytes are activated, 5-LOX translocates to the nuclear membrane and associates with FLAP, an integral membrane protein that facilitates AA to 5-LOX interaction (Evans et al., 2008). Drugs that inhibit FLAP block LT production. A two-step reaction is catalyzed by 5-LOX: oxygenation of AA to form 5-HPETE followed by dehydration to an unstable epoxide, LTA_4. LTA_4 is transformed by distinct enzymes to LTB_4 or LTC_4. Extracellular metabolism of the peptide moiety of LTC_4 generates LTD_4 and LTE_4 (Peters-Golden and Henderson, 2007). Collectively, LTC_4, LTD_4, and LTE_4 are the *CysLTs*. LTB_4 and LTC_4 are actively transported out of the cell. LTA_4, the primary product of the 5-LOX pathway, is metabolized by 12-LOX to form LXA_4 and LXB_4. These mediators also can arise through 5-LOX metabolism of 15-HETE.

Products of CYPs

The CYP epoxygenases, primarily CYP2C and CYP2J, metabolize AA to EETs (Fleming, 2014). In endothelial cells, EETs function as EDHFs, particularly in the coronary circulation. EET biosynthesis can be altered by pharmacological, nutritional, and genetic factors that affect CYP expression.

Other Pathways

The isoeicosanoids, a family of eicosanoid isomers, are generated by nonenzymatic free radical catalyzed oxidation of AA. Unlike PGs, these compounds are initially formed esterified in phospholipids and released by PLs; the isoeicosanoids then circulate and are metabolized and excreted into urine. Their production is not inhibited in vivo by inhibitors of COX-1 or COX-2, but their formation is suppressed by antioxidants. Isoprostanes correlate with cardiovascular risk factors, and increased levels are found in a large number of clinical conditions (Milne et al., 2015). Their relevance as biologically active mediators remains unclear. A series of compounds, *LXs, maresins, resolvins,* when synthesized and administered to certain models of inflammation, hasten its resolution. It remains to be established whether the endogenous compounds are formed in quantities sufficient to exert this effect in vivo (Skarke et al., 2015).

Inhibitors of Eicosanoid Biosynthesis

Inhibition of PLA_2 decreases the release of the precursor fatty acid and the synthesis of all its metabolites. PLA_2 may be inhibited by drugs that reduce the availability of Ca^{2+}. *Glucocorticoids* inhibit PLA_2 indirectly by inducing the synthesis of a group of proteins termed *annexins* that modulate PLA_2

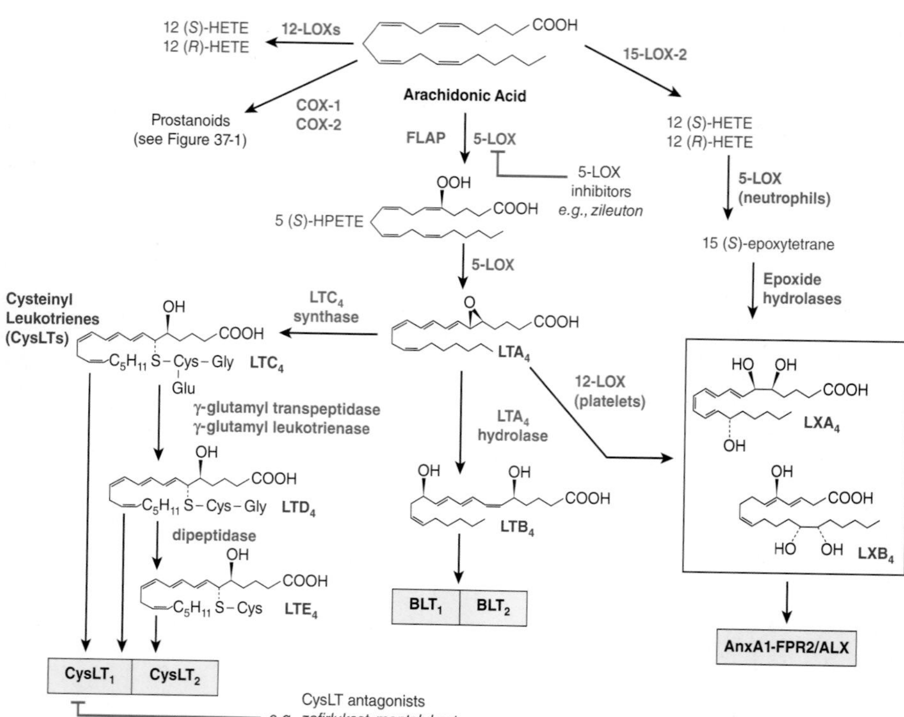

Figure 37–2 *Lipoxygenase pathways of AA metabolism.* FLAP presents AA to 5-LOX, leading to the generation of the LTs and CysLTs. LXs (boxed) are products of cellular interaction via a 5-LOX–12-LOX pathway or via a 15-LOX–5-LOX pathway. Biological effects are transduced via membrane-bound receptors (blue boxes). While its biological relevance remains controversial, LXA_4 can activate a GPCR also activated by Annexin A1 and by the formyl peptide. This GPCR is termed the AnxA1-Formyl peptide receptor 2/ALX receptor (AnxA1-FPR2/ALX) to reflect the range of its putative ligands. Zileuton inhibits 5-LOX but not the COX pathways (expanded in Figure 37–1). CysLT antagonists prevent activation of the $CysLT_1$ receptor. See the text and the Abbreviations list for further definitions.

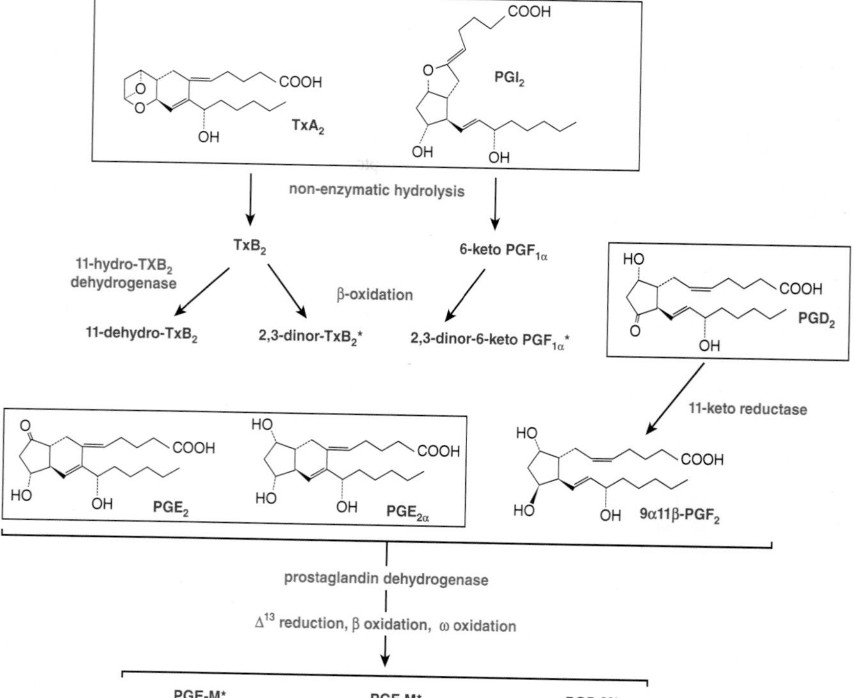

Figure 37–3 *Major pathways of prostanoid degradation.* Active metabolites are boxed. *Major urinary metabolites (M). See the text and the Abbreviations list for further definitions.

activity. Glucocorticoids also downregulate induced expression of COX-2 but not of COX-1 (see Chapter 46). Aspirin and NSAIDs inhibit the COX, but not the POX, moiety of both COX enzymes and thus the formation of downstream prostanoids. These drugs do not inhibit LOXs and may cause increased formation of LTs by shunting of substrate to the LOX pathway. Dual inhibitors of COX and 5-LOX have proven effective in some models of inflammation and tissue injury (Minutoli et al., 2015; Oak et al., 2014). LTs may contribute to the GI side effects associated with NSAIDs (Janusz et al., 1998; Xu et al., 2009).

Differences in the sensitivity of COX-1 and COX-2 to inhibition by certain anti-inflammatory drugs led to the development of selective inhibitors of COX-2, including the coxibs (Grosser et al., 2010) (see Chapter 38). These drugs were hypothesized to offer therapeutic advantages over older NSAIDs (many of which are nonselective COX inhibitors) because COX-2 was thought to be the predominant source of PGs in inflammation, whereas COX-1 is the major source of cytoprotective PGs in the GI tract. Randomized trials of selective COX-2 inhibitors reported their superiority in GI safety over nonselective NSAID comparators.

However, there now is compelling evidence that COX-2 inhibitors confer a spectrum of cardiovascular hazards (myocardial infarction, stroke, systemic and pulmonary hypertension, congestive heart failure, and sudden cardiac death) (Grosser et al., 2010). The hazards can be explained sufficiently by suppression of cardioprotective COX-2–derived PGs, especially PGI_2, and the unrestrained effects of endogenous stimuli, such as platelet COX-1–derived TxA_2, on platelet activation, vascular proliferation and remodeling, hypertension, and atherogenesis.

Because LTs mediate inflammation, efforts have focused on development of LT receptor antagonists and selective inhibitors of the LOXs. *Zileuton*, an inhibitor of 5-LOX, and selective $CysLT_1$ receptor antagonists (*zafirlukast*, *pranlukast*, and *montelukast*) have established efficacy in the treatment of mild-to-moderate asthma (see Chapter 40). These treatments remain, however, less effective than inhaled corticosteroids. A common polymorphism in the gene for LTC_4 synthase that correlates with increased LTC_4 generation may be associated with higher asthma risk in some populations and with the efficacy of anti-LT therapy. Interestingly, although polymorphisms in the genes encoding 5-LOX or FLAP have yet to be linked to asthma, studies have demonstrated an association of these genes with myocardial infarction, stroke, and atherosclerosis (Peters-Golden and Henderson, 2007); thus, inhibition of LT biosynthesis may eventually prove to be useful in the prevention of cardiovascular disease.

Eicosanoid Degradation

Most eicosanoids are efficiently and rapidly inactivated (Figure 37–3). The enzymatic catabolic reactions are of two types:

- a rapid initial step, catalyzed by widely distributed PG-specific enzymes, wherein PGs lose most of their biological activity; and
- a second step in which these metabolites are oxidized, probably by enzymes identical to those responsible for the β and ω oxidation of fatty acids.

The lung, kidney, and liver play prominent roles in the enzymatically catalyzed reactions. Metabolic clearance requires an energy-dependent cellular uptake PG transporter and possibly other transporters (Schuster et al., 2002). The initial step is the oxidation of the 15-OH group to the corresponding ketone by PGDH. PGI_2 and TxA_2, however, undergo spontaneous hydrolysis as a first degradative step. LTC_4 degradation also occurs in the lungs, kidney, and liver but may also occur in LTC_4 via CYP4F enzymes. Inactivation of 15-hydroxyprostaglandin dehydrogenase, which elevates the capacity of tissues to form PGE_2, enhances tissue regeneration after hematopoietic stem cell transplantation and after hemihepatectomy (Zhang et al., 2015).

Pharmacological Properties

The eicosanoids function through activation of specific GPCRs (Table 37–1) that couple to intracellular second-messenger systems to modulate cellular activity (Figure 37–4).

Prostaglandin Receptors

The PGs activate membrane receptors locally near their sites of formation. Eicosanoid receptors interact with G_s, G_i, and G_q to modulate the activities of adenylyl cyclase and PLC (see Chapter 3). Single-gene products have been identified for the receptors for PGI_2 (the IP), $PGF_{2\alpha}$ (the FP), and TxA_2 (the TP). Four distinct PGE_2 receptors (EP_{1-4}) and two PGD_2 receptors (DP_1 and DP_2—also known as $CRTH_2$) have been cloned. Additional isoforms of the TP (α and β), FP (A and B), and EP_3 (I-VI, e, f) receptors can arise through differential messenger RNA splicing (Smyth et al., 2009; Woodward et al., 2011). The prostanoid receptors appear to derive from an ancestral EP receptor and share high homology. Phylogenetic comparison of this receptor family reveals three subclusters (Figure 37–4):

- the relaxant receptors EP_2, EP_4, IP, and DP_1, which increase cellular cyclic AMP generation;
- the contractile receptors EP_1, FP, and TP, which increase cytosolic levels of Ca^{2+}; and
- EP_3, which can couple to both elevation of cytosolic $[Ca^{2+}]$ and inhibition of adenylyl cyclase.

The DP_2 receptor is an exception and is unrelated to the other prostanoid receptors; rather, it is a member of the fMLP receptor superfamily.

Leukotriene Receptors

Two receptors exist for both LTB_4 (BLT_1 and BLT_2) and $CysLT_1$ and $CysLT_2$ (Bäck et al., 2011, 2014). The fMLP-2 receptor also binds LXA_4, but the functional importance of this ligand in vivo remains controversial. All are GPCRs and couple with G_q and other G proteins, depending on the cellular context. BLT_1 is expressed predominantly in leukocytes, thymus, and spleen, whereas BLT_2, the low-affinity receptor for LTB_4, is found in spleen, leukocytes, ovary, liver, and intestine.

$CysLT_1$ binds LTD_4 with higher affinity than LTC_4, while $CysLT_2$ shows equal affinity for both LTs. Both receptors bind LTE_4 with low affinity. Activation of G_q, leading to mobilization of intracellular Ca^{2+}, is the primary signaling pathway reported. Studies also have placed G_i downstream of $CysLT_2$. $CysLT_1$ is expressed in lung and intestinal smooth muscle, spleen, and peripheral blood leukocytes, whereas $CysLT_2$ is found in heart, spleen, peripheral blood leukocytes, adrenal medulla, and brain.

Other Agents

Other AA-derived products (e.g., isoprostanes, EETs) have potent biological activities, and there is evidence for distinct receptors for some of these substances. An orphan receptor, GPR31, has been identified as a receptor for 12(S)-HETE (Powell and Rokach, 2015). Specific receptors for the HETEs and EETs have been proposed, and evidence that the orphan receptor GPR75 functions as a receptor for 20-HETE has recently been provided (Garcia et al 2017).

Physiological Actions and Pharmacological Effects

The widespread biosynthesis and myriad pharmacological actions of eicosanoids are reflected in their complex physiology and pathophysiology. Knowledge of the distribution of the major eicosanoid receptors helps to put the complexity into perspective (Figure 37–1). The development of mice with targeted disruptions of genes regulating eicosanoid biosynthesis and eicosanoid receptors has revealed unexpected roles for these autacoids and has clarified hypotheses about their function (see Table 37–1). These topics, summarized here, were well reviewed by Smyth et al. (2011).

Cardiovascular System

Because of their short $t_{1/2}$, prostanoids act locally and generally are considered not to affect systemic vascular tone directly. They may modulate vascular tone locally at their sites of biosynthesis or through renal or other indirect effects. PGI_2, the major arachidonate metabolite released from the vascular endothelium, is derived primarily from COX-2 in humans. PGI_2 generation and release is regulated by shear stress and by both vasoconstrictor and vasodilator autacoids. In most vascular beds, PGE_2, PGI_2, and PGD_2 elicit vasodilation and a drop in blood pressure; physiologically,

TABLE 37–1 ■ HUMAN EICOSANOID RECEPTORS

RECEPTOR	LIGANDS 1° (2°)	PRIMARY COUPLING	MAJOR PHENOTYPE IN KNOCKOUT MICE
DP_1	PGD_2	G_s	↓ Allergic asthma
DP_2/$CHRT_2$	PGD_2 (15d-PGJ_2)	G_i	↑ or ↓ Allergic airway inflammation
EP_1	PGE_2 (PGI_2)	G_q	↓ Response of colon to carcinogens
EP_2	PGE_2	G_s	Impaired ovulation and fertilization Salt-sensitive hypertension
EP_3 I–VI, e, f	PGE_2	G_i; G_s; G_q	Resistance to pyrogens ↓ Acute cutaneous inflammation
EP_4	PGE_2	G_s	Patent ductus arteriosus ↓ Bone mass/density in aged mice ↑ Bowel inflammatory response ↓ Colon carcinogenesis
$FP_{A,B}$	$PGF_{2\alpha}$ (IsoPs)	G_q	Failure of parturition
IP	PGI_2 (PGE_2)	G_s	↑ Thrombotic response ↓ Response to vascular injury ↑ Atherosclerosis ↑ Cardiac fibrosis Salt-sensitive hypertension ↓ Joint inflammation
$TP_{\alpha\beta}$	TxA_2 (IsoPs)	G_q, G_i, $G_{12/13}$, G_{16}	↑ Bleeding time ↓ Response to vascular injury ↓ Atherosclerosis ↑ Survival after cardiac allograft
BLT_1	LTB_4	G_{16}, G_i	Some suppression of inflammatory response
BLT_2	LTB_4 [12(*S*)-HETE, 12(*R*)-HETE]	G_q-like, G_i-like, G_z-like	? (Reports of altered inflammatory processes)
$CysLT_1$	LTD_4 (LTC_4/LTE_4)	G_q	↓ Innate and adaptive immune vascular permeability response ↑ Pulmonary inflammatory and fibrotic response
$CysLT_2$	LTC_4/LTD_4 (LTE_4)	G_q	↓ Pulmonary inflammatory and fibrotic response

This table lists the major classes of eicosanoid receptors and their signaling characteristics. Splice variants for EP_3, TP, and FP are indicated.

these responses are quite local because endogenous prostanoids are paracrine mediators that do not circulate (Smyth et al., 2009). Responses to $PGF_{2\alpha}$ is a potent constrictor of both pulmonary arteries and veins. TxA_2 is a potent vasoconstrictor and a mitogen in smooth muscle cells.

Prostaglandin E_2 can also cause vasoconstriction through activation of EP_1 and EP_3. Infusion of PGD_2 in humans results in flushing, nasal stuffiness, and hypotension. Local subcutaneous release of PGD_2 contributes to dilation of the vasculature in the skin, which causes facial flushing associated with niacin treatment in humans. Subsequent formation of F-ring metabolites from PGD_2 may result in hypertension. PGI_2, the major prostanoid released from the vascular endothelium, relaxes vascular smooth muscle, causing hypotension and reflex tachycardia on intravenous administration. PGI_2 limits pulmonary hypertension induced by hypoxia and systemic hypertension induced by AngII and lowers pulmonary resistance in patients with pulmonary hypertension.

Cyclooxygenase 2–derived PGE_2, acting via the EP_4 maintains the ductus arteriosus patent until birth, when reduced PGE_2 levels (a consequence of increased PGE_2 metabolism) permit closure. The traditional NSAIDs induce closure of a patent ductus in neonates (see Chapter 38). Contrary to expectation, animals lacking the EP_4 die with a patent ductus during the perinatal period (Table 37–1) because the mechanism for control of the ductus in utero, and its remodeling at birth, is absent.

Infusion of PGs of the E and F series generally increases cardiac output. Weak, direct inotropic effects have been noted in various isolated preparations. In the intact animal, however, increased force of contraction and increased heart rate are, in large measure, a reflex consequence of a fall in total peripheral resistance. PGI_2 and PGE_2, acting on the IP or the EP_3, respectively, protect against oxidative injury in cardiac tissue.

Studies suggest a role for COX-2 in cardiac function. PGI_2 and PGE_2, acting on the IP or the EP_3, respectively, protect against oxidative injury in cardiac tissue. IP deletion augments myocardial ischemia/reperfusion injury, and both mPGE synthase-1 (mPGES-1) deletion and cardiomyocyte-specific deletion of the EP_4 exacerbate the decline in cardiac function after experimental myocardial infarction. COX-2–derived TxA_2 contributed to oxidant stress, isoprostane generation, and activation of the TP, and also possibly the FP, to increase cardiomyocyte apoptosis and fibrosis in a model of heart failure. Selective deletion of COX-2 in cardiomyocytes results in mild heart failure and a predisposition to arrhythmogenesis (Wang et al., 2009).

Leukotriene C_4 and LTD_4 can constrict or relax isolated vascular smooth muscle preparations, depending on the concentrations used and the vascular bed (Bäck et al., 2011). Although LTC_4 and LTD_4 have little effect on most large arteries or veins, nanomolar concentrations of these agents contract coronary arteries and distal segments of the pulmonary artery. The renal vasculature is resistant to this constrictor action, but the mesenteric vasculature is not. LTC_4 and LTD_4 act in the microvasculature to increase permeability of postcapillary venules; they are about 1000-fold more potent than histamine in this regard. At higher concentrations, LTC_4 and LTD_4 can constrict arterioles and reduce exudation of plasma. There is evidence for a role of the LTs in cardiovascular disease (Peters-Golden and Henderson, 2007). Human genetic studies have demonstrated a link

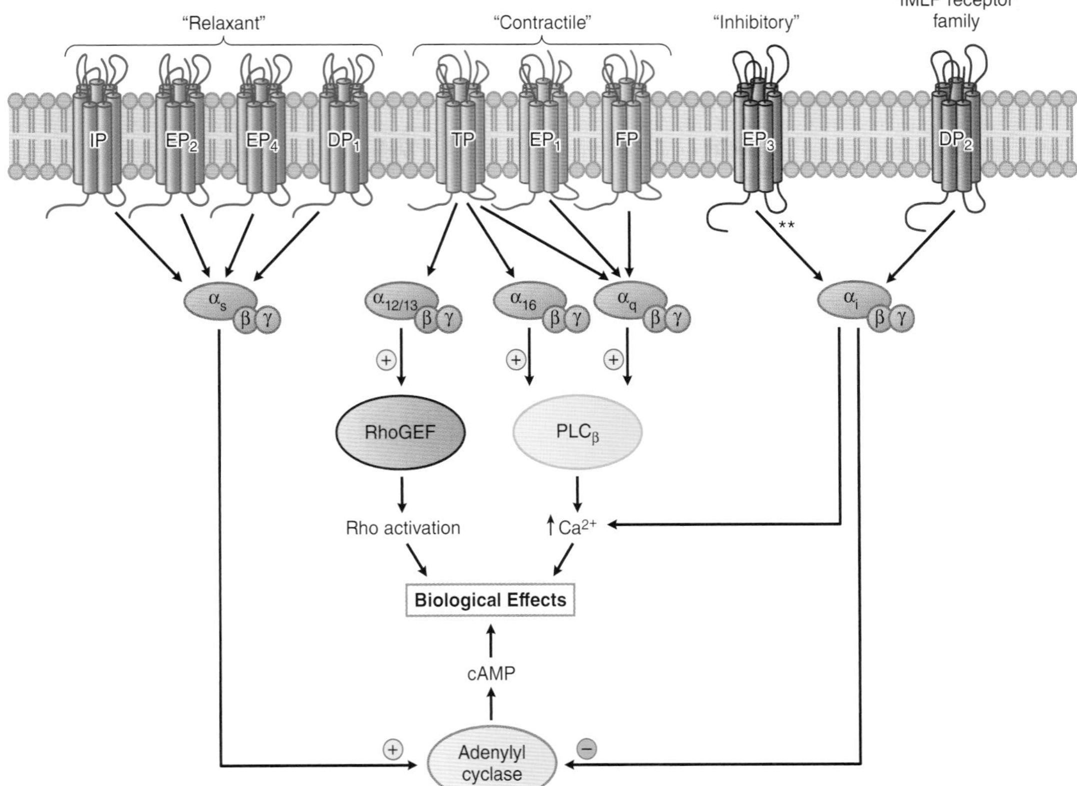

Figure 37–4 *Prostanoid receptors and their primary signaling pathways.* Prostanoid receptors are heptaspanning GPCRs. The terms *relaxant*, *contractile*, and *inhibitory* refer to the phylogenetic characterization of their primary effects. All EP_3 isoforms couple through G_i; some can also activate G_s or $G_{12/13}$ pathways. RhoGEF, Rho Guanine nucleotide Exchange Factor.

between cardiovascular disease and polymorphisms in the LT biosynthetic enzymes and FLAP.

The EETs cause vasodilation in a number of vascular beds by activating the large conductance Ca^{2+}-activated K^+ channels of smooth muscle cells, thereby hyperpolarizing the smooth muscle and causing relaxation. EETs likely also function as EDHFs, particularly in the coronary circulation. Endogenous biosynthesis of EETs is increased in human syndromes of hypertension.

Platelets

Platelet aggregation leads to activation of membrane phospholipases, with the release of AA and consequent eicosanoid biosynthesis. In human platelets, TxA_2 and 12-HETE are the two major eicosanoids formed, although eicosanoids from other sources (e.g., PGI_2 derived from vascular endothelium) also affect platelet function. Mature platelets express only COX-1. TxA_2, the major product of COX-1 in platelets, induces platelet aggregation and amplifies the signal for other, more potent platelet agonists, such as thrombin and ADP. The importance of the TxA_2 pathway is evident from the efficacy of platelet COX-1 inhibition with low-dose aspirin in the secondary prevention of myocardial infarction and ischemic stroke. The total biosynthesis of TxA_2, as determined by excretion of its urinary metabolites, is augmented in clinical syndromes of platelet activation, including unstable angina, myocardial infarction, and stroke. Deletion of the TP in the mouse prolongs bleeding time, renders platelets unresponsive to TP agonists, and blunts the response to vasopressors and the proliferative response to vascular injury (Smyth et al., 2009). TxA_2 induces platelet shape change, through G_{12}/G_{13}-mediated Rho/Rho kinase–dependent regulation of myosin light-chain phosphorylation, and aggregation through G_q-dependent activation of PKC. The actions of TxA_2 on platelets are restrained by its short $t_{1/2}$ (~30 sec), by rapid TP desensitization, and by endogenous inhibitors of platelet function, including NO and PGI_2.

Low concentrations of PGE_2, via the EP_3, enhance platelet aggregation. In contrast, higher concentrations of PGE_2, acting via the IP or possibly EP_2 or EP_4 inhibit platelet aggregation. Both PGI_2 and PGD_2 inhibit the aggregation of platelets. PGI_2 limits platelet activation by TxA_2, and disaggregates preformed platelet clumps. The increased incidence of myocardial infarction and stroke in patients receiving selective inhibitors of COX-2, explained by inhibition of COX-2–dependent PGI_2 formation, supports this concept (Grosser et al., 2010).

Inflammation and Immunity

Eicosanoids play a major role in inflammatory and immune responses. LTs generally are pro-inflammatory and interact with PGs to promote and sustain inflammation (Ricciotti and FitzGerald, 2011), although there are some exceptions, such as the inhibitory actions of PGE_2 on mast cell activation. PGs and LXs and related compounds may also contribute to the resolution of inflammation (Buckley et al., 2014). COX-2 is the major source of prostanoids formed during and after an inflammatory response.

Prostaglandin E_2 and PGI_2 are the predominant pro-inflammatory prostanoids as a result of increased vascular permeability and blood flow in the inflamed region. TxA_2 can increase platelet-leukocyte interaction. PGD_2 may contribute to the resolution of inflammation. Lymphocytes have a minimal capacity to form PGs, yet they are a primary target of their action. PGs generally inhibit lymphocyte function and proliferation, suppressing the immune response. PGE_2 depresses the humoral antibody response by inhibiting the differentiation of B lymphocytes into antibody-secreting plasma cells. PGE_2 acts on T lymphocytes to inhibit mitogen-stimulated proliferation and lymphokine release by sensitized cells. PGE_2 and TxA_2 also may play a role in T-lymphocyte development by regulating apoptosis of immature thymocytes. PGE_2, acting via EP2 and EP4, has been shown to interact with the programmed cell death ligand to restrain cytotoxic T-cell function and survival during chronic infection in mice (Chen et al., 2015). The COX-2/mPGES-1/PGE2 pathway can regulate PD-L1 expression in tumor infiltrating myeloid cells (Prima et al 2017). Given the efficacy of blockade of this pathway in a range of cancers, the possibility that blockade of PGE2 synthesis or action might augment this effect has been suggested. PGD_2 is a potent leukocyte chemoattractant, primarily through the DP_2.

The LTs are potent mediators of inflammation. Deletion of either 5-LOX or FLAP reduces inflammatory responses in model systems. LTB_4 is a potent chemotactic agent for neutrophils, T lymphocytes, eosinophils, monocytes, dendritic cells, and possibly also mast cells (Bäck et al., 2011). LTB_4 stimulates the aggregation of eosinophils and promotes degranulation and the generation of superoxide. LTB_4 promotes adhesion of neutrophils to vascular endothelial cells and their transendothelial migration and stimulates synthesis of pro-inflammatory cytokines from macrophages and lymphocytes.

The CysLTs are chemotaxins for eosinophils and monocytes. They also induce cytokine generation in eosinophils, mast cells, and dendritic cells. At higher concentrations, these LTs also promote eosinophil adherence, degranulation, cytokine or chemokine release, and oxygen radical formation. In addition, CysLTs contribute to inflammation by increasing endothelial permeability, thus promoting migration of inflammatory cells to the site of inflammation.

Bronchial and Tracheal Muscle

A complex mixture of autacoids is released when sensitized lung tissue is challenged by the appropriate antigen, including COX-derived bronchodilator and bronchoconstrictor substances. Amongst these, TxA_2, $PGF_{2\alpha}$, and PGD_2 contract, and PGE_2 and PGI_2 relax, bronchial and tracheal muscle. PGI_2 causes bronchodilation in most species; human bronchial tissue is particularly sensitive. PGI_2 antagonizes bronchoconstriction induced by other agents. PGD_2 appears to be the primary bronchoconstrictor prostanoid of relevance in humans. Polymorphisms in the genes for PGD_2 synthase and the TP have been associated with asthma in humans.

Roughly 10% of people given aspirin or NSAIDs develop bronchospasm. This appears attributable to a shift in AA metabolism to LT formation. This substrate diversion appears to involve COX-1, not COX-2. CysLTs are bronchoconstrictors that act principally on smooth muscle in the airways and are a thousand times more potent than histamine. They also stimulate bronchial mucus secretion and cause mucosal edema.

The CysLTs probably dominate during allergic constriction of the airway. Deficiency of 5-LOX leads to reduced influx of eosinophils in airways and attenuates bronchoconstriction. Furthermore, unlike COX inhibitors and histaminergic antagonists, CysLT receptor antagonists and 5-LOX inhibitors are effective in the treatment of human asthma (see Inhibitors of Eicosanoid Biosynthesis). The relatively slow LT metabolism in lung contributes to the long-lasting bronchoconstriction that follows challenge with antigen and may be a factor in the high bronchial tone that is observed in asthmatic patients in periods between acute attacks (see Chapter 40).

GI Smooth Muscle

Prostaglandin E_2 and PGF_2 stimulate contraction of the main longitudinal muscle from stomach to colon. PG endoperoxides, TxA_2, and PGI_2 also produce contraction but are less active. Circular muscle generally relaxes in response to PGE_2 and contracts in response to $PGF_{2\alpha}$. The LTs have potent contractile effects. PGs reduce transit time in the small intestine and colon. Diarrhea, cramps, and reflux of bile have been noted in response to oral PGE. PGEs and PGFs stimulate the movement of water and electrolytes into the intestinal lumen. Such effects may underlie the watery diarrhea that follows their oral or parenteral administration. PGE_2 appears to contribute to the water and electrolyte loss in cholera, a disease that is somewhat responsive to therapy with NSAIDs.

GI Secretion

In the stomach, PGE_2 and PGI_2 contribute to increased mucus secretion (*cytoprotection*), reduced acid secretion, and reduced pepsin content. PGE_2 and its analogues also inhibit gastric damage caused by a variety of ulcerogenic agents and promote healing of duodenal and gastric ulcers (see Chapter 49). Although COX-1 may be the dominant source of such cytoprotective PGs under physiological conditions, COX-2 predominates during ulcer healing. Selective inhibitors of COX-2 and deletion of the enzyme delay ulcer healing in rodents, but the impact of COX-2 inhibitors in humans is unclear. CysLTs, by constricting gastric blood vessels and enhancing production of pro-inflammatory cytokines, may contribute to the gastric damage.

Uterus

Strips of nonpregnant human uterus are contracted by $PGF_{2\alpha}$ and TxA_2 but are relaxed by PGEs. Sensitivity to the contractile response is most prominent before menstruation, whereas relaxation is greatest at midcycle. PGE_2, together with oxytocin, is essential for the onset of parturition. PGI_2 and high concentrations of PGE_2 produce relaxation. The intravenous infusion of low concentrations of PGE_2 or $PGF_{2\alpha}$ to pregnant women produces a dose-dependent increase in uterine tone and in the frequency and intensity of rhythmic uterine contractions. PGEs and PGFs are used to terminate pregnancy. Uterine responsiveness to PGs increases as pregnancy progresses but remains smaller than the response to oxytocin.

Kidney

Cyclooxygenase-2–derived PGE_2 and PGI_2 increase medullary blood flow, resulting in pressure diuresis, and inhibit tubular sodium reabsorption (Hao and Breyer, 2007). Expression of medullary COX-2 is increased during high salt intake. COX-1–derived products promote salt excretion in the collecting ducts. Cortical COX-2–derived PGE_2 and PGI_2 increase renal blood flow and glomerular filtration through their local vasodilating effects and as part of the tubuloglomerular feedback mechanism that controls renin release. Expression of COX-2 in macula densa cells increases in conditions of low distal tubular flow during low dietary salt intake or volume depletion. COX-2–derived PGE_2, and also possibly PGI_2, results in increased renin release, leading to sodium retention and elevated blood pressure.

TxA_2, generated at low levels in the normal kidney, has potent vasoconstrictor effects that reduce renal blood flow and glomerular filtration rate. Infusion of $PGF_{2\alpha}$ causes both natriuresis and diuresis. Conversely, $PGF_{2\alpha}$ may activate the renin-angiotensin system, contributing to elevated blood pressure. CYP epoxygenase products may regulate renal function. Both 20-HETE and the EETs are generated in renal tissue; 20-HETE constricts the renal arteries, while EETs mediate vasodilation and natriuresis.

Bartter syndrome is an autosomal recessive trait that manifests as hypokalemic metabolic alkalosis. The antenatal variant of Bartter syndrome is due to dysfunctional ROMK2 (Kir1.1), the K^+ channel that recycles K^+ into the tubular fluid. This syndrome also is known as *hyperPGE syndrome*. The relationship between dysfunctional ROMK2 and elevated PGE_2 synthesis is not clear; however, in patients with antenatal Bartter syndrome, inhibition of COX-2 ameliorates many of the clinical symptoms.

Eye

Prostaglandin $F_{2\alpha}$ induces constriction of the iris sphincter muscle, but its overall effect in the eye is to decrease intraocular pressure by increasing the aqueous humor outflow. A variety of FP agonists have proven effective in the treatment of open-angle glaucoma, a condition associated with the loss of COX-2 expression in the pigmented epithelium of the ciliary body (see Chapter 69).

Central Nervous System

Prostaglandin E_2 induces fever. The hypothalamus regulates the body temperature set point, which is elevated by endogenous pyrogens such as IL-1β, IL-6, TNF-α, and interferons (Morrison and Nakamura, 2011). The response is mediated by coordinate induction of COX-2 and mPGES-1 in the endothelium of blood vessels in the preoptic hypothalamic area to form PGE_2. PGE_2 can cross the blood-brain barrier and act on the EP_3 (and perhaps EP_1) on thermosensitive neurons, triggering the hypothalamus to elevate body temperature. Exogenous $PGF_{2\alpha}$ and PGI_2 induce fever but do not contribute to the endogenous pyretic response. PGD_2 appears to act on arachnoid trabecular cells in the basal forebrain to mediate an increase in extracellular adenosine that, in turn, facilitates induction of sleep. COX-2–derived prostanoids also have been implicated in the pathogenesis of several CNS degenerative disorders (e.g., Alzheimer disease, Parkinson disease; see Chapter 18).

Pain

Inflammatory mediators, including LTs and PGs, increase the sensitivity of nociceptors and potentiate pain perception. Centrally, both COX-1 and COX-2 are expressed in the spinal cord under basal conditions and release PGs in response to peripheral pain stimuli. Both PGE_2, through the EP_1 and EP_4 and PGI_2, via the IP, reduce the threshold to stimulation of nociceptors, causing "peripheral sensitization." PGE_2, and perhaps PGD_2, PGI_2, and $PGF_{2\alpha}$, can increase excitability in pain transmission neuronal pathways in the spinal cord, causing hyperalgesia and allodynia. LTB_4 also produces hyperalgesia. The release of these eicosanoids during the inflammatory process thus serves as an amplification system for the pain mechanism. The role of PGE_2 and PGI_2 in inflammatory pain is discussed in more detail in Chapter 38.

Endocrine System

The systemic administration of PGE_2 increases circulating concentrations of ACTH, growth hormone, prolactin, and gonadotropins. Other effects include stimulation of steroid production by the adrenals, stimulation of insulin release, and thyrotropin-like effects on the thyroid. PGE_2 works as part of a positive-feedback loop to induce oocyte maturation required for fertilization during and after ovulation. The critical role of $PGF_{2\alpha}$ in parturition relies on its ability to induce an oxytocin-dependent decline in progesterone levels. LOX metabolites also have endocrine effects. 12-HETE stimulates the release of aldosterone from the adrenal cortex and mediates a portion of the aldosterone release stimulated by AngII, but not that which occurs in response to ACTH.

Bone

Prostaglandins are strong modulators of bone metabolism. COX-1 is expressed in normal bone, while COX-2 is upregulated in settings such as inflammation and during mechanical stress. PGE_2 stimulates bone formation by increasing osteoblastogenesis and bone resorption via activation of osteoclasts.

Cancer

Pharmacological inhibition or genetic deletion of COX-2 restrains tumor formation in models of colon, breast, lung, and other cancers. Large human epidemiological studies reported that the incidental use of NSAIDs is associated with significant reductions in relative risk for developing these and other cancers. PGE_2 has been implicated as the primary pro-oncogenic prostanoid in multiple studies.

Therapeutic Uses

Inhibitors and Antagonists

The NSAIDs are used widely as anti-inflammatory drugs, whereas low-dose aspirin is employed frequently for cardioprotection (see Chapter 38). LT antagonists are useful clinically in the treatment of asthma, and FP agonists are used in the treatment of open-angle glaucoma (see Chapter 69). EP agonists are used to induce labor and to ameliorate gastric irritation owing to NSAIDs. DP_1 antagonists may be useful in offsetting the facial flushing associated with niacin. Orally active antagonists of LTC_4 and D_4, which block the $CysLT_1$ are used in the treatment of asthma that is mild to moderately severe (see Chapter 40). Their effectiveness in patients with aspirin-induced asthma also has been shown.

Prostanoids and Their Analogues

Prostanoids have a short $t_{1/2}$ in the circulation, and their systemic administration produces significant adverse effects. Nonetheless, several prostanoids are of clinical utility in the following situations.

Labor and Therapeutic Abortion. Prostaglandin E_2, $PGF_{2\alpha}$, and their analogues are used to induce labor at term and terminate pregnancy at any stage by promoting uterine contractions. These agents facilitate labor by promoting ripening and dilation of the cervix. Dinoprostone or misoprostol, synthetic analogues of PGE_2 and PGE_1, are used for cervical ripening and induction of labor and as abortifacients in the second trimester of pregnancy. Misoprostol, in combination with the antiprogesterone mifepristone (RU486), is highly effective in the termination of pregnancy. An analogue of $PGF_{2\alpha}$, carboprost tromethamine, is used to induce second-trimester abortions and to control postpartum hemorrhage that does not respond to conventional methods.

Maintenance of Patent Ductus Arteriosus. The ductus arteriosus in neonates is highly sensitive to vasodilation by PGE_1. Maintenance of a patent ductus may be important hemodynamically in some neonates with congenital heart disease. PGE_1 (alprostadil) is highly effective for palliative therapy to maintain temporary patency until surgery can be performed. Apnea is observed in about 10% of neonates treated, particularly those who weigh less than 2 kg at birth.

Gastric Cytoprotection. Several PG analogues are used to suppress gastric ulceration. Misoprostol, a PGE_1 analogue, is approved for prevention of NSAID-induced gastric ulcers and is about as effective as the proton pump inhibitor omeprazole (Chapter 49).

Impotence. Prostaglandin E_1 (alprostadil), given as an intracavernous injection or urethral suppository, is a second-line treatment of erectile dysfunction. Phosphodiesterase 5 inhibitors (e.g., sildenafil, tadalafil, vardenafil, and avanafil; see Chapter 45) have superseded PGE_1 as the preferred treatment of this condition.

Pulmonary Hypertension. Long-term therapy with PGI_2 (epoprostenol), via continuous intravenous infusion, improves symptoms and can delay or preclude the need for lung or heart-lung transplantation in a number of patients. Several orally available PGI_2 analogues with longer $t_{1/2}$ have been used clinically. Iloprost can be inhaled or delivered by intravenous administration (injectable form is not available in the U.S.). Treprostinil ($t_{1/2}$ ~ 4 h) may be delivered by continuous subcutaneous or intravenous infusion. Chapter 31 presents a comprehensive picture of the treatment of pulmonary artery hypertension.

Glaucoma. Latanoprost, a stable, long-acting $PGF_{2\alpha}$ derivative, was the first prostanoid used for glaucoma. Similar prostanoids with ocular hypotensive effects include bimatoprost, tafluprost, and travoprost. These drugs act as agonists at the FP and are administered as ophthalmic drops (see Chapter 69).

Platelet-Activating Factor

In 1971, Henson demonstrated that a soluble factor released from leukocytes caused platelets to aggregate. Benveniste and his coworkers characterized the factor as a polar lipid and named it *platelet-activating factor*. During this period, Muirhead described an antihypertensive polar renal lipid (APRL) produced by interstitial cells of the renal medulla that proved to be identical to PAF. Hanahan and coworkers then synthesized acetyl glyceryl ether phosphorylcholine (AGEPC) and determined that this phospholipid had chemical and biological properties identical to those of platelet activating factor (PAF). Independent determination of the structures of PAF and APRL showed them to be structurally identical to AGEPC. The commonly accepted name for this substance is PAF; however, its actions extend far beyond platelets.

Chemistry and Biosynthesis

Platelet-activating factor (1-*O*-alkyl-2-acetyl-*sn*-glycero-3-phosphocholine) represents a family of phospholipids because the alkyl group at position 1 can vary in length from 12 to 18 carbon atoms (Prescott et al., 2000). In human neutrophils, PAF consists predominantly of a mixture of the 16- and 18-carbon ethers, but its composition may change when cells are stimulated.

$$\begin{array}{l} {}^{1}CH_2-O-(CH_2)_n-CH_3 \\ CH_3-\underset{\|}{\overset{}{C}}(=O)-O-{}^{2}C-H \\ {}^{3}CH_2-O-P(=O)(O^-)-O-CH_2-CH_2-\overset{+}{N}(CH_3)_3 \end{array}$$

PLATELET-ACTIVATING FACTOR (n = 11 to 17)

Synthesis of eicosanoids and PAF depends on PLA_2 activity. The major biosynthetic pathway for PAF, the remodeling pathway, involves the precursor 1-*O*-alkyl-2-acyl-glycerophosphocholine, a membrane lipid; the 2-acyl substituents include AA. PAF is synthesized from this substrate in two steps (Figure 37–5). The rate-limiting step is the second one, acetyl-coenzyme-A-lyso-PAF acetyltransferase. The synthesis of PAF may be stimulated during antigen-antibody reactions or by a variety of agents, including chemotactic peptides, thrombin, collagen, and other autacoids; PAF also can stimulate its own formation. Both the PL and acetyltransferase are Ca^{2+}-dependent enzymes; thus, PAF synthesis is regulated by the availability of Ca^{2+}. The inactivation of PAF is catalyzed by PAF-AHs. PAF is inactivated by PAF-AH–catalyzed hydrolysis of the acetyl group, generating Lyso-PAF, which is then converted to a 1-*O*-alkyl-2-acyl-glycerophosphocholine by an acyltransferase (McIntyre et al., 2009; Stafforini et al., 2003).

Synthesis of PAF also can occur de novo by transfer of a phosphocholine substituent to alkyl acetyl glycerol by a lyso-glycerophosphate acetyl–coenzyme A transferase. This pathway may contribute to physiological levels of PAF for normal cellular functions. PAF-like molecules can be formed from oxidized phospholipids (oxPLs) (Stafforini et al., 2003). These compounds are increased in settings of oxidant stress, such as cigarette smoking, and differ structurally from PAF in that they contain a fatty acid at the *sn*-1 position of glycerol joined through an ester bond and various short-chain acyl groups at the *sn*-2 position. oxPLs mimic the structure of PAF, bind to its receptor, and elicit the same responses. Unlike the synthesis of PAF, which is highly controlled, oxPL production is unregulated. Degradation of oxPLs by PAF-AH is therefore necessary to suppress toxicity. Increased levels of plasma PAF-AH have been reported in colon cancer, cardiovascular disease, and stroke.

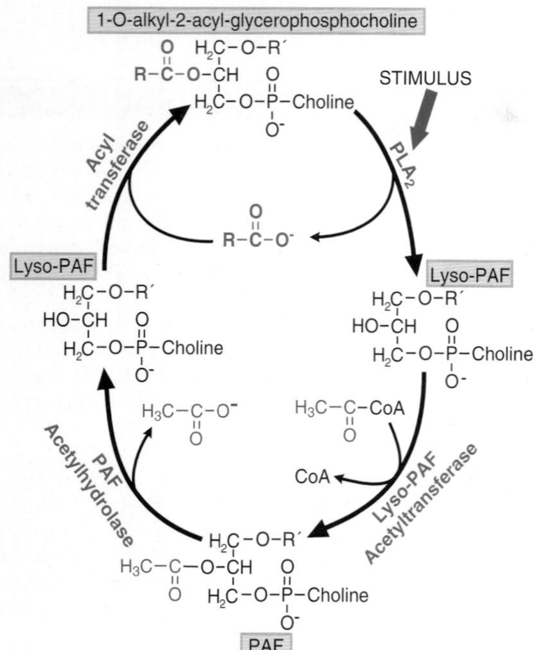

Figure 37–5 *Synthesis and degradation of PAF.* $RCOO^-$ is a mixture of fatty acids but is enriched in AA that may be metabolized to eicosanoids.

Sites of PAF Synthesis

Platelet-activating factor is not stored in cells but is synthesized in response to stimulation. PAF is synthesized by platelets, neutrophils, monocytes, mast cells, eosinophils, renal mesangial cells, renal medullary cells, and vascular endothelial cells. Depending on cell type, PAF can either remain cell associated or be secreted. For example, PAF is released from monocytes but retained by leukocytes and endothelial cells. In endothelial cells, PAF is displayed on the surface for juxtacrine signaling and stimulates adherent leukocytes.

Mechanism of Action of PAF

Extracellular PAF exerts its actions by stimulating a specific GPCR (Honda et al., 2002). The PAF receptor couples to Gq (to activate the PLC-IP_3–Ca^{2+} pathway) and to Gi (to inhibit adenylyl cyclase). Consequent activation of PLs A_2, C, and D gives rise to second messengers, including AA-derived PGs, TxA_2, or LTs, which may function as mediators of the effects of PAF.

In addition, p38 mitogen-activated protein kinase is activated downstream of the PAF-receptor–Gq interaction, while extracellular signal–regulated kinase activation can occur via interaction of activated PAF receptor with Gq, Go, or their $\beta\gamma$ subunits, or via transactivation of the EGF receptor, leading to nuclear factor kappa B activation. PAF exerts many of its important pro-inflammatory actions without leaving its cell of origin. For example, PAF is synthesized in a regulated fashion by endothelial cells stimulated by inflammatory mediators. This PAF is presented on the surface of the endothelium, where it activates the PAF receptor on juxtaposed cells, including platelets, PMNs, and monocytes, and acts cooperatively with P selectin to promote adhesion. This function of PAF is important for orchestrating the interaction of platelets and circulating inflammatory cells with the inflamed endothelium.

Physiological and Pathological Functions of PAF

Platelet-activating factor generally is viewed as a mediator of pathological events and has been implicated in allergic asthma, endotoxic shock, acute pancreatitis, certain cancers, dermal inflammation, and inflammatory cardiovascular diseases such as atherosclerosis.

Inflammatory and Allergic Responses

Experimental administration of PAF reproduces many of the signs and symptoms in anaphylactic shock. However, the effects of PAF antagonists in the treatment of inflammatory and allergic disorders have been disappointing. In patients with asthma, PAF antagonists partially inhibit the bronchoconstriction induced by antigen challenge but not by challenges by methacholine, exercise, or inhalation of cold air. These results may reflect the complexity of these pathological conditions and the likelihood that other mediators contribute to the inflammation associated with these disorders.

Cardiovascular System

Platelet-activating factor is a potent vasodilator in most vascular beds; when administered intravenously, it causes hypotension. PAF-induced vasodilation is independent of effects on sympathetic innervation, the renin-angiotensin system, or AA metabolism and likely results from a combination of direct and indirect actions. PAF may, alternatively, induce vasoconstriction depending on the concentration, vascular bed, and involvement of platelets or leukocytes. For example, the intracoronary administration of very low concentrations of PAF increases coronary blood flow by a mechanism that involves the release of a platelet-derived vasodilator. Coronary blood flow is decreased at higher doses by the formation of intravascular aggregates of platelets or the formation of TxA_2. The pulmonary vasculature also is constricted by PAF, and a similar mechanism is thought to be involved.

Intradermal injection of PAF causes an initial vasoconstriction followed by a typical wheal and flare. PAF increases vascular permeability and edema in the same manner as histamine and bradykinin. The increase in permeability is due to contraction of venular endothelial cells, but PAF is more potent than histamine or bradykinin by three orders of magnitude.

Platelets

The PAF receptor is constitutively expressed on the surface of platelets. PAF potently stimulates platelet aggregation. The intravenous injection of PAF causes formation of intravascular platelet aggregates and thrombocytopenia. Although this is accompanied by the release of TxA_2 and the granular contents of the platelet, PAF does not require the presence of TxA_2 or other aggregating agents to produce this effect. PAF antagonists fail to block thrombin-induced aggregation, even though they prolong bleeding time and prevent thrombus formation in some experimental models. Thus, PAF may contribute to thrombus formation, but it does not function as an independent mediator of platelet aggregation.

Leukocytes

Platelet-activating factor is a potent and common activator of inflammatory cells. PAF stimulates a variety of responses in PMNs (eosinophils, neutrophils, and basophils). PAF stimulates PMNs to aggregate, degranulate, and generate free radicals and LTs. PAF is a potent chemotactic for eosinophils, neutrophils, and monocytes and promotes PMN-endothelial adhesion contributing, along with other adhesion molecular systems, to leukocyte rolling, tight adhesion, and migration through the endothelial monolayer. PAF also stimulates basophils to release histamine, activates mast cells, and induces cytokine release from monocytes. In addition, PAF promotes aggregation of monocytes and degranulation of eosinophils.

Smooth Muscle

Platelet-activating factor contracts GI, uterine, and pulmonary smooth muscle. PAF enhances the amplitude of spontaneous uterine contractions; these contractions are inhibited by inhibitors of PG synthesis. PAF does not affect tracheal smooth muscle but contracts airway smooth muscle. When given by aerosol, PAF increases airway resistance as well as the responsiveness to other bronchoconstrictors. PAF also increases mucus secretion and the permeability of pulmonary microvessels.

Stomach

In addition to contracting the fundus of the stomach, PAF is the most potent known ulcerogen. When given intravenously, it causes hemorrhagic erosions of the gastric mucosa that extend into the submucosa.

Kidney

Platelet-activating factor decreases renal blood flow, glomerular filtration rate, urine volume, and excretion of Na^+ without changes in systemic hemodynamics. PAF exerts a receptor-mediated biphasic effect on afferent arterioles, dilating them at low concentrations and constricting them at higher concentrations. The vasoconstrictor effect appears to be mediated, at least in part, by COX products, whereas vasodilation is a consequence of the stimulation of NO production by endothelium.

Other

Platelet-activating factor, a potent mediator of angiogenesis, has been implicated in breast and prostate cancer. PAF-AH deficiency has been associated with small increases in a range of cardiovascular and thrombotic diseases in some human populations.

PAF Receptor Antagonists

Several experimental PAF receptor antagonists exist that selectively inhibit the actions of PAF in vivo and in vitro. None has proven clinically useful. Thus, synthetic PAF, when administered in sufficient quantities, exerts a broad spectrum of effects. However, the evidence of its importance as an endogenous mediator remains to be established. Interestingly, inhibition of PAF-AH, which would be expected to elevate endogenous levels of PAF, was pursued as the protein also functions as a lipoprotein-associated PLA_2. Trials of an inhibitor, darapladib, failed to establish either clinical efficacy attributable to eicosanoid suppression or an adverse effect profile potentially attributable to increased levels of PAF (O'Donoghue et al., 2014).

Acknowledgment: *Jason D. Morrow, L. Jackson Roberts II, and Anne Burke contributed to this chapter in earlier editions of this book. We have retained some of their text in the current edition.*

Drug Facts for Your Personal Formulary: *Eicosanoids*

Drug	Therapeutic Uses	Clinical Pharmacology and Tips
Prostanoids and Prostanoid Analogues: PGE_1/PGE_2		
Alprostadil (PGE_1)	• Erectile dysfunction • Temporary maintenance of patent ductus arteriosus in neonates	• Rapidly metabolized • Prolonged erection (4–6 h) in 4% of patients • Apnea in 10%–12% of neonates with congenital heart defects; ventilator assistance should be available during treatment
Misoprostol (PGE_1 analogue)	• Protection from NSAID-induced gastric toxicity	• Contraindicated for use in pregnant women; women who may become pregnant must use birth control when taking misoprostol • Combined with mifepristone to terminate early pregnancy
Dinoprostone (PGE_2)	• Labor induction	• Rapidly metabolized
Prostanoids and Prostanoid Analogues: PGI_2 (Prostacyclin)		
Epoprostenol (PGI_2)	• Pulmonary arterial hypertension	• Rapidly metabolized • Administered by intravenous infusion • Most common dose-limiting adverse effects are nausea, vomiting, headache, hypotension, and flushing
Iloprost (PGI_2 analogue)	• Pulmonary arterial hypertension	• Administered by inhalation • Synthetic PGI_2 analogue with longer $t_{1/2}$ • May increase risk of bleeding when used with anticoagulants or platelet inhibitors
Treprostinil (PGI_2 analogue)	• Pulmonary arterial hypertension	• May be administered by subcutaneous/intravenous infusion or by inhalation • Adverse events similar to Iloprost
Prostanoids and Prostanoid Analogues: $PGF_{2\alpha}$		
Carboprost tromethamine	• Abortifacient (second trimester) • Postpartum hemorrhage	• Common adverse effects are vomiting, diarrhea, nausea, fever, flushing

Drug Facts for Your Personal Formulary: *Eicosanoids(continued)*

Drug	Therapeutic Uses	Clinical Pharmacology and Tips
Prostanoids and Prostanoid Analogues: $PGF_{2\alpha}$		
Bimatoprost	• Ocular hypertension • Open-angle glaucoma • Hypotrichosis of the eyelashes	• Upper respiratory tract infections in about 10% of patients • May cause changes in pigmentation and hair growth
Latanoprost	• Ocular hypertension • Open-angle glaucoma	• Increased iris pigmentation with time
Tafluprost	• Ocular hypertension • Open-angle glaucoma	• Metabolized to active drug in the eye • May cause increased iris pigmentation
Travoprost	• Ocular hypertension • Open-angle glaucoma	• May cause increased iris pigmentation
Nonsteroidal Anti-Inflammatory Drugs		
Listed in Chapter 38		
Cysteinyl Leukotriene Receptor Antagonists/5-Lipoxygenase Inhibitors		
Listed in Chapter 40		

Bibliography

Bäck M, et al. International Union of Basic and Clinical Pharmacology. LXXXIV: leukotriene receptor nomenclature, distribution, and pathophysiological functions. *Pharmacol Rev,* **2011**, *63*:539–584.

Bäck M, et al. Update on leukotriene, lipoxin and oxoeicosanoid receptors: IUPHAR Review 7. *Br J Pharmacol,* **2014**, *171*:3551–3574.

Buckley CD, et al. Proresolving lipid mediators and mechanisms in the resolution of acute inflammation. *Immunity,* **2014**, *40*:315–327.

Chen JH, et al. Prostaglandin E_2 and programmed cell death 1 signaling coordinately impair CTL function and survival during chronic viral infection. *Nat Med,* **2015**, *4*:327–334.

Duchez AC, et al. Platelet microparticles are internalized in neutrophils via the concerted activity of 12-lipoxygenase and secreted phospholipase A2-IIA. *Proc Natl Acad Sci U S A,* **2015**, *112*:E3564–E3573.

Evans JF, et al. What's all the FLAP about? 5-Lipoxygenase-activating protein inhibitors for inflammatory diseases. *Trends Pharmacol Sci,* **2008**, *29*:72–78.

Fleming I. The pharmacology of the cytochrome P450 epoxygenase/soluble epoxide hydrolase axis in the vasculature and cardiovascular disease. *Pharmacol Rev,* **2014**, *66*:1106–1140.

Garcia, V et al. 20-HETE signals through G-protein–coupled receptor GPR75 (Gq) to affect vascular function and trigger hypertension. *Circ Res,* **2017**, *120*:1776–1788.

Grosser T, et al. Emotion recollected in tranquility: lessons learned from the COX-2 saga. *Annu Rev Med,* **2010**, *61*:17–33.

Haeggström JZ, Funk CD. Lipoxygenase and leukotriene pathways: biochemistry, biology, and roles in disease. *Chem Rev,* **2011**, *111*: 5866–5898.

Hao CM, Breyer MD. Physiologic and pathophysiologic roles of lipid mediators in the kidney. *Kidney Int,* **2007**, *71*:1105–1115.

Honda Z, et al. Platelet-activating factor receptor. *J Biochem,* **2002**, *131*:773–779.

Janusz JM, et al. New cyclooxygenase-2/5-lipoxygenase inhibitors. 1. 7-tert-buty1-2,3-dihydro-3-dimethylbenzofuran derivatives as gastrointestinal safe antiinflammatory and analgesic agents: discovery and variation of the 5-keto substituent. *J Med Chem,* **1998**, *41*:1112–1123.

McIntyre TM, et al. The emerging roles of PAF acetylhydrolase. *J Lipid Res,* **2009**, *50*(suppl):S255–S259.

Milne GL, et al. The isoprostanes-25 years later. *Biochim Biophys Acta,* **2015**, *1851*:433–445.

Minutoli L, et al. A dual inhibitor of cyclooxygenase and 5-lipoxygenase protects against kainic acid-induced brain injury. *Neuromolecular Med,* **2015**, *17*:192–201.

Morrison SF, Nakamura K. Central neural pathways for thermoregulation. *Front Biosci,* **2011**, *16*:74–104.

Oak NR, et al. Inhibition of 5-LOX, COX-1, and COX-2 increases tendon healing and reduces muscle fibrosis and lipid accumulation after rotator cuff repair. *Am J Sports Med,* **2014**, *42*:2860–2868.

O'Donoghue ML, et al. Effect of darapladib on major coronary events after an acute coronary syndrome: the SOLID-TIMI 52 randomized clinical trial. *JAMA,* **2014**, *312*:1006–1015.

Peters-Golden M, Henderson WR Jr. Leukotrienes. *N Engl J Med,* **2007**, *357*:1841–1854.

Prima V, et al. COX2/mPGES1/PGE2 pathway regulates PD-L1 expression in tumor-associated macrophages and myeloid-derived suppressor cells. *Proc Natl Acad Sci USA,* **2017**, *114*:1117–1122.

Powell WS, Rokach J. Biosynthesis, biological effects, and receptors of hydroxyeicosatetraenoic acids (HETEs) and oxoeicosatetraenoic acids (oxo-ETEs) derived from arachidonic acid. *Biochim Biophys Acta,* **2015**, *1851*:340–355.

Prescott SM, et al. Platelet-activating factor and related lipid mediators. *Annu Rev Biochem,* **2000**, *69*:419–445.

Ricciotti EI, FitzGerald GA. Prostaglandins and inflammation. *Arterioscler Thromb Vasc Biol,* **2011**, *5*:986–1000.

Rouzer CA, Marnett LJ. Cyclooxygenases: structural and functional insights. *J Lipid Res,* **2009**, *50*(suppl):S29–S34.

Schuster VL. Prostaglandin transport. *Prostaglandins Other Lipid Mediat,* **2002**, *68–69*:633–647.

Skarke C, et al. Bioactive products formed in humans from fish oils. *J Lipid Res,* **2015**, *56*:1808–20.

Smith WL, et al. Enzymes of the cyclooxygenase pathways of prostanoid biosynthesis. *Chem Rev,* **2011**, *111*:5821–5865.

Smyth EM, et al. Lipid-derived autacoids. In: Brunton L, Chabner B, Knollmann B, eds. *The Pharmacological Basis of Therapeutics.* 12th ed. McGraw-Hill, New York, **2011**, 942–948.

Smyth EM, et al. Prostanoids in health and disease. *J Lipid Res,* **2009**, *50*(suppl):S423–S428.

Stafforini DM, et al. Platelet-activating factor, a pleiotrophic mediator of physiological and pathological processes. *Crit Rev Clin Lab Sci,* **2003**, *40*:643–672.

Wang D, et al. Cardiomyocyte cyclooxygenase-2 influences cardiac rhythm and function. *Proc Natl Acad Sci USA,* **2009**, *109*:7548–7552.

Woodward DF, et al. International Union of Basic and Clinical Pharmacology. LXXXIII: classification of prostanoid receptors, updating 15 years of progress. *Pharmacol Rev,* **2011**, *63*:471–538.

Xu GL, et al. Anti-inflammatory effects and gastrointestinal safety of NNU-hdpa, a novel dual COX/5-LOX inhibitor. *Eur J Pharmacol,* **2009**, *611*:100–106.

Zhang Y, et al. Tissue regeneration. Inhibition of the prostaglandin-degrading enzyme 15-PGDH potentiates tissue regeneration. *Science,* **2015**, *348*:aaa2340.

Pharmacotherapy of Inflammation, Fever, Pain, and Gout

Tilo Grosser, Emer M. Smyth, and Garret A. FitzGerald

第三十八章 炎症、发热、疼痛和痛风的药物治疗

中文导读

本章主要介绍：炎症、疼痛和发热；非甾体抗炎药（NSAIDs），包括作用机制、治疗应用、NSAIDs治疗的不良反应、药物相互作用、儿童和老年人用药；NSAIDs的特性，包括阿司匹林及其他水杨酸类、对乙酰氨基酚、乙酸衍生物、丙酸衍生物、灭酸酯类、烯醇酸类（昔康类）、针对COX-2开发的选择性NSAIDs；病症缓解性抗风湿药；痛风的药物治疗，包括秋水仙碱、别嘌呤醇、非布司他、尿酸酶和促尿酸排泄药。

Abbreviations

AA: arachidonic acid
ACE: angiotensin-converting enzyme
ASA: acetylsalicylic acid/aspirin
AUC: area under the curve
COX: cyclooxygenase
CSF: cerebrospinal fluid
G6PD: glucose-6-phosphate dehydrogenase
GSH: glutathione
15(*R*)-HETE: 15(*R*)-hydroxyeicosatetraenoic acid
5-HIAA: 5-hydroxyindoleacetic acid
5HT: 5-hydroxytryptamine/serotonin
Ig: immunoglobulin
IL: interleukin
IM: intramuscular
IV: intravenous
LOX: lipooxygenase
LT: leukotriene
MI: myocardial infarction
NAC: *N*-acetylcysteine
NAPQI: *N*-acetyl-*p*-benzoquinone imine
NSAID: nonsteroidal anti-inflammatory drug
OAT: organic anion transporter
OTC: over the counter
PAF: platelet-activating factor
PG: prostaglandin
PGI_2: prostacyclin
PPI: proton pump inhibitor
TNF: tumor necrosis factor
Tx: thromboxane
UGT: uridine diphosphate glucuronosyltransferase
URAT: urate transporter
XO: xanthine oxidase

HISTORICAL PERSPECTIVE

The history of aspirin provides an interesting example of the translation of a compound from the realm of herbal folklore to contemporary therapeutics. The use of willow bark and leaves to relieve fever has been attributed to Hippocrates but was most clearly documented by Edmund Stone in a 1763 letter to the president of the Royal Society. Similar properties were attributed to potions from meadowsweet (*Spiraea ulmaria*), from which the name aspirin is derived. Salicin was crystallized in 1829 by Leroux, and Pina isolated salicylic acid in 1836. In 1859, Kolbe synthesized salicylic acid, and by 1874, it was being produced industrially. It soon was being used for rheumatic fever and gout and as a general antipyretic. However, its unpleasant taste and adverse GI effects made it difficult to tolerate for more than short periods. In 1899, Hoffmann, a chemist at Bayer Laboratories, sought to improve the adverse effect profile of salicylic acid (which his father was taking with difficulty for arthritis). Hoffmann came across the earlier work of the French chemist Gerhardt, who had acetylated salicylic acid in 1853, apparently ameliorating its adverse effect profile, but without improving its efficacy, and therefore abandoned the project. Hoffmann resumed the quest, and Bayer began testing acetylsalicylic acid (ASA) in animals by 1899 and proceeded soon thereafter to human studies and the marketing of aspirin.

Acetaminophen was first used in medicine by von Mering in 1893. However, it gained popularity only after 1949, when it was recognized as the major active metabolite of both acetanilide and phenacetin. Acetanilide is the parent member of this group of drugs. It was introduced into medicine in 1886 under the name antifebrin by Cahn and Hepp, who had discovered its antipyretic action accidentally. However, acetanilide proved to be excessively toxic. A number of chemical derivatives were developed and tested. One of the more satisfactory of these was phenacetin. It was introduced into therapy in 1887 and was extensively employed in analgesic mixtures until it was implicated in analgesic abuse nephropathy, hemolytic anemia, and bladder cancer; it was withdrawn in the 1980s.

This chapter describes the non-steroidal anti-inflammatory drugs (NSAIDs) used to treat inflammation, pain, and fever and the drugs used for hyperuricemia and gout. The NSAIDs are first considered by class, then by groups of chemically similar agents described in more detail. Many of the basic properties of these drugs are summarized in Tables 38–1, 38–2, and 38–3.

The NSAIDs act by inhibiting the prostaglandin (PG) G/H synthase enzymes, colloquially known as the cyclooxygenases (COXs) (see Chapter 37). There are two forms, COX-1 and COX-2. The inhibition of COX-2 is thought to mediate, in large part, the antipyretic, analgesic, and anti-inflammatory actions of NSAIDs. Adverse reactions are largely caused by the inhibition of COX-1 and COX-2 in tissues in which they fulfill physiological functions, such as the GI tract, the kidney, and the cardiovascular system. Aspirin is the only irreversible inhibitor of the COX enzymes in clinical use. All other NSAIDs bind the COXs reversibly and act either by competing directly with arachidonic acid (AA) at the active site of COX-1 and COX-2 or by changing their steric confirmation in a way that alters their ability to bind arachidonic acid. Acetaminophen (paracetamol) is effective as an antipyretic and analgesic agent at typical doses that partly inhibit COXs and has only weak anti-inflammatory activity. Purposefully designed selective inhibitors of COX-2 (celecoxib, etoricoxib) are a subclass of NSAIDs; several of the older traditional NSAIDs, such as diclofenac and meloxicam (see Figure 38–1) also selectively inhibit COX-2 at therapeutic doses.

Inflammation, Pain, and Fever

Inflammation

The inflammatory process is the immune system's protective response to an injurious stimulus. It can be evoked by noxious agents, infections, and physical injuries, which release damage- and pathogen-associated molecules that are recognized by cells charged with immune surveillance (Tang et al., 2012). The ability to mount an inflammatory response is essential for survival in the face of environmental pathogens and injury. In some situations and diseases, inflammation may be exaggerated and sustained without apparent benefit and even with severe adverse consequences (e.g., hypersensitivity, automimmune diseases, chronic inflammation). The inflammatory response is characterized mechanistically by

- transient local vasodilation and increased capillary permeability;
- infiltration of leukocytes and phagocytic cells; and
- resolution with or without tissue degeneration and fibrosis.

Many molecules are involved in the promotion and resolution of the inflammatory process. Histamine, bradykinin, 5HT, prostanoids, LTs, PAF, and an array of cytokines are important mediators (see Chapters 34, 37, and 39). Prostanoid biosynthesis is significantly increased in inflamed tissue. PGE_2 and prostacyclin (PGI_2) are the primary prostanoids that mediate inflammation. They increase local blood flow,

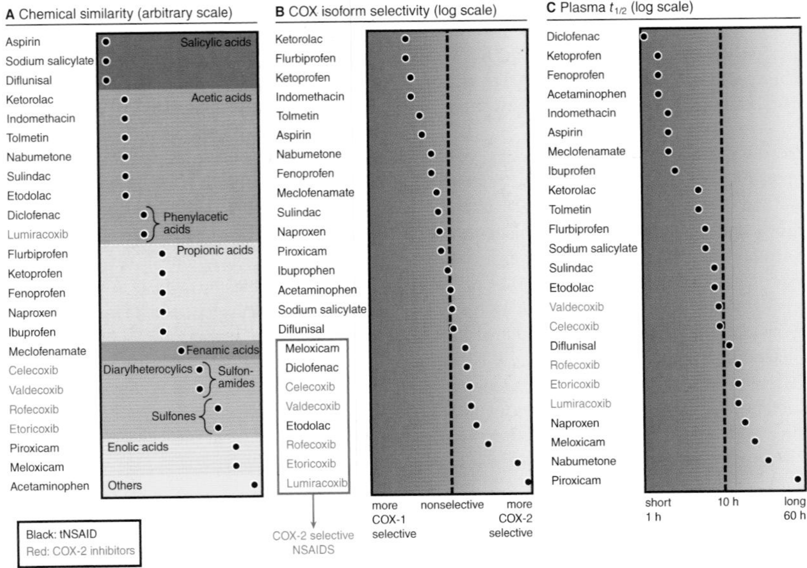

Figure 38–1 *Classification of NSAIDs by chemical similarity* (**A**), *COX isoform selectivity* (**B**), *and plasma* $t_{1/2}$ (**C**). The COX selectivity chart is plotted from data published in Warner T., et al. Nonsteroid drug selectivities for cyclooxygenase-1 rather than cyclooxygenase-2 are associated with human gastrointestinal toxicity: a full in vitro analysis. *Proc Natl Acad Sci U S A*, **1999**, *96*:7563–7568; and FitzGerald GA, Patrono C. The coxibs, selective inhibitors of cyclooxygenase-2. *N Engl J Med*, **2001**, *345*:433–442.

vascular permeability, and leukocyte infiltration through activation of their respective receptors, EP_2 and IP. PGD_2, a major product of mast cells, contributes to inflammation in allergic responses, particularly in the lung.

Activation of endothelial cells plays a key role in recruiting circulating cells to inflammatory sites (Muller, 2011). Endothelial activation results in leukocyte rolling and adhesion as the leukocytes recognize newly expressed selectins, integrins, and adhesion molecules. PGE_2 and TxA_2 enhance leukocyte chemoattraction and endothelial adhesion.

The recruitment of inflammatory cells to sites of injury also involves the concerted interactions of the complement factors PAF, and eicosanoids such as LTB_4 (see Chapter 37). All can act as chemotactic agonists. Cytokines play essential roles in orchestrating the inflammatory process, especially TNF and IL-1. Several biological anti-inflammatory therapeutics target these cytokines or their signaling pathways (see Chapter 35). Other cytokines and growth factors (e.g., IL-2, IL-6, IL-8, granulocyte-macrophage colony-stimulating factor) contribute to manifestations of the inflammatory response. The concentrations of many of these factors are increased in the synovia of patients with inflammatory arthritis. Glucocorticoids interfere with the synthesis and actions of cytokines, such as IL-1 or TNF-α (see Chapter 35). Although some of the actions of these cytokines are accompanied by the release of PGs and TxA_2, COX inhibitors appear to block primarily their pyrogenic effects.

Pain

Nociceptors, peripheral terminals of primary afferent fibers that sense pain, can be activated by various stimuli, such as heat, acids, or pressure. Inflammatory mediators released from nonneuronal cells during tissue injury increase the sensitivity of nociceptors and potentiate pain perception. Among these mediators are bradykinin, H^+, 5HT, ATP, neurotrophins (nerve growth factor), LTs, and PGs. PGE_2 and PGI_2 reduce the threshold to stimulation of nociceptors, causing *peripheral sensitization*. Reversal of peripheral sensitization is thought to represent the mechanistic basis for the peripheral component of the analgesic activity of NSAIDs. NSAIDs may also have important central actions in the spinal cord and brain. Both COX-1 and COX-2 are expressed in the spinal cord under basal conditions and release PGs in response to peripheral pain stimuli.

Centrally active PGE_2 and perhaps also PGD_2, PGI_2, and $PGF_{2\alpha}$ contribute to *central sensitization*, an increase in excitability of spinal dorsal horn neurons that causes hyperalgesia and allodynia in part by disinhibition of glycinergic pathways (Chen et al., 2013). Central sensitization reflects the plasticity of the nociceptive system that is invoked by injury. This usually is reversible within hours to days following adequate responses of the nociceptive system (e.g., in postoperative pain). However, chronic inflammatory diseases may cause persistent modification of the architecture of the nociceptive system, which may lead to long-lasting changes in its responsiveness. These mechanisms contribute to chronic pain.

Fever

The hypothalamus regulates the set point at which body temperature is maintained. This set point is elevated in fever, reflecting an infection, or resulting from tissue damage, inflammation, graft rejection, or malignancy. These conditions all enhance formation of cytokines such as IL-1β, IL-6, TNF-α, and interferons, which act as endogenous pyrogens. The initial phase of the thermoregulatory response to such pyrogens may be mediated by ceramide release in neurons of the preoptic area in the anterior hypothalamus (Sanchez-Alavez et al., 2006). The second phase is mediated by coordinate induction of COX-2 and formation of PGE_2 (Engblom et al., 2003). PGE_2 can cross the blood-brain barrier and acts on EP_3 and perhaps EP_1 receptors on thermosensitive neurons. This triggers the hypothalamus to elevate body temperature by promoting an increase in heat generation and a decrease in heat loss. NSAIDs suppress this response by inhibiting COX-2–dependent PGE_2 synthesis.

Nonsteroidal Anti-inflammatory Drugs

The NSAIDs are mechanistically classified as *isoform nonselective NSAIDs*, which inhibit both COX-1 and COX-2, and *COX-2-selective NSAIDs* (FitzGerald and Patrono, 2001). Most NSAIDs are competitive, noncompetitive, or mixed reversible inhibitors of the COX enzymes. Aspirin (ASA) is a noncompetitive, irreversible inhibitor because it acetylates the isozymes in the AA-binding channel. Acetaminophen, which is antipyretic and analgesic but largely devoid of anti-inflammatory activity, acts as a noncompetitive reversible inhibitor by reducing the peroxide site of the enzymes.

The majority of NSAIDs are organic acids with relatively low pK_a values. As organic acids, the compounds generally are well absorbed orally, highly bound to plasma proteins, and excreted either by glomerular filtration or by tubular secretion. They also accumulate in sites of inflammation, where the pH is lower, potentially confounding the relationship between plasma concentrations and duration of drug effect. Most COX-2–selective NSAIDs have a relatively bulky side group, which aligns with a large side pocket in the AA-binding channel of COX-2 but hinders its optimal orientation in the smaller binding channel of COX-1 (Smith et al., 2011). Both isoform nonselective NSAIDs and the COX-2–selective NSAIDs generally are hydrophobic drugs, a feature that allows them to access the hydrophobic AA-binding channel and results in shared pharmacokinetic characteristics. Again, aspirin and acetaminophen are exceptions to this rule.

Mechanism of Action

Cyclooxygenase Inhibition

The principal therapeutic effects of NSAIDs derive from their ability to inhibit PG production. The first enzyme in the PG synthetic pathway is COX, also known as PG G/H synthase. This enzyme converts AA to the unstable intermediates PGG_2 and PGH_2 and leads to the production of the prostanoids, TxA_2, and a variety of PGs (see Chapter 37). COX-1, expressed constitutively in most cells, is the dominant source of prostanoids for housekeeping functions, such as hemostasis. Conversely, COX-2, induced by cytokines, shear stress, and tumor promoters, is the more important source of prostanoid formation in inflammation and perhaps in cancer (see Chapter 37). However, both enzymes contribute to the generation of autoregulatory and homeostatic prostanoids with important functions in normal physiology (see Chapter 37). The indiscriminant inhibition of both inflammatory and homeostatic prostanoids by NSAIDs explains mechanistically most adverse reactions to this drug class. For example, inhibition of COX-1 accounts largely for the gastric adverse events and bleeding that complicate therapy because COX-1 is the dominant cytoprotective isoform in gastric epithelial cells and forms TxA_2 in platelets, which amplifies platelet activation and constricts blood vessels at the site of injury. Similarly, COX-2–derived products play important roles in blood pressure regulation and act as endogenous inhibitors of hemostasis. Inhibition of COX-2 can cause or exacerbate hypertension and increases the likelihood of thrombotic events.

While the functional COX enzymes are sequence homodimers, they are configured as conformational heterodimers in which one of the monomers functions as the catalytic subunit with heme bound and the other, without heme, serves as the allosteric subunit. Most NSAIDs inhibit the catalytic subunits of COX-1 and COX-2. However, COX-2 inhibition by naproxen, and flurbiprofen occurs primarily on the allosteric subunit (Dong et al., 2011; Zou et al., 2012).

Irreversible Cyclooxygenase Inhibition by Aspirin

Aspirin covalently acetylates the catalytic subunits of the COX-1 and COX-2 dimers, irreversibly inhibiting COX activity. This is an important distinction from all the other NSAIDs because the duration of aspirin's effects is related to the turnover rate of the COXs in different target tissues.

The importance of enzyme turnover in recovery from aspirin action is most notable in platelets, which, being anucleate, have a markedly limited capacity for protein synthesis. Thus, the consequences of inhibition of platelet COX-1 last for the lifetime of the platelet. Inhibition of platelet COX-1–dependent TxA_2 formation therefore is cumulative with repeated doses of aspirin (at least as low as 30 mg/d) and takes 8–12 days (the platelet turnover time) to recover fully once therapy has been stopped. Importantly, even a partially recovered platelet pool—just a few days after the last aspirin dose—may afford recovery of sufficient hemostatic integrity for some types of elective surgery to be performed. However, such a partial platelet function also may predispose noncompliant patients on low-dose aspirin for antiplatelet therapy to thrombotic events. The unique sensitivity of platelets to inhibition by low doses of aspirin is related to their presystemic inhibition in the portal circulation before aspirin is deacetylated to salicylate on first pass through the liver (Pedersen and FitzGerald, 1984). In contrast to aspirin, salicylic acid has no acetylating capacity. It is a relatively weak, reversible inhibitor of COX. Salicylic acid derivates, rather than the acid, are available for clinical use.

The COXs are configured such that the active site is accessed by the AA substrate via a hydrophobic channel. Aspirin acetylates serine 529 of COX-1, located high up in the hydrophobic channel. Interposition of the bulky acetyl residue prevents the binding of AA to the active site of the enzyme and thus impedes the ability of the enzyme to make PGs. Aspirin acetylates a homologous serine at position 516 in COX-2. Although covalent modification of COX-2 by aspirin also blocks the COX activity of this isoform, an interesting property not shared by COX-1 is that acetylated COX-2 synthesizes 15(*R*)-HETE. This may be metabolized, at least in vitro, by 5-LOX to yield 15-epi-lipoxin A_4, which has anti-inflammatory properties in model systems (see Chapter 37).

Selective Inhibition of Cyclooxygenase 2

The chronic use of the NSAIDs is limited by their poor GI tolerability. Selective inhibitors of COX-2 were developed to afford efficacy similar to traditional NSAIDs with better GI tolerability (FitzGerald and Patrono, 2001). Six such COX-2 inhibitors, the coxibs, were initially approved for clinical use: celecoxib, rofecoxib, valdecoxib (approved in the U.S.) and its prodrug parecoxib, etoricoxib, and lumiracoxib. Most coxibs have been either restricted in their use or withdrawn from the market in view of their adverse cardiovascular risk profile (Grosser et al., 2010). Celecoxib currently is the only COX-2 inhibitor licensed for use in the U.S. Some older NSAID compounds—diclofenac, etodolac, meloxicam, and nimesulide (the last not available in the U.S.)—exhibit selectivity for COX-2 that is close to that of celecoxib (Figure 38–1).

ADME

Absorption. The NSAIDs are rapidly absorbed following oral ingestion, and peak plasma concentrations are reached within 2–3 h. The poor aqueous solubility of most NSAIDs often is reflected by a less-than-proportional increase in the AUC of plasma concentration–time curves, due to incomplete dissolution, when the dose is increased. Food intake may delay absorption and systemic availability (i.e., fenoprofen, sulindac). Antacids, commonly prescribed to patients on NSAID therapy, variably delay absorption. Some compounds (e.g., diclofenac, nabumetone) undergo first-pass or presystemic elimination. Aspirin begins to acetylate platelets within minutes of reaching the presystemic circulation (Pedersen and FitzGerald, 1984).

Distribution. Most NSAIDs are extensively bound (95%–99%) to plasma proteins, usually albumin. Conditions that alter plasma protein concentration may result in an increased free drug fraction with potential toxic effects. Highly protein bound NSAIDs have the potential to displace other drugs if they compete for the same binding sites. Most NSAIDs are distributed widely throughout the body and readily penetrate arthritic joints, yielding synovial fluid concentrations in the range of half the plasma concentration (i.e., ibuprofen, naproxen, piroxicam) (Day et al., 1999). Most NSAIDs achieve sufficient concentrations in the CNS to have a central analgesic effect. Celecoxib is particularly lipophilic and moves readily into the CNS. Multiple NSAIDs are marketed in formulations for topical application on inflamed or injured joints. However, direct transport of topically applied NSAIDs into inflamed tissues and joints appears to be minimal, and detectable concentrations in synovial fluid of some agents (i.e., diclofenac) following topical use are primarily attained via dermal absorption and systemic circulation. Methods designed to enhance transdermal delivery, such as iontophoresis or chemical penetration enhancers, are under investigation. Topical application is also being explored as a delivery route for drug combinations containing narcotics and NSAIDs.

Metabolism and Excretion. Hepatic biotransformation and renal excretion are the principal routes of metabolism and elimination of the majority of NSAIDs. Plasma $t_{1/2}$ varies considerably among NSAIDs. Ibuprofen, diclofenac, and acetaminophen have a $t_{1/2}$ of 1–4 h, while piroxicam has a $t_{1/2}$ of about 50 h at steady state. Naproxen has a comparatively long but highly variable $t_{1/2}$ ranging from 9 to 25 h. Genetic variation in the major metabolizing enzymes and variation in the composition of intestinal microbiota may contribute to variability in metabolism and elimination. Elimination pathways frequently involve oxidation or hydroxylation. Acetaminophen, at therapeutic doses, is oxidized only to a small degree to form traces of the highly reactive metabolite NAPQI. Following overdose, however, the principal metabolic pathways are saturated, and hepatotoxic NAPQI concentrations can be formed (see Figure 4–5). Several NSAIDs or their metabolites are glucuronidated or otherwise conjugated. In some cases, such as the propionic acid derivatives naproxen and ketoprofen, the glucuronide metabolites can hydrolyze back to form the active parent drug when the metabolite is not removed efficiently due to renal insufficiency or competition for renal excretion with other drugs. This may prolong elimination of the NSAID significantly. In general, NSAIDs are not recommended in the setting of advanced hepatic or renal disease due to their adverse pharmacodynamic effects. NSAIDs usually are not removed by hemodialysis due to their extensive plasma protein binding; salicylic acid is an exception to this rule.

Therapeutic Uses

The NSAIDs are antipyretic, analgesic, and anti-inflammatory, with the exception of acetaminophen, which is antipyretic and analgesic but is largely devoid of anti-inflammatory activity.

Inflammation

The NSAIDs provide mostly symptomatic relief from pain and inflammation associated with musculoskeletal disorders, such as rheumatoid arthritis and osteoarthritis. Some NSAIDs are approved for the treatment of ankylosing spondylitis and gout. Patients with more debilitating disease may not respond adequately to full therapeutic doses of NSAIDs and may require aggressive therapy with second-line agents.

Pain

The NSAIDs are effective against inflammatory pain of low-to-moderate intensity. Although their maximal efficacy is generally less than the opioids, NSAIDs lack the unwanted adverse effects of opiates in the CNS, including respiratory depression and the potential for development of physical dependence. Coadministration of NSAIDs can reduce the opioid dose needed for sufficient pain control and reduce the likelihood of adverse opioid effects. For example, acetaminophen can be prescribed in combination with hydrocodone. NSAIDs do not change the perception of sensory modalities other than pain. NSAIDs are particularly effective when inflammation has caused sensitization of pain perception (see other discussion in this section on inflammation, pain, and fever). Thus, postoperative pain or pain arising from inflammation, such as arthritic pain, is controlled well by NSAIDs, whereas pain arising from the hollow viscera usually is not relieved. An exception to this is menstrual pain. Treatment of menstrual pain with NSAIDs has met with considerable success because cramps and other symptoms of primary dysmenorrhea are caused by the release of PGs by the endometrium during menstruation. NSAIDs are commonly used to treat migraine attacks and can be combined with drugs such as the triptans or with antiemetics to aid relief of the associated nausea. NSAIDs generally lack efficacy in neuropathic pain.

Fever

Antipyretic therapy is reserved for patients in whom fever in itself may be deleterious and for those who experience considerable relief when fever is lowered. NSAIDs reduce fever in most situations, but not the circadian variation in temperature or the rise in response to exercise or increased ambient temperature.

Fetal Circulatory System

The PGs are implicated in the maintenance of patency of the ductus arteriosus, and indomethacin, ibuprofen, and other NSAIDs have been used in neonates to close the inappropriately patent ductus. Conversely, infusion of prostandoid analogues maintains ductal patency after birth (see Chapter 37).

Cardioprotection

Ingestion of aspirin prolongs bleeding time. This effect is due to irreversible acetylation of platelet COX and the consequent inhibition of platelet function. It is the permanent suppression of platelet TxA_2 formation that is thought to underlie the cardioprotective effect of aspirin.

Aspirin reduces the risk of serious vascular events in high-risk patients (e.g., those with previous myocardial infarction) by 20%–25%. The reduction of subsequent thrombotic strokes is somewhat less, roughly 10%–15% (Antithrombotic Trialists' Collaboration et al., 2009). Low-dose aspirin (≤100 mg/d) is associated with a lower risk for GI adverse events than higher doses (e.g., 325 mg/d) and is often used following percutaneous coronary intervention (Xian et al., 2015). Low doses of aspirin are associated with a small (roughly 2-fold) but detectable increase in the incidence of serious GI bleeds and intracranial bleeds in placebo-controlled trials. The benefit from aspirin, however, outweighs these risks in the case of secondary prevention of cardiovascular disease. The issue is much more nuanced in patients who have never had a serious atherothrombotic event (primary prevention); here, prevention of myocardial infarction by aspirin is numerically balanced by the serious GI bleeds it precipitates (Patrono, 2015). Given their relatively short $t_{1/2}$ and reversible COX inhibition, most other NSAIDs are not thought to afford cardioprotection. Data suggest that cardioprotection is lost when combining low-dose aspirin with NSAIDs through a drug-drug interaction at the aspirin target site in platelet COX-1 (Catella-Lawson et al., 2001; Farkouh et al., 2004; Li et al., 2014). COX-2–selective NSAIDs are devoid of antiplatelet activity, as mature platelets do not express COX-2.

Other Clinical Uses

Systemic Mastocytosis. Systemic mastocytosis is a condition in which there are excessive mast cells in the bone marrow, reticuloendothelial system, GI system, bones, and skin (Theoharides et al., 2015). In patients with systemic mastocytosis, PGD_2, released from mast cells is the major mediator of severe episodes of flushing, vasodilation, and hypotension; this PGD_2 effect is resistant to antihistamines. The addition of aspirin or ketoprofen (off-label use) may be beneficial in patients with high levels of urinary PGD metabolites who have flushing and angioedema. However, NSAIDs can cause degranulation of mast cells, so blockade with histamine receptor antagonists should be established before NSAIDs are initiated.

Niacin Tolerability. Large doses of niacin (nicotinic acid) effectively lower serum cholesterol levels, reduce low-density lipoprotein, and raise high-density lipoprotein (see Chapter 33). However, niacin induces intense facial flushing mediated largely by release of PGD_2 from the skin, which can be inhibited by treatment with aspirin (Song et al., 2012).

Bartter Syndrome. Bartter syndrome includes a series of rare disorders (frequency ≤ 1/100,000 persons) characterized by hypokalemic, hypochloremic metabolic alkalosis with normal blood pressure and hyperplasia of the juxtaglomerular apparatus. Fatigue, muscle weakness, diarrhea, and dehydration are the main symptoms. Distinct variants are caused by mutations in a Na^+-K^+-$2Cl^-$ cotransporter, an apical ATP-regulated K^+ channel, a basolateral Cl^- channel, a protein (barttin) involved in cotransporter trafficking, and the extracellular Ca^{2+}-sensing receptor. Renal COX-2 is induced, and biosynthesis of PGE_2 is increased. Treatment with indomethacin, combined with potassium repletion and spironolactone, is associated with improvement in the biochemical derangements and symptoms. Selective COX-2 inhibitors also have been used (Nusing et al., 2001).

Cancer Chemoprevention. Epidemiological studies suggested that daily use of aspirin is associated with a 24% decrease in the incidence of colon cancer (Rothwell et al., 2010). Similar observations have been made with NSAID use in this and other cancers. NSAIDs have been used in patients with familial adenomatous polyposis, an inherited disorder characterized by multiple adenomatous colon polyps developing during adolescence and the inevitable occurrence of colon cancer by the sixth decade.

Adverse Effects of NSAID Therapy

Adverse events common to aspirin and NSAIDs are outlined in Table 38–1. To minimize potential adverse events of NSAIDs, the lowest effective dose should be used for the shortest feasible length of time. Age generally is correlated with an increased probability of developing serious adverse reactions to NSAIDs, and caution is warranted in choosing a lower starting dose for elderly patients. NSAIDs are labeled with a black-box warning related to cardiovascular risks and are specifically contraindicated following coronary artery bypass graft (CABG) surgery.

Gastrointestinal

The most common symptoms associated with these drugs are GI (~40% of patients), including dyspepsia, abdominal pain, anorexia, nausea, and diarrhea. However, these symptoms are not predictive of gastric or intestinal lesions such as subepithelial hemorrhages, erosions, and ulcers, which can be endoscopically detected in about 30%–50% of NSAID users, but are often asymptomatic and tend to heal spontaneously. Serious complications—bleeding, perforation, or obstruction—occur at an annual rate of 1%–2% in regular NSAID users. Many patients who develop a serious upper GI adverse event while receiving NSAID therapy are asymptomatic prior to diagnosis. The risk is particularly high in those with *Helicobacter pylori* infection, heavy alcohol consumption, or other risk factors for mucosal injury, including the concurrent use of glucocorticoids. All selective COX-2 inhibitors are less prone to induce gastric ulcers than equally efficacious doses of isoform nonselective NSAIDs (Sostres et al., 2013).

Several mechanisms contribute to NSAID-induced GI complications (see Chapter 37). Inhibition of COX-1 in gastric epithelial cells depresses mucosal cytoprotective PGs, especially PGI_2 and PGE_2. These eicosanoids inhibit acid secretion by the stomach, enhance mucosal blood flow, and promote the secretion of cytoprotective mucus in the intestine. COX-2 also contributes to constitutive formation of these PGs by human gastric epithelium, and products of COX-2 may contribute to ulcer healing. Another factor that may play a part in the formation of ulcers is the local irritation from contact of orally administered NSAIDs—most of which are organic acids—with the gastric mucosa. However, the incidence of serious GI adverse events is not significantly reduced by formulations devised to limit drug contact with the gastric mucosa, such as enteric coating or efferent solutions, suggesting that the contribution of direct irritation to the overall risk is minor. Platelet inhibition by NSAIDs increases the likelihood of bleeds when mucosal damage has occurred. Coadministration of proton pump inhibitors or H_2 antagonists in conjunction with NSAIDs reduces the rate of duodenal and gastric ulceration (see Chapter 49, Figure 49-1).

Cardiovascular

The COX-2–selective NSAIDs were developed to improve GI safety. However, COX-2 inhibitors depress formation of PGI_2 but do not inhibit the COX-1–catalyzed formation of platelet TxA_2. PGI_2 inhibits platelet aggregation and constrains the effect of prothrombotic and atherogenic stimuli by TxA_2 (Grosser et al., 2006, 2010, 2017), and renal PGI_2 and PGE_2 formed by COX-2 contribute to arterial pressure homeostasis (see Chapter 37). Genetic deletion of the PGI_2 receptor, IP, in mice augments the thrombotic response to endothelial injury, accelerates experimental atherogenesis, increases vascular proliferation, and adds to the effect of hypertensive stimuli (Cheng et al., 2002, 2006; Egan et al., 2004; Kobayashi et al., 2004). Tissue-specific genetic deletion of COX-2 in the vasculature accelerates the response to thrombotic stimuli and raises blood pressure (Yu et al., 2012). Together, these mechanisms would be expected to alter the cardiovascular risk of humans, as COX-2 inhibition in humans depresses PGI_2 synthesis (Catella-Lawson et al., 1999; McAdam et al., 1999). Indeed, a human mutation of the IP, which disrupts its signaling, is associated with increased cardiovascular risk (Arehart et al., 2008).

Clinical trials—with celecoxib, valdecoxib (withdrawn), and rofecoxib (withdrawn)—revealed an increase in the incidence of myocardial infarction, stroke, and vascular death by approximately 1.4-fold (Coxib and

TABLE 38–1 ■ SOME SHARED ADVERSE EFFECTS OF NSAIDS[a]

SYSTEM	MANIFESTATIONS
Gastrointestinal	Abdominal pain, bleeding, constipation, diarrhea, dyspepsia, dysphagia, eructation,[b] esophageal stricture/ulceration, esophagitis, flatulence, gastritis, hematemesis,[b] melena,[b] nausea, odynophagia, perforation, pyrosis, stomatitis, ulcers, vomiting, xerostomia[b]
Platelets	Inhibited platelet activation,[b] propensity for bruising,[b] increased risk of hemorrhage,[b] platelet dysfunction,[b] thrombocytopenia[b]
Renal	Azotemia,[b] cystitis,[b] dysuria,[b] hematuria, hyponatremia, interstitial nephritis, nephrotic syndrome,[b] oliguria,[b] polyuria,[b] renal failure, renal papillary necrosis, proteinuria, salt and water retention, hypertension, worsening of renal function in renal/cardiac/cirrhotic patients, ↓ effectiveness of antihypertensives and diuretics, hyperkalemia,[b] ↓ urate excretion (especially with aspirin)
Cardiovascular	Edema,[b] heart failure,[c] hypertension, MI,[c] palpitations,[b] premature closure of ductus arteriosus, sinus tachycardia,[b] stroke,[c] thrombosis,[c] vasculitis[b]
Neurologic	Anorexia,[b] anxiety,[b] aseptic meningitis, confusion,[b] depression, dizziness, drowsiness,[b] headache, insomnia,[b] malaise,[b] paresthesias, tinnitus, seizures,[b] syncope,[b] vertigo[b]
Reproductive	Prolongation of gestation, inhibition of labor, delayed ovulation
Hypersensitivity	Anaphylactoid reactions, angioedema, severe bronchospasm, urticaria, flushing, hypotension, shock
Hematologic	Anemia, agranulocytosis, aplastic anemia,[b] hemolytic anemia,[b] leukopenia[b]
Hepatic	Elevated enzymes, hepatitis, hepatic failure,[b] jaundice
Dermatologic	Diaphoresis,[b] exfoliative dermatitis, photosensitivity,[b] pruritus, purpura,[b] rash, Stevens-Johnson syndrome, toxic epidermal necrolysis, urticaria
Respiratory	Dyspnea,[b] hyperventilation (salicylates)
Other	Alopecia,[b] blurred vision,[b] conjunctivitis,[b] epistaxis,[b] fever,[b] hearing loss,[b] pancreatitis,[b] paresthesias, visual disturbance,[b] weight gain[b]

[a]Refer to product label for specific information.
[b]Reported for most, but not all, NSAIDs.
[c]With the exception of low-dose aspirin.

Traditional NSAID Trialists' Collaboration et al., 2013). The risk extends to diclofenac, which is almost as COX-2 selective as celecoxib, and to some of the other older NSAIDs. An exception in some individuals may be naproxen. There is considerable between-person variation in the $t_{1/2}$ of naproxen, and platelet inhibition might be anticipated throughout the dosing interval in some, but not all, individuals on naproxen (Capone et al., 2005). While this is supported by randomized controlled trials (Coxib and Traditional NSAID Trialists' Collaboration et al., 2013), identifying individuals who fall into the long-acting group is currently not practical in clinical routine. The FDA has determined that the data differentiating the risk between distinct NSAIDs is not sufficient to distinguish between drugs on the regulatory level; thus, a cardiovascular risk warning is included on the label of all NSAIDs (U.S. Food and Drug Administration, 2015). Similarly, all NSAIDs share a class black-box warning contraindicating their use for the treatment of perioperative pain in the setting of CABG surgery.

The NSAIDs with selectivity for COX-2 should be reserved for patients at high risk for GI complications. The cardiovascular risk appears to be conditioned by factors influencing drug exposure, such as dose, $t_{1/2}$, degree of COX-2 selectivity, potency, and treatment duration. Thus, the lowest possible dose should be prescribed for the shortest possible period.

Blood Pressure and Renal Adverse Events

All NSAIDs have been associated with renal and renovascular adverse events. Up to 5% of regular NSAID users can be expected to develop hypertension. Clinical studies suggest that hypertensive complications occur more commonly in patients treated with COX-2–selective than with nonselective NSAIDs. Heart failure risk is roughly doubled.

The NSAIDs have little effect on renal function or blood pressure in healthy human subjects because of the redundancy of systems that regulate renal function. In situations that challenge the regulatory systems, such as dehydration, hypovolemia, congestive heart failure, hepatic cirrhosis, chronic kidney disease, and other states of activation of the sympathoadrenal or renin-angiotensin systems, regulation of renal function by PG formation becomes crucial (see Chapter 37). NSAIDs impair the PG-induced inhibition of both the reabsorption of Cl^- and the action of antidiuretic hormone, which may result in the retention of salt and water. Inhibition of COX-2–derived PGs that contribute to the regulation of renal medullary blood flow may lead to a rise in blood pressure, increasing the risk of cardiovascular thrombotic events and heart failure. NSAIDs promote reabsorption of K^+ as a result of decreased availability of Na^+ at distal tubular sites and suppression of the PG-induced secretion of renin. The last effect may account in part for the usefulness of NSAIDs in the treatment of Bartter syndrome (see Bartter Syndrome section).

Analgesic Nephropathy. Analgesic nephropathy is a condition of slowly progressive renal failure, decreased concentrating capacity of the renal tubule, and sterile pyuria. Risk factors are the chronic use of high doses of combinations of NSAIDs and frequent urinary tract infections. If recognized early, discontinuation of NSAIDs may permit recovery of renal function.

Pregnancy

Myometrial COX-2 expression and levels of PGE_2 and $PGF_{2\alpha}$ increase markedly in the myometrium during labor. Prolongation of gestation by NSAIDs has been demonstrated in humans. Some NSAIDs, particularly indomethacin, have been used off label to stop preterm labor. However, this use is associated with closure of the ductus arteriosus and impaired fetal circulation in utero, particularly in fetuses older than 32 weeks of gestation. COX-2–selective inhibitors have been used off label as tocolytic agents; this use has been associated with stenosis of the ductus arteriosus and oligohydramnios. Low-dose aspirin (81 mg/d) reduces the risk of preeclampsia by 24% when used as (off-label) preventive medication after 12 weeks of gestation in women who are at high risk (LeFevre and Force, 2014).

Hypersensitivity

Hypersensitivity symptoms to aspirin and NSAIDs range from vasomotor rhinitis, generalized urticaria, and bronchial asthma to laryngeal edema, bronchoconstriction, flushing, hypotension, and shock. Aspirin intolerance (including aspirin-associated asthma) is a contraindication to therapy with any other NSAID because of cross sensitivity. Although less common in children, this cross sensitivity may occur in 10%–25% of patients with asthma, nasal polyps, or chronic urticaria and in 1% of apparently healthy individuals. It is provoked by even low doses (<80 mg) of aspirin and apparently involves COX inhibition. Treatment of aspirin hypersensitivity is similar to that of other severe hypersensitivity reactions, with support of vital organ function and administration of epinephrine.

Aspirin Resistance

All forms of treatment failure with aspirin have been collectively called *aspirin resistance*, but pharmacological resistance to aspirin is rare. Pseudoresistance, reflecting delayed and reduced drug absorption, complicates enteric-coated, but not immediate-release aspirin administration (Grosser et al., 2013).

Hepatotoxicity

Liver injury occurs in 17% of adults with unintentional acetaminophen overdose (Blieden et al., 2014). Liver toxicity from therapeutic doses of acetaminophen is extremely rare (see Acetaminophen section). By contrast, therapeutic dosing of diclofenac may be complicated by hepatotoxicity. While the entire class of NSAIDs has a rate of less than 1 liver injury per 100,000 patients on average, chronic consumption of diclofenac is associated with a risk of 6–11 liver injuries per 100,000 users (Bjornsson et al., 2013; de Abajo et al., 2004) (see Diclofenac section). NSAIDs are not recommended in advanced hepatic or renal disease.

Reye Syndrome

Due to the possible association with Reye syndrome, aspirin and other salicylates are contraindicated in children and young adults less than 20 years of age with viral illness–associated fever (Schrör, 2007). Reye syndrome, a severe and often fatal disease, is characterized by the acute onset of encephalopathy, liver dysfunction, and fatty infiltration of the liver and other viscera. Although a mechanistic understanding is lacking, the epidemiologic association between aspirin use and Reye syndrome is sufficiently strong that aspirin and bismuth subsalicylate labels must indicate the risk. As the use of aspirin in children has declined dramatically, so has the incidence of Reye syndrome. Acetaminophen and ibuprofen have not been implicated in Reye syndrome and are the agents of choice for antipyresis in children and youths.

Drug Interactions

Refer to the individual product labels for a comprehensive listing of NSAID drug-drug interactions.

Concomitant NSAIDs and Low-Dose Aspirin

Many patients consume both an NSAID for chronic pain and low-dose aspirin for cardioprevention. Epidemiological studies suggest that this combination therapy increases significantly the likelihood of GI adverse events over either class of NSAID alone. In addition, prior occupancy of platelet COX-1 by the NSAID can impede access of aspirin to its acetylation target Ser 529 and prevents irreversible inhibition of platelet function (Catella-Lawson et al., 2001). This has been unequivocally shown to occur with ibuprofen and naproxen and may also affect other isoform nonselective NSAIDs (Li et al., 2014). This drug-drug interaction may undermine the cardioprotective effect of aspirin. Celecoxib is unlikely to cause this drug-drug interaction in vivo, but confers a direct cardiovascular hazard (Grosser et al., 2017). Thus, pain management in patients with preexisting cardiovascular disease remains a particular challenge because of the cardiovascular adverse effects of NSAIDs and the risk of drug-drug interactions that might undermine the antiplatelet effects of aspirin.

Other Drug-Drug Interactions

The ACE inhibitors act, at least partly, by preventing the breakdown of kinins that stimulate PG production (see Figure 39–4). Thus, NSAIDs may attenuate the effectiveness of ACE inhibitors by blocking the production of vasodilator and natriuretic PGs. The combination of NSAIDs and ACE inhibitors also can produce marked hyperkalemia, leading to cardiac arrhythmia, especially in the elderly and in patients with hypertension, diabetes mellitus, or ischemic heart disease. Corticosteroids and selective serotonin reuptake inhibitors may increase the frequency or severity of GI complications when combined with NSAIDs.

The NSAIDs may augment the risk of bleeding in patients receiving warfarin both because almost all NSAIDs suppress normal platelet function temporarily during the dosing interval and because some NSAIDs also increase warfarin levels by interfering with its metabolism. Thus, concurrent administration should be avoided.

Many NSAIDs are highly bound to plasma proteins, so they may displace other drugs from their binding sites. Such interactions can occur in patients given salicylates or other NSAIDs together with warfarin, sulfonylurea hypoglycemic agents, or methotrexate; the dosage of such agents may require adjustment to prevent toxicity. Patients taking lithium should be monitored because NSAIDs, including aspirin, reduce the renal excretion of this drug and can lead to toxicity.

Pediatric and Geriatric Use

Therapeutic Uses in Children

Therapeutic uses for NSAIDs in children include fever (acetaminophen, ibuprofen); pain (acetaminophen, ibuprofen); postoperative pain (ketorolac injection [single-dose only]); inflammatory disorders, such as juvenile arthritis (celecoxib, etodolac, meloxicam, naproxen, oxaprozin, tolmetin) and Kawasaki disease (off-label high-dose aspirin); and relief of ocular itching due to seasonal allergic rhinitis and postoperative inflammation after cataract extraction (ketorolac ophthalmic solution).

Kawasaki Disease. Aspirin generally is avoided in pediatric populations due to its potential association with Reye syndrome (see Reye Syndrome). However, high doses of aspirin (30–100 mg/kg/d) are used to treat children during the acute phase of Kawasaki disease, followed by low-dose antiplatelet therapy in the subacute phase.

Pharmacokinetics in Children

The NSAID dosing recommendations frequently are based on extrapolation of pharmacokinetic data from adults or children older than 2 years, and there are often insufficient data for dose selection in younger infants. For example, the pharmacokinetics of the most commonly used NSAID in children, acetaminophen, differ substantially between the neonatal period and older children or adults. The systemic bioavailability of rectal acetaminophen formulations in neonates and preterm babies is higher than in older patients. Acetaminophen clearance is reduced in preterm neonates, probably due to their immature glucuronide conjugation system (sulfation is the principal route of biotransformation at this age). Therefore, acetaminophen dosing intervals need to be extended (8–12 h) or daily doses reduced to avoid accumulation and liver toxicity.

Aspirin elimination also is delayed in neonates and young infants compared to adults, raising the risk of accumulation. Disease also may affect NSAID disposition in children. For example, ibuprofen plasma concentrations are reduced and clearance increased (~80%) in children with cystic fibrosis. This is probably related to the GI and hepatic pathologies associated with this disease. Aspirin's kinetics are markedly altered during the febrile phase of rheumatic fever or Kawasaki vasculitis. The reduction in serum albumin associated with these conditions causes an elevation of the free salicylate concentration, which may saturate renal excretion and result in salicylate accumulation to toxic levels. In addition to dose reduction, monitoring of the free drug may be warranted in these situations.

Pharmacokinetics in the Elderly

The clearance of many NSAIDs is reduced in the elderly due to changes in hepatic metabolism and creatine clearance. NSAIDs with a long $t_{1/2}$ and primarily oxidative metabolism (i.e., piroxicam, tenoxicam, celecoxib) have elevated plasma concentrations in elderly patients. For example, plasma concentrations after the same dose of celecoxib may rise up to 2-fold higher in patients older than 65 years than in patients younger than 50 years of age, warranting dose adjustment. The capacity of plasma albumin to bind drugs is diminished in older patients and may result in higher concentrations of unbound NSAIDs. For example, free naproxen concentrations are markedly increased in older patients, although total plasma concentrations essentially are unchanged, and the higher susceptibility of older patients to GI complications may be due in part to elevated total or free NSAID concentrations. Generally, it is advisable to start most NSAIDs at a low dosage in the elderly and increase the dosage only if the therapeutic efficacy is insufficient.

Specific Properties of Individual NSAIDs

General properties shared by NSAIDs were considered in the section, Nonsteroidal Anti-inflammatory Drugs. In this section, important characteristics of individual substances are discussed. NSAIDs are grouped by their chemical similarity, as in Figure 38–1.

Aspirin and Other Salicylates

The salicylates include aspirin, salicylic acid, methyl salicylate, diflunisal, salsalate (an unapproved marketed drug in the U.S.), olsalazine, sulfasalazine, balsalazide, choline magnesium trisalicylate (an unapproved marketed drug in the U.S.), magnesium salicylate, mesalamine, and salicylamide (a carboxamide derivative of salicylic acid contained as an ingredient in some OTC combination pain relievers). Salicylic acid is so irritating that it can only be used externally; therefore, the various derivatives of this acid have been synthesized for systemic use. For example, aspirin is the acetate ester of salicylic acid (ASA). Aspirin is a widely consumed analgesic, antipyretic, and anti-inflammatory agent. Because aspirin is so available, the possibility of misuse and serious toxicity is underappreciated, and it remains a cause of fatal poisoning in children.

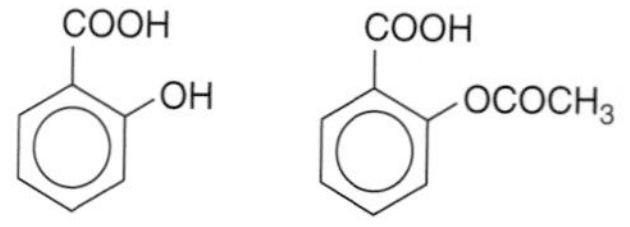

COOH, OH — SALICYLIC ACID; COOH, $OCOCH_3$ — ASPIRIN

Table 38–2 summarizes the clinical pharmacokinetic properties of two salicylates, aspirin and diflunisal.

Mechanism of Action

The effects of aspirin are largely caused by its capacity to acetylate proteins, as described in Irreversible Cyclooxygenase Inhibition by Aspirin. Other salicylates generally act by virtue of their content of salicylic acid, which is a relatively weak inhibitor of the purified COX enzymes. Salicylic acid may also suppress inflammatory upregulation of COX-2 by interfering with transcription factor binding to the COX-2 promoter.

ADME

Absorption. Orally ingested salicylates are absorbed rapidly, partly from the stomach, but mostly from the upper small intestine. The peak plasma level is reached in about 1 h. The rate of absorption is determined by disintegration and dissolution rates of the tablets administered, the pH at the mucosal surface, and gastric emptying time. Even though salicylate is more ionized as the pH is increased, a rise in pH also increases the solubility of salicylate and thus dissolution of the tablets. The overall effect is to enhance absorption. The presence of food delays absorption of salicylates. Rectal absorption of salicylate usually is slower than oral absorption and is incomplete and inconsistent.

Salicylic acid is absorbed rapidly from the intact skin, especially when applied in oily liniments or ointments, and systemic poisoning has occurred from its application to large areas of skin. Methyl salicylate likewise is speedily absorbed when applied cutaneously; however, its GI absorption may be delayed many hours, making gastric lavage effective for removal even in poisonings that present late after oral ingestion.

Enteric coating delays and reduces the bioavailability of aspirin by roughly half and renders absorption more variable in the presence of food (Bogentoft et al., 1978), which is likely the cause of "pseudoresistance" to aspirin (see Aspirin Resistance).

TABLE 38–2 ■ NSAIDS: SALICYLATES, ACETAMINOPHEN, AND ACETIC ACID DERIVATIVES

CLASS/DRUG	PHARMACOKINETICS	DOSING	COMMENTS	COMPARED TO ASPIRIN
Salicylates				
Aspirin	Peak C_p, 1 h Protein binding, 80–90% Metabolite, Salicyluric acid $t_{1/2}$, therapeutic, 2–3 h $t_{1/2}$, toxic dose, 15–30 h	Antiplatelet, 40–80 mg/day Pain/fever, 325–650 mg 4–6 h Rheumatic fever, Children 1 g/ 4–6 h or 10 mg/kg 4–6 h	Permanent platelet COX-1 inhibition Adverse effects: GL, ↑clotting time hypersensitivity Avoid in children with acute febrile illness (Reye syndrome)	
Diflunisal	Peak C_p, 2–3 h Protein binding, 99% Metabolite, Glucuronide $t_{1/2}$, 8–12 h	250–500 mg every 8–12 h (maximum = 1 g/dose and 4 g/d); children <12 y: 10–15 mg/kg every 4 h (maximum 5 doses/24 h) IV (>50 kg): 1000 mg every 6 h or 650 mg every 4 h; (<50 kg): 15 mg/kg every 6 h or 12.5 mg/kg 4h	Not metabolized to salicylic, competitive COX inhibitor, excreted into breast milk.	Analgesic and anti-inflammatory, 4–5 × more potent Antipyretic, weaker Fewer platelet and GI side effects.
Para-aminophenol derivative				
Acetaminophen	Peak C_p, 30–60 min Protein binding, 20–50% Metabolites, Glucuronides (60%); sulfates (35%) $t_{1/2}$, 2 h	650 mg or less every 4 h (maximum of 4000 mg/24 h)	Weak nonspecific COX inhibitor at common doses Potency may be modulated by peroxidase Overdose ⇒ toxic metabolite, (NAPQI) liver necrosis	Analgesic/antipyretic, equivalent Anti-inflammatory, GI, and platelet effects < aspirin at 1000 mg/day
Acetic acid derivatives				
Indomethacin	Peak C_p, 1–2 h Protein binding, 99% Metabolites, *O*-demethyl (50%); unchanged (20%) $t_{1/2}$, 2 h	25 mg 2–3 times/day; 75–100 mg at night	Side effects (3–50%); frontal headache, neutropenia, thrombocytopenia; 20% discontinue	10–40 × more potent; intolerance typically limits dose
Sulindac (sulfoxide prodrug)	Peak C_p 1–2 h; active metabolite 8 h, extensive enterohepatic circulation Metabolites, sulfone/conjugates (30%); sulindac/conjugate (25%) $t_{1/2}$, 7 h; 18 h for active sulfone metabolite	150–200 mg twice/day	20% GI side effects; 10% CNS side effects (headache, dizziness rash)	Efficacy comparable
Etodolac	Peak C_p, 1 h Protein binding, 99% Metabolism, Hepatic $t_{1/2}$, 7 h	200–400 mg 3–4 times/day, max: 1200 mg/d or 1000 mg/d (extended release) > 6 years (extended release): 400 mg/d (20–30 kg); add 200 mg/15 kg more wgt.	Some COX-2 selectivity in vitro Adverse effects similar to sulindac, but ~ half as frequent	100 mg etodolac efficacy ≈ 650 mg of aspirin, may be better tolerated
Tolmetin	Peak C_p, 20–60 min Protein binding, 99% Metabolites, Carboxylate conjugates $t_{1/2}$, 5 h	Adults: 400–600 mg 3 times/d Children > 2 y: 20 mg/kg/d in 3–4 divided doses	Food delays anti decreases peak absorption. May persist in synovial fluid ⇒ biological efficacy >plasma $t_{1/2}$	Efficacy similar; 25–40% develop side effects; 5–10% discontinue drug
Ketorolac	Peak C_p, 30–60 min Protein binding, 99% Metabolite, Glucuronide (90%) $t_{1/2}$, 4–6 h	See FDA Package insert	Parenterally (60 mg IM, then 30 mg every 6 h, or 30 mg IV every 6 h) Available as ocular prep	Potent analgesic, poor anti-inflammatory

(Continued)

TABLE 38–2 ■ NSAIDS: SALICYLATES, ACETAMINOPHEN, AND ACETIC ACID DERIVATIVES (CONTINUED)

CLASS/DRUG	PHARMACOKINETICS	DOSING	COMMENTS	COMPARED TO ASPIRIN
Diclofenac	Peak C_p, 1 h; extended release, 5 h Protein binding, 99% Metabolites, Glucuronide and sulfide (renal 65%, bile 35%) $t_{1/2}$ 1.2–2 h (immediate-release tabs); 12 h (topical epolamine patch)	50 mg 3 times/day or 75 mg twice/day	As topical gel, ocular solution, oral tablets combined with misoprostol First-pass effect; oral bioavailability, 50%	More potent; 20%, side effects; 2% discontinue; 15%, elevated liver enzymes Substrate for CYPs 2C9 are 3A4
Nabumetone (6-methoxy-2-napthylacetic acid prodrug)	Peak C_p, ~3 h Protein binding, 99% Metabolites, conjugates $t_{1/2}$, 19–26 h; 22–38 h (elderly)	500–1000 mg 1–2 times/d (maximum 2000 mg/d); Patients < 50 kg less likely to require more than 1000 mg/d	First-pass effects, 35% conversion of prodrug to active metabolite; preferential COX-2 inhibition at low doses; Adverse effects (13%): GI upset, abdominal pain	Less fecal blood loss during short-term therapy

Time to peak plasma drug concentration C_p is after a single dose. In general, food delays absorption but does not decrease peak concentration. The majority of NSAIDs undergo hepatic metabolism, and the metabolites are excreted in the urine. Major metabolites or disposal pathways are listed. Typical $t_{1/2}$ is listed for therapeutic doses; if $t_{1/2}$ is much different with the toxic dose, this is also given. Typical adult oral doses are listed unless otherwise noted. Refer to the current product labeling for complete prescribing information, including current labeled pediatric indications

Distribution. After absorption, salicylates are distributed throughout most body tissues and transcellular fluids, primarily by pH-dependent processes. Salicylates are transported actively out of the CSF across the choroid plexus. The drugs readily cross the placental barrier. Ingested aspirin mainly is absorbed as such, but some enters the systemic circulation as salicylic acid after hydrolysis by esterases in the GI mucosa and liver. Roughly 80%–90% of the salicylate in plasma is bound to proteins, especially albumin; the proportion of the total that is bound declines as plasma concentrations increase. Hypoalbuminemia, as may occur in rheumatoid arthritis, is associated with a proportionately higher level of free salicylate in the plasma. Salicylate competes with a variety of compounds for plasma protein-binding sites; these include thyroxine, triiodothyronine, penicillin, phenytoin, sulfinpyrazone, bilirubin, uric acid, and other NSAIDs, such as naproxen. Aspirin is bound to a more limited extent; however, it acetylates human plasma albumin in vivo by reaction with the ε-amino group of lysine and may change the binding of other drugs to albumin. Aspirin also acetylates other plasma and tissue proteins, but there is no evidence that this contributes to clinical efficacy or adverse events.

Metabolism and Excretion. Aspirin is rapidly deacetylated to form salicylic acid by spontaneous hydrolysis or esterases located in the intestinal wall, red blood cells, and the liver. The three chief metabolic products are salicyluric acid (the glycine conjugate), the ether or phenolic glucuronide, and the ester or acyl glucuronide. Salicylates and their metabolites are excreted in the urine. The excretion of free salicylates is variable and depends on the dose and the urinary pH. For example, the clearance of salicylate is about four times as great at pH 8 as at pH 6, and it is well above the glomerular filtration rate at pH 8. High rates of urine flow decrease tubular reabsorption, whereas the opposite is true in oliguria. The plasma $t_{1/2}$ for aspirin is about 20 min, and for salicylate is 2–3 h at antiplatelet doses, rising to 12 h at usual anti-inflammatory doses. The $t_{1/2}$ of salicylate may rise to 15–30 h at high therapeutic doses or when there is intoxication. This dose-dependent elimination is the result of the limited capacity of the liver to form salicyluric acid and the phenolic glucuronide, resulting in a larger proportion of unchanged drug being excreted in the urine at higher doses. Salicylate metabolism shows high intersubject variability due to the variable contribution of different metabolic pathways. Women frequently exhibit higher plasma concentrations, perhaps due to lower intrinsic esterase activity and gender differences in hepatic metabolism. Salicylate clearance is reduced and salicylate exposure is significantly increased in the elderly. The plasma concentration of salicylate is increased by conditions that decrease the glomerular filtration rate or reduce proximal tubule secretion, such as renal disease, or the presence of inhibitors that compete for the transport system (e.g., probenecid). In case of an overdose, hemodialysis and hemofiltration techniques remove salicylic acid effectively from the circulation.

Monitoring of Plasma Salicylate Concentrations. Aspirin is one of the NSAIDs for which plasma salicylate can provide a means to monitor therapy and toxicity. Intermittent analgesic-antipyretic doses of aspirin typically produce plasma aspirin levels of less than 20 μg/mL and plasma salicylate levels of less than 60 μg/mL. The daily ingestion of anti-inflammatory doses of 4–5 g of aspirin produces plasma salicylate levels in the range of 120–350 μg/mL. Optimal anti-inflammatory effects for patients with rheumatic diseases require plasma salicylate concentrations of 150–300 μg/mL. Significant adverse effects can be seen at levels greater than 300 μg/mL. At lower concentrations, the drug clearance is nearly constant (despite the fact that saturation of metabolic capacity is approached) because the fraction of drug that is free, and thus available for metabolism or excretion, increases as binding sites on plasma proteins are saturated. The total concentration of salicylate in plasma is therefore a relatively linear function of dose at lower concentrations. At higher concentrations, however, as metabolic pathways of disposition become saturated, small increments in dose can disproportionately increase plasma salicylate concentration. Failure to anticipate this phenomenon can lead to toxicity.

Therapeutic Uses

Systemic Uses. The *analgesic-antipyretic* dose of aspirin for adults is 325–1000 mg orally every 4–6 h. It is only rarely used for inflammatory diseases such as *arthritis, spondyloarthropathies,* and *systemic lupus erythematosus;* NSAIDs with a better GI safety profile are preferred. The anti-inflammatory doses of aspirin, as might be given in rheumatic fever, range from 4 to 8 g/d in divided doses. The maximum recommended daily dose of aspirin for adults and children 12 years or older is 4 g. The rectal administration of aspirin suppositories may be preferred in infants or when the oral route is unavailable. Aspirin suppresses clinical signs and improves tissue inflammation in acute rheumatic fever. Other salicylates available for systemic use include salsalate (salicylsalicylic acid), magnesium salicylate, diflunisal, and a combination of choline salicylate and magnesium salicylate (choline magnesium trisalicylate).

Diflunisal is a difluorophenyl derivative of salicylic acid that is not converted to salicylic acid in vivo. It is a competitive inhibitor of COX and a potent anti-inflammatory drug but is largely devoid of antipyretic effects, perhaps because of poor penetration into the CNS. The drug has been used primarily as an analgesic in the treatment of osteoarthritis and musculoskeletal strains or sprains; in these circumstances, it is about three to four times more potent than aspirin. For rheumatoid arthritis or osteoarthritis, 250–1000 mg/d is administered in two divided doses; maintenance dosage should not exceed 1.5 g/d. Diflunisal may produce fewer auditory side effects (see Ototoxic Effects) and appears to cause fewer and less-intense GI and antiplatelet effects than does aspirin.

Local Uses. Mesalamine (5-aminosalicylic acid) is a salicylate that is used for its local effects in the treatment of *inflammatory bowel disease* (see Figure 51–4). Oral formulations that deliver drug to the lower intestine are efficacious in the treatment of inflammatory bowel disease (in particular, ulcerative colitis). These preparations rely on pH-sensitive coatings and other delayed-release mechanisms such as linkage to another moiety to create a poorly absorbed parent compound that must be cleaved by bacteria in the colon to form the active drug. Mesalamine is available as a rectal enema for treatment of mild-to-moderate ulcerative colitis, proctitis, and proctosigmoiditis and as a rectal suppository for the treatment of active ulcerative proctitis. Mesalamine derivatives in clinical use include *balasalazide*, *sulfasalazine*, and *olsalazine*. Sulfasalazine (salicylazosulfapyridine) contains mesalamine linked covalently to sulfapyridine, and balsalazide contains mesalamine linked to the inert carrier molecule 4-aminobenzoyl-β-alanine. Sulfasalazine and olsalazine have been used in the treatment of rheumatoid arthritis and ankylosing spondylitis. Some OTC medications to relieve indigestion and diarrhea agents contain bismuth subsalicylate and have the potential to cause salicylate intoxication, particularly in children.

The keratolytic action of free salicylic acid is employed for the local treatment of warts, corns, fungal infections, and certain types of eczematous dermatitis. After treatment with salicylic acid, tissue cells swell, soften, and desquamate. Methyl salicylate (oil of wintergreen) is a common ingredient of ointments and deep-heating liniments used in the management of musculoskeletal pain; it also is available in herbal medicines and as a flavoring agent. The cutaneous application of methyl salicylate can result in pharmacologically active, and even toxic, systemic salicylate concentrations and has been reported to increase prothrombin time in patients receiving warfarin.

Adverse Effects and Toxicity

Respiration. Salicylates increase O_2 consumption and CO_2 production (especially in skeletal muscle) at anti-inflammatory doses, a result of uncoupling oxidative phosphorylation. The increased production of CO_2 stimulates respiration. Salicylates also stimulate the respiratory center directly in the medulla. Respiratory rate and depth increases, the $P\text{CO}_2$ falls, and respiratory alkalosis ensues.

Acid-Base and Electrolyte Balance and Renal Effects. Therapeutic doses of salicylate produce definite changes in the acid-base balance and electrolyte pattern. Compensation for the initial event, respiratory alkalosis, is achieved by increased renal excretion of bicarbonate, which is accompanied by increased Na^+ and K^+ excretion; plasma bicarbonate is thus lowered, and blood pH returns toward normal. This stage of compensatory renal acidosis was often seen in adults given intensive salicylate therapy before the development of safer alternatives. Today, it is an indicator of ensuing intoxication (see Salicylate Intoxication). Salicylates can cause retention of salt and water, as well as acute reduction of renal function in patients with congestive heart failure, renal disease, or hypovolemia. Although long-term use of salicylates alone rarely is associated with nephrotoxicity, the prolonged and excessive ingestion of analgesic mixtures containing salicylates in combination with other NSAIDs can produce papillary necrosis and interstitial nephritis (see Analgesic Nephropathy).

Cardiovascular Effects. Low-dose aspirin (≤100 mg daily) lowers cardiovascular risk and is recommended for the prevention of myocardial infarction and stroke in patients at elevated risk (see Cardioprotection section) (Patrono, 2015). At high therapeutic doses (≥3 g daily), salt and water retention can lead to an increase (≤20%) in circulating plasma volume and decreased hematocrit (via a dilutional effect). There is a tendency for the peripheral vessels to dilate because of a direct effect on vascular smooth muscle. Cardiac output and work are increased. Those with carditis or compromised cardiac function may not have sufficient cardiac reserve to meet the increased demands, and congestive cardiac failure and pulmonary edema can occur. High doses of salicylates can produce noncardiogenic pulmonary edema, particularly in older patients who ingest salicylates regularly over a prolonged period.

GI Effects. Ingestion of salicylates may result in epigastric distress, heartburn, dyspepsia, nausea, and vomiting. Salicylates also may cause erosive gastritis and GI ulceration and hemorrhage. These effects occur primarily with acetylated salicylates (i.e., aspirin). Because nonacetylated salicylates lack the ability to acetylate COX and thereby irreversibly inhibit its activity, they are weaker inhibitors than aspirin.

Aspirin-induced gastric bleeding sometimes is painless and, if unrecognized, may lead to iron-deficiency anemia. The daily ingestion of anti-inflammatory doses of aspirin (3–4 g) results in an average fecal blood loss of between 3 and 8 mL/d, as compared with about 0.6 mL/d in untreated subjects. Gastroscopic examination of aspirin-treated subjects often reveals discrete ulcerative and hemorrhagic lesions of the gastric mucosa; in many cases, multiple hemorrhagic lesions with sharply demarcated areas of focal necrosis are observed.

Hepatic Effects. Salicylates can cause hepatic injury, usually after high doses that result in plasma salicylate concentrations greater than 150 μg/mL. The injury is not an acute effect; rather, the onset characteristically occurs after several months of high-dose treatment. The majority of cases occur in patients with connective tissue disorders. There usually are no symptoms, simply an increase in serum levels of hepatic transaminases, but some patients note right upper quadrant abdominal discomfort and tenderness. Overt jaundice is uncommon. The injury usually is reversible on discontinuation of salicylates. However, the use of salicylates is contraindicated in patients with chronic liver disease. Considerable evidence implicates the use of salicylates as an important factor in the severe hepatic injury and encephalopathy observed in Reye syndrome. Large doses of salicylates may cause hyperglycemia and glycosuria and deplete liver and muscle glycogen.

Uricosuric Effects. The effects of salicylates on uric acid excretion are markedly dependent on dose. Low doses (1 or 2 g/d) may decrease urate excretion and elevate plasma urate concentrations; intermediate doses (2 or 3 g/d) usually do not alter urate excretion. Larger-than-recommended doses (>5 g/d) induce uricosuria and lower plasma urate levels; however, such large doses are tolerated poorly. Even small doses of salicylate can block the effects of probenecid and other uricosuric agents that decrease tubular reabsorption of uric acid.

Hematologic Effects. Irreversible inhibition of platelet function underlies the cardioprotective effect of aspirin. If possible, aspirin therapy should be stopped at least 1 week before surgery; however, preoperative aspirin often is recommended prior to cardiovascular surgery and percutaneous interventions. Patients with severe hepatic damage, hypoprothrombinemia, vitamin K deficiency, or hemophilia should avoid aspirin because the inhibition of platelet hemostasis can result in hemorrhage. Salicylates ordinarily do not alter the leukocyte or platelet count, the hematocrit, or the hemoglobin content. However, doses of 3–4 g/d markedly decrease plasma iron concentration and shorten erythrocyte survival time. Aspirin can cause a mild degree of hemolysis in individuals with a deficiency of G6PD.

Endocrine Effects. Long-term administration of salicylates decreases thyroidal uptake and clearance of iodine, but increases O_2 consumption and the rate of disappearance of thyroxine and triiodothyronine from the circulation. These effects probably are caused by the competitive displacement by salicylate of thyroxine and triiodothyronine from transthyretin and the thyroxine-binding globulin in plasma (see Chapter 43).

Ototoxic Effects. Hearing impairment, alterations of perceived sounds, and tinnitus commonly occur during high-dose salicylate therapy and are sometimes observed at low doses. Ototoxic symptoms are caused by increased labyrinthine pressure or an effect on the hair cells of the cochlea, perhaps secondary to vasoconstriction in the auditory microvasculature. Symptoms usually resolve within 2 or 3 days after withdrawal of the drug. As most competitive COX inhibitors are not associated with hearing loss or tinnitus, a direct effect of salicylic acid rather than suppression of PG synthesis is likely.

Salicylates and Pregnancy. Infants born to women who ingest salicylates for long periods may have significantly reduced birth weights. When administered during the third trimester, there also is an increase in perinatal mortality, anemia, antepartum and postpartum hemorrhage, prolonged gestation, and complicated deliveries; thus, its use during this period should be avoided. NSAIDs during the third trimester of pregnancy also can cause premature closure of the ductus arteriosus and should be avoided.

Local Irritant Effects. Salicylic acid is irritating to skin and mucosa and destroys epithelial cells.

Salicylate Intoxication. Salicylate poisoning or serious intoxication most often occurs in children and sometimes is fatal. CNS effects, intense hyperpnea, and hyperpyrexia are prominent symptoms. Death has followed use of 10–30 g of sodium salicylate or aspirin in adults, but much larger amounts (130 g of aspirin in one case) have been ingested without a fatal outcome. The lethal dose of methyl salicylate (also known as oil of wintergreen, sweet birch oil, gaultheria oil, betula oil) is considerably less than that of sodium salicylate. As little as a 4 mL (4.7 g) of methyl salicylate may cause severe systemic toxicity in children. Mild chronic salicylate intoxication is called *salicylism*. When fully developed, the syndrome includes headache, dizziness, tinnitus, difficulty hearing, dimness of vision, mental confusion, lassitude, drowsiness, sweating, thirst, hyperventilation, nausea, vomiting, and occasionally diarrhea.

Neurological Effects. In high doses, salicylates have toxic effects on the CNS, consisting of stimulation (including convulsions) followed by depression. Confusion, dizziness, tinnitus, high-tone deafness, delirium, psychosis, stupor, and coma may occur. Salicylates induce nausea and vomiting, which result from stimulation of sites that are accessible from the CSF, probably in the medullary chemoreceptor trigger zone.

Respiration. The respiratory effects of salicylates contribute to the serious acid-base balance disturbances that characterize poisoning by this class of compounds. Salicylates stimulate respiration indirectly by uncoupling of oxidative phosphorylation and directly by stimulation of the respiratory center in the medulla (described previously). Uncoupling of oxidative phosphorylation also leads to excessive heat production, and salicylate toxicity is associated with hyperthermia, particularly in children. Prolonged exposure to high doses of salicylates leads to depression of the medulla, with central respiratory depression and circulatory collapse, secondary to vasomotor depression. Because enhanced CO_2 production continues, respiratory acidosis ensues. Respiratory failure is the usual cause of death in fatal cases of salicylate poisoning. Elderly patients with chronic salicylate intoxication often develop noncardiogenic pulmonary edema, which is considered an indication for hemodialysis.

Acid-Base Balance and Electrolytes. High therapeutic doses of salicylate are associated with a primary respiratory alkalosis and compensatory metabolic acidosis. The phase of primary respiratory alkalosis rarely is recognized in children with salicylate toxicity. They usually present in a state of mixed respiratory and metabolic acidosis, characterized by a decrease in blood pH, a low plasma bicarbonate concentration, and normal or nearly normal plasma P_{CO_2}. Direct salicylate-induced depression of respiration prevents adequate respiratory hyperventilation to match the increased peripheral production of CO_2. Consequently, plasma P_{CO_2} increases and blood pH decreases. Because the concentration of bicarbonate in plasma already is low due to increased renal bicarbonate excretion, the acid-base status at this stage essentially is an uncompensated respiratory acidosis.

Superimposed, however, is a true metabolic acidosis caused by accumulation of acids as a result of three processes. First, toxic concentrations of salicylates displace plasma bicarbonate. Second, vasomotor depression caused by toxic doses of salicylates impairs renal function, with consequent accumulation of sulfuric and phosphoric acids; renal failure can ensue. Third, salicylates in toxic doses may decrease aerobic metabolism as a result of inhibition of various enzymes. This derangement of carbohydrate metabolism leads to the accumulation of organic acids, especially pyruvic, lactic, and acetoacetic acids.

The same series of events also causes alterations of water and electrolyte balance. The low plasma P_{CO_2} leads to decreased renal tubular reabsorption of bicarbonate and increased renal excretion of Na^+, K^+, and water. Water also is lost by salicylate-induced sweating (especially in the presence of hyperthermia) and hyperventilation. Dehydration, which can be profound, particularly in children, rapidly occurs. Because more water than electrolyte is lost through the lungs and by sweating, the dehydration is associated with hypernatremia.

Cardiovascular Effects. Toxic doses of salicylates lead to an exaggeration of the unfavorable cardiovascular responses seen at high therapeutic doses, and central vasomotor paralysis occurs. Petechiae may be seen due to defective platelet function.

Metabolic Effects. Large doses of salicylates may cause hyperglycemia and glycosuria and deplete liver and muscle glycogen; these effects are partly explained by the release of epinephrine. Such doses also reduce aerobic metabolism of glucose, increase glucose-6-phosphatase activity, and promote the secretion of glucocorticoids. There is a greater risk of hypoglycemia and subsequent permanent brain injury in children. Salicylates in toxic doses cause a significant negative nitrogen balance, characterized by an aminoaciduria. Adrenocortical activation may contribute to the negative nitrogen balance by enhancing protein catabolism. Salicylates reduce lipogenesis by partially blocking incorporation of acetate into fatty acids; they also inhibit epinephrine-stimulated lipolysis in fat cells and displace long-chain fatty acids from binding sites on human plasma proteins. The combination of these effects leads to increased entry and enhanced oxidation of fatty acids in muscle, liver, and other tissues and to decreased plasma concentrations of free fatty acids, phospholipid, and cholesterol; the oxidation of ketone bodies also is increased.

Management of Salicylate Overdose. Salicylate poisoning represents an acute medical emergency, and death may result despite maximal therapy. Monitoring of salicylate levels is a useful guide to therapy but must be used in conjunction with an assessment of the patient's overall clinical condition, acid-base balance, formulation of salicylate ingested, timing, and dose. There is no specific antidote for salicylate poisoning.

Drug Interactions

The plasma concentration of salicylates generally is little affected by other drugs, but concurrent administration of aspirin lowers the concentrations of indomethacin, naproxen, ketoprofen, and fenoprofen, at least in part by displacement from plasma proteins. Important adverse interactions of aspirin with warfarin, sulfonylureas, and methotrexate were mentioned previously (in Drug Interactions). Other interactions of aspirin include the antagonism of spironolactone-induced natriuresis and the blockade of the active transport of penicillin from CSF to blood. Magnesium-aluminum hydroxide antacids can alkalize the urine enough to increase salicylic acid clearance significantly and reduce steady-state concentrations. Conversely, discontinuation of antacid therapy can increase plasma concentrations to toxic levels.

Acetaminophen

Acetaminophen (paracetamol; *N*-acetyl-*p*-aminophenol) is the active metabolite of phenacetin.

HO H N

ACETAMINOPHEN

Acetaminophen raises the threshold to painful stimuli, thus exerting an analgesic effect against pain due to a variety of etiologies. Acetaminophen is available without a prescription and is used as a common household analgesic by children and adults. It also is available in fixed-dose combinations containing narcotic and nonnarcotic analgesics (including aspirin and other salicylates), barbiturates, caffeine, vascular headache remedies, sleep aids, toothache remedies, antihistamines, antitussives, decongestants, expectorants, cold and flu preparations, and sore throat treatments. Acetaminophen is well tolerated; however, overdosage—two-thirds of which are intentionally induced—can cause severe hepatic damage (see Figure 4–4); it leads to nearly 80,000 emergency department visits and 30,000 hospitalizations annually in the U.S. (Blieden et al., 2014). The maximum FDA-recommended dose of acetaminophen is 4 g/d.

Mechanism of Action

Acetaminophen has analgesic and antipyretic effects similar to those of aspirin, but only weak anti-inflammatory effects. It is a nonselective COX inhibitor, which acts at the peroxide site of the enzyme and is thus distinct among NSAIDs. The presence of high concentrations of peroxides, as occur at sites of inflammation, reduces its COX-inhibitory activity.

ADME

Oral acetaminophen has excellent bioavailability. Peak plasma concentrations occur within 30–60 min, and the $t_{1/2}$ in plasma is about 2 h. Acetaminophen is relatively uniformly distributed throughout most body fluids. Binding of the drug to plasma proteins is variable, but less than with other NSAIDs. Some 90%–100% of drug may be recovered in the urine within the first day at therapeutic dosing, primarily after hepatic conjugation with glucuronic acid (~60%), sulfuric acid (~35%), or cysteine (~3%); small amounts of hydroxylated and deacetylated metabolites also have been detected (see Table 38–2). Children have less capacity for glucuronidation of the drug than do adults. A small proportion of acetaminophen undergoes CYP-mediated *N*-hydroxylation to form NAPQI, a highly reactive intermediate. This metabolite normally reacts with sulfhydryl groups in GSH and thereby is rendered harmless. However, after ingestion of large doses of acetaminophen, the metabolite is formed in amounts sufficient to deplete hepatic GSH and contributes significantly to the toxic effects of overdose (see Acetaminophen Intoxication).

Therapeutic Uses

Acetaminophen is suitable for analgesic or antipyretic uses; it is particularly valuable for patients in whom aspirin is contraindicated (e.g., those with aspirin hypersensitivity, children with a febrile illness, patients with bleeding disorders). The conventional oral dose of acetaminophen is 325–650 mg every 4–6 h; total daily doses should not exceed 4 g (2 g/d for chronic alcoholics). Single doses for children 2–11 years old depend on age and weight (~10–15 mg/kg); no more than five doses should be administered in 24 h. An injectable preparation is available. Particular attention is warranted due to the availability of a wide variety of prescription and nonprescription multi-ingredient medications that represent potentially toxic overlapping sources of acetaminophen.

Adverse Effects and Toxicity

Acetaminophen usually is well tolerated. Therapeutic doses of acetaminophen have no clinically relevant effects on the cardiovascular and respiratory systems, platelets, or coagulation. The GI adverse effects are less common than with therapeutic doses of NSAIDs. Rash and other allergic reactions occur occasionally, but sometimes these are more serious and may be accompanied by drug fever and mucosal lesions. Patients who show hypersensitivity reactions to the salicylates only rarely exhibit sensitivity to acetaminophen. The most serious acute adverse effect of overdosage of acetaminophen is a potentially fatal hepatic necrosis (Graham et al., 2005). Hepatic injury with acetaminophen involves its conversion to the toxic metabolite NAPQI. The glucuronide and sulfate conjugation pathways become saturated, and increasing amounts undergo CYP-mediated *N*-hydroxylation to form NAPQI. This is eliminated rapidly by conjugation with GSH and then further metabolized to a mercapturic acid and excreted into the urine. In the setting of acetaminophen overdose, hepatocellular levels of GSH become depleted. The highly reactive NAPQI metabolite binds covalently to cell macromolecules, leading to dysfunction of enzymatic systems and structural and metabolic disarray. Furthermore, depletion of intracellular GSH renders the hepatocytes highly susceptible to oxidative stress and apoptosis. Renal tubular necrosis and hypoglycemic coma also may occur.

In adults, hepatotoxicity may occur after ingestion of a single dose of 10–15 g (150–250 mg/kg) of acetaminophen; doses of 20–25 g or more are potentially fatal. Conditions of CYP induction (e.g., heavy alcohol consumption) or GSH depletion (e.g., fasting or malnutrition) increase the susceptibility to hepatic injury, which has been documented, albeit uncommonly, with doses in the therapeutic range. Plasma transaminases become elevated, sometimes markedly so, beginning about 12–36 h after ingestion. Symptoms that occur during the first 2 days of acute poisoning by acetaminophen reflect gastric distress (e.g., nausea, abdominal pain, anorexia) and belie the potential seriousness of the intoxication. Clinical indications of hepatic damage manifest within 2–4 days of ingestion of toxic doses, with right subcostal pain, tender hepatomegaly, jaundice, and coagulopathy. Renal impairment or frank renal failure may occur. Liver enzyme abnormalities typically peak 72–96 h after ingestion. Biopsy of the liver reveals centrilobular necrosis with sparing of the periportal area. In nonfatal cases, the hepatic lesions are reversible over a period of weeks or months.

Management of Acetaminophen Intoxication. Severe liver damage occurs in 90% of patients with plasma concentrations of acetaminophen greater than 300 μg/mL at 4 h or 45 μg/mL at 15 h after the ingestion of the drug. Activated charcoal, if given within 4 h of ingestion, decreases acetaminophen absorption by 50%–90% and should be administered if the ingested dose is suspected to exceed 7.5 g. NAC is indicated for those at risk of hepatic injury. NAC functions by detoxifying NAPQI. It both repletes GSH stores and may conjugate directly with NAPQI by serving as a GSH substitute. In addition to NAC therapy, aggressive supportive care is warranted. This includes management of hepatic and renal failure, if they occur, and intubation if the patient becomes obtunded. Hypoglycemia can result from liver failure, and plasma glucose should be monitored closely. Fulminant hepatic failure is an indication for liver transplantation.

Acetic Acid Derivatives

Diclofenac

Diclofenac, a phenylacetic acid derivative, is among the most commonly used NSAIDs in Europe. Diclofenac has analgesic, antipyretic, and anti-inflammatory activities. Its potency is substantially greater than that of other NSAIDs. Although it was not developed to be a COX-2 selective drug, the selectivity of diclofenac for COX-2 resembles that of celecoxib (see Figure 38–1).

ADME. Diclofenac displays rapid absorption, extensive protein binding, and a $t_{1/2}$ of 1–2 h (see Table 38–2). The short $t_{1/2}$ makes it necessary to give doses of diclofenac considerably higher than would be required to inhibit COX-2 fully at peak plasma concentrations to afford sustained COX inhibition throughout the dosing interval. Thus, both COX isoforms are inhibited for the first phase of the dosing interval. However, as plasma levels decrease, diclofenac behaves like a COX-2 inhibitor in the later phase of the dosing interval. There is a substantial first-pass effect, such that only about 50% of diclofenac is available systemically. The drug accumulates in synovial fluid after oral administration, which may explain why its duration of therapeutic effect is considerably longer than its plasma $t_{1/2}$. Diclofenac is metabolized in the liver by a member of the CYP2C subfamily to 4-hydroxydiclofenac, the principal metabolite, and other hydroxylated forms; after glucuronidation and sulfation, the metabolites are excreted in the urine (65%) and bile (35%).

Therapeutic Uses. Diclofenac is approved in the U.S. for the long-term symptomatic treatment of rheumatoid arthritis, osteoarthritis, ankylosing spondylitis, pain, primary dysmenorrhea, and acute migraine. Multiple oral formulations are available, providing a range of release times; the usual daily oral dosage is 50–150 mg, given in several divided doses. For acute pain such as migraine, a powdered form for dissolution in water and a solution for intravenous injection are available. Diclofenac also is available in combination with misoprostol, a PGE_1 analogue; this combination retains the efficacy of diclofenac while reducing the frequency of GI ulcers and erosions. A 1% topical gel, a topical solution, and a transdermal patch are available for short-term treatment of pain due to minor strains, sprains, and bruises. A 3% gel formulation is indicated for topical treatment of actinic keratosis. In addition, an ophthalmic solution of diclofenac is available for treatment of postoperative inflammation following cataract extraction and for the temporary relief of pain and photophobia in patients undergoing corneal refractive surgery.

Adverse Effects. Diclofenac produces side effects (particularly GI) in about 20% of patients. The incidence of serious GI adverse effects, hypertension, and myocardial infarction are similar to the COX-2-selective inhibitors (Cannon et al., 2006). Hypersensitivity reactions have occurred following topical application and systemic administration. Severe liver injury occurs in 6–11 per 100,000 regular users annually (Bjornsson et al., 2013; de Abajo et al., 2004). Elevation of hepatic transaminases in plasma by more than three times the upper normal limit, indicating significant liver damage, occurs in about 4% of patients (Rostom et al., 2005). Transaminases should be monitored during the first 8 weeks of therapy with diclofenac. Other untoward responses to diclofenac include CNS effects, rashes, fluid retention, edema, and renal function impairment. The drug is not recommended for children, nursing mothers, or pregnant women.

Diclofenac is extensively metabolized. One metabolite, 4′-hydroxy diclofenac, can form reactive benzoquinone imines (similar to acetaminophen's metabolite NAPQI) that deplete hepatic GSH. Another highly reactive metabolite, diclofenac acyl glucuronide, is primarily catalyzed by UGT2B7 (King et al., 2001). Genetic variation that causes higher catalytic activity of UGT2B7 is associated with an increased risk of hepatotoxicity among patients taking diclofenac (Daly et al., 2007).

Indomethacin

Indomethacin is a methylated indole derivative indicated for the treatment of moderate-to-severe rheumatoid arthritis, osteoarthritis, and ankylosing spondylitis; acute gouty arthritis; and acute painful shoulder. Although indomethacin is still used clinically, mainly as a steroid-sparing agent, toxicity and the availability of safer alternatives have limited its use.

Indomethacin is a potent nonselective inhibitor of the COXs. It also inhibits the motility of polymorphonuclear leukocytes, depresses the biosynthesis of mucopolysaccharides, and may have a direct, COX-independent vasoconstrictor effect. Indomethacin has prominent anti-inflammatory and analgesic-antipyretic properties similar to those of the salicylates.

ADME. Oral indomethacin has excellent bioavailability. Peak concentrations occur 1–2 h after dosing (Table 38–2). The concentration of the drug in the CSF is low, but its concentration in synovial fluid is equal to that in plasma within 5 h of administration. There is enterohepatic cycling of the indomethacin metabolites and probably of indomethacin itself. The $t_{1/2}$ in plasma is variable, perhaps because of enterohepatic cycling, but averages about 2.5 h.

Therapeutic Uses. While indomethacin is estimated to be about 20 times more potent than aspirin, a high rate of intolerance limits its use. An intravenous formulation of indomethacin is approved for closure of persistent patent ductus arteriosus in premature infants. The regimen involves intravenous administration of 0.1–0.25 mg/kg every 12 h for three doses, with the course repeated one time if necessary. Successful closure can be expected in more than 70% of neonates treated. The principal limitation of treating neonates is renal toxicity, and therapy is interrupted if the output of urine falls significantly (<0.6 mL/kg/h). An injectable formulation of ibuprofen is an alternative for the treatment of patent ductus arteriosus.

Adverse Effects. A very high percentage (35%–50%) of patients receiving indomethacin experience adverse drug reactions. GI adverse events are common and can be fatal; elderly patients are at significantly greater risk. Diarrhea may occur and sometimes is associated with ulcerative lesions of the bowel. Acute pancreatitis has been reported, as have rare, but potentially fatal, cases of hepatitis. The most frequent CNS effect is severe frontal headache. Dizziness, vertigo, light-headedness, and mental confusion may occur. Seizures have been reported, as have severe depression, psychosis, hallucinations, and suicide. Caution is advised when administering indomethacin to elderly patients or to those with underlying epilepsy, psychiatric disorders, or Parkinson disease because they are at greater risk for the development of serious CNS adverse effects. Hematopoietic reactions include neutropenia, thrombocytopenia, and rarely aplastic anemia.

The total plasma concentration of indomethacin plus its inactive metabolites is increased by concurrent administration of probenecid. Indomethacin antagonizes the natriuretic and antihypertensive effects of furosemide and thiazide diuretics and blunts the antihypertensive effect of β receptor antagonists, AT_1-receptor antagonists, and ACE inhibitors.

Sulindac

Sulindac is a congener of indomethacin. Sulindac is a prodrug whose anti-inflammatory activity resides in its sulfide metabolite, which is more than 500 times more potent than sulindac as an inhibitor of COX but less than half as potent as indomethacin (see Figure 38–1). ADME data are summarized in Table 38–2. Sulindac is used for the treatment of rheumatoid arthritis, osteoarthritis, ankylosing spondylitis, painful shoulder, and gouty arthritis. Its analgesic and anti-inflammatory effects are comparable to those achieved with aspirin. The most common dosage for adults is 150–200 mg twice a day. Although the incidence of toxicity is lower than with indomethacin, adverse reactions to sulindac are common. The typical NSAID GI side effects are seen in nearly 20% of patients. CNS side effects as described for indomethacin are seen in 10% or fewer of patients. Rash occurs in (3%–9%) of patients, and pruritus occurs in 1%–3% of patients. Transient elevations of hepatic transaminases in plasma are less common. The same precautions that apply to other NSAIDs regarding patients at risk for GI toxicity, cardiovascular risk, and renal impairment also apply to sulindac.

Etodolac

Etodolac is an acetic acid derivative with some degree of COX-2 selectivity (see Table 38–2, Figure 38–1). A single oral dose (200–400 mg) of etodolac provides postoperative analgesia that lasts for 6–8 h. Etodolac also is effective in the treatment of osteoarthritis, rheumatoid arthritis, and mild-to-moderate pain, and the drug appears to be uricosuric. Sustained-release preparations are available. Etodolac is relatively well tolerated. About 5% of patients who have taken the drug for 1 year or less discontinue treatment because of GI side effects, rashes, and CNS effects.

Tolmetin

Tolmetin is approved for the treatment of osteoarthritis, rheumatoid arthritis, and juvenile rheumatoid arthritis and has been used in the treatment of ankylosing spondylitis. ADME and comparison to aspirin are in Table 38–2. Tolmetin recommended doses for adults (200–600 mg three times/d) are typically given with meals, milk, or antacids to lessen abdominal discomfort. However, peak plasma concentrations and bioavailability are reduced when the drug is taken with food. Side effects occur in 25%–40% of patients who take tolmetin. GI side effects are the most common (~15%), and gastric ulceration has been observed. CNS side effects similar to those seen with indomethacin and aspirin occur, but they are less common and less severe.

Ketorolac

Ketorolac is a potent analgesic but only a moderately effective anti-inflammatory drug. The use of ketorolac is limited to 5 days or less for acute pain and can be administered orally, intravenously, intramuscularly, or intranasally. Typical doses are 30–60 mg (intramuscular), 15–30 mg (intravenous), 10–20 mg (oral), and 31.5 mg (intranasal). Pediatric patients aged between 2 and 16 years may receive a single intramuscular (1 mg/kg up to 30 mg) or intravenous (0.5 mg/kg up to 15 mg) dose of ketorolac for severe acute pain. Ketorolac has a rapid onset of action and a short duration of action (see Table 38–2). It is widely used in postoperative patients, but it should not be used for routine obstetric analgesia. Topical (ophthalmic) ketorolac is approved for the treatment of seasonal allergic conjunctivitis and postoperative ocular inflammation. Ketorolac in a fixed-dose combination with phenylephrine is indicated as an irrigation during cataract or intraocular lens replacement surgery to maintain pupil size, prevent miosis, and reduce postoperative pain. Side effects of systemic ketorolac include somnolence (6%), dizziness (7%), headache (17%), GI pain (13%), dyspepsia (12%), nausea (12%), and pain at the site of injection (2%). Serious adverse GI, renal, bleeding, and hypersensitivity reactions to ketorolac may occur. Patients receiving greater than recommended doses or concomitant NSAID therapy, and the elderly, appear to be particularly at risk.

Nabumetone

Nabumetone is the prodrug of 6-methoxy-2-naphthylacetic acid. Nabumetone is approved for the treatment of rheumatoid arthritis and osteoarthritis. Its comparative pharmacokinetic properties are summarized in Table 38–2. Nabumetone is associated with crampy lower abdominal pain (12%) and diarrhea (14%). Other side effects include rash (3%–9%); headache (3%–9%); dizziness (3%–9%); heartburn, tinnitus, and pruritus (3%–9%).

Propionic Acid Derivatives

The propionic acid derivatives *ibuprofen, naproxen, flurbiprofen, fenoprofen, ketoprofen*, and *oxaprozin* are available in the U.S. (see Table 38–3). Ibuprofen is the most commonly used NSAID in the U.S. and is available with or without a prescription. Naproxen, also available with or without a prescription, has a longer but variable $t_{1/2}$. Oxaprozin also has a long $t_{1/2}$ and may be given once daily.

Mechanism of Action

Propionic acid derivatives are nonselective COX inhibitors with the effects and side effects common to other NSAIDs. Some of the propionic acid derivatives, particularly naproxen, have inhibitory effects on leukocyte function, and some evidence suggests that naproxen may have slightly better efficacy with regard to analgesia and relief of morning stiffness. This suggestion of benefit accords with the longer $t_{1/2}$ of naproxen in comparison to other propionic acid derivatives.

Therapeutic Uses

Propionic acid derivatives are approved for use in the symptomatic treatment of rheumatoid arthritis, juvenile arthritis, and osteoarthritis. Some also are approved for pain, ankylosing spondylitis, acute gouty arthritis, tendinitis, bursitis, headache, postoperative dental pain and swelling, and primary dysmenorrhea. These agents may be comparable in efficacy to aspirin for the control of the signs and symptoms of rheumatoid arthritis and osteoarthritis.

Drug Interactions

Ibuprofen and naproxen have been shown to interfere with the antiplatelet effects of aspirin (Catella-Lawson et al., 2001; Li et al., 2014). Propionic acid derivatives have not been shown to alter the pharmacokinetics of the oral hypoglycemic drugs or warfarin. Refer to the full product labeling for a comprehensive listing of other drug interactions.

Ibuprofen

ADME. Table 38–3 summarizes the comparative pharmacokinetics of ibuprofen. Ibuprofen is absorbed rapidly, bound avidly to protein, and undergoes hepatic metabolism (90% is metabolized to hydroxylate or carboxylate derivatives) and renal excretion of metabolites. The $t_{1/2}$ is about 2 h. Slow equilibration with the synovial space means that its antiarthritic effects may persist after plasma levels decline. In experimental animals, ibuprofen and its metabolites readily cross the placenta.

Therapeutic Uses. Ibuprofen is supplied as tablets, chewable tablets, capsules, caplets, and gelcaps containing 50–600 mg; as oral drops; and as an oral suspension. An injectable formulation of ibuprofen is approved to close patent ductus arteriosus in premature infants. Solid oral dosage forms containing 200 mg or less are available without a prescription. Ibuprofen is licensed for marketing alone and in fixed-dose combinations with antihistamines, decongestants, famotidine, oxycodone, and hydrocodone. It is short acting, with a $t_{1/2}$ of about 2 h. The usual dose for mild-to-moderate pain is 400 mg every 4–6 h as needed.

Adverse Effects. Ibuprofen is better tolerated than aspirin and indomethacin and has been used in patients with a history of GI intolerance to other NSAIDs. Nevertheless, 5%–15% of patients experience GI side effects. Less-frequent adverse effects of ibuprofen include rashes (3%–9%), thrombocytopenia (<1%), headache (1%–3%), dizziness (3%–9%), blurred vision (<1%), and, in a few cases, toxic amblyopia (<1%), fluid retention (1%–3%), and edema (1%–3%). Patients who develop ocular disturbances should discontinue the use of ibuprofen and have an ophthalmic evaluation. Ibuprofen can be used occasionally by pregnant women; however, the concerns apply regarding third-trimester effects, including delay of parturition. Excretion into breast milk is thought to be minimal, so ibuprofen also can be used with caution by women who are breastfeeding.

Naproxen

Naproxen is supplied as tablets, delayed-release tablets, extended-release tablets, gelcaps, and caplets containing 200–500 mg of naproxen or naproxen sodium and as an oral suspension and suppositories. Solid oral dosage forms containing 200 mg or less are available without a prescription. Naproxen is licensed for marketing alone and in fixed-dose combinations with pseudoephedrine, diphenhydramine, esomeprazole, and sumatriptan; it is copackaged with lansoprazole. Naproxen is indicated for juvenile and rheumatoid arthritis, osteoarthritis, ankylosing spondylitis, pain, primary dysmenorrhea, tendonitis, bursitis, and acute gout.

ADME. Naproxen is absorbed fully after oral administration. Naproxen also is absorbed rectally but more slowly than after oral administration. Naproxen is almost completely (99%) bound to plasma proteins after normal therapeutic doses. The $t_{1/2}$ of naproxen in plasma is variable, 9 to 25 h. Age plays a role in the variability of the $t_{1/2}$ because of the age-related decline in renal function (and consequently longer $t_{1/2}$) (see Table 38–3). Low doses should be prescribed in the elderly. Naproxen is extensively metabolized in the liver. About 30% of the drug undergoes 6-desmethylation, and most of this metabolite, as well as naproxen itself, is excreted as the glucuronide or other conjugates. Metabolites of naproxen are excreted almost entirely in the urine. Naproxen crosses the placenta and appears in the milk of lactating women at about 1% of the maternal plasma concentration.

Adverse Effects. Although the best available data were consistent with the suggestion that naproxen is an NSAID that is not associated with an increase in myocardial infarction rate (Coxib and Traditional NSAID Trialists' Collaboration et al., 2013), the FDA in 2015, based on the advisory committee recommendations, has issued a warning that NSAIDs can cause heart attacks and strokes, and that there is inconclusive evidence regarding whether the particular risk of any NSAID is definitively higher or lower than another NSAID (https://www.fda.gov/Drugs/DrugSafety/ucm451800.htm).

About 1%–10% of patients taking naproxen experience GI adverse effects that include heartburn, abdominal pain, constipation, diarrhea, nausea, dyspepsia, and stomatitis. Adverse effects with naproxen occur at approximately the same frequency as with indomethacin and other NSAIDs (see Table 38–1). CNS side effects include drowsiness (3%–9%), headache (3%–9%), dizziness (≤9%), vertigo (<3%), and depression (<1%). Other common reactions include pruritus (3%–9%) and diaphoresis (<3%). Rare instances of jaundice, impairment of renal function, angioedema, thrombocytopenia, and agranulocytosis have been reported.

Fenamates

The fenamates (anthranilic acids) include *mefenamic acid, meclofenamate*, and *flufenamic acid*. The pharmacological properties of the fenamates are those of typical NSAIDs, and therapeutically, they have no advantages over others in the class (see Table 38–3). Mefenamic acid and meclofenamate sodium are used in the short-term treatment of pain in soft-tissue injuries, dysmenorrhea, and rheumatoid and osteoarthritis. These drugs are not recommended for use in children or pregnant women. Roughly 5% of patients develop a reversible elevation of hepatic transaminases. Diarrhea, which may be severe and associated with steatorrhea and inflammation of the bowel, also is relatively common. Autoimmune hemolytic anemia is a potentially serious but rare side effect.

Enolic Acids (Oxicams)

The oxicam derivative *piroxicam* is the nonselective COX inhibitor with the longest $t_{1/2}$. *Meloxicam* shows modest COX-2 selectivity comparable to celecoxib (see Figure 38–1) and was approved as a COX-2–selective NSAID in some countries. These agents are similar in efficacy to aspirin, indomethacin, or naproxen for the long-term treatment of rheumatoid

TABLE 38–3 ■ COMPARISON OF REPRESENTATIVE NSAIDS: FENAMATES AND PROPIONIC ACID DERIVATIVES

CLASS/DRUG	PHARMACOKINETICS	DOSING	COMMENTS	COMPARED TO ASPIRIN
Fenamates				
Mefenamic acid	Peak C_p, 2–4 h Protein binding, >90% Metabolism, CYP2C9 oxidation; glucuronidation of parent drug and metabolites $t_{1/2}$, 2–4 h	500 mg load, then 250 mg every 6 h	Therapy usually should not exceed 7 days or 2–3 days (dysmenorrhea); 15% elevated liver enzymes; excreted in breast milk	Efficacy similar
Meclofenamate	Peak C_p, 0.5–2 h; 3–4 h (with food) Protein binding, 99% Metabolism, Oxidation to 3-OH (~20% activity of parent) $t_{1/2}$, 0.8–2.1 h (parent); 0.5–4 h (active metabolite)	50–100 mg 4–6 times/d (maximum 400 mg/d)	Side effects: CNS, GI, and rash (all > 10%); administration with food ↓ rate/extent of absorption	Efficacy similar
Propionic acid derivatives				
Ibuprofen	Peak C_p, 2 h (tablets) , 1 h (chewable tablets), 0.75 h (liquid) Protein binding, 99% Metabolites, CYP2C9 oxidation to 2- and 3-hydroxylates; conjugation to acyl glucuronides $t_{1/2}$, 2–4 h (adults); 23–75 h (premature infants); 0.9–2.3 h (children)	200–800 mg 3–6 times/d with food (maximum 3.2 g/d); Canadian and U.S. pediatric max 2.4 g/d Children: 4–10 mg/kg/dose, 3–4 times/d	10%–15% discontinue; may increase risk of aseptic meningitis; excreted in breast milk Racemate: 60% of R-enantiomer converts to S-ibuprofen	Equipotent
Naproxen	Peak C_p, 2–4 h (base tabs); 1–4 h (liquid); 1–2 h (sodium salt); 4–12 h (delayed-release tabs) Protein binding, 99% (↑ free fraction in elderly) Metabolism, CYPs 2C9, 1A2, 2C8 oxidation to 6-O-desmethyl and other metabolites $t_{1/2}$, 9–25 h	250 mg 3–4 times/d; 250–550 mg 2 times/d; 750–1000 mg daily (extended release) Children: 5 mg/kg 2 times/d (max 15 mg/kg/d)	Peak anti-inflammatory effects after 2–4 weeks; ↑ free fraction and ↓ excretion ⇒ ↑ risk of toxicity in elderly; may increase risk of aseptic meningitis; excreted in breast milk; variably prolonged $t_{1/2}$ may afford cardioprotection in some individuals	Usually better tolerated
Fenoprofen	Peak C_p, 2 h Protein binding, 99% Metabolites, 4-OH metabolite; glucuronide conjugates $t_{1/2}$, 2.5–3 h	200 mg 4–6 times/d or 300–600 mg 3–4 times/d (max 3.2 g/d)	Peak anti-inflammatory effects after 2–3 weeks; 15% experience side effects; few discontinue use; excreted in breast milk	Generally better tolerated
Ketoprofen	Peak C_p, 1.2 h; 6.8 h (extended-release) Protein binding, 99% Metabolites, Glucuronide conjugates; enterohepatic recirculation? $t_{1/2}$, 0.9–3.3 h	25–50 mg 3–4 times/d; 75 mg 3 times/d; 200 mg daily (extended release); max 300 mg/d Anti-inflammatory, 50–75 mg, 3–4/d	30% develop side effects (usually GI, usually mild); ~13% liver function abnormalities; unbound fraction, systemic exposure, and $t_{1/2}$ ↑ with age in elderly; excreted in breast milk	Generally better tolerated; biological efficacy > plasma $t_{1/2}$
Flurbiprofen	Peak C_p, ~2 h Protein binding, 99% Metabolism, CYP2C9 oxidation, UGTB7 glucuronidation of parent and 4′-OH metabolite $t_{1/2}$, 7.5 h	200–300 mg/d in 2–4 divided doses (maximum 100 mg/dose)	Racemate; excreted in breast milk; available for ophthalmic use	Generally better tolerated

(*Continued*)

TABLE 38–3 ■ COMPARISON OF REPRESENTATIVE NSAIDS: FENAMATES AND PROPIONIC ACID DERIVATIVES (*CONTINUED*)

CLASS/DRUG	PHARMACOKINETICS	DOSING	COMMENTS	COMPARED TO ASPIRIN
Oxaprozin	Peak C_p, 2.4–3 h Protein binding, 99% Metabolism, 65% oxidates, 35% glucuronides $t_{1/2}$, 41–55 h	600–1200 mg daily (maximum 1800 mg); children > 21 kg: 600–1200 mg daily based on weight (maximum 1200 mg)	Slow onset, not indicated for fever or acute pain; dose in elderly adjusted on the basis of weight; expected to be excreted in breast milk	Generally better tolerated

Time to peak plasma drug concentration C_p is after a single dose. In general, food delays absorption but does not decrease peak concentration. The majority of NSAIDs undergo hepatic metabolism, and the metabolites are excreted in the urine. Major metabolites or disposal pathways are listed. Typical $t_{1/2}$ is listed for therapeutic doses; if $t_{1/2}$ is much different with the toxic dose, this is also given. Typical adult oral doses are listed unless otherwise noted. Refer to the current product labeling for complete prescribing information, including current labeled pediatric indications.

arthritis or osteoarthritis. The main advantage suggested for these compounds is their long $t_{1/2}$, which permits once-a-day dosing (see comparative pharmacokinetic and dosing data in Table 38–4).

Piroxicam

Piroxicam may inhibit activation of neutrophils, apparently independently of its ability to inhibit COX; hence, additional modes of anti-inflammatory action have been proposed, including inhibition of proteoglycanase and collagenase in cartilage.

Piroxicam is approved for the treatment of rheumatoid arthritis and osteoarthritis. Due to its slow onset of action and delayed attainment of steady state, it is less suited for acute analgesia but has been used to treat acute gout.

ADME. The pharmacokinetics of piroxicam are described in Table 38–4. The usual daily dose is 20 mg. Piroxicam is absorbed completely after oral administration and undergoes enterohepatic recirculation. Estimates of the $t_{1/2}$ in plasma have been variable; the average is about 50 h. Steady-state blood levels are reached in 7–12 days. Less than 5% of the drug is excreted into the urine unchanged. The major metabolic transformation in humans is hydroxylation of the pyridyl ring (predominantly by an isozyme of the CYP2C subfamily), and this inactive metabolite and its glucuronide conjugate account for about 60% of the drug excreted in the urine and feces.

Adverse Effects. Approximately 20% of patients experience side effects

TABLE 38–4 ■ REPRESENTATIVE NSAIDS: ENOLIC ACID DERIVATIVES AND COXIBS

CLASS/ DRUG	PHARMACOKINETICS	DOSING	COMMENTS	COMPARED TO ASPIRIN
Enolic acid derivatives				
Piroxicam	Peak C_p, 3–5 h Protein binding, 99% Metabolites, CYP2C9 hydroxylation, conjugation, *N*-demethylation $t_{1/2}$, ~50 h	20 mg daily	20% side effects; 5% discontinue; slow onset, not indicated for fever or acute pain; excreted in breast milk	Equipotent with lower incidence of minor GI effects
Meloxicam	Peak C_p, 4–5 h (and 12–14 h due to biliary recycling) Protein binding, 99% Metabolism, Hydroxylation $t_{1/2}$, 15–20 h	7.5 mg daily (maximum 15 mg/d); Children ≥ 2: lowest effective dose, 0.125 mg/kg daily (maximum 7.5 mg daily)	Some COX-2 selectivity, especially at lower doses; elderly females have higher systemic exposure and peak plasma concentrations than men and young women; excretion in breast milk unknown	—
Diaryl heterocyclic nsaids (*COX-2 selective*)				
			Evidence for cardiovascular adverse events	Decrease in GI side effects and in platelet effects
Celecoxib	Peak C_p, ~3 h Protein binding, 97% Metabolism, CYPs 2C9 (major) and 3A4 (minor), glucuronide $t_{1/2}$, 11.2 h	100–200 mg 1–2 times/d; 400 mg followed by 200 mg if needed on first day (acute pain); maximum, 800 mg/d. Children > 2 y: 50 mg (10–25 kg) or 100 mg (>25 kg) 2 times/d	CYP2D6 and CYP2D8 inhibitor; Adverse effects: GI complaints (5%); aseptic meningitis and methemoglobinemia have been reported; disseminated intravascular coagulation risk in pediatric patients; 40% higher systemic exposure in blacks and elderly females; excreted in breast milk	Usually better tolerated; does not usually prolong bleeding time

Time to peak plasma drug concentration C_p is after a single dose. In general, food delays absorption but does not decrease peak concentration. The majority of NSAIDs undergo hepatic metabolism, and the metabolites are excreted in the urine. Major metabolites or disposal pathways are listed. Typical $t_{1/2}$ is listed for therapeutic doses; if $t_{1/2}$ is much different with the toxic dose, this is also given. Typical adult oral doses are listed unless otherwise noted. Refer to the current product labeling for complete prescribing information, including current labeled pediatric indications.

with piroxicam, and about 5% of patients discontinue use because of these effects. Piroxicam may be associated with more GI and serious skin reactions than other nonselective NSAIDs. In 2007, the European Medicines Agency reviewed the safety of orally administered piroxicam and concluded that its benefits outweigh its risks, but advised it should no longer considered a first-line agent or be used for the treatment of acute (short-term) pain and inflammation.

Meloxicam

Meloxicam is approved for use in osteoarthritis, rheumatoid arthritis, and juvenile rheumatoid arthritis. The recommended adult dose of meloxicam is 7.5–15 mg once daily. Meloxicam demonstrates some COX-2 selectivity (see Figure 38–1). There is significantly less gastric injury compared to piroxicam (20 mg/d) in subjects treated with 7.5 mg/d of meloxicam, but the advantage is lost with a dosage of 15 mg/d (Patoia et al., 1996).

Purpose-Developed COX-2 Selective NSAIDs

Selective inhibitors of COX-2 are molecules with side chains that fit within its hydrophobic pocket but are too large to block COX-1 with equally high affinity. Celecoxib is the only purposefully developed COX-2 inhibitor still approved in the U.S. (see its clinical pharmacokinetic properties and precautions in Table 38–4). As mentioned, other, older compounds (diclofenac, etodolac, meloxicam, nimesulide) have been retrospectively found to have a certain degree of selectivity for COX-2 (see Figure 38–1). Etoricoxib is approved in several countries, but restricted in its indications; rofecoxib, valdecoxib, and lumiracoxib were withdrawn worldwide because of the cardiovascular complications caused by suppression of cardioprotective COX-2–derived PGs, especially PGI_2, and the unrestrained effects of endogenous stimuli, such as platelet COX-1–derived TxA_2, on platelet activation, vascular proliferation and remodeling, hypertension, and atherogenesis. COX-2–selective NSAIDs should be avoided in patients prone to cardiovascular or cerebrovascular disease. While the purposefully developed COX-2 inhibitors have generally been shown to reduce severe GI complications when compared to isoform nonselective compounds, none of the COX-2–selective NSAIDs has established superior efficacy.

Celecoxib

ADME. The bioavailability of oral celecoxib is not known; peak plasma levels occur at 2–4 h after administration. The elderly (≥65 years of age) may have up to 2-fold higher peak concentrations and AUC values than younger patients (≤55 years of age). Celecoxib is bound extensively to plasma proteins. Most is excreted as carboxylic acid and glucuronide metabolites in the urine and feces. The elimination $t_{1/2}$ is about 11 h. The drug commonly is given once or twice daily during chronic treatment. Plasma concentrations are increased in patients with mild and moderate hepatic impairment, requiring reduction in dose. Celecoxib is metabolized predominantly by CYP2C9 and inhibits CYP2D6. Clinical vigilance is necessary during coadministration of drugs that are known to inhibit CYP2C9 and drugs that are metabolized by CYP2D6.

Therapeutic Uses. Celecoxib is used for the management of acute pain for the treatment of osteoarthritis, rheumatoid arthritis, juvenile rheumatoid arthritis, ankylosing spondylitis, and primary dysmenorrhea. The recommended dose for treating osteoarthritis is 200 mg/d as a single dose or divided as two doses. In the treatment of rheumatoid arthritis, the recommended dose is 100–200 mg twice daily. Due to cardiovascular hazard, physicians are advised to use the lowest possible dose for the shortest possible duration.

Adverse Effects. Celecoxib confers a risk of myocardial infarction and stroke, and this appears to relate to dose and the underlying risk of cardiovascular disease. Effects attributed to inhibition of PG production in the kidney—hypertension and edema—occur with nonselective COX inhibitors and also with celecoxib. Selective COX-2 inhibitors lose their GI advantage over other NSAIDs alone when used in conjunction with aspirin. Chronic use of celecoxib may decrease bone mineral density, particularly in older male patients. There is some suggestion that celecoxib may slow fracture healing and tendon-to-bone healing.

Etoricoxib

Etoricoxib is a COX-2–selective inhibitor with selectivity second only to that of lumiracoxib (see Figure 38–1). Etoricoxib is incompletely (~80%) absorbed and has a long $t_{1/2}$ of 20–26 h. It is extensively metabolized before excretion. Patients with hepatic impairment are prone to drug accumulation. Renal insufficiency does not affect drug clearance. Etoricoxib is used for symptomatic relief in the treatment of osteoarthritis, rheumatoid arthritis, and acute gouty arthritis, as well as for the short-term treatment of musculoskeletal pain, postoperative pain, and primary dysmenorrhea. The drug is associated with the increased risk of heart attack and stroke. Etoricoxib is not available in the U.S.

Disease-Modifying Antirheumatic Drugs

Rheumatoid arthritis is an autoimmune disease that affects about 1% of the population. The pharmacological management of rheumatoid arthritis includes symptomatic relief through the use of NSAIDs. However, although they have anti-inflammatory effects, NSAIDs have minimal, if any, effect on progression of joint deformity. Disease-modifying antirheumatic drugs (DMARDs), on the other hand, reduce the disease activity of rheumatoid arthritis and retard the progression of arthritic tissue destruction. DMARDs include a diverse group of small-molecule nonbiological and biological agents (mainly antibodies or binding proteins), as summarized in Table 38–5.

Biological DMARDs remain reserved for patients with persistent moderate or high disease activity and indicators of poor prognosis. Therapy is tailored to the individual patient, and the use of these agents must be weighed against their potentially serious adverse effects. The combination of NSAIDs with these agents is common.

Pharmacotherapy of Gout

Gout results from the precipitation of urate crystals in the tissues and the subsequent inflammatory response. Acute gout usually causes painful distal monoarthritis and can cause joint destruction, subcutaneous deposits (tophi), and renal calculi and damage. Gout affects 3% of the adult population of Western countries.

The pathophysiology of gout is incompletely understood. Hyperuricemia, while a prerequisite, does not inevitably lead to gout. Uric acid, the end product of purine metabolism, is relatively insoluble compared to its hypoxanthine and xanthine precursors, and normal serum urate levels (~5 mg/dL, or 0.3 mM) approach the limit of solubility. In most patients with gout, hyperuricemia arises from underexcretion rather than overproduction of urate. Mutations of one of the renal URATs, URAT-1, are associated with hypouricemia. Urate tends to crystallize as monosodium urate in colder or more acidic conditions. Monosodium urate crystals activate monocytes/macrophages via the toll-like receptor pathway mounting an innate immune response. This results in the activation of the cryopyrin inflammasome, the secretion of cytokines, including IL-1β and TNF-α, endothelial activation, and attraction of neutrophils to the site of inflammation. Neutrophils secrete inflammatory mediators that lower the local pH and lead to further urate precipitation. The aims of treatment are to:

- decrease the symptoms of an acute attack;
- decrease the risk of recurrent attacks; and
- lower serum urate levels.

The following substances are available for these purposes:

- Drugs that relieve inflammation and pain (NSAIDs, colchicine, glucocorticoids)
- Drugs that prevent inflammatory responses to crystals (colchicine and NSAIDs)
- Drugs that act by inhibition of urate formation (e.g., allopurinol, febuxostat) or to augment urate excretion (probenecid)

TABLE 38–5 ■ DISEASE-MODIFYING ANTIRHEUMATIC DRUGS

DRUG	CLASS OR ACTION	CHAPTER NUMBER
Small molecules		
Methotrexate	Antifolate	66
Leflunomide	Pyrimidine synthase inhibitor	66
Hydroxychloroquine	Antimalarial	53
Minocycline	5-Lipoxygenase inhibitor, tetracycline antibiotic	37, 59
Sulfasalazine	Salicylate	38, 51
Azathioprine	Purine synthase inhibitor	66
Cyclosporine	Calcineurin inhibitor	35
Cyclophosphamide	Alkylating agent	66
Penicillamine	Chelating agent	71
Auranofin	Gold compound	71
Biologicals		
Adalimumab	Ab, TNF-α antagonist	34, 35
Golimumab	Ab, TNF-α antagonist	
Etanercept	Ab, TNF-α antagonist	
Infliximab	IgG-TNF receptor fusion protein (anti-TNF)	
Certolizumab	Fab fragment toward TNF-α	
Abatacept	T-cell costimulation inhibitor (binds B7 protein on antigen-presenting cell)	34, 35
Rituximab	Ab toward CD20 (cytotoxic toward B cells)	67
Anakinra	IL-1 receptor antagonist	35, 67
Tocilizumab	IL-6 receptor antagonist	35, 67
Tofacitinib	Janus kinase inhibitor	67

The NSAIDs have been discussed previously. Glucocorticoids are discussed in Chapter 46. This section focuses on *colchicine, allopurinol, febuxostat, pegloticase, rasburicase*, and the uricosuric agents *probenecid* and *benzbromarone*. Some other drugs used off label to reduce uric acid levels or treat gout include losartan, fenofibrate, and canakinumab; in 2011, the FDA denied a license application for canakinumab, citing an unfavorable risk-versus-benefit safety profile.

Colchicine

Colchicine is one of the oldest available therapies for acute gout. Plant extracts containing colchicine were used for joint pain in the 6th century. Colchicine is considered second-line therapy because it has a narrow therapeutic window and a high rate of side effects, particularly at higher doses.

Mechanism of Action

Colchicine exerts a variety of pharmacological effects, but how these relate to its activity in gout is partially understood (Leung et al., 2015). It has antimitotic effects, arresting cell division in G_1 by interfering with microtubule and spindle formation (an effect shared with vinca alkaloids). This effect is greatest on cells with rapid turnover (e.g., neutrophils, GI epithelium). Depolymerization of microtubules by colchicine reduces neutrophil recruitment to inflamed tissue and neutrophil adhesion. Colchicine may alter neutrophil motility and decreases the secretion of chemotactic factors and superoxide anions by activated neutrophils. Colchicine limits monosodium urate crystal–induced NALP3 inflammasome activation and subsequent formation of IL-1β and IL-18. This mechanism may explain its therapeutic activity in familial Mediterranean fever and other inflammatory diseases. Colchicine inhibits the release of histamine-containing granules from mast cells, the secretion of insulin from pancreatic β cells, and the movement of melanin granules in melanophores.

Colchicine also exhibits a variety of other pharmacological effects. It lowers body temperature, increases the sensitivity to central depressants, depresses the respiratory center, enhances the response to sympathomimetic agents, constricts blood vessels, and induces hypertension by central vasomotor stimulation. It enhances GI activity by neurogenic stimulation, but depresses it by a direct effect, and alters neuromuscular function.

ADME

Absorption of oral colchicine is rapid but variable. Peak plasma concentrations occur 0.5–2 h after dosing. Food does not affect the rate or extent of colchicine absorption. In plasma, 39% of colchicine is protein bound, primarily to albumin. The formation of colchicine-tubulin complexes in many tissues contributes to its large volume of distribution. There is significant enterohepatic circulation. The exact metabolism of colchicine in humans is unknown, but in vitro studies indicated that it may undergo oxidative demethylation by CYP3A4; glucuronidation may also be involved. In healthy volunteers, 40%–65% of the total absorbed oral dose of colchicine is recovered unchanged in the urine. The kidney, liver, and spleen also contain high concentrations of colchicine, but it apparently is largely excluded from heart, skeletal muscle, and brain. Colchicine is a substrate of P-glycoprotein efflux. The plasma $t_{1/2}$ of colchicine is about 31 h. The drug is contraindicated in patients with hepatic or renal impairment requiring concomitant therapy with CYP3A4 or P-glycoprotein inhibitors. Colchicine is not removed by hemodialysis.

Therapeutic Uses

The dosing regimen for colchicine must be individualized on the basis of age, renal and hepatic function, concomitant use of other medications, and disease severity. A minimum of 3 days, but preferably 7–14 days, should elapse between courses of gout treatment with colchicine to avoid cumulative toxicity. Patients with hepatic or renal disease and dialysis patients should receive reduced doses or less-frequent therapy. For elderly patients, adjust the dose for renal function. For those with cardiac, renal, hepatic, or GI disease, NSAIDs or glucocorticoids may be preferred.

Acute Gout. Colchicine dramatically relieves acute attacks of gout. It is effective in roughly two-thirds of patients if given within 24 h of attack onset. Pain, swelling, and redness abate within 12 h and are completely gone within 48–72 h. The regimen approved for adults recommends a total of two doses taken 1 h apart: 1.2 mg (2 tablets) at the first sign of a gout flare followed by 0.6 mg (1 tablet) 1 h later. Patients with severe renal or hepatic dysfunction and patients receiving dialysis should not receive repeat courses of therapy more frequently than every 2 weeks.

Prevention of Acute Gout. Colchicine is used in the prevention of recurrent gout, particularly in the early stages of antihyperuricemic therapy. The typical dose for prophylaxis in patients with normal renal and hepatic function is 0.6 mg taken orally 3 or 4 days/week for patients who have less than 1 attack per year, 0.6 mg daily for patients who have more than 1 attack per year, and 0.6 mg up to two times daily for patients who have severe attacks.

Adverse Effects

Exposure of the GI tract to large amounts of colchicine and its metabolites via enterohepatic circulation and the rapid rate of turnover of the GI mucosa may explain why the GI tract is particularly susceptible to colchicine toxicity. Nausea, vomiting, diarrhea, and abdominal pain are the most common untoward effects and the earliest signs of impending colchicine toxicity. Drug administration should be discontinued as soon as these symptoms occur. There is a latent period, which is not altered by dose, of several hours or more between the administration of the drug and the onset of symptoms. A dosing study demonstrated that one dose initially and a single additional dose after 1 h was much less toxic than the traditional hourly dosing regimen for acute gout flares. Acute intoxication causes hemorrhagic gastropathy.

Other serious side effects of colchicine therapy include myelosuppression, leukopenia, granulocytopenia, thrombopenia, aplastic anemia, and rhabdomyolysis. Life-threatening toxicities are associated with administration of concomitant therapy with P-glycoprotein or CYP3A4 inhibitors. The FDA suspended the U.S. marketing of all injectable dosage forms of colchicine in 2008. Colchicine is marketed in a fixed-dose combination with probenecid for the management of frequent recurrent gout attacks.

Allopurinol

History

Allopurinol initially was synthesized as a candidate antineoplastic agent but was found to lack antineoplastic activity. Subsequent testing showed it to be an inhibitor of XO that was useful clinically for the treatment of gout.

Allopurinol inhibits XO and prevents the synthesis of urate from hypoxanthine and xanthine. Allopurinol is used to treat hyperuricemia in patients with gout and to prevent it in those with hematological malignancies about to undergo chemotherapy (acute tumor lysis syndrome). Even though underexcretion rather than overproduction is the underlying defect in most gout patients, allopurinol remains effective therapy.

Allopurinol is an analogue of hypoxanthine. Its active metabolite, oxypurinol, is an analogue of xanthine.

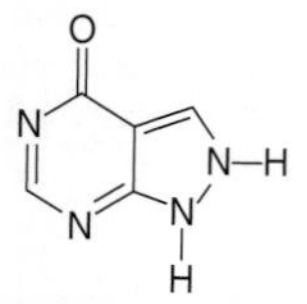

ALLOPURINOL 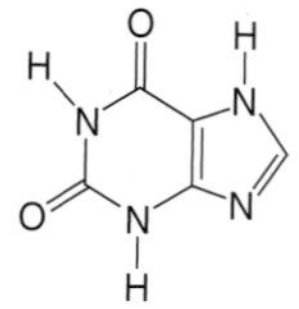 XANTHINE 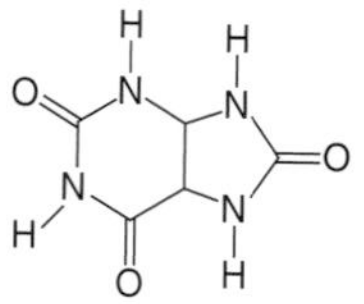 URIC ACID

Mechanism of Action

Both allopurinol and its primary metabolite, oxypurinol (alloxanthine), reduce urate production by inhibiting XO, which converts xanthine to uric acid. Allopurinol competitively inhibits XO at low concentrations and is a noncompetitive inhibitor at high concentrations. Allopurinol also is a substrate for XO; the product of this reaction, oxypurinol, also is a noncompetitive inhibitor of the enzyme. The formation of oxypurinol, together with its long persistence in tissues, is responsible for much of the pharmacological activity of allopurinol.

In the absence of allopurinol, the dominant urinary purine is uric acid. During allopurinol treatment, the urinary purines include hypoxanthine, xanthine, and uric acid. Because each has its independent solubility, the concentration of uric acid in plasma is reduced and purine excretion is increased, without exposing the urinary tract to an excessive load of uric acid. Despite their increased concentrations during allopurinol therapy, hypoxanthine and xanthine are efficiently excreted, and tissue deposition does not occur. There is a small risk of xanthine stones in patients with a very high urate load before allopurinol therapy, which can be minimized by liberal fluid intake and urinary alkalization.

Allopurinol facilitates the dissolution of tophi and prevents the development or progression of chronic gouty arthritis by lowering the uric acid concentration in plasma below the limit of its solubility. The formation of uric acid stones virtually disappears with therapy, which prevents the development of nephropathy. Once significant renal injury has occurred, allopurinol cannot restore renal function but may delay disease progression. The incidence of acute attacks of gouty arthritis may increase during the early months of allopurinol therapy as a consequence of mobilization of tissue stores of uric acid. Coadministration of colchicine helps suppress such acute attacks. In some patients, the allopurinol-induced increase in excretion of oxypurines is less than the reduction in uric acid excretion; this disparity primarily is a result of reutilization of oxypurines and feedback inhibition of de novo purine biosynthesis.

ADME

Allopurinol is absorbed relatively rapidly after oral ingestion, and peak plasma concentrations are reached within 60–90 min. About 20% is excreted in the feces in 48–72 h, presumably as unabsorbed drug, and 10%–30% is excreted unchanged in the urine. The remainder undergoes metabolism, mostly to oxypurinol. Oxypurinol is excreted slowly in the urine by glomerular filtration, counterbalanced by some tubular reabsorption. The plasma $t_{1/2}$ of allopurinol and oxypurinol is about 1–2 h and about 18–30 h (longer in those individuals with renal impairment), respectively. This allows for once-daily dosing and makes allopurinol the most commonly used antihyperuricemic agent. Allopurinol and its active metabolite oxypurinol are distributed in total tissue water, with the exception of brain, where their concentrations are about one-third of those in other tissues. Neither compound is bound to plasma proteins. The plasma concentrations of the two compounds do not correlate well with therapeutic or toxic effects.

Therapeutic Uses

Allopurinol is available for oral and intravenous use. Oral therapy provides effective therapy for primary and secondary gout, hyperuricemia secondary to malignancies, and calcium oxalate calculi. The goal of therapy is to reduce the plasma uric acid concentration to less than 6 mg/dL (<360 μmol/L) and typically less than 5 mg/dL (<297 μmol/L) in patients with tophi to accelerate the clearance of monosodium urate. In the management of gout, it is customary to antecede allopurinol therapy with colchicine and to avoid starting allopurinol during an acute attack. Fluid intake should be sufficient to maintain daily urinary volume greater than 2 L; slightly alkaline urine is preferred. An initial daily dose of 100 mg in patients with estimated glomerular filtration rates greater than 40 mg/min is increased by 100-mg increments at weekly intervals. Most patients can be maintained on 300 mg/d. Patients with reduced glomerular filtration require a lower dose to achieve the targeted uric acid concentration, and their clinical and pharmacological response needs be monitored frequently. Those with hematological malignancies may need up to 800 mg/d beginning 2–3 days before the start of chemotherapy. Daily doses greater than 300 mg should be divided.

The usual daily dose in children with secondary hyperuricemia associated with malignancies is 150–300 mg, depending on age. Allopurinol also is useful in lowering the high plasma concentrations of uric acid in patients with Lesch-Nyhan syndrome (orphan designation) and thereby prevents the complications resulting from hyperuricemia; there is no evidence that it alters the progressive neurological and behavioral abnormalities that are characteristic of the disease. Other orphan uses for allopurinol include Chagas disease and the ex vivo preservation of cadaveric kidneys prior to transplantation.

Adverse Effects

Allopurinol generally is well tolerated. The most common adverse effects are hypersensitivity reactions that may manifest after months or years of therapy. Serious hypersensitivity reactions preclude further use of the drug. The cutaneous reaction caused by allopurinol is predominantly a pruritic, erythematous, or maculopapular eruption, but occasionally the lesion is urticarial or purpuric.

Rarely, toxic epidermal necrolysis or Stevens-Johnson syndrome occurs, which can be fatal. The risk for Stevens-Johnson syndrome is limited primarily to the first 2 months of treatment. Because the rash may precede severe hypersensitivity reactions, patients who develop a rash should discontinue allopurinol. If indicated, desensitization to allopurinol can be carried out starting at 10–25 μg/d, with the drug diluted in oral suspension and doubled every 3–14 days until the desired dose is reached. This is successful in approximately half of patients.

Oxypurinol has orphan drug status and is available for compassionate use in the U.S. for patients intolerant of allopurinol. Fever, malaise, and myalgias also may occur in about 3% of patients, more frequently in those with renal impairment. Transient leukopenia or leukocytosis and eosinophilia are rare reactions that may require cessation of therapy. Hepatomegaly and elevated levels of transaminases in plasma and progressive renal insufficiency also may occur.

Allopurinol is contraindicated in patients who have exhibited serious adverse effects or hypersensitivity reactions to the medication and in nursing mothers and children, except those with malignancy or certain inborn errors of purine metabolism (e.g., Lesch-Nyhan syndrome). Allopurinol generally is used in patients with hyperuricemia posttransplantation. It can be used in conjunction with a uricosuric agent.

Drug Interactions

Allopurinol increases the $t_{1/2}$ of probenecid and enhances its uricosuric effect, while probenecid increases the clearance of oxypurinol, thereby increasing dose requirements of allopurinol. Allopurinol inhibits the enzymatic inactivation of mercaptopurine and its derivative azathioprine by XO. Thus, when allopurinol is used concomitantly with oral mercaptopurine or azathioprine, dosage of the antineoplastic agent must be reduced to 25%–33% of the usual dose (see Chapters 35 and 66). This is of importance when treating gout in the transplant recipient. The risk of bone marrow suppression also is increased when allopurinol is administered with cytotoxic agents that are not metabolized by XO, particularly cyclophosphamide. Allopurinol also may interfere with the hepatic inactivation of other drugs, including warfarin. Although the effect is variable, increased monitoring of prothrombin activity is recommended in patients receiving both medications.

It remains to be established whether the increased incidence of rash in patients receiving concurrent allopurinol and ampicillin should be ascribed to allopurinol or to hyperuricemia. Hypersensitivity reactions have been reported in patients with compromised renal function, especially those who are receiving a combination of allopurinol and a thiazide diuretic. The concomitant administration of allopurinol and theophylline leads to increased accumulation of an active metabolite of theophylline, 1-methylxanthine; the concentration of theophylline in plasma also may be increased (see Chapter 40).

Febuxostat

Febuxostat is an XO inhibitor approved for treatment of hyperuricemia in patients with gout.

Mechanism of Action

Febuxostat is a nonpurine inhibitor of XO. Unlike oxypurinol, the active metabolite of allopurinol, which inhibits the reduced form of XO, febuxostat forms a stable complex with both the reduced and oxidized enzymes and inhibits catalytic function in both states.

ADME

Febuxostat is rapidly absorbed with maximum plasma concentrations at 1–1.5 h postdose. The absolute bioavailability is unknown. Magnesium hydroxide and aluminum hydroxide delay absorption by about 1 h. Food reduces absorption slightly. Febuxostat, $t_{1/2}$ of 5–8 h, is extensively metabolized by both conjugation via UGT enzymes, including UGT1A1, UGT1A3, UGT1A9, and UGT2B7, and oxidation by CYPs 1A2, 2C8, and 2C9 and non-CYP enzymes and has elimination by both hepatic and renal pathways. Mild-to-moderate renal or hepatic impairment does not affect its elimination kinetics relevantly.

Therapeutic Use

Febuxostat is approved for hyperuric patients with gout attacks but is not recommended for treatment of asymptomatic hyperuricemia. It is available in 40- and 80-mg oral tablets. A dose of 40-mg/d febuxostat lowered serum uric acid to similar levels as 300-mg/d allopurinol. More patients reached the target concentration of 6.0 mg/dL (360 μmol/L) on 80-mg/d febuxostat than on 300-mg/d allopurinol. Thus, therapy should be initiated with 40 mg/d and the dose increased if the target serum uric acid concentration is not reached within 2 weeks.

Adverse Events

The most common adverse reactions in clinical studies were liver function abnormalities, nausea, joint pain, and rash. Liver function should be monitored periodically. An increase in gout flares was frequently observed after initiation of therapy, due to reduction in serum uric acid levels resulting in mobilization of urate from tissue deposits. Concurrent prophylactic treatment with an NSAID or colchicine is usually required. There was a higher rate of myocardial infarction and stroke in patients on febuxostat than on allopurinol. Whether there is a causal relationship between the cardiovascular events and febuxostat therapy or whether these were due to chance is not clear. Meanwhile patients should be monitored for cardiovascular complications.

Drug Interactions

Plasma levels of drugs metabolized by XO (e.g., theophylline, mercaptopurine, azathioprine) will increase when administered concurrently with febuxostat. Thus, febuxostat is contraindicated in patients on azathioprine or mercaptopurine; care should be exercised with concomitant administration of theophylline due to a 400-fold increase in the urinary excretion of the 1-methylxanthine metabolite.

Uricase

Pegloticase is a pegylated uricase (urate oxidase) that catalyzes the enzymatic oxidation of uric acid into allantoin, a more soluble and inactive metabolite. The recombinant enzyme, based on the porcine uricase, is administered by infusion. Pegloticase is used for the treatment of severe, treatment-refractory, chronic gout or when use of other urate-lowering therapies is contraindicated.

The drug's efficacy may be hampered by the production of antibodies against the drug. Pegloticase antibodies develop in nearly 90% of people, and high titers are associated with loss of the urate-lowering effect and with an elevated risk for infusion reactions. Anaphylactic reactions, and hemolysis in G6PD-deficient patients, have been associated with the use of pegloticase. Other frequently observed adverse reactions include vomiting, nausea, chest pain, constipation, diarrhea, and erythema, pruritus, and urticaria.

Rasburicase is a recombinant uricase that has been shown to lower urate levels more effectively than allopurinol. It is indicated for the initial management of elevated plasma uric acid levels in pediatric and adult patients with leukemia, lymphoma, and solid tumor malignancies who are receiving anticancer therapy expected to result in tumor lysis and significant hyperuricemia. The experience with rasburicase for treatment of gout is limited because of the formation of activity-limiting antibodies against the drug. Hemolysis in G6PD-deficient patients, methemoglobinemia, acute renal failure, and anaphylaxis have been associated with the use of rasburicase. Other frequently observed adverse reactions include vomiting, fever, nausea, headache, abdominal pain, constipation, diarrhea, and mucositis. Rasburicase causes enzymatic degradation of the uric acid in blood samples, and special handling is required to prevent spuriously low values for plasma uric acid in patients receiving the drug.

Uricosuric Agents

Uricosuric agents increase the excretion of uric acid. These agents are typically reserved for patients who underexcrete uric acid relative to their plasma levels. In humans, urate is filtered, secreted, and reabsorbed by the kidneys. Reabsorption is robust, such that the net amount excreted usually is about 10% of that filtered. Reabsorption is mediated by an OAT family member, URAT-1, which can be inhibited.

Urate is exchanged by URAT-1 for either an organic anion such as lactate or nicotinate or less potently for an inorganic anion such as chloride. Uricosuric drugs such as probenecid, benzbromarone (not available in the U.S.), and losartan compete with urate for the transporter, thereby inhibiting its reabsorption via the urate–anion exchanger system. However, transport is bidirectional, and depending on dosage, a drug may either decrease or increase the excretion of uric acid.

There are two mechanisms by which a drug may nullify the uricosuric action of another. First, the drug may inhibit the secretion of the uricosuric agent, thereby denying it access to its site of action, the luminal aspect of the brush border. Second, the inhibition of urate secretion by one drug may counterbalance the inhibition of urate reabsorption by the other.

Probenecid

Probenecid is a highly lipid-soluble benzoic acid derivative (pK_a 3.4).

$(CH_3CH_2CH_2)_2NSO_2-C_6H_4-COOH$

PROBENECID

Mechanism of Action. ***Inhibition of Organic Acid Transport.*** The actions of probenecid are confined largely to inhibition of the transport of organic acids across epithelial barriers. Probenecid inhibits the reabsorption of uric acid by OATs, principally URAT-1. Uric acid is the only important endogenous compound whose excretion is known to be increased by probenecid. The uricosuric action of probenecid is blunted by the coadministration of salicylates.

Inhibition of Transport of Miscellaneous Substances. Probenecid inhibits the tubular secretion of a number of drugs, such as methotrexate and the active metabolite of clofibrate. It inhibits renal secretion of the inactive glucuronide metabolites of NSAIDs such as naproxen, ketoprofen, and indomethacin and thereby can increase their plasma concentrations. Probenecid inhibits the transport of 5-HIAA and other acidic metabolites of cerebral monoamines from the CSF to the plasma. The transport of drugs such as penicillin G also may be affected, and probenecid is used therapeutically to elevate and prolong plasma β-lactam levels. Probenecid depresses the biliary secretion of certain compounds, including the diagnostic agents indocyanine green and bromosulfophthalein. It also decreases the biliary secretion of rifampin, leading to higher plasma concentrations.

ADME. Probenecid is absorbed completely after oral administration. Peak plasma concentrations are reached in 2–4 h. The $t_{1/2}$ of the drug in plasma is dose dependent and varies from less than 5 to more than 8 h. Between 85% and 95% of the drug is bound to plasma albumin; the 5%–15% of unbound drug is cleared by glomerular filtration and active secretion by the proximal tubule. A small amount of probenecid glucuronide appears in the urine. It also is hydroxylated to metabolites that retain their carboxyl function and have uricosuric activity.

Therapeutic Uses. Probenecid is marketed for oral administration, alone and in combination with colchicine. The starting dose is 250 mg twice daily, increasing over 1–2 weeks to 500–1000 mg twice daily. Probenecid increases urinary urate levels. Liberal fluid intake therefore should be maintained throughout therapy to minimize the risk of renal stones. Probenecid should not be used in gouty patients with nephrolithiasis or with overproduction of uric acid. Concomitant colchicine or NSAIDs are indicated early in the course of therapy to avoid precipitating an attack of gout, which may occur in 20% or fewer of gouty patients treated with probenecid alone. After 6 months, if serum uric acid levels are within normal limits and there have been no gout attacks, the dose of probenecid may be tapered off by 500 mg every 6 months.

Combination With Penicillin. Higher doses of probenecid (1–2 g/d) are used as an adjuvant to prolong the dwell time of penicillin and other β-lactam antibiotics in the body (see Chapter 57).

Adverse Effects. Probenecid is well tolerated. Approximately 2% of patients develop mild GI irritation. The risk is increased at higher doses. It is ineffective in patients with renal insufficiency and should be avoided in those with creatinine clearance of less than 50 mL/min. Hypersensitivity reactions usually are mild and occur in 2%–4% of patients. Substantial overdosage with probenecid results in CNS stimulation, convulsions, and death from respiratory failure.

Benzbromarone

Benzbromarone is a potent uricosuric agent that has been marketed in several countries since 1970. It is a reversible inhibitor of the urate–anion exchanger in the proximal tubule. Hepatotoxicity reported in conjunction with its use has limited its availability. The drug is absorbed readily after oral ingestion; peak plasma levels are achieved in about 4 h. It is metabolized to monobrominated and dehalogenated derivatives, both of which have uricosuric activity, and is excreted primarily in the bile.

As the micronized powder, it is effective in a single daily dose ranging from 25 to 100 mg. It is effective in patients with renal insufficiency and may be prescribed to patients who are either allergic or refractory to other drugs used for the treatment of gout. Preparations that combine allopurinol and benzbromarone are more effective than either drug alone in lowering serum uric acid levels, in spite of the fact that benzbromarone lowers plasma levels of oxypurinol, the active metabolite of allopurinol. The uricosuric action is blunted by aspirin or sulfinpyrazone.

Lesinurad

Lesinurad is FDA approved for combination therapy with an XO inhibitor in treating hyperuricemia.

Mechanism of Action. Lesinurad inhibits the URAT-1 and OAT-4 transporters, thereby reducing renal uric acid reabsorption.

ADME. Lesinurad is rapidly absorbed after oral administration and has bioavailability of about 100%. Lesinurad is largely bound to plasma albumin and other plasma proteins (<98%). The elimination $t_{1/2}$ is about 5 h (clearance ~ 6 L/h). CYP2C9 is the major metabolizing enzyme. Lesinurad (30% unchanged) and its metabolites are excreted in the urine (>60% of dose) and feces. Renal impairment increases exposure, and lesinurid should not be used when the renal function is severely reduced (estimated creatinine clearance < 45 mL/min).

Therapeutic Uses. Lesinurad (200 mg/d) is marketed for the treatment of gout in patients who have not achieved the target serum uric acid levels with an XO inhibitor alone. It should not be used for the treatment of asymptomatic hyperuricemia or as monotherapy.

Adverse Effects. Lesinurad has been labeled with a black-box warning because of a risk of acute renal failure that is more common when it is used without an XO inhibitor. Increases in blood creatinine levels (1.5- to 2-fold) were observed with a frequency of approximately 4% during combination therapy and 8% during monotherapy. Renal failure occurred in less than 1% of patients during combination therapy and approximately 9% during monotherapy. Similarly, the risk of nephrolithiasis is increased when lesinurad is given alone. Thus, if treatment with the XO inhibitor is interrupted, lesinurid dosing should also be interrupted. Other adverse reactions reported by patients during clinical trials include headache (~5%), influenza-like symptoms (~5%), and gastroesophageal reflux (~3%).

Acknowledgment: *Jason D. Morrow, L. Jackson Roberts II, and Anne Burke contributed to this chapter in earlier editions of this book. We have retained some of their text in the current edition.*

Drug Facts For Your Personal Formulary: *NSAIDs* (see also Tables 38–1, 38–2, and 38–3)

Drugs	Therapeutic Uses	Clinical Pharmacology and Tips
Salicylates • Used to treat pain, fever, inflammation • Adverse Effects: Primarily GI and CV, salicylate intoxication		
Aspirin	• Vascular indications • Pain/fever • Rheumatoid disease / Rheumatic fever	• Irreversible COX inhibitor ⇒ long-acting inhibition of platelet function at low doses • At higher concentrations, small increments in dose disproportionately ↑ C_p and toxicity • Use in children: limited due to Reye's syndrome association • Reduces the risk of recurrent adenomas in persons with a history of colorectal cancer or adenomas • Prolongs bleeding time for ~ 36 h after a dose
Salsalate	• Arthritis • Rheumatic disorders	• Prodrug of salicylic acid • Not approved in the US
Diflunisal	• Mild to moderate pain • Osteoarthritis/Rheumatoid arthritis	• Salicylic acid derivative • Largely devoid of antipyretic effects • $t_{1/2}$ prolonged with renal impairment
Mesalamine (5-aminosalicylic acid)	• Inflammatory bowel disease	• Oral formulation delivers 5-aminosalicylic acid to lower GI tract; relative bowel specificity reduces side effects • May cause an acute intolerance syndrome (difficult to discern from an exacerbation)
Sulfasalazine	• Rheumatoid arthritis • Inflammatory bowel disease	• Active metabolite 5-aminosalicylic acid (see mesalamine) released by colonic bacteria • With G6PD deficiency: susceptibility to hemolytic anemia
Olsalazine	• Inflammatory bowel disease	• Active metabolite 5-aminosalicylic acid (see mesalamine) is released by colonic bacteria.
Balsalazide	• Inflammatory bowel disease	• Active metabolite, 5-aminosalicylic acid (see mesalamine), is released by colonic bacteria.
Para-Aminophenol Derivative • Only acetaminophen remains on the market		
Acetaminophen	• Pain • Fever	• Weak nonspecific COX inhibitor at common doses • Low anti-inflammatory activity • Little effect on platelets • Overdose results in formation of hepatotoxic metabolite (NAPQI) • Toxicity risk ↑ with liver impairment, ethanol consumption ≥3 drinks/day, or malnutrition
Acetic Acid Derivatives		
Indomethacin	• Acute pain • Arthritis, inflammatory conditions • Patent ductus arteriosus	• Potent anti-inflammatory with frequent adverse events (20% discontinue) • High-risk medication in patients ≥ 65 years
Sulindac	• Inflammatory diseases including osteoarthritis, rheumatoid arthritis, acute gouty arthritis, ankylosing spondylitis, acute painful shoulder	• Sulfoxide prodrug
Etodolac	• Pain, osteoarthritis, rheumatoid arthritis, juvenile arthritis	• Some COX-2 selectivity
Tolmetin	• Osteoarthritis, rheumatoid arthritis, juvenile arthritis	• ~33% of patients experience side effects
Ketorolac	• Moderate-to-severe acute pain • Off label: pericarditis, migraine • Ocular pain, seasonal allergic conjunctivitis	• Potent analgesic, poor anti-inflammatory • Max total systemic therapy: 5 days • Oral, IM, IV, nasal, and ophthalmic administration

Drug Facts For Your Personal Formulary: *NSAIDs* (see also Tables 38–1, 38–2, and 38–3)(*continued*)

Drugs	Therapeutic Uses	Clinical Pharmacology and Tips
Acetic Acid Derivatives		
Diclofenac	• Pain • Dysmenorrhea • Migraine (oral solution) • Osteoarthritis, rheumatoid arthritis • Ankylosing spondylitis	• Some COX-2 selectivity • Short $t_{1/2}$ requires relatively high doses to extend dosing interval • Rate of CV toxicity similar to that of COX-2 inhibitors • Liver toxicity (4%); severe liver injury in ~8 per 100,000 regular users annually
Nabumetone	• Osteoarthritis, rheumatoid arthritis	• Some COX-2 selectivity • 6-methoxy-2-napthylacetic acid prodrug
Fenamates • Anthranilic acids; Nonselective COX inhibitors with effects similar to other NSAIDs		
Mefenamic acid	• Pain • Dysmenorrhea	• For patients ≥ 14 years and ≤ 7 days of treatment • ↑ hepatic enzymes in 5%
Meclofenamate	• Pain/fever, dysmenorrhea • Osteoarthritis, rheumatoid arthritis, juvenile arthritis • Ankylosing spondylitis, acute gouty arthritis, acute painful shoulder	• For patients ≥ 14 years • ↑ hepatic enzymes in 5%
Propionic Acid Derivatives • Nonselective COX inhibitors with the effects and side effects common to other NSAIDs		
Ibuprofen	• Pain/fever, dysmenorrhea • Osteoarthritis, rheumatoid arthritis • Inflammatory diseases • Patent ductus arteriosus	• Over-the-counter NSAID • Injectable solution available • $t_{1/2}$: 2–4 h (adults); 23–75 h (premature infants); 0.9–2.3 h (children) • Interacts with aspirin's antiplatelet effect
Naproxen	• Pain, dysmenorrhea • Osteoarthritis, rheumatoid arthritis, ankylosing spondylitis; gout; juvenile arthritis, inflammatory diseases • Patent ductus arteriosus	• Over-the-counter NSAID • $t_{1/2}$ variable (9–25 h), age-related • FDA warning: naproxen may not have a lower risk of CV side effects compared to other NSAIDs • Interacts with aspirin's antiplatelet effect
Fenoprofen	• Pain • Osteoarthritis, rheumatoid arthritis	
Ketoprofen	• Pain, dysmenorrhea • Osteoarthritis, rheumatoid arthritis	• 30% develop side effects (usually GI, usually mild) • ↑ hepatic enzymes ~1%
Flurbiprofen	• Osteoarthritis, rheumatoid arthritis	• ↑ hepatic enzymes > 1%
Oxaprozin	• Osteoarthritis, rheumatoid arthritis, juvenile arthritis	• $t_{1/2}$: 41-55 h • Slow onset, not indicated for fever or acute pain
Enolic Acid Derivatives		
Piroxicam	• Osteoarthritis, rheumatoid arthritis	• nonselective COX inhibitor with the longest $t_{1/2}$ ~50 h • Slow onset, not indicated for fever or acute pain • Adverse effects, 20%, 5% of patients discontinue; more GI and serious skin reactions than other NSAIDs
Meloxicam	• Osteoarthritis, rheumatoid arthritis, juvenile arthritis	• Some COX-2 selectivity • $t_{1/2}$: 15-20 h
Diaryl Heterocyclic NSAIDs		
Celecoxib	• Pain • Dysmenorrhea • Osteoarthritis, rheumatoid arthritis, juvenile arthritis • ankylosing spondylitis • Off label use: gout	• COX-2 selective • Sulfonamide • Risk of myocardial infarction observed in randomized placebo controlled trials.

Drug Facts For Your Personal Formulary: *Gout*

Drugs	Therapeutic Uses	Clinical Pharmacology and Tips
Drugs that relieve inflammation and pain		
NSAIDs	• *See* NSAIDs, above	• *See* NSAIDs, above
Glucocorticoids	• *See* Chapter 46	• *See* Chapter 46
Colchicine	• Prophylaxis and the treatment of acute gout flares	• Depolymerizes microtubules ⇒ ↓neutrophil migration into inflamed area • Narrow therapeutic index; toxic effects related to antimitotic activity • $t_{1/2}$: 31 h (21–50 h) • Individualize dose on the basis of age, hepatic and renal function • Contraindicated in patients with GI, renal, hepatic or cardiac disorders • Adverse effects: primarily GI • Drug interactions with P-gp and CYP3A4 inhibitors
Xanthine oxidase (XO) inhibitors • Inhibit urate synthesis		
Allopurinol	• Hyperuricemia in patients with gout gout • Calcium oxalate calculi • Hyperuricemia associated with cancer treatment	• active metabolite: oxypurinol • $t_{1/2}$: allopurinol 1–2 h, oxypurinol 18–30h; adjust dose in renal impairment • Rash, diarrhea, nausea frequent • Risk of gout attacks during the early months of therapy (tissue urate mobilization) • Serum [urate] usually ↓ in 24–48 h, normal 1–3 weeks
Febuxostat	• Hyperuricemia	• non-purine • more selective for XO than allopurinol • $t_{1/2}$: 5 to 8 h • Liver function abnormalities (5–7%)
Uricase • Oxidizes uric acid to allantoin (more soluble and inactive metabolite)		
Pegloticase	• Chronic gout refractory to conventional therapy	• $t_{1/2}$, 14 days • ↓Blood urate within hours of initial administration • Antibody development against drug may limit efficacy, cause hypersensitivity reactions • Adverse effects: bruising (11%), urticaria (11%), nausea (11%), gout flare during early therapy (74%), chest pain (6%)
Rasburicase	• Hyperuricemia associated with malignancy (pediatric and adult patients)	• $t_{1/2}$: 16 to 23 h • ↓Uric acid levels within hours of initial administration • Not suitable for chronic gout; activity-limiting antibodies form against the drug.
Uricosuric drugs–Inhibit of reabsorption of uric acid by organic anion transporters, thereby increasing excretion of uric acid		
Probenecid	• Hyperuricemia associated with gout (but not for acute attacks) • Prolongation and elevation of beta-lactam plasma levels	• Interferes with renal tubular handling of organic acids • $t_{1/2}$: 6-12 h (dose–dependent) • Risk of gout attacks during the early months of therapy (tissue urate mobilization) • ineffective in patients with renal insufficiency
Lesinurad	• Gout in patients who have not achieved the target serum uric acid levels with XO inhibitor alone	• $t_{1/2}$: 5 h • CYP2C9 substrate, so caution is recommended in patients who are CYP2C9 poor metabolizers • Must be used together with XO inhibitor due to renal failure risk

Bibliography

Antithrombotic Trialists' Collaboration, et al. Aspirin in the primary and secondary prevention of vascular disease: collaborative meta-analysis of individual participant data from randomised trials. *Lancet*, **2009**, *373*:1849–1860.

Arehart E, et al. Acceleration of cardiovascular disease by a dysfunctional prostacyclin receptor mutation: potential implications for cyclooxygenase-2 inhibition. *Circ Res*, **2008**, *102*:986–993.

Bjornsson ES, et al. Incidence, presentation, and outcomes in patients with drug-induced liver injury in the general population of Iceland. *Gastroenterology*, **2013**, *144*:1419–1425, 1425, e1411–e1413; quiz e1419–e1420.

Blieden M, et al. A perspective on the epidemiology of acetaminophen exposure and toxicity in the United States. *Expert Rev Clin Pharmacol*, **2014**, *7*:341–348.

Bogentoft C, et al. Influence of food on the absorption of acetylsalicylic acid from enteric-coated dosage forms. *Eur J Clin Pharmacol*, **1978**, *14*:351–355.

Cannon CP, et al. Cardiovascular outcomes with etoricoxib and diclofenac in patients with osteoarthritis and rheumatoid arthritis in the Multinational Etoricoxib and Diclofenac Arthritis Long-term (MEDAL) programme: a randomised comparison. *Lancet*, **2006**, *368*:1771–1781.

Capone ML, et al. Pharmacodynamic interaction of naproxen with low-dose aspirin in healthy subjects. *J Am Coll Cardiol*, **2005**, *45*:1295–1301.

Catella-Lawson F, et al. Cyclooxygenase inhibitors and the antiplatelet effects of aspirin. *N Engl J Med*, **2001**, *345*:1809–1817.

Catella-Lawson F, et al. Effects of specific inhibition of cyclooxygenase-2 on sodium balance, hemodynamics, and vasoactive eicosanoids. *J Pharmacol Exp Ther*, **1999**, *289*:735–741.

Chen L, et al. Prostanoids and inflammatory pain. *Prostaglandins Other Lipid Mediat*, **2013**, 104–105 58–66.

Cheng Y, et al. Role of prostacyclin in the cardiovascular response to thromboxane A_2. *Science*, **2002**, *296*:539–541.

Cheng Y, et al. Cyclooxygenases, microsomal prostaglandin E synthase-1, and cardiovascular function. *J Clin Invest*, **2006**, *116*:1391–1399.

Coxib and Traditional NSAID Trialists' Collaboration, et al. Vascular and upper gastrointestinal effects of non-steroidal anti-inflammatory drugs: meta-analyses of individual participant data from randomised trials. *Lancet*, **2013**, *382*:769–779.

Daly AK, et al. Genetic susceptibility to diclofenac-induced hepatotoxicity: contribution of UGT2B7, CYP2C8, and ABCC2 genotypes. *Gastroenterology*, **2007**, *132*:272–281.

Day RO, et al. Pharmacokinetics of nonsteroidal anti-inflammatory drugs in synovial fluid. *Clin Pharmacokinet*, **1999**, *36*:191–210.

de Abajo FJ, et al. Acute and clinically relevant drug-induced liver injury: a population based case-control study. *Br J Clin Pharmacol*, **2004**, *58*:71–80.

Dong L, et al. Human cyclooxygenase-2 is a sequence homodimer that functions as a conformational heterodimer. *J Biol Chem*, **2011**, *286*:19035–19046.

Egan KM, et al. COX-2-derived prostacyclin confers atheroprotection on female mice. *Science*, **2004**, *306*:1954–1957.

Engblom D, et al. Microsomal prostaglandin E synthase-1 is the central switch during immune-induced pyresis. *Nat Neurosci*, **2003**, *6*(11):1137–1138.

Farkouh ME, et al. Comparison of lumiracoxib with naproxen and ibuprofen in the Therapeutic Arthritis Research and Gastrointestinal Event Trial (TARGET), cardiovascular outcomes: randomised controlled trial. *Lancet*, **2004**, *364*:675–684.

FitzGerald GA, Patrono C. The coxibs, selective inhibitors of cyclooxygenase-2. *N Engl J Med*, **2001**, *345*:433–442.

Graham GG, et al. Tolerability of paracetamol. *Drug Saf*, **2005**, *28*: 227–240.

Grosser T, et al. Drug resistance and pseudoresistance: an unintended consequence of enteric coating aspirin. *Circulation*, **2013**, *127*:377–85.

Grosser T, et al. Biological basis for the cardiovascular consequences of COX-2 inhibition: therapeutic challenges and opportunities. *J Clin Invest*, **2006**, *116*:4–15.

Grosser T, et al. The Cardiovascular Pharmacology of Nonsteroidal Anti-Inflammatory Drugs. *Trends Pharmacol Sci*, **2017**, *38*:733–748.

Grosser T, et al. Emotion recollected in tranquility: lessons learned from the COX-2 saga. *Annu Rev Med*, **2010**, *61*:17–33.

King C, et al. Characterization of rat and human UDP-glucuronosyltransferases responsible for the in vitro glucuronidation of diclofenac. *Toxicol Sci*, **2001**, *61*:49–53.

Kobayashi T, et al. Roles of thromboxane A_2 and prostacyclin in the development of atherosclerosis in apoE-deficient mice. *J Clin Invest*, **2004**, *114*:784–794.

LeFevre ML, Force U. Low-dose aspirin use for the prevention of morbidity and mortality from preeclampsia: U.S. Preventive Services Task Force recommendation statement. *Ann Intern Med*, **2014**, *161*:819–826.

Leung YY, et al. Colchicine—update on mechanisms of action and therapeutic uses. *Semin Arthritis Rheum*, **2015**, *45*:341–350.

Li X, et al. Differential impairment of aspirin-dependent platelet cyclooxygenase acetylation by nonsteroidal antiinflammatory drugs. *Proc Natl Acad Sci U S A*, **2014**, *111*:16830–16835.

McAdam BF, et al. Systemic biosynthesis of prostacyclin by cyclooxygenase (COX)-2: the human pharmacology of a selective inhibitor of COX-2. *Proc Natl Acad Sci U S A*, **1999**, *96*:272–277.

Muller WA. Mechanisms of leukocyte transendothelial migration. *Annu Rev Pathol*, **2011**, *6*:323–344.

Nusing RM, et al. Pathogenetic role of cyclooxygenase-2 in hyperprostaglandin E syndrome/antenatal Bartter syndrome: therapeutic use of the cyclooxygenase-2 inhibitor nimesulide. *Clin Pharmacol Ther*, **2001**, *70*:384–390.

Patoia L, et al. A 4-week, double-blind, parallel-group study to compare the gastrointestinal effects of meloxicam 7.5 mg, meloxicam 15 mg, piroxicam 20 mg and placebo by means of faecal blood loss, endoscopy and symptom evaluation in healthy volunteers. *Br J Rheumatol*. **1996**, *35*(suppl 1):61–67.

Patrono C. The multifaceted clinical readouts of platelet inhibition by low-dose aspirin. *J Am Coll Cardiol*, **2015**, *66*:74–85.

Pedersen AK, FitzGerald GA. Dose-related kinetics of aspirin. Presystemic acetylation of platelet cyclooxygenase. *N Engl J Med*, **1984**, *311*:1206–1211.

Rostom A, et al. Nonsteroidal anti-inflammatory drugs and hepatic toxicity: a systematic review of randomized controlled trials in arthritis patients. *Clin Gastroenterol Hepatol*, **2005**, *3*:489–498.

Rothwell PM, et al. Long-term effect of aspirin on colorectal cancer incidence and mortality: 20-year follow-up of five randomised trials. *Lancet*, **2010**, *376*(9754):1741–1750.

Sanchez-Alavez M, et al. Ceramide mediates the rapid phase of febrile response to IL-1beta. *Proc Natl Acad Sci U S A*, **2006**, *103*:2904–2908.

Schrör K. Aspirin and Reye syndrome: a review of the evidence. *Paediatr Drugs*, **2007**, *9*:195–204.

Smith WL, et al. Enzymes of the cyclooxygenase pathways of prostanoid biosynthesis. *Chem Rev*, **2011**, *111*: 5821–5865.

Song WL, et al. Niacin and biosynthesis of PGD(2)by platelet COX-1 in mice and humans. *J Clin Invest*, **2012**, *122*:1459–1468.

Sostres C, et al. Nonsteroidal anti-inflammatory drugs and upper and lower gastrointestinal mucosal damage. *Arthritis Res Ther*, **2013**, *15*(suppl 3):S3.

Tang D, et al. PAMPs and DAMPs: signal 0s that spur autophagy and immunity. *Immunol Rev*, **2012**, *249*:158–175.

Theoharides T, et al. Mast cells, mastocytosis, and related disorders. *N Engl J Med*, **2015**, *373*:163–172.

U.S. Food and Drug Administration. FDA Drug Safety Communication: FDA strengthens warning that non-aspirin nonsteroidal anti-inflammatory drugs (NSAIDs) can cause heart attacks or strokes. **2015**. Available at: http://www.fda.gov/Drugs/DrugSafety/ucm451800.htm. Accessed June 1, 2016.

Warner T, et al. Nonsteroid drug selectivities for cyclo-oxygenase-1 rather than cyclo-oxygenase-2 are associated with human gastrointestinal toxicity: a full in vitro analysis. *Proc Natl Acad Sci U S A*, **1999**, *96*:7563–7568.

Xian Y, et al. Association of discharge aspirin dose with outcomes after acute myocardial infarction: insights from the Treatment With ADP Receptor Inhibitors: Longitudinal Assessment of Treatment Patterns and Events After Acute Coronary Syndrome (TRANSLATE-ACS) study. *Circulation*, **2015**, *132*:174–181.

Yu Y, et al. Vascular COX-2 modulates blood pressure and thrombosis in mice. *Sci Transl Med*, **2012**, *4*:132–154.

Zou H, et al. Human cyclooxygenase-1 activity and its responses to COX inhibitors are allosterically regulated by nonsubstrate fatty acids. *J Lipid Res*, **2012**, *53*:1336–1347.

Histamine, Bradykinin, and Their Antagonists

Randal A. Skidgel

第三十九章 组胺和缓激肽及其拮抗药

中文导读

本章主要介绍：组胺，包括组胺的分布和生物合成、内源性组胺的释放和功能、生理和药理效应；组胺受体拮抗药，包括H_1受体拮抗药、H_2受体拮抗药、H_3受体拮抗药和H_4受体拮抗药；缓激肽、胰激肽及其拮抗药，包括内源性激肽释放酶–激肽原–激肽系统、激肽释放酶抑制药、缓激肽和血管紧张等转换酶抑制药的作用、激肽受体拮抗药。

Endogenous histamine plays a role in the immediate allergic response and is an important regulator of gastric acid secretion. More recently, a role for histamine as a modulator of neurotransmitter release in the central and peripheral nervous systems has emerged. The cloning of four receptors for histamine and the development of subtype-specific receptor antagonists have enhanced our understanding of the physiological and pathophysiological roles of histamine. Competitive antagonists of H_1 receptors are used therapeutically in treating allergies, urticaria, anaphylactic reactions, nausea, motion sickness, and insomnia. Antagonists of the H_2 receptor are effective in reducing gastric acid secretion.

The peptides bradykinin and kallidin, released after activation of the kallikrein-kinin system, have cardiovascular effects similar to those of histamine and play prominent roles in inflammation and nociception. Icatibant, a competitive antagonist of the bradykinin B_2 receptor, and ecallantide, a specific plasma kallikrein inhibitor, are approved for the treatment of acute episodes of edema in patients with hereditary angioedema.

Histamine

Histamine is a hydrophilic molecule consisting of an imidazole ring and an amino group connected by an ethylene group; histamine is biosynthesized from histidine by decarboxylation (Figure 39–1). Histamine acts through four classes of receptors, designated H_1 through H_4. The four histamine receptors, all GPCRs, can be differentially activated by analogues of histamine (Figure 39–2) and inhibited by specific antagonists (Table 39–1).

Distribution and Biosynthesis

Distribution

Almost all mammalian tissues contain histamine in amounts ranging from less than 1 to more than 100 μg/g. Concentrations in plasma and other body fluids are generally very low, but they are significant in human CSF. The concentration of histamine is particularly high in tissues that contain

Abbreviations

ACE: angiotensin I converting enzyme
ACh: actetylcholine
ADHD: attention-deficit/hyperactivity disorder
Ang: angiotensin
AT: angiotensin receptor
AV: atrioventricular
CNS: central nervous system
CPM/N: carboxypeptidase M/N
CSF: cerebrospinal fluid
EDHF: endothelial-derived hyperpolarizing factor
EET: epoxyeicosatrienoic acid
eNOS: endothelial nitric oxide synthase
GABA: gamma-aminobutyric acid
GPCR: G protein–coupled receptor
HMW: high molecular weight
5HT: serotonin
IgE: immunoglobulin E
IL-1: interleukin 1
iNOS: inducible nitric oxide synthase
IP_3: inositol triphosphate
JNK1/2: c-Jun N-terminal kinase1/2
LMW: low molecular weight
MAO: monoamine oxidase
PAF: platelet-activating factor
PG: prostaglandin
TNF-α: tumor necrosis factor alpha

HISTORY

Histamine was first prepared synthetically in 1907 and isolated from ergot extracts in 1910 (Emanuel, 1999). It was identified as a natural constituent of mammalian tissues in 1927 by Best and colleagues and named *histamine* after the Greek word for tissue, *histos*. Dale and Laidlaw made the crucial observation that histamine injection into mammals caused a shock-like reaction and proposed its role in mediating symptoms of anaphylaxis (Emanuel, 1999).

large numbers of mast cells, such as skin, bronchial mucosa, and intestinal mucosa.

Synthesis, Storage, and Metabolism

Histamine is formed by the decarboxylation of histidine by the enzyme *L-histidine decarboxylase* (Figure 39–1). Mast cells and basophils synthesize histamine and store it in secretory granules. At the secretory granule pH of about 5.5, histamine is positively charged and ionically complexed with negatively charged acidic groups on other granule constituents, primarily proteases and heparin or chondroitin sulfate proteoglycans. The turnover rate of histamine in secretory granules is slow (days to weeks). Non–mast cell sites of histamine formation include the epidermis, enterochromaffin-like cells of the gastric mucosa, neurons within the CNS, and cells in regenerating or rapidly growing tissues. Turnover is rapid at these non–mast cell sites because the histamine is released continuously rather than stored. Non–mast cell sites of histamine production contribute significantly to the daily excretion of histamine metabolites in the urine. Because L-histidine decarboxylase is an inducible enzyme, the histamine-forming capacity at such sites is subject to regulation. Histamine that is released or ingested is rapidly metabolized by either ring methylation catalyzed by *histamine-N-methyltransferase* or oxidative deamination catalyzed by *diamine oxidase* (Figure 39–1), and the metabolites are eliminated in the urine.

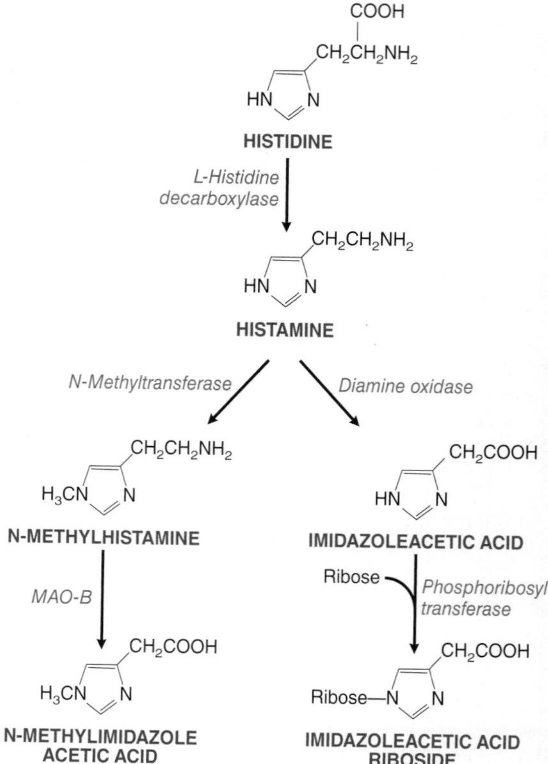

Figure 39–1 *Pathways of histamine synthesis and metabolism in humans.* Histamine is synthesized from histidine by decarboxylation. Histamine is metabolized via two pathways, predominantly by methylation of the ring followed by oxidative deamination (left side of figure) and secondarily by oxidative deamination and then conjugation with ribose.

Release and Functions of Endogenous Histamine

Histamine is released from storage granules as a result of the interaction of antigen with IgE antibodies on the mast cell surface. Histamine plays a central role in immediate hypersensitivity and allergic responses. The actions of histamine on bronchial smooth muscle and blood vessels account for many of the symptoms of the allergic response. Histamine is a leukocyte chemoattractant, plays a major role in regulating gastric acid secretion, and modulates neurotransmitter release. In addition, some drugs act directly on mast cells to release histamine, causing untoward effects.

Role in Allergic Responses

The principal target cells of immediate hypersensitivity reactions are mast cells and basophils (Schwartz, 1994). As part of the allergic response to an antigen, IgE antibodies are generated and bind to the surfaces of mast cells and basophils via specific high-affinity F_c receptors. This receptor, FcεRI, consists of α, β, and two γ chains (see Chapter 34). Antigen bridges the IgE molecules and via FcεRI activates signaling pathways in mast cells or basophils involving tyrosine kinases and subsequent phosphorylation of multiple protein substrates within 5–15 sec of contact with antigen. These events trigger the exocytosis of the contents of secretory granules that, in addition to histamine, includes serotonin, proteases, lysosomal enzymes, cytokines, and proteoglycans (Schwartz, 1994).

Release of Other Autacoids

Stimulation of IgE receptors also activates PLA_2, leading to the production of a host of mediators, including PAF and metabolites of arachidonic acid such as leukotrienes C_4 and D_4, which contract bronchial smooth muscle

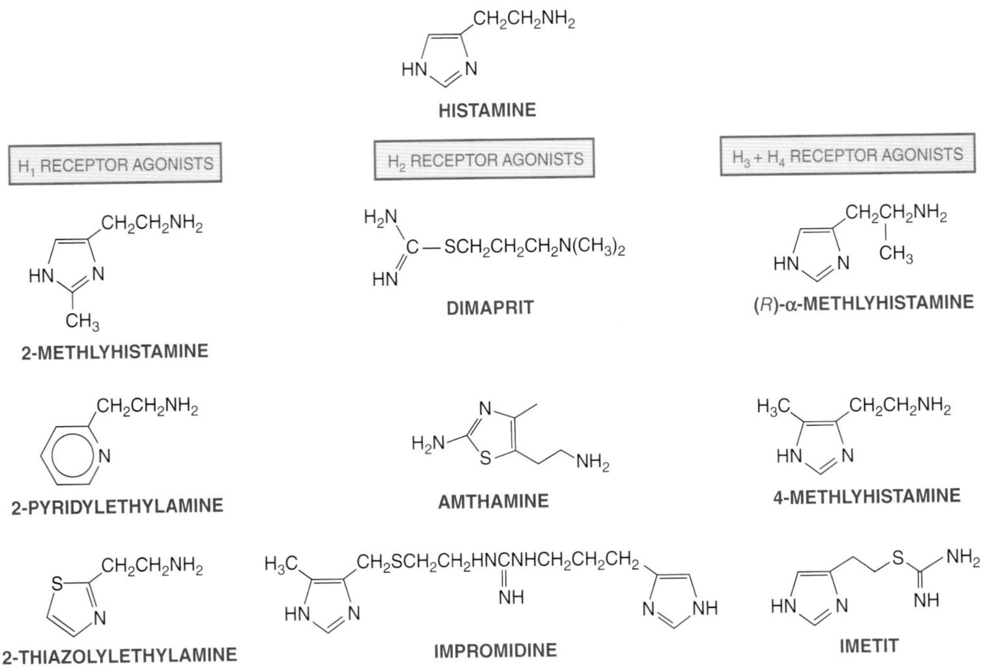

HISTAMINE

H_1 RECEPTOR AGONISTS

2-METHLYHISTAMINE

2-PYRIDYLETHYLAMINE

2-THIAZOLYLETHYLAMINE

H_2 RECEPTOR AGONISTS

DIMAPRIT

AMTHAMINE

IMPROMIDINE

$H_3 + H_4$ RECEPTOR AGONISTS

(*R*)-α-METHLYHISTAMINE

4-METHLYHISTAMINE

IMETIT

Figure 39–2 *Structure of histamine and some H_1, H_2, H_3, and H_4 agonists.* Dimaprit and 4-methylhistamine, originally identified as specific H_2 agonists, have a much higher affinity for the H_4 receptor; 4-methylhistamine is the most specific available H_4 agonist, with about 10-fold higher affinity than dimaprit, a partial H_4 agonist. Impromidine not only is among the most potent H_2 agonists but also is an antagonist at H_1 and H_3 receptors and a partial agonist at H_4 receptors. (R)-α-Methylhistamine and imetit are high-affinity agonists of H_3 receptors and lower-affinity full agonists at H_4 receptors.

(Chapters 37 and 40). Kinins also are generated during some allergic responses. Thus, the mast cell secretes a variety of inflammatory mediators in addition to histamine, each contributing to aspects of the allergic response (see discussion that follows).

Histamine Release by Drugs, Peptides, Venoms, and Other Agents

Mechanical injury and many compounds, including a large number of therapeutic agents, stimulate the release of histamine from mast cells directly and without prior sensitization. Responses of this sort are most likely to occur following intravenous injections of certain categories of substances, particularly organic bases. Tubocurarine, succinylcholine, morphine, some antibiotics, radiocontrast media, and certain carbohydrate plasma expanders also may elicit the response. The phenomenon is one of clinical concern and may account for unexpected anaphylactoid reactions. Basic polypeptides often are effective histamine releasers, and over a limited range, their potency generally increases with the number of basic groups. For example, bradykinin is a poor histamine releaser, whereas kallidin (Lys-bradykinin) and substance P, with more positively charged amino acids, are more active (Johnson and Erdos, 1973). Some venoms, such as that of the wasp, contain potent histamine-releasing peptides. Basic polypeptides released on tissue injury constitute pathophysiological stimuli for secretion from mast cells and basophils.

Within seconds of the intravenous injection of a histamine liberator, human subjects experience a burning, itching sensation. This effect, most marked in the palms of the hand and in the face, scalp, and ears, is soon followed by a feeling of intense warmth. The skin reddens, and the color rapidly spreads over the trunk. Blood pressure falls, the heart rate accelerates, and the subject usually complains of headache. After a few minutes, blood pressure recovers, and crops of hives usually appear

TABLE 39–1 ■ CHARACTERISTICS OF HISTAMINE RECEPTORS

	H_1	H_2	H_3[a]	H_4
Size (amino acids)	487	359	329–445	390
G protein coupling (second messengers)	$G_{q/11}$ (↑ Ca^{2+}; ↑ NO and ↑ cGMP)	G_s (↑ cAMP)	$G_{i/o}$ (↓ cAMP; ↑ MAP kinase)	$G_{i/o}$ (↓ cAMP; ↑ Ca^{2+})
Distribution	Smooth muscle, endothelial cells, CNS	Gastric parietal cells, cardiac muscle, mast cells, CNS	CNS: pre- and post-synaptic	Cells of hematopoietic origin
Representative agonist	2-CH_3-histamine	Amthamine	(*R*)-α-CH_3-histamine	4-CH_3-histamine
Representative antagonist	Chlorpheniramine	Ranitidine	Tiprolisant	JNJ7777120

[a]At least 20 alternately spliced H_3 isoforms have been detected at the mRNA level. Eight of these isoforms, ranging in size from 329 to 445 residues, were found to be functionally competent by binding or signaling assays (see Esbenshade et al., 2008).

on the skin. Colic, nausea, hypersecretion of acid, and moderate bronchospasm also frequently occur. The effect becomes less intense with successive administration of the secretagogue as mast cell stores of histamine are depleted. Histamine liberators do not deplete histamine from non–mast cell sites. The mechanism by which basic secretagogues release histamine likely involves their direct interaction with G proteins or activation of a mast cell–specific cell surface GPCR named MRGRX2 (Seifert, 2015).

Increased Proliferation of Mast Cells and Basophils; Gastric Carcinoid Tumors

In urticaria pigmentosa (cutaneous mastocytosis), mast cells aggregate in the upper corium and give rise to pigmented cutaneous lesions that sting when stroked. In systemic mastocytosis, overproliferation of mast cells is also found in other organs. Patients with these syndromes suffer a constellation of signs and symptoms attributable to excessive histamine release, including urticaria, dermographism, pruritus, headache, weakness, hypotension, flushing of the face, and a variety of GI effects, such as diarrhea or peptic ulceration. A variety of stimuli, including exertion, insect stings, exposure to heat, allergens (including drugs to which a patient is allergic), can activate mast cells and cause histamine release, as can organic bases (many drugs) that cause histamine release directly. In myelogenous leukemia, elevation of blood basophils can result in histamine content high enough to cause flushing, pruritus, and hypotension. Management of these patients can be complicated by a large release of histamine after cytolysis, causing shock. Gastric carcinoid tumors secrete histamine, which is responsible for episodes of vasodilation as part of the patchy "geographical" flush.

Gastric Acid Secretion

Histamine acting at H_2 receptors is a powerful gastric secretagogue, evoking copious secretion of acid from parietal cells (see Figure 49–1); it also increases the output of pepsin and intrinsic factor. The secretion of gastric acid from parietal cells also is caused by stimulation of the vagus nerve and by the enteric hormone gastrin. However, histamine is the dominant physiological mediator of acid secretion; blockade of H_2 receptors not only antagonizes acid secretion in response to histamine but also inhibits responses to gastrin and vagal stimulation (see Chapter 49).

CNS

Histamine-containing neurons affect both homeostatic and higher brain functions, including regulation of the sleep-wake cycle, circadian and feeding rhythms, immunity, learning, memory, drinking, and body temperature. However, no human disease has yet been directly linked to dysfunction of the brain histamine system. Histamine, histidine decarboxylase, enzymes that metabolize histamine, and H_1, H_2, and H_3 receptors are distributed widely but nonuniformly in the CNS. H_1 receptors are associated with both neuronal and nonneuronal cells and are concentrated in regions that control neuroendocrine function, behavior, and nutritional state. Distribution of H_2 receptors is more consistent with histaminergic projections than that of H_1 receptors, suggesting that they mediate many of the postsynaptic actions of histamine. H_3 receptors are concentrated in areas known to receive histaminergic projections, consistent with their function as presynaptic autoreceptors. Histamine inhibits appetite and increases wakefulness via H_1 receptors.

Physiological and Pharmacological Effects

Receptor-Effector Coupling and Mechanisms of Action

Histamine receptors are GPCRs, coupling to second-messenger systems and producing effects (Simons, 2004) as noted in Table 39–1. H_1 receptors couple to $G_q/_{11}$ and activate the PLC-IP_3-Ca^{2+} pathway and its many possible sequelae, including activation of PKC, Ca^{2+}-calmodulin–dependent enzymes (eNOS and various protein kinases), and PLA_2. H_2 receptors link to G_s to activate the adenylyl cyclase–cyclic AMP–PKA pathway; H_3 and H_4 receptors couple to $G_i/_o$ to inhibit adenylyl cyclase and decrease cellular cyclic AMP. Activation of H_3 receptors also can activate MAP kinase and inhibit the Na^+/H^+ exchanger; activation of H_4 receptors can mobilize stored Ca^{2+} (Simons and Simons, 2011). H_3 and H_4 receptors have about 1000-fold higher affinity for histamine (low nanomolar range) than do H_1 and H_2 receptors (low micromolar range). Activation of H_1 receptors on vascular endothelium stimulates eNOS to produce NO, which diffuses to nearby smooth muscle cells to increase cyclic GMP and cause relaxation. Stimulation of H_1 receptors on smooth muscle will mobilize Ca^{2+} and cause contraction, whereas activation of H_2 receptors on the same smooth muscle cell will link via G_s to enhanced cyclic AMP accumulation, activation of PKA, and then to relaxation.

Pharmacological definition of H_1, H_2, and H_3 receptors was possible through the use of relatively specific agonists and antagonists. Because the H_4 receptor exhibits 35%–40% homology to isoforms of the H_3 receptor, the two were initially harder to distinguish pharmacologically, but this has been resolved by the development of several H_3- and H_4-selective antagonists (Sander et al., 2008; Thurmond, 2015). 4-Methylhistamine and dimaprit, previously identified as specific H_2 agonists, are actually more potent H_4 agonists.

H_1 and H_2 Receptors

H_1 and H_2 receptors are distributed widely in the periphery and in the CNS and their activation by histamine can exert local or widespread effects (Simons and Simons, 2011). For example, histamine causes itching and stimulates secretion from nasal mucosa. It contracts many smooth muscles, such as those of the bronchi and gut, but markedly relaxes others, including those in small blood vessels. Histamine also is a potent stimulus of gastric acid secretion. Other, less-prominent effects include formation of edema and stimulation of sensory nerve endings. Bronchoconstriction and contraction of the gut are mediated by H_1 receptors. In the CNS, H_1 activation inhibits appetite and increases wakefulness. Gastric secretion results from the activation of H_2 receptors. Some responses, such as vascular dilation, are mediated by both H_1 and H_2 receptor stimulation.

H_3 and H_4 Receptors

The H_3 receptors are expressed mainly in the CNS, especially in the basal ganglia, hippocampus, and cortex (Haas et al., 2008). Presynaptic H_3 receptors function as autoreceptors on histaminergic neurons, inhibiting histamine release and modulating the release of other neurotransmitters. H_3 receptors are also found postsynaptically, especially in the basal ganglia, but their function is still being unraveled (Ellenbroek and Ghiabi, 2014). H_3 agonists promote sleep, and H_3 antagonists promote wakefulness.

The H_4 receptors primarily are found in eosinophils, dendritic cells, mast cells, monocytes, basophils, and T cells but have also been detected in the GI tract, dermal fibroblasts, CNS, and primary sensory afferent neurons (Thurmond, 2015). Activation of H_4 receptors has been associated with induction of cellular shape change, chemotaxis, secretion of cytokines, and upregulation of adhesion molecules, suggesting that H_4 antagonists may be useful inhibitors of allergic and inflammatory responses (Thurmond, 2015).

Although specific H_3 and H_4 receptor antagonists have been developed, none of these agents has yet been FDA-approved for clinical use. Based on the functions of H_3 receptors in the CNS, H_3 antagonists have potential in the treatment of sleeping disorders, ADHD, epilepsy, cognitive impairment, schizophrenia, obesity, neuropathic pain, and Alzheimer disease. Because of the unique localization and function of H_4 receptors, H_4 antagonists are promising candidates to treat inflammatory conditions such as allergic rhinitis, asthma, rheumatoid arthritis, and possibly pruritus and neuropathic pain.

Feedback Regulation of Release

Stimulation of H_2 receptor increases cyclic AMP and leads to feedback inhibition of histamine release from mast cells and basophils, whereas activation of H_3 and H_4 receptors has the opposite effect by decreasing cellular cyclic AMP. Activation of presynaptic H_3 receptors inhibits histamine release from histaminergic neurons. Because H_3 receptors have high constitutive activity, histamine release is tonically inhibited. H_3 inverse agonists thus reduce receptor activation and increase histamine release from histaminergic neurons.

Cardiovascular System

Histamine dilates resistance vessels, increases capillary permeability, and lowers systemic blood pressure. In some vascular beds, histamine constricts veins, contributing to the extravasation of fluid and edema formation upstream in capillaries and postcapillary venules.

Vasodilation. Vasodilation is the most important vascular effect of histamine in humans and can result from activation of either the H_1 or H_2 receptor. H_1 receptors have a higher affinity for histamine and cause Ca^{2+}-dependent activation of eNOS in endothelial cells; NO diffuses to vascular smooth muscle, increasing cyclic GMP (see Table 39–1) and causing rapid and short-lived vasodilation. By contrast, activation of H_2 receptors on vascular smooth muscle stimulates the cyclic AMP–PKA pathway, causing dilation that develops more slowly and is more sustained. As a result, H_1 antagonists effectively counter small dilator responses to low concentrations of histamine but blunt only the initial phase of larger responses to higher concentrations of the amine.

Increased Capillary Permeability. Histamine's effect on small vessels results in efflux of plasma protein and fluid into the extracellular spaces and an increase in lymph flow, causing edema. H_1 receptor activation on endothelial cells is the major mediator of this response, leading to G_q-mediated activation of RhoA and ROCK, which stimulates the contractile machinery of the cells and disrupts interendothelial junctions (Mikelis et al., 2015). The gaps between endothelial cells also may permit passage of circulating cells recruited to tissues during the mast cell response. Recruitment of circulating leukocytes is enhanced by H_1 receptor–mediated expression of adhesion molecules (e.g., P-selectin) on endothelial cells.

Triple Response of Lewis. If histamine is injected intradermally, it elicits a characteristic phenomenon known as the *triple response*. This consists of the following:

- a localized "reddening" around the injection site, appearing within a few seconds, and maximal at about 1 min;
- a "flare" or red flush extending about 1 cm beyond the original red spot and developing more slowly; and
- a "wheal" or swelling that is discernible in 1–2 min at the injection site.

The initial red spot (a few millimeters) results from the direct vasodilating effect of histamine (H_1 receptor–mediated NO production). The flare is due to histamine-induced stimulation of axon reflexes that cause vasodilation indirectly, and the wheal reflects histamine's capacity to increase capillary permeability (edema formation).

Heart. Histamine affects both cardiac contractility and electrical events directly. It increases the force of contraction of both atrial and ventricular muscle by promoting the influx of Ca^{2+}, and it speeds heart rate by hastening diastolic depolarization in the SA node. It also directly slows AV conduction to increase automaticity and, in high doses, can elicit arrhythmias. The slowed AV conduction involves mainly H_1 receptors, while the other effects are largely attributable to H_2 receptors and cyclic AMP accumulation. The direct cardiac effects of histamine given intravenously are overshadowed by baroreceptor reflexes stimulated by reduced blood pressure.

Extravascular Smooth Muscle

Histamine directly contracts or, more rarely, relaxes various extravascular smooth muscles. Contraction is due to activation of H_1 receptors on smooth muscle to increase intracellular Ca^{2+}, and relaxation is mainly due to activation of H_2 receptors. Although the spasmogenic influence of H_1 receptors is dominant in human bronchial muscle, H_2 receptors with dilator function also are present. Thus, histamine-induced bronchospasm in vitro is potentiated slightly by H_2 blockade. Patients with bronchial asthma and certain other pulmonary diseases are much more sensitive to the bronchoconstrictor effects of histamine.

Peripheral Nerve Endings

Histamine stimulates various nerve endings, causing sensory effects. In the epidermis, it causes itch; in the dermis, it evokes pain, sometimes accompanied by itching. Stimulant actions on nerve endings, including autonomic afferents and efferents, contribute to the "flare" component of the triple response and to indirect effects of histamine on the bronchi and other organs.

Histamine Shock

Histamine given in large doses or released during systemic anaphylaxis causes a profound and progressive fall in blood pressure. As the small blood vessels dilate, they trap large amounts of blood, their permeability increases, and plasma escapes from the circulation. These effects, resembling surgical or traumatic shock, diminish effective blood volume, reduce venous return, and greatly lower cardiac output.

Histamine Toxicity From Ingestion

Histamine is the toxin in food poisoning from spoiled scombroid fish such as tuna. Symptoms include severe nausea, vomiting, headache, flushing, and sweating. Histamine toxicity also can follow red wine consumption in persons with a diminished ability to degrade histamine. The symptoms of histamine poisoning can be suppressed by H_1 antagonists.

Histamine Receptor Antagonists

H_1 Receptor Antagonists

HISTORY

Antihistamine activity was first demonstrated by Bovet and Staub in 1937 with one of a series of amines with a phenolic ether moiety. The substance, 2-isopropyl-5-methylphenoxy-ethyldiethyl-amine, protected guinea pigs against several lethal doses of histamine but was too toxic for clinical use. By 1944, Bovet and his colleagues had described *pyrilamine maleate*, an effective histamine antagonist of this category. The discovery of highly effective *diphenhydramine* and *tripelennamine* soon followed. In the 1980s, nonsedating H_1 histamine receptor antagonists were developed for treatment of allergic diseases. Despite success in blocking allergic responses to histamine, the H_1 antihistamines failed to inhibit a number of other responses, notably gastric acid secretion. The discovery of H_2 receptors and H_2 antagonists by Black and colleagues provided a new class of agents that antagonized histamine-induced acid secretion (Black et al., 1972); the pharmacology of these drugs (e.g., *cimetidine, famotidine*) is described in Chapter 49.

Pharmacological Properties

All the available H_1 receptor "antagonists" are actually inverse agonists (see Chapter 3) that reduce constitutive activity of the receptor and compete with histamine binding to the receptor (Simons, 2004). The pharmacological actions and therapeutic applications of these antagonists can be largely predicted from knowledge of the location and mode of signaling of the histamine receptors.

Chemistry. Like histamine, many H_1 antagonists contain a substituted ethylamine moiety (the black portion on the figure that follows). Unlike histamine, which has a primary amino group and a single aromatic ring, most H_1 antagonists have a tertiary amino group linked by a two- or three-atom chain to two aromatic substituents (in red) and conform to the general formula:

$$\begin{matrix} Ar_1 \diagdown & & | & & | & & \diagup \\ & X - & C & - & C & - N & \\ Ar_2 \diagup & & | & & | & & \diagdown \end{matrix}$$

where Ar is aryl and X is a nitrogen or carbon atom or a —C—O— ether linkage to the β-aminoethyl side chain. Sometimes, the two aromatic rings are bridged, as in the tricyclic derivatives, or the ethylamine may be part of a ring structure. Figure 39–3 shows the varied structures of representative

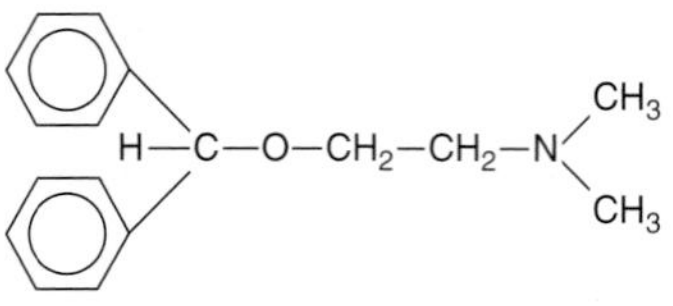

DIPHENHYDRAMINE (an ethanolamine)

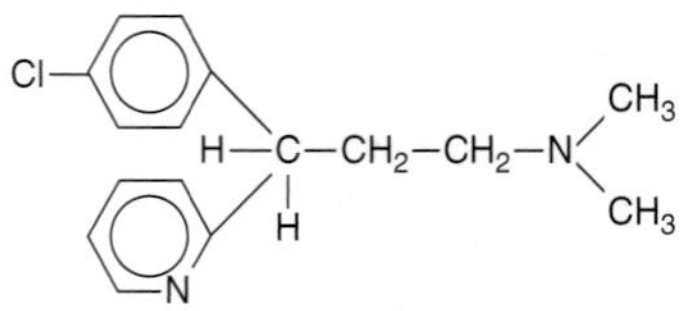

CHLORPHENIRAMINE (an alkylamine)

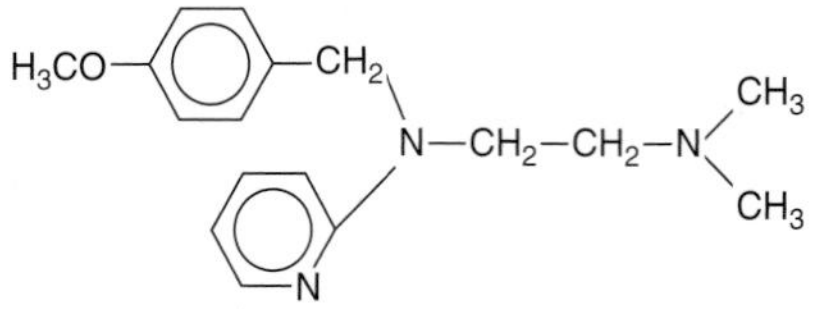

PYRILAMINE (an ethylenediamine)

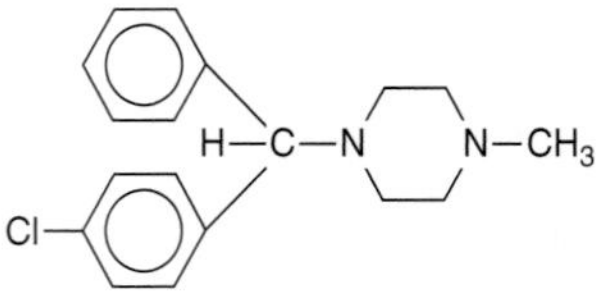

CHLORCYCLIZINE (a piperazine)

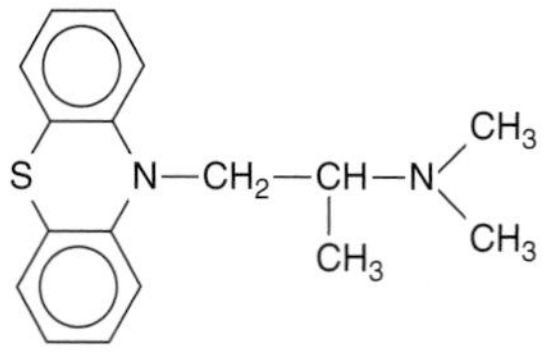

PROMETHAZINE (a phenothiazine)

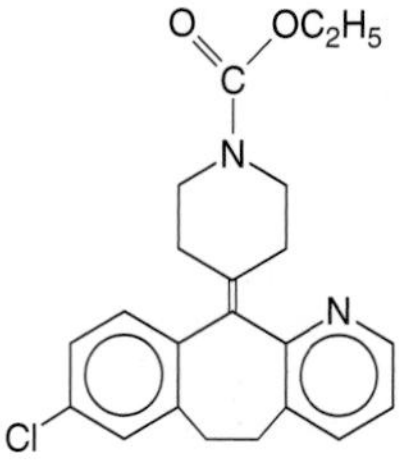

LORATADINE (a tricyclic piperidine)

Figure 39–3 *Representative H_1 antagonists.*

H_1 antagonists built around this framework and constitute the several generations of compounds.

Effects on Physiological Systems

Smooth Muscle. The H_1 antagonists inhibit most of the effects of histamine on smooth muscles, especially the constriction of respiratory smooth muscle. H_1 antagonists inhibit the more rapid vasodilator effects mediated by activation of H_1 receptors on endothelial cells (synthesis/release of NO and other mediators) at lower doses of histamine. They also inhibit venous constriction seen in some vascular beds.

Capillary Permeability. H_1 antagonists strongly block the increased capillary permeability and formation of edema and wheal caused by histamine.

Flare and Itch. H_1 antagonists suppress the action of histamine on nerve endings, including the flare component of the triple response and the itching caused by intradermal injection.

Exocrine Glands. H_1 antagonists do not suppress gastric secretion. However, the antimuscarinic properties of many H_1 antagonists may contribute to lessened secretion in cholinergically innervated glands and reduce ongoing secretion in, for example, the respiratory tree.

Immediate Hypersensitivity Reactions: Anaphylaxis and Allergy. During hypersensitivity reactions, histamine is one of the many potent autacoids released, and its relative contribution to the ensuing symptoms varies widely with species and tissue. The protection afforded by H_1 antagonists varies accordingly. In humans, edema formation and itch are effectively suppressed. Other effects, such as hypotension, are less well antagonized. H_1 antagonists are ineffective in blocking bronchoconstriction due to asthma.

Mast Cell–Stabilizing and Anti-inflammatory Properties. Many second-generation H_1 antagonists (e.g., cetirizine, desloratadine, fexofenedine, olopatadine, ketotifen, alcaftadine, and others) exhibit mast cell–stabilizing effects, resulting in reduced release of mast cell mediators during an allergic response (Levi-Schaffer and Eliashar, 2009). These agents also have anti-inflammatory properties, which can include reduced cytokine secretion, decreased adhesion molecule expression, and inhibition of eosinophil infiltration. These effects can be both H_1 receptor dependent and independent, but precise mechanisms are still unclear, and it is unknown what role they play at normal therapeutic doses of these drugs. There is some evidence that H_1 antagonists with these additional properties may be more effective in the topical treatment of allergic conjunctivitis (Abelson et al., 2015).

CNS. The first-generation H_1 antagonists can both stimulate and depress the CNS (Simons and Simons, 2011). Stimulation occasionally is encountered in patients given conventional doses; the patients become restless, nervous, and unable to sleep. Central excitation also is a striking feature of overdose, which commonly results in convulsions, particularly in infants. Central depression, on the other hand, usually accompanies therapeutic doses of the older H_1 antagonists. Diminished alertness, slowed reaction times, and somnolence are common manifestations. Patients vary in their susceptibility and responses to individual drugs. The ethanolamines (e.g., diphenhydramine) are particularly prone to causing sedation. Because of the sedation that occurs with first-generation antihistamines, these drugs cannot be tolerated or used safely by many patients except at bedtime. Even then, patients may experience an antihistamine "hangover" in the morning, resulting in sedation with or without psychomotor impairment. Second-generation H_1 antagonists are termed *nonsedating* because they do not cross the blood-brain barrier appreciably. This is due to their decreased lipophilicity and because they are substrates of P-glycoprotein, which pumps them out of the blood-brain barrier capillary endothelial cells and back into the capillary lumen (see Chapter 5 and Simons and Simons, 2011).

Many antipsychotic agents are H_1 and H_2 receptor antagonists, but it is unclear whether this property plays a role in the antipsychotic effects of these agents. In test systems, the atypical antipsychotic agent *clozapine* is an effective H_1 antagonist, a weak H_3 antagonist, and an H_4 receptor agonist. The H_1 antagonist activity of typical and atypical antipsychotic drugs is responsible for the propensity of these agents to cause weight gain.

Anticholinergic Effects. Many of the first-generation H_1 antagonists tend to inhibit muscarinic cholinergic responses and may be manifest during clinical use (Simons and Simons, 2011). Some H_1 antagonists also can be used to treat motion sickness (see Chapters 9 and 50), probably as a result of their anticholinergic properties. Indeed, promethazine has perhaps the strongest muscarinic-blocking activity among these agents and is the most effective H_1 antagonist in combating motion sickness. The second-generation H_1 antagonists have no effect on muscarinic receptors (Simons and Simons, 2011).

Local Anesthetic Effect. Some H_1 antagonists have local anesthetic activity, and a few are more potent than procaine. Promethazine is especially active. However, the concentrations required for this effect are much higher than those that antagonize histamine's interactions with its receptors.

ADME. The H_1 antagonists are well absorbed from the GI tract. Following oral administration, peak plasma concentrations are achieved in 1–3 h, and effects usually last 4–6 h for first-generation agents; however, some of the drugs are much longer acting, as are most second-generation H_1 antagonists (del Cuvillo et al., 2006; Simons, 2004) (Table 39–2). These agents are distributed widely throughout the body, including the CNS for the first-generation agents. Peak concentrations of these drugs in the skin may persist long after plasma levels have declined. Thus, inhibition of "wheal-and-flare" responses to the intradermal injection of histamine or allergen can persist for 36 h or more after initial treatment and up to 7 days after discontinuation of treatment in patients who regularly use an H_1 antagonist for 1 week or more (del Cuvillo et al., 2006).

All first-generation and most second-generation H_1 antagonists are metabolized by CYPs and little, if any, is excreted unchanged in the urine; most appears there as metabolites (Bartra et al., 2006; Simons, 2004). Exceptions are cetirizine and acrivastine (<40% metabolized) and fexofenadine, levocetirizine, and epinastine (<10% metabolized). Cetirizine, levocetirizine, and acrivastine are excreted primarily into the urine; fexofenadine is mainly excreted in the feces, and epinastine is excreted in both urine (55%) and feces (30%).

The H_1 antagonists that are metabolized are eliminated more rapidly by children than by adults and more slowly in those with severe liver disease. These antagonists also have higher potential for drug interactions. For example, plasma levels of H_1 antagonists may be reduced when coadministered with drugs that induce CYP synthesis (e.g., benzodiazepines) or elevated when taken with drugs that compete with or inhibit the same CYP isoform (e.g., erythromycin, ketoconazole, antidepressants) (Bartra et al., 2006; Simons, 2004). Clinically relevant interactions are more likely with first-generation than second-generation drugs, which have a higher therapeutic index. However, two second-generation H_1 antagonists marketed previously, *terfenadine* and *astemizole*, were found in rare cases to prolong the QTc interval and induce a potentially fatal arrhythmia, torsade de pointes, due to their capacity to inhibit a cardiac K^+ channel, I_{Kr}, when their metabolism was impaired and their plasma concentrations rose too high, due, for instance, to liver disease or to drugs that inhibited the CYP3A family (Bartra et al., 2006; Simons, 2004) (see Chapter 30). This led to the withdrawal of terfenadine and astemizole from the market. Astemizole and an active hydroxylated metabolite naturally have very long half-lives. Terfenadine is a prodrug, metabolized by hepatic CYP3A4 to fexofenadine, which is its replacement and lacks noticeable cardiotoxicity. In vitro testing for a new drug's capacity to inhibit I_{Kr} is now available.

Therapeutic Uses

The H_1 antagonists are used for treatment of various immediate hypersensitivity reactions. The central properties of some of the drugs also are of therapeutic value for suppressing motion sickness or for sedation.

Allergic Diseases. H_1 antagonists are useful in acute types of allergy that present with symptoms of rhinitis, urticaria, and conjunctivitis (Simons and Simons, 2011). Their effect is confined to the suppression of symptoms attributable to the histamine released by the antigen-antibody reaction. In bronchial asthma, histamine antagonists have limited efficacy and are not used as sole therapy (see Chapters 38 and 40). In the treatment of systemic anaphylaxis, where autacoids other than histamine are important, the mainstay of therapy is *epinephrine*; histamine antagonists have only a subordinate and adjuvant role. The same is true for severe angioedema, in which laryngeal swelling constitutes a threat to life (see Chapter 12).

Certain allergic dermatoses respond favorably to H_1 antagonists. The benefit is most striking in acute urticaria. H_1 antagonists are also first-line therapy for chronic urticaria but may require doses up to four times higher than that approved for treating rhinitis; patients refractory to high-dose H_1 antagonists should be switched to drugs targeting the immune response (Viegas et al., 2014). H_1 antagonists have a place in the treatment of pruritus. Some relief may be obtained in many patients with atopic and contact dermatitis (although topical corticosteroids are more effective) and in such diverse conditions as insect bites and poison ivy. The urticarial and edematous lesions of serum sickness respond to H_1 antagonists, but fever and arthralgia often do not.

Common Cold. H_1 antagonists are without value in combating the common cold. The weak anticholinergic effects of the older agents may tend to lessen rhinorrhea, but this drying effect may do more harm than good, as may their tendency to induce somnolence.

Motion Sickness, Vertigo, and Sedation. Scopolamine, the muscarinic antagonist, given orally, parenterally, or transdermally, is the most effective drug for the prophylaxis and treatment of motion sickness. Some H_1 antagonists are useful for milder cases and have fewer adverse effects. These drugs include dimenhydrinate and the piperazines (e.g., cyclizine, meclizine). Promethazine, a phenothiazine, is more potent and more effective, and its additional antiemetic properties may be of value in reducing vomiting; however, its pronounced sedative action usually is disadvantageous. Whenever possible, the various drugs should be administered about 1 h before the anticipated motion. Treatment after the onset of nausea and vomiting rarely is beneficial. Some H_1 antagonists, notably dimenhydrinate and meclizine, often are of benefit in vestibular disturbances such as Ménière disease and in other types of true vertigo. Only promethazine is useful in treating the nausea and vomiting subsequent to chemotherapy or radiation therapy for malignancies; however, other, more effective, antiemetic drugs (e.g., $5HT_3$ antagonists) are available (see Chapter 50). Diphenhydramine can reverse the extrapyramidal side effects caused by antipsychotics (see Chapter 16). The tendency of some H_1 receptor antagonists to produce somnolence has led to their use as hypnotics. H_1 antagonists, principally diphenhydramine, often are present in various proprietary over-the-counter remedies for insomnia. The sedative and mild antianxiety activities of hydroxyzine contribute to its use as an anxiolytic.

Adverse Effects

The most frequent side effect of first-generation H_1 antagonists is sedation. Concurrent ingestion of alcohol or other CNS depressants produces an additive effect that impairs motor skills. Other untoward central actions include dizziness, tinnitus, lassitude, incoordination, fatigue, blurred vision, diplopia, euphoria, nervousness, insomnia, and tremors. Other potential side effects, including loss of appetite, nausea, vomiting, epigastric distress, and constipation or diarrhea, may be reduced by taking the drug with meals. H_1 antagonists such as cyproheptadine may increase appetite and cause weight gain. Other side effects, owing to the antimuscarinic actions of some first-generation H_1 antagonists, include dryness of the mouth and respiratory passages (sometimes inducing cough), urinary retention or frequency, and dysuria. These effects are not observed with second-generation H_1 antagonists. Allergic dermatitis is not uncommon; other hypersensitivity reactions include drug fever and photosensitization. Hematological complications, such as leukopenia, agranulocytosis, and hemolytic anemia, are very rare.

Because H_1 antihistamines cross the placenta, caution is advised for women who are or may become pregnant (Simons and Simons, 2011).

TABLE 39–2 ■ PREPARATIONS AND DOSAGE OF REPRESENTATIVE H_1 RECEPTOR ANTAGONISTS[a]

CLASS *Generic name*	DURATION OF ACTION (h)[b]	PREPARATIONS[c]	SINGLE DOSE (adult)
First-generation agents			
Tricyclic dibenzoxepins			
Doxepin HCl	6–24	O, L, T	10–150 mg; insomnia: 6 mg (O) Pruritus: thin film 4 times/d (T)
Ethanolamines			
Carbinoxamine maleate	3–6	O, L	4–8 mg; 6–16 mg (SR)
Clemastine fumarate	12	O, L	1.34–2.68 mg
Diphenhydramine HCl	12	O, L, I, T	25–50 mg (O/L/I)
Dimenhydrinate[d]	4–6	O, I	50–100 mg
Ethylenediamines			
Pyrilamine maleate (only in combination products)	4–6	O, L	7.5–30 mg
Alkylamines			
Chlorpheniramine maleate	24	O, L, I, SR	4 mg, 12 mg (SR)
Brompheniramine maleate	4–6	O, L, I, SR	2 mg
Piperazines			
Hydroxyzine HCl	6–24	O, L, I	25–100 mg
Hydroxyzine pamoate	6–24	O, L (not in the U.S.)	25–100 mg
Cyclizine HCl	4–6	O	50 mg
Cyclizine lactate (not in the U.S.)	4–6	I	50 mg
Meclizine HCl	12–24	O	25–50 mg
Phenothiazines			
Promethazine HCl	4–6	O, L, I, S	12.5–50 mg
Piperidines			
Cyproheptadine HCl[e]	4–6	O, L	1–6.5 mg
Second-generation agents			
Tricyclic dibenzoxepins			
Olopatadine HCl	6–12	T	2 sprays/nostril; 1 drop/eye
Alkylamines			
Acrivastine[f]	6–8	O	8 mg
Piperazines			
Cetirizine HCl[f]	12–24	O, L	5–10 mg
Levocetirizine HCl	12–24	O, L	2.5–5 mg
Piperidines			
Alcaftadine	16–24	T	1 drop/eye
Bepotastine besilate	8	T	1 drop/eye
Desloratadine	24	O, L	5 mg
Fexofenadine HCl	12–24	O, L	60–180 mg
Ketotifen fumarate	8–12	T	1 drop/eye
Loratadine	24	O, L	10 mg
Other second-generation drugs			
Azelastine HCl[f]	12–24	T	2 sprays/nostril; 1 drop/eye
Emedastine	8–12	T	1 drop/eye
Epinastine	8–12	T	1 drop/eye

[a]For a discussion of phenothiazines, see Chapter 16.
[b]Duration of action of H_1 antihistamines by objective assessment of suppression of histamine- or allergen-induced symptoms is longer than expected from measurement of plasma concentrations or terminal elimination $t_{1/2}$ values.
[c]Preparations are designated as follows: O, oral solids; L, oral liquids; I, injection; S, suppository; SR, sustained release; T, topical. Many H_1 receptor antagonists also are available in preparations that contain multiple drugs. SR forms dissuade pseudoephedrine extraction for methamphetamine production.
[d]Dimenhydrinate is a combination of diphenhydramine and 8-chlorotheophylline in equal molecular proportions.
[e]Also has antiserotonin properties.
[f]Has mild sedating effects.

Several antihistamines (e.g., azelastine, hydroxyzine, fexofenadine) had teratogenic effects in animal studies, whereas others (e.g., chlorpheniramine, diphenhydramine, cetirizine, loratadine) did not. A recent systematic review concluded that antihistamines are unlikely to be strong risk factors for major birth defects (Gilboa et al., 2014). A combination drug consisting of the H_1 antagonist doxylamine and vitamin B_6 (pyridoxine) was approved in 1956 for treating the nausea and vomiting of pregnancy and then voluntarily removed in 1983 due to concerns over birth defects. Subsequent analyses showed the drug caused no increased risk of birth defects, and in 2013 it was reapproved for the same indication in a fixed-dose, delayed-release formulation. Antihistamines can be excreted in small amounts in breast milk, and first-generation antihistamines taken by lactating mothers may cause symptoms such as irritability, drowsiness, or respiratory depression in the nursing infant.

In acute poisoning with first-generation H_1 antagonists, their central excitatory effects constitute the greatest danger. The syndrome includes hallucinations, excitement, ataxia, incoordination, athetosis, and convulsions, fixed, dilated pupils with a flushed face, together with sinus tachycardia, urinary retention, dry mouth, and fever. The syndrome exhibits a remarkable similarity to that of atropine poisoning. Terminally, there is deepening coma with cardiorespiratory collapse and death usually within 2–18 h. Treatment is along general symptomatic and supportive lines. Overdoses of second-generation H_1 antagonists have not been associated with significant toxicity (Simons and Simons, 2011).

Pediatric and Geriatric Indications and Problems. Although little clinical testing has been done, second-generation antihistamines are preferred for elderly patients (>65 years of age), especially those with impaired cognitive function, because of the sedative and anticholinergic effects of first-generation drugs (Simons, 2004). In addition, a recent prospective study in participants 65 years old and older without dementia showed a significant 10-year cumulative dose-response relationship between use of anticholinergics (first-generation H_1 antagonists among the most common) and risk of dementia, primarily Alzheimer disease (Gray et al., 2015).

First-generation antihistamines are not recommended for use in children because their sedative effects can impair learning and school performance. The second-generation drugs have been approved by the FDA for use in children and are available in appropriate lower-dose formulations (e.g., chewable or rapidly dissolving tablets, syrup). Use of over-the-counter cough and cold medicines (containing mixtures of antihistamines, decongestants, antitussives, expectorants) in young children has been associated with serious side effects and deaths. In 2008, the FDA recommended that they should not be used in children less than 2 years of age, and drug manufacturers affiliated with the Consumer Healthcare Products Association voluntarily relabeled products "do not use" for children less than 4 years of age.

Available H_1 Antagonists

Summarized next are notable properties of a number of H_1 antagonists, grouped by their chemical structures. Representative preparations are listed in Table 39–2.

First-Generation Dibenzoxepin Tricyclic (Doxepin). Doxepin is marketed as a tricyclic antidepressant (see Chapter 15). It also is one of the most potent H_1 antagonists and has significant H_2 antagonist activity, but this does not translate into greater clinical effectiveness. It can cause drowsiness and is associated with anticholinergic effects. Doxepin is better tolerated by patients with depression than those who are not depressed, for whom even small doses may cause disorientation and confusion.

Second-Generation Dibenzoxepin Tricyclic (Olopatadine). Olopatadine is a topical H_1 antagonist with additional mast cell–stabilizing and anti-inflammatory properties. In drop form, it is an effective treatment of allergic conjunctivitis and as a spray helps reduce the nasal symptoms of allergic rhinitis.

Ethanolamines (Prototype: Diphenhydramine). The ethanolamines possess significant antimuscarinic activity and have a pronounced tendency to induce sedation. About half of those treated acutely with conventional doses experience somnolence. The incidence of GI side effects, however, is low with this group.

Ethylenediamine (Prototype: Pyrilamine). Pyrilamine is among the most specific H_1 antagonists. Although its central effects are relatively feeble, somnolence occurs in a fair proportion of patients. GI side effects are common.

First-Generation Alkylamines (Prototype: Chlorpheniramine). The first-generation alkylamines are among the most potent H_1 antagonists. The drugs are less prone to produce drowsiness and are more suitable for daytime use, but a significant proportion of patients still experience sedation. Side effects involving CNS stimulation are more common than with other groups.

Second-Generation Alkylamine (Acrivastine). The second-generation alkylamine is a derivative of the first-generation alkylamine triprolidine and may exhibit a somewhat higher incidence of mild sedation than other second-generation H_1 antagonists.

First-Generation Piperazines. Hydroxyzine is a long-acting compound that is used widely for skin allergies; its considerable CNS-depressant activity may contribute to its prominent antipruritic action, and it is also used as a sedative and antianxiety agent. Cyclizine and meclizine have been used primarily to counter motion sickness, although promethazine and diphenhydramine are more effective (as is the antimuscarinic scopolamine).

Second-Generation Piperazines (Cetirizine). Cetirizine has minimal anticholinergic effects. It also has negligible penetration into the brain but is associated with a somewhat higher incidence of drowsiness than most other second-generation H_1 antagonists. The active enantiomer levocetirizine has slightly greater potency and may be used at half the dose with less resultant sedation. Cetirizine and levocetirizine have additional mast cell–stabilizing and anti-inflammatory properties.

Phenothiazines (Prototype: Promethazine). Promethazine, which has prominent sedative and considerable anticholinergic effects, and its many congeners are used primarily for their antiemetic effects (see Chapter 50).

First-Generation Piperidine (Cyproheptadine). Cyproheptadine uniquely has both antihistamine and antiserotonin activity by antagonizing the $5HT_{2A}$ receptor. Cyproheptadine causes drowsiness; it also has significant anticholinergic effects and can increase appetite.

Second-Generation Piperidines (Prototype: Loratadine). Terfenadine and astemizole, early second-generation drugs, are no longer marketed because of their potential for causing a rare, but potentially fatal, arrhythmia, torsade de pointes (see previous discussion). Terfenadine was replaced by fexofenadine, an active metabolite that lacks the toxic side effects of terfenadine, is not sedating, and retains the antiallergic properties of the parent compound. Another antihistamine of this class developed using this strategy is *desloratadine*, an active metabolite of loratadine. These agents lack significant anticholinergic actions and penetrate poorly into the CNS. Taken together, these properties appear to account for the low incidence of side effects of piperidine antihistamines. All members of this class have mast cell–stabilizing and anti-inflammatory properties. Although the therapeutic significance of these additional effects are unclear for the drugs administered orally, they appear to provide additional benefit when used in topical formulations to treat allergic conjunctivitis. Alcaftadine has additional antagonist activity on H_4 receptors, which likely explains its superiority to other topical H_1 antagonists in reducing the ocular itch of allergic conjunctivitis (Thurmond, 2015).

Other Second-Generation H_1 Antagonists. Drugs in this group (azelastine, emedastine, and epinastine) have divergent structures with therapeutic efficacy and side effects similar to other second-generation H_1 antagonists. They all are marketed as topical eye drops for the treatment of allergic conjunctivitis; azelastine is also available as a nasal spray for treating symptoms of allergic or vasomotor rhinitis. Epinastine has both H_1 and H_2 antagonist activity, which may help reduce eyelid edema. Epinastine and azelastine exhibit mast cell–stabilizing and anti-inflammatory properties. Emedastine is a highly selective H_1 antagonist without these additional actions.

H_2 Receptor Antagonists

The pharmacology and clinical utility of H_2 antagonists (e.g., cimetidine, ranitidine) for inhibiting gastric acid secretion in the treatment of GI disorders are described in Chapter 50.

H_3 Receptor Antagonists

The H_3 receptors are presynaptic autoreceptors on histaminergic neurons that originate in the tuberomammillary nucleus in the hypothalamus and project throughout the CNS, most prominently to the hippocampus, amygdala, nucleus accumbens, globus pallidus, striatum, hypothalamus, and cortex (Haas et al., 2008; Sander et al., 2008). The activated H_3 receptor depresses neuronal firing at the level of cell bodies/dendrites and decreases histamine release from depolarized terminals. Thus, H_3 agonists decrease histaminergic transmission, and antagonists increase it.

The H_3 receptors also are presynaptic heteroreceptors on a variety of neurons in brain and peripheral tissues, and their activation inhibits transmitter release from noradrenergic, serotoninergic, GABAergic, cholinergic, and glutamatergic neurons, as well as pain-sensitive C fibers. H_3 receptors in the brain have significant constitutive activity in the absence of agonist; consequently, inverse agonists reduce this constitutive activity, withdraw inhibition of transmitter release, and thereby promote transmitter release (activation of these neurons).

The H_3 antagonists/inverse agonists have a wide range of central effects; for example, they promote wakefulness, improve cognitive function (e.g., enhance memory, learning, and attention), and reduce food intake. As a result, there is considerable interest in developing H_3 antagonists for possible treatment of sleeping disorders, ADHD, epilepsy, cognitive impairment, schizophrenia, obesity, neuropathic pain, and Alzheimer disease (Haas et al., 2008; Sander et al., 2008). Thioperamide was the first "specific" H_3 antagonist/inverse agonist available experimentally, but it was equally effective at the H_4 receptor. A number of other imidazole derivatives have been developed as H_3 antagonists, including clobenpropit, ciproxifan, and proxyfan, but the imidazole ring enhances binding to the H_4 receptor and CYPs. Because of this, more selective nonimidazole H_3 antagonists/inverse agonists (e.g., tiprolisant) were developed (Haas et al., 2008; Sander et al., 2008), and some are now in phase 2 and 3 clinical trials.

H_4 Receptor Antagonists

The H_4 receptors are expressed on cells with inflammatory or immune functions and can mediate histamine-induced chemotaxis, induction of cell shape change, secretion of cytokines, and upregulation of adhesion molecules (Thurmond et al., 2008). The H_4 receptors also have a role in pruritus and neuropathic pain. Because of the unique localization and function of H_4 receptors, H_4 antagonists are promising candidates to treat inflammatory conditions and possibly pruritus and neuropathic pain (Thurmond, 2015). The H_4-specific antagonist JNJ-39758979 has been tested in phase 1 and 2 clinical trials for treatment of persistent asthma, pruritis, dermatitis, and rheumatoid arthritis.

The H_4 receptor has the highest homology with the H_3 receptor and binds many H_3 ligands, especially those with imidazole rings, although sometimes with different effects (Thurmond et al., 2008). For example, thioperamide is an effective inverse agonist at both H_3 and H_4 receptors, whereas H_3 inverse agonist clobenpropit is a partial agonist of the H_4 receptor; impentamine (an H_3 agonist) and iodophenpropit (an H_3 inverse agonist) are both neutral H_4 antagonists.

Bradykinin, Kallidin, and Their Antagonists

In the 1920s and 1930s, Frey, Kraut, and Werle characterized a hypotensive substance in urine, which was also found in other fluids and tissues, and named this material *kallikrein* after a Greek synonym for the pancreas, an especially rich source (Werle, 1970). It was established that kallikrein generates a pharmacologically active substance from an inactive precursor present in plasma; the active substance, *kallidin*, proved to be a polypeptide cleaved from a plasma globulin (Werle, 1970). Rocha e Silva, Beraldo, and associates later reported that trypsin and certain snake venoms acted on plasma globulin to produce a substance that lowered blood pressure and caused a slowly developing contraction of the gut (Rocha e Silva et al., 1949); they named it *bradykinin*, derived from the Greek words *bradys*, meaning "slow," and *kinein*, meaning "to move." In 1960, bradykinin, a nine amino acid peptide, was isolated and synthesized; shortly thereafter, kallidin was identified as bradykinin with an additional N-terminal Lys residue. The kinins have short half-lives because they are destroyed by plasma and tissue peptidases (Erdös and Skidgel, 1997). Two types of kinin receptors, B_1 and B_2, were identified based on the rank order of potency of kinin analogues and later validated by cloning (Leeb-Lundberg et al., 2005). The development of receptor-specific antagonists and receptor knockout mice have furthered our understanding of the role of kinins in the regulation of cardiovascular homeostasis and inflammatory processes (Leeb-Lundberg et al., 2005).

Tissue damage, allergic reactions, viral infections, and other inflammatory events activate a series of proteolytic reactions that generate bradykinin and kallidin in tissues. These peptides contribute to inflammatory responses as autacoids that act locally to produce pain, vasodilation, and increased vascular permeability but can also have beneficial effects, for example, in the heart, kidney, and circulation (Bhoola et al., 1992). Much of their activity is due to stimulation of the release of potent mediators such as prostaglandins, NO, or EDHF.

The Endogenous Kallikrein-Kininogen-Kinin System

The nonapeptide bradykinin and decapeptide kallidin (*lysyl-bradykinin*) (Table 39–3) are cleaved from α_2 globulins termed *kininogens* (Figure 39–4). There are two kininogens: HMW kininogen and LMW kininogen. A number of serine proteases will generate kinins, but the two highly specific proteases that release bradykinin and kallidin from the kininogens are termed *kallikreins*.

TABLE 39–3 ■ STRUCTURE OF KININ AGONISTS AND ANTAGONISTS

NAME	STRUCTURE	FUNCTION
Bradykinin	Arg-Pro-Pro-Gly-Phe-Ser-Pro-Phe-Arg	Agonist, B_2
Kallidin	Lys-Arg-Pro-Pro-Gly-Phe-Ser-Pro-Phe-Arg	Agonist, B_2
[des-Arg^9]-Bradykinin	Arg-Pro-Pro-Gly-Phe-Ser-Pro-Phe	Agonist, B_1
[des-Arg^{10}]-Kallidin	Lys-Arg-Pro-Pro-Gly-Phe-Ser-Pro-Phe	Agonist, B_1
des-Arg^{10}-[Leu^9]-Kallidin	Lys-Arg-Pro-Pro-Gly-Phe-Ser-Pro-Leu	Antagonist, B_1
NPC-349	[D-Arg]-Arg-Pro-Hyp-Gly-Thi-Ser-D-Phe-Thi-Arg	Antagonist, B_2
HOE-140	[D-Arg]-Arg-Pro-Hyp-Gly-Thi-Ser-Tic-Oic-Arg	Antagonist, B_2
[des-Arg^{10}]-HOE-140	[D-Arg]-Arg-Pro-Hyp-Gly-Thi-Ser-Tic-Oic	Antagonist, B_1
FR173657	See Figure 32–3 of the 12th edition	Antagonist, B_2
FR190997		Agonist, B_2
SSR240612		Antagonist, B_1

Hyp, trans-4-hydroxy-Pro; Thi, β-(2-thienyl)-Ala; Tic, [D]-1,2,3,4-tetrahydroisoquinolin-3-yl-carbonyl; Oic, (3as,7as)-octahydroindol-2-yl-carbonyl.

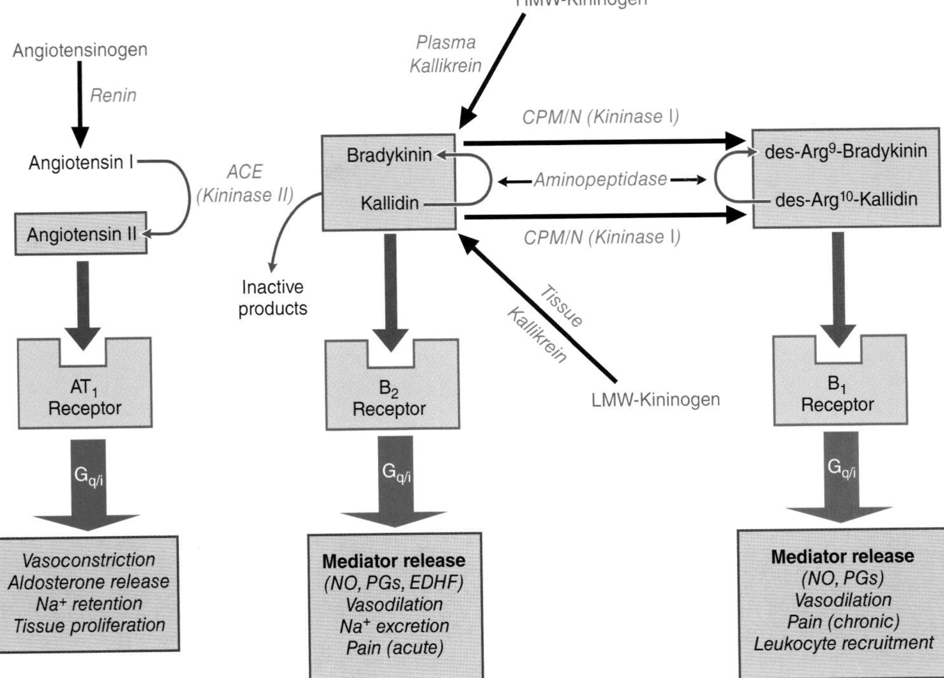

Figure 39–4 *Synthesis and receptor interactions of active peptides generated by the kallikrein-kinin and renin-angiotensin systems.* Bradykinin is generated by the action of plasma kallikrein on HMW kininogen, whereas kallidin (Lys1-bradykinin) is released by the hydrolysis of LMW kininogen by tissue kallikrein. Kallidin and bradykinin are the natural ligands of the B_2 receptor but can be converted to corresponding agonists of the B_1 receptor by removal of the C-terminal Arg by kininase I–type enzymes: the plasma membrane–bound CPM or soluble plasma CPN. Kallidin or [des-Arg^{10}]-kallidin can be converted to the active peptides bradykinin or to [des-Arg^9]-bradykinin by aminopeptidase cleavage of the N-terminal Lys residue. In a parallel fashion, the inactive decapeptide AngI is generated by the action of renin on the plasma substrate angiotensinogen. By removal of the C-terminal His-Leu dipeptide, ACE generates the active peptide AngII. These two systems have opposing effects. AngII is a potent vasoconstrictor that also causes aldosterone release and Na^+ retention via activation of the AT_1 receptor; bradykinin is a vasodilator that stimulates Na^+ excretion by activating the B_2 receptor. ACE generates active AngII and, at the same time, inactivates bradykinin and kallidin; thus, its effects are prohypertensive, and ACE inhibitors are effective antihypertensive agents. The B_2 receptor mediates most of bradykinin's effects under normal circumstances, whereas synthesis of the B_1 receptor is induced by inflammatory mediators in inflammatory conditions. Both B_1 and B_2 receptors couple through G_q to activate PLC and increase intracellular Ca^{2+}; the physiological response depends on receptor distribution on particular cell types and occupancy by agonist peptides. For instance, on endothelial cells, activation of B_2 receptors results in Ca^{2+}-calmodulin–dependent activation of eNOS and generation of NO, which causes cyclic GMP accumulation and relaxation in neighboring smooth muscle cells. However, in endothelial cells under inflammatory conditions, B_1 receptor stimulation results in prolonged NO production via G_i and an acute MAP kinase–dependent activation of iNOS. On smooth muscle cells, activation of kinin receptors coupling through G_q results in an increased $[Ca^{2+}]$i and contraction. B_1 and B_2 receptors also can couple through G_i to activate PLA_2, causing the release of arachidonic acid and the local generation of prostanoids (PGs) and other metabolites such as EDHF. Kallikrein also plays a role in the intrinsic blood coagulation pathway (see Chapter 32).

Kallikreins

Bradykinin and kallidin are cleaved from HMW or LMW kininogens by plasma or tissue kallikrein, respectively (see Figure 39–4). Plasma kallikrein and tissue kallikrein are distinct enzymes that are activated by different mechanisms (Bhoola et al., 1992). Plasma prekallikrein is an inactive protein of about 88 kDa that complexes with its substrate, HMW kininogen. The ensuing proteolytic cascade is normally restrained by the protease inhibitors present in plasma, most importantly the activated first component of complement (C1-INH) and α_2 macroglobulin. Under experimental conditions, the kallikrein-kinin system is activated by the binding of factor XII (*Hageman factor*) to negatively charged surfaces. Bound factor XII, a protease that is common to both the kinin and the intrinsic coagulation cascades (see Chapter 32), slowly undergoes autoactivation and, in turn, activates prekallikrein. Importantly, kallikrein rapidly further activates factor XII, thereby exerting a positive feedback on the system. In vivo, the order of this process can be reversed. The binding of the HMW kininogen–prekallikrein heterodimer to a multiprotein-receptor complex on endothelial cells leads to activation of the prekallikrein-HMW kininogen complex by either heat shock protein 90 (Hsp90) or prolylcarboxypeptidase to generate kallikrein, which can then activate factor XII to start the positive-feedback loop, and cleave HMW kininogen to generate bradykinin (Kaplan and Joseph, 2014). This process may contribute to the symptoms of hereditary angioedema in patients that lack C1-INH.

Human tissue kallikrein is 1 of 15 gene family members with high sequence identity that are clustered at chromosome 19q13.4 (Prassas et al., 2015). However, the classical "tissue kallikrein," hK1, is the only family member to readily generate kallidin from LMW kininogen. Tissue kallikrein is synthesized as a 29-kDa preproprotein in the epithelial cells or secretory cells in several tissues, including salivary glands, pancreas, prostate, and renal distal nephron (Bhoola et al., 1992). Tissue kallikrein also is expressed in human neutrophils; it acts locally near its sites of origin. The synthesis of tissue prokallikrein is controlled by a number of factors, including aldosterone in the kidney and salivary gland and androgens in certain other glands. The activation of tissue prokallikrein to kallikrein requires proteolytic cleavage to remove a seven–amino acid propeptide, which can be accomplished in vitro by plasma kallikrein and by some serine and metalloproteases. However, the activating enzyme(s) in vivo is unknown.

Kininogens

The two substrates for the kallikreins, HMW kininogen (120 kDa) and LMW kininogen (66 kDa), are derived from a single gene by alternative splicing. The first 401 amino acids are identical (through the bradykinin sequence and 12 additional residues) and then the sequences diverge, with HMW kininogen containing a 56-kDa C-terminal light chain and LMW kininogen a 4-kDa light chain (Bhoola et al., 1992). HMW kininogen is cleaved by both plasma and tissue kallikrein to yield bradykinin and kallidin, respectively, whereas LMW kininogen is cleaved only by tissue kallikrein to produce kallidin.

Metabolism of Kinins

The decapeptide kallidin is about as active as the nonapeptide bradykinin, even without conversion to bradykinin, which occurs when the N-terminal lysine residue is removed by an aminopeptidase (see Figure 39–4). The $t_{1/2}$ of kinins in plasma is only about 15 sec; 80%–90% of the kinins may be destroyed in a single passage through the pulmonary vascular bed by enzymes present on the large endothelial surface area of the lung (Erdös and Skidgel, 1997). Plasma concentrations of bradykinin are difficult to measure because inadequate inhibition of kininogenases or kininases in the blood can lead to artifactual formation or degradation of bradykinin during blood collection. When care is taken to inhibit these processes, the reported physiological concentrations of bradykinin in blood are in the picomolar range.

The principal catabolizing enzyme in the lung and other vascular beds is kininase II, or ACE, a membrane-anchored peptidase on the surface of endothelial cells (see Chapter 26). Removal of the C-terminal dipeptide by ACE or neutral endopeptidase 24.11 (neprilysin) inactivates kinins (Figure 39–5) (Erdös and Skidgel, 1997). A slower-acting plasma enzyme, carboxypeptidase N (lysine carboxypeptidase, kininase I), releases the C-terminal arginine residue, producing [desArg^9]-bradykinin or [des-Arg^{10}]-kallidin (see Table 39–3 and Figures 39–4 and 39–5) (Skidgel and Erdös, 2007), either of which no longer activate B_2 receptors but are potent B_1 receptor agonists. Carboxypeptidase N is expressed in the liver and constitutively secreted into the blood. A rare familial carboxypeptidase N deficiency was associated with angioedema or urticaria, possibly due to increased bradykinin (Skidgel and Erdös, 2007). Carboxypeptidase M, which cleaves the C-terminal Arg of bradykinin about 3-fold faster than carboxypeptidase N, is a widely distributed plasma membrane–bound enzyme that is also found on lung microvascular endothelial cells (Zhang et al., 2013a). Finally, aminopeptidase P is a membrane enzyme on epithelial and endothelial cells that can cleave the N-terminal arginine of bradykinin, rendering it inactive and susceptible to further cleavage by dipeptidyl peptidase IV (Erdös and Skidgel, 1997) (Figure 39–5).

Kinin Receptors and Their Signaling Pathways

The B_1 and B_2 kinin receptors are GPCRs whose signaling mediates most of the biological effects of the kallikrein-kinin system (Leeb-Lundberg et al., 2005). The B_2 receptor is expressed in most normal tissues, where it selectively binds intact bradykinin and kallidin (see Table 39–3 and Figure 39–4). The B_2 receptor mediates the effects of bradykinin and kallidin under normal circumstances, whereas synthesis of the B_1 receptor is induced by inflammatory conditions. The B_1 receptor is activated by the C-terminal des-Arg metabolites of bradykinin and kallidin produced by the actions of carboxypeptidases N and M. Interestingly, carboxypeptidase M and the B_1 receptor interact on the cell surface to form an efficient signaling complex that enhances B_1 receptor agonist affinity and can lead to allosteric activation of B_1 receptor signaling by substrate binding to carboxypeptidase M (Zhang et al., 2013a, 2013b). B_1 receptors are normally absent or expressed at low levels in most tissues. B_1 receptor expression is upregulated by tissue injury and inflammation and by cytokines, endotoxins, and growth factors. Carboxypeptidase M expression also is increased by cytokines, to such a degree that B_1 receptor effects may predominate over B_2 effects (Zhang et al., 2013a).

Both B_1 and B_2 receptors couple through G_q to activate PLC and increase intracellular Ca^{2+}; the physiological response depends on receptor distribution on particular cell types, the cell environment, and mediators generated (Leeb-Lundberg et al., 2005). For example, on normal endothelial cells, activation of B_2 receptors results in G_q and Ca^{2+}-calmodulin–dependent activation of eNOS and short-term generation of NO, which causes cyclic GMP accumulation and relaxation in neighboring smooth muscle cells. However, direct activation of B_1 or B_2 receptors on smooth muscle cells leads to coupling through G_q and increased $[Ca^{2+}]_i$, resulting in contraction.

Inflammatory conditions alter receptor signaling in endothelial cells, such that B_2 receptor stimulation leads to prolonged eNOS-derived NO that depends on G_i-mediated activation of MEK1/2 and JNK1/2, whereas B_1 receptor activation couples through G_i and MAP kinase activation to cause ERK1/2-mediated phosphorylation and activation of iNOS, which generates prolonged, high-output NO (Kuhr et al., 2010; Lowry et al., 2013). Both B_1 and B_2 receptor stimulation activate the pro-inflammatory transcription factor NF-κB coupled through $G\alpha_q$ and βγ subunits and also activate the MAP kinase pathway (Leeb-Lundberg et al., 2005). B_1 and B_2 receptors also can couple through G_i to activate PLA_2, causing the release of arachidonic acid and the local generation of metabolites such as prostaglandins and vasodilator EETs (Campbell and Falck, 2007).

The B_1 and B_2 receptors differ in their time courses of downregulation after agonist stimulation; the B_2 receptor response is rapidly desensitized, whereas the B_1 response is not (Leeb-Lundberg et al., 2005). This likely

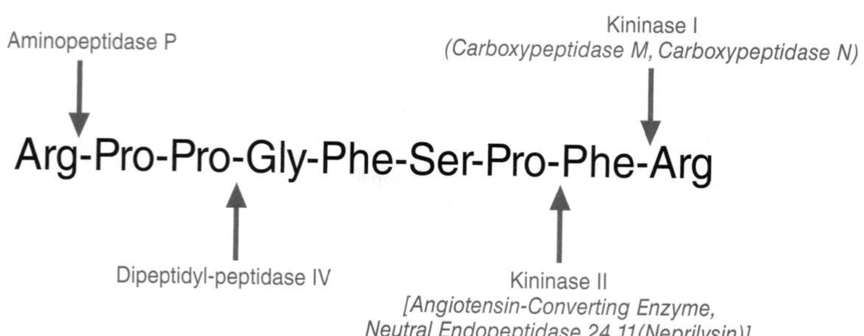

Figure 39–5 *Schematic diagram of the degradation of bradykinin.* Arrows denote the primary cleavage sites in bradykinin. Bradykinin and kallidin are inactivated in vivo primarily by kininase II (ACE). Neutral endopeptidase 24.11 (neprilysin) cleaves bradykinin and kallidin at the same Pro-Phe bond as ACE and also is classified as a kininase II–type enzyme. In addition, aminopeptidase P can inactivate bradykinin by hydrolyzing the N-terminal Arg1-Pro2 bond, leaving bradykinin susceptible to further degradation by dipeptidyl peptidase IV. Bradykinin and kallidin are converted to their respective des-Arg^9 or des-Arg^{10} metabolites by kininase I–type carboxypeptidases M and N. Unlike the parent peptides, these kinin metabolites are potent ligands for B_1 kinin receptors but not B_2 kinin receptors.

is due to modification at a Ser/Thr-rich cluster present in the C-terminal tail of the B_2 receptor that is not conserved in the B_1 receptor sequence. However, the B_1 receptor can heterodimerize with the B_2 receptor and in this form can be cross desensitized by activation of the B_2 receptor with agonist (Zhang et al., 2015).

Functions and Pharmacology of Kallikreins and Kinins

The utility of specific kinin receptor antagonists currently is being investigated in diverse areas such as pain, inflammation, chronic inflammatory diseases, and the cardiovascular system (Campos et al., 2006). The beneficial effects of ACE inhibitor therapy rest in part on enhancing bradykinin activity (e.g., on the heart, kidney, blood pressure; see Chapter 26); this has led to the suggestion that kinin agonists could be therapeutically beneficial (Heitsch, 2003).

Pain. The kinins are powerful algesic agents that cause an intense burning pain when applied to the exposed base of a blister. Bradykinin excites primary sensory neurons and provokes the release of neuropeptides such as substance P, neurokinin A, and calcitonin gene–related peptide. Although there is overlap, B_2 receptors generally mediate acute bradykinin algesia, whereas the pain of chronic inflammation appears to involve increased numbers and activation of B_1 receptors.

Inflammation. Kinins participate in a variety of inflammatory conditions (Bhoola et al., 1992; Leeb-Lundberg et al., 2005). Plasma kinins increase permeability in the microcirculation, acting on the small venules to cause disruption of the interendothelial junctions. This, together with an increased hydrostatic pressure gradient, causes edema. Edema, coupled with stimulation of nerve endings, results in a wheal-and-flare response to intradermal injection. In acute attacks of hereditary angioedema, excess bradykinin is formed, as reflected by depletion of the upstream components of the kinin cascade, and is a primary mediator of swelling, laryngeal edema, and abdominal pain (Walford and Zuraw, 2014).

The B_1 receptors on inflammatory cells (e.g., macrophages) can elicit production of the inflammatory mediators IL-1 and TNF-α. Kinin levels are increased in a number of chronic inflammatory diseases and may be significant in gout, disseminated intravascular coagulation, inflammatory bowel disease, rheumatoid arthritis, or asthma. In addition, kinins and their receptors are associated with a variety of neuroinflammatory disorders, including neuropathic pain in diabetes, autoimmune encephalomyelitis, and Alzheimer disease. Kinins may contribute to the skeletal changes seen in chronic inflammatory states; kinins stimulate bone resorption through B_1 and possibly B_2 receptors, perhaps by osteoblast-mediated osteoclast activation (see Chapter 44).

Respiratory Disease. The kinins have been implicated in allergic airway disorders such as asthma and rhinitis (Abraham et al., 2006). Inhalation of kinins causes bronchospasm mimicking an asthma attack in asthmatic patients but not in normal individuals. This bradykinin-induced bronchoconstriction is blocked by anticholinergic agents but not by antihistamines or cyclooxygenase inhibitors. Similarly, nasal challenge with bradykinin is followed by sneezing and glandular secretions in patients with allergic rhinitis, but not normal individuals or those with nonallergic, noninfectious perennial rhinitis.

Cardiovascular System. Infusion of bradykinin causes vasodilation and lowers blood pressure. Bradykinin causes vasodilation by activating its B_2 receptor on endothelial cells, resulting in the generation of NO, prostacyclin, and a hyperpolarizing EET that is a CYP-derived metabolite of arachidonate (Campbell and Falck, 2007). The endogenous kallikrein-kinin system plays a minor role in the regulation of normal blood pressure, but it may be important in hypertensive states. Urinary kallikrein concentrations are decreased in individuals with high blood pressure.

The kallikrein-kinin system is cardioprotective. Many of the beneficial effects of ACE inhibitors on heart function are attributable to enhancement of bradykinin effects, such as their antiproliferative activity or ability to increase tissue glucose uptake (Heitsch, 2003; Madeddu et al., 2007). Bradykinin contributes to the beneficial effect of preconditioning to protect the heart against ischemia and reperfusion injury. Bradykinin also stimulates tissue plasminogen activator release from the vascular endothelium and may contribute to the endogenous defense against some cardiovascular events, such as myocardial infarction and stroke (Heitsch, 2003; Madeddu et al., 2007).

Kidney. Renal kinins act in a paracrine manner to regulate urine volume and composition. Kallikrein is synthesized and secreted by the connecting cells of the distal nephron. Tissue kininogen and kinin receptors are present in the cells of the collecting duct. Like other vasodilators, kinins increase renal blood flow. Bradykinin also causes natriuresis by inhibiting Na^+ reabsorption at the cortical collecting duct. Treatment with mineralocorticoids, ACE inhibitors, and neutral endopeptidase (neprilysin) inhibitors increases renal kallikrein.

Other Effects. Kinins promote dilation of the fetal pulmonary artery, closure of the ductus arteriosus, and constriction of the umbilical vessels, all of which occur in the transition from fetal to neonatal circulation. Kinins also affect the CNS, disrupting the blood-brain barrier and allowing increased CNS penetration. Kinins and kinin receptor signaling have been associated with neuroinflammatory disorders, such as neuropathic pain in diabetes, autoimmune encephalomyelitis and Alzheimer disease.

Kallikrein Inhibitors

Aprotinin is a natural proteinase inhibitor that inhibits mediators of the inflammatory response, fibrinolysis, and thrombin generation following cardiopulmonary bypass surgery, including kallikrein and plasmin. Aprotinin was employed clinically to reduce blood loss in patients undergoing coronary artery bypass surgery, but unfavorable survival statistics in retrospective and prospective studies resulted in its discontinuation.

Ecallantide is a synthetic plasma kallikrein inhibitor approved for the treatment of acute attacks of hereditary angioedema in patients 12 years and older. It is administered by a healthcare professional (with appropriate medical support to manage possible anaphylaxis) subcutaneously at a total dose of 30 mg, divided into three 10-mg injections of 1 mL each. An additional dose of 30 mg may be administered within a 24-h period if the attack persists. The most common side effects (~3%–8% of patients) include headache, nausea, diarrhea, fever, injection site reactions, and nasopharyngitis. Safety has not been tested in pregnant or nursing women. Anaphylaxis has been reported in about 4% of treated patients, occurring within 1 h after dosing. Approximately 20% of patients treated with ecallantide develop antibodies to the drug and may be at a higher risk of hypersensitivity reactions on subsequent exposure. Ecallantide is currently being investigated as a potential treatment of other forms of angioedema (Zuraw et al., 2013).

Bradykinin and the Effects of ACE Inhibitors

The ACE inhibitors, widely used in the treatment of hypertension, congestive heart failure, and diabetic nephropathy, block the conversion of AngI to AngII and also block the degradation of bradykinin by ACE (see Figure 39–4 and Chapter 26). Numerous studies demonstrated that bradykinin contributes to many of the protective effects of ACE inhibitors (Heitsch, 2003; Madeddu et al., 2007). The search is on to find a suitable stable B_2 agonist for clinical evaluation that provides cardiovascular benefit without pro-inflammatory effects.

A rare side effect of ACE inhibitors is angioedema, which is likely due to the inhibition of kinin metabolism by ACE (Zuraw et al., 2013). A common side effect of ACE inhibitors that may be related to enhanced kinin levels is a chronic, nonproductive cough that dissipates when the drug is stopped. Bradykinin may also contribute to the therapeutic effects of the AT_1 receptor antagonists. During AT_1 receptor blockade, AngII signaling through the unopposed AT_2 subtype receptor is enhanced, causing an increase in bradykinin concentrations, which has beneficial effects on cardiovascular and renal function (Padia and Carey, 2013). However, the increase in bradykinin levels is likely more modest than that achieved by ACE inhibitors, as reflected by the lower incidence of angioedema in patients taking AT_1 receptor antagonists (Zuraw et al., 2013).

Kinin Receptor Antagonists

The selective B_2 receptor antagonist *icatibant* has been approved in the E.U. and recently in the U.S. for treatment of acute episodes of swelling in patients more than 18 years of age with hereditary angioedema. It is administered by a healthcare professional, or self-administered by the patient after training, at a dose of 30 mg in 3 mL of solution by subcutaneous injection in the abdomen. Additional doses may be administered at intervals of at least 6 h if the response is inadequate or symptoms recur, not to exceed three doses in any 24-h period. A common side effect experienced by most patients is a local reaction at the injection site (e.g., redness, bruising, swelling, burning, itching, etc.). A small percentage of patients experienced fever, elevated transaminase, dizziness, nausea, headache, or rash. Safety has not been tested in pregnant or nursing women. Although icatibant has the potential to attenuate the antihypertensive effects of ACE inhibitors, it is unclear if this is clinically significant, since patients taking ACE inhibitors were excluded from clinical trials with icatibant. Icatibant is currently being investigated as treatment of ACE inhibitor–induced angioedema, and initial results of small trials and individual case reports indicate that it is effective (Zuraw et al., 2013). Other forms of angioedema are under investigation for responsiveness to icatibant.

Acknowledgment: *Nancy J. Brown, L. Jackson Roberts II, Ervin G. Erdös, and Allen P. Kaplan contributed to this chapter in earlier editions of this book. We have retained some of their text in the current edition.*

Drug Facts for Your Personal Formulary: *H_1 Antagonists*

Drugs	Therapeutic Uses	Clinical Pharmacology and Tips
First-Generation Antihistamines: H_1 receptor inverse agonists • Most have central and anticholinergic effects • Use with caution in children and in adults > 65 years of age		
Doxepin	• Tricyclic antidepressant • Insomnia • Pruritis (topical cream) • Pruritis (atopic dermatitis, eczema, lichen simplex) (cream)	• Causes significant sedation/drowsiness • Anticholinergic effects • Increased risk of suicidal thoughts (children, adolescents, and young adults)
Carbinoxamine Clemastine Diphenhydramine Dimenhydrinate	• Symptoms of allergic response • Mild urticaria • Insomnia (diphenhydramine) • Motion sickness (dimenhydrinate, diphenhdramine)	• Pronounced tendency to cause sedation • Significant anticholinergic effects • GI side effects are low • Carbinoxamine and diphenhydramine: adjunct to epinephrine for anaphylaxis
Pyrilamine (only available as an ingredient in OTC combination preparations)	• Symptoms of allergic response	• Anticholinergic effects • Central effects < other first-generation drugs • GI side effects are quite common
Chlorpheniramine Dexchlorpheniramine Brompheniramine Dexbrompheniramine (component of cold medicine)	• Allergic conjunctivitis • Allergic rhinitis • Anaphylaxis (adjunct), histamine-mediated angioedema, dermatographism, pruritus, sneezing, urticaria (brompheniramine) • Symptoms of allergic response	Less drowsiness than other first-generation drugs; CNS stimulation side effects more common
Hydroxyzine	• Pruritis • Sedation • Antianxiety • Atopic dermatitis • Antiemetic • Urticaria	• CNS depressant action may contribute to antipruritic effects
Cyclizine (discontinued in the U.S.) Meclizine (not for use in children)	• Motion sickness • Nausea/vomiting • Vertigo	• Antinausea properties due to prominent anticholinergic effects • Less likely to cause drowsiness than other first-generation drugs • Meclizine, most used, long effect (≥8 h)
Promethazine	• Antiemetic • Motion sickness • Pruritus • Sedation • Symptoms of allergic response (off-label use)	• Risk of fatal respiratory depression in children, especially < 2 years • May lower seizure threshold • Has local anesthetic activity • Most potent antihistamine antiemetic
Cyproheptadine	• Allergic conjunctivitis • Allergic rhinitis • Anaphylaxis • Histamine-mediated angioedema • Pruritus, allergy • Vasomotor rhinitis • Urticaria • Dermatographism	• May increase appetite, cause weight gain • Has significant anticholinergic activity • Also blocks serotonin effects by antagonizing the $5HT_{2A}$ receptor

Drug Facts for Your Personal Formulary: H_1 *Antagonists(continued)*

Drugs	Therapeutic Uses	Clinical Pharmacology and Tips
Second-Generation Antihistamines: H_1 receptor inverse agonists • Lack significant central and anticholinergic effects		
Olopatadine (nasal and ophthalmic only)	• Allergic conjunctivitis • Allergic rhinitis • Ocular pruritus • Rhinorrhea • Sneezing	• Approved for once-daily dosing • Eye drops may cause headaches in some • Nasal spray can cause epistaxis and nasal ulceration or septal perforation • Some increase in risk of somnolence with nasal spray • Nasal spray minor side effects include bitter taste and headache
Acrivastine (only marketed in combination with pseudoephedrine)	• Allergic rhinitis • Nasal congestion • Allergic symptoms	• ~40% metabolized by CYPs, reducing potential for drug interactions • Somewhat higher risk of mild sedation than other second-generation drugs
Cetirizine Levocetirizine	• Allergic rhinitis • Atopic dermatitis (cetirizine) • Urticaria (chronic idiopathic)	• Somewhat higher risk of mild sedation than other second-generation drugs; more potent levocetirizine can be used at lower dose with less risk of sedation • Only ~30% (cetirizine) or ~1% (levocetirizine) metabolized by CYPs, reducing potential for drug interactions
Loratadine Desloratadine	• Allergic rhinitis • Chronic idiopathic urticaria • Exercise-induced bronchospasm prophylaxis (loratadine) • Pruritus (desloratadine)	• Desloratadine is the active metabolite of loratadine • 24-h duration of activity so only once-a-day dosing is required
Fexofenadine	• Allergic rhinitis • Chronic idiopathic urticaria	• Is the active metabolite of terfenadine (withdrawn from the market due to risk of torsades de pointes) • Only ~8% metabolized by CYPs, reducing potential for drug interactions
Alcaftadine (ophthalmic only)	• Allergic conjunctivitis • Ocular pruritus	• In addition to mast cell–stabilizing and anti-inflammatory properties, its H_4 antagonist activity may give superior relief from ocular itching • Approved for once-daily dosing • Most common adverse reactions (<4%) are eye irritation, redness, and pruritis
Bepotastine (ophthalmic only)	• Allergic conjunctivitis • Ocular pruritus	• Has mast cell–stabilizing and anti-inflammatory properties • Most common (~25%) adverse reaction is mild taste • Other minor (2%–5%) reactions are eye irritation, headache, and nasopharyngitis
Ketotifen (ophthalmic only)	• Allergic conjunctivitis • Ocular pruritus	• Has mast cell–stabilizing and anti-inflammatory properties • Most common (~10%–25%) adverse reactions are red eyes and mild headache or rhinitis
Azelastine (nasal and ophthalmic only)	• Allergic conjunctivitis • Allergic rhinitis (alone and combined with fluticasone) • Ocular pruritus • Vasomotor rhinitis	• Has mast cell–stabilizing and anti-inflammatory properties • Eye drops may cause transient eye burning/stinging • Some increase in risk of somnolence with nasal spray • Minor side effects with eye drops and nasal spray include bitter taste and headache
Emedastine (ophthalmic only)	• Allergic conjunctivitis • Ocular pruritus	• Lacks mast cell–stabilizing and anti-inflammatory properties • Common side effect: headache (~11%) • Minor reactions (<5%): abnormal dreams, bad taste, eye irritation
Epinastine (ophthalmic only)	• Allergic conjunctivitis • Ocular pruritus	• In addition to mast cell–stabilizing and anti-inflammatory properties, its H_2 antagonist activity may reduce eyelid edema • Common side effect (~10%): symptoms of upper respiratory infection • Minor ocular reactions: burning sensation, folliculosis, hyperemia, and pruritis

Bibliography

Abelson MB, et al. Advances in pharmacotherapy for allergic conjunctivitis. *Expert Opin Pharmacother*, **2015**, *16*:1219–1231.

Abraham WM, et al. Peptide and non-peptide bradykinin receptor antagonists: role in allergic airway disease. *Eur J Pharmacol*, **2006**, *533*:215–221.

Bartra J, et al. Interactions of the H_1 antihistamines. *J Investig Allergol Clin Immunol*, **2006**, *16*(suppl 1):29–36.

Bhoola KD, et al. Bioregulation of kinins: kallikreins, kininogens, and kininases. *Pharmacol Rev*, **1992**, *44*:1–80.

Black JW, et al. Definition and antagonism of histamine H_2-receptors. *Nature*, **1972**, *236*:385–390.

Campbell WB, Falck JR. Arachidonic acid metabolites as endothelium-derived hyperpolarizing factors. *Hypertension*, **2007**, *49*:590–596.

Campos MM, et al. Non-peptide antagonists for kinin B_1 receptors: new insights into their therapeutic potential for the management of inflammation and pain. *Trends Pharmacol Sci*, **2006**, *27*:646–651.

del Cuvillo A, et al. Comparative pharmacology of the H_1 antihistamines. *J Investig Allergol Clin Immunol*, **2006**, *16*(suppl 1):3–12.

Ellenbroek BA, Ghiabi B. The other side of the histamine H_3 receptor. *Trends Neurosci*, **2014**, *37*:191–199.

Emanuel MB. Histamine and the antiallergic antihistamines: a history of their discoveries. *Clin Exp Allergy*, **1999**, *29*(suppl 3):1–11.

Erdös EG, Skidgel RA. Metabolism of bradykinin by peptidases in health and disease. In: Farmer SG, ed. *The Kinin System*. Academic Press, London, **1997**, 111–141.

Esbenshade TA, et al. The histamine H_3 receptor: an attractive target for the treatment of cognitive disorders. *Br J Pharmacol*, **2008**, *154*: 1166–1181.

Gilboa SM, et al. Antihistamines and birth defects: a systematic review of the literature. *Expert Opin Drug Saf*, **2014**, *13*:1667–1698.

Gray SL, et al. Cumulative use of strong anticholinergics and incident dementia: a prospective cohort study. *JAMA Intern Med*, **2015**, *175*: 401–407.

Haas HL, et al. Histamine in the nervous system. *Physiol Rev*, **2008**, *88*:1183–1241.

Heitsch H. The therapeutic potential of bradykinin B_2 receptor agonists in the treatment of cardiovascular disease. *Expert Opin Investig Drugs*, **2003**, *12*:759–770.

Johnson AR, Erdos EG. Release of histamine from mast cells by vasoactive peptides. *Proc Soc Exp Biol Med*, **1973**, *142*:1252–1256.

Kaplan AP, Joseph K. Pathogenic mechanisms of bradykinin mediated diseases: dysregulation of an innate inflammatory pathway. *Adv Immunol*, **2014**, *121*:41–89.

Kuhr F, et al. Differential regulation of inducible and endothelial nitric oxide synthase by kinin B_1 and B_2 receptors. *Neuropeptides*, **2010**, *44*:145–154.

Leeb-Lundberg LM, et al. International union of pharmacology. XLV. Classification of the kinin receptor family: from molecular mechanisms to pathophysiological consequences. *Pharmacol Rev*, **2005**, *57*:27–77.

Levi-Schaffer F, Eliashar R. Mast cell stabilizing properties of antihistamines. *J Invest Dermatol*, **2009**, *129*:2549–2551.

Lowry JL, et al. Endothelial nitric-oxide synthase activation generates an inducible nitric-oxide synthase-like output of nitric oxide in inflamed endothelium. *J Biol Chem*, **2013**, *288*:4174–4193.

Madeddu P, et al. Mechanisms of disease: the tissue kallikrein-kinin system in hypertension and vascular remodeling. *Nat Clin Pract Nephrol*, **2007**, *3*:208–221.

Mikelis CM, et al. RhoA and ROCK mediate histamine-induced vascular leakage and anaphylactic shock. *Nat Commun*, **2015**, *6*:6725.

Padia SH, Carey RM. AT_2 receptors: beneficial counter-regulatory role in cardiovascular and renal function. *Pflugers Arch*, **2013**, *465*: 99–110.

Prassas I, et al. Unleashing the therapeutic potential of human kallikrein-related serine proteases. *Nat Rev Drug Discov*, **2015**, *14*:183–202.

Rocha e Silva M, et al. Bradykinin, a hypotensive and smooth muscle stimulating factor released from plasma globulin by snake venoms and by trypsin. *Am J Physiol*, **1949**, *156*:261–273.

Sander K, et al. Histamine H_3 receptor antagonists go to clinics. *Biol Pharm Bull*, **2008**, *31*:2163–2181.

Schwartz LB. Mast cells: function and contents. *Curr Opin Immunol*, **1994**, *6*:91–97.

Seifert R. How do basic secretagogues activate mast cells? *Naunyn Schmiedebergs Arch Pharmacol*, **2015**, *388*:279–281.

Simons FE. Advances in H_1-antihistamines. *N Engl J Med*, **2004**, *351*: 2203–2217.

Simons FE, Simons KJ. Histamine and H1-antihistamines: celebrating a century of progress. *J Allergy Clin Immunol*, **2011**, *128*:1139–1150.

Skidgel RA, Erdös EG. Structure and function of human plasma carboxypeptidase N, the anaphylatoxin inactivator. *Int Immunopharmacol*, **2007**, *7*:1888–1899.

Thurmond RL. The histamine H_4 receptor: from orphan to the clinic. *Front Pharmacol*, **2015**, *6*:65.

Thurmond RL, et al. The role of histamine H_1 and H_4 receptors in allergic inflammation: the search for new antihistamines. *Nat Rev Drug Discov*, **2008**, *7*:41–53.

Viegas LP, et al. The maddening itch: an approach to chronic urticaria. *J Investig Allergol Clin Immunol*, **2014**, *24*:1–5.

Walford HH, Zuraw BL. Current update on cellular and molecular mechanisms of hereditary angioedema. *Ann Allergy Asthma Immunol*, **2014**, *112*:413–418.

Werle E. Discovery of the most important kallikreins and kallikrein inhibitors. In: Erdös EG, ed. *Handbook of Experimental Pharmacology. Vol. 25*. Springer-Verlag, Heidelberg, **1970**, 1–6.

Zhang X, et al. Carboxypeptidase M augments kinin B_1 receptor signaling by conformational crosstalk and enhances endothelial nitric oxide output. *Biol Chem*, **2013a**, *394*:335–345.

Zhang X, et al. Carboxypeptidase M is a positive allosteric modulator of the kinin B1 receptor. *J Biol Chem*, **2013b**, *288*:33226–33240.

Zhang X, et al. Downregulation of kinin B_1 receptor function by B_2 receptor heterodimerization and signaling. *Cell Signal*, **2015**, *27*:90–103.

Zuraw BL, et al. A focused parameter update: hereditary angioedema, acquired C1 inhibitor deficiency, and angiotensin-converting enzyme inhibitor-associated angioedema. *J Allergy Clin Immunol*, **2013**, *131*: 1491–1493.

Pulmonary Pharmacology

Peter J. Barnes

第四十章 肺脏药理学

中文导读

本章主要介绍：哮喘发病机制；慢性阻塞性肺疾病（COPD）的发病机制；肺部给药途径，包括吸入给药、口服给药和非肠道途径给药；支气管舒张药，包括β_2-肾上腺素能受体激动药、甲基黄嘌呤、毒蕈碱胆碱能拮抗药、新型支气管舒张药；糖皮质激素，包括其作用机制、在哮喘中的抗感染作用、对β_2-肾上腺素能反应的影响、药物动力学、给药及给药途径、不良反应、治疗选择、未来的研发；克罗蒙斯（Cromones）；磷酸二酯酶抑制药；介质拮抗药，包括抗组胺药和抗白三烯药；免疫调节治疗，包括免疫抑制治疗、抗IgE受体治疗和特异性免疫治疗；针对呼吸道疾病的新药研发，包括新型介质拮抗药、蛋白酶抑制药、新型抗感染药、黏液调节药、黏液溶解药和祛痰药；镇咳药，包括阿片类、右美沙芬、局部麻醉药、神经调节药、其他药物和新型镇咳药；治疗呼吸困难和通气控制药，包括治疗呼吸困难的药物、通气刺激药。

Abbreviations

AC: adenylyl cyclase
ACh: acetylcholine
ALT: alanine aminotransferase
BDP: beclomethasone dipropionate
cAMP: cyclic adenosine monophosphate
CCR3: C-C chemokine receptor type 3
COMT: catechol-*O*-methyl transferase
COPD: chronic obstructive pulmonary disease
CRTh2: chemokine receptor homologous molecule expressed on Th2 lymphocytes
CXCR2: C-X-C motif chemokine receptor 2
cys-LT: cysteinyl-leukotriene
DPI: dry powder inhaler
FDA: Food and Drug Administration
FEV_1: forced expiratory volume in 1 second
FFA: free fatty acid
GABA: γ-aminobutyric acid
GR: glucocorticoid receptor
HDAC2: histone deacetylase 2
HFA: hydrofluoroalkane
ICS: inhaled corticosteroid
Ig: immunoglobulin
IL: interleukin
ILC2: innate type 2 lymphocyte
IM: intramuscular
IP_3: inositol 1,4,5-trisphosphate
IV: intravenous
LABA: long-acting inhaled β_2 agonist
LAMA: long-acting muscarinic antagonist
5-LO: 5′-lipoxygenase
LT: leukotriene
MAO: monoamine oxidase
MDI: metered-dose inhaler
MMAD: mass median aerodynamic diameter
MMP: matrix metalloproteinase
MOR: μ opioid receptor
NF-κB: nuclear factor kappa B
NMDA: *N*-methyl-D-aspartate
PAF: platelet-activating factor
PDE: phosphodiesterase
PG: prostaglandin
PKA: protein kinase A
PLC: phospholipase C
pMDI: pressurized metered-dose inhaler
SABA: short-acting β_2 agonists
SAMA: short-acting muscarinic antagonist
TAS2R: taste 2 receptor
Tc1 cell: cytotoxic T lymphocyte
Th17: T helper-17 cell
T_H2: T helper 2 lymphocyte
TNF: tumor necrosis factor
TRP: transient receptor potential
VIP: vasoactive intestinal polypeptide

Pulmonary pharmacology concerns understanding how drugs act on the lung and the pharmacological therapy of pulmonary diseases. Much of pulmonary pharmacology is concerned with the effects of drugs on the airways and the therapy of airway obstruction, particularly asthma and COPD, which are among the most common chronic diseases in the world. Both asthma and COPD are characterized by chronic inflammation of the airways, although there are marked differences in inflammatory mechanisms and response to therapy between these diseases (Barnes, 2008b; Postma and Rabe, 2015). This chapter discusses the pharmacotherapy of obstructive airways disease, particularly therapy with bronchodilators, which act mainly by reversing airway smooth muscle contraction, and anti-inflammatory drugs, which suppress the inflammatory response in the airways. This chapter focuses on the pulmonary pharmacology of β_2 adrenergic agonists and corticosteroids; the basic pharmacology of these classes of agents is presented elsewhere (Chapters 12 and 46).

This chapter also discusses other drugs used to treat obstructive airway diseases, such as mucolytics and respiratory stimulants, and covers the drug therapy of cough, the most common respiratory symptom. Drugs used in the treatment of pulmonary hypertension (Chapter 31) or lung infections, including tuberculosis (Chapter 60), are covered elsewhere.

Mechanisms of Asthma

Asthma is a chronic inflammatory disease of the airways that is characterized by activation of *mast cells*, infiltration of *eosinophils, T helper 2 (T_H2) lymphocytes, and innate type 2 lymphocytes (ILC2)* (Figure 40–1) (Barnes, 2011b; Lambrecht and Hammad, 2015). Mast cell activation by allergens and physical stimuli releases *bronchoconstrictor mediators*, such as *histamine, LTD_4, and prostaglandin D_2*, which cause bronchoconstriction, microvascular leakage, and plasma exudation. Increased numbers of mast cells in airway smooth muscle are a characteristic of asthma.

Many of the symptoms of asthma are due to airway smooth muscle contraction, and therefore bronchodilators are important as symptom relievers. Whether airway smooth muscle is intrinsically abnormal in asthma is not clear, but increased contractility of airway smooth muscle may contribute to airway hyperresponsiveness, the physiological hallmark of asthma.

The mechanism of chronic inflammation in asthma is still not well understood. It may initially be driven by allergen exposure, but it appears to become autonomous so that asthma is essentially incurable. The inflammation may be orchestrated by dendritic cells that regulate T_H2 cells that drive eosinophilic inflammation and also IgE formation by B lymphocytes.

Airway epithelium plays an important role through the release of multiple inflammatory mediators and through the release of growth factors

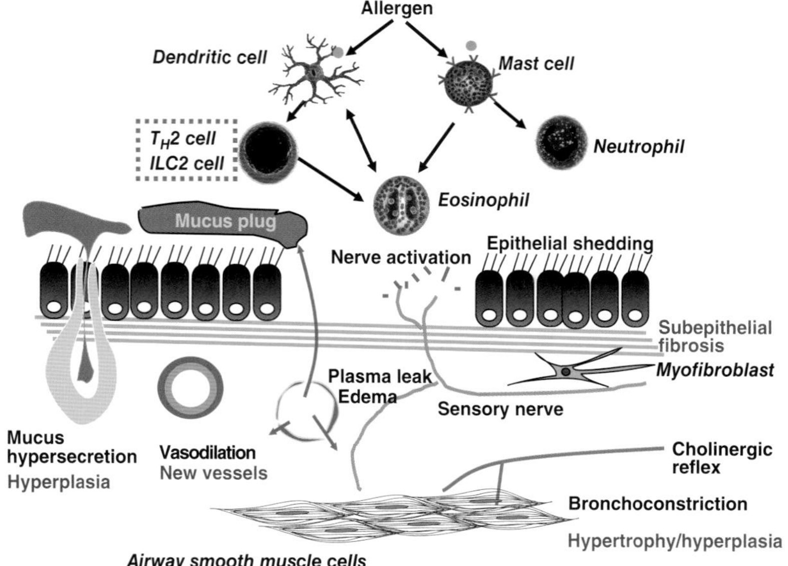

Figure 40–1 *Cellular mechanisms of asthma.* Myriad inflammatory cells are recruited and activated in the airways, where they release multiple inflammatory mediators, which can also arise from structural cells. These mediators lead to bronchoconstriction, plasma exudation and edema, vasodilation, mucus hypersecretion, and activation of sensory nerves. Chronic inflammation leads to structural changes, including subepithelial fibrosis (basement membrane thickening), airway smooth muscle hypertrophy and hyperplasia, angiogenesis, and hyperplasia of mucus-secreting cells.

in an attempt to repair the damage caused by inflammation. The inflammatory process in asthma is mediated through the release of more than 100 inflammatory mediators (Hall and Agrawal, 2014). Complex cytokine networks, including chemokines and growth factors, play important roles in orchestrating the inflammation process (Barnes, 2008a).

Chronic inflammation may lead to structural changes (remodeling) in the airways, including an increase in the number and size of airway smooth muscle cells, blood vessels, and mucus-secreting cells. A characteristic histological feature of asthma is collagen deposition (fibrosis) below the basement membrane of the airway epithelium (Figure 49–1). This appears to be the result of eosinophilic inflammation and is found even at the onset of asthmatic symptoms. The complex inflammation of asthma is suppressed by corticosteroids in most patients, but even if asthma is well controlled, the inflammation and symptoms return if corticosteroids are discontinued. Asthma usually starts in early childhood, then may disappear during adolescence and reappear in adulthood. It is characterized by variable airflow obstruction and typically shows a good therapeutic response to bronchodilators and corticosteroids. Asthma severity usually does not change, so that patients with mild asthma rarely progress to severe asthma and patients with severe asthma usually have this from the onset, although some patients, particularly with late-onset asthma, show a progressive loss of lung function like patients with COPD. Patients with severe asthma may have a pattern of inflammation more similar to COPD and are characterized by reduced responsiveness to corticosteroids (Trejo Bittar et al., 2015).

Mechanisms of COPD

Chronic obstructive pulmonary disease involves inflammation of the respiratory tract with a pattern that differs from that of asthma. In COPD, there is a *predominance of neutrophils, macrophages, cytotoxic T lymphocytes (Tc1 cells), and T helper-17 (Th17) cells*. The inflammation *predominantly affects small airways*, resulting in progressive small-airway narrowing and fibrosis (chronic obstructive bronchiolitis) and destruction of the lung parenchyma with destruction of the alveolar walls (emphysema) (Figure 40–2) (Barnes et al., 2015). These pathological changes result in airway closure on expiration, leading to air trapping and hyperinflation, particularly on exercise (dynamic hyperinflation). This accounts for shortness of breath on exertion and exercise limitation that are characteristic symptoms of COPD.

Bronchodilators reduce air trapping by dilating peripheral airways and are the mainstay of treatment in COPD. In contrast to asthma, the airflow obstruction of COPD tends to be progressive. The inflammation in the peripheral lung of patients with COPD is mediated by multiple inflammatory mediators and cytokines, although the pattern of mediators differs from that of asthma (Barnes, 2004). In contrast to asthma, the inflammation in patients with COPD is largely corticosteroid resistant, and there are currently no effective anti-inflammatory treatments. Many patients with COPD have comorbidities, including ischemic heart disease, hypertension, congestive heart failure, diabetes, osteoporosis, skeletal muscle wasting, depression, chronic renal disease, and anemia (Barnes and Celli, 2009). These diseases may occur together as part of multimorbidity, as diseases of accelerated aging with common pathogenetic mechanisms (Barnes, 2015).

Routes of Drug Delivery to the Lungs

Drugs may be delivered to the lungs by oral or parenteral routes and also by inhalation. The choice depends on the drug and on the respiratory disease.

Inhaled Route

Inhalation (Figure 40–3) is the preferred mode of delivery of many drugs with a direct effect on airways, particularly for asthma and COPD (Sanchis et al., 2013). It is the only way to deliver some drugs, such as cromolyn sodium and anticholinergic drugs, and is the preferred route of delivery for β_2 agonists and corticosteroids to reduce systemic side effects. Antibiotics may be delivered by inhalation in patients with chronic respiratory sepsis (e.g., in cystic fibrosis). The major advantage of inhalation is the delivery of drug to the airways in doses that are effective with a much lower risk of systemic side effects. This is particularly important with the

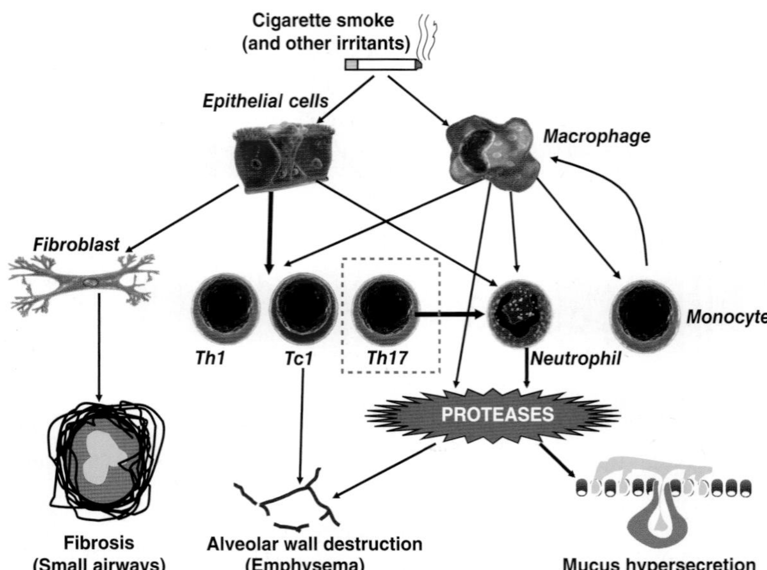

Figure 40–2 *Cellular mechanisms in COPD.* Cigarette smoke and other irritants activate epithelial cells and macrophages in the lung to release mediators that attract circulating inflammatory cells, including monocytes (which differentiate to macrophages within the lung), neutrophils, and T lymphocytes (T_H1, T_C1, and Th17 cells). Fibrogenic factors released from epithelial cells and macrophages lead to fibrosis of small airways. Release of proteases results in alveolar wall destruction (emphysema) and mucus hypersecretion (chronic bronchitis).

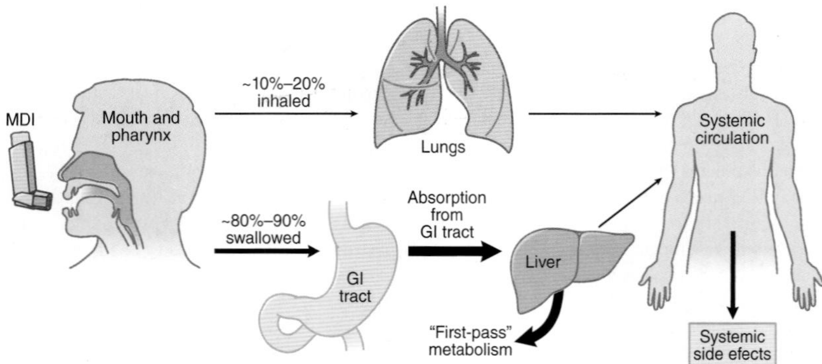

Figure 40–3 *Schematic representation of the deposition of inhaled drugs (e.g., corticosteroids, β_2 agonists).* Inhalation therapy deposits drugs directly, but not exclusively, in the lungs. Distribution between lungs and oropharynx depends mostly on the particle size and the efficiency of the delivery method. Most material will be swallowed and absorbed, entering systemic circulation after undergoing the first-pass effect in the liver. Some drug will also be absorbed into the systemic circulation from the lungs. Use of a large-volume spacer will reduce the amount of drug deposited on the oropharynx, thereby reducing the amount swallowed and absorbed from the GI tract, thus limiting systemic effects.

use of ICS, which largely avoids systemic side effects. In addition, inhaled bronchodilators have a more rapid onset of action than when taken orally.

Particle Size

The size of particles for inhalation is of critical importance in determining the site of deposition in the respiratory tract. The optimum size for particles to settle in the airways is 2- to 5-μm MMAD. Larger particles settle out in the upper airways, whereas smaller particles remain suspended and are therefore exhaled. There is increasing interest in delivering drugs to small airways, particularly in COPD and severe asthma (Usmani and Barnes, 2012). This involves delivering drug particles of about 1-μm MMAD, which is now possible using drugs formulated in HFA propellant.

Pharmacokinetics

Of the total drug delivered, only 10%–20% enters the lower airways with a conventional pMDI. Drugs are absorbed from the airway lumen and have direct effects on target cells of the airway. Drugs may also be absorbed into the bronchial circulation and then distributed to more peripheral airways. Drugs with higher molecular weights tend to be retained to a greater extent in the airways. Nevertheless, several drugs have greater therapeutic efficacy when given by the inhaled route. The ICS *ciclesonide* is a prodrug activated by esterases in the respiratory tract to the active principle des-ciclesonide. More extensive pulmonary distribution of a drug with a smaller MMAD increases alveolar deposition and thus is likely to increase absorption from the lungs into the general circulation, resulting in more systemic side effects. Thus, although HFA pMDIs deliver more ICS to smaller airways, there is also increased systemic absorption, so that the therapeutic ratio may not be changed.

Delivery Devices

Pressurized Metered-Dose Inhalers. Drugs are propelled from a canister in the pMDI with the aid of a propellant, previously with a chlorofluorocarbon (Freon) but now replaced by an *HFA* that is "ozone friendly." These devices are convenient, portable, and typically deliver 50–200 doses of drug.

Spacer Chambers. Large-volume spacer devices between the pMDI and the patient reduce the velocity of particles entering the upper airways and the size of the particles by allowing evaporation of liquid propellant. This reduces the amount of drug that impinges on the oropharynx and increases the proportion of drug inhaled into the lower airways. Application of spacer chambers is useful in the reduction of the oropharyngeal deposition of ICS and the consequent reduction in the local side effects of these drugs. Spacer devices are also useful in delivering inhaled drugs to small children who are not able to use a pMDI. Children as young as 3 years of age are able to use a spacer device fitted with a face mask.

Dry Powder Inhalers. Drugs may also be delivered as a dry powder using devices that scatter a fine powder dispersed by air turbulence on inhalation. Children less than 7 years of age find it difficult to use a DPI. DPIs have been developed to deliver peptides and proteins, such as insulin, systemically but have proved to be problematic because of consistency of dosing.

Nebulizers. Two types of nebulizer are available. *Jet nebulizers* are driven by a stream of gas (air or oxygen), whereas *ultrasonic nebulizers* use a rapidly vibrating piezoelectric crystal and thus do not require a source of compressed gas. The nebulized drug may be inspired during tidal breathing, and it is possible to deliver much higher doses of drug compared with a pMDI. Nebulizers are therefore useful in treating acute exacerbations of asthma and COPD, for delivering drugs when airway obstruction is extreme (e.g., in severe COPD), for delivering inhaled drugs to infants and small children who cannot use the other inhalation devices, and for giving drugs such as antibiotics when relatively high doses must be delivered.

Oral Route

Drugs for treatment of pulmonary diseases may also be given orally. The oral dose is much higher than the inhaled dose required to achieve the same effect (typically by a ratio of about 20:1), so that systemic side effects are more common. *When there is a choice of inhaled or oral route for a drug (e.g., β_2 agonist or corticosteroid), the inhaled route is always preferable*, and the oral route should be reserved for the few patients unable to use inhalers (e.g., small children, patients with physical problems such as severe arthritis of the hands). Theophylline is ineffective by the inhaled route and therefore must be given systemically. Corticosteroids may have to be given orally for parenchymal lung diseases (e.g., in interstitial lung diseases).

Parenteral Route

The intravenous route should be reserved for delivery of drugs in the severely ill patient who is unable to absorb drugs from the GI tract. Side effects are generally frequent due to the high plasma concentrations.

Bronchodilators

Bronchodilator drugs relax constricted airway smooth muscle in vitro and cause immediate reversal of airway obstruction in asthma in vivo (Cazzola et al., 2012). They also prevent bronchoconstriction (and thereby provide bronchoprotection). Three main classes of bronchodilator are in current clinical use:

- β_2 Adrenergic agonists (sympathomimetics)
- Theophylline (a methylxanthine)
- Anticholinergic agents (muscarinic receptor antagonists)

Drugs such as *cromolyn sodium*, which prevent bronchoconstriction, have no direct bronchodilator action and are ineffective once bronchoconstriction has occurred. *Anti-LTs* (LT receptor antagonists and 5′-lipoxygenase inhibitors) have a small bronchodilator effect in some asthmatic patients and appear to prevent bronchoconstriction. *Corticosteroids*, although gradually improving airway obstruction, have no direct effect on contraction of airway smooth muscle and are not therefore considered to be bronchodilators.

β_2 Adrenergic Agonists

Inhaled β_2 agonists are the bronchodilator treatment of choice in asthma because they are the most effective bronchodilators and have minimal side effects when used correctly. Systemic, short-acting, and nonselective β agonists, such as isoproterenol (isoprenaline) or metaproterenol, should only be used as a last resort.

Chemistry

The development of β_2 agonists is based on substitutions in the catecholamine structure of norepinephrine and epinephrine (see Chapters 8 and 12). The catechol ring consists of hydroxyl groups in the 3 and 4 positions of the benzene ring. Norepinephrine differs from epinephrine only in the terminal amine group; in general, further modification at this site confers β receptor selectivity. Many β_2-selective agonists have now been introduced, and although there may be differences in potency, there are no clinically significant differences in selectivity. Inhaled β_2-selective drugs in current clinical use have a similar duration of action (3–6 h).

The inhaled LABAs, salmeterol and formoterol, have a much longer duration of effect, providing bronchodilation and bronchoprotection for more than 12 h (Cazzola et al., 2013b). Formoterol has a bulky substitution in the aliphatic chain and has moderate lipophilicity, which appears to keep the drug in the membrane close to the receptor, so it behaves as a slow-release drug. Salmeterol has a long aliphatic chain, and its long duration may be due to binding within the receptor binding cleft ("exosite") that anchors the drug in the binding cleft. Once-daily β_2 agonists, such as indacaterol, vilanterol, and olodaterol, with a duration of action more than 24 h have now been developed.

Mode of Action

Occupation of β_2 receptors by agonists results in the activation of the G_s-adenylyl cyclase-cAMP-PKA pathway, resulting in phosphorylative events leading to bronchial smooth muscle relaxation (Figure 40–4). β_2 Receptors are localized to several different airway cells, where they may have additional effects. β_2 Agonists may cause bronchodilation also *indirectly* by inhibiting the release of bronchoconstrictor mediators from inflammatory cells and of bronchoconstrictor neurotransmitters from airway nerves. These mechanisms include the following:

- Prevention of mediator release from isolated human lung mast cells (via β_2 receptors)
- Prevention of microvascular leakage and thus the development of bronchial mucosal edema after exposure to mediators, such as histamine, LTD_4, and prostaglandin D_2
- Increase in *mucus secretion* from submucosal glands and *ion transport* across airway epithelium (may enhance mucociliary clearance, reversing defective clearance found in asthma)
- *Reduction in neurotransmission* in human airway *cholinergic nerves* by an action at presynaptic β_2 receptors to inhibit ACh release

Although these additional effects of β_2 agonists may be relevant to the prophylactic use of these drugs against various challenges, their rapid bronchodilator action is probably attributable to a direct effect on smooth muscle of all airways.

Anti-inflammatory Effects

Whether β_2 agonists have anti-inflammatory effects in asthma is controversial. The inhibitory effects of β_2 agonists on mast cell mediator release and microvascular leakage are clearly anti-inflammatory, suggesting that β_2 agonists may modify *acute* inflammation. However, β_2 agonists do not appear to have a significant inhibitory effect on the *chronic* inflammation of asthmatic airways, which is suppressed by corticosteroids. This has now been confirmed by several biopsy and bronchoalveolar lavage studies in patients with asthma who are taking regular β_2 agonists (including LABAs), that demonstrated no significant reduction in the number or activation in inflammatory cells in the airways, in contrast to resolution of the inflammation that occurs with ICS. This may be related to the fact

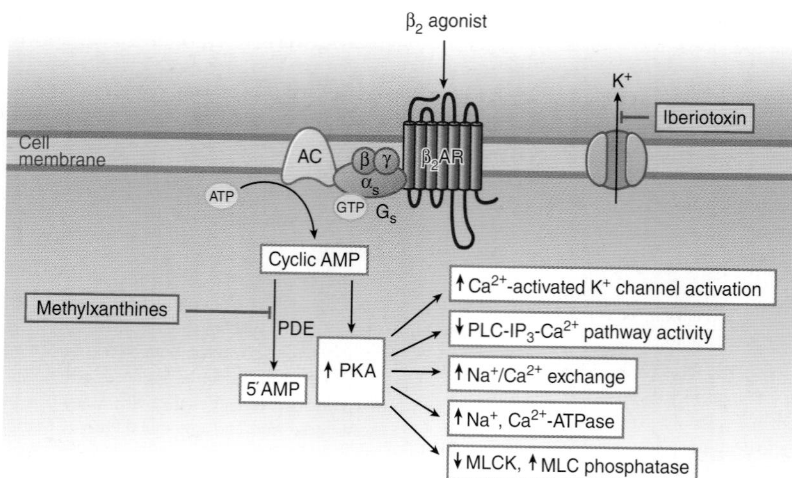

Figure 40–4 *Molecular actions of β_2 agonists to induce relaxation of airway smooth muscle cells.* Activation of β_2 receptors (β_2AR) results in activation of AC via G_s, leading to an increase in intracellular cAMP and activation of PKA. PKA phosphorylates a variety of target substrates, resulting in opening of Ca^{2+}-activated K^+ channels (K_{Ca}), thereby facilitating hyperpolarization, decreased PI hydrolysis, increased Na^+/Ca^{2+} exchange, increased Na^+, Ca^{2+}-ATPase activity, and decreased myosin light chain kinase (MLCK) activity and increased myosin light chain (MLC) phosphatase. β_2 Receptors may also couple to K_{Ca} via G_s. PDE, cyclic nucleotide phosphodiesterase.

that effects of β_2 agonists on macrophages, eosinophils, and lymphocytes are rapidly desensitized.

Clinical Use

Short-Acting β_2 Agonists. Inhaled SABAs are the most widely used and effective bronchodilators in the treatment of asthma due to their functional antagonism of bronchoconstriction. When inhaled from pMDIs or DPIs, they are convenient, easy to use, rapid in onset, and without significant systemic side effects. These agents are effective in protecting against various asthma triggers, such as exercise, cold air, and allergens. SABAs are the bronchodilators of choice in treating acute severe asthma. The nebulized route of administration is easier and safer than intravenous administration and just as effective. Inhalation is preferable to oral administration because systemic side effects are less. *SABAs, such as albuterol, should be used "as required" by symptoms and not on a regular basis in the treatment of mild asthma; increased use indicates the need for more anti-inflammatory therapy.*

Oral β_2 agonists are occasionally indicated as an additional bronchodilator. Slow-release preparations (e.g., slow-release albuterol and bambuterol [not available in the U.S.]) may be indicated in nocturnal asthma; however, these agents have an increased risk of side effects. Several SABAs are available; they are resistant to uptake and enzymatic degradation by COMT and MAO; all are usable by inhalation and orally, have a similar duration of action (~3–4 h; less in severe asthma), and similar side effects. Differences in β_2 receptor selectivity have been claimed but are not clinically important. Drugs in clinical use include *albuterol (salbutamol), levalbuterol, metaproterenol, terbutaline, pirbuterol,* as well as several not available in the U.S. (*fenoterol, tulobuterol, and rimiterol*).

Long-Acting Inhaled β_2 Agonists. The LABAs *salmeterol, formoterol,* and *arformoterol* have proved to be a significant advance in asthma and COPD therapy. These drugs have a bronchodilator action of more than 12 h and also protect against bronchoconstriction for a similar period (Cazzola et al., 2013b). They improve asthma control (when given twice daily) compared with regular treatment with SABAs (four to six times daily). Once-daily LABAs, such as *indacaterol, vilanterol,* and *olodaterol,* with a duration of over 24 h have now been developed and are more effective in patients with COPD than twice-daily LABAs and more frequent SABAs.

Tolerance to the bronchodilator effect of formoterol and the bronchoprotective effects of formoterol and salmeterol have been demonstrated but is of doubtful clinical significance. Although both formoterol and salmeterol have a similar duration of effect in clinical studies, there are differences. Formoterol has a more rapid onset of action and is an almost-full agonist, whereas salmeterol is a partial agonist with a slower onset of action. These differences might confer a theoretical advantage for formoterol in more severe asthma, whereas it may also make it more likely to induce tolerance. However, no significant clinical differences between salmeterol and formoterol have been found in the treatment of patients with severe asthma (Nightingale et al., 2002).

In COPD, LABAs are effective bronchodilators that may be used alone or in combination with anticholinergics or ICSs. LABAs improve symptoms and exercise tolerance by reducing both air trapping and exacerbations. *In patients with asthma, LABAs should never be used alone because they do not treat the underlying chronic inflammation, and this may increase the risk of life-threatening and fatal asthma exacerbations; rather, LABAs should always be used in combination with an ICS in a fixed-dose combination inhaler.* LABAs are an effective add-on therapy to ICSs and are more effective than increasing the dose of an ICS when asthma is not controlled at low doses.

Combination Inhalers. Combination inhalers that contain a LABA and a corticosteroid (e.g., *fluticasone/salmeterol, budesonide/formoterol*) are now widely used in the treatment of asthma and COPD. In asthma, combining a LABA with a corticosteroid offers complementary synergistic actions (Barnes, 2002). The combination inhaler is more convenient for patients, simplifies therapy, and improves adherence with the ICS. Also, delivering the two drugs in the same inhaler ensures they are delivered simultaneously to the same cells in the airways, allowing the beneficial molecular interactions between LABAs and corticosteroids to occur. Combination inhalers are now the preferred therapy for patients with persistent asthma. These combination inhalers are also more effective in patients with COPD than a LABA and an ICS alone, but the mechanisms accounting for this beneficial interaction are less well understood than in patients with asthma.

Stereoselective β_2 Agonists. Albuterol is a racemic mixture of active *R*- and inactive *S*-isomers. Although *R*-albuterol (levalbuterol) was more potent than racemic *R/S*-albuterol in some studies, careful dose responses showed no advantage in terms of efficacy and no evidence that the

S-albuterol is detrimental in asthmatic patients (Lotvall et al., 2001). Because levalbuterol is usually more expensive than normally used racemic albuterol, this therapy has no clear clinical advantage. Stereoselective formoterol (*R,R*-formoterol, arformoterol) has now been developed as a nebulized solution but also appears to offer no clinical advantage over racemic formoterol in patients with COPD (Loh et al., 2015).

β_2 Receptor Polymorphisms. Several single-nucleotide polymorphisms and haplotypes of the human *ADRβ2*, which affect the structure of β_2 receptors, have been described. The common variants are $Gly^{16}Arg$ and $Gln^{27}Glu$, which have in vitro effects on receptor desensitization, but clinical studies have shown inconsistent effects on the bronchodilator responses to SABAs and LABAs (Hawkins et al., 2008). Some studies have shown that patients with the common homozygous $Arg^{16}Arg$ variant have more frequent adverse effects and a poorer response to SABAs than heterozygotes or $Gly^{16}Gly$ homozygotes, but overall these differences are small, and there appears to be no clinical value in measuring *ADRβ2* genotype. No differences have been found with responses to LABA between these genotypes (Bleecker et al., 2007).

Side Effects. Unwanted effects are dose related and due to stimulation of extrapulmonary β receptors (Table 40–1 and Chapter 12). Side effects are not common with inhaled therapy but quite common with oral or intravenous administration.

- *Muscle tremor* due to stimulation of β_2 receptors in skeletal muscle is the most common side effect. It may be more troublesome with elderly patients and so is a more frequent problem in patients with COPD.
- *Tachycardia* and *palpitations* are due to reflex cardiac stimulation secondary to peripheral vasodilation, from direct stimulation of atrial β_2 receptors (human heart has a relatively high proportion of β_2 receptors; see Chapter 12), and possibly also from stimulation of myocardial β_1 receptors as the doses of β_2 agonist are increased.
- *Hypokalemia* is a potentially serious side effect. This is due to β_2 receptor stimulation of potassium entry into skeletal muscle, which may be secondary to a rise in insulin secretion. Hypokalemia might be serious in the presence of hypoxia, as in acute asthma, when there may be a predisposition to cardiac arrhythmias (Chapter 30). In practice, however, significant arrhythmias after nebulized β_2 agonists are rarely observed in acute asthma or patients with COPD.
- *Ventilation-perfusion* V/Q *mismatch* due to pulmonary vasodilation in blood vessels previously constricted by hypoxia results in the shunting of blood to poorly ventilated areas and a fall in arterial oxygen tension. Although in practice the effect of β_2 agonists on Pao_2 is usually very small (<5 mm Hg fall), occasionally in severe COPD it can be large, although it may be prevented by giving additional inspired oxygen.
- *Metabolic* effects (increase in free fatty acid, insulin, glucose, pyruvate, and lactate) are usually seen only after large systemic doses.

Tolerance. Continuous treatment with an agonist often leads to tolerance, which may be due to downregulation of the receptor (Chapter 12). Tolerance of nonairway β_2 receptor–mediated responses, such as tremor and cardiovascular and metabolic responses, is readily induced in normal and asthmatic subjects. In asthmatic patients, tolerance to the bronchodilator effects of β_2 agonists has not usually been found. However, tolerance develops to the bronchoprotective effects of β_2 agonists, and this is more marked with indirect bronchoconstrictors that activate mast cells (e.g., adenosine, allergen, and exercise) than with direct bronchoconstrictors, such as histamine and methacholine. The reason for the relative resistance of airway smooth muscle β_2 responses to desensitization remains uncertain but may reflect the large receptor reserve: More than 90% of β_2 receptors may be lost without any reduction in the relaxation response. The high level of *ADRβ2 expression* in airway smooth muscle compared with peripheral lung may also contribute to the resistance to tolerance because a high rate of β receptor synthesis is likely. In addition, the expression of GRK2, which phosphorylates and inactivates occupied β_2 receptors, is very low in airway smooth muscle (Penn et al., 1998). By contrast, there is no receptor reserve in inflammatory cells, GRK2 expression is high, and tolerance to β_2 agonists rapidly develops at these sites.

Experimental studies have shown that corticosteroids prevent the development of tolerance in airway smooth muscle and prevent and reverse the fall in pulmonary β receptor density (Mak et al., 1995). However, ICSs fail to prevent the tolerance to the bronchoprotective effect of inhaled β_2 agonists, possibly because they do not reach airway smooth muscle in a high enough concentration.

TABLE 40–1 ■ SIDE EFFECTS OF β_2 AGONISTS

- Muscle tremor (direct effect on skeletal muscle β_2 receptors)
- Tachycardia (direct effect on atrial β_2 receptors, reflex effect from increased peripheral vasodilation via β_2 receptors)
- Hypokalemia (direct β_2 effect on skeletal muscle uptake of K^+)
- Restlessness
- Hypoxemia (↑ $\dot{V}/\dot{Q}$ mismatch due to reversal of hypoxic pulmonary vasoconstriction)
- Metabolic effects (↑ FFA, glucose, lactate, pyruvate, insulin)

Long-Term Safety. Because of a possible relationship between adrenergic drug therapy and the rise in asthma deaths in several countries during the early 1960s, doubts were cast on the long-term safety of β agonists. A particular β_2 agonist, fenoterol, was linked to the rise in asthma deaths in New Zealand in the early 1990s because significantly more of the fatal cases were prescribed fenoterol than the case-matched control patients (Beasley et al., 1999). An epidemiological study examining the links between drugs prescribed for asthma and death or near death from asthma attacks found a marked increase in the risk of death with high doses of all inhaled β_2 agonists. The risk was greater with fenoterol, but when the dose is adjusted to the equivalent dose for albuterol, there is no significant difference in the risk for these two drugs.

The link between high β_2 agonist usage and increased asthma mortality does not prove a causal association because patients with more severe and poorly controlled asthma, who are more likely to have an increased risk of fatal attacks, are more likely to be using higher doses of β_2 agonist inhalers and less likely to be using effective anti-inflammatory treatment. Indeed, in the patients who used regular inhaled steroids, there was a significant reduction in risk of death.

Regular use of inhaled β_2 agonists has also been linked to increased asthma morbidity. Regular use of fenoterol was associated with worse asthma control and a small increase in airway hyperresponsiveness compared with patients using fenoterol "on demand" for symptom control over a 6-month period (Sears, 2002). However, this was not found in a study with regular albuterol (Dennis et al., 2000). There is some evidence that regular inhaled β_2 agonists may increase allergen-induced asthma and sputum eosinophilia (Gauvreau et al., 1997).

SABAs should only be used on demand for symptom control, and if they are required frequently (more than three times weekly), an ICS is needed.

The safety of LABAs in asthma remains controversial. A large study of the safety of salmeterol showed an excess of respiratory deaths and near deaths in patients prescribed salmeterol, but these deaths occurred mainly in African Americans living in inner cities who were not taking ICSs (Nelson and Dorinsky, 2006). Similar data have also raised concerns about formoterol. However, concomitant treatment with an ICS appears to obviate such risk, so it is recommended that LABAs should only be used when ICSs are also prescribed (preferably in the form of a combination inhaler so that the LABAs can never be taken without the ICSs) (Cates et al., 2014). All LABAs approved in the U.S. carry a black-box warning cautioning against overuse. There are fewer safety concerns with LABA use in COPD. No major adverse effects were reported in several large and prolonged studies and no evidence of cardiovascular problems (Kew et al., 2013).

Future Developments

The β agonists will continue to be the bronchodilators of choice for asthma because they are effective in all patients and have few or no side effects when used in low doses. When used as required for symptom control, inhaled β_2 agonists appear safe. Use of large doses of inhaled β_2 agonists indicates poor asthma control; such patients should be assessed and appropriate controller medication used. LABAs are a useful option for long-term control in asthma and COPD. In patients with asthma, LABAs should probably only be used in a fixed combination with an ICS to prevent the potential danger associated with LABAs alone. There is little advantage to be gained by improving β_2 receptor selectivity because most of the side effects of these agents are due to β_2 receptor stimulation (muscle tremor, tachycardia, hypokalemia). Once-daily inhaled β_2 agonists are useful in patients with COPD and may have additive effects with LAMAs.

Methylxanthines

Methylxanthines, such as theophylline, which are related to caffeine, have been used in the treatment of asthma since 1930, and theophylline is still widely used in developing countries because it is inexpensive. Theophylline became more useful with the introduction of reliable slow-release preparations. However, inhaled β_2 agonists are far more effective as bronchodilators, and ICSs have a greater anti-inflammatory effect. In patients with severe asthma and COPD, it still remains a useful drug as an add-on therapy (Barnes, 2013c).

THEOPHYLLINE ADENOSINE CYCLIC AMP

Chemistry

Theophylline is a methylxanthine similar in structure to the common dietary xanthines caffeine and theobromine. Several substituted derivatives have been synthesized, but only two appear to have any advantage over theophylline: *Enprofylline* is a more potent bronchodilator and may have fewer toxic effects because it does not antagonize adenosine receptors; *doxofylline*, a novel methylxanthine available in some countries, has an inhibitory effect on PDEs similar to that of theophylline but is less active as an adenosine antagonist and has a more favorable side-effect profile (Akram et al., 2012).

Many salts of theophylline have also been marketed; the most common is aminophylline. Other salts do not have any advantage. Theophylline remains the major methylxanthine in clinical use.

Mechanism of Action

The mechanisms of action of theophylline are still uncertain. In addition to its bronchodilator action, theophylline has many nonbronchodilator effects that may be relevant to its effects in asthma and COPD (Figure 40–5). Several molecular mechanisms of action have been proposed:

- *Inhibition of PDEs.* Theophylline is a nonselective PDE inhibitor, but the degree of inhibition is relatively minimal at concentrations of theophylline that are within the therapeutic range. PDE inhibition and the concomitant elevation of cellular cAMP and cyclic GMP likely account for the bronchodilator action of theophylline. Several isoenzyme families of PDE have now been recognized, and those important in smooth muscle relaxation include PDE3, PDE4, and PDE5.
- *Adenosine receptor antagonism.* Theophylline antagonizes adenosine receptors at therapeutic concentrations. Adenosine causes bronchoconstriction in airways from asthmatic patients by releasing histamine and LTs. Antagonism of A_1 receptors may be responsible for serious side effects, including cardiac arrhythmias and seizures.
- *Interleukin 10 release.* IL-10 has a broad spectrum of anti-inflammatory effects, and there is evidence that its secretion is reduced in asthma. IL-10 release is increased by theophylline, and this effect may be mediated via inhibition of PDE activities, although this has not been seen at the low doses that are effective in asthma.
- *Effects on gene transcription.* Theophylline prevents the translocation of the pro-inflammatory transcription factor NF-κB into the nucleus, potentially reducing the expression of inflammatory genes in asthma and COPD (Ichiyama et al., 2001). However, these effects are seen at high concentrations and may be mediated by inhibition of PDE.
- *Effects on apoptosis.* Prolonged survival of granulocytes due to a reduction in apoptosis may be important in perpetuating chronic inflammation in asthma (eosinophils) and COPD (neutrophils). Theophylline promotes apoptosis in eosinophils and neutrophils in vitro. This is associated with a reduction in the antiapoptotic protein Bcl-2 (Chung et al., 2000). This effect is not mediated via PDE inhibition, but in neutrophils may be mediated by antagonism of adenosine A_{2A} receptors (Yasui et al., 2000). Theophylline also induces apoptosis in T lymphocytes via PDE inhibition.
- *Histone deacetylase activation.* Recruitment of HDAC2 by GRs switches off inflammatory genes. Therapeutic concentrations of theophylline activate HDAC, thereby enhancing the anti-inflammatory effects of corticosteroids (Cosio et al., 2004). This mechanism appears to be mediated by inhibition of PI_3-kinase-δ, which is activated by oxidative stress (To et al., 2010).

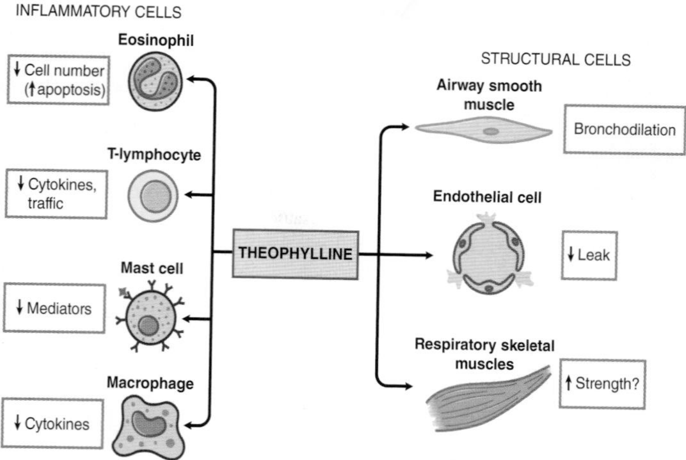

Figure 40–5 *Theophylline affects multiple cell types in the airway.*

Nonbronchodilator Effects

Theophylline has clinical benefit in asthma and COPD at plasma concentrations less than 10 mg/L, sufficiently low that such effects are unlikely to be explained by theophylline's bronchodilator action. There is increasing evidence that theophylline has anti-inflammatory effects in asthma (Barnes, 2013c). In patients with mild asthma, chronic oral treatment with theophylline inhibits the late response to inhaled allergen and reduces infiltration of eosinophils and CD4+ lymphocytes into the airways after allergen challenge (Lim et al., 2001). In patients with COPD, theophylline reduces the total number and proportion of neutrophils in induced sputum, the concentration of IL-8, and neutrophil chemotactic responses (Culpitt et al., 2002). Theophylline withdrawal in patients with COPD results in worsening of disease. In vitro theophylline is able to increase responsiveness to corticosteroids and to reverse corticosteroid resistance in cells from subjects with COPD (Cosio et al., 2004).

Pharmacokinetics and Metabolism

Theophylline has antiasthma effects other than bronchodilation below 10 mg/L, so the therapeutic range is now taken as 5–15 mg/L. The dose of theophylline required to give these therapeutic concentrations varies among subjects, largely because of differences in clearance of the drug. In addition, there may be differences in bronchodilator response to theophylline; furthermore, with acute bronchoconstriction, higher concentrations may be required to produce bronchodilation. Theophylline is rapidly and completely absorbed, but there are large interindividual variations in clearance due to differences in hepatic metabolism. Theophylline is metabolized in the liver, mainly by CYP1A2; myriad factors influence hepatic metabolism and clearance of of theophylline (see Table 40–2).

Because of these variations in clearance, individualization of theophylline dosage is required, and plasma concentrations should be measured 4 h after the last dose with slow-release preparations when steady state has been achieved. There is no significant circadian variation in theophylline metabolism, although there may be delayed absorption at night related to supine posture.

Preparations and Routes of Administration

Intravenous aminophylline, an ethylene diamine ester of theophylline that is water soluble, has been used for many years in the treatment of acute severe asthma. The recommended dose is 6 mg/kg given intravenously over 20–30 min, followed by a maintenance dose of 0.5 mg/kg per hour. If the patient is already taking theophylline, or there are any factors that decrease clearance, these doses should be halved and the plasma level checked more frequently. Nebulized β_2 agonists are now preferred over intravenous aminophylline for acute exacerbations of asthma and COPD.

Oral immediate-release theophylline tablets or elixirs, which are rapidly absorbed, give wide fluctuations in plasma levels and are not recommended. Several sustained-release preparations are now available that are absorbed at a constant rate and provide steady plasma concentrations over a 12- to 24-h period. Both slow-release aminophylline and theophylline are available and are equally effective (although the ethylene diamine component of aminophylline has been implicated in allergic reactions). For continuous treatment, twice-daily therapy (~8 mg/kg twice daily) is needed. For nocturnal asthma, a single dose of slow-release theophylline at night is often effective. Once optimal doses have been determined, routine monitoring of plasma concentrations is usually not necessary unless a change in clearance is suspected or evidence of toxicity emerges.

TABLE 40–2 ■ FACTORS AFFECTING CLEARANCE OF THEOPHYLLINE

Increased clearance

- Enzyme induction (mainly CYP1A2) by coadministered drugs (e.g., rifampicin, barbiturates, ethanol)
- Smoking (tobacco, marijuana) via CYP1A2 induction
- High-protein, low-carbohydrate diet
- Barbecued meat
- Childhood

Decreased clearance

- CYP inhibition (cimetidine, erythromycin, ciprofloxacin, allopurinol, fluvoxamine, zileuton, zafirlukast)
- Congestive heart failure
- Liver disease
- Pneumonia
- Viral infection and vaccination
- High-carbohydrate diet
- Old age

Clinical Use

In patients with acute asthma, intravenous aminophylline is less effective than nebulized β_2 agonists and should therefore be reserved for those patients who fail to respond to, or are intolerant of, β agonists. Theophylline should not be added routinely to nebulized β_2 agonists because it does not increase the bronchodilator response and may increase their side effects. Theophylline has been used as a controller in the management of mild persistent asthma, although it is usually found to be less effective than low doses of ICSs. Addition of low-dose theophylline to an ICS in patients who are not adequately controlled provides better symptom control and lung function than doubling the dose of inhaled steroid (Lim et al., 2001). LABAs are more effective as an add-on therapy, but theophylline is considerably less expensive and may be the only affordable add-on treatment when the costs of medication are limiting.

Theophylline is still used as a bronchodilator in COPD, but inhaled anticholinergics and β_2 agonists are preferred. Theophylline tends to be added to these inhaled bronchodilators in patients with more severe disease and has been shown to give additional clinical improvement when added to a LABA.

Side Effects

Unwanted effects of theophylline are usually related to plasma concentration and tend to occur at C_p greater than 15 mg/L. The most common side effects are headache, nausea, and vomiting (due to inhibition of PDE4), abdominal discomfort, and restlessness (Table 40–3). There may also be increased acid secretion (due to PDE inhibition) and diuresis (due to inhibition of adenosine A_1 receptors). Theophylline may lead to behavioral disturbance and learning difficulties in schoolchildren. At high concentrations, cardiac arrhythmias may occur as a consequence of inhibition of cardiac PDE3 and antagonism of cardiac A_1 receptors. At very high concentrations, seizures may occur due to central A_1 receptor antagonism. Use of low doses of theophylline, targeting plasma concentrations of 5–10 mg/L, largely avoids side effects and drug interactions.

Summary and Future Developments

Theophylline use has been declining, partly because of the problems with side effects, but mainly because more effective therapy with β_2 agonists and ICSs have been introduced. Oral theophylline remains a useful

TABLE 40–3 ■ SIDE EFFECTS OF THEOPHYLLINE AND MECHANISMS

SIDE EFFECT	PROPOSED MECHANISM
Nausea and vomiting	PDE4 inhibition
Headaches	PDE4 inhibition
Gastric discomfort	PDE4 inhibition
Diuresis	A_1 receptor antagonism
Behavioral disturbance (?)	?
Cardiac arrhythmias	PDE3 inhibition, A_1 receptor antagonism
Epileptic seizures	A_1 receptor antagonism

A, adenosine.

HISTORY

Datura stramonium (jimson weed) and related species of the nightshade family contain a mixture of muscarinic antagonists (atropine, hyoscyamine, scopolamine) and were smoked for relief of asthma two centuries ago. Subsequently, the purified plant alkaloid atropine was introduced for treating asthma. Due to the significant side effects of atropine, particularly drying of secretions, less-soluble quaternary compounds, such as atropine methylnitrate and ipratropium bromide, have been developed. These compounds are topically active and are not significantly absorbed from the respiratory or GI tracts.

add-on treatment in some patients with difficult asthma and appears to have effects beyond those provided by steroids. Rapid-release theophylline preparations are the only affordable antiasthma medication in some developing countries. There is increasing evidence that theophylline has some antiasthma effect at doses that are lower than those needed for bronchodilation, and plasma levels of 5–15 mg/L are recommended.

Muscarinic Cholinergic Antagonists

The basic pharmacology of the antimuscarinic agents is presented in Chapter 9.

Mode of Action

As competitive antagonists of endogenous ACh at muscarinic receptors, these agents inhibit the direct constrictor effect on bronchial smooth muscle mediated via the M_3-G_q-PLC-IP_3-Ca^{2+} pathway (see Chapters 3 and 9). The efficacy stems from the role played by the parasympathetic nervous system in regulating bronchomotor tone. The effects of ACh on the respiratory system include bronchoconstriction and tracheobronchial mucus secretion. Thus, antimuscarinic drugs antagonize these effects of ACh, resulting in bronchodilation and reduced mucus secretion.

Acetylcholine may also be released from other airway cells, including epithelial cells (Wessler and Kirkpatrick, 2008). The synthesis of ACh in epithelial cells is increased by inflammatory stimuli (such as TNF-α), which increase the expression of choline acetyltransferase, which could contribute to cholinergic effects in airway diseases. Muscarinic receptors are expressed in airway smooth muscle of small airways that do not appear to be significantly innervated by cholinergic nerves; these receptors may be a mechanism of cholinergic narrowing in peripheral airways that could be relevant in COPD, responding to locally synthesized, nonneuronal ACh.

Myriad mechanical, chemical, and immunological stimuli elicit reflex bronchoconstriction via vagal pathways, and cholinergic pathways may play an important role in regulating acute bronchomotor responses in animals. Anticholinergic drugs will only inhibit reflex ACh-mediated bronchoconstriction and have no blocking effect on the *direct* effects of inflammatory mediators, such as histamine and LTs, on bronchial smooth muscle. Furthermore, cholinergic antagonists probably have little or no effect on mast cells, microvascular leak, or the chronic inflammatory response.

Clinical Use

In asthmatic patients, anticholinergic drugs are less effective as bronchodilators than β_2 agonists and offer less-efficient protection against bronchial challenges. Anticholinergics are currently used as an additional bronchodilator in asthmatic patients not controlled on a LABA. Nebulized anticholinergic drugs are effective in acute severe asthma but less effective than β_2 agonists. In the acute and chronic treatment of asthma, anticholinergic drugs may have an additive effect with β_2 agonists and should therefore be considered when control of asthma is not adequate with nebulized β_2 agonists. A muscarinic antagonist should be considered when there are problems with theophylline or when inhaled β_2 agonists cause a troublesome tremor in elderly patients.

In COPD, anticholinergic drugs may be as effective as or even superior to β_2 agonists. Their relatively greater effect in COPD than in asthma may be explained by an inhibitory effect on vagal tone, which, although not necessarily increased in COPD, may be the only reversible element of airway obstruction and one that is exaggerated by geometric factors in the narrowed airways of patients with COPD (Figure 40–6). Anticholinergic drugs reduce air trapping and improve exercise tolerance in patients with COPD.

Therapeutic Choices

The *SAMA* ipratropium bromide is available as a pMDI and nebulized preparation. The onset of bronchodilation is relatively slow and is usually maximal 30–60 min after inhalation but may persist for 6–8 h. It is usually given by MDI three or four times daily on a regular basis, rather than intermittently for symptom relief, in view of its slow onset of action, but has now been replaced by *LAMAs*, such as tiotropium bromide.

Long-Acting Muscarinic Antagonists

Several LAMAs have now been developed from the treatment of COPD and, more recently, severe asthma. *Tiotropium bromide* is a long-acting anticholinergic drug that is suitable for once-daily dosing as a DPI (Spiriva) or via a soft mist mininebulizer device and was more effective than *ipratropium* four times daily in several studies; it also significantly reduces exacerbations (Cheyne et al., 2015). Tiotropium binds to all muscarinic receptor subtypes but dissociates slowly from M_3 and M_1 receptors, giving it a degree of kinetic receptor selectivity for these receptors compared with M_2 receptors, from which it dissociates more rapidly. Thus, compared with ipratropium, tiotropium is less likely to antagonize M_2-mediated inhibition of ACh release (the resulting increase in ACh could counteract the blockade of M_3 receptor–mediated bronchoconstriction) (Chapter 9). Over a 4-year period, tiotropium improved lung function and health status and reduced exacerbations and all-cause mortality, although there was no effect on disease progression (Tashkin et al., 2008).

Glycopyrronium bromide and *umeclidinium bromide* are also once-daily LAMAs with very similar clinical effects to tiotropium, whereas *aclidinium bromide* has to be given twice daily (Cazzola et al., 2013a). LAMAs are now becoming the bronchodilators of choice for patients with COPD. LAMAs are also effective as additional bronchodilators in patient with asthma not adequately controlled with maximal ICS/LABA therapy, although not all patients respond (Kerstjens et al., 2015).

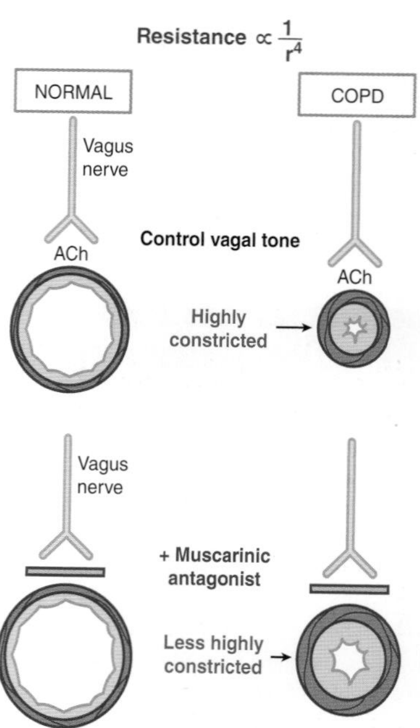

Figure 40–6 *Anticholinergic drugs inhibit vagally mediated airway tone, thereby producing bronchodilation.* This effect is small in normal airways but is greater in airways of patients with COPD, which are structurally narrowed and have higher resistance to airflow because airway resistance is inversely related to the fourth power of the radius r.

Combination Inhalers

There are additive bronchodilator effects between anticholinergics and β_2 agonists in patients with COPD, which has led to the development of fixed-dose combinations. SABA/SAMA combinations, such as *albuterol/ipratropium*, are popular. Several studies have demonstrated additive effects of these two drugs, thus providing an advantage over increasing the dose of β_2 agonist in patients who have side effects.

LABA/LAMA dual combination inhalers have also been developed, including *indacaterol/glycopyrronium, vilanterol/umeclidinium bromide, olodaterol/tiotropium bromide* (all once daily), and *formoterol/glycopyrronium bromide, formoterol/aclidinium bromide* (twice daily), which all sow beneficial effects on lung function compared with either LABA or LAMA alone, although they may not be clearly beneficial in terms of reducing exacerbations (Calzetta et al., 2016).

Adverse Effects

Inhaled anticholinergic drugs are generally well tolerated. On stopping inhaled anticholinergics, a small rebound increase in airway responsiveness has been described. Systemic side effects after SAMA or LAMA are uncommon during normal clinical use because there is little systemic absorption. Because cholinergic agonists can stimulate *mucus secretion*, there has been concern that anticholinergics may reduce secretion and lead to more viscous mucus. However, ipratropium bromide and tiotropium bromide, even in high doses, have no detectable effect on mucociliary clearance in either normal subjects or in patients with airway disease. A significant unwanted effect is the unpleasant *bitter taste* of inhaled ipratropium, which may contribute to poor compliance. Nebulized ipratropium bromide may precipitate *glaucoma* in elderly patients due to a direct effect of the nebulized drug on the eye. This may be prevented by nebulization with a mouthpiece rather than a face mask.

Reports of *paradoxical bronchoconstriction* with ipratropium bromide, particularly when given by nebulizer, were largely explained as effects of the hypotonic nebulizer solution and by antibacterial additives, such as benzalkonium chloride and EDTA. This problem has not been described with tiotropium bromide or other LAMAs. Occasionally, bronchoconstriction may occur with ipratropium bromide given by MDI. It is possible that this is due to blockade of prejunctional M_2 receptors on airway cholinergic nerves that normally inhibit ACh release.

LAMAs cause dryness of the mouth in 10%–15% of patients, but this usually disappears during continued therapy. Urinary retention is occasionally seen in elderly patients.

Future Developments

The LABA/LAMA fixed-combination inhalers are likely to become the bronchodilators of choice in patients with COPD, and LAMAs are added to ICS/LABA combinations in severe asthma. Some triple inhalers that have the ICS/LABA/LAMA combination, such as *budesonide/formoterol/glycopyrronium, mometasone/indacaterol/glycopyrronium*, and *fluticasone furoate/umeclidinium/vilanterol*, are in development for use in patients with severe asthma and asthma-COPD overlap. Dual-action drugs that are both muscarinic antagonists and β_2 agonist are also in clinical development, but it has proved difficult to balance the β agonist and anticholinergic activities (Ray and Alcaraz, 2009).

Novel Classes of Bronchodilator

Currently, the most effective bronchodilators are LABAs for asthma and a LAMA for COPD. Inventing new classes of bronchodilator has been difficult; several agents have had problems with vasodilator side effects because they relax vascular smooth muscle to a greater extent than airway smooth muscle. Nonetheless, there are several classes of bronchodilators under development, as described next.

Magnesium Sulfate

Magnesium sulfate ($MgSO_4$) is useful as an additional bronchodilator in children and adults with acute severe asthma. Intravenous or nebulized $MgSO_4$ benefits adults and children with severe exacerbations ($FEV_1 < 30\%$ of predicted value), giving improvement in lung function when added to nebulized β_2 agonist and a reduction in hospital admissions (Kew et al., 2014). The treatment is cheap and well tolerated, although the clinical benefit appears small. Side effects include flushing and nausea but are usually minor. Magnesium sulfate appears to act as a bronchodilator and may reduce cytosolic Ca^{2+} concentrations in airway smooth muscle cells. The concentration of magnesium is lower in serum and erythrocytes of asthmatic patients than in normal controls and correlates with airway hyperresponsiveness, although the improvement in acute severe asthma after magnesium does not correlate with plasma concentrations. The effects of intravenous $MgSO_4$ in COPD are minimal, and there are too few studies to make any firm recommendation (Shivanthan and Rajapakse, 2014).

Potassium Channel Openers

The K^+ channel openers such as *cromakalim* or *levcromakalim* (the *levo*-isomer of cromakalim) open ATP-dependent K^+ channels in smooth muscle, leading to membrane hyperpolarization and relaxation of airway smooth muscle. This suggests that K^+ channel activators may be useful as bronchodilators (Pelaia et al., 2002). Clinical studies in asthma, however, have been disappointing, with no bronchodilation or protection against bronchoconstrictor challenges. The cardiovascular side effects of these drugs (postural hypotension, flushing) limit the oral dose; furthermore, inhaled formulations are problematic. New developments include K^+ channel openers that open Ca^{2+}-activated large conductance K^+ channels (maxi-K channels) that are also opened by β_2 agonists; these drugs may be better tolerated. Maxi-K channel openers also inhibit mucus secretion and cough, and they may be of particular value in the treatment of COPD. So far, none of these drugs has been studied in patients with airway disease.

Vasoactive Intestinal Polypeptide Analogues

Vasoactive intestinal polypeptide is a peptide that has 28 amino acids; it binds to two GPCRs, $VPAC_1$ and $VPAC_2$, both of which couple primarily to G_s to stimulate the adenylyl cyclase-cAMP-PKA pathway leading to relaxation of smooth muscle. VIP is a potent dilator of human airway smooth muscle in vitro but is not effective in patients because it is rapidly metabolized (plasma $t_{1/2} \sim 2$ min); in addition, VIP causes vasodilator side effects. More stable analogues of VIP, such as Ro 25-1533, which selectively stimulates VIP receptors in airway smooth muscle (via $VPAC_2$), have been synthesized. Inhaled Ro 25-1533 has a rapid bronchodilator effect in asthmatic patients, but it is not as prolonged as formoterol (Linden et al., 2003).

Bitter Taste Receptor Agonists

Bitter taste receptors (TAS2R) are GPCRs that are expressed in airway smooth muscle and mediate bronchodilation in response to agonists, such as *quinine* and *chloroquine*, even after β_2 receptor desensitization (An et al., 2012). However, these agonists are weak, so more potent drugs are needed.

Other Inhibitors of Smooth Muscle Contraction

Agents that inhibit the contractile machinery of airway smooth muscle, including rho kinase inhibitors, inhibitors of myosin light chain kinase, and myosin inhibitors, are also in development. Because these agents also cause vasodilation, it will be necessary to administer them by inhalation.

Corticosteroids

The introduction of *ICSs*, as a way of reducing the requirement and side effects of oral steroids, has revolutionized the treatment of chronic asthma (Barnes et al., 1998b). Because asthma is a chronic inflammatory disease, ICSs are considered first-line therapy in all but patients with the mildest disease. In marked contrast, ICSs are much less effective in COPD and should only be used in patients with severe disease who have frequent exacerbations. Oral corticosteroids remain the mainstay of treatment of several other pulmonary diseases, such as sarcoidosis, interstitial lung diseases, and pulmonary eosinophilic syndromes. The general pharmacology of corticosteroids is presented in Chapter 46.

Mechanism of Action

Corticosteroids enter target cells and bind to GRs in the cytoplasm (Chapter 46). There is only one type of GR that binds corticosteroids and no evidence for the existence of subtypes that might mediate different aspects of corticosteroid action (Barnes, 2011a). The steroid-GR complex moves into the nucleus, where it binds to specific sequences on the upstream regulatory elements of certain target genes, resulting in increased (or, rarely, decreased) transcription of the gene, with subsequent increased (or decreased) synthesis of the gene products.

The GRs may also interact with protein transcription factors and coactivator molecules in the nucleus and thereby influence the synthesis of certain proteins independently of any direct interaction with DNA. The repression of transcription factors, such as AP-1 and NF-κB, is likely to account for many of the anti-inflammatory effects of steroids in asthma. In particular, corticosteroids reverse the activating effect of these pro-inflammatory transcription factors on histone acetylation by recruiting HDAC2 to inflammatory genes that have been activated through acetylation of associated histones (Figure 40–7). GRs are acetylated when corticosteroids are bound and bind to DNA in this acetylated state as dimers, whereas the acetylated GR has to be deacetylated by HDAC2 to interact with inflammatory genes and NF-κB (Ito et al., 2006).

There may be additional mechanisms that are also important in the anti-inflammatory actions of corticosteroids. Corticosteroids have potent inhibitory effects on MAP kinase signaling pathways through the induction of MAP kinase phosphatase 1, which may inhibit the expression of multiple inflammatory genes (Clark, 2003)

Anti-inflammatory Effects in Asthma

Corticosteroids have widespread effects on gene transcription, increasing the transcription of several anti-inflammatory genes and suppressing transcription of many inflammatory genes. Steroids have inhibitory effects on many inflammatory and structural cells that are activated in asthma and prevent the recruitment of inflammatory cells into the airways (Figure 40–8). In patients with mild asthma, the inflammation may be completely resolved after inhaled steroids.

Steroids potently inhibit the formation of multiple inflammatory cytokines, particularly cytokines released from T_H2 cells. Corticosteroids also decrease eosinophil survival by inducing apoptosis. Corticosteroids inhibit the expression of multiple inflammatory genes in airway epithelial cells, probably the most important action of ICSs in suppressing asthmatic inflammation. Corticosteroids also prevent and reverse the increase in vascular permeability due to inflammatory mediators and may therefore lead to resolution of airway edema. Steroids have a direct inhibitory effect on mucus glycoprotein secretion from airway submucosal glands, as well as indirect inhibitory effects by downregulation of inflammatory stimuli that stimulate mucus secretion.

Corticosteroids have no direct effect on contractile responses of airway smooth muscle; improvement in lung function after ICSs is presumably due to an effect on the chronic airway inflammation, edema, and airway hyperresponsiveness. A single dose of an ICS has no effect on the early response to allergen (reflecting the ICSs lack of effect on mast cell mediator release) but inhibits the late response (which may be due to an effect on macrophages, eosinophils, and airway wall edema) and also inhibits the increase in airway hyperresponsiveness.

The ICSs have rapid anti-inflammatory effects, reducing airway hyperresponsiveness and inflammatory mediator concentrations in sputum within a few hours (Erin et al., 2008). However, it may take several weeks or months to achieve maximal effects on airway hyperresponsiveness, presumably reflecting the slow healing of the damaged inflamed airway. It is important to recognize that corticosteroids *suppress* inflammation in the airways but do not cure the underlying disease. When steroids are withdrawn, there is a recurrence of the same degree of airway hyperresponsiveness, although in patients with mild asthma it may take several months to return.

Effect on β_2 Adrenergic Responsiveness

Steroids potentiate the effects of β agonists on bronchial smooth muscle and prevent and reverse β receptor desensitization in airways in vitro *and* in vivo (Barnes, 2002; Black et al., 2009). At a molecular level,

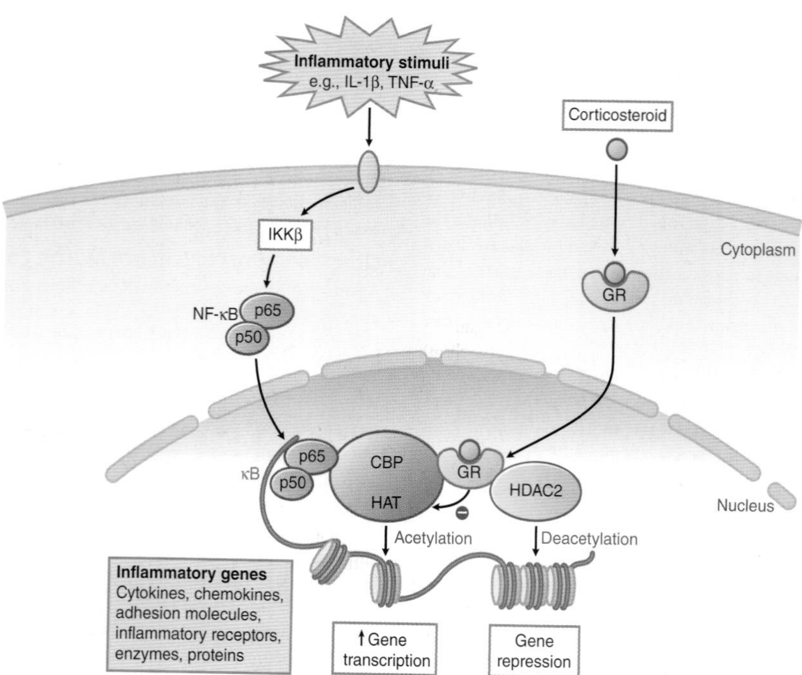

Figure 40–7 *Mechanism of anti-inflammatory action of corticosteroids in asthma.* Inflammatory stimuli (IL-1β, TNF-α, etc.) activate IKKβ, which activates the transcription factor NF-κB. A dimer of p50 and p65 NF-κB proteins translocates to the nucleus and binds to specific κB recognition sites and to coactivators, such as the CREB-binding protein (CBP), which have intrinsic histone acetyltransferase (HAT) activity. This results in acetylation of core histones and consequent increased expression of genes encoding multiple inflammatory proteins. Cytosolic GRs bind corticosteroids; the receptor-ligand complexes translocate to the nucleus and bind to coactivators to inhibit HAT activity in two ways: directly and, more importantly, by recruiting HDAC2, which reverses histone acetylation, leading to the suppression of activated inflammatory genes.

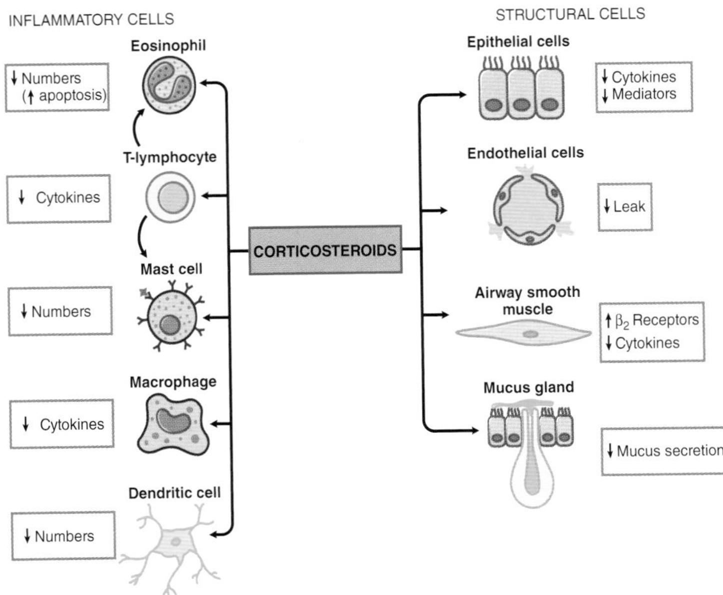

Figure 40–8 *Effect of corticosteroids on inflammatory and structural cells in the airways.*

corticosteroids increase the transcription of the β_2 receptor gene in human lung in vitro and in the respiratory mucosa in vivo and also increase the stability of its messenger RNA. They also prevent or reverse uncoupling of β_2 receptors to G_s. In animal systems, corticosteroids prevent downregulation of β_2 receptors.

β_2 Agonists also enhance the action of GRs, resulting in increased nuclear translocation of liganded GR receptors and enhancing the binding of GRs to DNA. This effect has been demonstrated in sputum macrophages of asthmatic patients after an ICS and inhaled LABA (Barnes, 2011a). This suggests that β_2 agonists and corticosteroids enhance each other's beneficial effects in asthma therapy.

Pharmacokinetics

The pharmacokinetics of oral corticosteroids are described in Chapter 46. The pharmacokinetics of ICSs are important in relation to systemic effects (Barnes et al., 1998b). The fraction of steroid that is inhaled into the lungs acts locally on the airway mucosa but may be absorbed from the airway and alveolar surface. Thus, a portion of an inhaled dose reaches the systemic circulation. Furthermore, the fraction of inhaled steroid that is deposited in the oropharynx is swallowed and absorbed from the gut. The absorbed fraction may be metabolized in the liver (first-pass metabolism) before reaching the systemic circulation (Figure 40–3). The use of a spacer chamber reduces oropharyngeal deposition and therefore reduces systemic absorption of ICSs, although this effect is minimal in corticosteroids with a high first-pass metabolism. Mouth rinsing and discarding the rinse have a similar effect, and this procedure should be used with high-dose dry powder steroid inhalers when spacer chambers cannot be used.

Beclomethasone dipropionate and *ciclesonide* are prodrugs that release the active corticosteroid after the ester group is cleaved by esterases in the lung. Ciclesonide is available as an MDI for asthma and as a nasal spray for allergic rhinitis. *Budesonide* and *fluticasone propionate* have a greater first-pass metabolism than BDP and are therefore less likely to produce systemic effects at high inhaled doses.

Routes of Administration and Dosing

Inhaled Corticosteroids in Asthma

Inhaled corticosteroids are recommended as first-line therapy for patients with persistent asthma. They should be started in any patient who needs to use a β_2 agonist inhaler for symptom control more than twice weekly. They are effective in mild, moderate, and severe asthma and in children as well as adults (Barnes et al., 1998b).

Most of the benefit may be obtained from doses of less than 400 μg BDP or equivalent. However, some patients (with relative corticosteroid resistance) may benefit from higher doses (up to 2000 μg/d). For most patients, ICSs should be used twice daily, a regimen that improves adherence once control of asthma has been achieved (which may require four-time daily dosing initially or a course of oral steroids if symptoms are severe). Administration once daily of some steroids (e.g., budesonide, mometasone, and ciclesonide in mild asthma and fluticasone furoate in all patients) is effective when doses of 400 μg or less are needed. If a dose greater than 800 μg daily via pMDI is used, a spacer device should be employed to reduce the risk of oropharyngeal side effects. ICSs may be used in children in the same way as in adults; at doses of 400 μg/d or less, there is no evidence of significant growth suppression (Pedersen, 2001). The dose of ICS should be the minimal dose that controls asthma; once control is achieved, the dose should be slowly reduced (Hawkins et al., 2003). Nebulized corticosteroids (e.g., budesonide) are useful in the treatment of small children who are not able to use other inhaler devices.

Inhaled Corticosteroids in COPD

Patients with COPD occasionally respond to steroids, and these patients are likely to have concomitant asthma. Corticosteroids do not appear to have any significant anti-inflammatory effect in COPD; there appears to be an active resistance mechanism, which may be explained by impaired activity of HDAC2 as a result of oxidative stress (Barnes, 2013a). ICSs have no effect on the progression of COPD, even when given to patients with presymptomatic disease; in addition, ICSs have no effect on mortality (Yang et al., 2012). ICSs reduce the number of exacerbations in patients with severe COPD ($FEV_1 < 50\%$ predicted) who have frequent exacerbations and are recommended in these patients, although there is debate about whether these effects are due to inappropriate analysis of the data (Ernst et al., 2015). Oral corticosteroids are used to treat acute exacerbations of COPD, but the effect is very small (Niewoehner et al., 1999).

Patients with cystic fibrosis and bronchiectasis, which involve chronic neutrophilic inflammation of the airways, are also resistant to high doses of ICS.

Systemic Steroids

Intravenous steroids are indicated in acute asthma if lung function is less than 30% predicted and in patients who show no significant improvement with nebulized β_2 agonist. *Hydrocortisone* is the steroid of choice because it has the most rapid onset (5–6 h after administration), compared with 8 h with *prednisolone.* It is common to give hydrocortisone 4 mg/kg initially, followed by a maintenance dose of 3 mg/kg every 6 h. *Methylprednisolone* is also available for intravenous use. Intravenous therapy is usually given until a satisfactory response is obtained, and then oral prednisolone may be substituted. *Oral prednisone or prednisolone* (40–60 mg) has a similar effect to intravenous hydrocortisone and is easier to administer. A high dose of *inhaled fluticasone propionate* (2000 μg daily) is as effective as a course of oral prednisolone in controlling acute exacerbations of asthma in a family practice setting and in children in an emergency department setting, although this route of delivery is more expensive (Manjra et al., 2000).

Prednisone and *prednisolone* are the most commonly used oral steroids. Maximal beneficial effect is usually achieved with 30–40 mg prednisone daily, although a few patients may need 60–80 mg daily to achieve control of symptoms. The usual maintenance dose is about 10–15 mg/d. Short courses of oral steroids (30–40 mg prednisolone daily for 1–2 weeks) are indicated for exacerbations of asthma; the dose may be tapered over 1 week after the exacerbation is resolved (the taper is not strictly necessary after a short course of therapy, but patients find it reassuring). Oral steroids are usually given as a single dose in the morning because this coincides with the normal diurnal increase in plasma cortisol and produces less adrenal suppression than if given in divided doses or at night.

Adverse Effects

Corticosteroids inhibit corticotropin and cortisol secretion by a negative-feedback effect on the pituitary gland (see Chapter 46). Hypothalamic-pituitary-adrenal (HPA) axis suppression depends on dose and usually only occurs with doses of prednisone greater than 7.5–10 mg/d. Significant suppression after short courses of corticosteroid therapy is not usually a problem, but prolonged suppression may occur after several months or years. *Steroid doses after prolonged oral therapy must be reduced slowly.* Symptoms of "steroid withdrawal syndrome" include lassitude, musculoskeletal pains, and, occasionally, fever. HPA suppression with inhaled steroids is usually seen only when the daily inhaled dose exceeds 2000 μg BDP or its equivalent daily.

Side effects of long-term oral corticosteroid therapy include fluid retention, increased appetite, weight gain, osteoporosis, capillary fragility, hypertension, peptic ulceration, diabetes, cataracts, and psychosis. Their frequency tends to increase with age. Very occasionally adverse reactions (such as anaphylaxis) to intravenous hydrocortisone have been described, particularly in aspirin-sensitive asthmatic patients.

The incidence of systemic side effects after ICSs is an important consideration, particularly in children (Lipworth, 1999) (Table 40–4). Initial studies suggested that adrenal suppression occurred only with inhaled doses greater than 1500–2000 μg/d. More sensitive measurements of systemic effects include indices of bone metabolism, such as serum osteocalcin and urinary pyridinium cross-links, and in children, knemometry,

TABLE 40–4 ■ SIDE EFFECTS OF INHALED CORTICOSTEROIDS

Local side effects
- Dysphonia
- Oropharyngeal candidiasis
- Cough

Systemic side effects
- Adrenal suppression and insufficiency
- Growth suppression
- Bruising
- Osteoporosis
- Cataracts
- Glaucoma
- Metabolic abnormalities (glucose, insulin, triglycerides)
- Psychiatric disturbances (euphoria, depression)
- Pneumonia

which may be increased with inhaled doses as low as 400 μg/d BDP in some patients. The clinical relevance of these measurements is not yet clear, however. Nevertheless, it is important to reduce the likelihood of systemic effects by using the lowest dose of inhaled steroid needed to control the asthma and by use of a large-volume spacer to reduce oropharyngeal deposition.

Several systemic effects of inhaled steroids have been described and include dermal thinning and skin capillary fragility (relatively common in elderly patients after high-dose inhaled steroids). Other side effects, such as cataract formation and osteoporosis, are reported but often in patients who are also receiving courses of oral steroids. There is some evidence that use of high-dose ICSs is associated with cataract and glaucoma, but it is difficult to dissociate the effects of ICS from the effects of courses of oral steroids that these patients usually require. There has been particular concern about the use of inhaled steroids in children because of growth suppression (Zhang et al., 2014).

The ICSs may have *local side effects* due to the deposition of inhaled steroid in the oropharynx. The most common problem is hoarseness and weakness of the voice (dysphonia) due to atrophy of the vocal cords following laryngeal deposition of steroid; it may occur in up to 40% of patients and is noticed particularly by patients who need to use their voices during their work (lecturers, teachers, and singers). Throat irritation and coughing after inhalation are common with MDIs and appear to be due to additives because these problems are not usually seen if the patient switches to a DPI. There is no evidence for atrophy of the lining of the airway. Oropharyngeal candidiasis occurs in about 5% of patients. There is no evidence for increased lung infections, including tuberculosis, in patients with asthma. Growing evidence suggests that high doses of ICSs increase the risk of pneumonia in patients with COPD (Finney et al., 2014); the risk appears to be higher with fluticasone propionate than budesonide.

Corticosteroid MDIs with HFA propellants produce smaller aerosol particles and may have a more peripheral deposition, making them useful in treating patients with more severe asthma.

Therapeutic Choices

Numerous ICSs are now available, including *BDP, triamcinolone, flunisolide, budesonide, hemihydrate, fluticasone propionate, mometasone furoate, ciclesonide,* and *fluticasone furoate.* All are equally effective as antiasthma drugs, but there are differences in their pharmacokinetics: Budesonide, fluticasone, mometasone, and ciclesonide have a lower oral bioavailability than BDP because they are subject to greater first-pass hepatic metabolism; this results in reduced systemic absorption from the fraction of the inhaled drug that is swallowed (Derendorf et al., 2006) and thus reduced adverse effects. At high doses (>1000 μg), budesonide and fluticasone propionate have fewer systemic effects than BDP and triamcinolone (not marketed in the U.S.), and they are preferred in patients who need high doses of ICSs and in children. Ciclesonide is another choice; it is a prodrug that is converted to the active metabolite by esterases in the lung, giving it low oral bioavailability and a high therapeutic index (Derendorf, 2007). Fluticasone furoate has the longest duration of action and is suitable for once-daily dosing (Woodcock et al., 2011).

When doses of inhaled steroid exceed 800 μg BDP or equivalent daily, a large-volume spacer is recommended to reduce oropharyngeal deposition and systemic absorption in the case of BDP. All currently available ICSs are absorbed from the lung into the systemic circulation, so that some systemic absorption is inevitable. However, the amount of drug absorbed does not appear to have clinical effects in doses of less than 800 μg BDP equivalent. Although there are potency differences among corticosteroids, there are relatively few comparative studies, partly because dose comparison of corticosteroids is difficult due to their long time course of action and the relative flatness of their dose-response curves.

Future Developments

Early treatment with ICSs in both adults and children may give a greater improvement in lung function than if treatment is delayed (Busse et al., 2008), likely reflecting the fact that corticosteroids are able to modify the underlying inflammatory process and prevent structural changes (fibrosis, smooth muscle hyperplasia, etc.). ICSs are currently recommended for patients with persistent asthmatic symptoms (e.g., need for an inhaled β_2 agonist more than twice a week).

Developing new corticosteroids with fewer systemic effects is desirable. It has been possible to develop corticosteroids that dissociate the DNA-binding effect of corticosteroids (which mediates most of the adverse effects) from the inhibitory effect on transcription factors such as NF-κB (which mediates much of the anti-inflammatory effect). Such "dissociated steroids" or selective GR agonists should, theoretically, retain anti-inflammatory activity but have a reduced risk of adverse effects; achieving this separation of desired and adverse effects is difficult in vivo (Belvisi et al., 2001). Nonsteroidal selective GR agonists are now in development.

Corticosteroid resistance is a major barrier to effective therapy in patients with severe asthma, in asthmatic patients who smoke, and in patients with COPD and cystic fibrosis (Barnes, 2013a; Barnes and Adcock, 2009). "Steroid-resistant" asthma is thought to be due to reduced anti-inflammatory actions of corticosteroids. In those with COPD and some patients with severe asthma, there is a reduction in HDAC2 expression that reduces corticosteroid responsiveness; this is potentially reversible by existing treatments, such as low-dose theophylline and nortriptyline.

Cromones

Cromolyn sodium (*sodium cromoglycate*) is a derivative of *khellin*, an Egyptian herbal remedy, and was found to protect against allergen challenge without any bronchodilator effect. A structurally related drug, *nedocromil sodium*, which has a similar pharmacological profile to cromolyn, was subsequently developed. Although cromolyn was popular in the past because of its good safety profile, its use has sharply declined with the more widespread use of the more effective ICSs, particularly in children.

Phosphodiesterase Inhibitors

The PDE inhibitors relax smooth muscle and inhibit inflammatory cells through an increase in cellular cAMP. PDE4 is the predominant PDE isoform in inflammatory cells, including mast cells, eosinophils, neutrophils, T lymphocytes, macrophages, and structural cells such as sensory nerves and epithelial cells (Hatzelmann et al., 2010), suggesting that PDE4 inhibitors could be useful as an anti-inflammatory treatment in both asthma and COPD.

In animal models of asthma, PDE4 inhibitors reduce eosinophil infiltration and responses to allergen, whereas in COPD they are effective against smoke-induced inflammation and emphysema. In COPD, an oral PDE4 inhibitor, *roflumilast*, has been approved for patients with COPD with severe disease ($FEV_1 < 50\%$ predicted, frequent exacerbations, and chronic bronchitis). Given once daily by mouth, it reduces exacerbations but has little effect on symptoms and lung function (Calverley et al., 2009), although it is effective on top of long-acting bronchodilators and ICSs (Martinez et al., 2015). The relatively weak efficacy is due to dose limitations as a result of side effects, particularly diarrhea, headaches, and nausea.

Of the four subfamilies of PDE4, PDE4D is the major form whose inhibition is associated with vomiting; inhibition of PDE4B is important for anti-inflammatory effects. Thus, selective PDE4B inhibitors may have a greater therapeutic index. Inhaled PDE4 inhibitors, to reduce systemic absorption and adverse responses, have proved to be ineffective. A dual PDE3/4 inhibitor gives bronchodilation in patients with COPD when given by nebulization, but it is uncertain whether there are significant anti-inflammatory effects (Franciosi et al., 2013).

Mediator Antagonists

Both H_1 antihistamines and anti-LTs have been applied to airway disease, but their added benefit over β_2 agonists and corticosteroids is slight (Barnes, 2004; Barnes et al., 1998a).

Antihistamines

Histamine mimics many of the features of asthma and is released from mast cells in acute asthmatic responses, suggesting that antihistamines may be useful in asthma therapy. There is little evidence that histamine H_1 receptor antagonists provide any useful clinical benefit, as demonstrated by a meta-analysis (van Ganse et al., 1997). Newer antihistamines, including *cetirizine* and *azelastine*, have some beneficial effects, but this may be unrelated to H_1 receptor antagonism. Antihistamines are not recommended in the routine management of asthma.

Antileukotrienes

There is considerable evidence that cys-LTs are produced in asthma and that they have potent effects on airway function, inducing bronchoconstriction, airway hyperresponsiveness, plasma exudation, mucus secretion, and eosinophilic inflammation (Figure 40–9; also see Chapter 37). These findings led to the development of 5′-lipoxygenase (5-LO) enzyme inhibitors (of which *zileuton* is the only drug marketed) and several antagonists of the cys-LT_1 receptor, including *montelukast* (s, *zafirlukast*, and *pranlukast* (not available in the U.S.).

Clinical Studies

In patients with mild-to-moderate asthma, anti-LTs cause a significant improvement in lung function and asthma symptoms, with a reduction in the use of rescue inhaled β_2 agonists. Several studies showed evidence for a bronchodilator effect, with an improvement in baseline lung function, suggesting that LTs are contributing to the baseline bronchoconstriction in asthma, although this varies among patients. However, anti-LTs are considerably less effective than ICSs in the treatment of mild asthma and cannot be considered the treatment of first choice (Chauhan and Ducharme, 2012). Anti-LTs are indicated as an add-on therapy in patients who are not well controlled on ICSs. The added benefit is small, equivalent to doubling the dose of ICS, and less effective than adding a LABA. Anti-LTs have a beneficial effect in allergic rhinitis and have a similar efficacy to antihistamines (Grayson and Korenblat, 2007).

In patients with severe asthma who are not controlled on high doses of ICS and LABA, anti-LTs do not appear to provide any additional benefit (Robinson et al., 2001). Theoretically, anti-LTs should be of particular

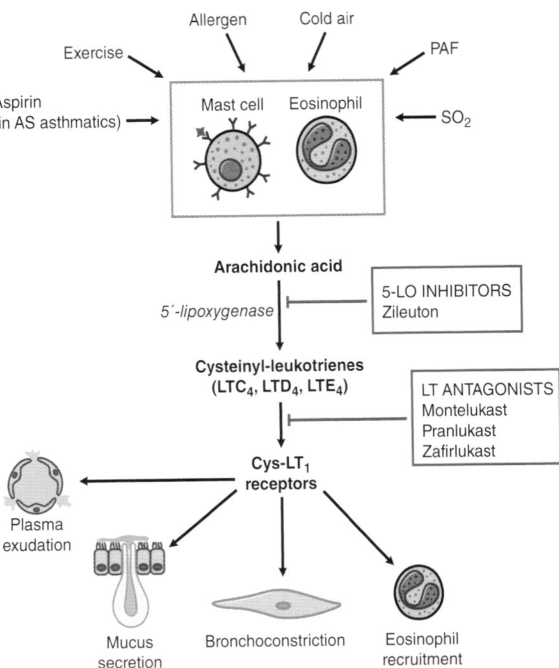

Figure 40–9 *Effects of cysteinyl-LTs on the airways and their inhibition by anti-LTs.* AS, aspirin sensitive.

value in patients with aspirin-sensitive asthma because they block the airway response to aspirin challenge; however, their benefit is no greater here than in other types of asthma.

Anti-LTs are effective in preventing exercise-induced asthma, with efficacy similar to that of LABAs (Coreno et al., 2000). Anti-LTs appear to act mainly as antibronchoconstrictor drugs, and they are clearly less broadly effective than β_2 agonists because they antagonize only one of several bronchoconstrictor mediators.

The cys-LT_1 receptor antagonists have no role in the therapy of COPD. By contrast, LTB_4, a potent neutrophil chemoattractant, is elevated in COPD, indicating that 5-LO inhibitors that inhibit LTB_4 synthesis may have some potential benefit by reducing neutrophil inflammation. However, a pilot study failed to indicate any clear benefit of a 5-LO inhibitor in patients with COPD (Bernstein et al., 2011).

Adverse Effects

Zileuton, zafirlukast, and montelukast are all associated with rare cases of hepatic dysfunction; thus, liver-associated enzymes should be monitored. Several cases of Churg-Strauss syndrome have been associated with the use of zafirlukast and montelukast. Churg-Strauss syndrome is a rare vasculitis that may affect the heart, peripheral nerves, and kidney and is associated with increased circulating eosinophils and asthma. Cases of Churg-Strauss syndrome have been described in patients on anti-LTs who were not on concomitant corticosteroid therapy, suggesting there is a causal link (Nathani et al., 2008).

Future Developments

One of the major advantages of anti-LTs is their effectiveness in tablet form. This may increase compliance with chronic therapy and makes treatment of children easier. Montelukast is effective as a once-daily preparation (10 mg in adults, 5 mg in children). In addition, oral administration may treat concomitant allergic rhinitis. However, the clinical studies indicated a modest effect on lung function and symptom control. This is not surprising. There are many mediators besides cys-LTs involved in the pathophysiology of asthma, and anti-LTs are unlikely to be as effective as a β_2 agonist, which will counteract bronchoconstriction regardless of the spasmogen. It is likely that anti-LTs will be used less in the future because combination inhalers are the mainstay of asthma therapy.

Some patients appear to show better responses than others, suggesting that LTs may play a more important role in some patients. The variability in response to anti-LTs may reflect differences in production of or responses to LTs in different patients, and this in turn may be related to polymorphisms of 5-LO, LTC_4 synthase, or cys-LT_1 receptors that are involved in the synthesis of LTs (Tantisira and Drazen, 2009).

Immunomodulatory Therapies

Immunosuppressive Therapy

Immunosuppressive therapy (e.g., *methotrexate, cyclosporine A, gold, intravenous immunoglobulin*) has been considered in asthma when other treatments have been unsuccessful or to reduce the dose of oral steroids required. However, immunosuppressive treatments are less effective and have a greater propensity for side effects than oral corticosteroids and therefore cannot be routinely recommended.

Anti-IgE Receptor Therapy

Increased specific IgE is a fundamental feature of allergic asthma. *Omalizumab* is a humanized monoclonal antibody that blocks the binding of IgE to high-affinity IgE receptors (FcεR1) on mast cells and thus prevents their activation by allergens (Figure 40–10). It also blocks binding on IgE to low-affinity IgE receptors (FcεRII, CD23) on other inflammatory cells, including T and B lymphocytes, macrophages, and possibly eosinophils, to inhibit chronic inflammation. *Omalizumab* also reduces levels of circulating IgE.

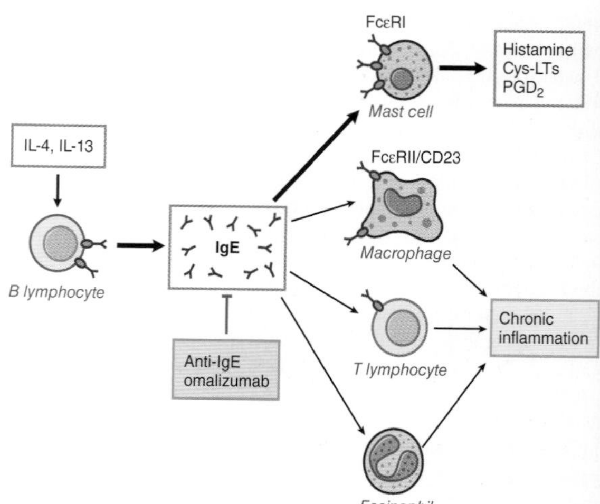

Figure 40–10 *Immunoglobulin E plays a central role in allergic diseases.* Blocking IgE using an antibody, such as omalizumab, is a rational therapeutic approach. IgE may activate high-affinity receptors (FcεRI) on mast cells as well as low-affinity receptors (FcεRII, CD23) on other inflammatory cells. Omalizumab prevents these interactions and the resulting inflammation..

Clinical Use

Omalizumab is used for the treatment of patients with severe asthma (Humbert et al., 2014). The antibody is administered by subcutaneous injection every 2–4 weeks, and the dose is determined by the titer of circulating total IgE. Omalizumab reduces the requirement for oral and ICSs and markedly reduces asthma exacerbations. Not all patients respond, and there are no clear clinical predictors of clinical response, necessitating a trial of therapy (usually over 4 months). Because of its high cost, this treatment is generally used only in patients with very severe asthma who are poorly controlled even on oral corticosteroids and in patients with very severe concomitant allergic rhinitis (Normansell et al., 2014). It may also be of value in protecting against anaphylaxis during specific immunotherapy. A recent study suggested that omalizumab may be effective in preventing asthma exacerbations if administered prior to the exacerbation season (Teach et al., 2015); this is linked to increased expression of type I interferons, which boost antiviral immunity. The major side effect of omalizumab is an anaphylactic response, which is uncommon (<0.1%).

Specific Immunotherapy

Although specific immunotherapy is effective in allergic rhinitis due to single allergens, there is little evidence that desensitizing injections to common allergens are effective in controlling chronic asthma (Rolland et al., 2009). Specific immunotherapy induces the secretion of the anti-inflammatory cytokine IL-10 from regulatory helper T lymphocytes, and this blocks costimulatory signal transduction in T cells (via CD28) so that they are unable to react to allergens presented by antigen-presenting cells (Ozdemir et al., 2016). Applying an understanding of the cellular processes involved might lead to safer and more effective approaches in the future. More specific immunotherapies may be developed with cloned allergen epitopes, T-cell peptide fragments of allergens, CpG oligonucleotides, and vaccines of conjugates of allergen and toll-like receptor 9 to stimulate T_H1 immunity and suppress T_H2 immunity (Broide, 2009).

New Drugs in Development for Airway Disease

Several new classes of drug are in development for asthma and COPD, but clinical development has been slow, and many treatments have either proved to be ineffective or are limited by toxicology and side-effect profiles (Barnes, 2012, 2013b)

Novel Mediator Antagonists

Blocking the receptors or synthesis of inflammatory mediators is a logical approach to the development of new treatments for asthma and COPD. However, in both diseases many different mediators are involved, and therefore blocking a single mediator is unlikely to be effective unless it plays a unique and key role in the disease process. Several specific mediator antagonists have been found to be ineffective in asthma, including antagonists/inhibitors of thromboxane, platelet-activating factor, bradykinin, and tachykinins. However, these blockers have often not been tested in COPD, in which different mediators are involved. A number of other approaches are under study, as noted next.

CRTh2 Antagonists

The chemotactic factor for T_H2 cells has been identified as prostaglandin D_2, which acts on a DP_2 receptor (Chapter 37). Several DP2/CRTh2 antagonists are now in development for asthma, with some promising initial results in patients with eosinophilic inflammation (Townley and Agrawal, 2012).

Antioxidants

Oxidative stress is important in severe asthma and COPD and may contribute to corticosteroid resistance. Existing antioxidants include vitamins C and E and *N*-acetyl-cysteine. These drugs have weak effects, but more potent antioxidants are in development, including activators of the transcription factor Nrf2 (Kirkham and Barnes, 2013).

Cytokine Modifiers

Cytokines play a critical role in perpetuating and amplifying the inflammation in asthma and COPD, suggesting that anticytokines may be beneficial as therapies (Barnes, 2008a). Although most attention has focused on inhibition of cytokines, some cytokines are anti-inflammatory and may have therapeutic potential. Several cytokine or cytokine receptor–blocking antibodies are in clinical development for asthma (Chung, 2015), but there has been less progress in COPD.

Interleukin 5 plays a pivotal role in eosinophilic inflammation and is also involved in eosinophil survival and priming. Anti–IL-5 and anti–IL-5 receptor (IL-5Rα) antibodies inhibit eosinophilic inflammation and airway hyperresponsiveness in patients with mild asthma but has no effect on allergen challenge (Leckie et al., 2000) or clinical benefits in unselected asthmatic patients (Flood-Page et al., 2007). In carefully selected patients with severe asthma and persistent eosinophilia despite high doses of corticosteroids, there is a significant reduction in exacerbations and sparing or oral steroids with an anti–IL-5 antibody, *mepolizumab* (Castro et al., 2014; Pavord et al., 2012). *Mepolizumab* has now been FDA approved for use in highly selected patients with severe asthma.

Blocking IL-4, which determines IgE synthesis and eosinophilic inflammation, has been ineffective in clinical studies. However, blocking IL-13 or its shared receptor with IL-4 (IL-4Rα) provides some clinic benefit and reduces exacerbations but is not yet approved (Hanania et al., 2015; Wenzel et al., 2013).

Production of TNF-α is increased in asthma and COPD and may play a key role in amplifying airway inflammation, through the activation of NF-κB, AP-1, and other transcription factors. However, in patients with COPD and in patients with severe asthma, anti–TNF-α blocking antibodies have been ineffective, at the expense of increasing infections and malignancies (Rennard et al., 2007; Wenzel et al., 2009).

Chemokine Receptor Antagonists

Many chemokines are involved in asthma and COPD and play a key role in recruitment of inflammatory cells, such as eosinophils, neutrophils, macrophages, and lymphocytes, into the lungs. Chemokine receptors are attractive targets because they are GPCRs; small-molecule inhibitors are now in development (Donnelly and Barnes, 2006). In asthma, *CCR3 antagonists*, which should block eosinophil recruitment into the airways, are the most favored target, but several small-molecule CCR3 antagonists have failed in development because of toxicity. In COPD, CXCR2 antagonists, which prevent neutrophil and monocyte chemotaxis due to CXC chemokines, such as CXCL1 and CXCL8, have been effective in animal models of COPD and in neutrophilic inflammation in normal subjects, but in clinical trials in patients with COPD, an oral CXCR2 antagonist provided little clinical benefit (Rennard et al., 2015).

Protease Inhibitors

Several proteolytic enzymes are involved in the chronic inflammation of airway diseases. Mast cell tryptase has several effects on airways, including increasing responsiveness of airway smooth muscle to constrictors, increasing plasma exudation, potentiating eosinophil recruitment, and stimulating fibroblast proliferation. Some of these effects are mediated by activation of protease-activated receptor, PAR2. Tryptase inhibitors have so far proved to be disappointing in clinical studies.

Proteases are involved in the degradation of connective tissue in COPD, particularly enzymes that break down elastin fibers, such as neutrophil elastase and MMPs, which are involved in emphysema. Neutrophil elastase inhibitors have been difficult to develop, and there are no positive clinical studies in patients with COPD. MMP9 appears to be the predominant elastolytic enzyme in emphysema, and several selective inhibitors are now in development.

New Anti-inflammatory Drugs

NF-κB Inhibitors

An important role is played by NF-κB in the orchestration of chronic inflammation (Figure 40–7); many of the inflammatory genes that are expressed in asthma and COPD are regulated by this transcription factor. This has prompted a search for specific blockers of these transcription factors. NF-κB is naturally inhibited by IκB, which is degraded after activation by specific kinases. Small-molecule inhibitors of the IκB kinase IKK2 (or IKKβ) are in clinical development (Ziegelbauer et al., 2005). These drugs may be of particular value in COPD, for which corticosteroids are largely ineffective. However, there are concerns that inhibition of NF-κB may cause side effects such as increased susceptibility to infections, which has been observed in gene disruption studies when components of NF-κB are inhibited.

Mitogen-Activated Protein Kinase Inhibitors

The MAP kinase pathways are involved in chronic inflammation. There has been particular interest in the p38 MAP kinase pathway that is blocked by a novel class of drugs, such as *losmapimod* (Norman, 2015). These drugs inhibit the synthesis of many inflammatory cytokines, chemokines, and inflammatory enzymes. The p38 MAP kinase inhibitors are in development for the treatment of asthma (they inhibit T_H2 cytokine synthesis) and for COPD (they inhibit neutrophilic inflammation and signaling of inflammatory cytokines and chemokines). However, clinical studies have given disappointing results in patients with COPD, and the dose is limited by side effects (MacNee et al., 2013). Several inhaled p38 inhibitors are in development to reduce the risk of side effects (Millan, 2011).

Mucoregulators

Mucus hypersecretion occurs in chronic bronchitis, COPD, cystic fibrosis, and asthma (Fahy and Dickey, 2010). In chronic bronchitis, mucus hypersecretion is related to chronic irritation by cigarette smoke and may involve neural mechanisms and the activation of neutrophils to release enzymes such as neutrophil elastase and proteinase 3 that have powerful stimulatory effects on mucus secretion. Mast cell–derived chymase is also a potent mucus secretagogue. This suggests that several classes of drugs may be developed to control mucus hypersecretion. Mucus secretion is regulated by epidermal growth factor receptors, which lead to increased mucin gene *MUC5AC* expression, but a nebulized epidermal growth factor receptor inhibitor has been ineffective in COPD (Woodruff et al., 2010).

Systemic anticholinergic drugs appear to reduce mucociliary clearance, but this is not observed with either ipratropium bromide or tiotropium bromide, presumably reflecting their poor absorption from the respiratory tract. β_2 Agonists increase mucus production and mucociliary clearance and have been shown to increase ciliary beat frequency in vitro. Because inflammation leads to mucus hypersecretion, anti-inflammatory treatments should reduce mucus hypersecretion; ICSs are very effective in reducing increased mucus production in asthma.

Mucolytics

Several agents can reduce the viscosity of sputum in vitro. One group consists of derivatives of cysteine that reduce the disulfide bridges that bind glycoproteins to other proteins, such as albumin and secretory IgA. These drugs also act as antioxidants and may therefore reduce airway inflammation. Only *N-acetylcysteine* is available in the U.S.; *carbocysteine, methylcysteine, erdosteine*, and *bromhexine* are available elsewhere. Orally administered, these agents are relatively well tolerated, but clinical studies in chronic bronchitis, asthma, and bronchiectasis have been disappointing. A large controlled study of oral *N*-acetylcysteine in patients with COPD showed no effect in disease progression or in preventing exacerbations, although there was some benefit in the patients not treated with ICSs (Decramer et al., 2005), as confirmed in a subsequent studies of carbocysteine and *N*-acetylcysteine in patients with COPD not treated with other medications (Zheng et al., 2008, 2014). *N*-Acetylcysteine is not currently recommended for COPD management.

DNAse (dornase alfa) reduces mucus viscosity in sputum of patients with cystic fibrosis and is indicated if there is significant symptomatic and lung function improvement after a trial of therapy (Henke and Ratjen, 2007). There is no evidence that dornase alfa is effective in COPD or asthma, however.

Expectorants

Expectorants are oral drugs that are supposed to enhance the clearance of mucus. Although expectorants were once commonly prescribed, there is little or no objective evidence for their efficacy. Such drugs are often emetics that are given in subemetic doses on the basis that gastric irritation may stimulate an increase in mucus clearance via a reflex mechanism. Lacking evidence for their efficacy, the FDA has removed most expectorants from the market in a review of over-the-counter drugs. With the exception of *guaifenesin*, no agents are approved as expectorants in the U.S. In patients who find it difficult to clear mucus, adequate hydration and inhalation of steam may be of some benefit.

Antitussives

Despite the fact that cough is a common symptom of airway disease, its mechanisms are poorly understood, and current treatment is unsatisfactory (Pavord and Chung, 2008). Viral infections of the upper respiratory tract are the most common cause of cough; postviral cough is usually self-limiting and commonly patient medicated. Their wide use notwithstanding, over-the-counter cough medications are largely ineffective (Dicpinigaitis et al., 2014). Because cough is a defensive reflex, its suppression may be inappropriate in bacterial lung infection. Before treatment with antitussives, it is important to identify underlying causal mechanisms that may require therapy.

Whenever possible, treat the underlying cause, not the cough. Asthma commonly presents as cough, and the cough will usually respond to ICSs. A syndrome characterized by cough in association with sputum eosinophilia but no airway hyperresponsiveness, termed *eosinophilic bronchitis*, also responds to ICSs (Birring et al., 2003). Nonasthmatic cough does not respond to ICSs but sometimes responds to anticholinergic therapy. The cough associated with postnasal drip of sinusitis responds to antibiotics (if warranted), nasal decongestants, and intranasal steroids. The cough associated with ACE inhibitors (in ~ 15% of patients treated) responds to lowering the dose or withdrawal of the drug and substitution of an AT_1 receptor antagonist (see Chapter 26). Gastroesophageal reflux is a common cause of cough through a reflex mechanism and occasionally as a result of acid aspiration into the lungs. This cough may respond to suppression of gastric acid with an H_2 receptor antagonist or a proton pump inhibitor (see Chapter 49). Some patients have a chronic cough with no obvious cause, and this chronic idiopathic cough or cough hypersensitivity syndrome may be due to airway sensory neural hyperesthesia (Haque et al., 2005). There are several treatments that have been assessed in the treatment of refractory cough (Gibson et al., 2016).

Opiates

Opiates have a central mechanism of action on MORs in the medullary cough center, but there is some evidence that they may have additional peripheral action on cough receptors in the proximal airways. *Codeine* and *pholcodine* (not available in the U.S.) are commonly used, but there is little evidence that they are clinically effective, particularly on postviral cough; in addition, they are associated with sedation and constipation. *Morphine* and *methadone* are effective but indicated only for intractable cough associated with bronchial carcinoma.

Dextromethorphan

Dextromethorphan is a centrally active NMDA receptor antagonist. It may also antagonize opioid receptors. Despite the fact that it is in numerous over-the-counter cough suppressants and used commonly to treat cough, it is poorly effective. In children with acute nocturnal cough, it is not significantly different from placebo in reducing cough (Dicpinigaitis et al., 2014). It can cause hallucinations at higher doses and has significant abuse potential.

Local Anesthetics

Benzonatate, a local anesthetic, acts peripherally by anesthetizing the stretch receptors located in the respiratory passages, lungs, and pleura. By dampening the activity of these receptors, benzonatate may reduce the cough reflex. The recommended dose is 100 mg, three times per day, and up to 600 mg/d, if needed. Although clinical studies shortly after its approval showed some efficacy, benzonatate (200 mg) was not effective in suppressing experimentally induced cough (Dicpinigaitis et al., 2009). Side effects include dizziness and dysphagia. Seizures and cardiac arrest have occurred following an acute ingestion. Severe allergic reactions have been reported in patients allergic to *para-aminobenzoic acid*, a metabolite of benzonatate.

Neuromodulators

Gabapentin and *pregabalin* are GABA analogues that inhibit neurotransmission and have been used in neuropathic pain syndromes. They have been shown to benefit chronic idiopathic cough, which also involved neural hypersensitivity (Gibson and Vertigan, 2015). Side effects of somnolence and dizziness are common at higher doses, so it is usual to initiate therapy at lower doses.

Other Drugs

Several other drugs reportedly have small benefits in protecting against cough challenges or in reducing cough in pulmonary diseases. These drugs include *moguisteine* (not available in the U.S.), which acts peripherally and appears to open ATP-sensitive K^+ channels. *Theobromine*, a naturally occurring methylxanthine, reduces cough induced by tussive agents. Although the expectorant *guaifenesin* is not typically known as a cough suppressant, it is significantly better than placebo in reducing acute viral cough and inhibits cough-reflex sensitivity in patients with upper respiratory tract infections (Dicpinigaitis et al., 2009).

Novel Antitussives

There is clearly a need to develop new, more effective therapies for cough, particularly drugs that act peripherally to avoid sedation. There are close analogies between chronic cough and sensory hyperesthesia, so new therapies with novel antitussives are likely to arise from pain research.

Transient Receptor Potential Antagonists

Several types of TRP ion channels have been described on airway sensory nerves and may be activated by various mediators and physical factors, resulting in cough. TRPV1 (previously called the *vanilloid receptor*) is activated by capsaicin, H^+, and bradykinin, all of which are potent tussive agents. *TRPV1 inhibitors* block cough induced by capsaicin and bradykinin and are effective in some models of cough (McLeod et al., 2008). In a clinical study of an oral TRPV1 inhibitor, there was protection against capsaicin-induced cough but no clinical improvement in chronic idiopathic cough after long-term treatment (Khalid et al., 2014). A side effect of these drugs is loss of temperature regulation and hyperthermia, which has prevented clinical development.

Transient receptor potential A1 is emerging as a more promising novel target for antitussives (Grace and Belvisi, 2011). This channel is activated by oxidative stress and many irritants and may be sensitized by inflammatory cytokines (Bonvini et al., 2015). Several selective TRPA1 antagonists are now in development. TRPV4 may also activate cough and may be activated by ATP (Bonvini et al., 2016).

ATP Receptor Antagonists

Adenosine triphosphate is a potent tussive agent and stimulates cough in patients with asthma and COPD via activation of P2X3 receptors on afferent nerves (Basoglu et al., 2015). A *P2X3 antagonist* (AF-219) is effective in reducing chronic idiopathic cough, although abnormal taste (dysgeusia) is a frequent side effect (Abdulqawi et al., 2015).

Drugs for Dyspnea and Ventilatory Control

Drugs for Dyspnea

Bronchodilators should reduce breathlessness in patients with airway obstruction. Chronic oxygen use may have a beneficial effect, but in a few patients dyspnea may be extreme. Drugs that reduce breathlessness may also depress ventilation in parallel and may therefore be dangerous in severe asthma and COPD. Some patients show a beneficial response to dihydrocodeine and diazepam; however, these drugs must be used with great caution because of the risk of ventilatory depression (Currow et al., 2014). Slow-release morphine tablets may also be helpful in patients with COPD with extreme dyspnea (Currow and Abernethy, 2007). Nebulized morphine may also reduce breathlessness in COPD and could act in part on opioid receptors in the lung. Nebulized furosemide has some efficacy in treating dyspnea from a variety of causes, but the evidence is not yet sufficiently convincing to recommend this as routine therapy (Newton et al., 2008).

Ventilatory Stimulants

Selective respiratory stimulants are indicated if ventilation is impaired as a result of overdose with sedatives, in postanesthetic respiratory depression, and in idiopathic hypoventilation. Respiratory stimulants are rarely indicated in COPD because respiratory drive is already maximal, and further stimulation of ventilation may be counterproductive because of the increase in energy expenditure caused by the drugs.

Doxapram

At low doses (0.5 mg/kg IV), doxapram stimulates carotid chemoreceptors; at higher doses, it stimulates medullary respiratory centers. Its effect is transient; thus, intravenous infusion (0.3–3 mg/kg per min) is needed for sustained effect. Unwanted effects include nausea, sweating, anxiety, and hallucinations. At higher doses, increased pulmonary and systemic pressures may occur. Both the kidney and the liver participate in the clearance of doxapram, which should be used with caution if hepatic or renal function is impaired. In COPD, the infusion of doxapram is restricted to 2 h. The use of doxapram to treat ventilatory failure in COPD has now largely been replaced by noninvasive ventilation.

Almitrine

Almitrine bismesylate is a piperazine derivative that appears to selectively stimulate peripheral chemoreceptors and is without central actions. Almitrine stimulates ventilation only when there is hypoxia. Long-term use of almitrine is associated with peripheral neuropathy, limiting its availability in most countries, including the U.S.

Acetazolamide

The carbonic anhydrase inhibitor acetazolamide (see Chapter 25) induces metabolic acidosis and thereby stimulates ventilation, but it is not widely used because the metabolic imbalance it produces may be detrimental in the face of respiratory acidosis. It has a small beneficial effect in respiratory failure in patients with COPD. The drug has proved useful in prevention of high-altitude (mountain) sickness (Faisy et al., 2016).

Naloxone

Naloxone is a competitive opioid antagonist that is indicated only if ventilatory depression is due to overdose of opioids.

Flumazenil

Flumazenil is a benzodiazepine receptor antagonist that can reverse respiratory depression due to overdose of benzodiazepines (Veiraiah et al., 2012).

Acknowledgment: *Bradley J. Undem and Lawrence M. Lichtenstein contributed to this chapter in earlier editions of this book. We have retained some of their text in the current edition.*

Drug Facts for Your Personal Formulary: *Asthma and COPD Therapeutics*

Drug	Therapeutic Uses	Clinical Tips
Short-Acting β_2 Agonists: Inhaled bronchodilators for symptom relief and acute bronchodilation		
Albuterol (salbutamol)	• Asthma, COPD, and exercise-induced bronchospasm • Inhaled: 180 µg (2 puffs) every 4 to 6 h as needed • Nebulized: 2.5 mg via oral inhalation every 6–8 h as needed over 5 to 15 min • Oral: 2–4 mg by mouth every 6–8 h	• Also available nebulized and inhaled as levalbuterol (active isomer, so half the dose) • May need to be nebulized with oxygen in severe exacerbation • Adverse effects: tachycardia, palpitations, muscle tremors, and hyperkalemia
Levalbuterol (L-albuterol)	• Bronchodilator • Inhaled (MDI nebulizer)	• Half of doses of racemic albuterol • No advantage over racemic albuterol • Adverse effects: tachycardia, palpitations, muscle tremors, and hyperkalemia
Pirbuterol	• 400 µg (2 puffs) every 4–6 h as needed • Inhaled (MDI nebulizer)	• Similar to albuterol • Adverse effects: tachycardia, palpitations, muscle tremors, and hyperkalemia

Drug Facts for Your Personal Formulary: *Asthma and COPD Therapeutics (continued)*

Drug	Therapeutic Uses	Clinical Tips
Long-Acting β_2 Agonists: Add-on therapy to ICSs in asthma; can be used alone in COPD		
Formoterol	• Asthma as add-on to ICS • Maintenance and treatment of severe COPD • Inhaled: 12 μg (contents of 1 capsule) every 12 h • Nebulized 20 μg in 2 mL, twice per day	• Used as maintenance, usually in a combination with an ICS • Can also be used as a reliever of bronchospasm • Adverse effects: tachycardia, palpitations, muscle tremors, and hyperkalemia
Arformoterol Salmeterol Indacaterol Olodaterol	• Arformoterol for severe COPD • Maintenance treatment for COPD • Arformoterol, inhaled (nebulized), 15 μg in 2 mL twice daily • Salmeterol, inhaled 50 μg twice daily • Indacaterol, inhaled (DPI) 75 cetazolamide once daily • Olodaterol, inhaled 2.5 cetazolamide once daily	• Cannot be used as a reliever, only for maintenance treatment for COPD • Adverse effects: tachycardia, palpitations, muscle tremors, and hyperkalemia
Anticholinergics: Muscarinic receptor antagonists inhaled as bronchodilators		
Ipratropium bromide Albuterol/ipratropium combination	• Inhaled, 2 puffs (17 μg/puff) 3–4 times/d • Combination albuterol 103 μg/ipratropium 18 μg/puff; 2 puffs 4 times daily	• Largely replaced by LAMAs • Avoid spraying in eyes • Adverse effects include dry mouth, tachycardia, urinary retention, glaucoma • Combination with albuterol may be used as a reliever
Tiotropium Bromide	• 2.5 μg via oral inhalation (2 puffs of 1.25 μg/actuation) once daily	• Caution in patients with urinary retention or glaucoma history
Umeclidinium bromide	• Inhaled (DPI) 62.5 μg (1 puff) once daily	
Aclidinium bromide	• Inhaled (DPI) 400 μg (1 puff) twice daily	
Glycopyrrolate	• Inhaled (DPI) 1 capsule (15.6 μg) inhaled twice daily	
LAMA-LABA Combination Inhalers: Maintenance treatment for COPD		
Glycopyrrolate/indacaterol	• Inhaled (DPI) 1 inhalation (glycopyrrolate 15.6 μg/indacaterol 27.5 μg) twice daily	• Side effects of anticholinergics and β_2 agonists as above • Maintenance treatment for COPD
Umeclidinium/vilanterol	• Inhaled (DPI) 1 inhalation (umeclidinium 62.5 μg/25 μg vilanterol) once daily	
Tiotropium/olodaterol	• Inhaled (mist inhaler), 2 inhalations (containing 2.5 μg tiotropium/2.5 μg of olodaterol per inhalation) once daily	
Inhaled Corticosteroids: Maintenance treatment for asthma		
Beclomethasone dipropionate (BDP)	• Inhaled (MDI, DPI); 88 μg (1 spray = 44 μg) twice daily • Not to exceed 440 μg twice daily	• More systemic effects than other ICSs: orally bioavailable BDP is converted to an active metabolite, beclomethasone monopropionate, following absorption • Local effects: hoarse voice, candidiasis • Systemic effects: growth suppression, bruising, adrenal suppression
Fluticasone propionate	• Inhaled (MDI, DPI); 50, 100, 250 μg 2 puffs, twice daily • Do not exceed 1000 μg daily	• Fewer systemic effects than BDP • Local: hoarse voice, candidiasis
Budesonide	• Inhaled via jet nebulizer either once daily or divided into 2 doses (maximum daily dose 0.5 mg/d)	• Fewer systemic effects than BDP • Used in children less than 8 who cannot use PDI • Local: hoarse voice, candidiasis
Ciclesonide	• Inhaled (MDI) 80 μg twice daily	• Least-systemic effects of all ICSs; may be effective once daily • Local: hoarse voice, candidiasis
ICS/LABA Combination Inhalers: Maintenance treatment in asthma and COPD		
Fluticasone propionate/salmeterol	• Inhaled (DPI) • Starting dosage based on asthma severity	• Use lowest dose that maintains asthma control • Use only in severe COPD or asthma-COPD overlap • Adverse effects as for ICSs and LABAs
Budesonide/formoterol	• Inhaled (MDI) (80 μg budesonide and 4.5 μg formoterol per inhalation) twice daily	
Fluticasone furoate/vilanterol	• Inhaled (DPI) 1 inhalation (fluticasone furoate 100 μg/vilanterol 25 μg) once daily	

Drug Facts for Your Personal Formulary: *Asthma and COPD Therapeutics (continued)*

Drug	Therapeutic Uses	Clinical Tips
Systemic Corticosteroids: Short course or oral maintenance for asthma (and COPD)		
Prednisone Prednisolone	• Oral: 40–80 mg once daily or divided dose for 3–10 days for acute exacerbation • Minimal dose for maintenance	• Prednisone converted to prednisolone in the liver • Bruising, weight gain, edema, osteoporosis, diabetes, cataracts, adrenal suppression (see Chapter 46)
Hydrocortisone succinate	• IM/IV: 100–500 mg every 12 h for acute severe asthma	• Only if patient not able to take oral steroids
Methylprednisolone	• IV: 100–1000 mg for acute severe asthma	• Rarely indicated because of steroid side effects
Antileukotrienes (Leukotriene Modifiers) for Asthma Maintenance		
Montelukast (10 Zafirlukast) Zileuton	• Oral: montelukast (10 mg once/d); zafirlukast (20 mg twice/d); zileuton (600 mg four times/d or 1200 mg twice/d)	• Less effective than ICS in asthma • Headache, Churg-Strauss syndrome • Zileuton may cause hepatic dysfunction (do not use if ALT increased)
Methylxanthines: Add-on maintenance treatment of severe asthma and COPD		
Theophylline (oral) Aminophylline (IV)	• Aminophylline (IV) is indicated for severe exacerbation that does not respond to nebulized β agonists; shorter action than theophylline	• Interaction with drugs that affect CYP450 • Nausea, headaches, diuresis, arrhythmias, seizures
Phosphodiesterase 4 Inhibitor: Maintenance for severe COPD		
Roflumilast	• Severe COPD • Oral administration 500 μg once daily	• Add to maximal inhaled therapy if severe disease with acute exacerbations and chronic bronchitis
Anti-IgE: Maintenance Treatment for severe asthma		
Omalizumab	• Severe asthma • Subcutaneous administration • Dose depends on total IgE; given every 2–4 weeks	• Expensive, so mainly indicated in severe asthma that is difficult to control • Well tolerated; occasional headache • Occasional anaphylaxis

Bibliography

Abdulqawi R, et al. P2X3 receptor antagonist (AF-219) in refractory chronic cough: a randomised, double-blind, placebo-controlled phase 2 study. *Lancet*, **2015**, *385*:1198–1205.

Akram MF, et al. Doxofylline and theophylline: a comparative clinical study. *J Clin Diagnos Res*, **2012**, *6*:1681–1684.

An SS, et al. TAS2R activation promotes airway smooth muscle relaxation despite beta(2)-adrenergic receptor tachyphylaxis. *Am J Physiol*, **2012**, *303*:L304–L311.

Barnes PJ. Scientific rationale for combination inhalers with a long-acting β2-agonists and corticosteroids. *Eur Respir J*, **2002**, *19*:182–191.

Barnes PJ. Mediators of chronic obstructive pulmonary disease. *Pharm Rev*, **2004**, *56*:515–548.

Barnes PJ. Cytokine networks in asthma and chronic obstructive pulmonary disease. *J Clin Invest*, **2008a**, *118*:3546–3556.

Barnes PJ. Immunology of asthma and chronic obstructive pulmonary disease. *Nat Immunol Rev*, **2008b**, *8*:183–192.

Barnes PJ. Glucocorticosteroids: current and future directions. *Br J Pharmacol*, **2011a**, *163*:29–43.

Barnes PJ. Pathophysiology of allergic inflammation. *Immunol Rev*, **2011b**, *242*:31–50.

Barnes PJ. New drugs for asthma. *Semin Respir Crit Care Med*, **2012**, *33*:685–694.

Barnes PJ. Corticosteroid resistance in patients with asthma and chronic obstructive pulmonary disease. *J Allergy Clin Immunol*, **2013a**, *131*: 636–645.

Barnes PJ. New anti-inflammatory treatments for chronic obstructive pulmonary disease. *Nat Rev Drug Discov*, **2013b**, *12*:543–559.

Barnes PJ. Theophylline. *Am J Respir Crit Care Med*, **2013c**, *188*:901–906.

Barnes PJ. Mechanisms of development of multimorbidity in the elderly. *Eur Respir J*, **2015**, *45*:790–806.

Barnes PJ, Adcock IM. Glucocorticoid resistance in inflammatory diseases. *Lancet*, **2009**, *342*:1905–1917.

Barnes PJ, et al. Chronic obstructive pulmonary disease. *Nat Rev Primers*, **2015**, *1*:1–21.

Barnes PJ, Celli BR. Systemic manifestations and comorbidities of COPD. *Eur Respir J*, **2009**, *33*:1165–1185.

Barnes PJ, et al. Inflammatory mediators of asthma: an update. *Pharmacol Rev*, **1998a**, *50*:515–596.

Barnes PJ, et al. Efficacy and safety of inhaled corticosteroids: an update. *Am J Respir Crit Care Med*, **1998b**, *157*: S1–S53.

Basoglu OK, et al. Effects of aerosolized adenosive 5′-triphosphate in smokers and patients with chronic obstructive pulmonary disease. *Chest*, **2015**, *148*:430–435.

Beasley R, et al. Beta-agonists: what is the evidence that their use increases the risk of asthma morbidity and mortality? *J Allergy Clin Immunol*, **1999**, *104*:S18–S30.

Belvisi MG, et al. Therapeutic benefit of a dissociated glucocorticoid and the relevance of in vitro separation of transrepression from transactivation activity. *J Immunol*, **2001**, *166*:1975–1982.

Bernstein JA, et al. MK-0633, a potent 5-lipoxygenase inhibitor, in chronic obstructive pulmonary disease. *Respir Med*, **2011**, *105*:392–401.

Birring SS, et al. Eosinophilic bronchitis: clinical features, management and pathogenesis. *Am J Respir Med*, **2003**, *2*:169–173.

Black JL, et al. Molecular mechanisms of combination therapy with inhaled corticosteroids and long-acting beta-agonists. *Chest*, **2009**, *136*:1095–1100.

Bleecker ER, et al. Effect of ADRB2 polymorphisms on response to long-acting beta2-agonist therapy: a pharmacogenetic analysis of two randomised studies. *Lancet*, **2007**, *370*:2118–2125.

Bonvini SJ, et al. Transient receptor potential cation channel, subfamily V, member 4 and airway sensory afferent activation: role of adenosine triphosphate. *J Allergy Clin Immunol*, **2016**, *138*:249–261.

Bonvini SJ, et al. Targeting TRP channels for chronic cough: from bench to bedside. *Naunyn Schmiedebergs Arch Pharmacol*, **2015**, *388*:401–420.

Broide DH. Immunomodulation of allergic disease. *Annu Rev Med*, **2009**, *60*:279–291.

Busse WW, et al. The Inhaled Steroid Treatment As Regular Therapy in Early Asthma (START) study 5-year follow-up: effectiveness of early intervention with budesonide in mild persistent asthma. *J Allergy Clin Immunol*, **2008**, *121*:1167–1174.

Calverley PM, et al. Roflumilast in symptomatic chronic obstructive pulmonary disease: two randomised clinical trials. *Lancet*, **2009**, *374*:685–694.

Calzetta L, et al. A systematic review with meta-analysis of dual bronchodilation with LAMA/LABA for the treatment of stable COPD. *Chest*, **2016**, *149*:1181–1196.

Castro M, et al. Benralizumab, an anti-interleukin 5 receptor alpha monoclonal antibody, versus placebo for uncontrolled eosinophilic asthma: a phase 2b randomised dose-ranging study. *Lancet Respir Med*, **2014**, *2*:879–890.

Cates CJ, et al. Safety of regular formoterol or salmeterol in adults with asthma: an overview of Cochrane reviews. *Cochrane Database Syst Rev*, **2014**, (2):CD010314.

Cazzola M, et al. Long-acting muscarinic receptor antagonists for the treatment of respiratory disease. *Pulm Pharmacol Ther*, **2013a**, *26*:307–317.

Cazzola M, et al. Pharmacology and therapeutics of bronchodilators. *Pharmacol Rev*, **2012**, *64*:450–504.

Cazzola M, et al. beta2-Agonist therapy in lung disease. *Am J Respir Crit Care Med*, **2013b**, *187*:690–696.

Chauhan BF, Ducharme FM. Anti-leukotriene agents compared to inhaled corticosteroids in the management of recurrent and/or chronic asthma in adults and children. *Cochrane Database Syst Rev*, **2012**, (5): CD002314.

Cheyne L, et al. Tiotropium versus ipratropium bromide for chronic obstructive pulmonary disease. *Cochrane Database Syst Rev*, **2015**, (9):CD009552.

Chung KF. Targeting the interleukin pathway in the treatment of asthma. *Lancet*, **2015**, *386*:1086–1096.

Chung IY, et al. The downregulation of bcl-2 expression is necessary for theophylline-induced apoptosis of eosinophil. *Cell Immunol*, **2000**, *203*:95–102.

Clark AR. MAP kinase phosphatase 1: a novel mediator of biological effects of glucocorticoids? *J Endocrinol*, **2003**, *178*:5–12.

Coreno A, et al. Comparative effects of long-acting beta2-agonists, leukotriene receptor antagonists, and a 5-lipoxygenase inhibitor on exercise-induced asthma. *J Allergy Clin Immunol*, **2000**, *106*:500–506.

Cosio BG, et al. Theophylline restores histone deacetylase activity and steroid responses in COPD macrophages. *J Exp Med*, **2004**, *200*:689–695.

Culpitt SV, et al. Effect of theophylline on induced sputum inflammatory indices and neutrophil chemotaxis in COPD. *Am J Respir Crit Care Med*, **2002**, *165*:1371–1376.

Currow DC, et al. Opioids for chronic refractory breathlessness: right patient, right route? *Drugs*, **2014**, *74*:1–6.

Currow DC, Abernethy AP. Pharmacological management of dyspnoea. *Curr Opin Support Palliat Care*, **2007**, *1*:96–101.

Decramer M, et al. Effects of *N*-acetylcysteine on outcomes in chronic obstructive pulmonary disease (Bronchitis Randomized on NAC Cost-Utility Study, BRONCUS): a randomised placebo-controlled trial. *Lancet*, **2005**, *365*:1552–1560.

Dennis SM, et al. Regular inhaled salbutamol and asthma control: the TRUST randomised trial. *Lancet*, **2000**, *355*: 1675–1679.

Derendorf H. Pharmacokinetic and pharmacodynamic properties of inhaled ciclesonide. *J Clin Pharmacol*, **2007**, *47*:782–789.

Derendorf H, et al. Relevance of pharmacokinetics and pharmacodynamics of inhaled corticosteroids to asthma. *Eur Respir J*, **2006**, *28*: 1042–1050.

Dicpinigaitis PV, et al. Inhibition of cough-reflex sensitivity by benzonatate and guaifenesin in acute viral cough. *Respir Med*, **2009**, *103*:902–906.

Dicpinigaitis PV, et al. Antitussive drugs—past, present, and future. *Pharmacol Rev*, **2014**, *66*:468–512.

Donnelly LE, Barnes PJ. Chemokine receptors as therapeutic targets in chronic obstructive pulmonary disease. *Trends Pharmacol Sci*, **2006**, *27*:546–553.

Erin EM, et al. Rapid anti-inflammatory effect of inhaled ciclesonide in asthma: a randomised, placebo-controlled study. *Chest*, **2008**, *134*:740–745.

Ernst P, et al. Inhaled corticosteroids in COPD: the clinical evidence. *Eur Respir J*, **2015**, *45*:525–537.

Fahy JV, Dickey BF. Airway mucus function and dysfunction. *N Engl J Med*, **2010**, *363*:2233–2247.

Faisy C, et al. Effect of acetazolamide vs placebo on duration of invasive mechanical ventilation among patients with chronic obstructive pulmonary disease: a randomized clinical trial. *JAMA*, **2016**, *315*:480–488.

Finney L, et al. Inhaled corticosteroids and pneumonia in chronic obstructive pulmonary disease. *Lancet Respir Medicine*, **2014**, *2*:919–932.

Flood-Page P, et al. A study to evaluate safety and efficacy of mepolizumab in patients with moderate persistent asthma. *Am J Respir Crit Care Med*, **2007**, *176*:1062–1071.

Franciosi LG, et al. Efficacy and safety of RPL554, a dual PDE3 and PDE4 inhibitor, in healthy volunteers and in patients with asthma or chronic obstructive pulmonary disease: findings from four clinical trials. *Lancet Respir Med*, **2013**, *1*:714–727.

Gauvreau GM, et al. Effect of regular inhaled albuterol on allergen-induced late responses and sputum eosinophils in asthmatic subjects. *Am J Respir Crit Care Med*, **1997**, *156*:1738–1745.

Gibson P, et al. Treatment of unexplained chronic cough: CHEST guideline and expert panel report. *Chest*, **2016**, *149*:27–44.

Gibson PG, Vertigan AE. Gabapentin in chronic cough. *Pulm Pharmacol Ther*, **2015**, *35*:145–148.

Grace MS, Belvisi MG. TRPA1 receptors in cough. *Pulm Pharmacol Ther*, **2011**, *24*:286–288.

Grayson MH, Korenblat PE. The role of antileukotriene drugs in management of rhinitis and rhinosinusitis. *Curr Allergy Asthma Rep*, **2007**, *7*:209–215.

Hall S, Agrawal DK. Key mediators in the immunopathogenesis of allergic asthma. *Int Immunopharmacol*, **2014**, *23*:316–329.

Hanania NA, et al. Lebrikizumab in moderate-to-severe asthma: pooled data from two randomised placebo-controlled studies. *Thorax*, **2015**, *70*:748–756.

Haque RA, et al. Chronic idiopathic cough: a discrete clinical entity? *Chest*, **2005**, *127*:1710–1713.

Hatzelmann A, et al. The preclinical pharmacology of roflumilast—a selective, oral phosphodiesterase 4 inhibitor in development for chronic obstructive pulmonary disease. *Pulm Pharmacol Ther*, **2010**, *23*:235–256.

Hawkins G, et al. Stepping down inhaled corticosteroids in asthma: randomised controlled trial. *BMJ*, **2003**, *326*:1115.

Hawkins GA, et al. Clinical consequences of ADRbeta2 polymorphisms. *Pharmacogenomics*, **2008**, *9*:349–358.

Henke MO, Ratjen F. Mucolytics in cystic fibrosis. *PaediatrRespir Rev*, **2007**, *8*:24–29.

Humbert M, et al. Omalizumab in asthma: an update on recent developments. *J Allergy Clin Immunol Pract*, **2014**, *2*:525–536.e521.

Ichiyama T, et al. Theophylline inhibits NF-κB activation and IκBα degradation in human pulmonary epithelial cells. *Naunyn Schmied Arch Pharmacol*, **2001**, *364*:558–561.

Ito K, et al. Histone deacetylase 2-mediated deacetylation of the glucocorticoid receptor enables NF-κB suppression. *J Exp Med*, **2006**, *203*:7–13.

Kerstjens HA, et al. Tiotropium or salmeterol as add-on therapy to inhaled corticosteroids for patients with moderate symptomatic asthma: two replicate, double-blind, placebo-controlled, parallel-group, active-comparator, randomised trials. *Lancet Resp Med*, **2015**, *3*:367–376.

Kew KM, et al. Intravenous magnesium sulfate for treating adults with acute asthma in the emergency department. *Cochrane Database Syst Rev*, **2014**, (5):CD010909.

Kew KM, et al. Long-acting beta2-agonists for chronic obstructive pulmonary disease. *Cochrane Database Syst Rev*, **2013**, (10):CD010177.

Khalid S, et al. Transient receptor potential vanilloid 1 (TRPV1) antagonism in patients with refractory chronic cough: a double-blind randomized controlled trial. *J Allergy Clin Immunol*, **2014**, *134*:56–62.

Kirkham PA, Barnes PJ. Oxidative stress in COPD. *Chest*, **2013**, *144*:266–273.

Lambrecht BN, Hammad H. The immunology of asthma. *Nature Immunol*, **2015**, *16*:45–56.

Leckie MJ, et al. Effects of an interleukin-5 blocking monoclonal antibody on eosinophils, airway hyperresponsiveness and the late asthmatic response. *Lancet*, **2000**, *356*:2144–2148.

Lim S, et al. Low-dose theophylline reduces eosinophilic inflammation but not exhaled nitric oxide in mild asthma. *Am J Respir Crit Care Med*, **2001**, *164*:273–276.

Linden A, et al. Bronchodilation by an inhaled VPAC(2) receptor agonist in patients with stable asthma. *Thorax*, **2003**, *58*:217–221.

Lipworth BJ. Systemic adverse effects of inhaled corticosteroid therapy: a systematic review and meta-analysis [see comments]. *Arch Intern Med*, **1999**, *159*:941–955.

Loh CH, et al. Review of drug safety and efficacy of arformoterol in chronic obstructive pulmonary disease. *Exp Opinion Drug Safety*, **2015**, *14*:463–472.

Lotvall J, et al. The therapeutic ratio of R-albuterol is comparable with that of RS-albuterol in asthmatic patients. *J Allergy Clin Immunol*, **2001**, *108*:726–731.

MacNee W, et al. Efficacy and safety of the oral p38 inhibitor PH-797804 in chronic obstructive pulmonary disease: a randomised clinical trial. *Thorax*, **2013**, *68*:738–745.

Mak JCW, et al. Protective effects of a glucocorticoid on down-regulation of pulmonary β_2 adrenergic receptors in vivo. *J Clin Invest*, **1995**, *96*:99–106.

Manjra AI, et al. Efficacy of nebulized fluticasone propionate compared with oral prednisolone in children with an acute exacerbation of asthma. *Respir Med*, **2000**, *94*:1206–1214.

Martinez FJ, et al. Effect of roflumilast on exacerbations in patients with severe chronic obstructive pulmonary disease uncontrolled by combination therapy (REACT): a multicentre randomised controlled trial. *Lancet*, **2015**, *385*:857–866.

McLeod RL, et al. TRPV1 antagonists as potential antitussive agents. *Lung*, **2008**, *186 (Suppl 1)*:S59–S65.

Millan DS. What is the potential for inhaled p38 inhibitors in the treatment of chronic obstructive pulmonary disease? *Future Med Chem*, **2011**, *3*:1635–1645.

Nathani N, et al. Churg-Strauss syndrome and leukotriene antagonist use: a respiratory perspective. *Thorax*, **2008**, *63*:883–888.

Nelson HS, Dorinsky PM. Safety of long-acting beta-agonists. *Ann Intern Med*, **2006**, *145*:706–710.

Newton PJ, et al. Nebulized furosemide for the management of dyspnea: does the evidence support its use? *J Pain Symptom Manage*, **2008**, *36*:424–441.

Niewoehner DE, et al. Effect of systemic glucocorticoids on exacerbations of chronic obstructive pulmonary disease. *N Engl J Med*, **1999**, *340*:1941–1947.

Nightingale JA, et al. Comparison of the effects of salmeterol and formoterol in patients with severe asthma. *Chest*, **2002**, *121*:1401–1406.

Norman P. Investigational p38 inhibitors for the treatment of chronic obstructive pulmonary disease. *Expert Opin Investig Drugs*, **2015**, *24*:383–392.

Normansell R, et al. Omalizumab for asthma in adults and children. *Cochrane Database Syst Rev*, **2014**, (1):CD003559.

Ozdemir C, et al. Mechanisms of aeroallergen immunotherapy: subcutaneous immunotherapy and sublingual immunotherapy. *Immunol Allergy Clin North Am*, **2016**, *36*:71–86.

Pavord ID, Chung KF. Management of chronic cough. *Lancet*, **2008**, *371*:1375–1384.

Pavord ID, et al. Mepolizumab for severe eosinophilic asthma (DREAM): a multicentre, double-blind, placebo-controlled trial. *Lancet*, **2012**, *380*:651–659.

Pedersen S. Do inhaled corticosteroids inhibit growth in children? *Am J Respir Crit Care Med*, **2001**, *164*:521–535.

Pelaia G, et al. Potential role of potassium channel openers in the treatment of asthma and chronic obstructive pulmonary disease. *Life Sci*, **2002**, *70*:977–990.

Penn RB, et al. Mechanisms of acute desensitization of the beta2AR-adenylyl cyclase pathway in human airway smooth muscle. *Am J Respir Cell Mol Biol*, **1998**, *19*:338–348.

Postma DS, Rabe KF. The asthma-COPD overlap syndrome. *N Engl J Med*, **2015**, *373*:1241–1249.

Ray NC, Alcaraz L. Muscarinic antagonist-beta-adrenergic agonist dual pharmacology molecules as bronchodilators: a patent review. *Expert Opin Ther Pat*, **2009**, *19*:1–12.

Rennard SI, et al. CXCR2 antagonist MK-7123—a phase 2 proof-of-concept trial for chronic obstructive pulmonary disease. *Am J Respir Crit Care Med*, **2015**, *191*:1001–1011.

Rennard SI, et al. The safety and efficacy of infliximab in moderate-to-severe chronic obstructive pulmonary disease. *Am J Respir Crit Care Med*, **2007**, *175*:926–934.

Robinson DS, et al. Addition of an anti-leukotriene to therapy in chronic severe asthma in a clinic setting: a double-blind, randomised, placebo-controlled study. *Lancet*, **2001**, *357*:2007–2011.

Rolland JM, et al. Allergen-related approaches to immunotherapy. *Pharmacol Ther*, **2009**, *121*:273–284.

Sanchis J, et al. Inhaler devices—from theory to practice. *Respir Med*, **2013**, *107*:495–502.

Sears MR. Adverse effects of beta-agonists. *J Allergy Clin Immunol*, **2002**, *110*:S322–S328.

Shivanthan MC, Rajapakse S. Magnesium for acute exacerbation of chronic obstructive pulmonary disease: a systematic review of randomised trials. *Ann Thorac Med*, **2014**, *9*:77–80.

Tantisira KG, Drazen JM. Genetics and pharmacogenetics of the leukotriene pathway. *J Allergy Clin Immunol*, **2009**, *124*:422–427.

Tashkin DP, et al. A 4-year trial of tiotropium in chronic obstructive pulmonary disease. *N Engl J Med*, **2008**, *359*:1543–1554.

Teach SJ, et al. Preseasonal treatment with either omalizumab or an inhaled corticosteroid boost to prevent fall asthma exacerbations. *J Allergy Clin Immunol*, **2015**, *136*:1476–1485.

To Y, et al. Targeting phosphoinositide-3-kinase-δ with theophylline reverses corticosteroid insensitivity in COPD. *Am J Respir Crit Care Med*, **2010**, *182*:897–904.

Townley RG, Agrawal S. CRTH2 antagonists in the treatment of allergic responses involving TH2 cells, basophils, and eosinophils. *Ann Allergy Asthma Immunol*, **2012**, *109*:365–374.

Trejo Bittar HE, et al. Pathobiology of severe asthma. *Annu Rev Pathol*, **2015**, *10*:511–545.

Usmani OS, Barnes PJ. Assessing and treating small airways disease in asthma and chronic obstructive pulmonary disease. *Ann Med*, **2012**, *44*:146–156.

van Ganse E, et al. Effects of antihistamines in adult asthma: a meta-analysis of clinical trials. *Eur Respir J*, **1997**, *10*:2216–2224.

Veiraiah A, et al. Flumazenil use in benzodiazepine overdose in the UK: a retrospective survey of NPIS data. *Emerg Med J*, **2012**, *29*: 565–569.

Wenzel S, et al. Dupilumab in persistent asthma with elevated eosinophil levels. *N Engl J Med*, **2013**, *368*:2455–2466.

Wenzel SE, et al. A randomized, double-blind, placebo-controlled study of TNF-α blockade in severe persistent asthma. *Am J Respir Crit Care Med*, **2009**, *179*:549–558.

Wessler I, Kirkpatrick CJ. Acetylcholine beyond neurons: the non-neuronal cholinergic system in humans. *BrJ Pharmacol*, **2008**, *154*: 1558–1571.

Woodcock A, et al. Efficacy in asthma of once-daily treatment with fluticasone furoate: a randomized, placebo-controlled trial. *Respir Res*, **2011**, *12*:132.

Woodruff PG, et al. Safety and efficacy of an inhaled epidermal growth factor receptor inhibitor (BIBW 2948 BS) in chronic obstructive pulmonary disease. *Am J Respir Crit Care Med*, **2010**, *181*:438–445.

Yang IA,et al. Inhaled corticosteroids for stable chronic obstructive pulmonary disease. *Cochrane Database Syst Rev*, **2012**, (7):CD002991.

Yasui K, et al. Theophylline induces neutrophil apoptosis through adenosine A_{2A} receptor antagonism. *J Leukoc Biol*, **2000**, *67*:529–535.

Zhang L, et al. Inhaled corticosteroids in children with persistent asthma: effects on growth. *Cochrane Database Syst Rev*, **2014**, (7):CD009471.

Zheng JP, et al. Effect of carbocisteine on acute exacerbation of chronic obstructive pulmonary disease (PEACE Study): a randomised placebo-controlled study. *Lancet*, **2008**, *371*:2013–2018.

Zheng JP, et al. Twice daily *N*-acetylcysteine 600 mg for exacerbations of chronic obstructive pulmonary disease (PANTHEON): a randomised, double-blind placebo-controlled trial. *Lancet Respir Med*, **2014**, *2*:187–194.

Ziegelbauer K, et al. A selective novel low-molecular-weight inhibitor of IkappaB kinase-beta (IKK-beta) prevents pulmonary inflammation and shows broad anti-inflammatory activity. *Br J Pharmacol*, **2005**, *145*:178–192.

Hematopoietic Agents: Growth Factors, Minerals, and Vitamins

Kenneth Kaushansky and Thomas J. Kipps

第四十一章　造血因子：生长因子、矿物质和维生素

中文导读

本章主要介绍：造血；生长因子生理学；红细胞生成刺激因子，包括红细胞生成素；骨髓生长因子，包括粒细胞-巨噬细胞集落刺激因子、粒细胞集落刺激因子；血小板生长因子，包括白细胞介素-11、血小板生成素受体激动药；缺铁和其他低色素性贫血，包括铁的生物利用度、铁代谢、铁的需求和饮食中铁的利用、铁缺乏的治疗，以及铜、维生素B_6和核黄素；维生素B_{12}、叶酸和巨幼细胞贫血，包括维生素B_{12}和叶酸的细胞作用、维生素B_{12}与人类健康、叶酸与人类健康。

Abbreviations

BFU: burst-forming units
BFU-E: BFU erythrocyte
CFU: colony-forming units
CFU-E: CFU erythrocyte
CFU-GEMM: CFU granulocyte, erythrocyte, monocyte and megakaryocyte
CFU-GM: CFU granulocyte and macrophage
CFU-Meg: CFU megakaryocyte
CH_3B_{12}: methylcobalamin
$CH_3H_4PteGlu_1$: methyltetrahydrofolate
CSF: colony stimulating factor
dTMP: thymidylate
dUMP: deoxyuridylate
EPO: erythropoietin
ESA: erythropoiesis-stimulating agent
FIGLU: formiminoglutamic acid
FL: FLT3 (FMS tyr kinase 3) ligand
FMS3: FMS tyr kinase 3
G-CSF: granulocyte colony-stimulating factor
GM-CSF: granulocyte-macrophage colony-stimulating factor
GVHD: graft-versus-host disease
HAART: highly active antiretroviral therapy
HFE: high Fe, hemochromatosis protein
HIF: hypoxia-inducible factor
HIV: human immunodeficiency virus
IFN: interferon
IL: interleukin
LAK: lymphokine-activated killer cell
M-CSF: monocyte-/macrophage-stimulating factor
NK: natural killer
PBSC: peripheral blood stem cell
PteGlu: pteroylglutamic acid, folic acid
SAM: S-adenosylmethionine
SCF: stem cell factor
TcII: transcobalamin II
TRA: thrombopoietin receptor agonist

HISTORICAL PERSPECTIVE

Modern concepts of hematopoietic cell growth and differentiation derive from experiments done in the 1950s. Till and McCulloch demonstrated that individual hematopoietic cells could form macroscopic hematopoietic colonies in the spleens of irradiated mice, thereby establishing the concept of discrete hematopoietic stem cells (i.e., the presence of a multilineage clonal splenic colony appearing 11 days after transplantation implied that a single cell lodged and expanded into several cell lineages). This concept now has been expanded to include normal human marrow cells. Moreover, such cells now can be prospectively identified.

The basis for identifying soluble growth factors was provided by Sachs and independently by Metcalf, who developed clonal, in vitro assays for hematopoietic progenitor cells. Such hematopoietic colonies first developed only in the presence of conditioned culture medium from leukocytes or tumor cell lines. Individual growth factors then were isolated based on their activities in clonal in vitro assays, assays that were instrumental in purifying a hierarchy of progenitor cells committed to individual and combinations of mature blood cells (Kondo et al., 2003).

In 1906, Paul Carnot postulated the existence of a circulating growth factor that controls red blood cell development. He observed an increase in the red cell count in rabbits injected with serum obtained from anemic animals and postulated the existence of a factor that he called hemopoietin. Only in the 1950s did Reissmann, Erslev, and Jacobsen and coworkers define the origin and actions of the hormone, now called erythropoietin. Subsequently, extensive studies of erythropoietin were carried out in patients with anemia and polycythemia, leading to the purification of erythropoietin from urine and the subsequent cloning of the erythropoietin gene. The high-level expression of erythropoietin in cell lines has allowed for its purification and use in humans with anemia.

Similarly, the existence of specific leukocyte growth factors was suggested by the capacity of different conditioned culture media to induce the in vitro growth of colonies containing different combinations of granulocytes and monocytes. An activity that stimulated the production of both granulocytes and monocytes was purified from murine lung-conditioned medium, leading to cloning of GM-CSF, first from mice (Gough et al., 1984) and subsequently from humans (Wong et al., 1985). Finding an activity that stimulated the exclusive production of neutrophils permitted the cloning of G-CSF (Welte et al., 1985). Subsequently, a megakaryocyte colony-stimulating factor termed thrombopoietin was purified and cloned (Kaushansky, 1998).

Growth factors that support lymphocyte growth were identified using assays that measured the capacity of the cytokine to promote lymphocyte proliferation in vitro. This permitted the identification of the growth-promoting properties of IL-7, IL-4, or IL-15 for all lymphocytes, B cells, or NK cells, respectively (Goodwin et al., 1989; Grabstein et al., 1994). Recombinant expression of these complementary DNAs permitted production of sufficient quantities of biologically active growth factors for clinical investigations, allowing for the demonstration of the potential clinical utility of such factors.

Hematopoiesis

The finite life span of most mature blood cells requires their continuous replacement, a process termed *hematopoiesis*. New cell production must respond to basal needs and states of increased demand. Erythrocyte production can increase more than 20-fold in response to anemia or hypoxemia, leukocyte production increases dramatically in response to systemic infections, and platelet production can increase 10- to 20-fold when platelet consumption results in thrombocytopenia.

The regulation of blood cell production is complex. Hematopoietic stem cells are rare marrow cells that manifest self-renewal and lineage commitment, resulting in cells destined to differentiate into the 10 or more distinct blood cell lineages. For the most part, this process occurs in the marrow cavities of the skull, vertebral bodies, pelvis, and proximal long bones; it involves interactions among hematopoietic stem and progenitor cells and the cells and complex macromolecules of the marrow stroma and is influenced by a number of soluble and membrane-bound hematopoietic growth factors. Several hormones and cytokines have been identified and cloned that affect hematopoiesis, permitting their production in quantities sufficient for research and, in some cases, therapeutic use. Clinical applications range from the treatment of primary hematologic diseases (e.g., aplastic anemia, congenital neutropenia) to use as adjuncts in the treatment of severe infections and in the management of patients with kidney failure or those undergoing cancer chemotherapy or marrow transplantation.

Hematopoiesis also requires an adequate supply of minerals (e.g., iron, cobalt, and copper) and vitamins (e.g., folic acid, vitamin B_{12}, pyridoxine, ascorbic acid, and riboflavin); deficiencies generally result in characteristic anemias or, less frequently, a general failure of hematopoiesis (Hoffbrand and Herbert, 1999). Therapeutic correction of a specific deficiency state depends on the accurate diagnosis of the anemic state and on knowledge about the correct dose, the use of these agents in appropriate combinations, and the expected response.

Growth Factor Physiology

Steady-state hematopoiesis encompasses the tightly regulated production of more than 400 billion blood cells each day. The hematopoietic organ also is unique in adult physiology in that several mature cell types are derived from a much smaller number of multipotent progenitors, which develop from a more limited number of pluripotent hematopoietic stem cells. Such cells are capable of maintaining their own number and differentiating under the influence of cellular and humoral factors to produce the large and diverse number of mature blood cells.

Our understanding of stem cell differentiation owes much to the in vitro culture of marrow cells. Using the results from clonal cultures in semisolid medium, stem cell differentiation can be described as a series of developmental steps that produce mixed blood cell lineage colonies, which give rise to large, immature and small, mature single-lineage burst-forming units (BFUs) and colony-forming units (CFUs), respectively, for each of the major blood cell types. These early progenitors (BFUs and CFUs) are capable of further proliferation and differentiation, increasing their number by some 30-fold. It is at this most mature stage of development that the lineage-committed growth factors (G-CSF, M-CSF, erythropoietin, and thrombopoietin) exert their primary proliferative and differentiative effects. Overall, proliferation and maturation of the CFU for each cell line can amplify the resulting mature cell product by another 30-fold or more, generating more than 1000 mature cells from each committed stem cell.

Hematopoietic and lymphopoietic growth factors are glycoproteins produced by a number of marrow cells and peripheral tissues. They are active at very low concentrations and typically affect more than one committed cell lineage. Most interact synergistically with other factors and stimulate production of additional growth factors, a process termed *networking*. Growth factors generally exert actions at several points in the processes of cell proliferation and differentiation and in mature cell function. However, the network of growth factors that contributes to any given cell lineage depends absolutely on a nonredundant, lineage-specific factor, such that absence of factors that stimulate developmentally early progenitors is compensated for by redundant cytokines, but loss of the lineage-specific factor leads to a specific cytopenia.

Some of the overlapping and nonredundant effects of the more important hematopoietic growth factors are illustrated in Figure 41–1 *and* Table 41–1.

Erythropoiesis-Stimulating Agents

Erythropoiesis-stimulating agent (ESA) is the term given to a pharmacological substance that stimulates red blood cell production.

Erythropoietin

Erythropoietin is the most important regulator of the proliferation of committed erythroid progenitors (CFU-E) and their immediate progeny. In its absence, severe anemia is invariably present, commonly seen in patients with renal failure. Erythropoiesis is controlled by a feedback system in which a sensor in the kidney detects changes in oxygen delivery to modulate the erythropoietin secretion. The sensor mechanism is now understood at the molecular level (Haase, 2010).

Hypoxia-inducible factor, a heterodimeric (HIF-1α and HIF-1β) transcription factor, enhances expression of multiple hypoxia-inducible genes, such as vascular endothelial growth factor and erythropoietin. HIF-1α is labile due to its prolyl hydroxylation and subsequent polyubiquitination and degradation, aided by the von Hippel-Lindau (VHL) *protein*. During states of hypoxia, the prolyl hydroxylase is inactive, allowing the accumulation of HIF-1α and activating erythropoietin expression, which in turn

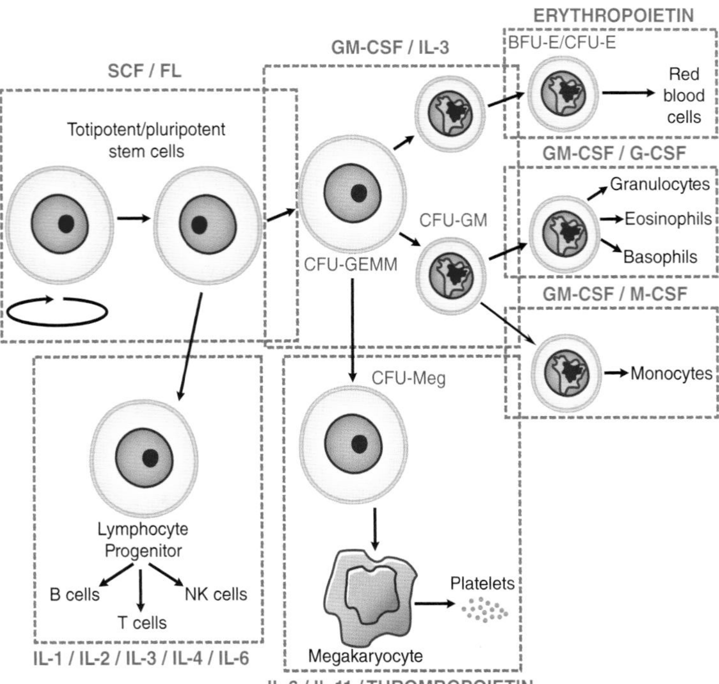

Figure 41–1 *Sites of action of hematopoietic growth factors in the differentiation and maturation of marrow cell lines.* A self-sustaining pool of marrow stem cells differentiates under the influence of specific hematopoietic growth factors to form a variety of hematopoietic and lymphopoietic cells. SCF, FL, IL-3, and GM-CSF, together with cell-cell interactions in the marrow, stimulate stem cells to form a series of BFUs and CFUs: CFU-GEMM, CFU-GM, CFU-Meg, BFU-E, and CFU-E. After considerable proliferation, further differentiation is stimulated by synergistic interactions with growth factors for each of the major cell lines—G-CSF, M-CSF, thrombopoietin, and erythropoietin. Each of these factors also influences the proliferation, maturation, and in some cases the function, of the derivative cell line (Table 41–1).

TABLE 41–1 ■ HEMATOPOIETIC GROWTH FACTORS

Erythropoietin (EPO) • Stimulates proliferation and maturation of committed erythroid progenitors to increase red cell production
Stem cell factor (SCF, c-kit ligand, Steel factor) and FLT 3 ligand (FL) • Act synergistically with a wide range of other colony-stimulating factors and interleukins to stimulate pluripotent and committed stem cells • FL also stimulates both dendritic and NK cells (antitumor response) • SCF also stimulates mast cells and melanocytes
Interleukins *IL-1, IL-3, IL-5, IL-6, IL-9, and IL-11* • Act synergistically with each other and SCF, GM-CSF, G-CSF, and EPO to stimulate BFU-E, CFU-GEMM, CFU-GM, CFU-E, and CFU-Meg growth • Numerous immunologic roles, including stimulation of B-cell and T-cell growth *IL-5* • Controls eosinophil survival and differentiation *IL-6* • IL-6 stimulates human myeloma cells to proliferate • IL-6 and IL-11 stimulate BFU-Meg to increase platelet production *IL-1, IL-2, IL-4, IL-7, and IL-12* • Stimulate growth and function of T cells, B cells, NK cells, and monocytes • Costimulate B, T, and LAK cells *IL-8 and IL-10* • Numerous immunological activities involving B- and T-cell functions • IL-8 acts as a chemotactic factor for basophils and neutrophils
Granulocyte-macrophage colony-stimulating factor (GM-CSF) • Acts synergistically with SCF, IL-1, IL-3, and IL-6 to stimulate CFU-GM and CFU-Meg to increase neutrophil and monocyte production • With EPO may promote BFU-E formation • Enhances migration, phagocytosis, superoxide production, and antibody-dependent cell-mediated toxicity of neutrophils, monocytes, and eosinophils • Prevents alveolar proteinosis
Granulocyte colony-stimulating factor (G-CSF) • Stimulates CFU-G to increase neutrophil production • Enhances phagocytic and cytotoxic activities of neutrophils
Monocyte/macrophage colony-stimulating factor (M-CSF, CSF-1) • Stimulates CFU-M to increase monocyte precursors • Activates and enhances function of monocyte/macrophages
Macrophage colony-stimulating factor (M-CSF) • Stimulates CFU-M to increase monocyte/macrophage precursors • Acts in concert with tissues and other growth factors to determine the proliferation, differentiation, and survival of a range of cells of the mononuclear phagocyte system
Thrombopoietin (TPO, *Mpl* ligand) • Stimulates the self-renewal and expansion of hematopoietic stem cells • Stimulates stem cell differentiation into megakaryocyte progenitors • Selectively stimulates megakaryocytopoiesis to increase platelet production • Acts synergistically with other growth factors, especially IL-6 and IL-11

stimulates rapid expansion of erythroid progenitors. Specific alteration of VHL leads to an oxygen-sensing defect, characterized by constitutively elevated levels of HIF-1α and erythropoietin, with resultant polycythemia (Gordeuk et al., 2004). A second isoform of HIF, HIF-2α, is an important regulator of the expression of genes that contribute to iron absorption (Mastrogiannaki et al., 2013); a genetic gain-of-function mutation in HIF-2α also induces erythrocytosis in patients (Percy et al., 2008).

Erythropoietin is expressed primarily in peritubular interstitial cells of the kidney. Erythropoietin contains 193 amino acids, of which the first 27 are cleaved during secretion. The final hormone is heavily glycosylated and has a molecular mass of about 30 kDa. After secretion, erythropoietin binds to a receptor on the surface of committed erythroid progenitors in the marrow and is internalized. With anemia or hypoxemia, synthesis rapidly increases by 100-fold or more, serum erythropoietin levels rise, and marrow progenitor cell survival, proliferation, and maturation are dramatically stimulated. This finely tuned feedback loop can be disrupted by kidney disease, marrow damage, or a deficiency in iron or an essential vitamin. With an infection or an inflammatory state, erythropoietin secretion, iron delivery, and progenitor proliferation all are suppressed by inflammatory cytokines, but this accounts for only part of the resultant anemia; interference with iron metabolism also is an effect of inflammatory mediator effects on the hepatic protein *hepcidin* (Drakesmith and Prentice, 2012). Loss of hepcidin-producing liver mass or genetic or acquired conditions that repress hepcidin production by the liver may lead to iron overload (Pietrangelo, 2016).

Preparations

Preparations of recombinant human erythropoietin include *epoetin alfa, epoetin beta, epoetin omega*, and *epoetin zeta*, which differ almost exclusively in carbohydrate modifications due to manufacturing differences and are supplied in single-use vials or syringes containing 500–40,000 units for intravenous or subcutaneous administration. When injected intravenously, epoetin alfas are cleared from plasma with a $t_{1/2}$ of 4–8 h. However, the effect on marrow progenitors lasts much longer, and once-weekly dosing can be sufficient to achieve an adequate response. An engineered epoetin alfa, darbepoetin, which displays a longer circulatory half-life, is also available for use in patients with indications similar to those for other epoetins. Based on phage display technology, small peptide agonists of the erythropoietin receptor were identified and developed into clinical agents by coupling to polyethylene glycol. One such erythropoiesis-stimulating peptide, peginesatide, was approved for the treatment of anemia due to chronic kidney disease; postmarketing reports of serious hypersensitivity reactions and anaphylaxis necessitated its removal from the market.

Recombinant human erythropoietin (*epoetin alfa*) is nearly identical to the endogenous hormone. The carbohydrate modification pattern of epoetin alfa differs slightly from the native protein, but this difference apparently does not alter kinetics, potency, or immunoreactivity of the drug. Modern assays can detect these differences and thereby identify athletes who use the recombinant product for "blood doping."

Therapeutic Uses, Monitoring, and Adverse Effects

Recombinant erythropoietin therapy, in conjunction with adequate iron intake, can be highly effective in a number of anemias, especially those associated with poor erythropoietic response. Epoetin alfa is effective in the treatment of anemias associated with surgery, AIDS, cancer chemotherapy, prematurity, and certain chronic inflammatory conditions. Darbepoetin alfa also has been approved for use in patients with anemia associated with chronic kidney disease. A Cochrane analysis could not demonstrate the superiority of one form of ESA over any another.

During erythropoietin therapy, absolute or functional iron deficiency may develop. Functional iron deficiency (i.e., normal ferritin levels but low transferrin saturation) presumably results from the inability to mobilize iron stores rapidly enough to support the increased erythropoiesis. Supplemental iron therapy is recommended for all patients whose serum ferritin is less than 100 μg/L or whose serum transferrin saturation is below 20%. During initial therapy and after any dosage adjustment, the hematocrit is determined once a week (patients infected with HIV and those with cancer) or twice a week (patients with renal failure) until it has stabilized in the target range and the maintenance dose has been established; the hematocrit then is monitored at regular intervals. If the hematocrit increases by more than 4 points in any 2-week period, the dose should be decreased. Due to the time required for erythropoiesis and the erythrocyte half-life, hematocrit changes lag behind dosage adjustments by 2–6 weeks. The dose of darbepoetin should be decreased if the hemoglobin increase exceeds 1 g/dL in any 2-week period because of the association of excessive rate of rise of hemoglobin with adverse cardiovascular events.

During hemodialysis, patients receiving epoetin alfa or darbepoetin may require increased anticoagulation. The risk of thrombotic events is higher in adults with ischemic heart disease or congestive heart failure receiving epoetin alfa therapy with the goal of reaching a normal hematocrit (42%) than in those with a lower target hematocrit of 30% (Bennett et al., 2008). ESA use is associated with increased rates of cancer recurrence and decreased on-study survival in patients in whom the drugs are administered for cancer-induced or for chemotherapy-induced anemia (Bohlius et al., 2009). The most common side effect of epoetin alfa therapy is aggravation of hypertension, which occurs in 20%–30% of patients and most often is associated with a rapid rise in hematocrit. ESAs should not be used in patients with preexisting uncontrolled hypertension. Patients may require initiation of, or increases in, antihypertensive therapy. Hypertensive encephalopathy and seizures have occurred in patients with chronic renal failure treated with epoetin alfa. Headache, tachycardia, edema, shortness of breath, nausea, vomiting, diarrhea, injection site stinging, and flu-like symptoms (e.g., arthralgias and myalgias) also have been reported in conjunction with epoetin alfa therapy.

Anemia of Chronic Renal Failure Patients with anemia secondary to chronic kidney disease are ideal candidates for epoetin alfa therapy as the disease represents a true hormone deficiency state. The response in predialysis, peritoneal dialysis, and hemodialysis patients depends on the severity of the renal failure, the erythropoietin dose and route of administration, and iron availability (Besarab et al., 1999; Kaufman et al., 1998). The subcutaneous route of administration is preferred over the intravenous route because absorption is slower and the amount of drug required is reduced by 20%–40%. The dose of epoetin alfa should be adjusted to obtain a gradual rise in the hematocrit over a 2- to 4-month period to a final hematocrit of 33%–36%. Treatment to hematocrit levels greater than 36% is not recommended.

Patients are started on doses of 80–120 units/kg of epoetin alfa, given subcutaneously, three times a week. The final maintenance dose of epoetin alfa can vary from 10 units/kg to more than 300 units/kg, with an average dose of 75 units/kg, three times a week. Children less than 5 years of age generally require a higher dose. Resistance to therapy is common in patients who develop an inflammatory illness or become iron deficient, so close monitoring of general health and iron status is essential. Less-common causes of resistance include occult blood loss, folic acid deficiency, carnitine deficiency, inadequate dialysis, aluminum toxicity, and osteitis fibrosa cystica secondary to hyperparathyroidism. Darbepoetin alfa is approved for use in patients who are anemic secondary to chronic kidney disease. The recommended starting dose is 0.45 μg/kg administered intravenously or subcutaneously once weekly or 0.75 μg/kg administered every 2 weeks, with dose adjustments depending on the response. Like epoetin alfa, side effects tend to occur when patients experience a rapid rise in hemoglobin concentration; a rise of less than 1 g/dL every 2 weeks generally is considered safe.

Anemia in Patients With AIDS Epoetin alfa therapy has been approved for the treatment of HIV-infected patients, especially those on zidovudine therapy (Fischl et al., 1990). Excellent responses to doses of 100–300 units/kg, given subcutaneously three times a week, generally are seen in patients with zidovudine-induced anemia. However, a more recent analysis of erythropoietin therapy in patients with HIV infection failed to support its routine use (Martí-Carvajal et al., 2011). The reason for the difference between 1990 and 2011 may lay in far more effective therapy for HIV in the HAART era, such that the origin of anemia in HIV-infected individuals today is different from what it was at the onset of the AIDS epidemic.

Cancer-Related Anemias Epoetin alfa therapy, 150 units/kg three times a week or 450–600 units/kg once a week, can reduce the transfusion requirement in patients with cancer undergoing chemotherapy as well as lead to reduced anemia-related symptoms. Previous therapeutic guidelines (Rizzo et al., 2002) recommended the use of epoetin alfa in patients with chemotherapy-associated anemia when hemoglobin levels fall below 10 g/dL, basing the decision to treat less-severe anemia (hemoglobin 10–12 g/dL) on clinical circumstances. For anemia associated with hematologic malignancies, the guidelines support the use of recombinant erythropoietin in patients with low-grade myelodysplastic syndrome. In this setting, neutropenia often dictates the use of G-CSF, which frequently augments the erythroid response to erythropoietin. In responding patients, the response duration is usually 2–3 years. A baseline serum erythropoietin level may help to predict the response; most patients with blood levels greater than 500 IU/L are unlikely to respond to any dose of the drug. Most patients treated with epoetin alfa experience an improvement in their anemia and their sense of well-being (Littlewood et al., 2001). Following these recommendations, case reports suggested a direct effect of both epoetin alfa and darbepoetin alfa in stimulation of tumor cells. A meta-analysis of a large number of patients and clinical trials estimated the risk at about 10% higher than for cancer patients not treated (Bohlius et al., 2009). Following on these results, new guidelines were issued (Rizzo et al., 2010). This finding is continuing to be evaluated by the FDA and warrants serious attention.

Use in Perioperative Patients Epoetin alfa has been used perioperatively to treat anemia (hematocrit 30%–36%) and reduce the need for allogeneic erythrocyte transfusion in nonanemic patients during and following surgery in patients with moderate or large anticipated blood loss. Patients undergoing elective orthopedic and cardiac procedures have been treated with 150–300 units/kg of epoetin alfa once daily for the 10 days preceding surgery, on the day of surgery, and for 4 days after surgery. As an alternative, 600 units/kg can be given on days 21, 14, and 7 before surgery, with an additional dose on the day of surgery. Using these dosing regimens, an average of four units of autologous blood can be obtained for postoperative use in a typical, nonanemic patient.

Other Uses Epoetin alfa has received orphan drug status from the FDA for the treatment of the anemia of prematurity, HIV infection, and myelodysplasia. In the last case, even very high doses (>1000 units/kg two to three times a week) sometimes have limited success. Highly competitive athletes have used epoetin alfa to increase their hemoglobin levels ("blood doping") and improve performance. Unfortunately, this misuse of the drug has been implicated in the deaths of several athletes and is strongly discouraged.

Myeloid Growth Factors

The myeloid growth factors are glycoproteins that stimulate the proliferation and differentiation of one or more myeloid cell types. Recombinant forms of several growth factors have been produced, including GM-CSF, G-CSF, IL-3, M-CSF or CSF-1, and stem cell factor (SCF) (see Table 41–1), although only G-CSF and GM-CSF have found meaningful clinical applications.

Myeloid growth factors are produced naturally by a number of different cells, including fibroblasts, endothelial cells, macrophages, and T cells (Figure 41–2). These factors are active at extremely low concentrations and act via membrane receptors of the cytokine receptor superfamily to activate the Jak/STAT signal transduction pathway. GM-CSF can stimulate proliferation, differentiation, and function of a number of the myeloid cell lineages (see Figure 41–1). It acts synergistically with other growth factors, including erythropoietin, at the level of the BFU. GM-CSF stimulates CFU-GM, CFU-M, CFU-E, and CFU-Meg to increase cell production. GM-CSF also enhances the migration, phagocytosis, superoxide production, and antibody-dependent cell-mediated toxicity of neutrophils, monocytes, and eosinophils (Weisbart et al., 1987).

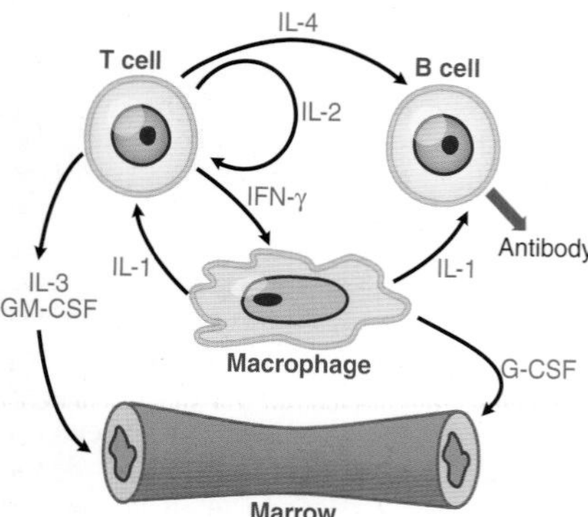

Figure 41–2 *Cytokine-cell interactions.* Macrophages, T cells, B cells, and marrow stem cells interact via several cytokines (IL-1, IL-2, IL-3, IL-4, IFN-γ, GM-CSF, and G-CSF) in response to a bacterial or a foreign antigen challenge. See Table 41–1 for the functional activities of these various cytokines.

The activity of G-CSF is restricted to neutrophils and their progenitors, stimulating their proliferation, differentiation, and function. It acts primarily on CFU-G, although it also can play a synergistic role with IL-3 and GM-CSF in stimulating other cell lines. G-CSF enhances phagocytic and cytotoxic activities of neutrophils. G-CSF reduces inflammation by inhibiting IL-1, tumor necrosis factor, and interferon gamma. G-CSF also mobilizes primitive hematopoietic cells, including hematopoietic stem cells, from the marrow into the peripheral blood (Sheridan et al., 1992). This observation has virtually transformed the practice of stem cell transplantation, such that more than 90% of all such procedures today use G-CSF–mobilized peripheral blood cells as the donor stem cell product.

Granulocyte-Macrophage Colony-Stimulating Factor

Recombinant human GM-CSF (*sargramostim*) is a glycoprotein with 127 amino acids. The primary therapeutic effect of sargramostim is to stimulate myelopoiesis.

The initial clinical application of sargramostim was in patients undergoing autologous marrow transplantation. By shortening the duration of neutropenia, transplant morbidity was significantly reduced without a change in long-term survival or risk of inducing an early relapse of the malignant process (Brandt et al., 1988).

The role of GM-CSF therapy in allogeneic transplantation is less clear. Its effect on neutrophil recovery is less pronounced in patients receiving prophylactic treatment of graft-versus-host disease (GVHD). However, it may improve survival in transplant patients who exhibit early graft failure (Nemunaitis et al., 1990).

It also has been used to mobilize CD34-positive progenitor cells for peripheral blood stem cell (PBSC) collection for transplantation after myeloablative chemotherapy (Haas et al., 1990). Sargramostim has been used to shorten the period of neutropenia and reduce morbidity in patients receiving intensive cancer chemotherapy (Gerhartz et al., 1993). It also stimulates myelopoiesis in some patients with cyclic neutropenia, myelodysplasia, aplastic anemia, or AIDS-associated neutropenia.

Sargramostim is administered by subcutaneous injection or slow intravenous infusion at doses of 125–500 μg/m²/d. Plasma levels of GM-CSF rise rapidly after subcutaneous injection and then decline with a $t_{1/2}$ of 2–3 h. When given intravenously, infusions should be maintained over 3–6 h. With the initiation of therapy, there is a transient decrease in the absolute leukocyte count secondary to cell margination and pulmonary vascular sequestration. This is followed by a dose-dependent, biphasic increase in leukocyte counts over the next 7–10 days. Once the drug is discontinued, the leukocyte count returns to baseline within 2–10 days. When GM-CSF is given in lower doses, the response is primarily neutrophilic, whereas monocytosis and eosinophilia are observed at larger doses. After hematopoietic stem cell transplantation or intensive chemotherapy, sargramostim is given daily during the period of maximum neutropenia until a sustained rise in the granulocyte count is observed. Frequent blood counts are essential to avoid an excessive rise in the granulocyte count. Higher doses are associated with more pronounced side effects, including bone pain, malaise, flu-like symptoms, fever, diarrhea, dyspnea, and rash. An acute reaction to the first dose, characterized by flushing, hypotension, nausea, vomiting, and dyspnea, with a fall in arterial oxygen saturation due to granulocyte sequestration in the pulmonary circulation, occurs in sensitive patients. With prolonged administration, a few patients may develop a capillary leak syndrome, with peripheral edema and pleural and pericardial effusions. Other serious side effects include transient supraventricular arrhythmia, dyspnea, and elevation of serum creatinine, bilirubin, and hepatic enzymes.

Granulocyte Colony-Stimulating Factor

Recombinant human G-CSF, *filgrastim*, is a glycoprotein with 175 amino acids. The principal action of filgrastim is the stimulation of CFU-G to increase neutrophil production (see Figure 41–1). Several forms of G-CSF are now available, including two longer-acting pegylated forms, pegfilgrastim and lipegfilgrastim.

Filgrastim is effective in the treatment of severe neutropenia after autologous hematopoietic stem cell transplantation and high-dose cancer chemotherapy (Lieschke and Burgess, 1992). Like GM-CSF, filgrastim shortens the period of severe neutropenia and reduces morbidity secondary to bacterial and fungal infections (Hammond et al., 1989). G-CSF also is effective in the treatment of severe congenital neutropenias. Filgrastim therapy can improve neutrophil counts in some patients with myelodysplasia or marrow damage (moderately SAA or tumor infiltration of the marrow). The neutropenia of patients with AIDS receiving zidovudine also can be partially or completely reversed.

Filgrastim is routinely used in patients undergoing PBSC collection for stem cell transplantation. It promotes the release of CD34⁺ progenitor cells from the marrow, reducing the number of collections necessary for transplant. G-CSF–induced mobilization of stem cells into the circulation also has the potential to enhance repair of other damaged organs in which PBSCs might play a role. PBSC grafts have a higher cell dose and somewhat more committed progenitor cells than steady-state marrow grafts, resulting in faster engraftment and faster immunological reconstitution.

Filgrastim is administered by subcutaneous injection or intravenous infusion over at least 30 min at doses of 1–20 μg/kg/d. The usual starting dose in a patient receiving myelosuppressive chemotherapy is 5 μg/kg/d. The distribution and clearance rate from plasma ($t_{1/2}$ of 3.5 h) are similar for both routes of administration. The recommended dose for pegfilgrastim is fixed at 6 mg for patients weighing more than 20 kg, administered subcutaneously once per chemotherapy cycle. As with GM-CSF therapy, G-CSF administered after hematopoietic stem cell transplantation or intensive cancer chemotherapy will increase granulocyte production and shorten the period of severe neutropenia. Frequent blood cell counts should be obtained to determine the effectiveness of the treatment and guide dosage adjustment. In patients who received intensive myelosuppressive cancer chemotherapy, daily administration of G-CSF for 14–21 days or more may be necessary to correct the neutropenia.

Adverse Reactions

Adverse reactions to filgrastim include mild-to-moderate bone pain in patients receiving high doses over a protracted period, local skin reactions following subcutaneous injection, and rare cutaneous necrotizing vasculitis. Patients with a history of hypersensitivity to proteins produced by *Escherichia coli* should not receive the drug; the same holds for patients with sickle cell anemia, as it has been known to precipitate severe crises and even death. Mild-to-moderate splenomegaly has been observed in patients on long-term therapy.

Patients with sickle cell anemia should not be administered G-CSF as it is reported to trigger severe crises. In 2004 and 2006, two papers were published suggesting that previously healthy stem cell donors receiving human G-CSF for mobilization displayed marrow cell changes concerning for the development of future malignancy. Previous studies have shown an increase in myeloid leukemia in patients with breast cancer receiving G-CSF for neutropenia. However, careful follow-up has failed to reveal any meaningful increase in myeloid leukemia in normal stem cell donors administered G-CSF.

Thrombopoietic Growth Factors

Interleukin 11

Interleukin 11 is a cytokine that stimulates hematopoiesis, intestinal epithelial cell growth, and osteoclastogenesis and inhibits adipogenesis. IL-11 also enhances megakaryocyte maturation in vitro. Recombinant human IL-11, *oprelvekin*, $t_{1/2}$ about 7 h, leads to a thrombopoietic response in 5–9 days when administered daily to normal subjects.

The drug is administered to patients at 25–50 μg/kg per day subcutaneously. Oprelvekin is approved for use in patients undergoing chemotherapy for nonmyeloid malignancies with severe thrombocytopenia (platelet count $< 20 \times 10^9$/L), and it is administered until the platelet count returns to more than 100×10^9/L. The major complications of therapy are fluid retention and associated cardiac symptoms, such as tachycardia, palpitation, edema, and shortness of breath; this is a significant concern in elderly patients and often requires concomitant therapy with diuretics. Also reported are blurred vision, injection site rash or erythema, and paresthesias.

Thrombopoietin Receptor Agonists

Thrombopoietin

Thrombopoietin, a glycoprotein produced by the liver, marrow stromal cells, and other organs, is the primary regulator of platelet production. Two forms of recombinant thrombopoietin have been tested for clinical use. One is a truncated version of the native protein, termed recombinant human megakaryocyte growth and development factor (rHuMGDF) that is covalently modified with polyethylene glycol to increase the circulatory $t_{1/2}$. The second is the full-length polypeptide termed recombinant human thrombopoietin (rHuTPO).

While use in thrombocytopenic clinical trial subjects was found to be safe, the use of rHuMGDF in a clinical trial of normal platelet donors, designed to boost the quantity of donated platelets, led to donor thrombocytopenia in several subjects due to the immunogenicity of this agent (Li et al., 2001). This experience led to both agents being abandoned for clinical use and to the development of small-molecular mimics of recombinant thrombopoietin, termed TRAs. Two of these agents are FDA approved for use in patients with immune thrombocytopenia (ITP), and one of the TRAs is also approved for use in patients with severe aplastic anemia (SAA) who have failed to respond to more conventional treatments. *Romiplostim* contains four copies of a small peptide that binds with high affinity to the thrombopoietin receptor, grafted onto an immunoglobulin scaffold. Romiplostim is safe and efficacious in patients with ITP (Kuter et al., 2008). The drug is administered weekly by subcutaneous injection, starting with a dose of 1 μg/kg, titrated to a maximum of 10 μg/kg, until the platelet count increases above 50×10^9/L. *Eltrombopag* is a small organic TRA that is administered orally; the recommended starting dose is 50 mg/d, titrated to 75 mg depending on platelet response. These and additional TRAs are undergoing clinical trials, in ITP and SAA, as well as in chemotherapy-induced thrombocytopenia and in several marrow disorders, including myelodysplastic syndromes.

Iron Deficiency and Other Hypochromic Anemias

The Bioavailability of Iron

Iron exists in the environment largely as ferric oxide, ferric hydroxide, and polymers. In this state, its biological availability is limited unless solubilized by acid or chelating agents. For example, bacteria and some plants produce high-affinity chelating agents that extract iron from the surrounding environment. Most mammals have little difficulty in acquiring iron; this is explained by ample iron intake and perhaps also by a greater efficiency in absorbing iron. Humans, however, appear to be an exception. Although total dietary intake of elemental iron in humans usually exceeds requirements, the bioavailability of the iron in the diet is limited.

HISTORICAL PERSPECTIVE

The modern understanding of iron metabolism began in 1937 with the work of McCance and Widdowson on iron absorption and excretion and Heilmeyer and Plotner's measurement of iron in plasma (Beutler, 2002). In 1947, Laurell described a plasma iron transport protein that he called *transferrin* (Laurell, 1951). Around the same time, Hahn and coworkers used radioisotopes to measure iron absorption and define the role of the intestinal mucosa to regulate this function (Hahn, 1948). In the next decade, Huff and associates initiated isotopic studies of internal iron metabolism. The subsequent development of practical clinical measurements of serum iron, transferrin saturation, plasma ferritin, and red cell protoporphyrin permitted the definition and detection of the body's iron store status and iron-deficient erythropoiesis. In 1994, Feder and colleagues identified the HFE gene, which is mutated in type 1 hemochromatosis (Feder et al., 1996). Subsequently, Ganz and colleagues discovered a peptide produced by the liver, which was termed *hepcidin* (Park et al., 2001), now known to be the master regulator of iron homeostasis and to play a role in anemia of chronic disease (Ganz and Nemeth, 2011).

Iron deficiency is the most common nutritional cause of anemia in humans. It can result from inadequate iron intake, malabsorption, blood loss, or an increased requirement, as with pregnancy. When severe, it results in a characteristic microcytic, hypochromic anemia. In addition to its role in hemoglobin, iron is an essential component of myoglobin, heme enzymes (e.g., cytochromes, catalase, and peroxidase), and the metalloflavoprotein enzymes (e.g., xanthine oxidase and α-glycerophosphate oxidase). Iron deficiency can affect metabolism in muscle independently of the effect of anemia on O_2 delivery. This may reflect a reduction in the activity of iron-dependent mitochondrial enzymes. Iron deficiency also has been associated with behavioral and learning problems in children, abnormalities in catecholamine metabolism, and possibly impaired heat production.

Metabolism of Iron

The body store of iron is divided between essential iron-containing compounds and excess iron, which is held in storage (Table 41–2). *Hemoglobin* dominates the essential fraction. Each hemoglobin molecule contains four atoms of iron, amounting to 1.1 mg (20 μmol) of iron/mL of red blood cells. Other forms of essential iron include *myoglobin* and a variety of heme and nonheme iron-dependent enzymes. *Ferritin* is a protein-iron storage complex that exists as individual molecules or as aggregates. *Apoferritin* (MW ~ 450 kDa) is composed of 24 polypeptide subunits that form an outer shell around a storage cavity for polynuclear hydrous ferric oxide phosphate. More than 30% of the weight of ferritin may be iron (4000 atoms of iron per ferritin molecule). Ferritin aggregates, referred to as *hemosiderin* and visible by light microscopy, constitute about one-third of normal stores. The two predominant sites of iron storage are the reticuloendothelial system and the hepatocytes.

Internal exchange of iron is accomplished by the plasma protein *transferrin*, a 76-kDa glycoprotein that has two binding sites for ferric iron. Iron is delivered from transferrin to intracellular sites by means of specific

TABLE 41–2 ■ THE BODY CONTENT OF IRON

	BODY WEIGHT, mg/kg	
	MALE	FEMALE
Essential iron		
Hemoglobin	31	28
Myoglobin and enzymes	6	5
Storage iron	13	4
Total	50	37

transferrin receptors in the plasma membrane. The iron-transferrin complex binds to the receptor, and the ternary complex is internalized through clathrin-coated pits by receptor-mediated endocytosis. A proton-pumping ATPase lowers the pH of the intracellular vesicular compartment (the endosomes) to about 5.5. Iron subsequently dissociates, and the receptor returns the apotransferrin to the cell surface, where it is released into the extracellular environment. Cells regulate their expression of transferrin receptors and intracellular ferritin in response to the iron supply (De Domenico et al., 2008). The synthesis of apoferritin and transferrin receptors is regulated posttranscriptionally by two iron-regulating proteins, IRP1 and IRP2. These IRPs are cytosolic RNA-binding proteins that bind to iron-regulating elements (IREs) present in the 5′ or 3′ untranslated regions of mRNA encoding apoferritin or the transferrin receptors, respectively. Binding of these IRPs to the 5′ IRE of apoferritin mRNA represses translation, whereas binding to the 3′ IRE of mRNA encoding the transferrin receptors enhances transcript stability, thereby increasing protein production.

The flow of iron through the plasma amounts to a total of 30–40 mg/d in the adult (~0.46 mg/kg of body weight). The major internal circulation of iron involves the erythron and reticuloendothelial cells (Figure 41–3). About 80% of the iron in plasma goes to the erythroid marrow to be packaged into new erythrocytes; these normally circulate for about 120 days before being catabolized by the reticuloendothelial system. At that time, a portion of the iron is immediately returned to the plasma bound to transferrin, while another portion is incorporated into the ferritin stores of reticuloendothelial cells and returned to the circulation more gradually. With abnormalities in erythrocyte maturation, the predominant portion of iron assimilated by the erythroid marrow may be rapidly localized in the reticuloendothelial cells as defective red cell precursors are broken down; this is termed *ineffective erythropoiesis*. The rate of iron turnover in plasma may be reduced by half or more with red cell aplasia, with all the iron directed to the hepatocytes for storage.

The human body conserves its iron stores to a remarkable degree. Only 10% of the total is lost per year by normal men (i.e., ~ 1 mg/d). Two-thirds of this iron is excreted from the GI tract as extravasated red cells, iron in bile, and iron in exfoliated mucosal cells. The other third is accounted for by small amounts of iron in desquamated skin and in the urine. Additional losses of iron occur in women due to menstruation. Although the average loss in menstruating women is about 0.5 mg per day, 10% of menstruating women lose more than 2 mg per day. Pregnancy and lactation impose an even greater requirement for iron (Table 41–3). Other causes of iron loss include blood donation, the use of anti-inflammatory drugs that cause

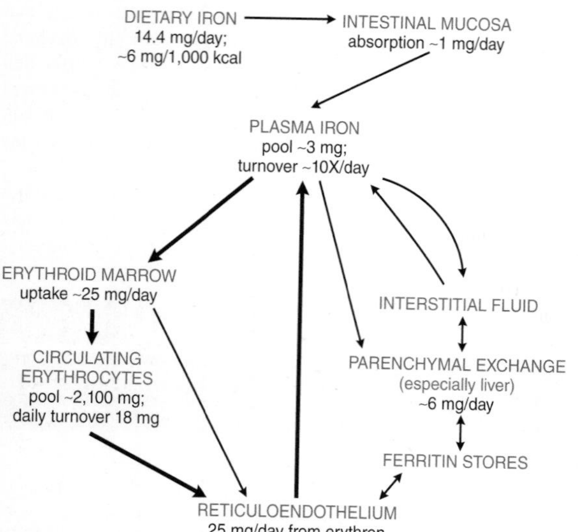

Figure 41–3 *Iron metabolism in humans (excretion omitted).*

TABLE 41–3 ■ IRON REQUIREMENTS FOR PREGNANCY

	AVERAGE (mg)	RANGE (mg)
External iron loss	170	150–200
Expansion of red cell mass	450	200–600
Fetal iron	270	200–370
Iron in placenta and cord	90	30–170
Blood loss at delivery	150	90–310
Total requirement[a]	980	580–1340
Cost of pregnancy[b]	680	440–1050

[a]Blood loss at delivery not included.
[b]Iron lost by the mother; expansion of red cell mass not included.
Source: Council on Foods and Nutrition. Iron deficiency in the United States. *JAMA*, **1968**, *203*:407–412. Used with permission.

bleeding from the gastric mucosa, and GI disease with associated bleeding.

The limited physiological losses of iron point to the primary importance of absorption in determining the body's iron content (Garrick and Garrick, 2009). After acidification and partial digestion of food in the stomach, iron is presented to the intestinal mucosa as either inorganic iron or heme iron. A ferrireductase, duodenal cytochrome B, located on the luminal surface of absorptive cells of the duodenum and upper small intestine, reduces the iron to the ferrous state, which is the substrate for divalent metal (ion) transporter 1 (DMT1, SLC11A2). DMT1 transports the iron to the basolateral membrane, where it is taken up by another transporter, *ferroportin* (Fpn; SLC40A1), and subsequently reoxidized to Fe^{3+}, primarily by *hephaestin* (Hp; *HEPH*), a transmembrane copper-dependent ferroxidase. Apotransferrin binds the resultant oxidized Fe^{3+}. The hepatic protein, hepcidin, binds to ferroportin, inducing its internalization and degradation, thus limiting the amount of iron released into the blood (Camaschella, 2013). Conditions that enhance the levels of hepcidin, such as inflammation, can result in decreased gut iron absorption, reduced serum iron, and inadequate iron available for developing red blood cells. Conversely, when hepcidin levels are low, such as in hemochromatosis, iron overload occurs due to excessive ferroportin-mediated iron influx.

Genetic polymorphism and consequent dysfunction in hepcidin or in proteins regulating its expression can result in inadequate levels of hepcidin and cause hereditary hemochromatosis (Pietrangelo, 2016). This can be due to polymorphism in *HFE*, resulting in a Cys→Tyr change at position 282 (C282Y) in the HFE protein, or pathogenic mutations in hepcidin (*HAMP*), ferroportin (*FPN*), hemojuvelin (*HJV*), or transferrin receptor 2 (*TfR2*). The phenotype may vary, ranging from severe, as in *HJV*– or *HAMP*–juvenile-onset hemochromatosis, to relatively milder forms of adult-onset hemochromatosis, resulting from defects in *FPN* or *TfR2*. Acquired hemochromatosis can result from excessive amounts of parenteral iron, such as may occur in multiple transfusions for hereditary anemia or acquired aplastic anemia, from loss of hepcidin-producing liver mass, or with disease factors such as hepatitis C or chronic alcoholism that impair the production of hepcidin.

Iron Requirements; Availability of Dietary Iron

Adult men must absorb only 13 μg of iron/kg of body weight/d (~1 mg/d), whereas menstruating women require about 21 μg/kg (~1.4 mg) per day. In the last two trimesters of pregnancy, requirements increase to about 80 μg/kg (5–6 mg) per day; infants have similar requirements due to their rapid growth (Table 41–4).

The difference between dietary supply and requirements is reflected in the size of iron stores, which are low or absent when iron balance is precarious and high when iron balance is favorable. In infants after the third month of life and in pregnant women after the first trimester, stores of iron are negligible. Menstruating women have approximately one-third the stored iron found in adult men (see Table 41–2).

TABLE 41–4 ■ DAILY IRON ABSORPTION REQUIREMENT

SUBJECT	IRON REQUIREMENT (μg/kg)	AVAILABLE IRON POOR DIET–GOOD DIET (μg/kg)	SAFETY FACTOR: AVAILABLE/REQUIREMENT
Infant	67	33–66	0.5–1
Child	22	48–96	2–4
Adolescent (male)	21	30–60	1.5–3
Adolescent (female)	20	30–60	1.5–3
Adult (male)	13	26–52	2–4
Adult (female)	21	18–36	1–2
Mid-to-late pregnancy	80	18–36	0.22–0.45

The numbers in columns 2 and 3 refer to iron absorption via the GI tract in micrograms per kilogram body weight. As noted in Figure 41–3, of 14.4 mg of dietary iron presented to the GI tract each day, only about 1 mg is absorbed. See text concerning factors influencing iron absorption and differential absorption of heme versus nonheme iron.

Although the iron content of the diet obviously is important, of greater nutritional significance is the bioavailability of iron in food. Heme iron, which constitutes only 6% of dietary iron, is far more available and is absorbed independent of the diet composition; it therefore represents 30% of iron absorbed (Conrad and Umbreit, 2000). The nonheme fraction represents the larger amount of dietary iron ingested by the economically underprivileged. In a vegetarian diet, nonheme iron is absorbed poorly because of the inhibitory action of a variety of dietary components, particularly phosphates. Ascorbic acid and meat facilitate the absorption of nonheme iron. In developed countries, the normal adult diet contains about 6 mg of iron per 1000 calories, providing an average daily intake for adult men of between 12 and 20 mg and for adult women of between 8 and 15 mg. Foods high in iron (>5 mg/100 g) include organ meats such as liver and heart, brewer's yeast, wheat germ, egg yolks, oysters, and certain dried beans and fruits; foods low in iron (<1 mg/100 g) include milk and milk products and most nongreen vegetables. Iron also may be added from cooking in iron pots. In assessing dietary iron intake, it is important to consider not only the amount of iron ingested but also its bioavailability.

Iron Deficiency

The prevalence of iron deficiency anemia in the U.S. is on the order of 1%–4% and depends on the economic status of the population (McLean et al., 2009). In developing countries, up to 20%–40% of infants and pregnant women may be affected. Better iron balance has resulted from the practice of fortifying flour, the use of iron-fortified formulas for infants, and the prescription of medicinal iron supplements during pregnancy.

Iron deficiency anemia results from dietary intake of iron that is inadequate to meet normal requirements (nutritional iron deficiency), blood loss, or interference with iron absorption (Camaschella, 2015). More severe iron deficiency is usually the result of blood loss, either from the GI tract or, in women, from the uterus. Finally, treatment of patients with erythropoietin can result in a functional iron deficiency. Iron deficiency in infants and young children can lead to behavioral disturbances and can impair development, which may not be fully reversible. Iron deficiency in children also can lead to an increased risk of lead toxicity secondary to pica and an increased absorption of heavy metals. Premature and low-birthweight infants are at greatest risk for developing iron deficiency, especially if they are not breast fed or do not receive iron-fortified formula (Finch, 2015). After the age of 2–3 years, the requirement for iron declines until adolescence, when rapid growth combined with irregular dietary habits again increase the risk of iron deficiency. Adolescent girls are at greatest risk; the dietary iron intake of most girls ages 11–18 is insufficient to meet their requirements.

Treatment of Iron Deficiency

General Therapeutic Principles

The response of iron deficiency anemia to iron therapy is influenced by several factors, including the severity of anemia, the ability of the patient to tolerate and absorb medicinal iron, and the presence of other complicating illnesses. Therapeutic effectiveness is best measured by the resulting increase in the rate of production of red cells. The magnitude of the marrow response to iron therapy is proportional to the severity of the anemia (level of erythropoietin stimulation) and the amount of iron delivered to marrow precursors.

The patient's ability to tolerate and absorb medicinal iron is a key factor in determining the rate of response to therapy. The small intestine regulates absorption and, with increasing doses of oral iron, limits the entry of iron into the bloodstream. This provides a natural ceiling on how much iron can be supplied by oral therapy. In the patient with moderately severe iron deficiency anemia, tolerable doses of oral iron will deliver, at most, 40–60 mg of iron per day to the erythroid marrow. This is an amount sufficient for production rates of two to three times normal.

Clinically, the effectiveness of iron therapy is best evaluated by tracking the reticulocyte response and the rise in the hemoglobin or the hematocrit. An increase in the reticulocyte count is not observed for at least 4–7 days after beginning therapy. A measurable increase in the hemoglobin level takes even longer. A decision regarding the effectiveness of treatment should not be made for 3–4 weeks after the start of treatment. An increase of 20 g/L or more in the concentration of hemoglobin by that time should be considered a positive response, assuming that no other change in the patient's clinical status can account for the improvement and that the patient has not been transfused.

If the response to oral iron is inadequate, the diagnosis must be reconsidered. A full laboratory evaluation should be conducted, and poor compliance by the patient or the presence of a concurrent inflammatory disease must be explored. A source of continued bleeding obviously should be sought. If no other explanation can be found, an evaluation of the patient's ability to absorb oral iron should be considered. There is no justification for merely continuing oral iron therapy beyond 3–4 weeks if a favorable response has not occurred.

Once a response to oral iron is demonstrated, therapy should be continued until the hemoglobin returns to normal. Treatment may be extended if it is desirable to replenish iron stores. This may require a considerable period of time because the rate of absorption of iron by the intestine will decrease markedly as iron stores are reconstituted. The prophylactic use of oral iron should be reserved for patients at high risk, including pregnant women, women with excessive menstrual blood loss, and infants. Iron supplements also may be of value for rapidly growing infants who are consuming substandard diets and for adults with a recognized cause of chronic blood loss. Except for infants, in whom the use of supplemented formulas is routine, the use of over-the-counter mixtures of vitamins and minerals to prevent iron deficiency should be discouraged.

Therapy With Oral Iron

Orally administered ferrous sulfate is the treatment of choice for iron deficiency. Ferrous salts are absorbed about three times as well as ferric salts. Variations in the particular ferrous salt have relatively little effect on bioavailability; the sulfate, fumarate, succinate, gluconate, aspartate, other ferrous salts, and polysaccharide-ferrihydrite complex are absorbed to approximately the same extent. The effective dose of all of these preparations is based on iron content.

Other iron compounds have utility in fortification of foods. Reduced iron (metallic iron, elemental iron) is as effective as ferrous sulfate, provided that the material employed has a small particle size. Large-particle ferrum reductum and iron phosphate salts have much lower bioavailability. Ferric edetate has been shown to have good bioavailability and to have advantages for maintenance of the normal appearance and taste of food. The amount of iron in iron tablets is important. It also is essential that the coating of the tablet dissolve rapidly in the stomach. Delayed-release preparations are available, but absorption from such preparations varies. Ascorbic acid (≥200 mg) increases the absorption of medicinal iron by at least 30%. However, the increased uptake is associated with an increase in the incidence of side effects. Preparations that contain other compounds with therapeutic action, such as vitamin B_{12}, folate, or cobalt, are not recommended because the patient's response to the combination cannot easily be interpreted.

The average dose for the treatment of iron deficiency anemia is about 200 mg of iron per day (2–3 mg/kg), given in three equal doses of 65 mg. Children weighing 15–30 kg can take half the average adult dose; small children and infants can tolerate relatively large doses of iron (e.g., 5 mg/kg). When the object is the prevention of iron deficiency in pregnant women, for example, doses of 15 to 30 mg of iron per day are adequate. Bioavailability of iron is reduced with food and by concurrent antacids. For a rapid response or to counteract continued bleeding, as much as 120 mg of iron may be administered four times a day.

The duration of treatment is governed by the rate of recovery of hemoglobin (Table 41–5) and the desire to create iron stores. The former depends on the severity of the anemia. With a daily rate of repair of 2 g of hemoglobin per liter of whole blood, the red cell mass usually is reconstituted within 1–2 months. Thus, an individual with a hemoglobin of 50 g per liter may achieve a normal complement of 150 g/L in about 50 days, whereas an individual with a hemoglobin of 100 g/L may take only half that time. The creation of stores of iron requires many months of oral iron administration. The rate of absorption decreases rapidly after recovery from anemia, and after 3–4 months of treatment, stores may increase at a rate of not much more than 100 mg/month. Much of the strategy of continued therapy depends on the estimated future iron balance. Patients with an inadequate diet may require continued therapy with low doses of iron. If the bleeding has stopped, no further therapy is required after the hemoglobin has returned to normal. With continued bleeding, long-term, high-dose therapy clearly is indicated.

Untoward Effects of Oral Preparations of Iron. Side effects of oral iron preparations include heartburn, nausea, upper gastric discomfort, and diarrhea or constipation. A good policy is to initiate therapy at a small dosage and then gradually to increase the dosage to that desired. Only individuals with underlying disorders that augment the absorption of iron run the hazard of developing iron overload (hemochromatosis).

Iron Poisoning. Large amounts of ferrous salts are toxic, but fatalities are rare in adults. Most deaths occur in children, particularly between the ages of 12 and 24 months. As little as 1–2 g of iron may cause death, but 2–10 g usually is ingested in fatal cases. All iron preparations should be kept in childproof bottles. Signs and symptoms of severe poisoning may occur within 30 min after ingestion or may be delayed for several hours. They include abdominal pain, diarrhea, or vomiting of brown or bloody stomach contents containing pills. Of particular concern are pallor or cyanosis, lassitude, drowsiness, hyperventilation due to acidosis, and cardiovascular collapse. If death does not occur within 6 h, there may be a transient period of apparent recovery, followed by death in 12–24 h. The corrosive injury to the stomach may result in pyloric stenosis or gastric scarring.

In the evaluation of a child thought to have ingested iron, a color test for iron in the gastric contents and determination of the concentration of iron in plasma can be performed. If the latter is less than 63 μmol (3.5 mg/L), the child is not in immediate danger. However, vomiting should be induced when there is iron in the stomach, and an X-ray should be taken to evaluate the number of pills remaining in the small bowel (iron tablets are radiopaque). When the plasma concentration of iron is greater than the total iron-binding capacity (63 μmol; 3.5 mg/L), *deferoxamine* should be administered (see Chapter 71). The speed of diagnosis and therapy is important. With early treatment, the mortality from iron poisoning can be reduced from 45% to about 1%. *Deferiprone* and *deferasirox* are oral iron chelators approved by the FDA for treatment of patients with thalassemia who have iron overload.

TABLE 41–5 ■ AVERAGE RESPONSE TO ORAL IRON

TOTAL DOSE OF IRON (mg/d)	ESTIMATED ABSORPTION %	ESTIMATED ABSORPTION mg	INCREASE IN BLOOD HEMOGLOBIN (g/L/d)
35	40	14	0.7
105	24	25	1.4
195	18	35	1.9
390	12	45	2.2

Therapy With Parenteral Iron

When oral iron therapy fails, parenteral iron administration may be an effective alternative. Common indications are iron malabsorption (e.g., sprue, short-bowel syndrome), severe oral iron intolerance, as a routine supplement to total parenteral nutrition, and in patients who are receiving erythropoietin. Parenteral iron can be given to iron-deficient patients and pregnant women to create iron stores, something that would take months to achieve by the oral route. The indications for parenteral iron therapy include documented iron deficiency and intolerance or irresponsiveness to oral iron.

The rate of hemoglobin response is determined by the balance between the severity of the anemia (the level of erythropoietin stimulus) and the delivery of iron to the marrow from iron absorption and iron stores. When a large intravenous dose of iron dextran is given to a severely anemic patient, the hematologic response can exceed that seen with oral iron for 1–3 weeks. Subsequently, however, the response is no better than that seen with oral iron.

Parenteral iron therapy should be used only when clearly indicated because acute hypersensitivity, including anaphylactic and anaphylactoid reactions, can occur. Other reactions to intravenous iron include headache, malaise, fever, generalized lymphadenopathy, arthralgias, urticaria, and, in some patients with rheumatoid arthritis, exacerbation of the disease.

Several iron formulations are available in the U.S. (Larson and Coyne, 2014). These include iron dextran, sodium ferric gluconate, ferumoxytol, iron sucrose, and ferric carboxymaltose. Ferumoxytol is a semisynthetic carbohydrate-coated superparamagnetic iron oxide nanoparticle approved for treatment of iron deficiency anemia in patients with chronic kidney disease; the ferumoxytol has to be administered safely as a 1.02-g infusion over a relatively short infusion time of 15 min (Auerbach et al., 2013). Indications for ferric gluconate and iron sucrose are limited to patients with chronic kidney disease and documented iron deficiency, although broader applications are being advocated (Larson and Coyne, 2014).

Iron Dextran. Iron dextran injection is a colloidal solution of ferric oxyhydroxide complexed with polymerized dextran (molecular weight ~ 180,000 Da) that contains 50 mg/mL of elemental iron. The use of low-molecular-weight iron dextran has reduced the incidence of toxicity relative to that observed with high-molecular-weight preparations. Iron dextran can be administered by intravenous (preferred) or intramuscular injection. Injection of a therapeutic dose should be initiated only after a test dose of 0.5 mL (25 mg of iron). Given intravenously in a dose less than 500 mg, the iron dextran complex is cleared with a plasma $t_{1/2}$ of 6 h. When 1 g or more is administered intravenously as total-dose therapy, reticuloendothelial cell clearance is constant at

10–20 mg/h.

Intramuscular injection of iron dextran should be initiated only after a test dose of 0.5 mL (25 mg of iron). If no adverse reactions are observed, the injections can proceed. The daily dose ordinarily should not exceed 0.5 mL (25 mg of iron) for infants weighing less than 4.5 kg, 1 mL (50 mg of iron) for children weighing less than 9 kg, and 2 mL (100 mg of iron) for other patients. However, local reactions and the concern about malignant change at the site of injection make intramuscular administration inappropriate except when the intravenous route is inaccessible. The patient should be observed for signs of immediate anaphylaxis and for an hour after injection for any signs of vascular instability or hypersensitivity, including respiratory distress, hypotension, tachycardia, or back or chest pain. Delayed hypersensitivity reactions also are observed, especially in patients with rheumatoid arthritis or a history of allergies. Fever, malaise, lymphadenopathy, arthralgias, and urticaria can develop days or weeks following injection and last for prolonged periods of time. Use iron dextran with extreme caution in patients with rheumatoid arthritis or other connective tissue diseases and during the acute phase of an inflammatory illness. Once hypersensitivity is documented, iron dextran therapy must be abandoned.

With multiple total-dose infusions such as those sometimes used in the treatment of chronic GI blood loss, accumulations of slowly metabolized iron dextran stores in reticuloendothelial cells can be impressive. The plasma ferritin level also can rise to levels associated with iron overload. It seems prudent, however, to withhold the drug whenever the plasma ferritin rises above 800 μg/L.

Sodium Ferric Gluconate. Sodium ferric gluconate is an intravenous iron preparation with a molecular size of about 295 kDa and an osmolality of 990 $mOsm/kg^{-1}$. Administration of ferric gluconate at doses ranging from 62.5 to 125 mg during hemodialysis is associated with transferrin saturation exceeding 100%. Unlike iron dextran, which requires processing by macrophages that may require several weeks, about 80% of sodium ferric gluconate is delivered to transferrin within 24 h. Sodium ferric gluconate also has a lower risk of inducing serious anaphylactic reactions than iron dextran (Sengolge et al., 2005).

Iron Sucrose. Iron sucrose is a complex of polynuclear iron (III)-hydroxide in sucrose (Beguin and Jaspers, 2014). Following intravenous injection, the complex is taken up by the reticuloendothelial system, where it dissociates into iron and sucrose. Iron sucrose is generally administered in daily amounts of 100–200 mg within a 14-day period to a total cumulative dose of 1000 mg. Like sodium ferric gluconate, iron sucrose appears to be better tolerated and to cause fewer adverse events than iron dextran (Hayat, 2008). This agent is FDA-approved for the treatment of iron deficiency in patients with chronic kidney disease. Chronic use has the potential to cause renal tubulointerstitial damage (Agarwal, 2006).

Ferric Carboxymaltose. Ferric carboxymaltose is an iron complex consisting of a ferric hydroxide core and a carbohydrate shell (Keating, 2015). With this preparation, a replenishment dose of up to 1000 mg of iron can be administered in 15 min. Intravenous administration results in transient elevations in serum iron, serum ferritin, and transferrin saturation, with subsequent correction in hemoglobin levels and replenishment of depleted iron stores. Ferric carboxymaltose is rapidly cleared from the circulation, becoming distributed (~80%) in the marrow, as well as the liver and spleen. Common reported drug-related adverse effects include headache, dizziness, nausea, abdominal pain, constipation, diarrhea, rash, and injection site reactions. However, the incidence of drug-related adverse events appears similar to those of patients treated with oral ferrous sulfate. Ferric carboxymaltose is FDA-approved for therapy of iron deficiency anemia.

Copper, Pyridoxine, and Riboflavin

Copper

Copper has redox properties similar to those of iron, which simultaneously are essential and potentially toxic to the cell. Cells have virtually no free copper. Instead, copper is stored by metallothioneins and distributed by specialized chaperones to sites that make use of its redox properties. Transfer of copper to nascent cuproenzymes is performed by individual or collective activities of P-type ATPases, ATP7A and ATP7B, which are expressed in all tissues (Nevitt et al., 2012). In mammals, the liver is the organ most responsible for the storage, distribution, and excretion of copper. Mutations in ATP7A or ATP7B that interfere with this function have been found responsible for Wilson disease or Menkes syndrome (steely hair syndrome) (de Bie et al., 2007), respectively, which can result in life-threatening hepatic failure.

Copper deficiency is extremely rare; the amount present in food is more than adequate to provide the needed body complement of slightly more than 100 mg. Even in clinical states associated with hypocupremia (sprue, celiac disease, and nephrotic syndrome), effects of copper deficiency usually are not demonstrable. Anemia due to copper deficiency has been described in individuals who have undergone intestinal bypass surgery, in those who are receiving parenteral nutrition, in malnourished infants, and in patients ingesting excessive amounts of zinc (Willis et al., 2005). Copper deficiency interferes with the absorption of iron and its release from reticuloendothelial cells. In humans, the prominent findings have been leukopenia, particularly granulocytopenia, and anemia. Concentrations of iron in plasma are variable, and the anemia is not always microcytic. When a low plasma copper concentration is determined in the presence of leukopenia and anemia, a therapeutic trial with copper is appropriate. Daily doses up to 0.1 mg/kg of cupric sulfate have been given by mouth, or 1–2 mg per day may be added to the solution of nutrients for parenteral administration.

Pyridoxine

Patients with either hereditary or acquired sideroblastic anemia characteristically have impaired hemoglobin synthesis and accumulate iron in the perinuclear mitochondria of erythroid precursor cells, so-called ringed sideroblasts. Hereditary sideroblastic anemia is an X-linked recessive trait with variable penetrance and expression that results from mutations in the erythrocyte form of δ-aminolevulinate synthase.

Oral therapy with pyridoxine is of proven benefit in correcting the sideroblastic anemias associated with the antituberculosis drugs isoniazid and pyrazinamide, which act as vitamin B_6 antagonists. A daily dose of 50 mg of pyridoxine completely corrects the defect without interfering with treatment, and routine supplementation of pyridoxine often is recommended (see Chapter 56). In contrast, if pyridoxine is given to counteract the sideroblastic abnormality associated with administration of levodopa, the effectiveness of levodopa in controlling Parkinson disease is decreased. Pyridoxine therapy does not correct the sideroblastic abnormalities produced by chloramphenicol or lead. Patients with idiopathic acquired sideroblastic anemia generally fail to respond to oral pyridoxine, and those individuals who appear to have a pyridoxine-responsive anemia require prolonged therapy with large doses of the vitamin, 50–500 mg/d. The occasional patient who is refractory to oral pyridoxine may respond to parenteral administration of pyridoxal phosphate. However, oral pyridoxine in doses of 200–300 mg per day produces intracellular concentrations of pyridoxal phosphate equal to or greater than those generated by therapy with the phosphorylated vitamin.

Riboflavin

The spontaneous appearance in humans of red cell aplasia due to riboflavin deficiency undoubtedly is rare, if it occurs at all. Riboflavin deficiency has been described in combination with infection and protein deficiency, both of which are capable of producing hypoproliferative anemia. However, it seems reasonable to include riboflavin in the nutritional management of patients with gross, generalized malnutrition.

Vitamin B_{12}, Folic Acid, and the Treatment of Megaloblastic Anemias

Vitamin B_{12} and folic acid are dietary essentials. A deficiency of either vitamin impairs DNA synthesis in any cell in which chromosomal replication and division are taking place. Because tissues with the greatest rate of cell turnover show the most dramatic changes, the hematopoietic system is especially sensitive to deficiencies of these vitamins.

Cellular Roles of Vitamin B_{12} and Folic Acid

The major roles of vitamin B_{12} and folic acid in intracellular metabolism are summarized in Figure 41–4. Intracellular vitamin B_{12} is maintained as two active coenzymes: *methylcobalamin* and *deoxyadenosylcobalamin*.

Methylcobalamin (CH_3B_{12}) supports the *methionine synthetase* reaction, which is essential for normal metabolism of folate (Weissbach, 2008). Methyl groups contributed by methyltetrahydrofolate ($CH_3H_4PteGlu_1$) are used to form methylcobalamin, which then acts as a methyl group donor for the conversion of homocysteine to methionine. This folate-cobalamin interaction is pivotal for normal synthesis of purines and pyrimidines, and therefore of DNA. The methionine synthetase reaction is largely responsible for the control of the recycling of folate cofactors; the maintenance of intracellular concentrations of folylpolyglutamates; and, through the synthesis of methionine and its product *SAM*, the maintenance of a number of methylation reactions.

Deoxyadenosylcobalamin (deoxyadenosyl B_{12}) is a cofactor for the *mitochondrial mutase* enzyme that catalyzes the isomerization of l-methylmalonyl CoA to succinyl CoA, an important reaction in carbohydrate and lipid metabolism. This reaction has no direct relationship to the metabolic pathways that involve folate.

Because methyltetrahydrofolate is the principal folate congener supplied to cells, the transfer of the methyl group to cobalamin is essential for the adequate supply of tetrahydrofolate ($H_4PteGlu_1$). Tetrahydrofolate is a precursor for the formation of intracellular folylpolyglutamates; it also acts as the acceptor of a one-carbon unit in the conversion of serine to glycine, with the resultant formation of 5,10-methylenetetrahydrofolate (5,10-$CH_2H_4PteGlu$). The last derivative donates the methylene group to dUMP for the synthesis of dTMP—an extremely important reaction in DNA synthesis. In the process, the 5,10-$CH_2H_4PteGlu$ is converted to dihydrofolate ($H_2PteGlu$). The cycle then is completed by the reduction of the $H_2PteGlu$ to $H_4PteGlu$ by dihydrofolate reductase, the step that is blocked by folate antagonists such as methotrexate (see Chapter 66). As shown in Figure 41–4, other pathways also lead to the synthesis of 5,10-methylenetetrahydrofolate. These pathways are important in the metabolism of FIGLU and purines and pyrimidines.

Deficiency of either vitamin B_{12} or folate decreases the synthesis of methionine and SAM and consequently interferes with protein biosynthesis, a number of methylation reactions, and the synthesis of polyamines. In addition, the cell responds to the deficiency by redirecting folate metabolic pathways to supply increasing amounts of methyltetrahydrofolate; this tends to preserve essential methylation reactions at the expense of nucleic acid synthesis. With vitamin B_{12} deficiency, methylenetetrahydrofolate reductase activity increases, directing available intracellular folates into the methyltetrahydrofolate pool (not shown in Figure 41–4). The methyltetrahydrofolate then is trapped by the lack of sufficient vitamin B_{12} to accept and transfer methyl groups, and subsequent steps in folate metabolism that require tetrahydrofolate are deprived of substrate. This process provides a common basis for the development of megaloblastic anemia with deficiency of either vitamin B_{12} or folic acid.

The mechanisms responsible for the neurological lesions of vitamin B_{12} deficiency are less well understood (Solomon, 2007). Damage to the myelin sheath is the most obvious lesion in this neuropathy. This observation led to the early suggestion that the deoxyadenosyl B_{12}–dependent methylmalonyl CoA mutase reaction, a step in propionate metabolism, is related to the abnormality. However, other evidence suggests that the deficiency of methionine synthetase and the block of the conversion of methionine to SAM are more likely to be responsible.

HISTORY

The discovery of vitamin B_{12} and folic acid is a dramatic story that began almost 200 years ago and includes two Nobel Prize–winning discoveries. Beginning in 1824, Combe and Addison wrote a series of case reports describing what must have been megaloblastic anemias (still known as Addisonian pernicious anemia). Austin Flint in 1860 first described a severe gastric atrophy and called attention to its possible relationship to the anemia. After Whipple's observation in 1925 that liver is a source of a potent hematopoietic substance for iron-deficient dogs, Minot and Murphy carried out Nobel Prize–winning experiments that demonstrated the effectiveness of the feeding of liver to reverse pernicious anemia. Soon thereafter, Castle defined the need for both intrinsic factor, a substance secreted by the parietal cells of the gastric mucosa, and extrinsic factor, the vitamin-like material provided by crude liver extracts. Nearly 20 years passed before Rickes and coworkers and Smith and Parker isolated and crystallized vitamin B_{12}; Dorothy Hodgkin received the Nobel Prize for determining its X-ray crystal structure.

As attempts were being made to purify extrinsic factor, Wills and her associates described a macrocytic anemia in women in India that responded to a factor present in crude liver extracts but not in the purified fractions known to be effective in pernicious anemia. This factor, first called Wills' factor and later vitamin M, is now known to be folic acid. The term *folic acid* was coined by Mitchell and coworkers in 1941, after its isolation from leafy vegetables. From more recent work, we know that neither vitamin B_{12} nor folic acid as purified from foodstuffs is the active coenzyme in humans. During extraction, active labile forms are converted to stable congeners of vitamin B_{12} and folic acid, cyanocobalamin and PteGlu, respectively. These congeners must be modified in vivo to be effective. Despite our knowledge of the intracellular metabolic pathways in which these vitamins function as required cofactors, many questions remain, among them, What is the relationship of vitamin B_{12} deficiency to the neurological abnormalities that occur in megaloblastic anemia?

Vitamin B_{12} and Human Health

Humans depend on exogenous sources of vitamin B_{12} (see structure in Figure 41–5). In nature, the primary sources are certain microorganisms that grow in soil or the intestinal lumen of animals that synthesize the vitamin. The daily nutritional requirement of 3–5 μg must generally be obtained from animal by-products in the diet. However, some vitamin B_{12} is available from legumes, which are contaminated with bacteria that can synthesize vitamin B_{12}, and vegetarians often fortify their diets with a wide range of vitamins and minerals; thus, strict vegetarians rarely develop vitamin B_{12} deficiency. The terms *vitamin B_{12}* and *cyanocobalamin* are used interchangeably as generic terms for all of the cobamides active in humans. Preparations of vitamin B_{12} for therapeutic use contain either cyanocobalamin or hydroxocobalamin because only these derivatives remain active after storage.

Metabolic Functions. The active coenzymes methylcobalamin and 5-deoxyadenosylcobalamin are essential for cell growth and replication. Methylcobalamin is required for the conversion of homocysteine to methionine and its derivative S-adenosylmethionine. In addition, when concentrations of vitamin B_{12} are inadequate, folate becomes "trapped" as methyltetrahydrofolate to cause a functional deficiency of other required intracellular forms of folic acid. The hematologic abnormalities in vitamin B_{12}–deficient patients result from this process. Deoxyadenosylcobalamin is required for the rearrangement of methylmalonyl CoA to succinyl CoA.

ADME and Daily Requirements

In the presence of gastric acid and pancreatic proteases, dietary vitamin B_{12} is released from food and salivary-binding protein and bound to gastric intrinsic factor. When the vitamin B_{12}–intrinsic factor complex reaches the ileum, it interacts with a receptor on the mucosal cell surface and is actively transported into circulation. Vitamin B_{12} deficiency in adults is rarely the result of a deficient diet per se; rather, it usually reflects a defect in one or

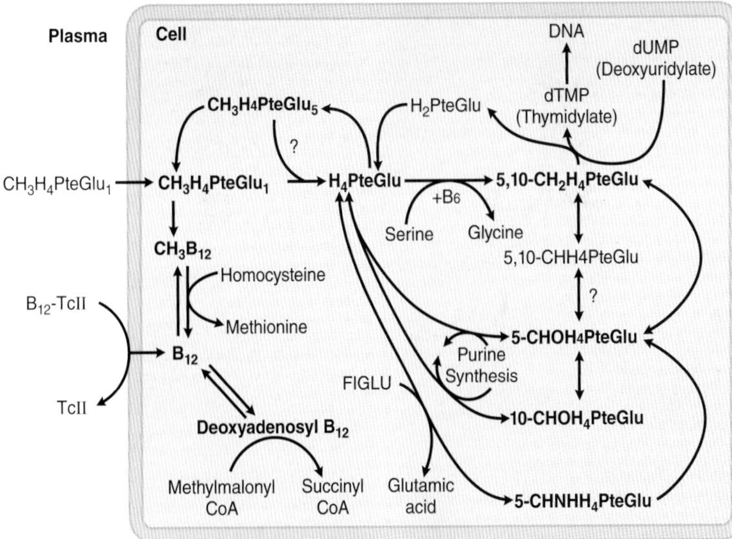

Figure 41–4 *Interrelationships and metabolic roles of vitamin B_{12} and folic acid.* See text for explanation and Figure 41–5 for structures of the various folate coenzymes. FIGLU, formiminoglutamic acid, which arises from the catabolism of histidine; TcII, transcobalamin II.

another aspect of this complex sequence of absorption (Figure 41–6). Antibodies to parietal cells or intrinsic factor complex also can play a prominent role in producing a deficiency. Several intestinal conditions can interfere with absorption, including pancreatic disorders (loss of pancreatic protease secretion), bacterial overgrowth, intestinal parasites, sprue, and localized damage to ileal mucosal cells by disease or as a result of surgery.

Absorbed vitamin B_{12} binds to transcobalamin II, a plasma β globulin, for transport to tissues. The supply of vitamin B_{12} available for tissues is directly related to the size of the hepatic storage pool and the amount of vitamin B_{12} bound to transcobalamin II (see Figure 41–6). Vitamin B_{12} bound to transcobalamin II is rapidly cleared from plasma and preferentially distributed to hepatic parenchymal cells. As much as 90% of the body's stores of vitamin B_{12}, from 1 to 10 mg, is in the liver. Vitamin B_{12} is stored as the active coenzyme with a turnover rate of 0.5–8 μg per day. The recommended daily intake of the vitamin in adults is 2.4 μg. Approximately 3 μg of cobalamins are secreted into bile each day, 50%–60% of which is not destined for reabsorption. Interference with reabsorption by intestinal disease can progressively deplete hepatic stores of the vitamin.

Vitamin B_{12} Deficiency

The plasma concentration of vitamin B_{12} is the best routine measure of B_{12} deficiency and normally ranges from 150 to 660 pM (~200–900 pg/mL). Deficiency should be suspected whenever the concentration falls below 150 pM. The correlation is excellent except when the plasma concentrations of transcobalamin I and III are increased, as occurs with hepatic disease or a myeloproliferative disorder. Inasmuch as the vitamin B_{12} bound to these transport proteins is relatively unavailable to cells, tissues can become deficient when the concentration of vitamin B_{12} in plasma is normal or even high. In subjects with congenital absence of transcobalamin II, megaloblastic anemia occurs despite relatively normal plasma concentrations of vitamin B_{12}; the anemia will respond to parenteral doses of vitamin B_{12} that exceed the renal clearance.

Vitamin B_{12} deficiency is recognized clinically by its impact on the hematopoietic and nervous systems. The sensitivity of the hematopoietic system relates to its high rate of cell turnover. Other tissues with high rates of cell turnover (e.g., mucosa and cervical epithelium) also have high requirements for the vitamin. As a result of an inadequate supply of

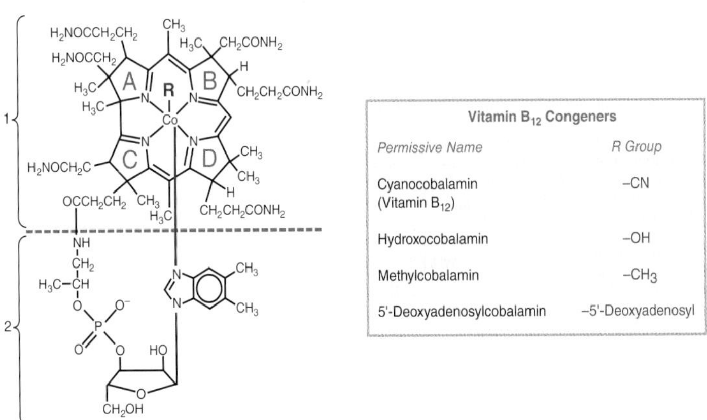

Vitamin B_{12} Congeners	
Permissive Name	R Group
Cyanocobalamin (Vitamin B_{12})	–CN
Hydroxocobalamin	–OH
Methylcobalamin	$-CH_3$
5'-Deoxyadenosylcobalamin	–5'-Deoxyadenosyl

Figure 41–5 *The structures and nomenclature of vitamin B_{12} congeners.* The vitamin B_{12} molecule has three major portions: (1) a planar group porphyrin-like ring structure with four reduced pyrrole rings (A–D) linked to a central cobalt atom and extensively substituted with methyl, acetamide, and propionamide residues; (2) a 5,6-dimethylbenzimidazolyl nucleotide, which links almost at right angles to the planar nucleus with bonds to the cobalt atom and to the propionate side chain of the C pyrrole ring; and (3) a variable R group—the most important of which are found in the stable compounds cyanocobalamin and hydroxocobalamin and the active coenzymes methylcobalamin and 5-deoxyadenosylcobalamin.

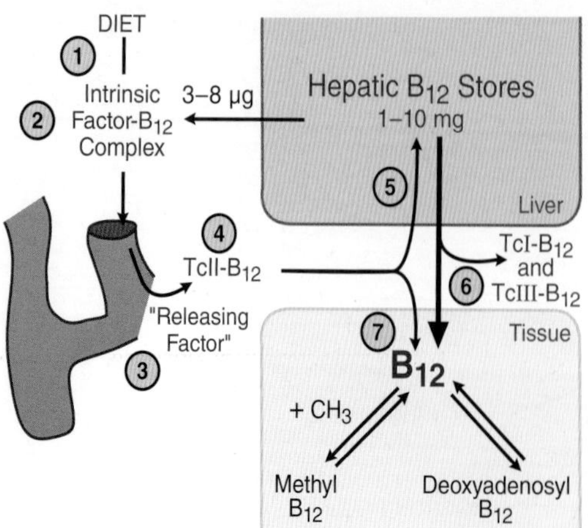

Figure 41–6 *Absorption and distribution of vitamin B_{12}.* Deficiency of vitamin B_{12} can result from a congenital or acquired defect in (1) inadequate dietary supply; (2) inadequate secretion of intrinsic factor (classical pernicious anemia); (3) ileal disease; (4) congenital absence of TcII; or (5) rapid depletion of hepatic stores by interference with reabsorption of vitamin B_{12} excreted in bile. The utility of measurements of the concentration of vitamin B_{12} in plasma to estimate supply available to tissues can be compromised by liver disease and (6) the appearance of abnormal amounts of TcI and TcIII in plasma. The formation of methylcobalamin requires (7) normal transport into cells and an adequate supply of folic acid as $CH_3H_4PteGlu_1$.

vitamin B_{12}, DNA replication becomes highly abnormal. Once a hematopoietic stem cell is committed to enter a programmed series of cell divisions, the defect in chromosomal replication results in an inability of maturing cells to complete nuclear divisions while cytoplasmic maturation continues at a relatively normal rate. This results in the production of morphologically abnormal cells and death of cells during maturation, a phenomenon referred to as *ineffective hematopoiesis*. Severe deficiency affects all cell lines, and pronounced pancytopenia results.

The diagnosis of a vitamin B_{12} deficiency usually can be made using measurements of the serum vitamin B_{12} or serum methylmalonate (which is somewhat more sensitive and useful in identifying metabolic deficiency in patients with normal serum vitamin B_{12} levels). In managing a patient with severe megaloblastic anemia, a therapeutic trial using very small doses of the vitamin can be used to confirm the diagnosis. Serial measurements of the reticulocyte count, serum iron, and hematocrit are performed to define the characteristic recovery of normal red cell production. The *Schilling test* can be used to measure the absorption of the vitamin and delineate the mechanism of the disease. By performing the Schilling test with and without added intrinsic factor, it is possible to discriminate between intrinsic factor deficiency by itself and primary ileal cell disease. *Vitamin B_{12} deficiency can irreversibly damage the nervous system.* Because the neurological damage can be dissociated from the changes in the hematopoietic system, vitamin B_{12} deficiency must be considered in elderly patients with dementia or psychiatric disorders, even if they are not anemic (Spence, 2016).

Vitamin B_{12} Therapy

Vitamin B_{12} has an undeserved reputation as a health tonic and has been used for a number of disease states. A number of multivitamin preparations are marketed either as nutritional supplements or for the treatment of anemia; many are supplemented with intrinsic factor. Although the combination of oral vitamin B_{12} and intrinsic factor would appear to be ideal for patients with an intrinsic factor deficiency, such preparations are not reliable.

Vitamin B_{12} is available for injection or oral administration; combinations with other vitamins and minerals also can be given orally or parenterally. The choice of a preparation always depends on the cause of the deficiency. Oral administration cannot be relied on for effective therapy in the patient with a marked deficiency of vitamin B_{12} and abnormal hematopoiesis or neurological deficits. The treatment of choice for vitamin B_{12} deficiency is cyanocobalamin administered by intramuscular or subcutaneous injection, never intravenously. Cyanocobalamin is administered in doses of 1–1000 μg. Tissue uptake, storage, and utilization depend on the availability of transcobalamin II. Doses greater than 100 μg are cleared rapidly from plasma into the urine, and administration of larger amounts of vitamin B_{12} will not result in greater retention of the vitamin. Administration of 1000 μg is of value in the performance of the Schilling test. After isotopically labeled vitamin B_{12} is administered orally, the compound that is absorbed can be quantitatively recovered in the urine if 1000 μg of cyanocobalamin is administered intramuscularly. This unlabeled material saturates the transport system and tissue binding sites, so more than 90% of the labeled and unlabeled vitamin is excreted during the next 24 h.

Effective use of the vitamin B_{12} depends on accurate diagnosis and an understanding of the following general principles of therapy:

- Vitamin B_{12} should be given prophylactically only when there is a reasonable probability that a deficiency exists or will exist (i.e., dietary deficiency in the strict vegetarian, the predictable malabsorption of vitamin B_{12} in patients who have had a gastrectomy, and certain diseases of the small intestine) (Del Villar Madrigal et al., 2015). When GI function is normal, an oral prophylactic supplement of vitamins and minerals, including vitamin B_{12}, may be indicated. Otherwise, the patient should receive monthly injections of cyanocobalamin.
- The relative ease of treatment with vitamin B_{12} should not prevent a full investigation of the etiology of the deficiency. The initial diagnosis usually is suggested by macrocytic anemia or an unexplained neuropsychiatric disorder.
- Therapy always should be as specific as possible. Although a large number of multivitamin preparations are available, the use of shotgun vitamin therapy in the treatment of vitamin B_{12} deficiency can be dangerous: Sufficient folic acid may be given to result in a hematologic recovery that can mask continued vitamin B_{12} deficiency and permit neurological damage to develop or progress.
- Although a classical therapeutic trial with small amounts of vitamin B_{12} can help confirm the diagnosis, acutely ill elderly patients may not be able to tolerate the delay in the correction of a severe anemia. Such patients require supplemental blood transfusions and immediate therapy with folic acid and vitamin B_{12} to guarantee rapid recovery.
- Long-term therapy with vitamin B_{12} must be evaluated at intervals of 6–12 months in patients who are otherwise well. If there is an additional illness or a condition that may increase the requirement for the vitamin (e.g., pregnancy), reassessment should be performed more frequently.

Treatment of the Acutely Ill Patient. The therapeutic approach depends on the severity of the illness. In uncomplicated pernicious anemia, in which the abnormality is restricted to a mild or moderate anemia without leukopenia, thrombocytopenia, or neurological signs or symptoms, the administration of vitamin B_{12} alone will suffice. Moreover, therapy may be delayed until other causes of megaloblastic anemia have been excluded and sufficient studies of GI function have been performed to reveal the underlying cause of the disease. In this situation, a therapeutic trial with small amounts of parenteral vitamin B_{12} (1–10 μg per day) can confirm the presence of an uncomplicated vitamin B_{12} deficiency.

In contrast, patients with neurological changes or severe leukopenia or thrombocytopenia associated with infection or bleeding require emergency treatment. Effective therapy must not wait for detailed diagnostic tests. Once the megaloblastic erythropoiesis has been confirmed and sufficient blood collected for later measurements of vitamin B_{12} and folic acid, the patient should receive intramuscular injections of 100 μg of cyanocobalamin and 1–5 mg of folic acid. For the next 1–2 weeks, the patient should receive daily intramuscular injections of 100 μg of cyanocobalamin, together with a daily oral supplement of 1 to 2 mg of folic acid. Because an effective increase in red cell mass will not occur for 10–20 days, the patient with a markedly depressed hematocrit and tissue hypoxia also should receive a transfusion of 2–3 units of packed red blood cells. If congestive heart failure is present, diuretics can be administered to prevent volume overload.

The first objective hematologic change is the disappearance of the megaloblastic morphology of the marrow. As the ineffective erythropoiesis is corrected, the concentration of iron in plasma falls dramatically as the metal is used in the formation of hemoglobin, usually within the first 48 h. Full correction of precursor maturation in marrow with production of an increased number of reticulocytes begins about the second or third day and peaks 3–5 days later. Patients with complicating iron deficiency, an infection or other inflammatory state, or renal disease may be unable to correct their anemia. Therefore, it is important to monitor the reticulocyte index over the first several weeks. If it does not continue at elevated levels while the hematocrit is below 35%, plasma concentrations of iron and folic acid should again be determined and the patient reevaluated for an illness that could inhibit the response of the marrow. The degree and rate of improvement of neurological signs and symptoms depend on the severity and the duration of the abnormalities. Those that have been present for only a few months usually disappear relatively rapidly. When a defect has been present for many months or years, full return to normal function may never occur.

Long-Term Therapy With Vitamin B_{12}. Once begun, vitamin B_{12} therapy must be maintained for life. This fact must be impressed on the patient and family, and a system must be established to guarantee continued monthly injections of cyanocobalamin.

Intramuscular injection of 100 μg of cyanocobalamin every 4 weeks is usually sufficient. Patients with severe neurological symptoms and signs may be treated with larger doses of vitamin B_{12} in the period immediately after the diagnosis. Doses of 100 μg per day or several times per week may be given for several months with the hope of encouraging faster and more complete recovery. It is important to monitor vitamin B_{12} concentrations in plasma and to obtain peripheral blood counts at intervals of 3–6 months to confirm the adequacy of therapy. Because refractoriness to therapy can develop at any time, evaluation must continue throughout the patient's life. Intranasal preparations are available for maintenance following normalization of vitamin B_{12}-deficient patients without nervous system involvement.

Folic Acid and Human Health

Biochemical Roles of Folate

Pteroylglutamic acid (Figure 41–7) is the common pharmaceutical form of folic acid. It is not the principal folate congener in food or the active coenzyme for intracellular metabolism. After absorption, PteGlu is rapidly reduced at the 5, 6, 7, and 8 positions to *tetrahydrofolic acid* (H_4PteGlu), which then acts as an acceptor of a number of one-carbon units. These are attached at either the 5 or the 10 position of the pteridine ring or may bridge these atoms to form a new five-member ring. The most important forms of the coenzyme that are synthesized by these reactions are listed in Figure 41–4, and each plays a specific role in intracellular metabolism:

- *Conversion of Homocysteine to Methionine.* This reaction requires CH_3H_4PteGlu as a methyl donor and uses vitamin B_{12} as a cofactor.
- *Conversion of Serine to Glycine.* This reaction requires tetrahydrofolate as an acceptor of a methylene group from serine and uses pyridoxal phosphate as a cofactor. It results in the formation of 5,10-CH_2H_4PteGlu, an essential coenzyme for the synthesis of dTMP.
- *Synthesis of Thymidylate.* 5,10-CH_2H_4PteGlu donates a methylene group and reducing equivalents to dUMP for the synthesis of dTMP—a rate-limiting step in DNA synthesis.
- *Histidine Metabolism.* H_4PteGlu also acts as an acceptor of a formimino group in the conversion of FIGLU to glutamic acid.
- *Synthesis of Purines.* Two steps in the synthesis of purine nucleotides require the participation of 10-$CHOH_4$PteGlu as a formyl donor in reactions catalyzed by ribotide transformylases: the formylation of glycinamide ribonucleotide and the formylation of 5-aminoimidazole-4-carboxamide ribonucleotide. By these reactions, carbon atoms at positions 8 and 2, respectively, are incorporated into the growing purine ring.
- *Utilization or Generation of Formate.* This reversible reaction uses H_4PteGlu and 10-$CHOH_4$PteGlu.

Daily Requirements. Many food sources are rich in folates, especially fresh green vegetables, liver, yeast, and some fruits. However, lengthy cooking can destroy up to 90% of the folate content of such food. Generally, a standard U.S. diet provides 50–500 μg of absorbable folate per day, although individuals with high intakes of fresh vegetables and meats will ingest as much as 2 mg per day. In the normal adult, the recommended daily intake is 400 μg; pregnant or lactating women and patients with high rates of cell turnover (such as patients with a hemolytic anemia) may require 500–600 μg or more per day. For the prevention of neural tube defects, a daily intake of at least 400 μg of folate in food or in supplements beginning a month before pregnancy and continued for at least the first trimester is recommended. Folate supplementation also is being considered in patients with elevated levels of plasma homocysteine.

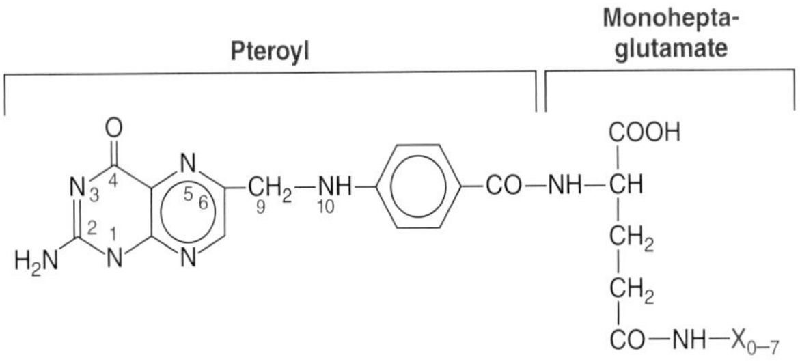

Pteroyl | Monohepta-glutamate

H_2N–pteridine (N1–N8; positions 1–6) –CH_2(9)–NH(10)–C_6H_4–CO–NH–CH(COOH)–CH_2–CH_2–CO–NH–X_{0-7}

Position	Radical	Congener	
N^5	—CH_3	CH_3H_4PteGlu	Methyltetrahydrofolate
N^5	—CHO	5-$CHOH_4$PteGlu	Folinic acid (citrovorum factor)
N^{10}	—CHO	10-$CHOH_4$PteGlu	10-Formyltetrahydrofolate
$N^{5,10}$	=CH—	5,10-CHH_4PteGlu	5,10-Methenyltetrahydrofolate
$N^{5,10}$	—CH_2—	5,10-CH_2H_4PteGlu	5,10-Methylenetetrahydrofolate
N^5	—CHNH	$CHNHH_4$PteGlu	Formiminotetrahydrofolate
N^{10}	—CH_2OH	CH_2OHH_4PteGlu	Hydroxymethyltetrahydrofolate

Figure 41–7 *The structures and nomenclature of PteGlu (folic acid) and its congeners.* X represents additional residues of glutamate; polyglutamates are the storage and active forms of the vitamin. The number of residues of glutamate is variable.

ADME. As with vitamin B_{12}, the diagnosis and management of deficiencies of folic acid depend on an understanding of the transport pathways and intracellular metabolism of the vitamin (Figure 41–8). Folates present in food are largely in the form of reduced polyglutamates, and absorption requires transport and the action of a *pteroylglutamyl carboxypeptidase* associated with mucosal cell membranes. The mucosae of the duodenum and upper part of the jejunum are rich in *dihydrofolate reductase* and can methylate most or all of the reduced folate that is absorbed. Because most absorption occurs in the proximal portion of the small intestine, it is not unusual for folate deficiency to occur when the jejunum is diseased. Both nontropical and tropical sprues are common causes of folate deficiency and megaloblastic anemia.

Once absorbed, folate is transported rapidly to tissues as CH_3H_4PteGlu. Although certain plasma proteins do bind folate derivatives, they have a greater affinity for nonmethylated analogues. The role of such binding proteins in folate homeostasis is not well understood. An increase in binding capacity is detectable in folate deficiency and in certain disease states, such as uremia, cancer, and alcoholism. A constant supply of CH_3H_4PteGlu is maintained by food and by an enterohepatic cycle of the vitamin. The liver actively reduces and methylates PteGlu (and H_2 or H_4PteGlu) and then transports the CH_3H_4PteGlu into bile for reabsorption by the gut and subsequent delivery to tissues. This pathway may provide 200 μg or more of folate each day for recirculation to tissues. The importance of the enterohepatic cycle was suggested by animal studies that showed a rapid reduction of the plasma folate concentration after either drainage of bile or ingestion of alcohol, which apparently blocks the release of CH_3H_4PteGlu from hepatic parenchymal cells.

Folate Deficiency. Folate deficiency is a common complication of diseases of the small intestine that interferes with the absorption of folate from food and the recirculation of folate through the enterohepatic cycle. The prevalence of folate deficiency in persons over age 65 is relatively high due to reduced dietary intake or intestinal malabsorption (Araujo et al., 2015). In acute or chronic alcoholism, daily intake of folate in food may be severely restricted, and the enterohepatic cycle of the vitamin may be impaired by toxic effects of alcohol on hepatic parenchymal cells; this is the most common cause of folate-deficient megaloblastic erythropoiesis and the most amenable to therapy, via reinstitution of a normal diet. Disease states characterized by a high rate of cell turnover, such as hemolytic anemias, also may be complicated by folate deficiency. In addition, drugs that inhibit dihydrofolate reductase (e.g., methotrexate and trimethoprim) or that interfere with the absorption and storage of folate in tissues (e.g., certain anticonvulsants and oral contraceptives) can lower the concentration of folate in plasma and may cause a megaloblastic anemia (Hesdorffer and Longo, 2015).

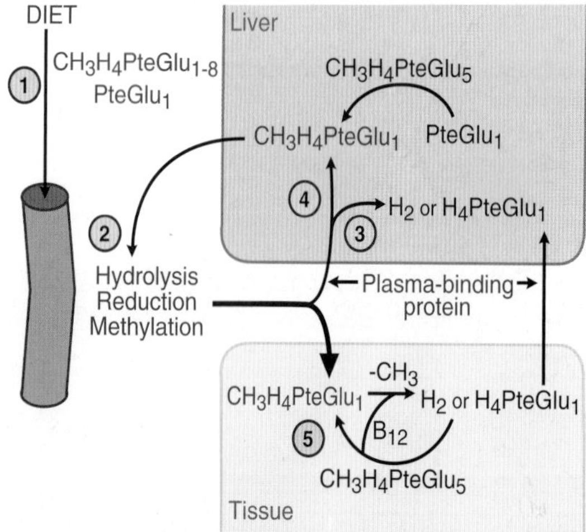

Figure 41–8 *Absorption and distribution of folate derivatives.* Dietary sources of folate polyglutamates are hydrolyzed to the monoglutamate, reduced, and methylated to $CH_3H_4PteGlu_1$ during GI transport. Folate deficiency commonly results from (1) inadequate dietary supply and (2) small intestinal disease. In patients with uremia, alcoholism, or hepatic disease, there may be defects in (3) the concentration of folate-binding proteins in plasma and (4) the flow of $CH_3H_4PteGlu_1$ into bile for reabsorption and transport to tissue (the folate enterohepatic cycle). Finally, vitamin B_{12} deficiency will (5) "trap" folate as CH_3H_4PteGlu, thereby reducing the availability of $H_4PteGlu_1$ for its essential roles in purine and pyrimidine synthesis.

Folate deficiency is recognized by its impact on the hematopoietic system. As with vitamin B_{12}, this fact reflects the increased requirement associated with high rates of cell turnover. The megaloblastic anemia that results from folate deficiency cannot be distinguished from that caused by vitamin B_{12} deficiency. In contrast to vitamin B_{12} deficiency, folate deficiency is rarely, if ever, associated with neurological abnormalities. After deprivation of folate, megaloblastic anemia develops much more rapidly than it does following interruption of vitamin B_{12} absorption (e.g., gastric surgery). This observation reflects the fact that body stores of folate are limited. Although the rate of induction of megaloblastic erythropoiesis may vary, a folate-deficiency state may appear in 1–4 weeks, depending on the individual's dietary habits and stores of the vitamin.

Folate deficiency is implicated in the incidence of neural tube defects (Wallingford et al., 2013). An inadequate intake of folate also can result in elevations in plasma homocysteine. Because even moderate hyperhomocysteinemia is considered an independent risk factor for coronary artery and peripheral vascular disease and for venous thrombosis, the role of folate as a methyl donor in the homocysteine-to-methionine conversion is receiving increased attention (Stanger and Wonisch, 2012).

General Principles of Therapy. The therapeutic use of folic acid is limited to the prevention and treatment of deficiencies of the vitamin. As with vitamin B_{12} therapy, effective use of the vitamin depends on accurate diagnosis and an understanding of the mechanisms that are operative in a specific disease state. The following general principles of therapy should be respected:

- Dietary supplementation is necessary when there is a requirement that may not be met by a "normal" diet. The daily ingestion of a multivitamin preparation containing 400–500 μg of folic acid has become standard practice before and during pregnancy to reduce the incidence of neural tube defects and for as long as a woman is breastfeeding. In women with a history of a pregnancy complicated by a neural tube defect, an even larger dose of 4 mg/d has been recommended. Patients on total parenteral nutrition should receive folic acid supplements as part of their fluid regimen because liver folate stores are limited. Adult patients with a disease state characterized by high cell turnover (e.g., hemolytic anemia) generally require 1 mg of folic acid given once or twice a day. The 1-mg dose also has been used in the treatment of patients with elevated levels of homocysteine.
- Any patient with folate deficiency and a megaloblastic anemia should be evaluated carefully to determine the underlying cause of the deficiency state. This should include evaluation of the effects of medications, the amount of alcohol intake, the patient's history of travel, and the function of the GI tract.
- Therapy always should be as specific as possible. Multivitamin preparations should be avoided unless there is good reason to suspect deficiency of several vitamins.
- The potential danger of mistreating a patient who has vitamin B_{12} deficiency with folic acid must be kept in mind. The administration of large doses of folic acid can result in an apparent improvement of the megaloblastic anemia, inasmuch as PteGlu is converted by dihydrofolate reductase to H_4PteGlu; this circumvents the methylfolate "trap." However, folate therapy does not prevent or alleviate the neurological defects of vitamin B_{12} deficiency, and these may progress and become irreversible.

Therapeutic Use of Folate. Folic acid is marketed as oral tablets containing PteGlu or l-methylfolate, as an aqueous solution for injection

(5 mg/mL), and in combination with other vitamins and minerals. Folinic acid (leucovorin calcium, citrovorum factor) is the 5-formyl derivative of tetrahydrofolic acid. The principal therapeutic uses of folinic acid are to circumvent the inhibition of dihydrofolate reductase as a part of high-dose methotrexate therapy and to potentiate fluorouracil in the treatment of colorectal cancer (see Chapter 66). It also has been used as an antidote to counteract the toxicity of folate antagonists such as pyrimethamine or trimethoprim. Folinic acid provides no advantage over folic acid, is more expensive, and therefore is not recommended. A single exception is the megaloblastic anemia associated with congenital dihydrofolate reductase deficiency.

Evaluation of the serum folate level can help exclude folate deficiency, but only in patients whose serum folate levels exceed 5.0 ng/mL; 2%–5% of healthy adults can have serum folate levels that are below this level. Red cell folate levels (reference range > 140 ng/mL) reflect chronic folate levels, are less affected by acute ingestion of folate than are serum levels, but are more time consuming and costly to measure. Serum folate concentrations more frequently show a higher correlation with serum homocysteine, which is a sensitive marker of deficiency (Farrell et al., 2013). In any case, a patient with a low serum or red cell folate level should have follow-up tests that include serum homocysteine (reference range 5–16 mmol/L), which is elevated in B_{12} and folate deficiency, and serum methylmalonic acid (reference range 70–270 mmol/L), which is elevated only in B_{12} deficiency.

Untoward Effects. There have been rare reports of reactions to parenteral injections of folic acid and leucovorin. Oral folic acid usually is not toxic. Folic acid in large amounts may counteract the antiepileptic effect of phenobarbital, phenytoin, and primidone and increase the frequency of seizures in susceptible children. The FDA recommends that oral tablets of folic acid be limited to strengths of 1 mg or less.

Acknowledgment*: Robert S. Hillman contributed to this chapter in a prior edition of this book. We have retained some of his text in the current edition.*

Bibliography

Agarwal R. Proinflammatory effects of iron sucrose in chronic kidney disease. *Kidney Int*, **2006**, *69*:1259–1263.

Araujo JR, et al. Folates and aging: role in mild cognitive impairment, dementia and depression. *Ageing Res Rev*, **2015**, *22*:9–19.

Auerbach M, et al. Safety and efficacy of total dose infusion of 1020 mg of ferumoxytol administered over 15 min. *Am J Hematol*, **2013**, *88*: 944–947.

Beguin Y, Jaspers A. Iron sucrose—characteristics, efficacy and regulatory aspects of an established treatment of iron deficiency and iron-deficiency anemia in a broad range of therapeutic areas. *Expert Opin Pharmacother*, **2014**, *15*:2087–2103.

Bennett CL, et al. Venous thromboembolism and mortality associated with recombinant erythropoietin and darbepoetin administration for the treatment of cancer-associated anemia. *JAMA*, **2008**, *299*:914–924.

Besarab A, et al. A study of parental iron regimens in hemodialysis patients. *Am J Kidney Dis*, **1999**, *34*:21–28.

Beutler E. History of iron in medicine. *Blood Cells Mol Dis*, **2002**, *29*:297–308.

Bohlius J, et al. Erythropoetin or darbepoetin for patients with cancer: meta-analysis based on individual patient data. *Cochrane Database Syst Rev*, **2009**, 3: CD007303. doi:10.1002/14651858. CD007303.pub2. Accessed July 23, 2017.

Brandt SJ, et al. Effect of recombinant human granulocyte-macrophage colony-stimulating factor on hematopoietic reconstitution after high-dose chemotherapy and autologous bone marrow transplantation. *N Engl J Med*, **1988**, *318*:869–876.

Camaschella C. Iron and hepcidin: a story of recycling and balance. *Hematology Am Soc Hematol Educ Program*, **2013**, *2013*:1–8.

Camaschella C. Iron-deficiency anemia. *N Engl J Med*, **2015**, *372*: 1832–1843.

Conrad ME, Umbreit JM. Iron absorption and transport - an update. *Am J Hematol*, **2000**, *64*:287–298

de Bie P, et al. Molecular pathogenesis of Wilson and Menkes disease: correlation of mutations with molecular defects and disease phenotypes. *J Med Genet*, **2007**, *44*:673–688.

De Domenico I, et al. The hepcidin-binding site on ferroportin is evolutionarily conserved. *Cell Metab*, **2008**, *8*:146–156.

Del Villar Madrigal E, et al. Anemia after Roux-en-Y gastric bypass. How feasible to eliminate the risk by proper supplementation? *Obes Surg*, **2015**, *25*:80–84.

Drakesmith H, Prentice AM. Hepcidin and the iron-infection axis. *Science*, **2012**, *338*:768–772.

Farrell CJ, et al. Red cell or serum folate: what to do in clinical practice? *Clin Chem Lab Med*, **2013**, *51*:555–569.

Feder JN, et al. A novel MHC class I-like gene is mutated in patients with hereditary haemochromatosis. *Nat Genet*, **1996**, *13*:399–408.

Finch CW. Review of trace mineral requirements for preterm infants: what are the current recommendations for clinical practice? *Nutr Clin Pract*, **2015**, *30*:44–58.

Fischl M, et al. Recombinant human erythropoietin for patients with AIDS treated with zidovudine. *N Engl J Med*, **1990**, *322*:1488–1493.

Ganz T, Nemeth E. Hepcidin and disorders of iron metabolism. *Annu Rev Med*, **2011**, *62*:347–360.

Garrick MD, Garrick LM. Cellular iron transport. *Biochim Biophys Acta*, **2009**, *1790*:309–325.

Gerhartz HH, et al. Randomized, double-blind, placebo-controlled, phase III study of recombinant human granulocyte-macrophage colony-stimulating factor as adjunct to induction treatment of high-grade malignant non-Hodgkin's lymphomas. *Blood*, **1993**, *82*:2329–2339.

Goodwin RG, et al. Human interleukin 7: molecular cloning and growth factor activity on human and murine B-lineage cells. *Proc Natl Acad Sci U S A*, **1989**, *86*:302–306.

Gordeuk VR, et al. Congenital disorder of oxygen sensing: association of the homozygous Chuvash polycythemia VHL mutation with thrombosis and vascular abnormalities but not tumors. *Blood*, **2004**, *103*:3924–3932.

Gough NM, et al. Molecular cloning of cDNA encoding a murine hematopoietic growth regulator, granulocyte-macrophage colony stimulating factor. *Nature*, **1984**, *309*:763–767.

Grabstein KH, et al. Cloning of a T cell growth factor that interacts with the β chain of the interleukin-2 receptor. *Science*, **1994**, *264*:965–968.

Haas R, et al. Successful autologous transplantation of blood stem cells mobilized with recombinant human granulocyte-macrophage colony-stimulating factor. *Exp Hematol*, **1990**, *18*:94–98.

Haase VH. Hypoxic regulation of erythropoiesis and iron metabolism. *Am J Physiol*, **2010**, *299*:F1–13.

Hahn PF. The use of radioactive isotopes in the study of iron and hemoglobin metabolism and the physiology of the erythrocyte. *Adv Biol Med Phys*, **1948**, *1*:287–319.

Hammond WPT, et al. Treatment of cyclic neutropenia with granulocyte colony-stimulating factor. *N Engl J Med*, **1989**, *320*:1306–1311.

Hayat A. Safety issues with intravenous iron products in the management of anemia in chronic kidney disease. *Clin Med Res*, **2008**, *6*:93–102.

Hesdorffer CS, Longo DL. Drug-induced megaloblastic anemia. *N Engl J Med*, **2015**, *373*:1649–1658.

Hoffbrand AV, Herbert V. Nutritional anemias. *Semin Hematol*, **1999**, *36*:13–23.

Kaufman JS, et al. Subcutaneous compared with intravenous epoetin in patients receiving hemodialysis. Department of Veterans Affairs Cooperative Study Group on Erythropoietin in Hemodialysis Patients. *N Engl J Med*, **1998**, *339*:578–583.

Kaushansky K. Thrombopoietin. *N Engl J Med*, **1998**, *339*:746–754.

Keating GM. Ferric carboxymaltose: a review of its use in iron deficiency. *Drugs*, **2015**, *75*:101–127.

Nevitt T, et al. Charting the travels of copper in eukaryotes from yeast to mammals. *Biochim Biophys Acta Mol Cell Res*, **2012**, *1823*:1580–1593.

Kondo M, et al. Biology of hematopoietic stem cells and progenitors: implications for clinical application. *Annu Rev Immunol*, **2003**, *21*:759–806.

Kuter DJ, et al. Efficacy of romiplostim in patients with chronic immune thrombocytopenic purpura: a double-blind randomised controlled trial. *Lancet*, **2008**, *371*:395–403.

Larson DS, Coyne DW. Update on intravenous iron choices. *Curr Opin Nephrol Hypertens*, **2014**, *23*:186–191.

Laurell CB. What is the function of transferrin in plasma? *Blood*, **1951**, 6:183–187.

Li J, et al. Thrombocytopenia caused by the development of antibodies to thrombopoietin. *Blood*, **2001**, *98*:3241–3248.

Lieschke GJ, Burgess AW. Granulocyte colony-stimulating factor and granulocyte-macrophage colony-stimulating factor (2). *N Engl J Med*, **1992**, *327*:99–106.

Littlewood TJ, et al. Effects of epoetin alfa on hematologic parameters and quality of life in cancer patients receiving nonplatinum chemotherapy: results of a randomized, double-blind, placebo-controlled trial. *J Clin Oncol*, **2001**, *19*:2865–2874.

Martí-Carvajal AJ, et al. Treatment for anemia in people with AIDS. *Cochrane Database Syst Rev*, **2011**, (10):CD004776. doi:10.1002/14651858. Accessed March 28, 2016.

Mastrogiannaki M, et al. The gut in iron homeostasis: role of HIF-2 under normal and pathological conditions. *Blood*, **2013**, *122*:885–892.

McLean E, et al. Worldwide prevalence of anaemia, WHO Vitamin and Mineral Nutrition Information System, 1993–2005. *Public Health Nutr*, **2009**, *12*:444–454.

Nemunaitis J, et al. Use of recombinant human granulocyte-macrophage colony-stimulating factor in graft failure after bone marrow transplantation. *Blood*, **1990**, *76*:245–253.

Park CH, et al. Hepcidin, a urinary antimicrobial peptide synthesized in the liver. *J Biol Chem*, **2001**, *276*:7806–7810.

Percy MJ, et al. Novel exon 12 mutations in the HIF2A gene associated with erythrocytosis. *Blood*, **2008**, *111*:5400–5402.

Pietrangelo A. Iron and the liver. *Liver Int*, **2016**, *36*(suppl 1):116–123.

Rizzo JD, et al. Use of epoetin in patients with cancer: evidence-based clinical practice guidelines of the American Society of Clinical Oncology and the American Society of Hematology. *Blood*, **2002**, *100*:2303–2320.

Rizzo JD, et al. American Society of Hematology and the American Society of Clinical Oncology clinical practice guideline update on the use of epoetin and darbepoetin in adult patients with cancer. *Blood*, **2010**, *116*:4045–4059.

Sengolge G, et al. Intravenous iron therapy: well-tolerated, yet not harmless. *Eur J Clin Invest*, **2005**, *35*(suppl 3):46–51.

Sheridan WP, et al. Effect of peripheral-blood progenitor cells mobilised by filgrastim (G-CSF) on platelet recovery after high-dose chemotherapy. *Lancet*, **1992**, *339*:640–644.

Solomon LR. Disorders of cobalamin (vitamin B_{12}) metabolism: emerging concepts in pathophysiology, diagnosis and treatment. *Blood Rev*, **2007**, *21*:113–130.

Spence JD. Metabolic B_{12} deficiency: a missed opportunity to prevent dementia and stroke. *Nutr Res*, **2016**, *36*:109–116.

Stanger O, Wonisch W. Enzymatic and non-enzymatic antioxidative effects of folic acid and its reduced derivates. *Subcell Biochem*, **2012**, *56*:131–161.

Wallingford JB, et al. The continuing challenge of understanding, preventing, and treating neural tube defects. *Science*, **2013**, *339*:1222002.

Weisbart RH, et al. Human GM-CSF primes neutrophils for enhanced oxidative metabolism in response to the major physiological chemoattractants. *Blood*, **1987**, *69*:18–21.

Weissbach H. The isolation of the vitamin B_{12} coenzyme and the role of the vitamin in methionine synthesis. *J Biol Chem*, **2008**, *283*:23497–23504.

Welte K, et al. Purification and biochemical characterization of human pluripotent hematopoietic colony-stimulating factor. *Proc Natl Acad Sci U S A*, **1985**, *82*:1526–1530.

Willis MS, et al. Zinc-induced copper deficiency: a report of three cases initially recognized on bone marrow examination. *Am J Clin Pathol*, **2005**, *123*:125–131.

Wong GG, et al. Human GM-CSF: molecular cloning of the complementary DNA and purification of the natural and recombinant proteins. *Science*, **1985**, *228*:810–815.

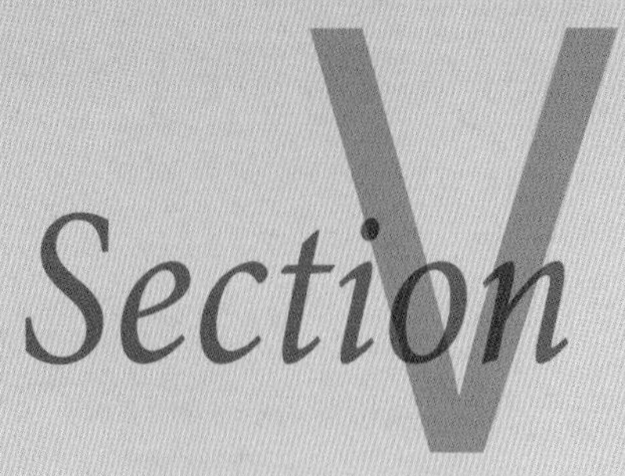

Hormones and Hormone Antagonists

第五篇　激素和激素拮抗药

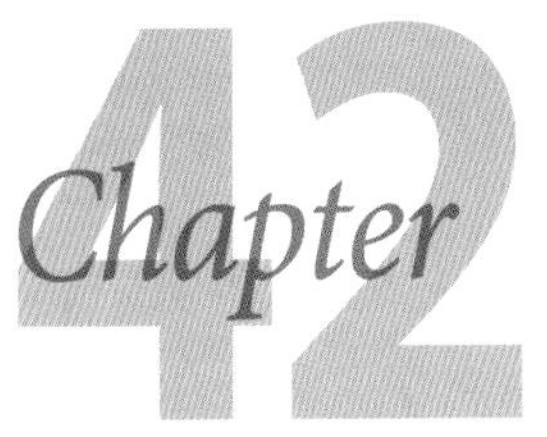

Introduction to Endocrinology: The Hypothalamic-Pituitary Axis

Mark E. Molitch and Bernard P. Schimmer

第四十二章　内分泌学导论：下丘脑-垂体轴

中文导读

本章主要介绍：内分泌学和激素的一般概念；下丘脑-垂体-内分泌腺轴；垂体激素及其下丘脑释放因子；生长激素和催乳素，包括生长激素和催乳素的结构、分泌的调节、发挥作用的分子和细胞学基础、生理学效应、病理生理学；生长激素和催乳素紊乱的药物治疗，包括生长激素过量的治疗、催乳素过量的治疗、生长激素缺乏的治疗；糖蛋白类激素（促甲状腺激素和促性腺激素），包括促性腺激素的结构-功能关系、促性腺激素的生理学、促性腺激素作用的分子和细胞基础；下丘脑-垂体-性腺轴的临床紊乱，包括性腺疾病的治疗和诊断；天然和重组促性腺激素，包括制剂、诊断用途和治疗应用；垂体后叶激素（催产素和升压素），包括催产素的生理学、作用部位及其临床应用。

Abbreviations

AC: adenylyl cyclase
ACTH: corticotropin, formerly adrenocorticotrophic hormone
CG: chorionic gonadotropin
CRH: corticotropin-releasing hormone
DA: dopamine
FSH: follicle-stimulating hormone, follitropin
GH: growth hormone
GHRH: growth hormone–releasing hormone
GnRH: gonadotropin-releasing hormone
GPCR: G protein –coupled receptor
hCG: human chorionic gonadotropin
5HT: 5-hydroxytryptamin serotonin
IGF-1: insulin-like growth factor 1
IGFBP: IGF-binding protein
IRS: insulin receptor substrate
LH: luteinizing hormone; lutropin
NPY: neuropeptide Y
OXTR: oxytocin receptor
POMC: pro-opiomelanocortin
PRL: prolactin
SC: subcutaneous
SHC: Src homology-containing protein
SHP2: Src-homology-2-domain-containing protein tyrosine phosphatase 2
SST: somatostatin
SSTR: SST receptor
TRH: thyrotropin-releasing hormone
TSH: thyroid-stimulating hormone, thyrotropin
VIP: vasoactive intestinal peptide

Endocrinology and Hormones: General Concepts

Endocrinology analyzes the biosynthesis of hormones, their sites of production, and the sites and mechanisms of their action and interaction. The term *hormone* is of Greek origin and classically refers to a chemical messenger that circulates in body fluids and produces specific effects on cells distant from the hormone's point of origin. The major functions of hormones include the regulation of energy storage, production, and utilization; the adaptation to new environments or conditions of stress; the facilitation of growth and development; and the maturation and function of the reproductive system. Although hormones were originally defined as products of ductless glands, we now appreciate that many organs not classically considered as "endocrine" (e.g., the heart, kidneys, GI tract, adipocytes, and brain) synthesize and secrete hormones that play key physiological roles. In addition, the field of endocrinology has expanded to include the actions of growth factors acting by means of autocrine and paracrine mechanisms, the influence of neurons—particularly those in the hypothalamus—that regulate endocrine function, and the reciprocal interactions of cytokines and other components of the immune system with the endocrine system.

Conceptually, hormones may be divided into two classes:

- Hormones that act predominantly via *nuclear receptors* to modulate transcription in target cells (e.g., steroid hormones, thyroid hormone, and vitamin D)
- Hormones that typically act via *membrane receptors* to exert rapid effects on signal transduction pathways (e.g., peptide and amino acid hormones)

The receptors for both classes of hormones provide tractable targets for a diverse group of compounds that are among the most widely used drugs in clinical medicine.

The Hypothalamic-Pituitary-Endocrine Axis

Many of the classic endocrine hormones (e.g., cortisol, thyroid hormone, sex steroids, GH) are regulated by complex reciprocal interactions among the hypothalamus, anterior pituitary, and endocrine glands (Table 42–1). The basic organization of the hypothalamic-pituitary-endocrine axis is summarized in Figure 42–1.

Discrete sets of hypothalamic neurons produce different releasing and inhibiting hormones, which are axonally transported to the median eminence. On stimulation, these neurons secrete their respective hypothalamic hormones into the hypothalamic-adenohypophyseal portal veins, which connect to the anterior pituitary gland. The *hypothalamic hormones* bind to membrane receptors on specific subsets of pituitary cells and regulate the secretion of the corresponding *pituitary hormones*. The pituitary hormones, which can be thought of as the *master signals*, circulate to the target endocrine glands or other tissues, where they activate specific receptors to stimulate the synthesis and secretion of the target *endocrine hormones or exert other tissue-specific effects*. These interactions are *feed-forward regulation* in which the master (signal) hormones stimulate the production of target hormones by the endocrine organs.

Superimposed on this positive feed-forward regulation is *negative-feedback* regulation, which permits precise control of hormone levels (see Figures 42–2 and 42–6). Typically, the endocrine target hormone circulates to both the hypothalamus and pituitary, where it acts via specific receptors to inhibit the production and secretion of both its hypothalamic-releasing hormone and the regulatory pituitary hormone. In addition, other brain regions have inputs to the hypothalamic hormone–producing neurons, further integrating the regulation of hormone levels in response to diverse stimuli.

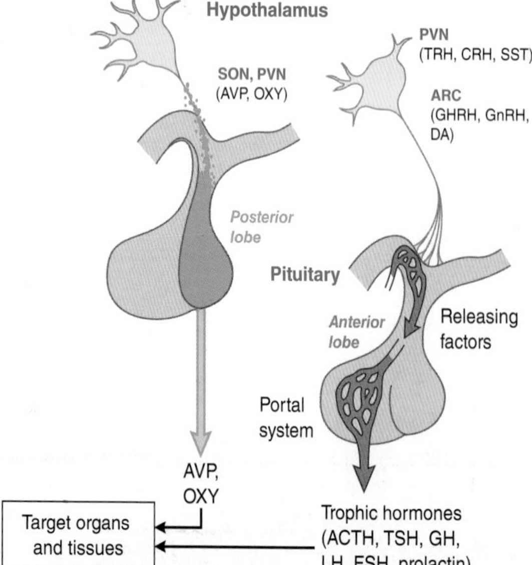

Figure 42–1 *Organization of the anterior and posterior pituitary gland.* Hypothalamic neurons in the supraoptic (SON) and paraventricular (PVN) nuclei synthesize arginine vasopressin (AVP) or oxytocin (OXY). Most of their axons project directly to the posterior pituitary, from which AVP and OXY are secreted into the systemic circulation to regulate their target tissues. Neurons that regulate the anterior lobe cluster in the mediobasal hypothalamus, including the PVH and the arcuate (ARC) nuclei. They secrete hypothalamic releasing hormones, which reach the anterior pituitary via the hypothalamic-adenohypophyseal portal system and stimulate distinct populations of pituitary cells. These cells, in turn, secrete the trophic (signal) hormones, which regulate endocrine organs and other tissues. ARC, arcuate; AVP, arginine vasopressin; OXY, oxytocin; PVN, paraventricular nuclei; SON, supraoptic nuclei; See Abbreviations list for other abbreviations.

TABLE 42–1 ■ HORMONES THAT INTEGRATE THE HYPOTHALAMIC-PITUITARY-ENDOCRINE AXIS

HYPOTHALAMIC HORMONE	EFFECT ON PITUITARY TROPHIC (SIGNAL) HORMONE	TARGET HORMONE(S)
Growth hormone-releasing hormone	↑↑ Growth hormone	IGF-1
Somatostatin	↓ Growth hormone ↓ Thyroid-stimulating hormone	
Dopamine	↓ Prolactin	—
Corticotropin-releasing hormone	↑ Corticotropin	Cortisol
Thyrotropin-releasing hormone	↑ Thyroid-stimulating hormone ↑ Prolactin	Thyroid hormone
Gonadotropin-releasing hormone	↑ Follicle-stimulating hormone ↑ Luteinizing hormone	Estrogen (f) Progesterone/estrogen (f) Testosterone (m)

f, female; m, male; ↑, increased production; ↓, decreased production.

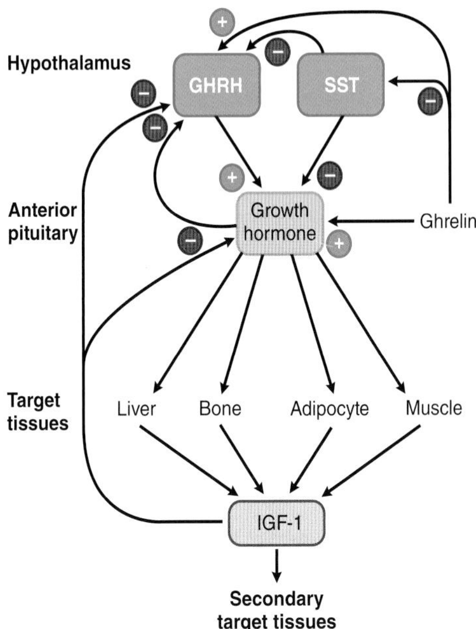

Figure 42–2 *Growth hormone secretion and actions.* Two hypothalamic factors, GHRH and SST, stimulate or inhibit the release of GH from the pituitary, respectively. IGF-1, a product of GH action on peripheral tissues, causes negative-feedback inhibition of GH release by acting at the hypothalamus and the pituitary. The actions of GH can be direct or indirect (mediated by IGF-1). See text for discussion of the other agents that modulate GH secretion and of the effects of locally produced IGF-1. Inhibition, –; stimulation, +.

Pituitary Hormones and Their Hypothalamic-Releasing Factors

The anterior pituitary hormones can be classified into three different groups based on their structural features (Table 42–2):

- POMC-derived hormones include *corticotropin* (ACTH) and α-MSH. These are derived from POMC by proteolytic processing (see Chapters 20 and 46).
- Somatotropic family of hormones *include GH* and *PRL*. In humans, the somatotropic family also includes placental lactogen.
- The glycoprotein hormones—*TSH* (also called thyrotropin), *LH* (also called lutropin), and *FSH* (also called follitropin). In humans, the glycoprotein hormone family also includes hCG.

The synthesis and release of *anterior pituitary hormones* are influenced by the CNS. Their secretion is positively regulated by a group of peptides referred to as *hypothalamic-releasing hormones* (see Figure 42–1). These include *CRH*, *GHRH*, *GnRH*, and *TRH*. *SST*, another hypothalamic peptide, negatively regulates secretion of pituitary GH and TSH. The neurotransmitter DA inhibits the secretion of PRL by lactotropes.

The *posterior pituitary gland*, also known as the neurohypophysis, contains the endings of nerve axons arising from the hypothalamus that synthesize either *arginine vasopressin* or *oxytocin* (see Figure 42–1). Arginine vasopressin plays an important role in water homeostasis (see Chapter 25); oxytocin plays important roles in labor and parturition and in milk letdown, as discussed in the sections that follow.

Growth Hormone and Prolactin

Growth hormone and PRL are structurally related members of the somatotropic hormone family and share many biological features. The somatotropes and lactotropes, the pituitary cells that produce and secrete GH and PRL, respectively, are subject to strong inhibitory input from hypothalamic neurons; for PRL, dopaminergic input is the dominant negative regulator of secretion. GH and PRL act via membrane receptors that belong to the cytokine receptor family and modulate target cell function via very similar signal transduction pathways (see Chapter 3).

Structures of GH and PRL

Table 42–2 presents some features of the somatotrophic family of hormones. GH is secreted by somatotropes as a heterogeneous mixture of peptides; the principal form is a single polypeptide chain of 22 kDa that has two disulfide bonds and is not glycosylated. Alternative splicing produces a smaller form (~20 kDa) with equal bioactivity that makes up 5%–10% of circulating GH. Recombinant human GH consists entirely of the 22-kDa form, which provides a way to detect GH abuse. In the circulation, a 55-kDa protein, which is derived from the extracellular domain of the proteolytically cleaved GHRH receptor, binds approximately 45% of the 22-kDa and 25% of the 20-kDa forms. A second protein unrelated to the GHR also binds approximately 5%–10% of circulating GH with lower affinity. Bound GH is cleared more slowly and has a biological $t_{1/2}$ about 10 times that of unbound GH, suggesting that the bound hormone may provide a GH reservoir that dampens acute fluctuations in GH levels associated with its pulsatile secretion.

TABLE 42–2 ■ PROPERTIES OF THE PROTEIN HORMONES OF THE HUMAN ADENOHYPOPHYSIS AND PLACENTA

CLASS Hormone	MASS (daltons)	PEPTIDE CHAINS	AMINO ACID RESIDUES	Comments
POMC-derived hormones[a]				
Corticotropin	4500	1	39	These peptides are derived by proteolytic processing of the common precursor, POMC.
α-Melanocyte–stimulating hormone	1650		13	
Somatotropic family of hormones				
Growth hormone	22,000		191	Receptors for these hormones belong to the cytokine superfamily.
Prolactin	23,000	1	199	
Placental lactogen	22,125		190	
Glycoprotein hormones				
Luteinizing hormone	29,400		β-121	These are heterodimeric glycoproteins with a common α subunit of 92 amino acids and unique β subunits that determine biological specificity and $t_{1/2}$.
Follicle-stimulating hormone	32,600	2	β-111	
Human chorionic gonadotropin	38,600		β-145	
Thyroid-stimulating hormone	28,000		β-118	

[a]See Chapter 46 for further discussion of POMC-derived peptides, including ACTH and α-MSH.

Human PRL is synthesized by lactotropes; a portion of the secreted hormone is glycosylated at a single Asn residue. In the circulation, multimeric forms of PRL occur, as do degradation products of 16 kDa and 18 kDa. As with GH, the biological significance of these polymeric and degraded forms is not known.

Human placental lactogen, structurally similar to GH and PRL, occurs in pregnant females, with maximal levels near term. Human placental lactogen alters the mother's metabolism to favor fetal nutrition (mainly elevated blood glucose, secondary to reduced maternal insulin sensitivity).

Regulation of Secretion

GH Secretion

Daily GH secretion varies throughout life. GH secretion is high in children, peaks during puberty, and then decreases in an age-related manner in adulthood. GH is secreted in discrete but irregular pulses. The amplitude of secretory pulses is greatest at night. GH secretion is stimulated by GHRH and ghrelin and subject to feedback inhibition by GH itself, SST, and IGF-1 (Figure 42–2).

Growth Hormone–Releasing Hormone. GHRH, a peptide with 44 amino acids produced by hypothalamic neurons, stimulates GH secretion (see Figure 42–2) by binding to a specific GPCR on somatotropes in the anterior pituitary. The stimulated GHRH receptor couples to G_s to raise intracellular levels of cAMP and Ca^{2+}, thereby stimulating GH synthesis and secretion. Loss-of-function mutations of the GHRH receptor cause a rare form of short stature in humans.

Ghrelin. Ghrelin, a 28-amino-acid peptide, stimulates GH secretion through actions on a GPCR called the GH secretagogue receptor. Ghrelin is synthesized predominantly in endocrine cells in the fundus of the stomach but also is produced at lower levels at a number of other sites, including the pituitary and hypothalamus. Hypothalamic ghrelin is thought to be a stimulus for GH release through actions on pituitary somatotrophs and hypothalamic GHRH-secreting neurons.

Both fasting and hypoglycemia increase circulating stomach-derived ghrelin levels, and this, in turn, stimulates appetite and increases food intake, apparently by central actions on NPY and agouti-related peptide neurons in the hypothalamus. The role of stomach-derived ghrelin in GH secretion is unclear because clinical studies attempting to correlate circulating levels of ghrelin with GH secretion have produced conflicting results (Nass et al., 2011).

Other Stimuli. Several neurotransmitters, drugs, metabolites, and other stimuli modulate the release of GHRH or SST and thereby affect GH secretion. DA, 5HT, and α_2 adrenergic receptor agonists stimulate GH release, as do hypoglycemia, exercise, stress, emotional excitement, and ingestion of protein-rich meals. In contrast, β adrenergic receptor agonists, free fatty acids, glucose, IGF-1, and GH itself inhibit release. Many of the physiological factors that influence PRL secretion also affect GH secretion. Thus, sleep, stress, hypoglycemia, exercise, and estrogen increase the secretion of both hormones.

Feedback Control of GH Secretion. Growth hormone and its major peripheral effector, *IGF-1*, act in negative-feedback loops to suppress GH secretion (Figure 42–2).

Insulin-like Growth Factor 1. The negative effect of IGF-1 is predominantly through direct effects on the anterior pituitary gland but also at the hypothalamus via stimulation of SST secretion. The negative-feedback action of GH is mediated in part by SST, synthesized in more widely distributed neurons (Ergun-Longmire and Wajnrajch, 2013).

After its synthesis and release, IGF-1 interacts with receptors on the cell surface that mediate its biological activities. The type 1 IGF receptor is closely related to the insulin receptor and consists of a heterotetramer with intrinsic tyrosine kinase activity. This receptor is present in essentially all tissues and binds IGF-1 and the related growth factor, IGF-2, with high affinity; insulin also can activate the type 1 IGF receptor but with an affinity approximately two orders of magnitude less than that of the IGFs. The signal transduction pathway for the insulin receptor is described in detail in Chapter 47.

Somatostatin. *Somatostatin* is synthesized as a 92-amino-acid precursor and processed by proteolytic cleavage to generate two peptides: SST-28 and SST-14 (Figure 42–3). SST exerts its effects by binding to and activating a family of five related GPCRs that signal through G_i to inhibit cAMP formation and to activate K^+ channels and protein phosphotyrosine phosphatases.

There are five SSTR subtypes. $SSTR_{1-4}$ bind the two forms of SST with approximately equal affinity; $SSTR_5$ has a 10- to 15-fold greater affinity for SST-28. $SSTR_2$ and $SSTR_5$ are the most important for regulation of GH secretion, and recent studies suggested that these two SSTRs form functional heterodimers with distinctive signaling behavior (Grant et al., 2008). SST exerts direct effects on somatotropes in the pituitary and indirect effects mediated via GHRH neurons in the arcuate nucleus.

PRL Secretion

Prolactin is unique among the anterior pituitary hormones in that hypothalamic regulation of its secretion is predominantly inhibitory. The major regulator of PRL secretion is DA, which interacts with the D_2 receptor, a GPCR on lactotropes, to inhibit PRL secretion (Figure 42–4). TRH and hypothalamic VIP have PRL-releasing properties, but their physiologic

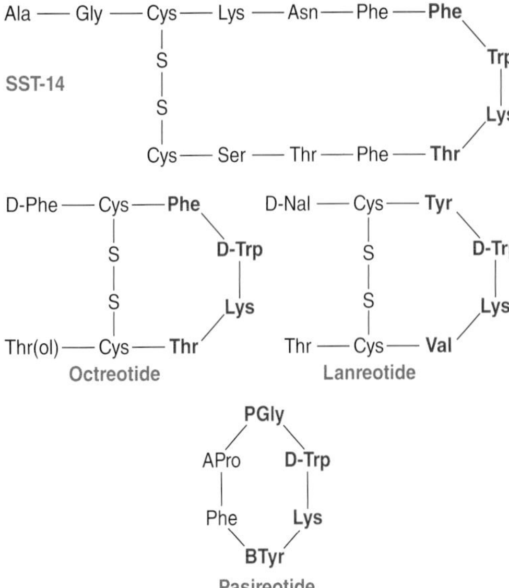

Figure 42–3 *Structures of SST-14 and selected synthetic analogues.* Residues that play key roles in binding to SST receptors are shown in red. Octreotide, lanreotide, and pasireotide are clinically available synthetic analogues of SST. APro, [(2-aminoethyl) aminocarboxyl oxy]-L-proline; D-Nal, 3-(2-napthyl)-D-alanyl; PGly, phenylglycine; BTyr, benzyltyrosine.

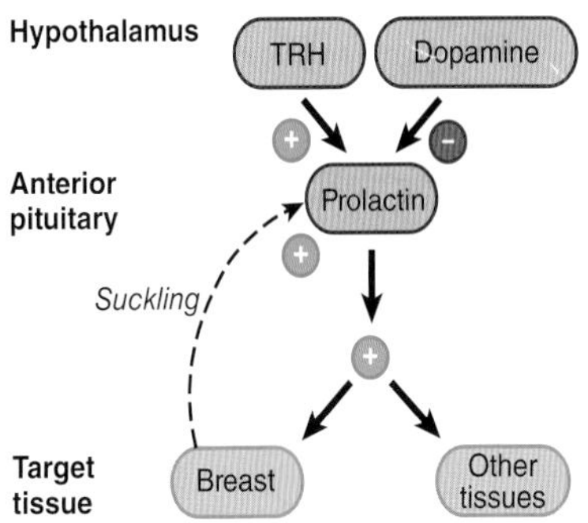

Figure 42–4 *Prolactin secretion and actions.* PRL is the only anterior pituitary hormone for which a unique stimulatory releasing factor has not been identified. TRH and VIP, however, can stimulate PRL release; DA inhibits it. Suckling induces PRL secretion, and PRL not only affects lactation and reproductive functions but also has effects on many other tissues. PRL is not under feedback control by peripheral hormones.

significance is uncertain. PRL acts predominantly in women, both during pregnancy and in the postpartum period in women who breastfeed. During pregnancy, the maternal serum PRL level starts to increase at 8 weeks of gestation, peaks to 150–250 ng/mL at term, and declines thereafter to prepregnancy levels unless the mother breastfeeds the infant. Suckling or breast manipulation in nursing mothers transmits signals from the breast to the hypothalamus via the spinal cord and the median forebrain bundle, causing elevation of circulating PRL levels. PRL levels can rise 10-fold within 30 min of stimulation. This response is distinct from milk letdown, which is mediated by oxytocin release from the posterior pituitary gland. The suckling response becomes less pronounced after several months of breastfeeding, and PRL concentrations eventually decline to prepregnancy levels. PRL also is synthesized by decidual cells early in pregnancy (accounting for the high levels of PRL in amniotic fluid during the first trimester of human pregnancy).

Molecular and Cellular Bases of GH and PRL Action

All of the effects of GH and PRL result from their interactions with specific membrane receptors on target tissues (Figure 42–5). Receptors for GH and PRL belong to the cytokine receptor superfamily and thus share structural similarity with the receptors for leptin, erythropoietin, granulocyte-macrophage colony-stimulating factor, and several of the interleukins. These receptors contain an extracellular hormone-binding domain, a single membrane-spanning region, and an intracellular domain that mediates signal transduction.

Growth hormone receptor activation results in the binding of a single GH to two receptor monomers to form a GH-[GHR]$_2$ ternary complex (initiated by high-affinity interaction of GH with one monomer of the GHR dimer [mediated by GH site 1], followed by a second, lower-affinity interaction of GH with the other GHR [mediated by GH site 2]). These interactions induce a conformational change that activates downstream signaling. The ligand-occupied GHR dimer lacks inherent tyrosine kinase activity but provides docking sites for two molecules of JAK2, a cytoplasmic tyrosine kinase of the Janus kinase family. The juxtaposition of the JAK2 molecules leads to *trans*-phosphorylation and autoactivation of JAK2, with consequent tyrosine phosphorylation of docking sites on the cytoplasmic segments of the GHR and of cytoplasmic proteins that mediate downstream signaling events (Figure 42–5; Chia, 2014). These include STAT proteins, SHC (an adapter protein that regulates the Ras/MAPK signaling pathway), and IRS-1 and IRS-2 (proteins that activate the PI3K pathway). One critical target of STAT5 is the gene encoding IGF-1, a mediator of many of the effects of GH (Figure 42–2). The fine control of GH action also involves feedback regulatory events that subsequently turn off the GH signal. As part of its action, GH induces the expression of a family of suppressor of cytokine signaling (SOC) proteins and a group of protein tyrosine phosphatases (including SHP2) that, by different mechanisms, disrupt the communication of the activated GHR with JAK2 (Flores-Morales et al., 2006).

Pegvisomant is a GH analogue with amino acid substitutions that disrupt the interaction at site 2; pegvisomant binds to the receptor and causes its internalization but cannot trigger the conformational change that stimulates downstream events in the signal transduction pathway.

The *effects of PRL* on target cells also result from interactions with a cytokine family receptor that is widely distributed and signals through many of the same pathways as the GHR (Bernard et al., 2015). Alternative splicing of the PRL receptor gene on chromosome 5 gives rise to multiple forms of the receptor that are identical in the extracellular domain but differ in their cytoplasmic domains. In addition, soluble forms that correspond to the extracellular domain of the receptor are found in circulation. Unlike human GH and placental lactogen, which also bind to the PRL receptor and thus are lactogenic, PRL binds specifically to the PRL receptor and has no somatotropic (GH-like) activity.

Physiological Effects of GH and PRL

The most striking physiological effect of GH is the stimulation of the longitudinal growth of bones. GH also increases bone mineral density after the epiphyses have closed. GH also increases muscle mass, increases the glomerular filtration rate, and stimulates preadipocyte differentiation into adipocytes. GH has potent anti-insulin actions in both the liver and peripheral tissues (e.g., adipocytes and muscle) that decrease glucose utilization and increase lipolysis, but most of its anabolic and growth-promoting effects are mediated indirectly through the induction of IGF-1. IGF-1 interacts with receptors on the cell surface that mediate its biological activities. Circulating IGF-1 is associated with a family of binding proteins (IGFBP) that serve as transport proteins and also may mediate certain aspects of IGF-1 signaling. Most IGF-1 in circulation is bound to IGFBP-3 and another protein called the acid-labile subunit.

The essential role of IGF-1 in growth is evidenced by patients with

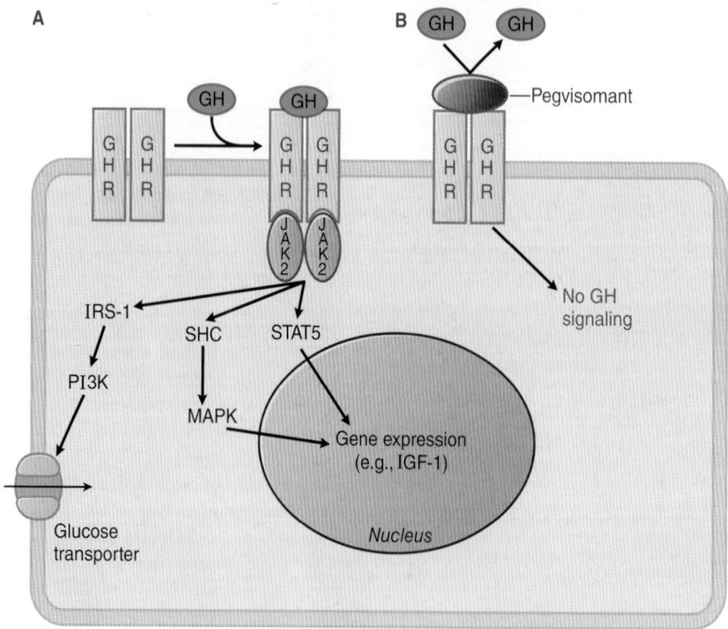

Figure 42–5 *Mechanisms of GH and PRL action and of GHR antagonism.* **A.** GH and two GHRs form a ternary complex that induces association and Tyr autophosphorylation of JAK2 and of docking sites on the cytoplasmic tail of GHRs. JAK2 phosphorylates cytoplasmic proteins that activate downstream signaling pathways, including STAT5 and mediators upstream of MAPK, which ultimately modulate gene expression. The structurally related PRL receptor also is a ligand-activated homodimer that recruits the JAK-STAT signaling pathway. GHR also activates IRS-1, which may mediate the increased expression of glucose transporters on the plasma membrane. **B.** Pegvisomant, a recombinant pegylated variant of human GH, is a high-affinity GH antagonist that interferes with GH binding.

loss-of-function mutations in both alleles of the *IGF1* gene, whose severe intrauterine and postnatal growth retardation is unresponsive to GH but responsive to recombinant human IGF-1, and by the association of mutations in the IGF-1 receptor with intrauterine growth retardation (Walenkamp and Wit, 2008).

The PRL effects are limited primarily to the mammary gland, where PRL plays an important role in inducing growth and differentiation of the ductal and lobuloalveolar epithelia and is essential for lactation. Target genes, by which PRL induces mammary development, include those encoding milk proteins (e.g., caseins and whey acidic protein), genes important for intracellular structure (e.g., keratins), and genes important for cell-cell communication (e.g., amphiregulin). PRL receptors are present in many other sites, including the hypothalamus, liver, adrenal, testes, ovaries, prostate, and immune system, suggesting that PRL may play multiple roles outside the breast. The physiological effects of PRL at these sites remain poorly characterized.

Pathophysiology of GH and PRL

Distinct endocrine disorders result from either excessive or deficient GH production. In contrast, PRL predominantly affects endocrine function when produced in excess.

Excess Production

Syndromes of excess secretion of GH and PRL typically are caused by somatotrope or lactotrope adenomas that oversecrete the respective hormones. These adenomas often retain some features of the normal regulation described previously, thus permitting pharmacological modulation of secretion—an important modality in therapy.

Clinical Manifestations of Excess GH. GH excess causes distinct clinical syndromes depending on the age of the patient. If the epiphyses are unfused, GH excess causes increased longitudinal growth, resulting in *gigantism*. In adults, GH excess causes *acromegaly*. The symptoms and signs of acromegaly (e.g., arthropathy, carpal tunnel syndrome, generalized visceromegaly, macroglossia, hypertension, glucose intolerance, headache, lethargy, excess perspiration, and sleep apnea) progress slowly, and diagnosis often is delayed. Mortality is increased at least 2-fold relative to age-matched controls, predominantly due to increased death from cardiovascular disease. Treatments that normalize GH and IGF-1 levels reverse this increased risk of mortality and ameliorate most of the other symptoms and signs.

Clinical Manifestations of Excess Prolactin. *Hyperprolactinemia* is a relatively common endocrine abnormality that can result from hypothalamic or pituitary diseases that interfere with the delivery of inhibitory dopaminergic signals, from renal failure, from primary hypothyroidism associated with increased TRH levels, or from treatment with DA receptor antagonists. Most often, hyperprolactinemia is caused by PRL-secreting pituitary adenomas. Manifestations of PRL excess in women include galactorrhea, amenorrhea, and infertility. In men, hyperprolactinemia causes loss of libido, erectile dysfunction, and infertility.

Diagnosis of Growth Hormone and Prolactin Excess. Although acromegaly should be suspected in patients with the appropriate symptoms and signs, diagnostic confirmation requires the demonstration of increased circulating GH or IGF-1. The "gold standard" diagnostic test for acromegaly is the oral glucose tolerance test. Whereas normal subjects suppress their GH level to less than 1 ng/mL in response to an oral glucose challenge (the absolute value may vary depending on the sensitivity of the assay), patients with acromegaly either fail to suppress or show a paradoxical increase in GH level.

In patients with hyperprolactinemia, the major question is whether conditions other than a PRL-producing adenoma are responsible for the elevated PRL level. A number of medications that inhibit DA signaling can cause moderate elevations in PRL (e.g., antipsychotics, metoclopramide), as can primary hypothyroidism, pituitary mass lesions that interfere with DA delivery to the lactotropes, and pregnancy. Thus, thyroid function and pregnancy tests are indicated, as is MRI to look for a pituitary adenoma or other defect that might elevate serum PRL.

Impaired Production

Clinical Manifestations of Growth Hormone Deficiency. Children with GH deficiency present with short stature, delayed bone age, and a low age-adjusted growth velocity. GH deficiency in adults is associated with decreased muscle mass and exercise capacity, decreased bone density, impaired psychosocial function, and increased mortality from cardiovascular causes. The diagnosis of GH deficiency should be entertained in children with height more than 2 to 2.5 standard deviations below normal, delayed bone age, a decreased growth velocity, and a predicted adult height substantially below the mean parental height. In adults, overt GH deficiency usually results from pituitary lesions caused by a functioning or nonfunctioning pituitary adenoma, secondary to trauma, or related to surgery or radiotherapy for a pituitary or suprasellar mass (Ergun-Longmire and Wajnrajch, 2013). Almost all patients with multiple deficits in other pituitary hormones also have deficient GH secretion.

Clinical Manifestations of Prolactin Deficiency. PRL deficiency may result from conditions that damage the pituitary gland. Inasmuch as the sole clinical manifestation of PRL deficiency is failure of postpartum lactation, PRL is not given as part of endocrine replacement therapy.

Pharmacotherapy of Disorders GH and PRL

Treatment of Growth Hormone Excess

The initial treatment modality in gigantism/acromegaly is selective removal of the adenoma by transsphenoidal surgery. Radiation and drugs that inhibit GH secretion or action are given if surgery does not result in cure (Katznelson et al., 2014). Pituitary irradiation may be associated with significant long-term complications, including visual deterioration and pituitary dysfunction. Thus, increased attention has been given to the pharmacological management of acromegaly.

Somatostatin Analogues

The development of synthetic analogues of SST has revolutionized the medical treatment of acromegaly. The goal of treatment is to decrease GH levels to less than 2.5 ng/mL after an oral glucose tolerance test and to bring IGF-1 levels to within the normal range for age and sex. The two SST analogues used widely are *octreotide* and *lanreotide*, synthetic derivatives that have longer half-lives than SST and bind preferentially to SST_2 and SST_5 receptors (see Figure 42–3).

Octreotide. Octreotide exerts pharmacologic actions similar to those of SST. Octreotide (100 μg) administered subcutaneously three times daily is 100% bioactive; peak effects are seen within 30 min, serum $t_{1/2}$ is about 90 min, and duration of action is about 12 h. An equally effective long-acting, slow-release form, *octreotide LAR*, is administered intramuscularly in a dose of 10, 20, or 30 mg once every 4 weeks. In addition to its effect on GH secretion, octreotide can decrease tumor size, although tumor growth generally resumes after octreotide treatment is stopped.

Lanreotide. Lanreotide autogel is a long-acting octapeptide SST analogue that causes prolonged suppression of GH secretion when administered by deep subcutaneous injection every 4 weeks. Its efficacy appears comparable to that of the long-acting formulation of octreotide. It is supplied in prefilled syringes containing 60, 90, or 120 mg.

Pasireotide. Pasireotide is a long-acting cyclohexapeptide SST analogue that is approved for the treatment of Cushing disease (excessive cortisol production triggered by increases in ACTH release due to a pituitary adenoma; see Chapter 46) in patients who are ineligible for pituitary surgery or in whom surgery has failed. Pasireotide binds to multiple SST receptors (1, 2, 3, and 5) but has its highest affinity for the SST_5 receptor. In a head-to-head study, a greater percentage of subjects administered pasireotide LAR reached treatment goals compared to those given octreotide LAR. Pasireotide LAR also is approved for treatment of acromegaly.

Adverse Effects. Gastrointestinal side effects—including diarrhea, nausea, and abdominal pain—occur in up to 50% of patients receiving all three SST analogues; the incidence and severity of these side effects are similar for the three analogues. The symptoms usually diminish over time and do not require cessation of therapy. Approximately 25% of patients receiving these drugs develop multiple tiny gallstones, presumably due to decreased gallbladder contraction and bile secretion. Bradycardia and QT prolongation may occur in patients with underlying cardiac disease. Inhibitory effects on TSH secretion rarely lead to hypothyroidism, but thyroid function should be evaluated periodically. Pasireotide suppresses ACTH secretion in Cushing disease and may lead to a decrease in cortisol secretion and to hypocortisolism. All SST analogues decrease insulin secretion, but the simultaneous reduction in GH levels results in a reduction in insulin resistance. For octreotide and lanreotide, most patients will experience no change in glucose tolerance; however, depending on the relative effects on insulin secretion versus resistance, some patients may experience a worsening and others an improvement in glucose tolerance. Pasireotide, in addition, decreases the secretion of glucagon-like peptide 1 and glucose insulinotropic peptide, two incretins that facilitate insulin secretion and inhibit glucagon secretion. As a result, glucose tolerance usually worsens significantly and antihyperglycemic therapy is often needed.

Other Therapeutic Uses. SST blocks not only GH secretion but also the secretion of other hormones, growth factors, and cytokines. Thus, the slow-release formulations of SST analogues have been used to treat symptoms associated with metastatic carcinoid tumors (e.g., flushing and diarrhea) and adenomas secreting VIP (e.g., watery diarrhea). Octreotide and lanreotide also can be used to treat patients who have failed surgery who have thyrotrope adenomas that oversecrete TSH. Octreotide is used for treatment of acute variceal bleeding and for perioperative prophylaxis in pancreatic surgery. Modified forms of octreotide labeled with indium or technetium have been used for diagnostic imaging of neuroendocrine tumors, such as pituitary adenomas and carcinoids; modified forms labeled with β emitters such as ^{90}Y have been used in selective destruction of SST_2 receptor-positive tumors.

Growth Hormone Antagonists

Pegvisomant. Pegvisomant is a GHR antagonist approved for the treatment of acromegaly. Pegvisomant binds to the GHR but does not activate JAK-STAT signaling or stimulate IGF-1 secretion (see Figure 42–5).

The drug is administered subcutaneously as a 40-mg loading dose, followed by administration of 10 mg/d. Based on serum IGF-1 levels, the dose is titrated at 4- to 6-week intervals to a maximum of 30 mg/d. Pegvisomant should not be used in patients with an unexplained elevation of hepatic transaminases, and liver function tests should be monitored in all patients. In addition, lipohypertrophy has occurred at injection sites, sometimes requiring cessation of therapy; this is believed to reflect the inhibition of direct actions of GH on adipocytes. Because of concerns that loss of negative feedback by GH and IGF-1 may increase the growth of GH-secreting adenomas, careful follow-up by pituitary MRI is strongly recommended.

Pegvisomant can also be given weekly, in addition to SST analogues, when IGF-1 levels are not fully controlled by the latter drugs (Lim and Fleseriu, 2017). Pegvisomant differs structurally from native GH and induces the formation of specific antibodies in about 15% of patients. Nevertheless, the development of tachyphylaxis due to these antibodies has not been reported.

Treatment of Prolactin Excess

The therapeutic options for patients with prolactinomas include transsphenoidal surgery, radiation, and treatment with DA receptor agonists that suppress PRL production via activation of D_2 receptors. Because of the very high efficacy of DA receptor agonists, they are generally regarded as the initial treatment of choice, with surgery and radiation reserved for patients who either do not respond or are intolerant of DA receptor agonists (Melmed et al., 2011).

Dopamine Receptor Agonists

Bromocriptine, *cabergoline*, and *quinagolide* effectively reduce PRL levels, thereby relieving the inhibitory effect of hyperprolactinemia on ovulation and permitting most patients with prolactinomas to become pregnant. Quinagolide should not be used when pregnancy is intended. These agents generally decrease both PRL secretion and the size of the adenoma. Over time, especially with cabergoline, the prolactinoma may decrease in size to the extent that the drug can be discontinued without recurrence of the hyperprolactinemia.

Bromocriptine. Bromocriptine is the DA receptor agonist against which newer agents are compared. Bromocriptine is a semisynthetic ergot alkaloid (see Chapter 13) that interacts with D_2 receptors to inhibit release of PRL; to a lesser extent, it also activates D_1 dopamine receptors. The oral dose of bromocriptine is well absorbed; however, only 7% of the dose reaches the systemic circulation because of extensive first-pass metabolism in the liver. Bromocriptine has a short elimination $t_{1/2}$ (between 2 and 8 h) and thus is usually administered in divided doses. To avoid the need for frequent dosing, a slow-release oral form is available outside the U.S. Bromocriptine may be administered vaginally (2.5 mg once daily), with fewer GI side effects.

Bromocriptine normalizes serum PRL levels in 70%–80% and decreases tumor size in more than 50% of patients with prolactinomas. Hyperprolactinemia and tumor growth recur on cessation of therapy in most patients. At higher concentrations, bromocriptine is used in the management of Parkinson disease (see Chapter 18). Bromocriptine mesylate (1.6–4.8 mg/d) is approved as an adjunct to diet and exercise to improve glycemic control in adults with type 2 diabetes mellitus.

Adverse Effects. Frequent side effects include nausea and vomiting, headache, and postural hypotension, particularly on initial use. Less frequently, nasal congestion, digital vasospasm, and CNS effects such as psychosis, hallucinations, nightmares, or insomnia are observed. These adverse effects can be diminished by starting at a low dose (1.25 mg) administered at bedtime with a snack and then slowly increasing the dose as needed by monitoring PRL levels. Patients often develop tolerance to the adverse effects.

Cabergoline. Cabergoline is an ergot derivative with a longer $t_{1/2}$ (~65 h), higher affinity, and greater selectivity for the DA D_2 receptor compared to bromocriptine. Cabergoline undergoes significant first-pass metabolism in the liver.

Cabergoline is the preferred drug for the treatment of hyperprolactinemia because of greater efficacy and lower adverse effects. Therapy is initiated at a dose of 0.25 mg twice a week or 0.5 mg once a week. The dose can be increased to 1.5–2 mg two or three times a week as tolerated; the dose should be increased only once every 4 weeks. Doses of 2 mg/week or less normalize PRL levels in 80% of patients. Cabergoline induces remission in a significant number of patients with prolactinomas. At higher doses, cabergoline is used in some patients with acromegaly alone or in conjunction with SST analogues.

Adverse Effects. Compared to bromocriptine, cabergoline has a much lower tendency to induce nausea, although it still may cause hypotension and dizziness. Cabergoline has been linked to valvular heart disease, an effect proposed to reflect agonist activity at the serotonin $5HT_{2B}$ receptor; however, this is seen primarily at the high doses used in patients being treated for Parkinson disease and is not seen in the conventionally used doses (≤2 mg/week) for patients with prolactinomas.

Quinagolide. Quinagolide is a nonergot D_2 receptor agonist with a $t_{1/2}$ of about 22 h. Quinagolide is administered once daily at doses of 0.1–0.5 mg/d. It is not approved for use in the U.S. but has been used in the E.U. and Canada.

Treatment of Growth Hormone Deficiency

Somatropin

Replacement therapy is well established in GH-deficient children (Richmond and Rogol, 2010) and is gaining wider acceptance for GH-deficient adults (Molitch et al., 2011).

Humans do not respond to GH from nonprimate species. In the past, when GH for therapeutic use was purified from human cadaver pituitaries, GH was available in limited quantities and was ultimately linked to the transmission of Creutzfeldt-Jakob disease. Currently, human GH is produced by recombinant DNA technology. *Somatropin* refers to the many GH preparations whose sequences match that of native GH.

Pharmacokinetics. As a peptide hormone, GH is administered subcutaneously, with a bioavailability of 70%. Although the circulating $t_{1/2}$ of GH is only 20 min, its biological $t_{1/2}$ is considerably longer, and once-daily administration is sufficient.

Indications for Treatment. GH deficiency in children is a well-accepted cause of short stature. With the advent of essentially unlimited supplies of recombinant GH, therapy has been extended to children with other conditions associated with short stature despite adequate GH production, including Turner syndrome, Noonan syndrome, Prader-Willi syndrome, chronic renal insufficiency, children born small for gestational age, and children with idiopathic short stature (i.e., > 2.25 standard deviations below mean height for age and sex but with normal laboratory indices of GH levels). Severely affected GH-deficient adults may benefit from GH replacement therapy. The FDA also has approved GH therapy for AIDS-associated wasting and for malabsorption associated with the short-bowel syndrome (based on the finding that GH stimulates the adaptation of GI epithelial cells). Adults considered for GH treatment should have organic etiologies for the GH deficiency and must demonstrate low GH production in response to standardized stimulation tests or have at least three other pituitary hormone deficiencies.

Contraindications. GH should not be used in patients with acute critical illness due to complications after open heart or abdominal surgery, multiple accidental trauma, or acute respiratory failure. GH also should not be used in patients who have any evidence of active malignancy. GH replacement does not cause regrowth of pituitary tumor remnants when given to patients whose tumors have been resected. Other contraindications include proliferative retinopathy or severe nonproliferative diabetic retinopathy. In treating Prader-Willi syndrome, GH therapy must be carefully supervised. Sudden death has been observed when GH was given to children who were severely obese or who had severe respiratory impairment.

Therapeutic Uses. In GH-deficient children, somatropin typically is administered in a dose of 25–50 μg/kg/d subcutaneously in the evening; higher daily doses (e.g., 50–67 μg/kg) are employed for patients with Noonan syndrome or Turner syndrome, who have partial GH resistance. In children with overt GH deficiency, measurement of serum IGF-1 levels sometimes is used to monitor initial response and compliance; long-term response is monitored by close evaluation of height, sometimes in conjunction with measurements of serum IGF-1 levels. GH is continued until the epiphyses are fused and also may be extended into the transition period from childhood to adulthood. Children with idiopathic rather than organic GH deficiency need retesting after growth has ceased before continuing GH treatment as adults; many with this diagnosis will have normal GH levels on stimulation testing as adults.

Benefits of GH treatment in GH-deficient adults include increases in muscle mass, exercise capacity, energy, bone mineral density, and quality of life and a decrease in fat mass. For adults, a typical starting dose is 150–300 μg/d (these doses may vary depending on brand product), with higher doses used in younger patients transitioning from pediatric therapy. Either an elevated serum IGF-1 level or persistent side effects mandates a decrease in dose; conversely, the dose can be increased (typically by 100–200 μg/d) if serum IGF-1 has not reached the normal range after 2 months of GH therapy. Because estrogen inhibits GH action, women taking oral—but not transdermal—estrogen may require larger GH doses to achieve the target IGF-1 level.

Adverse Effects. In children, GH therapy is associated with remarkably few side effects. Rarely, patients develop intracranial hypertension, with papilledema, visual changes, headache, nausea, or vomiting. Because of this, funduscopic examination is recommended at the initiation of therapy and at periodic intervals thereafter. The consensus is that GH should not be administered in the first year after treatment of pediatric tumors, including leukemia, or during the first 2 years after therapy for medulloblastomas or ependymomas. Because an increased incidence of type 2 diabetes mellitus has been reported, fasting glucose levels should be followed periodically during therapy. Finally, too-rapid growth may be associated with slipped epiphyses or scoliosis.

Side effects associated with the initiation of GH therapy in adults (peripheral edema, carpal tunnel syndrome, arthralgias, and myalgias) occur most frequently in older or obese patients and generally respond to a decrease in dose. Estrogens (e.g., birth control medications and estrogen supplements) inhibit GH action so that a larger dose is needed to maintain the same IGF-1 level. GH therapy can increase the metabolic inactivation of cortisol in the liver.

Drug Interactions. The effects of estrogen on GH therapy were noted above. This effect is much less marked with transdermal estrogen preparations. Recent studies suggested that GH therapy can increase the metabolic inactivation of glucocorticoids in the liver. Thus, GH may precipitate adrenal insufficiency in patients with occult secondary adrenal insufficiency or in patients receiving replacement doses of glucocorticoids. This has been attributed to the inhibition of the type 1 isozyme of steroid 11β-hydroxysteroid dehydrogenase, which normally converts inactive cortisone into the active 11-hydroxy derivative cortisol (see Chapter 46).

Insulin-like Growth Factor 1

Based on the hypothesis that GH predominantly acts via increases in IGF-1 (see Figure 42–2), IGF-1 has been developed for therapeutic use (Cohen et al., 2014). Recombinant human IGF-1 (*mecasermin*) and a combination of recombinant human IGF-1 with its binding protein, IGFBP-3 (*mecasermin rinfabate*), are FDA-approved. The latter formulation was subsequently discontinued for use in short stature due to patent issues, although it remains available for other conditions, such as severe insulin resistance, muscular dystrophy, and HIV-related adipose redistribution syndrome.

ADME. Mecasermin is administered by subcutaneous injection, and absorption is virtually complete. IGF-1 in circulation is bound by six proteins; a ternary complex that includes IGFBP-3 and the acid labile subunit accounts for more than 80% of the circulating IGF-1. This protein binding prolongs the $t_{1/2}$ of IGF-1 to about 6 h. Both the liver and kidney have been shown to metabolize IGF-1.

Therapeutic Uses. Mecasermin is FDA-approved for patients with impaired growth secondary to mutations in the GHR or postreceptor signaling pathway, patients who develop antibodies against GH that interfere with its action, and patients with IGF-1 gene defects that lead to primary IGF-1 deficiency. Typically, the starting dose is 40–80 μg/kg twice daily by subcutaneous injection, with a maximum of 120 μg/kg per dose twice daily. In patients with impaired growth secondary to GH deficiency or with idiopathic short stature, mecasermin stimulates linear growth but is less effective than conventional therapy using recombinant GH.

Adverse Effects. Side effects of mecasermin include hypoglycemia and lipohypertrophy. To diminish the frequency of hypoglycemia, mecasermin should be administered shortly before or after a meal or snack. Lymphoid tissue hypertrophy, including enlarged tonsils, also is seen and may require surgical intervention. Other adverse effects are similar to those associated with GH therapy.

Contraindications. Mecasermin should not be used for growth promotion in patients with closed epiphyses. It should not be given to patients with active or suspected neoplasia and should be stopped if evidence of neoplasia develops.

Growth Hormone–Releasing Hormone

Tesamorelin. Tesamorelin is a synthetic N-terminally modified form of human GHRH that is resistant to degradation by dipeptidyl peptidase 4 and therefore has a prolonged duration of action. Tesamorelin is able to increase the levels of GH and IGF-1, but its clinical effects are primarily to reduce visceral fat accumulation, with minimal effects on insulin resistance. Tesamorelin is FDA-approved for treatment of HIV-associated lipodystrophy but not for GH deficiency (Spooner and Olin, 2012).

The Glycoprotein Hormones: TSH and the Gonadotropins

The gonadotropins include *LH*, *FSH*, and *CG*. They are referred to as the gonadotropins because of their actions on the gonads. Together with TSH, they constitute the glycoprotein family of pituitary hormones (see Table 42–2). LH and FSH were named initially based on their actions on the ovary; appreciation of their roles in male reproductive function came later. LH and FSH are synthesized and secreted by gonadotropes, which make up about 10% of the hormone-secreting cells in the anterior pituitary. CG is produced by the placenta only in primates and horses. GnRH stimulates pituitary gonadotropin production, which is further regulated by feedback effects of the gonadal hormones (Figure 42–6; see Figure 44–2 and Chapters 44 and 45). TSH is measured in the diagnosis of thyroid disorders, and recombinant TSH (thyrotropin alfa) is used in the evaluation and treatment of well-differentiated thyroid cancer (see Chapter 43).

Structure-Function Aspects of the Gonadotropins

Each gonadotropic hormone is a glycosylated heterodimer containing a common α subunit and a distinct β subunit that confers specificity of action (see Table 42–2). The heterogeneity of glycosylation on the subunits produces myriad isoforms of these hormones and may affect receptor binding and signal transduction; terminal sialate residues seem to increase plasma half-lives of these gonadotropins (Mullen et al., 2013). Among the gonadotropin β subunits, that of CG is most divergent because it contains a carboxy-terminal extension of 30 amino acids and extra carbohydrate

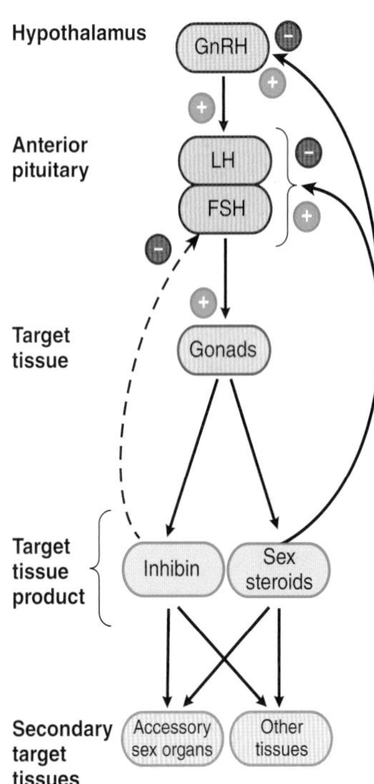

Figure 42–6 *The hypothalamic-pituitary-gonadal axis.* A single hypothalamic-releasing factor, GnRH, controls the synthesis and release of both gonadotropins (LH and FSH) in males and females. Gonadal steroid hormones (androgens, estrogens, and progesterone) exert feedback inhibition at the level of the pituitary and the hypothalamus. However, these feedback effects are dependent on sex, concentration, and time; the preovulatory surge of estrogen also can exert a stimulatory effect at the level of the pituitary and the hypothalamus. Inhibins, a family of polypeptide hormones produced by the gonads, specifically inhibit FSH secretion by the pituitary.

residues that prolong its $t_{1/2}$. The longer $t_{1/2}$ of hCG has some clinical relevance for its use in assisted reproduction technologies.

Physiology of the Gonadotropins

In men, LH acts on testicular Leydig cells to stimulate the de novo synthesis of androgens, primarily *testosterone*, from cholesterol. FSH acts on the Sertoli cells to stimulate the production of proteins and nutrients required for sperm maturation. In women, the actions of FSH and LH are more complex. FSH stimulates the growth of developing ovarian follicles and induces the expression of LH receptors on theca and granulosa cells. FSH also regulates the expression of aromatase in granulosa cells, thereby stimulating the production of *estradiol*. LH acts on the theca cells to stimulate the de novo synthesis of *androstenedione*, the major precursor of ovarian estrogens in premenopausal women (see Figure 44–1). LH also is required for the rupture of the dominant follicle during ovulation and for the synthesis of progesterone by the corpus luteum.

Regulation of Gonadotropin Synthesis and Secretion

The predominant regulator of gonadotropin synthesis and secretion is the hypothalamic peptide GnRH, a decapeptide with blocked amino and carboxyl termini derived by proteolytic cleavage of a precursor peptide with 92 amino acids.

Gonadotropin-releasing hormone release is pulsatile and is governed by a hypothalamic neural pulse generator (primarily in the arcuate nucleus) that controls the frequency and amplitude of GnRH release. Shortly before puberty, CNS inhibition decreases and the amplitude and frequency of GnRH pulses increase, particularly during sleep. As puberty progresses, the GnRH pulses increase further in amplitude and frequency until the normal adult pattern is established. The intermittent release of GnRH is crucial for the proper synthesis and release of the gonadotropins; the continuous administration of GnRH leads to desensitization and downregulation of GnRH receptors on pituitary gonadotropes.

Molecular and Cellular Bases of GnRH Action. GnRH signals through a specific GPCR on gonadotropes that activates the $G_{q/11}$-PLC-IP_3-Ca^{2+} pathway (see Chapter 3), resulting in increased synthesis and secretion of LH and FSH. Although cAMP is not the major mediator of GnRH action, binding of GnRH to its receptor also increases adenylyl cyclase activity. GnRH receptors also are present in the ovary, testis, and other sites, where their physiological significance remains to be determined.

Other Regulators of Gonadotropin Production. Gonadal steroids regulate gonadotropin production at the level of the pituitary and the hypothalamus, but effects on the hypothalamus predominate (see Figure 42–6). The feedback effects of gonadal steroids are dependent on sex, concentration, and time. In women, low levels of estradiol and progesterone inhibit gonadotropin production, largely through opioid action on the neural pulse generator. Higher and more sustained levels of estradiol have positive-feedback effects that ultimately result in the gonadotropin surge that triggers ovulation. In men, testosterone inhibits gonadotropin production, in part through direct actions and in part via its conversion by aromatase to estradiol. Gonadotropin production also is regulated by the *inhibins*, which are members of the bone morphogenetic protein family of secreted signaling proteins. *Inhibin A* and *B* are made by granulosa cells in the ovary and Sertoli cells in the testis in response to the gonadotropins and local growth factors. They act directly in the pituitary to inhibit FSH secretion without affecting that of LH. Inhibin A exhibits variation during the menstrual cycle, suggesting that it acts as a dynamic regulator of FSH secretion.

Molecular and Cellular Bases of Gonadotropin Action

The actions of LH and hCG on target tissues are mediated by the LH receptor; those of FSH are mediated by the FSH receptor. The FSH and LH receptors couple to G_s to activate the adenylyl cyclase–cAMP pathway. At higher ligand concentrations, the agonist-occupied gonadotropin receptors also activate PKC and Ca^{2+} signaling pathways via G_q-mediated effects on PLC_β. Most actions of the gonadotropins can be mimicked by cAMP analogues.

Clinical Disorders of the Hypothalamic-Pituitary-Gonadal Axis

Clinical disorders of the hypothalamic-pituitary-gonadal axis can manifest either as alterations in levels and effects of sex steroids (hyper- or hypogonadism) or as impaired reproduction. This section focuses on those conditions that specifically affect the hypothalamic-pituitary components of the axis and those for which gonadotropins are used diagnostically or therapeutically.

Deficient sex steroid production resulting from hypothalamic or pituitary defects is termed *hypogonadotropic hypogonadism* because circulating levels of gonadotropins are either low or undetectable. Hypogonadotropic hypogonadism in some patients results from GnRH receptor mutations; some of these mutations impair targeting of the GnRH receptor to the plasma membrane of gonadotropes, prompting efforts to develop pharmacological strategies to correct receptor trafficking and restore function (Conn et al., 2007). Many other disorders can impair gonadotropin secretion, including pituitary tumors, genetic disorders such as Kallmann syndrome, infiltrative processes such as sarcoidosis, and functional disorders such as exercise-induced amenorrhea.

In contrast, reproductive disorders caused by processes that directly impair gonadal function are termed *hypergonadotropic* because the impaired production of sex steroids leads to a loss of negative-feedback inhibition, thereby increasing the synthesis and secretion of gonadotropins.

- **Precocious Puberty.** Puberty normally is a sequential process requiring several years over which the GnRH neurons escape CNS inhibition and initiate pulsatile secretion of GnRH. This stimulates the secretion of gonadotropins and gonadal steroids, thus directing the development of secondary sexual characteristics appropriate for sex. Normally, the initial signs of puberty (breast development in girls and testes enlargement in boys) do not occur before age 8 in girls or age 9 in boys; the initiation of sexual maturation before this time is termed "precocious." GnRH-dependent excessive secretion of gonadotropins is rare and causes precocious puberty in children. This condition may be due to GnRH-producing hamartomas or other CNS abnormalities, but often no specific abnormality is found. This central precocious puberty must be differentiated from that due to hormone-producing tumors of the gonads, in which case gonadotropin levels will be low. GnRH-independent precocious puberty results from peripheral production of sex steroids in a manner not driven by pituitary gonadotropins; etiologies include adrenal or gonadal tumors, activating mutations of the LH receptor in boys, and congenital adrenal hyperplasia. Synthetic GnRH analogues play important roles in the diagnosis and treatment of GnRH-dependent precocious puberty (see further discussion). In contrast, drugs that interfere with the production of sex steroids, including ketoconazole and aromatase inhibitors, are used in patients with GnRH-independent precocious puberty (Shulman et al., 2008), with varying success.
- **Sexual Infantilism.** The converse of precocious puberty is a failure to initiate the processes of pubertal development at the normal time. This can reflect defects in the GnRH neurons or gonadotropes (secondary hypogonadism) or primary dysfunction in the gonads. In either case, induction of sexual maturation using sex steroids (estrogen followed by estrogen/progesterone in females, testosterone in males) is standard therapy. This suffices to direct sex differentiation in the normal manner. If fertility is the goal, then therapy with either GnRH or gonadotropins is needed to stimulate appropriate germ cell maturation.
- **Infertility.** Infertility, or a failure to conceive after 12 months of unprotected intercourse, is seen in up to 10%–15% of couples and is increasing in frequency as women choose to delay childbearing. When the infertility is due to impaired synthesis or secretion of gonadotropins (hypogonadotropic hypogonadism), various pharmacological approaches are employed. In contrast, when infertility results from intrinsic processes